ROCKWOOD AND GREEN'S
FRACTURES
IN ADULTS

VOLUME 1

THIRD EDITION

ROCKWOOD AND GREEN'S
FRACTURES
IN ADULTS

EDITED BY

Charles A. Rockwood, Jr., M.D.
Professor and Chairman Emeritus
Department of Orthopaedics
The University of Texas
Health Science Center at San Antonio
San Antonio, Texas

David P. Green, M.D.
Clinical Professor
Department of Orthopaedics
Former Chief, Hand Surgery Service
The University of Texas
Health Science Center at San Antonio
San Antonio, Texas

Robert W. Bucholz, M.D.
Professor and Chairman
Department of Orthopaedic Surgery
The University of Texas Southwestern Medical Center
Dallas, Texas

With 49 Contributors

1

J. B. Lippincott Company   **Philadelphia**
New York   London   Hagerstown

Acquisitions Editor: Darlene Barela Cooke
Developmental Editor: Delois Patterson
Project Editor: Virginia Barishek
Indexer: Ann Cassar
Design Coordinator: Kathy Kelley-Luedtke
Production Manager: Caren Erlichman
Production Coordinator: Caren Erlichman
Compositor: Tapsco, Inc.
Printer/Binder: Halliday Lithograph

3rd Edition

6   5   4   3   2

Library of Congress Cataloging-in-Publication Data

Rockwood and Green's fractures in adults/edited by Charles A.
  Rockwood, Jr., David P. Green, Robert W. Bucholz; with 48 con-
  tributors.—3rd ed.
      p.   cm.
    Rev. ed. of: Fractures in adults/edited by Charles A. Rockwood,
  Jr., and David P. Green; with 31 contributors. 2nd ed. c1984.
    Includes bibliographical references.
    Includes index.
    ISBN 0-397-50975-8 (set: v.1, 2, and 3)
    ISBN 0-397-51151-5 (set: v. 1 and 2)
    ISBN 0-397-51230-9 (v. 1)
    1. Fractures.   2. Dislocations.   I. Rockwood, Charles A.,
  1936–   .   II. Green, David P.   III. Bucholz, Robert
  W.   IV. Title: Fractures in adults.
    [DNLM: 1. Dislocations.   2. Fractures.   WE 175 R684]
  RD101.F739   1991
  617.1'5—dc20
  DNLM/DLC
  for Library of Congress   90-13697
                                                          CIP

The authors and publisher have exerted every effort to ensure that
drug selection and dosage set forth in this text are in accord with
current recommendations and practice at the time of publication.
However, in view of ongoing research, changes in government reg-
ulations, and the constant flow of information relating to drug therapy
and drug reactions, the reader is urged to check the package insert
for each drug for any change in indications and dosage and for added
warnings and precautions. This is particularly important when the
recommended agent is a new or infrequently employed drug.

*To our students, residents, and fellows,
by whom we continue to be taught*

Contributors

Lewis D. Anderson, M.D.
Professor and Chairman
Department of Orthopaedic Surgery
University of South Alabama
Mobile, Alabama

Daniel R. Benson, M.D.
Professor of Orthopaedics
University of California, Davis
Davis, California
Chief, Spinal Deformity Service
University of California, Davis Medical Center
Sacramento, California

Louis U. Bigliani, M.D.
Associate Professor, College of Physicians
  and Surgeons
Columbia University
Chief, Shoulder Service
Columbia Presbyterian Medical Center
New York, New York

Robert J. Brumback, M.D.
Associate Professor of Surgery (Orthopaedics)
University of Maryland School of Medicine
Attending Surgeon, Orthopaedic Surgery
Maryland Institute for Emergency Medical
  Services Systems
The Shock Trauma Center
Baltimore, Maryland

Robert W. Bucholz, M.D.
Professor and Chairman
Department of Orthopaedic Surgery
University of Texas Southwestern Medical Center
Dallas, Texas

Joseph A. Buckwalter, M.D.
University of Iowa Hospital
Department of Orthopaedic Surgery
Iowa City Veteran's Medical Center
Iowa City, Iowa

Andrew R. Burgess, M.D.
Assistant Professor of Surgery (Orthopaedics)
University of Maryland School of Medicine
Director, Orthopaedic Traumatology/Surgery
Maryland Institute for Emergency Medical
  Services Systems
The Shock Trauma Center
Baltimore, Maryland

Kenneth P. Butters, M.D.
Clinical Assistant Professor
Oregon Health Sciences University–Portland
Staff Orthopaedist
Sacred Heart Hospital
Eugene, Oregon

Michael W. Chapman, M.D.
Professor and Chairman
Department of Orthopaedic Surgery
University of California, Davis
Sacramento, California

William P. Cooney, M.D.
Professor of Orthopaedic Surgery
Chief, Section of Hand Surgery
Department of Orthopaedic Surgery
Mayo Clinic Foundation
Rochester, Minnesota

Edward V. Craig, M.D.
Associate Professor of Orthopaedic Surgery
University of Minnesota Medical School
Attending Staff Surgeon
University of Minnesota Hospital
Minneapolis, Minnesota

Richard L. Cruess, M.D.
Dean, Faculty of Medicine
McGill University
Professor of Surgery
McGill University
Senior Orthopaedic Surgeon
Royal Victoria Hospital and Shriner's Hospital
   for Crippled Children
Montreal, Quebec

Jesse C. DeLee, M.D.
Associate Professor
Department of Orthopaedics
The University of Texas
Health Science Center at San Antonio
San Antonio, Texas

James H. Dobyns, M.D.
Professor (Emeritus) of Orthopaedic Surgery
Mayo Medical School
Rochester, Minnesota
Consultant Associate
The Hand Center of San Antonio
San Antonio, Texas

Charles H. Epps, Jr., M.D.
Professor of Orthopaedic Surgery
Dean, College of Medicine
Howard University
Washington, D.C.

C. McCollister Evarts, M.D.
The Milton S. Hershey Medical Center
Pennsylvania State University
Hershey, Pennsylvania

Richard E. Grant, M.D.
Assistant Professor and Chief
Department of Orthopaedic Surgery
Howard University
Washington, D.C.

David P. Green, M.D.
Clinical Professor
Department of Orthopaedics
Former Chief, Hand Surgery Service
The University of Texas
Health Science Center at San Antonio
San Antonio, Texas

James W. Harkess, M.D.
Assistant Professor of Orthopaedic Surgery
University of Tennessee, Memphis
Active Staff, Campbell Clinic
Attending Orthopaedic Surgeon
Elvis Presley Memorial Trauma Center
Baptist Memorial Hospitals
Memphis, Tennessee

James W. Harkess, M.B., Ch.B.
Clinical Professor of Orthopaedic Surgery
University of Louisville School of Medicine
Louisville, Kentucky

James D. Heckman, M.D.
Professor and Chairman
Department of Orthopaedics
The University of Texas
Health Science Center at San Antonio
San Antonio, Texas

Mason Hohl, M.D.
Clinical Professor, Surgery/Orthopaedics
U.C.L.A. Medical School
Consultant in Orthopaedics
Wadsworth Veteran's Administration Hospital
Los Angeles, California

Robert N. Hotchkiss, M.D.
Clinical Assistant Professor
Department of Orthopaedics
The University of Texas
Health Science Center at San Antonio
The Hand Center of San Antonio
San Antonio, Texas

James Langston Hughes, Jr., M.D.
Professor and Chairman
Department of Orthopaedics
University of Mississippi Hospital
  and Medical Center
Jackson, Mississippi

John N. Insall, M.D.
Professor of Orthopaedic Surgery
Cornell University Medical College
Attending Orthopaedic Surgeon
The Hospital for Special Surgery
  and The New York Hospital
Director, The Knee Service
The Hospital for Special Surgery
New York, New York

L. Candace Jennings, M.D.
Clinical Fellow
Department of Orthopaedic Surgery
Division of Orthopaedic Oncology
Massachusetts General Hospital
Boston, Massachusetts

Eric E. Johnson, M.D.
Associate Professor of Orthopaedic Surgery
Chief of Orthopaedic Traumatology
University of California, Los Angeles
Staff Surgeon
Wadsworth Veteran's Hospital
Los Angeles, California

David Glen LaVelle, M.D.
Assistant Professor
Department of Orthopaedic Surgery
University of Tennessee
Staff, Campbell Clinic
Active Staff, Regional Medical Center
  and the Elvis Presley Memorial Trauma Center
Associate Staff, Baptist Memorial Hospital
Memphis, Tennessee

Ronald L. Linscheid, M.D.
Professor of Orthopaedic Surgery
Mayo Medical School
Consultant in Orthopaedic Surgery
  and Surgery of the Hand
Mayo Clinic
Rochester, Minnesota

Michael MacMillan, M.D.
Assistant Professor
Department of Orthopaedics
Chief, Division of Spinal Surgery
University of Florida
Gainesville, Florida

Frederick A. Matsen III, M.D.
Professor and Chairman
Department of Orthopaedics
University of Washington School of Medicine
Seattle, Washington

Frederick N. Meyer, M.D.
Assistant Professor, Orthopaedic Surgery
Chief, Division of Hand Surgery
University of South Alabama Medical Center
Mobile, Alabama

Pasquale X. Montesano, M.D.
Assistant Professor of Orthopaedic Surgery
University of California, Davis
Sacramento, California

Charles S. Neer II, M.D.
Professor of Clinical Orthopaedic Surgery
Columbia University College of Physicians
  and Surgeons
Attending Orthopaedic Surgeon and Chief of Adult
  Orthopaedic Service
New York Orthopaedic Hospital
Columbia-Presbyterian Medical Center
New York, New York

Vincent D. Pellegrini, Jr., M.D.
Associate Professor
Department of Orthopaedics
University of Rochester
Strong Memorial Hospital
Rochester, New York

William C. Ramsey, M.D.
Clinical Instructor
Orthopaedic Surgery
University of Louisville
Louisville, Kentucky

Charles A. Rockwood, Jr., M.D.
Professor and Chairman Emeritus
Department of Orthopaedics
The University of Texas
Health Science Center at San Antonio
San Antonio, Texas

Spencer A. Rowland, M.D., M.S.
Clinical Professor
Department of Orthopaedics
Hand Surgery Service
The University of Texas
Health Science Center at San Antonio
Consultant in Hand Surgery
Brooke Army Medical Center
San Antonio, Texas

Robert C. Russell, M.D., F.R.A.C.S., F.I.C.S.
Professor
Chief, Section of Microsurgery and Research
Southern Illinois University School of Medicine
Springfield, Illinois

Thomas Anthony Russell, M.D.
Assistant Professor of Orthopaedic Surgery
University of Tennessee
Campbell Clinic
Memphis, Tennessee

William E. Sanders, M.D.
Clinical Associate Professor of Orthopaedics
Department of Orthopaedics
The University of Texas
Health Science Center at San Antonio
San Antonio, Texas

Felix H. Savoie, M.D.
Clinical Assistant Professor of Orthopaedic Surgery
University of Mississippi Medical Center
Director, Shoulder and Upper Extremity Service
Mississippi Sports Medicine and Orthopaedic Center
Jackson, Mississippi

W. Norman Scott, M.D.
Associate Attending Surgeon
Chief of the Implant Service
Lenox Hill Hospital
New York, New York

Dempsey Springfield, M.D.
Visiting Orthopaedic Surgeon
Massachusetts General Hospital
Associate Professor in Orthopaedics
Harvard Medical School
Boston, Massachusetts

E. Shannon Stauffer, M.D.
Professor and Chairman
Orthopaedics and Rehabilitation
Southern Illinois University School of Medicine
Director of Spinal Injury Unit
Memorial Medical Center
Springfield, Illinois

J. Charles Taylor, M.D.
Chief of Orthopaedics
Regional Medical Center and the Elvis Presley
    Memorial Trauma Center
Memphis, Tennessee

Steven C. Thomas, M.D.
Orthopaedic Specialists of Nevada
Las Vegas, Nevada

Marvin Tile, M.D., F.R.C.S.
Professor of Surgery
University of Toronto
Surgeon-in-Chief
Attending Orthopaedic Surgeon
Sunnybrook Health Science Centre
Toronto, Canada

Robert A. Vander Griend, M.D.
Associate Professor
Department of Orthopaedics
University of Florida
Gainesville, Florida

Gerald R. Williams, M.D.
Attending Surgeon
Director of Resident Education
Department of Orthopaedic Surgery
Graduate Hospital
Philadelphia, Pennsylvania

Donald A. Wiss, M.D.
Associate Professor of Orthopaedic Surgery
University of Southern California
Director, Orthopaedic Trauma Service
Los Angeles County Hospital
Los Angeles, California

D. Christopher Young, M.D.
Staff Orthopaedic Surgeon
Brooke Army Medical Center
San Antonio, Texas

Preface

Dramatic changes have transpired in fracture treatment since the first edition of this book appeared in 1975. Even since the second edition, which was published in 1984, more aggressive operative treatment of open fractures and more sophisticated use of internal and external fixation techniques have radically changed the management of many fractures by North American orthopaedists. This is especially true in the lower extremity, and for this reason we enlisted the assistance of a third editor in the preparation of this new edition of *Fractures in Adults.* Dr. Robert W. Bucholz is a recognized expert in trauma and also a seasoned editor. He helped us select several new authors with extensive experience in the management of lower extremity fractures, and he then edited those chapters. We believe that his input has made this a better set of texts.

The basic format of the third edition is unchanged, and the details of time-proven nonoperative techniques of fracture management presented in the previous editions have been retained. However, all chapters have been extensively rewritten, and new authors have been added with appropriate updates in the section entitled Author's Preferred Methods of Treatment.

Charles A. Rockwood, Jr., M.D.
David P. Green, M.D.

Preface to the First Edition

Orthopaedists agree on the need for a comprehensive, up-to-date reference book on fractures. Texts that once filled this role are now either out of date or unavailable. Since the most recent of those books was published—a short span of some 14 years—significant advances have been made in the recognition and management of bone and joint injuries. For example, improved methods of external and internal fixation have been devised, a more sophisticated appreciation of the ligamentous anatomy of the knee has led to improved operative repair of damaged structures, and innovative thinking in regard to the management of spine injuries has revolutionized the management of patients with spinal cord injuries.

One cannot properly discuss fractures and exclude dislocations and ligamentous injuries and, indeed, our intent has been to cover the entire range of bone and joint injuries in adults.

We recognize that much controversy exists in the treatment of musculoskeletal injuries and that there may be several "correct" methods of treating any given injury. Realizing this, our goals in this book are (1) to present the historical background, diagnosis and pathological anatomy of virtually every bone and joint injury the orthopaedist is called upon to treat; (2) to offer a thorough discussion of the various alternative methods of treating each injury, discussing, when pertinent, the relative advantages and disadvantages of each; (3) to allow each author, chosen for his recognized competence in the management of the injuries about which he is writing, to present the methods he has come to prefer; and (4) to provide a comprehensive list of references at the end of each chapter, in order to give the reader as complete a compilation as possible of valuable sources for further study. It is our hope that we have succeeded.

Charles A. Rockwood, Jr., M.D.
David P. Green, M.D.

Contents

Index

Principles of Fractures and Dislocations

James W. Harkess
William C. Ramsey
James W. Harkess

DESCRIPTION OF FRACTURES

Fractures may be categorized in several ways: (1) by anatomical location (proximal, middle, or distal third of the shaft; supracondylar; subtrochanteric); (2) by the direction of the fracture line (transverse, oblique, spiral); and (3) by whether the fracture is linear or comminuted (ie, with multiple extensions, giving rise to many small fragments). Greenstick fractures, so common in children, are rarely, if ever, found in adults, but occasionally an incomplete fracture or infraction may be seen. When the shaft of a long bone is driven into its cancellous extremity, it is said to be "impacted." This is common in fractures of the upper humerus, but we believe that the so-called impacted fracture of the femoral neck is really a misnomer for an incomplete or partial fracture.

Fractures are termed "open" when the overlying soft tissues have been breached, exposing the fracture to the external environment, or "closed" when the skin is still intact. The archaic terms "compound" and "simple" have nothing to recommend them and should be dropped.

Although most fractures occur as the result of a single episode by a force powerful enough to fracture normal bone, there are two types of fractures in which this is not so: pathologic and stress fractures.

PATHOLOGIC FRACTURES

A *pathologic fracture* is one in which a bone is broken through an area weakened by preexisting disease by a degree of stress that would have left a normal bone intact. Osteoporosis, from whatever cause, may be a source of pathologic fracture and is one of the important factors implicated in the high incidence of fractures in the elderly. Although fractures through any type of lesion may reasonably be called pathologic, sometimes the term is used in a rather more restricted sense to denote a fracture through a malignant lesion, such as an osseous metastasis or a primary tumor (eg, myeloma). Pentecost and associates have suggested the term "insufficiency fracture" for those fractures occurring in bones affected with nontumorous disease.[344]

STRESS FRACTURES

Bone, as other materials, reacts to repeated loading. On occasion, it becomes fatigued and a crack develops, which may lead to a complete fracture—a *stress fracture*. These fractures are seen most frequently in military installations where recruits undergo rigorous training. However, they are sometimes found in ballet dancers and athletes, and no age group or occupation is immune.[121,122,157] Baker and associates[25] suggested that stress fractures occur only after muscle fatigue, and the absence of functioning muscles allows abnormal stress concentration with subsequent failure of the bone.

BIOMECHANICS OF FRACTURES

Biomechanics, for many people, is an inherently dry subject, but an understanding of some principles is necessary to treat fractures rationally. What follows constitutes a rather elementary review of the subject, which we hope will serve as an introduction for the uninitiated. Whether or not a bone fractures under stress depends on both extrinsic and intrinsic factors.

The extrinsic factors important in the production of fractures are the magnitude, duration, and direction of the forces acting on the bone, as well as the rate at which the bone is loaded.[145,155]

EXTRINSIC FACTORS

For the purposes of subsequent discussion, it might be well to define some terms. A *force* is an action or influence, such as a push or pull, which, when applied to a free body, tends to accelerate or deform it (force = mass × acceleration). Forces, having both magnitude and direction, may be represented by vectors. A *load* is a force sustained by a body. If no acceleration results from the application of a load, it follows that a force of equal magnitude and opposite direction (ie, a reaction), opposes it (Newton's third law).

Stress may be defined as the internal resistance to deformation or the internal force generated within a substance as the result of the application of an external load. Stress is calculated by the formula:

$$Stress = \frac{Load}{Area\ on\ which\ the\ load\ acts}$$

Stress cannot be measured directly. Both stress and force may be classified as tension, compression, or shear. *Tension* attempts to pull a substance or material apart; *compression* does the reverse. The stresses evoked by such forces resist the lengthening or squashing; because these stresses act at right angles to the plane under consideration, they are called *normal stresses*. A *shear stress* acts in a direction parallel to the plane being considered.

Stress is usually expressed as pounds per square inch (psi) or kilograms per square centimeter (kg/cm²). However, purists point out that kilograms and pounds are measurements of mass and not force, so that the rather clumsy terms "pound force" and "kilogram force" have been introduced to differentiate force from mass. To further complicate matters, other units of force have been created: dynes, poundals, newtons, kiloponds, and hectobars (see box).

Currently, stress is likely to be expressed in newtons/m² (1 newton/m² = 1 pascal) or as newtons/mm² (1 newton/mm² = 1 megapascal).

GLOSSARY

Dyne. That force which, if applied to 1 gram mass, gives it an acceleration of 1 centimeter per second per second (cm/sec²)

Poundal. That force which, if applied to 1 pound mass, gives it an acceleration of 1 foot per second per second (ft/sec²)

Newton. That force which, if applied to 1 kilogram mass, gives it an acceleration of 1 meter per second per second (m/sec²)

Kilopond (Kp). The force required to give 1 kilogram mass an acceleration of 9.80665 meters per second per second (9.8 m/sec²) or a force of 9.80665 newtons. "This force is equivalent to the weight of one kilogram mass under standard earth gravity; it represents the force with which this mass is attracted toward the center of the earth."

Hectobar. 1 Hectobar = 100 Bars and 1 Bar = 10⁶ dynes/cm² or 10⁵ pascals.

Strain is defined as the change in linear dimensions of a body resulting from the application of a force or a load. *Tensile strain* and *compression strain* are, respectively, the increase or decrease in length per unit of the starting length and may be expressed as inches per inch, centimeters per centimeter, or merely as a percentage of the starting length. Tensile and compressive strains are normal—that is, they act perpendicular to the cross section of the structure and are designated as ϵ (epsilon) (Fig. 1-1).

Shear strain has been defined as the relative movement of any two points perpendicular to the line joining them, expressed as a fraction of the length of that line, and it is produced when an external load is applied, producing an angular deformity (Fig. 1-2). This may be demonstrated by drawing a right angle on the surface of an object

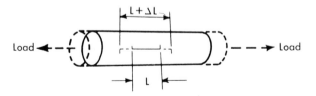

Fig. 1-1. Normal strain. (*Murphy, E. F., and Burstein, A. H.: Physical Properties of Materials Including Solid Mechanics. In A.A.O.S. Atlas of Orthotics: Biomechanical Principles and Application, p. 7. St. Louis, C.V. Mosby, 1975.*)

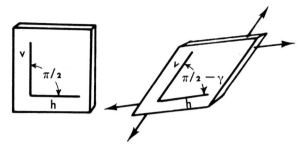

Fig. 1-2. Shear strain. *(Murphy, E. F., and Burstein, A. H.: Physical Properties of Materials Including Solid Mechanics. In A.A.O.S. Atlas of Orthotics: Biomechanical Principles and Application, p. 7. St. Louis, C.V. Mosby, 1975.)*

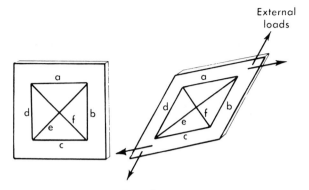

Fig. 1-4. Shear, tensile, and compressive strains. *(Murphy, E. F., and Burstein, A. H.: Physical Properties of Materials Including Solid Mechanics. In A.A.O.S. Atlas of Orthotics: Biomechanical Principles and Application, p. 8. St. Louis, C.V. Mosby, 1975.)*

and noting the angular change after load. This angle is denoted γ (gamma), and shear strain is defined as Tan γ. Because this is a small angle, it can be assumed that Tan γ is equal to the angle measured in radians ($360° = 2\pi$ radians or 1 radian = 57.3°).[314]

Normal and shear strains are not mutually exclusive. Tension and compression strains are always associated with shear strains. If a square is drawn on the surface of an object which is then subjected to a compression load (Fig. 1-3), the consequent shortening of sides a and c has changed the angles of the diagonals, thus demonstrating shear strain. Similarly, Figure 1-4 demonstrates strain produced by an oblique load. The angles of the square have changed, indicating shear strain, but diagonal f is shortened and e is lengthened, indicating compressive and tensile strain. However, these diagonals still intersect each other at 90°, indicating that there is no shear strain in these directions.[314]

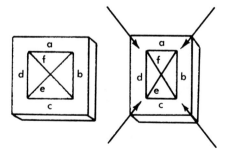

Fig. 1-3. Compressive and shear strain. *(Murphy, E. F., and Burstein, A. H.: Physical Properties of Materials Including Solid Mechanics. In A.A.O.S. Atlas of Orthotics: Biomechanical Principles and Application, p. 7. St. Louis, C.V. Mosby, 1975.)*

INTRINSIC FACTORS

Gaynor Evans[145] listed the properties of bone that are important in determining its susceptibility to fracture as energy-absorbing capacity, modulus of elasticity (Young's modulus), fatigue strength, and density.

Energy-Absorbing Capacity

Energy is the capacity to do work, and work is the product of a force moving through a displacement (ie, work = force × distance). Work and energy are measured in foot pounds (ft lbs), kilogram centimeters (kg cm), or Newton meters (Nm)

The unit of force in the SI system is the *Newton (N)*, which is the force required to give 1 kg mass an acceleration of 1 meter per second per second (m/sec²), and 1 kg force (kgf) is equal to 9.80665 Newtons. One Newton meter (Nm), which would be the unit of work or energy, has been named the *joule*, which is also the measure of energy represented by a current of 1 ampere at a voltage of 1 volt.

Strain energy is the energy a body is capable of absorbing by changing its shape under the application of an external load. The more rapidly a bone is loaded, the greater will be the energy absorption prior to failure. Thus fractures associated with slow loading are generally linear, whereas rapid loading infuses enormous strain energy so that an explosion of the bone takes place at failure, giving rise to the severe comminution of high-energy fractures.

According to Frankel and Burstein,[155] the energy absorbed to produce failure of a femoral neck has been found experimentally to be 60 kg cm. However, in falls, kinetic energy far in excess of this level is produced. This energy—if it can be dissipated by muscle action, elastic and plastic strain of the soft tissues, and other mechanisms—will not produce a fracture. In old age, these mechanisms become progressively impaired, and this is a potent factor in the production of fractures in the elderly.

Young's Modulus and Stress–Strain Curves[49,145,155,441]

When a rubber band is stretched, once the deforming force is removed, the band will revert to its resting length; in other words, there has been a stretch deformation which is recoverable, and this is known as *elastic strain.* However, if greater stress is applied to the material, its power to recover may be exceeded, and it remains permanently deformed. This is known as *plastic strain.* Eventually, if the strain increases, a point will come when the material fails. This is known as the *break point.*

If a specimen of a substance is subjected to a tensile stress and the strain is measured, the stress may be compared to the strain by plotting a graph. Figure 1-5 shows such a stress–strain curve for mild steel.

It can be seen that the first portion of this curve is linear; the strain increases proportionately to the stress, until point b is reached. Point b, known as the *yield point* or *limit of proportionality,* denotes the end of the elastic region of the curve. If at any point

along this gradient up to the point b the load is removed, the substance will regain its resting shape. The slope of this curve is a measure of the material's stiffness. The steeper the curve, the stiffer the material; the gradient is known as the *modulus of elasticity (E)* or *Young's modulus.*

The curve from point b to x (the break point where failure occurs) shows that strain increases much more rapidly with each increment of stress. This is the plastic region of the curve, where permanent strain or deformity has been produced in the material. If the load is removed at point c, there will be some recovery and the curve will parallel Young's modulus, but permanent deformity remains, represented by point e.

With the application of a load, a maximum stress will be achieved (point f). This is the *ultimate tensile strength* (UTS), the maximum stress the material can sustain before fracturing. Beyond this point, strain increases with diminished stress. This is because the material "necks"; that is, the cross section diminishes, owing to shear strains at 45° to the long axis. A material that undergoes plastic deformity is said to be *ductile,* and those that fail soon after the yield point are *brittle.*

The amount of energy absorbed by the material is represented by the area under the curve. In a comparison between two types of steel (Fig. 1-6), one can see that the hard steel has a much higher yield point and UTS than the soft ("mild") steel, but it is much more brittle and its ability to absorb

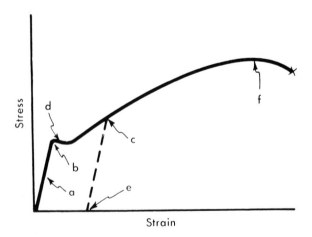

Fig. 1-5. Effect of simple tension of mild steel. (*Murphy, E. F., and Burstein, A. H.: Physical Properties of Materials Including Solid Mechanics. In A.A.O.S. Atlas of Orthotics: Biomechanical Principles and Application, p. 11. St. Louis, C.V. Mosby, 1975.*)

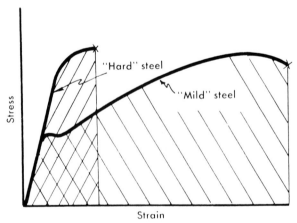

Fig. 1-6. Stress–strain curve for steel. (*Murphy, E. F., and Burstein, A. H.: Physical Properties of Materials Including Solid Mechanics. In A.A.O.S. Atlas of Orthotics: Biomechanical Principles and Application, p. 12. St. Louis, C.V. Mosby, 1975.*)

energy prior to failure is quite inferior; thus, the mild steel has greater "toughness." *Toughness* then is the amount of energy a material is able to absorb prior to failure and is measured in joules/m³ or ft lbs/inch³.

Fatigue Strength

When a material is subjected to repeated or cyclical stresses, it may fail, even though the magnitude of the individual stresses is much lower than the UTS of the material. This is known as *fatigue failure* (see Fig. 1-19C). In metal, the process starts as one or more cracks on the surface which gradually propagate until the cross-sectional area becomes so reduced that the metal fails by conventional overload mechanisms. The initial crack may start as a defect in the metal, a surface scratch, corrosion, or other stress riser. Once the crack has been initiated, it cannot be cured by resting. There is no self-healing mechanism in metals.

The fatigue strength of a metal may be illustrated by plotting the stress range against the number of cycles necessary to produce failure. From this curve the fatigue or endurance limit can be read. The *endurance limit* is the greatest repetitive stress for which the metal does not fail. Steel used in manufacturing orthopaedic implants may tolerate 1000 N/mm² for a single load but only half that amount when subjected to more than 100,000 cycles. Providing the stress level never rises above that of the endurance limit, a ferrous alloy can withstand an infinite number of cycles. This is not necessarily true of other metals, however, and aluminum alloys are particularly liable to fatigue. The endurance limit for a metal is between 30% and 50% of its yield strength, or about 0.4 times the UTS.[2]

BIOMECHANICAL PROPERTIES OF BONE

When compared to cast iron, bone is three times as light and ten times more flexible, but both materials have about the same tensile strength. Bone is a two-phase material consisting of matrix, which is mostly collagen, and bone mineral. Bone mineral (hydroxyapatite) is more rigid than bone with a modulus of 114 giganewtons/m² compared to 18 giganewtons/m² for bone (1 giganewton = 1 billion newtons) and is stronger in compression than in tension. Bone collagen, on the other hand, offers no resistance to compression, but has a tensile strength five times that of bone. It would seem that this composite owes its tensile strength to its col-

lagen and its rigidity and resistance to compression to its mineral content. Bone has a tensile strength of about 140 Nm/m² and a compression strength of 200 Nm/m².[2]

The arrangement of apatite crystals closely packed, but in discrete units, may protect bone from crack propagation, because a crack traversing a crystal will meet an interface, thus forming a T-shaped crack that dissipates energy and prevents the crack from extending (Cook-Gordon mechanism). This is the same mechanism seen when the propagation of a crack in a wooden structure is halted when a hole is drilled at the advancing end of the crack. Furthermore, stiffness and static strength increase with the degree of mineralization of bone so that its ultimate strength is three times greater at 70% mineralization than at 60%.

A stress–strain curve for bone shows that it is ductile; but, being anisotropic, its tensile strength and Young's modulus are greater when bone is loaded in its longitudinal axis than in other directions. Bone can be strained 0.75% before plastic deformity occurs, and the breaking strain is 2% to 4%. During plastic deformation it can absorb six times as much energy prior to fracture than during the elastic phase. As bone elongates, the cross section diminishes. This is known as the *Poisson effect,* and Poisson's ratio, change in diameter over change in length $\Delta d/\Delta L$, is said to be 0.2 to 0.3.

However, bone is not a simple elastic substance as is mild steel. If one loads a spring, the deformation will be immediate, and no matter how long the load is applied for, there will be no change in the strain unless the load is altered. Bone is a viscoelastic material, and the addition of viscosity introduces a rate-dependent element to the effects of loading.

The simplest model of a viscoelastic material is the combination of a dashpot and spring in parallel (Fig. 1-7).[156] A dashpot is a device for cushioning or dampening a movement to prevent sudden shock and consists of a cylinder filled with air or fluid and a piston. When a load is applied to the piston, it will move at a rate proportional to the load as long as the force is applied or until there is no more fluid to be displaced. A hypodermic syringe has the same mechanics as a dashpot. Owing to the viscosity of the fluid, the velocity with which it flows through the needle is proportional to the pressure applied to it, and much greater force must be applied to the plunger to inject quickly than slowly. The greater the viscosity of the fluid, the longer it takes to empty. Viscoelastic materials behave differently at different load and strain rates; the elastic element

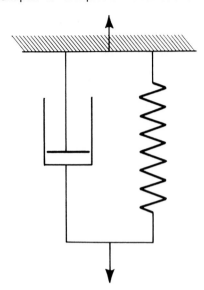

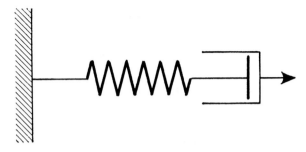

Fig. 1-8. A series combination of a Hookean body and a Newtonian body is known as a Maxwell body. *(Frankel, V. H., and Burstein, A. H.: Orthopaedic Biomechanics, p. 105. Philadelphia, Lea & Febiger, 1970.)*

Fig. 1-7. The Kelvin body is the parallel combination of a Newtonian body and a Hookean body. *(Frankel, V. H., and Burstein, A. H.: Orthopaedic Biomechanics, p. 102. Philadelphia, Lea & Febiger, 1970.)*

determines the maximum deformity and the viscous component the time that will be taken to reach it.

The spring, because it conforms to Hooke's law, is known as a ''Hookean body''; the dashpot, as a ''Newtonian body''; and the combination, hooked up in parallel, as a ''Kelvin body'' (see Fig. 1-7). A Hookean body and a Newtonian body in series is called a ''Maxwell body'' (Fig. 1-8).

Energy is required to deform both Hookean and Newtonian bodies; however, whereas the energy is recoverable in the former when the load is removed (ie, when the spring regains its former length), this is not true of the dashpot. There is no tendency to restitution in the Newtonian body, and the energy is lost.

Figure 1-9 shows the load deformation curves for a Kelvin body produced by a constantly increasing load and increasing strain. The straight-line portion of both these curves is equal to the spring constant. The first part of the curve on the left represents the immediate resistance of the Newtonian element.

If the loading direction is reversed under conditions of a constant-loading rate, the load defor-

Fig. 1-9. (Left) The load-deformation curve for a Kelvin body produced by a constantly increasing load. The curve is asymptotic to a line of slope k. **(Right)** Load-deformation characteristics for a Kelvin body under the application of a constant strain rate. *(Frankel, V. H., and Burstein, A. H.: Orthopaedic Biomechanics, p. 103. Philadelphia, Lea & Febiger, 1970.)*

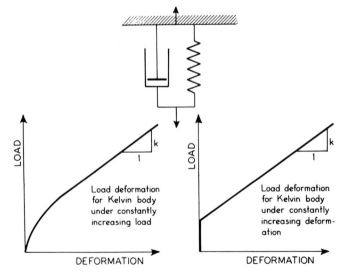

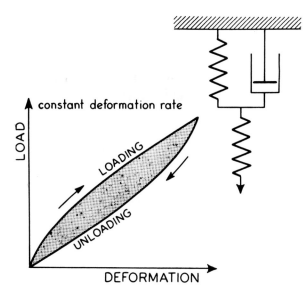

Fig. 1-10. Loading–unloading curve for constant strain rate. The shaded area is a hysteresis loop and represents energy loss during the loading and unloading cycle. *(Frankel, V. H., and Burstein, A. H.: Orthopaedic Biomechanics, p. 104. Philadelphia, Lea & Febiger, 1970.)*

(see Fig. 1-11). It is also evident that, unless the loading procedure is reversed, the model cannot return to its original dimensions.

Various rheological models for bone have been suggested by Sedlin, Piekarski, and Currey (Fig. 1-12).[109,352,409]

Because bone is a viscoelastic material, the rate of application of stress is a major factor in determining the degree of damage to both bone and soft tissues when fractures occur. The higher the loading speed, the greater the bone's ability to absorb energy; however, if the loading is carried to failure, the greatly enhanced amount of energy, when dissipated, wreaks havoc with the bone. Low-energy fractures are generally linear without much displacement, but with increasing amounts of energy the comminution and displacement of the fractures will increase, as will the damage to the soft tissue components of the extremity.

Fatigue (Stress) Fractures

Just as metal subjected to repeated stresses will fail, so will bone. Fatigue fractures are most commonly seen in military installations where recruits, unaccustomed to vigorous activity, are exercised. Such fractures are also seen in highly trained athletes, ballet dancers, and even greyhounds. Frankel[155] believes that a key factor in stress fractures is muscle fatigue, which leads to abnormal loading of the bones. Normally, muscles allow the body to shunt stress from the bones. This stress shielding is lost when the muscle action is no longer opti-

mation curve (Fig. 1-10) shows a "hysteresis loop," the area of which corresponds to the energy loss.

Similar curves are shown for the Maxwell body in Figure 1-11. As can be seen, deflection continues to increase without increase in load after the resistance generated by the Hookean body is taken up

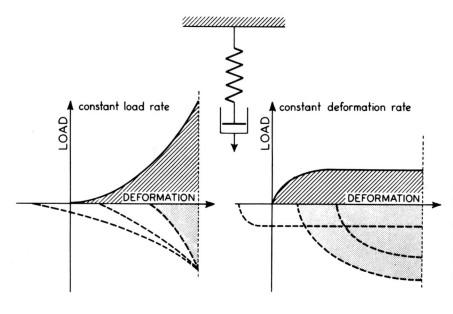

Fig. 1-11. **(Left)** The load deformation characteristics for a Maxwell body under a constantly increasing load. **(Right)** The load-to-deformation characteristics for a Maxwell body under constantly increasing deformation. *(Frankel, V. H., and Burstein, A. H.: Orthopaedic Biomechanics, p. 106. Lea & Febiger, 1970.)*

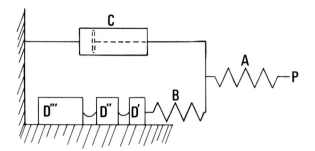

Fig. 1-12. Currey's model for the viscoelastic behavior of bone. *(Currey, J. D.: The Mechanical Properties of Bone. Clin. Orthop., 73:222, 1970.)*

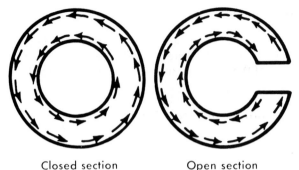

Closed section   Open section

Fig. 1-13. The effect of an open section on torsional stress patterns in the shaft of a bone. *(Murphy, E. F., and Burstein, A. H.: Physical Properties of Materials Including Solid Mechanics. In A.A.O.S. Atlas of Orthotics: Biomechanical Principles and Application, p. 222. St. Louis, C.V. Mosby, 1975.)*

mal.[121,122,211,303] It is likely that this is also a factor in stress fractures in the elderly.

Carter and Hayes[80] examined specimens of cortical bone that were fractured by a single flexural loading and compared them with flexural fatigue specimens. The pattern of fracture was similar in both groups: a transverse fracture formed on the tension side and an oblique fracture on the compression side. However, the oblique fracture surface was much greater in the fatigue specimens. Specimens that were not fatigued to complete fracture showed diffuse microscopic damage. Repeated loading caused a progressive loss of stiffness, a decrease in yield strength, and an increase in permanent deformation and hysteresis. The damage was most marked on the compressive side, where there was oblique cracking and longitudinal splitting. The damage on the tension side was more subtle and consisted mainly of separation at cement lines and interlamellar cement bonds.

Bone, when tested in the laboratory, has no endurance limit and ultimately will fail when subjected to enough cycles. But bone *in vivo,* unlike other materials, has the property of self repair, so that rest and protection from stress will allow these fractures to heal. Indeed, it has been suggested that Wolff's law might be contingent on the healing of microstress fractures, thus buttressing the regions of highest stress.

The strength of bone is dependent on the density of the bone, the mineral content, and the quality and amount of collagen. It follows that any condition that diminishes these attributes (osteoporosis, osteomalacia, scurvy, and so forth) will increase susceptibility to fracture. An increase in density alone, however, is no guarantee of strength. Osteopetrosis and Paget's disease are both associated with increased liability to fracture.

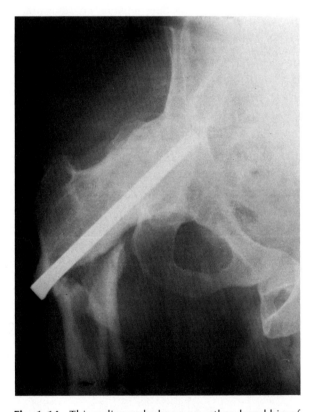

Fig. 1-14. This radiograph shows an arthrodesed hip of a middle-aged man who stumbled and fell in a restaurant. Because of the long lever arm of his lower extremity, considerable moments were applied in the region of the Smith-Peterson nail, which acted as a stress riser, resulting in a fracture below the nail.

Holes in Bone

Holes of any size significantly weaken bones,[31,54] but when the diameter of the hole is greater than 30% of the diameter of bone, the weakening effect becomes exponential. Worse still is the effect of an open section, as would result from the harvesting of a cortical bone graft or resection of a lesion from bone. After such procedures the affected bone must be protected from stress, and it is good practice to graft defects with cancellous bone after removing lesions. When an open section is left in the shaft of a bone and the bone is subjected to torsional stress, there is a redistribution of the shear stresses (Fig. 1-13) so that the more central stresses are in the same direction as the applied torque and, rather

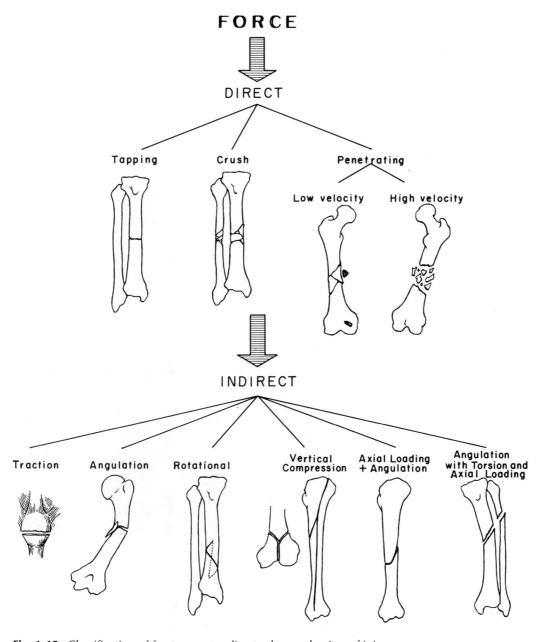

Fig. 1-15. Classification of fractures according to the mechanism of injury.

than resisting it, are additive.[155] Theoretically, sharp corners in a defect also act as stress risers, but this effect is negligible when compared to the effect of the open section. (For a more detailed discussion of the effects of holes in bone, see p. 101).

Effect of Metallic Implants

Orthopaedic implants weaken bone by stress shielding, but they also predispose to fracture by increasing the stiffness of a segment of bone so that there is an abrupt transition between the degree of elasticity of the supported and unsupported segments of bone. This is a *stress riser,* and fractures at the lower end of an implant are distressingly common (Fig. 1-14).

The strength of any structure depends not only on the material from which it is made, but also on how that material is distributed in relation to the forces that act on it. Thus one can take a ruler and bend it easily in one direction but, when one tries to angulate it across its broadest axis it will not deflect. The resistance to bending is related to the amount of material resisting the applied force and the distance of this material from the neutral axis. Resistance to bending can be calculated by the area moment of inertia; for a rectangular beam this resistance is calculated by the formula $BH^3/12$ where B = width and H = height.[155,314] For example, for a beam with a cross section of 2 inches by 4 inches, there will be an area moment of inertia of $(2 \times 64)/12 = 10.67$ in one axis, and $(4 \times 8)/12 = 2.67$ in the other, so that in one configuration the beam will be four times as resistant to bending than the other.[155,314]

It is also evident that a solid rod will have less resistance to bending than a hollow cylinder with

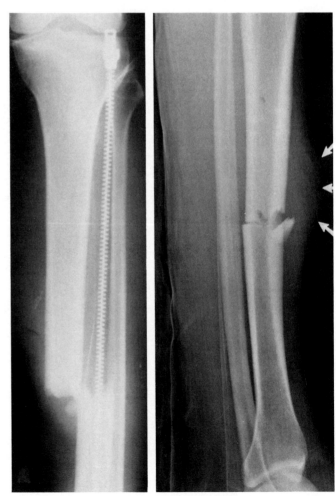

Fig. 1-16. Anteroposterior and lateral views of the left tibia, showing a typical tapping fracture. The fracture is transverse with comminution of one cortex, and the fibula is intact. Note the fracture hematoma overlying the point of impact *(arrows).*

a larger radius, even though the amount of material in each is the same. The area moment of inertia for a cylindrical structure is $(\pi r^3)/2$.[155,314] If the cylinder is hollow, the value would be diminished by subtracting $(\pi r_2^3)/2$, where r_2 is the radius of the hollow portion.

Because bending moments are proportional to the length of the lever, it follows that people with long, slender bones are at greater risk than those with short bones with large diameters. It follows too that fusion or ankylosis of the hip or knee will preclude a person from shortening the lever arm of the extremity in a fall. These factors, in addition to removing the energy-dissipating function of the mobile joint, predispose to fracture. Supracondylar fracture of the femur is a price that may be paid for arthrodesis of the knee, and subtrochanteric fracture for fusion of the hip.

Resistance to torsional stress is dependent on the distance of material from the neutral axis. It is described by the polar moment of inertia, which is calculated for a circular cross section by the formula $(\pi r^4)/2$.[155,314] (See fractures due to torsion p. 14.)

CLASSIFICATION OF FRACTURES BY THE MECHANISM OF INJURY

Deducing the probable mechanism of injury by interpreting the clinical and radiographic features of a fracture is not merely a sterile academic exercise. Knowing how a fracture was produced has therapeutic implications. Bones fracture both from direct and indirect forces, which may be classified (Fig. 1-15).

DIRECT TRAUMA

Perkins[345] divided fractures produced by direct application of the force to the fracture site into tapping fractures, crush fractures, and penetrating fractures. Essentially these are caused, respectively, by a small force acting on a small area, a large force acting on a large area, and a large force acting on a small area.

Tapping Fractures

Tapping fractures occur when a force of dying momentum is applied over a small area. The identifying features are a transverse fracture line and the frequent finding in the forearm or leg that only one bone is fractured. Because most of the energy is absorbed by the bone, there is very little soft tissue

damage, although a small area of overlying skin may be split or bruised. Tapping fractures frequently are inflicted by kicks on the shin or blows with nightsticks or other blunt weapons (Fig. 1-16).

Crush Fractures

Crush fractures are accompanied by extensive soft tissue damage. The bone is either extensively comminuted or broken transversely. In the forearm or leg, both bones fracture at the same level (Fig. 1-17).

Penetrating (Gunshot) Fractures

Penetrating fractures are produced by projectiles, and for all intents and purposes they can be called gunshot fractures. A distinction should be made between high-velocity and low-velocity missiles. There is some disagreement in the literature as to what constitutes a high-velocity weapon. Dimond and Rich,[124] quote the Wound Ballistics Manual of the Office of the Surgeon General as stating that a

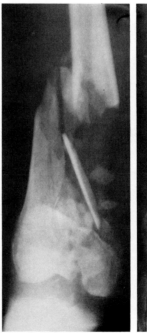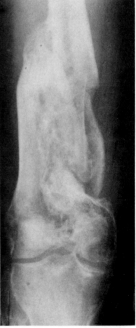

Fig. 1-17. (Left) A crush fracture of the distal end of the right femur. This woman attempted suicide by jumping from an overpass on an interstate highway and was struck by a speeding truck. Note the gross comminution of the fracture. **(Right)** The end result of this fracture after treatment by traction and active motion of the knee. After 8 months the defects in the femur were healed in by periosteal new bone.

muzzle velocity greater than 2500 feet per second constitutes high velocity. DeMuth and Smith[119] considered anything over 1800 feet per second high velocity, and Russotti and Sim[390] use 2000 feet per second as the cut-off point. Regardless of the precise definition of a high-velocity missile, however, the distinction has important implications in the management of gunshot wounds. Because the kinetic energy of the bullet varies directly with the square of its velocity and only linearly with its mass, any increase in velocity produces an exponential increase in tissue damage. For example, the M16 rifle has a muzzle velocity of 3250 feet per second, so that in spite of using a smaller projectile than a 0.300 caliber rifle, it has greatly increased destructive properties. Low-velocity missiles produce little in the way of soft tissue damage. They may splinter the shaft of a bone or embed themselves in cancellous ends (Figs. 1-18**A** and 1-19). High-velocity wounds from military rifles, on the other hand, involve extensive soft tissue damage, and the frag-ments of the bone, which disintegrates on being struck, become secondary missiles (Fig. 1-18**B**).

INDIRECT TRAUMA

Fractures produced by a force acting at a distance from the fracture site are said to be caused by indirect trauma.

Traction or Tension Fractures

The shaft of a long bone is most unlikely to be pulled apart by a traction or tension force, but this can happen to the patella or olecranon when the knee or elbow is forcibly flexed while the extensor muscles are contracting (Fig. 1-20). Similarly, the medial malleolus may be pulled off by the deltoid ligament in eversion and external rotation injuries of the ankle. The fracture line in tension fractures is transverse, which is what one would expect if the bone fibers fail under tension at right angles to

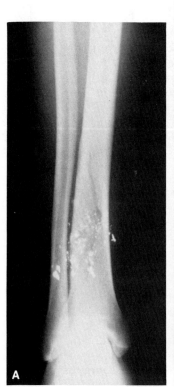
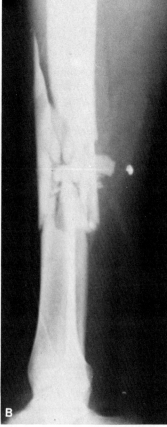

Fig. 1-18. (A) Low-velocity gunshot wound of the left tibia. The fracture line is linear without displacement, and the bullet has disintegrated on contact with the bone. **(B)** High-velocity gunshot wound sustained during a robbery attempt. The patient was shot by the police with an M-16 rifle. Note in this case the extreme comminution of the fracture fragments caused by the greater energy imparted to the bone.

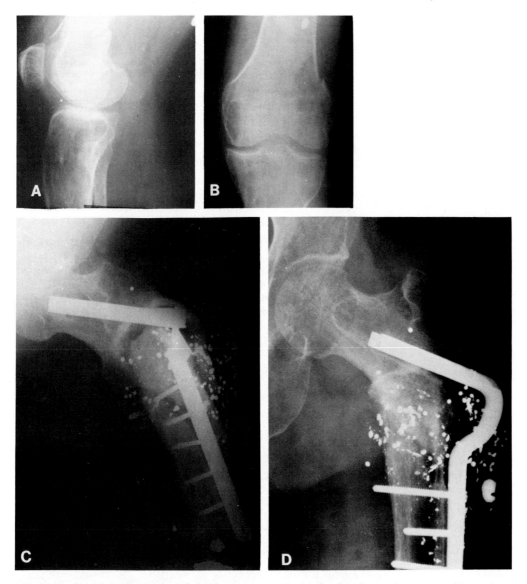

Fig. 1-19. (A, B) Radiographs of the knee in a patient who lived an adventurous life and was admitted with a fracture produced by a .22-caliber bullet. **(C)** An x-ray film of the ipsilateral hip demonstrated a nonunion of an old shotgun fracture fixed by a bladeplate assembly. Nonunion had resulted with breakage of the plate through the first screw hole. This type of fixation is inadequate for subtrochanteric fractures, which are better treated with a Zickel or similar type nail. **(D)** This fracture went on to union after the insertion of a compression plate device.

the direction of pull. Albright,[2] however, stated that the plane of fracture may be along shear lines at 45° to the direction of pull.

Angulation Fractures

When a lever is angulated (Fig. 1-21), the convexity is under a tension stress, the concavity is under compression, and somewhere in between there is a neutral plane under neither compression nor tension. The further from the neutral plane, the greater will be the magnitude of these stresses (Fig. 1-22), and in a bone with an asymmetric cross section these forces may be greater on one side than on the other (Fig. 1-23). Because bone is stronger in

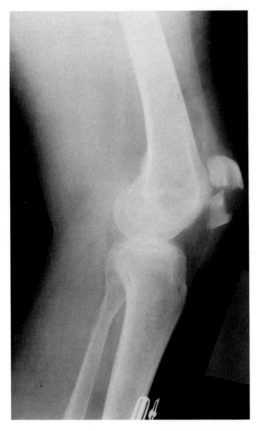

Fig. 1-20. Fractures of the patella may occur as the result of a flexion force being applied to the knee while the quadriceps is in contraction, leading to a separated transverse fracture.

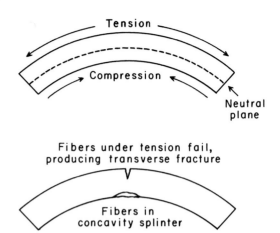

Fig. 1-21. Mechanism of an angulation fracture. If a bone is angulated, tension stresses will be present over the convexity, while compression stresses will be present in the concavity. Because bone is most likely to fail in tension, the fibers over the convexity will rupture first, throwing the stress onto the fibers immediately adjacent until a transverse fracture is produced. Commonly, the bone in the concavity of the angulation will fail in compression, causing some splintering of the cortex.

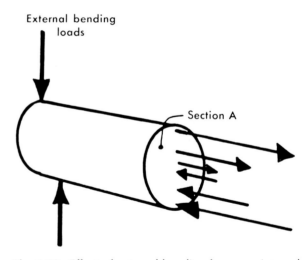

Fig. 1-22. Effect of external bending forces on internal forces within the beam. (*Murphy, E. F., and Burstein, A. H.: Physical Properties of Materials Including Solid Mechanics. In A.A.O.S. Atlas of Orthotics: Biomechanical Principles and Application, p. 15. St. Louis, C.V. Mosby, 1975.*)

compression than in tension, the fibers over the convexity fail first, thereby throwing more stress on the adjacent fibers, which in turn fail. By this progression a transverse fracture line is propagated (Fig. 1-24). Not uncommonly, however, the bone in the concavity which is under compression will fail in shear at an angle to the main fracture line, breaking off a triangular fragment of variable size.[11]

Rotational Fractures

When a piece of chalk is twisted until it breaks, a characteristic spiral fracture line is produced that makes one complete rotation around the circumference, each end of which is joined by a vertical component with or without some splintering (Fig. 1-25). Formerly it was contended that this spiral was caused by shear forces at 45° to the long axis, but this is not the case.[11] It is now generally agreed that the spiral is caused by failure in tension. Reilly

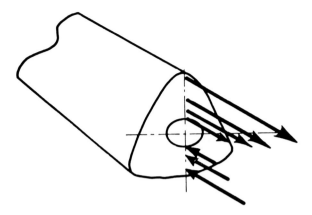

Fig. 1-23. Unequal effect of bending loads on the tibia. *(Murphy, E. F., and Burstein, A. H.: Physical Properties of Materials Including Solid Mechanics. In A.A.O.S. Atlas of Orthotics: Biomechanical Principles and Application, p. 15. St. Louis, C.V. Mosby, 1975.)*

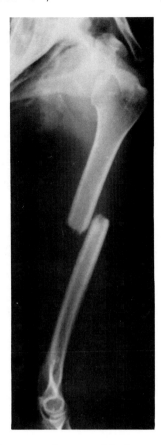

Fig. 1-24. Transverse fracture of the humerus secondary to an angulation force.

and Burstein have shown that the vertical component is a shear failure and initiates the fracture.

Netz and associates[320] described torsional fractures as occurring in two stages: in stage I, an increasing number of cracks occur in the cortex; in stage II, at maximum torque, ultimate failure is brought about by the sudden propagation of the cracks to form the spiral fracture. However, because all the fragments fit together without distortion, they believe that the nonlinear portion of the stress–strain curve does not result from viscoelasticity, but rather from the stage I cracking of the cortex.

If torque or a twisting force is applied to a bone, vertical and horizontal shear stresses result (Fig. 1-26). The horizontal shear can be resolved into compression and tension forces, which are maximal at 45° to the plane of maximum shear. Because bone is more liable to fail in tension, it is along this line that the fracture runs (Fig. 1-27).

Torsional stresses are greatest the further they are removed from the axis of rotation, but are inversely proportional to the polar moment of inertia $(\pi r^4)/2$, which explains why such fractures are more common in the distal third of the tibia than in the proximal third, even though the cortex of the former is much thicker and denser (Fig. 1-28).

Compression Fractures

If one were to take a uniform cylinder of a homogeneous material and load it axially until it failed, it would fracture along a linear plane at an angle of almost 45° (Fig. 1-29). However, long bones are not uniform cylinders or columns and are only rarely fractured by a pure compression force. When this happens, the hard shaft of the long bone is driven into the cancellous end, giving rise to the T- or V-shaped fracture (eg, at the lower end of the humerus or femur)[11] (Fig. 1-30). Experimentally, Currey[109] has shown that a compressive load applied in the long axis of a bone will produce a fracture in a plane 30° to the direction of force. He suggested that the fracture is initiated with the production of shear lines formed by buckling of lamellae that probably first appear in areas of stress concentration such as a vessel or resorption space. With increasing strain, the bone eventually cracks along these lines by a combination of compression and shear.

Less commonly, compression in the longitudinal axis of the tibia sometimes produces longitudinal fractures without displacement. Perkins has chris-

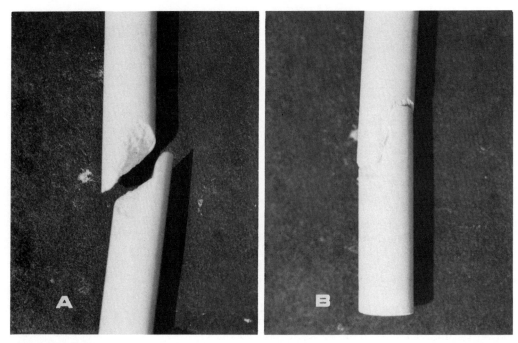

Fig. 1-25. **(A)** A model of a spiral fracture produced by torque. **(B)** The vertical fracture line joining the upper and lower extremities of the spiral fracture.

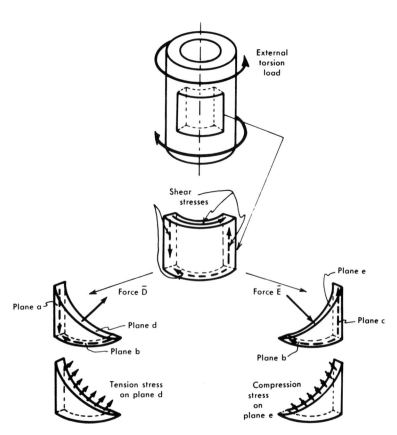

Fig. 1-26. Effect of torsion on shear and compressive stress. *(Murphy, E. F., and Burstein, A. H.: Physical Properties of Materials Including Solid Mechanics. In A.A.O.S. Atlas of Orthotics: Biomechanical Principles and Application, p. 11. St. Louis, C.V. Mosby, 1975.)*

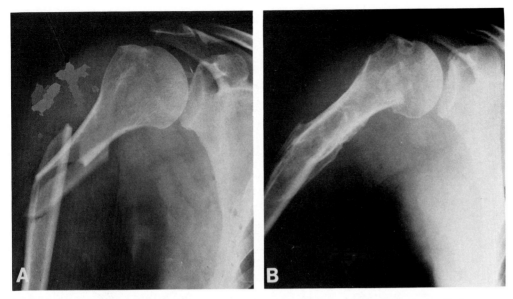

Fig. 1-27. **(A)** Radiograph of a spiral fracture of the left humerus with a loose butterfly fragment in a 67-year-old man. **(B)** Ten years later the fracture seems to be well healed. After a subsequent fall, he sustained an impacted fracture of the humeral neck.

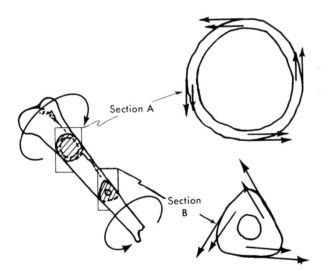

Fig. 1-28. Effect of torsional loading of the tibia. *(Murphy, E. F., and Burstein, A. H.: Physical Properties of Materials Including Solid Mechanics. In A.A.O.S. Atlas of Orthotics: Biomechanical Principles and Application, p. 17. St. Louis, C.V. Mosby, 1975.)*

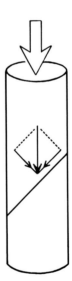

Fig. 1-29. If a column of a uniform material is vertically loaded, it will tend to fail in shear at an angle of 45° to the long axis of the column. If the force is resolved into two components, as shown here, the maximum shear force will be at 45° to the long axis of the column.

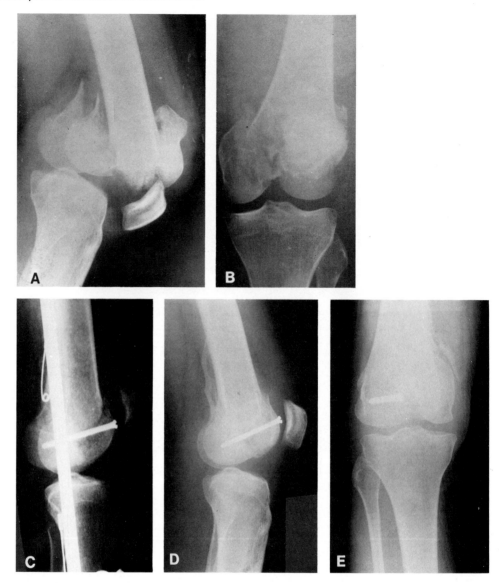

Fig. 1-30. (A, B) Compression fracture of the lower end of the femur where the femoral shaft has been driven through the condyles, giving rise to a supracondylar T fracture plus a vertical fracture of the lateral femoral condyle. **(C)** Open reduction was carried out with internal fixation of the lateral condyle by a screw. **(D, E)** Long-term follow-up showing healing of the fracture. This patient has a full range of motion of the knee in spite of a defect in the lateral femoral condyle.

tened these "teacup fractures," comparing them to a cracked cup that does not break and is still usable (Fig. 1-31A).[346] These fractures do not become displaced, need no treatment, and always heal. A similar fracture, "cleavage intercondylar fracture of the femur," has been described by Pogrund and associates,[355] which is also caused by a longitudinal force applied through the patella. This fracture too does not appear to displace. Fractures are usually produced by a combination of forces rather than by one acting alone. In his analysis of fracture mechanics, Alms[11] stated that when a beam is loaded axially with a force insufficient to cause failure and then angulated, this will result in the compressive

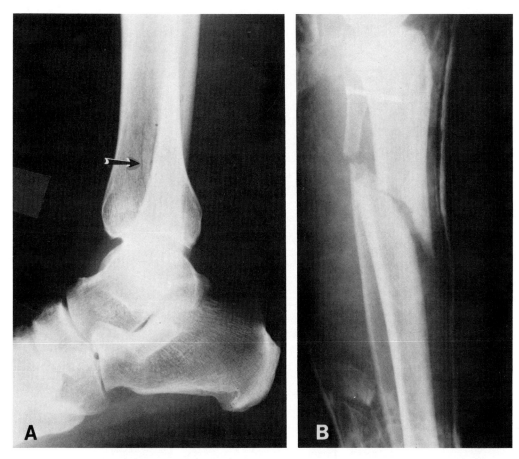

Fig. 1-31. **(A)** Radiograph of the ankle in a 45-year-old man who fell from a chair and landed heavily on his foot. Pain developed in his distal tibia and ankle. He has vertical fracture lines traversing the articular surfaces of the joint, but without displacement. This is a typical "teacup fracture," as described by Perkins. **(B)** Radiograph of the lower leg in a patient who was riding a motorcycle and sustained this fracture in a collision when his foot struck the ground. The fracture has both oblique and transverse elements, caused by a combination of vertical compression and angulation. The head of the fibula was also dislocated, and resection of the fibular shaft was necessary to reduce the dislocation and relieve the tension on the common peroneal nerve. The tibial fracture became very unstable and required stabilization by a plate.

force being diminished on the convex side of the beam and increased on the concave side. As a result, failure might start by shearing at an angle of 45° where the bone is under compression; alternatively, the failure may start at right angles to the shaft, owing to tension stress over the convexity. In either case, the resultant fracture line is curved, consisting of an oblique component caused by compression and a transverse component caused by angulation (Fig. 1-31**B**). The magnitude of each component will be proportional to the respective forces. Fre-

quently, the fragment of bone bearing the oblique surface is sheared off, forming a butterfly fragment.

Fractures Due to Angulation, Rotation, and Axial Compression

The result of combined angulation and rotation is the equivalent of an angulation about an oblique axis, which causes an oblique fracture.[10,11] If the shaft of a long bone is also loaded axially, the tendency to fracture is increased with a shear force at 45° to the long axis (Fig. 1-32). It could be argued,

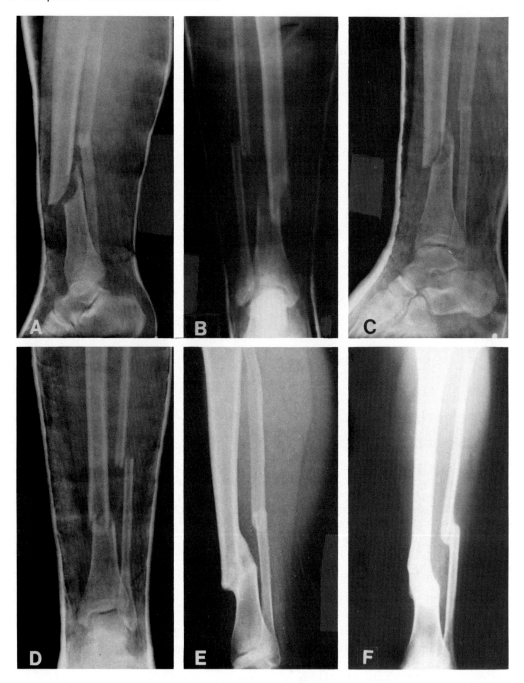

Fig. 1-32. **(A, B)** Anteroposterior and lateral views of an oblique fracture. The proximal fragment is shaped like a trowel. This reduction, obtained by a tyro, is inadequate. Note the large air space at the upper end of the tibia where the cast has lost contact with the tibia. **(C, D)** After remanipulation and the application of three-point fixation, the proximal and distal fragments are parallel in both planes, and there is little or no shortening. **(E, F)** The fracture has united by periosteal callus. In spite of the off-set, the cosmetic and functional results are excellent.

however, that these are merely angulation fractures around an oblique axis.

This type of fracture is sometimes confused with a spiral fracture. Perkins[346] stated that the broken ends of a spiral fracture are "long and sharp and pointed like pen nibs" (Fig. 1-33), whereas in oblique fractures they are "short, blunted and rounded like a garden trowel." Charnley[90] noted that, "if [a fracture is] truly spiral it will be impossible for a clear gap to be seen through the fracture by any orientation of the radiograph."

CLINICAL FEATURES OF FRACTURES

In the majority of fractures the diagnosis is self-evident, but the following signs and symptoms, alone or in combination, should alert the surgeon to the possibility of a fracture.

PAIN AND TENDERNESS

All fractures cause pain in neurologically intact people, although the intensity may vary considerably. Minor compression fractures of the vertebrae, for example, often go untreated because the pain is not severe enough for the patient to seek medical advice. On the other hand, pain and tenderness may be the only evidence of fracture (eg, fractured scaphoid and fatigue fractures). A possible exception to this rule is the finding of Grosher and associates[174] that, on examining military recruits with radioactive bone scans, some fatigue fractures were asymptomatic.

In an examination of the injured patient, gentle palpation will generally confirm the presence of tenderness, and once this has been established, there is little point in reconfirming the observation at the expense of the patient's discomfort.

LOSS OF FUNCTION

Function is lost owing to pain and the loss of a lever arm, in most, but not all fractures. In incomplete fractures of the femoral neck, for example, it is not uncommon for the patient to continue to walk or even ride a bicycle.

DEFORMITY

The hemorrhage resulting from fracture generally gives rise to perceptible swelling, and fractures

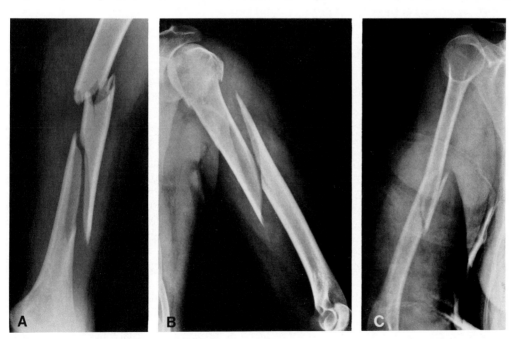

Fig. 1-33. **(A)** Radiograph of a fractured humerus in a girl who was riding the pillion of a motorcycle that ran off the road. The segmental fracture is produced by an oblique fracture proximally and a spiral fracture distally. **(B)** A combination of an impacted humeral neck proximally and spiral fracture distally as a result of a fall and torque to the humerus. **(C)** Spiral fracture of the humerus with butterfly fragment. Note the sharp ends of the fracture fragments "like pen-nibs" which, according to Perkins, characterize spiral fractures.

commonly produce angulation or rotational deformities and, especially where there is marked muscle spasm, shortening.

ATTITUDE

The attitude of a patient is sometimes diagnostic. The patient with a fractured clavicle generally supports the affected upper extremity with the opposite hand and rotates his head to the side of the fracture. When a patient sits up from the supine position holding his head with his hands, a fracture of the odontoid is very probably the cause.

ABNORMAL MOBILITY AND CREPITUS

When motion is possible in the middle of a long bone, there can be little doubt that it is fractured. Such motion may also provoke crepitus, the transmitted grating sensation of bone fragments rubbing on each other. Because eliciting these signs is painful to the patient and potentially dangerous, they should never be sought deliberately.

NEUROVASCULAR INJURY

No examination for suspected fracture is complete without careful evaluation of peripheral nerve function and vascularity. One must be particularly alert in supracondylar fractures of the humerus and femur, where both nerves and vessels are at serious risk.

RADIOGRAPHIC FINDINGS

Ultimately, the proof of the pudding is the radiographic demonstration of a fracture. There are pitfalls to avoid in this regard.[346] Fractures will be missed if the proper views are not requested. The x-ray films should include the joints at each end of the bone. Technically poor films should not be accepted. Fractures of the carpal bones may not show immediately or if the proper view has not been taken, and stress fractures may not be evident until a considerable time after the onset of pain (Fig. 1-34).

Fractures of the axial skeleton are the most likely to be missed, and cervical spine films should always be taken when patients have head injuries and are unconscious.

The introduction of computed tomograms (CT scans) has been of inestimable benefit in the evaluation of injuries to the spine and acetabulum, and increasingly so with three-dimensional reconstruction.

CLINICAL FEATURES OF DISLOCATIONS

A *dislocation* is a complete disruption of a joint so that the articular surfaces are no longer in contact (Fig. 1-35). *Subluxations* are minor disruptions of joints where articular contact still remains. Perkins[346] stated that most subluxations are associated with fractures of the joint, and we agree with this (Fig. 1-36**E**).

PAIN

Like other injuries, dislocations are associated with pain, which may be severe and persist until the joint is relocated.

LOSS OF NORMAL CONTOUR AND RELATIONSHIP OF BONY POINTS

In anterior dislocation of the shoulder, the flattening of the deltoid and the loss of the greater tuberosity as the most lateral point of the shoulder confirms the diagnosis. When the elbow is flexed 90°, the epicondyles and olecranon form an equilateral triangle. With the joint fully extended, the epicondyles and the olecranon form a straight line. These relationships are disrupted when the joint is dislocated.

LOSS OF MOTION

In all dislocations, both active and passive motion are grossly limited or impossible.

ATTITUDE

The position in which the limb is held is diagnostic in dislocations of the hip. The flexed, adducted, internal rotation deformity of the posterior dislocation, and the abducted, externally rotated lower extremity with apparent lengthening of an anterior dislocation are both diagnostic.

RADIOGRAPHIC FINDINGS

As in fractures, x-ray films are an indispensable part of the evaluation. If this step is omitted, catastrophes will occur, because associated fractures will go unrecognized. Radiographic examination without clinical examination is equally reprehensible. A distressingly high proportion of posterior dislocations of the shoulder go unrecognized, because the limitation of motion is not elicited and the ap-

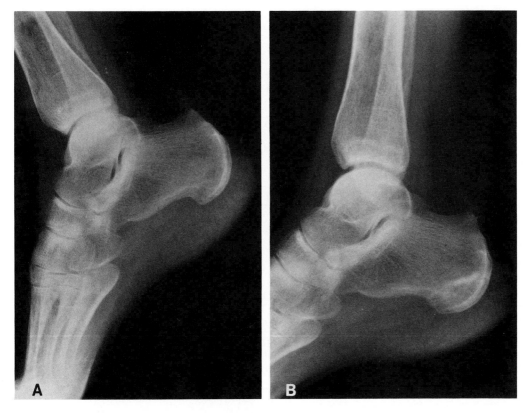

Fig. 1-34. (A) Lateral view of the foot in a woman who complained of severe pain in her heel reveals no evidence of fracture. **(B)** Films taken 1 month later show a linear density of endosteal callus in the posterior of the os calcis, indicating a healing fatigue fracture.

propriate axillary or angle-up views are not obtained.

NEUROVASCULAR INJURY

As in the case of fractures, a neurologic examination must be done. The incidence of neurologic damage is much higher with dislocations than with fractures. The sciatic nerve is often contused in posterior dislocations of the hip, with the common peroneal division taking the brunt. The common peroneal nerve is also pulled asunder by varus dislocations of the knee. Shoulder dislocations are often associated with brachial plexus or axillary nerve stretching, and radial head dislocations with injury to the posterior interosseous nerve. One must always be alert to the danger of occult vascular damage, particularly in dislocations of the knee where damage to the popliteal artery may vary from complete disruption to internal tears that initiate occlusion clots. An early arteriogram is indicated when there is any suspicion of vascular damage.

EMERGENCY MANAGEMENT OF FRACTURES

The treatment of fractures may be divided into three phases: emergency care, definitive treatment, and rehabilitation.

Unfortunately, physicians are rarely present to give the initial treatment at the site of the accident, and of necessity we have delegated this role to others. We cannot, however, completely abrogate our responsibility in this matter. The burden of teaching EMS technicians, ambulance attendants, firemen, policemen, and others must rest with the medical profession.

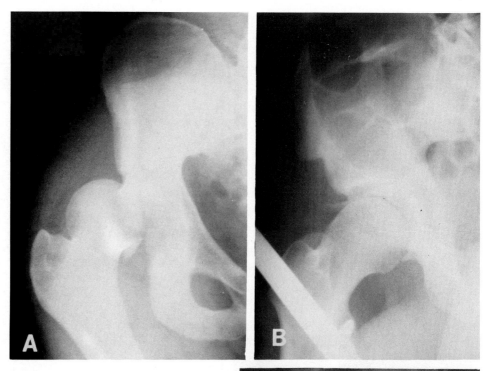

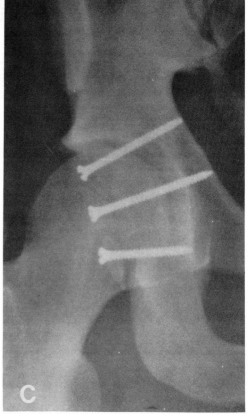

Fig. 1-35. **(A)** A classic posterior dislocation of the hip, with the hip held in the flexed, adducted, and internally rotated position. **(B)** On closed reduction bony fragments have been reduced into the acetabulum and the hip is unstable. **(C)** The result following open reduction and internal fixation of the fragments from the posterior lip.

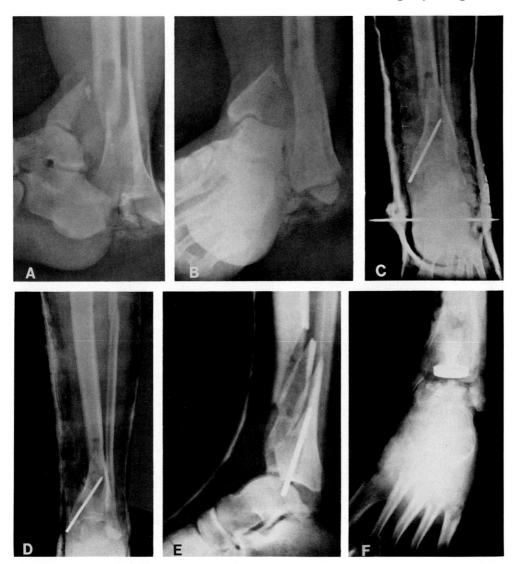

Fig. 1-36. (A, B) Views of the left ankle of a worker who fell 50 feet from a bosun's chair and plunged through a rooftop. He sustained a comminuted open fracture–dislocation of the ankle and had pitch from the rooftop embedded in the distal end of his tibia and fibula. **(C)** The immediate postoperative film after debridement and reconstruction of the ankle. Because of the instability of the ankle, transfixation pins were passed through the os calcis and proximal tibia to maintain stability. **(D, E)** Four months later, while the anteroposterior view looks reasonably good, the ankle shows anterior subluxation caused by the absence of the anterior lip of the tibia in spite of all efforts to keep it reduced. **(F)** Appearance of the ankle after bone grafting for nonunion and an attempt to reconstruct the ankle by a total joint prosthesis.

SPLINTING

. . . Not only should the technical use (of splints) be appreciated by the men, but it should also be appreciated that all unnecessary handling of the injured part without splinting should be avoided. It cannot be too strongly emphasized that a wound which may be of moderate seriousness may become greatly increased in importance by careless or incompetent handling in the transport to or from the hospital.*

* Joel E. Goldthwait, Lt. Col. M.C. In Jones, Robert (ed.): Orthopaedic Surgery of Injuries. London, Oxford Medical Publications. Published by the Joint Committee of Henry Frowde, Hodder, & Stoughton, 1921.

One of the most highly touted and least frequently obeyed maxims in emergency care is, "Splint them where they lie." London,[274] in his investigation of ambulance services in England, stated, "Little formal splintage was used; when questioned, crews often said that with a journey that was usually short they did not think that the time spent on applying splints was justifiable." In the same paper, London made the following observations: "Crews were encouraged to think in terms of comfortable support rather than splintage or immobilization. . . . What was disappointing was the infrequent use of inflatable splints."

What is true in England is, we believe, equally true in the United States. Even after being seen in emergency rooms, the majority of patients are shuffled off to radiology departments without splints. Even worse, those arriving with splints not infrequently have them removed before they are sent for x-ray studies. In an informal survey of five emergency rooms in Louisville, we found that fewer than 20% of patients with fractures had been splinted prior to being seen by an orthopaedist.

Adequate splinting is desirable for the following reasons:

1. Further soft tissue injury (especially to nerves and vessels) may be averted and, most importantly, closed fractures are saved from becoming open.
2. Immobilization relieves pain.
3. Splinting may well lower the incidence of clinical fat embolism and shock.
4. Patient transportation and radiographic studies are facilitated.

Improvised Splints

The excuse should never be used that no splints were available. Almost anything rigid can be pressed into service—walking sticks, umbrellas, slats of wood—padded by almost any material that is soft. Folded newspapers or magazines make admirable splints for the arm or forearm; and when all else fails, bandaging the lower extremities together or fixing the arm to the trunk will help. For injuries of the legs and ankles, a pillow pinned or bandaged around the injured limb immobilizes by its bulk.

Conventional Splints

BASSWOOD SPLINTS

Basswood splints, still found in first aid kits and some hospitals, are hallowed by tradition and really fall in the category of improvised splints.

UNIVERSAL SPLINTS

Universal arm and leg splints, rather ludicrous looking, are aluminum and prefabricated to fit the leg or upper limb. These splints look like portions of discarded armor and are designed to fit everyone, and so fit no one.

CRAMER WIRE SPLINTS

Cramer wire splints resemble miniature ladders with malleable metal uprights and wire rungs. They can be bent into appropriate shapes, padded, and bandaged to the extremities. They do not appreciably interfere with x-ray examinations and are most useful. This is the type of splinting advocated in *Emergency War Surgery,* the NATO handbook for armed forces.[137]

THOMAS SPLINTS

Thomas splints have a long and honorable history in the emergency care of lower extremity fractures. Their introduction in World War I by Sir Robert Jones reduced the horrendous mortality from fractures of the femur from 80% to 20%. Use of the Thomas splint was continued by the British Army into World War II where, with the addition of plaster of paris, it became the "Tobruk splint."

The Thomas splint and its modifications are still in widespread use. In most emergency services, the half-ring type is used, and in fact this is required ambulance equipment by national standards. Traction is usually accomplished by a padded hitch over the shoe with a Spanish windlass, and the leg is held firmly in place with Velcro fasteners. Such special accessories for the Thomas splint are not essential. We prefer to apply the splint with triangular bandages. A narrow-fold bandage made into a clove hitch and placed over the shoe or boot without constricting the ankle provides the traction. Devices, such as the Millbank clip, are used to grasp the heel of the shoe, and spats with traction tapes are also available. Broad-fold bandages are then tied at intervals along the splint to support the limb. The whole process takes only a few minutes.

INFLATABLE SPLINTS

Inflatable splints consist of a double-walled polyvinyl jacket with a zip fastener which is placed around the injured limb. A valve on the outer wall then allows the jacket to be inflated, either by mouth or by a pump.

These splints have been enthusiastically endorsed as being easy to apply, comfortable, effective, and safe. They are said to control swelling and bleeding, and are thought by some to be the splint of choice in fractured limbs that are burned.[466] We are considerably less enthusiastic about inflatable splints than most other authors. Frequently, we find that they have been applied to the leg to splint fractures of the femur, but barely reach the fracture site. Meanwhile the ambulance attendant or policeman believes he has splinted the fracture, and the patient is certainly no better—and perhaps even worse off—as a result of his ministrations. Although the air splints are excellent for forearm, wrist, and ankle injuries, the belief that they are the answer to all extremity injuries is unfounded.

Ashton[19] has shown that these splints, when inflated to a pressure of 40 mm Hg, markedly reduced blood flow in the limbs of all of 15 subjects tested, and that there was complete cessation of flow in six of them. Inflation to 30 mm Hg caused a similar but less pronounced reduction in flow, which was further aggravated by elevation of the extremity, so that five of the six subjects tested had complete cessation of flow. It would seem that when splints are inflated to pressures that are efficient, there is danger of circulatory embarrassment, and at lower pressures they are ineffective.

Shakespeare and associates[415] studied the application of pneumatic splints and their effects. They found that when trained ambulance attendants inflate the splints the median pressure is 25 mm Hg (range, 15–35 mm Hg). This pressure is transmitted directly into the limb and is added to the preexisting pressure within the soft tissue compartments. In contrast, when uneven pressure is applied to an extremity by a compressive dressing, direct transmission does not occur. These authors also noted that there is a gradual loss of pressure with time with pneumatic dressings. In numerical terms, if an initial pressure of 50–60 mm Hg is obtained with an air splint, 75% of this pressure is transmitted to the anterior compartment of a leg. It is likely that this pressure is an additive to the preexisting compartment pressure. The same stability could be obtained easily with a firm wool and crepe dressing, without the additive pressure to the anterior compartment.

Inflatable splints should not be applied over clothing, because folds can cause high-pressure points and blistering. We have also had trouble removing splints that had adhered to an area of abrasion and other exuding surfaces such as burns.

STRUCTURAL ALUMINUM MALLEABLE (SAM) SPLINTS

If one were to enumerate the properties of the ideal first-aid splint, they might be as follows: it should be efficient, light, inexpensive, easily applied to a variety of anatomical locations, easily stored or carried, and radiolucent.

Dr. Sam Scheinberg* invented such a splint—the structural aluminum malleable (SAM) splint—a strip of soft aluminum 0.02 inches thick and coated with polyvinyl. Subsequently he modified the splint by coating 0.016-inch-thick aluminum foil with low-density, closed-coil polyethylene foam. Cut into $34 \times 4\frac{1}{2}$–inch strips, this composite can be rolled up like a bandage or packed flat, weighs 5½ oz, takes up very little room, and is easily carried by soldiers, ski patrols, and ambulances. When folded longitudinally (the "structural bend"), these floppy, malleable strips change as if by magic to rigid members. The structural bend gives the splint a configuration like the slat from a venetian blind. Sugar-tong splints can be made to immobilize the forearm and humerus. A two-poster splint can be made to stabilize the cervical spine, and the femur can be splinted by an aluminum Liston splint. The excess length may either be folded on itself or easily trimmed with bandage scissors. Much to our surprise, we found that SAM splints could be used many times without developing fatigue fractures. They are self-padded, stain resistant, can be trimmed to size by scissors, and conform to any contour. Happily, they present no impediment to x-rays, and excellent radiographs can be obtained without removing them.

The U.S. Army is now using SAM splints and they have also been adopted by many EMS units. They do not seem to be adversely affected by extremes of climate, are water- and blood-repellent, and have been carried by an Everest expedition.

Splinting Open Fractures

Open fractures should be splinted exactly as closed fractures, except that the wound should be covered as early as possible. Even if sterile dressings are unavailable, a clean handkerchief over the wound is better than nothing. Gratuitous interference with wounds outside the operating room is the worst kind of meddling, and external bleeding is best managed by local pressure over the wound. We deprecate the undoing of dressings over open fractures, even in the emergency room. The only place to investigate such wounds is in the operating room under sterile conditions.

* Scheinberg, S.: Personal communication, 1974.

DEFINITIVE TREATMENT OF FRACTURES

Definitive treatment of fractures must be delayed until the general condition of the patient has stabilized. The establishment and maintenance of an adequate airway and the treatment of chest, abdominal, and other life-threatening injuries all take precedence over the management of fractures.

The fact that large volumes of blood may be lost even in closed fractures should not be forgotten. Fractures of the femur may be associated with a blood loss of 1 to 2.5 liters; tibial fractures, with 0.5 to 1.5 liters. Fractures of the pelvis are notoriously treacherous in this regard and may result in exsanguination. Any patient who has sustained multiple fractures has lost a lot of blood and should have blood drawn immediately for cross matching. Even if the patient appears in no great distress, it is circumspect in these cases to have a large needle or catheter in at least one vein to keep it open with saline or some other physiologic solution. Open fractures, of course, are even more dangerous from this point of view. It is good practice to estimate what the blood loss has been and to monitor the patient's physical signs, hemoglobin, and hematocrit.[94,95,96,148]

The objectives of the treatment of a fracture are to have the bone heal in such a position that the function and cosmesis of the extremity are unimpaired, and to return the patient to his vocation and avocations in the shortest possible time with the least expense. Unfortunately, these objectives are sometimes incompatible, and the goals which are to be stressed depend on the desires and needs of the patient.

It is customary to talk about the "conservative" and the "operative" treatment of fractures. Conservative does not necessarily mean nonoperative. The meaning of this word has become so corrupted by modern usage that this connotation should be dropped. We much prefer to talk of open and closed methods of treatment. Either may, on occasion, be radical or conservative, depending on one's point of view.

CLOSED TREATMENT

The closed treatment of fractures generally consists of some form of manipulation or "reduction," followed by the application of a device to maintain the reduction until healing has occurred.

Reduction

The sooner the reduction of a fracture is attempted the better, because swelling of the extremity tends to increase for 6 to 12 hours after the injury. This hemorrhage and edema in the soft tissues make them inelastic and pose a barrier to adequate reduction. While the closed fracture is never a surgical emergency—the late Dr. John Royal Moore deferred all of his closed reductions to one day a week—it is easier to effect a reduction early than late.

Prior to embarking on the manipulative reduction, adequate x-ray films must be obtained to determine what the objectives of the manipulation are to be or, if indeed a reduction is necessary. Perkins[346] stated that closed reduction is contraindicated when:

1. There is no significant displacement.
2. The displacement is of little concern (eg, humeral shaft).
3. No reduction is possible (eg, comminuted fracture of the head and neck of humerus).
4. The reduction, if gained, cannot be held (eg, compression fracture of the vertebral body).
5. The fracture has been produced by a traction force (eg, displaced fracture of the patella).

To achieve a reduction, the following steps usually are advised: (1) apply traction in the long axis of the limb; (2) reverse the mechanism that produced the fracture; and (3) align the fragment that can be controlled with the one that cannot.

TRACTION

Traction can achieve a reduction only when the fragments are connected by a soft tissue bridge (Fig. 1-37). Indeed, no manipulative reduction can be successful without some form of soft tissue linkage, and great care must be taken not to disrupt these soft tissue connections by ill-advised, overstrenuous manipulation. When traction is applied to a limb, the distal fragment, guided by the soft tissue hinge, falls into place.

Unhappily, traction by itself does not always achieve this result. Where bone fragments penetrate overlying muscles, it may be impossible to disengage the fragments, so that there is a soft tissue obstruction to reduction. One might suspect this to be so when no sensation of crepitus is present on manipulation.

A second obstruction to reduction by traction, described by Charnley,[90] is the presence of a large hematoma in the thigh with a fracture of the femur.

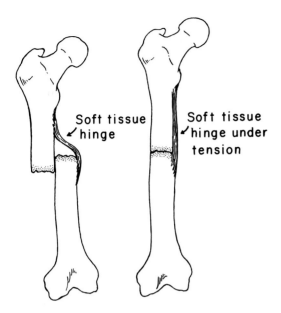

Fig. 1-37. In most fractures a soft tissue hinge will be present between the bone ends. This hinge will lie in the concavity of the angulation in a transverse fracture, or along the vertical component of a spiral fracture. This soft tissue hinge is the linkage that allows the fracture to be reduced, and under appropriate tension it will stabilize the fracture once it has been reduced.

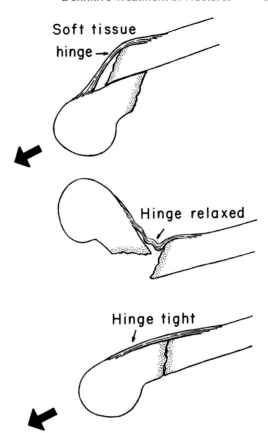

Fig. 1-38. The soft tissue hinge may act as an obstruction to reduction by traction when the fragment ends are interlocked. Excessive traction will rupture the soft tissue hinge, making further attempts at reduction fruitless. Under these circumstances the fracture should be angulated to relax the soft tissue hinge, and then further traction and angulation in the opposite direction will reduce and stabilize the fracture.

To accommodate this blood, the thigh becomes grossly swollen and tense with an increase in its transverse diameter. As a result, the elasticity of the soft tissues is grossly reduced, and the fragments cannot be pulled out to length owing to the soft tissue resistance.

A third mechanism, the description of which Charnley[90] ascribed to Beveridge Moore, is that of soft tissue interlocking (Fig. 1-38). In this circumstance, the bone ends are overlapped, and the soft tissue hinge then acts as an obstruction to the reduction. Traction, if pursued with vigor, will rupture the hinge, making the fracture completely unstable, and will lead to overdistraction. To reduce such a fracture, it must be "toggled" (ie, the angulation is increased until the bone ends disengage, after which the bone ends are latched on and the fracture is reduced by gentle traction and reversal of the angulation).

By and large, traction should be reserved for fractures that are overlapped (eg, fractures of the femur where the pull of the quadriceps shortens the bone). It must also be remembered that, unless the bone ends can be locked on and are stable, once traction is discontinued, the shortening will recur.

REVERSING THE MECHANISM OF INJURY

It seems axiomatic that if a fracture is produced by an external torque, it should be reduced by making the distal fragment retrace its steps—by twisting it internally. Similarly, angulation in one direction should be reduced by angulation in the opposite direction. An initial period of longitudinal traction may aid in fracture reduction by overcoming muscle pull and disimpacting the fracture, but the definitive reduction should be accomplished by reversing the mechanism of injury. For example, a Colles' fracture, which is produced by supination and dorsal angulation, should be reduced not by prolonged traction on the fingers but by pronating and flexing the distal fragment. Reduction by this method depends on the presence of a soft tissue linkage, which, when put on the stretch, stabilizes the reduction. In oblique and transverse fractures, the soft tissue hinge is in the concavity of the angulation, and in spiral fractures, it is in the region of the vertical fracture line. Where there is no soft tissue hinge, closed reduction is not feasible.

ALIGNING THE FRAGMENT
THAT CAN BE CONTROLLED

By and large, the recommendation to align the fragment that can be controlled with the one that cannot be is somewhat simplistic. Essentially, the fragment that can be controlled is the distal fragment, and this should be lined up with the proximal fragment. The proximal fragment adopts a position dictated by the pull of the muscles attached to it. In fractures of the forearm, the key to reduction is the position of the proximal radial fragment. If the fracture is through the proximal third, the proximal fragment will be strongly supinated by the supinator and biceps, and the forearm must be manipulated accordingly. A fracture at a lower level adds the action of the pronator teres, so that the proximal fragment is in a position midway between full supination and full pronation. A slavish adherence to this dictum may lead one astray on occasion and should be tempered by what the radiograph shows. Similarly, in the closed management of transverse subtrochanteric fractures, the proximal fragment is flexed, abducted, and externally rotated, and the distal fragment must be aligned with the proximal to effect a successful reduction.

Immobilization

Once a satisfactory reduction has been achieved, it must then be maintained until primary union has taken place. Immobilization may be provided by a cast, continuous traction, or some form of splint.

PLASTER-OF-PARIS CASTS*

The use of splints for the maintenance of fracture reduction has been practiced from times immemorial. Albucasis immobilized fractures by bandages made stiff with egg albumin. The genius who first impregnated a dressing with dehydrated gypsum to be used in the treatment of battlefield injuries was a Flemish military surgeon named

* Although the correct term is plaster-of-paris cases, or casings, it does seem rather pedantic, and we shall use the incorrect but common appellation, cast.

Antonius Mathijsen.[286] This invention, which eventually developed into the modern plaster bandage, is second in importance only to x-rays in the history of fracture treatment.

The plaster-of-paris bandage consists of a roll of muslin stiffened by dextrose or starch and impregnated with the hemihydrate of calcium sulfate. When water is added, the calcium sulfate takes up its water of crystallization ($CaSO_4 \cdot H_2O + H_2O \leftrightharpoons CaSO_4 \cdot 2H_2O$ + heat). This is an exothermic reaction, and after a few minutes the plaster-of-paris becomes a homogeneous, rocklike mass. Accelerator substances are added to the bandages to afford a spectrum of available setting rates ranging from slow to extra fast. Setting may be accelerated by increasing the temperature of the water or by adding alum and slowed by adding common salt.

Methods of Application.   Every orthopaedist has his own preferred method of applying plaster-of-paris casts, but in essence there are three schools.
Skin-Tight Cast.   The skin-tight cast was advocated by Böhler, the famous Viennese fracture surgeon. The plaster-of-paris bandage is applied directly to the skin without any intervening padding, in an effort to gain the most efficient immobilization possible. This type of cast is rarely (if ever) used now. It required a great deal of skill to apply and was fraught with the danger of pressure sores and circulatory embarrassment, and it was uncomfortable to remove because the patient's hair was incorporated into the cast.
Bologna Cast.   The Bologna cast, emanating from the Rizzoli Institute, was advocated by Charnley.[90] In contrast to Böhler's method, generous amounts of cotton wadding are applied to the limb and compressed by the plaster bandage with ''just the right amount of tension.'' This technique is said by Charnley to be demanding, so most surgeons (including us) split the difference and apply a padded cast without tension. We shall call this the ''third way.''
Third Way.   In the third way, most orthopaedists use stockinette, a tubular knitted stocking that stretches freely in diameter but sparingly in length. Stockinette may be applied over the entire member to be immobilized, but our preference is to apply just two segments, to cover the upper and lower ends of the casts (Fig. 1-39). This makes the cast look tidy and pads the sharp margins. It is probably best to avoid stockinette in postoperative casts where swelling is anticipated.

Sheet wadding is applied over the stockinette from the distal to the proximal end of the limb, as

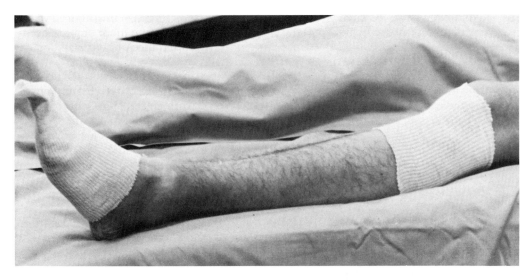

Fig. 1-39. It is necessary to use stockinette only at the upper and lower ends of the cast. Not only is this economical, but it prevents tension of the stockinette over bony prominences that may later give rise to burning pain and even pressure sores.

smoothly as possible. Each turn should be applied transversely, tearing the border that traverses the greater diameter of the limb so that it lies smoothly (Fig. 1-40). Various types of wadding are available; our preference is for the rather soft, quilted variety that can be stretched easily. The more densely compressed forms of wadding are more likely to exert a tourniquet effect if they become wadded or displaced. The amount of wadding to be used depends on how much swelling one anticipates after the application of the cast. Too much padding reduces the efficacy of the cast, and the more padding, the more plaster is necessary. Thighs are so well padded by nature that we apply the plaster directly on the stockinette without any padding. It is circumspect to apply a little extra padding to bony prominences such as the heel and malleoli. If felt pads are to be used, they must be applied as the most superficial layer, immediately under the plaster. Since they adhere to the plaster, they cannot displace. When not fixed by this means, pads may wander and give rise to embarrassing pressure sores.

The rolled plaster bandage must be thoroughly immersed in water until air bubbles stop rising. At this point the bandage is saturated with water and should be held with one end in each hand and gently squeezed. It never should be wrung out like a washcloth, since this tends to leave the plaster of paris in the pail rather than in the bandage. It is also prudent to unwrap the first 2 or 3 inches before wetting so that the tail of the bandage can be located

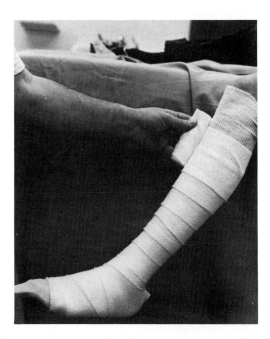

Fig. 1-40. Padding should be applied from distal to proximal, taking care to apply the padding evenly. Each turn should be overlapped by 50% of the succeeding turn.

easily. It has been our practice to use cold water only, especially when using extra-fast-setting plaster. This allows more time to mold the cast and rub the layers of the cast together. We formerly believed that cold water also gave us the strongest cast, but Callahan and associates[77] have showed this is not true. They found that when the dip water was 35°C, the resulting cast was stronger than when the dip water was 10°C. However, in their conclusions they felt that this difference in strength was not great enough to be of major importance clinically.

The largest bandage that can be handled should be used—8-inch for the thigh, 6-inch for the leg, 4-inch for the hand and forearm. When the plaster is applied with the bandage held vertically, the central core tends to drop out. This can be prevented by pushing it back at intervals with the opposite thumb. The plaster bandage should be rolled onto the limb in the same direction as the wadding. At all times the bandage should be in contact with the limb; if it is rolled on by the fingertips, it can never be too tight. Each turn of the bandage should overlap the preceding turn by half and the bandage should always be moving (Fig. 1-41). It is permissible to put two turns in the same place only at the upper and lower extremities of the cast. In this way the cast is uniformly thick throughout its length. Areas of uneven thickness act as stress risers; the cast tends to break at the juncture between thick and thin.

The bandage should always be laid on transversely, and tucks are taken in the lower border by the left hand to accommodate for the changing circumference of the limb. Each turn is smoothed by the left thenar eminence as it is laid down, and the bandage is smoothed by the palms of both hands after it is applied, so that every layer is melded with the other into a homogeneous whole. Where this

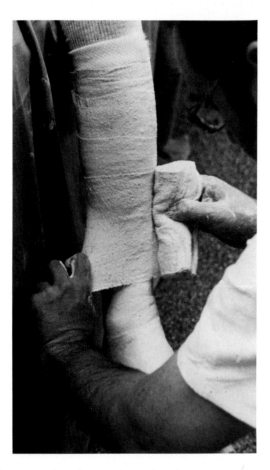

Fig. 1-41. The plaster-of-paris bandage should be applied in the same direction as the wadding. The roll should be applied with the fingertips and must never be removed from the extremity. In order to make the bandage conform to the varying circumferences of the arm or leg, tucks should be taken in it with the left hand.

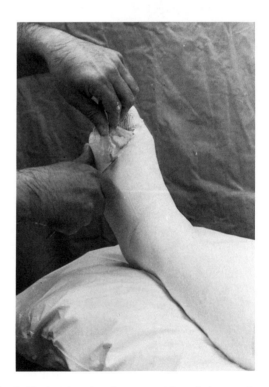

Fig. 1-42. In trimming the extremities of plaster-of-paris casts, a good method is to brace the thumb against the plaster and hold a sharp knife in the remaining four fingers. Tension is applied to the plaster to be removed by the other hand as the knife cuts.

is not done, the cast is lamellated and much weaker than it should be. A plaster bandage should never be reversed, as may be done when applying a gauze bandage. If one does so, the bandage runs against the grain and cannot be applied easily.

A plaster-of-paris cast should always be made too long and then trimmed to size with a sharp knife or a cast saw. We prefer a scalpel, which should be held with the four fingers and the palm while the thumb is braced against the cast to prevent slipping. The plaster to be removed is held in the left hand and pulled while the blade cuts (Fig. 1-42). After trimming, the stockinette is folded over the cut edge and fixed by a turn of bandage or by a plaster strip (Fig. 1-43).

In reducing fractures, it is often necessary to manipulate the fracture through the wet cast for the final adjustment. This requires the cast to be applied as quickly and as dexterously as possible. These manipulations must be done with the palms and thenar eminences (Fig. 1-44). On no account must the cast be indented by a fingertip, as this will almost certainly produce a pressure sore in the underlying skin. In molding the cast to achieve three-point fixation, one hand must exert pressure over the fracture site on the side opposite the soft tissue bridge, while the other hand gently massages the distal fragment in the proper direction to close the gap. As Charnley advised, "It takes a curved cast to produce a straight bone" (Fig. 1-45).

Once the plaster is felt to "set," all manipulations must be halted until the cast gains functional strength. During this "green period" it is very easy to crack the cast, and this defect can be remedied

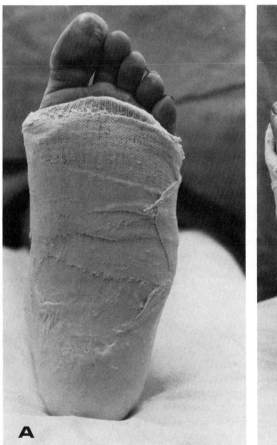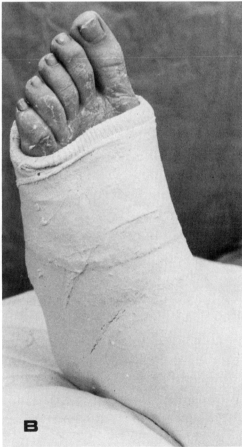

Fig. 1-43. (A, B) Casts should be trimmed so that the fingers and toes are free to move. The stockinette is then folded over the edges of the cast and anchored with a plaster-of-paris strip. Care should always be taken to make sure that the lateral border of the cast does not impinge on the fifth toe.

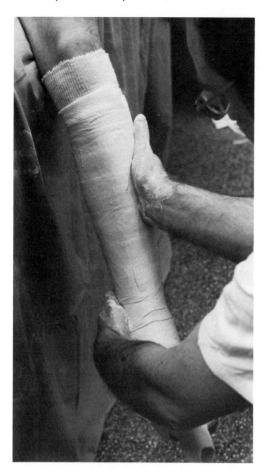

Fig. 1-44. When manipulating through a wet cast or rubbing in the turns of the bandage, always use the palms of the hands and thenar eminences and never the fingertips.

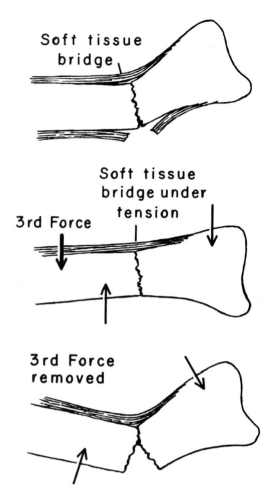

Fig. 1-45. In order to maintain the reduction of the fracture, a three-point system must be used. The cast should be molded so that the soft tissue bridge is under tension. This means that the forces must be applied as in this diagram. Should one of the three forces be removed, the system becomes unstable. (After Charnley)

only by the addition of further layers of plaster, making the cast heavier than desirable. The ultimate strength of the cast depends on its thickness, the degree to which the layers are fused together, and the smoothness of the finish. To achieve the maximum strength for a given amount of plaster, rubbing with wet hands is essential. The operator should always have the bucket near him so that he may easily dip his hands in the water. Rubber gloves are said to help make the cast smoother,[296] but they also make the bandage slippery and less easy to control. (The parsimonious senior author of this chapter [JWH] decries the use of rubber gloves merely to apply a cast and considers it effete, but he is a minority of one.)

The removal of troublesome plaster of paris ad-

hering to the hairs of the forearm can be facilitated by adding some sugar to the hands when washing.

For most purposes a cast that is ¼-inch thick will be adequate and, in general, upper extremity casts need much less plaster than do weight-bearing casts of the lower extremity. A forearm gauntlet cast can be applied with no more than one 4-inch bandage in a woman and a below-knee cast with three or four 6-inch bandages.

A cast that looks good might conceivably be wrong, but a cast that looks bad cannot be good. The expeditious, efficient application of plaster is as important a skill for the apprentice orthopaedist to acquire as the use of a scalpel, and an ill-applied cast can negate the results of an impeccable surgical procedure.

Upper-Extremity Casts. Casts on the upper extremity may extend above the elbow or be limited to the forearm and hand. In either case, the cast should be trimmed along the line of the knuckles on the dorsum and obliquely across the proximal flexion crease of the palm on the volar side to allow unrestricted motion of the fingers. A hole should be cut out around the thumb just large enough to allow unrestricted motion. The edges of this thumb hole must be carefully everted, so that the sharp edge does not cut the skin (see Fig. 1-62). Occasionally, the thumb may be included in the cast. Most surgeons prefer to treat fractured scaphoids with the thumb immobilized.

Lower-Extremity Casts. Long-leg casts may be applied with the knee flexed or extended, but if weight-bearing is to be allowed, the knee should be neutral or in 5° of flexion. The cast should be trimmed in line with the metatarsal heads on the plantar aspect and at the base of the toes dorsally. The fifth toe must be entirely free; this is a common site for a plaster sore (see Fig. 1-43). Perkins[345] stated that it is most important not to immobilize the forefoot in varus, and he left the metatarsal heads free to bear weight. If a toe plate is used the metatarsophalangeal joints must not be held in hy-

perextension. In fractures of the lower third of the tibia, dorsiflexion of the foot frequently causes angulation of the fracture. It is quite permissible under these circumstances to immobilize the foot in plantar flexion, although in fractures of the ankle this would be proscribed. When the foot is immobilized in plantar flexion and a walking heel is applied, the contralateral shoe should be raised to equalize leg lengths.

Böhler walking irons and rubber walking heels have largely become supplanted by plaster boots or cast shoes. These have the advantage of being removable at bedtime, and the patient walks with a better gait. The only indication for a rubber heel in our practice is when we employ early weight-bearing in a tibial fracture where the foot is in equinus.

Many orthopaedists reinforce their casts by applying splints to the posterior aspect of the cast. This adds weight without adding much strength. The same amount of plaster applied anteriorly as a fin strengthens the cast immeasurably, making fracture of the cast at the ankle virtually impossible (Fig. 1-46).

Patellar Tendon–Bearing Casts. Patellar tendon–bearing (PTB) casts were devised by Sarmiento[394] to immobilize fractures of the tibial shaft and at the same time allow the knee to bend. We have tended to use an above-knee cast, as recommended by Dehne, for the first 2 or 3 weeks following re-

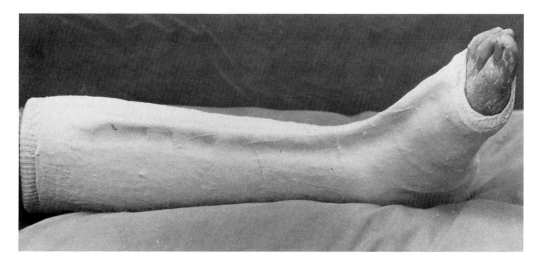

Fig. 1-46. To reinforce the cast with a splint, it is much better to apply it in the concavity of an angulation, as an I-beam or fin, than to apply it over a convexity, such as a lamina. Such a fin substantially increases the strength of the ankle, whereas the same amount of plaster applied posteriorly would have very little effect.

duction, then replacing it with a PTB cast.[21,115,116] This type of cast must be applied with care over minimal padding and is applied in segments. In applying the upper portion of the cast, the knee should be flexed to a right angle and the cast molded flat over the upper calf to give a triangular cross section. The cast is molded anteriorly around the patella, and an indentation is made over the patellar tendon (Fig. 1-47). The cast is trimmed to look like a PTB prosthesis, and it is most important to trim the cast like a wing-back chair around the femoral condyles to prevent rotation of the proximal tibia on weight-bearing (Figs. 1-47 and 1-48).

Cast Braces.   Cast braces enjoyed a considerable vogue during the 1970's for the management of femoral fractures and fractures of the tibial plateau. After preliminary treatment by traction, the cast brace is applied when the fracture is "stable and firm." In essence, a long-leg cast is applied over a long Spandex stocking, with the upper end molded to the shape of a quadrilateral socket, or a plastic socket is incorporated in the cast. The knee is then cut out and hinged. Although excellent results were obtained by this method of treatment, it required meticulous care and a great deal of supervision of the patient. Complications were common and the method is no longer so popular in the United States.

Hip and Shoulder Spicas.   We abhor the use of hip and shoulder spicas because they are large, heavy, and cumbersome and are highly inefficient in the immobilization of fractures in adults. In the past, patients were frequently sent home in hip spicas to make space in hospitals. In their home environment, if no one cares for them, they may lie unturned, soaking in their own urine and feces, and manufacturing immense decubitus ulcers. We have seen a paraplegic woman with a fractured spine transported in a double hip spica, who on arrival had bone showing over both iliac spines, both greater trochanters, and her sacrum (Fig. 1-49). It is hazardous to place patients in spicas when they lack sensation and it is only under the most unusual

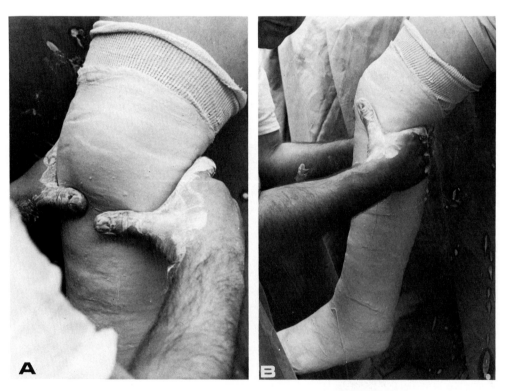

Fig. 1-47. (A, B) In the application of a patellar tendon–bearing cast, indentation must be made over the patellar tendon, and the cast must be carefully molded around the patella. At the same time, the posterior calf must be molded to make a triangular cross section at the upper end of the leg.

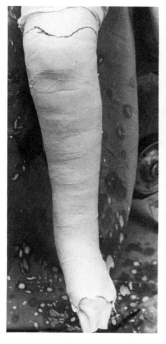

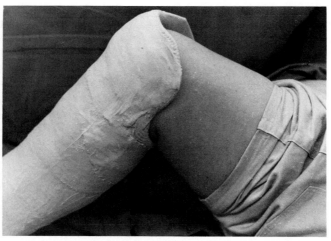

Fig. 1-48. The patellar tendon–bearing cast should be cut out to resemble a patellar tendon–bearing prosthesis, and it is particularly important to trim the lateral portion like a wing-back chair. When the knee is flexed, pressure is taken from the patellar tendon, but in full extension, pressure is exerted on the thick skin over the tendon.

circumstances that we would now advocate the use of the hip spica in adult fractures.

To reduce the weight of these casts and make the patient more comfortable, a substantial window should be cut out over the belly. This portion of the cast contributes nothing to its strength, but it should always be circular or oval and never rectangular, because corners act as stress risers. This means that the window is best cut with a knife. If one waits too long, cutting the hard plaster can be tedious. The task is made easier by outlining the window with the knife and then making a cross with the plaster saw within the circle. The free corners may then be pried up and the cutting of the circumference completed with ease (Fig. 1-50).

All orthopaedists at some time or other in our careers have been embarrassed by the disconcerting habit that spicas have of breaking at the hip. This is sometimes caused when a triangular area, commonly known as the ''intern's angle,'' at the junction of the limb and trunk does not receive its fair share of the plaster. It also results, as Strange[432] pointed out, from the juncture of the body and leg being an open section and thus very much weaker

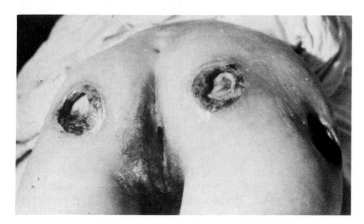

Fig. 1-49. This paraplegic woman was transported in a double hip spica. On arrival at her new hospital she had large decubiti over both ischial tuberosities, both greater trochanters, and both anterior superior iliac spines. The application of circular casts or spicas in patients without sensation is fraught with terrible danger and should rarely, if ever, be done.

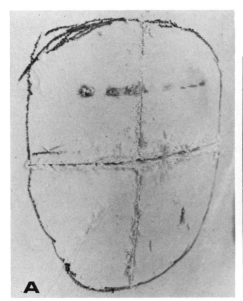
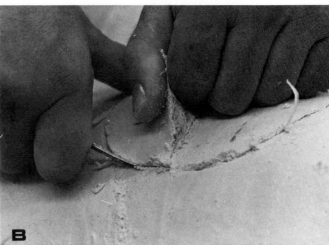

Fig. 1-50. (A, B) Cutting a belly hole in a plaster jacket or spica can be tedious, especially when the plaster is hard. The easiest method is to outline the dimensions of the hole with a pencil and then divide the area into four quadrants with a reciprocating plaster saw. The circle is then outlined with a knife along the pencil marks and the free edges of the quadrant can be pried upward and the periphery cut with the knife. It is always safer to brace the thumb against the cast to prevent the knife from slipping.

than the circular portions of the cast (Fig. 1-51). To strengthen this weak point, fin-like reinforcements are applied anteriorly, posteriorly, and laterally, much in the same way that a walking cast might be reinforced (see Fig. 1-46).

Wedging Plaster-of-Paris Casts.   After an attempted closed reduction and the application of a circular cast, there may be some residual varus or valgus angulation or posterior bow. Under these circumstances, it is quite permissible to make a transverse cut two thirds of the way around the cast (leaving a hinge opposite the convexity of the angulation) and open up the cut until the angulation is adequately corrected. The cut edges of the cast must then be everted with molders, or, if these are not available, pliers. Some surgeons place little blocks of wood or corks to hold the wedge open, but these are unnecessary and potentially dangerous because they may exert pressure on the underlying skin. We generally pack some sheet wadding in the defect and repair the cast while holding the limb in the corrected position. To gain the greatest mechanical advantage, the wedge should be made at the point where the central long axes of both fragments intersect; this point can be ascertained by drawing the appropriate lines on the x-ray film.[90] The ge-

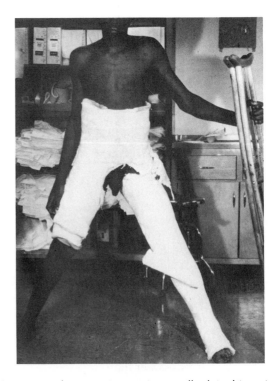

Fig. 1-51. This sporting patient walked in his spica, which failed at its weakest point, the open section of the thigh at the "intern's angle."

ometry and technique of wedging has been described in some detail by Husted.[219] It must be stressed, however, that wedging will correct only angulation, never lateral shift or rotation. We find the greatest use for wedging in fractures of the tibia, where the correction tends to be comparatively small. If large corrections are to be made, a combination of an opening wedge on the concave side and closing wedge on the convex side is safer, because a large opening wedge will elongate the cast and apply undue pressure on the dorsum of the foot. However, if large corrections are necessary, we usually apply a new cast.

Windows in Casts.   There are times when it is necessary to inspect wounds under casts, and making windows to do so seems reasonable. If at the time of cast application such a window is known to be necessary, it is a good plan to apply a large bolus of dressings over the wound, so that it sticks out. One may then take a sharp knife and cut around the periphery of this wad, leaving an oval hole. A rectangular hole cut with a saw makes the cast weak, because the corners act as stress risers. The cast might reasonably be reinforced by a dorsal fin to make up for the weakness of the open section.

Windows in casts are hazardous if left open, especially if there is any tendency for the limb to swell. The soft tissue may herniate through the hole, becoming grossly edematous, and the skin tends to break down from the pressure produced by the margins of the defect. To avoid this complication, we generally cut a piece of felt or sponge rubber to the size of the hole and bandage this snugly in place over the dressings with an elastic bandage to provide uniform compression.

PLASTER-OF-PARIS SPLINTS

Thus far we have been describing only circular casts, where the entire circumference of the anatomical part is encased. However, plaster-of-paris may be used in the form of splints, either as first aid or, in some cases, as the definitive treatment of fractures.

The two most common types of splint used in the upper extremity are the radial slab and the sugar tong. In adult fracture work, both of these splints may be used in the treatment of a Colles' fracture.

Radial Slab.   The radial slab consists of eight to ten thicknesses of 6-inch plaster with a thumb hole cut in it. No padding other than stockinette is used, and the wet plaster is applied to the radial side of the forearm, overlapping the dorsal and volar surfaces of the wrist and forearm. This splint is applied

with the forearm and hand strongly pronated and in as much ulnar deviation as possible. It is then wrapped with a wet gauze bandage (2- or 3-inch) and allowed to set. Owing to the tendency of the fingers to swell after Colles' fractures, we sometimes apply a hand dressing of fluffs or absorbent cotton on top of the splint with only the fingertips showing and elevate the arm. Should there be any circulatory embarrassment, the splint is easily removed with a pair of scissors.

Sugar Tong Splint.   Although the radial slab has not been popular in the United States, the sugar-tong splint has. After reduction of the fracture, a splint is run from the knuckles on the dorsum over the flexed elbow and the volar aspect of the forearm to the mid-palmar crease. Padding is applied either before the plaster or as a longitudinal strip along with the plaster. It is molded while setting and wrapped with gauze or an elastic wrap. This, of course, limits the motion of the elbow and, like the radial slab, is easily removed. We have an aversion to the sugar tong for Colles' fractures, probably because of our own ineptitude, but we never feel that we can adequately control the radial shift, which is the key to mastery of this troublesome fracture. We do not have the same reservations, however, about the treatment of fractures of the humeral shaft. A sugar tong running from the axilla medially to the shoulder laterally, combined with a collar and cuff or a stockinette Velpeau, is an admirable way to treat these fractures.

In the lower extremity, posterior splints are frequently used for the temporary splintage of fractures or for immobilization after open reduction when circular casts may be contraindicated because of the danger of postoperative swelling. When such splints are used, particularly when the knee is to be included, they must be made thick enough to support the load without breaking. Thick splints incur the danger of thermal injury so that one must take steps to prevent burns (see "Thermal Effects of Plaster" p. 53).

THE EFFICACY OF PLASTER IMMOBILIZATION

The object of applying a plaster-of-paris cast is to keep the bone ends in apposition and the fractures aligned until the fracture heals. It has been said that immobilization by plaster will work only where the soft tissue hinge is intact, where there is inherent stability of the reduced fracture, and where the cast is properly applied using a three-point system. When a bone is fractured and not widely separated, the soft tissue hinge in the concavity of the angulation or around the vertical fracture in a spiral fracture is, as we have seen, the linkage that allows us to reduce the fracture with manipulation. If no soft tissue bridge is present, reduction by manipulation is not feasible and a fracture will stay reduced only if the soft tissue bridge remains under tension. This requires three-point fixation, which is achieved by molding the wet cast in a similar manner to the way the fracture was reduced initially. Two of these three points, therefore, are applied by the hands. Two forces acting alone *cannot* stabilize a fracture; a third force must be present. This third force is supplied by the portion of the cast over the proximal portion of the limb (see Fig. 1-45). With overreduction the bridge is under the greatest tension and the reduction is even more stable—"a curved plaster is necessary in order to make a straight limb".[90]

Charnley[90] divided fractures into three categories: those with inherent stability against shortening (transverse fractures), those with potential stability against shortening (oblique fractures less than 45° to the long axis of the bone), and those with no stability against shortening (oblique, spiral, and comminuted fractures). Only the first two categories, he believed, are suitable for immobilization by casts alone.

However, there is another factor: the hydrodynamic effect of the cast. Because the soft tissues are semifluid, the hydrostatic pressure increases when they are compressed by a cast. This increased tension tends to keep the limb from shortening as it most certainly would do were it unsupported. We believe it is this factor that makes possible the success of the Dehne[115,116] method of early ambulation in fractures of the tibia. Initially, Sarmiento[394] believed that by the application of a PTB cast, he would be able to bypass the tibial fracture and transfer weight from the foot to the proximal tibia. After making a series of biomechanical studies, he no longer believes this and attributes the success of his cast to the "hydraulic container" effect.[395] More recently, Svend-Hansen and associates[438] have studied above-knee, below-knee, and PTB casts by measuring the load on the heel while weight-bearing. The results were identical for all three casts, and they concluded that there was no fracture-suspending effect produced by PTB casts.

We have treated many oblique, spiral, and indeed, comminuted fractures of the tibia with weight-bearing casts with no more than 1.25 cm of shortening after healing. We would admit, however, that some such fractures do need a little help with transfixation pins for 3 or 4 weeks to prevent undue shortening. However, this is now generally achieved by an external fixator rather than by pins and plaster. The need to resort to such measures is perhaps more related to the skill of the surgeon in applying the cast than to the inherent instability of the fracture.

It would be very naive to believe that absolute immobilization can ever be achieved by any type of external splint. Patients are often quite conscious of movement of the fracture fragments in the early days of treatment, but with the production of callus and its progressive stiffening, this disappears.

Hicks[197] applied casts to two lower limbs with simulated tibial fractures that had been amputated through the distal third of the femur. These casts were applied "more tightly than would ever have been risked in clinical practice." When he windowed the casts over the fracture sites, he was able to produce a lateral shift of 2.5 cm. in one and more than 3 cm in the other merely by pushing with his fingers. "Rotation to the extent of 20° and angulation to the extent of 6° were just as easily obtained."

Hicks[197] has also shown that plaster-of-paris casts applied ostensibly to immobilize fracture fragments may have the reverse effect and increase the amplitude of motion at the fracture site. A slavish obedience to the rule of immobilizing the joints proximal and distal to the fracture does not necessarily ensure better fixation of the fracture. In fractures of the forearm, an above-elbow cast prevents the muscles spanning the elbow from exerting their action on the elbow joint. As a result their pull is transmitted distally to the fracture sites. Sarmiento[393,396] has drawn attention to the deforming action of the brachioradialis in Colles' fractures, and Hughston[216] to its role in the displacement of Galeazzi fractures of the distal radius. London[275] has shown that when forearm fractures in children are treated with forearm casts, late redisplacement of the fractures does not occur. Although this method of treatment does not seem applicable to fractures of the forearm in adults, owing to their "inherent lack of stability," Sarmiento[397] reported on the management of 42 forearm fractures by a functional brace that allows "early freedom of motion of all joints." No one who has suffered through the travail of trying to achieve union in indolent supracondylar fractures of the humerus or femur with ankylosis of the elbow or knee can doubt that the immobilization of a joint has a deleterious effect on the healing of a contiguous fracture.

Furthermore, Hicks[197] has also demonstrated that if, in an amputated specimen with a fractured tibia, the action of the peroneal tendon is simulated, the subtalar joint is fixed by the cast and the lower fragment of the tibia is rotated externally. Similarly, simulated inverter action is accompanied by rotation of this fragment in the reverse direction. A total range of 12° rotation is produced by this means. This experimental evidence lends credence to the clinical observation of Sarmiento[394,395] that free motion of the foot and ankle is not deleterious in the treatment of tibial fractures.

It would appear, then, that for at least some fractures of the forearm and leg better immobilization is obtained by casts employing three-point fixation of the fractures and not of the joints.

FIBERGLASS CASTS

Until recently there had been no challenge to the plaster-of-paris bandage as the material to employ in the making of casts. Plastic materials requiring ultraviolet light to "cure" the casts gave a lightweight, durable product but were time-consuming and inconvenient to apply.[268] In recent years, however, a variety of knitted materials—cotton, rayon, and fiberglass—have been impregnated with polyurethane pre-polymer, which when soaked in water cures to form a light, durable, material that is radiolucent. The pre-polymer molecules have isocyanate end-groups which react with any molecule containing an active hydrogen,[489] and the chemical reaction is:

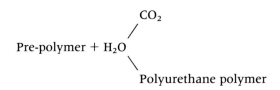

$$\text{Pre-polymer} + \text{H}_2\text{O} \Big\langle \begin{array}{c} \text{CO}_2 \\ \\ \text{Polyurethane polymer} \end{array}$$

The most popular bandage material is knitted fiberglass, and typically there is a ratio of 45% polyurethane resin to 55% fiberglass. The pre-polymer is methylene bisphenyl di-isocyanate (MDI), which converts to a nontoxic polymeric urea substance.[489] Although this is an exothermic reaction, the temperatures reached during curing pose no hazard of thermal injury.[356] Although this material is capable of burning, it is not readily set afire and the patient would be cognizant of the temperature long before the cast would ignite.[374]

The technique of applying fiberglass is somewhat different from that for plaster of paris. One cannot easily make the generous "tucks" of the plaster bandage, so bandages of smaller width should be used and the tucks eliminated. Rather than making turns of bandage at right angles to the limb, fiber-

glass conforms more easily if applied spirally, squaring the upper and lower ends by horizontal turns. We generally use 4-inch bandages for the leg (and even 3-inch in small women), 2-inch around the hand and forearm, and 3- or 4-inch around the arm.

It is permissible to apply fiberglass with a little more tension than plaster of paris since fiberglass is more elastic. Because fiberglass bandages cannot easily be trimmed with a knife, we try to limit the cast to what would be the trim lines of a plaster cast. This ensures a smooth edge, whereas trimming may produce an irregular, jagged border. When trimming cannot be avoided, Böhler's scissors are recommended when the cast is still "green," or a saw may be used after it has set. Either way, the edges should be everted by molders to prevent erosion of the skin. Reversing the bandage is permissible and helpful when bandaging around the hand and thumb.

Much to the dismay of penny-pinching Scotsmen, rubber gloves are mandatory for all who handle these bandages to prevent the monomer from polymerizing on the skin. Furthermore, the use of the specially designed nylon padding and stockinette is advised, so that if the cast becomes wet, it may easily be dried by the judicious use of a hair drier. We are, however, reluctant to advise patients that it is permissible to go swimming with such casts, particularly if there is a recent wound.

IMMOBILIZATION BY CONTINUOUS TRACTION

Some fractures are so unstable that maintenance of a reduction by plaster-of-paris casts is impossible, or casts may be, for one reason or another, impractical. In these circumstances the bone can be reduced and held to length by means of continuous traction, provided a soft tissue linkage still exists.

Traction has been shown to be a safe and dependable way of treating fractures for more than 100 years. It does, however, require constant care and vigilance, and it is costly in terms of the length of hospital stay. All of the hazards of prolonged bed rest—thromboembolism, decubiti, pneumonia, and atelectasis—must be considered when traction is used.

It does seem extraordinary that, although traction had been used for millenia in the reduction of fractures and dislocations, and many elaborate machines and devices were invented to apply it, continuous traction was not employed until the 19th century.[342]

Continuous traction may be applied through traction tapes attached to the skin by adhesives or by a direct pull through pins transfixing the skeleton.

Skin Traction.   Although Gurdon Buck did not invent skin traction (nor did he claim to have done so), isotonic skin traction has come to be known by his name. It was used extensively in the Civil War in the treatment of fractured femurs and later spread to Europe and Great Britain, where it was called "the American method."[342] Skin, however, is designed to bear compression forces and not shear. If much more than 8 pounds is applied for any length of time, the superficial layers of the skin are pulled off, leaving an irritated, exuding surface. The force exerted by skin traction is dissipated in the soft tissues, so that this form of traction in adult fracture work is used only as a temporary measure to make the patient comfortable while awaiting definitive therapy.

When skin traction is to be used, we prefer moleskin for the traction tape. Ordinary adhesive tape must never be used, because it is impervious to moisture and thus allows the underlying skin to become sodden with perspiration; the tape then creeps, pulling off the superficial layers of the skin, leaving a weeping, angry excoriation (Fig. 1-52). On no account should the limb be shaved. The su-

perficial layers of the skin have a protective function, and tape on shaved skin causes irritation and discomfort. Some surgeons believe that tincture of benzoin applied to the skin prior to the application of adhesive traction protects the skin, but there is no good evidence to support this contention.

The malleoli must be protected from the traction tape by padding proximal to them. Pressure sores may result from padding applied directly to the malleoli. The moleskin tapes should be applied evenly without wrinkles, and, if necessary, oblique cuts may be made in the borders to make them conform to the limb. The traction tapes are applied to a block or a spreader and through this to a cord, which passes over a pulley to an attached weight. The moleskin is held in place by an elastic bandage carefully applied from the ankle to the knee, which must be checked regularly to ensure that it does not exert a tourniquet effect by becoming disarranged (Fig. 1-53**A**).

A variety of prepackaged skin traction devices are available that can be applied easily and quickly. Some of these are adherent, whereas others exert their action by the friction of sponge rubber against the skin so that they may be removed and reapplied as often as is desired.

We seldom use skin traction in adults, and when

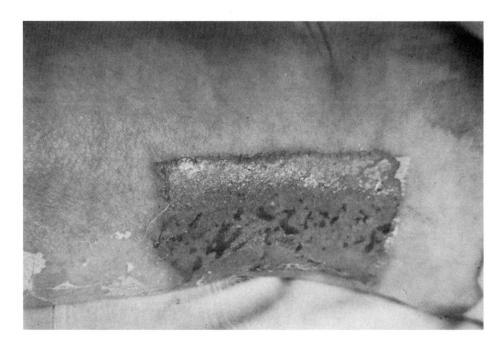

Fig. 1-52. When skin traction is applied using regular adhesive tape, superficial layers of the skin may be avulsed. The result is a weeping, angry excoriation.

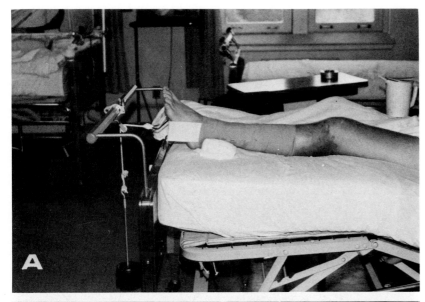

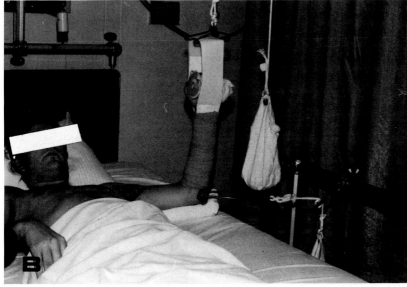

Fig. 1-53. (A) Skin traction should be applied only as a temporary expedient. Padding is applied *superior* to the malleoli, and the traction tapes are bandaged by an elastic bandage from the ankle to the knee. (B) Olecranon traction is sometimes used in the treatment of fractures of the humerus, especially supracondylar fractures. The pin is inserted through the ulnar shaft immediately distal to the olecranon, taking care to avoid the ulnar nerve. The forearm and hand are supported by skin traction.

we do, as a temporary measure in hip fractures, we tend to use the sponge rubber boot. In the elderly where the skin is fragile, great care must be exercised and no more than 5 pounds applied. There is also a great danger of friction burn to the heel so that we frequently place a water-filled rubber glove under the heel.

Skeletal Traction. Skeletal traction was first achieved by the use of tongs. As we know it today, skeletal traction is applied by a pin transfixing bone,

introduced by Fritz Steinmann. Kirschner also invented a similar device using a very fine wire that required a special traction bail to keep the wire under tension.[349] The idea of using a wire of small diameter that does minimal damage to the tissues is most attractive but, unhappily, Kirschner wires, especially over the long term, have a propensity for cutting through the bone like wire through cheese.

Our own preference is Steinmann pin traction, using a threaded pin rather than one that is smooth. Smooth pins tend to loosen rapidly, so they slip in and out, frequently leading to soft tissue infection and, on occasion, to osteomyelitis of the host bone. Recently, partially threaded Steinmann pins have been introduced. These combine the strength of the smooth pin with the holding power of the threaded, and this, we believe, is the best option for skeletal traction.

To insert Steinmann pins, the skin must be prepared as for any surgical procedure. Gloves are worn, the area is isolated with towels, and sterile precautions are observed.

Frequently the patient will be under general or spinal anesthesia, but there is no reason why the pins cannot be inserted under local infiltration anesthesia, provided care is taken to infiltrate the periosteum adequately.

In drilling a Steinmann pin, particularly when a skin incision has not been used, the skin may be caught by the pin and become puckered. If left like this it will slough, and tension should be relieved by nicking it with a knife at three points equidistant from each other.[90] The pin holes should be dressed by sponges impaled on the pins and soaked with tincture of benzoin or ace adherent or, if desired, by sponges soaked in an antiseptic such as Betadine.

In current American practice, the most common indication for skeletal traction is for fractures of the femur. Posterior bowing and late varus deformities in fractures of the femur owing to the pull of the adductors will plague the unwary, but abduction of the hip and the use of posterior pads do prevent these untoward deformities. Overdistraction of the fracture with consequent delayed union or nonunion is a major complication. With improvements in intramedullary fixation and the high cost of hospital care, continuous traction as primary treatment for femoral fractures is almost entirely passé in current practice.

Occasionally skeletal traction is indicated for humeral fractures in patients with multiple injuries. It is also commonly used in supracondylar fractures of the humerus and in tibial plateau fractures when these difficult fractures are to be treated with early motion (Apley's traction). On occasion, it is used in the treatment of tibial fractures, particularly where there are associated burns; however, because nonunion or delayed union of the tibia has been attributed to skeletal traction,[475] we are inclined to use an external fixator in such circumstances.

TRACTION FOR FEMORAL FRACTURES.   The proximal tibia is the site of choice for traction in femoral fractures. (Although one would imagine that traction through the distal femur would be much more efficient, it has the inherent disadvantage that the

pin may provoke binding down of the quadriceps, particularly when the pin tract becomes infected.)

The tibial tubercle is palpated, and the pin is drilled from the lateral to the medial side, 2 cm posterior to the tibial tubercle. In osteoporotic patients, it is prudent to go more distally into the bone of the shaft. This purchase is less likely to fail than one in the weak bone of the metaphysis.

Although femoral fractures may be treated by traction alone in the "90–90" position (ie, with both the hip and knee flexed to 90°) or merely over a pillow as Perkins[345] described, most fractures of the femur are treated with some form of additional splintage.

The most popular method is balanced suspension in a Thomas splint, or variant of it, with a Pearson attachment and isotonic traction with weights. Commonly, the reduction of these fractures is achieved by the traction and the secondary use of pads, slings, or pushers. We much prefer, whenever possible, to reduce the fracture by gentle manipulation under anesthesia and to hold the position gained by maintenance traction. This technique was also preferred by Charnley,[90] who made an excellent case for isometric traction in a straight Thomas splint.

Charnley[90] also recommended the use of a "traction unit," which is a short-leg cast incorporating a tibial Steinmann pin. Whenever a smooth Steinmann pin is used for traction, we believe that it should be anchored in plaster. Other advantages claimed for this "traction unit" are: (1) it prevents equinus of the foot; (2) the popliteal nerve and calf muscles are protected from the pressure of the slings of the splint; (3) external rotation of the foot and distal femur is controlled; (4) the tendocalcaneus is protected from pressure; (5) it is comfortable; and (6) fractures of the tibia and ipsilateral femur can be treated in this way.

Hugh Owen Thomas personally made his bed splints to fit the patient, but made-to-measure splints are a luxury not obtainable in many hospitals. In most institutions it is difficult to find a splint of exactly the right size. The leather covering the rings is often hard, dry, cracked, and, frequently, soiled by the last patient to use it. For this reason, the Harris splint (which has no ring) is useful, but we have had some problems with the medial upright impinging in the patient's perineum (Fig. 1-54).

Many hospitals use a variant of the Thomas splint with a half ring (Keller-Blake) that can be swiveled so that one splint can be used for both right and left extremities. When the ring is positioned pos-

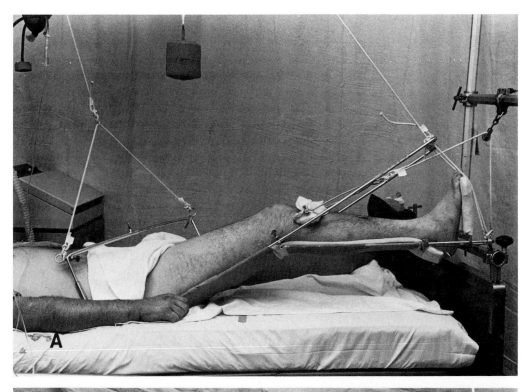

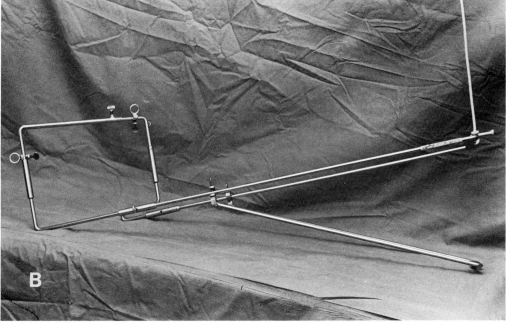

Fig. 1-54. (A, B) Balanced traction in a Harris splint with Pearson attachment. The entire system is counterbalanced by a 10-pound weight. Longitudinal traction is applied to a pin through the tibia, and the foot is kept out of equinus position by a plantar support. Care must be taken to see that the tendocalcaneus is well padded and that pressure over bony prominences or the peroneal nerve does not occur.

teriorly, the ring is uncomfortable and tends to collapse. If such a splint is used, it is better to place the solid half ring anteriorly and pass the webbing strap posteriorly over an abdominal pad.

In 1924, Hamilton Russell[384] described a method of treating fractures of the femur in which a single rope is attached to a sling, which supports the thigh and also exerts a longitudinal pull through a pulley on a foot plate. The traction applied to the femur is the result of the forces acting at the thigh sling and on the foot. By the arrangement of pulleys at the distal end, a 10-pound weight exerts a 20-pound pull. We believe the reason this method was popular was the perception of getting something for nothing—a 20-pound pull for 10. In practice, we find this traction a tedious business requiring continual readjustment and attention. However, a development of this traction is a method known as "split Russell's traction," where traction is applied through both a supracondylar pin and an os calcis pin attached to separate weights. Again, the pull on the femur is the result of these two forces.

Yet another modification (Litchman and Duffy[272]) employs two slings, one under the thigh and the other under the calf, and replaces the weights with a constant-force spring. This arrangement dispenses with the pillow under the limb as described by Russell. Although we use this arrangement for children, it can easily be modified for adults by using a pin through the os calcis.

We prefer to use another variation, invented by Kenneth G. Tomberlin and Orhan Alemdaroglu,* in which a Pearson attachment is attached to a tibial Steinmann pin and held in place by a traction bow. A pulley is braised to the end of this splint so that longitudinal traction is applied through the Pearson attachment. As in Russell's traction, a single rope provides traction in two planes: in an upward direction from the traction bow and longitudinally through the splint; the pull on the femur is the result of the two-plane traction. The traction rope runs from the traction bow to an overhead pulley, from there to a pulley on a bar at the end of the bed, then through the pulley on the splint, and finally through a second pulley at the end of the bed and to the weights. This pulley arrangement doubles the pull of the traction weights. Finally, a supportive sling is placed under the thigh with a 5- to 10-pound pull on it (Fig. 1-55).

Pressure over the tendoachilles or heel is a problem for patients in traction. We use a rubber glove, partially filled with water and tied, as a localized water bed for the heel. This is an invention of Dr. George Wright,* and we have used it for a number of years with success. It is important that the glove remain soft and not overdistended.

A most ingenious traction system for femoral fractures was invented by the late Alonzo Neufeld,[321] which he called the "dynamic method". A Steinmann pin is inserted through the proximal tibia, which is anchored in a plaster gaiter or below-knee cast. A half-ring Thomas splint with a Pearson attachment is applied with the half ring placed anteriorly. The distal end of the Thomas splint is cut off, making the assembly very similar to a Fisk splint. The leg is affixed to the Pearson attachment by more plaster of paris, and the leg and splint assembly is suspended by ropes attached to the splint at mid-leg and mid-thigh. These ropes are attached to the ends of a crossbar, which is suspended by a single rope at its midpoint. This single rope runs over a union traction pulley, which is free to run on an overhead bar. The weight for this traction is transmitted by the pulley over the foot of the bed and is between 10 and 20 pounds. Immediate knee motion is permitted with this apparatus, and in a short time the patient is able to stand up in bed. This traction has been used for patients aged 5 to 90 years.

DISTAL FEMORAL TRACTION. The main indication for distal femoral traction is where the ligaments of the knee have been injured on the ipsilateral side of a femoral fracture. In supracondylar fractures, where the posterior tilt of the distal fragment cannot be controlled by other means, a pin or a Kirschner wire may be inserted at the level of the superior border of the patella and the recalcitrant fragment pulled anteriorly (Fig. 1-56). The Steinmann pin is best inserted from the medial to the lateral side (to avoid any risk to the femoral vessels) and immediately proximal to the condyles.

CALCANEAL TRACTION. Traction through the os calcis may be used in the treatment of tibial or femoral fractures, but we tend to avoid it whenever possible, because osteomyelitis of the calcaneus is such a chronic and disabling condition. When it must be used, great care should be exercised to avoid skewering the subtalar joint. The preferred location is a point 2.5 cm posterior and 2.5 cm inferior to the lateral malleolus or, as Charnley[90] advised, "a point 1 inch superior and 1 inch anterior to the profile of the heel."

---

* Unpublished work.

* Unpublished work.

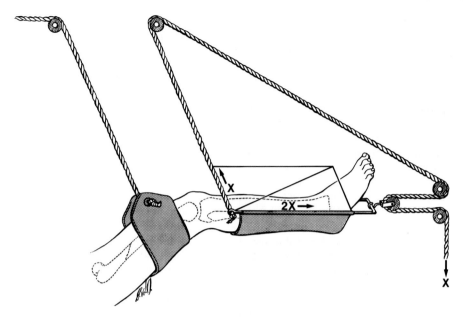

Fig. 1-55. Tomberlin's traction. The Steinmann pin in the tibia is subjected to a longitudinal pull through the Pearson attachment and a pull in a cephalad and vertical direction through the traction bow. The arrangement of two pulleys at the end of the bed and the pulley on the Pearson attachment doubles the effect of the applied weights. By adjusting the overhead pulley, the resultant pull is in the long axis of the femur, with a magnitude of 1.5 to 1.75 times the added weights. The thigh sling is for comfort and has a weight of 5 pounds to support the limb.

Traction Through the Olecranon. A medium or small threaded Steinmann pin is inserted from the medial side 1½ inches distal to the tip of the olecranon. The course of the ulnar nerve must be kept in mind. The flat posteromedial surface of the ulna is palpated, and the pin is drilled through. The traction may be in the side-arm position, or the humerus may be held vertically with the forearm supported by a felt sling. In the side-arm position, skin traction with a spreader may be used to support the forearm (Fig. 1-53*B*).

To avoid problems with the ulnar nerve, traction may be applied to the head of an AO spongiosa screw or a small screw hook inserted directly into the olecranon.

Traction by Plaster. Traction may also be applied by means of plaster-of-paris casts. In fractures of the humerus a very light "hanging" cast[76,431] is applied from the knuckles to a point no higher than 2.5 cm above the fracture site and suspended at the wrist from a string around the neck. The combined weight of the upper extremity and cast applies traction to the humeral fracture. Anteroposterior bow-

ing may be corrected by shortening or lengthening the string; varus or valgus angulation is addressed by altering the suspension point at the wrist.

Pins and Plaster. In very unstable fractures of the leg, particularly where there has been marked comminution, it may be impossible to prevent gross shortening in a conventional cast. Under these circumstances, pins may be inserted through the proximal tibia and os calcis. The fracture is pulled out to length and a cast is applied incorporating the pins, thereby applying continuous distraction of the fracture.

There are a variety of apparati designed to hold transfixation pins to immobilize a fracture while a cast is being applied. In Louisville, we have used the device invented by Dr. Arnold Griswold, a former professor of surgery at the University of Louisville, which worked extremely well (Fig. 1-57). After 3 or 4 weeks, when the fracture has gained some inherent stability, the pins are removed and a walking cast is applied. Weight-bearing is not permitted so long as the pins are *in situ,* owing to the danger of pin breakage.

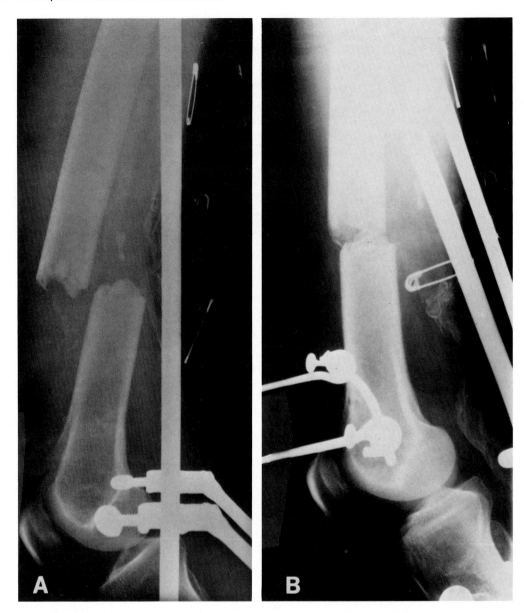

Fig. 1-56. (A, B) This femoral fracture could not be reduced by simple longitudinal traction alone. A better position was produced with the addition of a Steinmann pin through the distal fragment at the level of the upper border of the patella and anterior traction.

Pins and plaster have been advocated for a number of fractures other than those of the tibia, including the femur[160,408] and the distal end of the radius. Although this method works, it demands meticulous care and is complicated by nonunion or delayed union, pin tract infection, and, especially in the lower extremity, pin breakage.[412] At the present time, the combination of pins and plaster has been supplanted almost entirely by external fixators; the last vestige of this method still in current use is the Essex-Lopresti method of treating calcaneal fractures (Fig. 1-58).

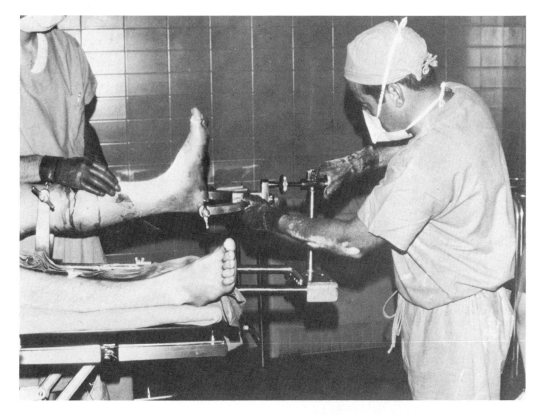

Fig. 1-57. Traction of the left tibia by the Griswold distraction machine. Pins have been applied to the proximal tibia and the os calcis, and the tibia was pulled out to length. Rotation and valgus and varus angulation may be adjusted by this machine, and when adequate reduction is achieved, a plaster-of-paris cast is applied, incorporating the Steinmann pins.

COMPLICATIONS OF PLASTER CASTS AND TRACTION

Many successful malpractice suits against orthopaedists and fracture surgeons are based on complications of plaster casts and traction.

Plaster Sores.   The skin is not designed to be compressed without relief over extended periods of time. When such pressure occurs for as little as 2 hours, irreversible damage may occur. The skin and the underlying fat, which has a poor blood supply, may necrose, and a plaster sore—nasty-smelling and usually infected—occurs.

These unhappy events do not occur without warning unless the patient is unconscious or the skin is insensate. Circular casts should be used with circumspection and trepidation in paraplegics or those who have impaired sensation (see Fig. 1-49). The patient harboring a potential plaster sore in-

variably complains of burning pain or discomfort, and these complaints must always be taken seriously. If neglected, the discomfort eventually disappears, but by then so has the skin and its nerve endings (Fig. 1-59). In all cases, the site of the patient's complaints should be inspected without delay. Irritating trips to the hospital in the middle of the night and the mutilation of one's elegant plaster casts can be avoided to some extent by paying attention to minor details during cast application.

It is not good practice to have your assistant support the lower extremity by holding the stockinette while you apply the plaster (Fig. 1-60). This creates pressure over the heel and burning pain. Similarly, in finishing the cast, pulling too vigorously on the stockinette may cause pressure on bony prominences.

Finger indentations on a cast produce high-pressure points to a much greater extent than do broad indentations made by the palm of the hand. In any

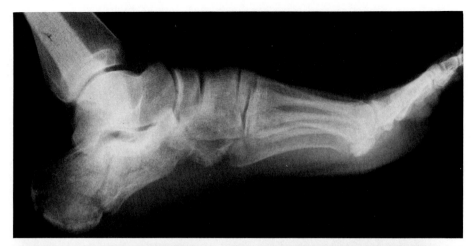

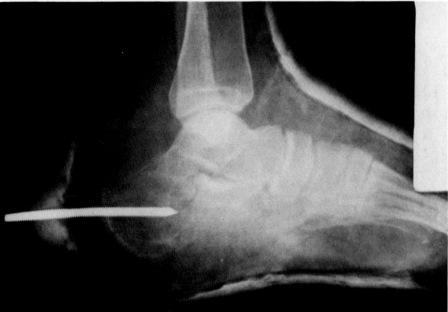

Fig. 1-58. Pins and plaster is still useful for the maintenance of calcaneal fractures. This patient's fracture was manipulated by the Essex-Lopresti method and the threaded pin incorporated in the cast.

case, indentations rarely occur when the cast is supported by the flat of the hand, and nurses and other helpers must be instructed accordingly (Fig. 1-61). After the cast is completed, it should not be allowed to rest on a sharp edge that will indent it but should be supported by a pillow or something soft.

The upper end of a cast may be unduly sharp and cause an excoriation. This is particularly common in the fold of the buttock, especially in obese pa-

tients. It can be avoided by bending out the upper edge of the cast with the fingers so that it flares. Not infrequently the patient may compound the difficulty by inserting tissues or something soft between the cast and the skin or by cutting away the offending plaster, often leaving a jagged edge that produces another sore. Patients should be told that if the cast cuts, the border should be bent out with a pair of pliers. This also applies to the margins of a thumb hole (Fig. 1-62).

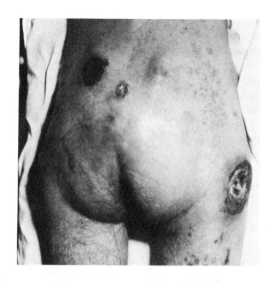

Fig. 1-59. This young man with multiple fractures was sent to convalesce at home in a plaster-of-paris spica. Although he did suffer some discomfort, his pain disappeared along with the skin over the trochanters, sacrum, and left posterosuperior iliac spine. All complaints of pain under plaster-of-paris casts must be taken seriously.

Immobilization of the metacarpophalangeal joints, especially in extension, must be avoided like the plague, owing to the danger of permanent stiffness (Fig. 1-63) (see Chapter 7).

On occasion, patients in casts will be seized by uncontrollable itching. In their efforts to get relief, they commonly unravel a wire coat hanger and use it to scratch under the cast. Not only do they produce excoriations but, by wadding up the padding, they may produce sores too.

Felt pads placed over bony prominences may migrate and have the opposite effect from that intended. To prevent this, the felt should be applied as the last layer of padding so that it adheres to the plaster.

The Tight Cast. Care should always be taken not to wrap a plaster bandage too tightly. However, even when a cast is not too tight when applied, if the limb swells, it may become tight later. Pain is the first and most constant complaint of the patient with a tight cast; even if the peripheral circulation appears unimpaired, the prudent course is to split the cast (Fig. 1-64). Garfin and co-workers[159] applied

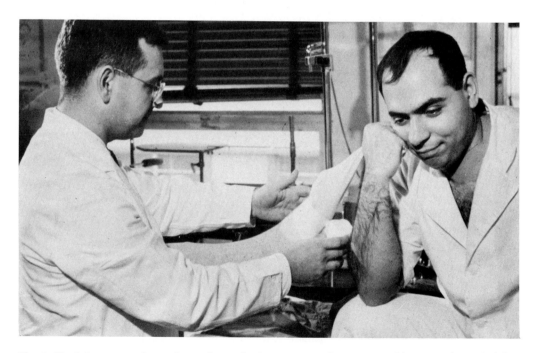

Fig. 1-60. It is not good practice to have the lower extremity supported by an assistant holding the stockinette. This inevitably causes undue pressure of the stockinette over the heel, and it may cause burning pain or even a sore. The same effect can be produced by pulling too vigorously on the stockinette when folding it over the sharp edges of the cast.

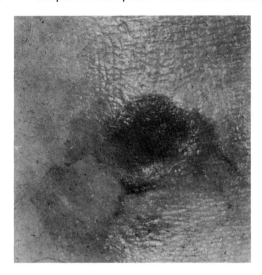

Fig. 1-61. The surgeon in this case inadvertently made an indentation with his thumb while modling the fractured ankle. The result was skin necrosis over the medial malleolus.

padded plaster-of-paris casts to the hind legs of dogs and monitored compartment pressures after the injection of autologous serum into the leg. When the casts were univalved (ie, a single cut made longitudinally), the intracompartmental pressures fell 30%; spreading the cut caused a 60% drop; and cutting the padding, a further 10%. Complete removal of the cast reduced the pressure by 85%.

Similar results were recorded when the padding was soaked in Betadine and blood or when the Webril had been soaked and dried, but the percentage drop was less.

In comparing the rise of pressure in the anterior compartments after injection in casted and non-casted legs, it was found that 40% less fluid was required in casted legs than in non-casted to produce the same increase in pressure.

It would seem logical that in a patient having symptoms from a tight cast, sequential decompression should be carried out until symptoms are relieved. However, blood-soaked padding appears to be as hard and as unyielding as the plaster of paris

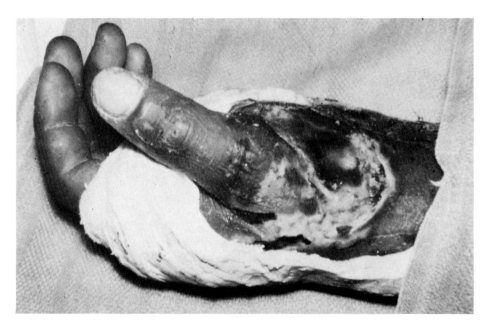

Fig. 1-62. This is the end result of pressure exerted by an improperly applied cast over the thumb metacarpal. The patient had a large, full-thickness skin slough and lost the abductor and extensor tendons of his thumb in the bargain. The sharp edges of the thumb hole must always be everted, and undue pressure over the base of the thumb metacarpal must be avoided.

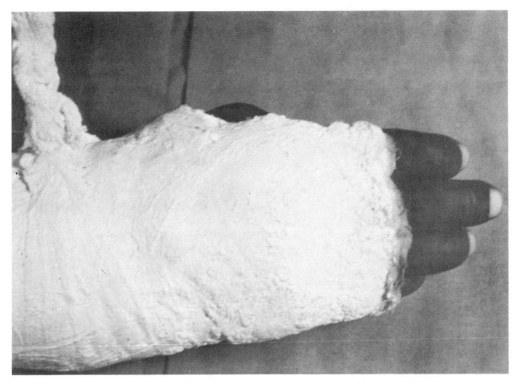

Fig. 1-63. This is the hand portion of a poorly applied hanging cast. Not only is this plaster rough and improperly applied, but by extending over the fingers, it limits their motion and holds the metacarpophalangeal joints in extension. Such a monstrosity, applied for even a short time, can cripple a hand.

itself, and one would never be wrong in bivalving the cast and cutting the padding to the skin.

Circular bandages of gauze or encircling adhesive tape should never be applied under a cast, because these, too, may have a tourniquet effect (Fig. 1-65).

Patrick and Levack[339] studied the pressure over the prominence of the distal radius after the application of a forearm cast. They found that the highest pressure was recorded immediately after the application of the cast. The pressure dropped over the next 2 or 3 hours, only to rise again to a submaximal peak at an average of 13 hours. Over the next 72 hours the pressure gradually fell, but at no time after the first hour did they record a pressure of more than 30 mm Hg. Five of the nine cases studied had edema of the hand and fingers after 48 to 72 hours. On the basis of this study they recommended initial immobilization by sugar tong splints rather than by circular casts.

Wherever possible after internally fixing fractures or where swelling is expected, we use a Jones-type dressing, with or without plaster reinforcements.

The Jones dressing is a bulky dressing usually applied after knee surgery. It consists of a thick layer of absorbent cotton wrapped with domett or elastic bandages followed by two more layers of cotton and bandage. We have modified this by using Kling or Kerlex bandages and cheap cotton batting instead of absorbent cotton and finishing the last layer with an elastic bandage. Where additional stability is required, slabs of plaster are placed on the medial and lateral sides of the limb as the most superficial layer under the last bandage. A similar sort of bulky dressing may also be used in the upper limb. This should not be called a compression dressing, because people will be encouraged to apply it too tightly. It should be applied without much tension and, if too tight, it is easily removed with scissors in seconds.

Thermal Effects of Plaster.   When dehydrated gypsum takes up its water of crystallization, an exothermic reaction takes place. How high the temperature becomes depends on the amount of plaster,

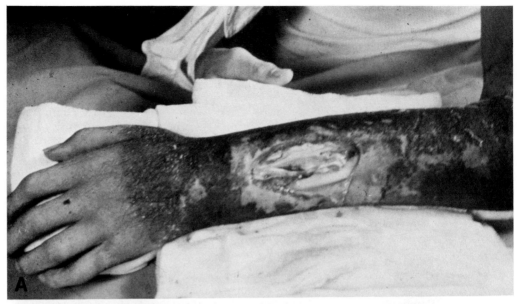

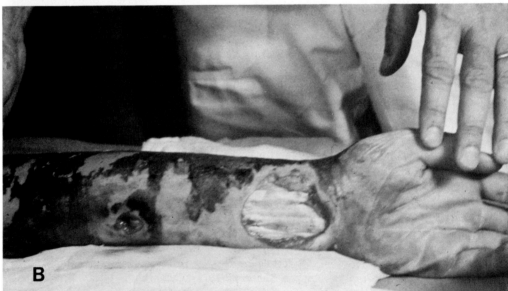

Fig. 1-64. (A, B) This young man had an open fracture of his left forearm treated by a plaster-of-paris cast. When, subsequently, the arm became infected and swollen, his complaints of pain were disregarded. Ultimately his entire forearm became necrotic. This is how it looked immediately prior to amputation.

its surface area, and the external environment's ability to allow the plaster to lose heat. Other factors such as chemical accelerators, temperature of the water, and the water content of the bandage are also important. While in most circumstances this exothermic reaction does nothing more than make the patient pleasantly warm, it is possible to produce thermal burns with the application of thick plaster-of-paris splints.[232] This is particularly so in preformed splints, 16-ply thick and backed by sponge padding to obviate the need of supplementary sheet wadding.

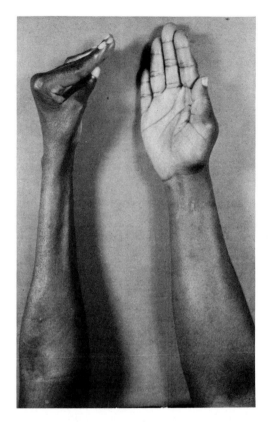

Fig. 1-65. The end result of circular constriction may be Volkmann's ischemic contracture, which in this case involved the intrinsic muscles of the left hand. This is the "main d'accoucheur." When a patient complains of pain, all encircling dressings and casts must be split.

Williamson and Scholtz[481] have shown that thermal injuries are temperature–time related and that second-degree burns will be produced by a temperature of 50°C after 12 minutes. Third-degree burns may result after a 50°C temperature has been maintained for 5 to 15 minutes.[123]

Occasionally temperatures as high as 82°C may be produced by curing plaster.[33]

Lavalette and associates[266] found that dip water warmer than 24°C, a cast thicker than eight ply, and the insulation of a pillow were conducive to temperatures hot enough to burn skin, especially when present in combination.

The circumspect orthopaedist should wet the plaster with water from the cold faucet; limit the thickness of splints or circular casts to the thinnest strong enough for his purpose; and leave the bandage manageably sloppy, because a dry bandage sets more quickly and is without the heat sink pro-

vided by the excess water. The danger is even more acute in comatose or unconscious patients or where the skin is insensitive. It is possible that, in shock, the lack of circulation in the skin might further impair the ability to dissipate heat. Furthermore, in these patients where emergency splintage is being applied, it makes sense to apply cast padding, a poor conductor, to the limb and to make sure that as much surface is exposed to the circulating air as possible.

Thrombophlebitis and Equinus Position.   Ochsner noted 30 years ago that thrombophlebitis or phlebothrombosis was uncommon in patients treated by lower extremity casts. He pointed out that, on a theoretical basis, one would expect to have more episodes rather than fewer when a lower limb was injured and immobilized. This comparative immunity, he believed, was related to the casted leg's being warmer than normal. Micheli,[302] however, reported six cases of patients with lower-extremity casts who developed pulmonary embolism in four instances and severe thrombophlebitis in two. Three of these patients had rupture of the tendocalcaneus and the others had a subtalar dislocation, a fractured tibial shaft, and a tibial plateau fracture, respectively. We have had two patients, treated for heel-cord rupture by immobilization in equinus, develop pulmonary embolism. We have attributed this to pooling of blood in the veins of the calf with subsequent clotting secondary to the loss of the "pumping" action of the triceps surae. In the extreme equinus position these muscles become so relaxed that they are unable to generate enough tension to strip the calf veins. Although we still treat fractures of the distal third of the tibia by a cast with the foot in equinus, we are careful not to overdo it, while at the same time not dorsiflexing the foot enough to angulate the fracture. The equinus position, contrary to popular belief, does not give rise to stiffness of the ankle in 2 or 3 weeks' time—unless there is also a fracture involving the mortise.

Hooper and associates[209] have studied fractures of the shaft of the tibia in which the fibula is intact. In these fractures there is an inherent tendency for the tibial fracture to collapse to the fibular side, producing a varus malalignment. This they attribute to the tibia's being displaced by dorsiflexion of the ankle. Although this can be averted by immobilization in equinus or by internal fixation, they prefer to osteotomize the fibula. The major lesson to be learned, however, is that extreme equinus is to be avoided.

The Cast Syndrome. In the past, compression fractures of the spine have been treated with hyperextension body jackets. Occasionally, patients treated in this way developed pernicious vomiting and electrolyte imbalance, and some even died. This "cast syndrome" is caused by an obstruction of the third portion of the duodenum resulting from constriction by the superior mesenteric vessels.[319] Few people now believe that immobilization of stable compression fractures of the spine is necessary, and certainly the position of extreme hyperextension should be avoided.

Some nervous people feel unduly constricted by any type of cast that encloses the body, a condition akin to claustrophobia. They, too, are liable to vomit and have a variety of psychosomatic complaints, which lead to the cast's having to be removed. The vomiting in such cases is rarely as severe and life-threatening as in the true cast syndrome.

Infection Secondary to Cast Application. It is rare to have wounds infected by contaminated plaster of paris, sheet wadding, or dip water, but such cases have been reported. It would seem that sterilization of plaster of paris or the use of distilled water for dip water is not indicated, but the circumspect surgeon will use sterile dressings and sheet wadding after surgery or where there is an open wound. It is also mandatory that plaster buckets be cleaned or replaced after use and not allowed to stand full of stagnant water as a potential culture medium.

The rather naive idea that one should be able to swim with a fiberglass cast on is potentially dangerous because this tends to promote maceration of the skin unless thorough drying by hot air is carried out and the padding is nylon. One case of ringworm has been reported under these circumstances,[283] and we have had an infection of a transcutaneous Kirschner wire in an operated foot which was dangled in a swimming pool. The absolute contraindication to this practice is the presence of a recent operative wound.

Allergic Reactions. We have never seen an allergic reaction to plaster of paris, but we have one patient with a sensitivity to cotton stockinette. There have, however, been two cases where sensitized patients have had allergic responses to the benzalkonium in the plaster bandage.[278,427]

Traction Hazards. Patients in traction develop pressure ulcers just as readily as those treated by plaster. The skin in contact with the ring of a Thomas splint, the sacrum, and other pressure areas must be inspected daily. In some high-risk patients, the sacrum should be protected by an "antigravity pad." A sheepskin, real or synthetic, or a commercially available "egg crate" foam pad is also helpful to preserve the back of a patient who will be in traction for extended periods. The heels and heel cords are particularly liable to develop decubiti and should be protected by heel cups, sponge rubber pads, or water-filled gloves.

If the foot is allowed to lie in the equinus position, a permanent drop-foot contracture may develop. This should be prevented by active exercise and the provision of some type of device to hold up the foot.

Circular bandages should be checked and reapplied as necessary to prevent constriction of the circulation and to assure that the skin tapes are not slipping. This is particularly true in children who are being treated by Bryant's or gallows traction. In general, this method is best used in very small children up to 20 pounds, and the absolute upper limit is 30 pounds. For larger children we advise Weber's method if catastrophic circulatory problems are to be avoided (Fig. 1-66).[399,476]

Under no circumstances should the lower extremity be allowed to rotate externally in a Thomas splint. This may cause pressure on the common peroneal nerve with subsequent paralysis.

In treatment of fractures of the cervical spine, traction by means of a head halter should be used only for a short time, as sores develop readily over the chin. Skull tongs should be inserted as early as possible (Fig. 1-67).

EXTERNAL FIXATION OF FRACTURES

> It is not wise to use external fixation everywhere and for everything.
>
> W. Taillard[444]

Although Alvin Lambotte has generally been given the credit for introducing, in 1907, the use of transfixing pins attached to an external frame to treat fractures, Seligson[413] has pointed out that Parkhill[337] was using such a device prior to 1897. Nevertheless, the European tradition of external fixation has been predicated on Lambotte's pioneer work.

In the United States, Roger Anderson[13] devised a frame with transfixion pins in 1934 that allowed him to line up difficult tibial fractures and then apply a cast that incorporated the pins. In cases where there was severe soft tissue trauma, he used the apparatus as the primary means of fixation.

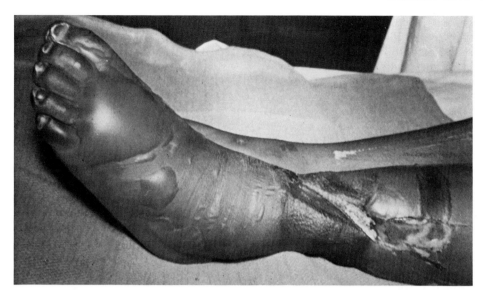

Fig. 1-66. This child had a fractured femoral shaft treated at home in Bryant's traction. Disarranged bandages acted as a ligature around the ankle, and the foot of the uninjured extremity had to be amputated.

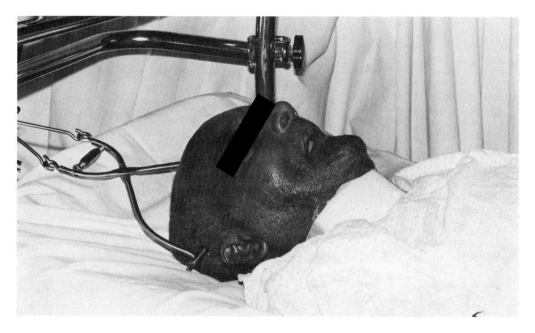

Fig. 1-67. Traction for injuries of the cervical spine should be by means of some type of skull tongs. The use of the head halter for more than a short period of time, especially if heavy weight is to be used, will give rise to excoriation of the skin over the chin.

Otto Stader,[426] a veterinarian, described an external fixator for use in animals in 1937, and this was adopted by surgeons treating people. While the use of external fixators declined in this country, probably owing to the complication of pin tract infection, its use continued in Europe.

The Hoffmann apparatus, originally described in 1939,[203] was modified and improved by Vidal and Ardrey,[470] and the excellent results achieved by surgeons in France, Switzerland, and elsewhere using this equipment sparked a revival of interest in this method worldwide. Many different types of fixators are now available, ranging from very expensive, elaborate machines to "do-it-yourself" frames of methymethacrylate.[16,222]

External fixators allow stabilization of a fracture at a distance from the fracture site without increasing soft tissue damage. They maintain the length and alignment of a fractured extremity without casting so that soft tissue wounds can be easily inspected and treated, and the stability engendered may allow early mobilization and activity.[35]

External fixation is particularly helpful in open fractures of the tibia, but it may be used under certain circumstances in the femur, pelvis, humerus, and other bones.

Types of External Fixation

In recent years there has been a plethora of external fixators described and advocated, and it would not be productive to give the details of every device in this discourse. Behrens[34] has divided these devices into two groups: pin fixators and ring fixators (Fig. 1-68). Pin fixators can be further subdivided into simple and clamp devices.

In ring fixators, a frame is built consisting of rings or partial rings and connecting rods that encompass the extremity, from which transfixion pins or wires suspend the bone. In pin fixators, the rigid pins are an intrinsic component of the frame as well as the means of anchorage to bone. In simple fixators, the pins are attached by independent articulations to a longitudinal rod, but in the other type of pin fixator, the pins are held by clamps which in turn are attached to the longitudinal rod by an articulation.

SIMPLE PIN FIXATORS

Examples of simple fixators are the Roger Anderson device and the AO/ASIF types. These devices provide much more latitude in pin placement than other fixators, both in the separation or spread of the pins and the angle of approach to the bone, which in turn enhances the rigidity of the frame. The number of configurations possible is legion and,

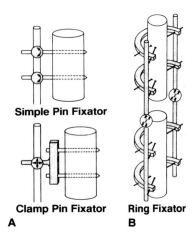

Simple Pin Fixator

Clamp Pin Fixator
A

Ring Fixator
B

Fig. 1-68. (A) Simple and clamp pin fixators. **(B)** Ring fixator. *(Behrens, F.: A Primer of External Fixation. Clin. Orthop., 241:8–9, 1989.)*

in the most difficult cases, we frequently will fall back on the very versatile Roger Anderson apparatus.

The major defect of simple fixators is that they allow very little adjustment after application, without replacing pins, so that the fracture must be reduced prior to the application of the frame.

CLAMP FIXATORS

Clamp fixators such as the Hoffman or Kronner devices allow for final reduction of the fracture after application of the device, but adjustments can be made by loosening the articulations. The pin spread and direction of the pins is dictated by the clamp, and the variety of frames that can be built is significantly abridged. Furthermore, gradual adjustment is not possible, and once the articulations are released, there is an inherent danger of losing the reduction.

RING FIXATORS

Ring fixators such as the Ilizarov or Ace-Fischer devices allow gradual and precise correction of angulatory and rotational deformity but, unlike pin fixators, tend to limit access to wounds of the extremities and make free tissue transfer difficult or impossible.

Simple Pin Fixators

THE ROGER ANDERSON SYSTEM

In the Roger Anderson system, multiple pins can be inserted either as transfixion pins or as half pins.

Each pin is connected to a clamp that also has a connection for an aluminum rod. There are also double connectors for the aluminum rods so that a frame can be built. The manufacturer's directions recommend using two or more pins in each fragment and having at least one pin through the widest possible part of the metaphysis. Half pins should be used only in locations where through-and-through transfixion is not anatomically feasible. They also recommend Crowe tip pins for cortical bone and tri-point pins for cancellous bones. The pins should be placed at an angle to each other in the same plane, but this angle should not exceed 60°. Before fixing the pins to the fracture rod, the ends should be moderately spread or compressed. Unlike other external fixators, the prescribed management is to supplement the device with a light plaster or back splint. We must confess that frequently we have transgressed and have not followed those directions to the letter. On occasion, we have tried to build an external frame of fracture rods in a series of triangles to make a more rigid frame, with some limited success (Figs. 1-69 and 1-70). In retrospect, we would have done better to insert more pins or to apply a second system, using half pins at right angles to the first. In spite of this, we have been pleased with the results we have achieved with this system.

Compression–distraction rods are also available with the Roger Anderson system, and although the system does not yield so stable a frame as the Hoffmann, it has been invaluable to us in the past. Where fractures are close to the end of a bone, we are able to get more pins in the smaller fragment than with the Hoffmann. We particularly like it for unstable Colles' fractures, where a quadrilateral frame is made with pins in the index and middle metacarpals and two pins in the radius.

THE WAGNER APPARATUS

The use of frames with transfixion pins for fractures of the femur is tedious and inherently dangerous. As a rule we prefer to fix femurs internally, but we have found the Wagner apparatus[215,428] helpful where internal fixation is not an option (eg, long-standing, shortened malunions and nonunions; infected, plated nonunions; fractures with large bone deficits; and neurovascular injuries) (Figs. 1-71 to 1-73).

It is probably best to line up the fracture by traction, inserting two Schanz screws proximally and distally, using a guide to keep them parallel. The screws should be inserted by hand. Alignment can be adjusted at the ends of the apparatus and the fracture distracted or compressed by turning the screw. This is particularly useful when a gradual reduction of a severe overlap is called for (Fig. 1-74).

THE ORTHOFIX FIXATOR
(DYNAMIC AXIAL FIXATOR)

The Wagner apparatus, while providing excellent axial fixation and the ability to compress or distract a fracture, must be applied to a fracture already reduced and allows little or no adjustment once applied. The Orthofix fixator provides the same advantages as the Wagner, but in addition allows the surgeon to carry out the reduction of the fracture after the application of the device and to make subsequent adjustments to correct angulatory and rotational discrepancies; it also allows dynamic axial compression after the appearance of callus.

The device is a single bar with a ball-and-socket joint at each end, to which is attached a clamp with five slots to provide a choice in the number and location of the anchoring pins (Fig. 1-75). These pins are self-tapping and are tapered, 5 mm at the point and 6 mm in the shaft. The body of the fixator contains a telescoping shaft controlled by a compression/distraction device. When the requisite degree of compression or distraction is reached, the shaft is locked, and the compression/distraction device removed. When dynamic axial compression is required, the shaft is unlocked.

The device is applied by inserting a screw through both cortices of one diaphyseal fragment after predrilling with a drill guide. Three more screws are inserted in a similar manner using a template for placement. In the tibia, the screws are inserted through the subcutaneous surface, and in the femur, a direct lateral approach is used.

After insertion of the screws, the bar is adjusted to the appropriate length and applied to the screws. When reduction of the fracture has been achieved, the pin clamps are locked by a cam arrangement at the ball joints and the telescopic central bar is locked in its sleeve. The joints allow 30° of angulation and free rotation. The positions of the locking cams are ascertained by pairs of markers on the camshaft end and the encasing collar. When these markers are aligned, the ball joint is unlocked. Locking occurs between 45° and 75° of rotation.

Chao and Hein[85] investigated the mechanical properties of this device and found it to be comparable to quadrilateral fixators with transfixing full pins and advised that multiple usage was permissible for four consecutive 6-month periods, providing that "careful inspection and routine replace-

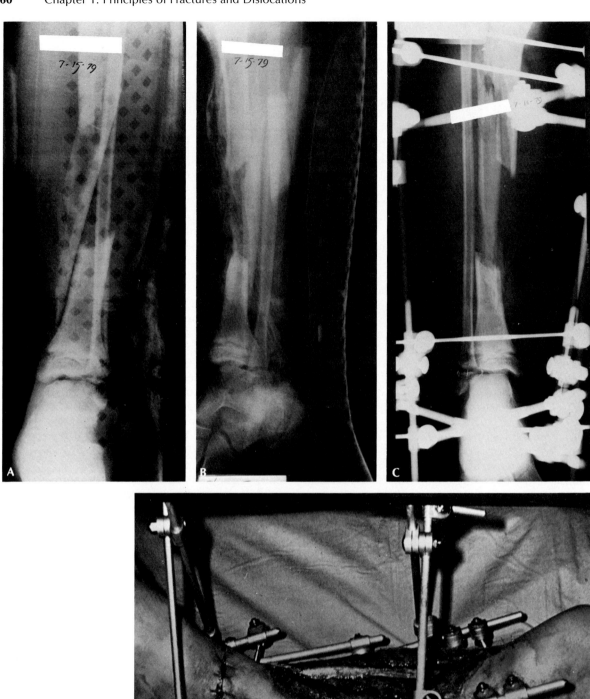

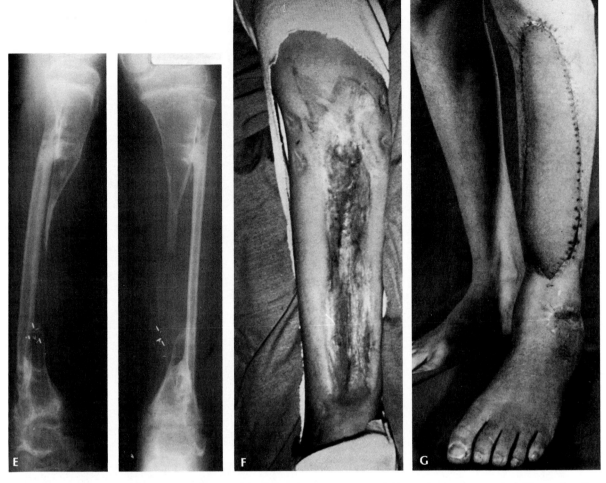

Fig. 1-69. Radiographs and clinical photos of the lower leg in a 10-year-old boy who inadvertently fell into a feeding augur and had his left leg chewed up. **(A, B)** The initial films show segmental fractures of the tibia and fibula and an open disruption of the ankle joint. **(C)** The leg after débridement and the application of a Roger-Anderson fixator. Unfortunately, the loose middle fragment became a sequestrum and had to be removed. **(D)** An intraoperative photograph at the time the fragment was removed. **(E)** The leg 2 years later, after multiple débridements and the creation of a tibiofibular synostosis proximally and distally by bone grafts. **(F)** A clinical photograph at this stage with split-thickness grafts covering the defect. These grafts were liable to break down with trauma and had to be replaced. **(G)** The leg after the application of a latissimus dorsi free flap.

ment of crucial parts is performed on the used apparatus before reapplication."

De Bastiani and associates[113] (in their initial report in English), treated 288 fresh fractures, of which 239 were closed and 49 were open; 117 were in the femur, 160 in the tibia, 44 in the humerus, 1 in the radius, and 16 in the pelvis. In closed fractures their success rates were 91% in the tibia and 98% in the femur and humerus. In open fractures their success rates for the tibia and femur were 88%

and 89%, respectively. Their pin tract infection rate was incredibly low; only 14 (in ten patients) of 1525 pins inserted. The average time taken to apply the apparatus was a mere 15 minutes.

THE AO/ASIF FIXATOR

The inventors of the AO/ASIF device[202] set out to provide a fixator that would be versatile, stable, and simple[8] (Fig. 1-76). It consists of four components: Steinmann pins, Schanz screws, a tube with an

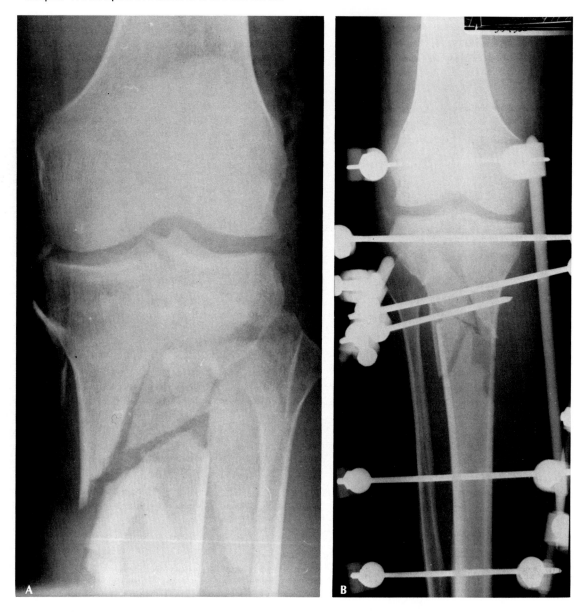

Fig. 1-70. (A to E) Radiographs of the knee in a man who drove his motorcycle off the road and sustained a severely comminuted fracture of the proximal end of the tibia with disruption of the ligamentum patellae and the pes anserinus. **(A)** The comminuted fracture. **(B, C)** The tibia after application of a Roger-Anderson external fixator. Note that the patella has also been included in the assembly. This allowed immediate mobilization of the knee, even in the presence of a repaired ligamentum patellae. During movements of the knee the patella was maintained in its proper relationship to the tibia by the external fixator.

(continued)

outer diameter of 11 mm, and an adjustable clamp to fix the pins to the tubes.

The tubes come in a variety of lengths from 100 to 600 mm and are approximately 2½ times as strong as the threaded bar of the earlier AO fixator.

The Steinmann pins are 5 mm in diameter (150–250 mm in length) and have a modified drill bit–point to eliminate thermal damage to the bone. The Schanz screws are also 5 mm in diameter and are available in lengths from 100 to 200 mm. These

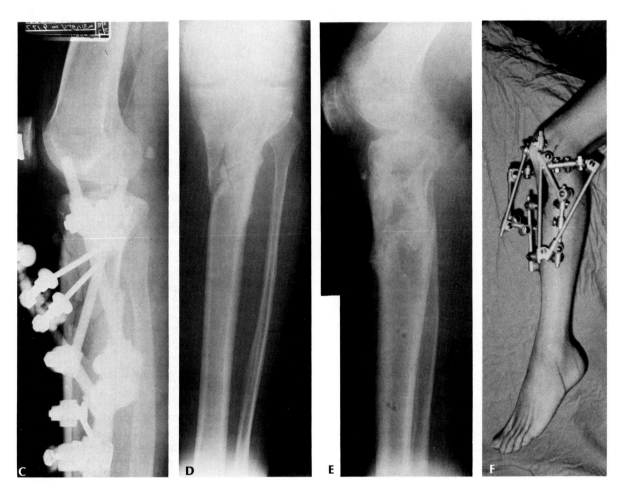

Fig. 1-70 (*continued*)
(D, E) The end result with complete healing of the fracture and the joint space well maintained. **(F)** Clinical photograph of a similar patient showing the external fixator with transfixion of the patella.

screws have been modified by making the threaded portion only 18 mm long so that it engages only the far cortex, while the near cortex is occupied by the smooth, unthreaded 5-mm shaft.

The adjustable clamp connects the Steinmann pins or the Schanz screws to the tubes and allows for correction in all planes. To insert the pins and screws, 3.5-mm and 4.5-mm drill bits are necessary, as well as a 3.5-mm trocar and drill sleeves with inner diameters of 3.5 mm and 5 mm.

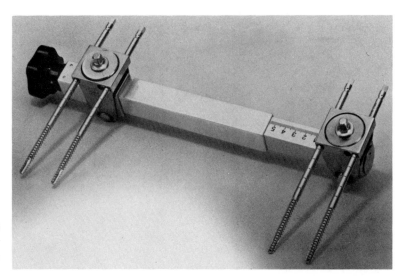

Fig. 1-71. The Hoffmann modification of the Wagner leg-lengthening apparatus. *(Courtesy of Howmedica, Inc., 1981.)*

To insert a Schanz screw, the drill sleeves and trocar are assembled and inserted through a stab wound until the trocar impinges on the surface of the bone. After removal of the trocar, both cortices of the bone are drilled through with a 3.5-mm drill. The 3.5-mm sleeve should then be removed and the near hole enlarged with the 4.5-mm drill. The Schanz screw is then introduced by a hand chuck and the 5-mm drill sleeve removed.

Steinmann pins are introduced in a similar fashion; the combined drill sleeves and trocar are introduced as before, but in this case, the trocar and 3.5-mm drill sleeve are both removed and both cortices drilled with the 4.5-mm bit. However, when quadrilateral or delta frames are applied, the aiming device should be used (Fig. 1-77). The aiming device ensures that the drills and subsequently the Steinmann pins pass accurately from the clamp on one tube to its companion on the other tube. In this case, the 3.5-mm sleeve of the aiming device is used to drill both cortices of the bone and then the aiming device is removed and the 4.5-mm drill is used to overdrill the 3.5-mm hole.

Although a large variety of configurations are possible using the AO components, three configurations are particularly recommended (Fig. 1-78): type I—unilateral frame; type II—bilateral frame; and type III—triangulated assembly.

Unilateral Frame.   The unilateral frame is particularly indicated where anatomical or functional conditions make the other frames inadvisable (eg, the humerus and forearm). It is also appropriate for open fractures of the femur and has been particu-larly advocated by Behrens and Solls for the management of tibial fractures. In the tibia, the pins are inserted in the tibial crest. A Schanz screw is placed in each fragment in the metaphysis close to the joint. Four (or six) clamps are placed on a tube of appropriate length that is fixed to the Schanz screws. A closed reduction of the fracture is then carried out, and the clamps are tightened. It is essential that rotational alignment be achieved at this juncture. Screws are then inserted through the remaining clamps and the assembly tightened. The closer the tube is placed to the tibial crest, the more rigid the fixation will be, and it may be further enhanced by adding a second tube. If a second tube is added, it must be done before the third and fourth screws are inserted, so that the screws can be inserted through each pair of clamps simultaneously. The frame may be made even stiffer by applying two unilateral frames at an angle to each other and cross linking the tubes.

Bilateral Frame.   The bilateral AO/ASIF configuration is used primarily in fractures of the tibia. The first Steinmann pin is inserted through the distal tibia, anterior to the fibula, and parallel to the ankle joint. If the bone is hard, it should be predrilled with the 3.5-mm drill and then with the 4.5-mm. In osteoporotic bone, however, predrilling with the 3.5-mm drill is adequate and the 5-mm Steinmann pin is inserted. Insertion of a proximal pin is carried out from lateral to medial immediately anterior to the fibula while an assistant applies traction and corrects rotational malalignment of the leg. The pins should be parallel and be inserted by

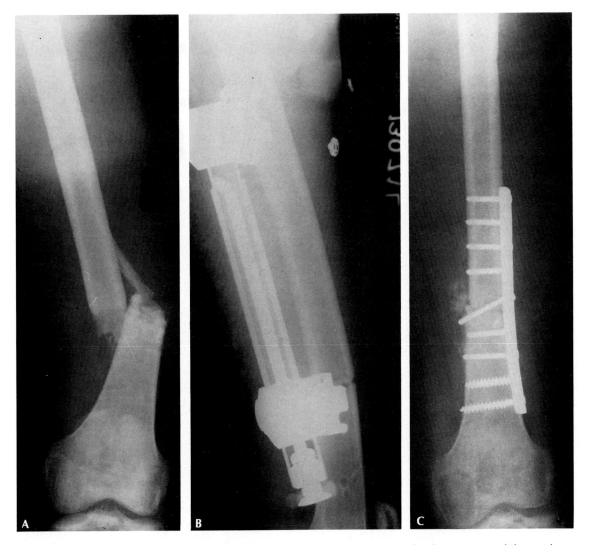

Fig. 1-72. Radiographs of the femur in a 20-year-old blind man who was involved in an automobile accident. He sustained an open fracture of the left tibia, a closed fracture of the right tibia, a crushing injury of the right foot that necessitated a Syme's amputation, and a fracture of the right femur. The right femur was temporarily stabilized with a Wagner apparatus and then plated. The use of the Wagner apparatus enabled this patient to be mobilized and facilitated the treatment of his leg injuries until the definitive treatment of the femur was performed. **(A)** The preoperative condition of the femur. **(B)** The Wagner apparatus, rather inexpertly applied, with the lower pins too close to the fracture site. **(C)** The femur with a plate on the tension side and an oblique screw through the fracture site to achieve satisfactory interfragmental compression. The ipsilateral tibia was treated with a Roger-Anderson fixator and bone grafting. Both fractures healed.

a hand chuck. Clamps corresponding to the number of pins desired are threaded on the longitudinal tubes and care is taken to place them in such a manner that their broad part lies anterior to the Steinmann pins, and the tube posterior to them. The clamps should be tightened minimally to allow later final reduction of the fracture. The screws are then tightened and the remaining Steinmann pins inserted using the pin guide to make the drill holes.

If the definitive treatment of the fracture is to be by fixator, pins should be inserted close to the fracture site; if internal fixation is planned for later, the pins should be inserted as far as possible from the fracture.

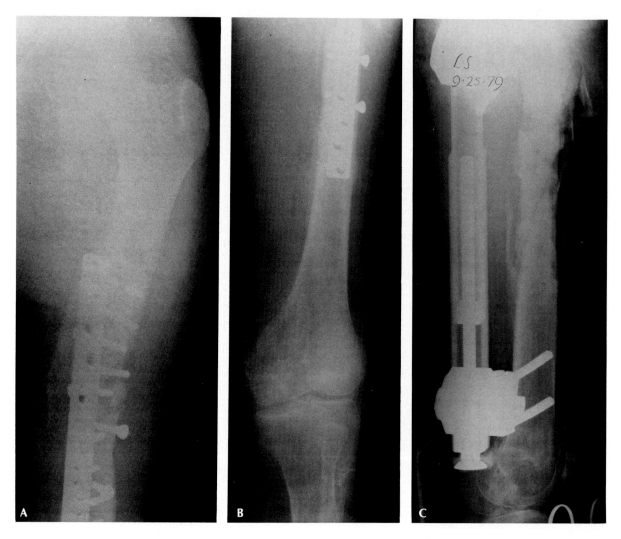

Fig. 1-73. Radiographs of the leg in a 16-year-old boy who sustained a femoral shaft fracture that was treated by the application of a plate. **(A, B)** Anteroposterior and lateral films of the femur show that the plate has been applied to the anterior aspect of the femur instead of the lateral side, and the fracture at this point is infected with loose internal fixation and broken screws. **(C)** Because the internal fixation was performing no useful function, it was removed and a Wagner external fixator applied. Cancellous bone grafting was performed during the operation.

(continued)

When this frame is used and there is adequate bony contact, axial compression may be exerted on the fracture site by preloading the Steinmann pins (ie, bending them toward the fracture) (Fig. 1-79). On the other hand, if there is a bony defect or no inherent stability because of comminution, the Steinmann pins should be preloaded within each fragment by bending the pins toward each other (see Fig. 1-79).

This preloading may be produced by applying the AO compressor or a Verbrugge clamp, or by one's fingers.

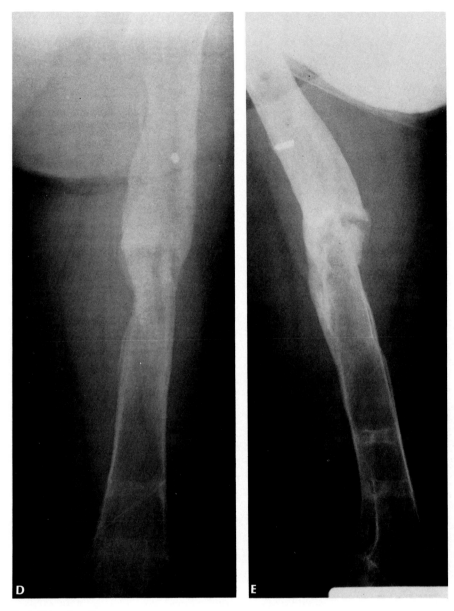

Fig. 1-73 *(continued)*
(D, E) The end result 16 months later, after having been maintained in the Wagner apparatus for 13 months.

Triangulated Assembly. The axial and lateral stability are about the same in type II and type III AO/ASIF configurations, but the triangulated assembly has greater torsional stability than is achieved by fewer anchoring pins in the bone. It is mostly used in the tibia, where fewer pins pierce the anterolateral compartment, but is sometimes indicated in fractures of the distal femur.

To build this frame, one Steinmann pin is inserted proximally and one distally in the same manner as when applying the type II bilateral frame. Three clamps are applied to each tube and the tubes are

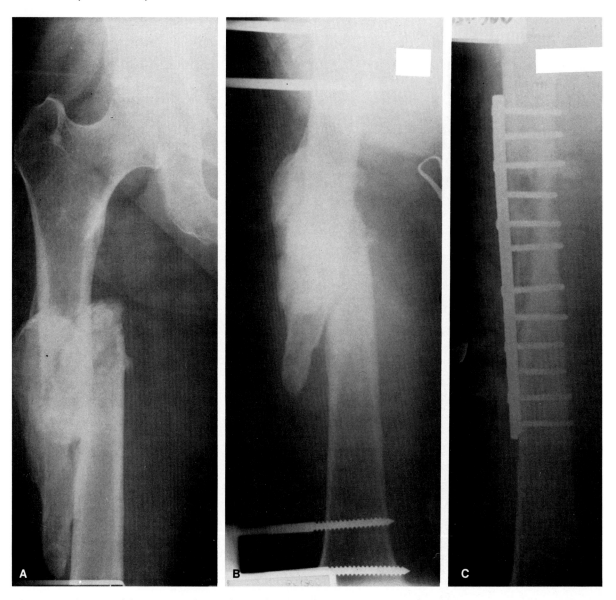

Fig. 1-74. The use of the Wagner device for gradual lengthening. A 44-year-old man fractured his femur when he overturned a tractor. He was treated at a military installation by a cast–brace. After removal of the cast–brace he developed pain in his thigh, but kept walking anyway. He was seen by four orthopaedists for disability evaluation, all of whom reported different leg-length discrepancies, which they believed to be secondary to shortening with malunion. **(A)** This x-ray film shows that no union had been achieved. **(B)** The femur was pulled out to length gradually by a Wagner apparatus. **(C)** Internal fixation by a plate after the femur had been pulled out to length.

applied to the Steinmann pins loosely. After reducing the fracture the clamps are tightened and one Schanz screw is inserted anteroposteriorly in each fragment. A third tube with four clamps attached is fitted to the Schanz screws, and the lateral tubes are cross linked to the sagittal tube using Steinmann pins and the previously applied clamps. As in the type II frame, the Steinmann pins in the bone are preloaded (see Fig. 1-78).

Clamp Fixators

THE HOFFMANN SYSTEM

The Hoffmann system is a clamp fixator. The resurgence of interest in external fixation was sparked

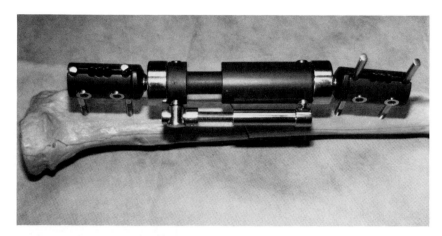

Fig. 1-75. The Orthofix fixator. (*Courtesy of EBI Medical Systems, Inc., 1989.*)

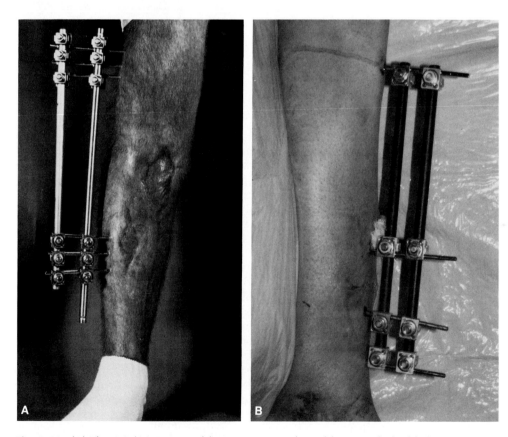

Fig. 1-76. (A) The AO/ASIF external fixator, type I unilateral frame with double bar. Note that the upper pins are in the distal femur to reduce a comminuted plateau fracture by ligamentotaxis and to stabilize a comminuted fracture of the shaft. **(B)** Immobilization of a tibial fracture by an anterior unilateral frame with double bars (Trauma Fix). Note that these bars are made of a radiolucent fiber composite.

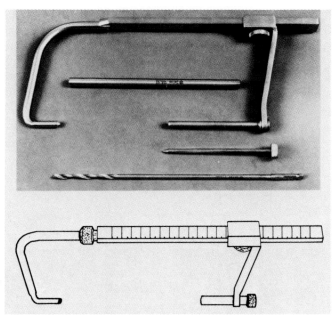

Fig. 1-77. The AO aiming device. *(Hierholzer, G.; Rüedi, T.; Allgöwer, M.; and Schatzker, J.: Manual on the AO/ASIF Tubular External Fixator. New York, Springer-Verlag, 1985, p. 27.)*

by Vidal and colleagues' utilization of the quadrilateral frame in conjunction with an improved Hoffmann system.[470]

The system consists of a number of components: ball joints, articulating couplings, connecting and adjustable connecting rods, and threaded transfixion pins and half-pins (4-mm, 5-mm, and 6-mm) that come in 200-mm, 250-mm and 300-mm lengths (Figs. 1-80 to 1-86). Mini-Hoffmann fixators are also available for use in forearm, hand, and foot fractures.

In Connes'[102] description of the technique of fixing a tibia, a guide is placed along the long axis of the bone and, if necessary, the anterior and posterior surfaces are palpated by a fine, sharp-pointed probe. A lancet or scalpel is placed through the guide, and a skin incision, at least 1 cm in length, is made. The pin selected is then passed through the guide and drilled with a hand drill until it protrudes through the skin on the opposite side, where a counterincision is made and the pin is advanced until the threads gain a purchase in each cortex. Connes warns against using a power drill, because high speeds can induce thermal necrosis; Mears[296] recommends using power for introducing the pin up to its threaded portion to minimize the pressure on the fragment; but perhaps the best method is to predrill with a 3.5-mm drill point. At any rate, at least three pins should be drilled in each fragment, and more if the bone is osteoporotic or if additional

stability is needed. The pins should be inserted in such a manner that both sets of pins are in the same horizontal plane when the fracture is reduced. After the pins are inserted, the notched points may be broken off.

The universal ball joints, which have clamps lined with Bakelite, are attached to the transfixion pins to ensure that the ball joint is placed on the far side from the fracture line. Two compression bars of appropriate length are selected, and the knurled knob is adjusted to the midposition. These bars are inserted into the universal points, a preliminary reduction is made, and the joints are tightened. The lower frame is then assembled by adding articulation couplings to the rods on the universal joint, and the rods are prevented from slipping off by the use of a spring clip. Two more compression bars are added, and the nut on the articulation coupling is tightened, completing the frame. Traction is applied to the tibia, final adjustments are made, and the nuts are tightened. To make the final adjustments with the compression bars, the two-sided screw (L) must be tightened, and the other four-sided screw (M) should be loose. Compression or distraction of the rod will be achieved by turning the knurled nut. When turned in the direction of the arrow, distraction will result. (At least one manufacturer in the United States has reversed the direction of this arrow, so it is important to be sure just how the apparatus works.) By altering the

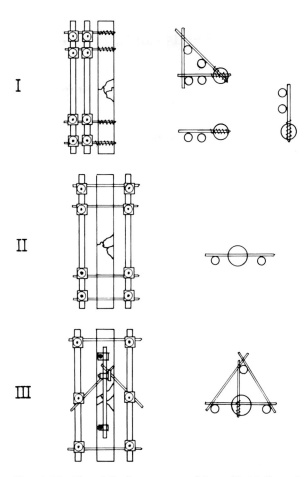

Fig. 1-78. The AO fixator assemblies. **(I)** Unilateral frame, one-plane and two-plane (V-shaped). **(II)** Bilateral frame. **(III)** Triangulated frame. *(Hierholzer, G.; Rüedi, T.; Allgöwer, M.; and Schatzker, J.: Manual on the AO/ASIF Tubular External Fixator. New York, Springer-Verlag, 1985, p. 31.)*

lengths of the rods, final adjustments may be made; angular deformities should be corrected by lengthening the short side. When a satisfactory alignment has been obtained, all the nuts should be tightened and the pinholes inspected to ensure that there is no tension on the skin. Hardaker and associates[179] suggested that cruciate incisions be made to obviate skin necrosis.

Half pins may be inserted into floating fragments and fixed to the frame. In inserting half pins, Connes recommends the use of a generous stab wound, alignment with the guide, and tapping the end of the pin with the T-wrench to engage the point in the cortex, thus facilitating the insertion

by the drill brace. However, predrilling with a 3.5-mm drill is better because it mitigates thermal damage to the bone.

While the quadrilateral frame provides excellent stability to axial compression, it is less effective in torsion and lateral flexion and it is much less effective against anteroposterior stresses.

When compared to a V-mounting (see below), the quadrilateral frame is 15 times less effective in resisting anteroposterior stresses. Vidal and colleagues have, over a 15-year period, amended the quadrilateral frame to increase its rigidity.[469] They have found that both lateral and torsional stiffness are enhanced by a six-pin configuration, but that any increase derived from the use of more than eight pins is negligible. Spreading the pins increases bending stiffness but does not influence torsional or axial stiffness, and the stiffness of the assembly is not affected by the distance the pin assemblies are displaced from the fracture site.

When the pin assemblies are loaded, the upper and lower pins take most of the stress, and the middle pin is loaded only in torsion.

The closer the connecting rods are moved to the limb, the more rigid the construct becomes; by decreasing this distance from 6 cm to 3 cm, the stiffness of the frame will be increased 40%.

When bone stability and axial compression can be achieved, the load on the pins is decreased and the stiffness (in bending torsion and axial loading) is enhanced.

Vidal and associates[469] have increased the rigidity of the quadrangular frame by increasing the pin diameter from 4 mm to 6 mm, by adding transverse couplings, and by the addition of half pins at an angle to the transfixion pins. These new configurations are known as the "triple frames" (Fig. 1-87).

THE TRIPLE FRAME

The triple frame is constructed by adding an anterior frame to the quadrangular frame. Two anterior transverse connecting rods, one on the upper frame and the other on the lower, are applied, from which a fifth longitudinal rod is attached immediately anterior to the tibial crest. From this fifth rod, two half pins are mounted which are inserted close to the fracture site anteriorly (see Fig. 1-87). By this means, almost all secondary motion in the sagittal plane is suppressed, and stiffness under torsional and bending loads is enhanced. The torsional stability achieved with this construct is comparable to that achieved by an eight-hole plate.[473]

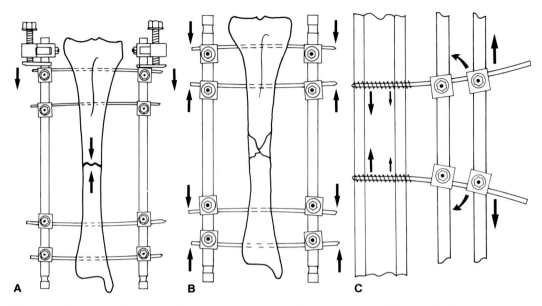

Fig. 1-79. To prevent loosening, Steinmann pins and Schanz screws should be preloaded. **(A)** Where compression of the fracture site is indicated, the pins are bent toward the fracture. **(B)** Loading Steinmann pins within each fragment by bending them toward each other. **(C)** Preloading Schanz screws within the same fragment. *(Hierholzer, G.; Rüedi, T.; Allgöwer, M.; and Schatzker, J.: Manual on the AO/ASIF Tubular External Fixator. New York, Springer-Verlag, 1985, p. 54, 58, 68.)*

THE TRIANGULATE TRIPLE FRAME (CHALET FRAME)

In the triangulate triple frame, two groupings of three or four 5-mm transfixing pins are attached to Versailles ball joints, which are connected by one longitudinal rod on each side of the leg. A third connecting rod is added to this frame by oblique couplings, giving a triangular appearance similar to that of a chalet roof (see Fig. 1-87). Half pins are inserted into the tibial crest and attached to the anterior connecting rod.

This frame is similar to the original quadrilateral frame in its resistance to axial, lateral, and torsional loads, but under bending loads it is 14 times stiffer. This mounting is simple to apply and is much less bulky than the quadrilateral frame.

CARBON-FIBER FIXATORS

One of the irritating aspects of external fixation is the difficulty in making serial radiographs of a fracture that is obscured by a metal frame. Witschger and Wegmüller[487] have addressed this problem by experimenting with a variety of materials to replace the metal longitudinal bars (plastics reinforced with fiberglass, kevlar, nylon, and carbon-reinforced epoxy). Of these alternatives, carbon-reinforced epoxy was found to be the most suitable, and Synthes has marketed a fixator made of this material under the trade name TraumaFix (see Fig. 1-76**B**).

The carbon rod is more rigid than the metal tube and is 40% lighter. It is also more resistant to fatigue. With an applied torque of 20 N, a metal tube breaks after 32,000 cycles whereas the carbon rod withstands up to 100,000 cycles without failure. The manufacturers recommend this fixator for single use, although the rod could reasonably be used more than once, and it comes, prepackaged and sterile, complete with 5-mm Schanz screws, 3.5-mm drill with drill sleeve, depth gauge, and an 11-mm wrench. The clamps are aluminum and have captive nuts, and the entire assembly weighs 12.3 oz.

A very similar, disposable, carbon-fiber fixator is marketed by the Howmedica Company under the name of Ultrafix (Fig. 1-88). In this system both single- and double-pin clamps are available as well as rod-to-rod clamps; all of these clamps allow 360° of rotation providing a great deal of versatility in pin placement and frame construction. Half pins 5 mm in diameter are used with this fixator, which is not designed to employ transfixion pins. It does

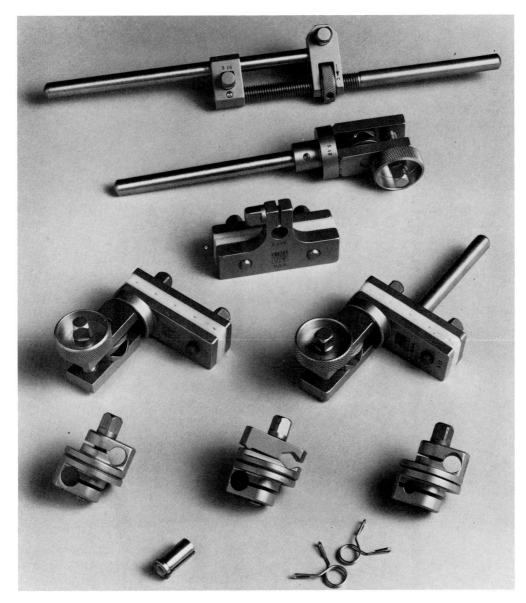

Fig. 1-80. Components of the Hoffmann fixator. (*Courtesy of Ace-Hoffmann, 1981.*)

allow two-plane fixation with linkage (delta frame) or double-bar unilateral fixation similar to the AO fixator.

Comparison of Pin Fixators

There has been a trend, certainly in the United States, away from quadrilateral frames. We have not used them in our practice for diaphyseal fractures during the last 5 years. Transfixing pins increase the hazard to neurovascular structures, and

in the tibia transfixion of the muscles of the anterior compartment is liable to interfere with ankle motion. Furthermore, insertion of pins through fleshy sites greatly increases the chances of pin tract infection.

While it might be argued that quadrilateral frames, especially with additions in other planes, are more rigid than unilateral frames, this disparity can be substantially reduced. In all pin fixators rigidity depends more on the pins than on any other

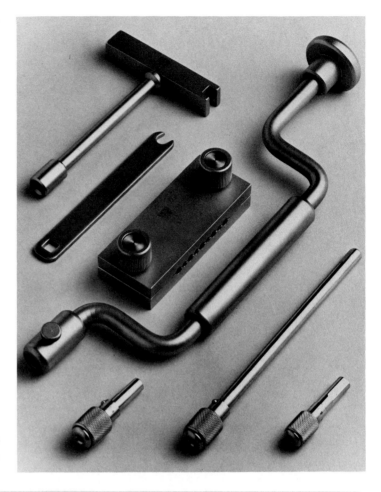

Fig. 1-81. Instruments for insertion of the Hoffmann fixator. *(Courtesy of Ace-Hoffmann, 1981.)*

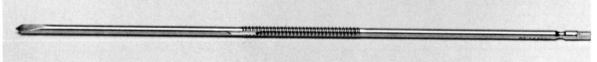

Fig. 1-82. A 4-mm transfixing pin with a 5-mm central thread. The thread prevents motion in the bone, and the smooth shank is stronger than a completely threaded pin. *(Courtesy of Ace-Hoffmann, 1981.)*

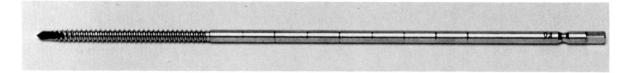

Fig. 1-83. A 4-mm half pin with continuous thread for cancellous bones.

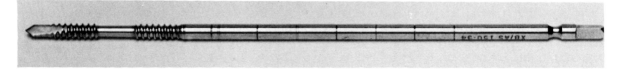

Fig. 1-84. A 4-mm half pin with interrupted thread for long bones.

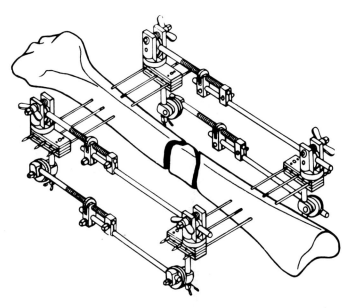

Fig. 1-85. Complete quadrilateral tibial frame (Hoffmann). *(Connes, H.: Hoffmann's External Anchorage, Edition GEAD, Paris, 1977.)*

factor.[79] Rigidity is greatly enhanced by increasing the number of pins, the size of pins, and their stiffness or modulus of elasticity.[37,79] It would be unwise, however, to increase the diameter of pins to more than 6 mm because of the weakening effects of a large hole in the bone (see p. 73). Greater stability is also gained by increasing the distance between pins and by having pins in different planes.

Behrens,[34-39] who has studied this problem extensively, compared the Hoffmann frame with a unilateral AO frame and found the AO frame to be stiffer in all planes. To add rigidity to frames employing half pins, he advised decreasing the distance between the bone and the longitudinal rod, increasing the pin-to-pin distance, use of two-plane configurations, and an anterior frame with two longitudinal bars. He stated that unilateral frames are more desirable because they provide better wound access, cause less joint stiffness, and diminish the chance of neurovascular damage.

Behrens found that, overall, the two-plane or delta configuration (see Fig. 1-78) was the stiffest, but exceeded the anterior, one-plane, double-bar (at 25 mm and 80 mm from the tibia) by only a negligible degree.[39] These principles do not apply to the AO system alone, but can be adapted to any pin fixation system (Fig. 1-89).

Ring Fixators

THE ILIZAROV FRAME

Several devices for external fixation using wires under tension suspended from metal rings have

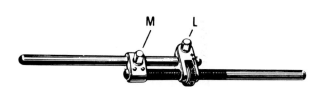

Fig. 1-86. The adjustable connecting rod for the Hoffmann device. To lengthen or compress, the two-sided screw *(L)* is locked and the square head *(M)* is loosened. In the original version, turning the knurled nut in the direction of the arrow will produce lengthening. When the desired effect is gained, *M* is locked. *(Connes, H.: Hoffmann's External Anchorage, Edition GEAD, Paris, 1977.)*

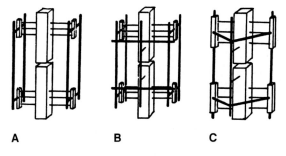

A   B   C

Fig. 1-87. **(A)** Original Hoffmann–Vidal quadrilateral double frame. **(B)** Quadrangular triple frame. **(C)** Triangular triple frame. *(Vidal, J.; Nakach, G.; and Orst, G.: New Biomechanical Study of Hoffmann® External Fixation. Orthopedics 7(4):654, 1984.)*

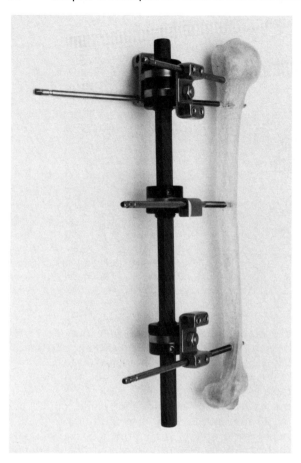

Fig. 1-88. The Ultra-X fixator, made of carbon fiber, does not obstruct radiographic monitoring of the fracture. *(Courtesy of Howmedica, Inc.)*

been designed. Both the Volkov-Oganesian and the Ilizarov[151,221,334,335,336] frames from the Soviet Union are examples of this method. Wires of small diameter (less than 2 mm) pass through the bone and are placed under tension of about 100 kg and secured to circumferential rings (Fig. 1-90). The stability of the apparatus has been demonstrated both clinically and in the laboratory. The smaller wires may cause less skin irritation and reduce pin tract infections. Two potential liabilities are the bulk of the frame and the resultant lack of access for soft tissue care.

The principles and apparatus of Ilizarov have created great interest and offer a substantially different approach to skeletal reconstruction following trauma. The fixator has been used for 35 years by its originator, Professor Gavriel Abramovich Ilizarov, who performs feats of legerdemain in an institute dedicated to his methods in Kurgan, Siberia. The primary focus in this country has been application of the technique in pseudarthrosis, bone defects, and deformity. However, in the Soviet Union the device has been used for years in the management of acute trauma and soft tissue defects.

The technical details and use of the frame are quite complex and beyond the scope of this chapter. For fractures that require stabilization or correction of deformity, the frame is applied to maintain alignment allowing early weight-bearing and longitudinal loading. End-to-end compression is applied when the fracture configuration allows. If deformity is present, the apparatus can be used to realign the fragments and maintain anatomic alignment. The use of the frame in this setting differs little from most external fixation devices.

In acute fractures with soft tissue defects, the principles of Ilizarov differ from the more traditional approach. Rather than maintain length with external fixation and treat the soft tissue loss with muscle flaps and bone grafting, the Soviets allow shortening at the site of bone and soft tissue loss in order to achieve primary healing, irrespective of acute limb shortening. A corticotomy and lengthening is then performed at a site *away* from the zone of injury to reestablish limb length. According to Ilizarov, the use of autogenous bone grafting and soft tissue coverage procedures are virtually eliminated. The experience with these methods in acute trauma in this country is limited and unreported at this time.

In comparing the Ilizarov with a variety of the common half-pin fixators, the Ilizarov is significantly less stiff in lateral bending than uniplanar fixators, comparable in anteroposterior bending and torsion, and 75% less stiff in axial loading.[151]

The frame is most stable when the Kirschner wire is inserted at a 90° angle to its mate at the same level, but anatomical constraints make this impractical. A 45°/135° placement decreases the stiffness in anteroposterior, but not lateral, bending. Increasing the wire tension from 900 N to 1300 N increases bending and axial stiffness but decreases torsional stiffness.[151]

The small diameter of the transfixion pins should not lull one into a sense of false security regarding their potential to damage neurovascular structures. One must pay the same meticulous attention to the anatomic hazards as when using larger transfixion pins. Partial rings to which large diameter half pins

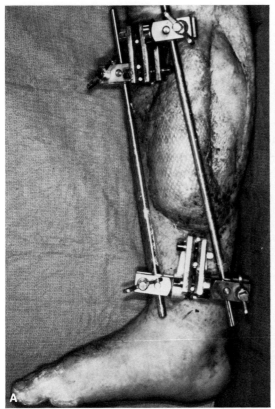 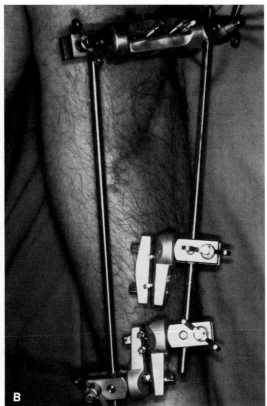

Fig. 1-89. (A) The Hoffmann uniaxial frame used in class III tibial fractures. **(B)** A comminuted open fracture of the tibia treated with a uniaxial Hoffmann frame with double bars and additional pins.

may be clamped are available. These are particularly helpful in anchorages to the upper end of the femur where transfixion wires are hazardous (Fig. 1-91).

THE MONTICELLI SPINELLI FIXATOR

The Monticelli Spinelli device is a modified Ilizarov frame and has been designed primarily for limb-lengthening procedures (Fig. 1-92). There are three sizes of color-coded rings: small (blue), medium (green), and large (grey). These rings are constructed by bolting two segments together—a ¾ ring and a ¼ ring. Each of these segments may be used separately in building a frame or combined to form a complete ring. A ¾ ring may be used in the proximal tibia to prevent the limiting of knee flexion that a full ring would engender. The ¼ ring may be used with half pins in the proximal femur in fixation of femoral fractures or in lengthenings.

THE ACE-FISCHER FIXATOR

The Ace-Fischer device is a ring fixator in which the rings are connected by rods that have universal joints at each end and are capable of either compression or distraction by rotating a compression wheel (one revolution equals 1 mm). Both ⅓ and ⅔ rings may be used and their fixation to bone is by transfixion pins, half pins, or Kirschner wires. The fixation pins are predrilled and are either fixed directly to the rings or through pin holders that accept up to three pins.

In fracture treatment two distractors are attached to a proximal and a distal ring and rotational deformity corrected with the universal joints unlocked. After correction, the joints are relocked. Angular deformity is then corrected by unlocking the universal joints in the plane of the required reduction and by lengthening and shortening the

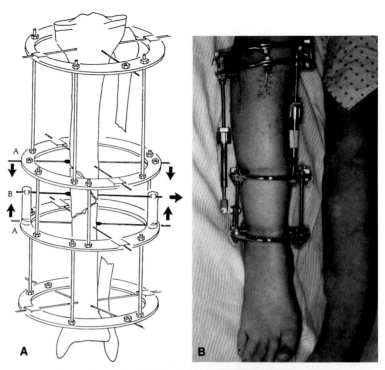

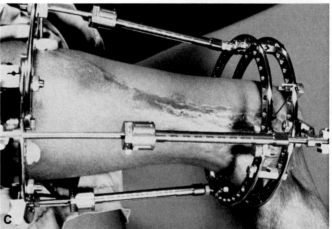

Fig. 1-90. The Ilizarov apparatus. **(A)** The frame for a fractured tibia. **(B)** Lengthening of the tibia after angular correction. **(C)** Lengthening of the femur. **(D)** During lengthening, the wire cuts through skin with immediate healing as the wire progresses.

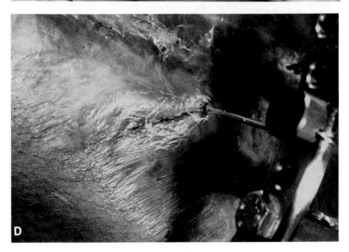

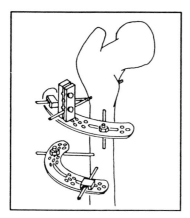

Fig. 1-91. Half rings carrying Steinmann pins for use where wires are not applicable. *(Courtesy of Richards Medical Company.)*

appropriate distractors. Similarly, displacement is corrected by loosening the four universal joints in the plane of displacement and manually correcting it. Following reduction, additional rods may be added and "dynamization" may be achieved by loosening the "fast-adjust" mechanism on the distraction rods. This allows axial loading without loss of reduction.

The Hex-Fix Fixator

The Hex-Fix fixator, recently introduced by the Richards Company, has features of simple, clamp, and ring fixators. It consists of a hexagonal longitudinal bar to which are attached "paddles" that hold 5-mm half pins. In the application of a unilateral, one-plane fixator, a swivel paddle is attached to each end of the hexagonal bar with two intervening single-pin paddles (Fig. 1-93). A trocar and drill sleeve are placed in the swivel paddle and introduced through a stab wound until they impinge on bone. Both cortices of the bone are drilled with a 3.5-mm drill, a depth gauge is used to determine the thread length of the screw, and a 5-mm pin is inserted by hand. When all of the terminal pins are inserted, the axial alignment is corrected and the paddles are locked using an Allen wrench.

Pins are then inserted through the single-pin paddles in the same way as before, and enter the bone 2 cm proximal and 2 cm distal to the fracture (see Fig. 1-93**A**). To provide two-plane fixation, the proximal single-pin paddle is replaced by a double-spool paddle, which allows two parallel pins to be inserted at an angle to the other pins (see Fig. 1-93**B**).

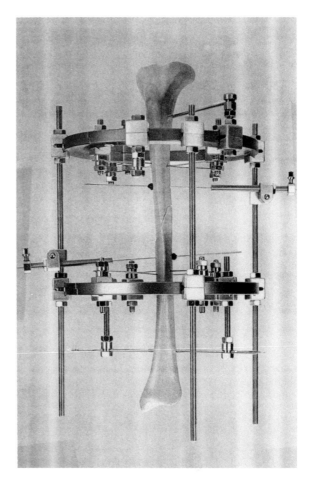

Fig. 1-92. Monticelli Spinelli external fixator. Note the stop-wires exerting interfragmentary compression. *(Courtesy of Richards Medical Company.)*

It is recommended that femoral fractures be managed by a single-axis frame mounting six pins (see Fig. 1-93**A**).

Where lengthening or segmental transport of bone is desired, a "drive unit" may be added, which is attached to an Ilizarov-type ring and allows distraction at a rate of 1 mm per turn of the screw (see Fig. 1-93**C**).

Combined Internal and External Fixation of Fractures

The stability of the frame, as we have seen, is greatly enhanced by contact of the bone ends of an inherently stable fracture, which allows compression to be applied. This desirable condition may also be achieved by limited open reduction and minimal

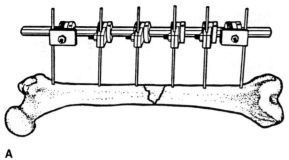

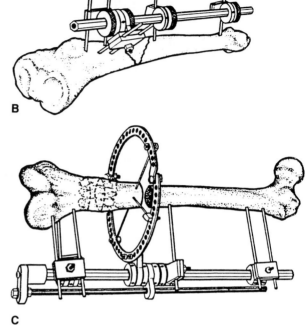

Fig. 1-93. The Hex-Fix fixator. **(A)** Uniplane fixation of femur. **(B)** Delta frame fixation of tibia. **(C)** Ilizarov model used for lengthening or bone transport. *(Courtesy of Richards Medical Company. "Hex-Fix" is a trademark of Richards Medical Company.)*

internal fixation with a screw or even cerclage (Fig. 1-94).[202]

What is not generally advocated in the literature on external fixation, but we have found most useful in unstable fractures of the tibia, is the principle of internally fixing the fibula as advocated by the late George Eggers. Even in the most catastrophic fractures of the leg, the skin over the fibula tends to be intact and one may plate the fibula with impunity. This immediately restores the length of the leg and supplements the stability of the external fixator (Fig. 1-95).

Another stratagem to increase stability where a segment of tibia has been lost was devised by Dr. Douglas Hanell* when he was a fellow in microsurgery in Louisville. In the case illustrated in Figure 1-96, an 18-month-old child sustained a shotgun blast to her leg resulting in a segmental loss of the tibia. She was treated by the application of a fixator and a latissimus dorsi free flap. In order to make the construct more stable, he inserted a hand-carved block of high-density polyethylene into the tibial defect. Later, when tissue homeostasis had been reached, this spacer was removed and replaced with

---

* Hanell, D.: Personal communication, 1984.

an adult radial allograft. Unhappily, the allograft lay inert in the leg for several months before we belatedly supplemented it with cancellous autograft. The end result has been most satisfactory.

We are not purists and have no compunction about combining external fixation with a supplementary fiberglass cast that need not incorporate the pins of the fixator. This has the advantage of preventing equinus deformity of the ankle and increases resistance to bending stresses (Fig. 1-97).

Complications of External Fixation

PIN TRACT INFECTION

The history of external fixation is rife with pin tract infection, which led to discontinuation of the technique in the past. It is said that Roger Anderson, when entertaining a group of visiting orthopaedists, was asked if there was not pus draining from a pin tract of one of his patients. "No, no," he said, "that's only a little serum." This apparently is the origin of the euphemism "Seattle serum" for pus.

Burny[69] stated that percutaneous implants in general are associated with infection and tissue proliferation. Smooth-surfaced implants undergo either marsupialization or deep sinus tract forma-

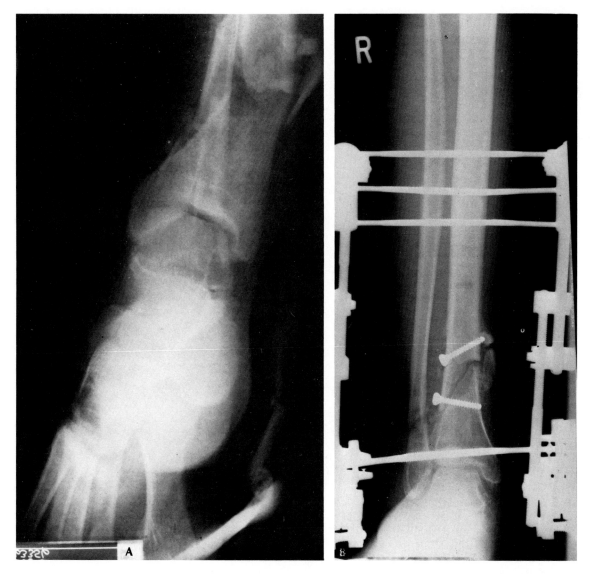

Fig. 1-94. Combination of external and internal fixation used to treat a young man who was involved in a motorcycle accident, and among other injuries sustained this fracture of the distal tibia and fibula, which was open. **(A)** The preoperative fracture. **(B, C)** The application of a Hoffmann external fixator and the insertion of two screws to coapt the loose butterfly fragment of the tibia.

(continued)

tion, and skin epithelium grows along the percutaneous portion of the implant and eventually surrounds it. Rough implants allow tissue ingrowth, providing a site for bacterial sequestration. Infection, commonly *Staphylococcus aureus,* originates on the body surface around the entry sites.

Pin tract infections may be classified, in ascending order of severity, as:

Grade I—Serous drainage
Grade II—Superficial cellulitis
Grade III—Deep infection
Grade IV—Osteomyelitis

As noted previously, placing pins through fleshy areas predisposes to infection, so pretibial placement is the site of choice in tibial fractures. Signif-

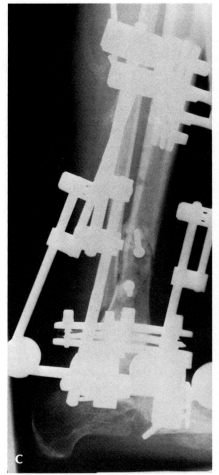 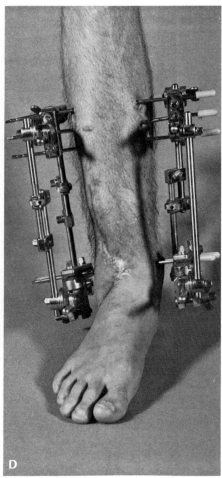

Fig. 1-94 (*continued*)
(D, E) Clinical photographs showing the patient bearing weight with the external fixator.

(*continued*)

icant infection of pins is infrequent with the Ilizarov system, perhaps owing to the small diameter of the transfixion pins; those infections that do occur tend to be grade I and are easily dealt with.[335]

Rommens and colleagues[377] reported a minor infection rate of 9.4% and a major infection rate of 9.1% in a series of 95 patients treated with the Vidal-Ardrey frame for tibial fractures, and Clifford and associates[98] had a 43% overall infection rate. However, in the latter report, when broken down into rates for transfixion and half pins, the infection rates were 78% and 17% respectively. De Bastiani and co-workers,[113] as we have seen, had a compar-

atively negligible infection rate; the reason for their unusual success is not obvious.

Prophylaxis consists of ensuring that pin incisions are adequate and that the threaded portion of a pin is not evident in the wound. Pin care (ie, the meticulous washing of the pin sites several times per day with soap and water and mechanical cleansing with cotton swabs) is the sheet anchor of pin management. Some surgeons use Betadine solution, which is fine, but we deprecate the use of hydrogen peroxide, which is a tissue poison.

When infection does supervene, free drainage by enlarging the wound and appropriate antibiotics

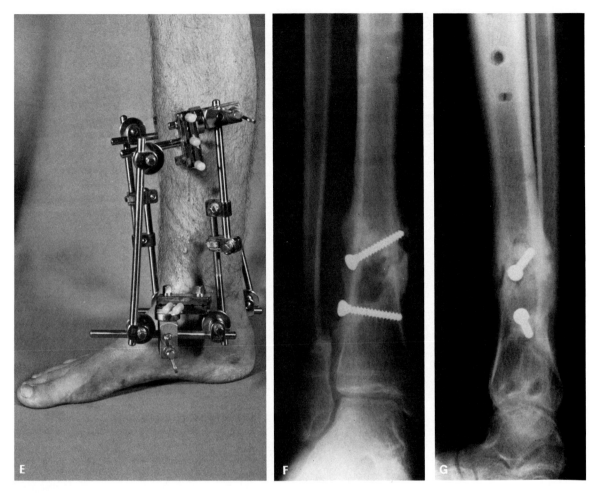

Fig. 1-94 (continued)
(F, G) Healing after removal of the external fixator.

are indicated. When this is ineffective, the pin should be removed and replaced, and curettage of the pin tract may be necessary to remove a sequestrum. We have no experience in the use of locally injected antibiotic solutions in pin tract infections and are somewhat skeptical regarding its utility.

PIN LOOSENING AND BREAKAGE

Pin loosening is inevitable if external fixators are on for long periods, and the loosening rate increases with time.

Pin anchorage is of prime importance; a loose pin is nonfunctional and, furthermore, contributes to pin tract infection.[69] Obviously the anchorage is dependent on the quality of the bone; cortical bone provides a better anchor than metaphyseal, and young healthy bone is better than osteoporotic bone. While we can do nothing about the quality of the bone, we can prevent the problems of improper pin insertion and select well-designed pins.

If bone is burned during pin insertion, a ring sequestrum forms, which can lead to infection and subsequent loosening.[69] Drilling bone with a Steinmann or other pin that does not allow the escape of bone chips increases the local temperature (see

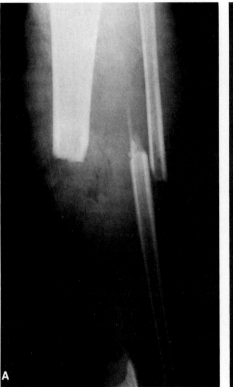

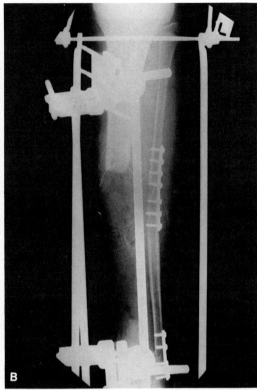

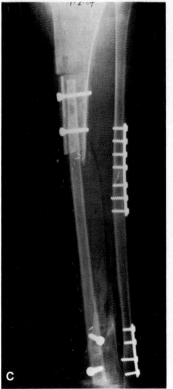

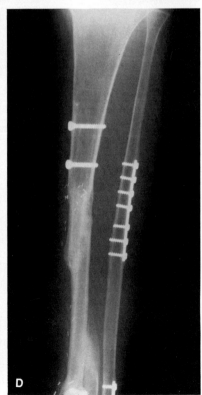

Fig. 1-95. In unstable fractures of the tibia, fibular plating enhances the stability of external fixation. Radiographs of the leg in a 15-year-old boy who was riding on a motorcycle and sustained ipsilateral femoral and tibial fractures. **(A)** On admission to hospital, the shaft of the tibia was missing. **(B)** The fibula was plated and an external fixator and Tomberlin traction were applied. **(C)** A vascularized fibular graft was used to bridge the defect in the tibia. **(D)** The end result.

p. 118). It follows that either the holes should be predrilled or a pin with a drill tip should be used. We prefer the former option and use a trocar with a drill-guide cannula to allow predrilling of the pin.

The best half pins are those with a small threaded region that engages only the far cortex, with the near hole occupied by the smooth shaft.[35] By this arrangement the effective stiffness of the pin is doubled, the bone fit is tighter, and the stress at the bone–pin interface is reduced. The use of tapered half pins that may be advanced to regain fixation is of doubtful utility and inevitably results in further protusion of the pin through the far cortex.

The bone–pin interface is subjected to compression because of bending of the pin and to shear stress because of tension and compression loads. Failure may occur from a simple overload or by fatigue. In 1173 tibial fractures treated by external fixation with 4-mm pins, Burny[71] reported a 0.5% incidence of interface fracture, and a 5.2% incidence of pin fracture.

Burny and his associates[70] investigated pin loosening by measuring the maximum torque at the time of pin removal and by the changes in the frequency of vibration of the external portion of the pin. They proposed the following clinical classification of loosening:

Stage 1—Perfect anchorage; no perceptible motion between pin and bone
Stage 2—Slight motion noticeable between pin and bone (sensation of "contact" on fast oscillations by hand)
Stage 3—Considerable motion between pin and bone (clinical loosening)
Stage 4—Possibility of manual extraction (or spontaneous pull out) of pin.

Because one of the major causes of pin loosening is failure at the pin–bone interface, it follows that early weight-bearing in unstable fractures is contraindicated, although this apparently does not apply to the Ilizarov method, where early weight-bearing is encouraged. Bone–pin stress is reduced by having the near hole occupied by the unthreaded, smooth shank of the fixation pin, and the pin breakage that occurs with early weight-bearing results from both overload and fatigue.[35]

The AO/ASIF group is of the opinion that straight pins under zero load cause bone resorption and loosening owing to micromovement and that this can be eliminated by preloading the pins. Their experiments show that bending paired Steinmann pins toward each other can reduce the linear displacement of each fragment by 45%; the horizontal displacement is also reduced, but to a lesser degree. This increase in stability decreases the pin loosening and the danger of slippage.[202]

LIMITATION OF JOINT MOTION

By transfixing muscles, the mobility of the contiguous joint may be limited, and this is particularly so where the muscles of the anterolateral compartment of the leg are involved. When a quadrilateral frame is applied to the tibia, the foot should be dorsiflexed to the neutral position before inserting the transfixing pins. Knee motion may also be limited by supracondylar pins or screws, and it is good practice to put the knee through a full range of motion to enlarge the puncture holes in the iliotibial tract.[202] Should a supracondylar pin become infected, there is some danger of the quadriceps scarring down to the underlying femur and permanently limiting knee flexion.

NEUROVASCULAR DAMAGE
AND COMPARTMENT SYNDROME

When applying an external frame, the surgeon should always have in the forefront of his mind the important anatomical structures at risk and the location of both safe and hazardous corridors for pin placement (Fig. 1-98). It is safer to place half pins than transfixion pins, but even half pins are not without risk, especially when the point of the pin protrudes in a hazardous area. One should always flex the knee when placing an anteroposterior penetrating pin in the proximal tibia to avoid damage to the posterior tibial neurovascular bundle.

The investing fascia converts the anterolateral compartment of the leg into a tight, unyielding box. A pin in this compartment, especially when the leg has been severely contused by a closed injury, may initiate enough bleeding to produce a compartment syndrome, so constant vigilance is necessary to prevent catastrophe.

MALALIGNMENT AND MALUNION

It is easy to apply a fixator to the tibia in malrotation, especially when the uninvolved leg, which might be used for comparison, is covered. Lining up the medial border of the patella with the first interdigital space is a good generalization, but there is a wide range of tibial torsion, and the safest plan is to make both legs match. Many frames allow little or no adjustment after application, and it saves

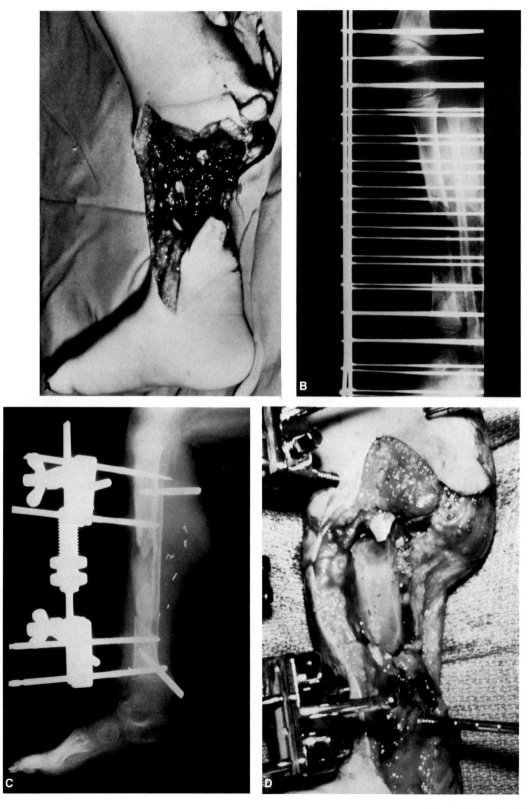

Figure 1-96 (*continued*)

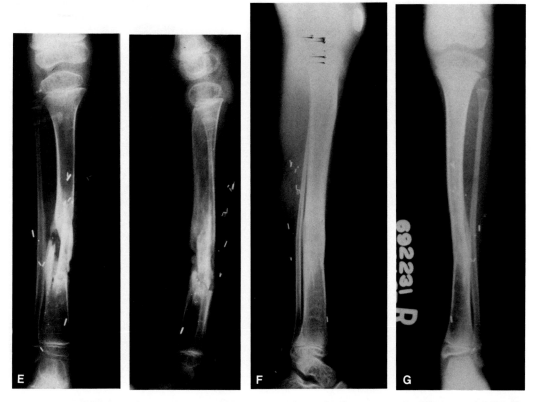

Fig. 1-96. An 18-month-old girl sustained an accidental close-range shotgun wound resulting in a massive soft tissue wound and loss of a portion of the shaft of the right tibia. **(A)** Clinical photograph of the leg. **(B)** Radiograph upon admission. **(C)** Application of an external fixator with a polyethylene spacer between the bone ends. **(D)** Intraoperative photograph showing the polyethylene spacer *in situ.* **(E)** The spacer was later removed and replaced with an allograft. **(F, G)** Radiographs of the end result.

a great deal of embarrassment to get it right the first time.

Even if the initial reduction has been perfect, pin loosening and weight-bearing may allow angular deformities to occur, so the circumspect surgeon checks alignment clinically and radiologically throughout the healing period.

DELAYED UNION OR NONUNION

Detractors of external fixation refer to frames as "nonunion machines," and indeed delayed union and nonunion are common with this form of treatment.

Rommens and associates[377] treated tibial fractures by a Vidal-Ardrey frame and reported that only 21% of the fractures healed within 4 months without other intervention. In 12.9% an overt pseudarthro-

sis developed, and 32.6% required a second procedure such as bone grafting, internal fixation, or both to achieve union.

Believing that the external fixator keeps the fracture distracted, some have advocated replacing the fixator with a cast after 6 weeks. But compression, *per se,* does not increase bone healing. Hart and his associates[187A] have shown experimentally that in the healing of osteotomies in dog tibias, compression increased the rigidity of fixation but not the rate of healing, and there was significantly more periosteal bone formation in noncompressed osteotomies.

Kenwright and Goodship[243,244] studied the effect of a short period of axial micromovement in simulated and clinical fractures of the tibia. Both in osteotomized sheep and in clinical cases treated by a Dynabrace fixator, healing was enhanced when

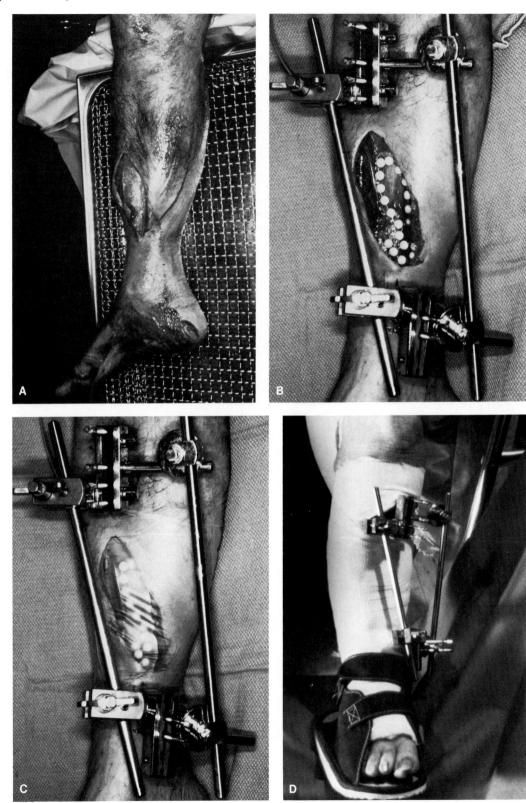

Figure 1-97 (*continued*)

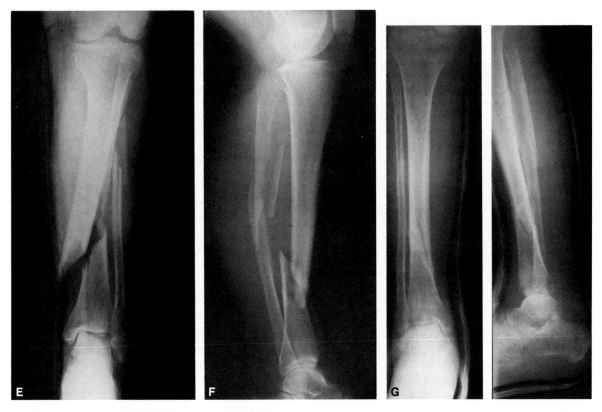

Fig. 1-97. Clinical and radiographic views of a fractured tibia in an elderly woman who had been inebriated when injured, was unattended until the following morning, and did not remember how she was hurt. **(A)** Condition of the leg upon admission. **(B)** After wound debridement and insertion of tobramycin beads and fixation by a one-plane, double-bar, Hoffmann fixator. **(C)** Bead pouch. **(D)** Cast supplementation of fixator. **(E, F)** Initial radiographs. **(G)** Early healing after 4 months.

500 cycles of micromovement were applied over 17 minutes at 0.5 Hz daily.

It now appears to be widely accepted that micromovement in the axial plane enhances bone formation and healing in externally fixed fractures. To achieve this axial micromotion, the frame may be destabilized by removal of pins; moving longitudinal bars further away from the bone; removing supplementary frames; or allowing the frame to telescope. In uniplanar fixation with two longitudinal bars or tubes, rigidity may be reduced by removing one of the bars or by replacing it with a shorter bar. This production of intermittent axial motion has come to be known as "dynamization," a neologism deprecated by Allgöwer[7] (a prejudice that we share), and has also been called "build down" by Behrens,[37] although this term would seem to be an oxymoron. Nonetheless, Melendez and Colon[299] treated 45 open tibial fractures (89%

type III) using an Orthofix frame and dynamized the fractures at 8 weeks. All of these fractures but one healed in 22.6 weeks, although 58% had supplementary bone grafting and the overall complication rate was 53%. DeBastiani,[113] using the same device, had a 91% success rate with tibial fractures that were dynamized when callus showed at 3 weeks. How long rigidity should be maintained or to what degree motion at the fracture site is beneficial is still to be determined. The process of destabilizing the frame and the timing of weight-bearing have been discussed by Allgöwer and Sequin[8] and Behrens and Johnson,[37] but no one presently has determined if motion other than axial—angulation, rotation, or both—is helpful or deleterious.

Nishimura[324] studied the stiffness of healing fractures by adding strain gauges to a longitudinal rod of a tibial fixator. The knee was extended against

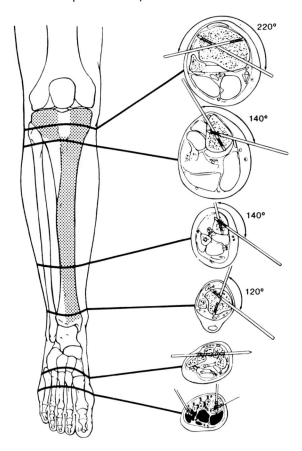

Fig. 1-98. "Safe corridors" and arcs of insertion in the leg. *(Behrens, F., and Searls, K.: External Fixation of the Tibia: Basic Concepts and Prospective Evaluation. J. Bone Joint Surg., 68B: 246–254, 1986.)*

1 kg and 2 kg loads and the strain measured. He established that there are five healing curves: normal, slow healing, nonunion, arrest in development, and breakage of callus. The strain on the connecting rod decreased hyperbolically as the callus strength and mass increased, and became constant when the strength reached a level equal to 50% of the intact bone. It would seem that this scale gives the surgeon an indication of whether or not a fracture is healing and provides a clue as to the appropriate time to "dynamize" the frame.

Indications for the Use of External Fixation

The prime indication for external fixation is when other means of fixation clearly are inappropriate. Fractures associated with extensive soft tissue injuries are the most common indication in the United States, and most class III and many class II injuries are treated by this means, which allows free access to the wounds and does not preclude free tissue transfer, cancellous grafting, or hydrotherapy. External fixation certainly has a role in grossly comminuted, unstable fractures; where there is a bony deficit; in fractures associated with burns; and in the preliminary fixation of pelvic fractures. We have also found it useful in comminuted metaphyseal fractures where the principle of "ligamentotaxis"[468] can be applied, as in Colles' fracture.[114,225,365,370] In our practice we also have found external fixation very useful in the management of the fractured calcaneus and in achieving preliminary reduction in pilon fractures (Fig. 1-99). An external frame is also useful to supplement an unstable osteosynthesis or in osteoporotic patients where conventional implants do not hold (Fig. 1-100).

The use of fixators for closed fractures of the tibia is more controversial, but Burny[71] has treated these fractures successfully by uniplane fixation and early weight-bearing.

In general, external fixators are a very useful means of treating a variety of complicated fractures. We see no virtue in using them in the treatment of most fractures where either plaster immobilization or internal fixation would be better. Healing is much quicker in fractures of the tibia managed by a cast and immediate weight-bearing, and intramedullary fixation of the femur generally is a better solution for combined closed fractures of the femoral and tibial shafts. External fixators do poorly in the management of epiphyseal or intra-articular fractures, except in Colles' fractures[114,225,365,370] and some tibial plateau fractures, where again the principle of ligamentotaxis[468] can be applied (see Fig. 1-99). On the other hand, we believe that open fractures with massive soft tissue damage can be handled much more expeditiously by external fixation. This allows the application of free flaps (latissimus dorsi or composite flaps with bone), so limbs that otherwise would have to be amputated are saved. Such wounds are easily inspected and redebrided and can be treated by hydrotherapy. In polytrauma this method allows instantaneous stabilization, especially where there is neurovascular injury, without subjecting a seriously ill patient to further trauma and blood loss. External fixation is also the only feasible means of fixation in infected fractures where the primary fixation is loose or broken and the bone is osteoporotic or necrotic.

We prefer to insert pins through viable skin whenever possible, but this is not mandatory and we have no compunction about placing pins through an open wound or denuded area if this is

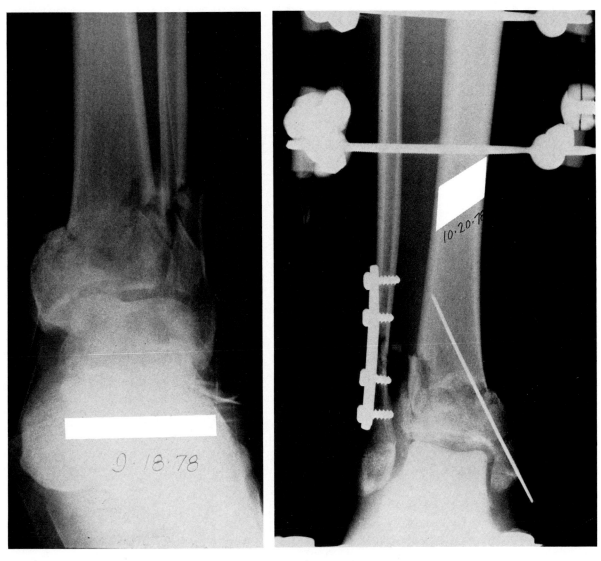

Fig. 1-99. An external fixator may be used to apply distraction across a joint, and by so doing, improve the alignment of an intra-articular fracture. **(Left)** Preoperative pilon fracture of the ankle. **(Right)** Intraoperative film showing an external fixator, which has realigned the shattered distal end of the tibia. This, however, was not adequate, *per se,* to retain the reduction indefinitely, and had to be supplemented with bone grafting of the tibia and plating of the fibula.

the only way. A little forethought in pin placement is necessary when soft tissue cover is going to be required, and access to the vascular bundles should not be obstructed.

It is not our purpose to advocate any particular fixator. The reader must make up his or her own mind regarding the competing claims of the manufacturers of the various devices and, indeed, the choice may be determined by what is available in one's own hospital. In our practice we are reluctant

to use the Ilizarov frame for acute trauma, especially in the multiply injured patient. The device requires a large inventory of parts, it is time-consuming to apply, and it precludes free tissue transfer; however, it undoubtedly will have an increasingly important role in the management of nonunion and segmental defects. Our experience with the Ilizarov frame has been entirely confined to leg-lengthening and the correction of angular deformities, where it has been enormously helpful. In general we believe that the

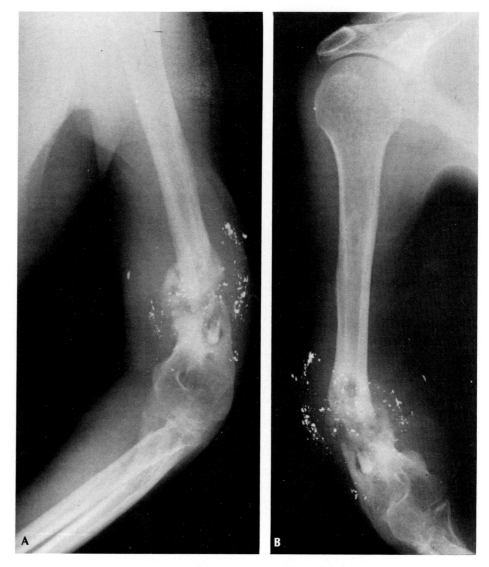

Fig. 1-100. Radiographs in a man who had been shot in the left arm and left leg in an altercation and was seen many months later with infected nonunions of both bones as well as a radial nerve deficit in the left arm. Several sequestrectomies of the humerus were required. Neither external nor internal fixation alone gave sufficient stability for healing, but the combination of both combined with cancellous grafting eventually produced a satisfactory union and an arm that no longer drained. **(A, B)** Views of the left humerus with sequestra and lead fragments from the bullet.

(continued)

best fixators are those that may be applied quickly, are applicable to a variety of fractures and anatomic sites, and supply adequate fixation.

INTERNAL FIXATION OF FRACTURES

Lord Lister repaired a fracture of the patella with silver wire, and Hugh Owen Thomas used silver wire ligatures in the treatment of open fractures of the mandible. However, it is probably true that the father of internal fixation of fractures in the English-speaking world was Sir Arbuthnot Lane.[200,264]

Mears[296] credits Hansmann with being the first to use metal plates and screws in 1886 and Gurlt with publishing a textbook showing patients treated by open reduction and internal fixation. The Lam-

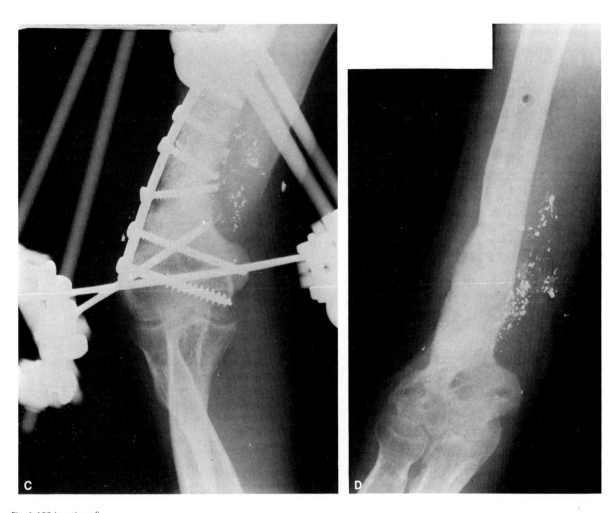

Fig. 1-100 (*continued*)
(C) A combination of plating and Roger-Anderson external fixation. **(D)** The end result. Similar techniques were employed for the nonunion of the tibia. Hyperbaric oxygen and antibiotic therapy were also used in the treatment of this man's infections.

botte brothers were early pioneers in continental Europe, and Albin Lambotte published treatises on open reduction and internal fixation.[296]

Initially, Lane used wire transfixion stitches or steel screws, but in 1907 he described the use of plates. These plates were made of German silver or steel in the beginning, but later he used only plates of steel. Unfortunately, the deleterious effects of metallic corrosion were not appreciated in those days, and loosened screws, broken plates, rarefying osteitis, and signs of inflammation were frequent. Lane himself ascribed these untoward complications to infection and incompetence on the part of the surgeon. To circumvent such infections, he invented his celebrated "no-touch technique," in which instruments were used instead of fingers, and the business ends of instruments were never touched by hand.[200]

The fact that metal appeared to produce serious reactions in the tissues tempted surgeons to use as little metal as possible, and implants were made so skimpy that their mechanical effectiveness was impaired. As recently as 1952 Watson-Jones[475] advocated the treatment of difficult comminuted fractures by the use of a single screw. Sherman,[416] in the United States, used his own plates, which were much stronger and larger. Lane did make his plates longer and stronger to take care of the serious fractures being sustained in World War I, but it was only after the introduction of stainless steel by Lange[296] and Vitallium by Venable and Stuck of San Antonio[464,465] that internal fixation came into its own.

Types of Internal Fixation

CIRCUMFERENTIAL WIRE FIXATION (CERCLAGE)

Although wire fixation was one of the earliest means of internally fixing fractures, it has not always been held in high repute. Charnley[90] decried the use of circumferential wiring. The evil effects, he believed, were caused by circumferential stripping of the periosteum and the encircling wire's obstruction of the bridging of periosteal callus. Furthermore, he maintained that the fixation provided by wiring oblique fractures was vastly inferior to that obtained by screws, and considered any success with such treatment "a tribute to the remarkable healing power of bone." In rebuttal of this view, Thunold[460] treated 18 oblique fractures of the tibia by cerclage, all of which went on to uncomplicated union without rarefaction or abnormal bone apposition around the wires. Rhinelander,[369] after making microcirculatory studies of the effects of cerclage, noted the following:

> This time-honored technique has been strongly condemned on the ground that a circumferential wire loop strangles bone. The periosteal blood supply, however, enters the cortex through innumerable small vessels. No periosteal arteries of the long bones run longitudinally to be pinched off with encircling wires. Callus grows abundantly over the wires, which are tight and hold the fracture reduced. It is only when the immobilization is insufficient that troubles arise.

It is generally agreed that Parhams's bands, since they cover a much greater area, do significantly interfere with periosteal circulation, particularly venous drainage, and they are best avoided.

We have used cerclage (Fig. 1-101) sparingly in the past but have used it increasingly for the fol-

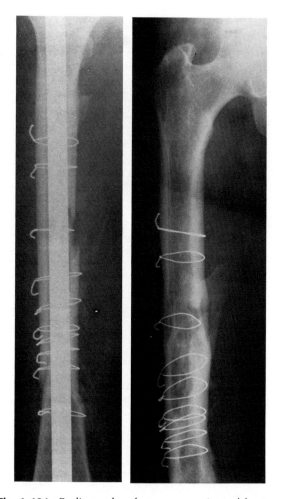

Fig. 1-101. Radiographs of a very comminuted fracture of the left femur. The patient had to be mobilized because she was developing a sacral decubitus and had had a pulmonary embolism. **(Left)** Postoperative views after intramedullary nailing and cerclage. If circumferential wires strangulate bone, this femur should have thoroughly garroted. **(Right)** Two years and nine months later there is excellent healing without impairment of the periosteal callus.

lowing purposes: temporary fixation during the plating of long bones; reattachment of osteotomized greater trochanters; cervical spine stabilization, and fractures of the olecranon, patella, and medial malleolus (Figs. 1-102 and 1-103). We have followed the AO "tension band" principle, and the results have been excellent. Before the introduction of interlocking nails we found cerclage particularly helpful as an adjunct to intermedullary nailing in the presence of one or more butterfly fragments (see Fig. 1-101).

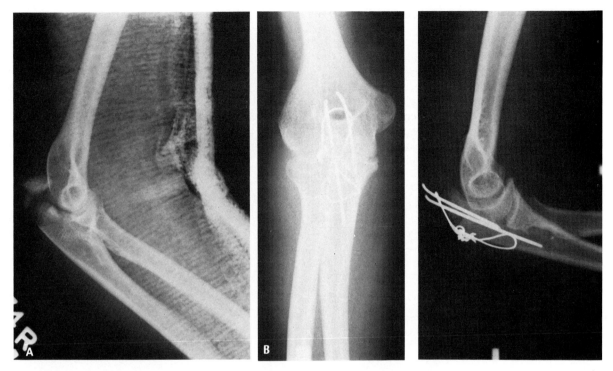

Fig. 1-102. A comminuted fracture of the olecranon. **(A)** Original x-ray film. **(B)** Loose fragments of bone were removed and the proximal fragment reattached to the ulna by longitudinal Kirschner wires and a tension band wire.

Fitzgerald and Southgate[150] agree with this approach and have reported 20 cases of fractured femurs treated by intramedullary nailing with supplementary cerclage. Sixteen of the fractures were in young people injured in vehicular accidents, but four were elderly women with long spiral fractures. They had no postoperative infection, and all of their patients had at least 120° of knee flexion.

We have also used the Luque technique to stabilize fracture–dislocations of the spine. In this stabilization system, wires are passed around the vertebral arches and tied around vertical rods on both sides of the midline. Although this technique has proved satisfactory, more recent devices may be more advantageous (Fig. 1-104).

The combination of Kirschner wires and cerclage is helpful in some fractures of the hand or to arthrodese an unsalvageable interphalangeal joint. Lister described the technique of interosseous wiring in the digital skeleton and Zimmerman and Weiland[493] used "ninety-ninety" wiring for fractures, arthrodeses, and fixation or replants in the hand.

Rüedi[379] has described the use of screws and wire cerclage in the management of metaphyseal fractures, especially of the proximal humerus. This combination in selected fractures obviates the need for bulky implants, but is contraindicated in patients with osteoporosis.

Cerclage must be carried out with care because excessive bending of the wire rapidly leads to fatigue failure. Notching or damaging the wire also reduces its strength, and the knot must be secure. Wang and associates[472] compared Vitallium wire with 16- and 18-gauge stainless steel wire as well as with three strands of 24-gauge stainless steel. The 18-gauge Vitallium proved to be strongest. They also compared the efficacy of twisting the wire, making a surgical knot, or tying a half hitch and then adding three or four twists. Twisting alone was the least effective and was prone to unravel. The other two methods were equally effective with stainless steel wire, but knotting was better when Vitallium wire was used.

These findings have largely been confirmed by Shaw and Daubert,[415] except that they found the most compressive force to be exerted by a modified square knot. The modified square knot is made by tightening the first hitch with a Harris wire tightener, then rotating the wire tightener 180° while

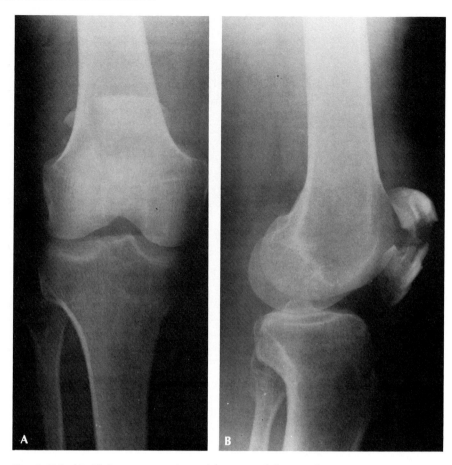

Fig. 1-103. (A, B) A very comminuted fracture of the patella.

(continued)

maintaining the tension. The second hitch is then tied. The least predictable method was that of twisting the wire. The wire was prone to break, and furthermore, in both twist knots and a half hitch with twist, turning down the twist to bone produced a loss of compression fixation.

These authors also compared Parham's bands, titanium cable, mersilene tape, and polypropylene and nylon ties with wire cerclage and found that 0.64-mm thick Parham's bands and titanium cable demonstrated the best fixation and greatest ultimate strength, but the physiologic effects of these systems *in vivo* were not tested. Rhinelander[309] stated:

> Parham's bands are flat and wide. In firm contact with the cortex, they block the efflux of venous blood circumferentially. They also block the approach of the extraosseous arterioles, and thereby impair callus formation. However, bone is a forgiving material so that these effects may not be critical in clinical practice. Nevertheless, it is well recognized that

Parham bands should be removed from the diaphysis of long bones during the remodelling stage.

Of the variety of wire tighteners on the market, we have used both the Harris and Rhinelander[368] instruments and have found them to be entirely satisfactory. Gadgets that merely twist wire without exerting tension are not worthwhile. The AO system has an efficient method using wires with a lasso end and their own wire tightener.

Another type of cerclage, introduced in 1976, is the Patridge band.[338] This is a nylon strap that is tensioned by a "gun" and locked. The undersurface has small projections which lift the strap away from the bone so that they do not interfere with venous drainage of the bone. These straps may be combined with special plates of nylon that have slots through which the straps are passed and metal spikes on the undersurface to hold the bone. These devices are used as an adjunct to intramedullary nailing in

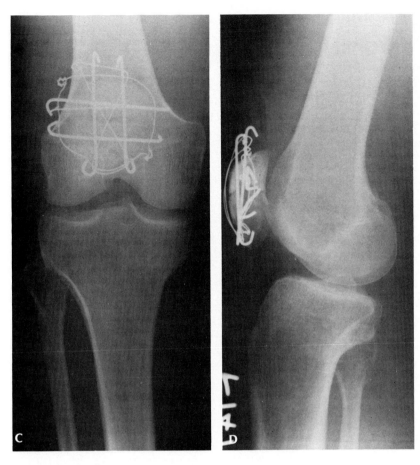

Fig. 1-103 (*continued*)
(C, D) It was possible to reassemble the patella with a "tic-tac-toe" arrangement of Kirschner wires and cerclage. (*Courtesy of John Johnson, M.D.*)

osteoporotic patients and to treat fractures in the vicinity of a hip prosthesis or femoral component of a total joint that preclude conventional plating.

Jones and associates[229] found that immersing these bands in calf serum for 4 days caused a 38% reduction in buckle strength and that the bands increased in length by 1.0%. Three cases of serious bone erosion underneath Partridge bands have been reported.[230] It would seem that Partridge bands and plates without intramedullary fixation are inadequate to stabilize femoral fractures, but the method may have some merit in the management of fractures around a prosthesis in the osteoporotic elderly patient.

FIXATION BY KIRSCHNER WIRES

Although Kirschner wires were originally designed to provide skeletal traction with minimal bone damage, they are virtually never used in this man-

ner now. Instead they are liberally used to provide fixation for fractures in the hand and to some extent in other locations. Such fixation is not likely to be intrinsically secure, even in fractures of the hand, and usually must be supplemented by some form of external splintage or reinforcement. If Kirschner wires are used alone, movement of the fracture fragments tends to occur, with possible backing out or failure of the wires.

When used as primary fixation, Kirschner wires should be supplemented by wire cerclage whenever possible. This combination is very useful in fractures of the olecranon, patella, phalanges, and on occasion the medial malleolus (see Figs. 1-102 and 1-103). We deprecate the use of Kirschner wires in other locations where they are unable to provide the necessary fixation to allow early movement. However, they are extremely useful in providing temporary ("provisional") fixation in complicated

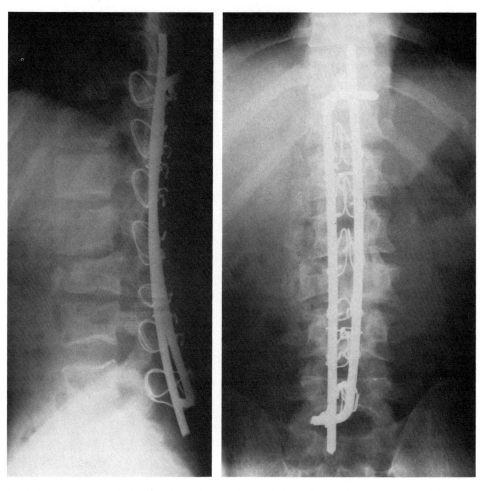

Fig. 1-104. Anteroposterior and lateral x-ray films of the spine with a comminuted fracture of L-3. This fracture has been reduced and held in a stable position by Luque rods and intersegmental wiring.

fractures while more rigid devices are being applied. In the hand, early AO minifragment fixation may provide rigid fixation stable enough to allow immediate active motion (Fig. 1-105), and in some respects this option is superior to Kirschner wire fixation (see Chapter 7).

FIXATION BY SCREWS AND PLATES

Machine Screws.   The screw most commonly used in orthopaedics is the machine screw, threaded from head to tip and with a blunt end. To insert these screws in bone, a preliminary drill hole must be made. Following this, threads may be cut by a tap prior to the insertion of the screw, or the screw may be designed to cut its own path with a fluted tip (ie, a self-tapping screw; Fig. 1-106). The head

of the screw may have a single slot to accommodate the screwdriver, but more commonly screws now have a cruciate or hex head.

The *pitch* of a screw is the distance between the threads, and the *lead* is the distance through which a screw advances with one turn. If the screw has only one thread, the pitch and lead are identical. However, if there is more than one thread, the lead of the screw is increased proportionately to the number of threads. A double-threaded screw has a lead double the pitch, and this allows the screw to be tightened more rapidly.[155]

The tensile strength of a screw, or its resistance to breaking, depends on its root diameter (ie, the diameter of the screw between the threads), whereas the pull-out strength depends on the outside diameter of the threads. Shear strength is pro-

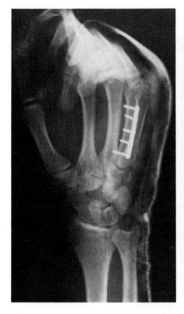
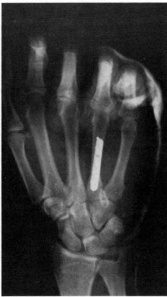

Fig. 1-105. Radiographs of the hand of a drummer for a jazz group that would have lost a great deal of money on their tour had he been unable to play. Following fixation by a mini-plate, he was able to play the same night.

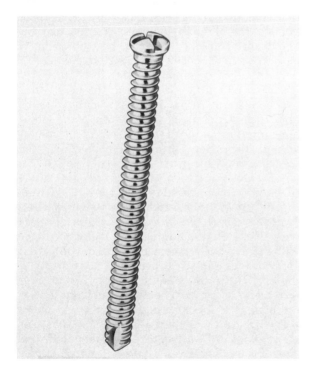

Fig. 1-106. Drawing of a typical machine screw, threaded from the head to the tip. The head is the cruciate- or Woodruff-type and there is a fluted end that indicates it is self-tapping. *(Courtesy of Zimmer, U.S.A.)*

portional to the cube of the root diameter, and tensile strength is proportional to its square. The number of threads per inch has no effect on the pull-out strength of the screw, provided five or six threads are in the cortex. In very osteoporotic bone with thin cortices, this may be a factor, in addition to the diminished strength of the bone.

Although Bechtol and Lepper[31] believed that thread configuration is of very little importance, Frankel and Burstein[155] disagreed. They said that the ability to resist stripping depends on the total cross-sectional area of material presented to the root of the thread (Fig. 1-107). Koranyi and associates[254] found no difference in the holding power of the V-threads of coarse and fine Sherman screws and the buttress threads of the ASIF screws, but in comparing the holding power of fluted ends of the fine and coarse Sherman screws with the shanks of the screws, they found a reduction of 17% and 24%, respectively.

When a screw is inserted into bone, torque is applied through the screw head so that the screw advances through its pretapped path, or cuts its way if it is self-tapping. With impingement of the screw head on the cortex or on the countersink of a plate, tension is generated in the screw. Torque stress is also induced in the screw to a varying degree, and this is enhanced by drilling too small a hole and by the increased friction engendered by a self-tapping screw. A screw's resistance to tensile stress will be reduced by a super-added torque shear, and *vice versa.* The strength of the screw is further impaired

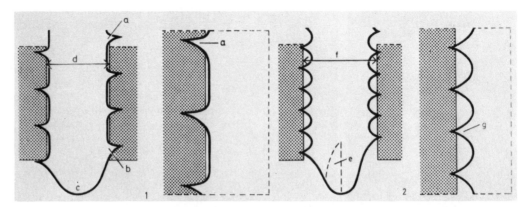

Fig. 1-107. (1) The thread of the AO screw, which is at right angles to the axis and has a greater purchase on the bone than the conventional self-tapping screw (2). *(Müller, M.E., Allgöwer, M., and Willenegger, H.: Manual of Internal Fixation, p. 35. New York, Springer-Verlag, 1970.)*

by bending moments induced by improper insertion. Screws should be inserted at 80% of the torque that would cause them to strip. Hughes and Jordan[214] have shown that stainless steel and titanium alloy (Ti-6Al-4V) screws have greater shear strength than those of pure titanium or Vitallium.

Schatzker and associates[401–403] made a series of studies on the holding power of screws in the living bone of dogs. Most other studies have been in bovine or cadaver bone or nonliving material. They compared the ''push-out'' rather than ''pull-out'' strength of 3.5-mm and 4.5-mm AO screws with that of Vitallium screws (a pretapped 4-mm buttress-thread screw and a 3.5-mm self-tapping screw). They showed that the predominant factor in the holding power of a screw, immediately after insertion, is the diameter of the screw thread. Other determinants such as thread profile, mode of insertion, and ratio of the drill hole to the external diameter of the screw were of minor importance.

The contention that a self-tapping screw, if removed and reinserted into the same hole, loses holding power by stripping its threads was also discredited by this study. Self-tapping screws inserted at 80% of their torque-out value were removed and reinserted 12 times without significant loss of holding power. Histologic studies showed no difference in the extent of bone death, splintering, or bone remodeling produced by tapped and self-tapped screws, or between Vitallium and stainless steel.

The mean values of holding power for all the screws tested increased between 150% and 190% at the end of 6 weeks, but declined to between 125% and 160% at the end of 12 weeks.

They also found that movement of screws in bone provoked bone resorption and marked fibrous tissue proliferation. A screw at rest, on the other hand, even when placed in a hole drilled too large, became enveloped in bone. This would suggest that bone resorption is caused by motion of the screw rather than screw loosening being secondary to resorption of bone. Furthermore, if a screw is stripped, it may be beneficial to leave it *in situ*, providing that no motion occurs between it and the bone.

The study also demonstrated that when a screw was inserted with overdrilling of the near cortex, new bone formed around the screw in the oversized hole. Granulation tissue did not form at the screw–bone interface in the far cortex, but the dead bone around the screw threads remodeled so that compression at the interface ultimately fell to zero.

AO Screws.   The AO cortical screw[296,312,313] has a thread diameter of 4.5 mm and a core diameter of 3 mm. The head, which has a diameter of 8 mm, has a deep hexagonal recess that mates accurately with the screwdriver, providing a large contact surface between the screw head and screwdriver for the efficient transfer of torque. The assembly of screw and instrument is stable and there is no mechanism to lock and unlock so that no time is wasted in loading the screwdriver (Fig. 1-108). The pilot hole is drilled (with the aid of a guide when a plate is used) with a 3.2-mm drill bit, the thread is precut with a 4.5-mm tap, and the screw is inserted. The tap and screwdriver may be operated by hand, but there are also attachments to the power drill to perform these functions more expeditiously. The length of the screw necessary is measured by a depth gauge prior to the tapping of the thread. When a lag effect is desired to provide interfragmentary compression, the near hole or glid-

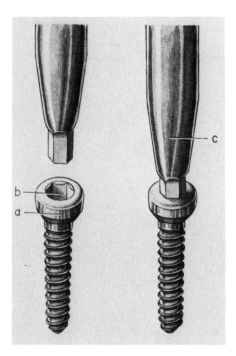

Fig. 1-108. The AO screw and screwdriver. The screw head has a shallow cylindrical flank that gives better contact with the hole in the plate, and the hexagonal screwdriver with matching recess in the screw gives a much larger surface area for transmission of the torque from the screwdriver to the screw. *(Müller, M. E.; Allgöwer, M.; and Willenegger, H.: Manual of Internal Fixation. New York, Springer-Verlag, 1970.)*

ing hole is overdrilled with a 4.5-mm drill bit. A drill sleeve with an outer diameter of 4.5 mm is inserted into this hole until it abuts on the far cortex. A 3.2-mm drill bit is inserted through the drill sleeve and the far or thread hole is bored (Fig. 1-109). This hole is then threaded with a tap—one with a smaller tapping length than the regular tap. Alternatively, the far hole may be drilled first, even prior to the reduction of the fracture. The fracture is then reduced, the far-hole guide is inserted in the hole, and the near hole is drilled (Fig. 1-110).

If the screw is not being inserted through a plate, a countersink cutter is inserted into the gliding hole to provide a recess for the spherical head of the screw. The depth gauge should be used after this step and not before if the screw is to be of optimal length.

In addition to the cortical screws, there are also spongiosa or cancellous screws. These screws have a smooth shank of 4.5 mm diameter and either a 16-mm or 32-mm thread length. The diameter of the thread is 6.5 mm, and the core diameter is 3 mm. Although these screws are primarily for use in cancellous bone, they may also be used for cortical fixation. The correct drill bits are 3.2 mm for cancellous bone and 4.5 mm for cortical bone. However, once inserted into cortical bone, the cancellous screw cannot cut its way back out and will have to be left in. These screws should not be tapped all the way, only the first few turns, because they gain much better purchase when they cut their own way into cancellous bone. In achieving interfragmentary compression, it is essential that the thread be inserted beyond the plane of the fracture so that only the smooth shank crosses it.

Malleolar screws have a sharper point than cancellous screws, with a core diameter of 3 mm and a thread diameter of 4.5 mm. Their use has been discontinued by AO/ASIF, having been superseded by small cancellous screws.

The AO system also includes a variety of smaller screws and implants in their small and mini-fragment sets. The smallest screws cannot encompass a hole for a hex-head screwdriver and consequently have cruciate slots.

In comparing AO screws with other types of screws, it is difficult to demonstrate marked superiority of the AO screw in any single parameter. Nevertheless, as Mears[296] has pointed out, where a measurable difference exists, it is always in the favor of the AO screw and, furthermore, it is part of a well-engineered, complete system of internal fixation. It is easier to insert and to take out; the head is unlikely to be injured by the screwdriver (this may be a problem with slotted screws, particularly those with Phillips heads); and it is much less likely to be overstressed by insertion through a plate.

The drilling of a hole in a bone immediately reduces its breaking strength. Bechtol and Lepper[31] stated that when the holes are placed in an area of tension, the weakening effect is greatest. The size of the hole has little effect on the breaking strength, so long as it is less than 20% of the diameter of the bone. When this size is exceeded, the degree of weakening is proportional to the size of the hole. The presence of a screw also weakens the bone to the same extent as an unfilled hole, but the effect diminishes with the production of new bone. Laurence[265] found that the bending moment required to fracture an intact tibia varied from 59 Nm to 226 Nm (mean = 137 Nm). When a 3-mm drill hole was made in the tibia, however, the moment required was reduced to 29 Nm to 147 Nm (mean = 98 Nm). Brooks and associates[54] studied the influence of drill holes on torsional fractures in paired

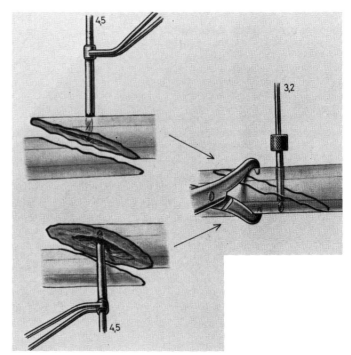

Fig. 1-109. Technique of lag screw fixation. Predrilling the gliding hole. **(Top left, bottom left)** A 4.5-mm hole is drilled in one cortex from inside or outside. Following reduction, the opposite cortex (thread hole) is drilled using the drill guide that has a 4.5-mm outer diameter and a 3.2-mm inner diameter. *(Müller, M. E.; Allgöwer, M.; Schneider, R.; and Willenegger, H.: Manual of Internal Fixation. Techniques Recommended by the AO Group, 2nd ed., p. 39. New York, Springer-Verlag, 1979.)*

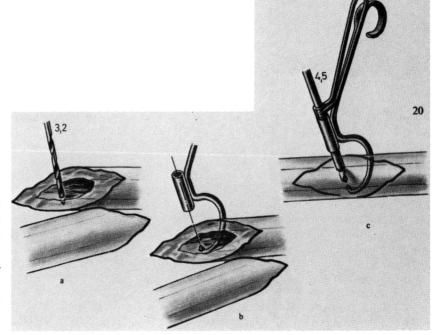

Fig. 1-110. Alternative technique of lag screw fixation. The thread hole may be drilled first and the gliding hole aligned with the far hole guide. *(Müller, M. E.; Allgöwer, M.; Schneider, R.; and Willenegger, H.: Manual of Internal Fixation. Techniques Recommended by the AO Group, 2nd ed., p. 39. New York, Springer-Verlag, 1979.)*

canine femurs. With a 2.8-mm hole and a load applied for 0.1 seconds, the mean reduction in energy absorption was 58.5%, and for 3.6-mm holes, 51.9%. Because the energy absorbed by these bones with holes is reduced, these fractures have less comminution (Fig. 1-111).

Burstein and associates,[72] at Case Western Reserve University, also found that a fresh screw hole weakened bone in bending and torsional loading. Whereas Bechtol found 20% to be the critical level, Burstein determined that the size of the screw hole had no effect on breaking strength until it exceeded 30% of the diameter of the bone. When torque was applied to the drilled bone, the stresses around the hole were 1.6 times greater than those over the remainder of the bone, and when failure occurred, the fracture line passed through the drill hole in more than 90% of the bones tested. With time, however, the strength of the bone increases even with the screw *in situ,* but after removal of the screw, the bone is again unduly susceptible to fracture. Rather surprisingly, in these latter cases the experimental fracture line passed through the screw hole in only 6 of 38 fractures.

Although the effects of having a screw in bone are mitigated by remodeling, once the screw is removed, the hole again becomes a stress riser. It follows then that the bone must be protected after the removal of screws at least until the defect heals. After removal of a screw, the hole remains evident on radiographs for an extended period of time. Just because there is a very obvious sclerotic margin, it does not mean that the hole has not healed. Histologic examination indeed will show that the defect is filled with woven bone in 6 to 8 weeks. Remedies for screw-hole weakness such as overdrilling or filling the holes with plastic plugs are not helpful. In our practice, we now protect forearms for 6 weeks with a forearm cast after removal of plates and screws, because over a 2-year period we had a 20% refracture rate. After removal of plates or screws in the lower extremities, we insist on protecting the limb by three-point crutch-walking for 6 weeks.

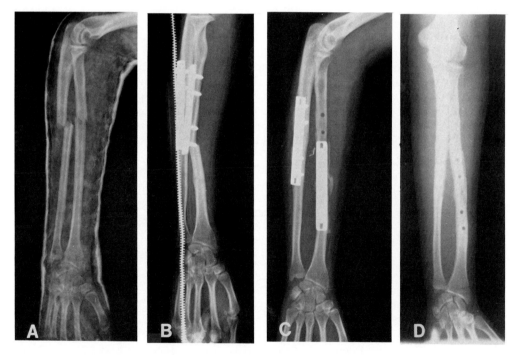

Fig. 1-111. (A) Radiograph showing fractures of both bones of the forearm in a 14-year-old girl. **(B)** Eight months after compression plating she sustained a refracture through the lower screw in the radius. **(C)** This fracture, too, was treated with a compression plate and the addition of an osteoperiosteal graft from her rib. **(D)** The appearance 4 months later, after removal of both plates. The holes in the bone persisted for a considerable time radiographically, but histologically the holes healed by woven bone after 6 weeks in spite of the radiographic appearance.

Fixation of fractures by screws alone is mechanically feasible only in long oblique and spiral fractures. To attempt to fix transverse or short oblique fractures with one or more screws is mechanically unsound. Although the medical literature is replete with x-ray films showing fractures fixed by screws inserted at right angles to the fracture line, this is the least secure configuration. Arzimanoglou and Skiadaressi[17] compared the results of fixing a standard fracture by screws inserted at right angles to the shaft, at right angles to the fracture line, and by a combination of the two. The greatest stability in compression was obtained by screws inserted at right angles to the shaft, and the least by those inserted perpendicular to the fracture line. Müller and associates[319] have endorsed this principle, but for treating spiral fractures with a loose butterfly fragment, they recommend fixing the two major fragments with a transverse screw and inserting the remaining screws at an angle midway between the perpendiculars to the shaft and the fracture line (Fig. 1-112). Although transverse screws give the greatest stability against compression, the combination position gives more protection against bending in an axis perpendicular to the screws.

There is general agreement that when machine screws are used in this manner, the near cortex should be overdrilled. This allows the screw head to be countersunk and, more importantly, produces a lag effect, which compresses the fracture line.

Wood Screws.   Wood screws have a taper and a sharp point. The neck portion is unthreaded, and these screws force their way into bone without needing a preliminary drill hole. They are not suitable for use in cortical bone, because they tend to split the cortex. They have been recommended for use in cancellous bone, although Venable[465] stated, "No screw holds well in cancellous bone. Wider threads to increase holding power intensify the concentration strain on the screw with an increasing absorption rate of calcium about the screw." Other lag screws have been developed by the AO group for use in cancellous bone and to fix femoral condyles and tibial plateaus. We would much sooner use these special AO screws, Knowles' pins, or cannulated lag screws than wood screws.

Plates.   Nearly 40 years ago, Peterson[350] laid down some basic principles to be observed in the plating of fractures. He cautioned that the plate should not be scratched or treated roughly; a screw hole should be drilled using a guide to center it and direct it at right angles to the shaft; and the length of the screw must be accurately determined by a depth gauge. Screws that are not centered properly do not fit the well in the plate so that unnecessary stress is placed on the screw head, making it more likely to fail. He also recommended that the screws should not be tightened all the way until the last screw is inserted, so that the tension on the screws is made as uniform as possible. The size of the drill hole, he believed, was of great importance. If it were too large, the screw would have no purchase; if too small, the screw would bind and perhaps split the cortex. On this point, Bechtol and Lepper[31] advised that the diameter of the drill be midway between that of the root of the screw and that of the thread.

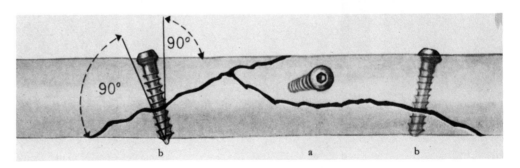

Fig. 1-112. This illustration demonstrates the AO method of fixing a spiral fracture by screws. The screw connecting the two major fragments is inserted at right angles to the long axis of the shaft while the remaining two screws holding the butterfly fragment in place are inserted at an angle bisecting the perpendiculars to the shaft and the fracture line. *(Müller, M. E.; Allgöwer, M.; and Willenegger, H.: Manual of Internal Fixation, p. 41. New York, Springer-Verlag, 1970.)*

They also believed that screws should be inserted by a torque equal to 75% of that required to strip the screw. The AO group advises 80% of stripping torque, but we are not sure how the operator gauges this. We insert the screw until it feels "snug."

Peterson[350] also warned that if it is necessary to bend a plate to make it conform to the contour of the bone, this should be done before application. Otherwise, the plate will be bent by the application of screws, which will then be under unequal tension and more likely to fail.

It has been recommended that plates be applied extraperiosteally to prevent devascularization of the bone and delayed union. We believe that this advice is predicated on a faulty conception of bone circulation and have seen no great advantage in doing so. However, we do make every effort to maintain the periosteal attachments of detached bone fragments.

In general, the most secure fixation and the best results are obtained with the heavier, stronger plates. When a fracture 'is plated, the bone itself carries the majority of the compression load. The resistance of a plate assembly to bending depends on the strength of the screw fixation, and in torsion the load is transmitted as a bending moment to the screws. The most secure fixation of all would be that achieved by having two plates on opposite sides of the bone; but this, although mechanically sound, may be biologically disastrous. Plating of shafts by two plates at 90°, advocated by Murray and associates[315] and Peterson and Reeder,[351] gives excellent fixation but is open to criticism because it requires excessive soft tissue dissection and periosteal stripping. However, bone is quite capable of healing without periosteal callus, provided the endosteal circulation is intact, and these authors reported excellent results (Fig. 1-113).

While the purpose of plates is to hold fractures together, sometimes they serve instead to hold the fragments apart. Eggers[133] invented slotted plates so that the fractures could be impacted at the time of surgery to prevent this difficulty (Fig. 1-114). The belief that these plates allow the fractures to impact later, after resorption at the fracture site, is not well founded.

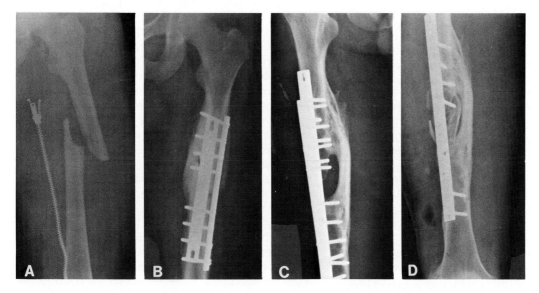

Fig. 1-113. (A) This spiral fracture of the femur was immobilized by an inflatable splint that barely reached the fracture site. **(B)** The end result after application of two plates at 90°. Proponents of rigid plating would not be pleased by the obvious periosteal callus. **(C)** Another patient treated by this method had resorption of a butterfly fragment. The stability of these rigid plates maintained the femur while a periosteal "flying buttress" formed. **(D)** The same femur after bone graft and the removal of one plate. If both plates are removed simultaneously, there is serious danger of refracture through screw holes.

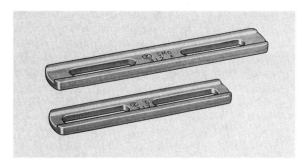

Fig. 1-114. Eggers compression plates with slots that theoretically allow impaction of the fracture prior to tightening the screws. *(Courtesy of Zimmer, U.S.A.)*

The AO System. Thirty years ago or so the AO or ASIF* group[312,313] introduced a system of rigid fixation by plates, screws, and other implants that revolutionized the management of long-bone fractures. Their objective was to make fixation so stable that external fixation was superfluous, allowing active exercise of muscles and joints to be initiated almost immediately. By so doing, they hoped to eliminate the so-called "fracture disease" (ie, chronic edema, soft tissue atrophy, osteoporosis, and joint stiffness). Unfortunately, in the United States, many surgeons bought the equipment without understanding the method and their results were unsatisfactory. This delayed the widespread acceptance of the AO method for some time.

Rigid fixation promotes "primary vascular bone healing," in which contact healing occurs across the apposed bone ends by cutting cones of revascularization that cross the fracture site. In such healing, periosteal callus is scant or absent. The appearance of external callus—"irritation callus"—is evidence that motion is occurring; motion leads to bone resorption, loosening of the screws, and failure.

To achieve stable fixation, interfragmemtary compression is produced by lag screws and axial compression by plates under tension. Interfragmentary fixation may be "static" or "dynamic." In *static compression* the force is applied solely by the implant (eg, a lag screw across a fracture interface). *Dynamic compression,* on the other hand, is achieved by harnessing normal physiologic loads to produce compression (ie, muscle tension). In cerclage of a transverse fracture of the patella, if the wire passes over the anterior surface and is tightened, the frac-

* ASIF (Association for the Study of Internal Fixation) is the English translation of AO (Arbeitsgemeinschaft für Osteosynthesefragen).

ture line gapes posteriorly. On flexing the knee, the tension of the quadriceps closes the gap and dynamic compression is exerted across the fracture gap. Similarly, when a long bone is plated, the plate is applied to the "tension side" with axial compression applied (ie, "the tension band principle"). Unfortunately, in fresh fractures it may be difficult to determine precisely which is the tension side.

An important attribute of the AO system is the provision of axial compression by pretensioning a plate. Initially substantial, rigid plates with round holes were used, but innovations in plate design have been made since those early days. Nonetheless, the basic premise and application of axial compression have remained unchanged. After reduction of the fracture, the plate is applied to the fracture and secured to one fragment. A drill guide for the compression device is inserted into the last hole of the opposite end of the plate, the hole is drilled and tapped, and the compression device is screwed to the bone. The compression device has a hook that fits into the last hole of the plate and, by turning a worm screw, the plate is pulled toward the device. The latest model, which has a direct-reading pressure gauge, has an excursicn of 20 mm in comparison with the 8 mm of the original model. (In the new version, the hook is reversible so that it may be used in a distraction mode for reducing an overlapped fracture.) This pretensioning causes the fracture to be compressed to an appropriate degree, following which the remaining screws are inserted (Fig. 1-115). Perren[347] has shown that bone can tolerate up to 300 kp/cm^2 without undergoing pressure necrosis, and that this compression enhances the rigidity of fixation. However, the level of the compression does not remain this high but gradually diminishes as the bone remodels and the fracture heals. After 2 months the compression falls to 50% of the initial level.

Plates may serve four functions: static compression, dynamic compression, neutralization, and buttressing.

Static compression does not utilize muscle load or other physiologic loads and is used mainly in fractures of the humerus. Compression on one side of the bone is liable to compress the near cortex and gap the far cortex. The pressure on the fracture can be evened up by prebending the plate slightly in the middle (Fig. 1-116) or by inserting a screw obliquely across the fracture (Fig. 1-117).

Dynamic compression is applied to the tension side of a bone, but is not appropriate in many acute fractures because the direction of tensile forces cannot be determined. In pseudarthroses of the

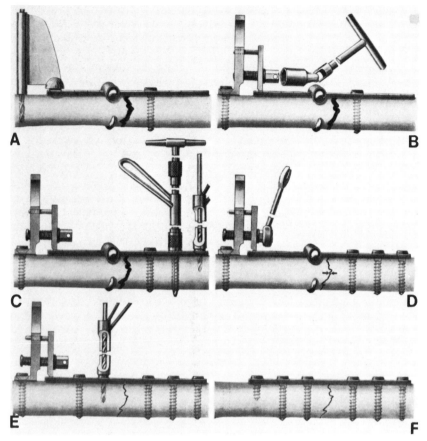

Fig. 1-115. These diagrams illustrate the steps in applying a straight tension band. **(A)** The plate is applied with a single screw and, using a guide, a hole is drilled for anchoring the tension device. **(B)** The tension device is applied and tightened until the reduction is complete. **(C)** The remaining screws are replaced in one end of the plate. The holes are predrilled using a centering device, after which the threads are tapped and the screw is inserted. **(D)** Extra compression is applied by means of an open-ended wrench. **(E)** The remaining screws are inserted on the other side of the fracture line. **(F)** The completed compression plating. The short screw gripping only one cortex is intended to smooth out the gradation between the normal elastic bone and the rigid segment deep to the plate. *(Müller, M. E.; Allgöwer, M.; and Willenegger, H.: Manual of Internal Fixation, p. 55. New York, Springer-Verlag, 1970.)*

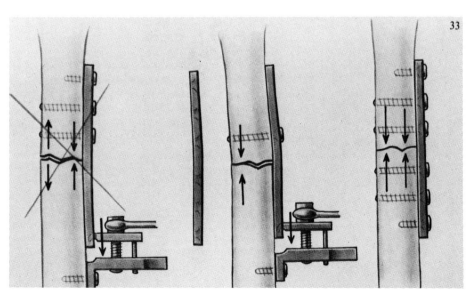

Fig. 1-116. Use of the tension device in transverse fractures. **(Left)** Tightening the tension band compresses the near cortex and gapes the far cortex. **(Center)** Prebending the plate equalizes the compression as shown on the **right**. *(Müller, M. E.; Allgöwer, M.; Schneider, R.; and Willenegger, H.: Manual of Internal Fixation, Techniques Recommended by the AO Group, 2nd ed., p. 57. New York, Springer-Verlag, 1979.)*

tibia, however, the plate must be applied over the convexity of the angulation, where it acts as a tension band.

Compression may also be applied to the fracture site by applying a straight plate to a concave surface (Fig. 1-118) or by bowing the plate (see Fig. 1-116).

In a *neutralization* mode, a plate is applied to protect interfragmentary screws from torsional, shear, and bending forces. The lag screws may be inserted independently or through holes in the plate. Any time a screw passes across a fracture plane, it should be lagged by overdrilling the near hole. Neutralization plates must be carefully contoured to fit the bone.

For *buttress* effect, plates are applied to prevent a cortex from collapsing or to protect a diaphyseal defect filled with bone graft.

Semitubular Plates.   Semitubular plates were introduced in 1960 and were originally designed to be used on the anterior crest and medial edge of the tibia. These plates are delicate (only 1 mm thick)

and easily deformed, but their semitubular conformation gives them much greater rigidity than a flat plate of similar dimensions. The semitubular plates have oval holes, so that by placing screws at the far end of the hole from the fracture line, the plate is self-compressing (Fig. 1-119). Although semitubular plates have been used for fractures of the forearm bones, they are easily broken, and we have largely given them up for this purpose, except occasionally in the proximal third of the radius in small forearm bones (Fig. 1-120). They are, however, useful in fibular fractures and in boot-top fractures of the tibia, where two plates are used to provide static compression. More recently, even more delicate plates (⅓ and ¼ tubular plates) have been introduced, which are fastened by 3.5-mm and 2.7-mm screws, respectively. These plates have their greatest usefulness in metatarsal and metacarpal fractures.

The Dynamic Compression Plate.   The dynamic compression plate (DCP)[9] is now the workhorse of

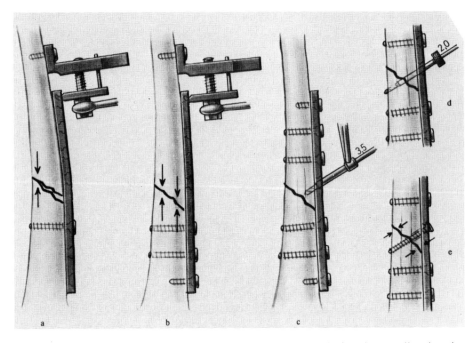

Fig. 1-117. Use of the tension device in oblique fractures. **(A)** The plate is affixed to the fragment whose spike is on the far cortex. **(B)** The spike of the other fragment is compressed into the reentrant formed by plate and bone. This prevents the shortening of bone that otherwise might result by compressing oblique surfaces. **(C, D, E)** Greater stability still is engendered by an oblique lag screw producing interfragmental compression. *(Müller, M. E.; Allgöwer, M.; Schneider, R.; and Willenegger, H.: Manual of Internal Fixation. Techniques Recommended by the AO Group, 2nd ed., p. 57. New York, Springer-Verlag, 1979.)*

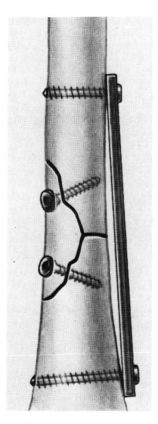

Fig. 1-118. Axial compression may be produced by mismatching a plate to a contoured surface. *(Müller, M. E.; Allgöwer, M.; Schneider, R.; and Willenegger, H.: Manual of Internal Fixation. Techniques Recommended by the AO Group, 2nd ed., p. 65. New York, Springer-Verlag, 1979.)*

the AO system. When introduced in 1965, it was made of titanium, but it is now fabricated from stainless steel (Fig. 1-121). It was hoped that the titanium plate, having a lower Young's modulus, would provide rigid internal fixation with more flexibility to diminish stress-shielding of the bone. Because titanium has a UTS of 80 kp/mm^2, titanium screws have a higher failure rate than screws of 316L steel (UTS, 90 kp/mm^2). For this reason, DCPs are now made of stainless steel. It is surprising that the titanium plate has not been used with stainless steel screws, which would solve the problem of screw breakage. However, as is discussed in the section on metallurgy (see p. 116), AO/ASIF apparently is experimenting with titanium implants, so it is likely that we shall see their reintroduction sometime in the future.[347] Titanium is so inert that one would not expect a battery effect when fixed by stainless steel screws.

The DCP derives its name from its ability to provide axial compression without the use of the tension device, although this may be used when necessary. Perhaps the term DCP is unfortunate, because it implies that it should be used for dynamic compression alone, although indeed it may be used as a static, neutralization, or buttress plate.

The DCP operates on the same basic principle as the Bagby plate,[23,24] which exerts its compression by the eccentric insertion of screws (Fig. 1-122). The slot for the screw has a sloping surface at one end. When the spherical head of the screw impinges on this surface, the plate moves away from the fracture, thereby compressing the fracture plane. The magnitude of this movement, and consequently of the compression, is determined by the drill guide that sites the screw hole (Fig. 1-123).

The load guide (see Fig. 1-123**B**), which is color-coded yellow, has an eccentrically placed hole. When this guide is used, the screw will meet the inclined load plane 1 mm from its end. When the fracture is accurately reduced, the horizontal displacement will produce 60 kp to 80 kp of axial, interfragmentary compression. When using the drill guide, it is very important to have the arrow engraved on the device pointing to the fracture site so that the screw is appropriately placed (see Fig. 1-123**B**). If more compression is necessary, subsequent screws may be inserted in the compression mode, but it is rarely necessary for more than two screws to be loaded. When additional compression is added, the tension on the initially inserted screws must be released by backing off one or two turns. Each screw is then tightened in turn when all the screws have been inserted.

The neutral drill guide (see Fig. 1-123**A**) is coded green. It is not quite neutral, because it is inserted eccentrically 0.1 mm along the load plane and thus exerts additional compression.

A third guide, the red-coded buttress guide, is no longer used by AO. This should never be used as a compression guide, because its greater excursion will overload the screw. If the DCP is to be used as a buttress plate, it is now recommended that the 58-mm long, 3.2-mm drill sleeve be used (see Fig. 1-123**C**). This drill-sleeve is inserted at the fracture end of the plate hole. Generally where a buttress effect is needed, one of the special plates—T, L, spoon, or cloverleaf—is appropriate.

Drill jigs are available to place the first two screw holes in exactly the same positions as they would be if they had been inserted in the plate with the load guide (Fig. 1-124). The jig is a helpful device. If a plate obscures the fracture line, the reduction

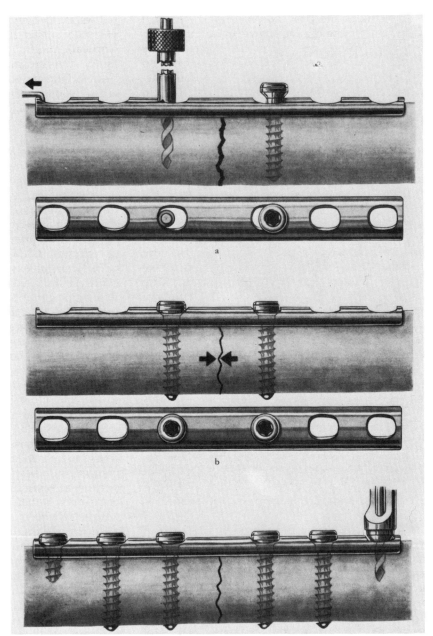

Fig. 1-119. Diagrammatic representation of the use of the semitubular plate of the AO system. The tightening up of eccentrically placed screws produces motion of the plate and compression at the fracture site. *(Müller, M. E.; Allgöwer, M.; and Willenegger, H.: Manual of Internal Fixation. Techniques Recommended by the AO Group, p. 67. New York, Springer-Verlag, 1970.)*

cannot be checked, but with the drill jig, the fracture line can be observed and the drill holes made. When the screws are inserted through the plate into the predrilled holes, the accurate reduction is preserved. There is a third drill guide in the jig (see Fig. 1-124) to allow the second screw hole from the fracture to be drilled in the compression mode, leaving the first hole in the plate to be used for a lag screw that passes obliquely through the fracture site. This should always be done in transverse and short

oblique fractures of the femur and tibia, but it is also advisable in the humerus and even in the forearm, although one has to be careful not to devascularize the tip of a spike in the radius or the ulna. This oblique screw ensures that the far cortex is under compression (Fig. 1-125).

The round holes in the original AO plates made perpendicular insertion of screws mandatory, and deviations mitigated the compression at the fracture site and stressed the screws. The design of the countersink of the DCP, however, allows cortical screws and spongiosa lag screws to be inserted at an angle without any deleterious effect, because the spherical head of the screw will mate with no angulation stress. By this means better interfragmentary compression may be achieved. Careful contouring of the DCP is essential and requires practice and skill. Not only are bends necessary (made with the bending press), but twists in the long axis must also be contrived with bending irons. This longitudinal twisting should be left until after all the other bends are made. This modeling of the plate is facilitated enormously by the use of a malleable, aluminum template which can be molded to the surface of the bone and then duplicated in the plate itself. Such "mutilation" of plates would formerly have been frowned upon, because it would have initiated cracks and thus would have significantly decreased the plate's fatigue life. The DCP, however, is annealed—that is, the grain size has been made larger by heating. This process makes the plate more malleable, and the subsequent "cold working" of the plate increases its strength and rigidity.

No matter which type of plate is used, having gaps in the bone owing to missing fragments will increase the stresses on the plate and screws. This should be obviated by accurate reduction of the fracture and the liberal use of cancellous or corticocancellous bone grafts.

For use in forearms and other sites where the regular plates are too large, smaller plates are available which are fastened by 3.5-mm screws. The instrumentation for these devices is color-coded in gold.

The 3.5-mm screw has recently been redesigned with a finer thread, an enlarged core diameter (increased from 1.9 to 2.4 mm), and a modified thread pitch (1.75 *versus* 1.25 mm). The tensile strength and bending moment at which plastic deformity begins are 62% higher than with the old screw.

This screw has increased holding power and is designed to be used with the 3.5-mm plates and pelvic reconstruction plates, as well as the ⅓ tubular plate. The 2.5-mm drill bit, tap, tap sleeve, and drill guide are brown to avoid confusion with the older instrumentation.

The old 3.5-mm screw is now designated as the 3.5-mm cancellous screw, and has been retained for use as a lag screw (medial malleolus) or for T-plates in the distal radius.

In addition to the regular AO plates, screws, and special plates, there are small and mini-plates and screws for use in the hands and feet. The small screws are 2.7 and 3.5 mm (cortical) and 4 mm (cancellous), and the mini-screws are 2 and 2.7 mm (cortical). All of these have appropriate instrumentation, and the smallest screws must of necessity have Phillips heads.

The Effects of Plating.   When a plated bone is subjected to flexural loading, the weakest configuration is obtained when the plate is under compression and the strongest when the bone is loaded from the side opposite to the plate. In the first instance the fracture tends to open up and the whole load is borne by the plate. On the other hand, loads which tend to close the fracture place the plate under tension and a significant portion of the load is supported by bone, thereby diminishing the bending moment on the plate. In this latter configuration, Bynum and associates[73] found that no benefit accrued from increasing either the breadth of the plate or the size of the screws, but when the plate was increased in length from 3 to 6 inches, the strength of the assembly was doubled.

Laurence and associates[265] studied the stress on the screws of a four-hole plate subjected to a load that tended to open up the fracture. Almost the entire load was carried by the two central screws on either side of the fracture. The stress on these two screws was unaffected by changing either the length of the plate or the distance between the screws. Even when an eight-hole plate was substituted for the four-hole, only the central two screws were significantly stressed. The remaining screws were under compression stress rather than tension. In this study, the load on the screws never exceeded their pull-out strength, so the plate became the vulnerable component of the assembly. They concluded that a four-hole plate is adequate to resist stresses that open up the fracture, even if the screws engage only one cortex.

The strength of a bone–plate assembly will be influenced by the character of the fracture. Transverse fractures are stronger under compression than oblique fractures; however, when tested in rotation, the reverse is true. Comminution, inadequate reduction, and missing fragments all contribute to weakness of the assembly. In plating metacarpal fractures in horses, Bynum[73] found that the maximum strength that could be achieved was 60% of that of the intact contralateral metacarpal. Because horses are obliged to stand up and are unable to run on three legs as dogs do, Bynum, in his clinical series, had only one successful outcome in 15 cases. Similarly, quiet walking in humans imposes a bending moment of 80 Nm on the tibia, and a tibia

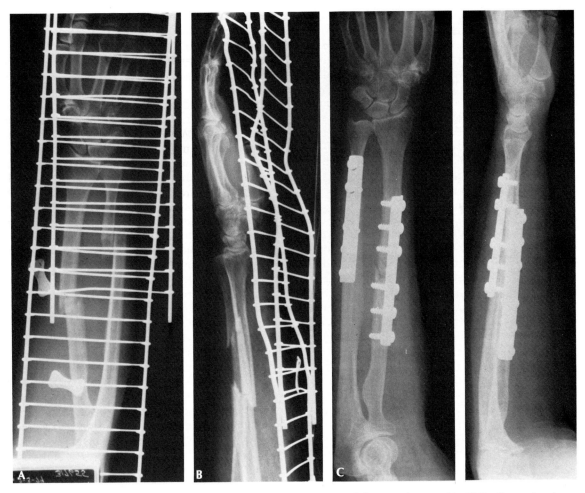

Fig. 1-120. Semitubular plates are occasionally used for very small forearm bones. **(A, B)** Radiographs show fractures of both bones of the forearm in a woman who fell on the ice. **(C)** The fractures were fixed with semitubular plates that were strong enough to immobilize her rather delicate bones.

(continued)

fixed with a Stamm plate fails at 24 Nm.[198] It is obvious that early, unrestricted weight-bearing is not feasible in plated fractures.

Rybicki and associates[387] have shown that in compression loading, the bone bears 80% of the load and the plate 20%. However, the stress is not evenly distributed across the bone so that the cortex on the plated side is protected from 75% of the applied stress, while on the opposite side the stress was 1½ times the applied value.

Wirth and associates[485] found that 80% of the fracture surfaces were not in contact when maximum compression was applied to a transverse fracture by an AO plate. Similarly, it has been shown

that by prebending the plate, a more even distribution of forces can be obtained at the fracture site and a significant enhancement of rigidity obtained. The same effect, however, can be obtained by an oblique screw across the fracture line, which is possible if a DCP is used.[312]

Hayes and Perren[129] determined the coefficient of friction for both titanium and stainless steel dynamic compression plates and found that there was no significant difference between these plates if the design was the same. They calculated that if a normal force of 200 kp would generate a frictional force of up to 75 kp at the plate–bone interface, this maximal friction force is commensurate with

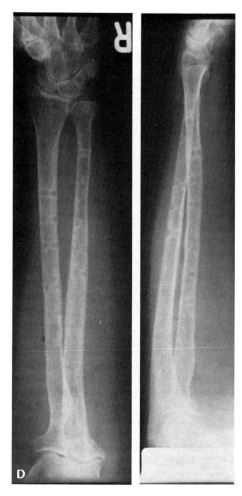

Fig. 1-120 (continued)
(D) The result after removal of the plates.

the total interfragmentary compressive forces (75 kp–135 kp) measured *in vivo* with instrumented compression plates. They concluded that frictional forces may transmit a significant proportion of the longitudinal, interfragmentary compressive force to a healing bone.

One must always temper the information gained from experimental data with equally valid information garnered from clinical experience. We know that four-hole plates have little place in the management of long-bone fractures, and it does appear that plates should have sufficient length to withstand bending and torsional moments, and screws strong enough to resist the tensile, shear, and angulatory stresses placed upon them.

On the basis of his experimental and clinical

studies, Hey-Groves[194] demonstrated that nonunions and infections were less common in plated fractures when large rigid implants were used. Hicks came to the same conclusion and claimed that his rigid lug plates were as efficacious as those of the AO.[198]

Superb studies of bone healing under rigid compression have been made by Schenk in collaboration with Willenegger.[312,313] They have shown that where bone is under compression so that there is no gap, dead bone is resorbed, and resorption cavities, produced by cutting cones of osteoclasts, traverse the fracture plane. Blood vessels accompanied by mesenchymal cells and osteoblast precursors soon follow to reconstitute the haversian systems.

If the axial compression opens up a gap in the cortex opposite the plate, usually about 200 microns, the healing process is a little different. Primary bone formation takes place, but the orientation of this bone is not longitudinal, but parallel to the fracture surface (gap healing). In the second stage of gap healing, the longitudinal haversian systems are reconstituted by "cutting cones" from each fragment, and the bone is united primarily without the need for ensheathing callus.

Clinically, the ideal end result of rigid plating is what Danis calls "soudure autogene" (ie, primary endosteal healing without perceptible periosteal callus).[312] The degree to which external callus forms is an index of the amount of motion at the fracture site. When ideal fixation is attained, there is no resorption of bone ends, and the fracture heals by revascularization of the bone ends and endosteal callus. Olerud and Danckwardt-Lilliestrōm[327] studied healing in dog tibias where a double osteotomy had been performed with removal of the loose segment to ensure its complete avascularity. When this loose fragment was replaced and fixed by a compression plate, they found that within 2 weeks 80% of the intermediate fragments had vessels in the haversian canals which were derived from the endosteal circulation. Both the intermediate fragment and the bone ends were being remodeled by simultaneous bone resorption and new bone formation in the haversian systems.

The provision of rigid internal fixation to facilitate primary healing exacts a price. The large, strong plates that eliminate micromotion at the fracture site also "stress-protect" the bone—that is, they bypass stresses that would normally be borne by the bone. If bone is not adequately stressed, it atrophies, and where plates have been *in situ* for some time the bone necks down and is vulnerable to re-

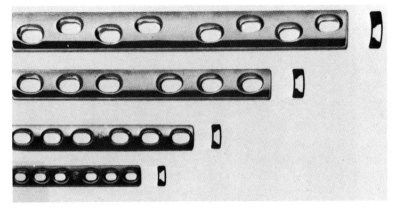

Fig. 1-121. Dynamic compression plates (DCP). **(A)** Broad—for humerus and femur. **(B)** Small—for the forearm, tibia, and pelvis. **(C)** Narrow. **(D)** For use with 2.7-mm screws. *(Müller, M. E.; Allgöwer, M.; Schneider, R.; and Willenegger, H.: Manual of Internal Fixation. Techniques Recommended by the AO Group, 2nd ed., p. 67. New York, Springer-Verlag, 1979.)*

fracture after removal of the metal[309,310] (Fig. 1-126). This further aggravates the problem of the empty screw holes.

Uhthoff and associates[460] studied dog femurs with transverse fractures treated by four-hole compression plates and found osteopenia, which was most pronounced in the cortex underlying the plate. There was subperiosteal resorption with a reduction in the caliber of the shaft. Histologically, there was a persistence of woven bone, but these changes reversed after removal of the plates.

Paavolainen and associates[332,333] also studied the healing of experimental fractures in rabbit tibiofibular bones that were fixed by six-hole, stainless steel

DCPs. These fractures were tested for torsional strength at intervals from 3 to 24 weeks postoperatively. During the first 9 weeks there was progressive improvement in maximum torque capacity, energy absorption, and torsional rigidity, reflecting the advancement of the union. From 9 to 24 weeks the torque capacity and energy absorption decreased while torsional rigidity reached a steady state. They concluded that, after healing, the continued presence of the implant has an adverse effect on the cortical bone, which loses strength. The rabbit normally obtains bony union at 6 to 8 weeks.

In histologic studies they found that after 9 weeks there was rapid excavation and breakdown of the

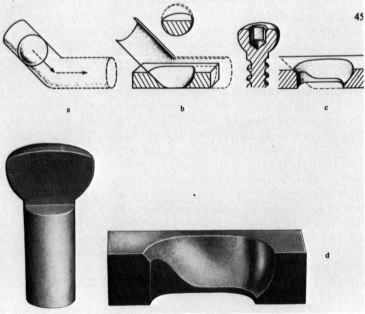

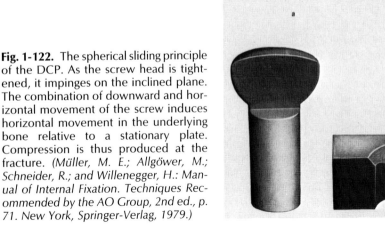

Fig. 1-122. The spherical sliding principle of the DCP. As the screw head is tightened, it impinges on the inclined plane. The combination of downward and horizontal movement of the screw induces horizontal movement in the underlying bone relative to a stationary plate. Compression is thus produced at the fracture. *(Müller, M. E.; Allgöwer, M.; Schneider, R.; and Willenegger, H.: Manual of Internal Fixation. Techniques Recommended by the AO Group, 2nd ed., p. 71. New York, Springer-Verlag, 1979.)*

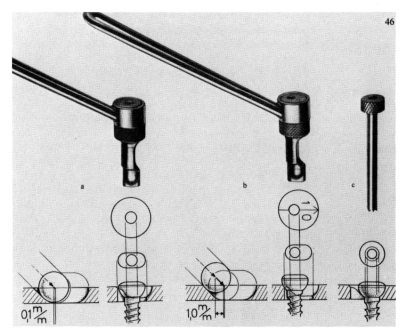

Fig. 1-123. Drill guides for dynamic compression plates. **(A)** Neutral guide. **(B)** Load guide. **(C)** The 58-mm drill sleeve. *(Müller, M. E.; Allgöwer, M.; Schneider, R.; and Willenegger, H.: Manual of Internal Fixation. Techniques Recommended by the AO Group, 2nd ed., p. 73. New York, Springer-Verlag, 1979.)*

cortical wall, and porosity increased from 9% to 37.5%. The osteoporosis was accompanied by new subperiosteal bone, giving rise to an increase in the overall diameter of the bone and the medullary cavity.

If the fixation is made even more perfect, the stress shielding is enhanced. Pilliar and associates[354]

applied a porous coating of cobalt-based alloy on the surface of 316L stainless steel plates. The powder was sintered to the plates in hydrogen at 1270°C. The control was a steel plate annealed at 1270°C for 3 hours. Six months after applying the plates in dogs, there was no difficulty in prying the control plates off, but the coated plates could be

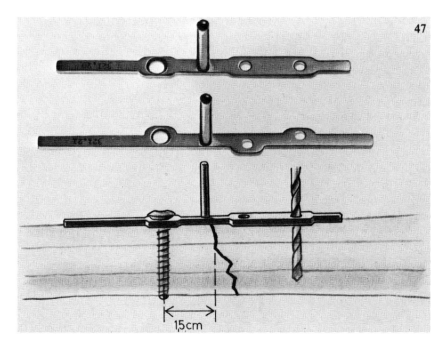

Fig. 1-124. Drill jigs for dynamic compression plates. *(Müller, M. E.; Allgöwer, M.; Schneider, R.; and Willenegger, H.: Manual of Internal Fixation. Techniques Recommended by the AO Group, 2nd ed., p. 73. New York, Springer-Verlag, 1979.)*

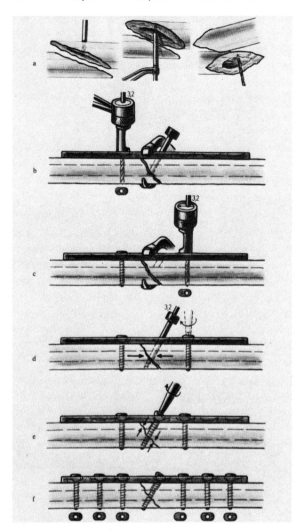

Fig. 1-125. Combination of axial and interfragmental compression using a DCP. Note that the first screw is inserted in the fragment whose spike is farthest from the plate. After axial compression is applied, an oblique lag screw is inserted for interfragmental compression. The remaining screws are inserted using the neutral guide. *(Müller, M. E.; Allgöwer, M.; Schneider, R.; and Willenegger, H.: Manual of Internal Fixation. Techniques Recommended by the AO Group, 2nd ed., p. 75. New York, Springer-Verlag, 1979.)*

removed only with great difficulty. There was much greater intracortical porosity and bone resorption on the side of the coated plate, evidently owing to the better bonding of the plate to bone, thereby increasing the stress shielding.

The current doctrine of the AO group is that osteoporosis under a plate is not secondary to "stress protection" but to disturbance of the blood supply,

and that it increases with increasing elasticity of the plate. Allgöwer[6] states that this osteoporosis secondary to vascular damage is rapidly reversible, but enough time should be allowed for cortical remodelling and restoration of structure. He recommends that the minimal times for the removal of a plate should be 1 year for the tibia, 18 months for the forearm and humerus, and 2 years for the femur.

When a plate is applied to bone, the modulus of the plated section is much higher than the rest of the bone, and there is an abrupt transition at the juncture of plated and unplated bone. This acts as a stress riser, and attempts have been made to mitigate this by tapered plates and the use of a unicortical screw in the last hole to smooth out the difference (see Fig. 1-119). Both problems could conceivably be solved by using plates that are less stiff. An attempt to do this was made by making the original dynamic compression plate out of pure titanium. Uthoff and co-workers[461] have compared stainless steel and titanium plates in the healing of osteotomies in beagles and found that the radiologic bone loss was 19% for stainless steel and only 3% for the titanium plates. The AO group, however, discontinued the use of their original titanium DCP because they felt it was unsatisfactory.[6] Plates of more flexible materials might be an answer, but too much flexibility may also interfere with the adequacy of fixation.

Recent experimental work in animals holds out some hope in this regard. Coutts and associates[108] compared stainless steel plates with plates made of a composite of carbon fibers laminated in polymethylmethacrylate. This was a short-term study on six mongrel dogs. The bending stiffness of the steel plates was 5.5×10^4 kg/cm^2, and of the composite, 6×10^3 kg/cm^2. There appeared to be no qualitative difference between the two plates in radiologic healing of the fractures, nor was there a difference in torque, deformation, or energy absorption at refracture. The computed maximal shear strengths were identical. Intracortical porosity, however, was 14% with steel plates and only 6.8% for the composite.

Carbon Fiber-Reinforced Plates. Tayton and his associates[449] have used semirigid, carbon fiber–reinforced plates (CFRP) both experimentally and in clinical practice. In sheep with both simple transverse and segmental osteotomies fixation with these plates was uniformly successful in achieving union.

The CFRP implants used clinically were of two varieties. In the first seven cases, a copy of the AO

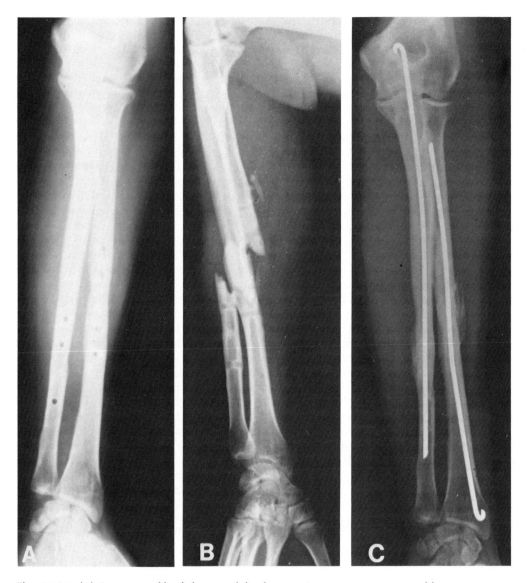

Fig. 1-126. (A) Fractures of both bones of the forearm in a young man treated by compression plates. It can be seen that there is some attenuation of the shaft of the radius where the plate has been. **(B)** Exactly 2 months later, following a trivial injury, refractures occurred through the upper screw hole in the ulna and through the attenuated area of the radius. **(C)** The appearance of the forearm 11 months later, after the insertion of Rush nails and the addition of osteoperiosteal grafts from the rib.

dynamic compression plate was used but the large, slotted holes were found to weaken the plate so much that the design was changed to an 8-hole, broad plate in which the holes were round. This latter plate was used in 13 patients.

The patients selected for the study had all sustained transverse or short oblique fractures of the midshaft of the tibia, some of which included but-

terfly fragments. Following surgery the patients were encouraged to walk with a cane as soon as they were comfortable (3 to 10 days).

Of the 7 patients in the initial AO DCP group, six went on to union while the seventh developed a hypertrophic nonunion after failure of the plate. Three of the patients with healed fractures complained of pain on weight-bearing.

All of the patients whose fractures were treated by the noncompressing, round-hole plates healed. Only two of these complained of pain and both were found to be harboring deep infections.

When the implants were removed from these 20 patients, they were tested by four-point bending to destruction. The round-hole plates were half as rigid as stainless steel and the DCPs one third as stiff, but both had greater fatigue strengths than metal. What was most interesting was the correlation between stiffness and the patients' complaints of pain. Most of those complaining had plates with a stiffness varying from 1 Nm to 1.7 Nm per degree. Tayton[448] concluded that the stiffness of tibial plates should therefore be greater than 1.75 Nm per degree and subsequently has used plates whose stiffness is 2 Nm per degree.

All of the fractures in this series healed with bridging callus. As Uhthoff[458] has observed, it is difficult to tell when a fracture has healed when held under rigid compression, and one must remove the implant after an arbitrary period of time. With flexible implants one can ascertain when healing has taken place, the area moment of inertia is increased, and, presumably, the stress-shielded osteoporosis should be less.

Plate Removal.   In our current practice, we have tended to accept the guidelines advised by the AO group for the removal of plates. They suggest that tibial plates may be removed after 1 year, femoral plates at 2 years, and forearm and humeral plates at 1.5 to 2 years.

TECHNIQUE OF DRILLING HOLES IN BONE

There is a paucity of information in the orthopaedic literature about drill-point design and the effects of drilling.[2,171,223,224,285] Most authorities, when they mention the subject at all, stress the importance of having a sharp drill point and recommend drilling at slow speeds and preferably by hand. Old-line purists tend to believe that orthopaedic trainees should serve an apprenticeship with hand tools even though power tools tend to be superior. It makes more sense to be able to concentrate entirely on controlling the direction of a cutting tool than to be diverted by also having to manipulate a brace or a ratchet. Indeed, no one can manipulate a hand drill without some degree of wobble, which produces an elliptical hole instead of a round one.

A drill point has two cutting edges, which are wedges and cut like the blade of a plane. The tip is cone-shaped and the angle subtended by the two cutting edges (point angle) is acute for cutting soft materials such as wood, and blunter for hard materials such as metal. Most bone drills have an angle of 90°. Leading from the cutting edge is a spiral channel or flute that carries the excised chips away from the cutting surface. Thus, the drill point must be kept rotating in a clockwise direction as it is withdrawn to prevent the bone fragments from being left in the hole. The edges of the flutes should not be sharp or the drill will act as a router and unduly enlarge the hole. By the same token, this makes the drill point a poor tool for enlarging the medullary cavity of the forearm bones to facilitate intramedullary nailing. The face of the terminal cone is ground so that it slants away from the cutting surface (ie, the clearance angle, which is 8° to 12°). This facilitates cutting, but, if overdone, it makes the cutting edge too delicate and prone to fracture. The *rake* or *helix angle* of the drill is the angle between the cutting edge and the leading edge of the helix. Bechtol[31] has advised that this angle should be 0° to prevent chipping of the bone as the drill point enters the cortex. The chisel edge of the drill is at the apex of the cone and is formed at the junction of the two clearance surfaces. Jacob[223,224] has advised that the most efficient drill point for bone is one with a point angle of 90° and a rake angle of 25° to 35° and that the drill point be inserted at a speed of 750 to 1250 rpm.

In drilling, two thirds of the energy is converted to heat, and the thermal energy transferred to bone will cause death of the bone if the temperature rises above 50°C.

Matthews and Hirsch[285] studied the heating effect of drilling bone with a 3.2-mm AO drill bit, by placing thermocouples 0.5, 1, 2, and 3 mm from the drill hole. They assessed such factors as sharpness of the drill point, drill pressure, and speed of rotation. The tests were conducted with rotational rates of 345, 885, and 2900 rpm and drill pressures of 2-, 6-, and 12-kg. The maximum temperature they recorded at 0.5 mm from the drill was 140°C. In general, the highest temperatures were produced at 2900 rpm and 2 kg force. By changing the drilling force from 2 kg to 6 or 12 kg, a significant drop in the duration of temperatures above 50°C occurred, but there was no significant difference between drill pressures of 6 and 12 kg. There was also no significant difference in maximum temperatures developed at the different drill speeds, but longer periods of elevation above 50°C were attained at low speeds.

Worn or blunt drills caused the greatest maximum temperatures and duration of high temperatures at all the thermocouple positions. When the holes were predrilled with 2.2-mm drills at 885 rpm with 6 kg force and then enlarged using 3.2-mm drills, the temperature never arose above 50°C. The use of drill guides did not cause elevation of temperature *per se,* but interfered with the other potent means of decreasing temperature—irrigation of the drill point.

Because heat is generated by friction and fragmentation of bone at the cutting edge, the total amount of heat generated is directly proportional to the number of revolutions it takes to complete the hole. Drilling with an increased force level causes the drill to cut deeper and thus the hole is completed with fewer revolutions. The cutting edge moves a shorter distance, and redistribution of heat to the chips may favor the decreased level and duration of temperature.

The lessons to be learned from this excellent study are obvious. Never use a dull or damaged drill bit, and discard a point after it has drilled 40 holes or if you are not making headway with it. Dull drill points have a way of returning to sets to bedevil the unwary. This can be obviated by bending them at the time of discard. Make sure the flutes are cleared of detritus with each insertion to allow the chips to escape and irrigate while drilling. Use a power drill with a right-angled guide, and apply sufficient pressure to enhance the rate of penetration.

Tungsten-steel drills are sharp but brittle. If these are used, do not angulate them or treat them roughly or they will snap off in the bone and become permanent monuments to your surgical ineptitude.

Green and Matthews[171] did a similar study on the heating effects of skeletal pins drilled into bone. They compared 4-mm pins with 3-facet trocar point, spade point, modified spade point (Hoffmann), and half drill (Matthews-Green) pins.

The highest temperature was generated by a trocar point at 700 rpm—180°C. Nearly all the pins produced temperatures in bone in excess of 55°C at 0.5 mm. Maximum bone temperature was almost independent of drill speed. Because there is no provision for chip removal with standard smooth pins, much greater friction is generated than with a drill point. The traditional trocar and spade pins produced the highest temperatures and durations, but the Matthews-Green pin, which provides for chip removal, performed significantly better. However, when predrilling with a 3.5-mm helical drill bit was performed before pin insertion, the maximum temperature for all the pins was reduced to less than 55°C. It is generally believed that the ring sequestrum produced by thermal necrosis leads to pin

loosening and infection. If this is so, the prudent surgeon should predrill the holes for the insertion of the fixation pins.

Christie[93] has described four patients' pin tract infections after Steinmann or Denham pins had been inserted by a power drill. In each case a draining sinus developed in the proximal tibia and x-ray films showed extensive bone necrosis around the pin tract. In three cases the infecting organism was *S. aureus* and in the other, *S. albus.* Two of these patients had fractures through the pin tracts and three required excision of the affected area. He attributed the thermal necrosis and the subsequent infection to the use of the power drill, but indeed the villain is the trocar point that grinds the chips into the hard bone and produces the heat. The friction and thermal damage can be just as readily produced by grinding away by hand.

Recently Jaquet Orthopédie S.A. has introduced a new external fixation pin with a helical flute design. It is self-tapping with diminished insertional torque, which allows the bone chips to escape. The manufacturer claims that these pins may be inserted by power without thermal damage. We have no first-hand experience with these pins.

INTRAMEDULLARY NAILING

Hey-Groves[194] inserted the first intramedullary nail in a femur during World War I and, writing in 1921 on ununited fractures, he stated:

> It occurred to me, therefore, to use a long internal peg or strut, such as would render unnecessary any further fixation and would afford absolute rigidity. I have used pegs of various shapes, cylindrical, cross-sectional, and solid rods; and I am inclined to think that the last named are the best, because they give maximum strength and there is an avoidance of hollows and crevices which form dead spaces.

Hey-Groves was defeated by inadequacies in metals, radiographs, and instrumentation, and it remained for Professor Gerhardt Küntscher[258] to rediscover and popularize intramedullary nailing of femoral shaft fractures. Although subsequent nail designs—including the Schneider,[406] Hanson-Street,[434] and Sampson[3] fluted rod—have enjoyed popularity, at best these were only applicable to transverse or short oblique fractures near the femoral isthmus. Their application in comminuted or distal fractures required supplementation by cerclage wires, screws, plates, methylmethacrylate, or postoperative traction and casting to prevent shortening and rotation.

In the 1970s, Klemm and Schellman[251] refined Küntscher's design to create an interlocking cloverleaf nail for use in comminuted femoral shaft

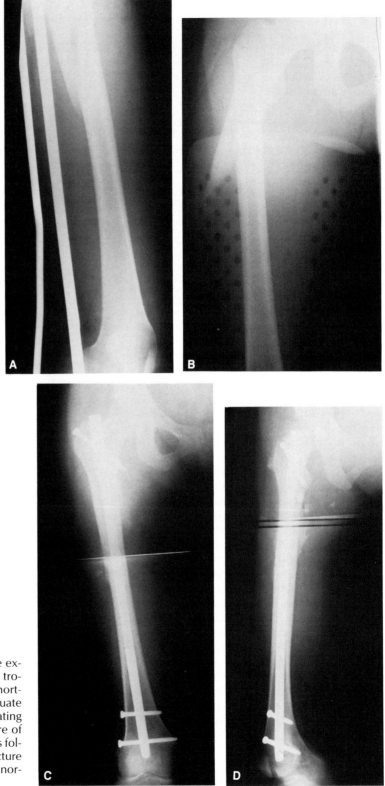

Fig. 1-127. (A, B) A spiral femur fracture extending to the inferior edge of the lesser trochanter. Standard nailing would allow shortening and rotation because of inadequate fixation in the proximal fragment. Plating would require an appliance and exposure of considerable length. **(C, D)** Three months following closed interlocking nailing, the fracture is united, and hip and knee motion are normal.

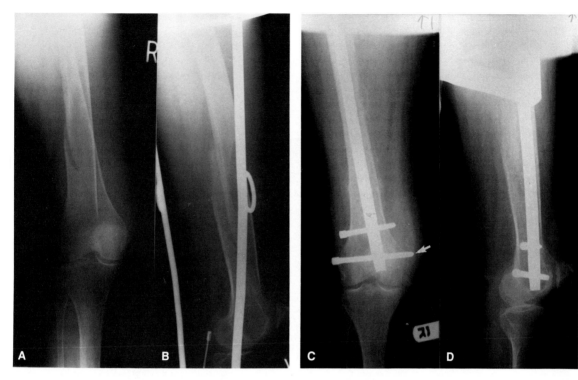

Fig. 1-128. (A, B) An elderly osteoporotic woman tumbled down a flight of stairs. The x-ray film shows a long spiral fracture of the distal femur extending to within 5 cm of the intercondylar notch. **(C, D)** Fixation with an interlocking nail inserted to the roof of the intercondylar notch. After 3 months, the fracture is healed and she lives independently. The distal screw *(arrow)* produced an adventitious bursa and limited knee motion. Prominent screws in this area are liable to cause symptoms.

fractures. The nail included an oblique proximal hole and two transverse distal holes which accepted interlocking screws. In France, Grosse and Kempf[241] later introduced their modification of the interlocking nail, and these devices became available in the United States in 1981. These modifications of Küntscher's technique, improved nail design, and the introduction of radiographic image intensification have broadened the applicability of intramedullary nailing and have made it the procedure of choice in the treatment of femoral shaft fractures[53,97,183,240,251,455,484,486,494] (Figs. 1-127 and 1-128). In a cost-conscious and litigious society, the diminished risk of nonunion and infection, shortened hospital stays, and rapid return to function have fostered the application of this technique to other long bones (Fig. 1-129).

Types of Nails. *Interlocking Nails.* The *Grosse-Kempf interlocking femoral nail*[131,240,455,494] comprises a proximal closed-section cylinder coupled with a cloverleaf distal section that is slotted posteriorly (Fig. 1-130). A threaded oblique hole for the proximal locking screw lies in the cylindrical segment so that separate right and left nails are required. Two transverse distal holes in the cloverleaf portion accept partially threaded screws, which capture only the far cortex. A threaded central hole has been made to accept the proximal targeting device. Distal targeting is accomplished either by image intensification or by a nail-mounted jig. The companion tibial nail is of a similar design with a gradual 20° proximal antecurvature to facilitate its insertion. Two proximal interlocking screws are directed in the anteroposterior plane.

The *Russell-Taylor femoral nail*[29,385] is a closed-section cloverleaf nail designed to provide improved rigidity in torsion (Fig. 1-131). Two crossed, unthreaded oblique holes for the proximal screw obviate the need for right and left nails, and the proximal and distal screws are interchangeable and fully threaded to prevent backing out (Fig. 1-132). The companion tibial nail has both proximal interlocking screws directed transversely to minimize the

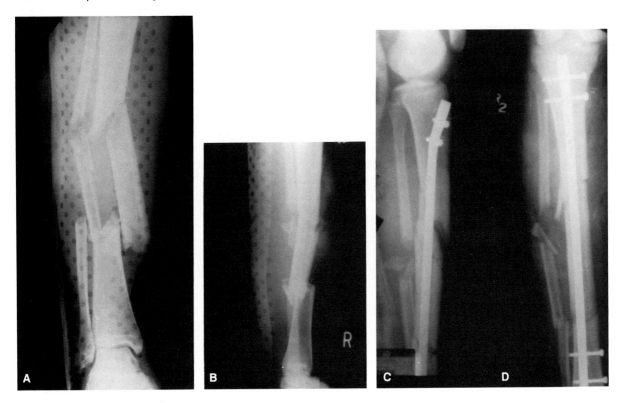

Fig. 1-129. (A, B) This motorcycle enthusiast suffered a segmental open tibial fracture, among other injuries. **(C, D)** An interlocking tibial nail provided excellent stability and facilitated early mobilization.

potential for posterior neurovascular injury. The recent introduction of a "delta" cross section and modulation of the wall thickness have allowed the fabrication of smaller-diameter nails for use in individuals with narrow medullary canals and in cases where medullary reaming is undesirable. Distal targeting and screw insertion are carried out through an image intensifier–assisted jig mounted on the proximal end of the nail.

Features of both the compression hip screw and the locked intramedullary nail have been incorporated into the *Russell-Taylor "reconstruction nail."* The proximal aspect of this nail has been enlarged to accept heavy, cannulated lag screws that are directed superiorly into the femoral head. Right and left nails are required to accommodate the normal anteversion of the femoral neck. A variety of comminuted intertrochanteric–subtrochanteric fractures and ipsilateral femoral neck and shaft fractures are amenable to treatment by this unique interlocking nail (Fig. 1-133).

The *AO/ASIF universal nail*[442,454] has recently been refined to allow interlocking (Fig. 1-134). The fully open-section cloverleaf nail is slotted anteriorly. The radius of curvature is smaller than in other nails, and the wall thickness is limited to increase flexibility, thereby lessening the likelihood of further comminution of the fracture. The proximal locking holes are transverse to allow use in both right and left femurs. A round and an oval hole are present proximally to allow either static or dynamic interlocking. The *AO tibial nail* has an additional anteroposterior hole distally to be used in difficult distal fractures. In both the femoral and tibial nails, distal screws are placed through a hand-held targeting device used with image-intensifier assistance.

The *Brooker-Wills nail* (Fig. 1-135) has a unique distal interlocking mechanism that obviates the necessity for a distal targeting device and the additional radiation exposure required for distal screw insertion.[52,53,183,484] Distal fins are deployed from within the nail for distal locking so that only a proximal exposure is required. The oblique proximal interlocking screw also prevents retraction of these distal fins into the nail after insertion. Both right and left nails are necessary.

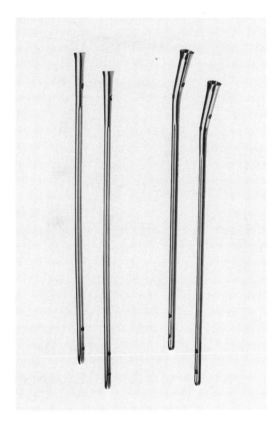

Fig. 1-130. Grosse-Kempf femoral **(left)** and tibial **(right)** nails. *(Courtesy of Howmedica, Inc.)*

The *Williams interlocking Y-nail*[192,193] is a modification of Küntscher's original Y-nail design. It consists of a trough-shaped femoral neck component that is fenestrated to allow passage of a cloverleaf nail down the medullary canal. The two components are locked together by a set screw, and the construct may be locked distally as well. The indications for its use include comminuted, unstable trochanteric fractures and ipsilateral trochanteric–femoral shaft fractures. This nail does not immobilize femoral neck fractures well and is difficult to insert.

The *Huckstep intramedullary compression nail*[212,213] has been in use for two decades. It differs from other nails in its quadrilateral cross section and titanium alloy composition. Holes along the length of the nail accept interlocking screws at multiple levels, and oblique proximal holes allow the insertion of lag screws up the femoral neck. Intraoperative radiographs are not routinely required, and, because the design is not amenable to closed nailing techniques, open reduction is mandatory.

Interlocking nails for humeral fracture fixation are currently in the developmental state and are not yet available for general use (Fig. 1-136). The ability to control rotation may expand the variety of humeral fractures amenable to medullary fixation.[473]

Specialized Nails. The *Zickel nail* was introduced in 1967 for the intramedullary fixation of traumatic and pathologic subtrochanteric fractures of the femur[112,311] (Fig. 1-137). A contoured cobalt-chrome alloy intramedullary rod is mated to a modified Smith-Petersen nail that gains a purchase in the femoral head and neck (Fig. 1-138). Open reduction with adjunctive internal fixation is often required in comminuted fractures, although closed insertion is possible. One should be aware that iatrogenic refracture of the femur can occur during removal of the device because of its shape and rigidity.[490]

The Zickel supracondylar device has been advocated for the treatment of supracondylar femoral fractures in elderly individuals with osteoporotic bone. This device consists of flexible nails that are

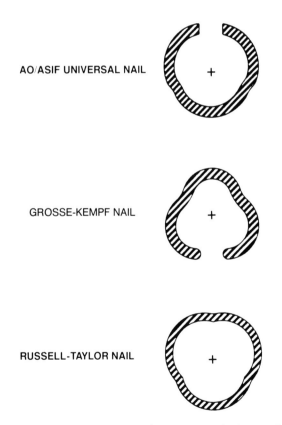

AO/ASIF UNIVERSAL NAIL

GROSSE-KEMPF NAIL

RUSSELL-TAYLOR NAIL

Fig. 1-131. Cross sections of current interlocking nail designs. *(Courtesy of Richards Medical Company.)*

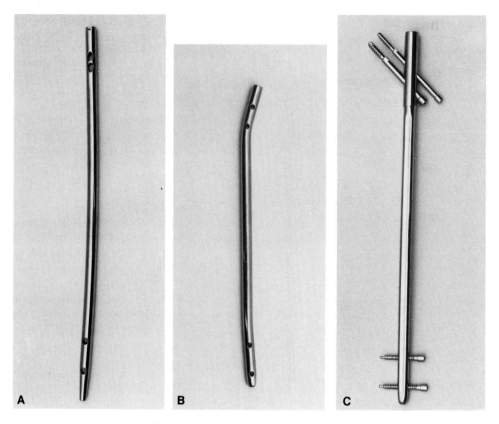

Fig. 1-132. Russell-Taylor nails. **(A)** Femoral. **(B)** Tibial. **(C)** Reconstruction. *(Courtesy of Richards Medical Company.)*

inserted through medial and lateral condylar portals.[492] The use of separate nails is to accommodate the differing configurations of the condyles (Fig. 1-139). Locking screws prevent backing out of the nails at the insertion sites, and medullary reaming is not required routinely.

Ender nails were originally introduced as condylocephalic nails for the fixation of intertrochanteric hip fractures.[136,138] These are flexible devices inserted through distal portals without exposure of the fracture site. The nails are prebent and depend on three-point contact in the medullary canal for fixation (Fig. 1-140). The rigidity of fixation is much less than with a compression hip screw.[175]

Flexible Ender nails have also been used in shaft fractures of the femur and tibia[62,287,301] and are rec-ommended for humeral fracture fixation in multiply injured patients[64,182] (Fig. 1-141). Fractures occurring distal to hip implants may also be treated with flexible nails[254] (Fig. 1-142).

The minimal surgical exposure and lack of reaming are decided advantages when these nails are used in the management of open fractures, but comminuted or unstable fractures may require open exposure and supplemental internal fixation, postoperative traction, or an orthosis to maintain reduction. Furthermore, the nails may back out at their insertion sites causing pain and stiffness in the adjacent joint.

Rush pins have been in use since 1936 and have been applied to virtually every fracture of long bones.[382] They have a round, solid cross section with

Fig. 1-133. Applications of reconstruction nails. **(A)** Ipsilateral fractures of femoral neck and shaft. **(B, C)** At 18 months both fractures are healed without evidence of avascular necrosis. **(D, E)** Comminuted subtrochanteric fracture with extension above the lesser trochanter. **(F, G)** Solid union 6 months following reconstruction nailing.

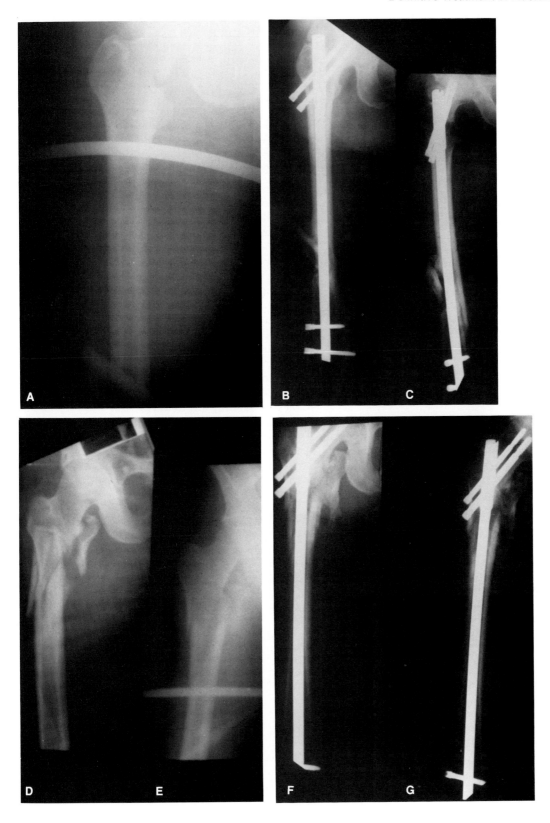

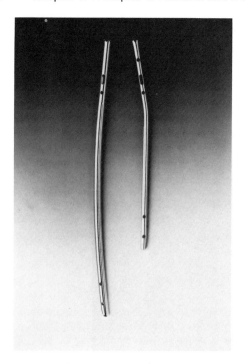

Fig. 1-134. AO/ASIF universal femoral **(left)** and tibial **(right)** nails. *(Courtesy of Synthes, USA.)*

a hook at one end and a sled-point runner at the other. Rush[383] reported a large series of femoral fractures treated with this device, but the applicability of Rush pins may be limited by fracture comminution, and they are subject to the same short-

comings as other flexible intramedullary nails (Fig. 1-143). They are, however, useful in fixation of fractures of the forearm and fibula (Fig. 1-144), where appropriate contouring of the pins is essential.

Fractures of the forearm are most often treated by compression plating, although specialized *forearm nails* that accommodate the complex anatomy of these bones have been devised. Triangular or square cross sectional nails, as designed by Sage[388] and Street,[433] provide improved rotational stability.

Biomechanics of Intramedullary Nails. During the period of fracture healing, internal fixation aids in transmission of forces from one end of the fractured bone to the other, thereby producing stresses in the implant. The mechanical behavior of the implant is determined both by its material and its geometry. The rigidity or stiffness of a cylindrical structure in bending and torsion is proportional to the fourth power of the radius (ie, the polar moment of inertia). The farther material is distributed from the bending or torsional axis, the stiffer the structure becomes. A 1-mm increase in the diameter of an intramedullary nail enhances its stiffness by 30% to 45%,[3] and a 25% increase in nail diameter doubles its bending strength.[263]

The original Küntscher nail had a cloverleaf cross section with a longitudinal slot. Küntscher believed that the open section would allow compression of the nail by the isthmus of the medullary canal, thereby providing greater rotational control. Plac-

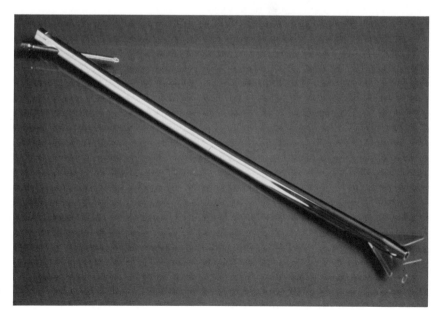

Fig. 1-135. Brooker-Wills nail. *(Courtesy of Bionet, Inc.)*

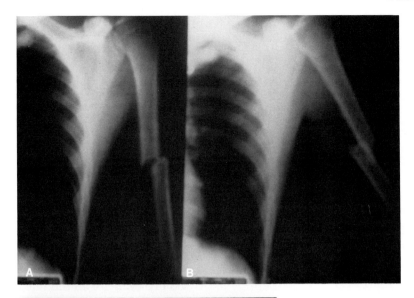

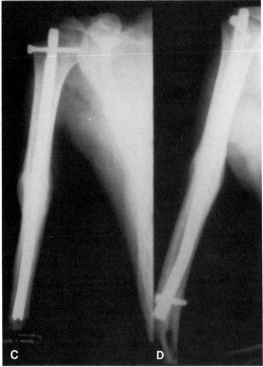

Fig. 1-136. Prototype interlocking humeral nail. **(A, B)** A multiply injured patient with a transverse humeral fracture. **(C, D)** Solid union following closed interlocking nail application.

ing the slot anteriorly on the tension side of the fracture provides the strongest configuration. When the slot is placed on the compression side, local buckling occurs with high bending loads.[4] An open section has little effect on the bending stiffness of a nail, but markedly reduces its stiffness in torsion. In a thin-walled cylinder, the addition of a narrow longitudinal slot reduces the torsional moment of inertia to 1/50 of its initial value.[4,263,445]

The *working length* of a nail is that portion of the nail that spans the fracture site between areas of fixation in the proximal and distal fragments (ie, the unsupported segment of the nail). This may vary from 1 mm to 2 mm in a transverse fracture at the

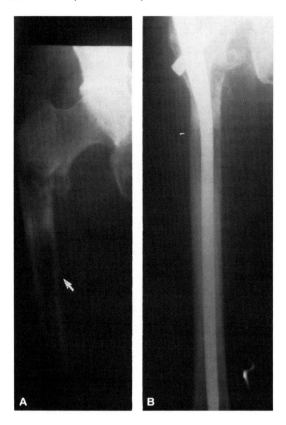

Fig. 1-137. (A) A 55-year-old man with multiple myeloma sustained a fracture through a subtrochanteric lesion following a trivial injury. Note the additional lytic lesion *(arrow)* at the level of the isthmus. **(B)** He was ambulatory and free of pain shortly after insertion of a Zickel nail. Both lesions were subsequently radiated and healed, although he succumbed to his disease 6 months later.

residual angular displacement after the load is released. *Gripping strength* is the resistance to slipping at the implant–bone interface and is essential for the transmission of torque between fracture fragments. Grip can be increased by cortical reaming to increase the length of cortical contact or by the addition of flutes.[3] Interlocking nails optimize grip by rigidly fixing the nail to the bone with screws.

Johnson and Tencer[228,452,453] have carried out extensive *in vitro* biomechanical evaluation of simulated comminuted subtrochanteric and femoral shaft fractures fixed by a variety of intramedullary nails. In three-point bending, fracture models with segmental subtrochanteric defects fixed with interlocking nails were 55% to 70% as stiff as intact femurs, and fractures fixed with Ender nails had less than 25% of the bending stiffness of an intact femur. Femurs with segmental defects of the shaft were significantly less rigid in bending for all intramedullary devices tested.

Models tested in axial loading showed wide variations. Ender nails failed by slippage of the nails

isthmus to several centimeters in a comminuted diaphyseal fracture. In a comminuted fracture fixed by a static-locked nail, the working length is the distance between the proximal and distal locking screws. The working length influences nail rigidity in both bending and torsion. In bending, the stiffness is inversely proportional to the square of the working length. A nail with a working length of 0.25 inches is 16 times more rigid in bending than a nail with a working length of 1 inch. In torsion, the stiffness is inversely proportional to the working length, so that doubling the working length will halve the torsional rigidity.[4] A short working length, therefore, improves nail rigidity both in bending and in torsion.

With torsional loading, a nail both twists and slips within the medullary canal. Slipping allows

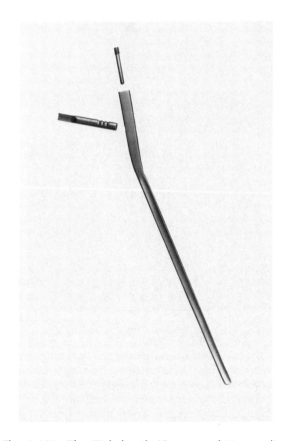

Fig. 1-138. The Zickel nail. *(Courtesy of Howmedica, Inc.)*

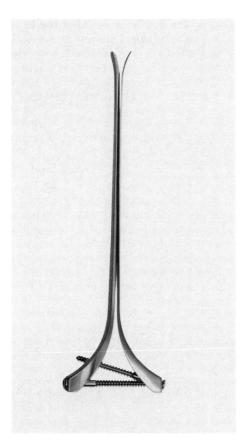

Fig. 1-139. The Zickel supracondylar device. *(Courtesy of Howmedica, Inc.)*

back through their insertion sites at loads less than body weight. Nails with deployable distal fins failed by the fins cutting out distally through metaphyseal bone at 1.5 times body weight, and nails with proximal and distal interlocking screws failed only at loads of nearly four times body weight. Failure in these cases occurred by fracture at the base of the femoral neck, by cutting out of the proximal screw, or by bending of the nail within the fracture site. No failure of the distal locking screws was reported.

All of the systems tested demonstrated low rigidity in torsion. Ender nails and open-section interlocking nails reestablish only 3% of the torsional stiffness of the intact femur, but with a closed section nail the torsional rigidity of the construct increases to about 50% of the intact femur.[457] Although torsional stiffness values for open-section nails are significantly lower than for closed-section nails, the bone–implant combination shows little residual angular displacement after testing. The nail deforms elastically and then springs back with only a minor slip in the bone. Deployable fins control

rotation as well as distal interlocking screws, even in those cases where deployment of both fins is incomplete. Ender nails, on the other hand, show a greater degree of slip, thus allowing residual rotational deformity after release of the load.

In animal models, variations in the rigidity of intramedullary fixation has been shown to affect fracture healing. Wang[471] studied the quality and strength of fracture callus in rabbit femurs fixed with rods of varying bending rigidity. Insufficient rigidity produced abundant callus but unreliable and widely variable bone healing. Excessive bending rigidity produced scant callus that demonstrated low energy absorption when stressed to failure. Callus formation and energy absorption to failure were optimal when the fracture was fixed by a rod of intermediate bending rigidity.

Torsional rigidity also influences fracture healing. Molster[306] studied healing of osteotomized rat femurs fixed with intramedullary rods with varying degrees of interlocking. Union was delayed in the femurs where rotational instability was the greatest. Woodward[488] reported differences in fracture healing of canine femoral fractures treated with rods of differing torsional rigidity. Closed-section rods were paired with open-section rods of equal bending but differing torsional rigidity, restoring 42% and 12% respectively of the torsional rigidity of the femur. Nonunion occurred in 50% of these femurs treated with slotted rods. All femurs treated by closed-section rods were united at 6 months.

Intramedullary nailing aligns fracture fragments and reduces motion at the fracture site, but does not provide the rigid internal fixation of a compression plate (gliding fixation). Fracture healing proceeds mainly by the formation of periosteal callus.[12,360] Medullary reaming disseminates particulate bone graft throughout the fracture hematoma, often resulting in huge amounts of bridging callus. Under these circumstances, it would seem prudent, therefore, to avoid further injury to the periosteal circulation. With current techniques of closed nailing using image intensification, exposure of the fracture site and further disturbance of the periosteal blood supply is seldom necessary. However, the endosteal circulation is inevitably destroyed and the biological consequences of medullary reaming and nail insertion continue to be of concern.

Medullary cortical reaming weakens a bone. Clawson[97] recommended removal of no more than 4 mm and cautioned that the cortex should not be reamed to less than half of its original thickness. Pratt[357] studied the effect of reaming on the torsional strength of cadaver femurs; reaming to 12 mm decreased the maximum torque to failure to

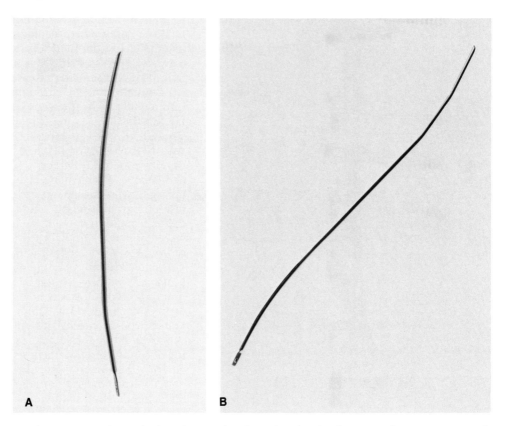

Fig. 1-140. Ender nails. **(A, B)** C- and S-shaped nails. The former is the most commonly used. *(Courtesy of Howmedica, Inc.)*

63% of matched controls, and further reaming to 16 mm decreased this value to 36%, with the largest increment occurring between 14 and 15 mm. He recommended reaming to less than half the bone's diameter at the midshaft. Molster[305] studied the effect of medullary reaming and nail insertion on intact rat femurs and found that reaming immediately reduced the strength of the femur by 15%, although the degree of cortical reaming was not specified. Femurs, after the introduction of rigid nails, remained weaker than matched controls without nails, indicating some degree of stress shielding by the nail. Current trends in nail design have been toward isoelasticity with bone, and stress shielding has not been a problem clinically. Refracture following removal of intramedullary nails has been infrequent, and this is in part related to the absence of multiple screw holes, which are stress risers.

Cortical reaming and nail insertion injure the medullary vascular system, and this results in avascularity of significant portions of the diaphyseal cortex.[111] The implications in open fractures are obvious, and the risk of infection must be carefully

weighed against the necessity of reaming. However, an implant that immobilizes the fracture facilitates early revascularization of the fracture site.[369] In studies of the canine tibia, fractures fixed with an intramedullary rod showed higher rates of whole bone and fracture-site blood flow than comparable fractures fixed with a plate, and they remained elevated for a longer period.[360] A delay in the maturation of callus was noted with intramedullary nails, but once union was achieved the biomechanical quality of union was similar in the two groups.

Current interlocking nails allow the surgeon to manage a variety of complex long-bone fractures without supplemental internal fixation of unstable fragments. If the fracture is stable to compressive forces, interlocking at each end of the nail may not be necessary. "Dynamic locking" refers to the placement of transfixing screws only in the shorter fragment, which is susceptible to rotational instability, and allows intermittent compression of the fracture during early weight-bearing. Dynamic fixation is used typically in fractures of the upper or

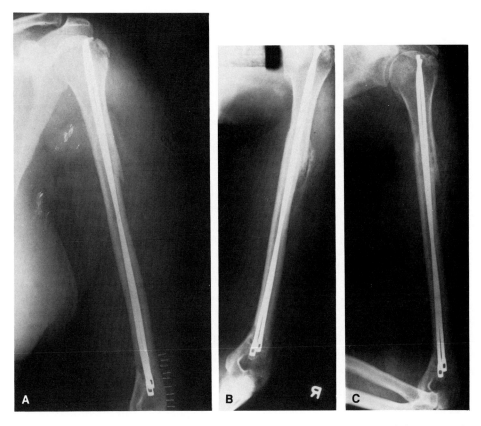

Fig. 1-141. Spiral fracture of the humerus in a multiply injured patient. **(A)** Retrograde fixation with Ender nails through a supracondylar portal. **(B, C)** At 3 months there is bridging callus. The patient has been able to use the extremity for limited activity, and shoulder and elbow motion are normal.

lower third of the shaft in the absence of comminution. When the fracture is comminuted or unstable to compressive or rotational forces, the interlocking screws must be placed above and below the fracture—"static locking." After early consolidation at the fracture site, interlocking screws can be removed from one fragment to allow compressive loading at the fracture site, and this procedure has been termed "dynamization." Early in the evolution of interlocking nails, there was concern that static locking might produce nonunion, and all nails were routinely dynamized. Subsequent series have shown similar high rates of union with both static and dynamic interlocking.[459] Currently, dynamization is carried out only when fracture callus fails to mature by 3 to 6 months.

Complications of Intramedullary Nailing. The introduction of interlocking nails has expanded the variety of long-bone fractures amenable to intramedullary fixation. Closed nailing techniques have

reduced blood loss, infection rates, and length of time in hospital. However, the added complexity of insertion has introduced new pitfalls and complications. Careful preoperative planning and operative technique, familiarity with instrumentation, and skilled radiographic monitoring are of the utmost importance.

Preoperative injury films must be carefully inspected for the fracture pattern, degree of comminution, canal size, deformity, and presence of associated injuries. Nondisplaced fractures of the femoral neck, butterfly fragments, and extensions into adjacent joints may not be appreciated intraoperatively with image intensification, and the discovery of such injuries on recovery-room films is at best an embarrassment.

Correct positioning on the fracture table allows easy access to the starting point for nail insertion and facilitates fracture reduction. In our experience, supine positioning for femoral nailing simplifies fracture reduction and the assessment of rotational

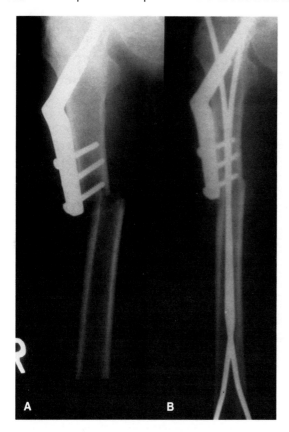

Fig. 1-142. (A) An intertrochanteric hip fracture in an elderly woman treated by a compression screw. Three months later another fall produced this transverse femoral shaft fracture at the distal end of the side plate. **(B)** Retrograde Ender nailing provided satisfactory stability without exposure of the fracture site or removal of the previous fixation device. Flexible nails can usually be manipulated around devices which do not completely fill the medullary canal.

alignment (Fig. 1-145) and is preferable in poly-traumatized patients. Lateral decubitus positioning allows easier access to the proximal starting point and facilitates distal interlocking, but care must be taken to avoid nailing distal third fractures in valgus.

For tibial nailing, the knee must be adequately flexed to allow access to the starting point without excessive pressure on the patellar tendon and skin. Perineal posts and knee bolsters must be adequately padded to prevent skin damage after application of traction.

Location of the proper starting point for nail insertion is a critical early step in closed nailing. An improper portal of entry will allow angular defor-

mity at the fracture site, or even worse, cause disastrous comminution during reaming or nail insertion (Fig. 1-146). In femoral nailings, an excessively medial starting point may compromise the vascularity of the femoral head or produce a stress riser in the femoral neck. A lateral portal directs the nail toward the medial cortex, causing varus angulation or medial comminution that may compromise the fixation of the proximal interlocking screw. Deformity and variations in anatomy make fixed anatomic reference points unreliable. The proper starting point is the one that allows access to the center of the medullary canal (Fig. 1-147).

Fracture reduction is remarkably simple when nailing is carried out within a few hours of injury. Subsequent hematoma formation in the thigh musculature makes maintenance of length progressively more difficult, so that if femoral nailing is delayed, a period of skeletal traction may be required. Preoperative radiographs should be made to confirm that the fracture fragments are out to length, or preferably slightly overdistracted. Excessive intraoperative traction to achieve length compromises skin and may produce stretch injury of the sciatic or peroneal nerves or pressure on the pudendal nerve. Operative reduction is facilitated by placement of an internal manipulator to lever the proximal fragment into position. Intramedullary reduction devices are available, although a smaller size nail works well. A knowledgeable, unscrubbed surgeon may provide additional assistance by external manipulation of the fracture with a crutch or similar device. However, an existence beneath the drapes, in a pool of blood, and in the path of the x-ray beam attracts few recruits.

Fracture reduction is maintained by the use of a guide wire over which cannulated, flexible reamers are used. A curved ball-tip guide wire is the type most easily passed across the fracture site. A guide wire should be advanced only a few millimeters at a time, and radiographic confirmation of intramedullary passage of the wire should be made in two planes each time the wire crosses a fracture site. Unrecognized advancement of the guide wire through soft tissues may produce neurologic or vascular injury, and the guide wire should be seated against subchondral bone in the distal fragment. With distal fractures, the guide wire can easily be inadvertently drawn back across the fracture site during reaming. When this occurs, replacement of the wire in the intramedullary location must always be confirmed before reaming is resumed. The first assistant should clamp and stabilize the guide wire during reaming to prevent migration.

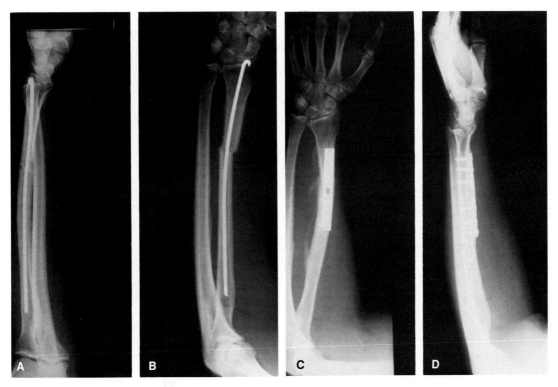

Fig. 1-143. (A, B) An improperly contoured Rush pin will not maintain fracture reduction. A 25-year-old mechanic was unable to work due to a complete loss of supination. **(C, D)** Normal motion was restored following recreation of the radial bow and application of a compression plate and autogenous bone graft.

Cannulated, flexible reamers are required to prepare a curved medullary canal. Reaming should progress in 1-mm increments until the cortex is reached and in 0.5-mm increments thereafter. Sharp reamers and gentle pressure will help avoid entrapment of the reamer. An incarcerated reamer can be extricated by withdrawing the ball tip of the guide wire against the reamer and gently disimpacting the guide wire with a vise grip and mallet. Conventional spring-type flexible reamers cannot be reversed or they will unwind within the medullary canal, a most chagrining experience.

The selection of the proper nail diameter and length is crucial. Never attempt to insert a nail larger than the last reamer used. Interlocking nails rely on transfixing screws for stabilization rather than tight endosteal contact, and slight overreaming allows greater ease of nail insertion with less implant deformation. Interlocking nails are over-reamed 0.5 to 1.5 mm, depending on the device being used.

A nail that is too long will cause soft tissue irritation and discomfort at the insertion site or, worse, penetrate the distal joint. The appropriate nail length is determined intraoperatively by direct measurement of the depth of guide wire insertion, but when the fracture is comminuted, the appropriate length may be difficult to determine. Preoperative scanograms may be of benefit, but these are exceedingly difficult to make when a patient is in skeletal traction. It is much easier to measure the uninjured side against nails of known length under the image intensifier and then adjust the traction on the injured side to "fit" this predetermined nail length. If both sides are fractured, then the least comminuted side is nailed first. An identical nail is used on the more comminuted side and the depth of insertion reproduced. With careful attention to detail, major limb-length inequality can be avoided.

During insertion, the nail should advance a few millimeters with each blow of the mallet. If no progress is being made, then the nail size, the adequacy of reaming, the starting point, and the reduction should be reevaluated. The use of excessive force may result in extensive additional commi-

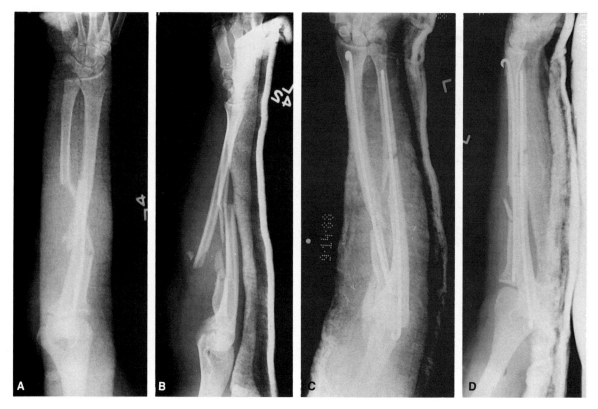

Fig. 1-144. (A, B) A comminuted forearm fracture complicated by an extensively contaminated volar soft tissue wound. Significant additional dissection would be required for compression plating. **(C, D)** Stabilization with Rush pins required little additional surgical trauma and greatly facilitated care of the soft tissues.

nution or incarceration of the nail. As the nail crosses the fracture site, its tip may impinge on the cortex of the distal fragment. If this occurs, the nail must be backed up slightly and the reduction improved before the nail is advanced.

Problems related to proximal screw insertion are infrequent, but care must be taken to seat the nail fully or the proximal screw will pass through the femoral neck rather than the dense cortex adjacent to the lesser trochanter. Nail-mounted proximal targeting jigs may loosen during driving of the nail and allow enough play to misdirect the drill bit anterior to posterior of the nail. In the Brooker-Wills system, the proximal screw is inserted after deployment of the distal fins. Reattaching the proximal targeting device can be difficult when the nail is already seated. This step can be omitted by inserting and partially withdrawing the proximal screw, then reinserting the screw after the distal fins are deployed.

Distal interlocking remains the most technically demanding step in intramedullary nailing. Every

attempt should be made to insert both distal screws, especially in distal fractures. A single distal screw allows excessive toggle.[66] Overlying soft tissues, particularly the iliotibial band, tend to deflect the drill bit and prevent precise drilling. The optimal site for distal femoral screw insertion is a limited area on the lateral cortex. Excessive external rotation of the nail, or torsional deformity of the nail on insertion, places the screw insertion site too far posterior. The cortex becomes much steeper in this area and the drill bit tends to walk posteriorly, making screw insertion all but impossible. If the Brooker-Wills nail is excessively rotated, the distal fins may extrude into the patellofemoral joint.

All of the targeting methods for distal screw insertion rely on the identification of a line passing through the center of the screw hole. When the image-intensifier beam is directed coincident with this line, the screw hole appears as a perfect circle. An experienced technologist is invaluable during this step. Several types of targeting devices are currently available; some are mounted on the image

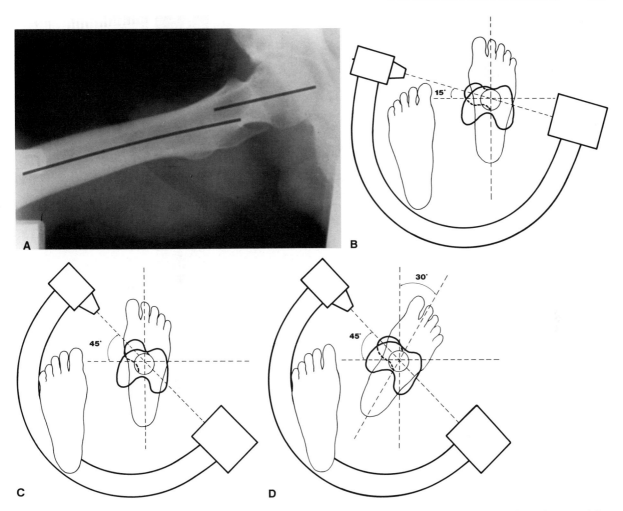

Fig. 1-145. Taylor technique for rotational alignment during supine femoral nailing. **(A)** A true lateral view of the hip is obtained with the image intensifier. In this view, the axes of the femoral neck and shaft are parallel, with a slight anterior offset of the femoral neck. The degree of external rotation of the proximal fragment is determined by the deviation of the image intensifier from a position parallel with the floor. **(B)** With the foot in neutral position, 15° external rotation of the proximal fragment restores normal femoral anteversion. **(C)** Muscular attachments may produce additional external rotation of the proximal fragment. This can be detected by finding the true lateral view of the hip. **(D)** The foot is externally rotated a corresponding amount to restore normal femoral anteversion. *(Courtesy of J. Charles Taylor, M.D.)*

intensifier and others on the proximal end of the nail. Significant play occurs at their attachments, but with a steady hand and some practice, they can be used in a time-efficient manner with limited radiation exposure. Hand-held targeting devices are commercially available for some nail systems,[442] and a simple, hand-held device can be constructed from a disposable suction catheter and a Steinmann pin.[281] Most surgeons, however continue to use freehand techniques, which may be applied to any nailing system (Fig. 1-148).

There has been considerable trepidation about the radiation exposure to the surgeon during the insertion of the distal screws. Interlocking via distal fins is completed without radiographic control and offers a clear advantage in this regard. Levin[270] has measured the radiation exposure to the surgeon's dominant hand during intramedullary nailings with freehand distal targeting. The average dose to the hand was 12 millirems. The exposure during nail insertion and proximal interlocking was 13 millirems. These figures are within the government

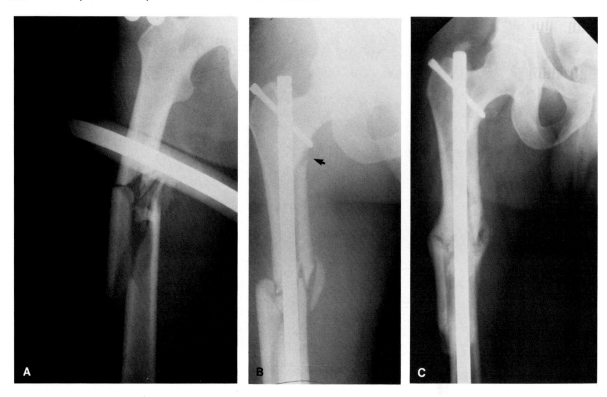

Fig. 1-146. (A) A 36-year-old man sustained a comminuted midshaft femur fracture in a motor vehicle accident. **(B)** An aberrant starting point directed the nail toward the anteromedial cortex, causing comminution up to the level of the lesser trochanter *(arrow)*. This new fracture was not detected intraoperatively with image intensification. **(C)** Fortunately, uneventful union occurred with a static locked nail.

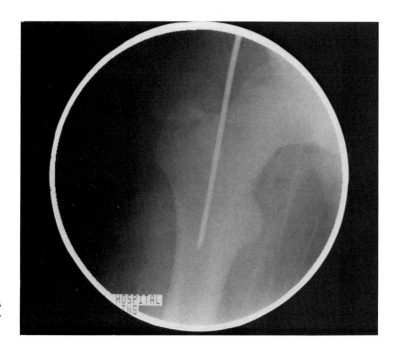

Fig. 1-147. The safest starting point allows direct access to the center of the medullary canal in both planes.

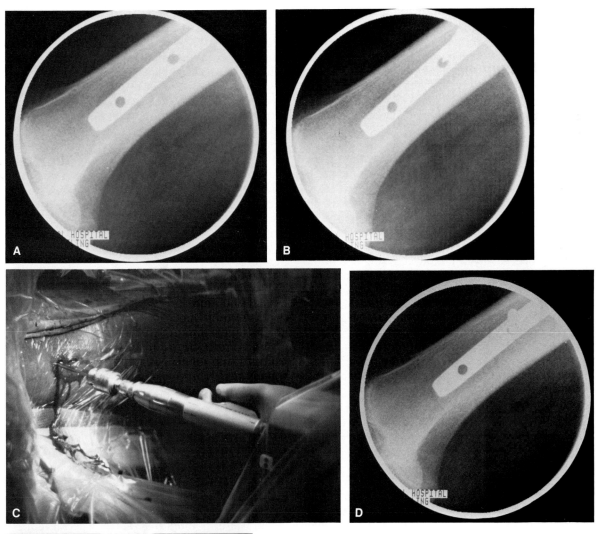

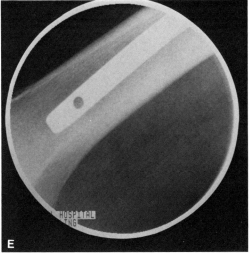

Fig. 1-148. Freehand distal screw insertion. **(A)** The image intensifier is aligned to produce "perfect circles." **(B)** A stab wound is made over the hole, and the tip of a pointed awl is placed precisely in the center of the hole. A dimple or unicortical hole is made. A long instrument helps keep the surgeon's hand distant from the radiation. **(C)** The drill bit is then aligned with the image intensifier in two planes. No radiographs are made while the surgeon's hand is in the path of the beam. **(D)** The drill chuck is removed and the position of the drill bit confirmed. **(E)** A screw of appropriate length is inserted and position again confirmed.

guidelines for radiation exposure during a 3-month period but many surgeons perform such procedures daily, and the long-term deleterious effects may be considerable. The surgeon must remain cognizant of his proximity to the radiation beam during all phases of the procedure, and the image intensifier should be used by necessity rather than by convenience. The use of a screen with memory is mandatory.

Postoperative shortening and loss of reduction may occur with dynamic interlocking nails. At the Baltimore Shock Trauma Center,[97] 10% of femoral fractures treated by dynamic intramedullary fixation had a postoperative loss of reduction, with an average of 2 cm of shortening. Overestimation of fracture stability by the surgeon was a factor in every case. Fracture comminution that is undetected preoperatively or produced during operation compromises the stability of dynamic fixation, particularly when the canal has been overreamed to facilitate nail insertion. All fractures with Winquist-Hansen grade 3 or 4 comminution require static locking, but even in less comminuted and apparently stable fractures, static locking should be considered or even used routinely.

Breakage of intramedullary nails is uncommon. In an extensive review of a series of intramedullary nails, Franklin[156] reported an aggregate incidence of breakage of 3.3% for the femur and 1% for the tibia. As would be expected, in a comminuted, unstable fracture pattern more stress is placed on the nail and breakage is more common. Prior to the use of interlocking nails, failure occurred at the original fracture site and could often be attributed to an undersized nail. In contrast, interlocking nails often fail in proximity to the proximal and distal interlocking mechanisms.

Partially slotted nails fail most frequently at the junction of the cylindrical and cloverleaf portions of the nail.[30,156,240,455] Initially this junction was welded, but currently such nails are produced in one piece[61] or have been redesigned with a full-length slot.[442] Distal screw holes may act as stress risers, and fatigue fracture through the more proximal of the holes may occur.[66,101] The close proximity of the fracture to this hole appears to increase the risk of breakage. Exacting technique during the distal screw insertion is required to prevent inadvertent scoring of the nail, which in turn produces an additional stress riser.

Bending occurs more readily in solid nails, whereas cloverleaf nails tend to break. Angulation of the nail predisposes to delayed union,[218] and it is wishful thinking to anticipate union before a bent nail finally breaks. A bent nail should always be replaced with a new one. The extremity may be manipulated immediately prior to exchange to facilitate removal, and specialized hooks have been devised for the removal of the distal portion of a broken nail.[156]

Deep infection following closed femoral nailing has been uncommon, in contrast to early series of open nailings. Most series report infection rates of 1% or less, and the majority of these fractures united after debridement with the nail left *in situ*.[97,183,240,250,455,480,484,486] Lhowe and Hansen[271] reported a deep infection rate of 5% in a series of open femoral shaft fractures treated by debridement and immediate reamed nailing. Similar rates have also been reported with delayed nailing of open fractures.[89,488]

Infection following tibial nailing has been more common than in the femur, particularly when open nailing techniques have been used.[46,134,250,287, 301,413,463] Open fractures treated by immediate reamed nailing or by delayed nailing following the removal of an external fixator are particularly at risk, but open tibial fractures treated with unreamed Lottes or Ender nails have yielded infection rates only slightly higher than closed fractures.[287,463] Unreamed interlocking nails are currently being evaluated and their use in open fractures appears promising.

While closed intramedullary nailing appears to be the management of choice for a variety of long-bone fractures, there still are those who advocate open nailing of femoral shaft fractures. Schatzker, in his paper in 1980 before blocked nails were in general use, pointed out that no special tables or image intensifiers are necessary, reduction of the fracture is easily attained and secured, and rotational reduction increases the inherent stability of the fracture. He was also of the opinion that the rate of infection is no higher in "properly executed" open reductions than in those treated by closed means. Be that as it may, there is agreement that the older technique of retrograde insertion of the nail is to be eschewed owing to the danger of fracture at the cervicotrochanteric junction. It is also mandatory that a nail of sufficient size and strength be used, and this usually requires intramedullary reaming, not only to allow a large nail to be inserted but also to increase the contact area between nail and bone. In the case depicted in Figure 1-149, the surgeon used a 9-mm Schneider nail, which did not fill the medullary cavity and was unequal to its task.

It did not provide rotational stability, so that a plate was added, threatening the vascularity of the cortical bone. Inevitably the internal fixation failed, with unhappy consequences for the patient.

Corrosion of Implants

When two dissimilar metals are in contact with each other in an electrolyte solution, one of these metals will be positive relative to the other, according to their positions in the electromotive series. Atoms from the anode go into solution as positively charged ions, leaving the anode negatively charged. Were there no cathode, the negative charge on the anode would tend to attract these metallic ions back. However, at the cathode another reaction is going on, which takes electrons from the cathode metal surface: $4e^- + O_2 + 2H_2O = 4OH^-$. With contact of the metal surfaces, there is a flow of electrons (ie, an electric current is produced, and the negative charge is reduced on the anode so that the attack on the anode continues). This is sometimes called a "battery effect," because it is essentially the same process that goes on in a galvanic cell. Even in a single metal, a battery effect can be produced. If a strip of iron is immersed in a salt solution, the portion nearest the surface, where the oxygen tension is greatest, becomes the cathode; the anode is a zone at a deeper level.

Where the cathode is large and the anode small, the corrosion[49,84,172,296] is greatest. If the cathode is a plate and the anode a screw, severe corrosion takes place (Fig. 1-150**B, C**). For this reason, different metals should not be used in the same assembly, especially if they are far apart in the electromotive series. However, Hicks and Cater[201] have shown that mixing of plates and screws made of the more inert metals such as Vitallium and titanium does not give rise to significant corrosion.

Mears[296,297] concurred with this view and pointed out that electrochemical techniques are available to test combinations of alloys and to classify them into three types:

1. Combinations that do not appreciably alter the corrosion resistance of either component
2. Combinations where the presence of one alloy improves the corrosion resistance of the other alloy by anodic protection, without deterioration of its own corrosion resistance
3. Combinations where an alloy improves the corrosion resistance of another alloy but simultaneously provokes more rapid corrosion of itself.

This latter principle was used to protect the copper sheathing of wooden ships by the addition of zinc, but it seems unlikely that this mechanism would have a useful role in orthopaedics.

Mears did not intend for orthopaedists to "mix and match" metals for themselves, but pointed out that combinations of alloys carefully selected by metallurgical methods will be useful for certain functions.

If a layer of oxide is present on the surface of the metals, it acts as a block to the passage of ions. The presence of molybdenum in a ferrous alloy helps in the formation of a passive oxide barrier, and stainless steel used in the manufacture of implants should contain 2.5% to 3.5% molybdenum. The oxide layer can be thickened artificially by treating it with nitric acid (passivation) or electrochemically (anodization).

Chloride ions interfere with oxidation and the formation of a passivation layer in stainless steel implants. The practice of steam sterilization of implants with saline in the environment gives rise to surface corrosion in both instruments and implants and should be prohibited.[296] Furthermore, rough usage and scratches will break the oxide film on the surface of an implant and be the nidus where corrosion, especially stress corrosion, may start. Implants should be handled with delicacy, never thrown around in basins or shaken together in a basket, or immersed in saline. Indeed, implants should be kept in their packages or placed in protective containers until the time of use.

In spite of the improvements in stainless steels, corrosion still occurs, and some of the mechanisms postulated to explain these cases are described below.

TRANSFER OF METALS FROM TOOLS TO IMPLANTS

Using radioactive tracer techniques, Bowden and associates[47] showed that significant amounts of metal were transferred from screwdrivers to screw heads and from drill bits to plates. This difficulty could be solved by using tools made from the same material as the implant, by making the screwdrivers harder, and by using drill guides to prevent contact between drill and plate. Hicks and Cater,[201] however, stated that this transfer of metal is not clinically significant.

CREVICE CORROSION

Differences in oxygen tension or concentrations of electrolytes or changes in pH in a confined space, such as in the crevices between a screw and a plate,

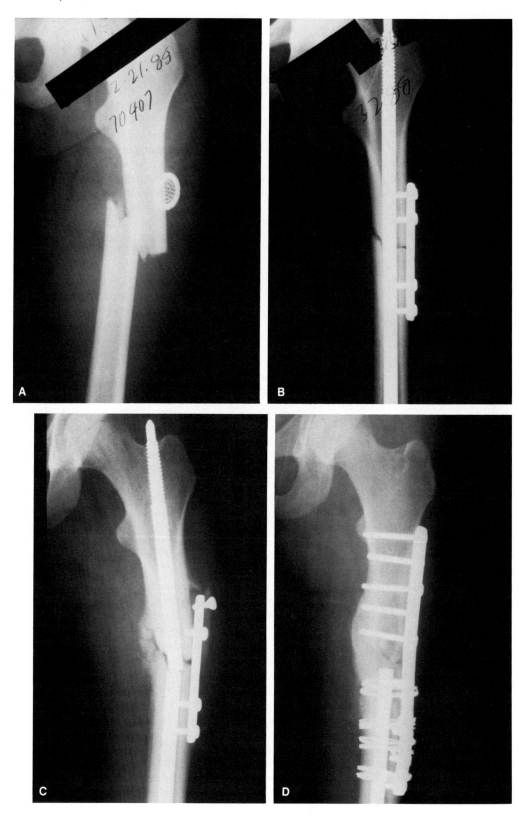

may result in local corrosion called "crevice corrosion" or "contact corrosion."[146]

FRETTING CORROSION

Cohen[100] subjected plate-and-screw assemblies to cyclic stress in saline solutions and found the greatest corrosion in the screw assemblies where the heads rubbed on the plate and where the nuts and washers were in contact. He believed that this was most probably secondary to abrasion of the metal surfaces removing the protective oxide coating (ie, fretting). Similar assemblies not subjected to the cyclical stresses did not show this marked effect.

STRESS-CORROSION CRACKING

Stress-corrosion cracking is a phenomenon in which a metal in certain environments, especially those rich in chlorides, is subjected to stress and fails at a much lower level than usual as a result of corrosion.[172]

In austenitic steels a process called "sensitization" may result when implants are subjected to heat treatments during manufacture. It is believed that some of the chromium becomes converted to chromium carbide, so that the grain boundaries of the metal lose their protective coating of chromium. This gives rise to increased corrosion because: (1) the metallic grains lose the passivation effect of chromium oxide; and (2) a galvanic effect accentuates corrosion because of differences in the composition of the grain itself and its boundary region. Stress accentuates this destructive effect, leading to failure.

Choice of Metals for Surgical Implants

If one could create the ideal implant material, it would be inert, nontoxic to the body, and absolutely corrosion-proof. It would be inexpensive, easily worked, and capable of being wrought in a variety of shapes without expensive manufacturing techniques. It would have great strength and high resistance to fatigue.

Unfortunately, this material is not available at the present time. Implants are made of stainless steel; cobalt, chromium, and molybdenum alloys (eg, Vitallium); and titanium. The characteristics of these materials have been detailed by Brettle[48,49] in his excellent reviews of this subject and more recently by Disegi and Wyss.[126]

Of the materials available, stainless steel has the best mechanical properties. It is strong and has good fatigue resistance. It is easily worked and cheap to manufacture, but it has the serious drawback of corrodability.

Vitallium has much better corrosion resistance than stainless steel, but it is in every way mechanically inferior. It has to be cast by the very complicated and expensive lost-wax process, and quality control is harder to achieve than with stainless steel. Vitallium also has a low ductility, and screws made of this material bond quite securely to bone. In removing a screw that has become securely anchored, it is easy to break the head off. Wrought Vitallium is a cobalt, chromium, nickel, and tungsten alloy with much more desirable mechanical properties than standard Vitallium and excellent corrosion resistance.

Titanium is the most inert of all. It is easily worked, and $\frac{1}{16}$-inch plates are radiolucent. Unfortunately, this admirable metal has an extremely low modulus of elasticity (15×10^6 psi, which is much less than the 28 to 30×10^6 psi for Vitallium and stainless steel) and has a lower tensile strength. Although titanium alloys may be used instead of titanium alone, it is Brettle's opinion that titanium's modulus of elasticity will not be appreciably altered. Titanium plates and implants, therefore, have to be bulkier than stainless steel in order to provide the same rigidity.

Titanium can be modified by alloying it with aluminum and vanadium (Ti-6Al-4V), and in the United States it is made into implants by the Zimmer Company, who market it under the trade name "Tivanium." They have given the implants a surface treatment that makes them gold colored for easy

---

Fig. 1-149. A 17-year-old girl sustained a fracture of the proximal third of the femur in an automobile accident. **(A)** The original radiograph. **(B)** The surgeon elected to insert a 9-mm Schneider nail, which did not fill the unreamed medullary cavity. Rotational stability could only be achieved by adding a four-hole unicortical plate. **(C)** Inevitably this small nail failed with disruption of the reduction and plate fixation. **(D)** The surgeon was unable to extract the distal fragment of the nail and elected to leave it *in situ*. This precluded the insertion of screws through the distal portion of the plate, which was then fixed with cerclage wires. This fixation was so insecure that a second surgeon applied a hip spica for 3 months, leaving the broken nail entombed in the medullary cavity of the femur.

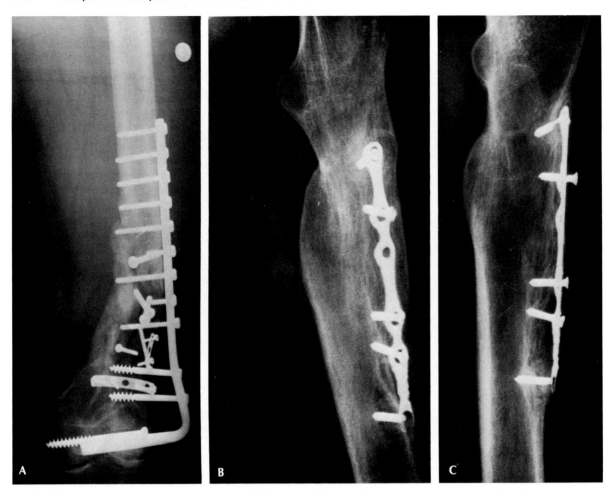

Fig. 1-150. Examples of inappropriate internal fixation. **(A)** Multiple injuries to a woman's left lower extremity including a comminuted fracture of the supracondylar region of the femur. This is the appearance of the bone 18 months after the injury, at which time she had a draining, immobile knee. The surgeon obviously embarked on the treatment of this fracture without a good preoperative plan. The reduction is inadequate, no bone grafts were used, and the use of the many screws and plates violated the principles of sound internal fixation. **(B, C)** This femoral fracture healed in spite of rather inadequate plating 50 years ago. There is advanced corrosion of the plate and screws that apparently is causing the patient no discomfort.

(continued)

identification. The alloy is said to have a greater tensile strength than either stainless steel or the chrome-cobalt alloys and has almost twice the fatigue strength of these materials. It is extremely hard and resistant to scratching, corrosion-proof, and has a ductility equal to that of stainless steel. It does have a low modulus of elasticity, so that if plates were to be made of it, they would have to be substantially thicker to provide the rigidity of stainless steel. On the other hand, by being less stiff, the problem of stress protection may be alleviated.

Perren and Pohler[347] echoed the opinions of others regarding the corrosion resistance and tissue tolerance of titanium and stressed that there have been no allergic reactions to titanium. Strength and ductility they say can be improved to satisfactory levels by cold work and the addition of traces of elements such as oxygen. They agree that the addition of aluminum and vanadium is controversial because vanadium, a soluble metal, is more toxic than nickel chloride. Such alloys as Ti-Al-Fe and Ti-Al-Ni are biologically well tolerated, but the plastic deformability is inferior to stainless steel.

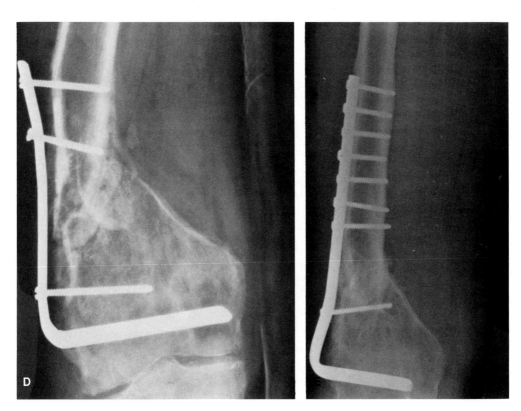

Fig. 1-150 (*continued*)
(D) A middle-aged man with rheumatoid arthritis sustained a supracondylar fracture of his right femur. An inadequate operation was performed with inadequate fixation producing this result. **(E)** When adequate fixation was inserted and union obtained, he wound up with a completely ankylosed knee.

The AO group has developed "a pure titanium of good strength and ductility." Implants made from this titanium have an electrochemically produced oxidation layer which gives the implants a golden appearance. Plates and screws of this titanium have been implanted in 5000 patients with good results. Other titanium alloys (ie, Ti-5Al-2.5Fe and Ti-6Al-7Nb) are also under investigation as implant materials. It has been suggested that titanium may be the metal of choice for upper extremity implants where the stresses are of a significantly lower order than in the lower limbs.

A number of alloys have been discovered that have "memory" (eg, gold–cadmium, copper–zinc, titanium–niobium).[28,178] If these metals are deformed at low temperatures they will recover their original configuration when the temperature is raised to the requisite level. Another such alloy is titanium–nickel. Originally discovered in the United States, this alloy (55% nickel and 45% titanium by weight) is known as "Nitinol," and implants have been made from this material, which is inert in the tissues.

Small changes in the composition of these alloys

may alter their behavior significantly, but in China a very similar alloy, Nitalloy (54% nickel and 46% titanium) has been used clinically.[262] A staple made of this material and deformed at 0°C may be implanted in bone. When heated to 34°C to 40°C it will regain its original configuration, allowing the staple to exert a compression force. In a similar manner, a rod or cable may be overstretched at low temperatures and then contract at body temperatures after implantation. It would seem that after further research a useful role for this or similar materials will be found.

A significant number of implant failures result from implants being used improperly or being applied in the wrong location. Even in the best-regulated circumstances, however, implant failure will sometimes occur. As Howard Rosen has said, "Any time metal is put into the body in the treatment of fracture, it's the start of a race between bone healing and implant failure." Obviously, quality control of implants is extremely important, and most manufacturers go to great lengths to make sure that their products are not defective.

However, Cahoon and Paxton[75] selected 35 implants at random from the stock of a hospital and subjected them to a rigorous examination. They found that more than 50% of these were unacceptable from a metallurgical viewpoint owing to large grain size, inclusions, porosity, cracks, pitting, and a molybdenum content below 2% in stainless steel. Molybdenum, of course, protects against pitting, corrosion, and fatigue failure and should be above the 2% level. They also found Jewett nails that had been manufactured by welding the nail to the side plate, so that large amounts of delta ferrite were formed, thereby reducing the implant's corrosion resistance.

Such studies should prompt the prudent orthopaedist to ensure that the manufacturer of the implants he uses adopts the recommended metallurgical standards, fabricates the implants with care, and maintains adequate testing facilities. In the increasingly litigious environment in which we live, it would be circumspect to retain a broken implant for subsequent metallurgical examination, if necessary. These words should not be taken in any way as an indictment of the orthopaedic implant industry. Indeed, we have been most impressed by the quality control provisions in the implant factories we have visited.

The reuse of implants is not permissible in the United States. Implants become seriously attenuated after being subjected to repeated stresses in the hostile environment of the body and are much more liable to fail with a second use. It may be permissible to allow their use in a country where implants are unavailable owing to their high cost, but even that is for purely economic reasons and certainly is not a desirable situation.

Allergic Responses to Implants

It has been known for some time that in certain individuals cutaneous eruptions will arise after implant surgery secondary to sensitivity to nickel, chrome, or cobalt. Kubba and associates,[266] in a prospective study, found 19 such patients. Six of these had transient exanthematic dermatitis, which was recurrent in two cases, and 13 had a persistent reaction.

In patients who have such problems it makes sense to use titanium implants, which are unlikely to evoke an allergic response.

Carcinogenic Effects of Metals

Recently there have been two articles in the lay press[43,404] regarding the possibility of metallic induction of malignant tumors. Such tumors have been reported in conjunction with total hip prostheses,[343,440] but only six cases have been reported where a tumor has arisen at the site of a metallic plate.[118,128,129,289,290,450] Of these plates, four were stainless steel and two cobalt-chrome. In one of these instances, a baby had bilateral derotational osteotomies carried out for congenital dislocation of the hip, which were fixed by stainless steel plates. After removal of the plates, a Ewing's sarcoma developed on one side. In all of these cases the association of malignancy and plates may well have been coincidental.

Black,[42] in his review of oncogenesis by metallic ions, summarized the experimental evidence regarding the release of cobalt, chromium, and nickel from implants and the induction of tumors. He stated that chromium may be released either in trivalent or hexavalent forms and that the latter is able to penetrate cell membranes and is probably a potent carcinogen.

Black's conclusions, and they pertain more to hip prostheses than plates and screws, were as follows:

1. There is adequate evidence to conclude that there is a finite, non-zero risk of oncogenesis in humans associated with the implantation of F75 alloy (chrome cobalt).
2. This risk increases with increasing dosage and increasing period of exposure.
3. It is prudent to act on these conclusions while awaiting a definite determination of risk.

It does seem that significant quantities of chromium, cobalt, and nickel may be liberated from metallic implants—especially when corrosion occurs. However, tumor induction would appear to be much more common in veterinary practice than it is in humans.[187,418] The cases cited, even if all *are* related to metallic tumor induction, represent an infinitesimal percentage of patients subjected to implant insertion. The risk perhaps is much greater in implants with sintered or pore-coated surfaces, where presumably the loss of ions will be much greater owing to the greatly enlarged surface area.

The circumspect fracture surgeon will avoid the use of stainless steel or chrome-cobalt where his patient has a demonstrated sensitivity to metal. On the other hand, the magnitude of the problem scarcely dictates eschewing stainless steel and chrome-cobalt in favor of titanium on this account alone.

SELECTION OF MODE OF TREATMENT

The question before the modern surgeon is not whether operative treatment is to supersede manipulative treatment. The problem before each of us is how can we improve our skill and technique in both manipulative and operative treatment and what means we must adopt in each individual case to give to our patients the surest, safest, and most complete restoration of function.

Those who have a large and varied experience of the manipulative treatment of deformity will probably have greater confidence in their ability to deal with deformities resulting from fractures by manipulation and external splinting. They will reserve direct operation for those cases in which they have found that their manipulative skill has not proved equal to returning the limb in a correct position until union of the fragments has taken place.

The crying evil of our art in these times is the fact that much of our surgery is too mechanical, our medical practice too chemical, and there is a hankering to interfere, which thwarts the inherent tendency to recovery possessed by all persons not actually dying. —H. O. Thomas, 1833

The case that starts botched up stays botched up. —Michael Rosco, 1967

In closed treatment of fractures an attempt is made to achieve adequate alignment of the fracture fragments. It is neither necessary, nor, in some cases, desirable to achieve an anatomical reduction. Lloyd Griffiths[173] gave the following reasons for reducing a fracture:

1. To ensure recovery of function of the limb where that is threatened by displacement of the fracture.
2. To prevent or to delay degenerative changes in joints, and particularly weight-bearing joints, which will result from persisting deformity.
3. To minimize the deforming effect of injury.

If closed reduction is unsuccessful, Griffiths stated, "the wrong technique may have been employed, or the fracture was unsuitable for closed reduction."

INDICATIONS FOR OPERATIVE TREATMENT

With the advent of improved metals and better designed implants, there has been an increasing trend, especially in continental Europe, to open reduction and internal fixation of fractures. The possible indications for such open reductions are outlined below.

Failure of Closed Methods

Failure of closed methods, as Lloyd Griffiths[173] has pointed out, may be secondary to the ineptitude of the surgeon, but undoubtedly closed reduction will fail in the hands of even the most expert if the fragments of bone are impaled in soft tissues or if an otherwise suitable fracture for closed manipulation has been seen too late. If bony apposition and adequate alignment cannot be achieved, open operation is indicated.

Known Contraindications to Closed Methods

Few would disagree that fractures of both bones of the forearm in adults or Monteggia and Galeazzi fractures are unlikely to be handled adequately by closed methods, so that open reduction and internal fixation is the method of choice. Similarly, fractures of the femoral neck would be poorly treated by traction or plaster immobilization.

Fractured and Displaced Articular Surfaces

Even minor incongruities in the articular surfaces of joints will result in derangements of function and the eventual appearance of degenerative arthritis. This is particularly so in the joints of the lower extremities. In studying the end results of tibial condylar fractures, Rasmussen[361] found that 4 to 11 years after injury 21% of his patients had demonstrable osteoarthritis of the affected knees, while the same patients had an incidence of 2% in their uninjured knees. Not all of this, however, could be ascribed to articular injury alone. Although bicondylar fractures gave the worst results and poor results were associated with persistent condylar widening, other factors, such as valgus and (even more so) varus deformity and instability, were also important. Rather surprisingly, neither age *per se* nor localized joint depression appeared to affect the end result significantly.

Proponents of open reduction of T-shaped fractures of the lower end of the humerus and fractures involving the knee joint claim better results in their series than could be obtained by closed methods,[83,144,168,238] whereas proponents of early motion without operation contend the reverse[15,245,345] (Figs.

1-151 and 1-152). By and large, it seems to us that the operative treatment of these injuries is difficult but, when performed well, gives the best results (see Fig. 1-30). On the other hand, the end results of poorly conceived and executed surgery are disastrous. Occasionally, unstable fractures of articular surfaces may be reduced by manipulation and fixed percutaneously (Fig. 1-153). The choice of treatment must depend to some extent on the skill and experience of the surgeon.

In injuries to joints where loose fragments are knocked off, the tendency has been to remove them. When this is done in the hip joints, degenerative

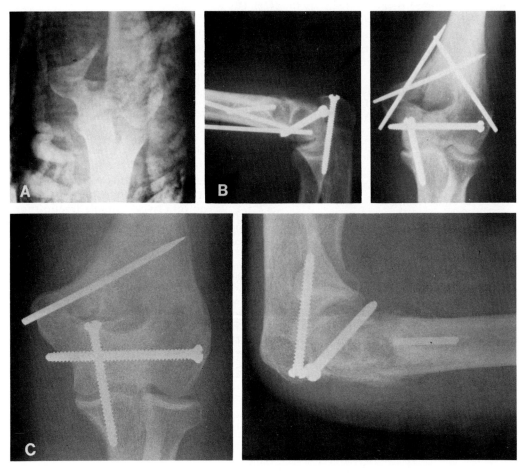

Fig. 1-151. (A) A 35-year-old woman fell on the point of her elbow, sustaining a comminuted T-shaped fracture of the lower end of the humerus. **(B)** The fracture was approached by osteotomizing the olecranon process, so that damage to the triceps muscle was minimized. The trochlea was reduced and fixed by a transverse screw, and the distal fragment was attached to the shaft by means of Steinmann pins. It would appear that one of the pins through the medial epicondyle is aberrant. **(C)** Two of the Steinmann pins were removed early because they presented under the skin and caused pain. The end result, however, was extremely good with almost a complete range of motion of the elbow.

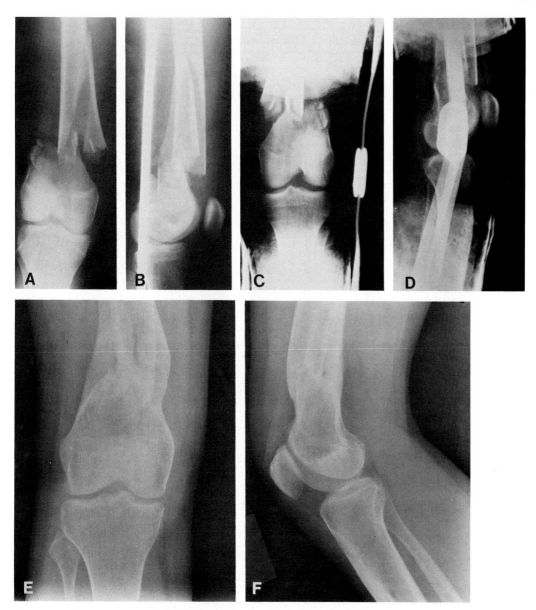

Fig. 1-152. **(A, B)** A 17-year-old girl sustained this fracture as the result of an accident on a motorcycle. In addition to the obvious fractures of the supracondylar region, she has an undisplaced fracture separating the condyles. **(C, D)** She was treated initially in traction followed by the application of a cast brace. **(E, F)** The final result; in spite of the fact that she does not have an anatomical reduction, she has a complete range of motion and no obvious cosmetic defect.

arthritis almost always supervenes early, so that primary arthroplasty has been recommended.[237] A review of fractures of the femoral head by Kelly[239] has shown that the best results were obtained when the loose fragment was reduced by manipulation. When this could not be accomplished, open operation with internal fixation of the fragment gave an end result much superior to excision of the fragment (Fig. 1-154).

Fractures Secondary to Tumor Metastasis

Fractures secondary to tumor metastasis is covered in Chapter 6. Internal fixation of such fractures relieves pain, makes nursing easier, and often allows

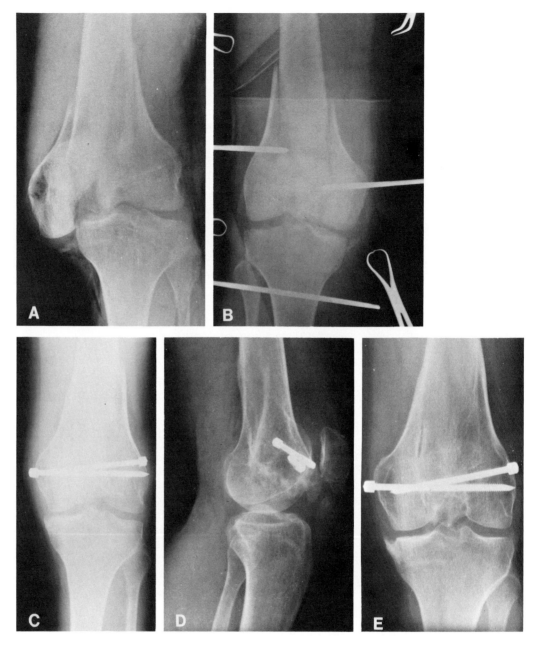

Fig. 1-153. **(A)** A man had his right leg smashed between the bumpers of two cars when one ran into the back of the other. He sustained a large popliteal laceration with complete division of his popliteal vessels. The vessels were repaired and the popliteal laceration was grafted. Further operative treatment of his fractures was deemed unwise. **(B)** Because an adequate reduction could not be obtained by traction alone, the fragments were manipulated percutaneously by Knowles pins and when satisfactory alignment had been obtained, the pins were driven across the femur. **(C)** The appearance of the femur 4 months later. **(D)** A lateral view shows a fragment anteriorly that united in malposition. **(E)** Seventeen months later there is an erosion of the medial plateau, but the patient has excellent range of motion and a painless joint. In spite of many invitations to have the aberrant fragment removed from his joint, he has steadfastly refused to have further surgery.

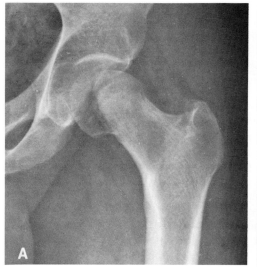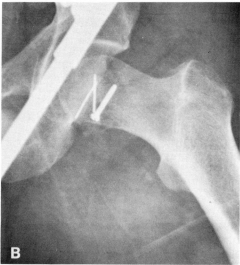

Fig. 1-154. **(A)** The hip of a policeman who suffered a posterior dislocation with an associated fracture of the femoral head. After reduction of the hip, his femoral head fragment was not adequately reduced so that open reduction and internal fixation were undertaken. **(B)** The postoperative film shows the fragment reattached by means of a countersunk screw and two Smillie pins. A medial (Ludloff) approach was used.

the patient to return home and spend precious time with his family.

Associated Arterial Injury

It has long been held that where an arterial injury has been suffered in conjunction with a fracture, fixation of the fracture is mandatory to protect the arterial repair. Doubt was thrown on this concept by Rich and associates[371] in their review of arterial injuries sustained in Vietnam. Of 29 patients who had simultaneous arterial repair and internal fixation of the associated fracture, ten later came to amputation. Five of these amputations were directly related to infection of the fracture and the anastomosis, and half of the patients had complications from the intramedullary nail that dictated its removal. Although a series of 29 patients is comparatively small, the amputation rate in these patients was 36%—compared to an overall rate of 13.5% in similar injuries treated without internal fixation—so this must be considered significant.

Connolly[104,105] carried out experiments on dogs where he fractured the femur, and, after dividing the femoral artery, repaired it with No. 6-0 silk. He found that an arterial anastomosis could withstand 40 lbs of tibial traction without disruption. Although one would expect traction to produce arterial spasm, studies with flow meters showed that blood flow in a 3- to 4-mm vessel was unaffected by 15 lbs of traction, provided the postrepair flow was no less than 50% of the original flow. From a review of the literature and 14 cases of popliteal artery injury associated with fracture from his own institution, he concluded, "This analysis. . . . does not substantiate the need for internal fracture fixation. A satisfactory and practical method of immobilizing fractures associated with arterial injury was 4.5 to 6.8 kilograms of skeletal traction." In our practice we tend to use external fixation rather than traction when fractures are complicated by an ipsilateral vascular injury.

Multiple Injuries

The association of several fractures makes it desirable to fix fractures internally for ease of nursing, for transportation, or to prevent joints from becoming stiff. Bilateral femoral fractures treated by traction present problems in using bedpans and in the prevention of decubiti. The common association of fractures of the femur and patella will almost certainly cause severe impairment of the knee when treated by traction, but early fixation or excision of the patella combined with intramedullary fixation of the femur gives much better results.[149]

Similarly, ipsilateral fractures of the femur and tibia require at least one of the bones, and probably both, to be fixed.[479] In our experience, the more fractures a patient has sustained, the more likely we are to open and internally fix the fractures. By so doing, the patient is made more independent and can be mobilized and transferred out of the hospital at an earlier date.

Meek and colleagues[298] compared two groups of patients with multiple injuries: one group treated early and aggressively by internal fixation and the other group treated "conservatively." The former group had a mortality rate of 4.5% and the latter, 28.5% in the 30 days following injury.

We have had extensive experience with the management of tibial fractures by closed reduction, plaster-of-paris immobilization, and early weight-bearing. Our failures, about 4%, have all been in patients with multiple injuries in whom early weight-bearing was not feasible. In the past 15 years we have become progressively more aggressive in the early internal fixation of the polytrauma patient.

Early Mobilization

Intertrochanteric fractures of the femur may be treated by traction with excellent healing of the fracture. However, this regimen requires skilled nursing if bed sores are to be avoided. Many elderly patients have pulmonary emphysema, heart disease, hiatus hernia, and other ailments that make it mandatory for them to sit up. Satisfactory internal fixation under these circumstances would appear to be the treatment of choice, especially when it allows them to be transferred to an extended care facility.

Devas,[120] in his excellent book, *Geriatric Orthopaedics,* underscores the desirability of restoring elderly people to function and walking at the earliest juncture and keeping them in the hospital as short a time as possible or, preferably, not at all. He advocates open reduction and internal fixation only if it will give them an early return to function. "Under no circumstances should any procedure be done for a fracture which does not allow the patient to be up and walking by the next day." The very old cannot walk with crutches or without weight-bearing. Intertrochanteric fractures must be firmly fixed, and in femoral neck fractures prostheses may be better than nails.

If open reduction is to be done, the strength of osteoporotic bone is such that screws will tend not to have a secure hold. Devas[120] recommends using longer plates and more screws to enhance fixation. He also recommends when plating femurs to place a high-density polyethylene plate on the opposite side of the bone. This plate should be 15 mm wide and 3 mm thick, and the screw holes should be predrilled with a drill bit one or two sizes smaller than that used for the bone. The screws holding on the plate engage the polythene plate, thus buttressing the attenuated cortex of the femur. We have not used this method, but it seems worthy of a trial.

Cost Reduction

It is easy to take a detached view of economics when the costs of treatment do not come out of one's own pocket. With the costs of hospital treatment rising daily, it makes good sense to keep patients in hospitals for the shortest time compatible with their well-being and a good ultimate result. Furthermore, the sooner a patient returns to a gainful occupation, the less financial strain will be placed upon the family. If this can be achieved by intramedullary nailing of the femur, then it is a reasonable indication. The factors to be considered in the selection of treatment are the risks involved, the danger of infection, the ultimate functional result, and cosmesis.

CHOICE OF OPERATIVE TREATMENT

It seems irrelevant to us whether bones unite by primary contact healing or by periosteal callus. What is important is whether or not the bone heals and how well the limb functions after it has healed. The surgeon must consider each particular patient's problem, assess the risks and merits of the alternatives, and decide on what will be safest and most expeditious in his hands. By and large, treatment by closed methods, skillfully applied, works well for many fractures and should not be arbitrarily discarded. On the other hand, we deprecate the term "conservative management" for closed treatment because it may, indeed, be quite radical. There is a widespread feeling that "closed is good" and "open is bad," on general principles, and this is nonsense.

When open methods are used, the implant should be selected by what is liable to work best in a particular situation and not by some rule of thumb or surgical dogma. The surgeon should have a clear plan before he starts, based on sound mechanical principles, and all the instruments and implants he needs to carry out the plan should be on hand before he starts. If he is circumspect, he will have a contingency plan for use if the original plan misfires. Haphazard, ill-conceived procedures are worse than no treatment at all (see Fig. 1-150).

We agree with Allgöwer and Spiegel[5] that better results can be obtained in forearm fractures, major intra-articular fractures, and fractures in the multiply injured patient by the use of open reduction and internal fixation. Now it is also evident that femoral and tibial fractures may do better with early and expert internal fixation.

On occasion, the choice must be made between plating and intramedullary nailing.[439] Intramedullary nails have the attraction of being inserted through small operative incisions or even blindly through stab wounds, whereas plates require an extensive operative exposure, especially when a compression device is to be used. Removal of an intramedullary nail can also be effected through a limited surgical incision while plate removal, unless it is on the subcutaneous surface of the tibia, requires the same incision that was necessary for insertion. Infection is much less likely to occur with nailing, but when it does it may spread from stem to stern in the bone and is a substantially greater problem than an infected plate.

The AO group prefers to call intramedullary nailing "internal splintage" rather than "internal fixation," and Perren[349] refers to intramedullary nails as "gliding splints" and plates as "non-gliding splints." Nails offer substantially better resistance to angulatory stresses but poorer resistance to torque, although this is improved by proximal and distal blocking. Plates, on the other hand, offer considerable resistance to torque but are much poorer in angulation. Stress shielding is minimal in nailed bones, so that full activity is resumed after removal of the nail and refracture is not frequent. Bone atrophy and screw-hole stress risers are a significant problem after plate removal, and protection of the bone must be continued over weeks or months.[310] After removing plates 60% of refractures occur in the first month and 80% within 2 months, but refracture may occur considerably later. It would seem, then, that intramedullary nailing would be the method of choice if one has the option, and this is particularly so now that interlocking nails have extended the use of intramedullary nailing to fractures formerly unfeasible for such treatment. Fractures of the distal third of the femur and tibia, which formerly were rotationally unstable after nailing, now may be very adequately controlled by distal blocking screws.

Svenningson and co-workers[439] compared the results of femoral platings and nailings. The nailings all healed (mean time, 15 weeks) and were bearing full weight at 8 weeks. There were 6 nonunions in the plated series, mean time to union was 8 weeks, and full weight-bearing was delayed until 15 weeks.

In forearm nailing, the lack of rotational stability makes the use of a cast mandatory, and it may be difficult or impossible to maintain the radial bow with an intramedullary nail (see Fig. 1-143). Plating allows early motion, and external splintage is unnecessary.

The humerus does not lend itself readily to intramedullary nailing, because transgression of the rotator cuff tends to lead to pain and limitation of motion of the shoulder, and the driving of a nail too far distally may be catastrophic. However, encouraging results have been reported by Ward and White[473] with the use of a blocked Küntscher nail (Fig. 1-136). We have been happy with the nailing of transverse humeral fractures by multiple Ender nails passed through an anterior cortical window. Plating of the humerus carries the risk of radial nerve injury, particularly at the time of plate removal. The safest and best treatment for most humeral fractures in our hands has been the Sarmiento brace, but in pathologic fractures of the humerus, for example, intramedullary nailing may be the only feasible solution.

After studying more than 700 tibial fractures, Nicoll[323] reported that nonunion rates were greatly influenced by four primary characteristics of the fracture: initial displacement, comminution, soft tissue wound, and infection. In comparing closed and open methods of management, he believed the former to be better and advocated plating only for the management of nonunion. This opinion is shared by Dehne[115] and the other advocates of his method of plaster immobilization and early weight-bearing. Although we continue to treat stable tibial fractures by closed means, we believe that unstable fractures may reasonably be managed by an interlocked nail and that fractures with severe soft tissue damage are best managed by external fixation.

TIMING OF OPEN REDUCTION

In 1959, Smith,[422] in a paper on the management of forearm fractures, noted that delay in operation appeared to have a beneficial effect on reducing the incidence of nonunion. Overall, those fractures operated on within the first 6 days had much worse results (17 nonunions in 78 fractures) than those operated after 7 days (no nonunions in 52 fractures). These results were not ostensibly skewed by such factors as open fracture or soft tissue damage, because both groups were of comparable severity.

Five years later Smith reported on the results of immediate and delayed operation in fractures of the femoral shaft.[421] Again he found that delayed fixation was better. There were 25 delayed unions and 20 nonunions in 85 femurs treated by early operation; but in 126 cases treated by delayed operation, there were 23 delayed unions and only one nonunion. On the basis of this study he concluded that the optimum time for open reduction of femoral shaft fractures was between 10 and 14 days.

He followed this up with a study of fractured tibial shafts in 1974.[423] In open fractures internally fixed on the day of injury, severe wound infection occurred in 20%, and there was a 12% incidence of osteitis. (The highest incidence of infection was in primary intramedullary nailings—33%.) The delayed union rate was 48%.

Delayed open reduction had significantly better results than operation within the first week after injury. From his data it would appear that open reduction should be deferred for at least 10 days to achieve the maximum union rate and the minimum incidence of infection.

Exponents of the AO method, on the other hand, advocate early surgery whenever possible, either before soft tissue swelling has occurred or immediately after its subsidence.

Rittman and associates[375] reported on 200 patients with 214 open fractures. Prophylactic antibiotics were given to the first 100 patients but were discarded later as being not worthwhile. The rationale for early fixation was restoration of normal anatomy, prevention of "fracture disease," and mobilization of the patient with polytrauma.

They were able to report excellent results, with 4.5% superficial infections and 3% deep infections, all of which were satisfactorily resolved. There was, however, a 7% incidence of osteitis, which in all cases became quiescent although there were secondary amputations in two patients. At time of review, 6 to 10 years after surgery, all patients but one were working.

Chapman and Mahoney[87] employed early internal fixation in the upper extremity of patients with polytrauma; in open fractures of massively traumatized limbs; some vascular injuries; and in major bone fractures in the elderly. All traumatic wounds were aggressively debrided and left open, internally fixed, and antibiotics given. Infection rates were 1.9% in type I wounds, 8% in type II wounds, and 41% in type III wounds, for an overall infection rate of 10.6%. However, there were no nonunions of long-bone fractures, and the authors believed that they had salvaged some limbs that otherwise would have been amputated.

Rüedi and Lüscher[380] managed 273 patients with 290 fractures of the shaft of the femur with primary plating as early after injury as possible. Eighty-five

percent were operated on within 24 hours of injury, and the remainder were delayed from 2 to 14 days. Of 103 closed comminuted fractures of the femur, six developed osteitis, as did two of the 28 open fractures. In all eight cases of osteomyelitis, bony union of the femur was obtained after further procedures, and all eight have remained without signs of infection since the removal of the implant. Nine patients required replacement of broken plates, and nine more had cancellous grafting for tardy union. Good and excellent results were achieved in 92%. Only two patients were believed to have poor or unacceptable results.

Magerl and associates[282] also have had excellent results from early fixation. Of 67 femoral shaft fractures, 51 were treated in the first 8 hours, and the rest at an average of 8.3 days. The results were: 45 excellent, 17 good, 3 fair, and 2 poor, with only 2 infections. Two patients suffered refracture, and there were nine broken plates. Erickson and Wallin[141] compared healing times and complications in 20 fractures of the femoral shaft treated by intramedullary nailing within 12 hours of injury with 47 fractures where the nailing was delayed 10 days or more. There were no significant differences between the two groups—signs of mild fat embolism occurred with the same frequency, and the only pulmonary embolism occurred in the delayed group. All of the fractures healed, but the immediately treated group returned to work 2 months earlier than the delayed group.

Christensen and associates[91] treated 96 displaced fractures of the tibia by early AO plating. Of these fractures, 40% were open and were operated on within 5 hours of injury. The closed fractures were operated on within 10 hours. The infection rate was 5.3% in the closed injuries and, rather surprisingly, no open fracture became infected, but 93% had antibiotic therapy started immediately after admission. More than 90% of the patients were back at work within 6 months, and there were no nonunions or refractures.

Christensen attributed these good results to the fact that all of the eight participating surgeons were experienced with the AO techniques, and no wound care was given in the emergency room. We would agree that AO methods improperly applied by those inexperienced in the technique almost inevitably lead to catastrophe.

Gustilo and co-workers[177] found that the incidence of adult respiratory distress syndrome (ARDS) and fat embolism syndrome was least in the polytraumatized patients who were operated on within the first week after injury; their most severely injured patients, of necessity, underwent surgery on the day of admission.

Obviously, there are cases where early stabilization is mandatory even if delayed union results. Perren and others[347] of the AO school have advanced the idea that firm skeletal fixation enhances soft tissue healing and may prevent infection, although other series would tend to dispute this contention.[14] In multifactorial problems such as this, only well-planned, prospective, documented studies will help us arrive at a rational solution. Obviously, ill-advised, inadequately fixed fractures will give the worst results of all, but this does not necessarily prove that rigid fixation, applied early, is also bad.

It does seem to us, however, that the advantages of early fixation of fractures far outweigh the dangers of delayed union or nonunion, if indeed they exist. We believe that the doctrine of ''delayed fixation'' is becoming increasingly untenable and that patients do best in institutions where they have immediate and thorough resuscitation, skilled anesthesia, and early and expeditious stabilization of their fractures. With the increasing, prohibitive cost of hospital care, 10 days of lying fallow is a luxury we can ill afford.

MATTERS RELATED TO FRACTURE CARE

JUDGING THE ADEQUACY OF REDUCTION

What constitutes adequate position must vary with the location of the fracture. Nothing short of anatomical restoration is adequate in the forearm, but in the humerus almost any position is compatible with good function. In general, one tries to line up the distal fragment with the proximal fragment. An overlap of 2 cm in the femur or tibia can be compensated for by pelvic tilt; but if it is greater than this, the shoe must be raised to avoid stress on the lumbar spine. It is said that valgus or varus angulation must be no more than 5° in the tibia to avoid shear stresses on the knee and ankle. However, in a follow-up study 29 years after fractures of the tibia, Merchant and Dietz[300] found that the magnitude of varus, valgus, and anteroposterior angulation made no appreciable difference to the incidence of arthritis of the knee or ankle. These surprising results are at variance with most of the opinions expressed in the literature and are of considerable medicolegal importance. Further studies of this nature are obviously indicated to assess to what degree malunion of the tibia is tolerable.

Late varus bow in the femur is not uncommon and gives surprisingly little trouble, but the upper limit of tolerance has not been established. However, valgus and varus deformities become progressively pernicious as they descend from proximal to distal in the femur. Fifteen degrees of coxa valga or vara is relatively inconsequential, but this amount of angulation is unacceptable in the supracondylar region.

Malrotation of the tibia leads to perceptible deformity and ruins the alignment of the knee and ankle. According to Perkins,[345] ''When the joint above the fracture is a ball and socket joint, correction (of rotation) is not essential.'' This is just as well, because one can only correct the rotation accurately at an operation where one can see exactly how the fragments fit and can maintain the reduction with a plate.

It would appear that some degree of malrotation occurs after both traction treatment and blind nailing of the femur. Although 10° of malrotation is common and asymptomatic, Sudmann[437] had one patient with 25° of malrotation who walked with an obvious external rotation deformity and had pain, presumably on this account.

Mayfield,[288] in his review of 75 femoral shaft fractures, discovered that 31 patients had an internal malrotation deformity. Those with severe deformity manifested a Trendelenberg sign and hip abductor weakness during walking owing to the functional reduction of the lever arm of the femoral neck.

It would appear that rotational malunions correct spontaneously in children. Brouwer[55] examined 55 patients 27 to 32 years after a childhood fracture and could find only one patient with significant rotational malalignment, and he was asymptomatic. Hägglund and associates[179] confirm that these malalignments correct spontaneously in 1 to 4.5 years even if the deformity is as much as 20°.

Connolly[103] has stressed that depending on two-dimensional radiographs alone in the management of three-dimensional fracture deformities is inadequate. Apparent valgus and varus deformity may be secondary to rotational malalignment and will not be cured in the tibia by wedging a cast. Overlapping finger deformities associated with fractures of the phalanx may not be evident on radiologic examination and is best prevented by ''buddy splinting'' to an adjacent digit (see Chapter 7).

Merwyn Evans[143] also made this point in his classic paper on rotational deformities of the radius in forearm fractures. Using the contour of the radial tuberosity as a marker, he compared films of the normal forearm in varying degrees of pronation and supination with those of the reduced, fractured forearm to make sure that the distal fragment was anatomically aligned (see Chapter 9).

One should also suspect malrotation when there is an abrupt change in diameter from one fragment to another at a fracture site where there is no comminution.[318]

Anterior or posterior bowing is compensated by the contiguous hinge joint and, except in the forearm, is innocuous. The main objections to such deformities are the cosmesis and shortening.

PREVENTION OF INFECTION

When an operation is undertaken, a closed fracture is converted into an open one with the potential danger of its becoming infected. This complication may be catastrophic. It can lead to the loss of a limb and, at best, it prolongs the period of morbidity, may make more operations necessary, and impairs the quality of the final result. It follows, then, that every precaution must be taken to prevent this dismal series of events.

Care of the Soft Tissues

A fracture was defined, we believe by Clay Ray Murray, as a "soft-tissue injury complicated by a break in a bone." The most important single factor in the management of fractures is the treatment of the overlying soft tissues[58,59,140,161,162]; in fractures of the tibia especially, this may determine the success or failure of treatment. Incisions made through traumatized, compromised skin may cause its demise. Early open reduction of the tibia, even in highly skilled hands, is associated with skin breakdown, delayed healing, and infection.[198,329]

There is still a tremendous compulsion for surgeons to close wounds primarily, even though it has been shown quite conclusively that delayed primary closure or secondary closure by skin grafting is much safer.[58,59] Certainly in well-debrided wounds seen early, where the soft tissue damage and contamination have not been severe, it is permissible to suture primarily. On the other hand, ill-advised attempts to provide skin cover for fractured tibias by suturing wounds under tension, by making "relaxing" incisions, and by the rotation of flaps is so fraught with danger that it should rarely be done.[58] If cover is mandatory, it has been suggested that Ger's technique, in which the bone is covered by a transposed muscle belly followed by skin grafting on the fifth postoperative day, is the best

means of achieving it.[161,162] We believe that this adds insult to injury in a severely traumatized limb and do not advocate it as an immediate measure. In Louisville we are most fortunate in having a number of highly skilled microsurgeons, so that tissue cover, in catastrophic soft tissue loss, is often provided by a latissimus dorsi or other composite free flap. This has revolutionized the management of leg injuries and has salvaged limbs which would inevitably have been amputated in other times. The timing of applying such composite, free grafts is a matter that has not been satisfactorily resolved. If the graft is delayed for more than 48 hours the recipient site becomes secondarily invaded by *Pseudomonas* and other undesirable opportunistic organisms, so immediate application of the graft after debridement is desirable. On the other hand, one hesitates to perform a procedure requiring several hours on a patient who is severely injured and who already may have been anesthetized for a considerable time. Furthermore, one is reluctant to compromise vessels in a traumatized limb until the total insult to the extremity can be accurately assessed. The full extent of tissue damage is sometimes not ascertainable and redebridement may be required later. Nevertheless, when conditions have been favorable, we have had excellent results from primary free tissue transfer.

Godina,[166] whose experience in covering exposed tibias was unrivalled, has shown that the results of cover in the first 48 hours is vastly superior to delayed cover. The infection rate, graft survival, and time in hospital are markedly better. He pointed out that edema and infection make the vascular anastomoses technically much more difficult, and so compromises the result. Furthermore, when the anterior tibial artery is transected it may be used as the donor artery only in the first 48 hours. After this time the flow in the vessel drops to 10% of normal and cannot sustain a free flap. (For a more extensive discussion of soft tissue management and free flaps, see Chapter 4).

A temporizing stratagem popularized by Seligson and Henry[191] is the "bead pouch." After debriding the wound, tobramycin- or other antibiotic-impregnated beads are placed in the wound and covered by Op-Site, is an adhesive plastic wound dressing which allows transpiration, and the closed space is drained by a small hemovac catheter. The wound is reexamined after 48 hours; if necessary, it is redebrided and new beads are inserted or, if the wound is clean, it is closed by whatever method is most appropriate (see Fig. 1-93).

Another promising method of temporary cover

of open wounds has recently been introduced from Europe.[252,253,478] This is the use of a synthetic skin substitute applied to the wound after debridement. This material, Epigard, is marketed by Synthes and consists of an outer coat of Gore-Tex and an inner layer of polyurethane mesh that absorbs the wound secretions. This dressing allows transpiration from the wound but blocks the ingress of bacteria. The dressing is cut to the shape and size of the wound and is bandaged in place. This material adheres to the wound bed and granulations grow into the interstices of the polyurethane mesh. Daily removal and reapplication of the dressing debrides the wound until it is ready for grafting or secondary closure.

All would agree that the most important predisposing causes of infection are the presence of dead or devitalized tissue, hematoma, dead space, and foreign bodies. It follows, therefore, that these conditions must be eliminated or controlled as far as possible. The management of open fractures and these problems is discussed in Chapter 3.

Prophylactic Antibiotics

The use of prophylactic antibiotics is still controversial, but interest in this subject has been renewed by the efforts to find means of averting the disaster of infected total hip and knee arthroplasties. If it can be shown that prophylactic antimicrobial therapy is efficacious for joint replacements, its application to fracture surgery is no less important. Unfortunately, the literature on this subject presents conflicting views. Many of the clinical studies are retrospective and poorly controlled, and even the laboratory studies are no more helpful.

Fogelberg and associates,[152] in their review of the subject, found that most studies concluded that prophylactic antibiotics either were of no value or enhanced the likelihood of postoperative infection. Stevens,[430] reviewing postoperative infections in Lexington, Kentucky, found that the infection rate increased significantly after procedures lasting more than 90 minutes and that prophylactic antibiotics in clean cases increased the incidence of sepsis.

In more recent studies by Scales and associates,[400] 1816 patients operated on at the Royal National Orthopaedic Hospital and the Queen Elizabeth II Hospital were reviewed. There was no correlation between the infection rate and such factors as age, sex, vacuum drainage, site of implant, weight-bearing, corrosion of metal, or chemical composition of the implant. Those patients given pre- and postoperative antibiotics for a total of 5 to 7 days had the lowest incidence of wound infection, while

those given antibiotics only after surgery had the highest rate of infection for the group.

Fogelberg and associates,[152] using pre- and postoperative penicillin for patients undergoing spinal surgery and mold arthroplasty of the hip were able to reduce the incidence of infection from 8.9% in the control group to 1.7% in the treated group. Similarly, Nach and Keim[317] found that prophylactic oxacillin, penicillin, or lincomycin given before, during, and after surgery was effective in reducing both major and minor infections. The treated group had an incidence of 1.6% major infection, while the control group had an 11.4% incidence of major infections and 3.8% of minor infections.

The use of local irrigants or aerosols containing antibiotics has also been shown to be effective in reducing the rate of postoperative infection.[153,248,474] Gingrass and associates,[163] in experimental studies, found that gentle scrubbing of contaminated wounds and irrigation with neomycin solution was superior to irrigation with saline or scrubbing with pHisoHex, either alone or in combination, in preventing infection in contaminated wounds. Parenteral neomycin, while ineffective by itself, did improve the results when used as an irrigant and was complemented by gentle scrubbing.

It is perhaps foolish to talk about prophylactic antibiotics in open fractures, because the organisms are already present in the wound and it is these microorganisms that most probably will be the source of subsequent infection. It makes sense, therefore, to send debrided soft tissue to the laboratory for culture and sensitivity in the management of open fractures. Quantitative Gram stain of this material is helpful in predicting subsequent wound infection.[106]

If antibiotics are to be used, they should be given early, and it is the routine practice in our emergency room for intravenous cephalosporins to be given in all open fractures and joint injuries. In the first edition of this book, we recommended cephalothin (Keflin) as the drug of choice, and indeed it appeared to be effective. There is no advantage in using second- or third-generation cepholosporins, and we generally use cephalothin (Keflin) or cephazolin (Kefzol). We administer an initial intravenous dose of 2 g and continue with 1 g intravenously every 4 hours for 48 hours. If there is no evidence of infection at that time, antibiotic therapy is discontinued. By limiting the duration of antibiotic therapy, we hope to reduce the incidence of drug-resistant organisms. We believe that if we have not killed off the organism within 48 hours, we shall probably not be able to do so with a longer exposure. Antibiotic therapy to prevent infection or nip it in the bud is still a controversial area; but until definitive studies show evidence to the contrary, we shall continue to use it in this manner.

When surgery is being performed on a previously open or infected fracture, we start antibiotics intravenously with the induction of anesthesia and continue them for 24 hours.

Internal Fixation and Infection

It used to be held that an internal fixation device, being a foreign body, in some way enhanced the chances of wound infection and was absolutely proscribed in the treatment of open fractures. This contention has been supported by published series. Gustilo and associates[177] analyzed 511 open fractures and found that of the 112 fractures treated by primary fixation, 11.6% became infected; whereas in the 299 without primary internal fixation, the infection rate was only 6.68%.

When infection occurred following internal fixation, it was formerly advised that the metal should be removed to control the sepsis. The idea that metal *per se* is responsible for infection is open to serious doubt.

McNeur[295] has shown that both in war wounds and open fractures in civilians adequate management of the soft tissue wound and the use of antibiotics allow the use of primary internal fixation without incurring prohibitively high infection rates. Of 145 cases treated at the Alfred Hospital, early skin healing was obtained in 125. Twelve patients had delayed wound healing and only five developed infection. In the total series, there were only six infected fractures (3.6%), and in none of these was the metal removed early. Four of the fractures went on to union in spite of infection.

Recent experience seems to confirm that when internal fixation is secure, it should not be removed; and with debridement, irrigation, and antibiotic therapy, union will eventually occur.[198,247,279,280] It may be that the optimum management of an infected nonunion is to combine aggressive treatment of the infection with secure, rigid, internal fixation.[277]

ANESTHESIA IN FRACTURE TREATMENT

Most fracture work is carried out under general or regional anesthesia administered by an anesthesiologist. The choice of method and agents under these circumstances must be left to the anesthe-

siologist and will be dictated by the age and condition of the patient as well as the experience of the person administering the anesthetic. It is axiomatic that the patient should be resuscitated and stabilized prior to the administration of anesthesia, and whenever possible anesthesia in a patient with a full stomach should be deferred to avoid the danger of aspiration pneumonia.

At Louisville General Hospital it was our practice, when anesthesia had to be induced to intubate the trachea with the patient awake, and this worked well. Spinal anesthesia in an acutely injured patient is hazardous and is best avoided.

On occasion the surgeon is obliged to work without the services of an anesthesiologist. Fractures of the tibia seen soon after injury may often be reduced and immobilized without anesthesia or under analgesics such as morphine or meperidine. When these drugs are used, we prefer to administer them intravenously (eg, 8 to 10 mg morphine or 75 to 100 mg meperidine), because their action is produced rapidly and predictably. They should be given slowly and should be well diluted. In general, fractures reduced without the services of an anesthesiologist tend to be minor ones in the upper extremity—especially of the wrist and hand.

The methods commonly used to provide such anesthesia are local infiltration of local anesthetics, intravenous regional anesthesia (Bier's block), and regional nerve block. Hypnosis or the use of ataractic drugs may also be employed.

LOCAL INFILTRATION

If a needle is introduced into a fracture hematoma, blood is easily aspirated, and analgesia may be obtained by injecting lidocaine, mepivicaine, or some similar drug into the hematoma.[125] This method is most frequently used in the treatment of Colles' fracture. The fracture is palpated and 10 ml of 1% lidocaine or a similar agent is injected into the hematoma. Another 5 ml must be injected around the ulnar styloid, or analgesia will be incomplete. Furthermore, at least 10 to 15 minutes should be allowed before starting to manipulate. Theoretically, this method would seem to carry the risk of infecting the hematoma, but in practice this rarely occurs. Case[81] treated a series of 136 Colles' fractures; 79 were anesthetized by infiltration of the hematoma, 30 by Bier's block, and 26 by general anesthesia. He found that there was no difference in the ease of reduction or in the end result, although the simplicity of induction and the economy of time in a busy casualty department made hematoma infiltration the method of choice. Case used 5 ml of 2% lignocaine and reduced the fracture after a 10- to 15-minute wait. There were no infections in his series.

INTRAVENOUS REGIONAL ANESTHESIA

Intravenous regional anesthesia, originally described by Bier in the 19th century, has been revived and is used in surgery of the forearm and hand, as well as in the leg and foot. A needle or venous catheter is inserted into a convenient superficial vein. The arm or leg is then elevated and exsanguinated by wrapping with an Esmarch or Ace bandage. A pneumatic tourniquet is inflated (250 mm Hg in the arm; 400 mm Hg in the leg), and the bandage is removed. In the arm 20 to 40 ml of 0.5% lidocaine is injected into the vein (for larger volumes, 0.25% solution can be used) and in the foot and leg 40 to 80 ml is required. Atkinson and associates[20] recommended that no more than 50 ml of 0.5% lidocaine should be used in the arm, and they used an average dose of 224 mg of lidocaine. Sorbie and Cracha[425] used no more than 200 mg in the arm and 400 mg in the leg. After this injection, anesthesia is usually produced within 5 minutes. At this point a second tourniquet is inflated distal to the first, and the original tourniquet, which is on unanesthetized skin, is deflated. Hollingsworth and associates[206] have recommended the use of bupivicaine as the agent of choice in this technique.

This method gives excellent anesthesia for an hour or more, although some patients complain of tourniquet pain. Should the tourniquet become deflated prior to 20 minutes after the injection, a toxic dose of lidocaine may be released into the general circulation. Great care should be taken to ensure that this does not happen, and drugs and equipment for dealing with reactions to local anesthetics must be on hand. No type of anesthetic should be undertaken without having another person in the room or at least within easy earshot. It goes without saying that no patient with a history of idiosyncrasy to local anesthetic agents should be treated by this method.

BRACHIAL BLOCK

Excellent anesthesia of the upper extremity can be produced by interscalene or supraclavicular brachial block. Because there is some danger inherent in both of these techniques, and because pneumothorax has been reported in up to 20% of supraclavicular blocks, we believe that these methods are best left to those skilled in their use. Brachial block by the axillary route, on the other hand, is a simple, efficient, and relatively risk-free means of producing upper-extremity anesthesia. This technique has been described well by Burnham, deJong, and others.[50,117,482] Kleinert and associates[249] reported the results of 647 blocks in 1963, and since that time axillary block has become our anesthetic of choice in the upper extremity. More than 90% of the hands operated on in Louisville are anesthetized in this manner, as well as Colles' fractures and other minor injuries of the upper extremity. A subsequent paper from the same authors reported their experience with more than 10,000 cases.[235]

Technique

The patient lies in the supine position, and the shoulder is externally rotated and abducted to 90°. The elbow is also flexed to a right angle, and the patient is placed in a comfortable position. After preparing the skin, the axillary artery is palpated where it lies under the cover of the pectoralis major. Using a 10-ml syringe and a ⅝-inch, 25-gauge needle, a wheal is raised in the skin overlying the artery, as high in the axilla as possible, and the needle is inserted into the neurovascular sheath (Figs. 1-155 to 1-157). A distinct sensation is felt as the sheath is pierced, and after detaching the syringe, the needle can be seen to pulsate owing to the proximity of the artery. At this point the patient should be questioned regarding paresthesias in the limb, which confirms that the sheath has been entered. To avert the hazard of intravascular injection, the needle should be aspirated before the anesthetic agent is injected. The duration of the block is enhanced by the addition of epinephrine, 1:200,000, to the anesthetic agent. If lidocaine is used, 20 ml of 1% solution may be adequate to produce anesthesia of the hand and forearm, and where more extensive anesthesia of the extremity is required, the dosage may be increased to 40 ml. Smaller doses may suffice if a tourniquet is placed around the arm prior to the insertion of the needle (Erickson technique) (see Fig. 1-156). This tourniquet prevents peripheral leakage and diffusion of the agent. To make sure that all three cords are blocked, two needles may be inserted, one above and one below the artery, but in general one needle is sufficient (see Fig. 1-157). A ⅝-inch needle is adequate for all but the most gargantuan arms, owing to the superficial location of the neurovascular bundle. If a longer needle is used, it is possible to inject the coracobrachialis muscle and produce no block at all. While there will inevitably be a small percentage of un-

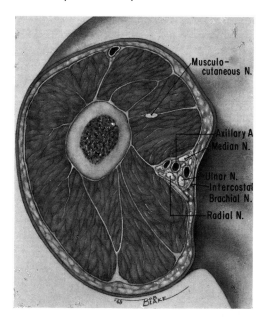

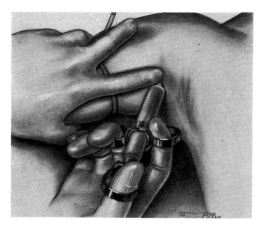

Fig. 1-155. A cross section of the axilla demonstrating the superficial position of the neurovascular bundle. *(Kasdan, M. L.; Kleinert, H. E.; Kasdan, A. P.; and Kutz, J. E.: Axillary Block Anesthesia for Surgery of the Hand. Plast. Reconstr. Surg., 46:256, 1970.)*

Fig. 1-156. The artery is palpated in the axilla, and the needle is passed close to the fingertips. A tourniquet prevents peripheral leakage and diffusion of the agent and allows the block to be produced by smaller dosages of local anesthetic. *(Kasdan, M. L.; Kleinert, H. E.; Kasdan, A. P.; and Kutz, J. E.: Axillary Block Anesthesia for Surgery of the Hand. Plast. Reconstr. Surg., 46:256, 1970.)*

successful blocks (Kasdan and associates[235] reported 90% success), the most common cause of failure is impatience. Although profound anesthesia may occur within 10 minutes, it may take 30 minutes. On occasion the patient awakes from general anesthesia with an excellent block because the surgeon was unwilling to wait.

In reported series of nerve blocks, the neurologic complication rate has been reported from 0% to greater than 5%. Most of the complications are minor and transitory and some, indeed, may be secondary to faulty positioning, complications of surgery or casting, tourniquet injury, or some other factor unrelated to the block *per se.* However, serious complications do occur, such as chronic pain, persistent loss of sensation, and paralysis.

Because modern anesthetic agents are unlikely to have direct toxic effects on nerves when used according to the manufacturer's directions, mechanical injury to the nerve by needling must be considered as a possible cause when untoward symptoms occur.

Selander and his group[411] have investigated this problem both clinically and experimentally. In the technique of axillary block, one may identify the major nerves by provoking paresthesia with the

probing needle and then injecting around the nerve. An alternative technique is the Eriksson method of inserting two needles in the axillary sheath and gauging their position by the transmitted pulsations of the artery. In his clinical study, Selander divided his patients into two groups: 290 were blocked by evoking paresthesias and 243 by the Eriksson technique. Of the latter group, 40% had paresthesia inadvertently evoked during the insertion of the needles. Eight complications resulted in the paresthesia

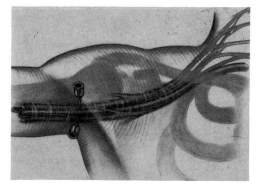

Fig. 1-157. The injection should be high in the axilla and a two-needle technique may be used to make sure that all three nerves are blocked. *(Kasdan, M. L.; Kleinert, H. E.; Kasdan, A. P.; and Kutz, J. E.: Axillary Block Anesthesia for Surgery of the Hand. Plast. Reconstr. Surg., 46: 256, 1970.)*

group (2.8%), and only 2 (0.8%) had complications in the other group.

Selander also investigated histologically the effects of puncturing sciatic nerves in rabbits, using needles with short bevels and needles with long bevels, 14° and 45°, respectively. The long-beveled needles were most likely to produce injury, but this depended on the orientation of the bevel to the long axis of the nerve. If the bevel was parallel to the nerve fascicles, comparatively little damage was done; but in other orientations, distortions or transections of nerve fibers resulted or perineural gaps were produced with herniation of fibers. Damage could be produced by short-beveled needles, but was less severe and independent of orientation.

It would seem, therefore, that the safest method of axillary block would be the Eriksson method, using 4-mm needles with 45° bevels.

D.B. Scott[407] has published a superb manual of regional anesthesia with detailed and explicit instructions and anatomical diagrams; this is an excellent guide for those who must do their own anesthesia.

INTRAVENOUS DIAZEPAM

Diazepam (Valium) is a benzodiazepine derivative that has ataractic and muscle relaxant properties. It is recommended by its manufacturer (Roche) for the treatment of anxiety and tension states. Valium is also used for the relief of skeletal muscle spasm such as in cerebral palsy, athetosis, and the stiff-man syndrome. This drug is contraindicated in patients with acute, narrow-angle glaucoma and should not be administered to patients in shock, coma, or acute alcohol intoxication who have depressed vital signs.

Bultitude and associates[67] reported on the use of intravenous diazepam as the sole anesthetic agent for the reduction of Colles' fractures. They advised a dose of 20 mg given intravenously, or 30 mg in heavy adults, administered over a period of seconds equal to twice the number of milligrams given (eg, 20 mg over 40 seconds). In their experience this was a useful anesthetic. They felt that the drug had little or no analgesic action but did induce transient amnesia. (One of our anesthesiologist friends has described this method as being the pharmacological equivalent of "biting the bullet.") Their patients were quick to recover, could sit up in 5 minutes, and were able to return home in 2 hours.

Of the 71 patients treated, only two 85-year-olds became unrousable for 2 minutes, and one of them had a fall in blood pressure for 10 minutes after the injection. Both of these patients made a full recovery. The only other complications reported in this study were pain at the injection site and thrombophlebitis. Others have noted respiratory depression following intravenous diazepam.

We have used this technique too, but have given somewhat smaller doses (10 to 20 mg). It has been useful in reducing dislocations of the shoulder and elbow as well as in minor fractures. Care must be taken with inebriated patients, because alcohol and diazepam appear to have a synergistic action. Diazepam or regional block should never be used where there is no one to help or if oxygen and some means of ventilating the patient are not easily available.

CHOICE OF AGENT

Most of the commonly used local anesthetic agents are effective, but bupivicaine (Marcaine) has the advantage of being extremely long-acting.[308] It lasts two to three times as long as lidocaine (Xylocaine) or mepivacaine (Carbocaine) and 20% to 25% longer than tetracaine (Pontocaine). It is relatively less toxic than other similar drugs, and in our hands 0.5% solutions have been excellent for both local infiltration and nerve blocks.

Etidocaine (Duranest)[207,273] is a long-acting agent that is comparable to bupivicaine in the duration of its action and is midway between lidocaine and bupivicaine in toxicity. An excellent axillary block may be obtained using 30 ml of 0.5% or 1.0% etidocaine with adrenaline, which will give 6 to 7 hours of surgical anesthesia. Onset of anesthesia occurs in 10 to 12 minutes and total recovery takes up to 10 hours.

At Louisville Jewish Hospital, where nearly 7000 blocks are done annually, the agent of choice is a mixture of etidocaine (30%) and bupivicaine (70%). This has been found to be more effective than either agent alone and capitalizes on the advantages of both drugs.

REHABILITATION FOLLOWING FRACTURES

The concept that rehabilitation is a process that should start after the healing of a fracture and may safely be delegated to physical therapists and physiatrists is fallacious. Rehabilitation is the business of the entire medical team, and it should start the minute the patient is admitted to the hospital.

The prime goals of rehabilitation in the fracture patient are: (1) to maintain or restore the range of motion of joints, (2) to preserve muscle strength and endurance, (3) to enhance the rate of fracture healing by activity, and (4) to return the patient to function and employment at the earliest juncture.

MAINTENANCE OF JOINT MOTION

The stiffness that results following immobilization of a joint is proportional to the length of time involved. The main factor in the production of this contracture is shortening of the surrounding musculature and, to a lesser degree, changes in the joint capsule. Intra-articular changes also occur—for example, proliferation of the subsynovial fatty tissue that encroaches on and may obliterate the synovial cleft. In time this soft tissue overgrowth may cover the articular cartilage and become confluent with it. Where articular surfaces are in contact, especially under pressure, fibrillation and degeneration occur, and fibrous adhesions or even bony fusion may result. The articular cartilage must depend on synovial fluid for its nutrition. The obliteration of the joint and the lack of motion to "pump" the fluid in and out may also add to the decrease in thickness of the cartilage.[56,139]

It follows that no joint should be immobilized unnecessarily and all joints should be put through a full range of motion every day. The elderly woman with a Colles' fracture should never be left to vegetate in a sling and develop a frozen shoulder and stiff fingers. Proper exercise (including the shoulder) is as much a part of her treatment as the application of the cast.

The shoulder is particularly liable to develop stiffness in people who are middle-aged and older, and circumduction exercises must be started as soon as they can be tolerated by patients with fractures of the humeral neck. When a frozen shoulder does develop, an active program of exercises may mobilize the shoulder. In recalcitrant cases, gentle manipulation under general anesthesia may be tried, keeping in mind the danger of fracturing an osteoporotic humerus. The manipulation is best carried out by stabilizing the scapula and abducting the shoulder by pressure on the proximal third of the humerus. No sudden stress should be applied, and on no account must the whole lever-arm of the humerus be used by grasping the elbow, nor should rotational stress be applied.

The elbow does not tolerate injury well and frequently becomes stiff. Early active motion in elbow injuries is desirable, and any attempt to force motion by passive manipulation is liable to incite myositis ossificans.

Limitation of knee motion following fractures of the femur is not infrequently caused by scarring down of the quadriceps to the underlying bone. Charnley[90] advised that this may be prevented by the early use of isometric quadriceps exercises, and others have devised means of starting active knee motion during treatment by traction. Nichols[322] has shown that in the Royal Air Force the average time off-duty following a fractured femoral shaft is 26 weeks when treated by early intramedullary nailing and 32 weeks after treatment by skeletal traction. This is a result, at least to some extent, of earlier resumption of knee motion. In comparing the results of intramedullary nailing with traction, Rokkanen[376] found that ultimately there was no significant difference in the range of knee motion in young people. However, patients older than 35 years who had been treated by intramedullary nails had significantly better motion than the traction group. We have followed the advice of the AO group by maintaining the knee in flexion for 48 hours after nailing or plating femoral fractures. Since we have adopted this regimen, regaining range of motion of the knee has not been a problem. Vigorous attempts to regain knee motion after femoral fracture may result in refracture. Reviewing the literature, O'Brien found incidences ranging from 4% to 16.6% in the published series.[326]

We have not found passive manipulation to be rewarding in restoring motion to stiff knees after fractures of the femur, and in fact it may produce a fracture of the patella. The procedure of choice where more motion is needed is a quadricepsplasty, and the results of this procedure are mediocre at best. In this regard, an ounce of prevention is worth a pound of cure.

Continuous Passive Motion

Salter,[389] in his presidential address to the Canadian Orthopaedic Society, reviewed the history of the management of bone and joint injuries and showed that most authorities favored rest and immobilization on a purely empiric basis. Hugh Owen Thomas, the father of British orthopaedics, advocated that immobilization should be "complete, prolonged, uninterrupted and enforced." This tradition dominated orthopaedic thinking, and Lucas-Champonniere alone, a late 19th-century French surgeon often castigated as a quack, promulgated the heresy of massage and motion to prevent muscle atrophy and joint stiffness in the treatment of fractures.

On the basis of experimental work on rabbits, Salter[391] has shown that continuous passive motion (CPM) enhances healing in both articular and ligamentous injuries of joints.

The practical application of this work has been the invention of passive motion devices to exercise the joints of both the upper and lower extremities following operation or injury.

Some devices on the market have variable speed controls, but Salter believes that the optimum rate is one cycle per 45 seconds and has designed his apparatus accordingly.

In all of these CPM machines the arc of motion may be preset to the needs of each patient and increased at will.

We have used such machines after internal fixation of complex knee injuries—floating knees, intra-articular fractures with and without patella fractures—and have been very happy with the results. Not only is joint range preserved, but pain is also alleviated by the motion. This would seem to contradict Blockey's observations[44] of muscles being inhibited by joint injury and pain being aggravated by passive motion.

MUSCLE EXERCISES

Muscle exercises may be isometric or isotonic. In isometric exercise, the length of the muscle does not change, the joint on which it acts does not move, but the tension of the muscle fibers increases (eg, quadriceps setting). Isotonic exercise, on the other hand, involves motion of the joint and shortening of the muscle fibers. The former is said to be more efficient in developing strength and is also indicated where joint motion causes pain and therefore secondary inhibition of the muscle. The latter is used to regain range of motion and to regain strength and endurance where the joint is not irritable. Either type of exercise may be modified by increasing the load against which the muscle must act as it grows stronger—progressive resistance exercises (PRE). To increase a muscle's strength, it is necessary to make it contract with its maximum power daily without overloading it. Endurance, on the other hand, is achieved by repetitive exercise stopping short of fatigue.

The strength of a muscle contraction is proportional to the starting length of its fibers. The therapist should use this principle by fully extending the muscle and even applying gentle passive stretch. Greater power will also be gained by preceding the exercise by a maximal contraction of the muscle's antagonist and by recruitment of additional anterior

horn cells by contracting additional muscles innervated by the same segment of the cord (eg, by dorsiflexing the ankle [L 4–5] while exercising the quadriceps [L 3–4]). Where muscles are so weak as to be nonfunctional, the exercises have to be assisted by the therapist or by eliminating gravity with hydrotherapy or supportive devices. At all costs a weak or partially innervated muscle should be protected from overstretching, because this greatly retards its recovery.

Profound change occurs in muscle following injury and immobilization, particularly when tendons have been allowed to heal in a lengthened position. Haggmark and co-workers have shown that the endurance of the triceps surae and the cross-sectional area of the muscle are greatly reduced when ruptures of the heelcord are treated nonoperatively, and this difference is not marked when the tendon is repaired operatively. However, there is no significant difference when the operative and nonoperative cases are tested on the Cybex II isokinetic dynometer. Another most interesting finding by this group is that immobilization of the knee following injury will reduce the proportion of type I fibers (slow twitch) in comparison to type II fibers in the involved quadriceps. This change, which is most pronounced in endurance athletes such as cross-country skiers, may be reversed by appropriate exercise and training.

Isokinetic Exercise

Currently in athletic circles there is great interest in exercise devices that control the rate of joint motion and vary the resistance with the strength of the subject's muscular effort (Cybex). The patient may push or pull as little or as much as he wants, but the cadence remains unchanged. This type of exercise is neither isometric nor isotonic, but, because its rate is constant, is isokinetic.[269,304]

It would appear that increase in muscular power (ie, the amount of work per unit time) can be achieved more efficiently by exercising muscles at higher speeds even if the loads are smaller and muscle endurance is similarly enhanced.

The newer models of Cybex have recording dynamometers that measure torque forces and give visual recordings of the tested muscles' activity.

Our own experience with this apparatus is favorable, and patients like it.

GAIT TRAINING

The value of early weight-bearing in closed treatment of tibial fractures has been firmly established in contemporary practice. However, without some supervision many patients develop undesirable gait patterns that persist even after removal of the cast.

It is best if ambulation is begun by having the patient stand in parallel bars to achieve standing balance equally distributed between the two feet. When this has been achieved, he should then practice weight transfer from one foot to the other. He must achieve balance on each foot before walking is commenced. From the parallel bars he should graduate to crutches or canes and, eventually (in some cases), to independent walking.

An even gait is impossible when there is marked discrepancy between leg lengths. For this reason we prefer an overshoe rather than a walking heel on a cast. This has the additional advantage of keeping the cast clean and dry. Alternatively, the shoe on the contralateral foot may be raised. This is particularly valuable in cast-bracing for femoral fractures, where it prevents late varus bowing. The patient should never be allowed to swivel on his walking foot by externally rotating at the hip, but should be encouraged to walk as closely as possible to a normal heel-and-toe gait.

AMBULATION AIDS

Most patients with lower-extremity fractures require some form of ambulation aid. While most rehabilitation centers appear to prefer other than simple axillary crutches, these have the advantage of being cheap and readily available. Because the large majority of patients uses them for only a short time, the expense of providing more sophisticated crutches does not seem reasonable. In adjusting these crutches, there should be a handbreadth between the pad of the crutch and the axilla. The pad is designed to take pressure on the lateral side of the chest and not in the axilla, where pressure on the brachial plexus can produce a "crutch palsy." The handpiece should allow the elbow to be flexed comfortably while bearing weight. To be able to use axillary crutches, the patient must have strong triceps, and preparatory exercises with dumbbells to strengthen these muscles while the patient is still confined to bed are useful. For comfort, the axillary portion and the handpiece should be padded with sponge rubber and, for safety, the largest rubber tips should be added.

Crutch Gaits

After having prescribed crutches, the most appropriate gait should be taught.

SWING-TO AND SWING-THROUGH GAIT

In swing-to and swing-through gait, both crutches are placed forward and the patient either pulls his body to the crutches or propels his body through them so that his feet are ahead of the crutch tips. The weight can be borne on both feet, as a paraplegic would, or on only one foot when weight-bearing is proscribed for the fractured side. This is by far the most rapid means of progression on crutches, and the most vigorous.

THREE-POINT GAIT

In three-point gait, the two crutches and the injured extremity are advanced together and bear weight simultaneously while the sound leg is advanced. The degree of weight-bearing on the injured extremity is controlled by the amount of weight borne by the hands.

TWO-POINT GAIT

In an alternating two-point gait, the crutch is advanced with the contralateral foot. This method is used in bilateral injuries where partial weight-bearing is desired.

FOUR-POINT GAIT

The four-point gait is similar to the two-point, but one crutch is advanced first, then the contralateral foot, followed by the second crutch, then the second foot. This is reserved for the most severely impaired or elderly patients.

Walkers

It is quite unrealistic to expect elderly patients to walk with crutches, because they have neither the strength nor the agility and coordination to use them. In such cases a simple walker made from tubular aluminum that they can lift up and place before them is the most stable and foolproof device. It is also unreasonable to prescribe non-weight-bearing ambulation for elderly people with fractured hips, and indeed, the work of Rydell and Frankel would seem to show that partial weight-bearing is more benign than many maneuvers carried out in bed. For this reason, in stable, well-fixed fractures of the hip we now start weight-bearing as soon as possible.

Canes

Canes are useful but less efficient than crutches for maintaining balance and relieving weight. The patient's natural tendency is to hold the cane with the hand on the side of the injury, which gives rise to a very awkward gait. He should be instructed to use the cane in the opposite hand and bear weight on the injured limb and cane simultaneously. The use of a solitary crutch should be discouraged, as it too gives rise to an ugly gait. By and large, if a patient needs one crutch, he needs two.

HEAT

In most departments of physical medicine, there are a number of expensive machines whose main purpose is to supply some form of heat to the tissues. We are not aware of any evidence that heat *per se* has any beneficial effect in rehabilitation after injury. Ultrasound has been shown to be more efficient in the heating of deep tissues, but the therapeutic benefits of this are somewhat nebulous. The daily application of ultrasound to neck injuries sustained in rear-end collisions seems to us to benefit mainly the owner of the machine.

The application of heat to painful joints and muscles does relieve pain and discomfort and is a useful preliminary measure to active exercises. In this regard, one method does not appear to be superior to another. Hot packs or immersion in warm water are as good as more sophisticated methods and have the advantage of being available at home. If short-wave diathermy is used, it must never be applied over implants, because it induces high temperatures in the metal with damage to the tissues.

Cold applications may also be used to reduce pain prior to exercise, but our preference is for heat and, where applicable, immersion in a Hubbard tank.

PURPOSEFUL EXERCISE

Exercise is dull, and most people prefer carrying out purposeful tasks. This fact is used by devising projects for patients that use the motion desired (eg, using a screwdriver to gain supination range and power). Such therapy not only achieves a therapeutic aim but is a diversion for the patient that breaks the tedium of a stay in the hospital.

It also is important to make the patient as self-sufficient as possible before he returns home. The use of the occupational therapist in supervising activities of daily living (ADL) is extremely helpful, but unfortunately these functions are rarely to be found outside rehabilitation centers and almost never in general or community hospitals.

MASSAGE

Massage is a time-honored treatment, but the laying on of hands has little place in the rehabilitation of patients with fractures, except as a means of softening up and mobilizing scars that are impeding joint motion. It is extremely unlikely that massage will dissipate edema or improve circulation to an extremity.

ORTHOTICS

Conventional bracing has very little place in the treatment of fractures. Long-leg braces with ischial seats or quadrilateral sockets and pelvic bands are sometimes prescribed to "protect" fractures of the femur or even fractures of the hip. Mechanically, such braces are ineffective and much inferior to cast braces. It has been shown that even subtrochanteric fractures may be treated by a skillfully applied cast brace, but this certainly would not be true of a long-leg caliper.

Sarmiento[394,395,397] has shown that fractures of the tibia may be managed with a patellar-bearing cast with a free ankle joint, and he has taken the process one step further by replacing the plaster of paris with Orthoplast, a plastic material that can be molded after heating. Such braces applied by an experienced orthotist are efficient, but factors such as cost and the availability of skilled orthotists make plaster casts the treatment of choice for most surgeons.

More recently Sarmiento has introduced prefabricated, polyethylene braces in the management of humeral[398] and radial and ulnar shaft fractures.[397] The management of humeral fractures by this means has been a great advance over hanging casts, sugar-tong splints, and Velpeau dressings, because it allows early motion of the shoulder and does not require the patient perpetually to sit up. We have our orthoses custom-made, as some of our more ample patients do not easily fit into the large size of the stock splint. We have no experience in the use of the ulnar splint and would be skeptical of orthoses designed for use in both bones of forearm fractures.

The major application for bracing in the treatment of fractures is to compensate for associated nerve injuries such as dropfoot secondary to peroneal palsy. Dynamic bracing also is frequently used in the after-treatment of hand injuries, both to compensate for nerve deficits and to stretch out contractures gently and restore joint motion.

INJURY AND THE LAW

A surgeon treating fractures must inevitably become involved with the law. On occasion patients sue for disabilities incurred; those injured at work are entitled to benefits under Workers' Compensation laws; and unhappily, some patients, discontented with the results of the surgeon's ministrations, may sue for malpractice. In addition, surgeons will also be asked to render independent medical opinions on patients treated by other surgeons.

Most physicians do not enjoy giving testimony in court and resent the time and effort in writing legal reports or filling out the routine reports for insurance companies. These duties can only be performed by physicians; and should they be carried out in a perfunctory manner, the patient will suffer, and the physician's professional competence may be brought into question in any ensuing litigation.

THE MEDICAL REPORT

For a variety of legal purposes, a medical report is necessary. Some examples of these reports do not support the contention that medicine is a learned profession. R.M. Fox,[154] a personal-injury attorney who has a somewhat slanted view of these matters, made a valid criticism: "No medical school in the United States today offers a course in medicolegal report writing, in spite of its obvious socioeconomic importance and the billions of dollars in the type of claim. Little, if any, postgraduate medical education on this subject is available."

A few words on the preparation of such reports would seem to be in order. If the report is on a patient other than our own, we make a practice of prefacing the report by naming the party who has requested the examination and the date on which this examination was performed. When the report is on our own patient, permission to release the information must be given by the patient.

History

Although the patient may give a lengthy account of the circumstances of the accident, only that which is germane to the assessment of his injury should be included in the report, and certainly no judgment as to culpability should appear in the medical report. Although the patient's account to a physician of the circumstances of the accident is inadmissible as evidence bearing on the actionable event itself, it will be admissible to the extent it is relevant in establishing the basis on which the physician's ultimate opinion is based. If, in some way, these notes are erroneous, they may damage the credibility of the patient or in some way influence the outcome of the case.

The past history of the patient must be recorded, especially where previous injury or disease is directly concerned in the production or aggravation of the problem being assessed. If the report is on a patient whom you have treated yourself, a detailed report of the initial examination and subsequent events should be included. The patient should be questioned regarding his current condition, and the nature, severity, duration, and frequency of his specific complaints should be listed and described.

Clinical Examination

The clinical examination is carried out in a meticulous manner. Notes are taken during the examination rather than depending on memory; care is taken to differentiate left from right. In most jurisdictions, the medical witness is permitted to refer to these notes to refresh his recollection, provided the notes were made at the time of the examination or shortly thereafter. Thorough notes can be invaluable for responding intelligently and consistently in the event of a far-reaching, extended cross examination. The sooner the formal report is dictated, the more accurate it will be. That which can be measured should be, with tape or goniometer. Scars should be noted, especially where they interfere with function or where cosmesis is important. Negative findings, where indicated, should also be noted.

Medical Assessment

After describing the medical findings in technical terms, we generally give a resumé of the findings in nontechnical, lay terms or translate the technical language as we go, depending on the complexity of the case. This is very helpful to the recipient of the report if he is a lawyer or other lay person. In the summation of the report the diagnoses should be listed, some opinion should be expressed about the compatibility of the patient's injuries with the patient's history of how they were incurred, and whether the complaints are consonant with the physical findings. There is no place, however, for gratuitous and unnecessarily pejorative remarks regarding the patient.

The prognosis should be discussed when it can be reasonably determined. No one can expect an absolutely accurate forecast of events, but an educated guess is much more helpful than saying that the prognosis is undetermined. The possible and probable end results and the length of time the patient is liable to be incapacitated should be estimated. If further surgery or rehabilitative treatment is necessary, this should be listed and justified.

Physical Impairment and Disability

In the event that the patient's condition is stable and no further treatment is indicated, many agencies and insurance companies will ask for an estimate of permanent disability, or permanent physical impairment expressed as a percentage. There is a distinction between these two terms. *Disability* is a measure of the loss of a person's ability to engage in his occupation or earn a living, and therefore is not a purely medical determination. *Physical impairment* is a measure of loss of function or assessment of anatomical defect, which is the same for all similar patients, irrespective of how they earn their living. To quote a hackneyed example: If two men each lost their left fifth fingers, their physical impairment would be identical. Were one a concert violinist and the other a manual laborer, their permanent disability would be vastly different. Obviously, disability has to be predicated on physical impairment, but the former is a legal determination and the latter, medical.

The physician is the final arbiter of physical impairment. He will be helped in this task by the use of various tables that have been devised by the American Medical Association, as well as other publications by authorities in the field.[27,246]

One should be prepared to show how the percentage of impairment was ascertained; it is not enough to pick a figure from the air or add another 20% because the patient is a sweet person or needs money badly. There are few functions undertaken by the orthopaedist that are more difficult and taxing than the fair, impartial determination of physical impairment.

TESTIMONY IN COURT

The large majority of personal-injury claims are settled out of court, and this process is facilitated in many instances by a comprehensive and lucid medical report. In those cases where settlement cannot be reached amicably, the surgeon will usually be asked to give a deposition prior to the formal trial. A *deposition* is a pretrial examination of a witness by the opposing attorneys without the presence of a judge. The proceedings are recorded by a court stenographer, and the evidence is given under oath. If the case goes to trial, the surgeon will answer the same or similar questions in more formal circumstances, or, in the event that he is unable to attend in person, the deposition may be entered as evidence. Should the medical witness give substantially different replies in court to similar questions asked in a deposition, one or either of the attorneys will pick up the discrepancy, and this will inevitably vitiate his testimony.

The attorney and physician who are brought together in litigation should have a common goal—to assist the court or jury in arriving at the truth. While this is a time-consuming and occasionally frustrating experience, it is absolutely necessary for the physician to educate the lawyer about the medical aspects of the case. Failure to do so may do a great disservice to the patient, because the lawyer may never ask the questions most pertinent to the case. Particularly close cooperation is essential when the physician's opinion, as is often the case, is based on a hypothetical question. The lawyer, in asking the hypothetical question on which the medical opinion will be based, must include all relevant material findings, including essential negative findings. On that assumed set of facts, the medical witness is asked, ''Do you have an opinion and, if so, what is that opinion?'' The most frequently encountered gambit in cross examination of the physician is to rephrase the hypothetical question with some omissions or possibly new inclusions. The experienced physician generally avoids these traps by paraphrasing the question by way of clarification (eg, ''Are you asking if my opinion would be different had the patient complained of sciatica at the time of my examination?'').

As a witness, one should testify to that which he believes to be true, and if he does not know the answer to the question or if it is beyond the area of his expertise, he should say so. Prior to a deposition the prudent physician refreshes his memory of the pertinent literature. While quotations from the medical texts or papers as such are not admissible as evidence, lawyers in many jurisdictions introduce such material in the process of cross examination and ask the medical witness if the authors are recognized authorities and if he agrees with the opinions they have expressed. The surgeon should be at least as well read as the attorney.

Not infrequently the attorney who has requested the surgeon to testify asks for a pretrial or predeposition conference in which he goes over the evidence, asks for clarifications, and reviews the questions he will ask. There is nothing unethical in such conferences, but the surgeon should not lose his objectivity and become a partisan for one side or the other. He is a witness, not an advocate.

In the adversary system of justice each attorney attempts to dispose of his opponent's arguments, and this may extend to discrediting the medical testimony, too. A lawyer is duty-bound to try to throw doubt on all evidence inimical to his case. This should not be construed as a personal attack by the medical witness.

It is sometimes said that lawyers try to make fools out of doctors on the witness stand. This they cannot do without generous help from the doctor himself. If he sticks to the facts of which he is sure, no lawyer will be able to shake his testimony. Many physicians go wrong by becoming advocates; they become emotionally involved. After losing their sangfroid on the witness stand, not only is their testimony suspect, but they look foolish, too. The duty of the medical witness is to state the facts of the case as he knows them, to offer his best medical opinion where he has sufficient grounds to formulate one, and to confine his testimony to what he is asked. Because juries are laymen, explanations should be as simple and straightforward as possible with a minimum of medical jargon. The witness's remarks should be addressed to the jury, because they, not the attorneys, are charged with the duty of determining the facts of the case and assessing the credibility of witnesses. In the rare event that a lawyer harries a medical witness, the opposing attorney or the judge will invariably intervene. To lose one's temper or argue with counsel is unprofessional and diminishes the value of one's testimony. At all times the medical witness should speak up clearly and distinctly and act like a member of a learned profession.

WORKERS' COMPENSATION

Workers' Compensation statutes vary from state to state, and the practicing physician should acquaint himself with the laws of his own state. In essence, these laws have been enacted to compensate employees injured while at work for loss of earnings and permanent disability. This compensation is paid by the employer or his insurance carrier, whether or not the employer was in any way negligent or whether the employee contributed to the accident by his own negligence. There is no attempt to compensate the employee for pain and suffering, but only for loss of earnings. Because Workers' Compensation claims are usually settled by a referee and the physician is normally not present at these hearings, the quality of the medical report is of major importance in the settlement of these claims.

PHYSICIAN LIABILITY

A physician is liable to be sued whenever a patient believes his treatment has been inadequate.

Whether these complaints have any substance is immaterial, and even the most careful and competent surgeon may be sued. It is commonly held by physicians that the present unhappy situation is related to the pernicious system of contingency payments to attorneys, but this overlooks the fact that the suit must be brought in the first place by a disgruntled patient. It seems to us that the causes for such actions are as outlined below.

Negligence

Many suits are related to the complications of tight or improperly applied casts, and precedents are so well established in such cases that the surgeon who does not take appropriate steps when a patient complains of pain under a cast is not only negligent, he is stupid. It is a pity that the five Ps of impending Volkmann's ischemia (pallor, pulselessness, pain, paresthesia, and paralysis) have been taught so well. The only one that is universally reliable is pain. Unreasonable pain in an immobilized limb must be investigated; the cast should be split to the degree that is necessary to relieve the patient's pain and, if necessary, the cast should be bivalved and the padding divided to the skin. If a compartment syndrome is likely, a decompression should be done without delay.

Another potent source of trouble is neglecting to make an x-ray examination of a painful area, so that a fracture goes undetected. The desire to spare the patient expense is a false economy, and the prudent surgeon makes such examinations even though he is reasonably sure that no fracture is present. He also must make sure that the examination is complete (eg, the hip and knee must be radiographed in fractures of the femur to rule out coexisting injuries of these joints). Furthermore, if the quality of the films is unsatisfactory, he must ensure that the examination is repeated and better films obtained. When a case is not progressing satisfactorily, the surgeon should not hesitate to call for assistance from more experienced or knowledgeable colleagues.

Undesirable Cosmetic or Functional Result

Even with the most assiduous care, it is impossible in all cases to restore an injured person to a condition comparable to that which he or she was in prior to the accident. The surgeon should make a realistic prognosis early on in his management so that no unrealistic expectations will be entertained by the patient or the patient's relatives. All operative procedures other than those life-saving measures that require action without delay should be discussed frankly with the patient and with the appropriate family members. The scope and aim of the procedure and a frank appraisal of the inherent risks should be explained, and this should be reflected in the operative permit that the patient signs.

Breakdown in Physician–Patient Rapport

Many suits, perhaps the majority, are engendered when a patient becomes angry because his doctor belittles or berates him or in some way shows a lack of concern, unapproachability, or off-handedness in his treatment. This may be of no importance when the result is good, but when the result is poor, it may be the factor that precipitates a suit. The patient should be treated as you would like your spouse or child to be treated in similar circumstances. A little kindness and encouragement costs nothing and improves rapport. Remember that the patient who irritates you the most is the one who is most liable to sue you. Gratuitous, pejorative descriptions of your patient in the chart will antagonize him if he reads it and may well identify you as a curmudgeon when read in court. In general, it is better to say that a patient "weighs 360 pounds" than to say that he is "grossly obese."

Remarks Critical of Treatment

The surgeon, another physician, or ancillary personnel can make remarks that can be construed as being critical of the treatment received. It goes without saying that everything that is said about treatment, especially that given by someone else, should be carefully worded, so that no pejorative inference may be picked up by the patient. Criticism of another without knowing all the circumstances is unfair and unjust, and the instigation of a lawsuit against another physician, unethical.

Medical Records

The best defense a surgeon has against groundless suits is obviously to give his patients competent, assiduous, and courteous service. The only way that this can be documented for legal purposes is by the completeness of the patient's records, both those in the hospital and in the surgeon's office. Voluminous notes may not prove the treatment has been excellent, but a paucity of records suggests a lack of care. In any case, the medical record may be the only evidence to corroborate the physician's story. The sooner these notes are written or dictated after the events they describe, the greater is their value. In many hospitals the dates of dictation and transcription appear on such documents as operative reports. Obviously an operative report dictated 3

months after the event does not carry as much weight in a court of law as one dictated immediately after the operation.

After a suit has been initiated, some misguided physicians attempt to doctor the record by additions or alterations. Almost always this is picked up by an alert attorney, and it damages the physician's case irreparably. Inevitably, errors creep into hospital records, owing to mistakes in transcription. When such errors are corrected, or when anything is added to the record, these additions should be dated and initialed. Considerable caution should be exercised where operative notes are dictated by an assistant. These should be read carefully, countersigned, and amended where necessary. It is even more prudent, however, for the surgeon to do his own dictation.

GOOD SAMARITAN LAWS

Some states have seen fit to enact legislation that exempts physicians from legal action as a result of their having given emergency medical treatment at the scene of an accident. Opinions vary as to whether such laws are really necessary. There is no legal compulsion for a physician to stop at any accident and give aid; but if he does so, he establishes a doctor–patient relationship and his conduct is then governed by what a reasonably prudent physician would do under similar circumstances. Suit being brought under these circumstances is highly unlikely and is even less likely to be sustained in a court of law, unless there has been gross mismanagement. The remote threat of a possible malpractice suit, at any rate, is a rather poor excuse for not carrying out one's obvious duty, and we feel that few physicians would refuse to render aid on this account.

REFERENCES

1. Adams, J.P.; Kenmore, P.I.; Russell, P.H.; and Haas, S.S.: Regional Anesthesia in the Upper Limb. *In* Adams, J.P. (ed.): Current Practice in Orthopaedic Surgery, Vol. 4, pp. 238–261. St. Louis, C.V. Mosby, 1969.
2. Albright, J.S.; Johnson, T.R.; and Saha, S.: Principles of Internal Fixation. *In* Ghista, D.N., and Roaf, R. (eds.): Orthopaedic Mechanics: Procedures and Devices, pp. 124–222. New York, Academic Press, 1978.
3. Allen, W.C.; Heiple, K.G.; and Burstein, A.H.: A Fluted Femoral Intramedullary Rod. J. Bone Joint Surg., 60A: 506–515, 1978.
4. Allen, W.C.; Piotrowski, G.; Burstein, A.H.; and Frankel, V.H.: Biomechanical Principles of Intramedullary Fixation. Clin. Orthop., 60:13–20, 1968.

5. Allgöwer, M., and Spiegel, P.: Internal Fixation of Fractures: Evolution of Concepts. Clin. Orthop., 138:26–29, 1979.

6. Allgöwer, M.: Modern Concepts of Fracture Treatment. AO/ASIF Dialogue, 1(1):1–3, 1985.

7. Allgöwer, M., and Sequin, F.: Dynamization of the AO/ASIF Tubular External Fixator. AO/ASIF Dialogue, 1(3):12–13, 1987.

8. Allgöwer, M.; Sequin, F.; and Ruedi, T.: Simplicity is the Rule of the Game: The AO/ASIF Tubular External Fixator. AO/ASIF Dialogue, 1(1):5–6, 1985.

9. Allgöwer, M.; Perren, S.; and Matter, P.: A New Plate for Internal Fixation—The Dynamic Compression Plate (DCP). Injury, 2:40–47, 1970.

10. Allum, R.L., and Mowbray, M.A.S.: A Retrospective Review of the Healing of Fractures of the Shaft of the Tibia with Special Reference to the Mechanism of Injury. Injury, 11:304–308, 1980.

11. Alms, M.: Fracture Mechanics. J. Bone Joint Surg., 43B:162–166, 1961.

12. Anderson, L.D.: Compression Plate Fixation and the Effect of Different Types of Internal Fixation on Fracture Healing. J. Bone Joint Surg., 47A:191–208, 1965.

13. Anderson, R.: An Automatic Method of Treatment for Fractures of the Tibia and the Fibula. Surg. Gynecol. Obstet., 58:639–646, 1934.

14. Anderson, J.T., and Gustilo, R.B.: Immediate Internal Fixation in Open Fractures. Orthop. Clin. North Am., 11(3):569–578, 1980.

15. Apley, A.G.: Fractures of the Lateral Tibial Condyle Treated by Skeletal Traction and Early Mobilization. J. Bone Joint Surg., 38B:699–708, 1956.

16. Aron, J.D.: Methylmethacrylate External Fixation Splints. Orthop. Rev., 9:35–44, 1978.

17. Arzimanoglou, A., and Skiadaressis, G.: Study of Internal Fixation by Screws of Oblique Fractures in Long Bones. J. Bone Joint Surg., 34A:219–223, 1952.

18. Ash, A.: Medico-legal Aspects of Traumatic Neurosis. Industrial Med. Surg., 37:30–36, 1968.

19. Ashton, H.: Effect of Inflatable Plastic Splints on Blood Flow. Br. Med. J., 2:1427–30, 1966.

20. Atkinson, D.I.; Modell, J.; and Moya, F.: Intravenous Regional Anesthesia. Anesth. Analg., 44:313–317, 1965.

21. Austin, R.T.: The Sarmiento Tibial Plaster: A Prospective Study of 145 Fractures. Injury, 13:10–22, 1981.

22. Bach, A.W., and Hansen, S.T., Jr.: Plate Versus External Fixation in Severe Open Tibial Fractures: A Randomized Trial. Clin. Orthop., 241:89–94, 1989.

23. Bagby, G.W., and Janes, J.M.: The Effect of Compression on the Rate of Fracture Healing Using a Special Plate. Am. J. Surg., 95:761–771, 1958.

24. Bagby, G.W.: Compression Bone-Plating: Historical Considerations. J. Bone Joint Surg., 59A:625–631, 1977.

25. Baker, J.; Frankel, V.H.; and Burstein, A.H.: Fatigue Fractures: Biomechanical Considerations (abstract). J. Bone Joint Surg., 54A:1345–46, 1972.

26. Barron, S.E.; Robb, R.A.; Taylor, W.F.; and Kelly, P.J.: The Effect of Fixation With Intramedullary Rods and Plates on Fracture-Site Blood Flow and Bone Remodeling in Dogs. J. Bone Joint Surg., 59A:376–385, 1977.

27. Bateman, J.E.: An Introduction to Disability Evaluation of the Extremities. Instr. Course Lect., XVII:332–336, 1960.

28. Baumgart, F.; Bensmann, G.; and Haaster, J.: Memory Alloys—New Material for Implantation in Orthopaedic Surgery. In Uhthoff, H.K. (ed.): Current Concepts of Internal Fixation of Fractures, pp. 122–127. New York, Springer-Verlag, 1980.

29. Beals, N.; Durham, G.; and Lynch, G.: Mechanical Characterizations of Interlocking Intramedullary Nails. Material Research Report ML-88-38, Richards Medical Company, Memphis, May 1988.

30. Beaupré, G.S.; Schneider, E.; and Perren, S.M.: Stress Analysis of a Partially Slotted Intramedullary Nail. J. Orthop. Res., 2:369–376, 1984.

31. Bechtol, C.O., and Lepper, H., Jr.: Fundamental Studies in the Design of Metal Screws for Internal Fixation of Bone (abstract). J. Bone Joint Surg., 38A:1385, 1956.

32. Beckenbaugh, R.D.: Colles' Fractures: A Closer Look. Cont. Ed., 13:19, 1980.

33. Becker, D.W., Jr.: Danger of Burns from Fresh Plaster Splints Surrounded by Too Much Cotton. Plast. Reconstr. Surg., 62:436–437, 1980.

34. Behrens, F.: A Primer of Fixator Devices and Configurations. Clin. Orthop., 241:5–14, 1989.

35. Behrens, F.: General Theory and Principles of External Fixation. Clin. Orthop., 241:15–23, 1989.

36. Behrens, F.: Unilateral External Fixation for Severe Lower Extremity Lesions: Experience with the ASIF (AO) Tubular Frame. In Seligson, D., and Pope, M.: Concepts in External Fixation, pp. 279–291. New York, Grune & Stratton, 1982.

37. Behrens, F., and Johnson, W.: Unilateral External Fixation: Methods to Increase and Reduce Frame Stiffness. Clin. Orthop., 241:48–56, 1989.

38. Behrens, F., and Searls, K.: External Fixation of the Tibia: Basic Concepts and Prospective Evaluation. J. Bone Joint Surg., 68B:246–254, 1986.

39. Behrens, F.; Johnson, W.D.; Koch, T.W.; and Kovacevic, N.: Bending Stiffness of Unilateral and Bilateral Fixator Frames. Clin. Orthop., 178:103–110, 1983.

40. Beyer, J.C. (ed.): Wound Ballistics. Dept. of the Army, Washington, D.C., Office of the Surgeon General, 1962.

41. Bielejeski, T., and Garrick, J.G.: Method of Cutting In Situ Metallic Appliances. J. Bone Joint Surg., 52A:585–587, 1970.

42. Black, J.: Metallic Ion Release and Its Relationship to Oncogenesis. In Fitzgerald, R.H., Jr (ed.): The Hip, pp. 199–213. St. Louis, C.V. Mosby, 1985.

43. Blakeslee, S.: New York Times, July 25, 1987:17–18.

44. Blockey, N.J.: An Observation Concerning the Flexor Muscles During Recovery of Function After Dislocation of the Elbow. J. Bone Joint Surg., 36A:833–840, 1954.

45. Bone, L.B.: Locked Intramedullary Nailing of Tibial Shaft Fractures. Techniques Orthop., 3:47–53, 1988.

46. Bone, L.B., and Johnson, K.D.: Treatment of Tibial Fractures by Reaming and Intramedullary Nailing. J. Bone Joint Surg., 68A:877–887, 1986.

47. Bowden, F.P.; Williamson, J.B.P.; and Laing, P.G.: The Significance of Metallic Transfer in Orthopaedic Surgery. J. Bone Joint Surg., 37B:676–690, 1955.

48. Brettle, J.: A Survey of the Literature on Metallic Surgical Implants. Injury, 2:26–39, 1970.

49. Brettle, J.; Hughes, A.N.; and Jordan, B.A.: Metallurgical Aspects of Surgical Implant Materials. Injury, 2:225–234, 1971.

50. Bromage, P.R.: Local Anaesthetic Procedures for the Arm and Hand. Surg. Clin. North Am., 44(4):919–923, 1964.

51. Brooker, A.F., Jr., and Edwards, C.C.: External Fixation: The Current State of the Art. Baltimore, Williams & Wilkins, 1979.

52. Brooker, A.F., Jr.: Brooker-Wills Nailing of Femoral Shaft Fractures. Techniques Orthop., 3:41–46, 1988.

53. Brooker, A.F., Jr., and Brumback, R.J.: Brooker-Wills Nails in Treatment of Infra-isthmal Injuries of the Femur. J. Trauma, 28:688–691, 1988.

54. Brooks, D.B.; Burstein, A.H.; and Frankel, V.H.: Biomechanics of Torsional Fractures: Stress Concentration Effect of a Drill Hole. J. Bone Joint Surg., 52A:507–514, 1970.

55. Brouwer, K.J.: Torsional Deformities After Fractures of the Femoral Shaft in Childhood: Retrospective Study, 27–32 Years After Trauma. Acta Orthop. Scand. (Suppl. 195), 52:79–163, 1981.

56. Brower, T.D.; Akahoshi, Y.; and Orlic, P.: The Diffusion of Dyes Through Articular Cartilage In Vivo. J. Bone Joint Surg., 44A:456–463, 1962.

57. Brown, P.W., and Urban, J.G.: Early Weight-Bearing Treatment of Open Fractures of the Tibia: An End Result of 63 Cases. J. Bone Joint Surg., 51A:59–75, 1969.

58. Brown, P.W.: The Fate of Exposed Bone. Am. J. Surg., 137:464–469, 1979.

59. Brown, R.F.: Compound Fractures of the Tibia—The Soft Tissue Defect. Proc. R. Soc. Med., 65:625–626, 1972.

60. Brown, S.A., and Mayor, M.B.: The Biocompatibility of Materials for Internal Fixation of Fractures. J. Biomed. Mater. Res., 12:67–82, 1978.

61. Browner, B.: Pitfalls, Errors, and Complications in the Use of Locking Kuntscher Nails. Clin. Orthop., 212:192–208, 1986.

62. Browner, B.D.; Burgess, A.R.; Robertson, R.J.; Baugher, W.H.; Freedman, M.T.; and Edwards, C.C.: Immediate Closed Antegrade Ender Nailing of Femoral Fractures in Polytrauma Patients. J. Trauma, 24:921–927, 1984.

63. Brumback, R.J.; Reilly, J.P.; Poka, A.; Lakatos, R.P.; Bathon, G.H.; and Burgess, A.R.: Intramedullary Nailing of Femoral Shaft Fractures: Part I. Decision-making Errors With Interlocking Fixation. J. Bone Joint Surg., 70A: 1441–52, 1988.

64. Brumback, R.J.; Bosse, M.J.; Poka, A.; and Burgess, A.R.: Intramedullary Stabilization of Humeral Shaft Fractures in Patients with Multiple Trauma. J. Bone Joint Surg., 68A:960–970, 1986.

65. Brumback, R.J.; Uwagie-Ero, S.; Lakatos, R.P.; Poka, A.; Bathon, G.H.; and Burgess, A.R.: Intramedullary Nailing of Femoral Shaft Fractures: Part II. Fracture-Healing With Static Interlocking Fixation. J. Bone Joint Surg., 70A: 1453–1462, 1988.

66. Bucholz, R.W.; Ross, S.E.; and Lawrence, K.L.: Fatigue Fracture of the Interlocking Nail in the Treatment of Fractures of the Distal Part of the Femoral Shaft. J. Bone Joint Surg., 69A:1391–99, 1987.

67. Bultitude, M.I.; Wellwood, J.M.; and Hollingsworth, R.P.: Intravenous Diazepam: Its Use in the Reduction of Fractures of the Lower End of the Radius. Injury, 3:249–253, 1972.

68. Burke, J.F.: The Effective Period of Preventive Antibiotic Action in Experimental Incisions and Dermal Lesions. Surgery, 50:161–168, 1961.

69. Burny, F.: The Pin as a Percutaneous Implant: General and Related Studies. Orthopedics, 7:610–615, 1984.

70. Burny, F.; Domb, M.; Donkerwolcke, M.; and Andrianne, Y.: Maximum Torque at the Time of Retrieval (MTR). Orthopedics, 7:627–628, 1984.

71. Burny, F.L.: Elastic External Fixation of Tibial Fractures: Study of 1421 Cases. *In* Brooker, A.F., and Edwards, C.C. (eds): External Fixation: The Current State of the Art, pp. 55–73, Baltimore, Williams & Wilkins, 1979.

72. Burstein, A.H.; Currey, J.; Frankel, V.H.; Heiple, K.G.; Lunseth, P.; and Vessely, J.C.: Bone Strength: The Effect of Screw Holes. J. Bone Joint Surg., 54A:1143–56, 1972.

73. Bynum, D., Jr.; Ray, D.R.; Boyd, C.L.; and Ledbetter, W.B.: Capacity of Installed Commercial Bone Fixation Plates. Am. J. Vet. Res., 32:783–791, 1971.

74. Byrd, H.S.; Cierny, G., III; and Tebbetts, J.B.: Management of Open Tibial Fractures with Associated Soft Tissue Loss: External Pin Fixation with Early Flap Coverage. Plast. Reconstr. Surg., 75:73–79, 1981.

75. Cahoon, J.R., and Paxton, H.W.: A Metallurgical Survey of Current Orthopaedic Implants. J. Biomed. Mater. Res., 4:223–244, 1970.

76. Caldwell, J.A.: Treatment of Fractures of the Shaft of the Humerus By Hanging Cast. Surg. Gynecol. Obstet., 70: 421–425, 1940.

77. Callahan, D.J.; Carney, D.J.; Daddario, N.; and Walter, N.E.: The Effect of Hydration Water Temperature on Orthopaedic Plaster Cast Strength. Orthopedics, 9:683–685, 1986.

78. Callahan, D.J.; Carney, D.J.; Daddario, N.; and Walter, N.E.: A Comparative Study of Synthetic Cast Material Strength. Orthopedics, 9:679–681, 1986.

79. Campbell, D., and Kempson, G.E.: Which External Fixation Device? Injury, 12:291–296, 1981.

80. Carter, D.R., and Hayes, W.C.: Compact Bone Fatigue Damage: A Microscopic Examination. Clin. Orthop., 127: 265–274, 1977.

81. Case, R.D.: Haematoma Block—A Safe Method of Reducing Colles' Fractures. Injury, 16:469–470, 1985.

82. Casey, M.J., and Chapman, M.W.: Ipsilateral Concomitant Fractures of the Hip and Femoral Shaft. J. Bone Joint Surg., 61A:503–509, 1979.

83. Cassebaum, W.H.: Open Reduction of T and Y Fractures of the Lower End of the Humerus. J. Trauma, 9:915–925, 1969.

84. Cater, W.H., and Hicks, J.H.: The Recent History of Corrosion in Metal Used for Internal Fixation. Lancet, 2:271, 871–873, 1956.

85. Chao, E.Y.S., and Hein, T.J.: Mechanical Performance of the Standard Orthofix External Fixator. Orthopedics, 11: 1057–69, 1988.

86. Chao, E.Y.S.; Aro, H.T.; Lewallen, D.G.; and Kelly, P.J.:

The Effect of Rigidity on Fracture Healing in External Fixation. Clin. Orthop., 241:24–35, 1989.

87. Chapman, M.W., and Mahoney, M.: The Role of Early Internal Fixation in the Management of Open Fractures. Clin. Orthop., 138:120–131, 1979.

88. Chapman, M.W.: The Use of Immediate Internal Fixation in Open Fractures. Orthop. Clin. North Am., 11(3):579–591, 1980.

89. Chapman, M.W.: The Role of Intramedullary Fixation in Open Fractures. Clin. Orthop, 212:26–34, 1986.

90. Charnley, J.: The Closed Treatment of Common Fractures, 3rd ed. Edinburgh, E. & S. Livingston, 1968.

91. Christensen, J.; Greiff, J.; and Rosendahl, S.: Fractures of the Shaft of the Tibia Treated with AO-Compression Osteosynthesis. Injury, 13:307–314, 1982.

92. Christensen, K.S.; Frautner, S.; Stickel, M.; and Nielsen, J.F.: Inflatable Splints: Do They Cause Tissue Ischaemia? Injury, 17:167–170, 1986.

93. Christie, J.: Surgical Heat Injury of Bone. Injury, 13:188–190, 1981.

94. Clarke, R.: Assessment of Blood Loss Following Injury. Br. J. Clin. Pract., 10:746–769, 1956.

95. Clarke, R.; Fisher, M.R.; Topley, E.; and Davies, J.W.L.: Extent and Time of Blood Loss After Civilian Injury. Lancet, 2:381–385, 1961.

96. Clarke, R.; Topley, E.; and Flear, C.T.G.: Assessment of Blood Loss in Civilian Trauma. Lancet, 1:629–638, 1955.

97. Clawson, D.K.; Smith, R.F.; and Hansen, S.T.: Closed Intramedullary Nailing of the Femur. J. Bone Joint Surg., 53A:681–692, 1971.

98. Clifford, R.P.; Lyons, T.J.; and Webb, J.K.: Complications of External Fixation of Open Fractures of the Tibia. Injury, 18:174–176, 1987.

99. Cochran, G. vanB.: Kilograms and Kilopounds: Mass Force or Weight? J. Bone Joint Surg., 53A:181–182, 1971.

100. Cohen, J.: Corrosion Testing of Orthopaedic Implants. J. Bone Joint Surg., 44A:307–316, 1962.

101. Cohn, B.T., and Bilfield, L.: Fatigue Fracture of a Tibial Interlocking Nail. Orthopedics, 9:1215–18, 1986.

102. Connes, H.: The Hoffman External Fixation Techniques: Indications and Results. Paris, Editions Gead, 1977.

103. Connolly, J.F.: Torsional Fractures and the Third Dimension of Fracture Management. South Med. J., 73:884–891, 1980.

104. Connolly, J.F.; Whittaker, D.; and Williams, E.: Femoral and Tibial Fractures Combined with Injuries to the Femoral or Popliteal Artery: A Review of the Literature and Analysis of 14 Cases. J. Bone Joint Surg., 53A:56–68, 1971.

105. Connolly, J.: Management of Fractures Associated with Arterial Injuries. Am. J. Surg., 120:331, 1970.

106. Cooney, W.P., III; Fitzgerald, R.H., Jr.; Dobyns, J.H.; and Washington, J.A., II: Quantitative Wound Cultures in Upper Extremity Trauma. J. Trauma 22:112–117, 1982.

107. Cornelissen, M.; Burny, F.; VanderPerre, G.; and Donkerwolcke, M.: Standardized Method to Measure the Fixation Quality of a Pin: Theoretical Derivation and Preliminary Results. Orthopedics, 7:623–626, 1984.

108. Coutts, R.E.; Adeson, W.H.; Woo, S.L.-Y; Matthews, J.V.; Gonsalves, M.; and Amiel, D.: Comparison of Stainless Steel and Composite Plates in the Healing of Diaphyseal Osteotomies of the Dog Radius. Orthop. Clin. North Am., 7:223–229, 1976.

109. Currey, J.D.: The Mechanical Properties of Bone. Clin. Orthop., 73:210–231, 1970.

110. Danckwardt-Lillieström, G.: Reaming of the Medullary Cavity and Its Effect on Diaphyseal Bone. Acta Orthop. Scand. (Suppl.), 128: 1969.

111. Danckwardt-Lillieström, G.; Lorenzi, L.; and Olerud, S.: Intracortical Circulation After Intramedullary Reaming With Reduction of Pressure in the Medullary Cavity: A Microangiographic Study on the Rabbit Tibia. J. Bone Joint Surg., 52A:1390–1394, 1970.

112. Davis, A.D.; Meyer, R.D.; Miller, M.E.; and Killian, J.T.: Closed Zickel Nailing. Clin. Orhop., 201:138–146, 1985.

113. DeBastiani, G.; Aldeghiri, R.; and Brivio, L.R.: The Treatment of Fractures with a Dynamic Axial Fixator. J. Bone Joint Surg., 66B:538–545, 1984.

114. deBruijn, H.P.: Functional Treatment of Colles' Fracture. Acta Orthop. Scand., (Suppl. 223) 58: 1987.

115. Dehne, E.: Treatment of Fractures of the Tibial Shaft. Clin. Orthop., 66:159–173, 1969.

116. Dehne, E.; Deffer, P.A.; Hall, R.M.; Brown, P.W.; and Johnson, E.V.: The Natural History of the Fractured Tibia. Surg. Clin. North Am., 41:1495–1513, 1961.

117. DeJong, R.H.: Axillary Block of the Brachial Plexus. Anesthesiology, 22:215–225, 1961.

118. Delgado, E.R.: Sarcoma Following a Surgically Treated Fractured Tibia: A Case Report. Clin Orthop., 12:315–318, 1958.

119. DeMuth, W.E., and Smith, J.M.: High-Velocity Bullet Wounds of Muscle and Bone: The Basis of Rational Early Treatment. J. Trauma, 6:744–755, 1966.

120. Devas, M. (ed.): Geriatric Orthopaedics. New York, Academic Press, 1977.

121. Devas, M.B.: Stress Fractures. Practitioner, 197:70–76, 1966.

122. Devas, M.B.: Compression Stress Fractures in Man and the Greyhound. J. Bone Joint Surg., 43B:540–551, 1961.

123. Diacke, A.W.; Schultz, R.D.; and Nohlgren, J.E.: Technique for Quantifying Low-Temperature Burns. J. Surg. Res., 4: 270–274, 1964.

124. Dimond, F.C., Jr., and Rich, N.M.: M-16 Rifle Wounds in Vietnam. J. Trauma, 7:619–625, 1967.

125. Dinley, R.J., and Michelinakis, E.: Local Anaesthesia in the Reduction of Colles' Fracture. Injury, 4:345–346, 1973.

126. Disegi, J.A., and Wyss, H.: Implant Materials for Fracture Fixation: A Clinical Perspective. Orthopedics, 12:75–79, 1989.

127. Dodge, H.S., and Cady, G.W.: Treatment of Fractures of the Radius and Ulna With Compression Plates. J. Bone Joint Surg., 54A:1167–76, 1972.

128. Dodion, P.; Putz, P.; Amiri-Lamraski, M.H.; Efira, A.; deMartelaere, E.; and Heimann, R.: Immunoblastic Lymphoma at the Site of an Infected Vitallium Bone Plate. Histopathology, 6:807–813, 1982.

129. Dube, V.E., and Fisher, D.E.: Hemangioendothelioma of the Leg Following Metallic Fixation of the Tibia. Cancer, 30:1260–66, 1972.

130. Dugas, R., and D'Ambrosia, R.: Civilian Gunshot Wounds. Orthopedics, 8:1121–25, 1985.

131. Dugas, R., and D'Ambrosia, R.: The Grosse-Kempf Interlocking Nail: Technique of Femoral and Tibial Fractures. Orthopedics, 8:1363–70, 1985.

132. Edwards, C.C.; Jaworski, M.F.; Solana, J.; and Aronson, B.S.: Management of Compound Tibial Fractures Using External Fixation. Am. Surg., 45:190–203, 1979.

133. Eggers, G.W.N.: Internal Contact Splint. J. Bone Joint Surg., 30A:40–52, 1948.

134. Ekeland, A.; Thoresen, B.O.; Alho, A.; Strømsøe, K.; Folleras, G.; and Haukebø, A.: Interlocking Intramedullary Nailing in the Treatment of Tibial Fractures: A Report of 45 cases. Clin. Orthop., 231:205–215, 1988.

135. Ekholm, R.: Nutrition of Articular Cartilage: A Radioautographic Study. Acta Anat., 24:329–338, 1955.

136. Elabdien, B.S.Z.; Olerud, S.; and Karlström, G.: Ender Nailing of Pretrochanteric Fractures: Results at Follow-up Evaluation After One Year. Clin. Orthop., 191:53–63, 1984.

137. Emergency War Surgery (NATO Handbook). U.S. Dept. of Defense, Washington, D.C., United States Government Printing Office, 1958.

138. Ender, J., and Simon-Weidner, R.: Die Fixierung der trochantaren Brucke mit runden elastischen condylennagein. Acta Chir. Austriaca, 2:40–42, 1970.

139. Enneking, W.F., and Horowitz, M.: The Intra-articular Effects of Immobilization on the Human Knee. J. Bone Joint Surg., 54A:973–985, 1972.

140. Epps, C.H., Jr., and Adams, J.P.: Wound Management in Open Fractures. Am. Surgeon, 27:766–769, 1961.

141. Eriksson, E., and Wallin, C.: Immediate or Delayed Kuntscher-Rodding of Femoral Shaft Fractures. Orthopedics, 9:201–204, 1986.

142. Evans, E.B.; Eggers, G.W.N.; Butler, J.K.; and Blumel, J.: Experimental Immobilization of Rat Knee Joint. J. Bone Joint Surg., 42A:737–758, 1960.

143. Evans, E.M.: Fractures of the Radius and Ulna. J. Bone Joint Surg., 33B:548–561, 1951.

144. Evans, E.M.: Supracondylar-Y Fractures of the Humerus. J. Bone Joint Surg., 35B:381–385, 1953.

145. Evans, F.G.: Relation of the Physical Properties of Bone to Fractures. Instr. Course Lect., XVIII:110–121, 1961.

146. Ferguson, A.B., Jr., and Laing, P.G.: Corrosion and Corrosion-Resistant Metals in Orthopaedic Surgery. Instr. Course Lect., XV:96–103, 1958.

147. Finsterbush, A., and Friedman, B.: Reversibility of Joint Changes Produced by Immobilization in Rabbits. Clin. Orthop., 111:290–298, 1975.

148. Fisher, M.R.: Clinical Signs Following Injury in Relation to Red Cell and Total Blood Volume. Clin. Sci., 17:181–204, 1958.

149. Fitzgerald, J.A.W.: The Management of Fractures of Ipsilateral Patella and Femur. Injury, 1:287–292, 1970.

150. Fitzgerald, J.A.W., and Southgate, G.W.: Cerclage Wiring in the Management of Comminuted Fractures of the Femoral Shaft. Injury, 18:111–116, 1987.

151. Fleming, B.; Paley, D.; Kristiansen, T.; and Pope, M.: A Biomechanical Analysis of the Ilizarov External Fixator. Clin. Orthop., 241:95–105, 1989.

152. Fogelberg, E.V.; Zetzmann, E.K.; and Stinchfield, F.E.: Prophylactic Penicillin in Orthopaedic Surgery. J. Bone Joint Surg., 52A:95–98, 1970.

153. Forbes, G.B.: Staphylococcal Infection of Operation Wounds with Special Reference to Topical Antibiotic Prophylaxis. Lancet, 2:505–509, 1961.

154. Fox, R.M.: The Medicolegal Report Theory and Practice. Boston, Little, Brown, & Co., 1969.

155. Frankel, V.H., and Burstein, A.H.: Orthopaedic Biomechanics. Philadelphia, Lea & Febiger, 1970.

156. Franklin, J.L.; Winquist, R.A.; Benirschke, S.K.; and Hansen, S.R., Jr.: Broken Intramedullary Nails. J. Bone Joint Surg., 70A:1463–71, 1988.

157. Freeman, M.A.R.; Todd, R.C.; and Pirie, C.J.: The Role of Fatigue in the Pathogenesis of Senile Femoral Neck Fractures. J. Bone Joint Surg., 56B:698–702, 1974.

158. Gallinaro, P., and Biasibetti, A.: External Fixation—Why, Which, When? In Ilizarov Techniques: Manual for the Course Sponsored by the Program of Continuing Medical Education, University of Maryland School of Medicine, May 16–18, 1988.

159. Garfin, S.R.; Mubarak, S.J.; Evans, K.L.; Hargens, A.R.; and Akeson, W.H.: Quantification of Intracompartmental Pressure and Volume Under Plaster Cast. J. Bone Joint Surg., 63A:449–453, 1981.

160. Garland, D.E.; Chick, R.; Taylor, J.; and Salisbury, R.B.: Treatment of Proximal-Third Femur Fractures with Pins and Thigh Plaster. Clin. Orthop., 160:86–93, 1981.

161. Ger, R.: The Management of Pretibial Skin Loss. Surgery, 63:757–763, 1968.

162. Ger, R.: The Management of Open Fractures of the Tibia with Skin Loss. J. Trauma, 10:112–121, 1970.

163. Gingrass, R.P.; Close, A.S.; and Ellison, E.H.: The Effect of Various Topical and Parenteral Agents on the Prevention of Infection in Experimental Contaminated Wounds. J. Trauma, 4:763–783, 1964.

164. Gissane, W.: Symposium on the Treatment of Fractures of the Shafts of the Long Bones. Proc. R. Soc. Med., 52: 291–295, 1959.

165. Gleis, G.E.; Frederick, L.D.; and Johnson, J.R.: Biomechanical Stability of Distally Blocked Femoral Fractures: Is One Screw Enough? Techniques Orthop., 3:6–8, 1988.

166. Godina, M.: The Tailored Latissimus Dorsi Free Flap. Plast. Reconstr. Surg., 80:304–306, 1987.

167. Goto, M., and Ogata, K.: Experimental Study on Thermal Burns Caused by Plaster Bandage. Nippon Seikeigeka Gakkai Zasshi, 60:671–680, 1986.

168. Gottfries, A.; Hagert, C.G.; and Sorensen, S.E.: T- and Y-Fractures of the Tibial Condyles: A Follow-up Study of Cases Treated by Closed Reduction and Surgical Fixation With a Wire Loop. Injury, 3:56–63, 1971.

169. Grana, W.A., and Kopta, J.A.: The Roger Anderson Device in the Treatment of Fractures of the Distal End of the Radius. J. Bone Joint Surg., 61A:1234–38, 1979.

170. Grana, W.A.; Gruel, J.; Wedro, B.; and Hollingsworth, S.: Complications of Ipsilateral Femur and Tibia Fractures. Orthopedics, 7:825–828, 1984.

171. Green, C.A., and Matthews, L.S.: The Thermal Effects of Skeletal Fixation Pin Placement in Human Bone (abstract). Trans. Orthop. Res. Soc., 6:103, 1981.

172. Greener, E., and Lautenschlager, E.: Materials for Bioengineering Applications. *In* Brown, J.H.V.; Jacobs, J.E.; and Stark, L. (eds.): Biomedical Engineering, Philadelphia, F.A. Davis, 1971.

173. Griffiths, D.L.: Hazards of Closed Reduction of Fractures. Tex. Med., 642:46–50, 1968.

174. Groshar, D.; Lam, M.; Even-Sapir, E.; Israel, O.; and Front, D.: Stress Fractures and Bone Pain: Are They Closely Associated? Injury, 16:526–528, 1985.

175. Gurtler, R.A.; Jacobs, R.R.; and Jacobs, C.R.: Biomechanical Evaluation of the Ender's Pins, the Harris Nail, and the Dynamic Hip Screw for the Unstable Intertrochanteric Fracture. Clin. Orthop., 206:109–112, 1986.

176. Gustilo, R.B.: Use of Antimicrobials in the Management of Open Fractures. Arch. Surg., 114:805–808, 1979.

177. Gustilo, R.B.; Simpson, L.; Nixon, R.; Ruiz, A.; and Indeck, W.: Analysis of 511 Open Fractures. Clin. Orthop., 66:148–154, 1969.

178. Haasters, J.; Vensmann, G.; and Baumgart, F.: Memory Alloys—New Material for Implantation in Orthopaedic Surgery: Part II. *In* Uhthoff, H.K. (ed.): Current Concepts of Internal Fixation of Fractures, pp. 128–135. New York, Springer-Verlag, 1980.

179. Hägglund, G.; Hansson, L.T.; and Norman, O.: Correction by Growth of Rotational Deformity After Femoral Fracture in Children. Acta Orthop. Scand., 54:858–861, 1983.

180. Häggmark, T.; Eriksson, E.; and Jansson, E.: Muscle Fiber Type Changes in Human Skeletal Muscle After Injuries and Immobilization. Orthopedics, 9:181–185, 1986.

181. Häggmark, T.; Liedberg, H.; Ericksson, E.; and Wredmark, T.: Calf Muscle Atrophy and Muscle Function After Nonoperative vs Operative Treatment of Achilles Tendon Ruptures. Orthopedics, 9:160–164, 1986.

182. Hall, R.F., and Pankovich, A.M.: Ender Nailing of Acute Fracture of the Humerus. J. Bone Joint Surg., 69A:558–567, 1987.

183. Hanks, G.A.; Foster, W.C.; and Cardea, J.A.: Treatment of Femoral Shaft Fractures With the Brooker-Wills Interlocking Intramedullary Nail. Clin. Orthop., 226:206–218, 1988.

184. Hardaker, W.T., Jr.; Ward, W.T.; and Goldner, J.L.: External Fixation in the Management of Severe Musculoskeletal Trauma. Orthopaedics, 4:437–444, 1981.

185. Hardy, N.; Burny, F.; and Deutsch, G.A.: Pin Tract Histological Study: Preliminary Clinical Investigations. Orthopedics, 7:616–618, 1984.

186. Harris, J.D.; Kenwright, J.; Evans, M.; Tanner, K.E.; and Gwillim, J.: Control of Movement and Fracture Stiffness Monitoring With External Fixation. Orthopedics, 7:485–490, 1984.

187. Harrison, J.W.; McLain, D.L.; Holm, R.B.; Wilson, G.P., III; Chalman, J.A.; and MacGowan, K.N.: Osteosarcoma Associated With Metallic Implants: Report of Two Cases in Dogs. Clin. Orthop., 116:253–257, 1976.

187A. Hart, M.B.; Wu H.-J.; Chao, E.Y.S.; Kelly, P.J.: External Skeletal Fixation of Canine Tibial Osteotomies. Compression Compared With No Compression. J. Bone Joint Surg., 67A:598–605, 1985.

188. Hassard, H.: Medical Malpractice: Risks, Protection, Prevention. Oradell, NJ, Medical Economics Book Division, 1966.

189. Hayes, W.C., and Perren, S.M.: Plate-Bone Friction in the Compression Fixation of Fractures. Clin. Orthop., 89:236–240, 1972.

190. Heiple, K.G.; Brooks, D.B.; Samson, B.L.; and Burstein, A.H.: A Fluted Intramedullary Rod for Subtrochanteric Fractures: Biomechanical Considerations and Preliminary Clinical Result. J. Bone Joint Surg., 61A:730–737, 1979.

191. Henry, S.L.; Ostermann, P.A.W.; and Seligson, D.: Prophylactic Management of Open Fractures with the Antibiotic Bead Pouch Technique. Presented at the Orthopaedic Trauma Association Meeting, Dallas, Tex., Oct. 27, 1988. (In press.)

192. Henry, S.L., and Seligson, D.: The Küntscher Y-Nail for Trochanteric Fractures of the Hip. Semin. Orthop., 1:232–241, 1986.

193. Henry, S.L.; Williams, M.; and Seligson, D.: The Williams Interlocking Y-Nail for Fixation of Proximal Femoral Fractures. Techniques Orthop., 3:25–32, 1988.

194. Hey-Groves, E.W.: Methods and Results of Transplantation of Bone in the Repair of Defects Caused by Injury or Disease. Br. J. Surg., 5:185–242, 1918.

195. Hey-Groves, E.W.: Modern Methods of Treating Fractures. New York, William Wood, 1922.

196. Hicks, J.H.: Letter to the Editor. Injury, 4:361, 1973.

197. Hicks, J.H.: External Splintage as a Cause of Movement in Fractures. Lancet, 1:667–670, 1960.

198. Hicks, J.H.: High Rigidity in Fractures of the Tibia. Injury, 3:121–134, 1971.

199. Hicks, J.H.: The Fallacy of the Fractured Clavicle. Lancet, 1:131–132, 1958.

200. Hicks, J.H.: The Influence of Arbuthnot Lane on Fracture Treatment. Injury, 1:314–316, 1970.

201. Hicks, J.H., and Cater, W.H.: Minor Reactions Due to Modern Metals. J. Bone Joint Surg., 44B:122–128, 1962.

202. Hierholzer, G.; Rüedi, T.; Allgöwer, M.; and Schatzker, J.: Manual on the AO/ASIF Tubular External Fixator. New York, Springer-Verlag, 1985.

203. Hoffmann, R.: Retules à os pour la reduction dirigée, non saglante, des fractures (osteotaxis). Helv. Med. Acta, 5:844–850, 1938.

204. Höjer, H.; Gillquist, J.; and Liljedahl, S.-O.: Combined Fractures of Femoral and Tibial Shafts in the Same Limb. Injury, 8:206–212, 1977.

205. Holden, C.E.A.: The Role of Blood Supply to Soft Tissue in the Healing of Diaphyseal Fractures. J. Bone Joint Surg., 54A:993–1000, 1972.

206. Hollingsworth, A.; Wallace, W.A.; Dabir, R.; Ellis, S.J.; and Smith, A.F.M.: Comparison of Bupivacaine and Prilocaine Used in Bier Block: A Double-Blind Trial. Injury, 13:331–336, 1982.

207. Hollmen, A., and Mononen, P.: Axillary Plexus Block with Etidocaine. Acta Anaesth. Scand. (Suppl.), 60:25–28, 1975.

208. Holst-Nielson, F.: Dynamic Intramedullary Osteosynthesis in Fractures of the Femoral Shaft. Acta Orthop. Scand., 43:411–420, 1972.

209. Hooper, G.; Buxton, R.A.; and Gillespie, W.J.: Isolated

Fractures of the Shaft of the Tibia. Injury, 12:283–287, 1981.

210. Hooper, G.J., and Lyon, D.W.: Closed Unlocked Nailing for Comminuted Femoral Fractures. J. Bone Joint Surg., 70B:619–621, 1988.

211. Howse, A.J.G.: Orthopaedists Aid Ballet. Clin. Orthop., 89:52–63, 1972.

212. Huckstep, R.L.: The Huckstep Interlocking Nail for Difficult Humeral, Forearm, and Tibial Fractures and for Arthrodesis. Techniques Orthop., 3:77–87, 1988.

213. Huckstep, R.L.: The Huckstep Intramedullary Compression Nail: Indications, Technique, and Results. Clin. Orthop., 212:48–61, 1986.

214. Hughes, A.N., and Jordon, B.A.: The Mechanical Properties of Surgical Bone Screws and Some Aspects of Insertion Practice. Injury, 4:25–38, 1972.

215. Hughes, L.J., and Jackson, M.S.: Use of the Wagner Apparatus in Fractures of the Femur. Presented at the 46th Annual Meeting of the American Academy of Orthopaedic Surgeons, San Francisco, Feb. 22–24, 1979.

216. Hughston, J.C.: Fractures of the Distal Radial Shaft: Mistakes in Management. J. Bone Joint Surg., 39A:249–264, 1957.

217. Hughston, J.C.: Fractures of the Forearm: Anatomical Considerations. J. Bone Joint Surg., 44A:1664–67, 1962.

218. Hunter, S.G.: Deformation of Femoral Intramedullary Nails: A Clinical Study. Clin. Orthop., 171:83–86, 1982.

219. Husted, C.M.: Technique of Cast Wedging in Long Bone Fractures. Orthop. Rev., XV:373–378, 1986.

220. Hutzschenreuter, P.; Perren, S.M.; Steinemann, S.; Geret, V.; and Klebl, M.: Some Effects of Rigidity of Internal Fixation on the Healing Pattern of Osteotomies. Injury, 1:77–81, 1969.

221. Ilizarov, G.A., and Frankel, V.H.: The Ilizarov External Fixator: A Physiologic Method of Orthopaedic Reconstruction and Skeletal Correction. A Conversation with Prof. G.A. Ilizarov and Victor H. Frankel, M.D., Ph.D. Orthop. Rev., 17:1142–1154, 1988.

222. Inoue, S.A.; Ichida, M.; Imai, R.; Suzu, F.; Ohashi, J.; and Sakakida, K.: External Skeletal Fixation Using Methylmethacrylate-Technique and Indication with Clinical Report. Int. Orthop. (SICOT), 1:64–69, 1977.

223. Jacob, C.H.; Berry, J.T.; Pope, M.H.; and Hoaglund, F.T.: A Study of the Bone Machining Process Drilling. J. Biomech., 9:343–349, 1976.

224. Jacobs, C.H.; Pope, M.H.; Berry, J.T.; and Hoaglund, F.T.: A Study of the Bone Machining Process—Orthogonal Cutting. J. Biomech., 7:131–136, 1974.

225. Jenkins, N.H.; Jones, D.G.; Johnson, S.R.; and Mintowt-Czyz, W.J.: External Fixation of Colles' Fractures: An Anatomical Study. J. Bone Joint Surg., 69B:207–211, 1987.

226. Jensen, J.S.; Hansen, F.W.; and Johansen, J.: Tibial Shaft Fractures: A Comparison of Conservative Treatment and Internal Fixation with Conventional Plates or AO Compression Plates. Acta Orthop. Scand., 48:204–212, 1977.

227. Jensen, J.S.; Johansen, J.; and Morch, A.: Middle-Third Femoral Fractures Treated with Medullary Nailing or AO Compression Plates. Injury, 8:174–181, 1977.

228. Johnson, K.D.; Tencer, A.F.; Blumenthal, S.; August, A.; and Johnston, D.W.C.: Biomechanical Performance of Locked Intramedullary Nail Systems in Comminuted Femoral Shaft Fractures. Clin. Orthop., 206:151–161, 1986.

229. Jones, C.B.; Wright, K.J.W.; and Scott, W.A.: An In Vitro Investigation Into the Biomechanical Status of Nylon Cerclage Bands. J. Bone Joint Surg. (abstract), 66B:278, 1984.

230. Jones, D.G.: Bone Erosion Beneath Partridge Bands. J. Bone Joint Surg., 68B:476–477, 1986.

231. Jones, R.: An Orthopaedic View of the Treatment of Fractures. Am. J. Orthop. Surg., 11:314–335, 1913.

232. Kaplan, S.S.: Burns Following Application of Plaster Splint Dressings. Report of Two Cases. J. Bone Joint Surg., 63A:670–672, 1981.

233. Karlström, G., and Olerud, S.: Percutaneous Pin Fixation of Open Tibial Fractures. J. Bone Joint Surg., 57A:915–924, 1975.

234. Karlström, G., and Olerud, S.: Secondary Internal Fixation: Experimental Studies on Revascularization and Healing in Osteotomized Rabbit Tibias. Acta Orthop. Scand. (Suppl), 175: 1979.

235. Kasdan, M.L.; Kleinert, H.E.; Kasdan, A.P.; and Kutz, J.E.: Axillary Block Anesthesia for Surgery of the Hand. Plast. Reconstr. Surg., 46:256–261, 1970.

236. Kellam, J.F.: The Role of External Fixation in Pelvic Disruption. Clin. Orthop., 241:66–82, 1989.

237. Kelly, P.J., and Lipscomb, P.R.: Primary Vitallium-Mold Arthroplasty for Posterior Dislocation of the Hip with Fracture of the Femoral Head. J. Bone Joint Surg., 40A:675–680, 1958.

238. Kelly, R.P., and Griffin, T.W.: Open Reduction of T-Condylar Fractures of the Humerus Through an Anterior Approach. J. Trauma, 9(11):901–914, 1969.

239. Kelly, R.P., and Yarbrough, S.H., III: Posterior Fracture–Dislocation of the Femoral Head with Retained Medial Head Fragment. J. Trauma, 11(2):97–108, 1971.

240. Kempf, I.; Grosse, A.; and Beck, G.: Closed Locked Intramedullary Nailing: Its Application to Comminuted Fractures of the Femur. J. Bone Joint Surg., 67A:709–720, 1985.

241. Kempf, I.; Grosse, A.; and Lafforgue, D.: L'apport due verrouillage dans l'enclousage centre-medullaire des os longs. Rev. Chir. Orthop., 64:635–651, 1978.

242. Kempson, G.E., and Campbell, D.: The Comparative Stiffness of External Fixation Frames. Injury, 12:297–304, 1981.

243. Kenwright, J.; Goodship, A.; and Evans, M.: The Influence of Intermittent Micromovement Upon the Healing of Experimental Fractures. Orthopedics, 7:481–484, 1984.

244. Kenwright, J., and Goodship, A.E.: Controlled Mechanical Stimulation in the Treatment of Tibial Fractures. Clin. Orthop., 241:36–47, 1989.

245. Keon-Cohen, B.T.: Fractures at the Elbow. J. Bone Joint Surg., 48A:1623–39, 1966.

246. Kessler, H.H.: Disability-Determination and Evaluation. Philadelphia, Lea & Febiger, 1970.

247. Key, J.A., and Reynolds, F.C.: The Treatment of Infection After Medullary Nailing. Surgery, 35:749–757, 1964.

248. Kia, D., and Dragstedt, L.R., II: Prevention of Likely Wound Infections: Prophylactic Closed Antibiotic-Detergent Irrigation. Arch. Surg., 100:229–231, 1970.

249. Kleinert, H.E.; DeSimone, K.; Gaspar, H.E.; Arnold, R.E.; and Kasdan, M.L.: Regional Anesthesia for Upper Extremity Surgery. J. Trauma, 3:3–12, 1963.

250. Klemm, K.W., and Borner, M.: Interlocking Nailing of Complex Fractures of the Femur and Tibia. Clin. Orthop., 212:89–100, 1986.

251. Klemm, K., and Schellman, W.D.: Dynamische und Statische Verriegkling des margnagels. Unfallheikunde, 75:568–575, 1972.

252. Knapp, U.: Synthetic Skin Substitute in the Treatment of Wounds Marked by Loss of Substance. Chir. Praxis, 23:173–183, 1977–78.

253. Knapp, U., and Weller, S.: Care of Soft Tissues in Open Fractures. Akt. Traumatol. 8:319–327, 1978.

254. Kolmert, L.: A Method of Fixation of Femoral Fractures Below Previous Hip Implants. J. Trauma, 27:407–410, 1987.

255. Koranyi, E.; Bowman, C.E.; Knechi, C.D.; and Janssen, M.: Holding Power of Orthopaedic Screws in Bone. Clin. Orthop., 72:283–286, 1970.

256. Kubba, R.; Taylor, J.S.; and Marks, K.E.: Cutaneous Complications of Orthopaedic Implants: Two Year Prospective Study. Arch. Dermatol., 117:554–560, 1981.

257. Kumar, P.; Bryan, C.E.; Leech, S.H.; Mathews, R.; Bowler, J.; and D'Ambrosia, R.D.: Metal Hypersensitivity in Total Joint Replacement: Review of the Literature and Practical Guidelines for Evaluating Prospective Recipients. Orthopaedics 6:1455–1458, 1983.

258. Küntscher, G.: Die Marknagelung von Knochenbruchen. Tierexpinentaller Teil. Klin. Schr., 19:6–10, 1940.

259. Küntscher, G.: Practice of Intramedullary Nailing. Springfield, Ill., Charles C. Thomas, 1967.

260. Küntscher, G.: The Intramedullary Nailing of Fractures. Clin. Orthop., 60:5–12, 1968.

261. Küntscher, G.: The Küntscher Method of Intramedullary Fixation. J. Bone Joint Surg., 40A:17–26, 1958.

262. Kuo, P.O.; Yang, P.; Zhang, Y.; Yang, H.; Yu, Y.; Dai, K.; Hong, W.; Ke, M.; Cai, T.; and Tao, J.: The Use of Nickel–Titanium Alloy in Orthopaedic Surgery in China. Orthopedics, 12:111–116, 1984.

263. Kyle, R.F.: Biomechanics of Intramedullary Fracture Fixation. Orthopedics, 8:1356–1359, 1985.

264. Lane, W.A.: The Direct Fixation of Fractures (abstract). Trans. Clin. Soc. London, 27:167, 1894.

265. Laurence, M.; Freeman, M.A.R.; and Swanson, S.A.V.: Engineering Considerations in the Internal Fixation of Fractures of the Tibial Shaft. J. Bone Joint Surg., 51B:754–768, 1969.

266. Lavalette, R.; Pope, M.H.; and Dickstein, H.: Setting Temperatures of Plaster Casts. J. Bone Joint Surg., 64A:907–911, 1982.

267. Lawyer, R.B., and Lubbers, L.M.: Use of the Hoffman Apparatus in the Treatment of Unstable Tibial Fractures. J. Bone Joint Surg., 62A:1266–1273, 1980.

268. Leach, R.E.: New Fiber Glass Casting System. Clin. Orthop., 103:109–117, 1974.

269. Lesmes, G.R.; Costill, D.L.; Coyle, E.F.; and Fink, W.J.: Muscle Strength and Power Changes During Maximal Isokinetic Training. Med. Sci. Sports, 10:266–269, 1978.

270. Levin, P.E.; Schoen, R.W., Jr.; and Browner, B.D.: Radiation Exposure to the Surgeon During Closed Interlocking Intramedullary Nailing. J. Bone Joint Surg. 69A:761–766, 1987.

271. Lhowe, D.W., and Hansen, S.T.: Immediate Nailing of Open Fractures of the Femoral Shaft. J. Bone Joint Surg., 70A:812–820, 1988.

272. Litchman, H.M., and Duffy, J.: Lower Extremity Balanced Traction: A Modification of Russell Traction. Clin. Orthop., 66:144–147, 1969.

273. Loftström, B. (ed.): Clinical Experience with Long-Acting Local Anaesthetics. Acta Anaesthesiol. Scand. (Suppl.), 60: 1975.

274. London, P.S.: Observations on Medical Investigation of Ambulance Services. Injury, 3:225–238, 1972.

275. London, P.S.: Observations on the Treatment of Some Fractures of the Forearm by Splintage That Does Not Include the Elbow. Injury, 2:252–270, 1971.

276. Lottes, J.O.: Intramedullary Nail of the Tibia. Instr. Course Lect., XV:65–77, 1958.

277. Lottes, J.O.: Medullary Nailing of Infected Fractures of the Femur. Clin. Orthop., 60:99–101, 1968.

278. Lovell, C.R., and Staniforth, P.: Contact Allergy to Benzalkonium Chloride in Plaster of Paris. Contact Dermatitis, 7:343–344, 1981.

279. MacAusland, W.R.: Treatment of Sepsis After Intramedullary Nailing of Fractures of Femur. Clin. Orthop., 60: 87–94, 1968.

280. MacAusland, W.R., and Eaton, R.G.: The Management of Sepsis Following Fractures of the Femur. J. Bone Joint Surg., 45A:1643–1653, 1963.

281. MacMillan, M., and Gross, R.H.: A Simplified Technique of Distal Femoral Screw Insertion for the Grosse-Kempf Interlocking Nail. Clin. Orthop., 226:252–259, 1988.

282. Magerl, F.; Wyss, A.; Brunner, C.; and Bonder, W.: Plate Osteosynthesis of Femoral Shaft Fractures in Adults. Clin. Orthop., 138:62–73, 1979.

283. Marks, M.T.; Guruswamy, A.; and Gross, R.H.: Ringworm Resulting from Swimming With a Polyurethane Cast. J. Pediatr. Orthop., 3:511–512, 1983.

284. Massie, W.K.: Intramedullary Fixation of Tibial Shaft Fractures. Clin. Orthop., 2:147–160, 1953.

285. Mathews, L.S., and Hirsch, C.: Temperatures Measured in Human Cortical Bone when Drilling. J. Bone Joint Surg., 54A:297–308, 1972.

286. Mathijsen, A.: Plaster-of-Paris in the Treatment of Fractures. Liege, Granmont-Doners, 1854.

287. Mayer, L.; Werbie, T.; Schwab, J.P.; and Johnson, R.P.: The Use of Ender Nails in Fractures of the Tibial Shaft. J. Bone Joint Surg., 67A:446–455, 1985.

288. Mayfield, G.W.: Rotational Malunion of Femoral Shaft Fractures and Its Functional Significance (abstract). J. Bone Joint Surg., 56A:1309, 1974.

289. McDonald, I.: Malignant Lymphoma Associated With In-

ternal Fixation of Fractured Tibia. Cancer, 48:1009–1011, 1981.

290. McDougall, A.: Malignant Tumor at the Site of Bone Plating. J. Bone Joint Surg., 38B:709–713, 1956.

291. McMahon, A.J.; Wilson, N.I.L.; and Hamblen, D.L.: Compression-Fixation of Long Bone Fractures: Problems and Pitfalls Revisited. Injury, 20:84–86, 1989.

292. McMaster, W.C.: Closed Insertion Technique for the Pre-bent Sampson Femoral Rod. Clin. Orthop., 138:238–242, 1979.

293. McMaster, W.C.; Prietto, C.; and Rovner, R.: Closed Treatment of Femoral Fractures with the Fluted Sampson Intramedullary Rod. Orthop. Clin. North Am., 11(3):593–606, 1980.

294. McNeur, J.C.: Management of Open Skeletal Trauma with Particular Reference to Internal Fixation. J. Bone Joint Surg., 52B:54–60, 1970.

295. Meachim, G.; Pedley, R.B.; and Williams, D.F.: A Study of Sarcogenicity Associated with Co-Cr-Mo Particles Implanted in Animal Muscle. J. Biomed. Mater. Res., 16:407–416, 1982.

296. Mears, D.C.: Materials and Orthopaedic Surgery. Baltimore, Williams & Wilkins, 1979.

297. Mears, D.C.: The Use of Dissimilar Metals in Surgery. J. Biomed. Mater. Res., 9:133–148, 1975.

298. Meek, R.N.; Vivoda, E.E.; and Pirani, S.: Comparison of Mortality of Patients with Multiple Injuries According to Type of Fracture Treatment: A Retrospective Age- and Injury-Matched Series. Injury, 17:2–4, 1986.

299. Melendez, E.M., and Colón, C.: Treatment of Open Tibial Fractures with the Orthofix Fixator. Clin. Orthop., 241:224–230, 1989.

300. Merchant, T.C., and Dietz, F.R.: Long-Term Follow-Up After Fractures of the Tibial and Fibular Shafts. J. Bone Joint Surg., 71A:599–606, 1989.

301. Merianos, P.; Pazaridis, S.; Serenes, P.; Orfanidis, S.; and Smyrnis, P.: The Use of Ender Nails in Tibial Shaft Fractures. Acta Orthop. Scand., 53:301–307, 1982.

302. Micheli, L.J.: Thromboembolic Complications of Cast Immobilization for Injuries of the Lower Extremities. Clin. Orthop., 108:191–195, 1975.

303. Miller, E.H.; Schneider, H.J.; Bronson, J.L.; and McLain, D.: A New Consideration in Athletic Injuries. Clin. Orthop., 111:181–191, 1975.

304. Moffroid, M.T., and Whipple, R.H.: Specificity of Speed of Exercise. Phys. Ther., 50:1692–1700, 1970.

305. Molster, A.O.: Biomechanical Effects of Intramedullary Reaming and Nailing on Intact Femora in Rats. Clin. Orthop., 202:278–285, 1986.

306. Molster, A.O.: Effects of Rotational Instability on Healing of Femoral Osteotomies in the Rat. Acta Orthop. Scand., 55:632–636, 1984.

307. Mooney, V.; Nickel, V.L.; Harcey, J.P.; and Snelson, R.: Cast-Brace Treatment for Fractures of the Distal Part of the Femur: A Prospective Controlled Study of 150 Patients. J. Bone Joint Surg., 52A:1563–1578, 1970.

308. Moore, D.C.; Bridenbaugh, L.D.; Bridenbaugh, P.O.; and Tucker, G.T.: Bupivacaine: A Review of 2,077 Cases. J.A.M.A., 214(1):713–718, 1970.

309. Moyen, B. J.-L.; Lahey, P.J., Jr.; Weinberg, E.H.; and Harris, W.H.: Effects on Intact Femora of Dogs of the Application and Removal of Metal Plates: A Metabolic and Structural Study Comparing Stiffer and More Flexible Plates. J. Bone Joint Surg., 60A:940–947, 1978.

310. Moyen, B.; Comtet, J.J.; Roy, J.C.; Basset, R.; and de-Mourgues, G.: Refracture After Removal of Internal Fixation Devices: Clinical Study of 20 Cases and Physiopathologic Hypothesis. Lyon Chir., 76:153–157, 1980.

311. Mullen, J.O., and Tranovich, M.: A Simplified Technique for Zickel Nail Insertion. Clin. Orthop., 208:195–198, 1986.

312. Müller, M.E.; Allgöwer, M.; and Willenegger, H.: Manual of Internal Fixation. New York, Springer-Verlag, 1970.

313. Müller, M.E.; Allgöwer, M.; Schneider, R.; and Willenegger, H.: Manual of Internal Fixation Techniques Recommended by the AO Group. New York, Springer-Verlag, 1979.

314. Murphy, E.F., and Burstein, A.H.: Atlas of Orthotics: Biomechanical Principles and Application. Chicago, American Academy of Orthopaedic Surgeons, 1975.

315. Murray, W.R.; Lucas, D.B.; and Inman, V.T.: Treatment of Non-union of Fractures of the Long Bones by the Two-Plate Method. J. Bone Joint Surg., 46A:1027–1048, 1964.

316. Mustard, W.T., and Simmons, E.H.: Experimental Arterial Spasm in the Lower Extremities Produced by Traction. J. Bone Joint Surg., 35B:437–441, 1953.

317. Nach, D.C., and Keim, H.A.: Prophylactic Antibiotics in Spinal Surgery. Orthop. Rev. 2(6):27–30, 1973.

318. Naumark, A.; Kossoff; and Leach, R.E.: The Disparate Diameter: Sign of Rotational Deformity in Fractures. J. Can. Assoc. Radiol., 34:8–11, 1983.

319. Nelson, J.P.; Ferris, D.O.; and Ivins, J.C.: The Cast Syndrome: Case Report. Postgrad. Med., 42:457–461, 1967.

320. Netz, P.; Eriksson, K.; and Stromberg, L.: Non-Linear Properties of Diaphyseal Bone: An Experimental Study on Dogs. Acta Orthop. Scand., 50:130–143, 1979.

321. Neufeld, A.J.; Mays, J.D.; and Naden, C.J.: A Dynamic Method for Treating Femoral Shaft Fractures. Orthop. Rev., 1:19–21, 1972.

322. Nichols, P.J.R.: Rehabilitation After Fractures of the Shaft of the Femur. J. Bone Joint Surg., 45B:96–102, 1963.

323. Nicoll, E.A.: Fractures of the Tibial Shaft: A Survey of 705 Cases. J. Bone Joint Surg., 46B:373–387, 1964.

324. Nishimura, N.: Serial Strain Gauge Measurement of Bone Healing in Hoffman External Fixation. Orthopedics, 7:677–684, 1984.

325. Nunamaker, D.M., and Perren, S.M.: A Radiological and Histological Analysis of Fracture Healing Using Prebending of Compression Plates. Clin. Orthop., 138:167–174, 1979.

326. O'Brien, J.P.: The Femoral Shaft Refracture. Aust. N.Z. J. Surg., 39(2):194–197, 1969.

327. Olerud, S., and Danckwardt-Lilliestrom, G.: Fracture Healing in Compression Osteosynthesis. Acta Orthop. Scand. (Suppl), 137: 1971.

328. Olerud, S., and Karlström, G.: Secondary Intramedullary Nailing of Tibial Fractures. J. Bone Joint Surg., 54A:1419–28, 1972.

329. Olerud, A., and Karlström, G.: Tibial Fractures Treated by AO Compression Osteosynthesis. Acta Orthop. Scand. (Suppl.), 140: 1972.

330. Olix, M.L.; Klug, T.J.; Coleman, C.R.; and Smith, W.S.: Prophylactic Penicillin and Streptomycin in Elective Operations of Bones, Joints, and Tendons. Surg. Forum, 10: 818–819, 1959.

331. Oonshi, H.; Tatsumi, M.; and Hasegawa, T.: Biomechanical Studies on Framework and Insertion of Pins of External Fixation. Orthopedics 7:658–668, 1984.

332. Paavolainen, P.; Penttinen, R.; Slätis, P.; and Karaharju, E.: The Healing of Experimental Fractures by Compression Osteosynthesis: II. Morphometric and Chemical Analysis. Acta Orthop. Scand., 50:375–383, 1979.

333. Paavolainen, P.; Slätis, P.; Karaharju, E.; and Holmström, T.: The Healing of Experimental Fractures by Compression Osteosynthesis: I. Torsional Strength. Acta Orthop. Scand., 50:369–374, 1979.

334. Paley, D.: Ilizarov Fracture Reduction Method With Preconstruction. Manual for the Course Sponsored by the Program of Continuing Education, University of Maryland School of Medicine, May 16–18, 1988.

335. Paley, D.: Insertion and Fixation Tips for Ilizarov Wires. Manual for the Course Sponsored by the Program of Continuing Education, University of Maryland School of Medicine, May 16–18, 1988.

336. Paley, D.: The Biomechanics of the Ilizarov Fixator in Ilizarov Techniques. Manual for the Course Sponsored by the Program of Continuing Education, University of Maryland School of Medicine, May 16–18, 1988.

337. Parkhill, C.: A New Apparatus for the Fixation of Bones After Resection and in Fractures with a Tendency to Displacement. Trans. Am. Surg. Assoc., 15:251–256, 1897.

338. Partridge, A.J., and Evans, P.E.L.: The Treatment of Fractures of the Shaft of the Femur Using Nylon Cerclage. J. Bone Joint Surg., 64B:210–214, 1987.

339. Patrick, J.H., and Levack, B.: A Study of Pressures Beneath Forearm Plasters. Injury, 13:37–41, 1981.

340. Patzakis, M.J.; Harvey, J.P.; and Ivler, D.: The Role of Antibiotics in the Management of Open Fractures. J. Bone Joint Surg., 56A:532–541, 1974.

341. Pavel, A.; Smith, R.L.; Ballard, A.; and Larson, I.J.: Prophylactic Antibiotics in Elective Orthopaedic Surgery: Prospective Study of 1591 Cases. South. Med. J., 70(Suppl. 1):50–55, 1977.

342. Peltier, L.F.: A Brief History of Traction. J. Bone Joint Surg., 50A:1603–1617, 1968.

343. Penman, H.G., and Ring, P.A.: Osteosarcoma in Association with Total Hip Replacement. J. Bone Joint Surg., 66B:632–634, 1984.

344. Pentecost, R.L.; Murray, R.A.; and Brindley, H.H.: Fatigue, Insufficiency, and Pathologic Fractures. 187:1001–1004, 1964.

345. Perkins, G.: Fractures and Dislocations. London, Athlone Press, 1958.

346. Perkins, G.L.: The Ruminations of an Orthopaedic Surgeon. London, Butterworth, 1970.

347. Perren, S., and Pohler, O.: News From the Lab: Titanium as Implant Material. AO/ASIF Dialogue, 1(3):11–12, 1987.

348. Perren, S.M.: Physical and Biological Aspects of Fracture Healing With Special Reference to Internal Fixation. Clin. Orthop., 138:175–196, 1979.

349. Perren, S.M.: The Biomechanics and Biology of Internal Fixation Using Plates and Nails. Orthopedics, 12:21–33, 1989.

350. Peterson, L.T.: Principles of Internal Fixation with Plates and Screws. Arch. Surg., 64:345–354, 1952.

351. Peterson, L.T., and Reeder, O.S.: Dual Slotted Plates in Fixation of Fractures of the Femoral Shaft. J. Bone Joint Surg., 32A:532–541, 1950.

352. Piekarski, K.: Structure, Properties and Rheology of Bone. *In* Ghista, D.N., and Roaf, R. (eds.): Orthopaedic Mechanics: Procedures and Devices, pp. 1–20. New York, Academic Press, 1978.

353. Piekarski, K.; Wiley, A.A.; and Bartels, J.E.: The Effect of Delayed Internal Fixation on Fracture Healing: An Experimental Study. Acta Orthop. Scand., 40:543–551, 1969.

354. Pilliar, R.M.; Cameron, H.U.; Binnington, A.G.; Szivek, J.; and MacNab, I.: Bone Ingrowth and Stress Shielding With a Porous Surface Coated Fracture Fixation Plate. J. Biomed. Mater. Res., 13:799–810, 1979.

355. Pogrund, H.; Husseini, N.; Bloom, R.; and Finsterbush, A.: The Cleavage Intercondylar Fracture of the Femur. Clin. Orthop., 160:74–77, 1981.

356. Pope, M.H.; Callahan, G.; and Lavalette, R.: Setting Temperatures of Synthetic Casts. J. Bone Joint Surg., 67A: 262–264, 1985.

357. Pratt, D.J.; Papagiannoupoulos, G.; Rees, P.H.; and Quinnell, R.: The Effects of Intramedullary Reaming on the Torsional Strength of the Femur. Injury, 18:177–179, 1987.

358. Pringle, R.G.: Missed Fractures. Injury, 4:311–316, 1973.

359. Puno, R.M.; Teynor, J.T.; Nagano, J.; and Gustilo, R.B.: Critical Analysis of Results of Treatment of 201 Tibial Shaft Fractures. Clin. Orthop., 212:113–121, 1986.

360. Rand, J.A.; An, K.N.; Chao, E.Y.S.; and Kelly, P.J.: A Comparison of the Effect of Open Intramedullary Nailing and Compression-Plate Fixation on Fracture-Site Blood Flow and Fracture Union. J. Bone Joint Surg., 63A:427–442, 1981.

361. Rasmussen, P.S.: Tibial Condylar Fractures as a Cause of Degenerative Arthritis. Acta Orthop. Scand., 43:566–575, 1972.

362. Rattner, I.N.: Injury Ratings: How to Figure Dollar Values in the U.S.A. New York, Crescent Publishing, 1970.

363. Ray, D.R.; Ledbetter, W.B.; Bynum, D.; and Boyd, C.L.: A Parametric Analysis of Bone Fixation Plates on Fractured Equine 3rd Metacarpal. J. Biomech., 4:163–174, 1971.

364. Regan, L.J.: Doctor and Patient and the Law, 3rd ed. St. Louis, C.V. Mosby, 1956.

365. Regazzoni, P., and Brunner, R.: External Fixation of the Distal Radius. AO/ASIF Dialogue, 1(3):8–9, 1987.

366. Regazzoni, P.; Ruedi, T.; and Wright, F.S.: The AO/ASIF 3.5 mm Screw. AO/ASIF Dialogue, 1(1):3–4, 1985.

367. Rhinelander, F.W.: Vascular Proliferation and Blood Supply During Fracture Healing. *In* Uhthoff, H.K. (ed.): Current Concepts of Internal Fixation of Fractures, New York, Springer-Verlag, 1980.

368. Rhinelander, F.W.: Instruments for Use With Flexible Steel

Wire in Bone Surgery. J. Bone Joint Surg., 40A:365–374, 1958.

369. Rhinelander, F.W.: The Normal Microcirculation of Diaphyseal Cortex and Its Response to Fracture. J. Bone Joint Surg., 50A:784–800, 1968.

370. Ricciardi, L., and Diquigiovanni: The External Fixation Treatment of Distal Articular Fractures of the Radius. Orthopedics, 7:637–641, 1984.

371. Rich, N.M.; Metz, C.W., Jr.; Hutton, J.E., Jr.; Baugh, J.H.; and Hughes, C.W.: Internal Versus External Fixation of Fractures with Concomitant Vascular Injuries in Vietnam. J. Trauma, 11:463–473, 1971.

372. Riska, E.B.; von Bondsdorff, H.; Hakkinen, S.; Jaroma, H.; Kiviluoto, Ol; and Paavolain, T.: External Fixation of Unstable Pelvic Fractures. Int. Orthop., 3:183–188, 1979.

373. Riska, E.B.; von Bonsdorff, H.; Hakkinen, S.; Jaroma, H.; Kiviluoto, O.; and Paavolain, T.: Primary Operative Fixation of Long Bone Fractures in Patients with Multiple Injuries. J. Trauma, 17:111–121, 1977.

374. Ritchie, I.K.; Wytch, R.; and Wardlaw, D.: Flammability of Modern Synthetic Bandages. Injury, 19:31–32, 1988.

375. Rittman, W.W.; Schibli, M.; Matter, P.; and Allgöwer, M.: Open Fractures: Long-Term Results in Two Consecutive Cases. Clin. Orthop., 138:132–140, 1979.

376. Rokkanen, P.; Slatis, P.; and Vankka, E.: Closed or Open Intramedullary Nailing of Femoral Shaft Fractures? A Comparison With Conservatively Treated Cases. J. Bone Joint Surg., 51B:313–323, 1969.

377. Rommens, P.M.; Broos, P.L.O.; Stappaerts, K.; and Gruwez, J.A.: Internal Stabilization After External Fixation of Fractures of the Shaft of the Tibia: Sense or Nonsense? Injury, 19:432–435, 1989.

378. Rüedi, T.; Kolbow, H.; and Allgöwer, M.: Experiences with Dynamic Compression Plate (D.C.P.) in 418 Fresh Fractures of Tibial Shaft. Arch. Orthop. Unfallchir., 82:247–256, 1975.

379. Rüedi, T.: The Treatment of Displaced Metaphyseal Fractures with Screws and Wiring Systems. Orthopedics, 12:55–59, 1989.

380. Rüedi, Th.P., and Lüscher, J.N.: Results After Internal Fixation of Comminuted Fractures of the Femoral Shaft with DC Plates. Clin. Orthop., 138:74–76, 1979.

381. Rush, L.V.: Atlas of Rush Pin Technics: A System of Fracture Treatment. Meridian, Miss., Berivon, 1955.

382. Rush, L.V.: Atlas of Rush Pin Techniques. Meridian, Miss., Berivon, 1976.

383. Rush, L.V.: Dynamic Intramedullary Fracture Fixation of the Femur: Reflections on the Use of the Round Rod After 30 Years. Clin. Orthop., 60:21–27, 1968.

384. Russell, R.H.: Fracture of the Femur: A Clinical Study. Br. J. Surg., 11A:491–502, 1924.

385. Russell, T.A., and Taylor, J.C.: Interlocking Intramedullary Nailing of the Femur: Current Concepts. Semin. Orthop., 1:217–231, 1986.

386. Russotti, G.M., and Sim, F.H.: Missile Wounds of the Extremities: A Current Concept Review. Orthopedics, 8:1106–15, 1985.

387. Rybicki, E.F.; Simonen, F.A.; Mills, E.J.; Hassler, C.R.; Scoles, P.; Milne, D.; and Weis, E.B.: Mathematical and Experimental Studies on the Mechanics of Plated Transverse Fractures. J. Biomech., 7:377–384, 1974.

388. Sage, F.P.: Medullary Fixation of Fractures of the Forearm: A Study of the Medullary Canal of the Radius and a Report of Fifty Fractures of the Radius Treated With Prebent Triangular Nail. J. Bone Joint Surg., 41A:1489–1516, 1959.

389. Salter, R.B.: Presidential Address to the Canadian Orthopaedic Association. J. Bone Joint Surg., 64B:251–254, 1982.

390. Salter, R.B., and Field, P.: The Effects of Continuous Compression on Living Articular Cartilage: An Experimental Investigation. J. Bone Joint Surg., 42A:31–49, 1960.

391. Salter, R.B.; Clements, M.D.; Ogilvie-Harris, D.; Bogoch, E.R.; Wong, D.A.; Bell, R.S.; and Minster, R.: The Healing of Articular Tissues Through Continuous Passive Motion: Essence of the First 10 Years of Experimental Investigation (abstract). J. Bone Joint Surg., 64B:640, 1982.

392. Santavirta, S.; Karaharju, E.; and Korkalla, O.: The Use of Osteotaxis as a Limb Salvage Procedure in Severe Compound Injuries of the Upper Extremity. Orthopedics, 7:642–648, 1984.

393. Sarmiento, A.: A Functional Treatment of Forearm Fractures: Preliminary Report. Presented at the Annual Meeting of the American Academy of Orthopaedic Surgeons, Dallas, Tex., 1974.

394. Sarmiento, A.: A Functional Below-the-Knee Cast for Tibial Fractures. J. Bone Joint Surg., 49A:855–875, 1967.

395. Sarmiento, A.: Functional Bracing of Tibial and Femoral Shaft Fractures. Clin. Orthop., 82:2–13, 1972.

396. Sarmiento, A.: The Brachioradialis as a Deforming Force in Colles' Fractures. Clin. Orthop., 38:86–92, 1965.

397. Sarmiento, A.; Cooper, J.S.; and Sinclair, W.F.: Forearm Fractures: Early Functional Bracing—Preliminary Report. J. Bone Joint Surg., 57A:297–304, 1975.

398. Sarmiento, A.; Kinman, P.B.; Galvin, E.G.; Schmitt, R.H.; and Phillips, J.G.: Functional Bracing of Fractures of the Shaft of the Humerus. J. Bone Joint Surg., 59A:596–601, 1977.

399. Saxer, U.: Fractures of the Shaft of the Femur. In Weber, B.G.; Brunner, C.; and Freuler, F. (eds.): Treatment of Fractures in Children and Adolescents, pp. 268–293. New York, Springer-Verlag, 1980.

400. Scales, J.T.; Towers, A.G.; and Roantree, B.M.: The Influence of Antibiotic Therapy on Wound Inflammation and Sepsis Associated with Orthopaedic Implants: A Long-Term Clinical Survey. Acta Orthop. Scand., 43:85–100, 1972.

401. Schatzker, J.: Open Intramedullary Nailing of the Femur. Orthop. Clin. North Am., 11:623–631, 1988.

402. Schatzker, J.; Horne, J.G.; and Sumner-Smith, G.: The Effect of Movement on the Holding Power of Screws in Bone. Clin. Orthop., 111:257–262, 1975.

403. Schatzker, J.; Sanderson, R.; and Murnaghan, J.P.: The Holding Power of Orthopaedic Screws In Vivo. Clin. Orthop., 108:115–116, 1975.

404. Schatzker, J.; Horne, J.G.; and Sumner-Smith, G.: The Reaction of Cortical Bone to Compression by Screw Threads. Clin. Orthop., 111:263–265, 1975.

405. Scheer, L.: Asbestos Again? Forbes Magazine, June 12, 1989.

406. Schneider, H.W.: Use of the 4-Flanged Self-Cutting Intramedullary Nail for Fixation of Femoral Fractures. Clin. Orthop., 60:29–39, 1968.

407. Scott, D.B.: Introduction to Regional Anaesthesia. New York, Appleton and Lang, 1989.

408. Scudese, V.A.: Femoral Shaft Fractures: Percutaneous Multiple Pin Fixation, Thigh Cylinder Plaster Cast and Early Weight Bearing. Clin. Orthop., 77:164–178, 1971.

409. Sedlin, E.D., and Hirsch, C.: Factors Affecting the Determination of the Physical Properties of Femoral Cortical Bone. Acta Othop. Scand., 37:29–48, 1966.

410. Sedlin, E.D., and Zitner, D.T.: The Lottes Nail in the Closed Treatment of Tibia Fractures. Clin. Orthop., 192:185–192, 1985.

411. Selander, D.; Dhuner, K.-G.; and Lundborg, G.: Peripheral Nerve Injury Due to Injection Needles Used for Regional Anesthesia: An Experimental Study of the Acute Effects of Needle Point Trauma. Acta Anaesth. Scand., 21:182–188, 1977.

412. Seligson, D., and Harman, K.: Negative Experiences with Pins-in-Plaster for Femoral Fractures. Clin. Orthop., 138:243–245, 1979.

413. Seligson, D., and Pope, M.: Concepts in External Fixation, New York, Grune & Stratton, 1982.

414. Shakespeare, D.T.; Henderson, N.J.; and Sherman, K.P.: Transmission of Pressure Into the Human Limb From Pneumatic Splints. Injury, 16:38–40, 1984.

415. Shaw, J.A., and Daubert, H.B.: Compression Capability of Cerclage Fixation Systems. Orthopedics, 11:1169–74, 1988.

416. Sherman, W.O'N.: Vanadium Steel Bone Plates and Screws. Surg. Gynecol. Obstet., 14:629–634, 1912.

417. Simmons, E.H.: An Experimental and Clinical Study of Vascular Spasm. Arch. Surg., 73:625–634, 1956.

418. Sinibaldi, K.; Rosen, H.; Liu, S.K.; and De Angelis, M.: Tumours Associated with Metallic Implants in Animals. Clin. Orthop., 118:257–266, 1976.

419. Slätis, P.; Karaharju, E.; Holmström, T.; Ahonen, J.; and Paavolainen, P.: Structural Changes in Intact Tubular Bone After Application of Rigid Plates With and Without Compression. J. Bone Joint Surg., 60A:516–522, 1978.

420. Smith, H. (ed.): Introduction Symposium on Medullary Fixation of the Femur. Instr. Course Lect., VIII:1, 1951.

421. Smith, J.E.M.: The Results of Early and Delayed Internal Fixation of Fractures of the Shaft of the Femur. J. Bone Joint Surg., 46B:28–31, 1964.

422. Smith, J.E.M.: Internal Fixation in the Treatment of Fractures of the Shafts of the Radius and Ulna in Adults. J. Bone Joint Surg., 41B:122–131, 1959.

423. Smith, J.E.M.: Results of Early and Delayed Internal Fixation for Tibial Shaft Fractures. (A Review of 470 Fractures). J. Bone Joint Surg., 56B:469–477, 1974.

424. Solheim, K.: Tibial Fractures Treated According to the AO Method. Injury, 4:213–220, 1973.

425. Sorbie, C., and Chacha, P.: Regional Anaesthesia by the Intravenous Route. Br. Med. J., 1:957–960, 1965.

426. Stader, O.: A Preliminary Announcement of a New Method of Treating Fractures. North Am. Vet., 18:37–38, 1937.

427. Staniforth, P.: Allergy to Benzalkonium Chloride in Plaster of Paris After Sensitisation to Cetrimide: A Case Report. J. Bone Joint Surg., 62B:500–501, 1980.

428. Stein, H., and Makin, M.: Use of the Wagner Apparatus in Fractures of Lower Limb. Orthop. Rev., 9(7):96–99, 1980.

429. Stein, H.; Horer, D.; and Horesh, Z.: The Use of External Fixators in the Treatment and Rehabilitation of Compound Limb Injuries. Orthopedics, 7:707–709, 1984.

430. Stevens, D.B.: Postoperative Orthopaedic Infections: A Study of Etiological Mechanisms. J. Bone Joint Surg., 46A:96–102, 1964.

431. Stewart, J.J.: Fractures of the Humeral Shaft. Curr. Pract. Orthop. Surg., 2:140–162, 1964.

432. Strange, F.A.St. Clair: The Hip. London, Heinemann, 1965.

433. Street, D.M.: Intramedullary Forearm Nailing. Clin. Orthop., 212:219–230, 1986.

434. Street, D.M.: One Hundred Fractures of the Femur Treated by Means of the Diamond-Shaped Medullary Nail. J. Bone Joint Surg., 33A:659–669, 1951.

435. Street, D.M.; Hansen, H.H.; and Brewer, B.J.: The Medullary Nail, Presentation of a New Type and Report of a Case. Arch. Surg., 55:423–432, 1947.

436. Strömberg, L., and Dalen, N.: Influence of a Rigid Plate for Internal Fixation on the Maximum Torque Capacity of Long Bones. Acta Chir. Scand., 142:115–122, 1976.

437. Sudmann, E.: Rotational Displacement After Percutaneous, Intramedullary Osteosynthesis of Femur Shaft Fractures. Acta Orthop. Scand., 44:242–248, 1973.

438. Sven-Hansen, H.; Bremerskov, V.; and Ostri, P.: Fracture-Suspending Effect of the Patellar-Tendon-Bearing Cast. Acta Orthop. Scand., 50:237–239, 1979.

439. Svenningsen, S.; Nesse, O.; Finsen, V.; Harnes, O.B.; and Benum, P.: Intramedullary Nailing Versus A-O Plate Fixation in Femoral Shaft Fractures (abstract). Acta Scand. Orthop., 57:609, 1986.

440. Swann, M.: Malignant Soft-Tissue Tumour at the Site of a Total Hip Replacement. J. Bone Joint Surg., 66B:629–631, 1984.

441. Swanson, S.A.V.: Biomechanical Characteristics of Bone. *In* Kenedi, R.M. (ed.): Advances in Biomedical Engineering, Vol. 1, New York, Academic Press, 1971.

442. Swiontkowski, M.F., and Seiler, J.G., III: The AO/ASIF Universal Intramedullary Nail. Techniques Orthop., 3:33–40, 1988.

443. Tachdjian, M.O., and Compere, E.L.: Postoperative Wound Infections in Orthopaedic Surgery: Evaluation of Prophylactic Antibiotics. J. Int. Coll. Surg., 28:797–805, 1957.

444. Taillard, W.: External Fixation: Past, Present, Future: Introduction to the Tenth International Conference on Hoffman External Fixation. Orthopedics, 7:398–400, 1984.

445. Tarr, R.S., and Wiss, D.A.: The Mechanics and Biology of Intramedullary Fracture Fixation. Clin. Orthop., 212:10–17, 1986.

446. Taylor, A.R.: Wrinkle Corner: External Fixation of Fractures: A Simple Method. Injury, 12:258–259, 1980.

447. Taylor, D.C.; Salvian, A.J.; and Shackleton, C.R.: Crush Syndrome Complicating Pneumatic Antishock Garment (PASG) Use. Injury, 19:43–44, 1988.

448. Tayton, K., and Bradley, J.: How Stiff Should Semirigid Fixation of the Human Tibia Be? A Clue to the Answer. J. Bone Joint Surg., 65B:312–315, 1983.

449. Tayton, K.; Johnson-Nurse, C.; McKibben, B.; Bradley, J.; and Hastings, G.: Use of Semi-Rigid Carbon Fiber–Reinforced Plastic Plates for Fixation of Human Fractures: Results of Preliminary Trials. J. Bone Joint Surg., 64B:105–111, 1982.

450. Tayton, K.J.J.: Ewing's Sarcoma at the Site of a Metal Plate. Cancer, 45:413–415, 1980.

451. Teitz, C.C.; Carter, D.R.; and Frankel, V.H.: Problems Associated With Tibial Fractures With Intact Fibulae. J. Bone Joint Surg., 62A:770–776, 1980.

452. Tencer, A.F.; Johnson, K.D.; Johnston, D.W.C.; and Gill, K.: A Biomechanical Comparison of Various Methods of Stabilization of Subtrochanteric Fractures of the Femur. J. Orthop. Res., 2:297–305, 1984.

453. Tencer, A.F.; Johnson, K.D.; and Sherman, M.C.: Biomechanical Considerations in Intramedullary Nailing of Femoral Shaft Fractures. Techniques Orthop., 3:1–5, 1988.

454. The Universal Nailing System. Technique Guide. Synthes USA, Paoli, Pa.

455. Thoresen, B.O.; Alho, A.; Edeland, A.; Strømsøe, K.; Follerås, G.; and Haukebø, A.: Interlocking Intramedullary Nailing in Femoral Shaft Fractures: A Report of 48 Cases. J. Bone Joint Surg., 67A:1313–20, 1985.

456. Thunold, J.: Fractura Cruris: An Analysis of a Six-Year Material. Acta Chir. Scand., 135:611–614, 1969.

457. Thunold, J.; Varhaug, J.E.; and Bjerkeset, T.: Tibial Shaft Fractures Treated by Rigid Internal Fixation. Injury, 7:125–133, 1975.

458. Uhthoff, H.K.: Preface. In Uhthoff, H.K.: Current Concepts of Internal Fixation, New York, Springer-Verlag, 1980.

459. Uhthoff, H.K.: Mechanical Factors Influencing the Holding Power of Screws in Compact Bone. J. Bone Joint Surg., 55B:633–639, 1973.

460. Uhthoff, H.K., and Dubuc, F.L.: Bone Structure Changes in the Dog Under Rigid Internal Fixation. Clin. Orthop., 81:165–170, 1971.

461. Uhthoff, H.K.; Bardes, O.T.; and Liskova-Kiar, M.: The Advantages of Titanium Alloy Over Stainless Steel Plates for Internal Fixation of Fractures: Experimental Study in Dogs. J. Bone Joint Surg., 63B:427–434, 1981.

462. Van Der Linden, W., and Larsson, K.: Plate Fixation Versus Conservative Treatment of Tibial Shaft Fractures: A Randomized Trial. J. Bone Joint Surg., 61A:873–878, 1979.

463. Velazco, A.; Whitesides, T.A., Jr.; and Fleming, L.L.: Open Fractures of the Tibia Treated With the Lottes Nail. J. Bone Joint Surg., 65A:879–885, 1983.

464. Venable, C.S., and Stuck, W.G.: Electrolysis Controlling Factor in the Use of Metals in Treating Fractures. J.A.M.A., 111:1349–1352, 1938.

465. Venable, C.S., and Stuck, W.G.: Results of Recent Studies and Experiments Concerning Metals Used in the Internal Fixation of Fractures. J. Bone Joint Surg., 30A:247–250, 1948.

466. Vere–Nicoll, E.D.: Air Splints for the Emergency Treatment of Fractures. J. Bone Joint Surg., 46A:1761–1764, 1964.

467. Vidal, J., and Orst, G.: External and Internal Fixation as Complementary Procedures in the Treatment of Trauma. Orthopedics, 7:715–717, 1984.

468. Vidal, J.; Buscayret, C.; and Connes, H.: The Treatment of Articular Fractures by "Ligamentotaxis" with External Fixation. In Brooker, A.F., and Edwards, C.C. (eds): External Fixation: The Current State of the Art, pp. 75–81. Baltimore, Williams & Wilkins, 1979.

469. Vidal, J.; Nakach, G.; and Orst, G.: New Biomechanical Study of Hoffmann External Fixation. Orthopedics, 7:653–657, 1984.

470. Vidal, J.; Rabischong, P.; Bonnel, F.; and Ardry, J.: Étude Biomechanique du Fixateur Externe d' Hoffmann Dans les Fractures de Jambe. Montpellier Chir., 16:43–52, 1970.

471. Wang, G.J.; Reger, S.I.; Mabie, K.N.; Richman, J.A.; and Stamp, W.G.: Semirigid Rod Fixation for Long-Bone Fracture. Clin. Orthop., 192:291–298, 1985.

472. Wang, G.J.; Reger, S.I.; Jennings, R.L.; Mclaurin, C.A.; and Stamp, W.G.: Variable Strengths of the Wire Fixation. Orthopedics, 5(4):435–436, 1981.

473. Ward, E.F., and White, J.L.: Interlocked Intramedullary Nailing of the Humerus. Orthopedics, 12:135–141, 1989.

474. Waterman, N.G., and Pollard, N.T.: Local Antibiotic Treatment of Wounds. In Maibach, H.I., and Rovee, D.T., (eds.): Epidermal Wound Healing, pp. 267–280. Chicago, Year Book Medical Publishers, 1972.

475. Watson-Jones, R.: Fractures and Joint Injuries, Vol. 1. Baltimore, Williams & Wilkins, 1952.

476. Weber, B.G.: Fractures of the Femoral Shaft in Childhood. Injury, 1:65–68, 1969.

477. Weinstein, A.M.; Clemow, A.J.T.; Starkebaum, W.; Milicie, M.; Klawitter, J.J.; and Skinner, H.B.: Retrival and Analysis of Intramedullary Rods. J. Bone Joint Surg., 63A:1443–1448, 1981.

478. Weise, K.; Holz, U.; and Sauer, N.: Second and Third Degree Open Fractures of Long Hollow Bones: Therapeutic Management and Results of Treatment. Akt. Traumatol., 13:24–29, 1983.

479. Weissman, S.L., and Khermosh, O.: Orthopedic Aspects in Multiple Injuries. J. Trauma, 10:377–385, 1970.

480. White, G.M.; Healy, W.L.; Brumback, R.J.; Burgess, A.R.; and Brooker, A.F.: The Treatment of Fractures of the Femoral Shaft With the Brooker-Wills Distal Locking Intramedullary Nail. J. Bone Joint Surg., 68A:865–876, 1986.

481. Williamson, C.; and Scholtz, J.R.: Time Temperature Relationships in Thermal Blister Formation. J. Invest. Dermatol., 12:41–47, 1949.

482. Winnie, A.P.; and Collins, V.J.: The Subclavian Perivascular Technique of Brachial Plexus Anesthesia. Anesthesiology, 25:353–363, 1964.

483. Winquist, R.A., and Hansen, S.T., Jr.: Comminuted Frac-

tures of the Femoral Shaft Treated by Intramedullary Nailing. Orthop. Clin. North Am., 11:633–648, 1980.

484.   Winquist, R.A.; Hansen, S.T., Jr.; and Clawson, D.K.: Closed Intramedullary Nailing of Femoral Fractures: A Report of Five Hundred and Twenty Cases. J. Bone Joint Surg., 66A:529–539, 1984.

485.   Wirth, C.R.; Campbell, C.J.; Askew, M.J.; and Mow, V.C.: The Biomechanical Effects of Compression Plates Applied to Fractures. J. Trauma, 14:563–571, 1974.

486.   Wiss, D.A.; Fleming, C.H.; Matta, J.M.; and Clark, D.: Comminuted and Rotationally Unstable Fractures of the Femur Treated With Interlocking Nailing. Clin. Orthop., 212:35–47, 1986.

487.   Witschger, P., and Wegmüller, M.: Carbon Fiber Rods for the AO/ASIF External Fixator. AO/ASIF Dialogue, 1(3): 9–10, 1987.

488.   Woodard, P.L.; Self, J.; Calhoun, J.; Tencer, A.F.; and Evans, E.B.: The Effect of Implant Axial and Torsional Stiffness on Fracture Healing. J. Orthop. Trauma, 1:331–340, 1987.

489.   Wytch, R.; Mitchell, C.; Ritchie, I.K.; Wardlaw, D.; and Ledingham, W.: New Splinting Materials: Prosthet. Orthot. Int., II:42–45, 1987.

490.   Yelton, C., and Low, W.: Iatrogenic Subtrochanteric Fracture: A Complication of Zickel Nails. J. Bone Joint Surg., 68A:1237–1240.

491.   Zardiackas, L.D.; Black, R.J.; Hughes, J.L.; and Reeves, R.B.: Metallurgical Evaluation of Retrieved Implants and Correlation of Failures to Patient Record Data. Orthopedics, 12:85–92, 1989.

492.   Zickel, R.E.; Hobeika, P.; and Robbins, D.S.: Zickel Supracondylar Nails for Fractures of the Distal End of the Femur. Clin. Orthop., 212:79–88, 1986.

493.   Zimmerman, N.B., and Weiland, A.J.: Ninety-Ninety Intraosseous Wiring for Internal Fixation of the Digital Skeleton. Orthopedics, 12:99–103, 1989.

494.   Zuckerman, J.D.; Veith, R.G.; Johnson, K.D.; Bach, A.W.; Hansen, S.T.; and Solvik, S.: Treatment of Unstable Femoral Shaft Fractures With Closed Interlocking Intramedullary Nailing. J. Orthop. Trauma, 1:209–218, 1987.

2

Healing of the Musculoskeletal Tissues

Joseph A. Buckwalter
Richard L. Cruess

Surgeons can treat musculoskeletal injuries without extensive knowledge of tissue healing, but they are better able to inform the patient of the severity of the injury and the expected result of treatment if they have this knowledge. Furthermore, they can treat musculoskeletal injuries or the problems of failed or inadequate healing better when they are as skilled in applying knowledge of tissue healing to make treatment decisions as they are in using surgical techniques and fracture fixation devices to restore the anatomy of injured limbs.

The potential for healing musculoskeletal tissue injuries varies not only among species but among humans. Some animals rapidly heal large wounds of their musculoskeletal tissues without treatment, and under certain circumstances they regenerate amputated limbs including all the component tissues. To some extent human fetuses and possibly neonates have similar healing potential. Older humans lack these remarkable capacities, but they can heal mild traumatic injuries successfully with minimal or no treatment. Unfortunately, other injuries may fail to heal or result in healing that leaves the individual permanently disabled. Characteristics of the injury, the patient, and the tissue place a limit on the potential for healing a specific injury, but within this limit treatment influences healing (Fig. 2-1). The surgeon's goal is to select and apply the treatment that promotes optimal healing.

Treatment of acute musculoskeletal trauma usually focuses on fractures and therefore on the restoration of bone structure and function. However, injuries to the other primary musculoskeletal tissues

[the dense fibrous tissues (tendon, ligament, joint capsule, and fascia);[7,36,96] articular cartilage;[37,39] and muscle[51,52]] frequently occur in association with fractures and can affect the result of fracture treatment. In addition, an injury that fractures bone and disrupts other primary musculoskeletal tissues often damages the supporting soft tissues (peripheral nerve, blood vessels, and lymphatic vessels). Injuries to these tissues may be more difficult to treat and leave patients with more significant permanent disability than fractures.[149,178]

This chapter first describes the general principles of musculoskeletal tissue healing and the variables that influence healing. Subsequent sections review the structure, composition, and response to acute traumatic injury of bone, dense fibrous tissues, cartilage, and muscle, and examine how specific injury, patient, tissue, and treatment variables influence healing of the individual tissues. The purpose is to provide a framework for understanding the healing potential of human musculoskeletal tissues following acute traumatic injuries and the influence of treatment on healing of these tissues.

HEALING

The damage to cells and matrices plus the hemorrhage caused by acute traumatic injury initiate a tissue response that, in vascularized tissues (eg, bone, most dense fibrous tissues, and muscle) includes inflammation, repair, and remodeling (see Fig. 2-1). Inflammation, repair, and remodeling do

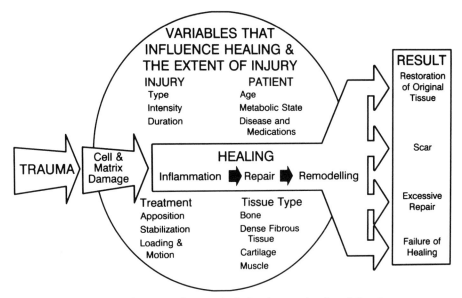

Fig. 2-1. A schematic diagram of musculoskeletal tissue healing following acute traumatic injury. Cell and matrix damage initiates the sequence of inflammation, repair, and remodeling. Healing may result in restoration of the original tissue, scar, excessive repair, or failure of repair depending on injury, tissue, patient, and treatment variables.

not occur as discrete events. Instead, tissue healing is a continuous sequence of cell, matrix, and vascular events initiated by injury that begins with the release of inflammatory mediators and ends when remodeling of the repair tissue ceases. Nonvascularized tissues (eg, cartilage and some regions of the menisci) do not generate a recognizable inflammatory response, but the tissue cells may attempt to repair tissue defects.[37–39]

Repetitive trauma causes a chronic tissue response similar to that seen following a single acute injury, but because repeated injuries interrupt healing, the tissue response to repetitive trauma does not progress through the sequence that follows an acute injury. Furthermore, when the repetitive trauma ceases, the result of healing may differ from that seen with a single acute injury.

INFLAMMATION, REPAIR, AND REMODELING

Inflammation

Inflammation, the cellular and vascular response to injury, includes release of inflammatory mediators, vasodilatation, exudation of plasma, and migration of inflammatory cells to the injury site. Clinically these tissue events appear as swelling, erythema, increased tissue temperature, pain, and impaired tissue function. Although inflammation

is not always beneficial, in many acute injuries it contributes to healing by facilitating removal of necrotic tissue and by stimulating repair.

Fetuses and neonates may heal wounds without an apparent inflammatory response or fibroblast recruitment to the injury site.[72] Mesenchymal cells appear to migrate from the surrounding tissues to the injury site and heal the wound. During the early stages of tissue growth and development, these cells normally are proliferating and can form bone, cartilage, fibrous tissue, muscle, fat, blood vessels, and probably other tissues (Fig. 2-2). Recognizable inflammation becomes part of healing later in development, perhaps when the normally proliferating mesenchymal cells in the immediate region of the injury no longer have the capacity to heal wounds. At this point inflammation may be critical in initiating effective repair by stimulating migration of mesenchymal cells to the injury site.

Because treatable musculoskeletal injuries in fetuses and neonates are rare, this chapter reviews healing as it occurs in individuals that respond to injuries of vascularized musculoskeletal tissue with inflammation. In these vascularized tissues inflammation begins immediately following injury. Release of vasoactive mediators from necrotic tissue may promote dilation and increased permeability of blood vessels near the injury. Blood escaping from damaged vessels forms a hematoma that tem-

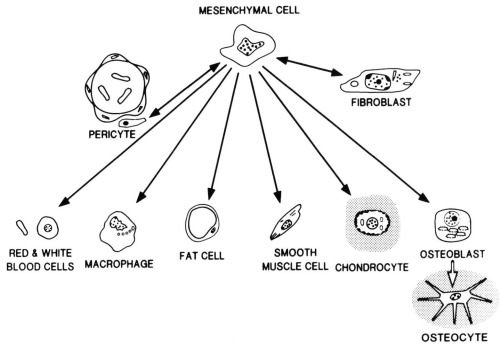

MESENCHYMAL CELL

PERICYTE

FIBROBLAST

RED & WHITE BLOOD CELLS MACROPHAGE FAT CELL SMOOTH MUSCLE CELL CHONDROCYTE OSTEOBLAST

OSTEOCYTE

Fig. 2-2. A diagrammatic representation of the potential of mesenchymal cells to differentiate into specialized connective tissue cells. *(Reproduced from Albright, J. A., and Brand, R. A. (eds.): The Scientific Basis of Orthopaedics, p. 3. Norwalk, Appleton Lange, 1987.)*

porarily fills the injury site. Within the hematoma fibrin forms and platelets bind to fibrillar collagen, thereby achieving hemostasis. With activation of the coagulation system and platelet adherence and aggregation, the platelets release potent vasoactive mediators including serotonin, histamine, and thromboxane A_2. Platelets also can release growth factors, specifically transforming growth factor beta (TGF-β), and platelet-derived growth factor. These small proteins, like other growth factors, can influence cell migration, proliferation, and differentiation, as well as matrix synthesis.[20,50,146,147,175,224,225,238]

Polymorphonuclear leukocytes are the first inflammatory cells to appear at the site of injury, followed by monocytes and T-lymphocytes. Endothelial cells of vessels near the injury proliferate and form new capillaries that extend into the injury site. Enzymes released from inflammatory cells may help remove necrotic tissue, and release of chemotactic and growth factors from monocytes and other inflammatory cells[171,218,224] may help stimulate vascular invasion of the injured tissue and the migration and proliferation of the mesenchymal cells that start the repair process. It appears that phagocytic, mesenchymal, and endothelial cells release growth factors that influence the other cells

as well as those that produce them. Blood vessel endothelial cells release platelet-derived growth factor, macrophages release platelet derived-growth factor and TGF-β, and fibroblasts may serve as sources of platelet-derived growth factor and TGF-β. In addition different cell types may respond to different growth factors. These observations may help explain the sequential appearance of the different cell types following injury.[171] According to this concept, each population of cells produces factors that attract and influence the function of the next population of cells.[171] When the fibroblasts appear, they continue to produce factors that influence fibroblast function.

Repair

Repair is the replacement of necrotic or damaged tissue by cell proliferation and synthesis of new matrix. In general repair cells are undifferentiated mesenchymal cells or fibroblasts that migrate to the injury site during inflammation. These repair cells have the capacity to form bone, cartilage, fibrous tissue, blood vessels, probably fat, and possibly muscle (see Fig. 2-2).[34] Their primary initial functions in most injuries are proliferation and synthesis of new matrix. Later they may differentiate into chondrocytes, osteoblasts, or other cell types. Signals within the injured tissue—including the types and concentrations of growth factors, hormones, and nutrients, as well as *p*H, oxygen tension, and the electrical and mechanical environment—control proliferation, matrix synthesis, and differentiation.

Remodeling

Repair of many acute injuries produces an excessive amount of cellular tissue with a poorly organized matrix. Remodeling reshapes the repair tissue by removing and replacing cells and matrix. As the cells reshape the repair tissue, they usually reorganize the matrix macromolecules. As remodeling progresses, cell density decreases, the cells remove excessive repair matrix, and frequently the repair tissue matrix collagen fibrils become more highly oriented along the lines of stress. Although most apparent remodeling ceases within months of injury, some removal and replacement of repair tissue may continue for years.

RESULTS OF HEALING

''Healing,'' as most patients and surgeons use the term, refers not to the sequence of cell and matrix events described above, but to the visible, palpable result of these events—that is, restoration of structural integrity to an injured tissue. As measured by this standard, the results of healing can be grouped into four overlapping categories: restoration of the original tissue; scar; excessive repair; and failure of repair (see Fig. 2-1).

To add to the complexity of understanding and treating musculoskeletal injuries, the result of healing as measured by the degree of restoration of tissue structure, composition, and function does not necessarily determine the functional outcome for the patient. Patients with nearly identical healing of type IIIA open tibia fractures may have different functional results as measured by return to work, ability to perform necessary activities of daily living, or ability to participate in recreational activities. These differences presumably are more closely related to social, economic, educational, and psychological factors than to the result of tissue healing.

VARIABLES THAT INFLUENCE HEALING

The result of healing (restoration of the original tissue, scar, excessive repair, or failure of healing) depends on the intrinsic tissue capacity for healing and the variables that influence healing. Animal experiments and clinical studies that have attempted to define the variables that influence healing show that they fall into four general categories: injury, tissue, patient, and treatment (see Fig. 2-1). Some of the specific injury, patient, and treatment variables have been well defined, some are presumed to influence healing based on clinical observations but have not been clearly defined, and others remain unknown.

The following sections provide a general description of the injury, tissue, patient, and treatment variables that influence healing of musculoskeletal tissues. Subsequent sections review current understanding of the effects of specific variables on tissue healing. Although injury, tissue, patient, and treatment variables influence the healing of all the musculoskeletal tissues, the specific effects of these variables have been more extensively studied for bone than for the other tissues. For this reason most of the chapter focuses on bone healing.

Injury Variables

TYPE OF INJURY

In general, acute mechanical injuries can be identified as blunt, penetrating, and/or tearing injuries. *Blunt injuries* compress and crush tissue and range from mild contusion to severe crushing. *Tearing injuries* range from minimal elongation or stretching to avulsion or tearing away of tissue. *Penetrating injuries* vary in depth and the extent to which they cleanly lacerate tissue or cause combinations of blunt and tearing injuries. Generally the extent of tissue damage from penetrating injuries can be relatively easily determined. It is more difficult to define the extent of cell and matrix injury from blunt or tearing trauma.

INTENSITY AND DURATION OF FORCE

If other factors are equal, including the type of injury and the condition and type of tissue, the intensity and duration of force applied to the tissue determine the severity of injury, that is, the extent of cell and matrix damage. For some injuries it is possible to estimate the energy transferred to the tissue. For example, the kinetic energy transferred to a tissue from a bullet can be calculated from knowledge of the mass of the bullet, its tumble, and the velocity at the time it struck the tissue. This information combined with knowledge of the tissue may make it possible to estimate the extent of cell and matrix damage. In other injuries, such as complex fractures with extensive soft tissue damage resulting from a high-speed automobile accident, determining the intensity and duration of force may not be possible.

Tissue Variables

The musculoskeletal tissues differ in their potential for healing. Fracture healing produces tissue that cannot be distinguished from uninjured bone. In contrast, clinically significant injuries to articular cartilage or transverse complete muscle lacerations usually heal by scar,[39,51,52] a form of repair that replaces lost cells and matrix with new cells and matrix consisting primarily of a dense collagen matrix and fibroblasts. Scar may restore the structural integrity of the tissue, but in cartilage and muscle it cannot restore the original structure, composition, and function. Following some acute injuries, excessive repair tissue may occur, (eg, scarring of tendons to surrounding tissue). Occasionally the repair phase of healing may fail to replace necrotic or lost tissue, leaving a structural defect containing granulation tissue, myxoid tissue, loose connective tissue, or fluid.

Even though bone and the primary musculoskeletal soft tissues differ in appearance, function, and material properties, they share common features that affect healing. They all have significant mechanical functions, respond to changes in loading with alterations of cell function, and have important cell matrix interactions that influence restoration of structure and function following injury.[34] Given these common characteristics it is not surprising that the mechanical environment or mechanical loading of these tissues following injury can significantly influence healing.

In all the musculoskeletal tissues the condition of the tissue at the time of injury and the presence or absence of other injuries influence healing. Ischemic tissues or the tissues of poorly nourished or aged patients usually suffer more severe damage from mechanical trauma than the normal tissues of well-nourished young patients. Although most acute musculoskeletal injuries are caused by mechanical damage, other types of acute injuries (eg, thermal, toxic, electrical, and radiation injuries) may occur in association with mechanical injuries. The extent of tissue damage from associated nonmechanical injuries can be deceptive in that cell death or injury may extend beyond the apparent mechanical damage. For example, a patient who contacts a high-voltage electrical wire and subsequently falls from a ladder suffering an open fracture may have far more extensive musculoskeletal injury than a similar patient who falls from a ladder but does not suffer the electrical injury.

Patient Variables

AGE

In general, younger people have the greatest healing potential and heal most rapidly. Animal experiments show that healing of injuries in fetuses and possibly neonates resembles the development and growth of the tissue and has the potential to restore the tissue to normal. There is little or no recognizable inflammatory response. The cells that migrate to the injury site and produce the repair matrix may be primarily normally proliferating mesenchymal cells.[72] In infants, injury causes an inflammatory response, and the cells that migrate to the injury site include acute and chronic inflammatory cells and undifferentiated mesenchymal cells that assume the form of fibroblasts. Failure of healing rarely occurs in infants and children. Healing of injuries in adults and the elderly follows the same sequence of inflammation, repair, and remodeling, but in the elderly healing may be slower and less effective and failure of healing occurs more frequently.

For some injuries the age-related differences in healing are great enough to alter the selection of treatment. For example, a minimally displaced closed femoral fracture in a 3-year-old child can heal within a month with restoration of near normal tissue structure and function. A similar fracture in a 70-year-old patient often requires 5 months or more to heal, and the restoration of normal structure and function is less predictable. For this reason treatment of many musculoskeletal injuries in older patients is likely to be more complex and the results often will be less satisfactory.

NUTRITION

Cell migration, proliferation, and matrix synthesis require substantial energy. Furthermore, to synthesize large volumes of collagens, proteoglycans, and other matrix macromolecules the cells need a steady supply of the components of these molecules: proteins and carbohydrates. As a result, the metabolic state of the patient can alter the outcome of injury, and in severely malnourished patients injuries that would heal rapidly in well-nourished individuals may fail to heal. Although few surgeons in economically developed countries see many severely malnourished patients, they may see relatively large numbers of patients with milder forms of protein–calorie malnutrition and other dietary deficiencies. Jensen and associates[124] found a 42.4% incidence of clinical or subclinical malnutrition in patients undergoing orthopaedic surgical procedures. Even the less obvious forms of malnutrition may adversely affect healing.[124]

Because trauma and major surgery can cause malnutrition and thereby decrease immunocompetence,[124] surgeons must pay careful attention to nutrition and metabolic balance in patients with multiple injuries.[160] Even in well-nourished patients, the nutritional demands of healing multiple injuries can exceed intake.[65,124] Leung and colleagues[141] reported that the adenosine triphosphate (ATP) content of a 2-week rabbit fracture callus was a thousand times greater than the ATP content of normal bone. Others have suggested that a single long-bone fracture can temporarily increase metabolic requirements 20% to 25%, and that multiple injuries and infection can increase metabolic requirements by 55%.[65,124] Failure to meet these increased nutritional needs may increase mortality and surgical complications including infection, wound dehiscence, impaired healing, and slower rehabilitation. An experimental study of fracture healing demonstrated that fracture callus does not achieve normal strength in states of dietary deficiency, and that a dietary deficiency of protein reduces fracture callus strength and energy storage capacity.[77] For these reasons, optimal treatment of injured patients requires assessment of their nutritional status and treatment, which may include nutritional support.[26,65,124,160]

SYSTEMIC AND LOCAL DISEASE

Systemic diseases including osteoporosis, diabetes, hypothyroidism, and renal failure and their associated medical treatments may adversely affect healing and increase the vulnerability of tissues to injury.[2,108,121,150] Localized diseases including neoplasms, infections, and developmental disorders or previous injuries may also weaken musculoskeletal tissues and compromise their capacity for healing.[3]

GENETIC DIFFERENCES

Some genetically determined diseases including Ehlers-Danlos syndrome, osteogenesis imperfecta, Marfan's disease, and osteopetrosis increase the vulnerability of the musculoskeletal tissues to injury and may adversely alter the healing response.[3] More subtle genetically determined differences also may affect healing, but these differences have not been well defined.

TREATMENT

Most other chapters of this book focus on the details of treating specific musculoskeletal injuries, in par-

ticular fractures and ligamentous injuries. They make clear that although many injuries can be satisfactorily treated by a variety of methods, all treatment of acute traumatic musculoskeletal injuries is based on common principles. Current surgical treatments do not improve the natural healing response; rather, they attempt to limit cell and matrix damage and provide the optimal environment for healing. Inappropriate treatment or complications of treatment may delay or even prevent healing.

The surgeon must select and apply treatment that creates the optimal biological and mechanical environment for healing. For some injuries, this consists of allowing healing to occur without treatment while providing relief of symptoms and protecting the injured tissue. Other injuries require nonsurgical or surgical intervention to create the optimal environment for healing. Examples of interventions include limiting progressive tissue damage from the injury; minimizing tissue damage caused by treatment; removing necrotic tissue; preventing infection; restoring and maintaining tissue alignment, apposition, and mechanical stability; restoring and maintaining the supporting nerves and blood vessels; and applying controlled loading and motion. Methods that are less well established or experimental include the use of electrical fields, growth factors, artificial matrices, and transplanted mesenchymal stem cells.

BONE

Structure and Composition

Like the other primary musculoskeletal tissues, bone[33,45,99,100] consists of mesenchymal cells imbedded within an abundant extracellular matrix. Unlike the matrices of the other tissues, bone matrix contains mineral that gives the tissue great strength and stiffness in compression and bending.[45] The organic component of the bone matrix, primarily type I collagen, gives bone great strength in tension.[45] Bone has an elaborate blood supply and contains nerves and lymphatics as well. The periosteum, consisting of two layers—an outer fibrous layer and an inner more cellular and vascular layer—covers the external bone surfaces and participates in healing of many types of fractures. The thicker, more cellular periosteum of infants and children has a more elaborate vascular supply than that of adults.[33,237] Perhaps because of these differences, the periosteum of children is more active in healing many fractures.

Human bones consist of two forms of bone tissue: *cortical or compact bone* and *cancellous or trabecular bone.* Long-bone diaphyses consist almost entirely of cortical bone. The metaphyses of long bones and most short and flat bones consist of relatively thin shells of cortical bone with large volumes of cancellous bone. These differences in the distribution of cortical and cancellous bone cause differences in the healing of fractures.[85,213,246]

Two types of bone can be distinguished by mechanical and biological properties: *woven or immature bone* and *lamellar or mature bone.* Woven bone forms the embryonic skeleton and is replaced by lamellar bone as the skeleton develops. Woven bone also forms the initial fracture repair tissue and is replaced by lamellar bone as the fracture remodels. Compared with lamellar bone, woven bone has a more rapid rate of deposition and resorption, an irregular woven pattern of matrix collagen fibrils consistent with its name, approximately four times the number of osteocytes per unit volume, and an irregular pattern of matrix mineralization. The frequent patchwork formation of woven bone and the spotty pattern of mineralization creates an irregular radiographic appearance that distinguishes the woven bone found in fracture callus from lamellar bone. Because of its lack of collagen fibril orientation, irregular mineralization and relatively high cell and water concentration, woven bone is less stiff and more easily deformed than lamellar bone.

Fracture Healing

A bone fracture initiates a sequence of inflammation, repair, and remodeling[25,116,157,218,249] (Figs. 2-1 and 2-3) that can restore the injured bone to its original state. Inflammation, the shortest phase of healing, begins immediately after injury and is followed rapidly by repair (see Fig. 2-3). After repair has replaced the lost and damaged cells and matrix, a prolonged remodeling phase begins. The energy requirements of fracture healing increase rapidly during inflammation and reach a peak during repair, when the cells in the fracture callus are proliferating and synthesizing large volumes of new matrix. The energy requirements of fracture healing

remain high until cell density and cell activity begin to decline as remodeling starts.[141]

INFLAMMATION

An injury that fractures bone not only damages the cells, blood vessels, and bone matrix (Fig. 2-4), but also the surrounding soft tissues, including the periosteum and muscle. A hematoma accumulates within the medullary canal, between the fracture ends and beneath elevated periosteum.[197] The damage to the bone blood vessels deprives osteocytes of their nutrition, and they die as far back as the junction of collateral channels, leaving the immediate ends of the fracture without living cells (see Fig. 2-4). Severely damaged periosteum and marrow, as well as other surrounding soft tissues, may also contribute necrotic material to the fracture site.

Inflammatory mediators released from platelets and from dead and injured cells cause blood vessels to dilate and exude plasma leading to the acute edema seen in the region of a fresh fracture.[20,50,116,171,218,224,225,238] Inflammatory cells migrate to the region, including polymorphonuclear leukocytes followed by macrophages and lymphocytes. As the inflammatory response subsides, necrotic tissue and exudate are resorbed, and fibroblasts appear and start producing a new matrix (see Fig. 2-3).

REPAIR

The factors that stimulate fracture repair probably include the chemotactic factors released during inflammation at the fracture site and bone matrix proteins exposed by disruption of the bone tissue. Electrical stimuli may also have a role. Electronegativity is found in the region of a fresh fracture and may stimulate osteogenesis.[28,89,140] This electronegativity depends on cell viability and, unlike the currents measured in intact bones, is not generated by stress. The degree of electronegativity slowly diminishes until the fracture is united.

Although the inflammation caused by a fracture

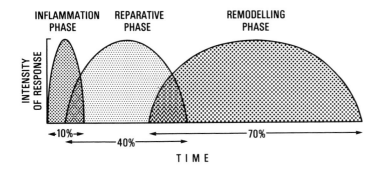

Fig. 2-3. An approximation of the relative intensities and duration of inflammation, repair, and remodeling in fracture healing. Notice that repair begins as inflammation starts to subside, and remodeling begins before repair is complete. The energy requirements of fracture healing reach the maximum during repair, corresponding with the most intense period of cell proliferation and matrix synthesis, and then gradually decrease during remodeling.

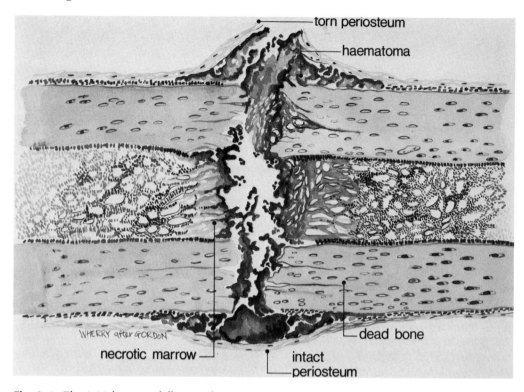

Fig. 2-4. The initial events following fracture of a long bone diaphysis. The periosteum is torn opposite the point of impact, and may remain intact on the other side. A hematoma accumulates beneath the periosteum and between the fracture ends. There is necrotic marrow and cortical bone close to the fracture line.

follows the same sequence for almost every fracture, the amount and composition of repair tissue may differ depending on whether the fracture occurs through primarily cancellous bone in the metaphysis or through primarily cortical bone in the diaphysis, whether the fracture is stable or unstable during repair, and the extent of soft tissue disruption surrounding the fracture. The summary of fracture repair that follows describes healing of diaphyseal fractures that are not rigidly stabilized and with intact soft tissues.

Disruption of blood vessels in the bone, marrow, periosteum, and surrounding tissue at the time of injury results in the extravasation of blood at the fracture site and the formation of a hematoma. Organization of this hematoma is usually recognized at the first step in fracture repair (Fig. 2-5). Open fractures or treatment of fractures by open reduction and internal fixation disrupts organization of the hematoma, but closing the soft tissue over the fracture allows formation of a new hematoma. The

fracture hematoma provides a fibrin scaffold that facilitates migration of repair cells. Growth factors and other proteins produced by cells in the fracture hematoma mediate the critical initial events in fracture repair including cell migration, proliferation, and synthesis of a repair tissue matrix.[20,116,157,171,218] At this stage, the microenvironment about the fracture is acidic,[228] which may affect cell behavior during the early phases of repair. As repair progresses, the pH gradually returns to neutral and then to a slightly alkaline level. When an alkaline pH is attained, the activity of the alkaline phosphatase enzyme is optimal and promotes mineralization of the fracture callus.

Although the volume of the vascular bed of an extremity increases shortly after fracture, the osteogenic response is limited largely to the zones surrounding the fracture itself.[264] It appears that, under ordinary circumstances, the periosteal vessels contribute the majority of capillary buds early in normal bone healing, with the nutrient medullary

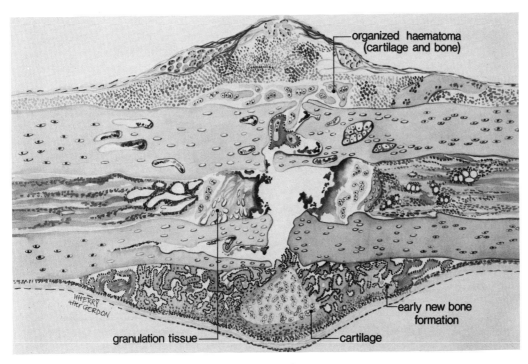

organized haematoma
(cartilage and bone)

early new bone
formation

granulation tissue

cartilage

WHERRY
after GORDON

Fig. 2-5. Early repair of a diaphyseal fracture of a long bone. There is organization of the hematoma, early woven bone formation in the subperiosteal regions, and cartilage formation in other areas. Periosteal cells contribute to healing this type of injury. If the fracture is rigidly immobilized or if it occurs primarily through cancellous bone and the cancellous surfaces lie in close apposition, there will be little evidence of fracture callus.

artery becoming more important later in the process.[202,203] Fibroblastic growth factors may be important mediators of the angiogenesis in fracture healing,[218,238] but the exact stimuli responsible for vascular invasion and endothelial cell proliferation have not been defined. When the surgeon interferes with the blood supply to the fracture site, either by stripping the periosteum excessively or by destroying the medullary system through the use of intramedullary nails, repair must proceed with vessels derived from the surviving system.[103,202,203]

The bone ends at the fracture site, deprived of their blood supply, become necrotic and are resorbed. The cells responsible for this function, the osteoclasts, come from a different cell line than the cells responsible for bone formation.[33,102] The osteoclasts are derived from circulating monocytes in the blood and monoblastic precursor cells from the local bone marrow,[33,216] whereas the osteoblasts appear to develop from the undifferentiated mesenchymal cells that migrate into the fracture site. The stimulus for bone resorption remains unclear, but prostaglandins have been identified in signifi-

cant amounts in the region of fresh fractures in experimental animals,[69] and these substances can increase osteoclast activity and cause recruitment of new osteoclasts.[74,205]

Pluripotential mesenchymal cells (see Fig. 2-2), probably of common origin, form the fibrous tissue, cartilage, and eventually bone at the fracture site. Some of these cells originate in the injured tissues, while others migrate to the injury site with the blood vessels. Cells from the cambium layer of the periosteum form the earliest bone.[237] Periosteal cells have an especially prominent role in healing childrens' fractures because the periosteum is thicker and more cellular in younger individuals.[33] With increasing age, the periosteum becomes thinner and its contribution to fracture healing becomes less apparent. Osteoblasts from the endosteal surface also participate in bone formation, but surviving osteocytes do not appear to form repair tissue.[236] The majority of cells involved directly in osteogenesis during fracture healing appear in the fracture site with the granulation tissue.[239] Although the appearance of the reparative cells appears to be associated with invasion of capillary loops, and these cells may be derived from the endothelial cells,[239] their precise source remains unknown.[15,239,268]

The mesenchymal cells at the fracture site proliferate, differentiate, and produce the tissue known as *fracture callus*, consisting of fibrous tissue, cartilage, and woven bone (Fig. 2-6). The bone formed initially at the periphery of the inflammatory reaction by intramembranous bone formation is called the *hard callus*. The new tissue that arises in regions of low oxygen tension in the center of the inflammatory reaction is primarily cartilage and is called the *soft callus*. Bone gradually replaces the cartilage through endochondral ossification, enlarging the hard callus and increasing the stability of the fracture fragments (see Fig. 2-6). This process continues until new bone bridges the fracture site, reestablishing continuity between the cortical bone ends.

The biochemical composition of the fracture callus matrix changes as repair progresses (Fig. 2-7).[243] The cells replace the fibrin clot with a loose fibrous matrix containing glycosaminoglycans, proteoglycans, and types I and III collagen. In many regions they convert this tissue to more dense fibrocartilage

or hyaline-like cartilage. With formation of hyaline-like cartilage, type II collagen, cartilage-specific proteoglycan and link protein content increase. During endochondral ossification and intramembranous bone formation the concentration of type I collagen, alkaline phosphatase, and bone-specific proteins[172] increases until the matrix mineralizes (see Fig. 2-7). Newly formed woven bone remodels to lamellar bone, and with remodeling the content of collagen and other proteins returns to normal levels.[243]

To synthesize the matrix proteins of fracture callus, chondrocytes and osteoblasts must activate the genes for these proteins. Analysis of fracture repair demonstrates a close correlation between the activation of genes for blood vessel, cartilage, and bone-specific proteins in the cells and the development of granulation tissue, cartilage, and bone (Fig. 2-8),[126,172,210] demonstrating that fracture repair depends on regulation of gene expression in the repair cells. The simultaneous occurrence of chondrogenesis, endochondral ossification, and intramembranous bone formation in different regions of the fracture callus suggests that local mediators and small variations in the microenvironment, in-

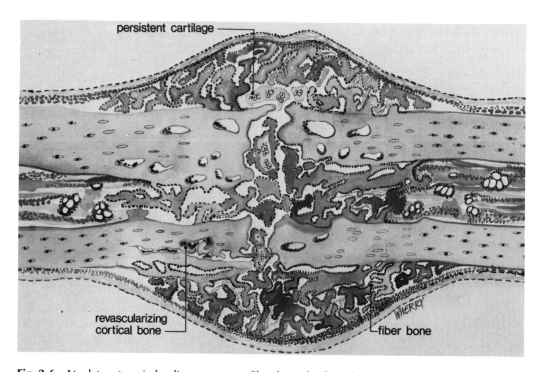

Fig. 2-6. At a later stage in healing, woven or fiber bone bridges the fracture gap. Cartilage remains in the regions most distant from ingrowing capillary buds. In many instances, the capillaries are surrounded by new bone. Vessels revascularize the cortical bone at the fracture site.

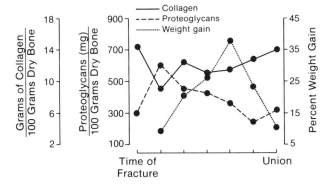

Fig. 2-7. A schematic representation of the changing composition and mass of fracture callus. Collagen formation precedes significant accumulation of mineral. After an initial rise, proteoglycan concentration falls gradually as fracture healing progresses. The total mass of the fracture callus increases during repair and then decreases during remodeling.

cluding stresses, determine what genes will be expressed and therefore the type of tissue the repair cells form. Compression discourages the formation of fibrous tissue. Intermittent shear forces promote normal calcification of newly formed fibrocartilage, whereas intermittent hydrostatic stress inhibits calcification.[18] Local mediators that may influence repair cell function include growth factors released from cells and platelets and oxygen tension. Acidic fibroblast growth factor (FGF), basic FGF, and TGF-β stimulate chondrocyte proliferation and cartilage formation, osteoblast proliferation, and bone synthesis.[125,168,171,175,224,225] TGF-β released from platelets immediately after injury may initiate formation of fracture callus. TGF-β synthesis is also associated with cartilage hypertrophy and calcification at the endochondral ossification front.[127] Tissue oxygen tension may help determine if bone or cartilage forms. In regions with low oxygen tension, possibly because of their distance from blood vessels,[202,203] cartilage forms.[11] Cells that receive enough oxygen and are subject to the necessary mechanical or electrical stimuli form bone.[11,13,18]

Mineralization of fracture callus results from an ordered sequence of cell activities. The cells synthesize a matrix with a high concentration of type I collagen fibrils[34,99,100,112] that have regular spaces called "hole zones"[99,100,112] (Fig. 2-9), and then create conditions that promote deposition of clusters of calcium hydroxyapatite crystals within the collagen fibrils.[99,100] Mineralization requires two cell functions. First, the cells must remove local conditions in the fibrocartilaginous callus matrix that inhibit mineralization, including high glycosaminoglycan concentrations. Fracture callus chondrocytes may accomplish this by secreting neutral proteoglycanases that degrade these molecules at the time of mineralization.[79] Second, after the cells prepare the matrix for mineralization, the chondrocytes, and later the osteoblasts, release "prepackaged" calcium phosphate complexes into the matrix by the budding of "matrix vesicles" from cell membranes (Figs. 2-10**A** and 2-10**B**).[29] These membrane-derived vesicles carry neutral proteases and alkaline phosphatase enzymes which degrade the proteoglycan-rich matrix and hydrolyze ATP

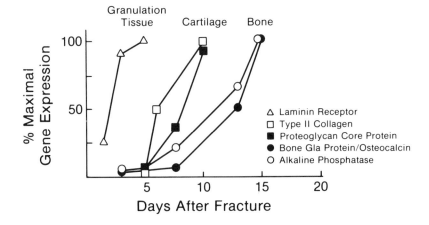

Fig. 2-8. Relative levels of protein gene expression during fracture repair in a rat. Expression of laminin receptor, a protein found in blood vessels, is increased during granulation tissue formation. Expression of genes for cartilage (type II collagen and proteoglycan core protein) and bone-associated proteins (bone Gla protein, osteocalcin, alkaline phosphatase) is increased when these tissues are forming in the callus. *(Contributed by Mark Bolander, Orthopaedic Research Unit NIAMS, National Institute of Health.)*

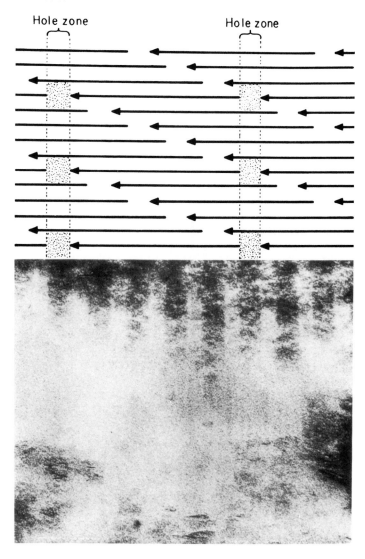

Fig. 2-9. The initial mineralization of the collagenous matrix appears to occur in the hole zone of collagen fibrils. *(Gilmcher, M.J.: A Basic Architectural Principle in the Organization of Mineralized Tissues. Clin. Orthop., 61:16–36, 1968.)*

and other high-energy phosphate-esters to provide phosphate ions for precipitation with calcium. Figure 2-11 shows the distribution of matrix vesicle enzyme activities over time. As callus begins to mineralize (approximately 14 to 17 days after fracture in the rat), neutral proteases and alkaline phosphatase show parallel increases and peaks in activity.[79]

As mineralization proceeds, the bone ends gradually become enveloped in a fusiform mass of callus containing increasing amounts of woven bone. The increasing mineral content correlates closely with increasing hardness of the fracture callus.[10] Stability of the fracture fragments progressively increases because of the internal and external callus formation, and eventually clinical union occurs—that is,

the fracture site becomes pain-free and radiographs show bone crossing the fracture site. However, at this stage the fracture healing is not complete. The immature fracture callus is weaker than normal bone, and it only gains full strength during remodeling.

REMODELING

During the final stages of repair (see Fig. 2-3), remodeling of the repair tissue begins with replacement of woven bone by lamellar bone and resorption of unneeded callus. Radioisotope studies have shown increased activity in fracture sites long after the patient has full restoration of function and plain radiographs show complete bone union,[256] demonstrating that fracture remodeling continues for

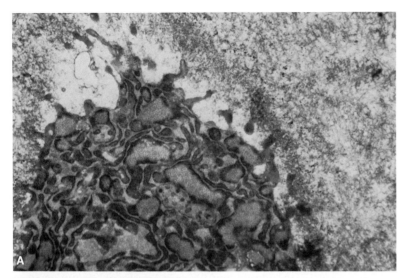

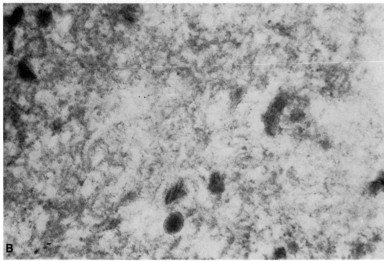

Fig. 2-10. The release of matrix vesicles from 14-day fracture callus chondrocytes. **(A)** Electron micrograph of half of a fracture callus chondrocyte showing portions of the membrane budding off and forming vesicular bodies. **(B)** In the matrix, these vesicles may mediate the deposition of calcium phosphate salts and their conversion to hydroxyapatite crystals. Notice the presence of dark material (amorphous mineral) within certain vesicles and needle-like structures (apatite crystals) in others. The background matrix is composed of collagen and glycosaminoglycans. *(Contributed by Thomas Einhorn, M.D., Mount Sinai School of Medicine, New York, N.Y.)*

years after clinical union. Remodeling of fracture repair tissue after all woven bone has been replaced presumably consists of osteoclastic resorption of superfluous or poorly placed trabeculae and formation of new struts of bone along lines of force.[92]

Electrical fields may influence fracture remodeling. When a bone is subjected to stress, electropositivity occurs on the convex surface and electronegativity on the concave surface.[13] Circumstantial evidence indicates that regions of electropositivity are associated with osteoclastic activity and regions of electronegativity with osteoblastic activity.[12] Thus the observation that changes in bone architecture are associated with changes in loading, often called *Wolff's law*,[260] may be explainable in terms of alterations in the electrical fields

that affect cellular behavior. The end result of fracture callus remodeling is bone that, even if it has not returned to its original form, has been altered to perform the function demanded of it.

Although fracture callus remodeling results from an elaborate sequence of cell and matrix changes, the important functional result for the patient is an increase in mechanical stability.[257] The progressive increase in fracture stability can be described as consisting of four stages. During stage I, a healing bone subjected to torsional testing fails through the original fracture site with a low-stiffness pattern. In stage II, the bone still fails through the fracture site, but the characteristics of failure indicate a high-stiffness, hard-tissue pattern. In stage III, the bone fails partly through the original fracture site and

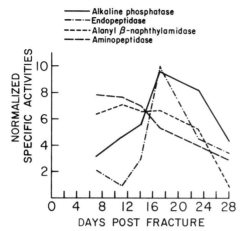

Fig. 2-11. Distribution of the activities of alkaline phosphatase and three different neutral proteases in matrix vesicles during fracture healing. Note that the enzyme responsible for degrading glycosaminoglycans (endopeptidase) and the enzyme responsible for calcifying the callus (alkaline phosphatase) are expressed in parallel and peak between 14 and 17 days. This is when fracture callus begins to mineralize. *(Reprinted with permission from Einhorn, T. A.; Hirschman, A.; Kaplan, C.; Nashed, R.; Devlin, V. J.; and Warman, J.: Neutral Protein-Degrading Enzymes in Experimental Fracture Callus. J. Orthop. Res., 7:792–805, 1989.)*

partly through the previously intact bone with a high-stiffness, hard-tissue pattern. Finally, in stage IV, the site of failure is not related to the fracture site, indicating that remodeling is complete as measured by restoration of the original mechanical properties of the injured tissues.

FRACTURE HEALING WITH RIGID STABILIZATION

As described above, when diaphyseal fractures are not rigidly stabilized, healing progressively stabilizes the fracture fragments by formation of callus. However, if a fracture is rigidly stabilized and if the bone surfaces are in contact, healing can occur without callus formation.[6,166,179,188–192,214,215] This type of fracture healing is commonly called *primary bone healing.*

Robert Danis, a Belgian surgeon, first described primary bone union and elucidated the principles of rigid internal fixation.[66] In 1958 a Swiss group, lead by Maurice E. Müller, formed the AO (Arbeitsgemeinschaft für Osteosynthesfragen) and put forward four "working hypotheses" that became the principles of internal fixation: (1) anatomical reduction; (2) rigid internal fixation; (3) atraumatic surgical technique; and (4) early, pain-free, active mobilization during the first 10 postoperative days.[6]

Schenk and Willenegger[214,215] described two stages of primary bone healing: gap healing and haversian remodeling. To some extent these stages correspond to the repair and remodeling phases of fractures that are not rigidly stabilized. Their examinations of fractures after compression plating showed that not all cortical bone ends are in close contact, leaving gaps of varying size at the fracture site, and that the mechanism, structure, and rate of new bone formation at the fracture site depends on the size of the gaps.[214,215] When there is direct contact between cortical bone ends, lamellar bone forms directly across the fracture line, parallel to the long axis of the bone, by direct extension of osteons.[188,191,214,215] A cluster of osteoclasts cuts across the fracture line, osteoblasts following the osteoclasts deposit new bone, and blood vessels follow the osteoblasts. The new bone matrix, enclosed osteocytes, and blood vessels form new haversian systems or "primary osteons." This process has been given the name "contact healing." In small gaps, 150 to 200 μm or approximately the outer diameter of the osteon, the cells form lamellar bone at right angles to the axis of the bone. In larger gaps, 200 μm to 1 mm, cells fill the defect with woven bone. Following gap healing, haversian remodeling begins, reestablishing normal cortical anatomy. Cutting cones consisting of osteoclasts followed by blood vessels and osteoblasts traverse the new bone in the fracture gap, depositing lamellar bone and reestablishing the cortical bone blood supply across the fracture site. Haversian remodeling presumably follows the paths of necrotic vessels and also cuts new vessel channels. If a large segment of cortical bone is necrotic, gap healing by direct extension of osteons still occurs, but at a slower rate, and areas of necrotic cortical bone remain unremodelled for a prolonged period.[179]

Perren and colleagues[188–192] noted that compression of a fracture eliminates the resorption of the cortical bone ends seen in spontaneous bone repair. They correlated the resorptive process with micromotion and resulting strain at the fracture site, and they demonstrated the importance of stability for primary bone formation. In the absence of stability, micromotion stimulates resorption by osteoclasts and inhibits contact healing and gap healing. Successful compression plating, by a combination of friction and preloading, eliminates micromotion and strain.

FAILURE OF FRACTURE HEALING

Despite the best treatment, some fractures heal slowly or fail to heal.[221] It is difficult to set the time when a given fracture should be united, but when healing progresses more slowly than average, the slow progress is referred to as *delayed union*. Watson-Jones[253] described a condition he called *slow union*, where the fracture line remains clearly visible radiographically, but there is no undue separation of the fragments, no cavitation of the surfaces, no calcification, and no sclerosis. This indolent fracture healing may be related to the severity of the injury, poor blood supply, the age of the patient, or other factors. It is not an ununited fracture, but rather a variation of normal healing. In contrast, a *nonunion* results from an arrest of the healing process. In a nonunion, a pseudarthrosis or fibrous tissue forms at the fracture site and does not progress to healing of the fracture.

VARIABLES THAT INFLUENCE FRACTURE HEALING

Occasionally delayed unions or nonunions occur without apparent cause, but in many instances injury, patient, and treatment variables that adversely influenced fracture healing can be identified. These variables include the following: severe soft tissue damage associated with open and comminuted fractures; infected fractures; segmental fractures; pathologic fractures; fractures with soft tissue interposition; poor local blood supply; systemic diseases, malnutrition; corticosteroids; and iatrogenic interference with healing. Many other variables have been reported to promote or retard bone healing (Table 2-1). Many of them exert an influence that can be measured in experimental studies, but in clinical practice relatively few of them cause detectable alterations in fracture healing.

Injury Variables.   *Severity.*   The significant soft tissue and bone damage found in severe fractures may be associated with large soft tissue wounds, loss of soft tissue, displacement and comminution of the bone fragments, loss of bone, and decreased blood supply to the fracture site. Displacement of the fracture fragments and severe trauma to the soft tissues retard fracture healing, probably because the extensive tissue damage increases the volume of necrotic tissue and hematoma, impedes the migration of mesenchymal cells and vascular invasion, decreases the number of viable mesenchymal cells, and disrupts the local blood supply.[202,203] Less severe injuries leave an intact soft tissue envelope that provides a ready source of mesenchymal cells, a tube that directs the repair efforts of these cells, and an internal splint that contributes to immobilization of the fragments.

Open Fractures.   Severe open fractures present the problem of soft tissue disruption, fracture displacement, and, in some instances, significant bone loss.[221] At the fracture site, extensive stripping of the soft tissue surrounding the fracture may disrupt the blood supply to large areas of bone, thereby impeding or preventing formation of a fracture hematoma and delaying formation of repair tissue. Exposed bone and soft tissue may become desiccated, further increasing the volume of necrotic tissue. Early use of vascularized soft tissue flaps to cover bone exposed by severe open fractures can facilitate healing of these injuries. (See Chapter 4.) In addition to the soft tissue damage, open fractures may become infected. Management of this complication usually includes debriding infected bone and soft tissue along with antibiotic treatment. In-

Table 2-1. Factors Influencing Bone Healing

Factors Claimed to Promote Bone Healing		Factors Claimed to Retard Bone Healing	
Factor	References	Factor	References
Growth hormone	107, 115, 133–135, 161, 174	Corticosteroids	64, 107, 219
Thyroid hormones	83, 133	Diabetes	108, 150, 265
Calcitonin	271	Anemia	207
Insulin	150, 220	Bone wax	114
Vitamin A	62, 242	Delayed manipulation	183
Vitamin D	62, 226	Denervation	201
Anabolic steroids	136, 137, 258	Anticoagulants	206, 227
Chondroitin sulphate	44, 109		
Hyaluronidase	22		
Electrical fields	11, 14, 28, 30, 91, 140		
Hyperbaric oxygen	63, 267		
Physical exercise	105		
Growth factors	20, 84, 146, 147, 167, 171, 175		
Demineralized bone matrix	19, 80, 168		
Bone marrow cells	48, 59		

fected fractures can unite if they are immobilized and the infection can be controlled.

Intra-articular Fractures.   Intra-articular extension of a fracture occasionally may adversely influence healing. Synovial fluid contains collagenases that can degrade the matrix of the initial fracture callus[138] and thereby retard the first stage in fracture healing. In addition, joint motion may cause movement of the fracture fragments. Most intra-articular fractures heal, but in some instances, especially if the fracture is not reduced or stabilized, healing may be delayed or nonunion may occur (Fig. 2-12).

Segmental Fractures.   A segmental fracture of a long bone impairs or disrupts intramedullary blood supply to the middle fragment. If there is severe soft tissue trauma, the periosteal blood supply to the middle fragment may also be compromised. Possibly because of this, the probability of delayed union or nonunion, proximally or distally, may be increased. When internal fixation of a segmental fracture is performed, the soft tissue attachments of the middle fragment should be preserved whenever possible.

Soft Tissue Interposition.   Interposition of soft tissue including muscle, fascia, tendon, and occasion-ally nerves and vessels between fracture fragments will compromise fracture healing. The presence of soft tissue interposition should be suspected when the bone fragments cannot be brought into apposition or alignment during attempted closed reduction. If this occurs, an open reduction may be necessary to extricate the interposed tissue and achieve an acceptable position of the fracture.

Inadequate Blood Supply.   Insufficient blood supply for successful fracture healing may result from a severe injury or from the normally limited blood supply to some bones or bone regions. For example, the vulnerable blood supplies of the femoral head, scaphoid, and talus may predispose these bones to delayed union or nonunion, even in the absence of severe soft tissue damage or fracture displacement.

Patient Variables.   *Age.*   Age is among the most important patient variables that influence fracture healing. Most fractures in children heal rapidly. The older a child is, the more the rate of fracture healing approaches that of an adult. One possible reason for the greater healing potential of children is that younger cells may differentiate more rapidly from the mesenchymal pool.[237] In addition, the rapid bone remodeling that accompanies growth allows correction of a greater degree of deformity in children.

Hormonal Effects.   A variety of hormones can influence fracture healing. Corticosteroids compromise fracture healing,[64,107,219] possibly by inhibiting differentiation of osteoblasts from mesenchymal cells[219] and by decreasing synthesis of bone organic matrix components[64] necessary for repair. Prolonged corticosteroid administration may also decrease bone density and increase the probability of rib and vertebral fractures.[2] Experimental work has shown that the rate of repair can be influenced by growth hormone,[115,133,161,174] but normal alterations in the level of circulating growth hormone probably have little effect on fracture healing. Thyroid hormone, calcitonin, insulin, and anabolic steroids have been reported in experimental situations to enhance the rate of fracture healing (see Table 2-1). Diabetes, castration, hypervitaminosis D, and rickets have been shown to retard fracture healing in experimental situations (see Table 2-1). Generally, in clinical practice fractures will heal in patients with hormonal disturbances, although union may be slower than normal.

Bone Necrosis.   Normally, healing proceeds from both sides of a fracture, but if one fracture fragment has lost its blood supply, healing depends entirely on ingrowth of capillaries from the living side. If a

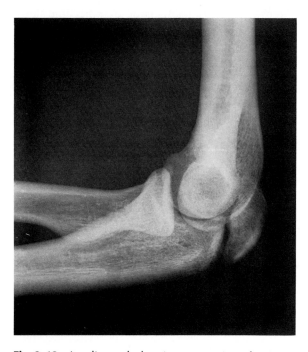

Fig. 2-12. A radiograph showing a nonunion of an intra-articular fracture of the olecranon. This 18-year-old man injured his elbow in a wrestling match. After the elbow was taped, he continued wrestling. Two years later he sought evaluation for persistent elbow pain and weakness of elbow extension.

fracture fragment is avascular the fracture can heal, but the rate is slower and the incidence of healing is lower[23] than if both fragments have a normal blood supply. If both fragments are avascular, the chances for union are decreased further. Traumatic or surgical disruption of blood vessels, infection, prolonged use of corticosteroids, and radiation treatment can cause bone necrosis. Irradiated bone, even when it is not obviously necrotic, often heals at a slower rate than normal bone. Nonunion may result,[101] probably because of radiation-induced cell death in the local region, thrombosis of vessels, and fibrosis of the marrow. These changes may reduce the population of cells that can participate in repair, increase the volume of necrotic tissue, and interfere with the ingrowth of capillaries and migration of fibroblasts into the fracture site. Figure 2-13 shows an example of impaired bone healing in a femur treated with radiation.

Infection.   For fracture healing to proceed at the maximum rate, the local cells must be devoted primarily to healing the fracture. If infection occurs following fracture or if the fracture occurs as a result of the infection, many cells must be diverted to attempt to wall off and eliminate the infection. Furthermore, infection may cause necrosis of normal tissue, edema, and thrombosis of blood vessels, thereby retarding or preventing healing.[8]

Tissue Variables.   *Form of Bone (Cancellous or Cortical).*   Healing of cancellous and cortical fractures differs,[85,213,246] probably because of the differences in surface area, cellularity, and vascularity.[33] Apposed cancellous bone surfaces usually unite rapidly, possibly because the large surface area of cancellous bone per unit volume creates many points of bone contact rich in cells and blood supply and because osteoblasts will form new bone directly on

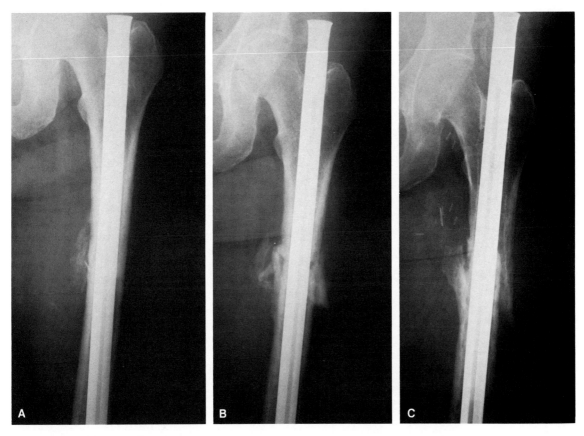

Fig. 2-13. Radiographs showing a nonunion of a femoral fracture associated with radiation treatment. This elderly patient had a sarcoma of her thigh treated by surgical resection followed by high-dose radiation therapy. **(A)** Five years after radiation treatment she slipped on her laundry room floor and suffered a transverse femoral fracture that was treated by intramedullary fixation. **(B)** Three months later the bone had fragmented at the fracture site. **(C)** Four years later the patient had been treated with bone grafts and a vascularized graft, but the bone continued to collapse and the nonunion persisted.

existing trabeculae. Because woven bone forms across points of contact, stable fractures located primarily in cancellous regions form little or no visible external callus[213] and rarely fail to heal. Where fractured cancellous bone surfaces are not in contact, new bone spreads from the points of contact to fill gaps.[54,213] When a gap is excessively large, two bone-forming fronts grow from the fracture fragments and eventually meet, but if excessive motion occurs, external callus (including cartilage) may develop. In contrast, cortical bone has a much smaller surface area per unit volume and generally a less extensive internal blood supply, and regions of necrotic cortical bone must be removed before new bone can form.[33]

Bone Disease.   Pathologic fractures occur through diseased bone and therefore require less force than that necessary to break normal bone. They may not heal if the cause of the decreased bone strength is not treated. Commonly recognized causes of pathologic fractures include osteoporosis, osteomalacia,

primary malignant bone tumors, metastatic bone tumors, benign bone tumors, bone cysts, osteogenesis imperfecta, fibrous dysplasia, Paget's disease, hyperparathyroidism, and infections.[2,3]

Fractures through bone involved with primary or secondary malignancies usually will not heal if the neoplasm is not treated. Subperiosteal new bone and fracture callus may form, but the mass of malignant cells impairs or prevents fracture healing, particularly if the mass of malignant cells continues to expand and destroy bone. Depending on the extent of bone involvement and the aggressiveness of the lesion, fractures through bones with nonmalignant conditions like simple bone cysts[169] (Fig. 2-14) and Paget's disease may heal.[173]

Treatment Variables.   *Apposition of Fracture Fragments.*   Decreasing the fracture gap decreases the volume of repair tissue needed to heal the fracture. Restoring fracture fragment apposition is especially important if the surrounding soft tissues have been

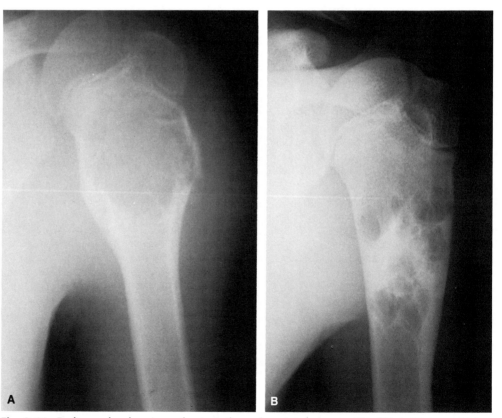

Fig. 2-14. Radiographs showing a fracture through a simple bone cyst. **(A)** A 12-year-old boy sustained a pathologic fracture through a simple bone cyst. The fracture healed within 6 weeks. **(B)** Eighteen months after injury the cyst has progressed towards healing.

disrupted or when soft tissues lie between the fracture fragments. When a significant portion of the periosteum and other soft tissue components remain intact or can be rapidly restored, lack of bone fragment apposition may not impair healing.

Loading of Fracture Callus.   The optimal mechanical conditions for fracture healing include at least some loading of the repair tissue. Based on the available evidence it seems likely that loading a fracture site stimulates bone formation or mineralization of fracture callus, perhaps through piezoelectric effects.[13] Experimentally, denervation can retard fracture healing, possibly by diminishing loading of the fracture[201] or by inhibiting the effect of growth factors that require activation by neurotransmitters. In contrast, exercise can increase the rate of repair,[105] and clinical experience shows that early or even immediate loading does not delay, and may even promote, fracture healing.[68,164,211]

Electrical Fields.   Under experimental conditions, electrical fields can alter cell proliferation and synthetic function. Electrical stimulation has not been shown to accelerate normal bone healing, but several reports indicate that the application of local electric current may stimulate healing of delayed unions and nonunions,[27,28,30,90,140] including fractures that failed to respond to other treatment.[30,90,91] Although reports of this clinical application of experimental work[12,13,28] describe encouraging results, defining the optimal clinical use of electrical fields to treat delayed unions and nonunions requires further study.

Fracture Stabilization.   Stabilization can facilitate fracture healing by preventing repeated disruption of repair tissue. Some fractures (eg, displaced intra-articular femoral neck and scaphoid fractures) rarely heal if they are not stabilized. Fracture stability appears to be particularly important for healing when there is extensive associated soft tissue injury or when the blood supply to the fracture site is marginal. For most fractures, excessive motion secondary to inappropriate or ineffective attempts at stabilization or repeated manipulation retards healing and may cause nonunion.[183] In these injuries it is probable that the repeated excessive motion disrupts the initial fracture hematoma or granulation tissue, delaying or preventing formation of fracture callus. If excessive motion continues, a cleft forms between the fracture ends, and a pseudarthrosis develops. Treatments that increase fracture stability include traction, cast immobilization, external fixation, and internal fixation.[53,190,221]

Despite the importance of stability for healing some fractures, instability may not impair healing of other fractures. During the early part of repair, motion occurs at most fractures except for those treated by rigid internal fixation. Fractures with intact surrounding soft tissues that provide some stability in a well-vascularized region of bone may heal rapidly even though palpable motion of the fracture site persists for weeks after injury. For example, closed rib, clavicle, many humeral diaphyseal, and some metacarpal fractures heal even though the fracture fragments remain mobile until fracture callus stabilizes them.

USE OF RIGID METALLIC IMPLANTS.   Rigid stabilization of fractures with metallic implants can maintain fracture reduction (thereby preventing malunion), permit patients to resume use of an injured limb sooner, and allow bone and soft tissue healing to occur without repetitive disruption of repair tissue.[6,189,190,221] Although rigid stabilization of a fracture makes possible direct bone repair without cartilage or connective tissue intermediates, it does not accelerate fracture healing.[188–191] Stable fixation of fractures and the resulting primary fracture repair have the advantages of allowing early motion and return to activity, thereby avoiding "fracture disease" (stiffness, loss of joint motion, and muscle weakness related to immobilization) and of making it possible to restore normal apposition of fracture fragments. This approach has proven especially beneficial in treatment of intra-articular fractures, unstable diaphyseal fractures of the radius and ulna, unstable spine fractures, hip fractures, and some types of femoral fractures.

The surgical procedure of stabilizing a fracture with a metallic implant causes acute and later chronic inflammation.[139] Repair follows with the production of scar that remodels to form mature fibrous tissue. For totally inert implants, this would be the end of the reaction. However, no metal is completely inert, because metals release ions that may cause a tissue response following the initial inflammatory reaction. In some patients, the fibrous tissue covering the implant thickens and becomes more vascular, and microscopic examination may demonstrate the presence of giant cells; however, these tissue reactions to implants have not been shown to alter fracture healing.

Although rigid stabilization of fractures with metallic implants has multiple potential advantages, it also has potential disadvantages. Rigid fixation can alter fracture remodeling and cause resorption of the surrounding bone because the stiffness of most implants differs from that of bone.[4,179,261,266] For example, steel is more than ten times as stiff as bone. When a fractured bone, rigidly fixed with a stiff implant, is loaded, the bone is not subjected to normal stress.[73,235,245] Regional loss of bone mass may occur (Fig. 2-15), which increases the probability of refracture following removal of the plate.[110,204,245] This problem might be avoided by use of less rigid plates (ie, plates that more closely approximate the modulus of elasticity of bone).[261,266] Attempts have been made to accomplish this by reducing the stiffness of the plate, either by decreasing its cross-sectional area or by choosing materials with a lower modulus of elasticity than stainless steel or chrome–cobalt–molybdenum.[4,244,261,262,270]

Attempted rigid stabilization of some fractures may require extensive surgical exposure that increases the risks of infection and of compromising the blood supply to injured tissues. In addition, at-

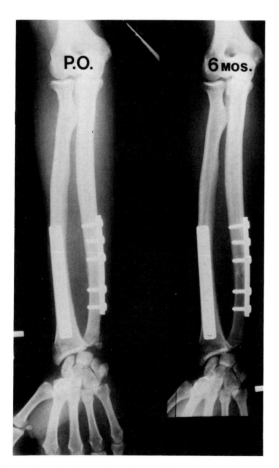

Fig. 2-15. Radiographs showing that rigid internal fixation can decrease bone density immediately beneath the compression plate. Immediately postoperatively (*P.O.*) the bone density appears normal, but 6 months later the bone density under the plate has decreased.

tempted rigid stabilization of fractures may adversely affect fracture healing when anatomic reduction and rigid fixation cannot be achieved. Formation of bone in the fracture gap depends on the width of the gap and the stability of fixation. When the gap is greater than 1 mm or there is motion at the fracture site, secondary osteons do not fill the gap with bone. Complex fracture patterns and multiple bone fragments caused by high-energy trauma or the weakness of osteoporotic bone may prevent the surgeon from obtaining anatomic alignment, fracture fragment compression, and rigid stabilization. If fixation devices hold a fracture site distracted or if rigid stability is not achieved after internal fixation, motion at the fracture site can result in resorption of bone in the fracture gap and the appearance of small amounts of external callus. Typically, this external callus is not adequate to stabilize the fracture site, and delayed union or nonunion may occur. Motion at the fracture site and protracted stress on the fixation device may cause failure of the device. For these reasons successful rigid stabilization of fractures requires careful planning and attention to surgical techniques.

Bone Grafting. Surgeons frequently use grafts of cancellous, cortical, or corticocancellous bone to stimulate fracture healing and replace lost bone.[43] In addition, vascularized bone grafts bring a new blood supply to the graft site. The genetic relationship between the donor and the recipient defines the four types of bone grafts:[209]

- *Autografts* are grafts transferred from a donor site to another site in the same person.
- *Isografts* are grafts transferred between people who have identical histocompatibility antigens (ie, identical twins).
- *Allografts* are grafts transferred between genetically dissimilar members of the same species.
- *Xenografts* are grafts transferred from a member of one species to a member of another species.

Currently surgeons commonly use nonvascularized and vascularized autografts, fresh allografts, and allografts prepared and preserved by several methods including freezing and freeze-drying. Autografts can be harvested, preserved, and then implanted later, but there are relatively few situations where this approach is used.

Fresh nonvascularized autografts contain cells that potentially can form new bone directly. In most grafts only cells close to the surface survive and retain the potential ability to form new bone.[1,46–48,55] For this to occur, the cells must be kept viable prior to implantation. The grafts should not be dried, exposed to solutions that kill cells, or maintained out of the body for prolonged periods. Following implantation, the graft cells must have a ready route of nutrition by diffusion. Diffusion of nutrients into the central regions of bone graft occurs if the particle size is not too large (5 mm is the maximum thickness that can be nourished in this fashion.)[198,199] Because cortical bone has a much smaller surface area per unit volume than cancellous bone, many cortical bone osteocytes lie far from the surface of the tissue[33] and cannot survive by diffusion. Replacement of these necrotic cells requires resorption of the bone surrounding them. In the process, osteoclasts resorb the graft, bringing granulation tissue and osteoblasts that form new bone using the graft material as a scaffold. For this reason small cancellous autografts are assumed to be the best source of cells that can form bone after transplantation.

Vascularized autografts have the advantages of maintaining the viability of bone cells and some of the surrounding soft tissue cells, including periosteal cells.[70,217,254] Large vascularized cortical autografts do not undergo the extensive resorption and remodeling seen in large nonvascularized cortical autografts, and they bring a new blood supply to the recipient site. These features of vascularized autografts may make them especially useful in promoting bone healing when the blood supply to the fracture site is limited or in healing large segmental defects.[70] The primary disadvantages of vascularized autografts are the technical difficulty of the surgical procedure and increased potential for surgical complications.

Fresh allografts have the potential to provide viable cells. Experimental studies indicate that viable cells from fresh allografts may participate in the repair process for about 2 weeks, but after this time they may invoke an inflammatory response that can obliterate the repair, a sequence similar to the graft rejection process described in other tissues.[21,81] For this reason, allografts usually are treated to decrease their antigenicity. Although many methods may be effective, in clinical practice freezing and freeze-drying are among the most common. The grafts may be taken and maintained under sterile conditions or sterilized with high-energy radiation.[47,55,106,117,240,241] The frozen, irradiated, or preserved allografts do not provide cells that form new bone and may stimulate an immunologic response. Nevertheless, their organic matrix may possess the ability to induce local bone formation,[47,48,248] and they can provide structural support.

Selection of a bone graft to promote fracture healing should be guided by evaluation of the problems presented by the fracture. Because there is no immunologic response on the part of the host, and because it may have the capacity to form new bone, an autograft containing cancellous bone represents the best choice to stimulate new bone formation. Cancellous bone has a large surface area per unit volume, and thus it need not be resorbed before new bone formation can begin and appositional new bone can form on the surface of necrotic cancellous bone.[130] Surgeons commonly use cancellous autografts to stimulate healing of fresh fractures, delayed unions, and nonunions with minimal fracture gaps. Massive cancellous autografts can heal fractures with large gaps, including large diaphyseal segmental defects, but during the prolonged healing period the cancellous grafts do not provide mechanical stability.[56]

In contrast, cortical bone autografts can provide immediate mechanical stability when they are used to replace lost diaphyseal bone segments. However, cortical bone must first be resorbed by osteoclasts before significant osteoblastic activity can take place. The resorption makes the graft porous and decreases its strength for months and possibly years after implantation.[70,82] The recipient site cells have a limited ability to resorb and replace massive cortical grafts. As a result, some massive cortical grafts persist as necrotic bone indefinitely,[259] and some are probably never completely replaced.

Use of vascularized autografts reduces the problems of cortical grafts from fracture healing and replacement of necrotic graft material to fracture healing at the ends of the vascularized bone graft, provided the vascular anastomoses remain patent until new blood vessels grow into the graft from the recipient site.[70,230,231,254] Free vascularized fibular or iliac crest grafts have been useful in treating fractures with extensive loss of bone.[70,230,231] These vascularized grafts incorporate rapidly and can hypertrophy in response to mechanical stress in their new anatomical location.

Cancellous and cortical allografts have not been widely used to promote fracture healing. Host bone will unite or bond with allograft bone, and allografts can replace segmental bone defects, but their efficacy in promoting fracture healing has not been clearly demonstrated.

Bone Transport.   Bone transport offers an alternative to bone graft treatment of a nonunion secondary to a segmental bone loss.[181] To replace a lost portion of a long-bone diaphysis the surgeon performs a corticotomy through normal bone, creating a mobile bone segment, and then uses an external fixation device to transport the segment across the defect. As the segment moves, a column of bone forms behind it and with time the bone that forms behind the advancing segment remodels to have a normal radiographic appearance, including a medullary cavity (Fig. 2-16). Most surgeons wait 10 to 14 days after the corticotomy to begin transporting the segment. The corticotomy should preserve the periosteum and the medullary cavity tissue and, if possible, should transect metaphyseal rather than diaphyseal bone. The fixation device must stabilize the bone fragments and guide the movement of the segment being transported. The rate of transport is usually 1 mm per day (0.25 mm q.i.d.). When the leading end of the transported segment reaches the end of the defect, the external fixation device can compress the nonunion site. If the fracture fails to heal it can be treated as a nonunion without a bone segmental defect.

A similar approach can be used to treat infected nonunions. The surgeon excises the infected nonunion site and transports a normal segment of bone across the defect. Although this procedure requires prolonged patient cooperation, it can be an effective method of treating nonunions secondary to bone loss and infection. The clinical results of bone transport treatment of nonunions have not been extensively reported in the English medical literature, but Ilizarov, who developed the procedure in the USSR, has described the principles of this technique,[118,119] and recently Paley[181] reported a 100% success rate in healing 25 tibial nonunions with bone loss.

Demineralized Bone Matrix, Growth Factors, and Autologous Bone Marrow Cells. Past improvements in treatment of fractures have occurred primarily

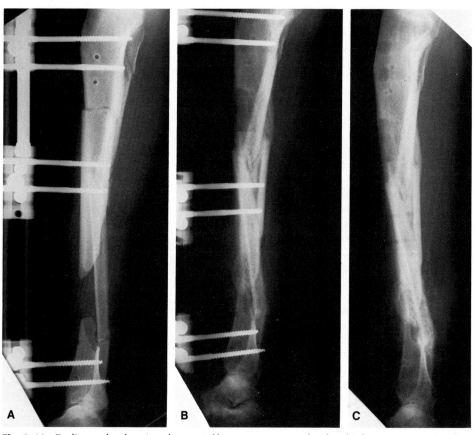

Fig. 2-16. Radiographs showing the use of bone transport to heal a tibial nonunion secondary to segmental bone loss. **(A)** This radiograph shows a bone defect of the distal tibia following an open fracture. A corticotomy has been performed in the proximal tibia and an external fixation device applied. **(B)** The external fixation device transports the proximal tibial bone across the defect. Notice the column of bone that formed behind the moving segment. **(C)** After the fracture healed, the external fixation device was removed and the bone continued to remodel. *(Contributed by J. Nepola and L. Marsh, University of Iowa Orthopaedics Department).*

through advances in mechanical stabilization, bone grafting, and surgical technique. New developments in cell and molecular biology have significantly increased understanding of healing and the potential for facilitating healing. In particular, demineralized bone matrix, proteins that stimulate bone formation, and autologous bone marrow cells have the potential to improve treatment of delayed unions and nonunions.[19,20,50,59,80,125,146,147,168,171,224,225,238]

Experimental implantation of demineralized bone matrix stimulates migration of undifferentiated mesenchymal cells to the implanted matrix and differentiation of these cells into chondrocytes that synthesize a cartilaginous matrix. The cartilage then undergoes enchondral ossification, leaving bone that subsequently remodels. This sequence of events duplicates the process of fracture healing, making the use of demineralized bone matrix a potentially attractive method of stimulating fracture healing by host cells.[19,80,168]

Growth factors help direct the growth, development, and healing of the musculoskeletal tissues. Bone matrix contains a number of growth factors that may promote fracture healing. Current investigations of growth factors are directed towards identifying specific molecules that might be used to stimulate fracture healing[20,146,147,168,224,225,238] and developing methods of delivering these factors to fracture sites.

Another approach to stimulating fracture healing is use of autologous bone marrow. Bone marrow contains cells that can contribute to bone formation,[48] and an experimental study[59] has shown that treatment of delayed unions in rabbits using bone marrow preparations improved bone healing. Based on these observations, investigators have used autologous bone marrow injections in an attempt to stimulate healing of human nonunions. The results appear encouraging, but this method of promoting fracture healing needs further investigation.

Inappropriate Treatment.   Most fractures will heal when treated by a number of different methods, and many will heal with minimal supportive treatment. Furthermore, the healing potential of many fractures, especially those in children, can overcome most treatment errors, but inappropriate or poorly performed surgical and nonsurgical interventions interfere with healing and may cause delayed union or nonunion. Inadequate immobilization of some fractures, separation of fracture fragments by surgical or nonsurgical treatment, repeated manipulations of a fracture, or excessive periosteal stripping or damage to other soft tissues during surgical exposure of a fracture may impair healing. Rigid fixation of fracture fragments in a distracted position,

infection following surgery, or failure to achieve acceptable apposition of fracture fragments or stable fixation may also cause delayed union or nonunion.

DENSE FIBROUS TISSUES

Structure and Composition

The musculoskeletal dense fibrous tissues form tough yet pliable sheets, bands, and cords with great tensile strength.[36,87,96] They consist of a matrix formed primarily from densely packed, highly oriented type I collagen fibrils and a sparse population of fibroblasts. Networks of blood vessels weave between dense bundles of collagen fibrils. Perivascular nerves accompany some vessels, and some regions contain peripheral nerve endings sensitive to mechanical loading. The specialized forms of dense fibrous musculoskeletal tissue include fascia, tendon, ligament, and joint capsule. These tissues differ in shape, location, form, composition, and function but share the ability to resist large tensile loads.

Dense Fibrous Tissue Healing

Like healing of bone, healing of dense fibrous tissue passes through inflammation, repair, and remodeling stages (see Figs. 2-1 and 2-17), and the repair matrix consists primarily of type I collagen. The primary difference is that the repair tissue formed following injury to dense fibrous tissue generally does not mineralize.

Although the specialized forms of dense fibrous tissue (tendon and ligament)[87,96] follow the same general pattern of healing, because of the differences in their structure and function the clinical problems of tendon healing differ from those of ligament and joint capsule.

Tendon

Tendons consist of three components: the bone insertion,[61,263] the substance of the tendon,[96] and the muscle–tendon junction.[95] Tendons contain relatively few cells, their level of metabolic activity is relatively low, and the cells in some tendon regions receive a significant proportion of their nutrition by diffusion.[113] Nonetheless, tendons deprived of their blood supply become necrotic.[194–196,222] In most regions the blood vessels that supply the tendon cells pass from the surrounding tissues through a mesotendon[58] to form a vascular network within the tendon substance.[24,31,36,42,58,96,184] The mesotendon consists of loose connective tissue and blood vessels so that as the tendon moves, the mesotendon

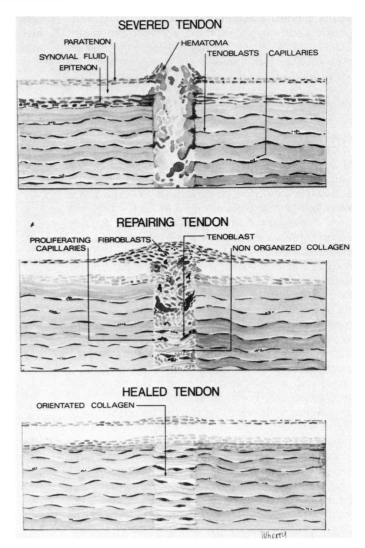

Fig. 2-17. The sequence of events following tendon laceration: A hematoma forms between the tendon ends. Stimulated by chemotactic factors, inflammatory cells migrate into the hematoma followed by blood vessels and fibroblasts. The fibroblasts synthesize a new matrix. They then remodel the repair tissue to restore the structure and function of the tendon. Healing of the other dense fibrous tissues follows the same pattern.

extends and recoils, thereby maintaining the blood supply to the substance of the tendon. In the sheathed portions of digital flexor tendons the mesotenon is especially important.

The specialized structure of tendons—and in some areas the structures surrounding tendons—make it possible to transmit the force of muscle contraction to bone, thereby producing joint motion. Complete disruption of a tendon allows the muscle to retract, increasing the gap at the injury site. For this reason restoration of tendon function following a complete disruption almost always requires surgical repair. Some tendons pass through well-defined synovial-lined sheaths and dense fibrous tissue pulleys. Healing lacerated digital flexor tendons within these tendon sheaths while pre-

serving the pulleys and the tendon motion presents a unique problem in the treatment of musculoskeletal injuries.[40,41,96] The cut tendon ends can be sutured and will heal, but if the repair tissue scars the tendon to the sheath or if the pulleys are damaged, the digit will lose active motion and healing of the tendon may not benefit the patient. Tendons without sheaths do not usually present this problem because scarring of their repair tissue to surrounding loose areolar tissue often will not severely restrict motion.

Most studies of tendon healing have concentrated on the problems of lacerated sheathed flexor tendons. Peacock[185,186] introduced the "one wound–one scar" concept, that is, a tendon laceration creates one wound including the skin, subcutaneous tissue, tendon, and tendon sheath and these tissues form a continuous mass of repair tissue. Potenza's[193,194] studies supported this view and led to the belief that tendon healing depends on migration of mesenchymal cells into the tendon laceration from the surrounding tissues. His work showed that tendon healing begins with inflammation including inflammatory cell infiltration, capillary budding, and exudation (see Fig. 2-17). Granulation tissue proliferates from outside the injury site, penetrating between the ends of the sutured tendons and depositing randomly oriented collagen fibrils. The density of fibroblasts increases up to 3 weeks after injury when a significant mass of granulation tissue surrounds the repaired area. If the tendon has been sutured, the suture material holds the tendon ends together until the fibroblasts have produced sufficient collagen to form a "tendon callus."[17] The tensile strength of the repaired tendon depends on the collagen concentration and the orientation of the collagen fibrils. The collagen fibrils become longitudinally oriented by about 4 weeks, and during the next 2.5 months the repair tissue remodels until it resembles normal tendon (see Fig. 2-17). The amount and density of the scar tissue adhesions between the tendon injury site and surrounding tissues depend on the intensity, extent, and duration of the inflammatory and repair phases of healing and whether or not the tendon is immobilized.

More recent work has emphasized the potential of intrinsic tendon cells to heal tendon injuries. Tendon cells produce collagen following injury, suggesting that they participate in tendon healing.[96,97,142–145,148,149,154] However, it is not clear that a lacerated tendon can be restored to its original strength by healing that does not include inflammation, vascular invasion, and migration of mesenchymal cells from outside the injury site.[36] It is clear that tendons can heal within their sheaths without a mass of repair tissue extending directly from the injury into the surrounding tissues. This observation is especially important, because restoring tendon function requires not only healing but preventing formation of excessive repair tissue that prevents motion.

Early controlled mobilization of repaired tendon can reduce scar adhesions between the tendon injury site and the surrounding tissue. The early use of motion and loading of a sutured tendon may also facilitate healing,[96,97,155,156] but excessive loading may disrupt the repair tissue. Thus, optimal tendon healing depends on surgical apposition and mechanical stabilization of the tendon ends without excessive soft tissue damage and on creating the optimal mechanical environment for healing. This mechanical environment includes sufficient motion to prevent adhesions and sufficient loading to stimulate remodeling of the repair tissue matrix along the lines of stress, but not so much motion or loading that the repair tissue is damaged.

Ligament and Joint Capsule

Ligaments and joint capsules[87] join adjacent bones with dense fibrous tissue to provide joint stability while allowing joint motion. Like tendons, ligaments and joint capsules consist primarily of highly oriented collagen fibrils, and they have well-developed bone insertions.[61,263] Unlike tendons they do not have elaborate synovial-lined sheaths or pulleys, and usually they move less relative to surrounding tissues. Furthermore, because there is no muscle-generated tension on ligaments and joint capsules when they rupture, the gap at the injury site is not increased by muscle pull and there is no direct muscle tension on the injury site.

Ligament and joint capsule healing follows the sequence described for tendon healing by extrinsic cells (see Fig. 2-17). Also as in tendon healing, early motion and loading of injured ligaments can stimulate healing.[7] Because controlled normal motion of a joint does not necessarily cause large forces in the ligaments and joint capsule, limited motion will not necessarily disrupt the repair of the tissue.

The most favorable condition for healing divided ligaments and joint capsules is direct apposition of the divided surfaces. Apposition and stabilization of the injury site decreases the volume of repair tissue required to heal the injury, minimizes scarring, and may help provide near-normal tissue length. A sutured ligament can heal with a minimal gap.[176,177] When tested under tension, sutured ligaments are stronger than those that heal with a significant length of scar tissue, and ligaments that heal with a gap between the cut ends may have decreased ability to stabilize the adjacent joint.[7,57,234] Joint instability owing to ligamentous laxity may compromise the function of the joint and increase the probability of subsequent joint injury and degenerative joint disease (Fig. 2-18). For this reason, restoration or maintenance of near-normal ligament and capsule length and maintenance of normal joint motion should be the objectives of treatment.

Failure of Dense Fibrous Tissue Healing

Occasionally dense fibrous tissue injuries fail to heal. Instead of firm scar aligned along the lines of stress, the injury site contains filmy loose connective tissue, myxoid tissue, or persistent granulation

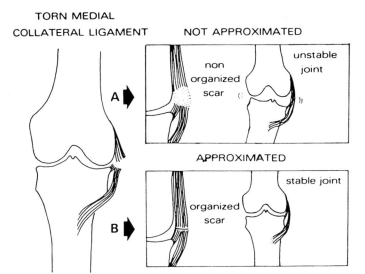

Fig. 2-18. Approximation of a torn ligament decreases the volume of the tissue defect. When a ligament heals with a significant gap, it may fail to provide joint stability.

tissue. The reasons for failure of healing are unclear in some instances, but identifiable causes include a large gap at the injury site, extensive damage to the surrounding tissue, excessive early loading of the repair tissue, and injury-related necrosis of the tissue. Surgical treatment may also contribute to poor healing. Extensive dissection can devascularize traumatized tissue, and inappropriate suture technique may also damage the blood supply to the injury site or place excessive tension on a sutured ligament.

Excessive Repair of Dense Fibrous Tissues

Not only may dense fibrous tissue injuries fail to heal and thereby not restore the structure and function of the tissue, they may heal with excessive scar that restricts motion between the injury site and the surrounding tissue. When this occurs following a ligament or joint capsule injury, it causes contracture of the adjacent synovial joint. When it occurs following tendon injury, it limits tendon excursion and can lead to weakness and joint contracture. In some patients the cause of excessive repair is not apparent and may result from a genetic predisposition to form exuberant repair tissue. Identifiable causes of excessive repair following dense fibrous tissue injuries include severe injuries and extensive surgery that increases the volume of injured tissue. Prolonged immobilization of injured fibrous tissues does not necessarily increase the extent of scar formation, but it can allow scar adhesions to form and mature. Therefore, the best methods of preventing excessive scar and scar

adhesions appear to be removing necrotic tissue and excessive hematoma when possible, minimizing surgical dissection, and use of early controlled loading and motion.[7,36,96]

Variables That Influence Dense Fibrous Tissue Healing

INJURY VARIABLES

Segmental loss of tissue, tendon injuries that disrupt tendon sheaths and pulleys, crushing injuries that compromise the vascular supply or damage surrounding tissues, and wide separation of the disrupted ends of tendon, ligament, or joint capsule make restoration of normal function difficult or impossible. Dense fibrous tissue injuries that produce relatively little loss of tissue and little damage to surrounding tissues and retain adequate vascular supply to the repair site have the potential for restoration of the original tissue function and near-normal tissue structure and composition.

PATIENT VARIABLES

The influence of patient variables on repair of the dense fibrous tissues has not been extensively studied. In general it appears that many of the variables that influence bone healing—including age, hormonal effects, and systemic disease—may be important.

TREATMENT VARIABLES

Surgical Repair. Optimal healing of dense fibrous tissue injuries occurs when there is a minimal volume of necrotic tissue that must be resorbed; viable ends of the damaged tissue lie in close apposition, minimizing the volume of tissue that must be replaced; and the injury site is mechanically stable, preventing disruption of the repair tissue. For tendon injuries the surgeon can accomplish this by irrigation and debridement followed by repair using a technique that provides apposition of viable tissue and adequate mechanical stability, but the surgical procedure should not significantly compromise the blood supply to the injury site or leave excessive suture material in the wound.[96,97] Obtaining the best results of many complete ligament and joint capsule disruptions also requires surgical repair, but for others healing will restore normal tissue function without operative repair.[7]

Loading and Motion.   Mechanical loading of dense fibrous tissues alters their normal organization and composition and in general tends to strengthen the tissues and increase their degree of matrix organization.[36] Investigations show that early loading and motion of the repair tissue promotes repair and matrix remodeling.[7,36,96] Use of early motion to promote repair and remodeling, decrease adhesions, and accelerate rehabilitation has become an accepted clinical practice for treatment of repaired tendons[96,97] and for some ligament and joint capsule injuries. However, excessive motion and loading can rupture or deform the repair tissue at a critical stage. For this reason loading and motion treatment of dense fibrous tissue injuries must be carefully controlled.

It is likely that the optimal motion and loading treatment differs among the types of dense fibrous tissues and among different types of injuries. For example, the optimal timing and intensity of loading and motion treatment of a clean laceration of a digital extensor tendon may differ from the optimal loading and motion treatment of a crushing avulsion of the Achilles tendon. Defining the optimal loading and motion treatment for different dense fibrous tissues, different injuries, and different forms of surgical or nonsurgical treatment should improve the predictability and quality of the results of healing of these tissues.

ARTICULAR CARTILAGE

Structure and Composition

Articular cartilage consists of sparsely distributed chondrocytes surrounded by an elaborate, highly organized macromolecular framework filled with water.[35,39] Three classes of molecules (collagens, proteoglycans, and noncollagenous proteins) form the macromolecular framework. Type II collagen fibrils give the cartilage its form and tensile strength, and a variety of quantitatively minor collagens help organize and maintain the meshwork of type II collagen fibrils. The interaction of proteoglycans with water gives the tissue its stiffness to compression and its resiliency and contributes to its durability.[165] The noncollagenous proteins are less well understood than the proteoglycans and collagens, but they appear to help organize and stabilize the matrix, attach chondrocytes to the matrix macromolecules, and possibly help stabilize the chondrocyte phenotype. Unlike the other primary musculoskeletal tissues, cartilage lacks a blood supply, a nerve supply, and a lymphatic supply.

Cartilage Healing

Because cartilage lacks blood vessels, it cannot respond to cell damage with inflammation. However, injuries that disrupt subchondral bone as well as cartilage initiate the fracture healing process, and the repair tissue from bone will fill an articular cartilage defect. Cartilage healing[37-39,151-153] then follows the sequence of inflammation, repair, and remodeling like that seen in bone or dense fibrous tissue. Unlike these tissues, the repair tissue that fills cartilage defects from subchondral bone initially differentiates towards articular cartilage rather than towards dense fibrous tissue or bone.[39]

In addition to mechanical injury, articular cartilage can sustain damage by disruption of the synovial membrane and exposure of articular cartilage. Because of these special features, acute traumatic injuries to articular cartilage and synovial joint injuries that damage cartilage can be separated into the following categories: (1) disruption of the soft tissues of the synovial joint without direct mechanical cartilage injury; (2) mechanical injury of articular cartilage limited to the cartilage; and (3) mechanical injury of articular cartilage that also disrupts bone.

DISRUPTION OF THE SYNOVIAL
JOINT SOFT TISSUES

Temporary exposure of cartilage by traumatic or surgical disruption of the joint capsule and synovial membrane can alter cartilage matrix composition by stimulating degradation of proteoglycans or suppressing synthesis of proteoglycans.[37,39,111,163] A decrease in matrix proteoglycan concentration decreases cartilage stiffness and may make the tissue more vulnerable to damage from impact loading. Prompt restoration of the synovial environment by closure of the synovial membrane will allow chondrocytes to repair the damage to the macromolecular framework of the matrix, and the tissue may regain its normal composition and function. However, if the exposure of the articular surface is prolonged and if the surface becomes desiccated, articular damage may be irreversible.[163]

It is not clear what duration of exposure causes irreversible damage. The available evidence, based on animal experiments, suggests that damage to the matrix macromolecular framework occurs with every disruption of the synovial membrane,[111] but clinical experience suggests that permanent progressive damage in human joints is relatively rare following temporary disruption of the synovial cavity.[37] Furthermore, cartilage can be restored to its normal condition if the loss of matrix proteoglycans does not exceed the amount the cells can replenish, if a sufficient number chondrocytes remain viable, and if the collagenous meshwork of the matrix remains intact.[37]

Exposure injury to cartilage can be minimized by decreasing the period of time that the cartilage is unprotected by synovium or other soft tissues. If cartilage must remain unprotected, keeping the surface moist with a physiologic solution may be helpful.[163] Because cartilage that has sustained exposure injury may be temporarily more vulnerable to mechanical injury, it seems advisable to minimize immediate impact loading of cartilage that has suffered this type of injury.[37]

MECHANICAL INJURY TO ARTICULAR CARTILAGE

Acute traumatic injury to articular cartilage may occur through several mechanisms. Osteochondral fractures mechanically disrupt cartilage and bone tissue at the fracture site, but in addition, osteochondral fractures may be associated with blunt trauma limited to cartilage, abrasions of the articular surface, or intracartilaginous fractures.[232] Alternatively, blunt trauma to a synovial joint may occur without an associated bone or cartilage fracture. Therefore, acute articular cartilage injuries can be separated into those caused by blunt trauma that does not disrupt or fracture tissue and those caused by blunt trauma or other mechanisms that mechanically disrupt or fracture the tissue. Injuries that fracture or disrupt cartilage can be further divided into those limited to articular cartilage and those affecting both cartilage and subchondral bone.[37–39]

Blunt Trauma Without Tissue Disruption. Although the effects of acute blunt trauma on articular cartilage have not been extensively studied clinically or experimentally,[75,200] blunt trauma to joints occurs frequently as an isolated injury or in association with a fracture or dislocation. Among the reasons for the limited number of studies are the lack of clearly defined clinically significant consequences of blunt trauma to cartilage, the ability of cartilage to withstand large acute loads without apparent immediate damage, lack of a clinically detectable injury and repair response in cartilage following blunt trauma, and difficulty in defining the relationship between the intensity of blunt trauma and the extent of cartilage injury.[37] Despite these limitations, current information suggests that acute blunt mechanical trauma to articular cartilage may damage the tissue even when there is no apparent tissue disruption.[37–39,75,200]

Physiologic levels of impact loading have not been demonstrated to produce cartilage injury, and clinical experience suggests that acute impact loading considerably greater than physiologic loading but less than that necessary to produce detectable fractures rarely causes significant articular cartilage injury. However, acute impact loading less than that necessary to produce visible tissue disruption may cause cartilage swelling and increased cartilage collagen fibril diameter and alter the relationships between collagen fibrils and proteoglycans.[75] This observation suggests that blunt trauma, under at least some conditions, may disrupt the macromolecular framework of the cartilage matrix and possibly injure cells without producing detectable fracture of the cartilage or bone. Presumably this tissue damage would make cartilage more vulnerable to subsequent injury if the cells could not rapidly restore the matrix. However, progressive deterioration of articular cartilage following acute blunt trauma that does not cause fracture of cartilage or bone has not been clearly demonstrated experimentally or reported as a common clinical occurrence.

Trauma that Disrupts Cartilage. *Injuries Limited to Articular Cartilage.* Lacerations, traumatically induced splits of articular cartilage perpendicular to the surface, or chondral fractures[232] kill chondrocytes at the site of the injury and disrupt the matrix. Viable chondrocytes near the injury may proliferate, form clusters of new cells, and synthesize new matrix.[37–39,151–153,158] They do not migrate to the site of the injury, and the matrix they synthesize does not fill the defect. A hematoma does not form, and inflammatory cells and fibroblasts do not migrate to the site of injury. This minimal response may be due to the inability of chondrocytes to respond effectively to injury, the inability of undifferentiated mesenchymal cells to invade the tissue defect, and the lack of a clot that attracts cells and gives them a temporary matrix to adhere to and replace with more permanent tissue. Although the response of chondrocytes to injury will not heal a clinically significant cartilage defect, most traumatic defects limited to small areas of articular cartilage do not progress.

Lacerations, fractures, or abrasions of the articular surface tangential or parallel to the surface presumably follow a similar course.[37,98,162] Cells directly adjacent to the injury site may die and others may show signs of increased proliferative or synthetic activity. A thin acellular layer of nonfibrillar material may form over an injured surface, but there is no evidence that the cell activity stimulated by the injury restores the articular cartilage to its original state.

Osteochondral Injury.   An articular cartilage injury that also damages subchondral bone stimulates fracture healing including inflammation, repair, and remodeling.[16,37–39,49,60,71,93,151–153] Blood from ruptured bone blood vessels fills the injury site with a hematoma that extends from the bony injury into the chondral defect. The clot may fill a small chondral defect, generally those less than several millimeters wide, but it usually does not completely fill larger defects.[39] Inflammatory cells migrate through the clot followed by fibroblasts that begin to synthesize a collagenous matrix. In the bone defect and the chondral defect some of the mesenchymal cells assume a rounded shape and begin to synthesize a matrix that closely resembles the matrix of articular cartilage.[39]

Within weeks of injury the repair tissue forming in the chondral portion of the defect and the tissue forming in the bony portion of the defect begin to differ.[39] That is, osteochondral injuries heal as though the bone and chondral injuries were different wounds. Tissue in the chondral defect has a higher proportion of repair cells and matrix that resemble hyaline cartilage, while the repair tissue in the bone defect has started to form new bone. Within 6 weeks of injury repair tissue in the two locations is distinguished by the new bone formed in the bone defect, the absence of bone in the chondral defect, and the higher proportion of hyaline cartilage repair tissue in the chondral defect.[39]

While the initial repair of an articular cartilage and bone defect is relatively predictable, subsequent changes in the cartilage repair tissue vary considerably among similar defects. In some chondral defects the production of a cartilaginous matrix continues and the cells may retain the appearance and some of the functions of chondrocytes, including production of type II collagen and proteoglycans. They rarely if ever restore the matrix to the original state but they may succeed in producing a form of fibrocartilaginous scar that maintains the integrity of the articular surface and provides clinically satisfactory joint function for years. Unfortunately, in many other injuries the cartilage repair tissue deteriorates rather than remodeling.[37] It becomes progressively more fibrillar, and the cells lose the appearance of chondrocytes and appear to become more fibroblastic. The fibrous matrix may begin to fibrillate and fragment, eventually leaving exposed bone. The reasons why healing of some osteochondral injuries results in formation of fibrocartilage that may provide at least temporary joint function, while others fail to repair, remain unknown.

VARIABLES THAT INFLUENCE CARTILAGE HEALING

Injury Variables.   The intensity of blunt trauma and involvement of subchondral bone have a significant influence on the result of cartilage healing. In addition, the volume and surface area of cartilage injury and the degree of disruption of joint congruity and stability can influence healing.[39,60] For example, small defects, those that are unlikely to alter joint function, tend to heal more successfully than larger, clinically significant defects.

Patient Variables.   As in other tissues, patient age may influence the healing potential of cartilage injuries. That is, infants or young children may have greater potential to heal and remodel chondral and osteochondral injuries than older individuals, although this has not been thoroughly investigated.[37] Other patient variables such as weight, activity level, and systemic disease may be clinically important, but their influence has not been demonstrated.

Treatment Variables.   *Apposition.*   Because experimental work indicates that smaller defects in articular cartilage tend to heal more successfully,[39,60] it seems reasonable to expect that treatments that decrease the volume and surface area of a chondral defect, such as open reduction and internal fixation of osteochondral fractures, will increase the probability of successful cartilage repair. Experimental work indicates that 1-mm defects tend to heal more successfully than larger defects,[39] and eliminating the gap between fragments of an osteochondral fracture results in better anatomic restoration of an articular surface. Therefore, it would seem that decreasing the width of an osteochondral fracture would increase the probability of a clinically acceptable result. However, depending on the location of the chondral injury within the joint and the presence or absence of other injuries to the joint, some separations of osteochondral fractures or loss of segments of the articular surface may not produce clinically significant disturbances of synovial joint function or rapid cartilage deterioration.

The clinical results of intra-articular fractures show that articular surfaces can sustain limited traumatic loss of cartilage without immediate disturbance of joint function and possibly without long-term consequences. An experimental study of osteochondral defects supports these observations.[170] Nelson and associates[170] made 6-mm diameter osteochondral defects in the weight-bearing regions of dog femoral condyles, destroying a significant portion of the width of the condylar surface. The authors found that the defects did not increase the cartilage stresses around the defects, and 11 months following injury there was no evidence of cartilage deterioration. Furthermore, the repair cartilage did not contribute to weight-bearing, suggesting that for some injuries the success or failure of cartilage repair may not significantly influence joint function. They concluded that articular cartilage can tolerate moderate incongruities without significant increases in cartilage pressure or obvious degeneration. However, the extent of tolerable loss of articular surface has not been defined and may vary among joints.

Loading and Motion. Prolonged immobilization of a joint following osteochondral fractures can lead to significant adhesions as well as deterioration of uninjured cartilage, resulting in poor synovial joint function.[37,129,182,233] Early motion during the repair and remodeling phases of healing can decrease or prevent adhesions and immobilization-induced deterioration of uninjured cartilage. However, loading and motion must be used carefully following injury, because these measures alone will not predictably restore normal articular cartilage structure and composition in clinically significant defects, and excessive loading and motion may damage chondral repair tissue and displace fracture fragments.

Restoration of Joint Congruity. Significant traumatically induced joint incongruity causes mechanical joint dysfunction including instability, locking, catching, and restricted range of motion, and may be associated with eventual deterioration of articular cartilage. It is not clear how much of the long-term cartilage deterioration following in-

juries that cause joint incongruity is secondary to the traumatic cartilage damage at the time of injury and how much is related to the long-term effects of incongruity. However, in most injuries restoration of acceptable joint congruity avoids immediate problems with mechanical joint dysfunction and may delay or decrease the severity and rate of cartilage deterioration.

Unfortunately, the degree of joint incongruity that can be tolerated without causing long-term joint deterioration has not been well defined. A study of contact stress aberrations following imprecise reduction of experimental human cadaver tibial plateau fractures showed that generally peak local cartilage pressure increased with increasing joint incongruity (fracture fragment step-off), but the results varied among joints.[32] In most specimens, cartilage pressure did not increase significantly until the fragment step-off exceeded 1.5 mm. When the step-off was increased to 3 mm, the peak cartilage pressure averaged 75% greater than normal. The authors estimated that the long-term pressure "tolerance level" of cartilage may be much higher, probably about twice the normal level, indicating that simple incongruities of several millimeters should not cause immediate or long-term problems. However, they also found that in some specimens even minor incongruities, as little as 0.25 mm, sometimes caused apparently deleterious peak local pressure elevations, suggesting that results may vary even among individuals with the same degree of articular incongruity.

Stabilization. Mechanical stabilization of an osteochondral injury in an acceptable position increases the likelihood of satisfactory healing by preventing disruption of the repair tissue and restoring articular cartilage congruity. An equally important potential benefit of stabilizing osteochondral injuries is that it allows early controlled loading and motion.

MUSCLE

Structure and Composition

Unlike bone, dense fibrous tissue, and cartilage, muscle[51,52,86,128] consists primarily of cells contained within a small volume of elaborate, highly organized matrix containing muscle-specific molecules. An elaborate system of blood vessels supports the high level of metabolic activity of muscle cells, and a complex network of nerves extends through the matrix to innervate every muscle cell. Normal function of skeletal muscle depends not only the integrity of the cells, matrix, and blood vessels, but also on the innervation of the tissue.

The cells of muscle (myofibers or muscle fibers) cluster into bundles called *fascicles*. Aggregates of fascicles form muscles. Each myofiber contains multiple nuclei, a unique form of endoplasmic reticulum termed the *sarcoplasmic reticulum,* and contractile proteins organized into cylindrical organelles termed *myofibrils.* Each myofibril consists of multiple sarcomeres, the contractile units of the organelle. Membranes of the sarcoplasmic reticulum encircle the myofibrils. The interfibrillar sarcoplasm contains the organelles found in other cells including mitochondria, lysosomes, and ribosomes.

Although the extracellular matrix makes up only a small fraction of the volume of muscle, it is critical for normal muscle function, maintenance of muscle structure, and healing. A basement membrane containing collagen, noncollagenous proteins, and muscle-specific proteoglycans surrounds each myofiber. The basement membranes, together with surrounding irregularly arranged fine collagen fibrils, form the *endomysium.* A thicker matrix sheath composed primarily of collagen fibrils and elastic fibers, the *paramysium,* covers muscle fasciculi. The *epimysium,* a more dense peripheral sheath of connective tissue, covers the entire muscle and is frequently continuous with the fascia overlying muscle.

The blood vessels and nerves supplying the myofibers lie within the extracellular matrix between muscle fasciculi. The vessels form rich capillary networks around individual myofibers, and the nerves penetrate the matrix surrounding the myofibers to form neuromuscular junctions with the cell membranes of the myofibers. The basement membrane serves as a specialized interface for attachment of the nerves. The extracellular matrix components bind myofiber membranes to the collagen fibrils of tendon and thereby transmit the contractile force generated by the myofibrils to the tendon.[95]

Muscle Healing

The same mechanisms of acute trauma that damage the cells and matrices of the other musculoskeletal tissues (ie, blunt trauma, lacerations, and tearing injuries) also damage muscle.[51,52,94,104] Because of its high level of metabolic activity and its contractile function, even temporary compromise of muscle vascular or nerve supply can cause permanent damage. Furthermore, unlike the other tissues, restoration of muscle function requires not only restoration of the original state of the tissue and its

blood supply, but restoration of its nerve supply and neuromuscular junctions. For these reasons classification of muscle tissue injuries differs from the classification of injuries to bone, dense fibrous tissue, and cartilage.

Although the healing of human skeletal muscle following acute trauma has not been extensively studied,[51,52] the available evidence shows that muscle healing, like healing of the other vascularized tissues, proceeds through inflammation, repair, and remodeling (see Fig. 2-1). The following description deals with these events in myofibers. As myofiber repair and remodeling proceed, other cells form and remodel fibrous tissue. In many types of muscle injuries the formation of fibrous tissue is the dominant form of muscle repair, and the result of healing is a tissue composed of scattered myofibers surrounded by scar.

INFLAMMATION

Damage to myofibers initiates inflammation, which includes migration of inflammatory cells into the injured muscle and, in most injuries, hemorrhage and formation of a hematoma. In addition to hematoma formation, an important part of the inflammatory process in skeletal muscle is the removal of damaged muscle fibers by phagocytic inflammatory cells that penetrate and fragment necrotic myofibers. After they enter damaged muscle fibers these cells phagocytize bundles of contractile filaments and other cytoplasmic debris. This macrophage activity not only removes damaged cell organelles, it may have an important role in stimulating regeneration of myofibers.[51]

REPAIR

As macrophages remove damaged or necrotic myofibers, spindle-shaped myogenic cells appear[251] and begin to proliferate and fuse with one another to form long syncytial myotubes with chains of central nuclei. Frequently several of these early regenerating myotubes form within the basement membrane tube of a single necrotic muscle fiber. As they enlarge, the myotubes construct their sarcoplasmic reticulum and begin to assemble organized bundles of contractile filaments. The central chains of nuclei break up and migrate to the periphery of the myotube, completing the transition of the myotube into a muscle fiber. Contractile proteins continue to accumulate and form myofibrils. To become functional, a regenerating muscle fiber must be innervated, including formation of a neuromuscular junction.

REMODELING

Once muscle fibers have appeared, the extracellular matrix continues to remodel. If the muscle cells are innervated, controlled muscle contraction and loading increases the strength of the injured muscle.

VARIABLES THAT INFLUENCE MUSCLE HEALING

Injury Variables.   Muscle injuries can be classified by the type or severity of injury and by the clinical mechanism of injury.[51]

Type of Muscle Tissue Injury.   Clinically significant acute muscle injuries can be grouped into three types that differ in their potential for healing based on the components of the muscle left intact.

A *type I muscle injury* damages muscle fibers but leaves the extracellular matrix, blood vessels, and nerve supply intact. Blunt trauma, mild stretching injuries, and temporary ischemia can cause a type I injury. The muscle fibers will be damaged but the basal lamina and other components of the extracellular matrix, the blood supply, and the nerve supply remain intact. These injuries occur frequently and can heal through spontaneous muscle fiber regeneration that restores the original structure, composition, and function of the muscle.

A *type II muscle injury* damages the nerve supply and may include damage to the myofibers, but leaves the extracellular matrix and blood supply intact. Type II injuries may result from isolated peripheral nerve damage, blunt trauma, or stretching of nerve and muscle. Because the matrix maintains the muscle structure, if regenerating nerve fibers reach intact neuromuscular junctions, the potential for restoration of function exists.

A *type III muscle injury* causes loss or necrosis of all muscle tissue components, including myofibers and extracellular matrix and/or prolonged loss of blood and nerve supply. Type III injuries result from severe blunt trauma, tearing, or penetrating trauma. If the vascular supply remains intact, the inflammatory response can remove the necrotic tissue, but some type III injuries compromise the blood supply, and the necrotic muscle is not removed and must be surgically debrided. If the necrotic tissue is removed, repair can begin. Cells capable of differentiating into myoblasts survive even severe injuries or migrate into the injury site. However, the lack of an extracellular matrix to guide regeneration of myofibers usually prevents formation of organized muscle tissue. Even if such tissue forms, lack of guidance for reinnervation prevents regenerated myofibers from regaining function. For these rea-

sons, the usual result of a type III muscle injury is healing by scar formation with scattered myoblasts attempting to form myofibers.

Clinical Mechanisms of Muscle Injury.   Mechanisms of acute mechanical muscle injury caused by application of an external load include blunt trauma, penetrating trauma, and tearing or stretching trauma. Muscles can also be injured by muscle contraction or muscle contraction against resistance.[51,52,88] Because this latter mechanism of muscle injury is not a form of direct mechanical trauma, it is not included in this chapter.

Blunt trauma to skeletal muscle occurs frequently as an isolated injury or in association with fractures. The results vary from type I to type III muscle injuries. Mild blunt trauma to skeletal muscle damages myofibers without disruption of extracellular matrix, nerves, or vessels—a type I muscle tissue injury. A slightly more severe injury ruptures blood vessels as well as myofibers, causing hemorrhage and inflammation. Healing of these injuries generally results in restoration of normal function. At the other extreme, blunt trauma can crush all components of skeletal muscle resulting in a type III muscle tissue injury that heals with scar tissue. If the area of the crushing injury is relatively small, muscle function may not be noticeably altered. However, following an extensive crushing injury, the cells replace large areas of the muscle with noncontractile regenerating myofibers and scar, permanently decreasing muscle strength.

Blunt trauma to muscle may also stimulate bone formation (ie, myositis ossificans).[120,208,252,269] A prospective study showed that 20% of patients with a quadriceps hematoma developed myositis ossificans,[208] suggesting that this type of muscle response to blunt trauma may occur frequently. The new bone can be contiguous with periosteum or lie entirely within muscle, free of any connection with underlying bone.[269] Although the clinical sequence of ossification within muscle following blunt trauma has been well described, the mechanism of this repair response has not been explained.

Most penetrating injuries of muscle result from lacerations or combinations of blunt trauma and lacerations. Because lacerations necessarily damage myofibrils, extracellular matrix, nerves, and blood vessels, they are type III tissue injuries. Given the highly organized structure of muscle with the parallel arrays of myofibrils, it would be expected that lacerations that parallel the long axes of the myofibrils would generally cause less damage than lacerations perpendicular to these axes. Muscles vary in the arrangement of their myofibrils from a simple longitudinal orientation in strap or fusiform muscles to the complex arrangement found in radial and multipennate muscles, thus, the result of a laceration transverse to the long axis of the muscle will vary among muscles depending on the arrangement of their myofibrils.[94] Experimental studies of complete and partial transverse muscle lacerations show that following complete laceration and suture repair the separated muscle fragments heal primarily by scar, with a small number of regenerated myotubes within the scar.[94] True regeneration of functional muscle tissue and nerves across complete lacerations has not been demonstrated, and muscle fragments separated from their nerve supply show the changes of denervation. Transected myofibers may form buds, but these buds fail to restore normal tissue across the laceration.

Tearing or stretching injuries range from mild muscle tissue damage, a type I injury, to avulsion of a segment of the muscle, a type III injury. These injuries may be deceptive in that the overlying soft tissue may remain intact over a severe internal disruption of the muscle.

Patient Variables.   Patient variables including age, nutrition, use of corticosteroids, and systemic diseases (eg, diabetes) may influence muscle healing, but they have not been well studied.

Treatment Variables.   Preventing or relieving ischemia gives muscle tissue an opportunity for healing and should be the first consideration. Restoring innervation as soon as possible and removing necrotic tissue also are important. Other treatments that may influence muscle healing, including removal of muscle hematoma,[104] temporary immobilization, and controlled loading and motion, may be important but their effects have not been fully investigated. For example, a study of crush injuries in rat striated muscle showed that early mobilization of injured muscles was associated with more rapid disappearance of the hematoma and inflammatory cells, more extensive and rapid muscle regeneration, and more rapid increase in tensile strength and stiffness.[122,123] Possible future treatments for type III muscle tissue injuries include creation of artificial matrices that might prevent the defect from filling with scar, allow myoblasts to form myofibers, provide a temporary framework for transmitting mechanical force, and stimulate directed growth of vessels and nerves.[51]

SUMMARY

To promote healing of acute musculoskeletal tissue injuries, surgeons must use their knowledge of musculoskeletal tissue healing to select and apply treatments that provide optimal biological and mechanical conditions for healing. This knowledge includes understanding of musculoskeletal tissue composition, structure and function, the healing process, and the variables that determine the result of the healing process. Among the most important are those associated with the tissue, the injury, the patient, and the treatment.

Each of the primary musculoskeletal tissues (bone, dense fibrous tissue, cartilage, and skeletal muscle) respond to an acute traumatic injury with a sequence of cellular actions that attempt to heal the injury—that is, to restore the structural integrity of the tissue. Damage to the cells of vascularized musculoskeletal tissues initiates a healing response that begins with inflammation (the cellular and vascular response to injury), proceeds through repair (the replacement of damaged or lost cells and matrices with new cells and matrices), and ends when remodeling (removal, replacement, and reorganization of the repair tissue, usually along the lines of mechanical stress) ceases. Injury to the nonvascularized tissue, articular cartilage, does not trigger an inflammatory response, but the chondrocytes respond to injury with an effort at cell proliferation and synthesis of new matrix. With the possible exception of small cartilage defects, this effort does not restore the structural integrity of the tissue.

The results of musculoskeletal tissue healing can be grouped into four overlapping categories: excessive repair, failure of repair, scar, and restoration of the original state of the tissue (see Fig. 2-1). Excessive repair occurs when the healing response produces exuberant scar that compromises musculoskeletal function, as in the fibrous ankylosis of synovial joints following intra-articular fractures or the scarring of tendon repair tissue to the tendon sheath. Occasionally healing may fail to restore the integrity of the tissue, leaving only thin, filmy connective tissue, poorly vascularized myxoid matrix, an organized hematoma, or other forms of structurally and functionally inadequate tissue. Examples of failure of healing include nonunions of bone or lack of functional repair following a complete ligamentous disruption. More often, musculoskeletal tissue damage heals by formation of scar consisting of a dense collagenous matrix containing primarily type I collagen and fibroblasts. Scar tissue may restore clinically acceptable function of injured tissue, especially in some tendon and ligament injuries and partial lacerations of skeletal muscle. The ideal result of the healing process—restoration of the original structure, function, and composition of the tissue—occurs frequently following bone fractures and may occur following certain dense fibrous tissue injuries and even some skeletal muscle injuries.

Currently the principles of treating acute musculoskeletal tissue injuries include preventing further cell and matrix damage following injury, removing necrotic tissue, preventing infection, rapidly restoring blood and nerve supply when necessary, and in some circumstances providing apposition, alignment, and stabilization of injured tissue. Controlled loading and motion of the repair and remodeling tissues improves healing of many injuries, but uncontrolled or excessive loading adversely affects healing. At the tissue level the effect of the mechanical environment on repair and the function of the repair tissue cells is not well understood, and at the clinical level the optimal protocols of loading and motion of musculoskeletal tissue injuries have not been well defined. Although future improvements in treatment of musculoskeletal tissue injuries, including motion and loading of repair and remodeling tissue and surgical restoration of apposition and mechanical stability of injured tissue, will undoubtedly be beneficial, it is not likely that they will restore the original state of the tissue for many severe musculoskeletal tissue injuries. In particular, large segmental losses or necrosis of bone and soft tissue and most clinically significant cartilage and muscle injuries present unsolved treatment problems. Future developments that may help promote healing of these injuries include creation and implantation of synthetic matrices and use of growth factors or implanted cells to guide and promote regeneration of musculoskeletal tissue.

The authors gratefully acknowledge the important suggestions, comments, criticisms, ideas, and figures contributed by Thomas Einhorn, M.D., Mount Sinai School of Medicine, New York, New York, and Mark Bolander, M.D., Orthopaedic Research Unit NIAMS, National Institutes of Health, Bethesda, Maryland.

REFERENCES

1. Abbott, L.C.; Schottstaedt, E.R.; Saunders, J.B.; and Bost, F.C.: The Evaluation of Cortical and Cancellous Bone as Grafting Material: A Clinical and Experimental Study. J. Bone Joint Surg., 29:381–414, 1947.

2. Adinoff, A.D., and Hollister, J.R.: Steroid Induced Fractures and Bone Loss in Patients with Asthma. N. Engl. J. Med., 309:265–268, 1983.

3. Aegerter, E., and Kirkpatrick, J.A., Jr.: Orthopaedic Diseases: Physiology, Pathology, Radiology, 3rd ed. Philadelphia, W.B. Saunders, 1968.

4. Akeson, W.H.; Woo, S.L.-Y.; Coutts, R.D.; Matthews, J.V.; Gonsalves, M.; and Amiel, D.: Quantitative Histological Evaluation of Early Fracture Healing of Cortical Bones Immobilized by Stainless Steel and Composite Plates. Calcif. Tissue Res., 19:27–37, 1975.

5. Allbrook, D.; Baker, W.; Kirkaldy-Willis, W.H.: Muscle Regeneration in Experimental Animals and in Man: The Cycle of Tissue Change That Follows Trauma in the Injured Limb Syndrome. J. Bone Joint Surg., 48B:153–169, 1966.

6. Allgöwer, M. and Spiegel, P.G.: Internal Fixation of Fractures: Evolution of Concepts. Clin. Orthop., 138:26–29, 1979.

7. Andriacchi, T.; Sabiston, P.; DeHaven, K.; Dahners, L.; Woo, S.; Frank, C.; Oakes, B.; Brand, R.; and Lewis, J.: Ligament Injury and Repair. *In* Woo, S.L. and Buckwalter J.A. (eds.): Injury and Repair of the Musculoskeletal Soft Tissues, pp. 103–127. Park Ridge, Ill., American Academy of Orthopaedic Surgeons, 1988.

8. Andriole, V.T.; Nagel, D.A.; and Southwick, W.O.: A Paradigm for Human Chronic Osteomyelitis. J. Bone Joint Surg., 55A:1511–1515, 1973.

9. Aripow, U.A.; Licmanowa, G.I.; Saatow, C.I.; and Chaitow, R.M.: Zu den Besonderheiten des Verlaufs der Reparation sprozesse bei der Einwirkung einiger physikalischer Faktoren auf den Organismus. Zentralbl. Chir., 92:1097–1101, 1967.

10. Aro, H.T.; Wippermann, B.W.; Hodgson, S.F.; Wahner, H.W.; Le Wallen, D.G.; and Chao, E.Y.S.: Prediction of Properties of Fracture Callus by Measurement of Mineral Density Using Micro-Bone Densitometry. J. Bone Joint Surg., 71A:1020–1030, 1989.

11. Bassett, C.A.L.: Current Concepts of Bone Formation. J. Bone Joint Surg., 44A:1217–1244, 1962.

12. Bassett, C.A.L.: Biophysical Principles Affecting Bone Structure. *In* Bourne, G.H. (ed.): The Biochemistry and Physiology of Bone, Vol. 3, 2nd ed., pp. 1–76. New York, Academic Press, 1971.

13. Bassett, C.A.L., and Becker, R.O.: Generation of Electric Potentials by Bone in Response to Mechanical Stress. Science, 137:1063–1064, 1962.

14. Becker, R.O.: Electrical Osteogenesis—Pro and Con. Calcif. Tissue Res., 26:93–97, 1978.

15. Becker, R.O., and Murray, D.G.: The Electrical Control System Regulating Fracture Healing in Amphibians. Clin. Orthop., 73:169–198, 1970.

16. Bennett, G.A., and Bauer, W.: Further Studies Concerning the Repair of Articular Cartilage in Dog Joints. J. Bone Joint Surg., 17:141–150, 1935.

17. Birdsell, D.C.; Tustanoff, E.R.; and Lindsay, W.K.: Collagen

Production in Regenerating Tendon. Plast. Reconstr. Surg., 37:504–511, 1966.

18. Blenman, P.R.; Carter, D.R.; and Bequpré, G.S.: Role of Mechanical Loading in the Progressive Ossification of a Fracture Callus. J. Orthop. Res., 7:398–407, 1989.

19. Bolander, M.E., and Balian, G.: The Use of Demineralized Bone Matrix in the Repair of Segmental Defects. J. Bone Joint Surg., 68A:1264–1274, 1986.

20. Bolander, M.E.; Joyce, M.E.; Terek, R.M.; and Jinguish, S.: Role of Transforming Growth Factor Beta in Fracture Healing. *In* Peiz, and Sporn, (eds.): Transforming Growth Factor Betas: Chemistry, Biology and Therapeutics. New York, New York Academy of Sciences, (In Press).

21. Bonfiglio, M.; Jeter, W.S.; and Smith, C.L.: The Immune Concept: Its Relation to Bone Transplantation. Ann. N.Y. Acad. Sci., 59:417–433, 1955.

22. Boni, M.; Lenzi, L.; Silva, E.; and Bolognani, L.: Action of Testicular Hyaluronidase Administered In Vivo on the Mineralization of Fracture Callus in Rats. Calcif. Tissue Res., 2(Suppl.):30–30A, 1968.

23. Boyd, H.B., and Salvatore, J.E.: Acute Fracture of the Femoral Neck: Internal Fixation or Prosthesis? J. Bone Joint Surg., 46A:1066–1068, 1964.

24. Braithwaite, F., and Brockis, J.G.: The Vascularisation of a Tendon Graft. Br. J. Plast. Surg., 4:130–135, 1951.

25. Brand, R.A., and Robin C.T.: Fracture Healing. *In* Albright, J.A., and Brand, R.A. (eds): The Scientific Basis of Orthopaedics, pp. 325–395. Norwalk, Appleton Lange, 1987.

26. Braun, R.M., and Schorr, R.: Surgical Nutrition in Patients with Multiple Injuries: Report of a Case. J. Bone Joint Surg., 65A:123–127, 1983.

27. Brighton, C.T.: The Semi-invasive Method of Treating Nonunion with Direct Current. Orthop. Clin. North Am., 15:33–45, 1984.

28. Brighton, C.T.; Hozach, W.J.; Brager, M.D.; Windsor, R.E.; Pollack, S.R.; Vreslovic, E.J.; and Kotwick, J.E.: Fracture Healing in the Rabbit Fibula—When Subjected to Various Capacitively Coupled Electrical Fields. J. Orthop. Res., 3:331–340, 1985.

29. Brighton, C.T., and Hunt, R.M.: Histochemical Localization of Calcium in Fracture Callus with Potassium Pyroantimonate. J. Bone Joint Surg., 68A:703–715, 1986.

30. Brighton, C.T., and Pollack, S.R.: Treatment of Recalcitrant Non-union with a Capacitively Coupled Electrical Field: A Preliminary Report. J. Bone Joint Surg., 67A:577–585, 1985.

31. Brockis, J.G.: The Blood Supply of the Flexor and Extensor Tendons of the Fingers in Man. J. Bone Joint Surg., 35B:131–138, 1953.

32. Brown, T.D.; Anderson, D.D.; Nepola, J.V.; Singerman, R.J.; Pedersen, D.R.; and Brand, R.A.: Contact Stress Aberrations Following Imprecise Reduction of Simple Tibial Plateau Fractures. J. Orthop. Res., 6:851–862, 1988.

33. Buckwalter, J.A., and Cooper, R.R.: Bone Structure and Function. Instr. Course Lect. XXXVI: 27–48, 1987.

34. Buckwalter, J.A., and Cooper, R.R.: The Cells and Matrices of Skeletal Connective Tissue. *In* Albright, J.A., and Brand, R.A. (eds.): The Scientific Basis of Orthopaedics, pp. 1–25. Norwalk, Appleton Lange, 1987.

35. Buckwalter, J.A.; Hunziker, E.; Rosenberg, L.; Coutts, R.; Adams, M.; and Eyre, D.: Articular Cartilage: Composition and Structure. *In* Woo, S.L., and Buckwalter, J.A. (eds.): Injury and Repair of the Musculoskeletal Soft Tissues, pp. 405–425. Park Ridge, Ill., American Academy of Orthopaedic Surgeons, 1988.

36. Buckwalter, J.A.; Maynard, J.A.; Vailas, A.C.: Skeletal Fibrous Tissues: Tendon, Joint Capsule and Ligament. *In* Albright, J.A., and Brand, R.A. (eds.): The Scientific Basis of Orthopaedics, pp. 387–405. Norwalk, Appleton Lange, 1987.

37. Buckwalter, J.A., and Mow, V.C.: Cartilage Repair as Treatment of Osteoarthritis. *In* Goldberg, V.M.; Mankin, H.J. (eds.): Osteoarthritis: Diagnosis and Management, 2nd ed. Philadelphia, W.B. Saunders, (In Press).

38. Buckwalter, J.A.; Rosenberg, L.; Coutts, R.; Hunziker, E.; Reddi, A.H.; and Moco, V.: Articular Cartilage Injury and Repair. *In* Woo, S.L., and Buckwalter, R.A. (eds.): Injury and Repair of the Musculoskeletal Soft Tissues, pp. 465–482. Park Ridge, Ill., American Academy of Orthopaedic Surgeons, 1988.

39. Buckwalter, J.A.; Rosenberg, L.C.; and Hunziker, E.: Articular Cartilage: Composition, Structure, Response to Injury and Methods of Facilitating Repair. *In* Ewing, J.W. (ed.): The Science of Arthroscopy, pp. 19–56. New York, Raven Press, 1990.

40. Bunnell, S.: Repair of Tendons in the Fingers and Description of Two New Instruments. Surg. Gynecol. Obstet., 26:103, 1918.

41. Bunnell, S.: Repair of Tendons in the Fingers. Surg. Gynecol. Obstet., 35:88–97, 1922.

42. Bunnell, S.: Surgery of the Hand, 3rd ed. Philadelphia, J.B. Lippincott, 1956.

43. Burchardt, H: The Biology of Bone Graft Repair. Clin. Orthop., 174:28–42, 1983.

44. Burger, M.; Sherman, B.S.; and Sobel, A.E.: Observations on the Influence of Chondroitin Sulphate on the Rate of Bone Repair. J. Bone Joint Surg., 44B:675–687, 1962.

45. Burstein, A.H.; Zika, J.M.; Heiple, K.G.; and Klein, L.: Contribution of Collagen and Mineral to the Elastic-Plastic Properties of Bone. J. Bone Joint Surg., 57A:956–961, 1975.

46. Burwell, R.G.: Studies in the Transplantation of Bone. VII: The Fresh Composite Homograft-Autograft of Cancellous Bone. J. Bone Joint Surg., 46B:110–140, 1964.

47. Burwell, R.G.: Studies in the Transplantation of Bone. VIII: Treated Composite Homograft-Autografts of Cancellous Bone: An Analysis of Inductive Mechanisms in Bone Transplantation. J. Bone Joint Surg., 48B:532–566, 1966.

48. Burwell, R.G.: The Function of Bone Marrow in the Incorporation of a Bone Graft. Clin. Orthop., 200:125–141, 1985.

49. Campbell, C.J.: The Healing of Cartilage Defects. Clin. Orthop., 64:45–63, 1969.

50. Canalis, E.; McCarthy, T.; and Centrella, M.: Growth Factors and the Regulation of Bone Remodeling. J. Clin. Invest., 81:277–281, 1988.

51. Caplan, A.; Carlson, B.; Faulkner, J.; Fischman, D.; and

Garrett, W.: Skeletal Muscle. *In* Woo, S.L., and Buckwalter, J.A. (eds): Injury and Repair of the Musculoskeletal Soft Tissues, pp. 213–291. Park Ridge, Ill., American Academy of Orthopaedic Surgeons, 1988.

52. Carlson, B.M., and Faulkner, J.A.: The Regeneration of Skeletal Muscle Fibers Following Injury: A Review. Med. Sci. Sports Excer. 15:187–198, 1983.

53. Chao, E. Y-S.: Biomechanics of External Fixation. *In* Lang, J.M. (ed): Fracture Healing, pp. 105–122. New York, Churchill-Livingstone, 1987.

54. Charnley, J., and Baker, S.L.: Compression Arthrodesis of the Knee. A Clinical and Historical Study. J. Bone Joint Surg., 34B:187–199, 1952.

55. Chase, S.W., and Herndon, C.H.: The Fate of Autogenous and Homogenous Bone Grafts: An Historical Review. J. Bone Joint Surg., 37A:809–841, 1955.

56. Christian, E.P.; Bosse, M.J.; and Robb, G.: Reconstruction of Large Diaphyseal Defects Without Free Fibular Transfer: In Grade IIIB Tibial Fractures. J. Bone Joint Surg., 71A: 994–1004, 1989.

57. Clayton, M.L., and Weir, G.J., Jr.: Experimental Investigations of Ligamentous Healing. Am. J. Surg., 98:373–378, 1959.

58. Colville, J.; Callison, J.R.; and White, W.L.: Role of the Mesotenon in Tendon Blood Supply. Plast. Reconstr. Surg., 43:53–60, 1969.

59. Connolly, J.; Guise, R.; Lippiello, L.; and Dehne, R.: Development of an Osteogenic Bone Marrow Preparation. J. Bone Joint Surg., 71A:684–691, 1989.

60. Convery, F.R.; Akeson, W.H.; and Keown, G.H.: The Repair of Large Osteochondral Defects: An Experimental Study in Horses. Clin. Orthop. 82:253–262, 1972.

61. Cooper, R.R., and Misol, S.: Tendon and Ligament Insertion. A Light and Electron Microscope Study. J. Bone Joint Surg., 52A:1–20, 1970.

62. Copp, D.H., and Greenberg, D.M.: Studies on Bone Fracture Healing. I: Effect of Vitamins A and D. J. Nutr., 29: 261–267, 1945.

63. Coulson, D.B.; Ferguson, A.B., Jr.; and Diehl, R.C., Jr.: Effect of Hyperbaric Oxygen on the Healing Femur of the Rat. Surg. Forum, 17:449–450, 1966.

64. Cruess, R.L., and Sakai, T.: Effect of Cortisone Upon Synthesis Rates of Some Components of Rat Bone Matrix. Clin. Orthop., 86:253–259, 1972.

65. Cuthbertson, D.P.: Further Observations of the Disturbance of Metabolism Caused by Injury, With Particular Reference to the Dietary Requirements of Fracture Cases. Br. J. Surg., 23:505–520, 1936.

66. Danis, R.: Theorie et Pratique de L'Osteosyntheses. Paris, Libraries de L'Academie de Medicine, 1949.

67. Danis, R.: Étude de l'Ossification Dans les Greffes de Moelle Osseuse. Acta Chir. Belg., 3(Suppl.):1–120, 1957.

68. Dehne, E.; Metz, C.W.; Deffer, P.A.; and Hall, R.M.: Non-operative Treatment of the Fractured Tibia by Immediate Weight Bearing. J. Trauma, 1:514–535, 1961.

69. Dekel, S.; Lenthall, G.; and Francis, M.J.O.: Release of Prostaglandins from Bone and Muscle after Tibial Fracture: An Experimental Study in Rabbits. J. Bone Joint Surg., 63B:185–189, 1981.

70. Dell, P.C.; Burchardt, H.; and Glowczewskie, F.P. Jr: A Roentgenographic, Biomechanical, and Histological Evaluation of Vascularized and Non-vascularized Segmental Fibular Canine Autografts. J. Bone Joint Surg., 67A:105–112, 1985.

71. DePalma, A.F.; McKeever, C.O.; and Subin, D.L.: Process of Repair of Articular Cartilage Demonstrated by Histology and Autoradiography with Tritiated Thymidine. Clin. Orthop., 48:229–242, 1066.

72. DePlama, R.L.; Krummel, T.M.; Durham, L.A., Michna, B.A.; Thomas, B.L.; Nelson, J.M.; and Diegelmann, R.F.: Characterization and Quantitation of Wound Matrix in the Fetal Rabbit. Matrix 9:224–231, 1989.

73. Diehl, K., and Mittelmeier, H.: Biomechanische Untersuchungen zur Erklä die, 112:235–243, 1974.

74. Dominguez, J., and Mundy, G.R.: Monocytes Mediate Osteo-clastic Bone Resorption by Prostaglandin Production. Calcif. Tissue Res., 31:29–33, 1980.

75. Donohue, J.M.; Buss, D.; Oegema, T.R.; and Thompson, R.C., Jr.: The Effects of Indirect Blunt Trauma on Adult Canine Articular Cartilage. J. Bone Joint Surg., 65A:948–957, 1983.

76. Duthie, R.B., and Barker, A.N.: The Histochemistry of the Preosseous Stage of Bone Repair Studied by Auto Radiography. J. Bone Joint Surg., 37B:691–710, 1955.

77. Einhorn, T.A.; Bonnarens, F.; and Burstein, A.H.: The Contributions of Dietary Protein and Mineral to the Healing of Experimental Fractures. A Biomechanical Study. J. Bone Joint Surg., 68A:1389–1395, 1986.

78. Einhorn, T.A.; Gundberg, C.M.; Devlin, V.J.; and Warman, J.: Fracture Healing: Osteocalcin Metabolism in Vitamin K Deficiency. Clin. Orthop., 237:219–225, 1988.

79. Einhorn, T.A.; Hirschman, A.; Kaplan, C.; Nashed, R.; Devlin, V.J.; and Warman, J.: Neutral Protein-Degrading Enzymes in Experimental Fracture Callus: A Preliminary Report. J. Orthop. Res., 7:792–805, 1989.

80. Einhorn, T.A.; Lane, J.M.; Burstein, A.H.; Kopman, C.R.; and Vigorita, V.J.: The Healing of Segmental Bone Defects Induced by Demineralized Bone Matrix. J. Bone Joint Surg., 66A:274–279, 1984.

81. Enneking, W.F.: Histological Investigation of Bone Transplants in Immunologically Prepared Animals. J. Bone Joint Surg., 39A:597–615, 1957.

82. Enneking, W.F.; Burchardt, H.; Puhl, J.J.; and Piotrowski, G.: Physical and Biological Aspects of Repair in Dog Cortical-Bone Transplants. J. Bone Joint Surg., 57A:237–252, 1975.

83. Ewald, F.; and Tachdjian, M.O.: The Effect of Thyrocalcitonin on Fractured Humeri. Surg. Gynecol. Obstet., 125: 1075–1080, 1967.

84. Finerman, G.A.M.; Gerth, N.; and Urist, M.R.: Effect of Growth Factors on Chondro-osseous Induction (abstract). Trans. Orthop. Res. Soc., 14:87, 1989.

85. Finnegan, M.A.; and Uhtoff, H.K.: Healing of Trabecular Bone. *In* Lang, J.M. (ed.): Fracture Healing, pp. 33–38. New York, Churchill Livingstone, 1987.

86. Fishman, D.A.: Myofibrillogenesis and the Morphogenesis of Skeletal Muscle. *In* Engel, A.E., and Banker, B.Q. (eds.): Myology, Vol. 1, pp. 5–37. New York, McGraw-Hill, 1986.

87. Frank, C.; Woo, S.L.; Andriacchi, T.; Brand, R.; Oakes, B.; Dahners, L.; De Haven U.; Lewis, J.; and Sabiston, P.: Normal Ligament: Structure, Function and Composition. *In* Woo, S.L., and Buckwalter, J.A. (eds.): Injury and Repair of the Musculoskeletal Soft Tissues, pp. 45–101. Park Ridge, Ill., American Academy of Orthopaedic Surgeons, 1988.

88. Friden, J.; Sjostrom, M.; and Ekbolm, B.: Myofibrillar Damage Following Intense Eccentric Exercise in Man. Int. J. Sports Med., 4:170–176, 1983.

89. Friedenberg, Z.B.; and Brighton, C.T.: Bioelectric Potentials in Bone. J. Bone Joint Surg., 48A:915–923, 1966.

90. Friedenberg, Z.B.; Brighton, C.T.: Biophysical Induction of Fracture Repair. *In* Lang, J.M. (ed.): Fracture Healing, pp. 75–80. New York, Churchill Livingstone, 1987.

91. Friedenberg, Z.B.; Harlow, M.C.; and Brighton, C.T.: Healing of Nonunion of the Medial Malleolus by Means of a Direct Current: A Case Report. J. Trauma, 11:883–885, 1971.

92. Frost, H.M.: Skeletal Physiology and Bone Remodeling. *In* Urist, M.R. (ed.): Fundamental and Clinical Bone Physiology, pp. 208–241. Philadelphia, J.B. Lippincott, 1980.

93. Furukawa, T.; Eyre, D.R.; Koide, S.; and Glimcher, M.J.: Biochemical Studies on Repair Cartilage Resurfacing Experimental Defects in the Rabbit Knee. J. Bone Joint Surg., 62A:79–89, 1980.

94. Garrett, W.E., Jr.; Seaber, A.V.; Boswich, J.; Urbaniak, J.R.; and Goldner, J.L.: Recovery of Skeletal Muscle After Laceration and Repair. J. Hand Surg. 9A:683–692, 1984.

95. Garrett, W., and Tidball, J.: Myotendinous Junction: Structure, Function and Failure. *In* Woo, S.L., and Buckwalter, J.A. (eds.): Injury and Repair of the Musculoskeletal Soft Tissues, pp. 171–207. Park Ridge, Ill., American Academy of Orthopaedic Surgeons, 1988.

96. Gelberman, R.; Goldberg, V.; An, K.-N.; and Banes, A.: Tendon. *In* Woo, S.L., and Buckwalter, J.A. (eds.): Injury and Repair of the Musculoskeletal Soft Tissues, pp. 5–40. Park Ridge, Ill., American Academy of Orthopaedic Surgeons, 1988.

97. Gelberman R.H.; Vande Berg, J.S.; Lundborg, G.N.; and Akeson, W.H.: Flexor Tendon Healing and Rotation of the Gliding Surface: An Ultrastructural Study in Dogs. J. Bone Joint Surg., 65A:70–80, 1983.

98. Ghadially, F.N.; Thomas, I.; Oryschak, A.F., and Lalonde, I.M.: Long-term Results of Superficial Defects in Articular Cartilage: A Scanning Electron Microscope Study. J. Pathol., 121:213–217, 1977.

99. Glimcher, M.J.: A Basic Architectural Principle in the Organization of Mineralized Tissues. Clin. Orthop., 61:16–36, 1968.

100. Glimcher, M.J.: Composition, Structure, and Organization of Bone and Other Mineralized Tissue and the Mechanism of Calcification. *In* Greep, R.O., and Astwood, E.B. (eds.): Handbook of Physiology, Section 7—Endocrinology. Washington, D.C., American Physiological Society, 7:25–116, 1976.

101. Goodman, A.H., and Sherman, M.S.: Postirradiation Fractures of the Femoral Neck. J. Bone Joint Surg., 45A: 723–730, 1963.

102. Göthlin, G., and Ericsson, J.L.E.: The Osteoclast: Review of Ultrastructure, Origin, and Structure–Function Relationship. Clin. Orthop., 120:201–231, 1976.

103. Göthman, L.: Vascular Reactions in Experimental Fractures. Microangiographic and Radioisotope Studies. Acta Chir. Scand., 248(Suppl.):1–34, 1961.

104. Heckman, J.D., and Levine, M.I.: Traumatic Closed Transection of the Biceps Brachia in the Military Parachutist. J. Bone Joint Surg., 60A:369–372, 1978.

105. Heikkinen, E.; Vihersaari; Penttinen, R.: Effect of Previous Exercise on Fracture Healing: A Biochemical Study with Mice. Acta Orthop. Scand., 45:481–489, 1974.

106. Heiple, K.G.; Chase, S.W.; and Herndon, C.H.: A Comparative Study of the Healing Process Following Different Types of Bone Transplantation. J. Bone Joint Surg., 45A: 1593–1616, 1963.

107. Herbsman, H.; Kwon, K.; Shaftan, G.W.; Gordon, B.; Fox, L.M.; and Enquist, I.F.: The Influence of Systemic Factors on Fracture Healing. J. Trauma, 6:75–85, 1966.

108. Herbsman, H.; Powers, J.C.; Hirschman, A.; and Shaftan, G.W.: Retardation of Fracture Healing in Experimental Diabetes. J. Surg. Res., 8:424–431, 1968.

109. Herold, H.Z., and Tadmor, A.: Chondroitin Sulphate in Treatment of Experimental Bone Defects. Isr. J. Med. Sci., 5:425–427, 1969.

110. Hidaka, S., and Gustilo, R.B.: Refracture of Bones of the Forearm After Plate Removal. J. Bone Joint Surg., 66A: 1241–1243, 1984.

111. Hoch, D.H.; Grodzinsky, A.J.; Kobb, T.J.; Albert, M.L.; and Eyre, E.R.: Early Changes in Material Properties of Rabbit Articular Cartilage after Meniscectomy. J. Orthop. Res., 1:4–12, 1983.

112. Hodge, D.E., and Peturska, J.A.: Collagen. *In* Ramachandran, G.N. (ed.): Aspects of Protein Structure. New York, Academic Press, 1963.

113. Hooper, G.; Davies, R.; and Tothill, P.: Blood Flow and Clearance in Dogs. J. Bone Joint Surg., 66B:441–448, 1984.

114. Howard, T.C., and Kelley, R.R.: The Effect of Bone Wax on the Healing of Experimental Rat Tibial Lesions. Clin. Orthop., 63:226–323, 1969.

115. Hsu, J.D., and Robinson, R.A.: Studies on the Healing of Long Bone Fractures in Hereditary Pituitary Insufficient Mice. J. Surg. Res., 9:535–536, 1969.

116. Hulth, A.: Current Concepts of Fracture Healing. Clin. Orthop., 249:265–284, 1989.

117. Hyatt, G.W., and Butler, M.C.: The Procurement, Storage and Clinical Use of Bone Homografts. Instr. Course Lect., XVII:133, 1957.

118. Ilizarov, G.A.: The Tension-Stress Effect of the Genesis and Growth of Tissues: Part I: The Influence of Stability of Fixation and Soft-Tissue Preservation. Clin. Orthop., 238:249–281, 1989.

119. Ilizarov, G.A.: The Tension-Stress Effect on the Genesis and Growth of Tissues: Part II: The Influence of Rate and Frequency of Distraction. Clin. Orthop., 239:263–285, 1989.

120. Jackson, D.W.; Feagin, J.A.: Quadriceps Contusions in Young Athletes: Relation of Severity of Injury to Treat-

ment and Prognosis. J. Bone Joint Surg., 55A:95–105, 1973.

121. Jacobs, S.J.; Gilbert, M.S.; and Einhorn, T.A.: The Treatment of Fractures in Uremic Bone Disease: Causes of Failure and Optimization of Healing. Contemp. Orthop., 18: 23–25, 1989.

122. Järvinen, M.: Healing of a Crush Injury in Rat Striated Muscle. 2. A Histological Study of the Effect of Early Mobilization and Immobilization on the Repair Processes. Acta Pathol. Microbiol. Immunol. Scand., 83:269–282, 1975.

123. Järvinen, M.: Healing of a Crush Injury in Rat Striated Muscle. 4. Effect of Early Mobilization and Immobilization on the Tensile Properties of Gastrocnemius Muscle. Acta Chir. Scand., 142:47–56, 1976.

124. Jensen, J.E.; Jensen, T.G.; Smith, T.K., Johnston, D.A.; and Dudrick, S.J.: Nutrition in Orthopaedic Surgery. J. Bone Joint Surg., 64A:1263–1272, 1982.

125. Jingushi, S.; Heydemann, A.; and Bolander, M.E.: Acidic FGF Injection Stimulates Cartilage Enlargement and Inhibits Cartilage Gene Expression in Rat Fracture Healing. J. Orthop. Res., 8:364–371, 1990.

126. Jingushi, S.; Heydemann, A.; Joyce, M.E.; and Bolander, M.E.: mRNA Expression for Type I Procollagen, Alkaline Phosphatase, Osteonectin, and bone GLA protein in soft callus during rat femur fracture healing. In Proceedings of Conference on Bone Grafts and Bone Substitutes. Tampa, Fla., January, 1989.

127. Jingushi, S.; Joyce, M.E.; Flanders, K.C.; Hjelmanland, L.; Robens, A.B.; Sporn, M.G.; Muniz, O.; Howell, D.; Dean, D.; and Bolander, M.E.: Distribution of Acidic Fibroblast Growth Factor, Basic Fibroblast Growth Factor and Transforming Growth Factor-β in rat growth plate. In Cohen; Glorieux; and Martin, (eds.): Proceedings of the First Joint ASBMR/ICCRH Congress. Amsterdam, Elsevier Science (In Press).

128. Jukl, P.: Muscle. In Albright, J.A., and Brand, R.A. (eds.): The Scientific Basis of Orthopaedics, pp. 407–422. Norwalk: Appleton Lange, 1987.

129. Jurvelin, J.; Kiviranta, I.; Tammi, M.; and Helminen, H.J.: Softening of Canine Articular Cartilage after Immobilization of the Knee Joint. Clin. Orthop., 207:246–252, 1986.

130. Kenzora, J.E.; Steele, R.E.; Yosipovitch, Z.H.; and Glimcher, M.J.: Experimental Osteonecrosis of the Femoral Head in Adult Rabbits. Clin. Orthop., 130:8–46, 1978.

131. Key, J.A.: Stainless Steel and Vitallium in Internal Fixation of Bone. Arch. Surg., 43:615–626, 1941.

132. Knoch, H.G.: Der Einfluss von Niedrund Hochfrequenzschwingungen auf das Kallusgewebe im Tierexperiment. Zentralbl. Chir., 92:1874–1799, 1967.

133. Koskinen, E.V.S.: The Repair of Experimental Fractures Under the Action of Growth Hormone, Thyrotropin and Cortisone: A Tissue Analytic, Roentgenologic and Autoradiographic Study. Ann. Chir. Gynaecol. Fenn., 48(Suppl)90:1–48, 1959.

134. Koskinen, E.V.S.: Effect of Endocrine Factors on Callus Development in Experimental Fractures. Symp. Biol. Hung., 7:315–322, 1967.

135. Koskinen, E.V.S.; Ryoppy, S.A.; and Lindholm, T.S.: Bone Formation by Induction Under the Influence of Growth Hormone and Cortisone. Isr. J. Med. Sci., 7:378–380, 1971.

136. Kowalewski, K.; Couves, C.M.; and Lang, A.: Protective Action of 17-Ethyl-19-Nortestosterone Against the Inhibition of Bone Repair in the Lathyrus-Fed Rat. Acta Endocrinol., 30:268–272, 1959.

137. Kowalewski, K., and Gort, J.: An Anabolic Androgen as a Stimulant of Bone Healing in Rats Treated with Cortisone. Acta Endocrinol., 30:273–276, 1959.

138. Lack, C.H.: Proteolytic Activity and Connective Tissue. Br. Med. Bull., 20:217–222, 1964.

139. Laing, P.G.; Ferguson, A.B., Jr.; and Hodge, E.S.: Tissue Reaction in Rabbit Muscle to Metallic Implants. J. Biomed. Mater. Res., 1:135–149, 1967.

140. Lavine, L.S., and Shamos, M.H.: Electric Enhancement of Bone Healing. Science, 175:118–121, 1972.

141. Leung, K.S.; Sher, A.H.; Lam, T.S.W., and Leung, P.C.: Energy Metabolism in Fracture Healing. J. Bone Joint Surg., 71B:567–660, 1989.

142. Lindsay, W.K., and Birch, J.R.: The Fibroblast in Flexor Tendon Healing. Plast. Reconstr. Surg., 34:223–232, 1964.

143. Lindsay, W.K., and McDougall, E.P.: Digital Flexor Tendons: An Experimental Study. Part III. The Fate of Autogenous Digital Flexor Tendon Grafts. Br. J. Plast. Surg., 13:293–304, 1961.

144. Lindsay, W.K., and Thomson, H.G.: Digital Flexor Tendons: An Experimental Study. Part I. The Significance of Each Component of the Flexor Mechanism in Tendon Healing. Br. J. Plast. Surg., 12:289–316, 1960.

145. Lindsay, W.K.; Thomson, H.G.; and Walker, F.G.: Digital Flexor Tendons: An Experimental Study. Part II. The Significance of a Gap Occurring at the Line of Suture. Br. J. Plast. Surg., 13:1–9, 1960.

146. Lucas, P.A.: Chemotactic Response of Osteoblast-like Cells to TGF-Beta (abstract). Trans. Orthop. Res. Soc., 14:86, 1989.

147. Lucas, P.A.; Syftestad, G.T.; and Caplan, A.I.: In Vivo Ectopic Induction of Cartilage and Bone by Water Soluble Proteins from Bone Matrix (abstract). Trans. Orthop. Res. Soc., 13:321, 1988.

148. Lundborg, G., and Rank, F.: Experimental Intrinsic Healing of Flexor Tendons Based Upon Synovial Fluid Nutrition. J. Hand Surg., 3:21–31, 1978.

149. Lundborg, G.; Rydevik, B.; Manthrope, M.; Varon, S.; and Lewis, J.: Peripheral Nerve: The Physiology of Injury and Repair. In Woo, S.L., and Buckwalter, J.A. (eds.): Injury and Repair of the Musculoskeletal Soft Tissue, pp. 297–352. Park Ridge, Ill., American Academy of Orthopaedic Surgeons, 1988.

150. Macy, L.D.; Kana, S.M.; Jingushi, S.; Terek, R.M.; Borretos, J.; and Bolander, M.D.: Defects of Early Fracture-Healing in Experimental Diabetes. J. Bone Joint Surg., 71A:722–733, 1989.

151. Mankin, H.J.: The Reaction of Articular Cartilage to Injury and Osteoarthritis: Part I. N. Engl. J. Med., 291:1285–1292, 1974.

152. Mankin, H.J.: The Reaction of Articular Cartilage to Injury

and Osteoarthritis: Part II. N. Engl. J. Med., 291:1335–1340, 1974.

153. Mankin, H.J.: The Response of Articular Cartilage to Mechanical Injury. J. Bone Joint Surg., 64A:460–466, 1982.

154. Manske, P.R.; Gelberman, R.H.; Vande Berg, J.S.; and Lester, P.A.: Intrinsic Flexor Tendon Repair: A Morphologic Study In Vitro. J. Bone Joint Surg., 66A:385–396, 1984.

155. Mason, M.L., and Allen, H.S.: The Rate of Healing of Tendons: An Experimental Study of Tensile Strength. Ann. Surg., 113:424–459, 1941.

156. Mason, M.L., and Shearon, C.G.: The Process of Tendon Repair: An Experimental Study of Tendon Suture and Tendon Graft. Arch. Surg., 25:615–692, 1932.

157. McKibbin, B.: The Biology of Fracture Healing in Long Bones. J. Bone Joint Surg., 60B:150–162, 1978.

158. Meachim, G.: The Effects of Scarification of an Articular Cartilage in the Rabbit. J. Bone Joint Surg., 45B:150–161, 1983.

159. Medawar, P.B.: Immunology of Transplantation. Harvey Lect., 50:114–116, 1957.

160. Michelsen, C.G., and Askanazi, J: Current Concepts Review: The Metabolic Response to Injury: Mechanism and Clinical Implantations. J. Bone Joint Surg., 68A:782–787, 1986.

161. Misol, S.; Samaan, N.; and Ponseti, I.V.: Growth Hormone in Delayed Fracture Union. Clin. Orthop., 74:206–208, 1971.

162. Mitchell, N., and Shephard, N.: Effect of Patellar Shaving in the Rabbit. J. Orthop. Res., 5:388–392, 1987.

163. Mitchell, N., and Shepard, N.: The Deleterious Effects of Drying on Articular Cartilage. J. Bone Joint Surg., 71A:89–95, 1989.

164. Mooney, V.; Nickel, V.; Harvey, J.P., Jr.; and Snelson, R.: Cast Brace Treatment for Fractures of the Distal Part of the Femur. J. Bone Joint Surg., 52A:1563–1578, 1970.

165. Mow, V., and Rosenwasser, M.: Articular Cartilage: Biomechanics. In Woo, S.C., and Buckwalter, J.A. (eds): Injury and Repair of the Musculoskeletal Soft Tissues, pp. 427–463. Park Ridge, Ill., American Academy of Orthopaedic Surgeons, 1988.

166. Müller, M.E.; Allgöwer, M.; and Willenegger, H.: Technique of Internal Fixation of Fractures. New York, Springer-Verlag, 1965.

167. Mulliken, J.B.; Kaban, L.B.; and Glowacki, J.: Induced Osteogenesis—the Biological Principle and Clinical Applications. J. Surg. Res., 37:487–496, 1984.

168. Muthukumaran, N., and Reddi, A.H.: Bone Matrix-Induced Local Bone Induction. Clin. Orthop., 220:159–164, 1984.

169. Neer, C.S.; Francis, K.C.; Marcove, R.C.; Terz, J.; and Carbonara, P.N.: Treatment of Unicameral Bone Cyst. J. Bone Joint Surg., 48A:731–745, 1966.

170. Nelson, B.H.; Anderson, D.D.; Brand, R.A.; and Brown, T.D.: Effect of Osteochondral Defects on Articular Cartilage: Contact Pressures Studied in Dog Knees. Acta Orthop. Scand., 59:574–579, 1988.

171. Nemeth, G.G.; Bolander, M.E.; and Martin, O.R.: Growth Factors and Their Role in Wound and Fracture Healing. In Barbule; Pines; Caldwell; and Hunt, (eds): Growth Factors and Other Aspects of Wound Healing: Biological and Clinical Implications, pp. 1–17. New York, Allen R. Liss, 1988.

172. Nemeth, G.G.; Heydemann, A.; Jingushi, S.; Terek, R.; and Bolander, M.E.: Temporal Activation and Abnormal Regulation of Cartilage and Bone Genes in Fracture Healing. In Proceedings of the Second International Conference on Molecular Biology and Pathology of Matrix, Philadelphia, June, 1988.

173. Nicholas, J.A., and Killoran, P.: Fracture of the Femur in Patients with Paget's Disease. J. Bone Joint Surg., 47A:450–461, 1965.

174. Nichols, J.T.; Toto, P.D.; and Choukas, N.C.: The Proliferative Capacity and DNA Synthesis of Osteoblasts during Fracture Repair in Normal and Hypophysectomized Rats. Oral Surg., 25:418–426, 1968.

175. Noda, M., and Camillier, J.J.: In Vivo Stimulation of Bone Formation by Transforming Growth Factor-β. Endocrinology, 124(6):2991–2994, 1989.

176. O'Donoghue, D.H.: Surgical Treatment of Fresh Injuries to the Major Ligaments of the Knee. J. Bone Joint Surg., 32A:721–738, 1950.

177. O'Donoghue, D.H.: An Analysis of End Results of Surgical Treatment of Major Injuries to the Ligaments of the Knee. J. Bone Joint Surg., 37A:1–13, 1955.

178. Oegema, T.; An, K.N.; Weiland, A.; Furcht, L.: Peripheral Blood Vessel. In Woo, S.C., and Buckwalter, J.A. (eds): Injury and Repair of the Musculoskeletal Soft Tissues, pp. 357–400. Park Ridge, Ill., American Academy of Orthopaedic Surgeons, 1988.

179. Olerud, S., and Danckwardt-Lillioeström, G.: Fracture Healing in Compression Osteosynthesis. An Experimental Study in Dogs with an Avascular, Diaphyseal, Intermedial Fragment. Acta Orthop. Scand., (Suppl.) 137: 1971.

180. O'Sullivan, M.E.; Chao, E.V.S.; and Kelly, P.J.: The Effects of Fixation on Fracture Healing. J. Bone Joint Surg., 71A:306–310, 1989.

181. Paley, D.; Catagni, M.D.; Argnani, F.; Villa, A.; Benedetti, G.B.; and Cattaneo, R: Ilizarov Treatment of Nonunions with Bone Loss. Clin. Orthop., 241:146–165, 1989.

182. Palmoski, M.J.; Perricone, D.; and Brandt, K.D.: Development and Reversal of a Proteoglycan Aggregation Defect in Normal Canine Knee Cartilage after Immobilization. Arthritis Rheum., 22:508–517, 1979.

183. Pappas, A.M., and Radin, E.: The Effect of Delayed Manipulation Upon the Rate of Fracture Healing. Surg. Gynecol. Obstet., 126:1287–1297, 1968.

184. Peacock, E.E., Jr.: A Study of the Circulation in Normal Tendons and Healing Grafts. Ann. Surg., 149:415–428, 1959.

185. Peacock, E.E., Jr.: Biological Principles in the Healing of Long Tendons. Surg. Clin. North Am., 45(2):461–476, 1965.

186. Peacock, E.E., Jr., and Van Winkle, W., Jr.: Surgery and Biology of Wound Repair. Philadelphia, W.B. Saunders, 1970.

187. Penttinen, R.: Biochemical Studies on Fracture Healing in the Rat. Acta Chir. Scand., (Suppl.) 432: 1972.

188. Perren, S.M.: Physical and Biological Aspects of Fracture Healing with Special Reference to Internal Fixation. Clin Orthop., 138:175–196, 1979.

189. Perren, S.M.: The Biomechanics and Biology of Internal Fixation Using Plates and Nails. Orthopedics, 12:21–34, 1989.

190. Perren, S.M.; Cordey, J.; and Gautier, E.: Rigid Internal Fixation Using Plates: Terminology, Principle and Early Problems. *In* Lang, J.M. (ed): Fracture Healing, pp. 139–151. New York, Churchill Livingstone, 1987.

191. Perren, S.M.; Huggler, A.; and Russenberger, S.: Cortical Bone Healing. Acta Orthop. Scand., (Suppl.) 125: 1969.

192. Perren, S.M.; Russenberger, M.; Steinmann, S.; Müller, M.E.; and Allgöwer, M.: A Dynamic Compression Plate. Acta Orthop. Scand., (Suppl.) 125:29–41, 1969.

193. Potenza, A.D.: Tendon Healing Within the Flexor Digital Sheath in the Dog. J. Bone Joint Surg., 44A:49–64, 1962.

194. Potenza, A.D.: Critical Evaluation of Flexor Tendon Healing and Adhesion Formation Within Artificial Digital Sheaths. J. Bone Joint Surg., 45A:1217–1233, 1963.

195. Potenza, A.D.: The Healing of Autogenous Tendon Grafts Within the Flexor Digital Sheath in Dogs. J. Bone Joint Surg., 46A:1462–1484, 1964.

196. Potenza, A.D.: Flexor Tendon Injuries. Orthop. Clin. North Am., 1:355–373, 1970.

197. Potts, W.J.: The Role of the Hematoma in Fracture Healing. Surg. Gynecol. Obstet., 57:318–324, 1933.

198. Ray, R.D.: Bone Grafting: Transplants and Implants. Instr. Course Lect., 13:177–186, 1956.

199. Ray, R.D., and Sabet, T.: Bone Grafts, Cellular Survival Versus Induction: An Experimental Study in Mice. J. Bone Joint Surg., 45A:337–344, 1963.

200. Repo, R.U., and Finlay, J.B.: Survival of Articular Cartilage After Controlled Impact. J. Bone Joint Surg., 59A:1068–1076, 1977.

201. Retief, D.H., and Dreyer, C.J.: Effects of Neural Damage on the Repair of Bony Defects in the Rat. Arch. Oral Biol., 12:1035–1039, 1967.

202. Rhinelander, F.W., and Baragry, R.A.: Microangiography in Bone Healing. I. Undisplaced Closed Fractures. J. Bone Joint Surg., 44A:1273–1298, 1962.

203. Rhinelander, F.W.; Phillips, R.S.; Steel, W.M.; and Beer, J.C.: Microangiography and Bone Healing. II. Displaced Closed Fractures. J. Bone Joint Surg., 50A:643–662, 1986.

204. Richon, A.; Livio, J.J.; and Saegesser, F.: Les Refractures Après Osteosynthèse par plaque á compression. Helv. Chir. Acta., 34:49–62, 1967.

205. Rifkin, B.R.; Baker, R.L.; and Coleman, S.J.: Effects of Prostaglandin E$_2$ on Macrophages and Osteoclasts in Cultured Fetal Long Bones. Cell Tissue Res., 207:341–346, 1980.

206. Rokkanen, P., and Slatis, P.: The Repair of Experimental Fractures During Long-Term Anticoagulant Treatment: An Experimental Study on Rats. Acta Orthop. Scand., 35: 21–38, 1964.

207. Rothman, R.H.: Effect of Anemia on Fracture Healing. Surg. Forum, 19:452–453, 1968.

208. Rothwell, A.G.: Quadriceps Hematoma: A Prospective Study. Clin. Orthop., 171:97–103, 1982.

209. Russell, P.S., and Monaco, A.P.: The Biology of Tissue Transplantation. Boston, Little, Brown, 1965.

210. Sandberg, M.; Aro, H.; Multimaki, P.; Aho, H.; and Vuorio, E.: In Situ Localization of Collagen Production by Chondrocytes and Osteoblasts in Fracture Callus. J. Bone Joint Surg., 71A:69–77, 1989.

211. Sarmiento, A.: A Functional Below-the-Knee Cast for Tibial Fractures. J. Bone Joint Surg., 49A:855–875, 1967.

212. Scales, J.T.; Winter, G.D.; and Shirley, H.T.: Corrosion of Orthopaedic Implants: Screws, Plates and Femoral Nail-Plates. J. Bone Joint Surg., 41B:810–820, 1959.

213. Schatzker, J.; Waddell, J.; and Stoll, J.E.: The Effects of Motion on the Healing of Cancellous Bone. Clin. Orthop., 245:282–287, 1989.

214. Schenk, R.K.: Cytodynamics and Histodynamics of Primary Bone Repair. *In* Lang, J.M. (ed): Fracture Healing, pp. 23–32. New York, Churchill Livingstone, 1987.

215. Schenk, R., and Willenegger, H.: Morphological Findings in Primary Fracture Healing: Callus Formation. Simposia Biologica Hungarica, 7:75–80, 1967.

216. Scheven, B.A.A.; Visser, J.W.M.; and Nijweide, P.J.: In Vitro Osteoclast Generation from Different Bone Marrow Fractions, Including a Highly Enriched Haematopoietic Stem Cell Population. Nature, 321:79–81, 1986.

217. Shaffer, J.W.; Field, G.A.; Goldberg, V.M.; and Davy, D.T.: Fate of Vascularized and Non-vascularized Autografts. Clin. Orthop., 197:32–43, 1985.

218. Simmons, D.J.: Fracture Healing Perspectives. Clin. Orthop., 200:101–113, 1985.

219. Simmons, D.J., and Kunvin, A.S.: Autoradiographic and Biochemical Investigations of the Effect of Cortisone on the Bones of the Rat. Clin. Orthop., 55:201–215, 1967.

220. Singh, R.H., and Udupa, K.N.: Some Investigations on the Effect of Insulin in Healing of Fractures. Indian J. Med. Res., 54:1071–1082, 1966.

221. Sisk, T.D.: General Principles of Fracture Treatment. *In* Crenshaw, A.H. (ed.), Campbell's Operative Orthopaedics, 7th ed., pp. 1557–2013. St. Louis, C.V. Mosby, 1987.

222. Skoog, T., and Persson, B.H.: An Experimental Study of the Early Healing of Tendons. Plast. Reconstr. Surg., 13: 384–399, 1954.

223. Smith, J.W.: Blood Supply of Tendons. Am. J. Surg., 109: 272–276, 1965.

224. Sporn, M.B., and Roberts, A.B.: Peptide Growth Factors are Multifunctional. Nature 332:217–219, March, 1988.

225. Sporn, M.B., and Roberts, A.B.: Transforming Growth Factor-β: Multiple Actions and Potential Clinical Applications. J.A.M.A., 262:938–941, 1989.

226. Steier, A.; Gedalia, I.; Schwarz, A.; and Rodan, A.: Effect of Vitamin D$_2$ and Fluoride on Experimental Bone Fracture Healing in Rats. J. Dent. Res., 46:675–680, 1967.

227. Stinchfield, F.E.; Sankaran, B.; and Samilson, R.: The Effect of Anticoagulant Therapy on Bone Repair. J. Bone Joint Surg., 38A:270–282, 1956.

228. Stirling, R.I.: Healing of Fractured Bones: Report of Investigation into Process of Healing of Fractured Bones, with Some Clinical Applications. Trans. R. Med. Chir. Soc. Edinb., 46:203–228, 1932.

229. Tarsoly, E.; Hájer, G.; and Urbán, I.: Uber die Heilung von Knochenfrakturen bei hypo-bzw hyperthyreotischen Tieren. Acta Chir. Acad. Sci. Hung., 6:435–445, 1965.

230. Taylor, G.I.; Miller, G.D.H.; and Ham, F.J.: The Free Vascularized Bone Graft: A Clinical Extension of Microvascular Techniques. Plast. Reconstr. Surg., 55:533–544, 1975.

231. Taylor, G.I., and Watson, N.: One-Stage Repair of Compound Leg Defects with Free, Revascularized Flaps of Groin Skin and Iliac Bone. Plast. Reconstr. Surg., 61:494–506, 1978.

232. Terry, G.G.; Flandry, F.; VanMangu, J.W.; and Norwood, L.A.: Isolated Chondral Fractures of the Knee. Clin. Orthop., 234:170–177, 1988.

233. Thaxter, T.H.; Mann, R.A.; and Anderson, C.E.: Degeneration of Immobilized Knee Joints in Rats: Histological and Autoradiographic Study. J. Bone Joint Surg., 47A:567–585, 1965.

234. Tipton, C.M.; Schild, R.J.; and Flatt, A.E.: Measurement of Ligamentous Strength in Rat Knees. J. Bone Joint Surg., 49A:63–72, 1967.

235. Tonino, A.J.; Davidson, C.L.; Klopper, P.J.; and Linclau, L.A.: Protection from Stress in Bone and its Effects: Experiments with Stainless Steel and Plastic Plates in Dogs. J. Bone Joint Surg., 58B:107–113, 1976.

236. Tonna, E.A.: An Electron Microscopic Study of Osteocyte Release During Osteoclasis in Mice of Different Ages. Clin. Orthop., 87:311–317, 1972.

237. Tonna, E.A., and Cronkite, E.P.: The Periosteum: Autoradiographic Studies on Cellular Proliferation and Transformation Utilizing Tritiated Thymidine. Clin. Orthop., 30:218–233, 1963.

238. Triffett, J.T.: Initiation and Enhancement of Bone Formation: A Review. Acta Orthop. Scand., 58:673–684, 1987.

239. Trueta, J.: The Role of the Vessels in Osteogenesis. J. Bone Joint Surg., 45B:402–418, 1963.

240. Turner, T.C.; Bassett, C.A.L.; Pate, J.W.; and Sawyer, P.N.: An Experimental Comparison of Freeze-Dried and Frozen Cortical Bone Graft Healing. J. Bone Joint Surg., 37A:1197–1205, 1955.

241. Turner, T.C.; Bassett, C.A.L.; Pate, J.W.; Sawyer, P.N.; Trump, J.G.; and Wright, K.: Sterilization of Preserved Bone Grafts by High Voltage Cathode Irradiation. J. Bone Joint Surg., 38A:862–884, 1956.

242. Udupa, K.N., and Gupta, L.P.: Role of Vitamin A in the Repair of Fracture. Indian J. Med. Res., 54:1122–1130, 1966.

243. Udupa, K.N., and Prasad, G.C.: Chemical and Histochemical Studies on the Organic Constituents in Fracture Repair in Rats. J. Bone Joint Surg., 45B:770–779, 1963.

244. Uhthoff, H.K.; Bardos, D.I.; and Liskova-Kiar, M.: The Advantages of Titanium Alloy Over Stainless Steel Plates for the Internal Fixation of Fractures: An Experimental Study in Dogs. J. Bone Joint Surg., 63B:427–434, 1981.

245. Uhthoff, H.K., and Dubuc, F.L.: Bone Structure Changes in the Dog Under Rigid Internal Fixation. Clin. Orthop., 81:165–170, 1971.

246. Uhthoff, H.K., and Rahn, B.A.: Healing Patterns of Metaphyseal Fractures. Clin. Orthop., 760:295–303, 1981.

247. Urbaniak, J.R.; Cahill, J.D.; and Mortenson, R.A.: Tendon Suturing Methods: Analysis of Tensile Strengths. American Academy of Orthopaedic Surgeons Symposium on Tendon Surgery in the Hand. pp. 70–80. St. Louis, C.V. Mosby, 1975.

248. Urist, M.R.; Iwata, H.; and Strates, B.S.: Bone Morphogenetic Protein and Proteinase. Clin. Orthop., 85:275–290, 1972.

249. Urist, M.R., and Johnson, R.W., Jr.: Calcification and Ossification. IV. The Healing of Fractures in Man Under Clinical Conditions. J. Bone Joint Surg., 25:375–426, 1943.

250. Venable, C.S.; Stuck, W.G.; and Beach, A.: The Effects on Bone of the Presence of Metals; Based Upon Electrolysis: An Experimental Study. Ann. Surg., 105:917–938, 1937.

251. Vracko, R., and Benditt, E.P.: Basal Lamina: The Scaffold for Orderly Cell Replacement: Observations on Regeneration of Injured Skeletal Muscle Fibers and Capillaries. J. Cell. Biol., 115:129–139, 1986.

252. Walton, M., and Rothwell, A.G.: Reactions of Thigh Tissues of Sheep to Blunt Trauma. Clin. Orthop., 176:273–281, 1983.

253. Watson-Jones, R.: Fractures and Joint Injuries, Vol. 2, 4th ed. Edinburgh, Livingstone, 1955.

254. Weiland, A.J., and Daniel, R.K.: Microvascular Anastomoses for Bone Grafts in the Treatment of Massive Defects in Bone. J. Bone Joint Surg., 61A:98–104, 1979.

255. Welsh, R.P.; MacNab, I.; and Riley, V.: Biomechanical Studies of Rabbit Tendon. Clin. Orthop., 81:171–177, 1971.

256. Wendeberg, B.: Mineral Metabolism of Fractures of the Tibia in Man Studied with External Counting of Strontium 85. Acta Orthop. Scand., 52(Suppl.):1–79, 1961.

257. White, A.A., III.; Panjabi, M.M.; and Southwick, W.O.: The Four Biomechanical Stages of Fracture Repair. J. Bone Joint Surg., 59A:188–192, 1977.

258. Wiancko, K.B., and Kowalewski, K.: Strength and Callus in Fractured Humerus of Rat Treated with Anti-anabolic and Anabolic Compounds. Acta Endocrinol., 36:310–318, 1961.

259. Wilson, P.D., Jr.: A Clinical Study of the Biomechanical Behavior of Massive Bone Transplants Used to Reconstruct Large Bone Defects. Clin. Orthop., 87:81–109, 1972.

260. Wolff, J.: Das Gaetz der Transformation: Transformation der Knocken. Berlin, Hirschwald, 1892.

261. Woo, S. L.-Y., and Akeson, W.H.: Appropriate Design Criteria for Less Rigid Plates. In Lang, J.M. (ed.): Fracture Healing, pp. 159–172. New York, Churchill Livingstone, 1987.

262. Woo, S.L.; Akeson, W.H.; Levenetz, B.; Coutts, R.D.; Matthews, J.V.; and Amiel, D.: Potential Application of Graphite Fiber and Methyl Methacrylate Resin Composites as Internal Fixation Plates. J. Biomed. Mater. Res., 8:321–338, 1974.

263. Woo, S.Y.; Maynard, J.; Butler, D.; Lyon, R.; Torzilli, P.; Akeson, W.; Cooper, R.; and Oakes, B.: Ligament, Tendon,

EDITORS' N(
Dr. Charles F.
one year after
of this book. H
first edition w
incisive, and a
remind us thai
great teachers
orthopaedics.
In the second
retained as wr
second part ad
Sigvard T. Ha
concepts. In th
combined the
However, the i
Gregory are re
chapter, in par
perspective, eti
(including wou

DEFINITIO

An *open fractur*
and underlyin
communicates
"Compound fra
because it is an
not be used in
fracture can be
a considerable
a wound occur

The most important and ultimate goal in the treatment of open fractures is to restore limb and patient function as early and as fully as possible. To achieve this goal, the surgeon must prevent infection, restore soft tissues, achieve bone union, avoid malunion, and institute early joint motion and muscle rehabilitation. Of these goals, the most important is to avoid infection, because infection is the most common event leading to malunion, nonunion, and loss of function.

HISTORICAL PERSPECTIVE

Hippocrates, it is said, considered war the most appropriate training ground for surgeons. His greatest contribution in this regard lay in his recognition that surgeons can only facilitate healing, they cannot impose it. He recognized the need to accept certain consequences of injury, like swelling, as essential and admonished against occlusive dressings before such swelling had occurred. He opposed frequent meddling with wounds, except to extrude purulent material, so long as the wound demonstrated progress in repairing itself. He further advocated "steel" or "iron" (actually the knife) in treating wounds that did not progress. His principal misconception is generally regarded as his aphorism, which held that diseases not curable by steel (knife) are curable by fire (cautery).

Galen and his followers also recognized purulence and admired it, considering it essential to the repair process. Frequent manipulations of a wound and a continuous search for medicaments that might be applied to enhance purulence were viewed as desirable to driving the wound to heal. Subsequently, most other schools represented one or the other of these viewpoints as a base for their particular methods of treatment.

Brunschwig and Botello, in the 15th and 16th centuries, advocated the removal of nonvital tissue from wounds that did not progress properly. It remained for Desault, in the 18th century, to establish the making of a deep incision to explore a wound, remove dead tissue, and provide drainage. It was he who adopted the term "débridement." His pupil, Larrey, extended the principle and included the issue of timing. The sooner débridement is done after wounding, he contended, the better the result.

Following Mathysen's development of plaster-of-paris bandages, the principle of occlusive dressings was reintroduced, only to lapse again because of untoward effects from misapplication.

Lister's introduction of carbolic acid dressings

seemed the ultimate item in the Galenist search for a magic medication that would persuade wounds to heal. Seized with alacrity, it too proved disappointing, likely because the principles of débridement were too soon forgotten or abandoned—an episode destined to be repeated so many times thereafter.

The imperative of débridement of missile wounds was reestablished more firmly during World War I, first by the German army and subsequently by the Allies. Thereafter, Trueta brought together the combination of débridement and an occlusive dressing that also served as a splint (the plaster cast) in the treatment of wounded extremities during the Spanish Civil War. By contrast with prior experience, his vast number of examples demonstrated the virtues of this method when properly applied.

World War II began just after the start of the sulfa era. Sulfa agents supplanted antiseptic solutions, but like them were applied directly to injured tissues. Antibiotics were available during the Korean War. Yet in each of these military endeavors, the primacy of débridement and the Hippocratic precept of leaving the wound open had to be relearned and then reestablished by directive. The Galenist hope that medicines might circumvent the need to leave wounds open in order for them to heal uneventfully was dashed again. To be sure, failure was often the result of technically inadequate débridement. Yet the open wound may heal despite that, but a closed wound seldom can, even aided by antibiotics.

It seems now that the two major schools of thought can finally be brought together. For the wound that is inadequately débrided and is left open (Hippocratic) may benefit additionally from an appropriate antibiotic (Galenist) introduced at the proper time. Such wounds probably have the best prospect for healing uneventfully, whatever their subsequent management.

ETIOLOGY

The post–World War II era saw a gradual but distinct rise in the incidence of trauma in general until the mid-1960s, when it could be said to have reached a quasi-epidemic level. Open fractures have continued to constitute a significant proportion of recorded injuries. Even as there was an absolute increase in the number of open fractures, so there has been an apparent increase in the magnitude of the injuries incurred.

Fractures occurring in two, three, or even all four limbs are no longer unusual. Moreover, one or more of the fractures is likely to be an open one.

Analyses of the patterns of injury that result from certain kinds of violence, plus some limited experimentation on the direct effects of controlled, violent forces have produced some useful information. Such knowledge of the mechanism of injury may alert the physician to seek evidence of obscure injury known to be associated with such mechanisms.

The essential equation underlying what is usually an unexpected application of a violent force to the human body is expressed as $K = MV^2/2$ where M represents mass and V the velocity of the wounding force. The contest thus arranged is a measure of how much kinetic energy (K) can be absorbed by the body's tissues before they are injured, or how much injury occurs when the kinetic energy exceeds the ability of body tissues to resist, or absorb and disperse it. Moreover, the kinds of tissue injuries that occur vary in relation to the source of the kinetic energy. The converse holds equally true when the body itself is in motion and the offending or wounding agent is essentially stationary. There are numerous examples of combinations of both.

Some of the common circumstances of injury can be measured fairly accurately; others cannot. Although the variety of conditions of injury are almost numberless, they fall in large measure into one of the following categories:

1. The body is stationary and struck by a moving object.
2. The body is in motion and strikes a stationary object.
3. The body is in motion and strikes another moving object or body.

In reviewing some examples of these three arrangements, certain other factors must be appreciated; among them the actual kinetic energy of moving objects—be it the object striking the body or the body itself, the size of the area of impact, and the capacity of the impacted tissue to absorb and disperse energy. Analyzing a few examples may be useful.

Open fracture of the tibia is a common injury often produced when a car strikes a pedestrian. Frequently, the initial contact is made over the posterior leg in the calf area. It is to be remembered that the force that remained great enough to fracture the tibia was transmitted first across the muscle bellies in the calf, even though the integument at that point had often remained intact. The muscles must have been damaged to some extent, and in-

deed we have found them on some occasions to be completely transected. The fractured bone ends are deflected anteriorly, against the rather thin, overlying soft tissue and skin, which then ruptures, creating the open fracture. In the course of débridement the surgeon who recognizes the potential damage to the posterior muscles may discover a communication between the fracture hematoma and the posterior compartment containing the damaged muscle. He must assume that contamination may have reached all parts of the wound, including the posterior compartment. He then faces a difficult decision. Should he confine his attentions to the anteriorly placed tissues, which are easily accessible, or should he consider entering the posterior compartment to deal with the injured tissue within?

In sharp contrast to the massive, relatively slow-moving car, which usually produces a broad area of impact when it strikes a body, a missile is a dense body of comparatively small mass. Yet, in accordance with the formula $K = MV^2/2$, the missile achieves a state in which it is highly freighted with kinetic energy. Moreover, it has a small impact area at contact, so that ordinarily its point of entry is small—approximately equal to its diameter. A number of factors enter into the pattern of subsequent effects, and they are worth a brief comment.

First, we must recall that gases are compressible and liquids are not. Should such a missile penetrate the chest wall and enter living tissue, it may pass through it, producing destruction only along its direct and immediate pathway (unless it should strike a bronchus or a large vessel). The air in the lung can be compressed momentarily as air in the flight path is pushed aside. On the contrary, when a rapidly moving missile strikes tissue with a high water content, such as the liver, it produces considerable displacement of the noncompressible liquid, creating in fact a significant momentary cavity.

An excellent illustration of this behavior can be easily contrived as follows: Make two targets, one a sealed can, empty except for atmosphere, and the other a sealed can of the same size, containing sauerkraut, which has a water content approximately equal to that of muscle or liver. Using a rifle with reasonably high-velocity bullets, hit each target from the same distance. If your marksmanship is equal to it, you will see the empty can jump from its resting place, and when it is examined it will demonstrate small holes of entry and exit with little other distortion. Next hit the target can of sauerkraut, and you will note that it virtually explodes. Often its ends will be blown loose and its seam split, the whole greatly distorted. The sauerkraut will be widely spread about the area.

Muscle behaves in a similar fashion when struck by a high-velocity missile, except that the cavity that permanently disrupted the rigid can tends to be only a momentary cavity in an animal or human limb. The surrounding elastic tissues recollapse the cavity walls, leaving only the small pathway of destruction made by actual contact of the missile with tissue as the residual identifiable wound. Two corollary events may also occur, events that will not be noted unless one is aware of the foregoing mechanism. First, the fluid wave that displaces tissue as the momentary cavity comes into existence may stretch or contuse adjacent nerves and blood vessels in the vicinity of the wave effect. Second, atmospheric air tends to rush into the momentary wound cavity in response to the rapidly produced vacuum and to sweep in with it whatever material lies adjacent to the entry wound. The material thus introduced may well contain bacteria. We shall consider the clinical significance of these observations later, and their importance will become evident.

Yet another example of the usefulness of knowledge regarding the etiology of an injury is the matter of close-range shotgun wounds.[62] The shotgun shell usually contains a large number of small pellets. Though they are intended to scatter at target distance, initially they move from the gun barrel in a rather dense group called a "shot cloud." If, while still quite closely packed, they strike a target, their collective impact may be somewhat like that of a bullet. However, each pellet has so much less kinetic energy than a bullet that they are soon expended. Thus many such injuries are only penetrating ones. Occasionally, some of the shot cloud emerges from the opposite side of the limb, producing a perforating wound. There is also a danger from shell wadding, a material that used to be made of jute and hair compressed with a binding agent. Wadding is impervious to gases and literally pushes the shot down the gun barrel ahead of it when the powder is ignited. The wadding is less dense but has greater mass and tends eventually to fall behind the shot cloud in flight, although remaining fairly close to the cloud and having the same trajectory for several feet. Thus, frequently the wadding enters the wound with the shot cloud, particularly in close-range shotgun injuries. Old-style wadding, which is still being used, is extremely irritating to tissues and incites a severe inflammatory response. Thus it must be removed. Often it is difficult to locate even when its presence is suspected, and indeed,

all too frequently it has been overlooked—to the ultimate detriment of the wound and the patient. Modern shotgun shells use a plastic plug in place of wadding and are therefore less damaging. However, in close-range wounds you must look for the plug.

Two other examples of somewhat special circumstances beset with hazards to the patient and surgeon are worth consideration. Not infrequently, a limb is caught in a violent compressive force, as often occurs when a motorcycle rider catches his leg between his machine and a car in a sideswipe collision. Sometimes the visible wound of the soft tissues is only modest, and the limb is not grossly deformed. Radiographs may confirm the diagnosis of fracture, but there is considerable increase in the separation between the tibia and fibula. This is a sign of severe soft tissue injury, which usually includes stripping of the extremely tough interosseous membrane. Intense swelling often follows, which, if it does not directly injure vessels, often produces compartment syndromes. Such swelling and its consequences can be anticipated by noting this tip-off in the x-rays, and measures may be taken to prevent trouble.

Wounds incurred in a tornado are virtually always contaminated by finely dispersed soil, which literally fills the air in this awesome phenomenon. Importantly, such soil often carries a variety of usual and unusual pathogens, many anaerobic. Recorded experience has indicated clearly that closing such wounds is likely to lead to serious infections, including those produced by clostridia.

Finally, injuries involving the rotary lawn mower are unique to our time. Though infrequent, people are sometimes struck by such unlikely a pseudomissile as a bit of wire or other metal set in flight by contact with a mower blade. The wounds produced are usually small, yet the pseudomissile may bury itself within a body cavity or even bone, which is some indication of the kinetic energy transferred to it by the mower blade. More importantly, it is an indication of the energy contained in the whirling tip of the mower blade itself, which in high-speed machines develops a significant, sustained blade-tip velocity. Coupled with its mass, it is capable of producing a great deal of kinetic energy.

As noted, unusual pathogenic bacteria are found in the wounds incurred by tornado victims. And in a very real sense, a wound produced by a mower blade is created in a minor tornado. The normally earthbound bacteria afloat with the detritus in the vacuum created in a mower casing may result in a wound inoculated by bacteria similar to those in a tornado. For the same reasons cited, we believe it wise never to close such wounds but to debride them and leave them open.

These few major examples of the multiple factors related to different kinds of injury illustrate the usefulness of knowing something about the "history" of how an injury was incurred. Though there are many others, of course, those mentioned should make the point. Moreover, they underscore the need for further investigation about wounding mechanisms and their immediate and late effects on tissues.

CLASSIFICATION

Classification of open fractures is important because it allows comparison of results in scientific publications, but more importantly because it gives the surgeon guidelines for prognosis and permits us to make some statements about methods of treatment. In North America and throughout most of the world, the wound classification system of Gustilo and Anderson[38] and the subsequent modification by Gustilo, Gruninger, and Davis[37,39,40] is the most widely accepted and quoted. This classification will be used throughout this chapter.

I find that there is wide variation in the interpretation and use of the Gustilo-Anderson classification, and generally there is too much emphasis on wound size. The critical factors in their classification system are (1) the degree of soft tissue injury, and (2) the degree of contamination. A devastating crush injury of the leg necessitating amputation may be associated with only a small

skin wound. The size of the skin wound is therefore a poor guide to the classification of the fracture. A very large wound caused by a sharp object such as a knife may have minimal associated soft tissue crush and therefore may carry a very good prognosis. The configuration of the fracture, particularly from the standpoint of the amount of displacement and comminution evident, often points to the amount of energy absorbed by the limb at the time of injury and is helpful in the classification, but is secondary to soft tissue considerations. For these reasons, I have chosen to clarify (rather than modify) the Gustilo-Anderson classification as I use it, in the hopes that the reader will find it easier to use and more accurate than descriptions presented elsewhere. Table 3-1 provides a quick reference to these guidelines.

A *type I wound* is caused by a low-energy injury that is usually less than 1 cm long (Fig. 3-1). It is generally caused by the bone piercing from the inside outward rather than by a penetrating injury. Unless the wounding occurs in a highly contaminated environment, the level of bacterial contamination usually is fairly low. A type I classification implies minimal or no muscle damage. As mentioned, a type I wound should not be judged by its size alone, because small wounds can be associated with dangerously contaminated wounds (eg, those occurring in a farmyard), and with high-energy trauma (eg, crush wounds of the tibia in pedestrians hit by automobiles). The surgeon must take all factors into account when classifying open fractures.

A *type II wound* is greater than 1 cm in length and has a moderate amount of soft tissue damage owing to a higher-energy injury (Fig. 3-2). These are generally outside-to-inside injuries. (This is a somewhat

Table 3-1. Classification of Open Fractures

Type	Wound	Level of Contamination	Soft Tissue Injury	Bone Injury
I	<1 cm long	Clean	Minimal	Simple, minimal comminution
II	>1 cm long	Moderate	Moderate, some muscle damage	Moderate comminution
III*				
A.	Usually >10 cm long	High	Severe with crushing	Usually comminuted soft tissue coverage of bone possible
B.	Usually >10 cm long	High	Very severe loss of coverage	Bone coverage poor; usually requires soft tissue reconstructive surgery
C.	Usually >10 cm long	High	Very severe loss of coverage plus vascular injury requiring repair	Bone coverage poor; usually requires soft tissue reconstructive surgery

* Segmental fractures, farmyard injuries, fractures occurring in a highly contaminated environment, shotgun wounds, or high-velocity gunshot wounds automatically result in classification as a type III open fracture.
(Chapman, M.W.: The Role of Intramedullary Fixation in Open Fractures. Clin. Orthop., 212:27, 1986.)

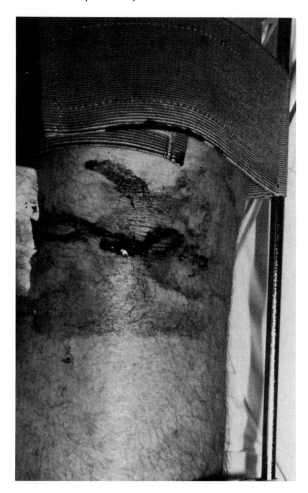

Fig. 3-1. Type I open fracture.

broad classification falling between type I and type III wounds.)

A *type III wound* results from a high-energy, outside-to-inside injury and is generally longer than 10 cm with extensive muscle devitalization. Generally, the fracture is widely displaced or comminuted, although this is not an essential component (Fig. 3-3). The following factors always make an open fracture a type III wound: a shotgun wound; a high-velocity gunshot wound; a segmental fracture with displacement; a fracture with diaphyseal segmental loss; a fracture with an associated major vascular injury requiring repair; a wound occurring in a farmyard or other highly contaminated environment; or a fracture caused by the crushing force from a fast-moving vehicle. The energy of the injury and the degree of soft tissue devitalization *must* be taken into account when applying this wound clas-

sification. Type III wounds can be further classified as follows:

A *type III-A open fracture* is one in which there is limited stripping of the periosteum and soft tissues from bone and bone coverage does not present any major problems. The overall soft tissue envelope about the fracture is usually fairly well preserved.

A *type III-B open fracture* is one in which there has been extensive stripping of soft tissues and periosteum from bone and where devitalization or loss of soft tissues usually requires plastic reconstructive procedures for closure.

A *type III-C open fracture* is one in which there is a major vascular injury requiring repair for salvage of the extremity.

EXAMINATION OF THE WOUND AND INITIAL EMERGENCY MANAGEMENT

Although an obvious open fracture may attract initial attention, you must first direct your efforts at

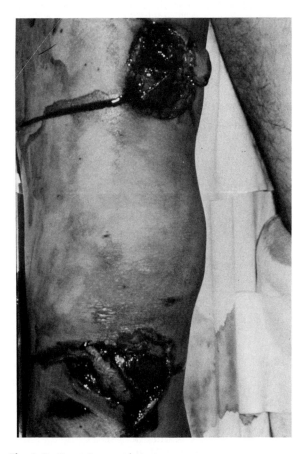

Fig. 3-2. Type II open fracture.

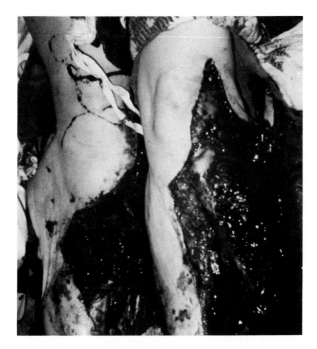

Fig. 3-3. Type III open fracture.

identifying life-threatening conditions and be as complete in the initial evaluation as the condition of the patient permits.[75] Address the "ABCs" of initial management: A—airway, B—bleeding, and C—circulation. Assure that the patient has an adequate airway and that ventilation and pulmonary function are adequate to sustain life. Apply compression dressings to control extremity hemorrhage. Evidence of inadequate circulation (shock) requires immediate fluid resuscitation, and in severe shock, administration of blood and an immediate search for hidden, life-threatening sources of hemorrhage in the abdomen or chest. When any immediate threat to the patient's life has been eliminated, perform a thorough, systematic examination of the patient, assess consciousness and central nervous system function, evaluate the cervical spine, and, in the multiply injured patient, apply a cervical collar until a lateral cervical spine film can be taken. Evaluate the thorax, abdomen, and genitourinary systems. Examine the spine and pelvis carefully for evidence of fractures and/or dislocations. Careful, meticulous examination of the apparently uninjured extremities is essential. Most patients require an immediate anteroposterior x-ray of the chest and pelvis. Initial sterile compression dressings and splints may be necessary prior to adequate evaluation of an open fracture wound

to stabilize the patient for life-salvaging procedures. As soon as possible, proceed to careful examination of the wound.

In major trauma centers surgeons from several surgical disciplines are often available for the initial resuscitation and care of the patient. This allows the orthopaedic surgeon to focus on the injuries of the musculoskeletal system. In smaller hospitals, however, the orthopaedic surgeon may be responsible for the complete care of the patient, including resuscitation and maintenance of life until a general surgeon or neurosurgeon can be summoned. In such cases, the measures outlined above are critical, so the surgeon can proceed with examination of the obviously injured extremity in a methodical and deliberate fashion, feeling comfortable that no other unrecognized or unassessed injury is likely to emerge suddenly or that the patient will be further compromised by neglect or oversight. This plea for a deliberate and orderly assessment underscores the fundamental principle that in dealing with the injured, one should take nothing for granted. To look offers the prospect to know—not to look is to guess. As an additional example (given by Gregory) even now one of the well-known triads of injury associated with fracture of the femoral shaft is still overlooked with distressing frequency: ipsilateral dislocation of the hip, fracture of the femoral neck, or ligamentous injury of the knee.

Initially, assess the circulation to the extremity and its neurologic function. If the limb is in a displaced or distorted position, I prefer to assess it before it is restored to its anatomic position to ensure that no neurovascular injury is caused by the manipulation. In most cases the limb will be in a reasonably normal position in a splint applied by emergency personnel in the field. Note the state of circulation to the limb as indicated by capillary blush, the filling of veins, and the status of peripheral pulses. Examine meticulously for the function of the peripheral nerves. Initial sensory examination to pressure and light touch gives a gross evaluation of the sensation in the limb, but examination for two-point discrimination is often necessary to detect more subtle losses, particularly in the upper extremity. Examination for motor function is difficult in the injured limb owing to pain and splinting secondary to muscle spasm. Often, the only valid motor evaluation is that done by the initial examiner. Once the patient learns how uncomfortable the examination may be, further cooperation may be blunted and the evaluation made inadequate. For this reason, the initial examiner must do a complete examination and record all findings. The normal side must be compared to the abnormal side and results recorded using the guidelines to motor strength illustrated in Table 3-2. This is vital, because a partial peroneal nerve palsy caused by the injury is often overlooked with an inadequate examination or inexact recording of the findings. Pain interfering with the examination can be minimized by good splinting of the fracture and stabilization of the joints not involved in the test for motor function. After the examination, if the limb is not in reasonably normal alignment, it should be returned to normal alignment with gentle traction, appropriately splinted, then reexamined.

Next, examine the skin around the wounds. Is it burned? Is it contaminated with usual or unusual agents—dirt, dust, petroleum products, fertilizer? Contaminants on the skin around the wound may also have invaded it. What are the dimensions and shape of the wound? Is the surrounding tissue badly abraded, contused, or flayed from its fascial bed? Examine the entire circumference of the wound, including the patient's entire back and buttocks. It is surprising how often significant wounds on the posterior side of the body are overlooked initially. The danger lies, of course, in not making provisions for dealing with them when formal treatment of the limb is undertaken. Polaroid photographs of the wound and limb which can be inserted directly into the medical record at the time they are taken are invaluable, both before and after formal wound débridement. Serial photographs throughout the treatment of the limb prove to be useful in educating the patient and his family, and are often vital in legal proceedings. If photography is not available, then a sketch of the limb and the wound often serves better than paragraphs of written description.

Because all open fractures will be formally débrided, there is little justification for exploration of

the wounds in the emergency area. Digital exploration provides little useful information, risks further contamination, and may precipitate profuse bleeding. Remove obvious foreign bodies with sterile forceps or a sterily gloved hand. If the patient will undergo formal débridement of the wound within an hour or so, then simply apply a sterile compression dressing. If a delay of more than 1 hour is expected, flush the wound gently with 1 to 2 liters of sterile saline poured from a container and then apply a sterile dressing. Some advocate application of povidone-soaked dressings; although I have no objection to this I am not certain that it has been proven to help. Patzakis[64,65] advocates a predébridement culture from the wound in the emergency area prior to administration of antibiotics or any antiseptics; again, I am not certain that this is helpful. The validity of these cultures will be discussed in more detail under Antibiotic Management (see p. 261). Start bactericidal intravenous antibiotics as soon as possible.

When a small wound in the skin overlies or is in the vicinity of a fracture, immediately the question arises as to whether the wound communicates with the fracture site, thus making it an open fracture. The safest way to answer this question is formal débridement of the wound, tracing it until its deepest extent is established. However, if the wound is treatable in the emergency room and the fracture or joint injury treatable by closed means, formal débridement, particularly of a very minor wound, in the operating room may not be necessary. In the case of joints, particularly the knee, this question can often be answered by injecting the joint with saline or methylene blue solution and looking for egress of the solution from the wound. Although this method is not 100% dependable in revealing whether there is communication, it has been used in our facility for the past 10 years with no apparent adverse outcomes. That is, we have not failed to formally débride a wound which has subsequently proven to have penetrated a joint. The same method can be used in the case of fractures by injecting saline or methylene blue through a sterile prepared area of intact skin into the underlying fracture hematoma. If this escapes through the wound, an open fracture is present. However, there is the hazard of contaminating a closed fracture hematoma, and as with joints, a ball-valve effect of the soft tissue may prevent leakage of the fluid when in fact a communication does exist. If there is any suspicion at all that a wound may communicate with a joint or adjacent fracture, perform formal débridement.

Table 3-2. Motor Strength Testing

Numerical Grade	Adjective Grade	Testing Parameters
0	Zero	No palpable muscle action
1	Trace	Muscle contraction palpable, produces no limb motion
2	Poor	Moves limb, but less than full range of motion against gravity
3	Fair	Moves limb segment through full range of motion against gravity
4	Good	Muscle strength better than fair but less than normal
5	Normal	Comparable to contralateral normal limb or expected normal strength in given individual

Having resuscitated the patient, saved his life, and carried out initial assessment, bandaging, and splinting of the fracture, it is appropriate to complete the patient's history and obtain as many details as possible about the injury.

PATIENT HISTORY

In severely injured patients it may not be possible to obtain more than the rudiments of an adequate history owing to altered mental status or the need to go immediately to the operating room. Obviously, as complete a history as possible must be obtained from the patient and from relatives, witnesses, ambulance attendants, or anyone who may have useful information.

Determine the patient's immunity to tetanus if at all possible. If the patient has been immunized against tetanus in the past 10 years, only toxoid may be needed as a booster. If the patient has not had a recent immunization, or if the history is uncertain, administer 250 to 500 units of tetanus human immune globulin and give tetanus toxoid as well.

Try to elicit all points in the medical history, but particularly those that may influence your decision in managing the open fracture wound, such as a history of diabetes mellitus, chronic steroid use, or the presence of other debilitating disease. A compromised immune system (particularly a history of active AIDS), may push one toward early amputation in a patient with a severe type III-C open fracture rather than risking a severe infection that could be life-threatening.

The complete history and physical examination and all information gathered to this point must be carefully and accurately recorded, including all measures taken in the treatment of the patient, the time they were carried out, and the patient's response to them.

RADIOGRAPHIC EXAMINATION

A discussion of x-ray examination of the open fracture has been delayed for the same reason that the taking of x-rays is usually delayed until the steps already discussed have been carried out. Several initial films are often critical to the care of the severely injured patient, including a lateral view of the cervical spine and anteroposterior views of the chest and pelvis. In well-equipped emergency rooms, these are taken by overhead-mounted machines in the resuscitation room. In less well-equipped emergency rooms, use of portable x-ray equipment in the resuscitation room may be necessary. Ideally, x-rays should be taken in a regular x-ray examination room rather than using portable equipment in the operating room, because the quality of films that can be obtained and the various views possible are much better.

Extremity radiographs can usually be deferred until the patient's general condition has been stabilized, life-threatening emergencies have been eliminated, and the wound has been inspected, dressed, and the fracture splinted as already outlined. Nothing annoys me more than to find a patient lying on an x-ray table with an open wound and an unsplinted, deformed limb. Radiographic examination is simply an adjunct to the initial evaluation of the patient, and obtaining x-rays under such conditions simply contributes to the patient's hemorrhage, contamination of the wound, and further soft tissue injury—to say nothing of the discomfort to the patient. Although well-padded plaster splints are the quickest and most effective way of immobilizing an open fracture, the plaster will interfere with the radiographic examination, particularly in injuries about joints. I encourage the use of radiolucent splints, if at all possible. Patients with multiple injuries may require a considerable number of x-rays, including cystograms, urethrograms, intravenous pyleograms, and multiple skeletal x-rays. CT scans of the head, abdomen, or pelvis may also be necessary. Careful planning to minimize the number of times the patient needs to be moved is not only more humane, but more efficient.

Good-quality anteroposterior and lateral x-rays of the fracture, including full visualization of the joints above and below, is the minimum examination necessary in any open fracture. Special views may be required to elucidate the full extent of the injury. In some dislocations and fracture–dislocations, adequate films can only be obtained after reduction. In such cases, a "scout" film may suffice for initial reduction, and then a more complete examination can be performed. A good example is a dislocation of the knee with compromised neurovascular function, where immediate reduction is essential. Perform a complete radiographic evaluation only after the fracture has been reduced and the neurovascular status has been reevaluated. In most cases of this type, immediate arteriography to rule out vascular injury is indicated. Also, in the ankle and subtalar joints persistent dislocation may threaten neurovascular structures or skin and adequate x-ray evaluation is rarely possible. After an initial scout film, closed reduction in the emergency room followed by splinting and complete radiographic examination is usually indicated. Reduction should be delayed *only* when closed reduction is not possible without a general or regional anesthetic.

Other useful findings, particularly in the soft tissues, may emerge on radiographic evaluation. Radiopaque foreign material may be seen, alerting the surgeon to seek it during débridement. Not uncommonly, air trapped in soft tissue planes may reveal a much more extensive injury than originally suspected. In addition, this finding may help interpret similar gas shadows found in a wound a few hours later, when gas-forming bacteria may be the only other logical explanation.

Finally, preoperative planning is essential for adequate care of the fracture, and complete radiographic examination is essential to this planning. It allows you to select the appropriate method for dealing with the fracture and may indicate the need to have more than one fracture stabilization system available.

You are now ready to proceed with formal surgical treatment of the open fracture.

PREPARATION FOR SURGICAL DÉBRIDEMENT

The reader is referred to the excellent text of Mast and coauthors[51] on preoperative planning. In preoperative planning, the order in which multiple fractures will be treated, the teams necessary to treat them, and the soft tissue and bone instruments needed are identified and made available. Open fractures often present unexpected surprises; therefore a full set of soft tissue and bone instruments must be immediately available. Plan for all contingencies. The full assortment of fixation devices that might be necessary to stabilize the fracture must be available. Determine the optimal position of the patient on the operating table and the need for an orthopaedic fracture table or fluoroscopy. Occasionally, in a clean type I open fracture where primary internal fixation is carried out (eg, a displaced fracture of the radial shaft in an adult) immediate cancellous bone grafting may be advisable. If so, plan a possible bone graft donor site.

Even the most grossly contaminated open fracture is not yet infected. In addition to eliminating the contaminating bacteria from the wound, it is critical to avoid further contamination by hospital-based organisms, which may prove to be far more virulent than those already in the wound. For this reason, irrigation and débridement must be carried out in a surgical suite and not in an emergency

room. The approach to the fracture must be the same as for all clean elective orthopaedic surgery from the standpoint of preparation and execution. An irrigation pan (Fig. 3-4) is very useful to collect the large volumes of fluid necessary for adequate irrigation while keeping the operative field dry.

Remove the emergency room splint and dressing, and while maintaining gentle traction to prevent further injury to soft tissues, elevate the limb for the surgical preparation. If possible, apply a tourniquet to the upper thigh or arm. Have a sterile tourniquet available in the event that the proximal extent of the wound precludes the use of a nonsterile tourniquet. A two-phase surgical preparation of the limb helps minimize further contamination of the wound and makes the surgical preparation most effective. With one prep set, wash the entire limb from the finger tips or toes to the tourniquet to eliminate gross contamination. Pour a liter of sterile saline over the wound and remove any obvious debris. Open a second preparation kit and then proceed with formal surgical preparation of the entire extremity. If profuse hemorrhage is encountered during the surgical preparation, inflation of the tourniquet will limit blood loss. Drape the limb free, being certain to cover the nonsterile table top with a plastic or other moisture-proof drape.

IRRIGATION AND DÉBRIDEMENT

Gregory noted that in discussions of débridement it is generally held that irrigation is the single most

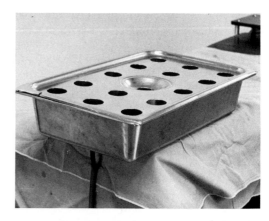

Fig. 3-4. When a limb is to be prepped or débridement is to be performed, placing the limb on the perforated surface of a pan facilitates the necessary rinsing and sluicing with considerable quantities of fluid; because a drainage tube vents the effluent into a pail on the floor, the operative field can be kept dry.

essential maneuver of the entire procedure. This is not quite true, of course, in that the critical aspect is the removal of all nonviable and contaminated tissue, and therefore the débridement itself is the essential maneuver. However, there are two adages that apply to open fracture irrigation: "If a little does some good, a lot will do a great deal more," and, "The solution to pollution is dilution." The importance of copious irrigation was emphasized by Gustilo and associates,[41] who showed that in a series where less than 10 liters of normal saline was used for irrigation there was a higher incidence of infection than in a series where more than 10 liters was used. Whether 10 liters should be run through every wound is less important than the fact that irrigation must be thorough and copious. I prefer to use irrigation and débridement simultaneously, as will be discussed. Some of the advantages of irrigation are:

1. Initial lavage by flushing away blood and other debris clears the wound for inspection, thus facilitating the removal of foreign material and débridement.
2. Irrigation fluid floats otherwise undetected and often necrotic fronds of fascia, fat, or muscle into the field where they can be seen and excised.
3. Lavage floats contaminated blood clots and loose pieces of tissue and debris from unseen recesses and tissue planes.
4. Lavage of the tissue restores its normal color and facilitates determination of viability.
5. Irrigation reduces the bacterial population.

Equally as important as the volume of irrigant used is the method of irrigation. Forceful streams such as those provided by a "Water Pik" may actually drive foreign material and bacteria into the tissue planes, which is obviously undesirable. Several mechanical irrigators are now widely available that pump aseptic irrigation fluids through shower heads in a pulsatile manner. These irrigators provide an ideal stream of irrigation solution over a broad area. They are far more effective than bulb syringes, and I recommend their routine use.

Because of the high volume of solution used, I generally do not include topical antibiotics in all of the irrigation solution. I do feel, however, that topical antibiotics are useful in the last 2 to 4 liters of irrigation solution. I usually add 50,000 units of bacitracin per 2-liter bag; however, the topical antibiotic must be selected case by case. Tissue cultures should be taken prior to using topical antibiotics.

Débridement (literal translation—"unbridling")

was once employed only in the treatment of infected wounds, as an incision to release the purulent contents of the wounds. Gradually it was realized that removal of necrotic tissue at the time of débridement was beneficial; and finally it was recognized that removal of wound debris and necrotic tissue is best carried out as early as possible after injury.

The objectives of débridement (and irrigation) are:

1. The detection and removal of foreign material, especially organic foreign material
2. The detection and removal of nonviable tissues
3. The reduction of bacterial contamination
4. The creation of a wound that can tolerate the residual bacterial contamination and heal without infection.

Proper use of a tourniquet in the débridement of open fractures is essential. Always have a tourniquet present, because it may be necessary to control severe hemorrhage encountered when a blood clot is removed from an unexpected major arterial injury. However, the tourniquet should not be inflated unless necessary to control bleeding, either for visualization or to limit blood loss, because the anoxia produced by the tourniquet interferes with evaluation of the viability of muscle (see p. 235). One major advantage of the tourniquet is that inflation for 10 minutes or so, followed by release, results in capillary flush of the skin distal to the tourniquet, which gives a good indication of the skin's viability. Thus, appropriate use of the tourniquet includes intermittent inflation during irrigation and débridement as indicated, but *not* constant inflation throughout the procedure.

SKIN AND SUBCUTANEOUS FAT

Use an extensile incision that will provide effective débridement and appropriate visualization of neurovascular structures, as needed, and the contaminated bone ends. Appropriate incisions require good judgment and a willingness to be innovative to avoid trapping oneself with a surgical approach that is not useful, or producing further damage such as distally based flaps that may become necrotic. Excise small puncture wounds or holes as well as small, ragged flaps that are not essential to closure (Fig. 3-5). The elliptical wound thus produced is usually easily closed by suture and can even be left open for spontaneous closure, leaving a simple linear scar. Avoid coring wounds, because this leaves a round hole that can only close by granulation and

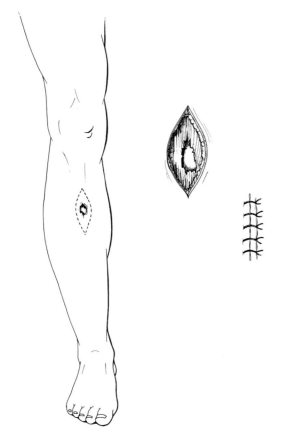

Fig. 3-5. An elliptical excision of the fracture wound permits proper inspection of the area of injury as well as better closure if the wound is sutured.

scar formation. The cicatrix thus produced often retracts and leaves an ugly, puckered wound. Consider the following points before proceeding with débridement of skin and making elective incisions:

1. The amount of gross loss of skin and subcutaneous fat
2. The extent of degloving that has occurred, which may influence the apparently viable skin remaining
3. The need to extend existing wounds for adequate exposure and the best directions for such extensions
4. The usefulness or dangers of connecting adjacent yet separate wounds
5. The prospect of survival for flaps created by the injury or by planned incisions
6. The amount of skin that can be sacrificed, if any, and its effect on subsequent closure
7. The usefulness of counter-incisions to facili-

tate adequate débridement, arrange bone coverage, or provide for wound drainage
8. The likelihood that a planned incision may transect a major superficial vein
9. The age of the patient and the state of skin and subcutaneous tissues
10. The need to develop a sufficiently wide wound that will allow thorough inspection of its deepest recesses.

By beginning with the skin and subcutaneous fat, initiate a methodical, layer-by-layer débridement of the traumatic wound. Be conservative in the excision of skin, particularly where it is at a premium (eg, over the tibia and in the foot and hand). In the hand, for example, particularly in stellate-type lacerations of the digits, excision of skin edges may be contraindicated. Where adequate skin is available, sharp excision of the contaminated and contused skin edge—1 to 2 mm into good-quality skin—with a sharp blade placed at right angles to the skin, removes contaminated and non-viable skin and provides a good wound edge for subsequent closure. This gives the best cosmetic result. The forceps used on skin should always be toothed and should be used with care to avoid further contusion. Frequent changing of the knife blade is necessary to assure a sharp, well-performed débridement.

The question of how much of an additional elective incision is required for deep exposure always arises. In wounds caused by high-energy injuries, a useful axiom is that the wound should be equal in length to the diameter of the limb at that level. A better guide is to expose the fracture site and then continue exposure until clean tissues are encountered and all areas of periosteal stripping have been identified. Although adequate débridement is obviously necessary, do not unnecessarily open uninvolved, clean, intact soft tissue planes. In particular, avoid detaching skin from its underlying fascial attachment as the vertical vessels to the skin necessary for survival will be damaged. Carry out meticulous hemostasis as débridement progresses, because considerable blood can be lost during débridement of even moderate-sized wounds.

A traumatic skin flap that has a base-to-length ratio of more than 1:2, particularly if distally based, will frequently have a nonviable tip. Ascertain this by looking for capillary flush after deflation of a tourniquet, as described above. Some advocate the injection of an ampule of fluorescein and visualization of the flap with a Woods lamp. Excise obviously nonviable portions, but leave any skin that is marginal; this can always be débrided later, and skin is not the major pabulum for infection from necrotic muscle. If very large wounds are produced by loss of skin and subsequent coverage is expected to be difficult, it may be possible to harvest skin from the excised flap. A Padgett dermatome works well, set at a 0.010- to 0.012-inch thickness. Run the graft through a 1-to-1½ or 1-to-3 skin mesher, then widely spread it. Often the graft can be applied immediately to viable muscle and fascia, because it does not actually result in closure of the wound and will rapidly epithelialize for coverage. Prior to making an elective incision, irrigate the wound with 2 or more liters of saline (depending on the size of the wound) until foreign debris and blood clot are no longer visible in the wound and the tissues appear clean and fresh. It is important to do this prior to making the elective incisions to minimize contamination of the elective portion of the wound. At each layer of the débridement, methodically irrigate the wound. At the level of muscle and bone, in grade II or higher open fractures, use at least 6 liters of saline. When combined with the initial 2 liters and the final 2 liters containing antibiotic solution, this results in a minimum irrigation of 10 liters for any type II or larger wound.

FASCIA

Excise any nonviable, damaged, or contaminated fascia. Leave no marginal fascia. In my opinion, limited fasciotomy is indicated in all open fractures secondary to high-energy injuries, and complete fasciotomy of all compartments is often indicated. This is discussed in more detail in the selection on fasciotomy (see p. 238).

MUSCLE

Whereas skin tends to tear or be punctured, and fascia to split or shred, muscle, because of its high water content, is subject to hydraulic damage by fluid waves when an injuring object impacts the limb. This is particularly true of high-velocity gunshot wounds. Of equal importance is that a high-energy fracture secondary to indirect rapid loading (eg, a high-velocity skiing injury) may result in comminution of the tibia or femur, where the bone literally explodes into many fragments. These fragments travel rapidly outward into the muscle and can cause significant muscle damage even when the outer envelope is seemingly undamaged. A small bone fragment may pierce the skin, producing what appears to be a very minor type I open fracture, when in fact there may be considerable deep muscle damage. This occurs because the more rapidly bone is loaded prior to fracture, the more energy is required to fracture it, and the more explosive the fracture is when it occurs. Because of this absence of direct physical trauma, it is easy to overlook nonvital muscle because it may not immediately be evident that it has been disturbed or damaged.

Necrotic muscle is the major pabulum for bacterial growth and poses a great danger in anaerobic infections. Make every effort to remove all nonvital muscle tissue, although often this will require careful judgment. In muscle débridement the approach of Brav[8] is the safest: "When in doubt, take it out." In type I, II, and III-A open fractures this may be taken literally, but in types III-B and III-C, débridement of an entire muscle or compartment may be necessary to meet this axiom. If the major arterial supply to a severely damaged muscle has been destroyed, the only recourse is total excision. It has been my experience, however, that if even 10% of a muscle belly and its attached tendon can be preserved, significant function is retained. For that reason, there may be an indication for leaving some marginal muscle at the time of initial débridement in severe open fractures, then returning within 24 to 48 hours for redébridement, at which time the muscle will have better declared its viability. The exception to this approach is in wartime or mass casualties where preservation of life takes precedence over the desire to preserve function.

Judgment of the viability of muscle is challenging, and the alliterative quartet provided by Gregory in his original chapter must be addressed by the surgeon: *color, consistency, contractility,* and *capacity to bleed.* Scully and associates,[73] in an attempt to correlate four features with histologic evidence of viability, concluded that consistency and capacity to bleed were the most significant. In my experience, contractility and consistency have been the most reliable, because color and capacity to bleed are easily misinterpreted. Remember that the hypoxemia associated with the use of a tourniquet, or in the presence of shock or injury to a major vessel of the involved limb, may make evaluation of these parameters difficult. Observe the following qualifications in the applications of these indications of viability.

Color

Color can be misleading and is generally a poor guide to viability. Muscle that is dark or even black on its surface may only represent a thin layer of blood lying beneath the myonesium or hemorrhage within the muscle substance which does not threaten viability. When freed of this thin layer, the underlying muscle may be found to be normal in color. In my experience, nonviable muscle generally is salmon, yellow, or gray in color and is distinctly different from the robust pink or red seen in normal muscle.

Consistency

Muscle consistency is a subjective evaluation and ranges from normal firm tissue to the stringy, friable, and even mushy state of severely damaged or disintegrating tissue. The firmer the muscle, the more certain it is viable. It is often useful to extend the wound to obviously uninjured viable muscle and compare its consistency to that in the injured area. Normal muscle, when pinched gently with a toothed forceps, immediately rebounds to its normal shape, leaving no marks from the sharp tips of the forceps. This is a delicate test, and crushing of the tissue must be avoided. When a gentle squeeze of the forceps leaves its mark in the muscle, viability is in question.

Contractility

Contractility clearly establishes muscle viability. Muscle tissue that vigorously retreats from the incising edge of a scalpel is obviously alive. Good-quality muscle will normally respond with a localized contraction to the gentle pinch of a toothed forceps, or to the stimulation from a nerve stimulator unit or Bovie set on a #1 or #2 setting. Normally, debridement should be carried out until all muscle remaining in the wound is contractile.

Capacity to Bleed

Vigorous bleeding may produce spurious evidence of viability. The muscle may be crushed, and there may be no substantial flow through the capillary beds of the muscle, yet the arterioles may continue to bleed vigorously when transected. On the contrary, gentle, persistent oozing from capillaries tends to demonstrate adequate local profusion, indicating that the muscle is probably viable. This distinction is subtle and demands your full attention.

TENDONS

Tendons, unless obviously severely damaged and contaminated, are not a major pabulum for infection, and if essential to function, should be preserved. Where coverage of tendons by some type of soft tissue will not be possible, preservation of the peritenon is essential for tendon survival. For that reason, I tend to not débride peritenon but rather copiously irrigate it. If tendon without peritenon must be left exposed in an open wound, a moist dressing must be applied and kept moist until coverage of the tendon can be obtained (see under Wound Closure, p. 258). If at all possible, try to swing some muscle, subcutaneous fat, or skin over tendon without peritenon.

BONE

Whereas muscle tissue may mount a defense against invading bacteria, bone tissue is essentially defenseless owing to its relatively poor blood supply. If judgments about muscle viability seem troublesome, judgments about what is to be done with bone fragments are perplexing. Generally speaking, remove small bits of cortical bone that are free of any soft tissue attachments. In areas of cancellous bone, a fracture may produce significant free, small fragments of cancellous bone. If these are not obviously contaminated, and if they contribute to the reconstruction of the fracture, they can be retained as bone graft. However, if a large cortical fragment constituting a significant segment of the injured bone is removed, the resulting gap will require bone grafting; this can pose treatment problems. If such a fragment has obvious soft tissue connections, and especially if its small vessels bleed on the exposed surface, retain it, even if you must trim the surfaces to eliminate minor contamination. Unless it is grossly contaminated, the fragment probably should be preserved. The major judgment problem lies with a bone fragment that has only a tenuous soft tissue attachment or is completely free. Its value as a bone graft, perfectly fitting the defect, is obvious. However, is it sufficiently free of contamination that it will be tolerated, or will it act as a foreign body, aggravating any infection that might occur? There are no absolute criteria, and judgment is based on experience. The inexperienced surgeon is wisest to débride the fragment. Although this risks delayed union or nonunion, it minimizes the risk of infection. There is no question that a delayed union or nonunion is a far less challenging complication than an infected nonunion.

In low-energy fractures where a major cortical bone fragment is essential to an internal fixation construct, where the surgeon is confident that the level of contamination is low, and adequate irrigation and débridement has been carried out, the fragment can be retained in the construct.[82] This allows for early redébridement if infection intervenes. In addition, retention of a large, segmental fragment of bone may lead to nonunion at one or both ends of the free fragment, and bridging of the nonviable fragment with onlay cancellous bone graft may be advisable at some time during treatment (see under Bone Grafting, p. 254). In the case of free butterfly fragments or segmental pieces in fractures where external fixation will provide the primary stabilization, interfragmentary screw fixation of the free fragment to the adjacent viable bone is usually indicated, followed by bone grafting across the junction site later.

As a general rule, bone débridement initially can be conservative; however, if infection intervenes, early aggressive redébridement of all nonviable bone is important. It is better to deal with the reconstruction of a large segmental defect than to allow chronic infection to result in chronic osteomyelitis, which may lead to even more bone loss. My most common judgment error in the management of infected open fractures has been the delayed excision of nonviable bone.

Determination of the viability of bone is difficult. Although I have personally not found them to be useful, (1) injection of fluorescein and observation of bone with a Woods lamp at the time of surgery, and (2) injection with a tetracycline label before redébridement and observation with a Woods lamp have been described as useful methods in determining bone viability. The best method may prove to be laser-doppler flowmetry to evaluate blood flow, but its efficacy in the débridement of open fractures has not yet been established.[77]

As described with tendons, bone without periosteum and not covered by soft tissue quickly desiccates and dies. It is critical, therefore, to preserve any periosteum attached to the bone where bone will not be immediately covered by muscle or subcutaneous fat and skin. It is usually better to thoroughly irrigate periosteum that is attached, rather than débride it, if coverage cannot be obtained (see under Wound Closure, p. 258).

JOINTS

Any wound that enters a joint mandates exploration. Débride the wound as described above down to the level of the joint. The traumatic wound itself may permit adequate exploration, or an extensile incision may be necessary. In many joints, however, adequate exploration through the arthrotomy will not be possible unless the excision is very large; this is particularly true in the knee and shoulder.

Under these circumstances, it may be better to combine débridement of the wound with arthroscopic examination of the joint. If fluid leakage through the wound is a problem, close the synovium and carry out arthroscopic inspection in the usual fashion. It is critical that the entire joint be adequately explored, because unexpected foreign bodies or osteochondral fractures are frequently found.

NERVES AND VESSELS

Brisk, small vessel or arterial bleeders encountered during débridement require immediate ligation or coagulation. Methodical, layer-by-layer hemostasis is important to limit blood loss. General oozing from capillary-sized vessels generally abates with time and compression. Major vessel injuries requiring repair are usually identified prior to surgery and appropriately planned for, but may be encountered unexpectedly during débridement. Because it is often difficult to know exactly how much time has lapsed from injury and loss of blood supply to the limb to the initiation of vascular repair, reinstitution of circulation is of primary importance. In my experience, loss of total blood supply to the limb for more than 8 hours always results in amputation. If there has been a significant delay, I prefer to do a very quick irrigation and débridement of the wound to remove the grossest contamination and then proceed with vascular repair. This is particularly important if the repair must be done through the open fracture wound. There are exceptions, however; for example, if the open fracture wound is anterior to the knee and repair of a popliteal artery requires an independent elective posteromedial exposure, perform appropriate initial surgical preparation of the limb using the two-phase method described previously; occlude the traumatic wound with a barrier drape and proceed immediately with the exposure for vascular repair. In the presence of arterial injury necessitating repair, preserve as much venous outflow as possible during the débridement.

In larger vessels, rather than carrying out immediate end-to-end anastomosis or vein grafting, it may be better to insert a temporary shunt. This permits irrigation and débridement and stabilization of the bone prior to final vascular repair. This may be important to establish proper limb length and avoid injury to the vessel during the bone repair.

When vascular repair is necessary, repeat débridement is frequently required, and easy visualization of the entire limb to assess circulation is important. For this reason, some advocate routine internal or external fixation in such situations. Others, notably Rich and associates[66] and Connolly[24] have shown that nonoperative immobilization works well—especially in a mass casualty situation. (The issue of internal fixation in open fractures will be dealt with later.)

Fasciotomy

Following arterial repair, massive swelling distal to the site of repair is very common, particularly in the forearm or leg. Because fasciotomy so often becomes necessary in such cases, I urge you to do it prophylactically in essentially every case. If there is any doubt about its indication, it probably should be done. Moreover, it is better done too early than too late.

In the forearm, both the volar and dorsal compartments must be relieved by two incisions placed at 180° to each other over the appropriate compartment. On the volar surface, the lacertus fibrosis (proximally) and carpal tunnel (distally) must be released.

In the leg, release all four compartments: anterior, lateral, superficial posterior, and deep posterior. In my opinion this is best done through one long incision over the lateral compartment. Exposure of the deep fascia for a short distance anterior and posterior to this incision, followed by a transverse incision through the fascia at the midpoint of the leg, allows easy identification of the vertical fascial planes separating the anterior, lateral, and posterior compartments. Release each compartment independently with a longitudinal incision extending the full length of the compartment. After release of the superficial posterior compartment, bluntly dissect posterior to the lateral compartment and release the fascia of the deep posterior compartment.[52]

Patman and Thompson[63] suggested four-compartment fasciotomy by resecting the fibular shaft through a single incision. I believe this is unnecessarily aggressive. Loss of the fibular shaft increases instability of the leg and removes an essential structure for reconstruction. I feel this method of compartment release is contraindicated.

In nearly all open fractures of grades II or above, or those with a crushing component, I advocate routine limited fasciotomy. This is easily accomplished by directing a pair of scissors subcutaneously to split the fascia longitudinally. Often this step will prevent a compartment syndrome, and it adds minimal, if any, morbidity. However, it is important to continue to observe for compartment syndrome, because a more complete fasciotomy may still be necessary.

After formal fasciotomy, do not close the skin because it may be as constricting as the fascia if severe swelling occurs. Frequently, skin grafts are required to provide coverage of such wounds because swelling recedes too slowly to permit suturing. However, this added morbidity pales in contrast with that visited on the patient who needs a compartment decompression but does not receive it.

FOREIGN BODIES

Foreign bodies, especially organic ones, must be sought and removed because they often lead to significant morbidity if left in the wound. Fragments of wood are especially troublesome, because they are easily buried in tissue, and after becoming blood-soaked, resemble adjacent muscle. Cloth and leather, on the other hand, are usually found in the planes between tissues but may find recesses remote from the site of injury. The intrinsic recesses, pits, or crevices of the foreign material may harbor pathogenic organisms or their spores. The foreign body itself, especially if organic, is likely to incite an inflammatory response.

Bullets, and especially pellets, usually are buried. Unless easily detected, surgical exploration to find them may entail more hazard by injury to the tissue disturbed than if they are left *in situ*. Remove shotgun pellets only as they are encountered during the débridement or if they have damaged a major blood vessel or nerve. Bullets in veins have been reported on rare occasions to become emboli. An exception to the matter of removing lead bullets or particles occurs if they lie, in whole or in part, within a joint or in the subarachnoid space. Joint or subarachnoid fluid acting on lead tends to break it down and, as Leonard[49] has reported, can induce serious synovitis as well as low-grade lead poisoning. Bullet fragments and pellets thought to be in joints are generally best sought for with the arthroscope, where possible; otherwise, open arthrotomy is indicated.

Shotgun wounds are less treacherous today than in the past in that horsehair wadding has been replaced by a plastic plug. However, both wadding and plugs should be sought and removed; this is most important if old shotgun shells have been used and horse hair wadding is present. Close-range shotgun wounds that perforate, and thereby create wounds of entrance and of exit, make access available to both wounds and thus facilitate thorough inspection and débridement. When the wound is simply penetrating (ie, no exit wound), thorough

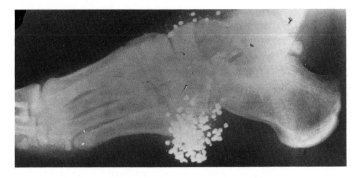

Fig. 3-6. The shot cloud has traversed this foot from its dorsal aspect, but has come to lie on the deep aspect of the plantar fascia. It serves as a clue to the location of any associated shell wadding that may also have entered the wound.

inspection is often difficult. Frequently, the shot cloud comes to lie against the fascia on the far side of the limb (Fig. 3-6). In this situation, a counter-incision is usually justified to remove the wadding or plastic plug.

Some advocate management of low-velocity, small-caliber gunshot wounds (eg, from small pistols), where the fracture is treatable by outpatient management, by local wound irrigation and débridement in the emergency room and oral antibiotics. Although acceptable results have been reported, I prefer to formally explore these in the operating room because foreign materials such as clothing commonly are dragged into the wound by the bullet.

IMMEDIATE OR EARLY AMPUTATION VERSUS LIMB SALVAGE

Immediate or early amputation through the fracture site may be indicated under the following circumstances:

1. When the limb is nonviable; that is, when there is a vascular injury that is nonreparable or is accompanied by warm ischemia time over 8 hours; or the limb is so severely crushed that there is minimal viable tissue remaining for revascularization;
2. When, even after revascularization, the limb is so severely damaged in whole or in part that function is less satisfactory than that afforded by a prosthesis;
3. In severely injured limbs in the presence of severe, debilitating, chronic disease where preservation of the limb is a threat to the patient's life (eg, a severe type III-C open fracture of the distal tibia in an elderly patient with severe di-

abetes with vascular disease and severe peripheral neuropathy);
4. In a limb where the severity of the injury will demand several operative procedures and a prolonged reconstruction time that is incompatible with the personal, sociological, and economic consequences the patient is willing to withstand (eg, a heavy equipment operator with multiple open fractures of the foot, where reconstruction, particularly of the soft tissues, may demand a year or more, and where the outcome is uncertain; a Symes amputation could return this patient to work within a few months);
5. In a military or mass casualty situation where salvage of life or transport of the injured victim, plus the need to direct attention to more severely injured patients, would justify amputation rather than the prolonged surgical effort necessary to salvage a severely injured extremity;
6. In a patient with severe, multiple-system injuries with an injury severity score* of approximately 20 or more, where salvage of a marginal extremity may result in a systemic load of necrotic tissue and inflammatory byproducts so high that it could induce pulmonary or multiple-organ failure and lead to death; and
7. In cases of replantation, where the function expected does not justify salvage (eg, amputation of a single finger through zone 2—the area of the proximal phalanx).

Lange and associates[48] have published absolute and relative indications for immediate amputation that are good guidelines. In fractures of the tibia their absolute indications for amputation are a type III-C fracture where vascular repair is required for

* The Abbreviated Injury Scale, rev. ed. Arlington Heights, Il., American Association for Automotive Medicine, 1985.

salvage of the extremity, the injury is accompanied by complete transection of the posterior tibial nerve, and the limb is nonviable. Relative indications are items 2 through 5 in the list above.

Often, the full extent of injury is not known prior to going to the operating room. If amputation is a serious consideration, it must be discussed with the patient prior to the initial débridement, if possible, and consent obtained for immediate amputation if it is determined to be indicated. In unconscious patients, or where appropriate informed consent is not obtainable, the limb should be amputated only if it is nonsalvageable or it is a threat to the patient's life. In such circumstances documentation by at least two other surgeons—preferably one from another specialty—accompanied by photographs placed in the medical record, is appropriate. If the limb appears to be salvageable, it may be best to complete the initial débridement, assess the extent of the injury, and then sit down with the patient under less harried and emotional circumstances to discuss rationally the pros and cons of reconstruction versus amputation of the limb. I believe it is critical, however, to make this decision early. It is a great disservice to the patient, and very costly to the patient and to society, to perform multiple surgical procedures over a 1- to 2-year period to salvage a badly mutilated limb, only to finally perform an amputation because the patient grows weary of the prolonged treatment, or the limb is simply not functional or is too painful.

STABILIZATION OF THE BONE

Once vascular repair has been completed and the limb salvaged, and/or irrigation and débridement have been done, stabilization of the bone is the next concern.

THE IMPORTANCE OF SKELETAL STABILITY

Achievement of stability means restoration of the fracture to as close to anatomic position as possible, with sufficient stability that multiple wound procedures will be possible and hopefully early function can be instituted. At the outset, reestablishment of good alignment realigns neurovascular structures, which provides optimal circulation to the injured extremity and minimizes the risk of compromising peripheral nerves. Restoration of normal length reduces the dead space in which blood can accumulate. Hematoma is avascular and is a pa-

bulum for infection. Restoration of normal anatomy improves venous and lymphatic return, thereby reducing soft tissue swelling. At the microscopic level, bone stability helps stabilize soft tissue planes. This facilitates capillary proliferation and ingrowth to revascularize devitalized bone and soft tissues. Early revascularization of devitalized structures improves local tissue resistance to infection. Stabilization and approximation of soft tissue planes also facilitates diffusion of nutrients and antibodies and facilitates white cell migration. All of these factors contribute to "local wound defense" against infection.

From the standpoint of the whole patient, fracture stability permits muscle rehabilitation and joint motion, which facilitates early return to function. The studies of Salter and associates[70] and Mitchell and Shepard[55] have shown that rigid internal fixation of osteochondral fractures and early restoration of joint motion are essential to achieve good cartilage healing and to prevent joint stiffness and intra-articular adhesions. In multiply injured patients, stabilization of major long-bone and axial skeletal fractures permits early mobilization, which facilitates cardiopulmonary care, may prevent thromboembolic phenomena, and has been shown to reduce morbidity and mortality.[6]

Stability can be achieved by traditional plaster-cast or traction immobilization, more functionally oriented cast bracing, cast-brace traction, pins and plaster, external fixation, internal fixation with devices including intramedullary rods, plates and screws, or combinations of the above.

Virtually all methods presently employed in the management of closed fractures can also be applied, within certain limits, to open fractures. However, in the open fracture, management of the bone fragments cannot logically be considered apart from the soft tissue wound. If the wound is minor, it is usually not much of a problem, but when the soft tissue injury is extensive, often including significant loss of skin and ensheathing muscle, it may make management of the fracture most formidable. Thus, what might be done with the fractured bone *per se* must often yield to what serves the best interest of the soft tissues—at least at the time of initial treatment. Whichever method of fracture treatment is chosen, it should meet certain criteria, including:

1. It should not compromise further the injured soft tissues;
2. It should maintain length of the bone, especially in the lower extremity and forearm; and
3. It should produce good alignment of bone frag-

ments, especially the joint surfaces in intra-articular fractures.

As in the treatment of closed fractures, it is difficult to be dogmatic about any one open fracture, and no one technique seems clearly superior to any other in *all* cases. For the surgeon who deals with open fractures only occasionally or on a temporary basis, the simpler the method, the better. Such a policy creates fewer problems for the first surgeon and provides greater latitude for definitive treatment by the last surgeon. However, the surgeon who treats open fractures on a regular basis must be aware of and consider the full range of available techniques, and even combine them or, when indicated, improvise.

Some open fractures seem to be open only "technically." A small, almost unnoticeable, wound may be associated with a minor fracture line in the underlying bone, whose fragments show no displacement on x-rays; this is indeed an open fracture. Such injuries are seductive in their appearance and treacherous. The danger of serious, even fatal infection proceeding from this circumstance has already been mentioned. The wound should receive the same consideration as any open fracture. The fracture as such may simply be splinted by a plaster slab or a cast. When the wound has healed, a definitive cast may be applied until the fracture is sufficiently united.

Larger wounds or those extended in the course of débridement and associated with displaced bone fragments frequently permit reduction under direct visualization. Yet the visualization is not always all that might be desired, because wounds, unlike incisions made for the purpose of exposure, are often neither appropriately located nor sufficiently extensive. At other times, of course, wounds are so large that the surgeon is distressed by how much of the fractured bone is so readily visible.

IMMOBILIZATION IN PLASTER

Plaster-of-paris casts have limitations in the treatment of open fractures because they may make access to the wound difficult and because they involve a circumferential hard dressing on a limb with the potential for swelling, which can cause compartment syndrome. In addition, a plaster cast may not provide the degree of fracture stability desired. On the other hand, in type I and low-grade type II open fractures where the wounds are moderate and manipulative reduction of the fracture fragments produces a stable, acceptable position, plaster-of-paris

cast immobilization may be quite appropriate, particularly in children. Apply the same type of cast used for closed management, incorporating the joints above and below the fracture.

Always make a full-length longitudinal cut in the cast with a cast saw after the plaster has dried to produce a univalved cast. A univalved cast is superior to a bivalved cast in that it can be spread to accommodate the limb without losing adequate fracture immobilization, and it provides more uniform decompression of the limb. A bivalved cast, when spread, provides decompression in only one axis of the limb, results in increased instability, and allows swelling of the skin between the bivalved portions of the cast that may produce blisters.

There should be a way to easily expose the wound in the cast to inspect it or to carry out delayed primary closure. Simply windowing the cast may be unsatisfactory because the window may not be accurately located over the wound, removal of the plaster and dressing may be difficult resulting in wound contamination, and the edges of the window (which are flush with the limb) may make application of dressings difficult. To avoid this, make a bubble in the cast directly over the wound; the bubble should be 1 to 2 inches in diameter larger than the widest part of the wound. This is accomplished by placing a bulky pad of loosely packed cast padding directly over the wound after the dressing and circumferential cast padding have been applied. The height of the bubble depends on the size of the wound. For a wound 2 inches long, a bubble 4 inches in diameter and approximately 2 inches high works well. This bubble has several advantages. First, it indicates precisely where the wound is located. Second, when the bubble is cut off by running the cast saw around the circumference of the bubble, it leaves a smooth lip on the cast which makes removal of the underlying dressings easy and avoids getting plaster debris in the wound. The cap of the bubble is easily removed without having to use cast spreaders and other instruments that might cause discomfort to the patient. When the cast padding in the bubble is removed, a cavity is produced which provides a nice elevated rim to protect the wound and a space in which dressing changes are easy to perform. Because the bubble produces no sharp edge against the skin, cast window edema and subsequent blistering are generally avoided. The cap can be replaced over the hole to provide a nice, protective hard shell over the dressing (Fig. 3-7).

Another clever aid suggested by Gregory is to outline the bubble on the cast with an indelible pencil. This ensures that a surgeon unfamiliar with

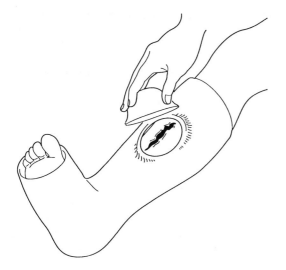

Fig. 3-7. Bubble in plaster-of-paris cast can be easily removed for wound care.

the patient will cut in the proper site. In addition, a drawing of the fracture and a brief description of the wound can be placed on the cast, thus providing an immediately available, accurate history for subsequent persons treating the patient. When the cap is replaced, if swelling is expected, it may be important to refill the void with loosely packed cast padding to produce uniform compression over the wound site.

PINS AND PLASTER

When I entered orthopaedic training in 1963, transverse through-and-through Steinmann pins or Kirschner wires incorporated in a plaster cast were standard methods of stabilizing unstable open fractures. Although the Roger-Anderson external fixator was available, for some reason it was used very little in open fractures. With the evolution of the external fixation frame to the currently popular single- and double-plane half-pin frames, pins and plaster have virtually disappeared as a method for immobilizing open fractures; in most cases, an external fixator can be applied more quickly. The external fixator offers the advantages of half-pin fixation, whereas pins and plaster nearly always require at least some through-and-through pins. In addition, the circumferential plaster presents problems in the swelling limb, limits wound care, and makes subsequent adjustments for fracture position difficult and certainly much more cumbersome than with most external fixation frames.

In spite of these disadvantages, pins and plaster have occasional indications. They are used frequently in third-world countries as a simple, inexpensive method for fracture immobilization where the cost of external fixators precludes their use. Another excellent and inexpensive fixator which I have seen used frequently in third-world countries involves simple Steinmann pins placed in a half-pin configuration and then incorporated into a bar of polymethylmethacrylate. Thus, a few comments about the technique of pins in plaster are merited.

Pins and plaster are most commonly indicated for the tibia. The most easily applied method uses Steinmann pins of sufficiently large dimension that *in vivo* bending of the pins will not occur. I find it best to use fully or partially threaded pins rather than smooth pins. Because the pin is incorporated in the cast and the cast tends to shift on the limb with changes in position, movement will be introduced in a smooth pin, making loosening and infection more likely. The disadvantage of a fully threaded pin is that it is more difficult to remove from the plaster cast. I find it easiest to place one through-and-through pin at approximately the level of the tibial tubercle in adults, and distal to the tibial tubercle in children to avoid injury to the physeal line. Place a second through-and-through pin approximately 1 inch proximal to the ankle joint. To avoid movement of the proximal fragment by the thigh musculature, place a third half pin extending just into, but not through, the posterior cortex (Fig. 3-8). With the knee flexed to 90°, hanging off the side of the operating table with the thigh supported, traction can then be applied to the distal pin and reduction of the fracture obtained. Apply an appropriate short-leg cast incorporating all three pins. For a secure hold, apply the plaster directly to the pin, leaving the pins extending beyond the leg for a distance on either side equal to the width of the leg at that level. If Kirschner wires are used, the Kirschner wire bow must be left in place to maintain tension on the wire. When the cast is removed it is easiest to cut around the base of the pin where it enters the cast to free the plaster on the pin from the remaining cast. After the cast is removed, the plaster cap on the wire can be screwed off or removed by cutting with the cast saw blade immediately against the pin. This cuts the plaster envelope in half, which will then drop off the pin.

Pins in plaster tend to produce relative distraction of the fracture site and therefore should be used only long enough to obtain sufficient healing at the

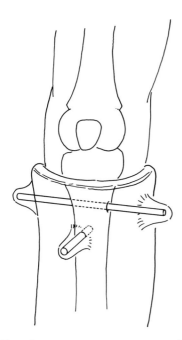

Fig. 3-8. Two Steinmann pins incorporated in plaster give good control against rotation of the proximal fragment. The anteroposterior pin should just engage the posterior cortex, not penetrate it, to avoid neurovascular injury. (Chapman, M. W.: Fractures of the Tibia and Fibula. In *Chapman, M. W. (ed.): Operative Orthopaedics, Vol. 1, p. 441. Philadelphia, J. B. Lippincott, 1988.)*

fracture site so that shortening and malrotation will not occur once the pins are removed. This healing generally is seen at 6 to 8 weeks after the fracture. At this time removal of the pins and conversion to a non–weight-bearing cast or weight-bearing plaster is appropriate. This technique is useful in the upper extremity as well for fractures of the distal radius and, on occasion, for the forearm. Through-and-through pins can be placed through the bases of the second and third metacarpals and the olecranon. Half pins can be used in the base of the metacarpals and into the shaft of the radius. Pins inserted into the radius must be inserted under direct vision to avoid injury to neurovascular structures and tendons.

Gregory described two other techniques for achieving temporary stability for cast application. In the tibia with a short, oblique fracture, the spike of one fragment can be inserted into the medullary canal of the other and placed into compression. This offers good stability, and if the obliquity is short, excessive shortening will not occur. An alternative is to reduce the fracture and percutaneously transfix

it with a smooth Kirschner wire or Steinmann pin. Place the pin through only one surface of the leg, not penetrating much beyond the cortex of the opposite side. After the cast is fully applied and dried, remove this smooth pin. Reduction will generally thereafter be maintained. Do not use a threaded pin for this method because it may become ensnared in the padding of the cast when removal is attempted (Fig. 3-9).

WEIGHT-BEARING CASTS

Dehne,[25] Brown and Urban,[10] and Sarmiento[71,72] have demonstrated the advantages and beneficial effects of early weight-bearing on the healing of fractures in the lower extremity. These advantages are equally true in the treatment of open fractures, but some practical considerations make immediate application of weight-bearing casts difficult. The wound care and potential for swelling encountered in most open fractures precludes immediate initial application of a weight-bearing cast. Once the wound has been closed, or is in a stable state where healing by secondary intention is acceptable, healing in the weight-bearing plaster may be quite appropriate. The threat of significant swelling must be passed prior to the application of one these close-fitting casts. In stable, minor type I open fractures the cast may be applied within a few days after the threat of swelling has passed. In more severe type II open fractures where external fixation has not been used, application of a total-contact cast may have to be delayed for up to 3 to 4 weeks. The risk of late wound complications and loss of reduction of the fracture can be minimized by seeing the patient weekly after initial application of the cast for repeat x-ray films and windowing of the cast or removal to check the wound as indicated by clinical findings.

It is not necessary to have a closed wound before application of a weight-bearing plaster. For many years it has been noted that wounds débrided properly may heal if left undisturbed under plaster. Henry's[44] pungent observations—"Wounds may stink their way to health in plaster"—is clearly underscored by the vast experience of Orr[59] and his contemporaries in the treatment of chronic bone infection. This was further emphasized by the extensive experience of Trueta,[79] who used Orr's method to manage fresh injuries in the Spanish Civil War, and Brown and Urban,[10] in the more recent Vietnam conflict. For success the principles of initial wound care must be meticulously followed.

Another consideration in the application of

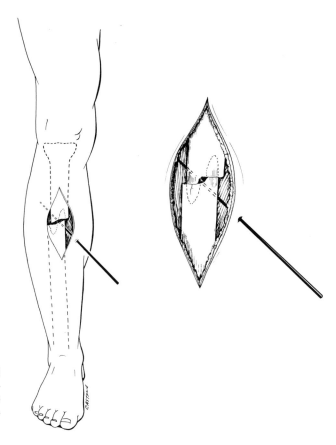

Fig. 3-9. (**Left**) General alignment can be achieved by a temporary transfixing pin. (**Right**) Note the resulting reciprocal cortical invagination. When the plaster has set, the pin may be removed by the technique outlined in the text.

weight-bearing casts for the treatment of open fractures is the problem of split-thickness skin grafts. No matter how skillfully a cast has been applied, some telescoping occurs when the nonunited fracture is subjected to weight-bearing. The telescoping produces friction between the skin and cast surfaces. Because split-thickness skin grafts are insensitive and have poor mobility, breakdown is common. This is particularly a problem where the split-thickness graft is applied over bone, such as the anterior subcutaneous border of the tibia, where there is virtually no mobility. Breakdown of the graft can occur very rapidly, necessitating at a minimum repeat grafting to attain coverage, and at worst exposure of bone that could lead to more serious, deep-seated infection. In patients with extensive split-thickness skin grafts it may be necessary to defer treatment in a weight-bearing plaster until sufficient early intrinsic stability is achieved, to minimize the risk of injury to the overlying skin. In some cases circumferential casts never become practical and some other means of treatment must be adopted. The evolution from weight-bearing casts to cast-braces and prefabricated braces has been well described by Sarmiento.[71,72]

SKELETAL TRACTION AND SUSPENSION

It is unusual for skeletal traction to be used as definitive treatment of open fractures in North America today because of the disadvantages of prolonged recumbency and because of the markedly increased costs of hospitalization compared with methods that allow earlier discharge from the hospital. However, traction is frequently used as a temporary means of fracture stabilization until more invasive methods are indicated, and as definitive treatment in third-world countries where internal or external fixation techniques are not readily available.

The most common indication for skeletal traction is an open fracture of the femur. In isolated open fractures of the femoral shaft, where early mobilization is not of concern, my practice has been to débride the fracture, leave the wound open, and place the leg in tibial pin traction with balanced suspension. After successful delayed primary closure of the wound, usually about 10 to 14 days post-injury, I carry out closed intramedullary nailing. Brumback and others[11] have recently shown that the infection rate after primary intramedullary nailing of type I open fractures of the femur is the same as for delayed nailing; therefore, I now carry out immediate fixation of these fractures (see under Internal Fixation, p. 250). In very unstable fractures I use a Thomas splint and Pearson attachment for suspension, but in more stable patterns where access to the wound may be important, I prefer modified skeletal Russell's traction (Fig. 3-10). The independent thigh sling permits easy access to wounds and also is more comfortable for the patient, making it much easier for nursing care and use of a bedpan. Because a large, threaded Steinmann pin is necessary to mount the patient on the fracture table used for closed intramedullary nailing, I prefer proximal tibial skeletal traction with a $\frac{3}{16}$ or $\frac{1}{4}$-inch fully threaded Steinmann pin with a bow. If intramedullary nailing is not contemplated, I prefer a Kirschner wire in the same location. I rarely use distal femoral traction unless there is a need to avoid pulling through injuries of the knee or a need for heavy traction for an acetabular or pelvic fracture. On occasion, 90°/90° traction does require a distal femoral pin (Fig. 3-11). Other than in children, my only indication for definitive treatment of a femoral fracture in traction is a decision by the patient not to proceed with internal or external fixation.

Gregory, in the first edition of this book, mentioned traction as a useful technique for the management of troublesome wounds, particularly on the proximal and posterior aspect of the thigh or buttocks. I have found external fixation, even fixation from the pelvis to the femur, to be superior to traction. In most circumstances it offers better stability, easier nursing care, and far better access to the wounds.

In injuries distal to the knee—in particular pilon fractures of the ankle—soft tissue swelling and injury of the skin may preclude early internal fixation. If you plan to perform internal fixation eventually, application of an external fixator may compromise later procedures, particularly if pin traction complications occur. For this reason, traction through a pin in the calcaneus with suspension of the leg in slings or support on a Böhler-Braun frame may be indicated. This also permits good visualization of the extremity where impending compartment syndrome requires full exposure and careful observation of the limb. Over the past 10 years I cannot recall a fracture of the diaphysis of the tibia that I have managed definitively with traction. However, occasionally there is an indication for definitive management of a pilon fracture of the tibia in traction.

In patients who can withstand prolonged recumbency, and in whom internal fixation of a displaced open pilon fracture is contraindicated by the quality of the skin or soft tissues, poor bone stock, or severe systemic disease, treatment in traction may be of

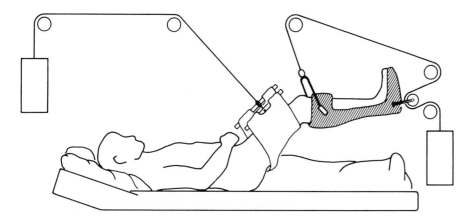

Fig. 3-10. The "Western boot" consists of modified Russell's traction using an independent thigh sling and a proximal tibial pin incorporated into a short-leg cast with an anterior section removed. The pulley on the foot is attached by a cord to the Steinmann pin. (Chapman, M. W., and Zickel, R. E.: Subtrochanteric Fractures of the Femur. In Chapman, M. W. (ed.): Operative Orthopaedics, Vol. 1, p. 364. Philadelphia, J. B. Lippincott, 1988.)

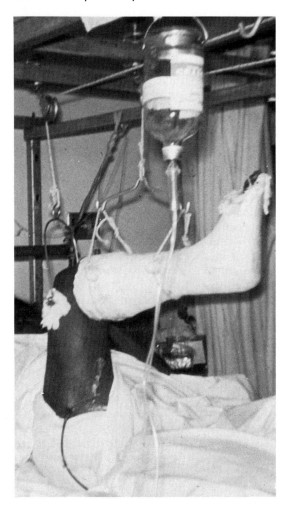

Fig. 3-11. Simple vertical traction on the femur (90°/90°, hip and knee) makes wounds located high on the posterior thigh or the buttock easier to manage. This traction must not be used longer than necessary in the adult because of its effect on the patellofemoral joint.

great advantage. Carry out closed reduction of the fracture or limited internal fixation of the articular surfaces, place a transverse traction pin through the calcaneus in alignment with the longitudinal axis of the tibia, and apply sufficient traction to produce slight distraction of the ankle joint. Early motion can then be instituted, which will help mold the fracture joint surfaces and preserve motion. After the threat of swelling has passed, it is sometimes useful to apply a set of mediolateral splints, or occasionally a gaiter-type cast to help stabilize metaphyseal area fragments. Unfortunately, treatment in traction often requires continuous traction for 6

to 12 weeks to obtain sufficient stability that subsequent treatment in plaster or a cast brace is possible.

Open fractures of the pelvis or acetabulum, particularly if definitive treatment has been delayed, may preclude internal fixation; external fixation may be inadequate, particularly in fractures of the pelvic ring with vertical instability and in fractures of the acetabulum. In these circumstances, definitive treatment in skeletal traction becomes necessary. Again, I prefer a proximal tibial pin, if possible, because this usually permits earlier motion at the hip and knee than does a distal femoral pin. Although some of these fractures may heal quickly enough to allow traction to be discontinued by 6 weeks, very unstable injuries may require traction for as long as 12 to 16 weeks.

Traction is now rarely indicated for open fractures of the upper extremity, except in the humerus. The instability found in open fractures of the humerus is so difficult to control with overhead traction that in the last 10 years I have treated all of these injuries with either primary internal fixation or external fixation.

EXTERNAL SKELETAL FIXATION

The popularity of external skeletal fixation for the treatment of open fractures has waxed and waned throughout the middle and latter parts of the 20th century. Stader popularized its use for the treatment of fractures in domestic animals. During World War II external fixation gained considerable popularity in the military and emerged for a time as a popular method in civilian practice. The Roger-Anderson frame was used commonly throughout the 1950s and early 1960s. For the most part, early external skeletal fixation frames used through-and-through pins, and their external structure did not provide much versatility. Little was known about the biomechanics of these frames in relation to fracture healing. Because of difficulties with external fixation and the emerging popularity of internal fixation, the external methods again waned until Vidal modified the Hoffmann fixator, which quickly gained wide popularity in the 1970s.[29] Although much more versatile than previous designs, the early Hoffmann fixators also used through-and-through pins.

External fixation finally became the fracture stabilization method of choice for the treatment of most open fractures of long bones with the emergence of half-pin frames, which were popularized by Fisher[30] and the AO group.[4] Many different external fixation devices are now available, each offering unique advantages and features. (See Chapter 1 for a more complete discussion of external fixation methods.) Today external fixation is the fracture stabilization method of choice in most type III open fractures of the tibia and fibula and in open fractures of the pelvis.[28]

External fixation devices offer the following advantages: for the most part, they are relatively easily and rapidly applied; excellent stability is obtained; and reasonably anatomical reduction of major fragments is possible. Minimal additional soft tissue trauma is required for placement, so the risk of infection is minimized. In most cases, sufficient stability is achieved to allow early joint motion and muscle rehabilitation. The patient is sufficiently mobile that cardiopulmonary care is facilitated in patients with multiple injuries.

The main disadvantage of external fixators is that in complex fractures with large wounds, application can be complex and time-consuming. Also, the pins may tie down musculotendon units and may interfere with soft tissue reconstructive surgery by preventing the mobilization of flaps. These problems are worse in the femur and humerus, which are covered by thick muscle envelopes, but can be minimized with the use of half-pin fixators. Although the risk of infection at the fracture site is minimized, inappropriate technique causing bone necrosis or early loosening of pins, can lead to pin tract infection. Loosening is more of a problem in osteopenic bone and cancellous bone. Prolonged use of external fixation devices, particularly non–weight-bearing, can lead to delayed union and nonunion of fractures. Many of these complications can be avoided by good surgical technique, which is discussed in other chapters in this text.

Regardless of the type of external fixation used, the following points about application apply:

1. A thorough irrigation and débridement of the fracture is essential.
2. The presence of the external fixator does not change the principles of wound management.
3. The frame must be applied to obtain as anatomical a reduction as possible and maximum contact between bone fragments.
4. Avoid bone necrosis by predrilling for the fixation pins using a water-cooled, sharp, drill point of the appropriate size. Insert the fixation pins by hand following the directions of the manufacturer.
5. Avoid injury to neurovascular structures and avoid tying down musculotendon units.

6. The stability of the fracture–external fixation frame construct is enhanced by:
   a. Using larger pins where the threaded portion is in the far cortex, and the smooth shank of the pin is within the near cortex;
   b. In a standard four-pin frame, two of the pins should be placed close to the fracture site and two remote to the fracture site, trying to locate all pins where sufficient cortical bone is present to provide good purchase for the pins; and
   c. Place the bar connecting the pins as close to the limb as practical. Further stability can be obtained by adding more bars to the single-plane, half-pin frame, by adding additional frames as close to 90° from the original frame as possible, and by cross-connecting these two frames.

Figure 3-12 illustrates a double half-pin frame used for an unstable open fracture of the tibia employing these principles.

Indications

In fractures where some type of internal or external fixation is required for stability, internal fixation generally is safest where the risk of infection is the lowest, and external fixation is indicated where the risk of infection is the highest.[35] Thus, internal fixation is safer in type I and low-grade type II open fractures, and external fixation is most strongly indicated in type III open fractures. In the upper extremity, the violence of trauma is likely to be less than in the lower extremity, and the wounds are generally of a lower grade. For this reason, internal fixation is used more commonly in the upper extremity than the lower.

In the humerus, internal fixation is well tolerated because of the large muscle envelope, and external fixation is less desirable. The neurovascular structures close to the humerus make insertion of external fixation pins by percutaneous or blind technique dangerous. It is necessary in most cases to expose the bone and insert the pins under direct vision to be safe, particularly around the radial nerve. In the humerus, I reserve external fixation for severe grade III open fractures and in those where comminution or poor bone quality makes internal fixation impractical or more hazardous. A single-plane, half-pin frame applied laterally works well.

One of the best indications for external fixation in the upper extremity is in the management of severe "side-swipe" type III open fractures of the

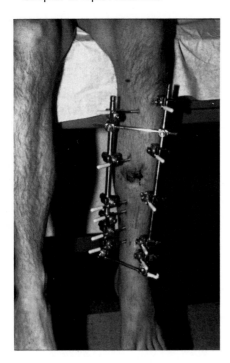

Fig. 3-12. AO half-pin frames placed in double config-uration and cross-connected. *(Chapman, M. W.: Fractures of the Tibia and Fibula. In Chapman, M. W. (ed.): Oper-ative Orthopaedics, Vol. 1, p. 444. Philadelphia, J. B. Lip-pincott, 1988.)*

elbow joint that result in major soft tissue injury, bone loss, and gross instability. A half-pin frame bridging the humerus and the ulna works quite well. The vast majority of open fractures of the ra-dius and ulna can be safely managed by primary internal fixation, with a very low complication rate.[15,17,19] As with the elbow, external fixation is most often indicated for unstable, open, commi-nuted, intra-articular fractures of the distal radius; external fixation from the dorsolateral radius to the second and/or third metacarpals works well.

External fixation also has been advocated for spine fractures; however, this has not gained wide acceptance. I have little experience with this method. Open fractures of the spine are rare and are nearly always secondary to penetrating trauma. Most authorities advocate internal fixation when immediate stabilization is needed in these injuries.

One of the strongest indications for external fix-ation is open fractures of the pelvis, where stability is essential to control hemorrhage, manage the soft tissues, and allow for early mobilization. Perineal wounds and ruptured viscus make the risk of in-fection in open fractures of the pelvis sufficiently

high that external fixation is generally the man-agement of choice. Fixators work well for control-ling the open-book pelvic injury, but are inadequate for the stabilization of pelvic ring fractures with vertical instability. Exotic and complicated frames have not proven to be adequate for pelvic ring frac-tures with vertical instability; therefore, simple frames using two pins in each iliac crest are suffi-cient for most injuries of the pelvic ring (Fig. 3-13). Those with vertical instability require supplemental skeletal traction or delayed posterior internal fix-ation. Complex open, unstable fractures of the ac-etabulum, knee, and ankle are well managed by external fixators bridging these joints.

In the femur, I now rarely use external fixation in fresh, open fractures. Internal fixation, particu-larly intramedullary nailing by closed or modified open technique, is possible immediately or on a delayed basis in most cases.[15] Type III open hip fractures are exceedingly rare. Most hip fractures are inside-to-outside injuries with pinpoint wounds, where primary internal fixation is usually reason-able. The vast majority of midshaft fractures can be nailed immediately or early (see under Internal Fixation, p. 250). I use external fixation for diaph-yseal fractures of the femur when intramedullary fixation is not possible or when there is an exceed-ingly dirty type III open fracture where the risk of infection is simply too high. Open fractures of the supracondylar region of the femur are usually sec-ondary to high-velocity trauma and carry a very high rate of infection, particularly after internal fixation where the rate of infection, in my experi-ence, is 15% to 20%. In these fractures, limited in-

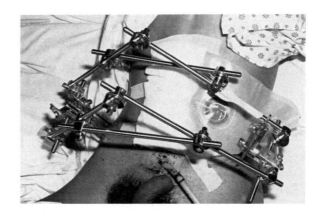

Fig. 3-13. External fixation of an open pelvic fracture. Note colostomy and suprapubic catheter. Internal fix-ation was not used because of risk of infection in this open fracture.

ternal fixation of the articular component with external fixation of the metaphyseal component is often wise. Subsequent conversion to internal fixation with a bone graft may be possible. In open fractures of the tibia, external fixation remains the preferred method of stabilization,[4] although recent reports suggest that non-reamed medullary nails may be as effective and have some advantages[19] (see under Internal Fixation, p. 250). The same rationale discussed for open supracondylar fractures of the femur applies to tibial plateau fractures and pilon fractures. In pilon fractures, a triangular-type frame with fixation to the calcaneus and the forefoot is advisable to avoid an equinus deformity and to assure adequate stabilization.

Postoperative Management

There are nearly as many formulas for care of external fixation pin sites after insertion as there are orthopaedists in the country. I have found that the primary cause of pin infection is loosening of the pin. The other causes are movement of the skin and soft tissues about the pin, causing soft tissue necrosis; the introduction of skin bacteria into the interface between the pin and deep soft tissues; and pressure necrosis of soft tissues owing to skin tension from improper insertion. Avoid these problems by taking the following steps: (1) Insert the pins into bone using the technique described above. (2) Be absolutely certain that there is no skin tension on the pin during or after insertion.

To avoid motion of the skin about the pin, I advocate using a #11 blade to make a puncture wound slightly smaller than the diameter of the pin. After insertion of the pin the skin grips the pin snugly, thereby preventing differential motion. One major disadvantage of this technique is that if great care is not taken, tension of the skin against the pin can easily occur. After insertion, if the skin is gathered on one side of the pin or another, release it by incising the tight side to ensure that no tension is present. Use a couple of sutures to close this incision to again produce snug application of the skin to the pin. Where longitudinal incisions have been used to insert the pin, differential motion of the skin about the pin can be limited by applying a compression dressing around the pin. This is nicely done by placing a couple of 2 × 2 gauze pads about the pin and then putting a rubber stopcock that has been incised or a plastic clip on the pin, which is then slid down to hold the 2 × 2 gauze pads against the skin.

The most effective method of skin care I have found is simple cleansing of the entire external fix-

ation frame, pin tracts, and skin daily with any standard commercial bathing soap to which the patient is not allergic. When the wounds are closed and any incisions around the pin sites have healed, this is easily accomplished during a daily shower by brushing down the frame with a surgical scrub brush and the pins and skin around the pins with a soft toothbrush. An effort must be made to remove all crusts and necrotic debris around the pin tracts. The frame and skin around the pins are then dried with a freshly laundered towel. I have found topical antiseptics to be unnecessary, and other ointments and antibiotic solutions are rarely, if ever, indicated. The minute any persistent drainage is noted from a pin, or persistent discomfort is present, loosening of the pin and infection must be suspected. In such cases, loosen the clamp holding the particular pin and carefully examine the pin. Frequently, loosening of the pin in the near cortex will be found; this can be confirmed by x-ray. Loose pins must never be left in place. Remove them and, if necessary, place a new pin in a new location. In some cases this may necessitate removal of the entire frame.

The timing of frame removal and type of subsequent fixation or mobilization are very complex issues and are beyond the scope of this chapter. Assuming that the external fixator allows good physiologic function of the extremity, I try to plan the treatment so that fracture union occurs in the fixator. This minimizes the risk of late deformity in a cast or brace, and eliminates the need for secondary internal fixation. In most cases, this involves altering the frame to allow progressive loading of the fracture site for enhanced fracture union. In the case of the tibia, for example, this requires altering the frame to assure fracture stability while permitting weight-bearing. Some frames allow for "dynamization," where alignment can be maintained while weight-bearing across the fracture site is permitted. As the fracture shows radiographic evidence of progression to union, the frame can be removed from the pins and the fracture checked for clinical stability. If the fracture is healed, the frame can be removed; if it is not healed, the frame can simply be replaced. In the tibia, conversion to a cast-brace or other type of removable brace is usually practical when the fracture is stable against shortening, cannot be translated, and its stiffness in bending is such that only 10° of motion in any given plane is possible.

Some advocate conversion of external fixation to internal fixation. The presence of infection in a pin tract, whether previous or current, dramatically increases the risk of infection in secondary internal fixation. Pin tract infection is a contraindication to conversion to internal fixation. In the absence of pin tract infection, the safest measure is to first remove the frame, temporarily immobilize the limb in a cast or in traction to allow for pin tract healing (generally 10 to 14 days), then proceed to internal fixation. The safest methods, of course, are those such as closed intramedullary nailing, where the pin tracts can be avoided.

INTERNAL FIXATION

The fear of infection has led to the traditionally accepted opinion that immediate internal fixation, or for that matter, any internal fixation, of open fractures is contraindicated. However, this attitude has changed markedly in the past 10 years. The prognosis in open fractures has improved dramatically since the two world wars. Military surgeons—particularly from the Korean and Vietnam wars—have effected a remarkable improvement in the infection rate by using early, meticulous, and aggressive wound débridement and irrigation; immobilizing with plaster casts or traction; and leaving wounds open, combined with parenteral bactericidal antibiotics. These advances have improved the overall prognosis and given surgeons more latitude in the treatment of open fractures.

Since 1970, reported infection rates in all types of open fractures have ranged from 2.1% to 9.4%.[37,38,39,40] Of more importance are the infection rates in each of the fracture types. In 1972, Gustilo and Anderson[38] reported no infections in type I open fractures, an incidence of 3.8% in type II, and 9% in type III. These were fractures treated without internal fixation. Their overall infection rate was 3.2%. In their later series,[37] the infection rate in type I open fractures was unchanged, in type II was 1.8%, and in type III was 18.4%, for an overall infection rate of 8.9%. They attributed this increase in infection rate to an increase in the percentage of severe type III open fractures in their practices. Of note is the 28% infection rate they encountered when type III fractures were internally fixed. The infection rate in type I open fractures approximates that of clean, elective orthopaedic surgery if a formal, meticulous débridement is carried out and the traumatic wound is left open. The indications for immediate internal fixation of open fractures have changed owing to the recent advances in wound care in open fractures, improved antibiotic therapy (and resultant improvement in infection rates), and the technical advances in internal fixation. Gristina and Rovere[36] have shown that the presence of metal *per se* does not promote bacterial growth *in vitro.* Few prospective, paired, randomized studies comparing internal fixation with external fixation for stabilizing open fractures have been reported. The older literature has three such studies (Table 3-3).[20,31,83] These studies showed that external fixation had a lower infection rate and higher rate of union compared with internal fixation. On this basis, one would conclude that internal fixation is contraindicated in open fractures. During the same period, however, Lottes and colleagues[50] and D'Aubigne and co-workers[24] showed excellent results using closed tibial nailing in the treatment of open fractures of the tibia. Lottes and colleagues had a 7% infection rate and no nonunions.

Studies of internal fixation of open fractures published in the 1980s, however, have shown remarkably good results. In the four series listed in Table 3-4, the average acute infection rate was 8.9% with only three cases going on to chronic osteomyelitis—a long-term infection rate of 0.8%. Although bone grafts were required to achieve union in a number of type III open fractures of the tibia, no nonunions occurred. All of the amputations reported occurred early in severe open fractures of the tibia in which an attempt at limb salvage was made—all cases that in the previous decade would have been amputated immediately. It is evident, however, that severe type III open fractures of the tibia remain a problem.

Table 3-3. Internal Fixation Versus External Immobilization

Authors	Internal Fixation			External Immobilization		
	No. Cases	% Nonunion	% Infection	No. Cases	% Nonunion	% Infection
Wade and Campbell[83]	51	27	14	58	9	0
Claffey[20]	48	17	35	70	0	0
Gallinaro and associates[31]	31	11	17	33	9	3
Totals	130			161		
Average Incidence		18%	33%		9%	3%

Of significance are the excellent functional results reported by Clancy and Hanson,[21] Rittmann and associates,[68] and LaDuca and associates.[47] Other than limb salvage, the most gratifying aspect of immediate internal fixation is the excellent functional results reported. The results in these series are comparable with, if not better than, studies using external fixation and nonoperative treatment. To achieve these results, however, the surgeon must be discriminating and use precise indications. The irrigation and débridement must be impeccable, and the technical execution of the internal fixation must be excellent. Meticulous postoperative care with good patient cooperation is essential. There is little room for misjudgment or error, because the consequences are usually more severe than the complications of external immobilization. There is little question that a role has been established for internal fixation in the treatment of open fractures. Because of the inherent and unavoidable risks of more extensive surgery, however, the gains to be made by internal fixation must justify its use.

Indications for Immediate Internal Fixation

When considering immediate internal fixation of an open fracture, take into account the "personality" of the fracture, your capabilities as a surgeon, the abilities of the operating room team, the adequacy of surgical equipment and implants available, and the particular situation within which the fracture must be treated. For example, will the operating room team be up to the task at 2 a.m., and will the patient's general condition permit extensive surgery? Bone quality must be sufficient to hold screws, and the fracture must not be so comminuted that internal fixation is impossible. You must be skilled with rigid internal fixation methods and perform them on a sufficiently frequent basis that the problem at hand will be adequately managed. Gentleness in the management of the soft tissues is as important as technical ability in fixing the fracture.

Internal fixation of open fractures may be indicated in intra-articular fractures, in certain diaphyseal fractures where internal fixation has proven to be equal to, or more effective than, external fixation, in fractures associated with vascular injuries, in major long-bone fractures in selected victims of multiple-system trauma, and in the elderly. In type I open fractures where internal fixation would be indicated if the fracture were closed, internal fixation can be carried out with minimal risk, but only after adequate irrigation and débridement. There are also social, psychiatric, and economic considerations in this decision-making process that may make internal fixation worth the additional risk.

INTRA-ARTICULAR FRACTURES

Mitchell and Shepard[55] have shown that interfragmentary compression may play a major role in the healing of cartilage in intra-articular fractures. Salter and colleagues[70] have shown that early institution of motion is probably necessary to achieve an optimal result. This requires rigid internal fixation of intra-articular fractures. This is especially true in weight-bearing joints, and clinical experience suggests that intra-articular fractures do best when anatomically reduced and treated with early motion for rehabilitation. These principles are applicable to open fractures as well as closed. The incidence of extensive soft tissue injuries associated with open fractures makes this more imperative for open fractures. Intra-articular fractures not requiring internal fixation are those that are anatomically reduced and stable, those in patients with limited life expectancies, or those in selected patients with neurologic diseases or paralysis. Severe comminution or underlying bone disease, which makes adequate fixation impossible, is also a contraindication to fixation.

The majority of open intra-articular fractures have type I wounds. The low infection rate in type I injuries makes it possible to immediately internally fix these fractures with a risk of infection

Table 3-4. Immediate Internal Fixation

Authors	No. Cases	Late Nonunions	Acute Infections†	Late Osteomyelitis	Secondary Amputation
Clancey and Hansen[21]	35	0	8	0	0
Rittmann and associates[68]	214	0	15	2	4*
Chapman and Mahoney[19]	101	0	10	1	1*
La Duca and associates[47]	42	0	2	0	
Totals	392	0	35	3	5
Average Incidence		0%	8.9%	0.8%	1.3%

* All in severe type III open fractures of the tibia.

† Up to a 40% infection rate in type III open fractures.[19]

roughly comparable with that of closed fractures *if* meticulous irrigation and débridement have been done. Because of the increased risk of infection in type II and type III open fractures, careful judgment is required. Simple, noncomminuted fractures, such as displaced medial and lateral malleolus fractures, are easily internally fixed with minimum fixation through the open fracture wound. Such a simple procedure adds little to soft tissue devitalization and accomplishes anatomical reduction and stability that greatly facilitates soft tissue management. Stabilization may even lower the infection rate rather than contribute to it.[67] In severe type II or type III open intra-articular fractures, staged surgery or limited internal fixation should be considered. Initially, irrigation and débridement are carried out and the wound is left open. The articular cartilage should be covered by soft tissue. At 5 days postinjury the patient is returned to the operating room, and if there is no evidence of infection, definitive internal fixation of the fracture can be carried out. After internal fixation, for ultimate safety, the wound can be left open initially and closed 5 days later. If bone grafting is required, it can be carried out at that time. Another approach at the time of initial débridement is to anatomically reduce the articular fragments and internally fix these alone, managing the metaphyseal portion of the fracture with external fixation. After successful primary closure, usually 14 to 21 days after injury, acute effects of soft tissue trauma have resolved and rigid internal fixation of the remainder of the fracture can be undertaken with less risk. This permits early joint mobilization. If the degree of soft tissue devitalization and contamination causes internal fixation to be delayed longer than 3 weeks after injury, or if the fracture is too comminuted to achieve rigid fixation, it is best to proceed with early joint mobilization in traction or a functional cast-brace.

An optimal end result in intra-articular fractures requires early joint mobilization and muscle rehabilitation. The worst management is to combine the risks of internal fixation with the complications of nonfunctional, external immobilization.

MASSIVELY TRAUMATIZED LIMBS

The recent increase in infection rates reported for open fractures is caused by surgeons' attempts to salvage limbs that a few years ago would never have been considered salvageable and would have been amputated. The advent of limb replantation with specialized microvascular repair techniques has been partly responsible for this change. The type III open fracture with extensive skin loss, severe muscle damage, and neurovascular injury, in which frequent operative intervention for soft tissue care is necessary, requires stabilization to achieve limb salvage and an acceptable, functional end result. Fractures of this type are often segmental, and loss of bone substance is common. This complicates the fixation problem and makes more challenging the reconstructive surgery necessary to achieve union. This situation is most frequently encountered in car-bumper crush injuries of the tibia and in high-velocity gunshot wounds. The high infection rate in these injuries is such that rigid stabilization with an external fixation device is generally preferred.[29] In many situations, however, external fixation devices are impractical, and internal fixation is necessary. External fixators may interfere with soft tissue management by preventing the use of muscle pedicle and skin flaps and by tying down musculotendon units. External fixators also may not offer adequate fixation for intermediate fragments.

Limited interfragmentary fixation with screws at the fracture site is often possible without additional soft tissue dissection; this adds to stability and may prevent the delayed union frequently encountered with external fixation devices. In massive injuries of the humerus where external fixation is impractical, my treatment of choice has been plate fixation. This usually works well because of the large soft tissue envelope around the humerus. Recently I have used non-reamed intramedullary nails (eg, a 3.5-mm Ender's pin), and in the past year, non-reamed, cross-locking nails have become available. Although the value of the latter has not been fully proven, it is a technique worthy of consideration. In the forearm, plate fixation is almost always the method of choice. In massive injuries, bone grafting early in treatment is nearly always necessary to avoid a nonunion.[17] In the femur, plate fixation works well because of the excellent muscle envelope covering this bone. If infection intervenes, it is usually less catastrophic than with reamed intramedullary nails, where infection frequently involves the entire length of the bone. Non-reamed nails, such as the Ender's, have a role to play because they are less threatening to the blood supply than reamed nails. Recent experience with immediate reamed nailing of severe open fractures of the femur indicates that the infection rate is three to four times higher than in closed or type I open fractures, but there are certain circumstances—particularly in the multiply traumatized patient—where this risk may be justified.[11,15] In the tibia, external fixation remains the preferred method of stabilization. Some[2,21,22,58] have advocated the use of plates in selected circumstances, but recent experience with non-reamed nails, particularly the Lottes nail[18,24,50] and Ender pins,[85] indicates they have a major role to play. They may be equal in efficacy, and in some ways superior, to external fixation. This past year has seen the introduction of non-reamed locking nails. Early experience indicates they are likely to be a valuable addition to our armamentarium. Experience is too limited at this point, however, to establish their role.

In the very elderly, or in nutritionally or immunologically compromised patients with multiple, severe injuries where the metabolic load of a massive injury is life-threatening, immediate amputation may be indicated.[41] This can be a life-saving measure.

VASCULAR INJURIES

In the presence of vascular injuries requiring repair, I usually stabilize the fracture with internal or external fixation. This is particularly true when bony impingement caused the vascular injury or residual instability threatens the repair. Because restoration of circulation to the limb is of primary concern, it is important that either vascular repair or temporary restoration of circulation be carried out before fixation. The presence of the fracture, in many instances, permits a repair through the open fracture wound that would otherwise not be possible. This is an additional reason for carrying out internal fixation after vascular repair. The surgeon must be sufficiently skilled and gentle in his technique that the vascular repair is not disrupted during internal fixation. Connolly,[23] through Vietnam war experience, has shown that internal fixation of fractures is not essential to protect vascular repairs; however, in open fractures with vascular injury accompanied by extensive soft tissue injury, the advantages of internal fixation are the same as those described for massively traumatized limbs.[66]

MULTIPLY INJURED PATIENTS

The contribution of multiple long-bone fractures to the demise of the multiply injured patient has only recently been appreciated.[6] Because the primary cause of death in victims of multiple trauma following successful resuscitation is respiratory failure, we have attributed these deaths to chest and abdominal trauma. Trunkey and associates[80] have shown that the most important factors predisposing to the adult respiratory distress syndrome are multiple long-bone fractures, shock on admission to the emergency room, voluminous blood replacement, and comminuted fractures of the pelvis.

Long-bone fractures contribute to this problem through hemorrhage, by adding to the initial quantity of injured muscle, and by preventing early mobilization because the patient is supine in bed with skeletal traction. Early stabilization of open fractures reduces hemorrhage, particularly in the pelvis. Irrigation and débridement of open fractures plus stabilization of long-bone fractures may reduce the ultimate metabolic load imposed on the patient. Pulmonary physiotherapy and achievement of a vertical chest by getting the patient out of bed are essential to avoid atelectasis and secondary infection in persistently dependent pulmonary segments.[47] Immediate stabilization of major long-bone fractures—particularly in the femur and in unstable fractures of the pelvis and spine—may be life-saving.

Any additional initial surgery in the extremities contributes to the total soft tissue trauma; therefore, the advantages of early internal fixation must be substantial, and thoughtful consultation among the orthopaedic surgeon, general surgeon, and anesthesiologist is essential. The femur most frequently requires fixation. Fractures of the upper extremity can usually be managed with plaster immobilization, with the exception of some unstable fractures of the humerus. Injuries below the knee also can be managed initially with external immobilization by plaster casts.

In some trauma centers it is thought that most pulmonary failure secondary to polytrauma has been eliminated by early, aggressive resuscitation and immediate internal fixation of all long-bone fractures.[6,47]

Although immediate internal fixation facilitates care in the intensive care unit, low tissue oxygen tensions during the immediate postinjury period may predispose to a higher wound complication rate. These advantages and disadvantages must be kept in mind when considering immediate internal fixation versus external fixation for open long-bone fractures in multiply injured patients.

ELDERLY PATIENTS

The same principles apply to open fractures in elderly patients as in the young, with some exceptions. The complications of enforced bed rest, particularly with pneumonia and thromboembolic disease, are far greater in the elderly and therefore early internal fixation to permit mobilization is even more important. As in multiply traumatized patients, the metabolic load of severe multiple injuries may necessitate early amputation to save a life.

SURGICAL TECHNIQUE

In the operating room, first direct your attention to meticulous irrigation and débridement of the open fracture. Plans for subsequent internal fixation should not divert your attention from this essential task. Plan extensile surgical incisions that permit adequate exposure, do not further compromise skin flaps, and permit soft tissue coverage of any implants that are to be placed. Internal fixation requires careful planning. Be certain that the bone quality and fracture configuration will permit fixation and that the skills of the operating room team will provide rapid, facile, and adequate application of the internal fixation appliances.

The fixation must provide absolute stability and as anatomical a reduction as possible. Internal fixation without good fracture-surface contact and excellent rigidity is worse than no fixation. The fixation should require minimal additional soft tissue dissection. The internal fixation is best applied through the open fracture wound and is placed so that soft tissue coverage is possible even if, biomechanically, the implant is not in the most advantageous position. This requires flexibility on the part of the surgeon. In general, primary wound closure should *not* be performed when immediate internal fixation of an open fracture is done. Partial muscle closure in the absence of tension to achieve coverage of the fracture site or implant is important, but the skin and deep fascia should always be left open. Plastic reconstructive procedures to obtain closure or coverage of an implant are rarely indicated at the time of the initial fixation.

The difficulties in determining viability, and the additional trauma from such surgery, often lead to necrosis of flaps. Flap or pedicle coverage is best achieved at the time of delayed primary closure, which is carried out at least 5 days after injury. Some authorities believe that flap coverage as early as 48 hours gives a higher success rate. This is discussed in much greater detail in Chapter 4. If the implant and bone cannot be covered immediately, meticulous wound care, keeping the bone and surroundings moist with physiologic saline or mild antiseptic solutions (eg, Dakin's solution) is important to prevent necrosis of exposed bone. Early full-thickness tissue coverage is important to enhance revascularization and limit the risk of infection. Although coverage can usually be achieved by local muscle pedicle flaps, microvascularized flaps are sometimes required. Try to achieve complete closure of the wound within 10 days, if possible.

Early vigorous muscle and joint rehabilitation is

important to achieve the maximum benefits from internal fixation. Immediate continuous passive motion is helpful, particularly in intraarticular fractures. In most cases the postinjury pain will subside in several days, and supervised range-of-motion and strengthening exercises can be undertaken. When the fixation permits, as with intramedullary nails in stable fractures, immediate weight-bearing is important.

Bone Grafting

Autogenous, *cancellous* bone grafts are used almost routinely in internal fixation of open fractures.[5] Because of the risk of infection, these bone grafts are rarely applied at the time of initial internal fixation. An exception is in type I and mild type II intra-articular fractures, where cancellous bone is necessary to fill defects for obtaining anatomical reduction and stable fixation. *All* bone defects, particularly in diaphyseal fractures, must be filled. There is a high incidence of delayed union in plate fixation of open diaphyseal fractures, so bone grafting should routinely be done to avoid premature plate failure from delayed union. Bone graft is best applied at the time of delayed primary closure. In high-risk cases, it may be done electively after successful delayed primary closure when infection is absent, usually 6 to 9 weeks after injury. Good-quality, abundant, cancellous bone graft is necessary; I usually take this from the posterior ilium in the region of the posterosuperior iliac spine. In rare cases where soft tissue coverage of the fracture site is impossible or infection has occurred, I use the open cancellous bone grafting technique described by Papineau.[61]

Special Considerations

FOOT AND HAND FRACTURES

The foot and hand in healthy, young adults have excellent blood supply; therefore, infection is not usually a major problem. Immediate internal fixation can be carried out according to the same indications used for closed fractures.[14,19] Most fixation is achieved with Kirschner wires, and the amount of additional soft tissue dissection required is minimal. In the massively traumatized hand, internal fixation that permits immediate motion is essential for restoration of hand function.

The indications for limited internal fixation of the calcaneus with pins and screws are the same as those in closed fractures. Displaced fractures of the body and neck of the talus should be reduced anatomically and immediately internally fixed.[42] In my experience, this has resulted in an almost uniform rate of union and a much lower incidence of avascular necrosis than previously reported.[42] A similar philosophy is applied to displaced fractures of the tarsonavicular joint.

ANKLE FRACTURE–DISLOCATIONS

Routine fractures of one malleolus, and bimalleolar, and trimalleolar fractures are usually best treated by primary internal fixation.[9] In type I and low-grade type II open fractures this can be achieved with no greater risk of infection than in closed fractures.[19,68] In severe type III open fractures of the ankle, extensive reconstruction that might require extensive plating at the time of initial débridement is best deferred. The articular surface can be reconstructed with wires and screws, and the remainder of the fracture may best be initially managed by external fixation or supportive hard dressing.

Internal fixation of routine ankle fractures presents few problems; however, pilon fractures are difficult to treat. Restoration of the articular surface with wires and screws to achieve anatomical position, and then temporary use of external fixation for the shaft portion of the fracture is a safe approach. After 5 to 10 days, and in the absence of infection, application of a buttress plate or other implants to achieve complete stability can be done more safely. It is also possible at this time to insert cancellous bone grafts. Regardless of the approach used, early motion to restore ankle function is essential.

In those fracture–dislocations where stability cannot be achieved with internal fixation, early motion can be instituted while the patient is in calcaneal pin traction. Stability can be augmented with a Delbet cast.

TIBIAL SHAFT FRACTURES

Immobilization in a functional weight-bearing cast provides good results in the majority of type I and mild type II open fractures of the tibia with stable fracture patterns.[10,71,72] In unstable fractures and in severe type II and type III open fractures, stabilization by external fixation is the current method of choice for fixation.[13,29,46] Stable fracture patterns can be adequately stabilized by a single-plane, half-pin frame; but more comminuted patterns, particularly those with segmental bone loss, may require double half-pin frames to enhance stability. Owing to the high rate of acute infection (up to 29% in the 1982 series of Gustilo) acute plate fixation is rarely indicated. Reasonably good results have been reported in some series[56,68] with the use of AO plates

combined with interfragmentary screws, and the incidence of nonunion and late osteomyelitis is quite low in these series (see Table 3-4).

Intramedullary nailing with non-reamed nails (eg, Lottes nail) has never been popular in spite of the excellent results reported by Lottes[50] and D'Aubigne.[24] Good results have been reported with the use of multiple flexible intramedullary nails without reaming.[60,86] In the past 2 years, acute fixation with non-reamed nails has gained popularity.[43] At the University of California, Davis, we just completed a randomized prospective study comparing the Lottes nail and AO external fixator in stable fracture patterns in all grades of open fractures.[76] We showed the rates of nonunion and infection to be nearly identical in the two groups, whereas the rate of malunion was substantially lower in the Lottes group. With the Lottes nails wound management was easier, application of the device was simpler, and patient acceptance was higher. Recent interest has developed in the use of non-reamed locking nails for more comminuted fractures, but their efficacy has not yet been proven. At this time, external skeletal fixation remains the treatment of choice, but non-reamed medullary nails no doubt have a major role to play.[54]

The role of Ilizarov fixation and techniques for the treatment of acute open fractures is not yet established in the Western world.[45] Through techniques of bone transportation, Ilizarov's method may prove to have a major role to play in the treatment of open fractures with segmental bone loss and in those complicated by osteomyelitis.

In comminuted fractures the tibia should not be shortened more than ½ inch to achieve good bone apposition, because the muscles below the knee do not accommodate well to shortening. Larger segmental defects can be bridged with bone grafts; segment transportation and restoration of full length provides optimal muscle function.

Because external fixation is the most commonly used method of fixation in the tibia, a few comments about management are merited. Unless the fracture pattern is stable and the frame is in compression, early weight-bearing, other than touch-down, usually is not possible. A dorsiflexion foot support to avoid an equinus deformity is important. If the fracture is not stable when the external fixation frame is removed, maintenance of position in a cast can be exceedingly difficult. For that reason, I try to keep the majority of tibial fractures in an external fixator until union occurs. I plan to adjust the frame to allow progressive weight-bearing through the fracture site as the fracture consolidates. I usually do not begin weight-bearing until some callus can be seen and the fracture has some early stability.

Early bone grafting is often indicated in open fractures of the tibia. In fractures with bone loss or with extensive soft tissue stripping, bone grafting should usually be performed early. In less severe cases, if the fracture is unstable and shows no evidence of callus formation by 12 weeks, then bone grafting is indicated. Another alternative would be the early institution of electrical stimulation, but the role of this method has not been established in fresh fractures or in delayed unions. I remove the frame and convert the patient to either a weight-bearing cast or cast-brace when the fracture is clinically stable. There is no problem testing this in the later stages of union by removing the fixation frame in the outpatient department. If the fracture is found to not yet be ready for conversion to a cast or brace, the frame is easily reapplied. Earlier conversion to a weight-bearing cast or brace may be necessary if pin complications mandate removal of the frame. Conversion to internal fixation is rarely necessary. In some cases where the fracture remains quite unstable but pin complications make early removal of the external fixator necessary, insertion of a non-reamed nail may be appropriate. To minimize the risk of infection, remove the fixator and allow the pin tracts to heal (this usually requires 10 to 20 days) prior to nailing, and use a closed technique. In my experience, conversion to a plate or reamed nail is too hazardous because of the high risk of infection.[53] This is particularly true if any of the pins of the external fixator have become infected.

When treating severe type III fractures of the tibia, particularly if complicated by infection or neurovascular injury, remember the indications for early amputation (see p. 239).

FRACTURES OF THE FEMUR

Type I open fractures of the shaft can be immediately internally fixed with intramedullary nails with an infection rate approaching that of closed fractures.[11,12] In grade II and III open fractures, the risk of infection rises substantially with acute nailing, and this is probably indicated only in patients who are victims of multiple trauma where the increased risk of infection is justified by the contribution of early stability of the femur to salvage of the patient's life.

In isolated open grade II or III fractures of the shaft, I prefer to irrigate and débride the fracture, leave the wound open, place the femur in traction,

and carry out delayed primary closure at 5 days. Approximately 10 to 14 days after injury, closed intramedullary nailing is done. Using this technique, I have had an infection rate of less than 1% and no nonunions.[16] In very severe, highly contaminated open fractures, particularly where soft tissue coverage may be a problem, external fixation may be indicated. I do not routinely use external fixation because the large soft tissue envelope around the femur makes internal fixation safer and external fixation more troublesome. I have not found the Wagner external fixator to be very useful because it places the fixation pins too distant from the fracture site; adequate stability cannot be obtained with this method unless the fracture pattern is very stable.[57] I prefer the versatility of single-plane, half-pin fixators such as the AO or Ultra-X. Although a single-plane frame can be used for initial fixation, long-term treatment with external fixation usually requires a biplane frame. In victims of multiple injuries, particularly if the patient has been placed on a regular operating table in the supine position, immediate intramedullary nailing may be difficult. In this circumstance, immediate plate fixation through the open fracture wound may be indicated. This can usually be accomplished rapidly and may be life-saving.

Although some type of skeletal fixation is used for the vast majority of open fractures of the femur in most trauma centers in the Western world, management by cast-braces also can work well, although the wound management is more difficult and the incidence of malunion is higher. Where fixation devices are not available, as in some third world countries, and in mass casualty situations where application of fixation may not be practical, immediate immobilization in a cast-brace or 1½ hip spica cast certainly serves a useful role. I can apply an external fixator much more rapidly than a good cast, however, and the advantages of the fixator over a cast are without question.

Fractures of the femur often occur in conjunction with severe ipsilateral knee injuries and fractures of the hip. In these situations, internal fixation is usually indicated.[12] Intra-articular fractures involving the knee are treated with the same principles used for fractures of the ankle (see p. 254). Rehabilitation of severe soft tissue injuries of the knee is usually inadequate in the presence of a femoral shaft fracture; therefore, internal fixation is usually indicated after successful delayed primary closure. Supracondylar fractures without intra-articular involvement can be successfully managed with a cast-brace, using early motion and weight-bearing. Enders pins are also useful for the treatment of difficult complex fractures of the femur.[13]

UPPER EXTREMITY LONG-BONE FRACTURES

The long bones of the upper extremity have good soft tissue coverage. This, combined with the fact that upper-extremity wounds usually involve less energy than lower-extremity wounds, makes the incidence of complications much lower.[17,19,68] In type I open fractures, internal fixation can be carried out with the same indications as in closed fractures. Stable type II and III open fractures of the humerus can often be managed with simple coaptation splints. In unstable fractures where the pull of the deltoid makes soft tissue management difficult, and in some fractures with associated neurovascular injury, immediate internal fixation should be considered.[81] I prefer plate fixation; however, Enders nails, Lottes nails, and newer interlocking nails are very useful. Intra-articular fractures in the upper extremity suitable for internal fixation are best fixed immediately. Fractures of the radius and ulna can be plated immediately, particularly when combined with a bone graft, with a high rate of union and low rate of infection.[17]

DEFINITIVE WOUND MANAGEMENT

The initial decision required in the treatment of open fractures is whether the limb should be salvaged or amputated. Once a decision to attempt salvage has been made, irrigation and débridement are required and then fracture stability must be obtained. Assuming that internal or external fixation has been employed, the final decision is how to manage the open fracture wound. The options available to the surgeon are[34]:

I. Primary Options for Definitive Wound Management
    A. Primary closure by suture
    B. Primary closure with autogenous skin graft or local or microvascularized full-thickness graft
    C. Wound left open
        1. gauze dressings
        2. biologic dressings—homografts, heterografts, or synthetic materials[3]

When the wound is left open, a series of secondary options must be considered.

II. Secondary Options for Definitive Wound Management
    A. Delayed primary closure by suture
    B. Delayed autogenous skin graft or local or microvascularized flap
    C. Secondary closure by suture or graft
    D. Healing by secondary intention
    E. Split-thickness skin graft with the intent of subsequent excision and closure by suture or flap

Although the foregoing lists include most options, they may at times be modified and are frequently combined for unusual situations.

PRIMARY CLOSURE

Primary closure is rarely, if ever, indicated. If it is to be done, the following criteria must be met:

1. The original wound must have been fairly clean and not have occurred in a highly contaminated environment.
2. All necrotic tissue and foreign material has been removed.
3. Circulation to the limb is essentially normal.
4. Nerve supply to the limb is intact.
5. The patient's general condition is satisfactory.
6. The wound can be closed without tension.
7. Closure will not create a dead space.
8. The patient does not have multiple-system injuries.

Type I open fracture wounds often meet these criteria; however, the type I wound is usually so small that closure by secondary intention is quite satisfactory. Type III wounds should never be closed primarily. Type II wounds require careful judgment and in general should be left open. The biggest risk of primary closure is gas gangrene, and this seems to occur in very benign-seeming wounds. If the surgeon is inexperienced or in doubt, it seems wise to invoke the axiom, "When in doubt, leave it open," or even better, "Leave all open fractures open."

On the other hand, there seems little question that fractured bones heal most rapidly when they are enclosed by infection-free, pliable, vascularized soft tissues. Thus, as Brav[8] has pointed out, one of the early objectives of treating an open fracture is to convert it to a closed one. This is probably best accomplished by delayed primary closure (see below). In most cases, the elective portion of the wound made by the surgeon can be closed, leaving the traumatic wound open. It is particularly im-

portant to cover primarily tendon without peritenon and bone not covered by periosteum, because
desiccation will result in the death of these structures. Usually some local muscle or fat can be drawn
across these structures, leaving the skin open. The
same rationale applies to open joints, where I usually close the capsule over a suction drain and leave
the remainder of the wound open.

DELAYED PRIMARY CLOSURE

In the healthy adult the wound healing process
proceeds for the first 5 days or so whether or not
the wound is closed. As long as closure is achieved
before the fifth day, wound strengths at 14 days
are comparable to those in wounds closed on the
first day. This is why closure prior to the fifth day
is termed "delayed primary closure." There are
several advantages to this approach: Leaving the
wound open minimizes the risk of anaerobic infection. Also, the delay allows the host to mount local
wound defensive mechanisms, which will permit
closure more safely than is possible on the first day.

LEAVING WOUNDS OPEN

There is a strong tendency for surgeons to put drains
into wounds that have been left open. For draining
an established abscess or tissue spaces that tend
naturally to reseal themselves (eg, palmar space,
subgluteal space), the reasons for and usefulness of
such drains are acknowledged. However, standard
mechanical drains (eg, the Penrose) may irritate
the tissues they contact and incite an innocent exudate. The trouble lies in the uncertainty that such
an exudate is in fact innocent. For major soft tissue
wounds that are to be left open after débridement,
gauze dressings inserted to a point just beneath the
fascia are sufficient, because the fascia and skin
usually create the most resistant barrier to the escape of accumulated purulent material. The dressing should just keep the fascial and skin edges separated. Do not pack wounds, because this often
produces an obturator effect and thus prevents exudate and serum from draining. Loosely placed
dressings conduct the exudate or transudate by
capillary action to the surface. When there is no
drainage, apart from the initial wound bleeding,
the blood soaks into the dressing, coagulates, and
may dry to a remarkable degree, leaving the dressing as a firm, rust-colored "blood shingle." Where
tendon and bone lack soft tissue coverage, it may
be useful to keep the wound moist by inserting a
catheter through which sterile fluid can be dripped.

Ordinarily, the wound is not exposed for inspection until the time of delayed primary closure—4
to 6 days after injury. Dressing changes in the patient's bed prior to that time are usually unnecessary, and simply increase the risk of nosocomial infection.

Should local symptoms of pain, odor, or obviously
excessive drainage appear early on, or should more
general signs of fever, leukocytosis or other problems be noted, early return to the operating room
for inspection and repeat irrigation and débridement are warranted. In type III open fractures and
those that occurred in a highly contaminated environment, early return to the operating room
within 36 to 48 hours may be indicated for wound
inspection and repeat irrigation and débridement,
particularly if the original irrigation and débridement were thought to be marginal.

When wound closure is not possible by about the
fifth day, particularly when there is residual necrotic tissue in the wound that would benefit from
dressing changes, then serial dressing changes in
the patient's bed may be necessary. This is particularly true if infection intervenes. I prefer wet to
dry dressing changes performed every 12 hours,
using either normal saline or half-strength Dakin's
solution. Place fine mesh gauze directly on the
wound and overlay it with moist 4 × 4 gauze pads.
Cover the wound lightly so the gauze can dry. When
the dressing is changed the overlying gauze is removed dry, thus débriding the wound, and a new
moist dressing is applied. When performed over
several days, this technique is remarkably effective
in removing superficial necrotic debris from wounds
and in encouraging granulation tissue.

WOUND CLOSURE

Closure by direct suturing is possible in most cases.
Place only the minimum amount of suture material
deep in the wound. Avoid tension in the closure
because this may produce necrosis of skin edges
and deeper soft tissues. If primary closure of the
wound without tension is not possible, alternatives
are "relaxing" incisions, split-thickness skin grafts,
and flaps.

Relaxing Incisions

A linear wound with minimal soft tissue loss may
be difficult to close because of underlying swelling.
When it is important to obtain full thickness coverage over bone or other structures, closure can
often be effected with a relaxing incision (Fig. 3-
14). It is important to understand that relaxing in-

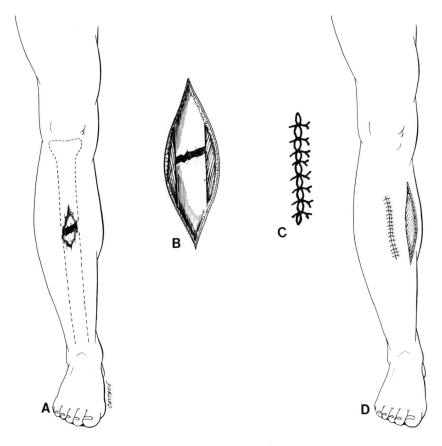

Fig. 3-14. (**A**) A rather significant loss of tissue directly over the crest of the tibia. (**B**) The degree of tissue loss after débridement. (**C**) The excessive tension at the wound margins that results when direct suture closure is attempted. (**D**) The principle of the relaxing incision. Care must be exercised to avoid making the interval bridge of skin (essentially a bipedicled flap graft) too narrow. The primary wound can now be closed for cover without tension at the suture line. The relaxing incision can communicate with the fracture to facilitate drainage.

cisions produce different types of local flaps, the most characteristic being a bipedicle flap. Exercise care to place these sufficiently distant from the original wound that the blood supply to the intervening skin is not threatened. This is particularly a problem if the skin between the two wounds has been injured. Be certain that the relaxing incision is long enough to allow closure of the primary wound without tension. Relaxing incisions are best suited to those areas in which there is some natural mobility of the skin and underlying tissue, such as the thigh and proximal leg, but less so where mobility is limited, as in the lower leg, ankle region, and about the wrist. Multiple, small, alternating relaxing incisions provide another technique of obtaining closure, but must be used cautiously, particularly when the surrounding skin has been damaged (Fig. 3-15).

Split-Thickness Skin Grafts

In most cases where the wound bed is composed of viable vascularized soft tissues, a split-thickness skin graft provides the best method of closure. This avoids the risk of a bipedicle flap and is better cosmetically because it leaves only one wound rather than two, as the opened relaxing incision requires split-thickness skin graft as well. In addition, when edema subsides, the skin graft will contract, and often the resulting wound will be much smaller and more cosmetically acceptable. If it is not, late excision and primary closure to produce a cosmetically acceptable wound may be possible.

Split-thickness skin grafts require support from host tissues on which they are deposited and do best when placed directly on viable muscle or well-formed granulation tissue. (Granulation tissue is not necessary as long as the underlying tissues are well vascularized.) Split grafts will not take on bare tendons or on bone not covered by periosteum. Their prospect for survival is somewhat less certain on tissues with a limited blood supply such as periosteum, fascia, and joint capsule.

Generally, relatively thin split-thickness skin grafts (0.010–0.012 inches) have demonstrated greater survival. The skin grafts mold to the wound site and drain much better if run through a 1 to 1½

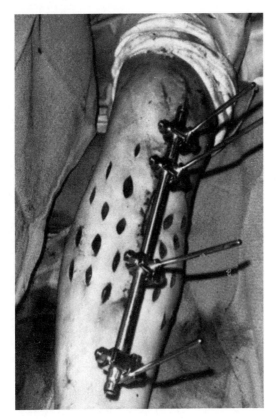

Fig. 3-15. Multiple 1-cm stab wounds allow closure of a longitudinal wound over the exposed anterior surface of the tibia. Note the spread and alternating pattern, which is necessary to avoid skin necrosis. Do not use this technique on contused or detached skin. (Chapman, M. W.: Fractures of the Tibia and Fibula. *In* Chapman, M. W. (ed.): Operative Orthopaedics, Vol. 1, p. 456. Philadelphia, J. B. Lippincott, 1988.)

mesher. The less the mesh is spread, the better the cosmetic result. If the wound is marginal, spreading the mesh widely enhances drainage.[78]

Flaps

When soft tissue loss is extensive and closure by primary suture or split-thickness skin graft is not possible, flaps become necessary. The types of flaps available are local fascial–cutaneous flaps, local muscle pedicle flaps, remote muscle pedicle flaps, and free microvascularized muscle flaps. This is a very extensive topic in itself and is described in detail in Chapter 4. Suffice it to say that surgeons treating open fractures must be skilled in using all of these flaps or have available a colleague with such skills. Generally flaps are not done at the time of initial irrigation and débridement, because it of-

ten is very difficult to predict the amount of progressive local tissue necrosis that may occur; a flap placed at this time may, in effect, result in primary closure of the wound. Where bone, tendon, and other structures require immediate coverage, I swing a local muscle flap without actually closing the entire wound. Otherwise, I believe most flaps are best done at about 5 days postinjury.

Most coverage problems occur in the tibia (Fig. 3-16), and the fracture surgeon should be familiar with the gastrocnemius, soleus, and flexor hallucis and flexor digitorum local muscle flaps[32] (see Chapter 4).

Biologic Dressings

When closure is not appropriate or cannot be carried out, and arrangements cannot be made for the

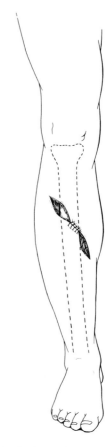

Fig. 3-16. A method of providing "cover" for an exposed medial surface of the tibial shaft while providing for drainage at either end of the wound. This is not suitable if very much skin has been lost, because tension may induce marginal necrosis of the distal edge at the sutured area.

covering of vulnerable tissues by the transposition of local tissues, biologic dressings of skin or synthetic material may be of value. Homologous human skin, heterologous porcine skin (prepared commercially), and synthetic dressings may suffice. My personal experience with these is very limited and they have not been used on our service on a routine basis; therefore, it is difficult for me to put their role into perspective. Baxter[3] has shown that these skin dressings have several advantages in the treatment of burn patients. Changing them is considerably less painful. They seem to be a deterrent to infection, and there is some evidence that existing infection may be suppressed or controlled. Because host granulation tissue invades such grafts, allowing them to take for varying periods, the biologic dressings can give evidence of the readiness of a wound bed for definitive autogenous grafting. Thus, such grafts need to be changed frequently. Salisbury[69] has shown that when granulation tissue from an autogenous graft donor site grows into a heterologous dressing, even if it is pulled away before any significant clinical take occurs, small bits of collagen from the heterologous dressing tissue remain in the host granulation tissue. This collagen apparently tends to incite a rather chronic inflammatory response, leading to some delay in epithelialization and an increase in inflammation. Because these dressings are not used commonly in the treatment of open fractures in North America, the reader is referred to the literature on this field.

ELEVATION

Perhaps there is no more critical point in the control of postdébridement swelling than the simple matter of elevation. Persistent, or increased, swelling may keep tissues turgid and wound surfaces moist, thereby preventing delayed primary closure. Edematous tissues increase tension in the suture line and may lead to marginal wound necrosis. Other disadvantages of swelling include a possible increase in the prospect of infection, a loss of reduction of fracture should swelling require a cast be split and spread, and probably an increased risk of thrombophlebitis.

Limbs must be elevated in a manner that is comfortable for the patient and guarantees continuous elevation at a level above the heart; however, elevation more than 10 cm above the heart does not enhance lymphatic or venous return, but does decrease the arterial input to the limb, which can be hazardous in impending compartment syndrome and in patients with peripheral vascular disease.

Under most circumstances, broad slings suspended from the overhead frame serve best.

ANTIBIOTICS

Antibiotics for open fracture wounds should not be considered prophylactic, but therapeutic, because these wounds are contaminated by bacteria. (Purists would argue that in the acute wound, infection is not present and therefore antibiotics *are* prophylactic, but I argue that many organisms are present in spite of adequate irrigation and débridement.) The role of antibiotics is to kill residual organisms and at least inhibit their growth to the point where host protective mechanisms will eradicate them.[87] Irrigation and débridement are by far the most important measures in preventing infection in open fractures, and antibiotics certainly cannot be relied on to prevent infection in an inadequately débrided wound.

Use of antibiotics in preventing infection in open fractures remains a controversial topic, particularly in discussions between North Americans and Europeans. In North America antibiotics are thought to be the standard of care, whereas in Europe many surgeons do not use antibiotics, and the infection rates reported are surprisingly comparable. Patzakis and associates[65] established the basis for current practices in North America. In their controlled, randomized, prospective study, they compared three groups: one received immediate administration of cephalothin, one immediate administration of penicillin and streptomycin, and the third group received no antibiotics. The infection rate in the cephalothin group was 2.3%, compared to 9.7% in the penicillin/streptomycin group, and 13.9% in the final group. It is on the basis of this study and subsequent clinical experience that cephalosporins remain the antibiotics of choice for the treatment of open fractures in North America. In addition, the data of Patzakis and associates strongly support that a culture taken from the wound before any treatment is likely to yield the organisms that will subsequently cause infection. The most common organism producing infection in their series was *Staphylococcus aureus;* most of these infections were resistant to penicillin.

Over the past decade, however, clinical experience has changed. As reflected in Gustilo's figures,[37,39] the overall infection rate in open fractures has risen somewhat, probably owing to the fact that the overall severity of open fractures has increased and we are now salvaging limbs that previously were amputated. Secondly, the spectrum of infecting organisms has changed. Although *S. aureus* remains a major player, gram-negative organisms have become very prevalent and mixed infections are common, particularly in type III open fractures. The precise cause for this change is not known. I hypothesize that three factors are playing a role: (1) The ubiquitous use of cephalosporins in open fractures probably is selecting out resistant gram-negative organisms; (2) Gram-negative organisms such as *Pseudomonas,* Enterobacter, and enterococcus, have become very prevalent nosocomial infective organisms; and (3) The severely traumatized limbs we try to salvage today may present to the population of bacteria a unique environment that was not readily available in the past, when we were more likely to amputate than to attempt limb salvage.

Thus, use of antibiotics has changed. In open fractures occurring in a reasonably clean environment, and for grades I or II fractures, most surgeons still use a cephalosporin—most commonly, cefazolin. In those fractures occurring in a highly contaminated environment, most add penicillin to prevent clostridial infection. In type III open fractures, aminoglycosides are frequently administered as well.[1,7,26]

The most important step a surgeon can take is to constantly monitor by cultures the organisms most frequently occurring in open fracture wounds in his institution, and those most commonly causing infection. Constant monitoring of the antibiotic sensitivities of these organisms should provide a good guide as to the appropriate antibiotics, doses, and routes of administration.

The use of topical antibiotics remains controversial. There is enough evidence to point to their effectiveness[33,84] that I routinely place topical antibiotics in the last 2-liter bag used for irrigation. In addition, the dressings can be soaked in these topical antibiotics. It seems to me that these agents remain in the wound long enough that some kill of remaining organisms will occur, thereby dropping the bacterial count in the wound. Many different antibiotics can be used for topical application; my advice regarding the selection of parenteral antibiotics applies to local antibiotics.

General principles to be followed in the use of antibiotics include: (1) Administer parenteral antibiotics as soon as possible. (2) Choose antibiotics that are bactericidal, and choose an antibiotic (or antibiotics) active against both gram-positive and gram-negative organisms. The drugs should produce bactericidal concentrations in blood, extracellular fluids, and joint fluids. They must be as hypoallergenic as possible and compatible with other antibiotics.

Antibiotic-Impregnated Beads

Numerous antibiotics can be incorporated in polymethylmethacrylate while maintaining their bactericidal activity. They leach out at sufficient rates that bactericidal levels are produced in the surrounding fluids and tissues.[18] Chains of methacrylate beads strung on stainless steel wire and impregnated with antibiotics have been used to treat infection, and more recently have been advocated for open fractures. Seligson[74] has produced what he calls a "bead pouch" by placing over the fracture site and beads an oxygen-permeable membrane (Opsite). Local wound levels of antibiotics produced are higher than those possible by the parenteral route.[27] This is suggested as a replacement for intravenous antibiotics, or in some cases as an adjunct. Although early results are promising, efficacy has not yet been firmly proven in open fractures.

REFERENCES

1. Antrum, R. M.; and Solomkin, J. S.: A Review of Antibiotic Prophylaxis for Open Fractures. Orthop. Rev., 16:246–254, 1987.
2. Bach, A. W.; and Solomkin, J. S.: Plates Versus External Fixation in Severe Open Tibial Shaft Fractures: A Randomized Trial. Clin. Orthop., 241:89–94, 1989.
3. Baxter, C. R.: Homografts and Heterografts as a Biological Dressing in the Treatment of Thermal Injury. Presented at the First Annual Congress of the Society of German Plastic Surgeons, September 28, 1970.
4. Behrens, F.; and Searls, K.: External Fixation of the Tibia: Basic Concepts and Prospective Evaluation. J. Bone Joint Surg., 68B:246–254, 1986.
5. Blick, S. S.; Brumback, R. J.; Lakatos, R.; Poka, A.; and Burgess, A. R.: Early Prophylactic Bone Grafting of High-Energy Tibial Fractures. Clin. Orthop., 240:21–41, 1989.
6. Bone, L. B.; Johnson, K. D.; Weigelt, J.; and Scheinberg, R.: Early Versus Delayed Stabilization of Femoral Fractures: A Prospective Randomized Study. J. Bone Joint Surg., 71A: 336–340, 1989.
7. Braun, R.; Enzler, M. A.; and Rittmann, W. W.: A Double-Blind Clinical Trial of Prophylactic Cloxacillin in Open Fractures. J. Orthop. Trauma, 1:12–17, 1987.
8. Brav, E. A.: Open Fractures: Fundamentals of Management. Postgrad. Med., 39:11–16, 1966.
9. Bray, T. J.; Endicott, M.; and Capra, S. E.: Treatment of Open Ankle Fractures: Immediate Internal Fixation Versus Closed Immobilization and Delayed Fixation. Clin. Orthop., 240:47–52, 1989.
10. Brown, P. W.; and Urban, J. G.: Early Weight-Bearing Treatment of Open Fractures of the Tibia: An End-Result Study of 63 Cases. J. Bone Joint Surg., 51:59–75, 1969.
11. Brumback, R. J.; Ellison, P. S., Jr.; Poka, A.; Lakatos, R.; Bathon, G. H.; and Burgess, A. R.: Intramedullary Nailing of Open Fractures of the Femoral Shaft. J. Bone Joint Surg., 71A:1324–1331, 1989.
12. Casey, M. J.; and Chapman, M. W.: Ipsilateral Concomitant

Fractures of the Hip and Femoral Shaft. J. Bone Joint Surg., 61A:503–509, 1979.

13. Caudle, R. J.; and Stern, P. J.: Severe Open Fractures of the Tibia. J. Bone Joint Surg., 69A:801–807, 1987.

14. Chapman, M. W.: The Use of Immediate Internal Fixation in Open Fractures. Orthop. Clin. North Am., 11(3):579–591, 1980.

15. Chapman, M. W.: The Role of Intramedullary Fixation in Open Fractures. Clin. Orthop., 212:26–34, 1986.

16. Chapman, M. W.; and Blackman, R. C.: Closed Intramedullary Nailing of Femoral-Shaft Fractures: A Comparison of Two Techniques (Proceedings) (abstract). J. Bone Joint Surg., 58A:732, 1976.

17. Chapman, M. W.; Gordon, J. E.; and Zissimos, A. G.: Compression-Plate Fixation of Acute Fractures of the Diaphyses of the Radius and Ulna. J. Bone Joint Surg., 71A: 159–169, 1989.

18. Chapman, M. W.; and Hadley, W. K.: The Effect of Polymethylmethacrylate and Antibiotic Combinations on Bacterial Viability: An In Vitro and Preliminary In Vivo Study. J. Bone Joint Surg., 58A:76–81, 1976.

19. Chapman, M. W.; and Mahoney, M.: The Role of Internal Fixation in the Management of Open Fractures. Clin. Orthop., 138:120–131, 1979.

20. Claffey, T.: Open Fractures of the Tibia (Proceedings) (abstract). J. Bone Joint Surg., 42B:407, 1960.

21. Clancey, G. J.; and Hansen, S. T., Jr.: Open Fractures of the Tibia: A Review of One Hundred and Two Cases. J. Bone Joint Surg., 60A:118–122, 1978.

22. Clifford, R. P.; Beauchamp, C. G.; Kellam, J. F.; Webb, J. K.; and Tile, M.: Plate Fixation of Open Fractures of the Tibia. J. Bone Joint Surg., 70:644–648, 1988.

23. Connolly, J.: Management of Fractures Associated With Arterial Injuries. Am. J. Surg., 120:331, 1970.

24. D'Aubigne, R. M.; Maurer, P.; Zucman, J.; and Masse, Y.: Blind Intramedullary Nailing for Tibial Fractures. Clin. Orthop., 105:267–275, 1974.

25. Dehne, E.: Treatment of Fractures of the Tibial Shaft. Clin. Orthop., 66:159–173, 1969.

26. Dellinger, E. P.; Caplan, E. S.; Weaver, L. D.; Wertz, M. J.; Droppert, B. M.; Hoyt, N.; Brumback, R.; Burgess, A.; Poka, A.; Benirschke, S. K.; Lennard, E. S.: Duration of Preventive Antibiotic Administration for Open Extremity Fractures. Arch. Surg., 123:333–339, 1988.

27. Eckman, J. B., Jr.; Henry, S. L.; Mangino, P. D.; and Seligson, D.: Wound and Serum Levels of Tobramycin With the Prophylactic Use of Tobramycin-Impregnated Polymethylmethacrylate Beads in Compound Fractures. Clin. Orthop., 237:213–215, 1988.

28. Edwards, C. C.; Simmons, S. C.; Browner, B. D.; and Weigel, M. C.: Severe Open Tibial Fractures: Results Treating 202 Injuries With External Fixation. Clin. Orthop., 230:98–115, 1988.

29. Edwards, C. C.; Jaworski, M. F.; Solana, J.; and Aronson, B. S.: Management of Compound Tibial Fractures Using External Fixation. Am. Surgeon, 45:190–203, 1979.

30. Fischer, D. A.: Skeletal Stabilization With a Multiplane External Fixation Device: Design Rationale and Preliminary Clinical Experience. Clin. Orthop., 180:50–62, 1983.

31. Gallinaro, P.; Crova, M.; and Denicolai, F.: Complications in 64 Open Fractures of the Tibia. Injury, 5:157–160, 1974.

32. Ger, R.: The Management of Open Fracture of the Tibia With Skin Loss. J. Trauma, 10:112–121, 1970.

33. Glotzer, D. J.; Goodman, W. S.; and Geronimus, L. H.: Topical Antibiotic Prophylaxis in Contaminated Wounds: Experimental Evaluation. Arch. Surg., 100:589–593, 1970.

34. Greene, T. L.; and Beatty, M. E.: Soft Tissue Coverage for Lower-Extremity Trauma: Current Practice and Techniques. A Review. J. Orthop. Trauma, 2:158–173, 1988.

35. Grewe, S. R.; Stephens, B. O.; Perlino, C.; and Riggins, R. S.: Influence of Internal Fixation on Wound Infections. J. Trauma, 27:1051–1054, 1987.

36. Gristina, A. G.; and Rovere, G. D.: An In Vitro Study of the Effects of Metals Used in Internal Fixation on Bacterial Growth and Dissemination. J. Bone Joint Surg. (Proceedings), 45A:1104, 1963.

37. Gustilo, R. B.: Current Concepts in the Management of Open Fractures. Instr. Course Lect., 36:359–366, 1987.

38. Gustilo, R. B.; and Anderson, J. T.: Prevention of Infection in the Treatment of One Thousand and Twenty-Five Open Fractures of Long Bones: Retrospective and Prospective Analyses. J. Bone Joint Surg., 58A:453–458, 1976.

39. Gustilo, R. B.; Gruninger, R. P.; and Davis, T.: Classification of Type III (Severe) Open Fractures Relative to Treatment and Results. Orthopedics, 10:1781–1788, 1987.

40. Gustilo, R. B.; Simpson, L.; Nixon, R.; Ruiz, A.; and Indeck, W.: Analysis of 511 Open Fractures. Clin. Orthop., 66:148–154, 1969.

41. Hansen, S. T., Jr.: The Type IIIC Tibial Fracture: Salvage or Amputation (Editorial). J. Bone Joint Surg., 69A:799–800, 1987.

42. Hawkins, L. G.: Fractures of the Neck of the Talus. J. Bone Joint Surg., 52A:991–1002, 1970.

43. Henlye, M. B.: Intramedullary Devices for Tibial Fracture Stabilization. Clin. Orthop., 240:87–96, 1989.

44. Henry, A. K.: Extensive Exposure, 1st ed. Edinburgh, E. & S. Livingstone, 1952.

45. Ilizarov, C. A.: Clinical Application of the Tension–Stress Effect for Limb Lengthening. Clin. Orthop., 250:8–26, 1990.

46. Johnson, K. D.; Bone, L. B.; and Scheinberg, R.: Severe Open Tibial Fractures: A Study Protocol. J. Orthop. Trauma, 2:175–180, 1988.

47. La Duca, J. N.; Bone, L. L.; Seibel, R. W.; and Border, J. R.: Primary Open Reduction and Internal Fixation of Open Fractures. J. Trauma, 20:580–586, 1980.

48. Lange, R. H.; Bach, A. W.; Hansen, S. T., Jr.; and Johansen, K. H.: Open Tibial Fractures With Associated Vascular Injuries: Prognosis for Limb Salvage. J. Trauma, 25:203–208, 1985.

49. Leonard, M. H.: The Solution of Lead by Synovial Fluid. Clin. Orthop., 64:255–261, 1969.

50. Lottes, J. O.; Hill, L. J.; and Key, J. A.: Closed Reduction, Plate Fixation and Medullary Nailing of Fractures of Both Bones of the Leg: A Comparative End-Result Study. J. Bone Joint Surg., 34A:861–877, 1952.

51. Mast, J.; Jakob, R.; and Ganz, R.: Planning and Reduction Technique in Fracture Surgery. New York, Springer-Verlag, 1989.

52. Matsen, F. A., III; Mayo, K. A.; Sheridan, G. W.; and Krugmire, R. B., Jr.: Monitoring of Intramuscular Pressure. Surgery, 79:702–709, 1976.

53. McGraw, J. M.; and Lim, E. V.: Treatment of Open Tibial-Shaft Fractures: External Fixation and Secondary Intramedullary Nailing. J. Bone Joint Surg., 70A:900–911, 1988.

54. Meléndez, E. M.; and Colón, C.: Treatment of Open Tibial Fractures with the Orthofix Fixator. Clin. Orthop., 241: 224–230, 1989.

55. Mitchell, N.; and Shepard, N.: Healing of Articular Cartilage in Intra-Articular Fractures in Rabbits. J. Bone Joint Surg., 62A:628–634, 1980.

56. Müller, M. E.; Allgöwer, M.; Schneider, R.; and Willenegger, H.: Manual of Internal Fixation: Technique Recommended by the AO Group, 2nd ed. New York, Springer-Verlag, 1979.

57. Murphy, C. P.; D'Ambrosia, R. D.; Dabezies, E. J.; Acker, J. H.; Shoji, H.; and Chuinard, R. G.: Complex Femur Fractures: Treatment with the Wagner External Fixation Device or the Grosse-Kempf Interlocking Nail. J. Trauma, 28: 1553–1561, 1988.

58. Olerud, S.; and Karlstrom, G.: Tibial Fractures Treated by AO Compression Osteosynthesis. Acta Orthop. Scand. [Suppl.], 140:3–104, 1972.

59. Orr, H. W.: The Treatment of Osteomyelitis by Drainage and Rest. J. Bone Joint Surg., 9:730–740, 1927.

60. Pankovich, A. M.; and Tarabishy, I.: Closed Ender Nailing of Tibial Shaft Fractures. Presented at 47th Annual Meeting of the American Academy of Orthopaedic Surgeons, Atlanta, February, 1980.

61. Papineau, L. J.; Alfageme, A.; Dalcourt, J. P.; and Pilon, L.: Chronic Osteomyelitis: Open Excision and Grafting after Saucerization [in French]. Int. Orthop. (SICOT), 3:165–176, 1979.

62. Paradies, L. H.; and Gregory, C. F.: The Early Treatment of Close-Range Shotgun Wounds to the Extremities. J. Bone Joint Surg., 48A:425–435, 1966.

63. Patman, R. D.; and Thompson, J. E.: Fasciotomy in Peripheral Vascular Surgery: Report of 164 Patients. Arch. Surg., 101:663–672, 1970.

64. Patzakis, M. J.: Management of Open Fracture Wounds. Instr. Course Lect., 36:367–369, 1987.

65. Patzakis, M. J.; Harvey, J. P., Jr.; and Ivler, D.: The Role of Antibiotics in the Management of Open Fractures. J. Bone Joint Surg., 56A:532–541, 1974.

66. Rich, N. M.; Baugh, J. H.; and Hughes, C. W.: Acute Arterial Injuries in Vietnam: 1,000 Cases. J. Trauma, 10:359–369, 1970.

67. Rittmann, W. W.; and Perren, S. M.: Cortical Bone Healing After Internal Fixation and Healing. New York, Springer-Verlag, 1974.

68. Ritmann, W. W.; Schibli, M.; Matter, P.; and Allgöwer, M.: Open Fractures: Long-Term Results in 200 Consecutive Cases. Clin. Orthop., 138:132–140, 1979.

69. Salisbury, R. E.; Wilmore, D. W.; Silverstein, P.; and Pruitt, B. A., Jr.: Biological Dressings for Skin Graft Donor Sites. Arch. Surg., 106:705–706, 1973.

70. Salter, R. B.; Simmonds, D. F.; Malcolm, B. W.; Rumble, E. J.; MacMichael, D.; and Clements, N. D.: The Biological Effect of Continuous Passive Motion on the Healing of Full-Thickness Defects in Articular Cartilage. J. Bone Joint Surg., 62A:1232–1251, 1980.

71. Sarmiento, A.: A Functional Below-the-Knee Cast for Tibial Fractures. J. Bone Joint Surg., 49A:855–875, 1967.

72. Sarmiento, A.; Sobol, P. A.; Sem Hoy, A. L.; Ross, S. D. K.; Racette, W. L.; and Tarr, M. S.: Prefabricated Functional Braces for the Treatment of Fractures of the Tibial Diaphysis. J. Bone Joint Surg., 66A:1328–1339, 1984.

73. Scully, R. E.; Artz, C. P.; and Sako, Y.: An Evaluation of the Surgeon's Criteria for Determining the Viability of Muscle During Debridement. Arch. Surg., 73:1031–1035, 1956.

74. Seligson, D.: Antibiotic-Impregnated Beads in Orthopaedic Infectious Problems. J. Ky. Med. Assoc., 82:25–29, 1984.

75. Shires, G. T.: Care of the Injured: The Surgeons Responsibility. Tenth Annual Scudder Oration. Bull. Am. Coll. Surg., 58:7–21, 1973.

76. Spiegel, J.; Bray, T.; Chapman, M.; and Swanson, T.: The Lottes Nail Versus AO External Fixation in Open Tibia Fractures (abstract). Ortho. Trans., 12(3):656, 1988.

77. Swiontkowski, M. F.; Ganz, R.; Schlegel, U.; and Perren, S. M.: Laser Doppler Flowmetry for Clinical Evaluation of Femoral Head Osteonecrosis: Preliminary Experience. Clin. Orthop., 218:181–185, 1987.

78. Tanner, J. C., Jr.; Vandeput, J.; and Olley, J. F.: The Mesh Skin Graft. Plast. Reconstr. Surg., 34:287–292, 1964.

79. Trueta, J.: The Principles and Practice of War Surgery with Reference to the Biological Method of the Treatment of War Wounds and Fractures. St. Louis, C. V. Mosby, 1943.

80. Trunkey, D. D.; Chapman, M. W.; Lim, R. C., Jr.; and Dunphy, E.: Management of Pelvic Fractures in Blunt Trauma Injury. J. Trauma, 14:912–923, 1974.

81. Vander Griend, R.; Tomasin, J.; and Ward, E. F.: Open Reduction and Internal Fixation of Humeral Shaft Fractures. Results Using AO Plating Techniques. J. Bone Joint Surg., 68A:430–433, 1986.

82. van Winkle, B. A.; and Neustein, J.: Management of Open Fractures With Sterilization of Large, Contaminated, Extruded Cortical Fragments. Clin. Orthop., 223:275–281, 1987.

83. Wade, P. A.; and Campbell, R. D., Jr.: Open Versus Closed Methods in Treating Fractures of the Leg. Am. J. Surg., 95:599–616, 1958.

84. Waterman, N. G.; Howell, R. S.; and Babich, M.: The Effect of a Prophylactic Antibiotic (Cephalothin) on the Incidence of Wound Infection. Arch. Surg., 97:365–370, 1968.

85. Wiss, D. A.: Flexible Medullary Nailing of Acute Tibial Shaft Fractures. Clin. Orthop., 212:122–132, 1986.

86. Wiss, D. A.; Segal, D.; Gumbs, V. L.; and Salter, D.: Flexible Medullary Nailing of Tibial Shaft Fractures. J. Trauma, 26: 1106–1112, 1986.

87. Worlock, P.; Slack, R.; Harvey, L.; and Mawhinney, R.: The Prevention of Infection in Open Fractures: An Experimental Study of the Effect of Antibiotic Therapy. J. Bone Joint Surg., 70A:1341–1347, 1988.

4

Bone and Soft Tissue Reconstruction

William E. Sanders
Robert C. Russell

This chapter is new to the text. It discusses recent advances in reconstruction of the soft tissue envelope and bony skeleton. Open fractures have long been the bane of the orthopaedic surgeon, and many articles in the literature attest to the high incidence of complications that accompany open injuries. Current techniques of soft tissue reconstruction make it possible to provide coverage for almost any open skeletal injury, primarily owing to the development of microsurgical techniques over the past 20 years. The use of experimental free flaps was reported in rats in 1967[533] and in pigs in 1973.[130] The first free flap in a human was done in 1973.[128,556] Despite early failure rates of more than 20%,[167] clinical trials continued and new types of flaps were developed. Daniel[127] credits McGregor's classic article on the groin flap[388] with stimulating microvascular surgeons to develop new flaps. By 1979, more than 618 free tissue transfers had been done.[253] Similarly, reconstruction of the bony skeleton by vascularized bone grafts has been added to our armamentarium since Ostrup[441] reported the first experimental vascularized bone grafts in dogs in 1975.

Early involvement of orthopaedic or plastic surgeons capable of soft tissue reconstruction is optimum.[146,209,519,626] Carpenter[86] stated, "If the soft tissues overlying the tibia are not preserved, hope of primary healing of the underlying fracture is gone forever." Open fractures are multisystem injuries, and soft tissue problems are an important aspect of treatment.[571] Free tissue transfer has revolutionized reconstruction of the soft tissue envelope.[373] Before soft tissue reconstruction was possible, the soft tissue defect usually determined the outcome of the fracture. If early soft tissue reconstruction is successful, the bone becomes the problematic area, and the results depend on the extent of bone devascularization and contamination.[240] The ability to reconstruct large soft tissue defects early, and in one stage, allows the treating orthopaedist to be more radical in the initial débridement.[365,608] Even if he or she is not trained in microsurgical techniques, knowledge of the prerequisites, timing, and availability of soft tissue and bone reconstruction will affect the initial treatment plan.[209] The microsurgeon should understand basic principles of fracture care and perfect replantation techniques before doing reconstructive microsurgery.[126] The literature provides more in-depth discussion of the history of microsurgery in orthopaedics.[552,553,594]

NOMENCLATURE

Flaps are classified by the tissue type (ie, skin, muscle, bone) or types (myocutaneous, osteocutaneous) transferred. Skin flaps are classified by their blood supply: cutaneous or random (from the surrounding skin), arterial or axial (based on a known arterial pedicle), and island (based on an arteriovenous pedicle).[124,130] A free flap is composed of any type of tissue (or several in a composite flap) that can be transferred by microvascular anastomosis of its pedicle. Bone grafts may be autografts (from the same individual) or allografts (cadaver bone transplants). Autogenous grafts may be cortical, cancellous, or both, and may be transferred without vascular supply (conventional bone graft) or as a vascularized bone graft either on a pedicle or as a free graft.[601]

ANATOMY

VASCULARITY OF SKIN

Cutaneous or *random flaps* derive their blood supply from small cutaneous vessels in the skin itself. In most instances, the flap cannot be longer than it is wide (1:1 ratio). *Arterial* or *axial flaps* have a named arterial supply and can be longer than they are wide (eg, 2:1 or 3:1 ratio). *Island flaps* are based on arteriovenous pedicles and can be rotated to a new position or transferred as free flaps with microvascular anastomosis.[130,177] *Fasciocutaneous flaps* contain skin, subcutaneous tissue, and the underlying fascia, and are typed according to their blood supply. Most of these rely on perforators or branches of some named artery and are therefore variants of axial or island flaps. Their length to width ratio can be as great as 3:1.[21,116,427,564]

VASCULARITY OF MUSCLE

Muscles available for transfer by rotation or as free flaps may be classified by their vascular supply (Table 4-1). Mathes and Nahai described five patterns based on: (1) the regional source of the pedicle(s); (2) the size of the pedicle(s); (3) the number of pedicles; (4) the location of the pedicle(s); and (5) the angiographic pattern of internal vessels.[177,371]

Within the muscle, the vessels of the pedicle arborize into a very rich capillary plexus.[365] The transfer of a muscle flap into a hypoxic wound to aid healing takes advantage of this important feature.

Table 4-1. Classification of Muscle Flaps by Vascularity

Type I	One vascular pedicle
Type II	Dominant vascular pedicles plus minor pedicles
Type III	Two dominant pedicles
Type IV	Segmental vascular pedicles
Type V	One dominant vascular pedicle and secondary segmental vascular pedicles

VASCULARITY OF BONE

The blood supply of an adult long bone comes from three sources: the nutrient artery, the metaphyseal arteries, and the periosteal arterioles.[120,473,474] In an immature long bone, the epiphysis has a separate supply. Bone necrosis (loss of vascularity) is of great significance in both fracture healing and osteomyelitis.[587] The effect of various internal fixation devices on bone blood supply, and the ability of the blood supply to adapt by collateral circulation, have been studied by several authors. The consensus is as follows:[203,271,473,474]

1. Afferent blood flow is normally from medullary to periosteal (ie, centrifugal).
2. The periosteal vessels are mainly efferent and normally supply *only* the outer third of the cortex.
3. In fracture healing, the callus is supplied with an extraosseous supply from the periosseous tissues.
4. Drainage occurs through an efferent venous system.
5. Intramedullary reaming and rod placement damage the medullary supply (from the nutrient and metaphyseal arteries). Until these vessels regenerate (10 days to 4 weeks), only the periosteal circulation is available.[203]
6. Fractures with displacement may tear the nutrient artery or its branches, and effectively devascularize a segment of cortex.[158]

Other studies have suggested that collaterals from the metaphyseal arteries fill the medullary circulation following loss of the nutrient artery.[569] Experimental studies in dogs suggest that the periosteal network can reverse flow and supply the entire cortex and medullary area.[596]

PHYSIOLOGY OF HEALING

WOUND HYPOXIA

Rhinelander stated, "Vascularity is the biological basis, and stability the biomechanical basis, of . . . healing."[204] Biologic considerations always take precedence over biomechanical ones. Stabilizing dead bone will not necessarily lead to healing. On the other hand, stabilizing a fracture prevents further damage to the soft tissue envelope. In evaluating the pathophysiology of soft tissue healing associated with fractures, Oestern and Tscherne[432] listed five important points:

1. All injuries, whether open or closed, lead to hypoxia in the damaged tissue.
2. Hypoxia and acidosis cause a further increase in vascular permeability.
3. The increased permeability leads to interstitial edema, swelling, and, by raising the interstitial pressure, to an amplification of the hypoxia and acidosis.
4. In severely injured patients with general hypoxia and acidosis, this tissue damage becomes protracted in the periphery.
5. Any mechanical constriction, whether caused by fascia or skin, causes further deterioration of the metabolic state in the injured tissue, predisposing to infection and hampering wound repair.

An *accurate evaluation of the soft tissue injury* is essential to the primary care of any wound. Soft tissue in hypoxic areas heals poorly and is more susceptible to infection. An open wound heals by granulation tissue that leads to fibrosis and impaired circulation.[57,115] Experimentally, anaerobic conditions increase the amount of aminoglycoside antibiotic required to inhibit bacterial growth by four to twenty times. Killing by cephalosporins is not affected, however. Increased local wound oxygenation does enhance the bactericidal potential of leukocytes.[136]

Thus, the two most important principles in management of open fractures are: (1) achievement of fracture stability, and (2) improvement of the vascular environment around the fracture site.[223] The methods and benefits of enhancement of the vascular environment are the subject of this chapter. Fracture stability is covered elsewhere in this text.

RESISTANCE TO INFECTION

The ability of various types of flaps to withstand infection has been studied. In dogs, musculocutaneous flaps were more resistant to infection than random-pattern skin flaps.[92] Oxygen tension was low in the random flaps and high in the muscle flaps. Muscle flaps resist necrosis, bring in a high oxygen concentration, and deliver host defense mechanisms including immunoglobulins and phagocytic cells.[366]

FRACTURE HEALING

Experimentally, ischemic bone will not revascularize until the surrounding soft tissue envelope has done so. Therefore, in open fractures, the vascularity of the remaining soft tissue envelope is of great importance. Experimentally, muscle tissue is the primary source of bone revascularization; therefore, absence or destruction of a viable muscular or soft tissue envelope delays bone healing.[281] Replacement by *muscle* tissue is superior to all types of skin flaps.[12,92,475] Omentum also revascularizes bone well.[16,249,302,435]

Many factors affect the healing of fractures and bone grafts.[121] Fractures may heal by external or endosteal callus, but the latter requires viable and stable fragments. In addition to the three normal sources of blood supply, fractures have an external vascularized callus supplied by extraosseous vessels, mainly from surrounding muscle.[75,622] True endosteal callus forms from the medullary supply.[474,568] Avascular fragments and conventional bone grafts are replaced by "creeping substitution." Poorly oxygenated, malnourished, multipotential mesenchymal cells are unlikely to undergo osteogenic induction.[27,270] The blood supply of fracture fragments is inversely proportional to the degree of initial displacement. Stripping of the periosteum by displacement or open reduction of the fracture may destroy the periosteal blood supply. If the nutrient artery is compromised by the fracture or by intramedullary nailing, the fragments become relatively avascular.[57,202,353] Soft tissue reconstruction aids fracture healing. In several clinical series of nonunited fractures with soft tissue defects treated by flaps, fracture union occurred without the need for bone grafting.[84,112,306,407] Both parasitic and vascularized flaps can have this effect.[84,112,306]

Decreased oxygen tension slows fracture healing and favors cartilage formation instead of bone, whereas increased tissue oxygen stimulates fracture healing.[424,625] Systemic hypoxia delays fracture healing and decreases its strength.[271] Because the ingrowth of vessels into fracture callus relies on the surrounding soft tissues (mainly muscle), areas not covered by a muscle envelope (eg, the distal third of the tibia) have lower healing potential.[202]

REVASCULARIZATION OF BONE GRAFTS

Weiland published an excellent overview including the history of bone grafting, revascularization of autogenous and allograft bone, and vascularized bone grafts.[594,595] Several very thorough and well-referenced review articles on the fate of bone grafts have also been written.[54,66,73,96,272,293,465] The exact mechanism of incorporation is not known, but the graft depends on the host bed for revascularization.

Two theories have been presented. The first suggests that osteogenic cells survive transplantation and contribute to new bone formation.[41,458] However, because only a small percentage of osteogenic cells survive, a second theory suggests that bone is formed as the bone graft induces the surrounding connective tissue to undergo metaplasia into bone.[121,578] Both mechanisms are probably involved. Conventional bone grafts depend on diffusion of nutrients from the surrounding tissue for viability of the osteogenic cells. Cancellous bone has an open structure that permits diffusion and vessel ingrowth with rapid incorporation, whereas cortical bone is relatively impenetrable and may never be completely revascularized.[63,64] Despite this, nonvascularized cortical grafts have been used with success, especially following tumor resection.[160] In either case, if the cells do not survive, the dead bone must first be resorbed and then replaced by new bone—the process known as "creeping substitution."[159,458,578] Obviously, a stable vascular recipient bed is necessary for this to occur,[66,270,594,599] and the rate of revascularization correlates strongly with clinical "success" of the graft. Autogenous cancellous grafts 5 mm thick are completely revascularized in 20 to 25 days.[121,535] Autogenous bone grafts replaced by creeping substitution are weaker structurally from 6 weeks to 6 months, but may be normal by 1 year.[159] For maximum osteocyte survival, bone grafts should be kept in chilled saline or blood and not exposed to air.[39,41,465]

ALLOGRAFTS

Allografts do not stimulate osteogenesis to the extent autografts do. Revascularization is slower and less complete than in autografts,[607] and, at least in freeze-dried grafts, no cells survive. However, allografts do not have the size limitations of autogenous grafts, and a joint or joint surface may be transferred. Therefore, they are especially useful in tumor surgery.[64,357]

FLAP RECONSTRUCTION

Several excellent articles review free flaps from their conception to final application. Those authored by Shaw[515,516] and Harii[253] are most concise. A great deal of progress has been made in a very short time. The first experimental free flaps were done in pigs and reported in 1973,[130] and free fibula transfer made the medicine section of *Time* in 1985.[313] Some references are best categorized by type of flap

(bone,[311,323,505,553,594] muscle,[12,182,370]) or site of application (upper[129] or lower extremity[75]). Three atlases on muscle and myocutaneous flaps have been published and are excellent references for the anatomy, dissection, and clinical application of these flaps.[364,369,383] Similar compilations of donor sites are also available.[75,100,126,251,368,384,427,582]

Only five reports of large series of flaps discussing indications, results, and complications were found in a thorough review of the literature.[74,617–619,631] Frequent reference will be made to these series.

Although a detailed discussion of all flaps used in orthopaedic reconstruction is beyond the scope of this chapter, the references for each flap are listed in the appropriate tables. References with detailed sections on anatomy and dissection or reports of significant clinical series are identified as such.

SOFT TISSUE RECONSTRUCTION

As a group, free flaps, rotational muscle flaps, and other methods of skin closure have advantages and disadvantages. Each individual flap also has specific inherent qualities that may make its use advantageous in a given situation, and advantages and indications become harder to separate. Table 4-2 lists the problems with conventional methods. Table 4-3 gives free flap advantages and disadvantages,

Table 4-2. Problems With Conventional Flaps

Local Flaps
  Small defects only[177,509]
  Limited areas[35,509]

Direct Distant (Cross-Leg)
  Moderate defects[509]
  May need delays[509]
  Long immobilization and hospital stay[509]
  Failure rate[509]
  Joint stiffness[35]

Indirect Distant (Tube) Flaps
  Multiple stages[509]
  Limited amount of tissue can be transferred[509]
  High cost, lengthy[509]
  Failure rate[509]
  Now obsolete[177]

Muscle Pedicle Flaps
  No help in distal third of limbs[177,509]
  Extensive surgical mobilization[509]
  Skin graft[509] usually needed
  Only useful for moderate defects in certain locations[35]

Myocutaneous Flaps
  Same as for muscle pedicle flaps
  Donor skin defect

Neurovascular Island Flaps (Plantar Foot and Dorsalis Pedis)
  Donor site problems[509]

Table 4-3. Advantages and Disadvantages of Free Flaps

Advantages	Disadvantages
General	
One-stage reconstruction[359,515,545]	About 10% reexploration rate (4% salvage)[255,515]
Variety and composite (multi-tissue) flaps possible[255,301,512,515]	Special equipment[515]
	Special training[512,515]
High success rate (≥93%)[512,515]	Need adequate recipient vessels, or must lengthen pedicle
Distant donor site[515]	with vein graft or arteriovenous fistula[180,515,553]
Independent blood supply not limited by pedicle length[512,515]	Donor site problems[515]
	Long OR time[359,515]
Freedom of design[515]	Risk of failure (5%)[515]
Shorter immobilization and improved patient comfort[255,301,359,545]	Requires match of donor site and defect, pedicle size and length, and operative position of patient[301,557]
Short hospital stay and earlier rehabilitation[255,301,545]	Close postoperative monitoring[301,499]
Increased vascularity[255,301,545]	Preoperative vascular evaluation (Doppler or
May be reinnervated[413,418]	angiogram)[215,301,500,552,553]
Scarring minimized at both donor and recipient sites[255,509]	Best done by two surgical teams[255,512]
No open wounds remain, so can combine with bone and tendon reconstruction[255]	
Elevation of limb allowed postoperatively[29]	
Free Skin Flaps—General	
Skin match[515]	Size limited[515]
No atrophy[515]	Ability to fight infection[515]
Higher tolerance for warm ischemia[515]	
Free Forearm	
Constant anatomy[415]	Donor scar, especially in females[415]
Large vessels, long pedicle[415]	Sacrifice of major vessel to hand (if not reconstructed)
Large, excellent skin area[415]	
Thin subcutaneous layer needs no defatting[415]	
Can be innervated[415]	
Small donor sites can be closed primarily[415]	
Free Groin	
Minimal donor defect[254,520]	Bulky at base[250]
Covers large defects[254]	Medial hair[250]
Brings in blood supply[29,254]	Short pedicle, small diameter (SCIA*)[250]
Provides acute coverage[254]	Anatomic variations common[250]
Single operation[29]	Microvascular team needed[254]
Patient comfort and easy mobilization[29]	Need healthy recipient vessels[254]
	Partial necrosis of groin flap based only on SCIA is common[255]
Free Muscle/Myocutaneous Flaps	
Skin larger than muscle territory[515]	Bulky if taken with skin[545]
Partial muscle flap leaves remaining function[515]	
Resists infection[301,365]	
Vascularizes bone well[301]	
Simple dissection[545]	
Good pedicle[545]	
Can be very large[545]	
Donor defect minimal[545]	
Free Omental Flap	
Long pedicle[301]	Laparotomy
Can be split into several areas	
Molds to fill defects[301]	
Free Bone Transfer—Free Fibula	
Skeletal reconstruction doesn't have to wait for soft tissue coverage[554]	Ipsilateral pedicle transfer limited to middle third of tibia[552]
May be done as a pedicle flap and avoid anastomoses[552]	Long OR time[557]
One stage[552,557]	Hard to monitor[38,43,102]
	Questionable donor morbidity

(continued)

Table 4-3. Advantages and Disadvantages of Free Flaps (*continued*)

Advantages	Disadvantages
Vascularized bone fights infection better[143,267,553]	May require major vessel sacrifice in donor or recipient site[552,557]
May use as a flow-through flap in reconstruction or trauma[143,553]	Can monitor with bone scan only during first week; must take skin or muscle island attached to monitor; difficult to monitor in deep locations[99,143,159,260,557,628]
Better fixation possible[552,557]	
May be internally fixed with plates and screws[129,617]	
Hypertrophy will occur[129]	Pedicle is short, anastomosis usually has to be end-to-end[260,594]
Epiphysis may be transferred[129,422,553,603]	
Can be taken with skin flap;[628] 5×15[99] or 10×20[99,260,617,628]	Skin territory small or leaves donor problems[553]
Matches size of radius and ulna[617]	Preoperative angiogram recommended[102,390,594]
Better osteocyte survival, heals faster[553,557,594]	Fixation may disturb blood supply if not done carefully[102]
Tolerates irradiation[553]	
Either medullary or periosteal circulation will maintain graft viability[553]	
Straight, compact, suitable for early weight-bearing[99,557]	
Other fibula may be left intact to help resist stress in recipient leg[557]	
If anastomosis fails, acts as a conventional graft[557]	
Better than conventional graft in traumatic, scar, or radiated areas[594]	
Free Iliac Osteocutaneous Flap	
Large skin flap possible[558]	Angiogram needed preoperatively; if obturator artery is abnormal, DCIA may be also[558]
Can be used as flow-through flap (DCIA)[558]	
One stage[558]	Must match curvature and vessel presentation to recipient site[558]
Composite (multi-tissue) reconstruction[554,558]	
DCIA matches leg vessels well, long pedicle[558]	Long OR time[558]
Skin island possible ($4.5-7.7 \times 18$ cm)[558]	Bulky[558]
Minimal donor morbidity[558]	Loss of lateral femoral cutaneous nerve[558]
Can reconstruct bone without having to wait for skin cover[554]	Curvature of the bone[553,558]
	Difficult disssection[215]

* SCIA = superficial circumflex iliac artery

and Table 4-4 defines indications and contraindications.

Conventional flaps can only be used in areas where adjacent tissue is available for transfer and the defect is small. Pedicle flaps require staged procedures. Rotational muscle flaps are not available in the distal aspects of the extremities (see Table 4-11). Free flaps offer one-stage reconstruction, a wide choice of tissue types, and closure of larger defects. Blood supply to the wound is enhanced (see Table 4-3). Many indications for free flaps have been identified, as well as a few contraindications. These are listed in detail in Table 4-4.

VASCULARIZED BONE GRAFTS

Pedicle Grafts

The first vascularized bone graft (VBG) was a pedicle fibula transfer reported by Huntington in 1905.[291] Several pedicle grafts have been identified, with blood supply maintained either through attached muscle tissue[20,90,134,138,536] or an arteriovenous pedicle.[90] The osteogenic potential, vascularity, and strength of these grafts is thought to be greater than conventional bone grafts.[135,267]

Free Vascularized Bone Grafts

Ostrup reported the first experimental free bone graft in 1974. In certain situations, a free vascularized bone graft (FVBG) offers significant advantages over a conventional graft. Large segments of bone can be transferred and revascularized by microvascular anastomosis. Osteogenic cells survive,[8,37] and repair is by the usual process of fracture healing between the graft and the recipient bone, rather than by creeping substitution.[441,597] Free bone grafts and segmental fractures heal in the same manner in experimental models.[616] Avascular, scarred, and radiated areas accept conventional grafts poorly, and especially benefit from new blood supply brought into the wound. Epiphyseal growth plates may be transferred, and if the epiphyseal blood supply is also reestablished, they grow almost normally.[53,422] Iliac crest, fibula, and rib are the

Table 4-4. Indications and Contraindications for Free Flaps

General Indications
Large defects[167,177,512,515,531,542]
Need for well-vascularized tissue; scar, radiation, poor wound bed (eg, ulcers, vasculitic wounds)[177,454,512,515]
Specialized tissue transfer (eg, functional muscle)[512,515]
Complex composite (multi-tissue) reconstruction needed[167,454,512,515]
Ends of extremities with insufficient adjacent tissue for transfer[167,177,512,515,520,531,542]
Replace nondurable tissue, perhaps before other surgery (eg, anterior tibia, foot, amputation stumps)[35,58,180,413,509]
Cover exposed joint, bone, nerve, tendon or prosthesis[35,62,177,416,509,540,542]
Failure (or expected failure) of conventional method[509,512]
Osteomyelitis[177,512,531,542]
Large defects that require more than one flap (staged reconstruction)[201,512]
Restore contour and form (esthetics)[509,512]
Innervation possible[167]
Reconstruct soft tissue envelope to prevent later complications such as amyloidosis and malignant degeneration of sinus tracts[68]

Contraindications
Other simpler and reliable means available[454,620]
Functional potential poor[620]

Specific Indications

Free Skin
Reinnervation of foot or hand[403,487]
Burns[254]
Unstable scar[254]

Free Muscle
Osteomyelitis[92,365,512]
Heel cover (with split thickness skin graft)[546]
Restoration of motion[296,359,360,503,512,548,561]
Defect of soft tissue and bone < 6 cm, flap and later conventional graft[512,606]
Soft tissue loss, moderate defect, proximal third of extremity[542]

Free Bone

FREE FIBULA INDICATIONS
Giant cell tumor of distal radius[97,492,600]
Congenital pseudarthrosis of forearm or tibia[97,102,139,188,200,237,310,330,406,440,461,554,594,598]
Ideal for long-bone defects secondary to trauma or tumor[102,129,330,594,617]
Conventional grafting unlikely to succeed[102,523,554]
Avascular bed secondary to chronic infection or radiation[102,454,554,603,617]
Defect size > 8 cm;[177,196,209,215,428,440,539,553,554,594,595,599,603,606,618–620] >4 cm;[196] >5 cm;[539] >6 cm;[177,428,440,554,594,595,599,618] 6–8 cm;[209,603] >10 cm;[619] >12 cm[215]
Large defect—free flap first, then free or ipsilateral fibula[201,215,512,553,620]
Only alternative is amputation[599,603]
Epiphyseal arrest injuries[151,330,553,570]
Congenital disorders[330]
For more aggressive débridement in treatment of osteomyelitis[209,462,618,619]
Excellent replacement for humerus, radius, and ulna[401,553]
After tumor resection; vascularized bone more resistant to radiation and chemotherapy[1,188,216,217,401,440,505,590,600]
Kyphosis[288]
Aseptic necrosis of femoral head[90,310]
Composite defects of skin/muscle and bone[440]
Established nonunion with gap and failure of conventional technique[440]
No available cancellous graft sites[462]
Defect <6 cm in poor bed[406]
Can be divided to make "double-barrel" bone graft (especially for femur)[217]

PEDICLE FIBULA
Many of the same indications[90,216]

FREE FIBULA CONTRAINDICATIONS
Lengthy OR, risk too great[617]
Conventional graft workable[617]

(continued)

Table 4-4. Indications and Contraindications for Free Flaps (*continued*)

Vascular disease[617]
Limb that should be amputated[617]
Not reliable in establishing primary union, secondary graft often needed[618]

FREE ILIAC OSTEOCUTANEOUS FLAP INDICATIONS
Bone defect 6–8 cm[196,209,539,553,619] >5 cm;[539] 4–10 cm[196]
Bone plus skin defect (larger than available from fibular osteocutaneous flap)[177,196,310,505,512,539,553,595,597,618]
Congenital pseudoarthrosis of tibia if defect < 7.5 cm[344]
Note: Some have abandoned this flap because of alignment and healing problems, and prefer staged soft tissue and later bone graft or free fibula.[102,606]

FIBULAR OSTEOCUTANEOUS FLAP INDICATIONS
Bone defect > 8–10 cm
Skin defect < 15 cm² [99,177,401,628]
Skin defect up to 10 × 20 cm;[99] up to 4.2 cm × 9 cm[401]
Taken with soleus muscle to fill soft tissue defect[30]
As a monitor for the fibula

OTHER
Free rib[597]
Tensor fascia lata and iliac osteocutaneous flaps have been used to aid fusion or fill short defects about the hip[90,310] or lower back[90]

most commonly used vascularized bone grafts. Each has advantages and disadvantages in certain situations. (See Table 4-3, sections on free fibula and free iliac osteocutaneous flap; and Table 4-4, under specific indications for free bone.)

The theoretical advantages of vascularized bone grafts include:

1. A greater percentage of osteogenic cells survive, especially centrally. The result is improved local vascularity and resistance to infection.[8,90,607]
2. Monitoring is possible by an attached skin island, or by bone scan during the first week for totally buried grafts. After the first week, the process of creeping substitution will show increased uptake, and the bone scan becomes useless for monitoring.[38,43]
3. If the vascular anastomoses fail, the graft acts as a conventional graft. However, the attached muscle or soft tissue envelope limits vessel ingrowth.[43]
4. Healing to recipient bone is by fracture union rather than creeping substitution.[148,150,440] Union occurs more often, more quickly, and with less infection than in controls.[267,429]
5. Rib and fibula grafts may be viable on both the medullary and periosteal supplies, or on either supply alone,[36,40,308,526] giving more options during reconstruction.

FUNCTIONAL MUSCLE TRANSFER

Experimental free muscle transfers were first reported in 1970.[548] The first clinical case was done in 1973.[358] The first reported clinical functional muscle transfer was done for facial paralysis.[257] Free functional muscle transfers replace selective function in extremities where tendon transfers are not possible (ie, after Volkmann's contracture or a severe crush injury).[359] The transfer must be performed before the capacity for reinnervation wanes, and must take into account:[124,294,358]

Donor loss;
Excursion and tension;[50]
Location and state of recipient nerve and vessels,
Monitoring; and
Soft tissue coverage needs.

Experimentally, the success rates of functional recovery of muscle fibers range from 25%[561] to as high as 60% to 80%,[294,295] and may take 6 to 24 months to occur. The gracilis (forearm),[295,359,360,362] pectoralis major (forearm),[295,296,360–362] latissimus dorsi, rectus femoris (forearm),[503,504] and tensor fascia lata (gastrocnemius/soleus) have all been used for functional transfer. These are well covered in texts on upper extremity reconstruction.[359] (References to reports of functional muscle transfers are listed in Table 4-5.)

RECONSTRUCTION OF OPEN FRACTURES

When Gustilo, author of the currently accepted classification system for open fractures, reported his large series of open fractures in 1976, he stated that

Table 4-5. Reports of Functional Muscle Transfers

	Reference Numbers	
Flap	Series	Anatomy/Dissection
Latissimus		25
Pectoralis major	362	
Gracilis	129, 362	
Rectus abdominis		62, 502
Serratus anterior		546

soft tissue loss, instability, and large areas of exposed bone remained unsolved problems.[231] In 1982 he reviewed 1400 open fractures and noted that the final outcome depended on:

Degree of soft tissue injury;
Adequacy of débridement;
Appropriate use of antibiotics;
Fracture stability; and
Early soft tissue coverage.[233]

In order to understand the place of muscle flaps and free tissue transfers in the management of open fractures, we need to trace the important advances in treatment during the past 200 years. We then can appreciate that this is not a radically new concept, but a *technique* allowing us to take another step in the development of a treatment plan for open fractures; one that has gradually changed over time and through three wars, but always in the direction of the earliest possible closure of the *adequately débrided* open fracture.

HISTORICAL REVIEW

Prior to aseptic wound management and antibiotics, abscess formation and granulation ("laudable pus") indicated a favorable outcome, whereas a watery, brown discharge was usually fatal. Therefore, the goal of treatment was to *produce* pus, a line of reasoning inappropriate today.[290] The modern era of wound surgery began in the 1700s when Desault first recommended débridement. Before the invention of the motorcycle and automobile, severe soft tissue loss associated with open fractures was almost always secondary to battlefield casualties. Amputation was standard treatment for severe extremity injury,[158] and history records that Larrey, Napoleon's battle surgeon, supervised more than 200 amputations in a 24-hour period during the battle of Borodino. The mortality rate was as high as 75% during that time, but Larrey lowered this to 25% using his techniques of early amputation, a radical

method of early closure of an adequately débrided open fracture. Mortality from open fractures remained significant into the early 1900s.[158]

During World War I, the standard treatment for open fractures was either amputation or débridement followed by plaster immobilization with healing by secondary intention (granulation). Orr advocated antisepsis, wide drainage by wound packing, and plaster immobilization, but did not stress débridement. Trueta advocated débridement and stated "sepsis will not follow if all devitalized tissue is removed."[75,158,566,567] Limb salvage was much greater than in the Napoleonic wars, but postfracture osteomyelitis was as high as 80%.[57] Unfortunately, the necessity of adequate débridement had to be relearned time and again.[55,210]

Better transportation of the injured, better surgical facilities, mandated débridement, and the arrival of antibiotics further improved the statistics during World War II.[108] During this period, the World War I treatment of plaster and granulation changed gradually to plaster and secondary closure, and later to plaster and delayed primary closure.[60,65,108,163,243] Flaps were occasionally used, and the importance of good soft tissue coverage in obtaining fracture healing was better understood.[479] The practice of a "second look" at 4 to 7 days to assess the potential for delayed primary wound closure or coverage was established.[65] The essential change during this time was conversion of the contaminated open fracture to a clean closed one as early as possible. As a result, the incidence of osteomyelitis and nonunion decreased to approximately 25%.[75]

The best histories of the treatment of open fractures are given by Saad,[491] Wagensteen,[589] Gustilo,[5,235] and Brown.[57] Brown advocated early soft tissue coverage, but lacked the techniques to accomplish it. He realized the hazards of open wound treatment, as illustrated in Figure 4-1. Gradually, the importance of the soft tissue envelope as a determinant of the final outcome was better appreciated.[86,210] Guidelines for débridement were estab-

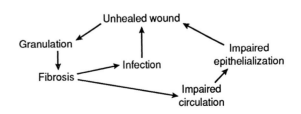

Fig. 4-1. The hazards of open wound treatment.

lished.[526] After adequate débridement, significant bone and soft tissue defects may be present, and if these are not closed, they may lead to chronic osteomyelitis and nonunion.[444] During the Vietnam era, radical débridement was practiced, and the fact that uncovered bone, fascia, and tendon would necrose was understood. Primary and delayed primary closure were used when possible.[244]

In 1956, Connelly noted that, "Everyone recognizes the value of immediate coverage in hand cases, but why we neglect immediate coverage in leg and foot problems is hard to understand"[113]—an observation echoed by others.[289] Inadequate débridement was identified as the major error in early wound closure.[65,132,289,583] This may explain the increased incidence of infection reported with closed wound management in some series.[162] Primary or secondary wound closure is an *elective* procedure that should only be done when the wound has been adequately débrided and is surgically clean.[65] Soft tissue reconstruction by pedicle, rotation, or free flap transfer enables the surgeon to be more radical and thorough in débridement.[405]

The last step in this direction was taken by Godina, whose series of early microsurgical reconstruction of complex extremity trauma was published posthumously in 1986.[193] He divided the wounds into those covered within 72 hours (group I), 3 days to 3 months (group II), and after 3 months (group III). The postoperative infection rate was lowest in wounds covered immediately, and highest in those covered between 3 days and 3 months. (See Table 4-13.)

Unfortunately, in our experience most free tissue transfers fall into group II. Godina found earlier operations easier to do because there was less fibrosis of adjacent tissues (especially vessels), and because bone fragments could be retained and would revascularize from the soft tissue envelope. Eighty percent of his transfers were done on the day of injury, and the low 1.5% infection rate attests to his skill in radical débridement. Duration of hospital stay was lowest in this group.

Thus, we see that the goals of treatment have changed through history—life preservation, limb preservation, preservation of function, and avoidance of osteomyelitis.[571] Recognition of the role of soft tissue reconstruction has been slow, and except in certain centers, the application of these techniques has not been routine. A 1983 textbook discussion of the management of infected nonunions did not mention free tissue transfer as an option.[225] Ironically, the pendulum is still swinging, and the initial infatuation with complex staged reconstruction is tempered by the financial and economic costs

when compared to early amputation—also a function-preserving option.[232,378]

INCIDENCE OF OPEN FRACTURES

Because of its location, the tibia is the most common site of open fractures, with the femur a close second.[67,219,232,235,338] Consequently, much of the literature on open fractures deals mainly or exclusively with tibial fractures. However, the *principles* learned from the treatment of open tibial fractures apply to any area. Special problems and solutions for other areas will be discussed separately.

SOFT TISSUE LOSS

In the upper extremity, except the elbow, wrist, and hand, there is thick muscle coverage over the skeleton. Soft tissue loss around the humerus, elbow, radius, and ulna usually can be managed by standard plastic surgery techniques, using skin grafting or pedicle flaps from the trunk and groin.[83,101,550] Free tissue transfer also remains an option for the wrist and hand. However, these are special situations, not within the scope of this chapter, and adequately covered in other publications.

SHOULDER AND HUMERUS

Small soft tissue defects can be managed by standard plastic surgery methods. Large degloving injuries as far distal as the elbow are often managed by a rotation or pedicled latissimus dorsi flap (Fig. 4-2). The arc of rotation of the flap may be extended by vein grafts.[496] The latissimus may be used to simultaneously restore elbow flexion and provide soft tissue coverage.[46,333,630] Other uses include defects with dead space in the shoulder area from infected prostheses or gunshot wounds[46] (Fig. 4-3). The pectoralis major has been rotated to treat sternoclavicular osteomyelitis.[52] A fasciocutaneous flap based on the posterior tibial artery has been used both to provide soft tissue coverage and reconstruct a brachial artery defect.[436]

Humeral nonunion and osteomyelitis are especially problematic, and free fibula transfer is a solution that allows restoration of length with all the advantages of vascularized tissue.[277,330,414,437,517,601–603,628] Fixation may be a problem, especially with long defects, and union is difficult to obtain.[617] The proximal epiphysis may be transferred with the fibula,[602] and it may be folded for

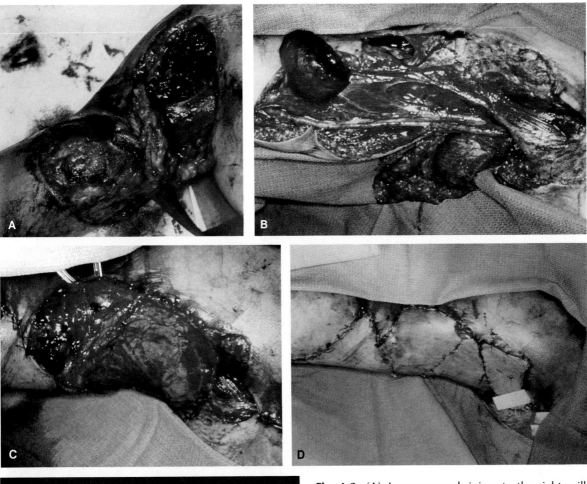

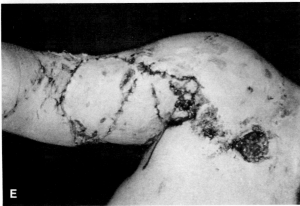

Fig. 4-2. (**A**) A severe crush injury to the right axilla and upper arm following a fall into a rock crusher. The arm was devascularized and the biceps completely avulsed. (**B**) Following débridement and vein grafting with the latissimus dorsi raised as a rotational flap. (**C**) Transposition of the flap for coverage of the defect. (**D**) Immediate application of split-thickness skin graft. (**E**) The wound at 3 weeks.

additional strength.[430] Iliac grafts have also been reported.[287]

ELBOW

Loss of the thin skin covering the posterior aspect of the elbow may occur from burns, "sideswipe" injuries, or olecranon bursa infections. Attempts to treat open elbow wounds without flap coverage have not been particularly successful.[133,275] Groin,[101,180] pedicle or free latissimus dorsi muscle,[295] free scapular,[26,242] and rectus abdominis flaps[502] have all been used for coverage (Fig. 4-4). The latissimus has been used to simultaneously re-

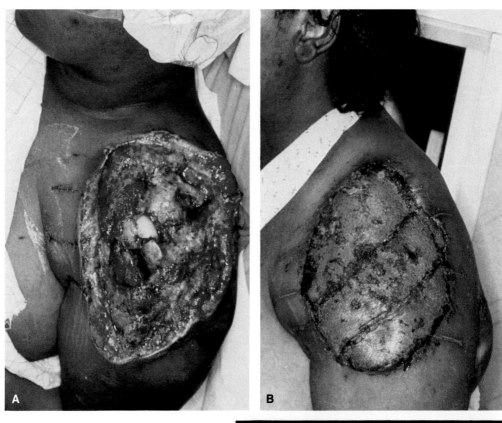

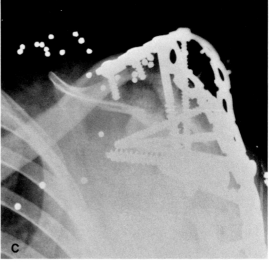

Fig. 4-3. (A) A close-range gunshot wound to the anterior aspect of the left shoulder with destruction of the glenohumeral joint. **(B)** Débridement and closure of the wound by rotational latissimus dorsi muscle flap and split-thickness skin graft coverage. **(C)** Subsequent bony reconstruction accomplished by scapulohumeral arthrodesis.

place posterior soft tissue and triceps function.[333] The brachioradialis may also be rotated anteriorly or laterally to cover small defects.[90] The flexor carpi ulnaris may be rotated proximally to cover the olecranon.[392] Fasciocutaneous and bipedicle chest wall flaps have been described for elbow coverage.[2,169] Release of severe elbow flexion contracture may require additional soft tissue.[398,510]

FOREARM AND WRIST

Soft Tissue

Soft tissue defects in the forearm or wrist are often manageable by standard plastic surgery techniques. Exposed muscle is covered by split-thickness skin graft. The distal forearm is similar anatomically to the lower third of the leg; local muscle flaps are not

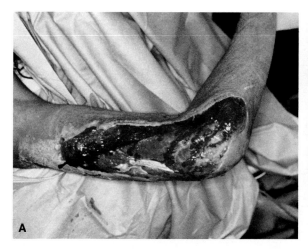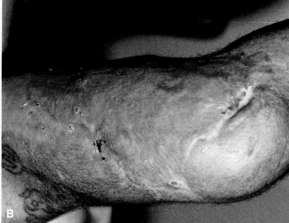

Fig. 4-4. (A) A degloving injury of the posteromedial arm and elbow treated by a large rotational latissimus dorsi flap. **(B)** These flaps will reach below the elbow for coverage.

available, and tendon, bone, and joint are often exposed. This area requires more aggressive management. Pedicle flaps are readily available from the chest and groin.[83,617] Advantages of free tissue transfer include:

1. Coverage for large defects;
2. Reconstruction of composite bone and soft tissue defects;
3. Elevation of the upper extremity, decreasing edema and scarring;
4. Earlier motion.

Skin flaps provide a cosmetic match for the forearm[101], and attached subcutaneous tissue may be wrapped around the tendons to decrease scar formation and to provide a gliding bed[26,494] (Fig. 4-5). The latissimus is often recommended for larger defects, but it is bulky and less cosmetic in women[129,295] (Fig. 4-6). The groin flap was formerly used but is less popular now.[180,295] The radial arm flap may be rotated distally to the wrist and hand, or may be transferred to the extensor surface of the forearm.[415]

Bone

Although conventional cancellous grafting and nonvascularized fibula transfers have enjoyed reasonable success in the forearm,[205,399,423] salvage procedures (synostosis or one-bone forearm) occasionally are required.[236,351,417] Free bone transfer has been recommended for several reasons, including:[603]

1. Size match to radius and ulna (fibula);
2. Long straight bone available (fibula);

3. Flow through vascular reconstruction via peroneal artery;[143,601] and,
4. Composite bone and soft tissue reconstruction (composite iliac osteocutaneous flap).[199,501]

Indications include:

1. Reconstruction following tumor resection (ie, giant cell tumor of the distal radius);[216,217,277,329,425,459,460,492,523,601,602]
2. Segmental defects following gun shot wounds or trauma;[99,284,285,400,440,462,494,601,602,628] a "double-barrel" fibula used to simultaneously reconstruct both the radius and ulna;[308]
3. Defects larger than 10 cm or with a poor soft tissue bed;[277]
4. Infected nonunion;[143,292,329]
5. For severe bone loss and instability, to create a one-bone forearm;[143] and,
6. To provide growth potential in children after trauma or in reconstruction of congenital anomalies.[570,602]

It has been suggested that the muscular envelope surrounding a free fibula flap may decrease the incidence of synostosis of the radius and ulna.[292] Although bone fixation should disturb the blood supply as little as possible,[277] in the forearm plate fixation is usually preferred over external fixation, even in an open fracture.[571] An infected, stable situation is preferable to an uninfected, unstable one. A temporary Kirschner-wire spacer bent into a bayonet configuration may be used to maintain length prior to final fixation.

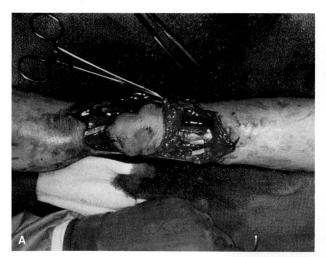
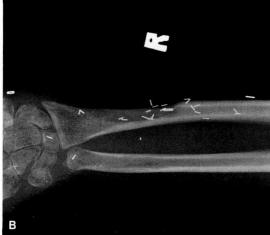
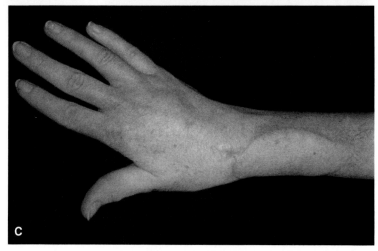

Fig. 4-5. (**A**) A 55-year-old female with epithelioid sarcoma of the first dorsal compartment. (**B**) Compartmental resection with 2-cm margins. X-ray following compartmental resection of the first and second dorsal compartments and saucerization of the radius. (**C**) Healed lateral arm flap, with excellent function.

FEMUR

Soft Tissue

Soft tissue loss is rarely a problem in the femur because of the thick muscle envelope. Rectus femoris, vastus lateralis, and rectus abdominis rotational muscle or myocutaneous flaps are available to cover the hip area.[12] Muscle pedicle bone grafts have been used to treat femoral neck fractures,[396,397] avascular necrosis of the femoral head,[20,138,339] hip fusion,[134] and following tumor resection.[345] The sartorius will cover narrow central defects.[621] The medial and lateral gastrocnemius will cover the knee and supracondylar area.[166,385] Viable muscle may be rotated into a femoral defect for the treatment of osteomyelitis.[172,484]

Bone

Femoral fractures with segmental bone loss have a high incidence of nonunion,[93] and in some series infected femoral nonunions are more common in the femur than in the tibia. Short segmental defects with a well-vascularized soft tissue envelope can be managed by conventional cancellous grafting (Fig. 4-7). Free fibula grafts are useful for long femoral defects, with the following advantages:

1. They can be harvested from the ipsilateral leg.
2. The graft is long and straight.
3. For lower-third defects and knee fusion, a *pedicle* fibula transfer may be possible.[216,217,550,554]

Vein grafts are often required because of the short peroneal pedicle and the deep location of the recipient vessels.[188,285,308,311,400,440,462,617] Problematic nonunions of the hip have been managed with this technique.[523] The iliac osteocutaneous flap has also been used.[501] The fibula may be divided and folded to increase the cross-sectional area of the graft.[188,430] Plating[571] and/or external fixation are used to support and align the graft. Monitoring is difficult be-

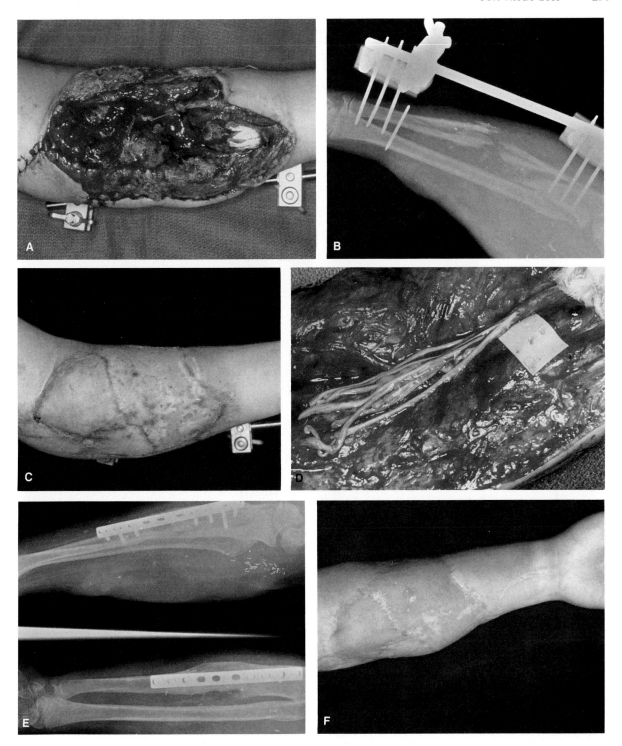

Fig. 4-6. (**A**) The arm of a 13-year-old boy who suffered a .270-caliber, high-velocity gunshot wound to the forearm resulting in an 8-cm loss of the median nerve and (**B**) a segmental fracture of the ulna. (**C**) Coverage by latissimus dorsi free flap and split-thickness skin graft. (**D**) Delayed interfascicular nerve graft of the median nerve 8 weeks later. The patient ultimately regained 6-mm, two-point discrimination. (**E**) The ulnar defect was bone grafted and healed without difficulty. (**F**) The final clinical result; note the atrophy of the flap—no defatting was done.

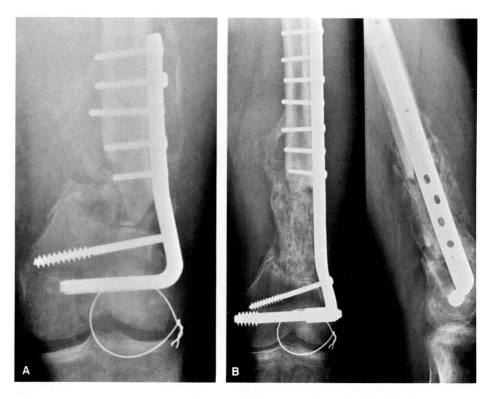

Fig. 4-7. (**A**) A 25-year-old man with a segmental femoral defect treated elsewhere by shortening of 8 to 9 cm and plating in external rotation. (**B**) The result following leg lenthening, secondary internal fixation, and cancellous grafting from both posterior iliac crests.

cause of the deep location, but the use of a skin island has been described.[628] The free fibula flap has been advocated in conjunction with core decompression and cancellous grafting to support and revascularize avascular necrosis of the femoral head.[178]

KNEE

Historically, cross-leg flaps have been used for knee coverage. Open treatment of open joint wounds works best when there is a good soft tissue envelope.[133] When additional tissue is needed, the medial and lateral gastrocnemius muscles are most widely used for coverage of the open knee joint, exposed patella, or femoral condyle (Figs. 4-8 and 4-9).[12,13,23,24,166,385,421,479,631] Exposed total knee prostheses have been salvaged in this way.[456,493]

Associated articular fractures may be managed by internal or external fixation.[480] The latissimus free muscle flap has been used to cover large popliteal defects,[467] and transferred with the serratus and vascularized rib for filling an osteomyelitis cavity about the knee.[258]

TIBIA

Anatomy

All orthopaedists who treat trauma would agree that a grave mistake was made in the design of the human tibia. One third of its circumference is subcutaneous and directly anterior where it is most susceptible to traumatic injury.[81,177,204,550,566,580] Numerous articles attest to the high incidence of complications including infection, nonunion, osteomyelitis, and poor skin coverage.[81,278,438] It has

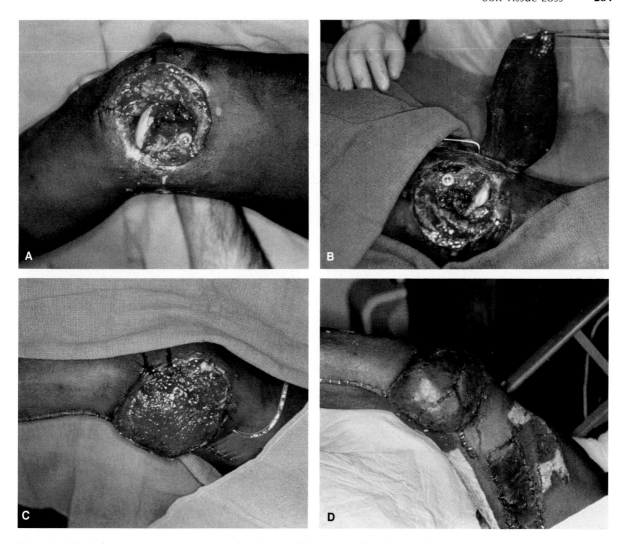

Fig. 4-8. (**A**) A close-range gunshot wound to the medial aspect of the knee with an open intra-articular fracture of the femoral condyles treated by AO lag-screw fixation. The joint was widely exposed. (**B**) An elevated medial gastrocnemius muscle rotation flap. (**C**) Coverage of the joint was obtained by removal of the deep tendon and epimysium and spreading of the muscle flap. A split-thickness skin graft was then applied. (**D**) Appearance of the flap and split-thickness skin graft coverage 2 weeks postoperatively. The patient had started knee range of motion.

been said that "Nowhere is an adequate knowledge of the vascularity of bone more important than in the management of fractures of the shaft of the tibia. . . ."[353] The nutrient artery enters the middle third and may be damaged by fractures, especially segmental ones. This makes the bone dependent on its soft tissue envelope for blood supply, and stripping of the soft tissues owing to trauma or surgical exposure may render the bone avascular.[120,204,474,577,610] The amount of apposition on the

initial x-ray is indicative of the degree of displacement sustained.[278]

The status of the soft tissue envelope is the single most important factor influencing the outcome.[86,577] Delayed closure for low-grade (I and II) open injuries works well in the proximal two thirds of the tibia because of the intact soft tissue envelope.[76] For grade III injuries in the proximal two thirds of the bone, local muscle flaps are available,[76] but in the lower third, pedicled or free tissue coverage is

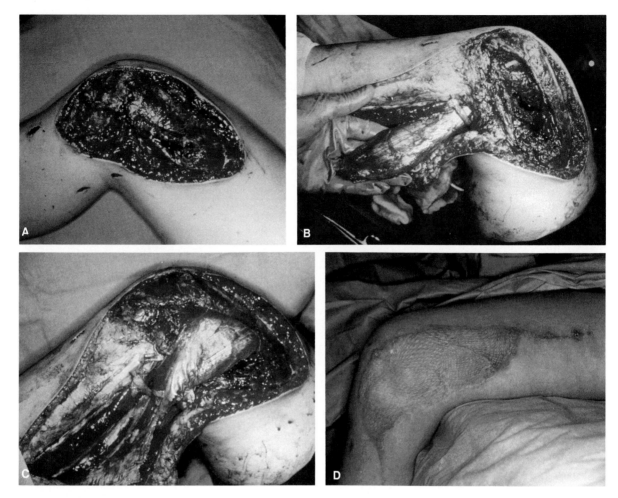

Fig. 4-9. (**A**) The knee joint of a 16-year-old female with a segmental femur fracture at the midshaft and supracondylar levels. The joint was exposed and was treated elsewhere by tight closure of the lateral capsule and extensor mechanism. This tight closure resulted in lateral subluxation of the patella. Coverage of the knee joint and restoration of alignment of the extensor mechanism was planned with intramedullary nailing of the segmental femur fracture. (**B**) A lateral gastrocnemius rotation flap was developed, the tendon and epimysium were removed, and the origin divided to allow a better arc of rotation. When the wound was débrided, the defect in the lateral joint capsule could be appreciated. (**C**) The defect is well covered by the muscle flap. (**D**) Final appearance of the wound following split-thickness skin grafting.

usually needed[454] to reconstruct the soft tissue envelope.

Mechanisms of Injury

Most civilian injuries of the tibia are from automobile or motorcycle accidents, and 30% of open fracture patients have polytrauma. The energy level of a 20-mph bumper injury is many times that of a high-velocity gunshot wound (Table 4-6).[168,221,230] Motorcycle-related tibial injuries have a high in-

cidence of bone and skin loss requiring reconstruction.[168]

Incidence of Complications

To adequately evaluate the efficacy of soft tissue reconstruction, one must compare the results with previous series treated by conventional methods. However, earlier reports lack sufficient detail to allow staging by current criteria,[56,140,141] and therefore comparison is difficult.[104] Perhaps many grade III

Table 4-6. Energy Level to the Tibia From Various Mechanisms of Injury*

Mechanism	Energy Level
Fall from a sidewalk	100 ft-lb
Skiing injury	300–500 ft-lb
High-velocity gunshot wound	2000 ft-lb
Motorcycle injury	80,040 ft-lb
Bumper injury at 20 mph	100,000 ft-lb

* Modified from Gustilo[221,230] and Findlay[168]

tibial injuries that we now attempt to reconstruct were amputated as "hopeless" in the past and may not have been included in statistics of nonunion and osteomyelitis. Conventional techniques have a high failure rate in these difficult situations.[76,89,158,482,565]

Gustilo[233] showed that the etiology of the type III injury had a pronounced effect on the complication rate (Table 4-7).

Godina[193] evaluated his patients according to the timing of soft tissue reconstruction (Table 4-8). His results demonstrated that those closed immediately had the best results—a tribute to the adequacy of his initial debridement.

Simultaneous free flap coverage and bone grafting may be feasible now that flap survival rates are greater than 90%. Although this will shorten the reconstruction time, it may increase the risk of complications.[336]

Classification

From his vast experience, Gustilo developed the most widely accepted classification system for open fractures.[221,230–232,234] (See Chapter 3.) The categorization of type III or "high-energy" fractures has been more difficult, and several subgroups have been added in an attempt to make comparison more meaningful. However, the exact definitions of grades III and IV vary from author to author.[44,76,77] The Gustilo system does have prognostic value, even

with "state-of-the-art" treatment.[88] Amputations, shotgun or high-velocity gunshot wounds, farm injuries, high-speed crush injuries, and segmental fractures or bone loss are always grade III or IV.[77,94] Other classification systems have been proposed, but these have not been widely accepted.[307,432] Oestern and Tscherne's classification takes into account fracture type and severity, and attempts to quantitate the degree of soft tissue damage and contamination.[432] To evaluate the effect of soft tissue reconstruction, better descriptions of the soft tissue wound would be helpful.

Current Concepts

"FEAR OF FAILURE"

Our concept of the optimum management of open tibial fractures has its foundation in historical experience and wisdom coupled with recent experience with early reconstruction of the soft tissue envelope.[44,57,76,104,106,117,158,201,204,209,226,321,336,571,626] Several authors have devised algorithms for the treatment of these injuries.[44,227–229,334] It is now possible to reconstruct the soft tissue envelope of even massive wounds, and if necessary, later reconstruct the underlying skeleton. Most problems in grade III tibial fractures are caused by "fear of failure." Faced with an open fracture of the tibia with severe soft tissue injury, the surgeon fails to adequately débride the tissue initially, fearing he will be unable to close the wound by delayed primary or secondary closure.[104,132,185,583] This leads to repeated dressing changes; the open wound period is extended, the bone remains exposed, and secondary infection occurs. If an external fixator is not used, cast immobilization will not adequately align and maintain the position of the fracture fragments because of the severe soft tissue injury and swelling. The incidence of delayed union and nonunion is increased. If an external fixator is used and the wound is not covered early, the pins may

Table 4-7. Complications in Various Categories of Type III Open Fractures, 1976–1979*[233]

Category	Number	Wound Infection	Chronic Infection	Delayed Union or Nonunion	Amputation
Gunshot wound	12	0	0	0	0
Farm injury	4	4 (100%)	3 (75%)	2 (50%)	1 (25%)
Segmental fracture	11	2 (18.18%)	0	2 (18.18%)	1 (9.09%)
Vascular injury	12	5 (41.66%)	2 (16.66%)	2 (16.66%)	5 (41.66%)
Extensive soft tissue injury	21	13 (61.90%)	8 (30.09%)	6 (28.57%)	4 (19.04%)

* All areas

eventually become infected and lose their purchase, with subsequent loss of stability, length, and possible pin tract osteomyelitis.

Devascularized bone fragments must be covered before bacterial colonization occurs if they are to be salvaged. Placement of a flap over necrotic or infected bone results in infection and occasionally loss of the flap.[117,155,206,381,513,539,543,572,605,606,618] (See Fig. 4-17.)

Débridement

Marginal wound débridement ignores the extended "zone of injury." Hypoxic tissue has poor resistance to infection, and inadequate débridement is the most common cause of complications.[113,432,513] (See Figs. 4-17 and 4-21.) Much of the tissue surrounding the open wound may not be viable, although it may appear so on initial inspection. Large degloved areas of tissue with no connection to the underlying fascia are usually nonviable,[94,409,626] as are free fragments of bone. If left in the wound, such tissues constitute a nidus for infection. Adequate débridement consists of removal of all nonviable and marginal tissue to establish a clean surgical wound; this is preparation for conversion of the open injury to a closed one by reconstruction of the soft tissue envelope.[235,373,472,482,513] Trimming back to viable bleeding tissue and the use of fluorescein injected intravenously may aid in deciding which tissues should be débrided and which left.[44,76,132,210,373,387] Obviously, any tissue that is severely crushed or contaminated with foreign material should be removed, with the exception of neurovascular structures, which are débrided and left intact, if possible. A second look at 24 to 48 hours allows identification and débridement of further nonviable tissue.[44,76,89,94,104,106,155,215,221,226,233,234,309,321,416,571] To allow primary closure by suture or immediate flap coverage, all dead bone and tissue must be removed and any dead space eliminated.[571] With experience, radical initial débridement can be followed immediately by coverage without a second look.[193]

Muscle débridement is done on the basis of Sculley's "four Cs": color, capacity to bleed, contractibility, and consistency.[44,94,210,231,506] It is more difficult to decide which bone fragments should be left in place and which should be removed. Standard x-rays do not assess the viability of bone, although bone scans can delineate avascular fragments. Magnetic resonance imaging ultimately may prove valuable in this regard. Retaining bone fragments that are potentially vascularized by soft tissue attachment has been recommended, while contaminated fragments with no attachment should be removed.[94,182,210,381,543] One must also remember that bone segments that are not loose or free may also be devascularized by loss of their intramedullary blood supply and/or periosteal covering. There is a high correlation between skin and soft tissue necrosis and the complication rate.[31,94,158,210,262,273,305,338,565]

ANTIBIOTICS

Antibiotics are "therapeutic," because all open wounds are by definition contaminated.[44] If antibiotics are continued beyond 48 to 72 hours, the

Table 4-8. Complex Extremity Trauma: Effect of Delay in Closure on Complication Rate[193]

Early Closure	Delayed Closure	Late Closure	Totals
Number of patients (%)			
134 (25.2)	167 (31.4)	231 (43.4)	532 (100)
Number of microsurgical procedure failures (%)			
1 (0.75)	20 (12)	22 (9.5)	43 (8)
Number of postoperative infections (%)			
2 (1.5)	29 (17.5)	14 (6)	45 (8.45)
Bone healing time (average)			
6.8 months (n = 33)	12.3 months (n = 95)	29 months (n = 78)	17.7 months (n = 206)
Hospitalization time (average)			
27 days	130 days	256 days	159 days
Number of anesthesias (average)			
1.3	4.1	7.8	5

emergence of resistant strains is enhanced.[231, 451,481,614] However, antibiotics never reach devascularized bone and soft tissue,[490] and are never a substitute for débridement.[220] Reconstruction of the soft tissue envelope brings blood supply and antibiotics to the injured area.[365]

RECONSTRUCTION OF THE SOFT TISSUE ENVELOPE

Healing by secondary intention has many disadvantages, including:

1. The open wound acts as a portal for the entry of secondary pathogens.[81,262,352]
2. Desiccation of bone and tendon occurs.
3. Fibrosis constricts vascularity on both macro- and microscopic levels. Wound hypoxia is detrimental to leukocyte and phagocyte function.[115,163,309,365]
4. A fibrotic granulating bed is not an optimum base for a skin graft.[115]

5. The resulting coverage (granulation and soft tissue skin graft) is nondurable and may later have to be replaced with a flap[115,289] (Fig. 4-10).

Reconstruction of the soft tissue envelope has many advantages and advocates.[44,76,77,104,158,184,209,215,235, 309,326,330,610,626] Advantages include:

1. Conversion of an open fracture to a closed one may be done.[77,95,472,482]
2. Earlier bone fixation or reconstruction is possible.
3. Vascular tissue resists necrosis, has a higher oxygen level, and brings in host defense mechanisms:[366] muscle is the most effective.[475]
4. More radical débridement is allowed.[580]

AMPUTATION VERSUS SALVAGE

Timely amputation is indicated for a severely injured limb which, following successful soft tissue

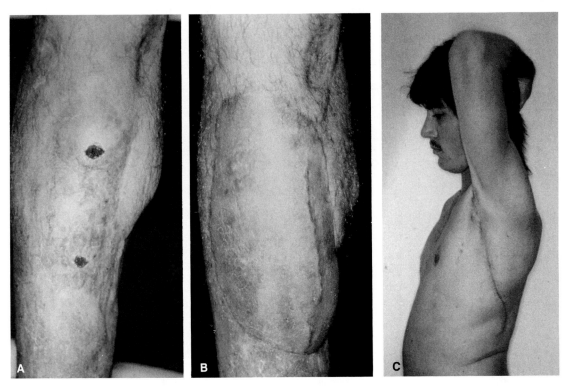

Fig. 4-10. (**A**) The leg of a 23-year-old patient following an open fracture of the tibia, which healed with some shortening and external rotation. The patient complained of continued breakdown of the nondurable epithelialized granulation tissue anteriorly because he frequently climbed a ladder in his occupation as a carpenter. (**B**) At 8 weeks following cover with a latissimus dorsi free flap and a split-thickness skin graft, durable full-thickness soft tissue reconstruction has been obtained. (**C**) The patient has full range of motion of the shoulder, and the donor scar is acceptable.

and bone reconstruction, would be less functional than a prosthesis. The problem is determining early what the ultimate outcome will be with or without attempts at salvage. We have treated several patients in whom multiple reconstructive attempts were made, and it was only obvious after some time that the limb was not as functional as would have been obtained by early amputation. Therefore, the decision to attempt salvage or to amputate is difficult. This depends on many factors, not the least of which is the expertise and judgment of the trauma surgeon.[42,88,118,211,246,332,334,335,352] With current techniques, salvage of a functional limb in a reasonable time span and at reasonable cost is possible. The following guidelines represent the consensus of authors who have studied this problem.[76,88,89,312]

Salvage should be attempted in children, even if replantation is necessary. If amputation is performed in a child, bony overgrowth through the soft tissue envelope is a common problem.[331,341] Equalization of leg lengths can be done later by lengthening or by contralateral epiphysiodesis.[280,286,579]

In the adult, salvage may be attempted either to preserve the entire leg or to reconstruct sufficient length to allow fitting of a below-knee rather than an above-knee prosthesis. Thus, complete amputations of the limb might be replanted not to preserve a functional leg and foot unit, but rather to provide a below-knee lever arm for adequate fitting of a prosthesis.[44,103] (See Figs. 4-20 and 4-21.)

In adults, entire limb reconstruction or salvage requires a sensate foot (intact posterior tibial nerve) that is or can be made viable.[161,229,232,283,335,381] Restoration of sensation by nerve repair after replantation of the foot has been reported, and is worth consideration in a sharp injury.[343,355]

An intact fibula or other reasonable method of maintaining nominal length (eg, external fixator) is necessary.[91,468,482,542] Treatment of the fibula is often neglected, but if aligned early by a Rush rod, maintenance of length and limb alignment are enhanced (Fig. 4-11). A healed fibula will preserve length and alignment, may allow earlier removal of the external fixator, and is often used for later bone reconstruction, especially in the "single-vessel" leg.[91,278,468,482,541,542] An intact or healed fibula greatly simplifies management.

Limb shortening of 2 cm or less is well tolerated and may obviate the need for skeletal and even soft tissue reconstruction.

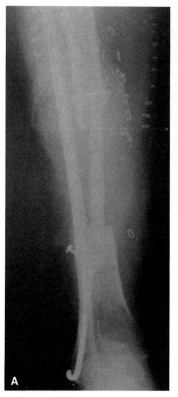

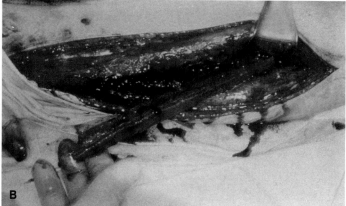

Fig. 4-11. (**A**) A segmental defect of the tibial shaft treated by free fibular bone graft. Note that length and alignment of the leg were maintained by Rush rod fixation of the fibular fracture. (**B**) The free fibula graft following its dissection from a lateral approach prior to division of the pedicle.

EXTERNAL VERSUS INTERNAL FIXATION

Hippocrates first used a crude external fixation device of padded rings about the knee and ankle, with bent tree branches for distraction. Fracture immobilization was by plaster or traction until trials of external fixation devices began during World War II. The incidence of infection and nonunion was so high that their use was forbidden by the armed forces.[108,337] With better understanding of the principles of their use, external fixators have enjoyed a rebirth in recent years. They are an extremely valuable adjunct to the treatment of open fractures,[33,94,220,315,338] especially when combined with current wound coverage techniques.[44,155–157,164,234,248,309,571]

Advantages of external fixation include:

1. Avoidance of additional soft tissue stripping or injury;[6,31,204,611]
2. Protection of a vessel repair;
3. Decreased incidence of infection and nonunion in grade III injury;[18,28,81,95,204,231,262,332,438,477,485,583]
4. Ease of dressing change, redébridement, and soft tissue care and reconstruction;[164,248]
5. Prevention of contractures of the foot and ankle;[44,157]
6. Less disruption of intramedullary blood supply than with intramedullary nailing;[6,202,203,226,473]
7. Use in infected nonunions to maintain length while allowing bone and soft tissue débridement;[206,224] and,
8. Ease of realignment, removal, and replacement.[156]

Pin placement requires early cooperation between the orthopaedist and the surgeon doing the soft tissue reconstruction. In most cases, a single frame directly anterior will allow access for most rotational and free tissue transfers, and not impale vascular structures or potential muscle flap donor sites (Fig. 4-12).[18,33,44,631]

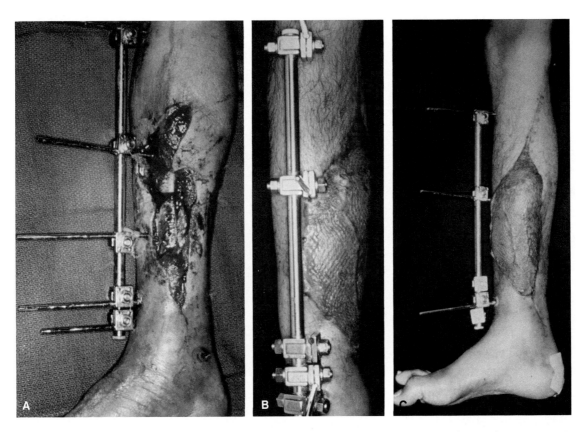

Fig. 4-12. (A) A 1-week-old open fracture of the tibia treated by débridement and a single anterior AO external fixator. **(B)** The result 6 weeks after coverage by a latissimus dorsi free flap plus a split-thickness skin graft. **(C)** Lateral view.

Use of intramedullary rods has been recommended,[266,349] but has the disadvantage of damage to the medullary circulation.[6,18,202,203,226,473,474,569] The use of small, non-reamed nails might be expected to preserve some blood supply while maintaining length and alignment. Pandiaphyseal infection is a severe potential complication of intramedullary nailing.[332] Plating of high-grade open fractures is usually not recommended because of the additional soft tissue stripping necessary. However, if the bone is already exposed, no additional trauma is caused by plate application. Plating has a higher infection rate, but an infected plate which has maintained fracture stability should be retained and covered with a well-vascularized flap. This frequently results in control of the infection. Plate fixation is especially useful in polytrauma patients.[6,477] Some patients tolerate exposed hardware remarkably well, and we have covered plates exposed for more than 6 weeks with free flaps, with no further drainage (Fig. 4-13).

Treatment Alternatives

SOFT TISSUE LOSS WITH OR WITHOUT FRACTURE

Acute or chronic loss of the skin and soft tissue envelope in the lower leg may be managed in many ways. These principles are presented here because of the high frequency of such injuries in the tibia, but are also applicable elsewhere. Many authors have reviewed the available procedures.[35,44,114,177,182,239,262,304,509,529,540,571,606]

Healing by Secondary Intention. Débridement, cast immobilization, and healing by secondary intention was the standard treatment regimen for soft tissue loss during World War I. Although many limbs were salvaged, the rate of osteomyelitis was high (approaching 80%) and seems unacceptable when other methods of treatment are available. The introduction of hyperbaric oxygen chambers has rekindled an interest in this method of treatment, with the belief that hyperbaric oxygenation will encourage rapid granulation of the wound, and a skin graft can then be applied. There are several problems with this concept:

1. Multiple hyperbaric oxygenation treatments are expensive and may require prolonged hospitalization.
2. Even if successful in closing the wound, the resultant coverage is not durable because the granulation tissue matures into scar that adheres directly to the underlying bone.[182,527] (See Fig. 4-10.)
3. If later skeletal reconstruction is required, an operation cannot be performed through this area, but must be done through an approach

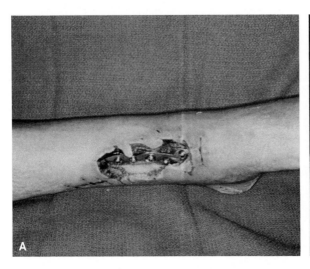 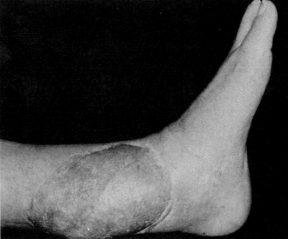

Fig. 4-13. (**A**) The leg of a 50-year-old patient who suffered necrosis of skin and overlying subcutaneous tissue after open reduction and internal fixation of a severe tibial plafond fracture. Coverage had to be delayed for 6 weeks because of a pulmonary embolus and the patient's consequent medical status. The wound was managed by local dressing changes, and a flap was applied at 6 weeks. (**B**) The latissimus dorsi free flap and split-thickness skin graft healed without incident, and there has been no subsequent drainage from the tibia over 3 years. The plafond fracture healed after one subsequent bone grafting procedure, carried out by lifting the posterior margin of the flap.

away from the scar.[55,77,107,162,163,182,210,225,226,231,337,527]

4. This method requires leaving the wound open for prolonged periods, which encourages fibrosis and delayed epithelialization.[163] The fracture site and external fixation pins are susceptible to secondary infection while healing occurs.

Delayed Closure. As mentioned earlier, during World War II immobilization and secondary closure (ie, closure after granulation tissue had begun to form) was gradually replaced by débridement and delayed primary closure. If there is sufficient skin and soft tissue present to cover denuded bone and tendon, then once the wound is clean and the fracture stabilized, closure within the first 5 to 7 days can produce a closed fracture and a healed wound. The injury has thus met the guidelines for stabilization of the fracture and early repair or reconstruction of the soft tissue envelope. Use of these methods, along with the introduction of antibiotics late in World War II, led to a decline in the incidence of osteomyelitis and nonunion to as low as 25%. Secondary closure may be possible after edema has subsided, but should not be done under tension, or marginal necrosis will occur.[55,107,114,158,162,210,219,221,231,234,244,472,571]

Split-Thickness Skin Graft. Skin grafts applied over well-vascularized muscle or subcutaneous tissue produce a durable repair.[177,409] However, even though split-thickness skin grafts may take over granulation, periosteum, and peritenon, the coverage is nondurable, cannot be operated through, and may require later resection and replacement by full-thickness tissue.[35,119,181,182,262,338] This may be done by staged excision and advancement, flaps, or tissue expansion.

Split-thickness skin grafting of secondarily granulated areas has several disadvantages. First, it requires that the wound be left open for a long period while granulation occurs. Second, the skin is placed on a fibroblastic bed which subsequently shrinks and becomes scar tissue. This provides poorly durable coverage over the anterior aspect of the tibia.[35,107,114,119,157,163,177,182,210,219,225,226,231,262,337,338,409]

Flap Reconstruction. *Rotation Flaps.* Cutaneous rotation flaps have a very high failure rate in the severely traumatized lower extremity because the skin receives its blood supply through perforators from the underlying fascia or muscle. High-energy trauma often damages this blood supply, and when

the flap is elevated, the result is often the loss of the flap and a larger soft tissue defect. Also, moving large portions of skin compromises the lymphatic drainage of the foot, most of which occurs in the subcutaneous tissue layer.[21,35,47,112,114,163,177,182,225,239,262,263,265,304,393,409,445,463,468,509,529,562,606] Fasciocutaneous flaps have a more abundant blood supply,[21,239,463,562,564] but still have a high complication rate.[146] Posterior midline relaxing incisions essentially form two large bipedicle flaps.[265,468]

Cross-Leg Flaps. The cross-leg flap is a viable alternative, probably safer in children than in adults.[279,528] Adults are prone to develop deep venous thrombosis, and they have problems tolerating the several weeks of immobilization required before division of the pedicle is possible.[613] Cross-leg flaps require lengthy periods of hospitalization with prolonged immobilization of the lower-extremity joints. They do not bring new blood supply into the area of the wound, because they are parasitic flaps (in fact on the "edge" of viability themselves).[137] They are worth considering in one-vessel extremities and as a salvage procedure following a failed free flap.[4,22,35,57,112,114,119,137,163,177,182,225,231,239,262,279,304,306,439,445,509,520,527–529,571,613] Myocutaneous or fasciocutaneous cross-leg flaps are more reliable.[439,627] Jump flaps carried in stages to the site of injury are of historical interest only.[84,114,509]

Rotational Muscle and Myocutaneous Flaps. In 1968, Ger first reported local muscle rotation flaps for coverage of wounds in the proximal and middle thirds of the tibia. Mathes and Nahai, as well as McCraw, beautifully expanded on this idea and published atlases of available muscle and myocutaneous flaps.[364,369,383] These rotation flaps can be very helpful when damage is confined to the anterior aspect of the leg and the posterior soft tissue structures remain intact (Fig. 4-14). Muscle flaps covered with split-thickness skin grafts are less bulky than myocutaneous flaps. Arnold described incising or excising the fascia or tendon to allow expansion of the muscle belly, and several other useful tricks.[13] Some function may be retained by separating the distal muscle belly but leaving the tendon intact,[370] or splitting the muscle.[241] Extension of these flaps with vein grafts has been reported.[317] Muscle tissue has been shown to revascularize bone better than skin flaps.[77]

Muscle rotation flaps provide coverage of small- to medium-sized defects in the proximal and middle thirds of the tibia, but have limited usefulness in the distal third of the tibia because the muscle bellies at that level are small and their blood supply is more tenuous. Therefore, for extremely large de-

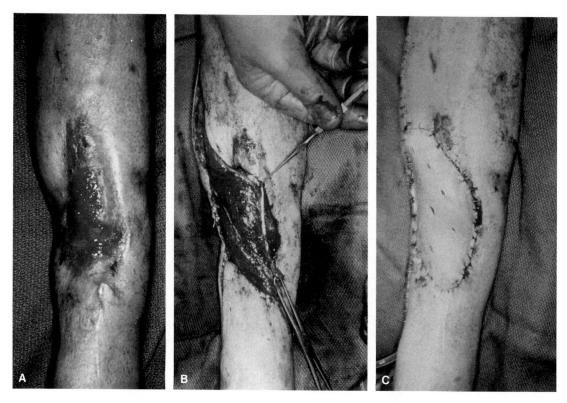

Fig. 4-14. (**A**) Open fracture of the tibia with a relatively small soft tissue defect in the middle third. Attempts at healing by granulation had this result at 8 weeks. (**B**) A soleus rotation flap was used to cover the wound. (**C**) Appearance of the flap following split-thickness skin grafting. The wound healed uneventfully without further drainage.

fects, and those involving the foot, ankle, and lower third of the tibia, rotational muscle flaps are not an acceptable solution.[10,12,13,15,24,35,145,157,166,172,177, 181–184,226,239,241,300,326,342,369,370,383,385,389,478,490,497, 509,563,571,581,582,621,623,627]

Free Tissue Transfer.   Daniel and Taylor reported the first free flap in 1973, and despite an early failure rate of approximately 25%, many investigators persevered in this area. Recent studies of free flap coverage of grade III fractures have reported success rates as high as 95%. Free tissue transfer has many attributes in the treatment of these wounds:

1. Because a wound of almost any size can be covered by appropriate free tissue transfer, free tissue transfer allows early and radical débridement of all damaged tissue (Fig. 4-15).
2. Because bony reconstruction is possible with vascularized bone grafts, even injuries with large segments of bone loss can be salvaged—providing the prerequisites of a sensate, viable foot and a method of maintaining length are met.
3. These flaps bring in blood supply and host defense mechanisms, provide antibiotics to the wound, and revascularize segments of exposed bone. The incidence of osteomyelitis and nonunion is decreased.[77,88,366]
4. Hospital stay is shortened, and the total cost of treatment may be less with this method.[508] However, free flaps do require an experienced microsurgical team. The initial cost of the procedures may well be justified by the possibility of improved function of the reconstructed limb and the decrease in hospitalization not only acutely, but also for secondary complications such as osteomyelitis and nonunion.[11,15,35,44,62,88,157,177,179,180,194,198,251,254,255, 316,340,347,366,374,375,380,413,431,433–435,466,508,509,515, 520,531,542,545,555,571,575,580,627]

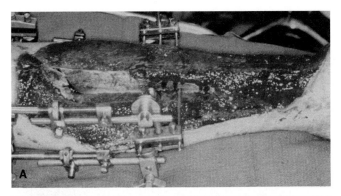

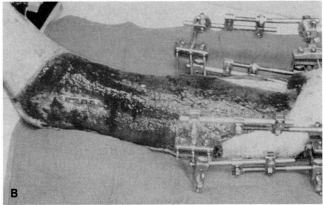

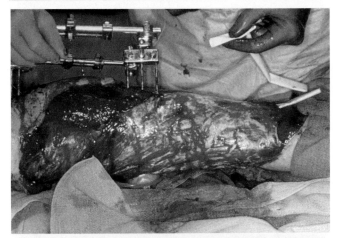

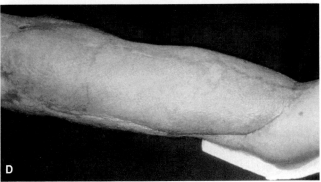

Fig. 4-15. (**A**) The right tibia 4 weeks following a degloving injury. A significant segment of the bone was exposed, and the only treatment had been débridement and hyperbaric oxygen. (**B**) Lateral view showing a plate on the fibula, which was also exposed. (**C**) This is the largest defect ever covered by the author (WES), and coverage required a combined medial gastrocnemius rotational flap and a latissimus dorsi free flap wrapped around to cover both the inferior exposed tibia and the exposed fibular plate. (**D**) The healed soft tissue envelope reconstruction.

Types of free flaps useful for tibial coverage include:

1. Skin[177,179,180,251,254,255,316,340,347,380,413,431,433,466,555,575]—many of these were groin flaps and the early failure rate was high;
2. Muscle and myocutaneous;[62,177,198,374,531,545] and
3. Omentum.[11,434,435]

There are several atlases of flap donor sites.[364,369,383,627] Also, the reader is referred to Tables 4-3 and 4-4 for a complete listing of flaps.

BONE LOSS

Cancellous and Cortical Grafts.   Selection of a bone graft depends on the state of the surrounding soft tissue envelope. Cancellous grafts are useful for short defects (<6 cm) in a well-vascularized, non-infected bed.[423,593,595] They have a higher success rate and are more completely revascularized than cortical grafts, which always contain areas of necrotic bone.[48,63,64,571] Defects larger than 9 cm long may exceed the supply of cancellous bone available.[208] Direct cancellous grafting of infected fractures with a healthy layer of granulation (Papineau technique) is an option when soft tissue coverage is absent.[223] Papineau grafts are excellent for filling large open metaphyseal defects in long bones (Fig.

4-16).[157] Posterolateral grafting techniques avoiding the area of soft tissue loss are superior to Papineau grafts in diaphyseal areas.[157]

Enneking has reported his results with cortical grafting of segmental defects; these serve as a basis for comparison of vascularized free bone grafting.[160]

Ipsilateral Fibular Transfers and Tibiofibular Synostosis.   The fibula plays an important role in reconstruction of segmental diaphyseal tibial defects. As previously mentioned, an intact or healed fibula in good alignment makes tibial reconstruction easier. In the severely injured or single-vessel extremity,[542] ipsilateral fibular transfer[82,89–91,98,131,147,291,395,449,552,593] or tibiofibular synostosis[80,190,213,391,395] may be safe methods of limb salvage (Fig. 4-17). Posterolateral bone grafting is a widely used type of tibiofibular synostosis, and may be done with relative safety in the presence of an open anterior wound.[157,176,259,338,469]

These procedures are also used following failure of free tissue or free bone transfer as the final salvage procedure before amputation.[542] Adjunctive cancellous grafting is usually required, even with fibular transposition. The dissection is best done from a posterior approach.[252,269]

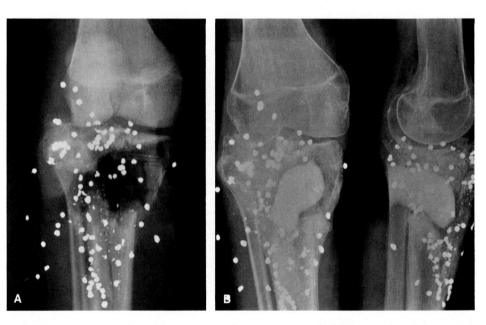

Fig. 4-16. (**A**) Radiograph of the knee joint of a 16-year-old male following a shotgun wound to the popliteal area. Revascularization was accomplished by vein bypass graft. The fractures were managed by an external fixator and healed, but a large cavity persisted in the proximal tibia. (**B**) Sinograms showing a large metaphyseal defect. Healing was accomplished by Papineau graft, done in two stages because of the size of the defect.

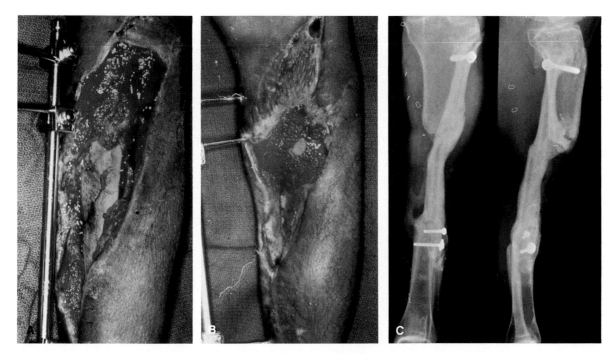

Fig. 4-17. (**A**) Clinical photo of a 25-year-old patient 3 weeks following a severe crush injury of both legs sustained while cleaning a commercial meat grinder. The AO frame was applied at another hospital and a butterfly fragment with no soft tissue attachment was left in place. (**B**) A latissimus dorsi free flap was done, but infection occurred and the distal half of the flap was lost. The cause of this was thought to be the retained necrotic bone fragment, and this fragment was subsequently removed. Once the wound had been redébrided and infection controlled, a second free tissue transfer was done using a rectus abdominis, and ultimately coverage was obtained. (**C**) Bone reconstruction by fibular transfer resulted in healing, and the patient is now ambulatory on both legs.

Free Iliac Bone Graft. For tibial reconstruction, vascularized iliac bone graft may be harvested on the deep circumflex iliac artery[188,251,287,454,501,553,558–560,595,619] the superficial circumflex iliac artery,[188,251,252] or both.[495] Varying amounts of bone, skin, fascia, and muscle tissue may be included.[251,495,553] Because of the curvature of the ilium, grafts larger than 10 to 12 cm are difficult to use unless an osteotomy of the graft is done.[525,542,553,558,560,597] The recipient vessels will dictate which crest is used.[558] A short bone defect associated with skin loss is the most common indication for this flap.[501,597,617,619] Hypertrophy and remodeling occur, but not as quickly as after free fibula transfer, and weight-bearing may have to be delayed.[501,553] The dissection is difficult, preoperative angiography is recommended, and hernia is a potential complication.[188,215,428,495,553,558,576] The outer table may be left to minimize donor site problems.[454] The reported success rate with this flap ranges from 87.5% to 90%, but up to one third of patients may require additional cancellous grafting.[525,595,617]

Free Fibula Bone Graft. Vascularized fibular transfer has been used extensively for reconstruction of segmental tibial defects, especially in the diaphyseal area (Fig. 4-18).[99,215,303,313,330,428,537,544,549,552,554,557] Several reports include significant numbers of fibular transfers.[188,260,400,525,553,595,604,620,628] The vascular anatomy has been thoroughly studied.[471] A lateral approach is preferred for harvest of the graft.[188,430,553,604,628] Monitoring may be done by bone scan or by an attached skin pedicle. Up to 10 × 20 cm of skin may be harvested with the fibula.[87,99,260,628] However, transfer of a large skin island creates a significant donor defect, and staged soft tissue and bone reconstruction may be preferable.[553,557] Up to 30 cm of fibula may be harvested. Only enough distal fibula to stabilize the lateral malleolus must be retained.[617] Reported union rates range from 62% to 89%. Secondary cancellous

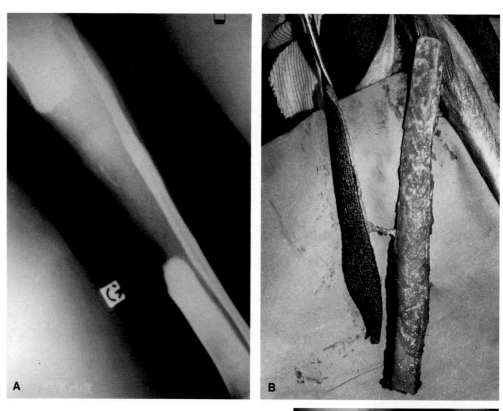

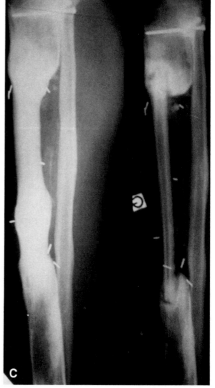

Fig. 4-18. (**A**) Radiograph of the lower leg in a 28-year-old man with chronic osteomyelitis following radical débridement of an infected tibia. (**B**) A free fibula graft raised with a skin island. (**C**) Immediate and 18-month postoperative x-ray films showing graft hypertrophy. *(Case courtesy of Alain Gilbert, M.D., Paris, France)*

grafting is often needed. The graft may be osteotomized and folded for greater strength,[430] and the
proximal growth plate may be transferred with the
fibula.[151,471]

Ilizarov Technique. Ilizarov recently reported reconstruction of segmental tibial defects by distrac-
tion-lengthening, or "bone transport."[298,299] The
amazing results of this technique have been confirmed by others, but secondary internal fixation
and bone grafting have occasionally been required
to achieve healing.[408,447,455] The technique is demanding, and an understanding of its biomechanical basis is mandatory.[14,207,298,299,446]

Other Options. Allografts are necessary in most
cases when an articular segment must be reconstructed. They are mainly used for tumor reconstruction, a subject beyond the scope of this chapter.[64,442,443] Vascularized allogenic bone transfer has
not been reported in clinical use.

Shortening of up to 3 cm may be accepted (or
produced) to avoid reconstruction of a segmental
defect, and may be compensated by a shoe lift.[15,196]

Reconstruction of a segmental tibial defect, especially when there is associated soft tissue loss, is
a major commitment for both the patient and the
surgeon. Reconstruction often requires more than
a year to complete, and psychological, financial,
and drug-related problems are common. Patients
should always be advised of the alternative of amputation, and if possible, be allowed to meet other
patients who use prostheses.[196,378]

Length Guidelines. In general, the better vascularized the bed, the more likely it is that a cancellous
graft will bridge the defect. Lengthy defects are better managed by vascularized grafting, but recommendations differ as to the minimum defect indicating the need for a vascularized graft. (See Table
4-4, under specific indications for free bone.) Mod-
ifying factors such as infection, scar, poor local vascularity, and radiation should be considered.[197]
Vascularized iliac grafts may be used for defects up
to 10 to 12 cm.[196,209,553,599,619] A vascularized fibula
may be used for any size defect as long as the nutrient artery or substantial periosteal supply is included.[177,196,209,428,440,541,553,554,599,619]

COMBINED BONE AND SOFT TISSUE LOSS

With both bone and soft tissue loss, reconstruction
may be done in several ways (Table 4-9). These
methods are useful in both acute and chronic defects.

Table 4-9. Methods of Reconstruction for Combined Soft Tissue and Bone Defects

Immediate Reconstruction
Composite bone and soft tissue flap
   Iliac[61,173,188,251,281,310,328,495,498,501,539,595,604,619]
   Fibula[30,99,260,401,595,619,628]
Soft tissue flap and cancellous graft
Double flap

Staged Reconstruction
Soft tissue coverage
Delayed cancellous graft
   Conventional
   Papineau
   Posterolateral bone graft
Delayed free vascularized bone graft
Fibula transposition[542]
Papineau graft and later split-thickness skin graft or soft
tissue flap

Immediate Reconstruction. The iliac osteocutaneous flap and vascularized fibula with skin or soleus muscle have been used for simultaneous reconstruction of combined bone and soft tissue
defects.[61,196,466,539,628] An anterolateral thigh flap
including iliac bone has been used for large defects.[328] Simultaneous soft tissue reconstruction and
cancellous bone grafting has been done in an attempt to decrease the prolonged recovery time required for such injuries.[15,114,255,336] The wound must
be thoroughly débrided and surgically clean, with
a low bacterial count, if this method is to be successful.

Double-flap reconstruction (rotational muscle flap
and free vascularized bone graft, or free soft tissue
and free bone graft) has been considered, but is felt
to be too demanding for routine use.

Staged Reconstruction. Primary soft tissue coverage with later cancellous grafting is probably the
most widely used method for short defects (Fig.
4-19).[117,215,513,606] The flap may be raised for placement of the graft, or a posterolateral graft may be
done.[469] Because the ability of the flap to revascularize bone diminishes with time, grafting should
be done within 6 to 8 weeks if possible.[486] Free
vascularized bone grafts are used when the defect
is more substantial. Iliac grafts provide a maximum
of 10 to 12 cm, but because these grafts are curved,
dissection and alignment are difficult.[215,428,495,501,595,606,619] The free fibula graft is easier to dissect
and provides up to 30 cm of length.[595,606,619,628] It
can be used for shorter defects by slotting it into
the ends of the nonunion. Rib has also been
used,[61,330,363,462] but significant hypertrophy does
not occur.[554]

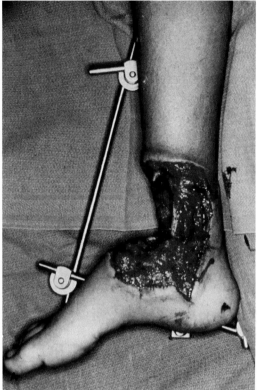
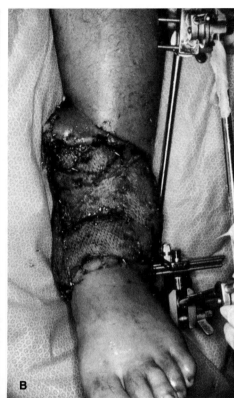
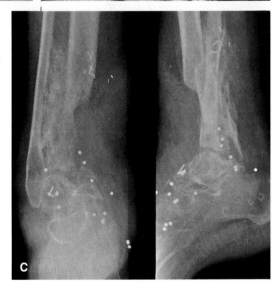

Fig. 4-19. (**A**) The foot of a 23-year-old woman who suffered a close-range shotgun wound with loss of the talar dome and distal 2 inches of the tibia. The posterior tibial neurovascular bundle was intact, but there was a large anterior soft tissue defect. (**B**) Anterior view of a latissimus flap and split-thickness skin graft 3 weeks postoperatively. (**C**) A posterolateral bone graft was performed, which healed proximally but not distally. Further grafting is planned.

Ipsilateral fibular transposition is often the final step in difficult cases, such as the one-vessel extremity. Therefore, a healed, straight fibula is a reconstructive asset. In cases where the soft tissue has not been replaced and bony defects are present with a well-vascularized bed, Papineau grafting may be effective. Large holes in metaphyseal areas are well suited to this technique. (See Fig. 4-16.) For cutaneous coverage, a skin graft or flap may be applied later.[225,226,394]

Authors' Preferred Methods of Treatment

OPEN FRACTURES

We believe that many of the problems and complications of open tibial fractures are secondary to delayed reconstruction of the soft tissue envelope. The treating orthopaedist has nothing to lose and everything to gain by débridement of the fracture, stabilization with an anterior single-frame external fixation device, and transfer of the patient as soon as other injuries permit to a facility where early reconstruction can be carried out. Once the wound has been covered, the patient can be returned to the treating orthopaedist for later bone grafting if the defect is short or, if necessary, free bone grafting can be done at the referral center.

Rotational gastrocnemius and soleus muscle flaps are within the armamentarium of many orthopaedists, and are especially useful with some grade II and smaller grade III injuries. We agree with recent studies that suggest a marked decrease in the complication rate with early soft tissue reconstruction. If radical débridement and early reconstruction are done (ie, within 3 to 5 days), it may be possible to retain even devascularized cortical fragments. However, to do this, closure of the wound by flap reconstruction must be done before the wound becomes contaminated. Flaps placed over infected necrotic pieces of bone are subject to infection and other complications. Treatment should be aggressive to accomplish healing in the shortest possible time. The limb should be amputated if the primary treatment is unsuccessful, and other options indicate a prolonged and uncertain course. The temptation to reconstruct a limb that will be less functional than a prosthesis must be vigorously resisted. Our indications for amputation will be discussed later.[106,117,155,334]

Protocol for Grade III Tibial Fractures. Our current protocol for a grade III fracture of the tibia is as follows.

Day of Injury. The wound should be evaluated by the orthopaedist and, if possible, the reconstructive surgeon. Débridement of all nonviable tissue with the exception of neurovascular structures is done, aided by fluorescein injection if necessary to determine viable versus nonviable skin. Débridement of muscle and periosteum is made on the basis of contractibility, color, and bleeding. Bone without soft tissue attachment is excised unless the fragments are surgically clean and immediate coverage is anticipated.

After 48 Hours. A dressing change and wound inspection are done; if redébridement is needed, it is done. If significant devitalized tissue is found, a second redébridement and dressing change are done at 96 hours postinjury. With adequate débridement, it should be possible to provide soft tissue coverage at either the first or second dressing change. This should be performed, if possible, within 5 days of injury.

Delayed primary closure is indicated only if it can be done without tension. Most significant injuries will require a local muscle flap with split-thickness skin graft. Free flaps are used when the defect is very large or cannot be covered adequately by a muscle rotation flap. Free tissue transfers are also necessary when the defect is in the lower third of the tibia, ankle, or foot area where adequate muscle rotation flaps are not available. A combination of these techniques may also be needed in the extensive wound where, for example, a medial gastrocnemius rotation flap might be combined with a latissimus dorsi free flap to cover an anterior degloving of the entire tibia. Exposed plates and other hardware necessary for treatment of the underlying injuries have been left in place without apparent difficulty in our experience.[631] Angiography, when required, may be done under anesthesia to lessen spasm in damaged recipient vessels if flap transfer is planned within a short period.[553] Contraindications to salvage will be discussed later.[334]

When the pedicle is short, vein grafts may be added on a back table, or an arteriovenous fistula first constructed. This will allow the anastomosis to be made out of the zone of injury.[553] Antibiotics (usually cephalosporins) are used for 48 to 72 hours, and restarted whenever the wound is manipulated. Aminoglycosides are added only if the wound is severely contaminated.[451] Prolonged use of antibiotics will encourage emergence of resistant organisms.[44,170,220,234,450–453] For established infection, infectious disease consultation and serum antibiotic levels are helpful.[117,614] Wound reconstruction by rotation or free flap coverage has many advantages and some disadvantages. These overlap with the indications and relative contraindications for the use of a specific flap. Many different flaps have been used in the reconstruction of orthopaedic injuries. Tables 4-10, 4-11, and 4-12 list these flaps and references for their use in orthopaedics. References that describe the anatomy or dissection in detail or report significant series of patients are so indicated. Detailed discussion of exact selection of a flap is beyond the scope of this chapter. However, it is worth noting that the latissimus dorsi free muscle flap is the "workhorse" for open fractures of the tibia. This muscle will provide a very large, well-vascularized envelope, and can even be extended to cover the fibula. (See Fig. 4-15.)

BONE LOSS

In the unusual case where there is segmental bone loss, but an intact and adequate soft tissue envelope, reconstruction of the defect depends on the length and location of the defect, and vascularity of the surrounding soft tissue envelope. The situation is analogous to a limb in which soft tissue reconstruction has been performed, and the wound is stable and ready for skeletal reconstruction by bone grafting. With a well-vascularized soft tissue envelope, cancellous bone grafting may be done up to 6 to 8 cm in length. (See Fig. 4-7.) The amount of cancellous graft required to fill a defect of this size requires harvest of both anterior or both posterior iliac crests. The surgeon should remember that if the graft fails, and a free vascularized bone graft is required, additional cancellous grafts are often needed. To strip the patient of all available cancellous bone graft sites in an attempt to heal a lengthy defect may create an insurmountable problem for the reconstructive surgeon.

Defects larger than 6 to 8 cm, or those in scarred, poorly vascularized, or irradiated beds are best treated by vascularized bone grafting. The free fibula is the preferred graft for the tibia, and donor site morbidity is low. (See Fig. 4-18.) Preoperative angiography of the injured limb is necessary. We often use Doppler studies as well to ensure that blood flow to the foot will be adequate with sacrifice of one of the three major vessels of the lower limb, if an end-to-end anastomosis is planned. Because damage to one or more extremity vessels is common, end-to-side anastomosis is most often used.[191,477] This requires planning because the fibular pedicle is short. An iliac vascularized bone graft can also be used, but this has significant disadvantages which have already been discussed. Dissection is difficult, and alignment and fixation of defects larger than 10 cm are difficult because of curvature of the graft. Remodeling and hypertrophy are not as marked as with fibular transfer. Well-vascularized metaphyseal defects are candidates for Papineau grafting.

Ipsilateral fibular transfer on a pedicle is often used. This is especially true when there has been massive damage to the limb, and only a single vessel or collaterals supply the foot. The fibula may be transferred and slotted into the distal and proximal ends of the nonunion, or proximally the head of the fibula may be decorticated and slotted into the tibial metaphysis. This is an exceptionally valuable salvage technique, and although it does not require

Table 4-10. Skin Flaps

Flap	Pedicle Length (cm)*	Pedicle Size (cm)*	Maximum Size (cm)*	Sensory Innervation Possible	Reference Numbers Series	Anatomy/Dissection
Groin	1 (SCIA)†	A:‡ 1–1.5 V: 1–2	10 × 25	No	29, 180, 252, 254, 255, 347, 388, 413, 431, 507, 509, 510, 520, 631	250, 252, 314, 388, 413, 433, 510, 512, 521, 555, 559
Medial thigh	5	2–5		Yes	19	19
Lateral thigh	10	2–5			19	19
Dorsalis pedis	5–10	A: 2–3 V: 2–3	8 × 15	Yes	386	356, 386
In-step			7 × 13		426	426
Scapular	4–15	A: 2–3 V: 4–6	12 × 24	No	26, 152, 153, 189, 242, 380, 509, 575	26, 152, 153, 189, 242, 323, 488
Parascapular				Yes	420	420
Radial forearm					175, 340, 415	346, 488
Ulnar forearm				Yes	350	350
Lateral arm				Yes	316	316
Deltoid	4–5	A: 2–3 V: 2–3	8 × 20	Yes	487	487, 488, 512

* Note: These numbers are based on adult anatomy; pedicles and maximum size of flaps are smaller in children.

† SCIA = superficial circumflex iliac artery.

‡ A = lumen diameter of artery; V = lumen diameter of vein.

microvascular anastomosis, the dissection must be carried out with the same skill and technique as for microvascular procedures. (See Fig. 4-17.)

A leg-length discrepancy of 2 to 3 cm is well tolerated by most patients. Therefore, small areas of bone loss may be made up by shortening. Loss in excess of 2 to 3 cm is unacceptable and requires reconstruction. Pending bone grafting, the limb must be aligned, rotation corrected, and length maintained by either internal or external fixation. External fixation is recommended, because plating has a high incidence of complications. Limited interfragmentary fixation of butterfly fragments or segmental defects is safe, however. Often, the tibia is aligned and protected with an external fixator, and the fibula is ignored. Several references have been made to the important role that the fibula may play in later reconstruction by ipsilateral transfer, or posterolateral bone grafting. Therefore, alignment of the fibula on a Rush rod, or plating if the fibular fracture is closed, should be considered. (See Fig. 4-11.) If the fibula heals, the external fixator may be removed earlier, decreasing the chance of pin tract osteomyelitis.

COMBINED BONE AND SOFT TISSUE LOSS

For bone loss under 10 cm accompanied by a moderate soft tissue defect, the iliac osteocutaneous flap or the free fibula with attached soft tissue can be utilized. However, the iliac dissection is difficult and the shortcomings of the iliac bone graft have been described. These shorter defects are within the range (ie, <8 cm) of cancellous bone grafting if an adequate soft tissue envelope is reconstructed. Therefore, a staged reconstruction is our most commonly used method at the present time. If the patient is seen immediately and can be managed from the onset, we consider immediate cancellous bone grafting beneath a free flap for defects less than 8 cm. However, in most cases we would obtain soft tissue coverage (usually with a latissimus free flap), and follow this with a cancellous bone graft, ipsilateral fibular transfer, or free vascularized fibula depending on the length of the defect, as described above.

Postoperative Care and Rehabilitation

Many patients with open tibial fractures have polytrauma, and resuscitation and early management should include maintenance of adequate hemoglobin and blood oxygen tension to ensure oxygenation of the peripheral tissues. Shock causes shunting of blood away from the extremities and aggravates local ischemia. The nutritional demands of these patients are extremely high, and nutritional supplements and management are indicated.[132,416,571]

Table 4-11. Muscle Flaps (Pedicle and Free)

Flap	Pedicle Length (cm)*	Pedicle Size (cm)*		Maximum size (cm)*	Reference Numbers	
					Series	*Anatomy/Dissection*
Latissimus	7–9	A:†	2–3	30 × 40	122, 194, 258, 374, 376, 496, 545, 606, 631	25, 194, 374, 488, 512, 627
		V:	3–4			
Serratus anterior				13 × 15	546	546
Rectus abdominis				8 × 30	62	62, 627
Tensor fascia lata	4–10	A:	1–2	15 × 35 (with skin)	79, 276, 336, 418, 419, 545	418, 419, 512
		V:	2–3			
Gracilis		A:	1.5–1.8		255, 256, 336, 366, 372, 631	372, 488, 627
		V:	1.5–2.0			
Gastrocnemius					13, 24, 145, 182, 317, 342, 581, 631	145, 183, 317, 627
Myocutaneous gastrocnemius				May extend skin 7–10 below muscle	166, 385, 497	497
Soleus					24, 181, 182, 241, 342, 421, 581, 623, 631	183, 627
Tibialis anterior					389, 478	
Flexor digitorum longus					24, 181, 581	183
Abductor hallucis					24, 181, 581	183
Flexor digitorum brevis					264, 581	264
Extensor digitorum brevis					24	

* Note: These numbers are based on adult anatomy; pedicles and maximum graft size are smaller in children.

† A = lumen diameter of artery; V = lumen diameter of vein.

In our experience, the hospital stay for a patient with a free flap to the tibia, when other injuries do not complicate the picture, is at least 10 to 14 days. After the flap procedure, the patient is kept at bed rest with the leg elevated for a minimum of 7 days. The vascular anastomosis is at risk of thrombosis, especially during the first 72 hours, and thrombo-prophylaxis (ie, dextran and aspirin) is routinely used for the first 5 days. Allowing the leg to be dependent before complete reendothelialization has occurred may lead to anastomotic problems. Therefore, patients are kept non-weight-bearing and the leg is elevated for a minimum of 4 to 6 weeks.

In fractures without segmental loss, weight-bearing is commenced at 6 weeks if the flap is healthy. Compressive dressings are used to decrease peripheral edema, to soften the flap, and to limit scar formation. When a segmental defect is present, weight-bearing is avoided until bone grafting procedures have been performed and early incorporation is noted. At that point, compression of the tibia with the external fixation device, or removal of the device and weight-bearing in a cast, is allowed.

Results and Cost of Treatment

There are significant variations within the category of grade III tibial injuries. Therefore, even with current classification systems, comparison of results is difficult. Gustilo's series of 1400 open fractures, in which there were 75 type III fractures, serves as a basis for comparison. Infection developed in 100% of farm-related injuries, 41% of those with vascular injuries, and 61% of patients with extensive soft tissue loss; amputation rates were 25%, 41%, and 19%, respectively. In a later report in 1982, he reviewed his cases from the previous 5 years, and noted infection in 2% to 14% of open fractures in general, and 10% to 50% of grade III fractures. Table 4-13 summarizes the complication rates (delayed union or nonunion and osteomyelitis) in reported series of open tibial fractures treated by early and delayed soft tissue reconstruction.

The staged reconstruction of a grade III tibial injury is a major undertaking that may require multiple operations, months of hospitalization, and 1 to 2 years of healing time. Lymphedema, chronic drainage, shortening, limitation of ankle motion, delayed union, and osteomyelitis all threaten the

Table 4-12. Bone Flaps

Flap	Pedicle Length (cm)*	Pedicle Size (cm)*	Maximum Size (cm)*	Sensory Innervation Possible	Difficulty	Reference Numbers	
						Series	Anatomy/Dissection
Fibula	2–5	A: 2–3 V: 2–3	30	N/A	2+	30, 126, 178, 188, 284, 285, 311, 330, 430, 525, 549, 551–554, 557, 570, 595–597, 599, 601, 603, 617, 619	Posterior approach: 269, 323, 552 Lateral approach: 30, 150, 187, 188, 284, 285, 390, 430, 390, 471, 553, 570, 576, 595, 603, 624
Osteocutaneous fibula	2–5	A: 2–3 V: 2–3	Bone: 30 Skin: 7 × 15 to 10 × 20	No	4+	98, 99, 260, 401, 628	87, 98, 99, 260, 628
Rib (bone only or rib osteocutaneous)	3–5	1–1.5	30 (curved)	Yes	4+	49, 61, 125, 126, 330, 363, 511, 554, 603, 619	9, 603
Iliac (bone only or osteocutaneous)	DCIA:‡ 7–9 SCIA:‡ 7–9	DCIA: A: 2–3 V: 4–5 SCIA: 0.8–3.0	Bone: 8–12 Skin: 8 × 18 to 16 × 30	Yes	4+	126, 287, 345, 466, 495, 498, 501, 539, 553, 554, 558, 560, 576, 595, 597, 599, 601, 603, 606, 617, 619	287, 323, 488, 495, 501, 512, 553, 558, 559, 560, 576, 595, 603, 624

* Note: These numbers are based on adult anatomy; pedicles and maximum graft size are smaller in children.

† A = lumen diameter of artery; V = lumen diameter of vein.

‡ DCIA = deep circumflex iliac artery; SCIA = superficial circumflex iliac artery.

result.[513] The costs to the patient need to be evaluated along with the potential benefits.

Open fractures have a significantly higher morbidity than closed ones. In one series,[307] hospitalization was almost four times as long (50 days versus 13 days) and time off work was more than twice as long (264 days versus 129 days). Other series report initial hospitalizations of up to 136 days,[477] with subsequent readmissions. Fractures with segmental loss are especially costly.[196] Several authors have noted that soft tissue reconstruction decreases the hospital time and cost of treatment, and results in better joint motion and better psychological status for the patient.[3,168,193,394,407] However, the additional cost of arteriography, hospitalization, and prolonged operating room time have been noted for free tissue transfer,[83] and we have been admonished not to abandon simpler flaps when applicable. The high cost of reconstruction versus amputation has also been documented.[247] In an early series consisting mainly of free groin flaps with a 23% failure rate, free flap transfer was still less costly than open treatment.[3]

Cierny and Byrd[76,266] reported that in patients whose wounds could be covered before 5 days, the hospital stay was 4.3 weeks, compared with 9 weeks for patients whose wounds could not be covered by that time. Findlay[168] noted that open tibial fractures secondary to motorcycles had a hospitalization time of 17.5 weeks compared to 1.8 weeks for other causes, and almost four times as many operative procedures. Even though the cross-leg flap was said

to reduce hospital stay in its day,[119] hospitalization of 62 to 81 days[186,509] has been noted with cross-leg flaps, compared to 32 days with free flaps.[509] Tube flaps, now of historical interest only, require periods of 6 months to 2 years for completion.[289,532] Staged reconstruction with free tissue transfer and later bone graft averaged 3-month hospitalizations in a military population.[513]

Osteomyelitis also requires prolonged hospitalization and multiple operative procedures. In one study, an average of 5.5 procedures was required to control bone infection.[491] Mathes, however, reported an average hospitalization of only 10 days for free flap coverage of osteomyelitis following débridement,[366] with no failures.

Hyperbaric oxygenation has been used to encourage and speed granulation of the wound prior to coverage with split-thickness skin graft. Davis and associates reported a large series of patients treated in this manner. The number of treatments ranged from 8 to 103, with an average of 48. At a cost of more than $300 per dive, the average cost for the hyperbaric treatments alone exceeded $15,000.

Complications

VASCULAR

The groin flap was the most popular early free flap. Because of small vessels and anatomic variations, the incidence of flap loss owing to vascular com-

Table 4-13. Open Fractures: Compiled Complication Rates of Series With Early Versus Delayed Soft Tissue Reconstruction

	Number of Fractures	Treatment/Coverage	Infection	Osteomyelitis	Delayed Union or Nonunion	Amputation	Hospitalization
Gustilo[233]	60	Open	40%	22%	20%	18%	—
Byrd[77]	38	Open	—	41%	29%	29%	—
		Acute flap	—	5%	14%	5%	—
Hallock[240]							
Cierny[104]	36	Delayed	67%	0%	17%	33%	9 weeks
		Early	12%	0%	4%	4%	4.2 weeks
Jones[309]	8	Early	—	—	0%	0%	—
Yaremchuk[626]	22	Delayed	14%	0%	0%†	9%	—
Godina[193]		By 72 hours	1.5%	—*	—*	—*	27 days
		3 days–3 months	17.5%				130 days
		After 3 months	6%				256 days
Caudle[88]							
IIIA	11		0	—	27%	0	—
IIIB	42		29%	—	43%	17%	—
Group 1	24	By 1 week	8%	—	23%	24%	—
Group 2	17	After 1 week	59%	—	77%	24%	—
IIIC	9			—	100%	78%	—

* Not clearly stated; article implies that none of these complications occurred.
† All healed after six had cancellous graft.

plications was initially high. However, use of flaps with larger and longer pedicles has markedly decreased the incidence of vascular complications. The failure rate in most series of elective free flaps is less than 5%, but in open tibial fractures, the incidence is as high as 20%. This is secondary to the extended zone of injury and to the pliability of the remaining vessels that must be used as recipient vessels. The incidence of vascular complications may be diminished by early coverage before changes occur in the recipient vessels, and by use of a long pedicle which extends to recipient vessels outside of the zone of injury. End-to-side anastomosis has also been credited in reducing the failure rate. Some patients will have to be returned to the operating room for revision of the anastomosis, and careful monitoring is required.

RECURRENT INFECTION

Radical débridement is the only sure way to control recurrent infection. This holds true for coverage of acute wounds, delayed wounds, and osteomyelitis. Many authors mention failure of adequate débridement as the etiology of subsequent infection. Failure to remove necrotic bone has especially been implicated as a cause of secondary infection.

NONUNION, GRAFT FRACTURE, AND NEED FOR ADDITIONAL CANCELLOUS BONE GRAFTING

Union rates of 70% to 90% have been obtained with vascularized bone grafting. However, to obtain these rates, secondary bone grafts are required in a high percentage of cases (10% to 60%). Graft fracture has been reported, but if the bone is viable, it usually heals with exuberant callus, and hypertrophy may be hastened.

DONOR MORBIDITY

Donor site morbidity has not been reported in detail in most articles. Russell and colleagues studied patients following latissimus free muscle transfer, and noted that 23 of their 24 patients were pleased with the procedure, but most had decreased shoulder range of motion and weakness that improved with time. Transient brachial plexus palsy and large wound hematomas were also seen.[376]

Donor morbidity with the iliac osteocutaneous flap includes contour defects, which may be lessened by splitting the crest and leaving the outer table,[454] and hernias in up to 20% of patients, although many of these are asymptomatic.[553,619]

Youdas and associates reported a detailed analysis of donor morbidity after vascularized fibula transfer, and found moderate gait changes before 10 months postoperatively, but minimal changes after 10 months. There was some impaired muscle strength in all patients, and the greater the length taken, the greater loss of ankle eversion strength.[629] Others have reported similar findings.[590] No lateral knee instability was noted following harvesting of the fibula with its epiphysis,[459] but peroneal palsy was seen in 3 of 60 patients following harvesting of a free fibula[620] and in 5 of 171 patients after tibiofibular synostosis.[80]

MALIGNANT DEGENERATION

A biopsy should always be taken when a chronic wound is débrided. Squamous cell carcinoma occurs with an incidence of 0.2% to 1.5% in chronic sinus tracts after a mean delay of 34 years.[587]

COMPARTMENT SYNDROME

Compartment syndromes may be seen with tibial fractures, and if missed, these may result in severe soft tissue necrosis.[142]

Salvage Replantation

The incidence of amputation secondary to vascular injury associated with open tibial fractures has been high.[222] However, early vein grafting and fasciotomy have dramatically lowered the amputation rate. As in other tibial arterial trauma,[514] bypass vein grafting is mandatory unless the limb is shortened.

Every attempt should be made to salvage a below-knee level, because the energy expenditure of ambulation is much lower than with an above-knee amputation.[591] In nonreplantable injuries just below the knee, a below-knee level may be salvaged by advancement of gastrocnemius muscle flaps[212] or early free tissue coverage. Attempts at limb salvage, including replantation and transplantation of bilaterally amputated parts, has been advocated.[94,103,110,286] Salvage is especially indicated in children;[280,412,579] this may avoid the problem of bone growth through the distal soft tissues after amputation.[331,341] Some authors believe that replantation is worth consideration even in adults, because sensation may be regained.[343,355] Replantation of the foot and ankle, even with severe shortening, may be indicated to maintain a functional below-knee stump length.

Fillet flaps of amputated parts have been reported both as free tissue transfers[44,103,110,489] and as neurovascular island flaps (Fig. 4-20).[500] A fillet of the posterior thigh for coverage of an above-knee amputation has been described.[174] These techniques may allow glabrous skin with the potential for reinnervation to be placed on weight-bearing areas of the stump (Fig. 4-21).

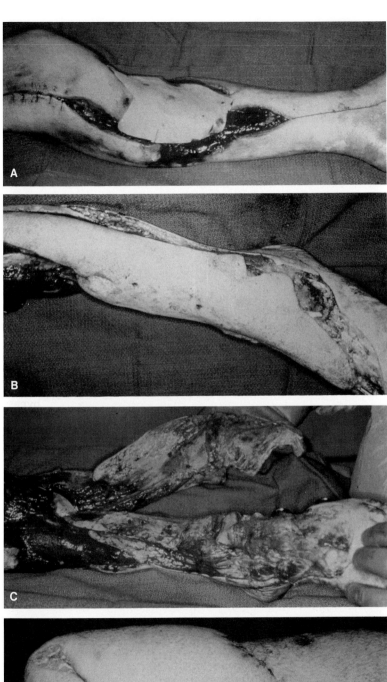

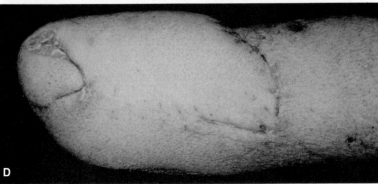

Fig. 4-20. (A) A large anterior soft tissue defect and segmental tibial defect. Amputation has been selected as definitive treatment. To provide durable sensate coverage to the stump, the dorsal skin of the foot will be filleted based on the anterior tibial artery—the only remaining blood supply to the foot. Note the posterior skin defect, which prevents use of a standard posterior flap. **(B)** Following application of the template to the dorsum of the foot, a flap exactly matching the defect is raised. **(C)** The flap has been raised, the deep surface is shown, and the amputation can be completed. **(D)** Appearance of the leg 8 weeks after amputation showing the full-thickness sensate coverage of the medial and anterior aspects of the tibial stump.

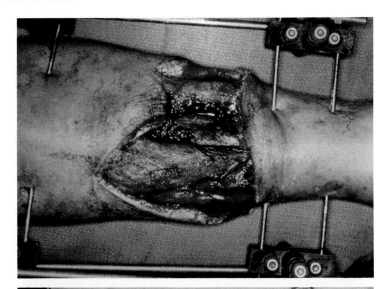

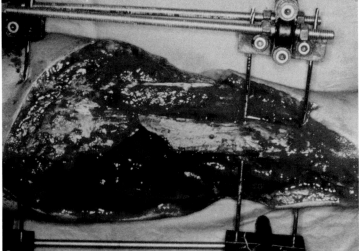

Fig. 4-21. (**A**) The leg of an 18-year-old patient 5 days following an open fracture of the tibia. The limb was severely contaminated with dirt, and a limited débridement and application of external fixation device had been performed at another hospital. The patient developed fever and foul-smelling drainage and was transferred for definitive care. (**B**) Appearance of the leg following radical débridement of the zone of injury and necrotic muscle and bone. Cultures subsequently grew clostridia. The patient was treated in a hyperbaric chamber and the infection was controlled. A bone scan showed significant devascularization of the exposed tibia and the only muscles to the foot were the posterior group. Therefore, amputation was elected. However, because there was inadequate soft tissue to cover the stump, an elective fillet flap of the foot was performed. (**C**) The posterior tibial artery was the only vessel intact to the foot. The perforating branch between the first and second metatarsals was preserved and the entire foot was filleted from the bone. It was then folded up to cover the stump.

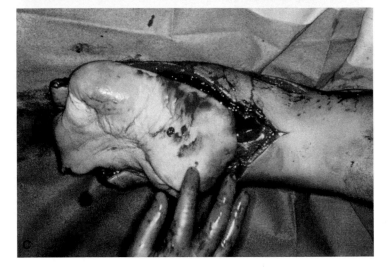

(continued)

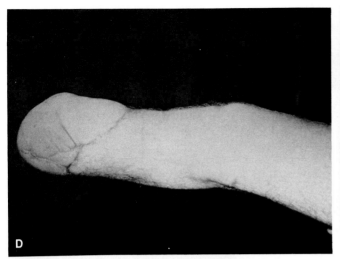

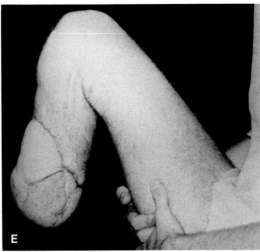

Fig. 4-21 *(continued)*
(D) Final result showing sensate durable coverage, and nearly full extension of the knee. **(E)** Flexion of the knee and a lateral view of the stump. **(F)** The patient fitted with his prosthesis.

Amputation

Before the availability of soft tissue reconstruction, skin necrosis and nonunion were the most common events leading to amputation.[273,338,491] Decision making has always been difficult in severe lower extremity injuries, and secondary amputation is especially hard on both patient and surgeon.[89,246,334,352] Criteria for salvage include a viable foot, sensate sole, intact fibula, and any body part in a child.[89,103,381] The incidence of eventual am-

putation in severe grade III injuries is high.[233,332,542] Proposed guidelines for immediate amputation include:[42,88,103,230,232,334,469]

Posterial tibial nerve loss;
Severe crush injury;
Warm ischemia longer than 6 hours;
Prolonged hypovolemic shock; and
Age greater than 50 years.

Now that soft tissue reconstruction is possible, blood

vessel and nerve injury have become the most common reasons for amputation.[77,161] Caudle and others recommended that vascularity should not be restored in grade IIIC injuries.[44,88] Others recommend that amputation be done only if an insensate foot is present or if reconstruction is deemed impossible.[469]

Point systems to predict the need for amputation have been devised[211,283,335] (Table 4-14). Browner studied the medical and economic impact of these injuries and concluded that there was an absence of objective parameters on which to base a decision.

Table 4-14. Mangled Extremity Syndrome Grading System[211]

Injury Severity Score (ISS)	
0–25	1
25–50	2
>50	3
Integument	
Guillotine	1
Crush/burn	2
Avulsion/degloving	3
Nerve	
Contusion	1
Transection	2
Avulsion	3
Vascular	
Artery	
Transsected	1
Thrombosed	2
Avulsed	3
Vein damage	1
Bone	
Simple fracture	1
Segmental fracture	2
Segmental comminuted fracture	3
Segmental comminuted fracture with bone loss < 6 cm*	4
Segmental fracture, intra- or extra-articular, with bone loss < 6 cm	5
Segmental fracture, intra- or extra-articular, with bone loss > 6 cm	6
Lag time	1 point for every hour > 6
Age (years)	
40–50	1
50–60	2
60–70	3
Preexisting disease	1
Shock	2

A score of less than 20 points suggests that salvage should be attempted. Conversely, amputation should be considered if the score is more than 20 points.

* Add 1 point for bone loss > 6 cm.

He also documented the marked increase in cost of secondary versus primary amputation.[42]

FOOT AND ANKLE

The foot and ankle are structures we take for granted until they are injured. Bipedal ambulation is necessary for the activities of daily living and most recreational endeavors, and traumatic injuries of the foot and ankle can drastically alter a patient's quality of life. The goal of surgical reconstruction is to restore form, and most importantly, foot and ankle function for ambulation. The surgeon must explain the treatment options to the patient and family, including the overall time required for rehabilitation. An amputation, instead of prolonged series of elaborate reconstructive procedures, may be the best treatment for some patients. Treatment plans must be developed on an individual basis with a goal of obtaining uncomplicated healing and optimal function.

Initial Evaluation

Evaluation of a complex foot and ankle injury should be carried out by physicians skilled in the treatment of bone and joint problems as well as soft tissue injuries. In most cases, this is best accomplished by a joint orthopaedic and plastic surgery consultation. The extent of the soft tissue injury and the status of the nerve and blood supply to the foot are determined. Loss of plantar sensibility owing to injury to the posterior tibial nerve may influence the choice of reconstruction. In an acute injury, the status of the vascular supply to the foot must be determined; if this is inadequate, it becomes a treatment priority. The degree of soft tissue loss and the status of the extrinsic tendons to the foot are assessed by direct observation, usually in the operating room under general anesthesia. Preoperative x-ray films are mandatory to assess the presence and severity of fractures and/or dislocations.

Initial Treatment

Complex ankle and foot wounds must be surgically débrided and all nonviable tissue and foreign bodies removed. This is best accomplished under tourniquet control with copious saline irrigation using a commercially available pressurized system. The wound is inspected and débrided from superficial to deep, region by region. Obviously nonviable tissues are débrided. The tourniquet can then be deflated and areas without adequate perfusion excised. Questionable areas should be retained at the initial débridement and examined at subsequent dressing changes.

Repair is begun by the orthopaedic service by reducing the fractures and dislocations. External fixation is preferred. Internal plates, screws, and Kirschner wires can be used in selected cases, but they may increase the risk of infection. Major vascular injuries are repaired primarily using interpositional vein grafts to avoid vascular compromise and improve healing. Nerve injuries are repaired primarily by microsurgical technique. Badly crushed or avulsed nerves with loss of nerve substance are held to length and repaired at a secondary procedure. Severe foot and ankle injuries often lack inadequate soft tissue for primary closure. Placement of sutures under tension is ill advised, especially in already traumatized tissues. Local flap coverage is also difficult to achieve in the ankle and foot because the extent of the surrounding "zone of injury" is unknown. After débridement, open wounds are covered with a biologic porcine xenograft dressing, which can be applied over exposed bone, nerve, tendon, and vessel. The wound is dressed with a bulky dressing and posterior splint. Bed rest and elevation of the injured limb decrease swelling and improve venous drainage. The patient is returned to the operating room every 2 to 3 days, and the wound is inspected under general anesthesia. Further débridement is performed until all nonviable tissue has been removed, infection is controlled, and the wound is ready for closure.

Reconstruction

PRINCIPLES

The biomechanics of foot and ankle motion after reconstruction must be considered in choosing the type of wound closure. During normal gait, the weight-bearing surface moves distally from heel strike to toe off. Immobility or instability of the bony skeleton allows abnormal, uneven force application to areas on the plantar surface, often leading to flap ulceration. Prospectively, it is difficult to anticipate how the foot and ankle will function after reconstruction, making decisions regarding flap coverage even more difficult. The choice of final wound closure is tailored to close the defect and provide maximum function. The dimensions of the wound are measured and a pattern is made to fit the defect. The desired location of the vascular pedicle and its direction from the pattern are noted. The pattern can then be moved to various donor sites to determine the best donor area. The aesthetic appearance of the foot or ankle after flap coverage

should also be considered. This is especially important in female patients and is a necessity to allow normal footwear.

TREATMENT ALTERNATIVES

Sommerlad[524] reported a series of 51 patients treated by a variety of techniques including split-thickness skin graft, full-thickness skin graft, local flaps, cross-leg flaps, and free tissue transfer. He concluded that no form of sole replacement was entirely satisfactory, but split-thickness skin graft had the worst results.

Cross-leg and pedicle flaps used for foot coverage include pedicled buttock flaps in children,[154,279] thigh and calf flaps,[34,404,508] and cross-leg instep flaps.[402]

Local flaps appear to be second in popularity after free flaps, judging by the number of articles in the literature. Reported techniques include:

Heel coverage by rotational flexor digitorum brevis muscle or myocutaneous transfer;[45,264,297,382,518,581]
Fasciocutaneous sole flap;[261,382,403,411,426,470]
Toe fillet;[382,522]
Dorsalis pedis island flap;[382,386]
Abductor hallucis and abductor digiti minimi for small ankle defects.[581]

Only the flexor digitorum brevis and instep flaps replace the heel with glabrous tissue.

Free tissue coverage options include skin, muscle, and myocutaneous flaps. Skin flaps may provide sensate coverage if reinnervation occurs.[327,615] The instep fasciocutaneous flap has been used both as an island and a free flap.[411,426] Omental,[435] groin,[29,58,101,180,476,508,592] radial forearm,[415] deltoid,[487] serratus anterior,[487] latissimus dorsi,[377,379] scapular,[26,380,483,575] tensor fascia lata,[483] and gracilis[377] flaps have been used.

An iliac osteocutaneous flap has been used to both reconstruct the calcaneus and provide coverage.[192,547]

DORSAL FOOT AND ANKLE

Wounds of the dorsal foot and dorsal and lateral ankle are best covered with a free fasciocutaneous flap or a muscle flap covered with a skin graft. Defects on the dorsal and lateral aspects of the foot and ankle are easily covered with a custom-designed muscle flap covered with a skin graft. The gracilis, rectus, or a segment of the latissimus dorsi muscle are ideal choices to close these defects (Fig. 4-22). The epimysial covering of the muscle flap is excised and the muscle spread over the defect. This thins

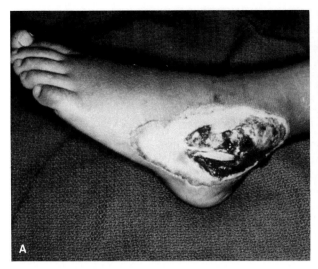
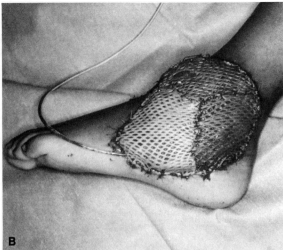

Fig. 4-22. (**A**) Exposure of the peroneal tendons, lateral malleolus, fibular physis, and ankle joint in a 6-year-old girl following a motorcycle chain avulsion injury. (**B**) Application of a latissimus dorsi free flap. Anastomosis was to the anterior tibial vessels end-to-side. The flap was trimmed and covered with mesh split-thickness skin graft. Partial necrosis of the flap occurred, but this was treated by watchful neglect and the muscle subsequently revascularized. Only repeat skin grafting was required to obtain durable full-thickness coverage.

the flap, allows it to cover a larger area, and improves the contour of the final reconstruction. Fasciocutaneous flaps, such as the deltoid or lateral arm flap, are also excellent choices for coverage of smaller defects (Fig. 4-23).

HEEL AND PLANTAR SURFACE

The plantar surface of the foot is the most difficult area to reconstruct. The plantar skin is thick and connected to the underlying bone by numerous fibrous septa which prevent shearing during ambulation. Glabrous skin is highly specialized and contains numerous sensory receptor sites found only in the hand and foot. This complex tissue is highly specialized and cannot be replaced. Therefore, every effort is made to preserve all viable glabrous skin during débridement.

Soft tissue loss in children can be treated by allowing the wound to granulate. With proper wound care, even extensive wounds in children granulate quickly, allowing coverage with a split-thickness skin graft. The graft contracts during healing, resulting in a smaller defect. In children, this technique has been used successfully even with plantar injuries.

In adults, avulsion injuries with exposed bone, joint, or tendon should be closed within 7 days, preferably using a free tissue transfer. Selection of the flap is based on the requirements of the trau-matic defect, including the vascularity of the remaining soft tissue, the integrity of the skeletal structures, and the need for sensibility and durability during weight-bearing. A muscle flap covered with skin graft is insensate and less durable than normal skin. However, muscle becomes firmly adherent to the underlying structures and is more resistant to shear stress generated during ambulation (Fig. 4-24). A fasciocutaneous flap, like the deltoid, has normal skin and can be reinnervated to provide sensibility, but the subcutaneous fat allows shear and is not suited to withstand the forces of ambulation. Flaps containing subcutaneous fat may thicken if the patient grows or gains weight and become too bulky for ordinary footwear. Skin flaps may be innervated and recover sensation. Return of some sensibility also has been noted in noninnervated flaps, presumably from peripheral innervation.[192]

Salvage Versus Amputation

The use of free tissue transfers has permitted salvage of foot and ankle injuries which previously would have resulted in amputation. The problem is to identify those injuries suitable for reconstruction and those which should be amputated. Unfortunately, the decision is not always easy or clear. Guidelines have already been discussed. (See p. 285.)

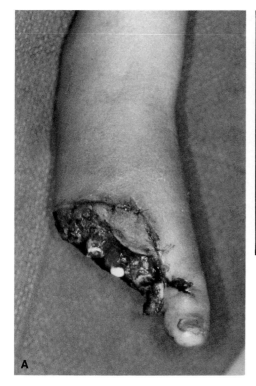

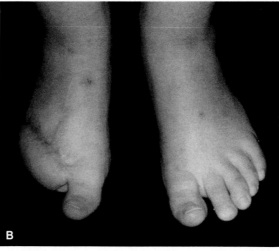

Fig. 4-23. (**A**) A 10-year-old with loss of all four lateral toes and adjacent soft tissue. (**B**) Durable coverage and maintenance of metatarsal length by a lateral arm free flap (1 year postoperatively). *(Case courtesy of Robert N. Hotchkiss, M.D., San Antonio, Texas)*

Rehabilitation

May and others have used gait analysis to study patients following foot flaps.[377] Renervation had no bearing on the success of the reconstruction. If any normal plantar skin remains after reconstruction, the patient will "walk toward" this surface instead of the reconstructed area during ambulation.[524]

"Walking away" from the flap coverage does help prevent flap breakdown, but can create other musculoskeletal problems. The most important aspect of postoperative care is the use of prosthetic and orthotic devices to provide stability or to diffuse the weight evenly over the plantar surface during ambulation. Each orthotic device must be custom made to fit the irregular shape and contour of the recon-

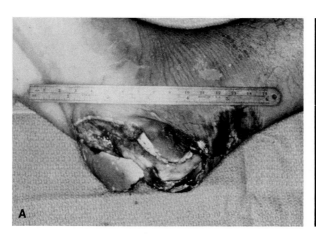

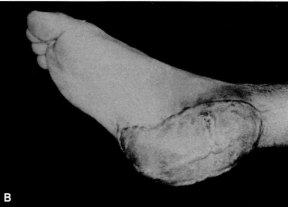

Fig. 4-24. (**A**) Complete avulsion of the heel pad in an illegal alien, suffered while jumping onto a train. (**B**) Appearance of the foot 4 weeks following a latissimus dorsi free flap and split-thickness skin graft.

structed foot. Most require frequent adjustments or tailoring throughout life. A good prosthetist is a necessity in the care of these patients after surgery.

OSTEOMYELITIS

CLASSIFICATION

Waldvogel classified osteomyelitis by etiology into three types:[584–587,609]

1. Hematogenous;
2. Secondary to a contiguous focus; and
3. Associated with peripheral vascular disease.

Until the advent of antibiotics, hematogenous staphylococcus osteomyelitis was the most common type, and was divided into acute, subacute, and chronic varieties.[85] However, now that this disease is generally controlled by antibiotics and appropriate surgical treatment, posttraumatic osteomyelitis (ie, secondary to a contiguous focus of infection) is now the most common type.[165] More gram-negative, aerobic, and mixed infections are now seen.[165,238,318] Criteria for diagnosis of osteomyelitis are listed in Table 4-15.

Weiland proposed a classification system based on the character of the wound (Table 4-16).

Kelly, in discussing infected nonunions of the femur and tibia, divided osteomyelitis into the following groups: hematogenous osteomyelitis, osteomyelitis plus united fracture, osteomyelitis plus nonunion, and postoperative osteomyelitis without

Table 4-15. Diagnostic Criteria for Osteomyelitis

Author	Criteria
Weiland[605]	Drainage for longer than 6 months with pus, infected granulation tissue, sequestra, draining sinus, resistant cellulitis
Irons[301]	Isolation of bacteria from deep tissue specimens plus x-ray changes consistent with osteomyelitis
May[375]	Exposed bone, drainage for longer than 6 weeks, positive culture, appropriate bone histology, x-ray films and/or bone scan consistent with osteomyelitis
Mathes[365]	Positive x-ray findings, histologic abnormalities in the bone, positive bone culture
Stark[530]	Draining sinuses, evidence of abscess or sequestra
Morrey[410]	Chronic osteomyelitis—present for at least 6 months, recurrence after one or more surgeries, recurrence after treatment with intravenous antibiotics

Table 4-16. Weiland's Classification of Osteomyelitis[605]

Type	Wound Characteristics
I	Open, exposed bone without evidence of osseous infection but with evidence of soft tissue infection
II	Circumferential, cortical, and endosteal infection; roentgenograms showing a diffuse inflammatory reaction, increased density, and spindle-shaped sclerotic thickening of the cortex in addition to areas of bone resorption; often an involucrum surrounding a sequestrum
III	Cortical and endosteal infection associated with a segmental bone defect

fracture. Mader and associates[354], in a study of conjunctive hyperbaric oxygen therapy, classified osteomyelitis as: I—medullary, II—superficial, III—localized, and IV—diffused. Modifiers were then attached for the physiologic state of the patient: A—normal host, B—host compromised by either systemic or local factors, and C—host in which treatment was worse than the disease. Thus, the classification would consist of a Roman numeral and a letter. This classification by Cierny and Mader[105,106] seems to offer the best characterization for each patient and allows meaningful comparison of various treatment modalities.

DÉBRIDEMENT

Tscherne noted that bone infection is usually secondary to local tissue hypoxia or anoxia, rather than primary bacterial contamination.[571] The wound in chronic osteomyelitis is hypoxic.[365] Necrotic, poorly vascularized tissue forms an interface between dead bone, and host defense mechanisms and blood-borne antibiotics.[59,60,117,322,464,484,530,584] Osteomyelitis persists because of the presence of: (1) necrotic and infected bone, (2) avascular and infected scar tissue, (3) dead space, (4) inadequate soft tissue coverage leading to recurrent ulceration and reinfection, and (5) relative wound ischemia.[75,185] All of these must be addressed if osteomyelitis is to be controlled.

It is difficult to determine the extent of bone involvement in osteomyelitis. Many procedures have been described to aid in the diagnosis of osteomyelitis, including:

1. Technetium and indium bone scans;[117]
2. Culture by biopsy[165] (peripheral culture and sensitivity unreliable owing to secondary contamination);

3. Sinogram;[60]
4. Bone biopsy to assess vascularity, either by open or needle technique; biopsy of the sinus tract for carcinoma should also be done in chronic wounds;
5. Operative assessment of punctate bleeding of the bone after removal of a thin layer with a slow-speed power burn;[123,245]
6. Fluorescein or tetracycline labeling of bone;[534]
7. Routine x-ray studies;
8. Laser Doppler studies to assess blood flow to bone;[543]
9. White cell count and sedimentation rate to follow progress of the disease.

Radical débridement of all necrotic bone and surrounding hypoxic scar is the cornerstone of treatment.[66,85,123,223,586] Unfortunately, mixed areas of necrotic and viable bone may be present, especially after healing of open fractures. Infection may recur after years of quiescence.[274] Control of recurrence, rather than a cure, is therefore the most realistic goal.

Earlier in this century, débridement followed by secondary granulation was the most common treatment. Closure was obtained using pedicle flaps, jump flaps, or split-thickness skin grafts to achieve a stable wound. Once the infection was under control, reconstruction was undertaken.[7,109,218,282,325,472] Flap reconstruction in osteomyelitis is a relatively new idea. A 1980 text did not mention flaps as an alternative in the treatment of osteomyelitis.[7] Most authors currently recommend the following:

1. Staged débridement aided by the studies mentioned above;
2. Coverage by well-vascularized tissue;
3. Adjunctive antibiotics with infectious disease consultation and serum blood levels, if needed;
4. Stabilization if nonunion is present; and
5. Delayed skeletal reconstruction when a defect is present.[75,184,229,301,318,319,321,366,405,457,464,484,563,605]

In the débridement of osteomyelitis, one must apply the principles used by tumor surgeons.[608] Free tissue transfer or rotational muscle flaps are of benefit because they allow more radical and complete débridement, fill dead space, and bring in vascularity, host defenses and antibiotics.[184,245,375,405,608,618] The same was said of split-thickness skin graft coverage in its time.[218]

Hyperbaric oxygenation, by improving the local vascularity, may help in the differentiation of viable bone, and aids leukocyte-killing mechanisms.[136,410,534] Improving the local blood supply by vascular reconstruction may be of benefit, especially if peripheral vascular disease is present.[608] Despite some advocates, suction irrigation following débridement has not been very successful in the management of osteomyelitis.[444,586]

TREATMENT ALTERNATIVES

Burri published an extensive review of the treatment of osteomyelitis in his monograph.[71] Although débridement has long been recognized as the cornerstone of treatment, lining, closing, or filling in the defect was always thought to be beneficial.[3,407,464,484] The results of these attempts prior to the advent of microvascular techniques are detailed in many articles from the first three quarters of this century.[7,17,59,66,67,72,78,109,228,229,268,282,318,348,444,612] Resection of infected bone is of primary importance, and osteomyelitis with significant medullary extension can therefore be controlled only by resection of all the involved bone.[542] Following débridement, various procedures have been advocated, as outlined below.

Healing by Primary or Secondary Closure

Authors who advocate healing by primary or secondary closure[59,60,69,322,464,472] note that the incidence of continued drainage is less than when the wound is allowed to heal by secondary intention.

Papineau Graft

The Papineau graft[66,67,78,144,208,228,229,268,464,538] is based on the concept of obtaining union first, then reconstructing the soft tissue envelope. It is most useful in the metaphysis, and most authors recommend that a well-vascularized bed be present prior to graft placement. However, other authors have advocated immediate cancellous grafting after débridement.[109,144,444]

Split-Thickness Skin Graft

The concept of split-thickness skin grafting[218,325,448,472] is to allow early granulation after débridement, and then obtain a closed wound with the split-thickness graft. Once the wound is stable and infection is under control, reconstructive plastic procedures may be done.

Cross-Leg and Pedicle Flaps

Although cross-leg and pedicle flaps[119,186,268,325] are not as common as they once were, they do permit either primary or secondary soft tissue envelope reconstruction. However, these flaps are parasitic and do not add vascularity to the wound as do pedicle or free vascularized flaps. However, they were efficacious in reducing the incidence of drainage and in leading to healing of problematic fractures.

Suction Irrigation

Although suction irrigation has been recommended,[67,70,149,165,195,320] most authors report very high rates of recurrence or failure.[67,111,224,444,584,586] Also, suction irrigation may allow the entrance of secondary organisms.[170] It works best when the wound can be closed over drains. Although once very popular, this technique is not commonly used now, and special codes for the procedure have been deleted from the AMA CPT codes.

Local Antibiotic Therapy

Silver ions, antibiotics delivered locally by pumps, and impregnated beads or cement have been used to fill dead space and provide a high local concentration of antibiotics. These methods avoid high systemic levels of antibiotics, with their associated complications.[32,171,214,324,457,574,588] As always, antibiotic therapy is *not* a substitute for adequate débridement.

Amputation

In the pre-antibiotic era, more than 50% of patients with osteomyelitis required amputation.[68] Even in recent series, the incidence of amputation is as high as 20%.[282] Amputation is always an alternative to a prolonged reconstructive attempt, especially when there are underlying systemic or host defense deficiencies. Malignant degeneration of sinus tracts surrounding osteomyelitic areas occurs with an incidence of 0.2% to 0.5%, and is an indication for amputation.[68] Theoretically, early soft tissue envelope reconstruction should diminish the chance of later malignant degeneration by obliterating the sinus tract.

Vascularized Reconstruction

Vascularized tissue transfer may itself be considered an adjunctive treatment.[245] Most authors believe that filling the defect that follows débridement with vascularized tissue will bring in blood supply and associated host defenses.[366] However, the ability of muscle flaps to deliver antibiotics to these wounds probably diminishes with time.[486]

Rotational muscle flaps are most useful in the upper and middle thirds of the tibia, and in other areas where large muscle bellies, which can be sacrificed, are found. They were in use prior to the advent of microvascular techniques, and are quite

effective.[51,75,105,184,185,245,366,405,407,490,519,530,631] However, the incidence of recurrent drainage is somewhat higher than in series utilizing free flaps;[608] this suggests that débridement was not as radical. Rotation flaps have size limitations that free flaps do not have, and their use should therefore be confined to smaller defects.

Free tissue transfer is indicated in the distal portion of extremities where rotational muscle flaps are not available, in large defects, and in poorly vascularized areas. The efficacy of free tissue coverage in controlling or "curing" osteomyelitis is well documented[16,75,245,301,366,367,375,405,480,519,531,542,605,608,631] (Table 4-17).

Skeletal Reconstruction

The alternatives for skeletal reconstruction in osteomyelitis are the same as those discussed in the section on bone grafting and reconstruction of tibial defects. (See p. 292.)

Hyperbaric Oxygenation

Adjunctive hyperbaric oxygenation may aid in the differentiation of viable and nonviable bone, and experimentally results in faster bone healing.[424,625] In one large series, 34 of 38 patients who were treated with hyperbaric oxygenation and allowed to heal had no drainage at an average of 34 months after treatment ended. An average of 6.1 operations was required, but the authors concluded that hyperbaric oxygenation prolonged the infection-free interval. The role of hyperbaric oxygenation in improving local vascularity also is helpful.

Systemic Antibiotics

Adjunctive antibiotics specific to the organisms cultured from bone biopsies, and periodic serum antibiotic levels are widely recommended. A thorough review of chronic osteomyelitis including

Table 4-17. Results of Flap Reconstruction of Osteomyelitis

Author	Flap Survival Rate (%)	Incidence of Recurrent Drainage (%)
Smith[519]	90	?
Irons[301]	76	12
May[375]	100	22
Mathes[365]	100	11
Weiland[605]	79	33
Hall[238]	80	?
Fitzgerald[172]	93	42
Weiland[608]	80	15–40
Zook[631]	93	23

current organisms and antibiotic therapy has recently been published.[573]

AUTHORS' PREFERRED METHODS OF TREATMENT

May and associates published an excellent review of the classification and treatment of osteomyelitis.[378] The classification system and protocol used at the University of Texas Medical Branch at Galveston for the treatment of osteomyelitis offer the most thorough discussion of current concepts and treatment. Several treatment algorithms are included.[105,106] This protocol includes the following principles:

1. The patient is evaluated thoroughly with special consideration given to local or systemic measures that compromise healing; malnutrition and other host problems are corrected prior to débridement.
2. Bone biopsy is done for culture, and biopsies of the wound and sinus tract are done to rule out malignant degeneration.
3. The surgical approach used is between myocutaneous territories to leave the option of rotational muscle flaps, especially in the proximal two thirds of the tibia.
4. Associated nonunions are stabilized rigidly.
5. A radical débridement is carried out using punctate bleeding of bone as a sign of viability. All scar and poorly vascularized tissue are excised. If this is not done, poorly durable coverage adjacent to a well-vascularized flap may allow further drainage (Fig. 4-25).
6. Culture-specific antibiotic therapy is used for 4 to 6 weeks with blood levels as indicated. Infectious disease consultation is usually warranted.
7. Staged débridements or "second looks" are done until the wound is clean. Adjunctive hyperbaric oxygenation may improve the ability to differentiate live from dead bone, and will improve the local oxygenation of the wound. If local blood flow is poor owing to vascular disease, this should be corrected using bypass grafting.
8. Once the infection is under control—as indicated by the appearance of the wound and a diminishing sedimentation rate and white count—coverage may be carried out using rotational muscle, myocutaneous flaps, or free tissue transfer. Muscle tissue is preferred because it fills the dead space well and revascularizes bone better than other soft tissue. In the

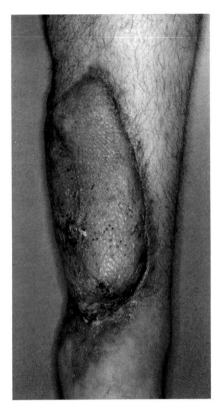

Fig. 4-25. Despite a successful free flap, inadequate excision of surrounding scar tissue resulted in a persistent sinus tract at the distal edge.

upper two thirds of the tibia, the gastrocnemius and soleus are useful for smaller defects. However, with larger defects, and in the distal third, free muscle flaps are preferred with the latissimus dorsi being the workhorse flap. The gracilis is the second most commonly used flap.

Nonunion

In nonunions, treatment of the bone defect may be done in several ways: (1) immediate or delayed cancellous grafting for short defects (ie, less than 4 to 6 cm); (2) delayed long-bone reconstruction by free vascularized iliac or fibular transfer; or, (3) tibiofibular synostosis or ipsilateral fibular transfer. Occasionally, a flap may add sufficient vascularity to the wound to allow healing without the need for later bone graft.[3] Most authors recommend delaying the bone graft until 3 to 6 months after the flap procedure.[531] However, if a vascularized bone graft is being done for nonunion with a small skin defect, or with adequate soft tissue coverage, the graft may be placed as soon as the wound is débrided and clean.[620]

Papineau grafts are another option, but we use these mainly for large, well-vascularized metaphyseal defects, and in limbs with either a single vessel or only collateral circulation.[206,208] (See Fig. 4-16.) Another reason to limit the length of defects treated with autogenous cancellous grafts is the limited availability of this material. A defect larger than 4 to 6 cm in diameter should probably be treated by free vascularized transfer, because many of these vascularized transfers require secondary cancellous grafting, and if all iliac graft sites have been used, future reconstructive options are limited.

Tibiofibular synostosis or ipsilateral fibular transfer are often useful for reconstruction of long-bone defects in limbs with severe injury.[147,319] The Ilizarov technique is a new option with which we have only limited experience.

Union

If the bone has healed, continued drainage may be related to sequestra, nondurable soft tissue coverage, retained foreign body, or malignant degeneration of the sinus tract. Osteomyelitis may be present up and down the medullary canal, and radical resection of the diaphysis may be required to control the infection. It may not be possible to remove all dead bone in these situations without compromising stability. A higher incidence of recurrent drainage has been noted in patients treated with flap reconstruction who had intact bone. This result is initially surprising, but débridement is more limited in these patients because of fear of producing a fracture. Some necrotic bone will probably be left behind because of the mixture of necrotic and viable bone in the healed fracture.[320,612] The review by May and colleagues offers a classification based on the tibial defect after débridement and the status of the fibula; treatment for each type is outlined.[378]

RESULTS

Using these methods, many patients may achieve control of drainage and a healed, functional limb. The survival rate for free tissue transfer is high if adequate débridement is done (Fig. 4-26).[319,531] Recurrent drainage ranges from 40%[608] to 93% stable coverage.[367] Smith attained wound healing in 37 of 53 patients with one operation, and 11 of 16 with a second operation. This left 5 patients out of 53 with continued problems, an incidence of approximately 10%. Of these, 2 continued to have drainage and 3 limbs were amputated.[519]

INDICATIONS FOR AMPUTATION

In some cases, all attempts at salvage fail. Indications for amputations include:

1. Extensive or systemic infection not controlled by débridement (ie, uncontrollable or life-threatening infections);
2. Situations where resection of the diseased bone would destroy function to the point that a prosthesis would give better function;
3. A patient having undergone multiple operative procedures and still draining;
4. Malignant change in the sinus tract;
5. Chronic arterial insufficiency not amenable to reconstructive vascular procedures;
6. An associated major nerve paralysis, such as the sciatic nerve, or an asensate foot;
7. Severe joint contractures in the affected limb;
8. Occasionally, to decrease the cost, psychological morbidity, lost work time, and hospitalization time of the patient.[7,85]

Late amputation is common because it is hard to recommend primary amputation. Needless conservative measures may continue until it is obvious to both patient and physician that amputation is the best choice. Unfortunately, this is costly in many ways.

The indications for amputation in open tibial fractures have already been discussed in detail. (See p. 285.)

MEDICOLEGAL CONSIDERATIONS

Salvage and reconstruction of a severely injured extremity are exceedingly costly not only to society and the insurance company, but to the patient as well. The advisability as well as the feasibility of surgery should be considered.[334] The cost of these procedures is measured by several factors. Reconstruction may require 2 to 3 years[94,378,608] with multiple operative procedures, long hospitalization, and prolonged disability. This often results in decimation of the patient's family, savings, self-image, and self-respect. Often, his or her job is lost as well.[117,196,247,334] Patients in whom a protracted course of reconstruction is predicted are best treated by primary amputation.[42] The prolonged use of external fixators has been noted to cause psychosocial problems.

Gregory and associates devised a severity grading system for multisystem injury of the extremity called the "mangled extremity syndrome" (see Ta-

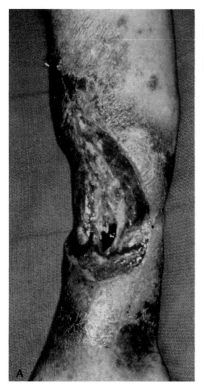 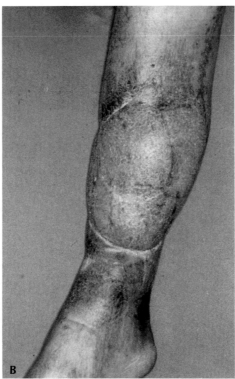

Fig. 4-26. (**A**) The leg of a patient who had 20 years of chronic drainage from a healed open tibia fracture with poorly durable scar directly overlying the tibia. The appearance of the wound following initial débridement of the scar and necrotic infected bone beneath the sinus tract. (**B**) Appearance of the leg 6 weeks after coverage was accomplished by a latissimus dorsi free flap plus a split-thickness skin graft. Four years postoperatively, no further drainage has occurred.

ble 4-14). Unfortunately, this rating scale is not widely used. It certainly would aid in decision making, and should be more widely applied so that further data can be collected. Otherwise, the patient is solely dependent on the experience of the treating physician. A "second opinion" is a wise precaution in this type of injury (whether reconstruction or amputation is considered), for the peace of mind and protection of both the patient and the physician. A high level of knowledge and experience on the part of the attending surgeon is necessary.[157,571] Orthopaedists are often not as well trained in the management of soft tissue wounds as in fractures, and early consultation should be considered either with other orthopaedists or with plastic surgeons who are experienced in soft tissue and bone reconstruction.

Finally, several experienced authors have noted the prolonged time necessary to complete reconstruction. Most of these have begun to recommend compression of the treatment plan in some manner. Options include early bone grafting of low-grade tibial fractures expected to have a high incidence of delayed or nonunion, combined coverage and bone grafting as a single procedure, and early amputation if reconstruction fails.[15,105,164,221,226,232,352,378,626]

REFERENCES

1. Aberg, M.; Rydholm, A.; Holmberg, J.; and Wieslander, J.B.: Reconstruction With a Free Vascularized Fibular Graft for Malignant Bone Tumor. Acta Orthop. Scand., 59(4):430–437, 1988.
2. Abu-Dalu, K.; Muggia, M.; and Schiller, M.: A Bipedicled Chest Wall Flap to Cover an Open Elbow Joint in a Burned Infant. Injury, 13:292–293, 1982.
3. Acland, R., and Smith, P.: Microvascular Surgical Techniques Used to Provide Skin Cover Over an Ununited Tibial Fracture. J. Bone Joint Surg., 58B:471–473, 1976.
4. Ambroggio, G.; Oberto, E.; and Teich-Alasia, S.: Twenty

Years' Experience Using the Cross-Leg Flap Technique. Ann. Plast. Surg., 9:152–163, 1982.

5. Anderson, J.T.: History of the Treatment of Open Fractures. *In* Gustilo, R.B. (ed.): Management of Open Fractures and Their Complications, 4th ed., pp. 1–11. Philadelphia, W.B. Saunders, 1982.

6. Anderson, J.T., and Gustilo, R.B.: Immediate Internal Fixation in Open Fractures. Orthop. Clin. North Am., 11: 569–578, 1980.

7. Anderson, L.D.: Infections. *In* Edmonson, A.S., and Crenshaw, A.H. (eds.): Campbell's Operative Orthopaedics, p. 1047. St. Louis, C.V. Mosby, 1980.

8. Arata, M.A.; Wood, M.B.; and Cooney, W.P., III: Revascularized Segmental Diaphyseal Bone Transfers in the Canine: An Analysis of Viability. J. Reconstr. Microsurg., 1:11–19, 1984.

9. Ariyan, S., and Finseth, F.J.: The Anterior Chest Approach for Obtaining Free Osteocutaneous Rib Grafts. Plast. Reconstr. Surg., 62:676–685, 1978.

10. Arnold, P.G., and Hodgkinson, D.: Extensor Digitorum Turn-Down Muscle Flap. Plast. Reconstr. Surg., 66:599–604, 1980.

11. Arnold, P.G., and Irons, G.B.: The Greater Omentum: Extensions in Transposition and Free Transfer. Plast. Reconstr. Surg., 67:169–176, 1981.

12. Arnold, P.G., and Irons, G.B.: Lower-Extremity Muscle Flaps. Orthop. Clin. North Am., 15:441–449, 1984.

13. Arnold, P.G., and Mixter, R.C.: Making the Most of the Gastrocnemius Muscles. Plast. Reconstr. Surg., 72:38–48, 1983.

14. Aronson, J.; Johnson, E.; and Harp, J.H.: Local Bone Transportation for Treatment of Intercalary Defects by the Ilizarov Technique: Biomechanical and Clinical Considerations. Clin. Orthop., 243:71–79, 1989.

15. Asco-Seljavaara, S.; Slatis, P.; Kannisto, M.; and Sundell, B.: Management of Infected Fractures of the Tibia With Associated Soft Tissue Loss: Experience With External Fixation, Bone Grafting and Soft Tissue Reconstruction Using Pedicle Muscle Flaps or Microvascular Composite Tissue Grafts. Brit. J. Plast. Surg., 38:546–555, 1985.

16. Azuma, H.; Kondo, T.; Mikami, M.; and Harii, K.: Treatment of Chronic Osteomyelitis by Transplantation of Autogenous Omentum With Microvascular Anastomosis. Acta Orthop. Scand. 47:271–275, 1976.

17. Bach, A.W., and Hansen, S.T., Jr.: Delayed Union, Nonunion, and Malunion of the Tibial Shaft. *In* Evarts, C.M. (ed.): Surgery of the Musculoskeletal System, Vol. 3, pp. 63–68. New York, Churchill Livingstone, 1983.

18. Bach, A.W., and Hansen, S.T., Jr.: Plates Versus External Fixation in Severe Open Tibial Shaft Fractures: A Randomized Trial. Clin. Orthop., 241:89–93, 1989.

19. Baek, S.M.: Two New Cutaneous Free Flaps: The Medial and Lateral Thigh Flaps. Plast. Reconstr. Surg., 71:354–363, 1983.

20. Baksi, D.P.: Treatment of Post-Traumatic Avascular Necrosis of the Femoral Head by Multiple Drilling and Muscle-Pedicle Bone Grafting: Preliminary Report. J. Bone Joint Surg., 65B:268–273, 1983.

21. Barclay, T.L.; Cardoso, E.; Sharpe, D.T.; and Crockett, D.J.: Repair of Lower Leg Injuries with Fascio-Cutaneous Flaps. Brit. J. Plast. Surg., 35:127–132, 1982.

22. Barclay, T.L.; Sharpe, D.T.; and Chisholm, E.M.: Cross-Leg Fasciocutaneous Flaps. Plast. Reconstr. Surg., 72:843–846, 1983.

23. Barfod, B., and Pers, M.: Gastrocnemius-Plasty for Primary Closure of Compound Injuries of the Knee. J. Bone Joint Surg., 52B:124–127, 1970.

24. Barfred, T., and Reumert, T.: Myoplasty for Covering Exposed Bone or Joint on the Lower Leg. Acta Orthop. Scand., 44:532–538, 1973.

25. Bartlett, S.P.; May, J.W., Jr.; and Yaremchuk, M.J.: The Latissimus Dorsi Muscle: A Fresh Cadaver Study of the Primary Neurovascular Pedicle. Plast. Reconstr. Surg., 67: 631–636, 1981.

26. Barwick, W.J.; Goodkind, D.J.; and Serafin, D.: The Free Scapular Flap. Plast. Reconstr. Surg., 69:779–785, 1982.

27. Bassett, C.A.L.: Current Concepts of Bone Formation. J. Bone Joint Surg., 44A:1217–1244, 1962.

28. Batten, R.L.; Donaldson, L.J.; and Aldridge, M.J.: Experience With the AO Method in the Treatment of 142 Cases of Fresh Fractures of the Tibial Shaft Treated in the United Kingdom. Injury, 10:108–114, 1978.

29. Baudet, J.; LeMaire, J.-M.; and Guimberteau, J.-C.: Ten Free Groin Flaps. Plast. Reconstr. Surg., 57:577–595, 1976.

30. Baudet, J.; Panconi, B.; Caix, P.; Schoofs, M.; Amarante, J.; and Kaddoura, R.: The Composite Fibula and Soleus Free Transfer. Int. J. Microsurg., 4:10–26, 1982.

31. Bauer, G.C.; Edwards, P.; and Widmark, P.H.: Shaft Fractures of the Tibia: Etiology of Poor Results in a Consecutive Series of 173 Fractures. Acta Chir. Scand., 124:386–393, 1962.

32. Becker, R.O., and Spadaro, J.A.: Treatment of Orthopaedic Infections with Electrically Generated Silver Ions: A Preliminary Report. J. Bone Joint Surg., 60A:871–881, 1978.

33. Behrens, F.: General Theory and Principles of External Fixation. Clin. Orthop., 241:15–23, 1989.

34. Bennett, J.E., and Kahn, R.A.: Surgical Management of Soft Tissue Defects of the Ankle–Heel Region. J. Trauma, 12:696–703, 1972.

35. Berger, A.: The Plastic Repair of Large Soft Tissue Defects. *In* Tscherne, H., and Gotzen, L. (eds.): Fractures With Soft Tissue Injuries, pp. 139–148. New York, Springer-Verlag, 1984.

36. Berggren, A.; Weiland, A.J.; and Dorfman, H.: Free Vascularized Bone Grafts: Factors Affecting Their Survival and Ability to Heal to Recipient Bone Defects. Plast. Reconstr. Surg., 69:19–29, 1982.

37. Berggren, A.; Weiland, A.J.; and Dorfman, H.: The Effect of Prolonged Ischemia Time on Osteocyte and Osteoblast Survival in Composite Bone Grafts Revascularized by Microvascular Anastomoses. Plast. Reconstr. Surg., 69:290–298, 1982.

38. Berggren, A.; Weiland, A.J.; and Ostrup, L.T.: Bone Scintigraphy in Evaluating the Viability of Composite Bone Grafts Revascularized by Microvascular Anastomoses,

Conventional Autogenous Bone Grafts and Free Non-Vascularized Periosteal Grafts. J. Bone Joint Surg., 64A: 799–809, 1982.

39. Berggren, A.; Weiland, A.J.; Ostrup, L.T.; and Dorfman, H.: The Effects of Storage Media and Perfusion on Osteoblast and Osteocyte Survival in Free Composite Bone Grafts. Microsurgery, 2:273–282, 1981.

40. Berggren, A.; Weiland, A.J.; Ostrup, L.T.; and Dorfman, H.: Microvascular Free Bone Transfer with Revascularization of the Medullary and Periosteal Circulation or the Periosteal Circulation Alone. J. Bone Joint Surg., 64A: 73–87, 1982.

41. Bohr, H.; Ravn, H.O.; and Werner, H.: The Osteogenic Effect of Bone Transplants in Rabbits. J. Bone Joint Surg., 50B:866–873, 1968.

42. Bondurant, F.J.; Cotler, H.B.; Buckle, R.; Miller-Crotchett, P.; and Browner, B.D.: The Medical and Economic Impact of Severely Injured Lower Extremities. J. Trauma, 28: 1270–1273, 1988.

43. Bos, K.E.: Bone Scintigraphy of Experimental Composite Bone Grafts Revascularized by Microvascular Anastomoses. Plast. Reconstr. Surg., 64:353–360, 1979.

44. Bosse, M.J.; Burgess, A.R.; and Brumback, R.J.: Evaluation and Treatment of the High-Energy Open Tibia Fracture. Adv. Orthop. Surg., 8:3–17, 1984.

45. Bostwick, J., III: Reconstruction of the Heel Pad by Muscle Transposition and Split Skin Graft. Surg. Gynecol. Obstet., 143:973–974, 1976.

46. Bostwick, J., III; Nahai, F.; Wallace, J.G.; and Vasconez, L.O.: Sixty Latissimus Dorsi Flaps. Plast. Reconstr. Surg., 63:31–41, 1979.

47. Bowen, J., and Meares, A.: Delayed Local Leg Flaps. Brit. J. Plast. Surg., 27:167–170, 1974.

48. Boyd, H.B.: The Treatment of Difficult and Unusual Non-Unions: With Special Reference to the Bridging of Defects. J. Bone Joint Surg., 25:535–552, 1943.

49. Bradford, D.S.: Anterior Vascular Pedicle Bone Grafting for the Treatment of Kyphosis. Spine, 5:328–323, 1980.

50. Brand, P.W.; Beach, R.B.; and Thompson, D.E.: Relative Tension and Potential Excursion of Muscles in the Forearm and Hand. J. Hand Surg., 6:209–219, 1981.

51. Briggs, J.G., Jr.; Huang, T.T.; and Lewis, S.R.: Use of Muscle Flaps in Treatment of Osteomyelitis of the Tibia. Tex. Med., 74:82–87, 1978.

52. Broadwater, J.R., and Stair, J.M.: Sternoclavicular Osteomyelitis: Coverage With a Pectoralis Major Muscle Flap. Surg. Rounds Orthop., September:47–50, 1988.

53. Brown, K.; Marie, P.; Lyszakowski, T.; Daniel, R.; and Cruess, R.: Epiphysial Growth After Free Fibular Transfer With and Without Microvascular Anastomosis: Experimental Study in the Dog. J. Bone Joint Surg., 65B:493–501, 1983.

54. Brown, K.L., and Cruess, R.L.: Bone and Cartilage Transplantation in Orthopaedic Surgery: A Review. J. Bone Joint Surg., 64A:270–279, 1982.

55. Brown, P.W.: The Prevention of Infection in Open Wounds. Clin. Orthop., 96:42–50, 1973.

56. Brown, P.W., and Urban, J.G.: Early Weight-Bearing Treatment of Open Fractures of the Tibia. J. Bone Joint Surg., 51A:59–75, 1969.

57. Brown, R.F.: The Management of Traumatic Tissue Loss in the Lower Limb, Especially When Complicated by Skeletal Injury. Brit. J. Plast. Surg., 18:26–50, 1965.

58. Brownstein, M.L.; Gordon, L.; and Buncke, H.J., Jr.: The Use of Microvascular Free Groin Flaps for the Closure of Difficult Lower Extremity Wounds. Surg. Clin. North Am., 57:977–985, 1977.

59. Buchman, J., and Blair, J.E.: Penicillin in the Treatment of Chronic Osteomyelitis: A Preliminary Report. Arch. Surg., 51:81–92, 1945.

60. Buchman, J., and Blair, J.E.: The Surgical Management of Chronic Osteomyelitis by Saucerization, Primary Closure, and Antibiotic Control: Preliminary Report on Use of Aureomycin. J. Bone Joint Surg., 33A:107–118, 1951.

61. Buncke, H.J., Jr.; Furnas, D.W.; Gordon, L.; and Achauer, B.M.: Free Osteocutaneous Flap From a Rib to the Tibia. Plast. Reconstr. Surg., 59:799–805, 1977.

62. Bunkis, J.; Walton, R.L.; and Mathes, S.J.: The Rectus Abdominis Free Flap for Lower Extremity Reconstruction. Ann. Plast. Surg., 11:373–380, 1983.

63. Burchardt, H.: The Biology of Bone Graft Repair. Clin. Orthop., 174:28–42, 1983.

64. Burchardt, H., and Enneking, W.F.: Transplantation of Bone. Surg. Clin. North Am., 58:403–427, 1978.

65. Burkhalter, W.E.: Open Injuries of the Lower Extremity. Surg. Clin. North Am., 53:1439–1457, 1973.

66. Burri, C.: Chronic Post-Traumatic Osteomyelitis. In Burri, C. (ed.): Post-Traumatic Osteomyelitis, pp. 163–243. Bern, Hans Huber, 1975.

67. Burri, C.: Results of Therapy. In Burri, C. (ed.): Post-Traumatic Osteomyelitis, pp. 245–280. Bern, Hans Huber, 1975.

68. Burri, C.: Complications of Post-Traumatic Osteomyelitis. In Burri, C. (ed.): Post-Traumatic Osteomyelitis, pp. 281–295. Bern, Hans Huber, 1975.

69. Burri, C.: Frequency and Contributing Factors in Post-Traumatic Osteomyelitis. In Burri, C. (ed.): Post-Traumatic Osteomyelitis. pp. 19–70. Bern, Hans Huber, 1975.

70. Burri, C.: Acute Post-Traumatic Osteomyelitis. In Burri, C. (ed.): Post-Traumatic Osteomyelitis, pp. 111–161. Bern, Hans Huber, 1975.

71. Burri, C.: Historical Review. In Burri, C. (ed.): Post-Traumatic Osteomyelitis, pp. 7–17. Bern, Hans Huber, 1975.

72. Burri, C.: Summary and Conclusions. In Burri, C. (ed.): Post-Traumatic Osteomyelitis, pp. 296–304. Bern, Hans Huber, 1975.

73. Burwell, R.G.: The Fate of Bone Grafts. In Apley, A.G. (ed.): Recent Advances in Orthopaedics, pp. 115–207. London, J & A Churchill, 1969.

74. Butt, W.P.: The Radiology of Infection. Clin. Orthop., 95: 20–30, 1973.

75. Byrd, H.S.: Lower Extremity Reconstruction. Sel. Read. Plast. Surg., 1:1–26, 1982.

76. Byrd, H.S.; Cierny, G., III; and Tebbetts, J.B.: The Management of Open Tibial Fractures With Associated Soft-

Tissue Loss: External Pin Fixation With Early Flap Coverage. Plast. Reconstr. Surg., 68:73–79, 1981.

77. Byrd, H.S.; Spicer, T.E.; and Cierny, G., III: The Management of Open Tibial Fractures. Plast. Reconstr. Surg., 76: 719–728, 1985.

78. Cabanela, M.E.: Open Cancellous Bone Grafting of Infected Bone Defects. Orthop. Clin. North Am., 15:427–440, 1984.

79. Caffee, H.H., and Asokan, R.: Tensor Fascia Lata Musculocutaneous Free Flaps. Plast. Reconstr. Surg., 68:195–200, 1981.

80. Campanacci, M., and Zanoli, S.: Double Tibiofibular Synostosis (Fibula Pro Tibia) for Non-Union and Delayed Union of the Tibia. J. Bone Joint Surg., 48A:44–56, 1966.

81. Campbell, R.D., Jr.: Treatment of Tibial Shaft Fractures. In Wade, P.A. (ed.): Surgical Treatment of Trauma, pp. 635–672. New York, Grune & Stratton, 1960.

82. Campbell, W.C.: Transference of the Fibula as an Adjunct to Free Bone Graft in Tibial Deficiency: Report of Three Cases. J. Orthop. Surg., 7:625–631, 1979.

83. Cannon, B.: Flaps Old and New. J. Hand Surg., 6:1–2, 1981.

84. Cannon, B.; Lischer, C.E.; Davis, W.B.; Chasko, S.; Moore, A.; Murray, J.E.; and McDowell, A.: The Use of Open Jump Flaps in Lower Extremity Repairs. Plast. Reconstr. Surg., 2:336–341, 1947.

85. Carnesale, P.G.: Osteomyelitis. In Crenshaw, A.H. (ed.): Campbell's Operative Orthopaedics, 7th ed., pp. 651–675. St. Louis, C.V. Mosby, 1987.

86. Carpenter, E.B.: Management of Fractures of the Shaft of the Tibia and Fibula. J. Bone Joint Surg., 48A:1640–1646, 1966.

87. Carr, A.J.; MacDonald, D.A.; and Waterhouse, N.: The Blood Supply of the Osteocutaneous Free Fibular Graft. J. Bone Joint Surg., 70B:319–321, 1988.

88. Caudle, R.J., and Stern, P.J.: Severe Open Fractures of the Tibia. J. Bone Joint Surg., 69A:801–807, 1987.

89. Chacha, P.B.: Salvage of Severe Open Fractures of the Tibia That Might Have Required Amputation. Injury, 2: 154–172, 1973.

90. Chacha, P.B.: Vascularized Pedicular Bone Grafts. Int. Orthop., 8:117–138, 1984.

91. Chacha, P.B.; Ahmed, M.; and Daruwalla, J.S.: Vascular Pedicle Graft of the Ipsilateral Fibula for Nonunion of the Tibia With a Large Defect: An Experimental and Clinical Study. J. Bone Joint Surg., 63B:244–253, 1981.

92. Chang, N., and Mathes, S.J.: Comparison of the Effect of Bacterial Inoculation in Musculocutaneous and Random-Pattern Flaps. Plast. Reconstr. Surg., 70:1–10, 1982.

93. Chapman, M.W.: Closed Intramedullary Bone-Grafting and Nailing of Segmental Defects of the Femur. J. Bone Joint Surg., 62A:1004–1008, 1980.

94. Chapman, M.W., and Hansen, S.T., Jr.: Open Fractures—Part II: Current Concepts in the Management of Open Fractures. In Rockwood, C.A., Jr., and Green, D.P. (eds.): Fractures in Adults, 2nd ed., pp. 199–218. Philadelphia, J.B. Lippincott, 1984.

95. Chapman, M.W., and Mahoney, M.: The Role of Early

96. Chase, S.W., and Herndon, C.H.: The Fate of Autogenous and Homogenous Bone Grafts: A Historical Review. J. Bone Joint Surg., 37A:809–885, 1955.

97. Chen, C.W.; Yu, Z.J.; and Wang, Y.: A New Method of Treatment of Congenital Tibial Pseudoarthrosis Using Free Vascularized Fibular Graft: A Preliminary Report. Ann. Acad. Med. Singapore, 8:465–473, 1979.

98. Chen, Z.W.; Chen, L.E.; Zhang, G.J.; and Yu, H.L.: Treatment of Tibial Defect With Vascularized Osteocutaneous Pedicled Transfer of Fibula. J. Reconstr. Microsurg., 2: 199–205, 1986.

99. Chen, Z.W., and Yan, W.: The Study and Clinical Application of the Osteocutaneous Flap of Fibula. Microsurgery, 4:11–16, 1983.

100. Chen, Z.W.; Yang, D.Y.; and Chang, D.S.: Free Muscle Transplantation. In Chen, C.W. (ed.): Microsurgery, pp. 232–260. New York, Springer Verlag, 1982.

101. Chen, Z.W.; Yang, D.Y.; and Chang, D.S.: Free Skin Flap Transfer. In Chen, C.W. (ed.): Microsurgery, pp. 198–231. New York, Springer Verlag, 1982.

102. Chen, Z.W.; Yang, D.Y.; and Chang, D.S.: Free Bone Grafting. In Chen, C.W. (ed.): Microsurgery, pp. 261–279. New York, Springer Verlag, 1982.

103. Chen, Z.W., and Yu, H.L.: Lower-Limb Replantation. In Urbaniak, J.R. (ed.): Microsurgery for Major Limb Reconstruction, pp. 67–73. St. Louis, C.V. Mosby, 1987.

104. Cierny, G., III; Byrd, H.S.; and Jones, R.E.: Primary Versus Delayed Soft Tissue Coverage for Severe Open Tibial Fractures: A Comparison of Results. Clin. Orthop., 178: 54–63, 1983.

105. Cierny, G., III, and Mader, J.T.: Management of Adult Osteomyelitis. In Evarts, C.M. (ed.): Surgery of the Musculoskeletal System, Vol. 4, pp. 15–35. New York, Churchill Livingstone, 1983.

106. Cierny, G., III; Mader, J.T.; and Pennick, J.J.: A Clinical Staging System for Adult Osteomyelitis. Contemporary Orthopaedics, 10:17–37, 1985.

107. Clancey, G.J., and Hansen, S.T., Jr.: Open Fractures of the Tibia: A Review of One Hundred and Two Cases. J. Bone Joint Surg., 60A:118–122, 1978.

108. Coates, J.B., Jr.; Cleveland, M.; and McFetridge, E.M.: Orthopedic Surgery in the European Theater of Operations, pp. 322–353. Office of the Surgeon General, Dept. of the Army, Washington, D.C., 1956.

109. Coleman, H.M.; Bateman, J.E.; Dale, G.M.; and Starr, D.E.: Cancellous Bone Grafts for Infected Bone Defects: A Single Stage Procedure. Surg. Gynecol. Obstet., 83:392–398, 1946.

110. Colen, S.R.; Romita, M.C.; Godfrey, N.V.; and Shaw, W.W.: Salvage Replantation. Clin. Plast. Surg., 10:125–131, 1983.

111. Compere, E.L.; Metzger, W.I.; and Mitra, R.N.: The Treatment of Pyogenic Bone and Joint Infections by Closed Irrigation (Circulation) With a Non-Toxic Detergent and One or More Antibiotics. J. Bone Joint Surg., 49A:614–624, 1967.

112. Connelly, J.R.: Pedicle Coverage in Non-Union of Fractures. Plast. Reconstr. Surg., 3:727–739, 1948.

113. Connelly, J.R.: Plastic Surgery in Bone Problems. Plast. Reconstr. Surg., 17:129–167, 1956.

114. Connelly, J.R.: Reconstructive Procedures of the Lower Extremity. *In* Grabb, W.C., and Smith, J.W. (eds.): Plastic Surgery—A Concise Guide to Clinical Practice, 2nd ed., pp. 914–930. Boston, Little, Brown, 1973.

115. Converse, J.M.: Early Skin Grafting in War Wounds of the Extremities. Ann. Surg., 115:321–335, 1942.

116. Cormack, G.C., and Lamberty, B.G.H.: A Classification of Fascio-Cutaneous Flaps According to Their Patterns of Vascularization. Brit. J. Plast. Surg., 37:80–87, 1984.

117. Coyler, R.A.: Infected Tibial Nonunions. Adv. Orthop. Surg., 10:201–206, 1987.

118. Crenshaw, A.H.: Delayed Union and Nonunion of Fractures. *In* Crenshaw, A.H. (ed.): Campbell's Operative Orthopaedics, 7th ed., pp. 2053–2118. St. Louis, C.V. Mosby, 1987.

119. Crikelair, G.F., and Symonds, C.F.: The Cross-Leg Pedicle in Chronic Osteomyelitis of the Lower Limb. Plast. Reconstr. Surg., 38:404–409, 1966.

120. Crock, H.V.: The Shafts of the Tibia and the Fibula. *In* Crock, H.V. (ed.): The Blood Supply of the Lower Limb Bones in Man, pp. 64–71. Edinburgh, E & S Livingstone, 1967.

121. Cruess, R.L.: Healing of Bone, Tendon, and Ligament. *In* Rockwood, C.A., Jr., and Green, D.P. (eds.): Fractures in Adults, 2nd ed., pp. 147–167. Philadelphia, J.B. Lippincott, 1984.

122. Dabb, R.W., and Conklin, W.T.: A Sensory Innervated Latissimus Dorsi Musculocutaneous Free Flap: Case Report. Microsurgery, 3:289–293, 1981.

123. Damholt, V.V.: Treatment of Chronic Osteomyelitis. Acta Orthop. Scand., 53:715–720, 1982.

124. Daniel, R.K.: Toward an Anatomical and Hemodynamic Classification of Skin Flaps. Plast. Reconstr. Surg., 56:330–332, 1975.

125. Daniel, R.K.: Free Rib Transfer by Microvascular Anastomoses. Plast. Reconstr. Surg., 59:737–738, 1977.

126. Daniel, R.K.: Clinical Microvascular Surgery and Free Tissue Transfers. *In* Grabb, W.C., and Smith, J.W. (eds.): Plastic Surgery, 3rd ed., pp. 660–684. Boston, Little, Brown, 1978.

127. Daniel, R.K., and May, J.W., Jr.: Free Flaps: An Overview. Clin. Orthop., 133:122–131, 1978.

128. Daniel, R.K., and Taylor, G.I.: Distant Transfer of an Island Flap by Microvascular Anastomoses: A Clinical Technique. Plast. Reconstr. Surg., 52:111–117, 1973.

129. Daniel, R.K., and Weiland, A.J.: Free Tissue Transfers for Upper Extremity Reconstruction. J. Hand Surg., 7:66–76, 1982.

130. Daniel, R.K., and Williams, H.B.: The Free Transfer of Skin Flaps by Microvascular Anastomoses—An Experimental Study and a Reappraisal. Plast. Reconstr. Surg., 52:16–31, 1973.

131. Davis, A.G.: Fibular Substitution for Tibial Defects. J. Bone Joint Surg., 25:229–237, 1944.

132. Davis, A.G.: Primary Closure of Compound-Fracture Wounds With Immediate Internal Fixation, Immediate Skin Graft, and Compression Dressings. J. Bone Joint Surg., 30A:405–415, 1948.

133. Davis, G.L.: Management of Open Wounds of Joints During the Vietnam War: A Preliminary Study. Clin. Orthop., 68:3–9, 1970.

134. Davis, J.B.: The Muscle-Pedicle Bone Graft in Hip Fusion. J. Bone Joint Surg., 36A:790–799, 1954.

135. Davis, J.B., and Taylor, A.N.: Muscle Pedicle Bone Grafts—Experimental Study. Arch. Surg., 65:330–336, 1952.

136. Davis, J.C.; Heckman, J.D.; DeLee, J.C.; and Buckwold, F.J.: Chronic Non-Hematogenous Osteomyelitis Treated with Adjuvant Hyperbaric Oxygen. J. Bone Joint Surg., 68A:1210–1217, 1986.

137. Dawson, R.L.: Complications of the Cross-Leg Flap Operation. Proc. R. Soc. Med., 65:2–5, 1972.

138. Day, B., and Shim, S.S.: Increased Femoral Head Vascularity After an Iliopsoas Muscle Pedicle Bone Graft. Surg. Forum., 30:494–496, 1979.

139. de Boer, H.H.; Verbout, A.J.; Nielsen, H.K.; and van der Eijken, J.W.: Free Vascularized Fibular Graft for Tibial Pseudarthrosis in Neurofibromatosis. Acta Orthop. Scand., 59:425–429, 1988.

140. Dehne, E.; Deffer, P.A.; Hall, R.M.; Brown, P.W.; and Johnson, E.V.: The Natural History of the Fractured Tibia. Surg. Clin. North Am., 41:1495–1513, 1961.

141. Dehne, E.; Metz, C.W.; Deffer, P.A.; and Hall, R.M.: Nonoperative Treatment of the Fractured Tibia by Immediate Weight Bearing. J. Trauma, 1:514–535, 1961.

142. DeLee, J.C., and Stiehl, J.B.: Open Tibia Fracture With Compartment Syndrome. Clin. Orthop., 160:175–184, 1981.

143. Dell, P.C., and Sheppard, J.E.: Vascularized Bone Grafts in the Treatment of Infected Forearm Nonunions. J. Hand Surg., 9A:653–658, 1984.

144. DeOliveira, J.C.: Bone Grafts and Chronic Osteomyelitis. J. Bone Joint Surg., 53B:672–683, 1971.

145. Dibbell, D.G., and Edstrom, L.E.: The Gastrocnemius Myocutaneous Flap. Clin. Plast. Surg., 7:45–50, 1980.

146. Dickson, W.A.; Dickson, M.G.; and Roberts, A.H.: The Complications of Fasciocutaneous Flaps. Ann. Plast. Surg., 19:234–237, 1987.

147. Doherty, J.H., and Patterson, R.L., Jr.: Fibular By-Pass Operation in the Treatment of Non-Union of the Tibia in Adults. J. Bone Joint Surg., 49A:1470–1471, 1967.

148. Doi, K.; Tominaga, S.; and Shibata, T.: Bone Grafts With Microvascular Anastomoses of Vascular Pedicles: An Experimental Study in Dogs. J. Bone Joint Surg., 54A:809–815, 1977.

149. Dombrowski, E.T., and Dunn, A.W.: Treatment of Osteomyelitis by Debridement and Closed Wound Irrigation–Suction. Clin. Orthop., 43:215–231, 1965.

150. Donski, P.K.; Buechler, U.; and Tschopp, H.M.: Surgical Dissection of the Fibula for Free Microvascular Transfer. Chir. Plast., 6:153–164, 1982.

151. Donski, P.K., and O'Brien, B.M.: Free Microvascular

Epiphyseal Transplantation: An Experimental Study in Dogs. Brit. J. Plast. Surg., 33:169–178, 1980.

152. dos Santos, L.F.: The Scapular Flap: A New Microsurgical Free Flap. Rev. Bras. Cir., 70:133–144, 1970.

153. dos Santos, L.F.: The Vascular Anatomy and Dissection of the Free Scapular Flap. Plast. Reconstr. Surg., 73:599–603, 1984.

154. Drabyn, G.A., and Avedian, L.: Ipsilateral Buttock Flap for Coverage of a Foot and Ankle Defect in a Young Child. Plast. Reconstr. Surg., 63:422–423, 1979.

155. Edwards, C.C.: Staged Reconstruction of Complex Open Tibial Fractures Using Hoffman External Fixation. Clin. Orthop., 178:130–161, 1983.

156. Edwards, C.C., and Jaworski, M.F.: Hoffman External Fixation in Open Tibial Fractures With Tissue Loss. Orthop. Trans., 3:261–262, 1979.

157. Edwards, C.C.; Simmons, S.C.; Browner, B.D.; and Weigel, M.C.: Severe Open Tibial Fractures: Results Treating 202 Injuries with External Fixation. Clin. Orthop., 230:98–115, 1988.

158. Edwards, P.: Fracture of the Shaft of the Tibia: 492 Consecutive Cases in Adults: Importance of Soft Tissue Injury. Acta Orthop. Scand. (Suppl.) 76:9–59, 1965.

159. Enneking, W.F.; Burchardt, H.; Puhl, J.J.; and Piotrowski, G.: Physical and Biological Aspects of Repair in Dog Cortical-Bone Transplants. J. Bone Joint Surg., 57A:237–252, 1975.

160. Enneking, W.F.; Eady, J.L.; and Burchardt, H.: Autogenous Cortical Bone Grafts in the Reconstruction of Segmental Skeletal Defects. J. Bone Joint Surg., 62A:1039–1058, 1980.

161. Epps, C.H., Jr.: Principles of Amputation Surgery in Trauma. In Evarts, C.M. (ed.): Surgery of the Musculoskeletal System, Vol. 4, pp. 7–23. New York, Churchill Livingstone, 1983.

162. Epps, C.H., Jr., and Adams, J.P.: Wound Management in Open Fractures. Am. Surg., 27:766–769, 1961.

163. Essex-Lopresti, P.: The Open Wound in Trauma. Lancet, 258:745–751, 1950.

164. Etter, C.; Burri, C.; Claes, L.; Kinzl, L.; and Raible, M.: Treatment by External Fixation of Open Fractures Associated With Severe Soft Tissue Damage of the Leg. Clin. Orthop., 178:80–88, 1983.

165. Evarts, C.M., and Mayer, P.J.: Complications. In Rockwood, C.A., Jr., and Green, D.P. (eds.): Fractures in Adults, 2nd ed., pp. 219–294. Philadelphia, J.B. Lippincott, 1984.

166. Feldman, J.J.; Cohen, B.E.; and May, J.W., Jr.: The Medial Gastrocnemius Myocutaneous Flap. Plast. Reconstr. Surg., 61:531–539, 1978.

167. Ferreira, M.C.; Monteiro, A.A.; and Besteiro, J.M.: Free Flaps for Reconstruction of the Lower Extremity. Ann. Plast. Surg., 6:475–481, 1981.

168. Findlay, J.A.: The Motor-cycle Tibia. Injury, 4:75–78, 1972.

169. Fisher, J.: External Oblique Fasciocutaneous Flap for Elbow Coverage. Plast. Reconstr. Surg., 75:51–61, 1985.

170. Fitzgerald, R.H., Jr.: The Epidemiology of Nosocomial Infections of the Musculoskeletal System. In Groschel, D. (ed.): Hospital-Associated Infections in the General Hospital Population and Specific Measures of Control, 3rd ed., pp. 25–35. New York, Dekker, 1979.

171. Fitzgerald, R.H., Jr.: Experimental Osteomyelitis: Description of a Canine Model and the Role of Depot Administration of Antibiotics in the Prevention and Treatment of Sepsis. J. Bone Joint Surg., 65A:371–380, 1983.

172. Fitzgerald, R.H., Jr.; Ruttle, Paul E.; Arnold, P.G.; Kelly, P.J.; and Irons, G.B.: Local Muscle Flaps in the Treatment of Osteomyelitis. J. Bone Joint Surg., 67A:175–185, 1985.

173. Fogdestam, I.; Hamilton, R.; and Markhede, G.: Microvascular Osteocutaneous Groin Flap in the Treatment of an Ununited Tibial Fracture With Chronic Osteitis: A Case Report. Acta Orthop. Scand., 51:175–179, 1980.

174. Foster, R.J.; Barry, R.J.; Holloway, A.; and Burney, D.W., III: A 50-cm Fillet Flap for Preservation of Maximal Lower Extremity Residual Limb Length. Clin. Orthop., 178:216–219, 1983.

175. Foucher, G.; van Genechten, F.; Merle, N.; and Michon, J.: A Compound Radial Artery Forearm Flap in Hand Surgery: An Original Modification of the Chinese Forearm Flap. Brit. J. Plast. Surg., 37:139–148, 1984.

176. Freeland, A.E., and Mutz, S.B.: Posterior Bone-Grafting for Infected Ununited Fracture of the Tibia. J. Bone Joint Surg., 58A:653–657, 1976.

177. Frykman, G.K., and Leung, V.C.L.: Free Vascularized Flaps for Lower Extremity Reconstruction. Orthopedics, 9:841–848, 1986.

178. Fujimaki, A., and Yamauchi, Y.: Vascularized Fibular Grafting for Treatment of Aseptic Necrosis of the Femoral Head—Preliminary Results in Four Cases. Microsurgery, 4:17–22, 1983.

179. Fujino, T., and Harashina, T.: Vascularized Free Flap Transfers. Clin. Orthop., 133:154–157, 1978.

180. Garrett, J.C., and Buncke, H.J., Jr.: Free Groin Flap Transfer for Skin Defects Associated With Orthopaedic Problems of the Extremities. Am. Surg., 45:597–601, 1979.

181. Ger, R.: The Management of Pretibial Skin Loss. Surgery, 63:757–763, 1968.

182. Ger, R.: The Management of Open Fractures of the Tibia With Skin Loss. J. Trauma, 10:112–121, 1970.

183. Ger, R.: The Technique of Muscle Transposition in the Operative Treatment of Traumatic and Ulcerative Lesions of the Leg. J. Trauma, 11:502–510, 1971.

184. Ger, R.: Muscle Transposition for Treatment and Prevention of Chronic Post-Traumatic Osteomyelitis of the Tibia. J. Bone Joint Surg., 59A:784–791, 1977.

185. Ger, R., and Efron, G.: New Operative Approach in the Treatment of Chronic Osteomyelitis of the Tibial Diaphysis: A Preliminary Report. Clin. Orthop., 70:165–169, 1970.

186. Ghormley, R.K., and Lipscomb, P.R.: The Use of Untubed Pedicle Grafts in the Repair of Deep Defects of the Foot and Ankle: Technique and Results. J. Bone Joint Surg., 26:483–488, 1944.

187. Gilbert, A.: Vascularized Transfer of the Fibular Shaft. Int. J. Microsurg., 1:100–102, 1979.

188. Gilbert, A.: Free Vascularized Bone Grafts. Int. Surg., 66:27–31, 1981.

189. Gilbert, A., and Teot, L.: The Free Scapula Flap. Plast. Reconstr. Surg., 69:601–604, 1982.

190. Girdlestone, G.R., and Foley, W.B.: Extensive Loss of Tibial Diaphysis: Tibio-Fibular Grafting. Brit. J. Surg., 20:467–471, 1933.

191. Godina, M.: Preferential Use of End-to-Side Arterial Anastomoses in Free Flap Transfers. Plast. Reconstr. Surg., 64:673–682, 1979.

192. Godina, M.: Discussion: The Free Scapula Flap. Plast. Reconstr. Surg., 69:786–787, 1982.

193. Godina, M.: Early Microsurgical Reconstruction of Complex Trauma of the Extremities. Plast. Reconstr. Surg., 78:285–292, 1986.

194. Godina, M.: The Tailored Latissimus Dorsi Free Flap. Plast. Reconstr. Surg., 80:304–306, 1987.

195. Goldman, M.A.; Johnson, R.K.; and Grossberg, N.M.: Artificial Circulation: A New Approach to Chronic Osteomyelitis. Am. J. Orthop., 2:63–66, 1960.

196. Goldstrohm, G.L.; Mears, D.C.; and Swartz, W.M.: The Results of 39 Fractures Complicated by Major Segmental Bone Loss and/or Leg Length Discrepancy. J. Trauma, 24:50–58, 1984.

197. Gordon, L.: Microsurgical Reconstruction of the Extremities, p. 81. New York, Springer-Verlag, 1988.

198. Gordon, L.; Buncke, H.J.; and Alpert, B.S.: Free Latissimus Dorsi Muscle Flap with Split-Thickness Skin Graft Cover: A Report of 16 Cases. Plast. Reconstr. Surg., 70:173–178, 1982.

199. Gordon, L.; Buncke, H.J.; Alpert, B.S.; Wilson, C.; and Koch, R.A.: Free Vascularized Osteocutaneous Transplants from the Groin for Delayed Primary Closure in the Management of Loss of Soft-Tissue and Bone in the Hand and Wrist. J. Bone Joint Surg., 67A:958–964, 1985.

200. Gordon, L.; Weulker, N.; and Jergesen, H.: Vascularized Fibular Grafting for the Treatment of Congenital Pseudarthrosis of the Tibia. Orthopedics, 9:825–832, 1986.

201. Gorman, P.W.; Barnes, C.L.; Fischer, T.J.; McAndrew, M.P.; and Moore, M.M.: Soft-Tissue Reconstruction in Severe Lower Extremity Trauma: A Review. Clin. Orthop., 243:57–64, 1989.

202. Gothman, L.: Arterial Changes in Experimental Fractures of the Rabbit's Tibia Treated With Intramedullary Nailing: A Microangiographic Study. Acta Chir. Scand., 120:289–302, 1960.

203. Gothman, L.: The Arterial Pattern of the Rabbit's Tibia After the Application of an Intramedullary Nail: A Microangiographic Study. Acta Chir. Scand., 120:211–220, 1961.

204. Gotzen, L., and Haas, N.: The Operative Treatment of Tibial Shaft Fractures with Soft Tissue Injuries. In Tscherne, H., and Gotzen, L. (eds.): Fractures With Soft Tissue Injuries, pp. 46–74. New York, Springer-Verlag, 1984.

205. Grace, T.G., and Eversmann, W.W.: The Management of Segmental Bone Loss Associated with Forearm Fractures. J. Bone Joint Surg., 62A:1150–1159, 1980.

206. Green, S.A.: Septic Nonunion. In Uhthoff, H. (ed.): Current Concepts of External Fixation of Fractures, pp. 221–233. New York, Springer-Verlag, 1982.

207. Green, S.A.: Ilizarov External Fixation Technical and Anatomic Considerations. Bull. Hosp. Jt. Dis. Orthop. Inst., 48:1:28–35, 1988.

208. Green, S.A., and Dlabal, T.A.: The Open Bone Graft for Septic Nonunion. Clin. Orthop., 180:117–124, 1983.

209. Greene, T.L., and Beatty, M.E.: Soft Tissue Coverage for Lower-Extremity Trauma: Current Practice and Techniques. A Review. J. Orthop. Trauma, 2:158–173, 1988.

210. Gregory, C.F.: Open Fractures—Part I. In Rockwood, C.A., Jr., and Green, D.P. (eds.): Fractures in Adults, 2nd ed., pp. 169–198. Philadelphia, J.B. Lippincott, 1984.

211. Gregory, R.T.; Gould, R.J.; Peclet, M.; Wagner, J.S.; Gilbert, D.A.; Wheeler, J.R.; Snyder, S.O.; Gayle, R.G.; and Schwab, C.W.: The Mangled Extremity Syndrome (M.E.S.): A Severity Grading System for Multisystem Injury of the Extremity. J. Trauma, 25:1147–1150, 1985.

212. Greminger, R.F., and Leather, R.P.: Knee Salvage Utilizing the Myocutaneous Principle. Plast. Reconstr. Surg., 73:131–136, 1984.

213. Griffiths, J.C.: Defects in Long Bones from Severe Neglected Osteitis. J. Bone Joint Surg., 50B:813–821, 1968.

214. Gruninger, R.P.; Tsukayama, D.T.; and Wicklund, B.: Antibiotic-Impregnated PMMA Beads in Bone and Prosthetic Joint Infections. In Gustilo, R.B.; Gruninger, R.P.; and Tsukayama, D.T. (eds.): Orthopaedic Infection: Diagnosis and Treatment, pp. 66–74. Philadelphia, W.B. Saunders, 1989.

215. Guba, A.M., Jr.: The Use of Free Vascular Tissue Transfers in Lower Extremity Injuries. Adv. Orthop. Surg., 7:60–68, 1983.

216. Guo, F., and Ding, B.F.: Vascularized Free Fibula Graft in Bone Tumors: Report of 3 Cases. Chin. Med. J., 93:745–752, 1980.

217. Guo, F., and Ding, B.F.: Vascularized Free Fibula Transfer in the Treatment of Bone Tumours: Report of Three Cases. Arch. Orthop. Trauma Surg., 98:209–215, 1981.

218. Gupta, R.C.: Treatment of Chronic Osteomyelitis by Radical Excision of Bone and Secondary Skin-Grafting. J. Bone Joint Surg., 55A:371–374, 1973.

219. Gustilo, R.B.: Management of Open Fractures: An Analysis of 673 Cases. Minn. Med., 54:185–189, 1971.

220. Gustilo, R.B.: Use of Antimicrobials in the Management of Fractures. Arch. Surg., 114:805–808, 1979.

221. Gustilo, R.B.: Principles of the Management of Open Fractures. In Sledge, C.B. (ed.): Management of Open Fractures and Their Complications, pp. 15–54. Philadelphia, W.B. Saunders, 1982.

222. Gustilo, R.B.: Open Fractures With Arterial and Nerve Injuries. In Sledge, C.B. (ed.): Management of Open Fractures and Their Complications, pp. 118–123. Philadelphia, W.B. Saunders, 1982.

223. Gustilo, R.B.: Management of Infected Nonunion. In Sledge, C.B. (ed.): Management of Open Fractures and Their Complications. pp. 159–182. Philadelphia, W.B. Saunders, 1982.

224. Gustilo, R.B.: Management of Infected Fractures. In Sledge, C.B. (ed.): Management of Open Fractures and Their Complications, pp. 133–158. Philadelphia, W.B. Saunders, 1982.

225. Gustilo, R.B.: Management of Infected Nonunion. In

Evarts, C.M. (ed.): Surgery of the Musculoskeletal System, Vol. 4, pp. 135–151. New York, Churchill Livingstone, 1983.

226. Gustilo, R.B.: Management of Infected Fractures. *In* Evarts, C.M. (ed.): Surgery of the Musculoskeletal System, Vol. 4, pp. 105–134. New York, Churchill Livingstone, 1983.

227. Gustilo, R.B.: Management of Acutely Infected Fractures. *In* Gustilo, R.B.; Gruninger, R.P.; and Tsukayama, D.T. (eds.): Orthopaedic Infection: Diagnosis and Treatment, pp. 123–138. Philadelphia, W.B. Saunders, 1989.

228. Gustilo, R.B.: Management of Infected Nonunion. *In* Gustilo, R.B.; Gruninger, R.P.; and Tsukayama, D.T. (eds.): Orthopaedic Infection: Diagnosis and Treatment, pp. 139–154. Philadelphia, W.B. Saunders, 1989.

229. Gustilo, R.B.: Management of Chronic Osteomyelitis. *In* Gustilo, R.B.; Gruninger, R.P.; and Tsukayama, D.T. (eds.): Orthopaedic Infection: Diagnosis and Treatment, pp. 155–165. Philadelphia, W.B. Saunders, 1989.

230. Gustilo, R.B.: Management of Open Fractures. *In* Gustilo, R.B.; Gruninger, R.P.; and Tsukayama, D.T. (eds.): Orthopaedic Infection: Diagnosis and Treatment, pp. 87–117. Philadelphia, W.B. Saunders, 1989.

231. Gustilo, R.B., and Anderson, J.T.: Prevention of Infection in the Treatment of One Thousand and Twenty-Five Open Fractures of Long Bones. J. Bone Joint Surg., 58A:453–458, 1976.

232. Gustilo, R.B.; Gruninger, R.P.; and Davis, T.: Classification of Type III (Severe) Open Fractures Relative to Treatment and Results. Orthopedics, 10:1781–1788, 1987.

233. Gustilo, R.B., and Mendoza, R.M.: Results of Treatment of 1400 Open Fractures. *In* Gustilo, R.B. (ed.): Management of Open Fractures and Their Complications, pp. 202–208. Philadelphia, W.B. Saunders, 1982.

234. Gustilo, R.B.; Mendoza, R.M.; and Williams, D.N.: Problems in the Management of Type III (Severe) Open Fractures: A New Classification of Type III Open Fractures. J. Trauma, 24:742–746, 1984.

235. Gustilo, R.B.; Simpson, L.; Nixon, R.; Ruiz, A.; and Indeck, W.: Analysis of 511 Open Fractures. Clin. Orthop., 66:148–154, 1969.

236. Haddad, R.J., Jr., and Drez, D.: Salvage Procedure for Defects in the Forearm Bones. Clin. Orthop., 104:183–190, 1974.

237. Hagan, K.F., and Buncke, H.J.: Treatment of Congenital Pseudarthrosis of the Tibia With Free Vascularized Bone Graft. Clin. Orthop., 166:34–44, 1982.

238. Hall, B.B.; Fitzgerald, R.H., Jr.; and Rosenblatt, J.E.: Anaerobic Osteomyelitis. J. Bone Joint Surg., 65A:30–35, 1983.

239. Hallock, G.: Cutaneous Coverage for the Difficult Lower Extremity Wound. Contemporary Orthopaedics, 10:17–26, 1985.

240. Hallock, G.: Severe Lower-Extremity Injury: The Rationale for Microsurgical Reconstruction. Orthop. Rev., 15:77–92, 1986.

241. Hallock, G.G.: Function Preservation With the Soleus Muscle Flap. Orthop. Rev., 14:472–477, 1985.

242. Hamilton, S.G., and Morrison, W.A.: The Scapular Free Flap. Brit. J. Plast. Surg., 35:2–7, 1982.

243. Hampton, O.P., Jr.: Delayed Internal Fixation of Compound Battle Fractures in the Mediterranean Theater of Operations: A Follow-Up Study in the Zone of Interior. Ann. Surg., 123:1–26, 1946.

244. Hampton, O.P., Jr.: Basic Principles in Management of Open Fractures. J.A.M.A. 159:417–419, 1955.

245. Hanel, D.P.: Vascularized Tissue Transfer: An Adjunct to the Treatment of Osteomyelitis. Orthop. Rev., 18:595–608, 1989.

246. Hansen, S.T., Jr.: The Type-IIIC Tibial Fracture: Salvage or Amputation (editorial). J. Bone Joint Surg., 69A:799–800, 1987.

247. Hansen, S.T., Jr.: Overview of the Severely Traumatized Lower Limb: Reconstruction Versus Amputation. Clin. Orthop., 243:17–19, 1989.

248. Hardaker, W.T., Jr.; Ward, W.T.; and Goldner, J.L.: External Fixation in the Management of Severe Musculoskeletal Trauma. Orthopedics, 5:437–444, 1981.

249. Harii, K.: Clinical Application of Free Omental Flap Transfer. Clin. Plast. Surg. 5:273–281, 1978.

250. Harii, K.: The Groin Flap. *In* Harii, K. (ed.): Microvascular Tissue Transfer, pp. 48–57. Tokyo, Igaku-Shoin, 1983.

251. Harii, K.: Microvascular Free Flaps for Skin Coverage: Indications and Selections of Donor Sites. Clin. Plast. Surg., 10:37–54, 1983.

252. Harii, K.: The Free Vascularized Bone Graft and Free Osteocutaneous Flap. *In* Harii, K. (ed.): Microvascular Tissue Transfer, pp. 157–176. Tokyo, Igaku-Shoin, 1983.

253. Harii, K.; Daniel, R.; Finseth, F.; and Ferreira, M.C.: Report of the Subcommittee on Microvascular Flaps. J. Hand Surg., 8:734–735, 1983.

254. Harii, K., and Ohmori, K.: Direct Transfer of Large Free Groin Skin Flaps to the Lower Extremity Using Microvascular Anastomoses. Chir. Plast., 3:1–14, 1975.

255. Harii, K., and Ohmori, K.: Free Skin Flap Transfer. Clin. Plast. Surg., 3:111–127, 1976.

256. Harii, K.; Ohmori, K.; and Sekiguchi, J.: The Free Musculocutaneous Flap. Plast. Reconstr. Surg., 57:294–303, 1976.

257. Harii, K.; Ohmori, K.; and Torii, S.: Free Gracilis Muscle Transplantation, With Microneurovascular Anastomoses for the Treatment of Facial Paralysis: A Preliminary Report. Plast. Reconstr. Surg., 57:133–143, 1976.

258. Harii, K.; Yamada, A.; Ishihara, K.; Miki, Y.; and Itoh, M.: A Free Transfer of Both Latissimus Dorsi and Serratus Anterior Flaps with Thoracodorsal Vessel Anastomoses. Plast. Reconstr. Surg., 70:620–629, 1982.

259. Harmon, P.H.: A Simplified Surgical Approach to the Posterior Tibia for Bone-Grafting and Fibular Transference. J. Bone Joint Surg., 27:496–498, 1945.

260. Harrison, D.H.: The Osteocutaneous Free Fibular Graft. J. Bone Joint Surg., 68B:804–807, 1968.

261. Harrison, D.H., and Morgan, B.D.: The Instep Island Flap to Resurface Plantar Defects. Brit. J. Plast. Surg., 34:315–318, 1981.

262. Harrison, S.H.: Fractures of the Tibia Complicated by Skin Loss. Brit. J. Plast. Surg., 21:262–276, 1968.

263. Harrison, S.H., and Saad, M.N.: The Sliding Transposition

Flap: Its Application to Leg Defects. Brit. J. Plast. Surg., 30:54–58, 1977.

264. Hartrampf, C.R., Jr.; Scheflan, M.; and Bostwick, J., III: The Flexor Digitorum Brevis Muscle Island Pedicle Flap: A New Dimension in Heel Reconstruction. Plast. Reconstr. Surg., 66:264–270, 1984.

265. Hartwell, S.W., and Evarts, C.M.: Secondary Coverage of Pretibial Skin Defects: Report of Four Representative Cases. Plast. Reconstr. Surg., 46:39–42, 1970.

266. Harvey, F.J.; Hodgkinson, A.H.T.; and Harvey, P.M.: Intramedullary Nailing in the Treatment of Open Fractures of the Tibia and Fibula. J. Bone Joint Surg., 57A:909–915, 1975.

267. Haw, C.S.; O'Brien, B.C.; and Kurata, T.: The Microsurgical Revascularization of Resected Segments of Tibia in the Dog. J. Bone Joint Surg., 60B:266–269, 1978.

268. Hazlett, J.W.: The Use of Cancellous Bone Grafts in the Treatment of Subacute and Chronic Osteomyelitis. J. Bone Joint Surg., 36B:584–590, 1954.

269. Henry, A.K.: Extensile Exposure, 2nd ed., pp. 241–276. London, E. Livingstone, 1966.

270. Hentz, V.R., and Pearl, R.M.: The irreplaceable Free Flap: Part I. Skeletal Reconstruction by Microvascular Free Bone Transfer. Ann. Plast. Surg., 10:36–42, 1983.

271. Heppenstall, R.B.; Goodwin, C.W.; and Brighton, C.T.: Fracture Healing in the Presence of Chronic Hypoxia. J. Bone Joint Surg., 58A:1153–1156, 1976.

272. Heslop, B.F.; Zeiss, I.M.; and Nisbet, N.W.: Studies on Transference of Bone. I. A Comparison of Autologous and Homologous Bone Implants With Reference to Osteocyte Survival, Osteogenesis and Host Reaction. Brit. J. Exp. Pathol., 441:269–287, 1960.

273. Hicks, J.H.: Amputation in Fractures of the Tibia. J. Bone Joint Surg., 46B:388–392, 1964.

274. Hicks, J.H.: Long-Term Follow-Up of a Series of Infected Fractures of the Tibia. Injury, 7:2–7, 1975.

275. Highsmith, L.S., and Phalen, G.S.: Sideswipe Fractures. Arch. Surg., 52:513–522, 1946.

276. Hill, H.; Nahai, F.; and Vasconez, L.O.: The Tensor Fascia Lata Myocutaneous Free Flap. Plast. Reconstr. Surg., 61:517–522, 1978.

277. Hirayama, T.; Suematsu, N.; Inoue, K.; Baitoh, C.; and Takemitsu, Y.: Free Vascularized Bone Grafts in Reconstruction of the Upper Extremity. J. Hand Surg., 10B:169–175, 1985.

278. Hoaglund, F.T., and States, J.D.: Factors Influencing the Rate of Healing in Tibial Shaft Fractures. Surg. Gynecol. Obstet. 124:71–76, 1967.

279. Hodgkinson, D.J., and Irons, G.B.: Newer Applications of the Cross-Leg Flap. Ann. Plast. Surg., 4:381–390, 1980.

280. Hoehn, J.G.; Jacobs, R.L.; and Karmody, A.: Replantation of the Foot. Surg. Rounds, 1:53–60, 1978.

281. Holden, C.E.: The Role of Blood Supply to Soft Tissue in the Healing of Diaphyseal Fractures. J. Bone Joint Surg., 54A:993–1000, 1972.

282. Horwitz, T.: Surgical Treatment of Chronic Osteomyelitis Complicating Fractures: A Study of 50 Patients. Clin. Orthop., 96:118–128, 1973.

283. Howe, H.R., Jr.; Poole, G.V., Jr.; Hansen, K.J.; Clark, T.; Plonk, G.W.; Koman, L.A.; and Pennell, T.C.: Salvage of Lower Extremities Following Combined Orthopedic and Vascular Trauma: A Predictive Salvage Index. Am. Surg., 53:205–208, 1987.

284. Hu, C.T.; Chang, C.W.; Su, K.L.; Shen, C.C.; and Shen, S.: Free Vascularised Bone Graft Using Microvascular Technique. Ann. Acad. Med. Singapore, 8:459–464, 1979.

285. Hu, Q.; Jiang, Q.; Su, G.; Shen, J.; and Shen, X.: Free Vascularized Bone Graft. Chin. Med. J., 93:753–757, 1980.

286. Huang, C.T.; Li, P.H.; and Kong, G.T.: Successful Restoration of a Traumatic Amputated Leg. Chin. Med. J., 84:641–645, 1965.

287. Huang, G.K.; Liu, Z.Z.; Shen, Y.L.; Hu, R.Q.; Miao, H.; and Yin, Z.Y.: Microvascular Free Transfer of Iliac Bone Based on the Deep Circumflex Iliac Vessels. Microsurgery, 2:113–120, 1980.

288. Hubbard, L.F.; Herndon, J.H.; and Buonanno, A.R.: Free Vascularized Fibula Transfer for Stabilization of the Thoracolumbar Spine: A Case Report. Spine, 10:891–893, 1985.

289. Hueston, J.T., and Gunter, G.S.: Primary Cross-Leg Flaps. Plast. Reconstr. Surg., 40:58–62, 1967.

290. Hunt, T.K., and Halliday, B.: Inflammation in Wounds: From "Laudable Pus" to Primary Repair and Beyond. In Hunt, T.K. (ed.): Wound Healing and Wound Infection: Theory and Surgical Practice, pp. 281–293. New York, Appleton-Century-Crofts, 1980.

291. Huntington, T.W.: A Case of Bone Transference: Use of a Segment of Fibula to Supply a Defect in the Tibia. Ann. Surg., 41:249–251, 1905.

292. Hurst, L.C.; Mirza, M.A.; and Spellman, W.: Vascularized Fibular Graft for Infected Loss of the Ulna: Case Report. J. Hand Surg., 7:498–501, 1982.

293. Hutchison, J.: The Fate of Experimental Bone Autografts and Homografts. Brit. J. Surg., 39:552–561, 1952.

294. Ikuta, Y.: Skeletal Muscle Transplantation in the Severely Injured Upper Extremity. In Serafin, D., and Buncke, H.J., Jr. (eds.): Microsurgical Composite Tissue Transplantation, pp. 587–604. St. Louis, C.V. Mosby, 1979.

295. Ikuta, Y.: Vascularized Free Flap Transfer in the Upper Limb. Hand Clin., 1:297–307, 1985.

296. Ikuta, Y.; Kubo, T.; and Tsuge, K.: Free Muscle Transplantation by Microsurgical Technique to Treat Severe Volkmann's Contracture. Plast. Reconstr. Surg., 58:407–411, 1976.

297. Ikuta, Y.; Murakami, T.; Yoshioka, K.; and Tsuge, K.: Reconstruction of the Heel Pad by Flexor Digitorum Brevis Musculocutaneous Flap Transfer. Plast. Reconstr. Surg., 74:86–94, 1984.

298. Ilizarov, G.A.: The Tension-Stress Effect on the Genesis and Growth of Tissues: Part II. The Influence of the Rate and Frequency of Distraction. Clin. Orthop. 239:263–285, 1989.

299. Ilizarov, G.A.: The Tension-Stress Effect on the Genesis and Growth of Tissues: Part I. The Influence of Stability of Fixation and Soft-Tissue Preservation. Clin. Orthop., 283:249–281, 1989.

300. Irons, G.B.; Arnold, P.G.; Masson, J.K.; and Woods, J.E.:

Experience With 100 Muscle Flaps. Ann. Plast. Surg., 4: 2–6, 1980.

301. Irons, G.B.; Fisher, J.; and Schmitt, E.H., III: Vascularized Muscular and Musculocutaneous Flaps for Management of Osteomyelitis. Orthop. Clin. North Am., 15:473–480, 1984.

302. Irons, G.B.; Witzke, D.J.; Arnold, P.G.; and Wood, M.B.: Use of the Omental Free Flap for Soft-Tissue Reconstruction. Ann. Plast. Surg., 11:501–507, 1983.

303. Ito, T.; Kohno, T.; and Kojima, T.: Free Vascularized Fibular Graft. J. Trauma, 24:756–760, 1984.

304. Jackson, I.T., and Scheker, L.: Muscle and Myocutaneous Flaps on the Lower Limb. Injury, 13:324–330, 1982.

305. Jackson, R.W., and MacNab, I.: Fractures of the Shaft of the Tibia: A Clinical and Experimental Study. Am. J. Surg., 97:543–557, 1959.

306. Jayes, P.H.: Cross-Leg Flaps: A Review of Sixty Cases. Brit. J. Plast. Surg., 3:1–5, 1950.

307. Johner, R., and Wruhs, O.: Classification of Tibial Shaft Fractures and Correlation With Results After Rigid Internal Fixation. Clin. Orthop., 178:7–25, 1983.

308. Jones, N.F.; Swartz, W.M.; Mears, D.C.; Jupiter, J.B.; and Grossman, A.: The Double Barrel Free Vascularized Fibular Bone Graft. Plast. Reconstr. Surg., 81:378–385, 1988.

309. Jones, R.E., and Cierny, G.C., III: Management of Complex Open Tibial Fractures With External Skeletal Fixation and Early Myoplasty or Myocutaneous Coverage. Can. J. Surg., 23:242–244, 1980.

310. Judet, H.; Judet, J.; and Gilbert, A.: Vascular Microsurgery in Orthopaedics. Int. Orthop., 5:61–68, 1981.

311. Jupiter, J.B.; Bour, C.J.; and May, J.W., Jr.: The Reconstruction of Defects in the Femoral Shaft With Vascularized Transfers of Fibular Bone. J. Bone Joint Surg., 69A: 365–374, 1987.

312. Jupiter, J.B.; Tsai, T.M.; and Kleinert, H.E.: Salvage Replantation of Lower Limb Amputations. Plast. Reconstr. Surg., 69:1–8, 1982.

313. Kalb, B.: Medicine—Making Bones as Good as New. Time. Jan. 14:62, 1985.

314. Karkowski, J., and Buncke, H.J.: A Simplified Technique for Free Flap Transfer of Groin Flaps, By Use of a Doppler Probe. Plast. Reconstr. Surg., 55:682–686, 1975.

315. Karlstrom, G., and Olerud, S.: Percutaneous Pin Fixation of Open Tibial Fractures. J. Bone Joint Surg., 57A:915–924, 1975.

316. Katsaros, J.; Schusterman, M.; Beppu, M.; Banis, J.C., Jr.; and Acland, R.D.: The Lateral Upper Arm Flap: Anatomy and Clinical Applications. Ann. Plast. Surg., 12:489–500, 1984.

317. Keller, A.; Allen, R.; and Shaw, W.: The Medial Gastrocnemius Muscle Flap: A Local Free Flap. Plast. Reconstr. Surg., 73:974–976, 1984.

318. Kelly, P.J.: Infections of Bones and Joints in Adult Patients. Instr. Course Lect. XXVI:3–13, 1977.

319. Kelly, P.J.: Infected Nonunion of the Femur and Tibia. Orthop. Clin. North Am., 15:481–490, 1984.

320. Kelly, P.J.; Martin, W.J.; and Coventry, M.B.: Chronic Osteomyelitis: II. Treatment with Closed Irrigation and Suction. J.A.M.A., 213:1843–1848, 1970.

321. Kenmore, P.I., and Garagusi, V.F.: Complications of Musculoskeletal Infections. In Epps, C.H., Jr. (ed.): Complications in Orthopaedic Surgery, 2nd ed., pp. 179–205. Philadelphia, J.B. Lippincott, 1986.

322. Key, J.A.: Sulfonamides in the Treatment of Chronic Osteomyelitis. J. Bone Joint Surg., 26:63–70, 1944.

323. Kleinert, H.E.: Bone and Osteocutaneous Microvascular Free Flaps. J. Hand Surg., 8:735–737, 1983.

324. Klemm, K.: Septopal—A New Way of Local Antibiotic Therapy. In van Rens, T.J.G., and Kayser, F.H. (eds.): Local Antibiotic Treatment in Osteomyelitis and Soft-Tissue Infections, pp. 24–37. Amsterdam, Excerpta Medica, 1981.

325. Knight, M.P., and Wood, G.O.: Surgical Obliteration of Bone Cavities Following Traumatic Osteomyelitis. J. Bone Joint Surg., 27:547–556, 1945.

326. Kojima, T.; Kohno, T.; and Ito, T.: Muscle Flap With Simultaneous Mesh Skin Graft for Skin Defects of the Lower Leg. J. Trauma, 19:724–729, 1979.

327. Koman, L.A.: Free Flaps for Coverage of the Foot and Ankle. Orthopedics, 9:857–862, 1986.

328. Koshima, I.; Fukuda, H.; and Soeda, S.: Free Combined Anterolateral Thigh Flap and Vascularized Iliac Bone Graft With Double Vascular Pedicle. J. Reconstr. Microsurg., 5:55–61, 1989.

329. Kumar, V.P.; Satku, K.; Helm, R.; and Pho, R.W.: Radial Reconstruction in Segmental Defects of Both Forearm Bones. J. Bone Joint Surg., 70B:815–817, 1988.

330. Kutz, J.E., and Thomson, C.B.: Free Vascularized Bone Grafts. In Urbaniak, J.R. (ed.): Symposium on Microsurgery: Practical Use in Orthopaedics, pp. 254–278. St. Louis, C.V. Mosby, 1979.

331. Lambert, C.N.: Amputation Surgery in the Child. Orthop. Clin. North Am., 3:473–482, 1972.

332. Lancaster, S.J.; Horowitz, M.; and Alonso, J.: Open Tibial Fractures: Management and Results. South. Med. J., 79: 39, 1986.

333. Landra, A.P.: The Latissimus Dorsi Musculocutaneous Flap Used to Resurface a Defect on the Upper Arm and Restore Extension to the Elbow. Brit. J. Plast. Surg., 32:275–277, 1979.

334. Lange, R.H.: Limb Reconstruction Versus Amputation Decision Making in Massive Lower Extremity Trauma. Clin. Orthop., 243:92–99, 1989.

335. Lange, R.H.; Bach, A.W.; Hansen, S.R., Jr.; and Johansen, K.H.: Open Tibial Fractures With Associated Vascular Injuries: Prognosis for Limb Salvage. J. Trauma, 25:203–208, 1985.

336. LaRossa, D.; Mellissinos, E.; Matthews, D.; and Hamilton, R.: The Use of Microvascular Free Skin–Muscle Flaps in Management of Avulsion Injuries of the Lower Leg. J. Trauma, 20:545–550, 1980.

337. Lawyer, R.B., Jr., and Lubbers, L.M.: Use of the Hoffman Apparatus in the Treatment of Unstable Tibial Fractures. J. Bone Joint Surg., 62A:1264–1273, 1980.

338. Leach, R.E.: Fractures of the Tibia and Fibula. In Rockwood, C.A., Jr., and Green, D.P. (eds.): Fractures in Adults, 2nd ed., pp. 1593–1663. Philadelphia, J.B. Lippincott, 1984.

339. Lee, C.K., and Rehmatullah, N.: Muscle-Pedicle Bone Graft

and Cancellous Bone Graft for the "Silent Hip" of Idiopathic Ischemic Necrosis of the Femoral Head in Adults. Clin. Orthop., 158:185–194, 1981.

340. Legre, R.; Kevorkian, B.; and Magalon, G.: Analysis of Sequelae Secondary to the Radial Forearm Flap: A Study of Twenty-Six Cases. Ann. Chir. Main, 5:208–212, 1986.

341. Lembert, C.N.: Amputation Surgery in the Child. Orthop. Clin. North Am., 3:473–482, 1972.

342. Lentz, M.W.; Noyes, F.R.; and Neale, H.W.: Muscle Flap Transposition for Traumatic Soft Tissue Defects of the Lower Extremity. Clin. Orthop., 143:200–210, 1979.

343. Lesavoy, M.A.: Successful Replantation of Lower Leg and Foot, With Good Sensibility and Function. Plast. Reconstr. Surg., 64:760–765, 1979.

344. Leung, P.C.: Congenital Pseudarthrosis of the Tibia: Three Cases Treated by Free Vascularized Iliac Crest Graft. Clin. Orthop., 175:45–50, 1983.

345. Leung, P.C., and Chow, Y.Y.: Reconstruction of Proximal Femoral Defects With a Vascular-Pedicled Graft. J. Bone Joint Surg., 66B:32–37, 1984.

346. Lin, S.D.; Lai, C.S.; and Chiu, C.C.: Venous Drainage in the Reverse Forearm Flap. Plast. Reconstr. Surg., 74:508–512, 1984.

347. Lister, G.D.: Letter #1989-41. ASSH Newsletter, April: 130–140, 1989.

348. Lord, J.P.: The Closure of Chronic Osteomyelitic Cavities by Plastic Methods. Surg. Gynecol. Obstet., 60:223–233, 1935.

349. Lottes, J.O.; Hill, L.J.; and Key, J.A.: Closed Reduction, Plate Fixation, and Medullary Nailing of Fractures of Both Bones of the Leg: A Comparative End-Result Study. J. Bone Joint Surg., 34A:861–877, 1952.

350. Lovie, M.J.; Duncan, G.M.; and Glasson, D.W.: The Ulnar Artery Forearm Free Flap. Brit. J. Plast. Surg., 37:486–492, 1984.

351. Lowe, H.G.: Radio-Ulnar Fusion for Defects in the Forearm Bones. J. Bone Joint Surg., 45B:351–359, 1962.

352. Lucas, K.; Fitzgibbon, G.M.; and Evans, E.M.: Discussion on Amputation in Relation to Severe Compound Fractures of the Tibia. J. Bone Joint Surg., 39B:158, 1957.

353. MacNab, I., and De Haas, W.G.: The Role of Periosteal Blood Supply in the Healing of Fractures of the Tibia. Clin. Orthop., 105:27–33, 1974.

354. Mader, J.T.; Hicks, C.A.; and Calhoun, J.: Bacterial Osteomyelitis Adjunctive Hyperbaric Oxygen Therapy. Orthop. Rev., 18:581–585, 1989.

355. Magee, H.R., and Parker, W.R.: Replantation of the Foot: Results After Two Years. Med. J. Aust., 1:751–755, 1972.

356. Man, D., and Acland, R.D.: The Microarterial Anatomy of the Dorsalis Pedis Flap and Its Clinical Applications. Plast. Reconstr. Surg., 65:419–423, 1980.

357. Mankin, H.K.; Doppelt, S.; and Tomford, W.: Clinical Experience With Allograft Implantation: The First Ten Years. Clin. Orthop., 174:69–86, 1983.

358. Manktelow, R.T.: Muscle Transplantation. In Serafin, D., and Buncke, H.J. (eds.): Microsurgical Composite Tissue Transplantation, pp. 369–390. St. Louis, C.V. Mosby, 1979.

359. Manktelow, R.T.: Free Muscle Transfers. In Green, D.P.

(ed.): Operative Hand Surgery, 2nd ed., pp. 1215–1244. New York, Churchill Livingstone, 1988.

360. Manktelow, R.T., and McKee, N.H.: Free Muscle Transplantation to Provide Active Finger Flexion. J. Hand Surg., 3:416–426, 1978.

361. Manktelow, R.T.; McKee, N.H.; and Vettese, T.: An Anatomical Study of the Pectoralis Major Muscle as Related to Functioning Free Muscle Transplantation. Plast. Reconstr. Surg., 65:610–615, 1980.

362. Manktelow, R.T.; Zuker, R.M.; and McKee, N.H.: Functioning Free Muscle Transplantation. J. Hand Surg., 9: 32–39, 1984.

363. Maruyama, Y.; Onishi, K.; Iwahira, Y.; Okajima, Y.; and Motegi, M.: Free Compound Rib–Latissimus Dorsi Osteomusculocutaneous Flap in Reconstruction of the Leg. J. Reconstr. Microsurg., 3:8–13, 1986.

364. Mathes, S., and Nahai, F.: Clinical Application for Muscle and Musculocutaneous Flaps. St. Louis, C.V. Mosby, 1982.

365. Mathes, S.J.: The Muscle Flap for Management of Osteomyelitis. N. Engl. J. Med., 306:294–295, 1982.

366. Mathes, S.J.; Alpert, B.S.; and Chang, N.: Use of Muscle Flap in Chronic Osteomyelitis: Experimental and Clinical Correlation. Plast. Reconstr. Surg., 69:815–829, 1982.

367. Mathes, S.J.; Feng, L.J.; and Hunt, T.K.: Coverage of the Infected Wound. Ann. Surg., 198:420–429, 1983.

368. Mathes, S.J.; McCraw, J.B.; and Vasconez, L.O.: Muscle Transposition Flaps for Coverage of Lower Extremity Defects—Anatomic Considerations. Surg. Clin. North Am., 54:1337–1354, 1974.

369. Mathes, S.J., and Nahai, F.: Clinical Atlas of Muscle and Musculocutaneous Flaps. St. Louis, C.V. Mosby, 1979.

370. Mathes, S.J., and Nahai, F.: Muscle Flap Transposition with Function Preservation: Technical and Clinical Considerations. Plast. Reconstr. Surg., 66:242–249, 1980.

371. Mathes, S.J., and Nahai, F.: Classification of the Vascular Anatomy of Muscles: Experimental and Clinical Correlation. Plast. Reconstr. Surg., 67:177–187, 1981.

372. Mathes, S.J.; Nahai, F.; and Vasconez, L.O.: Myocutaneous Free-Flap Transfer: Anatomical and Experimental Considerations. Plast. Reconstr. Surg., 62:162–166, 1978.

373. Maxwell, G.P., and Hoopes, J.E.: Management of Compound Injuries of the Lower Extremity. Plast. Reconstr. Surg., 63:176–185, 1979.

374. Maxwell, G.P.; Manson, P.N.; and Hoopes, J.E.: Experience With Thirteen Latissimus Dorsi Myocutaneous Free Flaps. Plast. Reconstr. Surg., 64:1–8, 1979.

375. May, J.W., Jr.; Gallico, G.G.; and Lukash, F.N.: Microvascular Transfer of Free Tissue for Closure of Bone Wounds of the Distal Lower Extremity. N. Engl. J. Med., 306:253–257, 1982.

376. May, J.W., Jr.; Gallico, G.G., III; Jupiter, J.; and Savage, R.C.: Free Latissimus Dorsi Muscle Flap With Skin Graft for Treatment of Traumatic Chronic Bony Wounds. Plast. Reconstr. Surg., 73:6411–649, 1984.

377. May, J.W., Jr.; Halls, M.J.; and Simon, S.R.: Free Microvascular Muscle Flaps With Skin Graft Reconstruction of Extensive Defects of the Foot: A Clinical and Gait Analysis Study. Plast. Reconstr. Surg., 75:627–639, 1985.

378. May, J.W., Jr.; Jupiter, J.B.; Weiland, A.J.; and Byrd,

H.S.: Clinical Classification of Post-Traumatic Tibial Osteomyelitis. J. Bone Joint Surg., 71A:1422–1428, 1989.

379. May, J.W., Jr.; Lukash, F.N.; and Gallico, G.G.: Latissimus Dorsi Free Muscle Flap in Lower Extremity Reconstruction. Plast. Reconstr. Surg., 68:603–607, 1981.

380. Mayou, B.J.; Whitby, D.; and Jones, B.M.: The Scapular Flap—An Anatomical and Clinical Study. Brit. J. Plast. Surg., 35:8–13, 1982.

381. McAndrew, M.P., and Lantz, B.A.: Initial Care of Massively Traumatized Lower Extremities. Clin. Orthop., 243:20–29, 1989.

382. McCraw, J.B.: Selection of Alternative Local Flaps in the Leg and Foot. Clin. Plast. Surg., 6:227–246, 1979.

383. McCraw, J.B., and Arnold, P.G.: McCraw and Arnold's Atlas of Muscle and Musculocutaneous Flaps. Norfolk, Va, Hampton Press, 1986.

384. McCraw, J.B.; Dibbell, D.G.; and Carraway, J.H.: Clinical Definition of Independent Myocutaneous Vascular Territories. Plast. Reconstr. Surg., 60:341–352, 1977.

385. McCraw, J.B.; Fishman, J.H.; and Sharzer, L.A.: The Versatile Gastrocnemius Myocutaneous Flap. Plast. Reconstr. Surg., 62:15–23, 1978.

386. McCraw, J.B., and Furlow, L.T., Jr.: The Dorsalis Pedis Arterialized Flap: A Clinical Study. Plast. Reconstr. Surg., 55:177–185, 1975.

387. McCraw, J.B.; Myers, B.; and Shanklin, K.D.: The Value of Fluorescein in Predicting the Viability of Arterialized Flaps. Plast. Reconstr. Surg., 60:710–719, 1977.

388. McGregor, I.A., and Jackson, I.T.: The Groin Flap. Brit. J. Plast. Surg., 25:3–16, 1972.

389. McHugh, M., and Prendiville, J.B.: Muscle Flaps in the Repair of Skin Defects Over the Exposed Tibia. Brit. J. Plast. Surg., 28:205–209, 1975.

390. McKee, N.H.; Haw, P.; and Vettese, T.: Anatomic Study of the Nutrient Foramen in the Shaft of the Fibula. Clin. Orthop., 184:141–144, 1984.

391. McMaster, P.E., and Hohl, M.: Tibiofibular Cross-Peg Grafting: A Salvage Procedure for Complicated Ununited Tibial Fractures. J. Bone Joint Surg., 47A:1146–1158, 1965.

392. Meals, R.A.: The Use of a Flexor Carpi Ulnaris Muscle Flap in the Treatment of an Infected Nonunion of the Proximal Ulna: A Case Report. Clin. Orthop., 240:168–172, 1989.

393. Mendes, J.E.; Cabral, A.T.; and Lima, C.: Open Fractures of the Tibia. Clin. Orthop., 156:98–104, 1981.

394. Meyer, S.; Weiland, A.J.; and Willenegger, H.: The Treatment of Infected Non-Union of Fractures of Long Bones: Study of Sixty-Four Cases With a Five to Twenty-One-Year Follow-Up. J. Bone Joint Surg., 57A:836–842, 1975.

395. Meyerding, H.W., and Cherry, J.H.: Tibial Defects With Nonunion Treated by Transference of the Fibula and Tibiofibular Fusion. Am. J. Surg., 52:397–404, 1941.

396. Meyers, M.H.: The Role of Posterior Bone Grafts (Muscle–Pedicle) in Femoral Neck Fractures. Clin. Orthop., 152:143–146, 1980.

397. Meyers, M.H.; Harvey, J.P., Jr.; and Moore, T.M.: Treatment of Displaced Subcapital and Transcervical Fractures of the Femoral Neck by Muscle-Pedicle–Bone Graft and Internal Fixation. A Preliminary Report on One Hundred and Fifty Cases. J. Bone Joint Surg., 55A:257–274, 1973.

398. Millard, D.R., Jr., and Ortiz, A.C.: Correction of Severe Elbow Contractures. J. Bone Joint Surg., 47A:1347–1354, 1965.

399. Miller, R.C., and Phalen, G.S.: The Repair of Defects of the Radius With Fibular Bone Grafts. J. Bone Joint Surg., 29:629–636, 1947.

400. Minami, A.; Kaneda, K.; Itoga, H.; and Usui, M.: Free Vascularized Fibular Grafts. J. Reconstr. Microsurg., 5:37–43, 1989.

401. Minami, A.; Usui, M.; Ogino, T.; and Minami, M.: Simultaneous Reconstruction of Bone and Skin Defects by Free Fibular Graft With a Skin Flap. Microsurgery, 7:38–45, 1986.

402. Mir y Mir, L.: Functional Graft of the Heel. Plast. Reconstr. Surg., 14:444–450, 1954.

403. Miyamoto, Y.; Ikuta, Y.; Shigeki, S.; and Yamura, M.: Current Concepts of Instep Island Flap. Ann. Plast. Surg., 19:97–102, 1987.

404. Mladick, R.A.; Pickrell, K.L.; Thorne, F.L.; and Royer, J.R.: Ipsilateral Thigh Flap for Total Plantar Resurfacing: Case Report. Plast. Reconstr. Surg., 43:198–200, 1969.

405. Moore, J.R., and Weiland, A.J.: Free Vascularized Bone and Muscle Flaps for Osteomyelitis. Orthopedics, 9:819–824, 1986.

406. Moore, J.R.; Weiland, A.J.; and Daniel, R.K.: Use of Free Vascularized Bone Grafts in the Treatment of Bone Tumors. Clin. Orthop., 175:37–44, 1983.

407. Morain, W.D.: Soft-Tissue Reconstruction of Below-Knee Defects. Am. J. Surg., 139:495–502, 1980.

408. Morandi, M.; Zembo, M.M.; and Ciotti, M.: Infected Tibial Pseudarthrosis: A 2-Year Follow-Up on Patients Treated by the Ilizarov Technique. Orthopedics, 12:497–508, 1989.

409. Morley, G.H.: Application of Plastic Surgery to the Care of the Injured. Brit. Med. J., 1:823–827, 1966.

410. Morrey, B.F.; Dunn, J.M.; Heimbach, R.D.; and Davis, J.: Hyperbaric Oxygen and Chronic Osteomyelitis. Clin. Orthop., 144:121–127, 1979.

411. Morrison, W.A.; Crabb, D.M.; O'Brien, B.M.; and Jenkins, A.: The Instep of the Foot as a Fasciocutaneous Island and as a Free Flap for Heel Defects. Plast. Reconstr. Surg., 72:56–63, 1983.

412. Morrison, W.A.; O'Brien, B.M.; and MacLeod, A.M.: Major Limb Replantation. Orthop. Clin. North Am., 8:343–348, 1977.

413. Morrison, W.A.; O'Brien, B.McC.; and MacLeod, A.: Clinical Experiences in Free Flap Transfer. Clin. Orthop., 133:132–139, 1978.

414. Moss, A.L.; Waterhouse, N.; and Townsend, P.: Free Vascularized Fibular Graft to Reconstruct Early a Traumatic Humeral Defect. Injury, 16:41–46, 1984.

415. Muhlbauer, W.; Herndl, E.; and Stock, W.: The Forearm Flap. Plast. Reconstr. Surg., 70:336–342, 1982.

416. Muhr, G.: Early Complications of Fractures With Soft Tissue Injuries. In Tscherne, H., and Gotzen, L. (eds.): Fractures With Soft Tissue Injuries, pp. 131–138. New York, Springer-Verlag, 1984.

417. Murray, R.A.: The One-Bone Forearm: A Reconstructive Procedure. J. Bone Joint Surg., 37A:366–370, 1955.

418. Nahai, F.; Hill, H.; and Hester, T.R.: Experiences With the Tensor Fascia Lata Flap. Plast. Reconstr. Surg., 63:788–799, 1979.

419. Nahai, F.; Silverton, J.S.; Hill, H.; and Vasconez, L.O.: The Tensor Fascia Lata Musculocutaneous Flap. Ann. Plast. Surg., 1:372–379, 1978.

420. Nassif, T.M.; Vidal, L.; Bovet, J.L.; and Baudet, J.: The Parascapular Flap: A New Cutaneous Microsurgical Free Flap. Plast. Reconstr. Surg., 69:591–600, 1982.

421. Neale, H.W.; Stern, P.J.; Kreilein, J.G.; Gregory, R.O.; and Webster, K.L.: Complications of Muscle-Flap Transposition for Traumatic Defects of the Leg. Plast. Reconstr. Surg., 72:512–515, 1983.

422. Nettelblad, H.; Randolph, M.A.; and Weiland, A.J.: Free Microvascular Epiphyseal Plate Transplantation: An Experimental Study in Dogs. J. Bone Joint Surg., 66A:1421–1429, 1984.

423. Nicoll, E.A.: The Treatment of Gaps in Long Bones by Cancellous Insert Grafts. J. Bone Joint Surg., 38B:70–82, 1956.

424. Niinikoski, J., and Hunt, T.K.: Oxygen Tensions in Healing Bone. Surg. Gynecol. Obstet. 134:746–750, 1972.

425. Noellert, R.C., and Louis, D.S.: Long-Term Follow-Up of Nonvascularized Fibular Autografts for Distal Radial Reconstruction. J. Hand Surg., 10:335–340, 1985.

426. Nohira, K.; Shintomi, Y.; Sugihara, T.; and Ohura, T.: Replacing Losses in Kind: Improved Sensation Following Heel Reconstruction Using the Free Instep Flap. J. Reconstr. Microsurg., 5:1–6, 1989.

427. Nunley, J.A.: Elective Microsurgery for Orthopaedic Reconstruction: Part I. Donor Site Selection for Cutaneous and Myocutaneous Free Flaps. Instr. Course Lect. XXXIII: 417–460, 1984.

428. Nusbickel, F.R.; Dell, P.C.; McAndrew, M.P.; and Moore, M.M.: Vascularized Autografts for Reconstruction of Skeletal Defects Following Lower Extremity Trauma: A Review. Clin. Orthop., 243:65–70, 1989.

429. O'Brien, B.M.: Microvascular Free Bone and Joint Transfer. In O'Brien, B.M. (ed.) Microvascular Reconstructive Surgery, pp. 267–289. New York, Churchill Livingstone, 1977.

430. O'Brien, B.M.; Gumley, G.J.; Dooley, B.J.; and Pribaz, J.J.: Folded Free Vascularized Fibula Transfer. Plast. Reconstr. Surg., 82:311–318, 1988.

431. O'Brien, B.M.; MacLeod, A.M.; Hayhurst, J.W.; and Morrison, W.A.: Successful Transfer of a Large Island Flap from the Groin to the Foot by Microsurgical Anastomoses. Plast. Reconstr. Surg., 52:271–278, 1973.

432. Oestern, H.-J., and Tscherne, H.: Pathophysiology and Classification of Soft Tissue Injuries Associated with Fractures. In Tscherne, H., and Gotzen, L. (eds.): Fractures with Soft Tissue Injuries, pp. 1–9. New York, Springer-Verlag, 1984.

433. Ohmori, K., and Harii, K.: Free Groin Flaps: Their Vascular Basis. Brit. J. Plast. Surg., 28:238–243, 1975.

434. Ohtsuka, H., and Shioya, N.: The Fate of Free Omental Transfers. Brit. J. Plast. Surg., 38:478–482, 1985.

435. Ohtsuka, H.; Torigai, K.; and Itoh, M.: Free Omental Transfer to the Lower Limbs. Ann. Plast. Surg., 4:71–78, 1980.

436. Okada, T.; Yasuda, Y.; Kitayama, Y.; and Tsukada, S.: Salvage of an Arm by Means of a Free Cutaneous Flap Based on the Posterior Tibial Artery. J. Reconstr. Microsurg., 1: 25–29, 1984.

437. Olerud, S.; Henriksson, T.G.; and Engkvist, O.: A Free Vascularized Fibular Graft in Lengthening of the Humerus With the Wagner Apparatus: Report of a Case in a Twenty-Year-Old Man. J. Bone Joint Surg., 65:111–114, 1983.

438. Olerud, S., and Karlstrom, G.: Tibial Fractures Treated by AO Compression Osteosynthesis: Experiences From a Five-Year Material. Acta Orthop. Scand. (Suppl.), 140:1–104, 1972.

439. Orticochea, M.: Immediate (Undelayed) Musculocutaneous Island Cross-Leg Flaps. Brit. J. Plast. Surg., 31:205–209, 1978.

440. Osterman, A.L., and Bora, F.W.: Free Vascularized Bone Grafting for Large-Gap Nonunion of Long Bones. Orthop. Clin. North Am., 15:131–142, 1984.

441. Ostrup, L.T., and Tam, C.S.: Bone Formation in a Free, Living Bone Graft Transferred by Microvascular Anastomoses. Scand. J. Plast. Reconstr. Surg., 9:101–106, 1975.

442. Ottolenghi, C.E.: Massive Osteoarticular Bone Grafts: Transplant of the Whole Femur. J. Bone Joint Surg., 48B: 646–659, 1966.

443. Ottolenghi, C.E.: Massive Osteo and Osteo-Articular Bone Grafts: Technic and Results of 62 Cases. Clin. Orthop., 87:156–164, 1972.

444. Overton, L.M., and Tully, W.P.: Surgical Treatment of Chronic Osteomyelitis in Long Bones. Am. J. Surg., 126: 736–741, 1973.

445. Padgett, E.C., and Gaskins, J.H.: The Use of Skin Flaps in the Repair of Scarred or Ulcerative Defects Over Bone and Tendons. Surg., 18:287–298, 1945.

446. Paley, D.: Bone Transport: The Ilizarov Treatment of Bone Defects. Surg. Rounds Orthop., 3:17–29, 1989.

447. Paley, D.; Catagni, M.A.; Argnani, F.; Villa, A.; Benedetti, G.B.; and Cattaneo, R.: Ilizarov Treatment of Tibial Nonunions With Bone Loss. Clin. Orthop., 241:146–165, 1989.

448. Papineau, L.J.; Alfageme, A.; Dalcourt, J.P.; and Pilon, L.: Chronic Osteomyelitis: Open Excision and Grafting After Saucerization. Int. Orthop., 3:165–175, 1979.

449. Parisien, V.: Fibular Transfer for Tibial Defect. Bull. Hosp. Joint Dis., 24:142–146, 1963.

450. Patzakis, M.J.; Harvey, J.P., Jr.; and Ivler, D.: The Role of Antibiotics in the Management of Open Fractures. J. Bone Joint Surg., 56A:532–541, 1974.

451. Patzakis, M.J., and Wilkins, J.: Factors Influencing Infection Rate in Open Fracture Wounds. Clin. Orthop., 243: 36–40, 1989.

452. Patzakis, M.J.; Wilkins, J.; and Moore, T.M.: Use of Antibiotics in Open Tibial Fractures. Clin. Orthop., 178:31–35, 1983.

453. Patzakis, M.J.; Wilkins, J.; and Moore, T.M.: Considerations in Reducing the Infection Rate in Open Tibial Fractures. Clin. Orthop., 178:36–41, 1983.

454. Pearl, R.M., and Hentz, V.R.: Irreplaceable Free Flaps in Reconstructive Surgery—Part II. Ann. Plast. Surg., 9:488–497, 1982.

455. Pearson, R.L., and Perry, C.R.: The Ilizarov Technique in the Treatment of Infected Tibial Nonunions. Orthop. Rev., 18:609–613, 1989.

456. Peled, I.J.; Frankl, U.; and Wexler, M.R.: Salvage of Exposed Knee Prosthesis by Gastrocnemius Myocutaneous Flap Coverage. Orthopedics, 6:1320–1322, 1983.

457. Perry, C.R.; Davenport, K.; and Vossen, M.K.: Local Delivery of Antibiotics Via Implantable Pump in the Treatment of Osteomyelitis. Clin. Orthop., 226:222–230, 1988.

458. Phemister, D.B.: The Fate of Transplanted Bone and Regenerative Power of Its Various Constituents. Surg. Gynecol. Obstet., 19:303–333, 1914.

459. Pho, R.W.H.: Free Vascularized Fibular Transplant for Replacement of the Lower Radius. J. Bone Joint Surg., 61B:362–365, 1979.

460. Pho, R.W.H.: Malignant Giant-Cell Tumor of the Distal End of the Radius Treated by a Free Vascularized Fibular Transplant. J. Bone Joint Surg., 63A:877–884, 1981.

461. Pho, R.W.H.; Levack, B.; Satku, K.; and Patradul, A.: Free Vascularized Fibular Graft in the Treatment of Congenital Pseudarthrosis of the Tibia. J. Bone Joint Surg., 67B:64–70, 1985.

462. Pho, R.W.H.; Vajara, R.; and Satku, K.: Free Vascularized Bone Transplants in Problematic Nonunions of Fractures. J. Trauma, 23:341–349, 1983.

463. Ponten, B.: The Fasciocutaneous Flap: Its Use in Soft Tissue Defects of the Lower Leg. Brit. J. Plast. Surg., 34:215–220, 1981.

464. Prigge, E.K.: The Treatment of Chronic Osteomyelitis by the Use of Muscle Transplant or Iliac Graft. J. Bone Joint Surg., 28:576–593, 1946.

465. Puranen, J.: Reorganization of Fresh and Preserved Bone Transplants: An Experimental Study in Rabbits Using Tetracycline Labelling. Acta Orthop. Scand. (Suppl.), 92:1–75, 1966.

466. Quillen, C.G.; Wiener, B.; Mendoza, L.; and Giampapa, V.: Experiences in the Use of Eight Cutaneous and Osteocutaneous Superficial and Deep Circumflex Iliac Free Flaps. J. Reconstr. Microsurg., 1:269–281, 1985.

467. Radici, G.; Donati, L.; Fox, U.; Candiani, P.; Signorini, M.; and Klinger, M.: Latissimus Myocutaneous Free Flap in the Reconstruction of Lower Limb Defects—Three Clinical Cases. Ann. Plast. Surg., 9:4–9, 1982.

468. Reckling, F.W., and Roberts, M.D.: Primary Closure of Open Fractures of the Tibia and Fibula by Fibular Fixation and Relaxing Incisions. J. Trauma, 10:835–866, 1970.

469. Reckling, F.W., and Waters, C.H., III: Treatment of Non-Unions of Fractures of the Tibial Diaphysis by Posterolateral Cortical Cancellous Bone-Grafting. J. Bone Joint Surg., 62A:936–941, 1980.

470. Reiffel, R.S., and McCarthy, J.G.: Coverage of Heel and Sole Defects: A New Subfascial Arterialized Flap. Plast. Reconstr. Surg., 66:250–260, 1980.

471. Restrepo, J.; Katz, D.; and Gilbert, A.: Arterial Vascularization of the Proximal Epiphysis and the Diaphysis of the Fibula. Int. J. Microsurg., 2:49–54, 1980.

472. Reynolds, F.C.: Open Fractures and War Wounds. In Conwell, H.E., and Reynolds, F.C. (eds.): Key and Conwell's Management of Fractures, Dislocations, and Sprains, 7th ed., pp. 158–182. St. Louis, C.V. Mosby, 1961.

473. Rhinelander, F.W.: Effects of Medullary Nailing on the Normal Blood Supply of Diaphyseal Cortex. Instr. Course Lect., XXII: 161–187, 1973.

474. Rhinelander, F.W.: Tibial Blood Supply in Relation to Fracture Healing. Clin. Orthop., 105:34–81, 1974.

475. Richards, R.R.; Orsini, E.C.; Mahoney, J.L.; and Verschuren, R.: The Influence of Muscle Flap Coverage on the Repair of Devascularized Tibial Cortex: An Experimental Investigation in the Dog. Plast. Reconstr. Surg., 79:946–956, 1987.

476. Rigg, B.M.: Transfer of a Free Groin Flap to the Heel by Microvascular Anastomoses. Plast. Reconstr. Surg., 55:36–40, 1975.

477. Rittmann, W.W.; Schibli, M.; Matter, P.; and Allgöwer, M.: Open Fractures: Long-term Results in 200 Consecutive Cases. Clin. Orthop., 138:132–140, 1979.

478. Robbins, T.H.: Use of Fascio-Muscle Flaps to Repair Defects in the Leg. Plast. Reconstr. Surg., 57:460–462, 1976.

479. Robinson, D.W.: Coverage Problem in Fractures of the Tibia. Arch. Surg., 63:53–59, 1951.

480. Rogge, D.: External Articular Transfixation for Joint Injuries With Severe Soft Tissue Damage. In Tscherne, H., and Gotzen, L. (eds.): Fractures with Soft Tissue Injuries, pp. 103–117. New York, Springer-Verlag, 1984.

481. Rojczyk, M.: Results of the Treatment of Open Fractures: Aspects of Antibiotic Therapy. In Tscherne, H., and Gotzen, L. (eds.): Fractures with Soft Tissue Injuries, pp. 33–38. New York, Springer-Verlag, 1984.

482. Rosenthal, R.E.; MacPhail, J.A.; and Ortiz, J.E.: Non-Union in Open Tibial Fractures: Analysis of Reasons for Failure of Treatment. J. Bone Joint Surg., 59A:244–248, 1977.

483. Roth, J.H.; Urbaniak, J.R.; Koman, L.A.; and Goldner, J.L.: Free Flap Coverage of Deep Tissue Defects of the Foot. Foot Ankle, 3:150–157, 1982.

484. Rowling, D.E.: The Positive Approach to Chronic Osteomyelitis. J. Bone Joint Surg., 41B:681–688, 1959.

485. Ruedi, T.; Webb, J.K.; and Allgöwer, M.: Experience With the Dynamic Compression Plate (DCP) in 418 Recent Fractures of the Tibial Shaft. Injury, 7:252–257, 1976.

486. Russell, R.C.; Graham, D.R.; Feller, A.M.; Zook, E.G.; and Mathur, A.: Experimental Evaluation of the Antibiotic Carrying Capacity of a Muscle Flap Into a Fibrotic Cavity. Plast. Reconstr. Surg., 81:162–168, 1988.

487. Russell, R.C.; Guy, R.J.; Zook, E.G.; and Merrell, J.C.: Extremity Reconstruction Using the Free Deltoid Flap. Plast. Reconstr. Surg., 76:586–595, 1985.

488. Russell, R.C.; Upton, J.; and Merrell, J.C.: Free Flap Donor Sites: Anatomical, Functional, and Technical Considerations. In Riley, W.B., Jr. (ed.): Plastic Surgery Educational Foundation: Instructional Courses, Vol. 1, pp. 316–360. St. Louis, C.V. Mosby, 1988.

489. Russell, R.C.; Vitale, V.; and Zook, E.C.: Extremity Reconstruction Using the "Fillet of Sole" Flap. Ann. Plast. Surg., 17:65–72, 1986.

490. Ruttle, P.E.; Kelly, P.J.; Arnold, P.G.; Irons, G.B.; and Fitzgerald R.H., Jr.: Chronic Osteomyelitis Treated With a Muscle Flap. Orthop. Clin. North Am., 15:451–459, 1984.

491. Saad, M.N.: The Problems of Traumatic Skin Loss of the Lower Limbs, Especially When Associated With Skeletal Injury. Brit. J. Surg., 57:601–615, 1970.

492. Salenius, P.; Santavirta, S.; Kiviluoto, O.; and Koskinen, E.V.: Application of Free Autogenous Fibular Graft in the Treatment of Aggressive Bone Tumors of the Distal End of the Radius. Arch. Orthop. Trauma Surg., 98:285–287, 1981.

493. Salibian, A.H., and Anzel, S.H.: Salvage of an Infected Total Knee Prosthesis with Medial and Lateral Gastrocnemius Muscle Flaps—A Case Report. J. Bone Joint Surg., 65A:681–684, 1983.

494. Salibian, A.H.; Anzel, S.H.; Mallerich, M.M.; and Tesoro, V.E.: Microvascular Reconstruction for Close-Range Gunshot Injuries to the Distal Forearm. J. Hand Surg., 9A:799–804, 1984.

495. Salibian, A.H.; Anzel, S.H.; and Salyer, W.A.: Transfer of Vascularized Grafts of Iliac Bone to the Extremities. J. Bone Joint Surg., 69A:1319–1327, 1987.

496. Salibian, A.H.; Tesoro, V.R.; and Wood, D.L.: Staged Transfer of a Free Microvascular Latissimus Dorsi Myocutaneous Flap Using Saphenous Vein Grafts. Plast. Reconstr. Surg., 71:543–547, 1983.

497. Salimbeni-Ughi, G.; Santoni-Rugiu, P.; and deVizia, G.P.: The Gastrocnemius Myocutaneous Flap (GMF): An Alternative Method to Repair Severe Lesions of the Leg. Arch. Orthop. Trauma Surg., 98:195–200, 1981.

498. Sanders, R., and Mayou, B.J.: A New Vascularized Bone Graft Transferred by Microvascular Anastomosis as a Free Flap. Brit. J. Plast. Surg., 66:787–788, 1979.

499. Sanders, W.E.: Principles of Microvascular Surgery. In Green, D.P. (ed.): Operative Hand Surgery, 2nd ed., pp. 1049–1103. New York, Churchill Livingstone, 1988.

500. Sanders, W.E., and Godsey, J.B.: Non-Invasive Vascular Testing in Candidates for Reconstructive Microsurgery. J. Vasc. Technol., 11:40–43, 1987.

501. Satoh, T.; Tsuchiya, M.; Kobayaski, M.; Nomoto, S.; Yasuwaki, Y.; Harii, K.; and Moriwaki, M.: Experience With Free Composite Tissue Transplantation Based on the Deep Circumflex Iliac Vessels. J. Microsurg., 3:77–84, 1981.

502. Sbitany, U., and Wray, R.C., Jr.: Use of the Rectus Abdominis Muscle Flap to Reconstruct an Elbow Defect. Plast. Reconstr. Surg., 77:988–989, 1986.

503. Schenck, R.R.: Free Muscle and Composite Skin Transplantation by Microneurovascular Anatomoses. Orthop. Clin. North Am., 8:367–375, 1977.

504. Schenck, R.R.: Rectus Femoris Muscle and Composite Skin Transplantation by Microneurovascular Anatomoses for Avulsion of Forearm Muscles: A Case Report. J. Hand Surg., 3:60–69, 1978.

505. Schuind, F.; Burny, F.; and Lejeune, F.J.: Microsurgical Free Fibula Bone Transfer: A Technique for Reconstruction of Large Skeletal Defects Following Resection of High-Grade Malignant Tumors. World J. Surg., 12:310–317, 1988.

506. Scully, R.E.; Artz, C.P.; and Sako, Y.: An Evaluation of the Surgeon's Criteria for Determining the Viability of Muscle During Debridement. Arch. Surg., 73:1031–1035, 1956.

507. Serafin, D., and Georgiade, N.G.: Microsurgical Composite Tissue Transplantation: A New Method of Immediate Reconstruction of Extensive Defects. Am. J. Surg., 133:752–757, 1977.

508. Serafin, D.; Georgiade, N.G.; and Smith, D.H.: Comparison of Free Flaps With Pedicled Flaps for Coverage of Defects of the Leg or Foot. Plast. Reconstr. Surg., 59:492–499, 1977.

509. Serafin, D., and Smith, D.H.: Composite Tissue Transplantation in Soft Tissue Reconstruction of the Lower Extremity. In Serafin, D., and Buncke, H. (eds.): Microsurgical Composite Tissue Transplantation. St. Louis, C.V. Mosby, 1979.

510. Serafin, D.; Villarreal-Rios, A.; and Georgiade, N.: Fourteen Free Groin Flap Transfers. Plast. Reconstr. Surg., 57:707–715, 1976.

511. Serafin, D.; Villarreal-Rios, A.; and Georgiade, N.G.: A Rib-Containing Free Flap to Reconstruct Mandibular Defects. Brit. J. Plast. Surg., 30:263–266, 1977.

512. Serafin, D., and Voci, V.E.: Reconstruction of the Lower Extremity: Microsurgical Composite Tissue Transplantation. Clin. Plast. Surg., 10:55–72, 1983.

513. Seyfer, A.E., and Lower, R.: Late Results of Free-Muscle Flaps and Delayed Bone Grafting in the Secondary Treatment of Open Distal Tibial Fractures. Plast. Reconstr. Surg., 83:77–84, 1989.

514. Shah, D.M.; Corson, J.D.; Karmody, A.M.; Fortune, J.B.; and Leather, R.P.: Optimal Management of Tibial Arterial Trauma. J. Trauma, 28:228–234, 1988.

515. Shaw, W.W.: Microvascular Free Flap—The First Decade. Clin. Plast. Surg., 10:3–20, 1983.

516. Shaw, W.W.: Microvascular Free Flaps: Survival, Donor Sites and Application. In Bunck, H.J., and Furnas, D.W. (eds.): Symposium on Clinical Frontiers in Reconstructive Microsurgery, Vol. 24, pp. 3–10. St. Louis, C.V. Mosby, 1984.

517. Silverton, J.S.; Nahai, F.; and Jurkiewicz, M.J.: The Latissimus Dorsi Myocutaneous Flap to Replace a Defect on the Upper Arm. Brit. J. Plast. Surg., 31:29–31, 1978.

518. Skef, Z.; Ecker, H.A., Jr.; and Graham, W.P., III: Heel Coverage by a Plantar Myocutaneous Island Pedicle Flap. J. Trauma, 23:466–472, 1983.

519. Smith, D.J., Jr., and Coyler, R.A.: An Aggressive Treatment Approach for Adult Osteomyelitis. Ann. Surg., 51:363–366, 1985.

520. Smith, D.J., Jr.; Loewenstein, P.W.; and Bennett, J.E.: Surgical Options in the Repair of Lower-Extremity Soft-Tissue Wounds. J. Trauma, 22:374–381, 1982.

521. Smith, P.J.; Foley, B.; McGregor, I.A.; and Jackson, I.T.: The Anatomical Basis of the Groin Flap. Plast. Reconstr. Surg., 49:41–47, 1972.

522. Snyder, G.B., and Edgerton, M.T., Jr.: The Principle of the Island Neurovascular Flap in the Management of Ulcerated Anesthetic Weightbearing Areas of the Lower Extremity. Plast. Reconstr. Surg., 36:518–528, 1965.

523. Solonen, K.A.: Free Vascularized Bone Graft in the Treatment of Pseudarthrosis. Int. Orthop., 6:9–13, 1982.

524. Sommerlad, B.C., and McGrouther, D.A.: Resurfacing the Sole: Long-Term Follow-Up and Comparison of Techniques. Brit. J. Plast. Surg., 31:107–116, 1978.

525. Sowa, D.T., and Weiland, A.J.: Clinical Applications of Vascularized Bone Autografts. Orthop. Clin. North Am., 18:257–273, 1987.

526. Speed, K.: A Textbook of Fractures and Dislocations Covering Their Pathology, Diagnosis and Treatment, pp. 79–83, 848–850. Philadelphia, Lea & Febiger, 1935.

527. Stark, R.B.: Cross-Leg Flap Procedure. Plast. Reconstr. Surg., 39:173–204, 1952.

528. Stark, R.B., and Kaplan, J.M.: Cross-Leg Flaps in Patients Over 50 Years of Age. Brit. J. Plast. Surg., 25:20–21, 1972.

529. Stark, R.B., and Kernahan, D.A.: Reconstructive Surgery of the Leg and Foot. Surg. Clin. North Am., 39:469–490, 1959.

530. Stark, W.J.: The Use of Pedicled Muscle Flaps in the Surgical Treatment of Chronic Osteomyelitis Resulting From Compound Fractures. J. Bone Joint Surg., 28:343–350, 1946.

531. Stern, P.J.; Neale, H.W.; Gregory, R.O.; and McDonough, J.J.: Functional Reconstruction of an Extremity by Free Tissue Transfer of the Latissimus Dorsi. J. Bone Joint Surg., 65A:729–737, 1983.

532. Stranc, M.F.; Labandter, H.; and Roy, A.: A Review of 196 Tubed Pedicles. Brit. J. Plast. Surg., 28:54–58, 1975.

533. Strauch, B., and Murray, D.E.: Transfer of Composite Graft With Immediate Suture Anastomosis of Its Vascular Pedicle Measuring Less Than 1 mm. in External Diameter Using Microsurgical Techniques. Plast. Reconstr. Surg., 40:325–329, 1967.

534. Strauss, M.B.: Chronic Refractory Osteomyelitis: Review and Role of Hyperbaric Oxygen. Hyperbaric Oxygen Rev., 1:231–256, 1980.

535. Stringa, G.: Studies of the Vascularisation of Bone Grafts. J. Bone Joint Surg., 39B:395–420, 1957.

536. Stuck, W.G., and Hinchey, J.J.: Experimentally Increased Blood Supply to the Head and Neck of the Femur. Surg. Gynecol. Obstet. 78:160–163, 1944.

537. Sudasna, S.; Thienprasit, P.; Poneprasert, S.; and Chiang-Thong, K.: Treatment of Massive Tibial Diaphyseal Defect With Free Fibular Transfer. J. Med. Assoc. Thai., 63:478–486, 1980.

538. Sudmann, E.: Treatment of Chronic Osteomyelitis by Free Grafts of Cancellous Autologous Bone Tissue: A Preliminary Report. Acta Orthop. Scand., 50:145–150, 1979.

539. Suematsu, N.; Hirayama, T.; Atsuta, Y.; and Takemitsu, Y.: Postoperative Course of Patients Treated with Iliac Osteocutaneous Free Flaps. A Two- to Five-Year Follow-Up Study. Clin. Orthop., 223:257–264, 1987.

540. Suren, E.G.: Guidelines for the Postoperative Management of Fractures With Severe Soft Tissue Injuries. *In* Tscherne, H., and Gotzen, L. (eds.): Fractures with Soft Tissue Injuries, pp. 118–130. New York, Springer-Verlag, 1984.

541. Swartz, W.M.: Discussion: Late Results of Free-Muscle Flaps and Delayed Bone Grafting in the Secondary Treatment of Open Distal Tibial Fractures. Plast. Reconstr. Surg., 83:83–84, 1989.

542. Swartz, W.M., and Mears, D.C.: The Role of Free-Tissue Transfers in Lower-Extremity Reconstruction. Plast. Reconstr. Surg., 76:364–373, 1985.

543. Swiontkowski, M.F.: Criteria for Bone Debridement in Massive Lower Limb Trauma. Clin. Orthop., 243:41–47, 1989.

544. Takami, H.; Doi, T.; Takahashi, S.; and Ninomiya, S.: Reconstruction of a Large Tibial Defect With a Free Vascularized Fibular Graft. Arch. Orthop. Trauma Surg., 102:203–205, 1984.

545. Takami, H.; Takahashi, S.; and Ando, M.: Microvascular Free Musculocutaneous Flaps for the Treatment of Avulsion Injuries of the Lower Leg. J. Trauma, 23:473–477, 1983.

546. Takayanagi, S., and Tsukie, T.: Free Serratus Anterior Muscle and Myocutaneous Flaps. Ann. Plast. Surg., 8:277–283, 1982.

547. Tamai, S.: Osteocutaneous Transplantation: Iliac Osteocutaneous Neurosensory Flap. *In* Serafin, D., and Buncke, H.F. (eds.): Microsurgical Composite Tissue Transplantation, pp. 391–397. St. Louis, C.V. Mosby, 1979.

548. Tamai, S.; Komatsu, S.; Sakamoto, H.; Sano, S.; Sasauchi, N.; Hori, Y.; Tatsumi, Y.; and Okuda, H.: Free Muscle Transplants in Dogs With Microsurgical Neurovascular Anastomoses. Plast. Reconstr. Surg., 46:219–225, 1970.

549. Tamai, S.; Sakamoto, H.; Hori, Y.; Tatsumi, Y.; Nakamura, Y.; Shimizu, T.; and Fukui, A.: Vascularized Fibula Transplantation: A Report of 8 Cases in the Treatment of Traumatic Bony Defect or Pseudarthrosis of Long Bones. Int. J. Microsurg., 2:205–212, 1980.

550. Taylor, G.I.: Tissue Defects in the Limbs: Replacement With Free Vascularized Tissue Transfers. Aust. N.Z.J. Surg., 47:276–284, 1977.

551. Taylor, G.I.: Free Bone Transfer. *In* Daniel, R.K., and Terzis, J.K. (eds.): Reconstructive Microsurgery, pp. 275–280. Boston, Little, Brown, 1977.

552. Taylor, G.I.: Microvascular Free Bone Transfer: A Clinical Technique. Orthop. Clin. North Am. 8:425–447, 1977.

553. Taylor, G.I.: The Current Status of Free Vascularized Bone Grafts. Clin. Plast. Surg., 10:185–209, 1983.

554. Taylor, G.I.; Buncke, H.J., Jr.; Watson, N.; and Murray, W.: Vascularized Osseous Transplantation for Reconstruction of the Tibia. *In* Serafin, D., and Buncke, H.J. (eds.): Microsurgical Composite Tissue Transplantation, pp. 713–742. St. Louis, C.V. Mosby, 1979.

555. Taylor, G.I., and Daniel, R.K.: The Anatomy of Several Free Flap Donor Sites. Plast. Reconstr. Surg., 56:243–253, 1973.

556. Taylor, G.I., and Daniel, R.K.: The Free Flap: Composite Tissue Transfer by Vascular Anastomosis. Aust. N.Z.J. Surg., 43:1–3, 1973.

557. Taylor, G.I.; Miller, G.D.H.; and Ham, F.J.: The Free Vascularized Bone Graft: A Clinical Extension of Microvascular Techniques. Plast. Reconstr. Surg., 55:533–544, 1975.

558. Taylor, G.I.; Townsend, P.; and Corlett, R.: Superiority of

the Deep Circumflex Iliac Vessels as the Supply for Free Groin Flaps—Clinical Work. Plast. Reconstr. Surg., 64:745–759, 1979.

559. Taylor, G.I.; Townsend, P.; and Corlett, R.: Superiority of the Deep Circumflex Iliac Vessels as the Supply for Free Groin Flaps: Experimental Work. Plast. Reconstr. Surg., 64:595–604, 1979.

560. Taylor, G.I., and Watson, N.: One-Stage Repair of Compound Leg Defects with Free, Revascularized Flaps of Groin Skin and Iliac Bone. Plast. Reconstr. Surg., 61:494–506, 1978.

561. Terzis, J.K.; Sweet, R.C.; Dykes, R.W.; and Williams, H.B.: Recovery of Function in Free Muscle Transplants Using Microneurovascular Anastomoses. J. Hand Surg., 3:37–59, 1978.

562. Thatte, R.L., and Laud, N.: The Use of the Fascia of the Lower Leg as a Roll-Over Flap: Its Possible Clinical Applications in Reconstructive Surgery. Brit. J. Plast. Surg., 37:88–94, 1984.

563. Tolhurst, D.E.: "Skin and Bone": The Use of Muscle Flaps to Cover Exposed Bone. Brit. J. Plast. Surg., 33:99–114, 1980.

564. Tolhurst, D.E.; Haeseker, B.; and Zeeman, R.J.: The Development of the Fasciocutaneous Flap and Its Clinical Applications. Plast. Reconstr. Surg., 71:597–605, 1983.

565. Tonnesen, P.A.; Heerfordt, J.; and Pers, M.: 150 Open Fractures of the Tibial Shaft—The Relation Between Necrosis of the Skin and Delayed Union. Acta Orthop. Scand., 46:823–835, 1975.

566. Trueta, J.: Treatment of War Wounds and Fractures With Special Reference to the Closed Method as Used in the War in Spain, pp. 1–150. London, W. Hamilton, 1939.

567. Trueta, J.: "Closed" Treatment of War Fractures. Lancet, 1:1452–1455, 1939.

568. Trueta, J.: Blood Supply and the Rate of Healing of Tibial Fractures. Clin. Orthop., 105:11–26, 1974.

569. Trueta, J., and Caladias, A.X.: A Study of the Blood Supply of the Long Bones. Surg. Gynecol. Obstet., 118:485–498, 1964.

570. Tsai, T.M.; Ludwig, L.; and Tonkin, M.: Vascularized Fibular Epiphyseal Transfer: A Clinical Study. Clin. Orthop., 210:228–234, 1986.

571. Tscherne, H.: The Management of Open Fractures. In Tscherne, H., and Gotzen, L. (eds.): Fractures with Soft Tissue Injuries, pp. 10–32. New York, Springer-Verlag, 1984.

572. Tscherne, H., and Gotzen, L.: Preface. In Tscherne, H., and Gotzen, L. (eds.): Fractures with Soft Tissue Injuries, pp. iii–iv. New York, Springer-Verlag, 1984.

573. Tsukayama, D.T.; Guay, D.R.; and Peterson, P.K.: Antibiotic Therapy of Chronic Osteomyelitis. In Gustilo, R.B.; Gruninger, R.P.; and Tsukayama, D.T. (eds.): Orthopaedic Infection: Diagnosis and Treatment, pp. 166–174. Philadelphia, W.B. Saunders, 1989.

574. Tsukayama, D.T.; Merkow, R.L.; and Gustilo, R.B.: The Use of Tobramycin-Impregnated Polymethlmethacrylate Beads in the Therapy of Deep Bone and Joint Infections. J. Orthop. Trauma, 1:263–264, 1987.

575. Urbaniak, J.R.; Koman, L.A.; Goldner, R.D.; Armstrong, N.B.; and Nunley, J.A.: The Vascularized Cutaneous Scapular Flap. Plast. Reconstr. Surg., 69:772–778, 1982.

576. Urbaniak, J.R., and Richards, R.R.: Complications in Microvascular Surgery. In Epps, C.H., Jr. (ed.): Complications in Orthopaedic Surgery, 2nd ed., pp. 845–864. Philadelphia, J.B. Lippincott, 1986.

577. Urist, M.R.; Mazet, R., Jr.; and McLean, F.C.: The Pathogenesis and Treatment of Delayed Union and Nonunion: A Survey of Eighty-Five Ununited Fractures of the Shaft of the Tibia and One Hundred Control Cases with Similar Injuries. J. Bone Joint Surg., 36A:931–967, 1954.

578. Urist, M.R., and McLean, F.C.: Osteogenic Potency and New-Bone Formation by Induction in Transplants to the Anterior Chamber of the Eye. J. Bone Joint Surg., 34A:443–467, 1952.

579. Usui, M.; Minami, M.; and Ishii, S.: Successful Replantation of an Amputated Leg in a Child. Plast. Reconstr. Surg., 63:613–617, 1979.

580. Varecka, T.F.: Soft Tissue Coverage in Open Fractures. In Gustilo, R.B.; Gruninger, R.P.; and Tsukayama, D.T. (eds.): Orthopaedic Infection: Diagnosis and Treatment. pp. 118–122. Philadelphia, W.B. Saunders, 1989.

581. Vasconez, L.O.; Bostwick, J., III; and McCraw, J.: Coverage of Exposed Bone by Muscle Transposition and Skin Grafting. Plast. Reconstr. Surg., 53:526–530, 1974.

582. Vasconez, L.O., and McCraw, J.B.: Reconstructive Procedures of the Lower Extremity. In Grabb, W.C., and Smith, J.W. (eds.): Plastic Surgery, 3rd ed., pp. 811–817. Boston, Little Brown, 1979.

583. Veliskakis, K.P.: Primary Internal Fixation in Open Fractures of the Tibial Shaft: The Problem of Wound Healing. J. Bone Joint Surg., 41B:342–354, 1959.

584. Waldvogel, F.A.; Medoff, G.; and Swartz, M.N.: Osteomyelitis: A Review of Clinical Features, Therapeutic Considerations and Unusual Aspects: Part II. N. Engl. J. Med., 282:260–266, 1970.

585. Waldvogel, F.A.; Medoff, G.; and Swartz, M.N.: Osteomyelitis: A Review of Clinical Features, Therapeutic Considerations and Unusual Aspects: Part I. N. Engl. J. Med., 282:198–206, 1970.

586. Waldvogel, F.A.; Medoff, G.; and Swartz, M.N.: Clinical Types of Osteomyelitis. In Waldvogel, F.A. (ed.): Osteomyelitis: Clinical Features, Therapeutic Considerations, and Unusual Aspects, pp. 13–62. Springfield, C.C. Thomas, 1971.

587. Waldvogel, F.A., and Vasey, H.: Osteomyelitis: The Past Decade. N. Engl. J. Med., 303:360–370, 1980.

588. Walenkamp, G.H.; Vree, T.B.; and van Rens, T.J.: Gentamicin-PMMA Beads: Pharmacokinetic and Nephrotoxicological Study. Clin. Orthop., 205:171–183, 1986.

589. Wangensteen, O.H.; Wangensteen, S.D.; and Klinger, C.F.: Wound Management of Ambroise Paré and Dominique Larrey, Great French Military Surgeons of the 16th and 19th Centuries. Bull. Hist. Med., 46:207–234, 1972.

590. Watari, S.; Ikuta, Y.; Adachi, N.; Murase, M.; and Tsuge, K.: Vascular Pedicle Fibular Transplantation as Treatment for Bone Tumor. Clin. Orthop., 133:158–164, 1978.

591. Waters, R.L.; Perry, J.; Antonelli, D.; and Hislop, H.: Energy Cost of Walking of Amputees: The Influence of Level of Amputation. J. Bone Joint Surg., 58A:42–46, 1976.

592. Watson, J.S.; Brough, M.D.; and Orton, C.: Simultaneous Coverage of Both Heels With One Free Flap. Plast. Reconstr. Surg., 63:269–270, 1979.

593. Weber, B.G., and Cech, O.: Pseudarthrosis: Pathophysiology, Biomechanics, Therapy, Results, pp. 1–60. New York, Grune & Stratton, 1976.

594. Weiland, A.J.: Current Concepts Review: Vascularized Free Bone Transplants. J. Bone Joint Surg., 63A:166–169, 1981.

595. Weiland, A.J.: Elective Microsurgery for Orthopaedic Reconstruction: Part III. Vascularized Bone Transfers. Instr. Course Lect., XXXIII: 446–460, 1984.

596. Weiland, A.J.; Berggren, A.; and Jones, L.: The Acute Effects of Blocking Medullary Blood Supply on Regional Cortical Blood Flow in Canine Ribs as Measured by the Hydrogen Washout Technique. Clin. Orthop., 165:265–272, 1982.

597. Weiland, A.J., and Daniel, R.K.: Microvascular Anastomoses for Bone Grafts in the Treatment of Massive Defects in Bone. J. Bone Joint Surg., 61A:98–104, 1979.

598. Weiland, A.J., and Daniel, R.K.: Congenital Pseudarthrosis of the Tibia: Treatment With Vascularized Autogenous Fibular Grafts: A Preliminary Report. Johns Hopkins Med. J., 147:89–95, 1980.

599. Weiland, A.J., and Daniel, R.K.: Clinical Techniques of Segmental Autogenous Bone Grafting on Vascular Pedicles. In Mears, D.C. (ed.): External Skeletal Fixation, pp. 646–679. Baltimore, Williams & Wilkins, 1983.

600. Weiland, A.J.; Daniel, R.K.; and Riley, L.H., Jr.: Application of the Free Vascularized Bone Graft in the Treatment of Malignant or Aggressive Bone Tumors. Johns Hopkins Med. J., 140:85–96, 1977.

601. Weiland, A.J.; Kleinert, H.E.; Kutz, J.E.; and Daniel, R.K.: Free Vascularized Bone Grafts in Surgery of the Upper Extremity. J. Hand Surg., 4:129–144, 1979.

602. Weiland, A.J.; Kleinert, H.E.; Kutz, J.E.; and Daniel, R.K.: Vascularized Bone Grafts in the Upper Extremity. In Serafin, D., and Buncke, H. (eds.): Microsurgical Composite Tissue Transplantation, pp. 605–625. St. Louis, C.V. Mosby, 1979.

603. Weiland, A.J., and Moore, J.R.: Vascularized Bone Grafts. In Green, D.P. (ed.): Operative Hand Surgery, 2nd ed., pp. 1245–1269. New York, Churchill Livingstone, 1988.

604. Weiland, A.J.; Moore, J.R.; and Daniel, R.K.: Vascularized Bone Autografts: Experience with 41 Cases. Clin. Orthop., 174:87–95, 1983.

605. Weiland, A.J.; Moore, J.R.; and Daniel, R.K.: The Efficacy of Free Tissue Transfer in the Treatment of Osteomyelitis. J. Bone Joint Surg., 66A:181–193, 1984.

606. Weiland, A.J.; Moore, J.R.; and Hotchkiss, R.N.: Soft Tissue Procedures for Reconstruction of Tibial Shaft Fractures. Clin. Orthop., 178:42–53, 1983.

607. Weiland, A.J.; Phillips, T.W.; and Randolph, M.A.: Bone Grafts: A Radiologic, Histolic, and Biomechanical Model Comparing Autographs, Allografts, and Free Vascularized Bone Grafts. Plast. Reconstr. Surg., 74:368–379, 1984.

608. Weiland, A.J.: Symposium: The Use of Muscle Flaps in the Treatment of Osteomyelitis in the Lower Extremity. Contemp. Orthop., 10:127–159, 1985.

609. Weinstein, A.J.: Classification of Adult Osteomyelitis and Antibiotic Therapy. In Evarts, C.M. (ed.): Surgery of the Musculoskeletal System, Vol. 4, pp. 5–13. New York, Churchill Livingstone, 1983.

610. Welch, M.C., and Miller, E.H.: Complications of Treatment of Fractures and Dislocations of the Tibia and Fibula. In Epps, C.H., Jr. (ed.): Complications in Orthopaedic Surgery, 2nd ed., pp. 585–597. Philadelphia, J.B. Lippincott, 1986.

611. Weller, S.: The External Fixator for the Prevention and Treatment of Infections. In Uhthoff, H. (ed.): Current Concepts of External Fixation of Fractures, pp. 215–220. New York, Springer-Verlag, 1982.

612. West, W.F.; Kelly, P.J.; and Martin, W.J.: Chronic Osteomyelitis: I. Factors Affecting the Results of Treatment in 186 Patients. J.A.M.A., 213:1837–1848, 1970.

613. White, W.L.; Dupertuis, S.M.; Gaisford, J.C.; Musgrave, R.H.; and Hanna, D.C.: Evaluation of 114 Cross-Leg Flaps. In Skoog, T., and Ivy, R.H. (eds.): Transactions of the First Congress of the International Society of Plastic Surgeons, pp. 516–524. Baltimore, Williams & Wilkins, 1955.

614. Williams, D.N.: Antibiotic Penetration Into Bones and Joints. In Gustilo, R.B.; Gruninger, R.P.; and Tsukayama, D.T. (eds.): Orthopaedic Infection: Diagnosis and Treatment, pp. 52–59. Philadelphia, W.B. Saunders, 1989.

615. Withers, E.H.; Bishop, J.O.; and Tullos, H.S.: Microvascular Free Flap Transfers to Foot and Ankle. Orthop. Rev., 14: 33–38, 1985.

616. Wood, M.B.: Comparison of Microsurgically Revascularized Diaphyseal Bone Grafts to Viable Segmental Long-Bone Fractures in the Canine: Blood Flow and Fluorochrome Uptake Quantitation. Orthop. Trans., 8:301–302, 1984.

617. Wood, M.B.: Free Vascularized Bone Transfers for Nonunions, Segmental Gaps and Following Tumor Resection. Orthopedics, 9:810–816, 1986.

618. Wood, M.B., and Cooney, W.P., III: Vascularized Bone Segment Transfers for Management of Chronic Osteomyelitis. Orthop. Clin. North Am., 15:461–472, 1984.

619. Wood, M.B.; Cooney, W.P., III; and Irons, G.B.: Posttraumatic Lower Extremity Reconstruction by Vascularized Bone Graft Transfer. Orthopedics, 7:255–262, 1984.

620. Wood, M.B.; Cooney, W.P., III; and Irons, G.B.: Skeletal Reconstruction by Vascularized Bone Transfer: Indications and Results. Mayo Clin. Proc., 60:729–734, 1985.

621. Woods, J.E.; Irons, G.B., Jr.; and Masson, J.K.: Use of Muscular, Musculocutaneous, and Omental Flaps to Reconstruct Difficult Defects. Plast. Reconstr. Surg., 59:191–199, 1977.

622. Wray, J.B.: Factors in the Pathogenesis of Nonunion. J. Bone Joint Surg., 47A:168–173, 1965.

623. Wright, J.K., and Watkins, R.P.: Use of the Soleus Muscle Flap to Cover Part of the Distal Tibia. Plast. Reconstr. Surg., 68:957–958, 1981.

624. Wright, P.E.: Microsurgery. In Crenshaw, A.H. (ed.):

Campbell's Operative Orthopaedics, 7th ed., pp. 509–594. St. Louis, C.V. Mosby, 1987.

625. Yablon, I.G., and Cruess, R.L.: The Effect of Hyperbaric Oxygen on Fracture Healing in Rats. J. Trauma, 8:186–202, 1969.

626. Yaremchuk, M.J.; Brumback, R.J.; Manson, P.N.; Burgess, A.R.; Poka, A.; and Weiland, A.J.: Acute and Definitive Management of Traumatic Osteocutaneous Defects of the Lower Extremity. Plast. Reconstr. Surg., 80:1–12, 1987.

627. Yaremchuk, M.J., and Manson, P.N.: Local and Free Flap Donor Sites for Lower-Extremity Reconstruction. *In* Yaremchuk, M.J.; Burgess, A.R.; and Brumback, R.J. (eds.): Lower Extremity Salvage and Reconstruction, pp. 117–157. New York, Elsevier Science Publishing, 1989.

628. Yoshimura, M.; Shimamura, K.; Iwai, Y.; Yamauchi, S.; and Ueno, T.: Free Vascularized Fibular Transplant: A New Method for Monitoring Circulation of the Grafted Fibula. J. Bone Joint Surg., 65:1295–1301, 1983.

629. Youdas, J.W.; Wood, M.B.; Cahalan, T.D.; and Chao, E.Y.: A Quantitative Analysis of Donor Site Morbidity After Vascularized Fibula Transfer. J. Orthop. Res., 6:621–629, 1988.

630. Zancolli, E., and Mitre, H.: Latissimus Dorsi Transfer to Restore Elbow Flexion. J. Bone Joint Surg., 55A:1265–1275, 1973.

631. Zook, E.G.; Russell, R.C.; and Asaadi, M.: A Comparative Study of Free and Pedicle Flaps for Lower Extremity Wounds. Ann. Plast. Surg., 17:21–33, 1986.

5

Complications

Vincent D. Pellegrini, Jr.
C. McCollister Evarts

SYSTEMIC COMPLICATIONS OF INJURY

Complications of musculoskeletal trauma can jeopardize life or limb depending on the severity of the local injury and the nature of the resultant systemic response. Even a "simple" femoral shaft fracture can trigger a life-threatening cascade of events culminating in multisystem failure, underscoring that rarely does there exist a truly "isolated" long bone extremity fracture.

HYPOVOLEMIA (SHOCK)

Shock is defined as a clinical state in which there is poor tissue perfusion with resultant tissue hypoxia threatening damage to the vital organs. Simeone[87] stated that "shock is a clinical condition in which, because of insufficient effective circulating blood volume or because of abnormal partitioning of cardiac output, the capillary blood flow in the vital tissues or in all tissues is reduced to levels below the minimum requirements for oxidative metabolism."

For centuries, shock has been recognized as a clinical entity. In 1872, Gross[42] defined shock as "a manifestation of root unhinging of the machinery of life." Many experimental studies have been performed to investigate the pathophysiologic mechanisms of shock.[15,16,22,23,25,28,31,43,44,54,64,65,72,88,94] Wig-gers[94] characterized shock as "a state of low cardiac output with decrease in total peripheral resistance." However, more recent investigators have shown that low cardiac output is not always present and that the hemodynamic pattern is directly related to the etiology of shock.[81,82,92]

CLASSIFICATION

In 1934, Blalock[14] suggested four categories of shock: hematogenic (oligemia); neurogenic (caused primarily by nervous influences); vasogenic (initially decreased vascular resistance and increased vascular capacity); and cardiogenic, owing to either failure of the heart as a pump or diminished cardiac output from various causes. Shires and coworkers[78] believed that shock invariably results from the loss of one or more of four separate but interrelated functions (ie, the heart, the volume of blood, the arteriolar resistance vessels, and the capacitance vessels).

Hemorrhagic (Hypovolemic) Shock

Hemorrhagic (hypovolemic) shock is the most common type of shock occurring in patients with multiple trauma and skeletal injury. The blood volume is low, resulting in tachycardia, low cardiac output, low central venous pressure, increased peripheral resistance, and hypotension.[95] A closed femoral shaft fracture can easily conceal a 2- to 3-unit blood loss in a swollen thigh without specific vascular injury. Half of all pelvic fractures result in blood loss sufficient to require transfusion therapy,

335

and hemorrhage is responsible for more than half of the reported mortality from pelvic fractures, ranging from 14% to 39%.[33,47] Injuries with a double break in the pelvic ring involving disruption of both anterior and posterior elements resulted in transfusion therapy in more than two thirds of patients, and replacement approached that of the entire circulating blood volume.[21,47] Therefore, the most common cause of circulatory failure in the trauma patient is hypovolemia, and the presence of shock in adult patients implies hypovolemia of 1 to 2 L of blood (Table 5-1). Smaller blood losses can produce shock in patients with pre-existing congestive heart failure. The compensatory mechanisms of venous vasoconstriction and increased myocardial contractility occur in the presence of hypovolemia so that adequate diastolic cardiac filling can take place at lower filling pressures. In a healthy adult, blood volume can be altered by 1 L without significant consequence. The patient who requires more than 2 to 3 L of blood during fluid resuscitation, after external bleeding has been stopped, should be further evaluated for an unrecognized source of internal blood loss.[17,19]

TREATMENT OF HYPOVOLEMIC SHOCK

The goal of treatment of hypovolemic shock is to safely restore adequate intravascular volume and oxygen-carrying capacity.[17,19,45,82] Because of the same mechanisms that attempt to maintain adequate diastolic cardiac filling (ie, venous vasoconstriction and increased myocardial contractility), there is a complex relationship between reinfused fluid volumes and these compensatory factors. In severe hypovolemic shock, it may be necessary to transfuse more than the normal blood volume to

establish adequate tissue perfusion. Thus the goal of fluid resuscitation should be to restore adequate tissue perfusion rather than to empirically correct an estimated specific deficit.[17,19,45,82]

Initial therapy for hypovolemic shock consists of the administration of normal saline solution followed by cross-matched whole blood. The patient who is quickly resuscitated following losses of 2 to 3 L of blood will do well. A two- to three-hour delay in resuscitation increases the potential mortality and morbidity because of subsequent multisystem failure. The number of clinical organ system failures observed relates directly to the length of time shock persists. It is important to restore blood pressure by increasing intravascular volume as rapidly as possible. Patients who have no blood pressure initially can receive transfusions of plasma or crystalloid solution. Ringer's lactate may be used until plasma or blood is obtained, but the calculated increase in intravascular volume will be only about one fourth to one fifth the volume of Ringer's lactate used; lactated Ringer's solution in excess of 3 to 4 L should not be used in place of plasma and blood.[19] If the initial hematocrit is greater than 35%, plasma expanders are preferable because of prompt increase in cardiac output. When the hematocrit is below 25%, whole blood is the treatment of choice.[24,86] In the absence of preexisting cardiopulmonary disease, the hematocrit should be maintained between 25% and 30% to create a satisfactory balance between adequate oxygen transport capacity and reduced viscosity to allow unimpeded flow in the microcirculation.[34,36,69,70,89] In acute *normovolemic* hemodilution during *elective* total hip replacement, a hematocrit of 21% was well tolerated in patients with normal cardiopulmonary function; increased

Table 5-1. Classes of Acute Hemorrhage

	Class I	Class II	Class III	Class IV
Blood loss (mL)	750	1,000–1,250	1,500–1,800	2,000–2,500
Blood loss (units)	1–2	2–3	3–4	5
Blood loss* (%)	15	20–25	30–35	40–50
Pulse rate† (b/min)	72–84	>100	>120	>140
Blood pressure‡ (mm Hg)	118/82	110/80	70–90/50–60	<50–60 systolic
Pulse pressure (mm Hg)	36	30	20–30	10–20
Capillary blanch test	Normal	Delayed	Delayed	Delayed
Respiratory rate	14–20	20–30	30–40	>35
Urine output (mL/hr)	30–35	25–30	5–15	Negligible
Central nervous system—mental status	Slightly anxious	Mildly anxious	Anxious and confused	Confused-lethargic
Fluid replacement	Crystalloid	Crystalloid	Crystalloid + Blood	Crystalloid + Blood

* = % of blood volume in a standard 70-kg male.
† = assume normal of 72/min.
‡ = assume normal of 120/80.
(Modified from Advanced Trauma Life Support Student Manual, p. 45. Chicago, American College of Surgeons, 1981.)[7]

cardiac output was the major compensatory factor in offsetting a decreased oxygen-carrying capacity to maintain nearly normal systemic oxygen transport.[52]

Blood Transfusion.   In an era of concern over the prevalence of human immunodeficiency virus (HIV) infection, any discussion of the use of blood products would be remiss without mention of this evolving crisis[1,50] (Fig. 5-1). Blood-soiled wounds, especially those with the sharp bone ends encountered in open fractures, should be handled using universal precautions to protect from direct contact with blood and other body fluids. Figures from the emergency department of one urban university hospital suggest that nearly 15% of victims with penetrating trauma presenting for treatment tested positive for HIV infection on serologic testing[35] (Fig. 5-2). Furthermore, increased risk of HIV transmission by pooled blood products from multiple donors should restrict their use to life-threatening situations until definitive testing methods can be universally employed.[34,70,89] Current estimates for contracting HIV infection from a unit of transfused blood range from 1:40,000 to 1:250,000 (Fig. 5-3), compared to a 1% risk of contracting non-A, non-B hepatitis with a subsequent chronic carrier rate of 30% to 50%.[20,34,37]

Although whole blood is the ideal replacement

substance in profound hypovolemic shock, its availability becomes a limiting factor in emergencies. A standard type and crossmatch, screening for ABO grouping, Rh typing, and antibody screening, requires approximately 1 hour to process. Total elapsed time between sending the sample to the laboratory and starting a fully matched transfusion is approximately one and a half hours. The safety factor against reaction is 99.9%. An abbreviated stat crossmatch requires 15 minutes and offers 99.8% safety. In an emergency, major grouping and Rh typing can be done in 10 minutes and offer 99% safety. The use of universal donor or group O Rh-negative blood is no quicker and somewhat less safe than specific blood and should be abandoned if possible.[48]

Massive transfusions replacing the entire circulating blood volume (10 or more units per 24 hours) expose the patient to special problems. Mortality has been reported at 10% to 80% and is largely related to the underlying injury requiring treatment. Conventional teaching holds that for every transfusion load of 10 units of whole blood or red cells, the patient should also be given 1 unit of fresh frozen plasma, a 10-pack of platelets, and 2 ampules of calcium.[91] The use of stored bank blood for patients in profound shock carries several risks and potential complications, including coagulation changes with secondary bleeding, depression of the

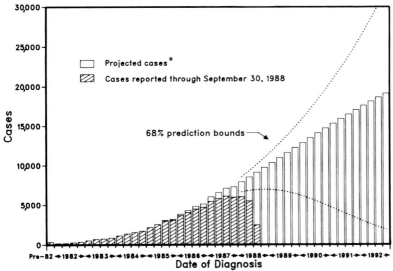

*Estimated numbers of cases diagnosed through December 1987 are reported cases adjusted for estimated reporting delays. Estimated numbers of cases for 1988-1992 are projected from cases diagnosed as of June 30, 1987, and reported as of March 31, 1988.

Fig. 5-1. Incidence of AIDS, by quarter and year of diagnosis, in the United States, pre-1982 to 1992.[1]

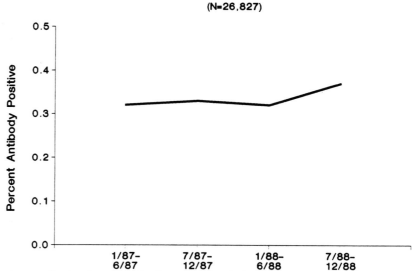

*Specimen collection began at the four pilot hospitals in 1/87; sufficient data (18 months or more) for trend analysis are expected from the next five hospitals by 9/89 and for the remaining 31 hospitals by 3/90.

Fig. 5-2. HIV–antibody prevalence in patients at four pilot sentinel hospitals,* from January 1987 to December 1988.[1]

oxygen-carrying capacity of the red blood cells, increased acid load, and introduction of cellular aggregates and debris causing pulmonary microemboli. Special filters are available for transfusion of stored bank blood, but their use is questionable when fresh blood is transfused. Olcott and Lim[71] have shown that from 20% to 40% of functioning platelets are removed by filters. This reduction of functioning platelets in filtered blood, although not significant in 1- or 2-unit transfusions, may become significant when 6 or more units are used. If filters are used, platelet transfusions may be necessary to compensate for the filter-trapped platelets. When fresh whole blood is used for massive blood re-

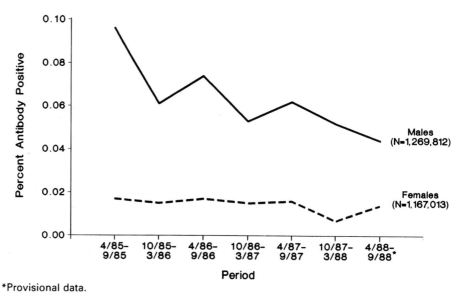

*Provisional data.

Fig. 5-3. HIV–antibody prevalence in first-time blood donors, by sex, as reported by the American Red Cross, from April 1985 to September 1988.[1]

placement in critically bleeding patients, filters should not be used.

Controversy remains in the choice of packed red blood cells and whole blood as transfusion therapy for hemorrhagic shock.[4,80,82] Following the development of techniques to prepare safe and effective blood components—including platelet concentrates, cryoprecipitate, fresh frozen plasma, albumin, gamma globulin, and other plasma protein fractions—pressure to use packed red cells in transfusion therapy has increased. Chaplin[25] believes that 80% of transfusion therapy needs in the United States can be met with packed red cells. Some clinicians believe that the only legitimate reason to use whole blood is for acute blood loss and, even then, specific component therapy is preferred for correction of the problem. Supporting this recommendation, many patients and laboratory animals have withstood acute blood loss with only crystalloid solutions administered for replacement.[34,40,41,89]

Although clotting times and hematocrits may be the same after resuscitation with either packed red blood cells or whole blood, significant differences are found when host defense parameters are measured.[26] Circulating plasma proteins known as opsonins facilitate clearance of particulate debris, such as bacteria and platelet–blood element microaggregates, from the intravascular space by the reticuloendothelial system.[75] In dogs subjected to controlled blood loss equal to 8% of their body weight, considerable depression of serum protein, C3, IgG, and total plasma opsonic activity was evident when the dogs were resuscitated with packed red cells in saline solution.[13] No such depression in serum components of opsonic activity was observed in identically bled dogs that were resuscitated with whole blood. When host defense parameters were measured, nearly 100% of serum opsonic activity returned in recipients of whole blood, but this activity fell to less than 25% of normal within 3 hours in dogs treated with packed red blood cells.[13]

Whole blood stored up to 21 days in acid citrate dextrose at 4°C contains all the components necessary for opsonization with only slight reduction of activity as compared with fresh whole blood.[59,60] Reconstituted packed red blood cells, however, contain only 30% of their volume as plasma components and, consequently, have a markedly reduced content of plasma opsonins.[26,59] Evidence suggests that low levels of opsonic proteins predispose a host to infection,[2,5,6,39,63] pulmonary dysfunction,[38] and multiorgan system failure[18]; impaired opsonization may be one of the most common causes of dysfunction of host defense mechanisms against infection.[25,68,93] Indeed, the use of cryoprecipitate as an opsonin-rich solution has been reported in the successful treatment of postburn sepsis[53] and the pulmonary dysfunction of severe adult respiratory distress syndrome.[74,75] Opsonic activity is important in the response to shock and trauma, and on this basis whole blood may be preferable to packed cells for resuscitation in acute hemorrhagic shock when the effect on repletion of circulating opsonic elements is considered. In the setting of severe shock, a significant decrease in host reticuloendothelial clearance occurs, and the failure of large-volume transfusion of packed red blood cells to reverse this deficiency may have considerable negative impact on ultimate survival.[13,14]

Crystalloid and Colloid.   Although primary treatment for hypovolemic shock consists of the administration of whole blood, crystalloid and colloid solutions can be used to restore intravascular volume if properly cross-matched blood is not immediately available. Ringer's lactate and normal saline solutions are the two most commonly used volume replacements. Both of these solutions are preferable to un-cross-matched blood, especially when the hematocrit is 35% or above, because the dilution provided by saline solutions will have beneficial effects on the microcirculation.[12,27,30,46,66,67,73,76,79,80,90] When large volumes of electrolyte solution are used for resuscitation, neither Ringer's lactate nor normal saline solution appears to produce harmful effects relative to acid-base balance.[55] Serum lactate levels and the acute chloride loads in patients receiving normal saline solution are handled well by trauma patients.[9,10] Lactate levels have actually been shown to decrease as cellular perfusion is increased, regardless of the solution given.[77] The critical factor is restoration of volume to enhance the microcirculation.

In patients with preexisting cardiorespiratory disease, 5% dextrose in water may be used alternately with sodium solution. It must be recognized that regardless of the fluid, be it Ringer's lactate, normal saline solution, or 5% dextrose in water, up to 90% of the volume eventually leaks into the interstitial water compartment. Therefore, colloid solutions may be theoretically more effective than crystalloid solutions in expanding and maintaining intravascular volume.

The basic colloid replacements commonly used are 5% albumin, plasmanate (a particular form of albumin), and dextran 40. The use of colloid as an adjunct to crystalloid has been reported beneficial in the treatment of hypovolemic shock.[8] The blood volume and the cardiorespiratory system show a much greater response to colloid administration than to crystalloid administration.[51,61,62,84,85] Colloid therapy tends to restore plasma volume without simultaneously expanding the interstitial water, minimizing the risk of pulmonary edema. The use of normal human serum albumin (25% albumin and 5% plasma protein fraction) has increased rapidly in recent years, and guidelines for its use have been previously defined. The following specific situations were designated appropriate indications for its use: shock, burns, retroperitoneal surgery, adult respiratory distress syndrome, ascites, and peritonitis.[3]

Of the available colloids, it appears that dextran 40 is the most effective in restoring plasma volume. Low-molecular-weight dextran (with an average molecular weight of 40,000) has been effective not only in expanding plasma volume, but also in decreasing blood viscosity and increasing microcirculatory flow.[32] Contrary to the theoretical advances of albumin, a large body of experimental and clinical evidence contraindicates the use of supplemental albumin therapy for hemorrhagic shock. Excessive concentrations of albumin given to patients in deep shock offer no advantage in resuscitation over the volume effects of dextran and in fact have proved harmful. Albumin extravasates into the lungs, heart, kidneys, and liver, thus increasing the likelihood of edema formation.[49] Although albumin can restore such levels as total serum protein and serum albumin to normal, it can also have a remarkably negative inotropic effect on the heart.[29] Administration of albumin also probably leads to impaired salt and water excretion and may contribute to central volume overload, respiratory failure, and acute renal failure.[57] Albumin has a detrimental effect on pulmonary function that may be caused by reduced saline diuresis, increased interstitial pulmonary water from trapped albumin, or impaired left ventricular function. Clinical trials examining the addition of albumin to the usual regimen of whole blood and balanced electrolyte solution for resuscitation from hypovolemic shock have been added to the experimental evidence in the indictment against the use of albumin in such situations. In addition, supplemental albumin added to standard resuscitative measures for hypovolemic shock increases the total serum protein and serum albumin levels to almost normal, while producing relative reduction in the globulins and other fractions. This results in decreased plasma fibrinogen levels and a prolonged prothrombin time, which may lead to significantly impaired coagulation in albumin-treated patients. The mild reduction in serum albumin concentration that occurs when shock is treated with whole blood and saline solution may actually be desirable. It therefore can now be concluded that supplemental albumin is contraindicated for patients in hypovolemic shock. Extra albumin (ie, more albumin than is given in the normal course of replacement of blood loss with blood) is not only unnecessary but also undesirable.[56,58]

Other Agents.   Vasopressors, hydrocortisone, and vasodilators are of questionable value in the treatment of hemorrhagic shock.[11] The response to these agents has been variable and unpredictable.[78,83]

For the patient in hypovolemic shock with open fractures and large wounds, the administration of prophylactic antibiotics is advisable.[51,63] Unless a patient has Addison's disease, has had an adrenalectomy, or has been receiving long-term corticosteroid therapy, the use of steroids in the management of hypovolemic shock is otherwise contraindicated.

MONITORING THE PATIENT IN SHOCK

In the patient being resuscitated, arterial blood pressure, pulse, central venous pressure (CVP), and urinary output must be monitored closely. These are all indirect measurements to help ascertain the patient's intravascular volume. Adequate venous access should be obtained by placement of several peripheral lines. An arterial line may be useful for continuous monitoring of blood pressure and frequent checks of arterial blood oxygenation. A CVP line, inserted through the internal jugular vein or the subclavian vein, should be placed so that the catheter tip is in or near the right atrium. A normal reading is 5 to 10 cm of water pressure; the CVP should not normally exceed 15 cm of water pressure. More accurate monitoring of intravascular volume and cardiac output can be obtained from a Swan-Ganz catheter. Data obtained from this device may be essential to the differentiation of cardiogenic from noncardiogenic pulmonary edema during fluid resuscitation.

Renal function must be monitored closely. The average adult should have a urinary output of 20 to 30 ml per hour as monitored by an indwelling Foley catheter, placed only after adequate rectal examination to investigate the possibility of urethral disruption. Renal function may be decreased by hemorrhagic shock, hyponatremia, urinary tract injury, or the use of pressors.

CARDIOPULMONARY ARREST

Standards and guidelines for cardiopulmonary resuscitation (CPR) and emergency cardiac care have been set by the American Heart Association.[115,116]

The major impetus for this was an increasing appreciation of premature cardiovascular mortality and morbidity. Resuscitation by CPR outside the hospital, followed by advanced measures in the hospital, has been effective in 40% to 60% of select subgroups of patients.[114,119,120]

The American Heart Association has recommended that competence in CPR be mandatory for physician reappointment to faculty.[116] Reviews of in-hospital resuscitation efforts show poor results, with a success rate of approximately 20%.[104] The practice of orthopaedic surgery encompasses numerous situations in which cardiac arrest may occur.[97,99,102,103,110,121,122,124] Our patient population includes many elderly, infirm patients who may have accompanying cardiopulmonary, renal, and metabolic diseases that predispose them to cardiac arrest.[109] Moreover, trauma frequently affects young people, who may suffer significant cardiopulmonary insult in addition to musculoskeletal injuries.[96,113] For these numerous reasons, the orthopaedic surgeon should be capable of instituting care in the management of cardiac arrest and must be proficient in the techniques of CPR and Advanced Cardiac Life Support (ACLS). Because it is beyond the scope of this text to cover this material in detail, the reader is referred to several excellent references for further study.[98,100,101,105-108,111,112,115-118,123]

FAT EMBOLISM SYNDROME

The fat embolism syndrome is a major cause of morbidity and mortality following fractures in the patient with multiple injuries. For more than a century the puzzling features of this entity have interested many. Its relationship to skeletal and soft tissue injury is well recognized, and many cases have been reported.[152,153,218] Fat embolism is an important cause of acute respiratory distress syndrome (ARDS).[142,159,224,248] However, the fat embolism syndrome is not always a sequela of trauma. It has been reported in association with a variety of nontraumatic entities, including hemoglobinopathy,[177] collagen disease,[185] diabetes,[156] burns,[158] severe infection,[205] inhalation anesthesia,[260] metabolic disorders,[186] neoplasms, osteomyelitis,[147,166] blood transfusion,[203] cardiopulmonary bypass,[211] renal infarction,[149] decompression owing to altitude,[184] and renal homotransplantation.[189] Since the mid-1960s a better understanding of the underlying pathophysiologic mechanisms of the fat embolism syndrome has developed,[151,162,176] and its relationship to acute respiratory distress syndrome has been clarified. Sproule and colleagues[243] identified the role of fat embolization in post-traumatic respiratory insufficiency. They established that fat embolism must be recognized as one of the acute respiratory distress syndromes. With prompt recognition, the treatment of the fat embolism syndrome has become more specific and less empiric, resulting in decreased morbidity and mortality. In more recent years, prevention of the fat embolism syndrome by early fracture fixation and patient mobilization has become the focus of a wave of clinical investigation.[144,145,164,173-175,188,204,225-227,229,230,236,246,249,264]

HISTORICAL ASPECTS

In 1861, Zenker[265] described fat droplets in the lung capillaries of a railroad worker who sustained a fatal thoracoabdominal crush injury. In 1865, Wagner[255] described the pathologic features of fat embolism. However, in 1873, Bergmann[140] became the first to establish the clinical diagnosis of fat embolism syndrome in a 38-year-old patient who sustained a comminuted fracture of the distal femur. Postmortem examination revealed a large amount of pulmonary fat. In 1875, Czerny[157] called attention to the symptoms associated with cerebral fat embolism and noted the importance of a funduscopic examination. In 1879, Fenger and Salisbury[165] from Cook County Hospital made the first clinical diagnosis of fat embolism syndrome in the United States in a patient who had a proximal femoral fracture. Autopsy examination revealed massive fat emboli in the lungs and brain.

In 1879, Scriba[234] reviewed and correlated the clinical, pathologic, and experimental observations of the fat embolism syndrome. In 1911, Benestad[136] and Grondahl[179] first described a petechial rash seen with fat embolism syndrome. Warthin[257] in 1913; Gauss[170] in 1916; Lehman and Moore[198] in 1927; Vance[253] in 1931; and Scuderi[235] in 1941 presented review papers and experimental evidence on the origin and nature of intravenous fat globules, the frequency and importance of fat embolism, and the clinical entity of cerebral fat embolism. In 1957, 1969, and 1971, Peltier[217,219,220] appraised the problem of fat embolism and has continued his investigations and established the importance of pulmonary fat embolism. Sproule and associates[243] were the first to report severe arterial hypoxemia in three patients with the fat embolism syndrome. In 1966, Ashbaugh and Petty[130] first described the use of corticosteroids in the treatment of the respiratory complications of fat embolism syndrome.

In 1973, Beck and Collins[135] published an extensive review of the theoretical and clinical aspects of the post-traumatic fat embolism syndrome. In

1982, Gossling and Pellegrini re-examined the pathophysiology and physiologic basis of treatment of the fat embolism syndrome.[176]

INCIDENCE

The exact incidence of and mortality caused by the fat embolism syndrome are not known; it is difficult to accumulate the data necessary to determine these statistics. Sutton[245] stated that 10% of battle casualties in World War I suffered fat emboli. In World War II a postmortem study of 60 patients who died of battle wounds revealed a 65% incidence of fat emboli.[263] In a study of 5,245 civilian accident victims, fat emboli occurred in 855 and contributed to death in more than half.[169] In Britain, an estimated 80 deaths resulting from highway accidents occur because of the fat embolism syndrome.[213] Recent clinical studies,[125,141,146,206,212,229,251,262] including a review of post-traumatic fat embolism in children,[160,261] have documented the frequent occurrence of this syndrome as a sequela to trauma, especially in patients with multiple fractures. It is apparent that increases in auto, motorcycle, and snowmobile accidents and in other types of trauma will lead to an increased frequency of the fat embolism syndrome. Also, the greatest risk of the fat embolism syndrome occurs with multiple fractures.[161] The mortality has been previously estimated to be as high as 50%. The fat embolism syndrome has become a frequent, serious, and often fatal complication of trauma, both on the battlefield and in civilian life. It has been estimated that more than 5,000 deaths annually are the result of the fat embolism syndrome.

The clinical signs and symptoms associated with the fat embolism syndrome are evident in 0.5% to 2% of patients with long bone fractures and in nearly 10% of patients with multiple skeletal fractures associated with unstable pelvic injuries.[176] Given the subjective clinical criteria essential for diagnosis of the syndrome, its exact incidence is difficult to define from the various reports in the literature. Fat embolization as a subclinical event, however, occurs with nearly all fractures of long bones, and its direct clinical effect is most readily quantitated by monitoring the arterial blood gas.[131] The clinically apparent fat embolism syndrome is, therefore, quite rare as compared to the subclinical fat embolization seen after nearly all lower extremity and pelvic trauma.[223] Clinical manifestations develop in children almost 100 times less frequently than they do in adults with comparable injuries, presumably because of a differing marrow fat content with a higher proportion of hematopoietic ele-

ments.[201] Myelodysplastic disorders, collagen vascular disease, osteoporosis, and extremity immobilization all cause medullary cavity enlargement and an increased liquid marrow fat content, thereby constituting an increased risk for development of fat embolism syndrome. Fat embolism following intramedullary reaming and nailing of long bones has been documented, especially when performed in situ for an impending pathologic fracture.[182,207,215,216,246,259] It has also been reported following fractures of the hip treated with prosthetic hemiarthroplasty.[178] In one controlled series of 854 patients with hip fractures treated without operation, the frequency of fat embolism syndrome ranged from 4% to 7%.[239] The clinical syndrome has also been reported following total hip and knee replacement.[137,197,223] We have had unfortunate experiences with acute fatal respiratory failure developing immediately after cemented total hip arthroplasty and intramedullary rodding of the intact femur with metastatic lytic lesions for impending pathologic fracture.[216] Postmortem examination revealed embolic marrow elements to the pulmonary capillary bed and embolic fat with small infarcts in the capillary bed of the brain.

PATHOGENESIS

The pathogenesis of the fat embolism syndrome is the subject of conjecture and controversy. The source of the embolic fat is thought by most to be the bone marrow.[171] Bone marrow elements have been demonstrated in lung sections, indicating that mechanical fat embolization does indeed occur.[129,183,209,258] The physicochemical theory of fat embolism postulates that the changes that occur in lipid stability after trauma and the alteration of the microcirculatory flow patterns combine to cause inadequate tissue perfusion, subsequent tissue hypoxia, and the fat embolism syndrome.[199,200,232,256] More than one possibility exists for the source of the embolic fat, and the causes are not mutually exclusive.

However, most investigators currently agree that bone marrow is the source of embolic fat seen in the lungs.[129,170,187,193,194,209,232] Considerably fewer agree on the exact role of this fat in the production of the clinical fat embolism syndrome.[134,139,181,191,199,200,250] Few investigators currently subscribe to Peltier's original hypothesis that lipase endogenous to the lung converts neutral fat to toxic free fatty acids.[217,220,221] Recent work by Barie and colleagues demonstrates that free fatty acids are rapidly bound by albumin and transported through the blood stream and lymphatic channels in this benign form.[134] However, one need not implicate conversion to free fatty acids to produce the clinically apparent respiratory failure seen in this syndrome.[176] An abundance of tissue thromboplastin is released with the marrow elements following long bone fracture. This activates the complement system and the extrinsic coagulation cascade via direct activation of factor VII.[137,181,195,231,242,250] Intravascular coagulation by-products such as fibrin and fibrin degradation products are then produced. These blood elements along with leukocytes, platelets, and fat globules combine to increase pulmonary vascular permeability, both by their direct actions on the endothelial lining and through release of numerous vasoactive substances.[155,176] Additionally, these same substances activate platelet aggregation. Suppression of the fibrinolytic system in the injured patient may then aggravate an ongoing accumulation of cellular aggregates, fat macroglobules, and clotting factors that are concentrated in the lung by virtue of its filtering action on venous blood before it is recycled to the systemic circulation.[155] It has become increasingly apparent that embolic marrow fat and other elements may only represent the catalyst for a single early step in a long chain of events leading to the final common pathway of increased pulmonary vascular permeability in response to many forms of systemic injury.

CLINICAL FINDINGS

The clinician must distinguish between the clinical entity of the fat embolism syndrome as the cause of acute respiratory insufficiency and the presence of intravascular fat emboli, which have been described in various conditions, including pancreatitis, osteomyelitis, diabetes, burns, and prolonged steroid therapy. The signs and symptoms of the fat embolism syndrome are predominantly those of the adult respiratory distress syndrome.

The most common etiologic factor associated with the fat embolism syndrome is a long bone fracture in a patient in the second or third decade of life, when tibial or femoral fractures are likely to occur, and in a patient in the sixth or seventh decade of life, when fractures of the hip are frequent. The onset of clinical symptoms may be immediate or may not occur for two or three days after trauma.[163] Sevitt[237] stated that 25 of 100 patients with fat embolism showed symptoms within the first 12 hours after injury; by 36 hours 75 patients and within 48 hours after injury, 85 patients demonstrated symptoms. In the earlier literature, however, emphasis was placed on the lucid interval; this interval may be more apparent than real. It is

difficult to diagnose a fulminating and rapidly progressing case that terminates in death and is associated with multiple fractures. Coma develops rapidly and is accompanied by marked respiratory distress. Occasionally, the patient may demonstrate hemoptysis, and pulmonary edema may become manifest. Often the symptoms and signs of fat embolism syndrome are masked by shock or coma or by an anesthetized state in a patient undergoing early operative treatment.

It is also likely that many cases of mild fat embolism syndrome are overlooked. The phenomenon called fracture fever, or hematoma fever, in the early postinjury state may be an unrecognized, mild variety of fat embolism syndrome.[163]

The enigma of the clinical fat embolism syndrome remains that although early diagnosis is extremely important in the management of the life-threatening pulmonary failure, the recognition of the fat embolism syndrome remains a diagnosis of exclusion dependent on the clinician's high index of suspicion. Certain features about fat embolism syndrome assist in its early clinical recognition. Symptoms are shortness of breath, which may begin relatively suddenly, followed by restlessness and confusion. The patient often becomes obstreperous and difficult to manage. Arterial hypoxemia is the hallmark. Other clinical signs associated with the fat embolism syndrome involve a flat temperature elevation to 39° to 40°C; tachypnea, with rates of 30 breaths per minute or higher; and tachycardia, with rates of 140 beats per minute or higher. Blood pressure does not vary widely and usually remains within normal limits. Another striking feature is the changing neurologic symptom: the onset of restlessness, disorientation followed by marked confusion, stupor, or coma.[196] Long tract signs may be present, with occasional extensor posturing and decerebrate rigidity and even focal seizures. These neurologic signs may change rapidly. Urinary incontinence may occur despite the patient's apparent well-being. In a young, healthy patient with a fracture, such a situation may indicate the onset of the fat embolism syndrome. Recovery may take several months, and permanent neurologic deficits have been reported, including severe mental retardation. Furthermore, it may be difficult to distinguish these neurologic manifestations of the fat embolism syndrome from those of primary craniocerebral trauma (Table 5-2).

The second or third day after injury, petechiae may be seen, characteristically located across the chest, the axilla, and the root of the neck and in the conjunctivae (Fig. 5-4). This appearance is in contrast to the petechial rash seen in patients with

Table 5-2. Comparison of Features of Cerebral Fat Embolism and Craniocerebral Trauma

Signs and Symptoms	Cerebral Fat Embolism	Craniocerebral Trauma
Lucid interval	18 to 24 h	6 to 10 h
Confusion	Severe	Moderate
Pulse rate	Rapid (140 to 160)	Slow
Respiration rate	Rapid	Slow
Onset of coma	Rapid	Slow
Localizing signs	Usually absent	Usually present
Decerebrate rigidity	Early	Terminal

(Evarts, C.M.: Diagnosis and Treatment of Fat Embolism. J.A.M.A., 194:899–901, 1965.)

subacute bacterial endocarditis. The petechial rash is fleeting and may last only a short while, fading rapidly (Fig. 5-5). It may occur periodically, with accompanying attacks of coma. The conjunctival lesions are sharp and distinct and can be seen by rolling back the eyelids (Fig. 5-6). Retinal lesions can be identified by funduscopic examination and appear as microinfarcts at the ends of the retinal arterioles.[192] There may be permanent changes in the optic nerve center after the fat embolism syndrome.

The clinical manifestations as described result from a reduced blood flow to vital organs, such as the lungs, demonstrating dyspnea and cyanosis; the cerebral cortex, with dyspnea, disorientation, and restlessness; and, occasionally, the kidneys, with resultant oliguria. Many injuries other than multiple fractures are associated with the fat embolism syndrome. The more common are intrathoracic, intra-abdominal, intracranial, and major arterial injuries. It is most important to identify all associated injuries, to institute corrective measures for their treatment, and to not overlook the blood loss that occurs with an associated injury as well as with the fracture.

LABORATORY FINDINGS

Unfortunately, a pathognomonic laboratory test for fat embolism syndrome does not exist, but arterial hypoxemia is the hallmark of fat embolism syndrome and should be sought immediately after trauma. It is most important to follow the arterial blood gas in patients suspected of having fat embolism syndrome with pulmonary insufficiency.[132,138,148,214] The measurement of arterial hypoxemia is a sensitive index of the degree of pulmonary fat embolism and monitors the response to treatment. Values of pO_2 of less than 60 mm Hg

indicate significant pulmonary hypoxemia. More sophisticated studies, such as the alveolar-arterial oxygen differences (A-a DO_2) measured after inhalation of 100% oxygen for 10 minutes, help determine physiologic shunting and also help identify the presence of pulmonary embolization. Serial determinations of the arterial pO_2 values can provide an index of the effectiveness of the treatment of the hypoxic state associated with pulmonary insufficiency accompanying the fat embolism syn-

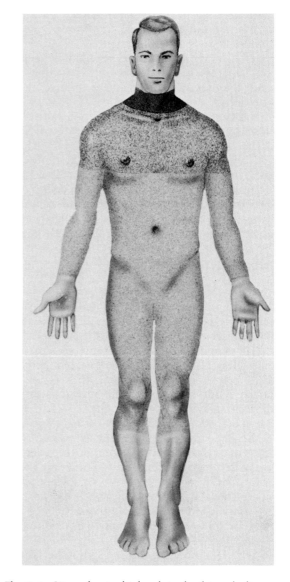

Fig. 5-4. Sites of petechial rash in the fat embolism syndrome. *(Evarts, C. M.: The Fat Embolism Syndrome: A Review. Surg. Clin. North Am., 50:493–507, 1970.)*

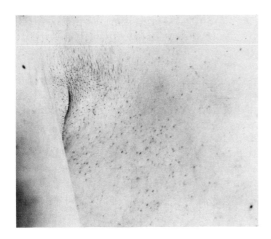

Fig. 5-5. Axillary petechiae. *(Evarts, C. M.: The Fat Embolism. A Review. Surg. Clin. North Am., 50:493–507, 1970.)*

drome. It has become clear that inapparent hypoxemia can occur in the patient without other clinical aspects of fat embolism. Symptoms directly referable to the respiratory system are often not present until the pO_2 falls below 65 mm Hg; tachypnea and cyanosis are present much less frequently and are seen only in the presence of severe oxygen desaturation.

In the early stages, thrombocytopenia may occur with platelet values of less than $150,000/mm^3$. The hematocrit value often decreases, sometimes with startling drops.[222]

Serial chest x-ray films should be obtained, because they demonstrate progressive snowstormlike pulmonary infiltrations in patients with fat embolism syndrome. The changes in chest x-ray films are characteristic but not specific (Fig. 5-7).[208] They frequently occur after the fat embolism syndrome is well under way.

Electrocardiographic changes may occur, demonstrating prominent S waves, arrhythmias, inversion of T waves, and a right bundle-branch block. However, these changes are not specific and reflect cardiac strain. Another helpful laboratory technique used for the identification of fat embolism syndrome is a cryostat-frozen section of clotted blood, which reveals the presence of fat. Pathologic fat in the venous circulating blood can be measured by filtering the blood through a microfilter with a pore size of 10 μ, allowing filtration of smaller fat globules but retaining the larger fat globules for staining. Gurd[180] reported that his test is of some value in the identification of the fat embolism syndrome.

If coma persists and there is no means of identifying the patient's problem, one author has suggested renal biopsy as a diagnostic aid in differentiating between coma that has occurred from cerebral trauma and coma secondary to fat embolism.[237] Lung biopsy has been suggested for the same reason, but its risk does not justify its widespread use. Biopsy of a skin petechial lesion can reveal the presence of embolic intravascular fat.[240] Analysis of the sputum or urine for fat has not proved to be accurate,[143] nor has the sizzle test of Scuderi.[235] Spinal fluid examination is not specifically diagnostic for fat embolism nor is electroencephalography.[167,247]

TREATMENT

Many forms of treatment have been suggested for patients with the fat embolism syn-

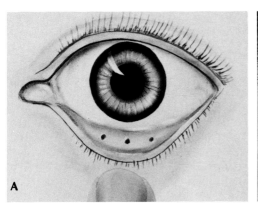
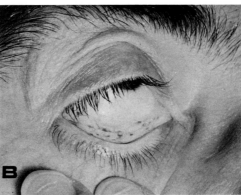

Fig. 5-6. **(A)** Diagram of conjunctival petechiae. **(B)** Clinical appearance of conjunctival petechiae. *(Evarts, C. M.: The Fat Embolism: A Review. Surg. Clin. North Am., 50:493–507, 1970.)*

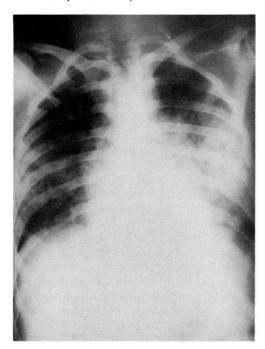

Fig. 5-7. X-ray showing pulmonary infiltrate in a patient with the fat embolism syndrome.

drome,[163,219,220,238] but unfortunately, many of these modes of therapy are derived from anecdotal studies without controls. Treatment can be considered in two categories: nonspecific, general measures and specific measures. As with all patients who have sustained multiple injuries, the following general management principles should be followed: the airway must be maintained, blood volume should be restored, fluid and electrolyte balance must be maintained, and unnecessary transportation should be avoided. The injured part or parts should be immobilized before any transportation is considered, because excess movement may cause further fat embolization.

Treatment of Hypoxemia

The initial (and perhaps the only specific) treatment of fat embolism is directed at decreasing the hypoxemia that occurs as a result of the respiratory distress. Oxygen should be administered immediately on admission to the emergency department. Accurate monitoring of blood gases is obviously critical in the management of pulmonary insufficiency. The arterial oxygen tension should be maintained at 90 mm Hg or higher. If the degree of hypoxemia is relatively mild, oxygen can be given by mask or nasal catheter, but this can be expected to deliver

only 40% or 50% oxygen concentration. If the degree of hypoxemia is severe and respiratory failure is impending, prompt mechanical ventilatory assistance is mandatory. Endotracheal intubation is the preferred method, because it provides suctioning and prevents aspiration. It has the disadvantage of causing tracheal necrosis when required for long-term use. A volume-cycled ventilator is used for mechanical ventilatory support in conjunction with positive end-expiratory pressure (PEEP) of 5 to 10 cm of water to assist in maintaining patency of small airways. The utmost caution should be taken in managing patients with hypoxemia; vigilance and meticulous attention to details are required if treatment is to be successful.

Specific Drug Therapy

The mystique of treatment of the fat embolism syndrome, however, currently surrounds the issues of specific drug therapy and the role and timing of definitive fracture fixation. Our vague understanding of the pathology of this process and difficulty in making an early clinical diagnosis have led to the development of a host of empirical therapies with a paucity of clinical and experimental justification for their use.[135,141,163,172,176,220,238]

ETHANOL

Ethanol was initially proposed as an emulsifying agent and later shown to function as a lipase inhibitor in suppressing the rise of free fatty acids in trauma patients. There has been some suggestion that intoxicated patients fare better following multiple skeletal injuries than those without a measurable blood alcohol level. Although Meyers and Taljaard have demonstrated a significant reduction in incidence of the syndrome with a blood alcohol level of 20 mg%, there have been no prospective controlled investigations of this agent.[210]

HEPARIN

Heparin was initially used for its ability to stimulate a circulating lipase that would break down the embolic neutral fats from the marrow. After free fatty acids were shown to be toxic to the lung parenchyma, rationale for continued use of this agent relied on its anticoagulant effects in decreasing platelet aggregation. No clinical trials have demonstrated any benefit, however, and indeed some have proven harmful effects.[127] Again, potential bleeding complications in the acutely injured patient and the demonstration of acute renal failure with this agent in hypovolemic laboratory animals have considerably tempered its use. No laboratory investigations have demonstrated its therapeutic value in this setting.

HYPERTONIC GLUCOSE

Hypertonic glucose has been suggested as an alternative metabolic fuel that would block the post-traumatic mobilization of free fatty acids.[241,244] Prospective clinical trials have demonstrated a significant improvement in levels of arterial oxygenation; when compared with controls, however, hypertonic glucose has not been shown to be effective in prevention of the full-blown fat embolism syndrome. Although numerous other treatment protocols have been followed, none has demonstrated efficacy in reducing the incidence of pulmonary failure following multiple fractures.

CORTICOSTEROIDS

Although few prospective studies exist, accumulating evidence supports the use of methylprednisolone in the treatment of the acute respiratory failure of fat embolism syndrome.[126,130,150,167,168,190,202,228,233,241,244,254] Ashbaugh and Petty first used 100-mg doses of cortisone intramuscularly in 1966, when they reported two successful cases with reversal of acute respiratory insufficiency following drug treatment.[130] Numerous laboratory investigations have demonstrated efficacy in the prevention of pulmonary failure when animals were pretreated prior to fatty acid injection to create a fat embolism model. In 1971, Fischer and associates documented a consistent pattern of improvement in respiratory failure following administration of Solu-Medrol in an uncontrolled series of 13 patients.[167] Arterial hypoxemia cleared within 12 hours, pulmonary compliance improved within 72 hours, and neurologic deficit resolved by three days after the start of methylprednisolone treatment. Rokkanen and associates were the first to treat prophylactically with steroids in dosages of 10 mg/kg of body weight every eight hours starting in the emergency room.[228] They noted a reduced incidence of fat embolism syndrome from 6 of 15 patients in the control group to 1 of 14 patients in the treatment group.

In 1977 Shier and colleagues reported on a series comparing fluid loading, hypertonic glucose, aspirin, steroids, and control groups.[241] Methylprednisolone was employed in dosages of 30 mg/kg of body weight every six hours starting on admission. No patients in the series demonstrated clinical fat embolism syndrome requiring respiratory support; however, the steroid-treated group had consistently better arterial oxygenation when compared with all other groups. Again, hypertonic glucose, methylprednisolone, and controls were compared in a study by Stoltenberg and Gustilo in 1979 with treatment commencing on admission.[244] Methylprednisolone was given in empiric dosages of 1 g every eight hours. Of 64 patients, clinical fat embolism syndrome developed in 3 in the glucose group and 2 in the control group following femoral shaft fractures. In no patient in the steroid group did the clinical syndrome develop; however, the study size was too small to prove statistical significance. There was statistically significant improvement in arterial oxygenation in all patients in the steroid-treated group when compared with the glucose and control groups. Alho and associates in 1978[126] and Schonfeld and colleagues in 1983[233] were the first to prove statistical significance in the protection offered by prophylactic administration of methylprednisolone in a dosage of 7 to 10 mg/kg of body weight four times daily. In the latter series, clinical fat embolism syndrome developed in 9 of 41 patients in the placebo group as compared with 0 of 21 patients in the steroid-treated group. A petechial rash was found in 5 of the 9 patients with fat embolism syndrome and was the only diagnostic criterion in this series that was specific for this condition. Complement activation as determined by C5A levels was found to be a nonspecific indicator of the syndrome, with a positive predictive value of only 41%.

In 1987, Lindeque and associates demonstrated improved arterial oxygenation in a methylprednisolone-treated group given 30 mg/kg of body weight twice on the day of admission.[202] Definition of fat embolism syndrome in this study was based largely on hypoxemia of less than 60 mm Hg without consideration of adjunctive physical findings. Petechial rash was seen in only 39% of the patients with arterial hypoxemia of less than 60 mm Hg. Again, serum C5A levels were elevated in almost all patients with long bone fractures, regardless of the development of fat embolism syndrome.

The mechanism of action of methylprednisolone remains the subject of discussion. Its general anti-inflammatory action is hypothesized to protect the capillary endothelium and preserve vascular integrity, stabilize granulocyte lysosomal membranes, reduce complement system activation, retard platelet aggregation and release of serotonin, and minimize transudation of interstitial edema. It has been postulated that blockade of vasoactive substances will relieve pulmonary vascular spasm and allow a rapid partial correction of ventilation-perfusion mismatch, thereby improving oxygenation. The late improvement in lung compliance and oxygenation is attributed to a gradual clearance of interstitial edema after the ongoing inflammatory process has been controlled by the steroids. Stabilization of the complement system may minimize the contribution of complement-mediated neutrophil activation in the production of increased pulmonary alveolar capillary permeability. Specific effects of methylprednisolone on the type II pneumocyte have been shown in laboratory animals to stimulate the proliferation and maturation of this cell line, resulting in increased surfactant production and restoration of a new cellular permeability barrier lining the alveolus.[150] Despite the multiplicity of potential sites of action of methylprednisolone, the astronomical inflation of steroid dosage in published series has been untested in controlled trials comparing various dosage regimens.

The Role of Fracture Stabilization

The second and most hotly contested issue in the treatment of the fat embolism syndrome is the role of operative fracture stabilization in the multiply injured patient. An increasingly large body of evidence supports early fracture fixation within 24 hours after injury based on a demonstrated decrease in the incidence of fat embolism syndrome and improvement in pulmonary function. This philosophy has notably evolved from a more conservative posture of delayed fracture fixation to these more aggressive current recommendations.

Analysis of comparative series of multitrauma patients is facilitated by the use of a common system of injury severity assessment. The Abbreviated Injury Scale (AIS) was first proposed in 1971 by the Committee on Medical Aspects of Automotive Safety and consisted of grading nonfatal injury to five body areas based on a 0 (no injury) to 5 (critical) rating system.[154] Baker and associates then observed that overall mortality increased in the presence of associated injury to a second or third body system but injury to a fourth system had little impact on survival.[133] Based on this information, the Injury Severity Score (ISS) was devised, consisting of the sum of the squares of the three highest AIS grades, with the maximum score being $3 \times (5)^2$, or 75. In 1980, the American College of Surgeons' Committee on Trauma modified the AIS and adopted the Hospital Trauma Index (HTI) by adding evaluation of cardiovascular injury and substituting objective diagnoses for subjective impressions in determining a specific injury grade in each body system.[128] Currently, the HTI includes injury assessment of six body systems: respiratory, cardiovascular, nervous, abdominal, extremity, and skin/subcutaneous tissues. The specific grading system applied to extremity trauma is included in Table 5-3. Subsequent application of the ISS to various series of multitrauma patients has confirmed the correlation between ISS and mortality rates and has demonstrated consistency of mortality figures for different ISS levels among the various studies. Although the ISS has significant short-comings in predicting injury survival by omitting age or patient-specific risk factors, it remains the best available system by which the efficacy and appropriateness of different treatments can be evaluated in the polytrauma patient.

The Finland experience with care of long bone fractures in the multiply injured patient documents a progressive decline in the incidence of fat embolism syndrome with the adoption in 1969 of a policy of rigid internal fracture fixation in these patients.[225–227] In the 3 years prior to 1970, 203 patients were seen with pelvis or long bone fractures, 24% had their fractures treated operatively, and there was an overall 29% incidence of the fat embolism syndrome. In contrast, in the 5 subsequent years from 1970 to 1974, 425 patients with pelvic or long bone fractures were seen, 46.2% had their fractures treated with internal fixation, and the fat embolism syndrome developed in only 7.8%. By 1974, two thirds of all fracture patients had their skeletal injuries treated operatively, and no cases of fat embolism syndrome were seen in 73 patients. During this same 5-year period, there were 47 patients with multiple injuries who had at least two long bone fractures treated by early internal fixation. In this subset, the fat embolism syndrome developed in nine patients (19%), and eight of these patients demonstrated this complication prior to the

Table 5-3. Hospital Trauma Index[128] Extremity Injury

Injury	Class	Index
No injury	No injury	0
Minor sprains and fractures—no long bones	Minor	1
Simple fractures: humerus, clavicle, radius, ulna, tibia, fibula, single nerve	Moderate	2
Fractures: multiple moderate, compound moderate, femur (simple), pelvic (stable), dislocation major, major nerve	Major	3
Fractures: two major, compound femur, limb crush or amputation, unstable pelvic	Severe	4
Fractures: two severe, multiple major	Critical	5

surgical intervention, which was in all cases undertaken within 2 weeks of the injury. In no patient was the respiratory status worsened by the surgery, which was done while the syndrome was still present. Overall, from 1967 through 1974, the incidence of clinical fat embolism syndrome was 22% in those patients with fractures treated by nonoperative means in comparison to 4.5% in those patients whose fractures were surgically fixed. These data prompted Riska[226,227] to adopt a more aggressive stance toward early operative fixation of fractures in the multiply injured patient. During the ensuing 4 years from 1975 to 1978, 211 patients with multiple injuries and long bone fractures were treated by "emergency surgery" with internal fixation in a primary stage. The resulting incidence of the clinical fat embolism syndrome was only 1.4%. In all patients the syndrome appeared postoperatively, petechiae were noted in 21 of 22 patients, only three patients required specific respiratory treatment because of hypoxemia, and only one patient died. In 1979 Hansen and Winquist provided similar data regarding the chronology of the fat embolism syndrome.[182] In reporting their first 300 cases of closed intramedullary rodding of femoral fractures, they noted clinical fat embolism syndrome requiring respiratory support in 9% of patients. In that study population, patients spent a minimum of five to seven days in traction preoperatively after the injury and all cases of fat embolism syndrome occurred during this interval. In no instance was the syndrome caused or, when already present, exacerbated by the operative procedure.

Subsequent research in dogs has demonstrated a significantly greater neutral fat release following intramedullary reaming of an intact femur in comparison to a fractured femur.[207] Neutral fat recovered from blood specimens from the ipsilateral femoral vein increased 500% in the intact bone compared with 25% in the fractured femur. Additionally, intramedullary pressure in the intact bones approached 200 torr in contrast to a level of only 50 torr reached in the fractured bones during reaming. Also, from Seattle in 1983, Talucci and coworkers compared patients in whom immediate intramedullary nailing of femoral shaft fractures was done within 24 hours of admission with patients in whom femoral rodding had been delayed a minimum of five days.[246] Fat embolism syndrome was not seen in the 57 patients who had immediate nailing; however, five patients (11%) who underwent delayed nailing had this complication, and four of these five were diagnosed during the pre-

operative interval. Even greater significance is attached to these data when one considers that, according to Baker, the average ISS in the group with immediate nailing was nearly twice that in the group with delayed nailing. However, "critical hypoxemia" was seen in 20% of patients in the former group as compared to 14% in the latter group; non–fat embolism adult respiratory distress syndrome occurred in 7% who had immediate nailing and 5% who had delayed nailing. The total incidence of pulmonary complications was 30% in both study groups. Although this is certainly cause to consider the contribution of intramedullary nailing to production of significant hypoxemia without the other classic findings of the fat embolism syndrome, the authors noted that a 27.8% incidence of critical hypoxemia was found in another group of 40 trauma patients without fractures having an ISS similar to that found in the group undergoing immediate nailing. They concluded that early intramedullary femoral nailing can be accomplished in severely injured patients without increasing the risk of fat embolism syndrome.

In 1985 Johnson and coworkers reported retrospectively on the occurrence of the adult respiratory distress syndrome in 132 multiply injured patients having undergone operative fracture stabilization at different intervals from the time of injury.[188] Injury to the central nervous system, overall ISS using the HTI, and the time to operative stabilization were all found to be significant in predicting the incidence of adult respiratory distress syndrome. The overall incidence of adult respiratory distress syndrome was increased more than fivefold in the group in whom pelvic and major long bone fracture stabilization was delayed more than 24 hours following injury, with the incidence increasing from 7% in the group receiving early fixation to 39% in the group receiving delayed fixation. The strength of this association increased, as did the severity of the injury. In those with an ISS of less than 30, no adult respiratory distress syndrome was seen in the group that underwent early stabilization as compared to an 8% incidence when orthopaedic surgery was delayed more than 24 hours; in those with an ISS exceeding 30, adult respiratory distress syndrome was found in 17% of those with early stabilization of fractures and in 75% of those who had a delay in operative fracture fixation. These data have been statistically significant for both the overall study group and the subset with an ISS of greater than 40.

Several other investigators have demonstrated the efficacy of early internal fracture stabilization in decreasing the duration of mechanical ventilatory support in multiply injured patients.[230,252,264] The main cause of death in polytrauma victims surviving 1 week beyond injury remains remote organ failure due to sepsis.[174] Early internal fracture fixation, optimizing pulmonary function and the mechanics of breathing by eliminating the enforced supine position, decompressing the fracture hematoma as an ongoing source of fat emboli and retained necrotic debris, and eliminating pain and physiologic stress associated with continued fracture motion, all likely contribute to reduced ventilatory dependence and, in turn, improved late survival. It has been shown that the pulmonary failure state following blunt multiple trauma lasts 48 to 72 hours on average, and prolongation of respiratory compromise is largely determined by the subsequent selection of specific therapy for the injured parts.[236] Additionally, planned postoperative mechanical ventilation used in conjunction with PEEP has been effective in preventing as well as treating adult respiratory distress syndrome in the patient with multiple trauma.[173,175,230,264] Goris has developed a prevention scale for adult respiratory distress syndrome (Table 5-4) by which the need for prophylactic ventilatory assistance is assessed; a score of 10 correlated with an ISS of 25 or two major fractures and identified patients receiving postoperative mechanical ventilation.[173] When considering the two variables of early internal fracture stabilization and prophylactic ventilatory support, both were found to independently reduce the incidence and severity of adult respiratory distress syndrome complicating the course of patients with polytrauma fractures. In a cohort of patients receiving planned mechanical ventilation, those with early operative treatment of fractures (ISS 39.4) had an 11% incidence of adult respiratory distress syndrome compared with 75% in the group with nonoperative fracture treatment (ISS 54.6).[175] When these two groups were normalized for injury severity and only those with scores greater than 50 were considered, mortality was 8% and the incidence of adult respiratory distress syndrome was 15% in the operatively treated group (ISS 56), whereas mortality was 50% and adult respiratory distress syndrome occurred in 80% of in the nonoperatively treated group (ISS 58). Furthermore, in those with ISS greater than 30, mortality from late sepsis was 6% and the mean duration of ventilation was 6 days in the operatively treated group, and mortality from late sepsis was 55% and the mean duration of ventilation was 11 days in survivors in the group without operative fracture treatment.[173,175]

The independent value of prophylactic mechanical ventilation was evidenced by an 11% incidence of adult respiratory distress syndrome in the ventilated, operatively treated fracture group as compared to a 50% incidence in the nonventilated, operatively treated fracture group; this was especially noteworthy in view of the higher average ISS of 39.4 in the ventilated group as compared to an ISS of 29.6 in the nonventilated group.[175] Also addressing the questions of prophylactic mechanical ventilation, Ruedi and Wolff reported a study group of 57 polytrauma patients all treated by early fracture stabilization; 2% of those prophylactically ventilated postoperatively acquired adult respiratory distress syndrome in contrast to 67% of those not mechanically ventilated following surgery.[230] In similar investigations, Seibel and associates found that in comparison to the multiply injured patient with an operatively treated femur fracture, ten days of skeletal traction for the fractured femur doubled the duration of ventilatory failure, increased the number of positive blood cultures by a factor of 10, and nearly quadrupled the number of fracture complications.[236] Thirty days of skeletal traction had proportionately greater detrimental effects: up to five times the duration of pulmonary failure, a 74-fold increase in positive blood cultures, and nearly 20 times the number of fracture complications. They concluded that traction for femoral shaft fractures in the patient with blunt multiple trauma should be avoided because it greatly increased the risk of multiple-system organ failure and the cost of care. In 1986 Lozman and associates reported that immediate fixation of all fractures in the mul-

Table 5-4. Prevention Scale for Adult Respiratory Distress Syndrome[173]

Injury	Value Points
Simple fracture of foot, ankle, wrist, rib, and mandible	1
Forearm, Le Fort II	2
Humerus, tibia, vertebra, Le Fort IV	3
Femur, pelvis	5
Ruptured spleen	3
Ruptured liver	4
Transfusion > 4 units of blood	3
Initial blood pressure < 80 mm Hg	4
P_aO_2 < 60 mm Hg	5
Flail chest, aspiration	10
Intestinal perforation	6
Contusio cerebri	4

Total score of 10 or more points indicates the need for mechanical ventilation prophylactically to reduce risk of adult respiratory distress syndrome.

tiply traumatized victim resulted in a significantly lower intrapulmonary shunt and a significant increase in the cardiac index in the four days following injury.[204] Other significant changes were a lower platelet count and greater fibrinogen concentration in the group receiving immediate fixation. Interestingly, the ability to demonstrate fat globules in pulmonary capillary blood samples was no different between the two groups. In a recently reported prospective series, Bone and coworkers noted a 43% incidence of adult respiratory distress syndrome in patients with polytrauma having a femoral fracture stabilized more than 48 hours following injury in contrast to a 3.3% incidence of adult respiratory distress syndrome when the femur was stabilized within 24 hours.[145]

This growing body of evidence would seem to construct an almost compelling case for early orthopaedic intervention in the care of the multiply traumatized patient. The mechanism of this beneficial effect from surgical fracture stabilization is likely dependent on improved patient positioning and better mechanics of breathing afforded during the postoperative period. Additionally, it has long been observed that the incidence of fat embolism syndrome is considerably less following open fractures than closed injuries. Perhaps the surgical decompression of the fracture hematoma diminishes intramedullary pressure sufficiently to reduce the escape of fat and thromboplastic material from the medullary canal into the systemic circulation. In any event, although this approach to fracture management contributes constructively to patient care, there are some shortcomings to be considered. In addition to logistical problems in maintaining access to the operating theater and availability of skilled orthopaedic surgeons to perform ''immediate'' fracture stabilization, the question of skeletal infection must be addressed. In 1977 Riska and associates noted that, in a group of 47 patients treated with rigid skeletal fixation, there were nine (19%) wound infections, which equaled the incidence of fat embolism syndrome in this same population.[227] Four cases were deep infection and five were superficial in nature, with three in each group occurring in open fractures. In 1985 Johnson and colleagues noted a 2.5-fold increase in the rate of ''major orthopaedic infection'' in the early fracture stabilization group (21%) as compared to the late or nonoperative group (8%).[188] Although this was not believed to be statistically significant, it is certainly cause for concern. Goris and associates reported a 7.7% incidence of ''post-traumatic osteitis'' in patients surviving polytrauma following early

operative fracture stabilization.[175] It would appear that this philosophy of management of skeletal injuries in the multiply traumatized patient must also be tempered by the traditional concern over osteomyelitis, which even in our current era of medical care frequently remains a lifelong disease.

PROGNOSIS

The prognosis for recovery of patients with fat embolism syndrome is poor in those who have marked pulmonary failure and coma. Mortality is high with these complications. Mild cases often go undetected, and mortality is low in patients without severe pulmonary insufficiency or cerebral manifestations. It is virtually impossible to perform a controlled prospective study to determine true mortality and morbidity. In the patient with severe, fulminating, and progressive fat embolism syndrome, treatment as outlined should begin early and promptly; without it the condition may be fatal.

In summary, fat embolization is a common complication of multiple skeletal injuries, and it may present as a clinical variant of adult respiratory distress syndrome. The clinical fat embolism syndrome is noted by the characteristic manifestations of fever, tachycardia, and confusion in association with arterial hypoxemia and other pertinent laboratory findings. Modern techniques in the management of respiratory distress have led to decreased mortality and morbidity. Recent clinical research suggests that steroid administration may aid in the treatment of fat embolism syndrome.[176] Early fracture fixation providing for rapid mobilization of the patient with polytrauma provides hope for prevention of the respiratory failure associated with the fat embolism syndrome in the polytrauma setting in which multiorgan system failure is often fatal.

HEMORRHAGIC COMPLICATIONS

This section was contributed by Charles W. Francis, M.D., Associate Professor, Division of Hematology, University of Rochester School of Medicine and Dentistry.

Hemorrhagic problems facing the orthopaedic surgeon usually fall into one of two categories. First, there are the problems related to the treatment, operative or conservative, of orthopaedic complications of congenital bleeding disorders, such as hemophilia. Second, there are those failures in the hemostatic mechanism that may arise during or after major surgical procedures or trauma. A detailed discussion of complex hemostatic disorders is beyond the scope of this section, which reviews three topics: the normal hemostatic mechanism, the diagnosis of the more common hemorrhagic disorders, and the principles of their treatment.[273]

NORMAL HEMOSTASIS

When a blood vessel is pierced or damaged, a series of events occurs to prevent loss of blood and repair the wound. This series consists of adhesion of platelets at the site of injury, aggregation of additional platelets to form a hemostatic plug, formation of fibrin to stabilize the platelet plug and form a clot, and removal of the clot and repair of damaged tissue. The events are described sequentially but overlap considerably. There is, of course, a limit to the size of the wound and the size of the vessel beyond which the normal hemostatic mechanism is ineffective without the addition of local pressure or mechanical closure.

Platelets and Vascular Phase

Local vasoconstriction occurs promptly following vascular damage, slowing or even stopping blood flow in the vessel and facilitating clot formation. Vessel wall damage also disrupts the normal endothelial cell lining, resulting in adherence of platelets to components of the subendothelium.[287,293] Release of adenosine diphosphate, thrombin, and other humoral agents causes the aggregation of additional platelets at the injury site. This enlarging platelet mass may be sufficient to initially stop the flow of blood from smaller vessels and to facilitate activation of the coagulation system to stabilize the hemostatic plug and form a fibrin clot.

Blood Coagulation

Activation of the coagulation system results in the formation of the proteolytic enzyme thrombin, which converts soluble fibrinogen to an insoluble fibrin clot. Local vascular damage initiates the extrinsic coagulation pathway (Fig. 5-8), which is activated through factor VII by exposure of blood to tissue factor, the one coagulation factor not present in blood but expressed on the membranes of many cells.[286] The intrinsic system functions solely with elements present in the blood. It is activated by interaction of factor XII with components of the subendothelium, which are exposed to the blood when the vessel is damaged. Both pathways must

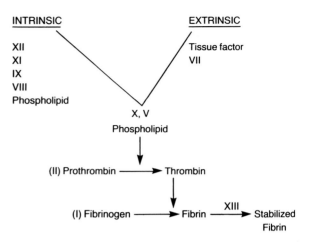

Fig. 5-8. A simplified scheme of the coagulation pathway.

function for normal hemostasis to occur; this is evident from the fact that a person deficient in factor VIII bleeds, despite having a normal extrinsic pathway, and conversely, factor VII deficiency results in a hemorrhagic diathesis, despite the presence of a normal intrinsic pathway. There are important connections between the two pathways. For example, in addition to activating factor X directly, factor VII and tissue factor can activate factor IX.[285] The components of the intrinsic system are required for a normal partial thromboplastin time (PTT), and the prothrombin time (PT) is used to assess the extrinsic system. Clotting is normally restricted to the local site of need by the combination of local activation at the site of vascular damage, binding of activated coagulation factors to platelets, and systemic inhibition of any activated coagulation factors by circulating inhibitors. These include antithrombin III, which inhibits the enzymatic activities of coagulation factors in reactions accelerated by heparin.[290] Protein C is a circulating zymogen converted by thrombin to activated protein C, a coagulation inhibitor that acts on factors V and VIII.[271] A lipoprotein-associated inhibitor of the extrinsic system has also been recently described.[289]

Fibrinolysis and Repair

After the leakage of blood has stopped, repair begins. The clot must first be removed by the fibrinolytic system (Fig. 5-9). The basic framework of this system is similar to that of coagulation, with a series of linked enzymatic reactions resulting in the production of the proteolytic enzyme plasmin.[272] Physiologic activators include tissue-type plasmin-

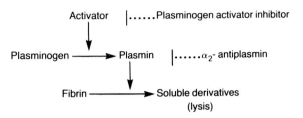

Fig. 5-9. The fibrinolytic system.

ogen activator and urokinaselike plasminogen activator, which differ in biochemical and immunologic properties.[266] Plasminogen activators are readily available at sites of clot formation or tissue damage, since they are present in most blood and in endothelial cells. Urokinase, a plasminogen activator normally found in the urine; streptokinase, an enzyme produced by bacteria; and tissue plasminogen activator (TPA), produced by recombinant DNA techniques, are available for systemic administration to treat thrombotic disorders by activation of the fibrinolytic system. As in coagulation, the fibrinolytic system is restricted to a local area through mechanisms of local activation, specific binding of plasminogen and plasmin to the fibrin clot, and systemic inhibition of fibrinolysis both by the plasmin inhibitor α_2-antiplasmin and by inhibitors of plasminogen activators. Repair of the vessel wall also involves the coagulation mechanisms, because factor XIII (fibrin-stabilizing factor) not only converts fibrin to a cross-linked, stabilized form, but also plays a role in local growth of fibroblasts.

PREOPERATIVE EVALUATION

The best defense against unexpected, excessive operative bleeding owing to hemorrhagic disorders is an adequate preoperative evaluation.[268,288] The history is the single most useful element to evaluate. Most adult patients have had major challenges to the integrity of the hemostatic system, such as tooth extraction, prior surgery, or trauma. A history of normal hemostasis with such procedures makes the presence of a significant congenital bleeding disorder unlikely, whereas a history of abnormal bleeding necessitates a more thorough hemostatic evaluation. The preoperative evaluation also reveals serious illnesses, such as liver or kidney disease, that may have important effects on hemostatic

competence. Laboratory testing is a useful supplement to this evaluation and is particularly important in patients in whom an adequate history cannot be obtained. An activated partial thromboplastin time (aPTT), to test the coagulation system, and an examination of a blood smear or a platelet count, to rule out thrombocytopenia, are the most useful tests. A PT is less useful but may occasionally detect unsuspected liver disease or oral anticoagulant use. If the history or the screening laboratory tests suggest an abnormality, more extensive evaluation is required.

HEMORRHAGIC DISORDERS AND LABORATORY TESTING

A derangement of any phases of hemostasis may lead to excessive bleeding. It is important to bear this in mind when considering the possible factors contributing to a hemorrhagic diathesis and the laboratory tests that may be used to elucidate its cause. In view of the complexity of the hemostatic process, the long list of causes of excessive bleeding should not be surprising. Discussion of each entity is beyond the scope of this section, but the common causes of hemorrhage and the more useful laboratory tests are considered as they relate to the several phases of hemostasis.

Platelet and Vascular Phase

Thrombocytopenia is the most common cause of a defect in the platelet and vascular phase. A general correlation exists between the degree of thrombocytopenia and the occurrence of hemorrhage. Hemostasis is usually normal at platelet counts above 100,000. Below this level, progressive impairment of hemostasis may be expected. When the platelet count is less than 20,000 mm³, spontaneous bleeding may occur, typically taking the form of bleeding into the skin and mucous membranes (eg, petechiae, purpura, and bruising). The more common causes of thrombocytopenia include reactions to drugs, idiopathic thrombocytopenic purpura, systemic lupus erythematosus, and the administration of cytotoxic drugs. Transfusion of large amounts of stored blood can be expected to lower the platelet count and can contribute to bleeding during surgery.[275]

Abnormal platelet function may also cause bleeding disorders. These conditions are associated with a normal platelet count but a prolonged bleeding time. The most common congenital disorder of this type is von Willebrand's disease, in which a prolonged bleeding time is caused by abnormal platelet function owing to deficiency or abnormality in a plasma protein, von Willebrand's factor. (Von Willebrand's disease is further discussed in a later section.) Uremia and severe liver disease are often associated with clinically significant platelet dysfunction, and many drugs, including aspirin and other nonsteroidal anti-inflammatory agents (NSAIDs), interfere with platelet function and may prolong the bleeding time. It is important to distinguish the antiplatelet effects of aspirin, lasting for the entire five- to ten-day life span of the irreversibly acetylated platelet, from those of the NSAIDs, which are reversible in the time necessary to clear the drug from the system, depending on its specific pharmacokinetics.

Simple laboratory tests may be used to ensure normal platelet number and function. Platelet number can be evaluated by examination of the blood smear, or a platelet count can be obtained. The bleeding time, an excellent screening test of the integrity of this phase of hemostasis, is usually normal with platelet counts above 100,000 and is increasingly prolonged with greater degrees of thrombocytopenia.[279] In the presence of a normal platelet count, a prolonged bleeding time is usually indicative of abnormal platelet function, which may be further evaluated by specialized tests in a coagulation laboratory.

Blood Coagulation

Abnormal coagulation may result from either a deficiency of one or more clotting factors or the presence of anticoagulant (inhibitor), which interferes with the function of the clotting factors. Deficiencies may be inherited or acquired. Inherited deficiencies usually involve a single factor, whereas most acquired abnormalities affect several factors. Hemophilia A, the most common hereditary hemorrhagic diathesis, is a sex-linked disorder caused by deficiency of factor VIII (antihemophilic factor, AHF).[281,282] The severity of the clinical manifestations is related to the level of circulating factor VIII, with severe disease occurring in the presence of a factor VIII level less than 1% of normal, resulting in frequent, apparently spontaneous bleeding into the joints and deep tissues. A level greater than 5% results in mild disease, with few spontaneous bleeding problems, but can cause serious hemorrhage after surgery or trauma. Factor VIII levels between 1% and 5% are associated with moderate disease of intermediate severity. Hemarthrosis is the major orthopaedic complication. It occurs almost invariably in the severe form of disease but rarely

in the mild form. After surgery or trauma, hemostasis may appear to be normal in hemophilia because platelet function is essentially normal. Excessive bleeding is typically delayed, beginning several hours after the operation.

Factor IX deficiency (Christmas disease, hemophilia B) is less common than hemophilia A but is clinically identical and is also inherited as a sex-linked disorder. Von Willebrand's disease, the second most common hereditary hemorrhagic disorder, is inherited as an autosomal dominant trait and has two associated abnormalities: deficiency of factor VIII and a prolonged bleeding time.[291] Both abnormalities are caused by a decreased plasma concentration or abnormal function of von Willebrand's factor. This high-molecular-weight plasma protein is synthesized in endothelial cells and is essential for normal platelet adherence to damaged subendothelium. Factor VIII circulates in plasma in association with von Willebrand's factor and is variably low in von Willebrand's disease as a result of the von Willebrand's factor abnormality. A wide spectrum of clinical syndromes may be seen. In the most severe form, spontaneous bleeding and hemarthrosis occur; in mild cases, hemostasis may be normal except after major surgery.

Acquired deficiencies of clotting factors are usually multiple. Deficiency of the vitamin K–dependent factors, II (prothrombin), VII, IX, and X can result from lack of intake of vitamin K (in newborns), malabsorption, liver disease, and administration of coumarin-containing drugs. Orthopaedic complications are rare. Deficiencies of several clotting factors, including platelets, factor VIII, and fibrinogen, may result from disseminated intravascular coagulation (DIC). This complex disorder of diverse etiology in which excessive activation of coagulation results in consumption of clotting factors is dealt with in more detail in another section.

Circulating anticoagulants (inhibitors) cause bleeding by interfering with the action of one or more coagulation factors.[292] The most common inhibitor is an antibody that develops in approximately 10% of patients with hemophilia and inactivates transfused factor VIII, greatly complicating therapy.[281,283] Spontaneous factor VIII inhibitors also occur occasionally in nonhemophiliacs. They may develop in the elderly without other apparent systemic disease, in the postpartum state, or in association with other immunologic disorders. The lupus anticoagulant is an antibody that interferes with the lipid used in coagulation testing in vitro and does not result in abnormal bleeding. Identification of a lupus inhibitor is important both as an explanation of the prolonged coagulation tests and because it is associated with an increased risk of thrombotic disease.[267] Heparin is so commonly used as an anticoagulant in hospitalized patients that it is a frequent cause of abnormal coagulation tests.

Laboratory evaluation of the coagulation system is simplified by the availability of screening tests, which are useful in identifying the presence of an abnormality and providing a basis for further investigation. The overall strategy is to begin with preliminary, screening-type tests and to use the results as a guide for more specific evaluation. The most useful screening tests are the aPTT and the PT. The aPTT involves the addition of a contact-activating substance, such as kaolin, and a platelet substitute (phospholipid) to the patient's plasma and measurement of the clotting time after adding calcium. It provides a sensitive evaluation of the intrinsic clotting pathway. The PT evaluates the extrinsic pathway and measures the time required for the patient's plasma to clot after the addition of tissue thromboplastin and calcium. The aPTT and PT evaluate both coagulation pathways and are sensitive to clinically significant abnormalities. Correction studies distinguish between a deficiency state and the presence of an anticoagulant and may also be used to identify the specific deficiency present. Their correct use and interpretation are predicated on the results of the preliminary studies.

Fibrinolysis and Repair

Excessive fibrinolysis may be primary or may occur as a secondary physiologic response to intravascular coagulation, or it may result from therapeutic administration of plasminogen activators such as urokinase, streptokinase, or TPA.[276,277] Primary fibrinolysis is an uncommon disorder but may lead to a hemorrhagic diathesis in patients with cirrhosis of the liver or prostatic carcinoma. In DIC, widespread microvascular thrombi form, and the fibrinolytic system is activated in response to maintain vascular patency. Laboratory testing may reveal evidence of heightened fibrinolysis, but this is usually of secondary clinical importance to the hemostatic derangements resulting from the consumption of coagulation factors. Hemorrhagic complications occur during fibrinolytic therapy, but normal hemostasis can be restored by discontinuing the drug and replacing consumed factors.

Laboratory evaluation can identify excessive fibrinolysis and help in distinguishing primary and secondary forms. In primary fibrinolysis, the euglobulin lysis time is shortened, reflecting excess circulating plasminogen activator, and serum fibrinogen degradation products are elevated as a result of fibrinogen and fibrin breakdown. In secondary fibrinolysis, these tests are also abnormal, and there is further evidence of consumption of coagulation factors, especially platelets.

TREATMENT

Hemorrhagic problems in orthopaedic disorders most frequently occur in two situations: (1) the orthopaedic problems associated with congenital hemorrhagic disorders, such as hemophilia, and (2) bleeding disorders occurring as a complication of operative procedures.

The hemostatic abnormality in hemophilia A is caused by deficiency of factor VIII. This can be reliably corrected with appropriate replacement therapy using factor VIII concentrates or cryoprecipitate.[269,282] Cryoprecipitate is the factor VIII-rich, cold, insoluble portion of a single unit of plasma. Its factor VIII content is somewhat variable but is usually between 70 and 100 units. The advantage of cryoprecipitate over factor VIII concentrate in replacement therapy is that the risk of transmission of hepatitis and other diseases is less, because there is exposure to fewer donors. Disadvantages include the inconvenience of administering multiple units, the problem of refrigerated storage, and less certainty regarding the amount of factor VIII infused. Commercial concentrates are prepared from large pools of donor blood. Their factor VIII content is assayed, and they are easy to store and can be quickly reconstituted for administration. Contamination of the blood supply with the HIV led to a high incidence of HIV infection and AIDS in hemophiliacs because of their frequent use of pooled plasma products and exposure to many blood donors. Currently available concentrates are prepared in ways that inactivate HIV. Desmopressin (DDAVP) causes release of von Willebrand's factor and factor VIII from storage sites and raises plasma concentrations. In selected patients with mild to moderate hemophilia A, it is currently the treatment of choice for limited surgical procedures since it has very few adverse side effects.[270,278]

Many hemophiliacs are on home transfusion programs that result in rapid treatment of bleeding episodes, less morbidity, and fewer hospital visits. Surgical procedures in the hemophiliac must be performed with adequate replacement therapy. The optimum factor VIII plasma level to ensure hemostasis is dependent on the extent of the surgical procedure.[282] Hemophiliacs with circulating inhibitors pose special problems, because they cannot usually be treated with factor VIII replacement alone. No completely adequate treatment is available at present, although plasmapheresis, cytotoxic agents, and prothrombin complex concentrates have been used successfully.[284] Administration of factor VII has also been effective in a few patients.[280]

Treatment of von Willebrand's disease requires replacement of von Willebrand's factor. In most cases this is best accomplished with the use of cryoprecipitate that is especially rich in high-molecular-weight, functional von Willebrand's factor. Therapy can normally be guided by the level of factor VIII coagulant activity, but sometimes more frequent transfusion to correct the bleeding time may also be necessary. Replacement therapy in von Willebrand's disease is further modified by the prolonged rise in factor VIII coagulant activity that follows transfusion in these patients. DDAVP has been used successfully to manage surgery and represents the treatment of choice in appropriate patients.[278]

Hemophilia B must be treated with factor IX replacement, using either plasma or prothrombin complex concentrates.[282] Replacement with plasma is difficult, because the large volumes that must be transfused may result in fluid overload. Prothrombin complex concentrates are convenient to use but are prepared from large donor pools and therefore carry a high risk of hepatitis and other disease transmission.

Treatment of complex, multifactorial, acquired hemostatic abnormalities is more complicated than that of congenital deficiencies. Vitamin K is specific therapy for deficiencies of this vitamin and may be used to correct overdoses of coumarin drugs. Deficiencies of vitamin K–dependent factors caused by liver disease rarely respond to vitamin K administration and are best treated with plasma. Treatment of DIC must be tailored to the individual patient, but the most effective treatment is aimed at correcting the underlying cause. Bleeding resulting from deficiencies of coagulation factors and platelets is best treated initially with plasma and platelet concentrates, but heparin administration may be required to stop the intravascular coagulation, especially when tissue ischemia from microvascular thrombosis becomes a problem.

Platelet concentrates for treatment of thrombocytopenia are available through most blood banks. They are especially effective in patients who have low platelet counts owing to defective production (eg, following cytotoxic drug therapy) or who have thrombocytopenia following massive transfusion.[274] They are generally ineffective in patients who have immunologically mediated thrombocy-

topenia (eg, idiopathic thrombocytopenic purpura), because the transfused platelets are rapidly destroyed.

In summary, normal function of the hemostatic system involves several elements acting in concert. Initial hemostasis is provided by platelets, which adhere to a site of vascular injury and aggregate to form a hemostatic plug. Activation of the coagulation system results in fibrin formation, which stabilizes the plug and provides a firm clot. The fibrinolytic system aids in remodeling the clot and eventually restores vascular patency. Defects in each of these phases of the hemostatic system may result in different bleeding problems and require separate laboratory evaluation.

In preoperative evaluation of the hemostatic system, the history is paramount. Laboratory testing is used to supplement the history and should include as a minimum an evaluation of platelet count, PT, and aPTT. More extensive investigation is required in patients with a history suggestive of a bleeding disorder.

Accurate diagnosis of and specific therapy for most congenital bleeding disorders are now available. Complex acquired hemostatic abnormalities resulting from systemic disease or following trauma or surgery are usually caused by deficient production or excessive consumption of platelets and multiple coagulation factors. A logical sequence of laboratory investigation of these disorders, beginning with screening tests and proceeding with more specific assays in consultation with a coagulation laboratory, is essential for optimum management. Successful management demands an understanding of underlying pathophysiology, laboratory evaluation to identify specific abnormalities, and familiarity with the products available for replacement therapy.

DISSEMINATED INTRAVASCULAR COAGULATION

This section was contributed by Charles W. Francis, M.D., Associate Professor, Division of Hematology, University of Rochester School of Medicine and Dentistry.

DIC is a syndrome of diverse etiology resulting in a complex derangement of hemostasis, with elements of vascular obstruction, consumption of coagulation factors, and heightened fibrinolysis, often leading to excessive bleeding.[297] It is not a primary diagnosis but rather develops as a manifestation of a serious underlying clinical condition that provides the inciting stimulus for activation of the coagulation system. The presentation and laboratory manifestations of DIC are modified by the wide variety of associated clinical conditions, such as those shown subsequently.[297,299,305,306] Several of these conditions, including malignancy, massive trauma, and septicemia, may be seen in routine orthopaedic practice. The surgeon must be prepared to recognize the manifestations, initiate laboratory investigations, and assist in difficult management decisions.

Widespread damage to the endothelium, such as occurs in endotoxemia, and entry of procoagulant proteins into the circulation, as may occur in disseminated malignancy or trauma, may be important inciting stimuli in DIC. The resultant excessive intravascular activation of coagulation results in varying degrees of microvascular obstruction, consumption of coagulation factors, and activation of fibrinolysis. The clinical and laboratory findings reflect these pathogenic processes. Vascular obstruction results in tissue ischemia and necrosis, with organ dysfunction. Consumption of coagulation factors results in thrombocytopenia and low levels of fibrinogen and other consumable coagulation proteins, leading to a bleeding tendency. The intense action of fibrinolysis that may occur can result in further consumption of coagulation factors and results in high circulating levels of fibrinogen or fibrin degradation products, which have anticoagulant properties that may exacerbate the hemostatic abnormality.[300]

Disorders Associated With Disseminated Intravascular Coagulation

Acute

  Septicemia
  Obstetric complication
    Amniotic fluid embolism
    Abruptio placentae
  Massive trauma
  Hemolytic transfusion reactions
  Snake bite

Chronic

  Malignancy
  Aortic aneurysm
  Retained dead fetus
  Giant cavernous hemangioma

CLINICAL FINDINGS

The clinical manifestations of DIC are microvascular thrombosis and bleeding superimposed on the underlying primary disorder. Platelet-fibrin thrombi occlude small blood vessels, resulting in tissue ischemia and organ dysfunction of variable extent and severity. Findings related to the skin, kidneys, and brain are most often recognized. Sharply demarcated hemorrhagic skin infarctions are easily recognized and give the dramatic picture of purpura fulminans in their severest form. Renal involvement usually presents as oliguria and acute renal failure, which may be worsened by coexisting shock. Nonspecific neurologic findings, such as delirium, convulsions, or coma, are more common than focal findings. Other organ systems frequently involved with severe DIC are the lungs, gastrointestinal tract, and adrenal glands.

The complex hemostatic dysfunction associated with DIC often results in a serious bleeding diathesis, possibly in the form of hemorrhage at the operative site during or after surgery. However, bleeding often occurs at nonoperative sites as well, and this is usually the first clear indication of the presence of a bleeding disorder. Thrombocytopenia and platelet dysfunction may result in petechiae and purpura. Bleeding from venipuncture sites, bleeding from gums, hematuria, and epistaxis often occur, as well as serious hemorrhage from arteriotomies. Gastrointestinal bleeding may complicate the course.

LABORATORY EVALUATION

Laboratory findings in DIC reflect the consumption of platelets and coagulation factors as well as heightened fibrinolysis.[305,306] Unfortunately, no single laboratory abnormality is diagnostic for DIC, and the diagnosis depends on a pattern of findings. In addition, the degree of abnormalities in coagulation tests is variable, depending on the severity of the process. In acute severe DIC, gross hemostatic abnormalities are easily identified; in the chronic form, findings are subtle.[302,304]

Laboratory Evaluation of Disseminated Intravascular Coagulation

Most Common Findings

1. Thrombocytopenia
2. Prolonged screening coagulation tests
    Prothrombin time
    Activated partial thromboplastin time
    Thrombin time
3. Decreased fibrinogen
4. Elevated serum fibrinogen degradation products

Other Abnormalities

1. Decreased factor levels (eg, factor V, factor VIII)
2. Decreased plasminogen
3. Shortened euglobulin lysis time
4. Decreased antithrombin III
5. Abnormal red cell morphology

A common feature in DIC is consumption of platelets, and some degree of thrombocytopenia is found in nearly all cases. A good estimate of platelet number may be readily obtained by examination of the peripheral blood smear, or a more precise platelet count can be obtained. Screening coagulation tests, such as the PT, aPTT, and thrombin clotting time, are typically prolonged, reflecting decreased coagulation factors and the anticoagulant effect of circulating fibrin(ogen) degradation products. The plasma concentration of fibrinogen is usually decreased in severe cases; however, fibrinogen is an acute phase reactant so that a normal level in an acutely ill patient may indicate a substantial decrease from the expected level. Serum fibrin(ogen) degradation products are usually elevated, sometimes to a striking degree.

Many additional abnormalities can be found in DIC, and some provide useful diagnostic help, particularly in difficult cases. Factor assays can be performed to verify the depression of consumable coagulation factors. Antithrombin III is consumed in the process of inactivating thrombin and is often low.[294,295,306] Heightened fibrinolysis is reflected by a decreased concentration of plasminogen and shortened euglobulin lysis time. Red blood cells may be damaged by their interaction with microvascular thrombi, and variable numbers of histocytes or red cell fragments are found on examination of the peripheral blood smear,[303] a finding that is not sensitive or specific for DIC.

On the basis of laboratory findings, it may be difficult to distinguish DIC, liver disease, and primary fibrinolysis. The presence of liver disease is usually evident from the typical clinical and laboratory findings; the hemostatic abnormalities, however, can closely mimic those of DIC. Primary fibrinolysis occurs less commonly than DIC, and the laboratory abnormalities reflect marked activation of fibrinolysis. In contrast to DIC, the platelet count is usually normal, whereas the fibrinogen level may be markedly decreased with higher levels of circulating fibrin(ogen) degradation products.[296,301]

TREATMENT

The most effective treatment for DIC is correction of the inciting disorder. If this can be done, the hemostatic abnormalities will improve without specific therapy. Because patients with DIC are often critically ill with shock and multiple organ dysfunction, aggressive supportive therapy is usually a critical factor in their successful management.

Therapy specifically designed for DIC is necessary when the underlying disorder cannot be reversed rapidly or when the hemostatic abnormalities assume major clinical significance. Treatment decisions should focus on the clinical manifestations and not aim solely to correct laboratory abnormalities. If microvascular thrombosis with tissue ischemia or organ dysfunction is the principal clinical finding, anticoagulation with heparin is the treatment choice.[298] Therapy is difficult to manage, because the usual laboratory tests employed to monitor its use are abnormal before therapy. Also, heparin may exacerbate any coexisting bleeding.[298] In addition to assessing the effect of heparin on the clinical abnormalities, monitoring the fibrinogen level, platelet counts, and serum fibrin(ogen) degradation products is useful. With successful treatment, consumption should decrease, resulting in a rise in fibrinogen and platelets and a fall in degradation products. Heparin should be given in the smallest dose that will improve tissue ischemia and hemostatic abnormalities. The necessary dose varies widely, but an infusion of 8 to 15 U/kg/hr is often successful.

If the primary manifestation of DIC is bleeding due to consumption of platelets and coagulation functions, then replacement therapy is the most appropriate first choice of treatment. In addition to plasma, cryoprecipitate can be given to replace fibrinogen and factor VIII, and platelet concentrates should be used to improve thrombocytopenia. If the underlying disorder cannot be corrected, replacement is unlikely to be adequate therapy, because consumption will continue or increase in intensity. A logical approach in this situation is to first stop the consumption by administration of heparin and then replace the necessary coagulation factors and platelets by transfusion.

In summary, DIC is a complex hemostatic disorder resulting from microvascular thrombosis, consumption of coagulation factors, and heightened fibrinolysis. The clinical manifestations are variable and include organ dysfunction and a generalized bleeding diathesis. Laboratory abnormalities include thrombocytopenia, prolonged screening coagulation tests, low fibrinogen, and increased fibrinogen degradation products. Prompt treatment of the underlying disorder and aggressive supportive therapy are critical in the management of DIC. Administration of heparin and appropriate transfusion therapy to replace coagulation factors and platelets may help correct the hemostatic abnormalities.

THROMBOEMBOLISM

Thromboembolic disease is one of the most common and dangerous of all complications in patients sustaining skeletal trauma and undergoing elective musculoskeletal surgery.[335,343,347,350,351,370,451,460] Despite some dissenting opinions, evidence exists that the incidence of pulmonary embolism is increasing and that a genuine rise in fatal pulmonary emboli has occurred.[346,394,414] Pulmonary embolism is the leading cause of hospital admissions for respiratory disease, excluding pneumonia. The threat of thromboembolism increases with the age of the patient, the extent and duration of the surgical procedure, the degree and length of immobilization, and the severity of the underlying systemic disease.[321,329,330,332,360,389,444,448] As more older patients have major joint replacements, the prevalence of the disease will rise.

To ascertain the true incidence of thromboembolic disease is difficult. It is probably higher in most European countries and North America than in Africa, Asia, and South America.[389,438] The frequency of the problem also varies within regions of the United States. Clinical investigators and, in particular, those using retrospective analysis have grossly underestimated the incidence of thromboembolic disease. Orthopaedic surgeons have tended to deny that thromboembolic disease is a major problem. Such an outlook is not only incorrect but also dangerous. In one autopsy study of 161 patients who died after hip fractures, 38% died from pulmonary emboli.[337,445] In direct contrast, pulmonary embolism was thought to be the cause of death in only 2% of 87 patients with hip fractures, when evaluated on clinical grounds only, without an autopsy. Table 5-5 illustrates the high incidence of thromboembolism associated with fractures of the hip or lower extremities and pelvis. It is important to recognize that general surgical patients are at less risk of thromboembolic disease than patients undergoing musculoskeletal surgery. Any study undertaken on the incidence, treatment, and prophylaxis of thromboembolic disease must be prospective, and the diagnosis must be established by phlebography. The magnitude of the problem is such that, in at least 50% of patients undergoing joint replacement surgery or having sustained fractures of the lower extremity, deep venous thrombosis develops; 10% of these patients run the risk of pulmonary emboli, and unless adequate protection is provided, 2% will die from fatal pulmonary emboli.[371,444] Of all patients with confirmed diagnosis of pulmonary embolism, 11% will not survive beyond one hour from the onset of symptoms; of the remaining patients, 8% will die despite appropriate anticoagulation, and mortality rises to 30% for those in whom the diagnosis is not made and no therapy is instituted.[424,432,453]

Preventing thromboembolism is much preferred to treating it, because anticoagulation therapy beginning after the diagnosis of deep venous thrombosis may not significantly decrease the incidence of pulmonary emboli.[403] Clearly, the most effective intervention is prophylactic rather than therapeutic.[360,380,420,425] The National Institutes of Health (NIH) Consensus Conference concluded that venous thromboembolic disease in orthopaedic patients "can be significantly reduced by prophylactic regimens, which should be used more extensively."[420] Despite the NIH conclusion that aspirin prophylaxis "has not been shown to be beneficial,"[420] a recent survey of practicing orthopaedic surgeons found aspirin to be the most popular agent for prophylaxis in adults undergoing elective hip surgery or repair of hip fracture.[425] Of some concern, this same survey also revealed that 15% to 25% of all orthopaedic surgeons do not employ prophylaxis in all patients undergoing hip surgery and 5% to 10% never use any form of prophylaxis, even in "high-risk" patients.[425] The accumulating evidence is now compelling that prevention of pulmonary embolism through prophylaxis of deep venous thrombosis is both cost-effective and reduces mortality from embolic complications.[420,424]

Thromboembolic disease has many enigmatic

Table 5-5. Thromboembolism Associated With Fractures of the Hip or Lower Extremities or Pelvis

Author	Injury	Number of Patients	Thromboembolism (%)
Sevitt and Gallagher[440]	Hip fractures	319	39.3
Tubiana and Duparc[451]	Hip fractures	389	15.0
Fagan[349]	Hip fractures	162	28.7
Solonen[446]	Fractures of lower extremities	178	21.3
Neu and associates[418]	Fractures of pelvis, lower extremities	100	20.0
Salzman and associates[436]	Hip fractures	184	26.0
Freeark and associates[357]	Hip fractures	70	42.0*
Hamilton and associates[366]	Hip fractures	38	48.0*
Sevitt and Gallagher[441]	Fractures	468	20.3
Golodner and associates[364]	Hip fractures	25	36.0

* Diagnosis of venous thrombosis confirmed by venography.

features: the initiating mechanisms are obscure, clinical recognition is elusive, the recurrence rate is high, and mortality is unpredictable.

THROMBOGENESIS

The basis for understanding thrombosis began more than a century ago, when Virchow[455] provided a conceptual framework for thrombogenesis. He stated that thrombosis may result from changes in the vessel wall, changes in the blood composition, or changes in blood flow promoting stasis. Early research emphasized the role of plasma coagulation factors in thrombus formation.[338] Two types of thrombi were proposed, each with a different pathogenesis: first, the red thrombus, composed primarily of erythrocytes and fibrin and characteristically forming in areas of venous stasis or retarded flow; second, the white thrombus, composed primarily of platelets and fibrin, relatively poor in erythrocytes, and found almost exclusively in areas of rapid arterial flow. The role of the platelet was thought to be secondary in the formation of red (venous) thrombus. Controversy existed as to whether the activation of a clotting mechanism preceded or followed the development of a mural platelet thrombus as the first stage of thrombus formation, not only in the arterial system but also in the venous system.[344] In addition, several studies have demonstrated abnormalities of platelet adhesiveness and survival time and alteration in fibrinolysis in patients with postoperative thromboembolism.[326,377,387,402] Hereditary deficiencies of normally occurring antithrombotic factors may contribute to a genetically determined increased risk of thrombosis in some patients.[404,407] The available evidence suggests that the activation of the venous thrombus may follow the formation of a small platelet nidus, thereby providing a common pathogenesis with its arterial counterpart.[382]

The cascade, or waterfall, mechanism for thrombus formation begins with adhesion of platelets to the exposed collagen in the damaged vessel wall. A series of morphologic and biochemical changes occur by way of a chain of enzymatic steps. Adenosine diphosphate is released, causing further platelet aggregation, and tissue factor lipoprotein in the endothelial cell membrane activates the extrinsic cascade. The clotting process then proceeds to thrombus formation (see Fig. 5-8).

The sequence of events leading to thrombus formation after trauma or musculoskeletal procedures is not completely understood. Little is known about the types of thrombi that are prone to pulmonary

emboli or that cause valvular damage and the postphlebitic syndrome. The pathogenesis of thrombosis remains elusive, despite extensive experimental work. More inquiry is required into the dynamics of peripheral clot formation.[311] The results of a study of 132 patients undergoing elective surgery showed that postoperative venous thrombosis developed in 40 patients.[387] Of the 40 clots, 14 disappeared within 72 hours of surgery and 26 persisted. All clots in the latter group originated with activity in the calf veins; 9 demonstrated proximal extension to the popliteal or femoral veins, and 4 of these resulted in pulmonary emboli. Venography, autopsy studies, and ^{125}I-labeled fibrinogen studies help to substantiate the viewpoint that thromboses primarily begin in the calf and later propagate into the popliteal and femoral veins. Flanc and associates[352] have shown that venous thrombosis is present in patients returning from elective surgery, strongly suggesting that the thrombotic process actually begins during surgery. In their study of 96 patients, the ^{125}I-labeled fibrinogen technique was employed for diagnosis, and the results were confirmed by venography. Thromboses developed in 35% of patients; 50% of the thromboses developed during the operative procedure. This indicates that greater attention should be given to the administration of prophylactic agents before—and certainly during—the operative procedure. It is known that changes in platelet adhesiveness occur after elective hip surgery as well as after trauma. In view of the primary role of platelet adhesion and aggregation in thrombus formation, an attempt can be made to alter these factors and suppress the development of thrombi. The usual anticoagulants, heparin and dicumarol, do not effectively suppress platelet surface reactions or adenosine diphosphate–induced platelet aggregation. These agents should theoretically be effective only in preventing the growth phase of the thrombus and in decreasing the diffuse clotting effect.[314,317,359,416]

DETECTION OF VENOUS THROMBOSIS

Because the clinical signs and symptoms of deep venous thrombosis are notoriously unreliable, the detection of venous thrombosis cannot be based on clinical findings alone.[348] However, accurate evaluation of possible clot formation requires careful clinical observation, including a check of the calf and the remainder of the lower extremity daily for pain, swelling, and tenderness, accompanied by an increase in temperature and pulse rate. Such signs, if present, cannot be ignored; they are an indication

Venography

Venography remains the standard of detection.[334,421,431] The lesser saphenous veins or subcutaneous veins of the foot provide excellent portals of entry to the venous system for the injection of the opaque medium used in venography. Current techniques allow for the identification of the soleal veins as well as the other calf veins and vessels of the lower extremity. The diagnosis of venous thrombosis depends on certain signs: (1) constant filling defects, (2) abrupt termination of the opaque contrast medium column occurring at a constant site, (3) nonfilling defects of the entire deep system, and (4) diversion of flow.[401] Rabinov and Paulin[431] believe that the most direct sign of thrombosis is demonstration of the thrombus itself. The other three signs reflect obstruction to venous flow and are indirect signs.[337] The artifacts that occur with phlebography include underfilling, dilution, and streamlining. A loose, potentially movable thrombus is thought to produce a ground-glass type of shadow, and the contrast medium can be seen between the thrombus and the vein wall. If the thrombus is old and fixed, the affected vein disappears on x-ray film and often dilated collateral veins appear more prominent. One study revealed that, despite careful clinical examination by members of the peripheral vascular disease department, 30 of 37 cases (81%) of postoperative venous thromboses were overlooked.[348] It remained for venography to demonstrate the presence of venous thrombosis in these patients. It should be recognized that there is a slight risk, less than 5%, of inducing thrombosis by venography. This test is not repeatable on a daily basis and therefore is not useful for frequent longitudinal follow-up examination. However, it reveals the position and extent of thrombus formation that in turn aids in the selection of therapeutic agents for treatment.

Radioactive Iodine-Labeled Fibrinogen

Another technique for the detection of venous thrombosis in the lower extremity employs radioactive iodine-labeled fibrinogen.[309,385,417,423] This method is based on the principle that if labeled fibrinogen is injected intravenously, it behaves in vivo as unlabeled fibrinogen and is converted into fibrin in any thrombotic process. The ^{125}I-labeled fibrinogen accumulates in the thrombus and can be detected by a scintillation counter placed over the affected area. However, this technique may give false-positive or false-negative results in the area of a femoral artery or venous pooling in the calf. It cannot be used in the vicinity of a large wound and hence is impractical after major hip surgery. It cannot detect thrombosis in the upper thigh, iliac, deep pelvic veins, which is a significant drawback. The risk of transmitting serum hepatitis is largely avoided in part by obtaining the human fibrinogen from a restricted pool of donors who are screened by laboratory testing to nearly eliminate the possibility of the presence of viral hepatitis.[322] The accuracy of the method in detecting thrombi in the legs, below the popliteal space, compares favorably with that of venography—90% to 95%. It has been used widely in Great Britain for the detection of venous thrombosis.

Ultrasound

Another screening test for the detection of deep venous thrombosis is based on the use of an ultrasound flowmeter using the Doppler effect, a noninvasive technique for detecting blood flow.[442,443] The patency of major veins can be examined. However, the obvious disadvantage is that small thrombi beginning in the calf or extending to the thigh veins cannot be detected. The test is also inaccurate for diagnosis of deep venous thrombosis in the large hip wound. Great sophistication is required in the technical aspects of its use, and the good results obtained by certain authors are not easily duplicated. The ultrasound technique is 76% to 93% accurate as recorded by various studies. Compression ultrasonography is not useful for detection of clots below the popliteal space but has been shown to have high specificity and sensitivity in thrombus detection in the thigh.[353,358,395,429] Color flow ultrasonography is a significant recent advance in ultrasound technology and offers promise for noninvasive thrombus detection in both the calf and thigh; however, considerably more clinical experience is needed before its role can be determined.[333]

Impedance Plethysmography

Impedance plethysmography is another method that has been suggested for the diagnosis of deep venous thrombosis.[378,459] This technique has been found to be inaccurate when compared with venography. It is most efficacious in detecting proximal disease above the knee but is technically difficult to perform on patients with hip pain and with a restricted range of hip motion. Combined use of I^{125}-fibrinogen scanning and impedance plethysmography has been suggested.[427] The impedance technique is only 53% to 88% accurate.

DIAGNOSIS OF PULMONARY EMBOLISM

As the techniques for the diagnosis of deep venous thrombosis have become more sophisticated, it has been recognized that the detection of pulmonary embolism is equally inaccurate when based on the usual clinical, x-ray, biochemical, and electrocardiographic criteria.[340,428,456] The diagnosis of pulmonary embolism during life is often impossible because of a lack of characteristic signs and symptoms or the explanation of certain signs and symptoms by alternative diagnosis. Smith and coworkers[445] estimated that pulmonary embolism is diagnosed before death in less than 50% of cases. A retrospective study showed that many deaths occurring from pulmonary embolism could have been prevented by anticoagulation.[430] Results of retrospective studies on pulmonary embolism are grossly inaccurate because of the inaccurate methods of routine autopsy. In 136 cases, Morrell and Dunnill[413] reported a 52% incidence of pulmonary emboli in 263 right lungs. In the same study they found that the incidence of pulmonary embolism increased with age and that there was a distinct association between pulmonary embolism and the operation. In 14% of the total number, death was entirely attributable to the embolism. The reported incidence in retrospective studies is approximately 10% to 18%. Hildner and Ormand[373] stated that most cases of pulmonary embolism were not identified by symptoms, physical findings, electrocardiographic examination, serum enzyme determinations, or chest x-ray films. Intraluminal interruption of the inferior vena cava has been employed for prevention of pulmonary embolism in high-risk patients or those with known deep venous thrombosis and contraindications to anticoagulation.[410]

Lung Scan

Radioisotope lung scanning has been employed to investigate the regional pulmonary blood flow to help determine the presence of perfusion defects.[327,400,409] However, it is difficult to differentiate the causes of such perfusion defects. If one combines a perfusion defect with a normal plain chest x-ray film, along with the symptoms and signs of a lowering of PaO_2 values, dyspnea, tachypnea, chest pain, cough, hemoptysis, cyanosis, tachycar-

dia, fever, and early heart failure, the combination is highly suggestive of pulmonary embolism. However, even in "low" and "high" probability scans there remains an error rate approaching 15%, resulting in a significant number of false-negative and false-positive interpretations, respectively, when confirmed by pulmonary angiogram.[400]

Pulmonary Angiography

Pulmonary angiography remains the most accurate diagnostic method of detecting pulmonary embolism.[319] The primary positive signs are the trailing edges of vascular occlusions within an arterial network of the lung and intraluminal defects outlined by contrast material within the lung vasculature. There are associated secondary signs, nonfilling of vessels, areas of slow perfusion, vascular tortuosity, and delayed clearance of contrast medium.

Greater emphasis must be placed on the identification of the presence of a pulmonary embolus. Blood gas studies should be obtained routinely. Chest x-ray films are obtained in all patients suspected of having a deep venous thrombosis or in patients with positive venograms or fibrinogen scans. If the chest x-ray films are normal, scintigrams of the lungs are obtained in an attempt to detect silent pulmonary emboli. If the diagnosis of pulmonary embolism can be made from the clinical picture, no further testing is necessary. If the chest x-ray films are abnormal, pulmonary angiography may be requested to detect the presence of pulmonary emboli. Angiography and lung scanning are complementary studies; both should be performed when necessary and correlated with the plain chest x-ray film.

TREATMENT

The hallmark of the treatment of thromboembolic disease is prevention. A profile of the orthopaedic patient in whom thromboembolic disease is likely to develop should be established. The archetype is an obese, elderly person with multiple injuries or operations and a history of associated cardiovascular or pulmonary disease who is about to undergo major musculoskeletal surgery.

Coumadin

It has been statistically proved that crystalline sodium warfarin (Coumadin), an anticoagulant, can reduce the risk of thromboembolic disease when given prophylactically.[348,470] Two regimens of Coumadin use are currently followed, and both require meticulous attention to detail.[307,356,371,450] Ten milligrams of Coumadin may be administered the evening before surgery. The PT must be obtained after surgery, and Coumadin is given the night following surgery, the usual dose being 5 to 10 mg. The daily maintenance dose ranges from 2 to 10 mg per day, administered orally. Previously, it was believed that the PT (protime) should be maintained at 2 to 2.5 times the control value; however, recent data suggest that prolongation of the protime by 3 to 5 seconds over control (ratio of 1.3 to 1.6) is equally effective in prevention of thrombus propagation.[375,376,379] In their studies of thromboembolism in orthopaedic surgery, Harris and associates[371] and Amstutz and coworkers[307] have shown that this method is effective in the prevention of thromboembolic disease. Alternatively, Coumadin may be administered in a low dose seven to ten days prior to an elective procedure to deplete essential vitamin K–dependent factors while maintaining the protime no greater than 14 seconds until after the planned procedure. Although requiring more preoperative planning, this method of administration is equally effective in preventing thrombus formation while minimizing postoperative bleeding complications.[356,450]

The use of Coumadin is contraindicated in patients with hemorrhagic disorders, peptic ulceration, active liver disease, hematuria, melena, hemoptysis, cerebral insufficiency, or a history of infarct. Increased risk of major bleeding has been demonstrated in patients over 65 years of age.[391] Many drugs decrease the effectiveness of Coumadin—for instance, aspirin, phenylbutazone, and barbiturates. Several other drugs such as aspirin and chloral hydrate will increase the protime by effectively displacing Coumadin from plasma proteins that act as the intravascular transport vehicle. After administration of Coumadin it is essential to obtain stool guaiac examinations periodically, hematocrit values three times per week, and PTs each day. Such complications as hemorrhage at the wound site, gastrointestinal bleeding, renal bleeding, and cerebral bleeding have occurred, along with the difficulty in administration and control of Coumadin anticoagulation. The incidence of major bleeding complications during outpatient therapy is 12% to 15%; the risk of major hemorrhage increases 80% for every 1.0 increase in the protime-to-control ratio.[392]

Dextran

The primary role of platelet adhesiveness and aggregation in thrombus formation has been emphasized previously. There is much to suggest that platelet activity underlies the initiation and propagation of certain venous thrombi.[339] In a search for safer and more reliable agents to prevent thromboembolism, attention was directed toward the dextran solutions. In 1944, Gronwall and Ingleman[365] developed fractionated dextran as a plasma volume expander. Bull and associates[323] confirmed the clinical value of dextran, and Bloom[318] prepared the first dextran in the United States and demonstrated its value as a blood volume expander. The dextrans represented a group of polysaccharides containing D-glucose units with predominantly 1:6 linkage. Clinical dextrans are glucose polymers containing a broad molecular-weight distribution composed of average molecular-weight fractions, either low-molecular-weight dextran (average molecular weight 40,000) or clinical dextran (average molecular weight 70,000).

The antithrombotic actions of dextran have been studied extensively, both experimentally[308,320,342,384] and clinically.[313,390,434,461] Dextrans decrease thrombus formation after arterial surgery. In experimentally damaged large veins, dextran decreased the incidence of thrombosis.[384] It has been demonstrated that low-molecular-weight dextran increases cardiac output and reduces the mean transit time.[345] These changes are the result of plasma volume expansion and the reduction of blood viscosity from hemodilution. Low-molecular-weight dextran causes a significant reduction in platelet adhesiveness, partly caused by adsorption to platelets and the alteration of their membranes, interaction of the plasma proteins, and coating of the endothelial walls. After intravenous administration of low-molecular-weight dextran, a change in electrophoretic mobility of the platelet occurs.[324,325] There appears to be no difference between antithrombotic effects of low-molecular-weight dextran in comparison with clinical dextran. The relative efficacy of low-molecular-weight dextran as a prophylactic agent against thromboemboli has been frequently studied in clinical trials.[315,316,348,393,437,449] Efficacy less than that found with Coumadin coupled with frequent complications related to volume expansion and fluid overload has made the use of low-molecular-weight dextran less popular in recent years.[316,424]

Absolute contraindications to the use of low-molecular-weight dextran are pulmonary edema, congestive heart failure, renal failure, severe dehydration, and allergic manifestations. Hypersensitivity reactions can range from mild cutaneous eruptions to generalized urticaria, nausea and vomiting, wheezing, and (rarely) anaphylactic shock. Such reactions almost always develop in the first few minutes after initiation of therapy. Therefore, the patient should be observed closely during the initial infusion. If any adverse symptoms or signs appear, the infusion should be stopped immediately. Therapy to counteract anaphylactoid shock, including epinephrine, steroids, and antihistamines, should be started promptly. If large amounts are given in the face of decreased urinary output, congestive heart failure and pulmonary edema may occur. A renal profile must be obtained preoperatively, and if chronic renal dysfunction is suspected, dextran administration should be avoided. Renal failure has occurred after the administration of low-molecular-weight dextran, and renal dialysis has been required in some patients.[348]

Aspirin

Other antiplatelet drugs, including aspirin, have been suggested to prevent thromboembolic disease.[338,422,457] Certain case reports and retrospective studies have suggested a beneficial action of aspirin.[368,383] Stamatakis and associates[447] found that aspirin failed to prevent postoperative deep venous thrombosis in patients undergoing total hip replacement. On the basis of published data, there is no persuasive evidence that aspirin is completely effective in the prophylaxis of venous thromboembolism in the musculoskeletal patient.[336,341,368,369,374,383,433,439,454] Its efficacy has not been proved for high-risk patients, especially women.[368]

Minidose Heparin

Much attention has again recently been given to the role of minidose heparin in the prevention of thromboembolic disease.[361,388,396,419] Following the identification of a potent, naturally occurring inhibitor, antithrombin III (AT III), to activated factor X and the recognition of the potentiated response by such a factor to minidose heparin, it was suggested that minidose heparin might prevent thrombus formation.[458] The anticoagulant effect of the inhibitor to activated factor X is markedly influenced by trace amounts of heparin in vitro. One microgram of the inhibitor, by neutralizing 32 units of activated factor X, indirectly prevents the generation of 1,600 NIH units of thrombin. Indeed, activated factor X may be a more potent thrombogenic agent than thrombin itself. However, in a study in which 5,000 international units (IU) of heparin were given subcutaneously 2 hours preoperatively, 5,000 IU postoperatively the night of surgery, and every 12 hours for the next seven to ten days, venous thrombosis developed in 7 of 25

patients.[347] Pulmonary embolism occurred in 6 of these patients undergoing total hip replacement. It was believed that the blood levels of heparin were not sufficiently high to exert a prophylactic effect.[398] In another study, low-dose heparin did not prevent deep venous thrombosis in 100 patients undergoing total hip replacement.[367] In contrast to the conclusions of individual reports, a statistical review of previously published studies of heparin prophylaxis in orthopaedic surgery suggests that collective consideration of all available data demonstrates a significant effect in prevention of deep venous thrombosis.[328] Furthermore, recent studies of heparin administered in conjunction with AT III following total hip and knee replacement have yielded incidences of venographically documented clots comparable to the best results previously reported with Coumadin.[354,355] Laboratory investigations suggest that musculoskeletal trauma results in a physiologic consumption of AT III, the naturally occurring antithrombotic substance to which heparin binds to produce its anticoagulant effect. Depletion of AT III following orthopaedic surgery may explain the apparent previous ineffectiveness of heparin in this setting without concurrent administration of AT III to restore normal circulating levels of the inhibitor.[363] Dihydroergotamine-heparin combination therapy has demonstrated efficacy in the prevention of orthopaedic thromboembolic disease comparable to other regimens, but its attendant risks of vasospasm in the elderly population with pre-existing vascular disease make it an unattractive choice for most patients.[312,386,406] Investigative use of a low-molecular-weight heparin has also shown promise in prevention of thrombosis following orthopaedic procedures.[412,452] Clearly, with this renewed interest in heparin, additional controlled studies with varying doses and in vivo measurement of both heparin and AT III levels are necessary before the efficacy of this agent in the prevention of orthopaedic thromboembolism can be ultimately determined.

Pneumatic External Compression Devices

Pneumatic external compression devices have recently been the focus of considerable interest in the prevention of thromboembolic disease because of their noninvasive nature and lack of associated drug-induced adverse effects.[372,426] Although overall efficacy appears comparable to that of other methods, a propensity for proximal thrombosis warrants further investigation before this modality can be recommended for general use (Pellegrini, V.; Francis, W.; and Marder, V., unpublished data, March, 1990). Other noninvasive mechanical methods of thrombosis prophylaxis, such as continuous passive motion, have yet to be proved efficacious.[399]

Authors' Preferred Method of Treatment

A confirmed diagnosis of deep vein thrombosis warrants serious consideration for further anticoagulant treatment.[397,411,415] Although virtually all clinically evident pulmonary emboli arise from proximal vein thrombi, 20% of all calf vein thrombi propagate to the proximal veins from which embolic events may then originate.[311,387,415,435] Because of documented clinically significant embolic complications from untreated deep system thrombosis distal to the knee, (Pellegrini, V.; Francis, W.; and Marder, V., unpublished data, May, 1990) we continue to treat all thromboembolic disease following orthopaedic injury and elective surgery. As soon as the diagnosis of deep venous thrombosis or pulmonary embolism is established, treatment should begin with 10,000 to 15,000 IU of heparin (aqueous heparin sodium injection) administered intravenously as a loading dose.[362] However, one should be cautioned against the indiscriminate use of intravenous heparin unless the diagnosis is *certain;* although rare, heparin-related thrombocytopenia and thrombosis may be life-threatening.[310] Given the limitations of most diagnostic studies, as previously described, this generally requires contrast venography of the lower extremities or pulmonary angiography. The administration of heparin is then converted to a continuous drip delivering 1,000 IU per hour and is adjusted to maintain the partial thromboplastin time at two to three times normal. This is continued for the next 72 hours, and Coumadin (5 to 15 mg per day) is begun. The heparin is discontinued after five days or when the PT has been prolonged to 1.3 to 1.8 times normal under the influence of Coumadin, whichever is longer.[375,376,379] During this initial period of anticoagulation, all physical therapy should be suspended and the patient maintained on bed rest. Coumadin is continued for 3 to 6 months in doses sufficient to maintain PTs 3 to 6 seconds greater than normal. Slightly greater prolongation to 1.6 to 1.8 times normal is indicated in the treatment of recurrent systemic embolism.[376] Infrequently, there may be certain indications for pulmonary embolectomy, namely, persistent hypotension, persistent cyanosis, and pulmonary arteriographic evidence of massive pulmonary embolism.[401,435] The initial treatment of a massive acute pulmonary embolism involves closed-chest cardiac massage, fluid resuscitation, and the immediate administration of heparin, positive-pressure ventilation, and vasopressors. If the patient survives, pulmonary embolectomy may be indicated. Again, although infrequently, there are certain indications for surgical venous interruption.[405,408] These involve suppurative venous thromboembolism, microembolic clots with cor pulmonale, and failure of anticoagulants to control thromboembolic episodes. In certain instances, when anticoagulants and antiplatelet agents are contraindicated, surgical venous interruption may be necessary.

In summary, it is imperative that the orthopaedic surgeon dealing with skeletal trauma and related disorders recognize the magnitude of the problem of thromboembolic disease. It is the most common disease following trauma or surgical procedures. Deep venous thrombosis develops in at least 50% of patients, and 2% of all untreated patients die of pulmonary embolism following elective hip surgery, including total hip replacement. A much higher percentage die of pulmonary embolism following trauma. A diagnosis of thromboembolism is best confirmed by venography or pulmonary angiography.

Prophylaxis remains the cornerstone of treatment. The prevention of thromboembolism depends on maintaining mobility and activity in the injured patient or the patient who has undergone operation, using graduated elastic compression stockings, elevating the lower limbs, and prescribing appropriate prophylactic anticoagulant therapy. The severity of thromboembolism is of great concern; appropriate attention should be given to the use of the most effective methods available to eliminate the occurrence of life-threatening complications. Meanwhile, the search continues for a noninvasive technique of identifying the patient whose blood is likely to clot and embolize, as well as identifying a safe oral agent that is uniformly effective in preventing thromboembolic disease.

REGIONAL COMPLICATIONS OF EXTREMITY INJURY

GAS GANGRENE

Gas gangrene is one of the most serious complications of traumatic wounds. Generally regarded as a disease associated with battlefield casualties, the high incidence of highway accidents and regional prevalence of farm injuries has refocused the attention of the orthopaedic surgeon on this devastating problem. MacLennan[490] has stated, "While true gas gangrene is an uncommon disease in civilian life, it is by no means so rare as is generally believed." Several authors have described the recognition and management of gas gangrene and have commented on the use of hyperbaric oxygen as an adjunct in the treatment of anaerobic infections.[471,484] Also, postoperative clostridial infections are being reported with increasing frequency.[473,474] Many anaerobic bacteria thought to be commensals have become invasive and produce gas gangrene in the face of host changes induced by extensive surgery or therapy with corticosteroids, cytotoxic agents, or antibiotics.[468,503]

Although the historical accounts of gas gangrene date to the Middle Ages, accurate descriptions of this entity became available beginning in the 18th century.[485] In 1871, Bottini[469] recognized the bacterial nature of the disease but did not isolate the invading organism. Further descriptions separated the various disease states, but these were somewhat ignored until World War I. World War II brought forth the recognition that the term *gas gangrene* should be limited to those invasive anaerobic infections of muscle characterized by profound toxemia, extensive edema, massive tissue necrosis, and gas production.[488] In 1945, Robb-Smith[497] proposed the name *anaerobic myonecrosis* to emphasize that the basic lesion is necrotic rather than inflammatory.

BACTERIOLOGY AND PATHOGENESIS

Clostridial Species Capable of Producing Gas Gangrene

C. perfringens (C. welchii)
C. novyi
C. septicum
C. histolyticum
C. bifermentans
C. fallax

The most important species in the preceding list is *Clostridium perfringens.* Identification is made on the basis of the morphology, the patterns of fermentation, and toxin production and its neutralization.[507] C. perfringens is a nonmotile, gram-positive, anaerobic bacillus without spores that produces marked milk fermentation with a lecithinase activity inhibited by *C. perfringens* antitoxin on a Nagler plate.[480,506] Such organisms are obligate anaerobes and cannot multiply in healthy tissues with high oxygen reduction potentials. Clostridia are

found widely distributed in fecal matter. *C. perfringens* is regarded as a ubiquitous organism also found in operating rooms, emergency departments, hospital corridors, and cart wheels and on shoes. It is a saprophytic commensal of the alimentary tract and can be isolated from skin in approximately 20% of patients.[495] The risk of clostridial contamination is always present in the operating room. The significant toxins associated with the clostridia are listed subsequently. When the cell wall (a lipoprotein complex containing a lecithin) is attacked by the α-toxin, a dermonecrotizing lecithinase, cell wall destruction and cell death occur.

Clostridial infections are caused not by the extra virulence of the organism but rather by unique local conditions. Oakley[492] discussed the factors required to establish a clostridial infection and pointed out that with ischemia and necrosis of muscle a decreased oxidation reduction potential promoted rapid advance of a highly lethal infection. The exact mechanism that converts the saprophytic state to the fulminating gangrenous state is not known. An unidentified lethal factor may contribute to the invasiveness and the toxemia that accompany gas gangrene.[491]

Histotoxins

Lecithinase (α-toxins)
Collagenase
Hyaluronidase
Leukocidin
Deoxyribonuclease
Protease
Lipase

It is easy to understand how trauma from the injury itself, surgery, tight casts, and so forth can lower the oxidation reduction potential values and create the proper environment for clostridial infection. Dirty wounds, especially those closed primarily without appropriate débridement, provide an ideal setting for the onset of gas gangrene.

The clinical course of gas gangrene depends on the spread of lethal toxins produced by clostridial organisms in a local lesion of dead tissue. The local lesion arises when toxicogenic clostridia are introduced into a deep wound of muscle, where under favorable conditions they multiply and produce toxins that diffuse into the surrounding tissues and devitalize them, allowing further colonization by the clostridial organisms.[472] Figure 5-10 illustrates the mode of action of clostridia with the production

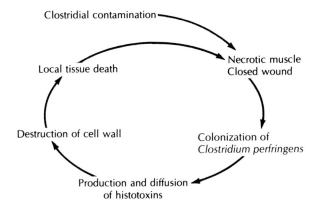

Clostridial contamination

Necrotic muscle
Closed wound

Local tissue death

Destruction of cell wall

Colonization of
Clostridium perfringens

Production and diffusion
of histotoxins

Fig. 5-10. Pathogenesis of clostridial myonecrosis.

and diffusion of the histotoxins. This vicious cycle promotes astonishingly rapid growth of the organisms and diffusion of the toxins. Although the activities of some of the toxins produced have been defined, the toxemia associated with gas gangrene is not clearly understood and has been attributed to release of the products of tissue necrosis, interference with cell enzyme systems, and acidosis.[504]

CLASSIFICATION

MacLennan[490] has provided a classification of the histotoxic infections in humans.

Histotoxic Infections

I. Traumatic wound infections
  A. Simple contamination
  B. Anaerobic cellulitis
  C. Anaerobic myonecrosis
    1. Clostridial myonecrosis
    2. Streptococcal myonecrosis
II. Nontraumatic infections
  A. Idiopathic
  B. Infected vascular gangrene

It is important to recognize the different categories of traumatic wound infections. The mere presence of anaerobic organisms in the wound and their multiplication do not cause pain or a systemic reaction, and such an infection is not often recognized. In a few instances the wound appears ragged and deep, with a watery, brown, seropurulent discharge. This represents simple contamination of a wound, and the surgeon need only remove the necrotic debris.

Anaerobic cellulitis necrotizing fasciitis is a clostridial infection of ischemic tissue, usually occurring after several days, in an inadequately débrided wound. Altemeier and Culbertson[463] commented on the rapidly spreading emphysematous infection along the fascial planes with extensive gas formation. Altemeier and Fullen[464] outlined the causes of crepitation in a wound.

Crepitant Nonclostridial Lesions

I. Bacterial
  A. Aerobic aerogenic infections
    1. Coliform
    2. Mixed
  B. Hemolytic staphylococcal fasciitis
  C. Hemolytic streptococcal gangrene
  D. Anaerobic streptococcal infections
  E. Infections with *Bacteroides* organism
II. Nonbacterial
  A. Mechanical effect of trauma
  B. Air hose injury
  C. Irrigation with hydrogen peroxide
  D. Benzine injection

(Altemeier, W.A., and Fullen, W.D.: Prevention and Treatment of Gas Gangrene. J.A.M.A., 217:806–813, 1971.)

Other common gas-forming organisms include the coliform bacteria, anaerobic streptococci, and the anaerobic bacteroides. In anaerobic cellulitis the onset is gradual; the toxemia is slight. The exudate is brown and seropurulent.[468,474,490] The gas formation is foul-smelling and abundant, but there remains no actual muscle invasion. There have been many needless amputations for anaerobic cellulitis, because it may be confused with gas gangrene. Table 5-6 presents the differential features.

The nontraumatic infections have been classified as idiopathic and infected vascular gangrene.[479] It is doubtful that true idiopathic gas gangrene occurs in humans, although it is well documented in veterinary medicine. It is more likely that the clostridial spores remain dormant in scar tissue for years after the original injury.

Infected vascular gangrene is a specific histotoxic infection of humans in which gas-producing anaerobes are found proliferating in gangrenous but anatomically intact muscle.[472] The organisms are saprophytes, not invaders in a limb that is ischemic. A line of demarcation is seen, and bacterial spread is limited. A foul smell and gas production occur, but rarely are the signs and symptoms of acute toxemia observed. Although a relatively benign form of infection, vascular gangrene, if neglected, can develop into a true clostridial myonecrosis.

INCIDENCE

The incidence of gas gangrene is not known. Reports have emphasized the continuing problem of clostridal myonecrosis in civilian practice.[493,496] The presence of clostridial organisms in a wound has been reported to be as high as 18% to 46%.[500] Anaerobic cellulitis may develop in approximately 5% of traumatic wounds. In a total series of 187,936 traumatic wounds, the overall incidence of gas gangrene was 1.76%.[465] The incidence of gas gangrene is related to the lapse of time between injury and surgical treatment. Also, the site of injury is significant. Clostridial myonecrosis occurs most frequently in wounds of the buttocks and thigh, then in the shoulder, and, finally, in the lower extremity. The mortality varied from more than 50% in World War I to less than 25% in World War II.[487] Treatment modalities, including the use of antibiotics and hyperbaric oxygen, have helped lower the morbidity and mortality.

CLINICAL FINDINGS

The third category of traumatic wound infection in MacLennan's classification is anaerobic myonecrosis, separated into clostridial and streptococcal myonecrosis.[475,478] Almost without exception the original wound involves injury to muscle—a deep, penetrating wound sealed off from ready access to the surface. The incubation period of clostridia is not long—12 to 24 hours after injury. The initial symptom is pain or a sense of heaviness in the affected area, followed by local edema and exudation of a thin, dark fluid. There is a dissociation between tachycardia and temperature elevation; the pulse rate is elevated but the temperature is not high initially. The progress of the disease is rapid and spectacular, with an increase in toxemia and local spread of the infection. Profound shock may occur. A peculiar bronze discoloration develops in the wound, along with a musty odor and a slight amount of gas production. A symptom characteristic of gas gangrene is the mental awareness marked by a terror of death in the face of profound toxemia. Shortly before death the patient usually becomes apathetic and coma ensues. It is difficult to determine the actual extent of muscle invasion and necrosis without surgical exploration. When examined, the muscle appears edematous, gray or dark red, and ischemic. Contractility is absent, and gas bubbles froth from the muscle fiber bundles.[477] Muscle involvement is invariably greater than the skin changes might indicate.

The other form of anaerobic myonecrosis is secondary to anaerobic streptococcal infection.[478,489] Most streptococcal myonecrosis infections have been located in either the perirectal or inguinal regions. Recent studies have indicated changes in the pattern of this illness, with a higher mortality reflecting increased longevity.[462] Superficially, this infection resembles clostridial gas gangrene; however, there is a slightly longer incubation period and the characteristic pain of clostridial myonecrosis is not present. Gas formation is slight, but there is a large amount of seropurulent discharge, in direct contrast to the discharge found in clostridial myonecrosis. Toxemia is less at the outset, and marked pain and septicemia do not occur except as terminal events. Important differential features of anaerobic cellulitis, streptococcal myonecrosis, and clostridial myonecrosis are listed in Table 5-6.

DIAGNOSIS

Diagnosis of clostridial myonecrosis can be made by its clinical features. The most important are se-

Table 5-6. Histotoxic Infections—Differential Diagnosis

Features	Anaerobic Cellulitis	Streptococcal Myonecrosis	Clostridial Myonecrosis
Incubation	>3 days	3 to 4 days	<3 days
Onset	Gradual	Subacute	Acute
Toxemia	Slight	Severe (late)	Severe
Pain	Absent	Variable	Severe
Swelling	Slight	Severe	Severe
Skin	Little change	Tense, copper colored	Tense, white
Exudate	Slight	Seropurulent	Serous, hemorrhagic
Gas	Abundant	Slight	Rarely abundant
Smell	Foul	Slight	Variable, "mousy"
Muscle	No change	Moderate	Severe

(DeHaven, K.E., and Evarts, C.M.: The Continuing Problem of Gas Gangrene: A Review and Report of Illustrative Cases. J. Trauma, 11:983–991, 1971.)

vere local pain and swelling associated with extensive tissue destruction and marked systemic toxemia. Gas formation is not a pathognomonic feature and in some instances may be scant.[466] Occasionally, jaundice, hemoglobinemia, and hemoglobinuria occur. Other differential features are listed in Table 5-6. Detection of gas may be obscured by the massive edema. Modern-day trauma can produce infections by other types of gas-forming organisms.

The radiographic interpretation of gas in the tissues is not specific for clostridial myonecrosis. Obviously, it can detect the presence of gas in the tissues, but it cannot identify the specific organism.[486]

The bacteriologic demonstration of pathogenic clostridia in infected tissues is also of limited significance, because the organisms, as previously mentioned, are commensal and widespread.[481] Type-specific identification takes a relatively long period—too long for lifesaving treatment to be delayed. However, a Gram stain of the exudate should be made. The common identifying features are listed in Table 5-7.

PROPHYLAXIS

The initial measure of prophylaxis is to recognize the predisposing causes of clostridial myonecrosis. These include deep penetrating wounds of the buttock and thigh, tight plaster casts, and loss of blood supply. The greatest problem in prophylaxis is delay of effective treatment. The fact that clostridial infections are caused not by uniquely pathologic strains but rather by uniquely local circumstances requires re-emphasis. The most important prophylactic step is early surgical treatment, which consists of meticulous and complete removal of any necrotic tissue.[508] The nonviable muscle must be removed; tight packing should be avoided, as should immediate primary suture if any possibility of clostridial infection remains. The prophylactic use of antibiotics for prevention of postoperative gas gangrene has been suggested in those patients thought to be at high risk for developing this complication.[494] Penicillin is the antibiotic of choice. However, there is no evidence that penicillin alone will prevent the

onset of clostridial myonecrosis in humans without proper surgical débridement and cleansing.

Although immunologic prophylaxis would be most desirable, no consistently effective preparation has been found for active immunization against *C. perfringens.* The use of antitoxin for passive immunization has largely been abandoned.[509]

TREATMENT

The success of the treatment of gas gangrene depends on early diagnosis and prompt surgical decompression and débridement. Surgery remains the cornerstone of treatment of clostridial myonecrosis.[472,484] Multiple incisions and fasciotomy for decompression and drainage of the fascial compartments, excision of the involved muscles, and open amputation constitute appropriate operative management.[490] Arrest of the infection can be accomplished without amputation if the diagnosis has been made early in the course of the disease.

Resuscitation must include careful scrutiny of fluid, blood, and electrolyte requirements; prompt replacement is mandatory. Fluid loss is marked, more so than with third-degree burns. Central venous pressure monitoring and urinary output measurements aid fluid replacement therapy.

Large intravenous dosages of penicillin, 3 million units every three hours, should be administered. In most patients who are allergic to penicillin, a cephalosporin or clindamycin would be effective treatment.[499] A second antibiotic, such as an aminoglycoside, is often given because of the common presence of organisms other than clostridial species.[482] Vigorous antibiotic therapy is an important adjunct to operative treatment.

A promising adjunct in the treatment of clostridial myonecrosis is the use of hyperbaric oxygen. In 1961 Boerema[467] developed a hyperbaric chamber and subsequently treated two patients with advanced gas gangrene, who recovered dramatically. Then, Brummelkamp and coworkers[470] reported its use in gas gangrene. The mechanism underlying the action of oxygen at high pressure appears complex. Experimental studies in vitro have demon-

Table 5-7. Analysis of Gram Stain of Exudate From Histotoxic Infections

Features	Anaerobic Cellulitis	Streptococcal Myonecrosis	Clostridial Myonecrosis
Leukocytes	Present	Present	±
Gram-positive rods	Present	Absent	Present
Flora	Varied	*Streptococcus*	Varied

strated both bacteriostatic and bactericidal effects of high oxygen tension on *C. perfringens*. Inhibition of toxin production and improvement of tissue oxygenation may also play a role.[464] Three atmospheric pressures are recommended for obtaining arterial oxygen tensions from 1,200 to 1,700 mm Hg. The patient should be placed in a hyperbaric chamber for 60 to 90 minutes every 8 to 12 hours as necessary. Usually four to six exposures result in maximum effect. There are distinct hazards in the use of hyperbaric oxygen therapy, including barotrauma, decompression sickness, convulsions, otitis media, claustrophobia, and oxygen poisoning.[502] Lung damage has been reported in animals. If a large hyperbaric oxygen chamber is available, the surgical treatment can be performed during the initial hyperbaric oxygen exposure. Few such chambers are available in the United States, and for most hospitals the cost of such a large chamber is prohibitive. Vital time may be lost transferring patients to facilities with hyperbaric oxygen.

Several reports have illustrated the efficacy of hyperbaric oxygenation in the treatment of clostridial myonecrosis.[476,482,483,498,501,505] It has been instrumental in arresting the progress of the clostridial infection and allows amputation at the most distal possible level. In patients with fulminating clostridial myonecrosis and those in whom ablative surgery is not feasible, the use of hyperbaric oxygen may be lifesaving.

The treatment regimen consists of four phases beginning immediately after the clinical diagnosis is made: (1) fluid and electrolyte replacement, (2) antibiotic administration, (3) meticulous surgical débridement and decompression, and (4) hyperbaric oxygenation. This regimen has resulted in a striking reduction of morbidity and mortality.

Illustrative Case[472]

A 10-year-old girl fell while horseback riding and sustained open fractures of both bones of her right forearm. Initial treatment consisted of blind surgical pinning of the ulna, primary suture of the open wound of the forearm, reduction, application of a long-arm cast, and administration of ampicillin and chloramphenicol.

Twenty-four hours after the injury the patient began to have severe pain in the forearm, followed by swelling of the hand and low-grade fever. Splitting the cast gave no relief, and the cast was removed. The forearm wound was foul and discolored, and a hemorrhagic exudate was present. Smear of the exudate showed gram-positive rods. The patient was given a large dose of penicillin and was transferred to a tertiary care facility.

On admission to the hospital, 90 hours after injury, she was in a toxic condition with a temperature of 40.6°C and tachycardia of 140. She was fearful of dying. Her right hand was white, swollen, anesthetic, and paralytic. The forearm wound was foul and necrotic, with a thin hemorrhagic exudate and bubbling gas. Smear of the exudate again revealed gram-positive rods, and cultures subsequently grew *C. perfringens*.

Treatment consisted of immediate débridement and decompression. There was extensive necrosis affecting all muscles of the volar aspect of the forearm, with associated thrombosis of major vessels, and there were pockets of gas within the muscle substance up to the level of the antecubital fossa. The wound was packed open, and the patient was placed in the hyperbaric oxygen chamber. In addition, she was given penicillin and polyvalent antitoxin intravenously. Three treatments with hyperbaric oxygen were administered.

Within six hours the patient's temperature was essentially normal and the toxemia cleared. It was subsequently necessary to perform an amputation below the elbow, after which she made an uneventful recovery.

The history of falling off a horse is significant and must not be disregarded; barnyard contamination is a real threat. Internal fixation of a forearm fracture in a 10-year-old child is not indicated in the presence of an open wound that is grossly contaminated from a barnyard accident. Débridement and drainage of the wound were inadequate, and primary suturing of such a wound is ill advised. Delayed primary suture or healing by secondary intention is safer and provides a satisfactory cosmetic result. A circular cast should be used during the first 48 to 72 hours only if necessary and should be immediately bivalved to allow for swelling. There was only a slight delay in recognition of the development of gas gangrene, but there was a significant delay in definitive treatment because of geographic separation from a hyperbaric oxygen treatment facility.

In conclusion, the incidence of anaerobic infections ranging from simple contamination to massive necrotizing muscle involvement is significant and may be increasing. The orthopaedic surgeon must be familiar with the diagnosis and management of the infections caused by the histotoxic anaerobic bacteria.

TETANUS

Tetanus is a potentially fatal disease but, unlike gas gangrene, a preventable one by appropriate immunization. It is a severe, infectious complication of wounds, especially lacerations, abrasions, or open fractures. In contrast to clostridial myonecrosis, which occurs in the patient with a neglected deep wound, tetanus may occur in the patient with a superficial wound or in the patient with no demonstrable wound.[534] Tetanus toxin must be produced by *C. tetani* organisms for tetanus to occur. In contrast to clostridial myonecrosis, tetanus immunization is available and effective, and complete primary immunization with tetanus toxoid provides a long-lasting protective antitoxin level.

Accurate descriptions of tetanus (lockjaw) are found in the works of Hippocrates[528] and Aretaeus.[511] In 1884, Carle and Rattone[514] produced the disease in rabbits. In 1889, Kitasato[533] obtained a pure culture of *C. tetani* and in 1890 described the toxins produced by this organism. The concept and use of tetanus toxoid for active immunization were presented by Ramon and Zoeller[545] in 1927. By 1946, tetanus immune globulin (human) was available from fractionated plasma. In 1966, 250 units of tetanus immune globulin (human)[535,538] was established as the routine prophylactic dose for passive immunization.

BACTERIOLOGY

C. tetani organisms and spores are found widespread in fecal matter of both domestic animals and humans. Soil fertilized with manure contains these anaerobes, whose function is to convert organic waste material into fertile soil. *C. tetani* are resistant and may be dormant for years, sealed in scar tissue. With subsequent injury, infection may occur. In direct distinction to *C. perfringens,* the tetanus organism is noninvasive and tends to remain localized. *C. tetani* is a large, gram-positive, motile bacillus, strictly anaerobic.[556] Spores cannot germinate in the presence of small amounts of oxygen.[547] *C. tetani* produces two exotoxins: tetanolysin and tetanospasmin.[559] Tetanolysin, a hemolysin, may contribute to the manifestations of clinical tetanus.[526] Tetanospasmin, a neurotoxin, is extremely toxic, and a very small amount can be lethal. Spores are resistant, and one to four hours of boiling is necessary to kill the organism. Autoclaving for about ten minutes at 120°C provides satisfactory sterilization.

The skin of humans, especially outdoor workers, is frequently contaminated, and any wound, however small, can carry *C. tetani* deep into the tissues. Three factors favor progression of the infection: deep wounds without exposure to air, wounds containing ischemic tissues, and wounds infected with other organisms. Once *C. tetani* begin to grow, the exotoxin tetanospasmin is produced and carried by way of the peripheral nerves to the central nervous system. In both the central and peripheral nervous tissues the toxin is bound with high affinity to the gangliosides.[532] The exact mechanism and site of action are not known, but experimental studies in the mouse demonstrate that tetanus toxin causes a presynaptic blockade of neuromuscular transmission and functional denervation of muscle.[518] Voluntary muscle is more sensitive to the toxin effects than involuntary smooth muscle.

Muscle spasm in humans is caused by hyperactivity of spinal motor neurons.[512] There is considerable evidence that tetanus toxin impairs cholinergic transmission in both the voluntary and autonomic nervous systems.[527,531,540,554] Morphologically, no tissue damage is done by the tetanus toxin; however, a critical feature of tetanus infection is the inability of the antitoxin to neutralize tissue-bound toxin.

INCIDENCE

Tetanus has been a major problem during wars. Despite the availability and widespread use of a highly effective toxoid vaccine, tetanus continues to be a serious health problem in the United States.[519] After continuously decreasing from 1955 through 1976, the number of reported cases of tetanus has remained stable (Fig. 5-11), a situation most likely related to inadequate vaccination levels in a portion of the population.[515] Figure 5-12 shows that people over age 60 have the highest incidence of tetanus, which again may result from inadequate vaccination coverage.[515,546] The incidence is highest in the lower Mississippi Valley and the Southeast. Recently, the case-to-fatality ratio has remained at about 60%. The hands and feet are the most common sites of injury, and injuries occurring at home accounted for more than 70% of all cases of tetanus infection.[534] The mean incubation period is about 1 week, and in one series of studies, 88% of the cases began within 14 days of injury. The length of the incubation period has been considered an indication of the prognosis with tetanus—a short period indicating a poor prognosis.[551] Tetanus involves all age groups but is more serious and often fatal in the neonate and the aged.

CLINICAL FINDINGS

Glenn[523] stated, "In my clinical experience I have never seen such a terrifying disease as tetanus." Tetanus may appear either locally or in a general

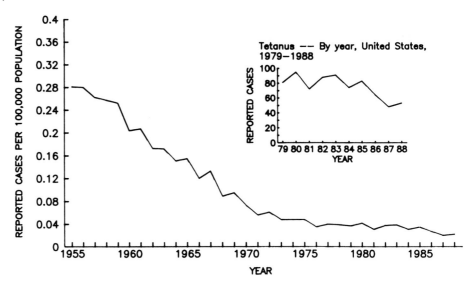

Fig. 5-11. Reported cases of tetanus in the United States from 1955 to 1988.[515]

form. Local spasm at the site of injury may be the first sign associated with this infection. The local form tends to be less serious.

The symptoms of generalized involvement are most commonly trismus, risus sardonicus, and difficulty in swallowing. The trismus is caused by muscle spasm, and the sustained contraction of the facial muscles produces a wry expression. Some patients have prodromal symptoms of restlessness and headaches. If the pharyngeal muscles are in spasm, swallowing is difficult. Opisthotonos is common,

especially in patients with severe tetanus. Other muscle groups become progressively involved, and muscle hyperirritability occurs.[542] Frequent toxic convulsions are part of the picture of *C. tetani* infection and are produced by minimal stimuli.[522] Death from tetanus infection may occur from the asphyxia associated with unremitting spasm of the laryngeal and respiratory muscles. During the disease the patient remains mentally clear. There is an associated tachycardia and often marked perspiration from hyperparasympathetic activity. The

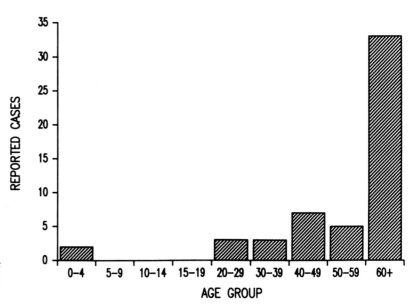

Fig. 5-12. Reported case rates of tetanus by age group in the United States in 1988.[515]

deep tendon reflexes are hyperactive, but no sensory changes are observed in tetanus. Death usually occurs within 2 weeks of the onset of the *C. tetani* infection. The mortality, although difficult to determine, is about 60%.

Diagnosis of *C. tetani* infection must be made from its clinical features. In one series of 160 cases, only 32% of the cultures were positive for *C. tetani*.[534] This finding is related to the very specific anaerobic growth requirements of *C. tetani*. Occasionally, bacterial overgrowth is thought to decrease the chance of recovery of the organism. Despite the lack of bacteriologic confirmation, the dramatic and characteristic symptoms and signs of tetanus in the presence of a wound or site of infection make possible the diagnosis. Other common laboratory studies are nonspecific in establishing the diagnosis of tetanus.

PROPHYLAXIS

Satisfactory active immunization exists for tetanus, and therefore the disease can be prevented. Progress has been made internationally to develop a standard tetanus toxoid.[529] Tetanus toxoid has been administered by intramuscular or subcutaneous injection. The experience in World War II demonstrates the efficacy of tetanus toxoid as a prophylactic agent.[536] Once the toxoid is administered, the immune reactions are sensitized so that subsequent doses of tetanus toxoid booster result in the production of circulating serum tetanus antitoxin. Allergic reactions to tetanus toxoid are unusual; when they occur, they are most often manifest as local edema and tenderness.[530,557] Hypersensitivity reactions to tetanus immune globulin (human) are rare.[520]

Tetanus toxoid is highly effective, and its administration results in excellent protection. The National Health Service Immunization Practices Advisory Committee has suggested that primary immunization with DTP—diptheria, tetanus toxoid, and pertussis vaccine—should be given to children 6 weeks to 6 years old. It should be given intramuscularly four times: three doses at 6-week intervals and a fourth dose 1 year after the first injection. For schoolchildren, a single DTP injection is recommended. Following the initial immunization, it is recommended that one dose of adult tetanus-diptheria toxoid be given every 10 years provided wound management is not required.[546]

The success of the prophylaxis of tetanus depends on early recognition and prompt surgical wound management. All wounds must be meticulously débrided and cleansed. The tissue care should be gentle, and wounds should not be closed primarily if there are questions about anaerobic conditions deep within the wound.

The Committee on Trauma of the American College of Surgeons has published a guide to prophylaxis.[510]

PROPHYLAXIS AGAINST TETANUS IN WOUND MANAGEMENT

General Principles

I. The attending physician must determine for each patient with a wound, individually, what is required for adequate prophylaxis against tetanus.

II. Regardless of the active immunization status of the patient, meticulous surgical care, including removal of all devitalized tissue and foreign bodies, should be provided immediately for all wounds. Such care is essential as part of the prophylaxis against tetanus.

III. Each patient with a wound should receive adsorbed tetanus toxoid* intramuscularly at the time of injury, either as an initial immunizing dose, or as a booster for previous immunization, unless he has received a booster or has completed his initial immunization series within the past five (5) years. As the antigen concentration varies in different products, specific information on the volume of a single dose is provided on the label of the package.

IV. Whether or not to provide passive immunization with tetanus immune globulin (human) must be decided individually for each patient. The characteristics of the wound, conditions under which it was incurred, its treatment, its age, and the previous active immunization status of the patient must be considered.

V. To every wounded patient, give a written record of the immunization provided, instructing him to carry the record at all times, and, if indicated, to complete active immunization. For precise tetanus prophylaxis, an accurate and immediately available history regarding previous active immunization against tetanus is required.

VI. Basic immunization with adsorbed tetanus toxoid requires three injections. A booster of adsorbed tetanus toxoid is indicated 10 years after the third injection or 10† years after an intervening wound booster. All individuals, including pregnant women, should have basic immunization and indicated booster injections.

Specific Measures for Patients With Wounds

I. Previously immunized individuals.

A. When the patient has been actively immunized within the past 10† years:

1. To the great majority, give 0.5 mL of adsorbed tetanus toxoid* as a booster unless it is certain that the patient has received a booster within the previous 5 years.

2. To those with severe, neglected, or old (more than 24 hours) tetanus-prone wounds, give 0.5 mL of adsorbed tetanus toxoid,* unless it is certain that the patient has received a booster within the previous year.

B. When the patient has been actively immunized more than 10† years previously:
   1. To the great majority, give 0.5 mL of adsorbed tetanus toxoid.*
   2. To those with severe, neglected, or old (more than 24 hours) tetanus-prone wounds:
      a. Give 0.5 mL of adsorbed tetanus toxoid.*‡
      b. Give 250 units of tetanus immune globulin (human).‡
      c. Consider providing oxytetracycline or penicillin.

II. Individuals not previously immunized.
   A. With clean minor wounds in which tetanus is most unlikely, give 0.5 mL of adsorbed tetanus toxoid* (initial immunizing dose).
   B. With all other wounds:
      1. Give 0.5 mL of adsorbed tetanus toxoid* (initial immunizing dose).‡
      2. Give 250 units§ of tetanus immune globulin (human).‡
      3. Consider providing oxytetracycline or penicillin

Precautions Regarding Passive Immunization With Tetanus Antitoxin (Equine)

If the patient is not sensitive to tetanus antitoxin (equine), and if the decision is made to administer it for passive immunization, give at least 3000 units.

Do not administer tetanus antitoxin (equine) except when tetanus immune globulin (human) is not available within 24 hours, and only if the possibility of tetanus outweighs the danger of reaction to heterologous tetanus antitoxin.

Before using tetanus antitoxin (equine), question the patient for a history of allergy and test for sensitivity. If the patient is sensitive to tetanus antitoxin (equine), do not use it, as the danger of anaphylaxis probably outweighs the danger of tetanus; rely on penicillin or oxytetracycline. Do not attempt desensitization, as it is not worthwhile.

---

* In 1981, the Public Health Service Immunization Practices Advisory Committee recommended DTP for basic immunization in infants and children from 6 weeks through the sixth year of age, and Td (combined tetanus and diphtheria toxoids: adult type) for basic immunization of those over 6 years of age. For the later group, Td toxoid was recommended for routine or wound boosters; but if there is any reason to suspect hypersensitivity to the diphtheria component, tetanus toxoid (T) should be substituted for Td.

† Some authorities advise 6 rather than 10 years, particularly for patients with severe, neglected, or old (more than 24 hours) tetanus-prone wounds.

‡ Use different syringes, needles, and sites of injection.

§ In severe, neglected, or old (more than 24 hours) tetanus-prone wounds, 500 units of tetanus immune globulin (human) are advisable.

There is no proof that the administration of antibiotics is effective in the prophylaxis of tetanus; antibiotics are known to have no effect against the toxin produced.[542] Antibiotics, especially penicillin and tetracycline, given immediately after injury may have a deterrent action against *C. tetani* infection by influencing the organisms that have not been removed surgically.[522] However, antibiotics cannot be used as a substitute for active or passive immunization.

TREATMENT

The treatment of tetanus involves both general supportive therapy and the specifics of wound care, passive immunization, sedation, and pulmonary ventilation.[513,516,517,520,521,525,544,552,553]

Patients with marked hyperirritability should be kept in a quiet, dark room, avoiding as many external stimuli as possible. Intensive nursing care should be provided. Proper fluid and electrolyte balance must be maintained.

A combination of penicillin, 2 million units intravenously every 6 hours, and streptomycin, 0.5 g intramuscularly every 12 hours, helps to decrease secondary invasive wound infections. The use of intrathecal injections of tetanus immune globulin has shown some promise.[524]

The management of the wound is important. If the tissues have been crushed, all devitalized tissue should be completely removed, and every attempt must be made to convert the wound from dirty to clean in every sense of the word.

Tetanus immune globulin (human) should be given early in doses of 500 to 1,000 units until a total dosage of 6,000 to 10,000 units is received.[537,539,543] Sedation is one of the keystones in the management of tetanus. Mild cases can be treated with phenobarbital, secobarbital, or paraldehyde.[551] In more severe cases thiopental sodium should be given by intravenous drip to quiet the patient and to lessen the number of convulsive attacks. The administration of muscle relaxants (D-tubocurarine and succinylcholine) should be supervised by an anesthesiologist, because improper administration may result in respiratory arrest.[555,558]

Maintaining an open airway and avoiding the complications associated with tracheostomy are a challenge for the surgeon. Proper emphasis on the prevention of respiratory problems is a recent advance in the management of tetanus.[548,550] Smythe presented a series of infants in whom the mortality was decreased to less than 20%. The good results were thought to be from the proper use of tracheostomy and intubation in the infant, the control of intermittent positive-pressure ventilation monitoring the CO_2 and the improvement in control of infection after instillation of penicillin and colistin into the tracheostomy tube.[549]

If pharyngospasm or laryngospasm develops in a patient, tracheostomy should be performed promptly and assisted mechanical ventilation instituted. Careful, continuous observation and monitoring of blood gases are vital in the management and treatment of respiratory infections.

Other measures, such as hyperbaric oxygen, have been tried in the treatment of tetanus, but these have not been helpful in preventing the toxemic state of an acute *C. tetani* infection.[541,542]

In summary, although the incidence of tetanus has decreased in the United States, it is a major potential problem for the orthopaedic surgeon dealing with traumatic wounds. Advances in the past century have made tetanus a preventable disease. It is the physician's responsibility to be aware of the prophylaxis and management of infections of all degrees caused by *C. tetani.*

OSTEOMYELITIS

There remains a significant failure rate in the treatment of bone infections despite advances in antibiotic therapy; thus osteomyelitis remains a great challenge to the orthopaedic surgeon. Continued interest and research have led to a better understanding of its etiology, pathogenesis, diagnosis, and treatment. A change in the character of osteomyelitis was suggested by Waldvogel and associates[658] in a comprehensive review in 1971. The majority of 248 cases reviewed were diagnosed as nonhematogenous osteomyelitis and occurred in an older age group, in contrast to a minority of cases of acute hematogenous osteomyelitis. The increase in injury to bone secondary to vehicular accident trauma, with subsequent infection, and the increase in major reconstructive orthopaedic surgical procedures have contributed to a definite rise in the incidence of nonhematogenous osteomyelitis.[571] Concurrently, the widespread use of antibiotics in the treatment of acute infections of bone has dramatically reduced the mortality from acute hematogenous osteomyelitis.[581,596,601,608] The most effective treatment of osteomyelitis remains its prevention, by meticulous wound care and débridement following open fractures.

Therefore, the orthopaedic surgeon is confronted not only with an increase in nonhematogenous osteomyelitis, but also with a different spectrum of bacterial organisms causing bone infection.[603,637,646] There are fewer staphylococcal infections and more gram-negative and mixed infections. The bacteriologic identification of the infecting organism(s) is vital to the selection of the appropriate antibiotic. The techniques of obtaining material for culture,

both soft tissue and bone, are even more important to the orthopaedic surgeon. He or she must face the complex management of open fractures, as well as the control of operating room environment and the possible selection and use of prophylactic antibiotics.[569,570,574,598]

CLASSIFICATION

Simply stated, bacterial osteomyelitis is a suppurative process in bone caused by a pyogenic organism. During the course of osteomyelitis, inflammation of the osteocytes and osteoblasts, their neurovascular components, and supportive connective tissue occurs within the confines of a mineral matrix. Bone matrix is destroyed by proteolytic enzymes, decalcified by hyperemia, and resorbed by osteoclasts.[563] Initially, osteomyelitis was classified as acute or chronic, according to the duration and severity of the infection. Clinically, the distinction between acute and chronic osteomyelitis can be difficult. Patients with acute osteomyelitis may have indolent, subclinical, chronic bone infection, whereas patients with chronic bone infections often experience acute exacerbations.

A classification modified from that of Waldvogel and associates[658] separates osteomyelitis into three groups on the basis of the pathogenesis of the lesion: (1) hematogenous osteomyelitis, (2) osteomyelitis secondary to a contiguous focus of infection, and (3) osteomyelitis from direct inoculation of bacteria at the time of injury or surgery.

INCIDENCE

Before the introduction of penicillin, osteomyelitis carried a high morbidity and mortality. The so-called golden era of antibiotics lasted from about 1944 to 1950. Penicillin was introduced during World War II, and the results were spectacular. During this period, penicillin-sensitive *Staphylococcus* and *Streptococcus* were the causative organisms in more than 90% of cases.[562] However, since 1951, penicillin-resistant staphylococcal infections have become more prevalent.[601,641] Acquired resistance has become a more common problem associated with antibiotic therapy. New types or modifications of organisms develop by mutation and subsequently prosper according to the law of survival of the fittest. Certain chemotherapeutic agents permit sufficient growth of the resistant organism to allow the development of a resistant strain. The exact mechanism likely involves genetic alteration. Ill-advised, subtherapeutic doses of chemotherapeutic agents contribute to the development of resistant pathogens. The result is that the orthopaedic surgeon continues to encounter an increase in penicillin-resistant staphylococcal infections. Fewer cases of hematogenous osteomyelitis have been reported, but more cases of septicemia in acute hematogenous osteomyelitis with multiple foci of involvement have been observed.[592,630] Osteomyelitis secondary to open fractures or major orthopaedic reconstructive procedures occurs more frequently. Overall, the mortality from osteomyelitis has decreased from 20% to 25% before the chemotherapeutic era to approximately 2% at present.[588,604,659]

PATHOPHYSIOLOGY

Hematogenous Osteomyelitis

Acute bone infection is a complex process that depends on many factors. The presence of bacteria alone within bone is not sufficient to cause infection. The bacteria must be localized, and the environment must support bacterial growth. The localization of acute hematogenous osteomyelitis has been outlined according to age by Kahn and Pritzker[616] (Table 5-8). In childhood the infectious process usually is localized in the metaphyseal portion of the long bones.[639] Hobo[613] studied the vascularity adjacent to the metaphyseal side of the growth plate and demonstrated that branches of the nutrient arteries in the metaphysis have straight, narrow capillaries, which in turn twist sharply back on themselves at the growth plate and terminate in veins with a much wider caliber than the capillaries. Trueta[656] believed that a decrease in blood flow occurred at the junction between the capillary side of the circulation and the larger-caliber veins on the venous side. He postulated that a relative stasis would increase the susceptibility to osteomyelitis. Other factors determining the selection of the lower extremity for hematogenous osteomyelitis may involve the mechanical stresses and subsequent injury that occur at the epiphyseal plates in the growing child.[639,645,651] Metaphyseal hemorrhage and necrosis might occur, thereby providing a suitable environment for bacterial growth. A defective phagocytic mechanism may exist in the metaphyseal region as compared with the diaphyseal areas.[613] Also, rapid metaphyseal growth may provide a fertile area for the development of osteomyelitis. Once a focus of infection in bone is established, the initial response is that of increased vascularity, leukocyte infiltration, and edema of the surrounding tissues. The suppurative process develops within a rigid-walled structure, and the resultant accumulation of pus exerts significant pressure on the surrounding tissues. The bacterial organisms liberate exotoxins, causing cell death and necrosis; these necrotic tissues serve in turn as a culture medium.[592,622] The infection may spread from the metaphysis along the path of least resistance into either the medullary canal or the subperiosteal space.[611] The nutrient artery supplying the inner two thirds of the cortex is compromised by the advancing infection. As the suppurative process spreads subperiosteally, the blood supply to the outer one third of the cortex is destroyed. It can thus be appreciated that untreated acute hematogenous osteomyelitis may extend to involve the entire bone. Furthermore, if the anatomic location of the metaphysis is intracapsular, the infection can rapidly become intra-articular (eg, the proximal femur).[595,616,639]

Nonhematogenous Osteomyelitis

As previously defined, nonhematogenous osteomyelitis is osteomyelitis secondary to a contiguous

Table 5-8. Characteristics of Hematogenous Osteomyelitis at Various Ages

Characteristics	Infancy (<1 yr)	Childhood (1 to 16 yr)	Adult (>16 yr)
Localization	Metaphysis	Metaphysis	Subchondral
Multiple foci	Frequent	Rare	—
Common organism	*Streptococcus* or *Staphylococcus*	*Staphylococcus*	Varied (*Staphylococcus*)
Spread	Joint space	Subperiosteal	Diaphysis
	Epiphysis	Diaphysis	Extraperiosteal
	Subperiosteal		Joint space
	Parosteal		
	Diaphysis		
Fistula	Rare	Frequent	Frequent
Periosteal involucrum formation	Marked	Moderate	Weak

(Kahn, D.S., and Pritzker, P.H.: The Pathophysiology of Bone Infection. Clin. Orthop., 96:12–19, 1973.)

focus of infection.[658] The pathophysiology of this type of osteomyelitis is different from that of acute hematogenous osteomyelitis. The bacterial organisms enter the bone directly through interrupted tissue planes as a result of fracture or surgical procedures.[610,652] Initially, the bacterial organisms in these adjacent deep structures elicit no response. However, the original injury causes hematoma formation that, during the period of contamination, serves as a fertile culture medium. As the bacterial organisms multiply and the inflammatory response is evoked, the bacterial organisms often extend through the hematoma and along the vascular planes to contact the bony surfaces. The amount of soft tissue damage, the extent of periosteal tearing and destruction, the amount of actual bone loss, and the degree of displacement of the fracture fragments all adversely influence the blood supply to the involved bone.[601,638] Internal fixation devices also change the blood supply. It is generally accepted that the external fixator provides optimal treatment of the injured soft tissues surrounding the open fracture while contributing least to further devascularization of bone during application of the device. However, a growing body of data warns against the delayed, or even late, conversion of an external fixator to a reamed intramedullary device owing to the extremely high rate of bone sepsis— especially if pin tract drainage existed prior to fixator removal.[628] In nonhematogenous osteomyelitis, the suppurative process is more confined than in acute hematogenous osteomyelitis. Less pressure develops, and consequently the process is less likely to spread through the intramedullary canal or along the subperiosteal space. A common finding is a chronic draining wound with sinus formation. The presence of foreign materials—metal, plastic, or bone cement—contributes to the nature, extent, and persistence of nonhematogenous osteomyelitis.

CLINICAL FINDINGS AND DIAGNOSIS

Signs and Symptoms

If a patient has severe pain, bone tenderness, high fever, headache, and vomiting, the diagnosis of this classic form of acute hematogenous osteomyelitis is not difficult.[601] However, this is a clinical picture not frequently observed. Often patients have vague symptoms and signs with an insidious onset.[608] Slight fever, few constitutional symptoms, and minimal complaints of pain may be present. A history of upper respiratory tract infection or mild trauma may be elicited. If a high index of suspicion

is not maintained, further examination of the musculoskeletal system will not be performed, and the diagnosis of osteomyelitis will be missed. Inappropriate use of antibiotics often obscures the clinical signs and symptoms, and the usual course of events associated with osteomyelitis is altered.

The clinical characteristics of osteomyelitis secondary to a direct infection occurring with an open fracture or a reconstructive orthopaedic procedure are somewhat different. The symptoms and signs are not those of severe sepsis. The patient may complain of pain or have a low-grade fever. The wound usually becomes edematous and erythematous and drains in most cases. The diagnosis is often obscure. Any attempt at aspiration of the involved area should be performed under sterile precautions and fluoroscopic control. If an early diagnosis of nonhematogenous osteomyelitis can be established, débridement can be initiated in conjunction with specific antibiotic therapy. Should a coexistent fracture nonunion be present, rigid immobilization must be achieved by any one of a number of available techniques.

The history and physical examination remain the keystones in diagnosis of osteomyelitis. They should at least raise the suspicion of an inflammatory process and instigate an effort to locate the site of infection and determine the offending organism. Early identification is of utmost importance, for early treatment (within 72 hours) drastically reduces the incidence of subsequent chronic osteomyelitis and osseous destruction.[659]

Laboratory Examination

Routine laboratory investigations are of only modest help in the diagnosis of acute osteomyelitis. Markedly elevated body temperature and white cell count are no longer common. Rather, some degree of leukocytosis, with a shift to the left, and mild anemia are often present. The serum calcium, phosphate, and alkaline phosphatase levels are usually normal. The erythrocyte sedimentation rate is usually elevated but is a nonspecific finding. It may be helpful in assessing activity during treatment; however, it has been shown to remain elevated for some time even at the end of a course of adequate treatment when the adjacent joint has been involved.[587] Antibodies to teichoic acid, a component of the cell wall of *Staphylococcus aureus*, are present in high titers in nearly all patients with endocarditis. They are present in low titers in some patients with staphylococcal osteomyelitis. Their determination may be helpful in equivocal cases.[657]

X-Rays

Diagnostic radiography is not effective in the early management of osteomyelitis.[572] The bone changes seen on x-ray films are delayed, first appearing 10 to 21 days after the onset of symptoms.[627] Soft tissue swelling with a loss of well-defined muscle planes and a diffuse haziness are usually the first radiographic signs. The earliest bone changes are hyperemia and demineralization. Actual changes in bone structure, such as lysis, are not visible on x-ray films until 40% of the bone substance has been destroyed. It is not common to observe massive periosteal reactive bone, although periosteal elevation appears simultaneously with the loss of bone. Bone sclerosis is a late radiographic sign and indicates chronicity of the osteomyelitis.[620] Antibiotic therapy given for the various forms of osteomyelitis has changed the radiographic features: the onset of bone changes is delayed, bone destruction is less, and multiple lytic defects are rare. The most common radiographic sign of early bone infection is rarefaction, representing diffuse demineralization secondary to inflammatory hyperemia.

Bone Scan

Difficulty in interpreting routine x-ray films or tomograms during the initial phase has been partly solved by improvements in radionuclide imaging. Technetium phosphate complexes reflect increased blood flow and metabolism, with the complex being adsorbed onto the hydroxyapatite crystals.[626] This is associated with a focal area of increased uptake, presenting as a hot spot on the bone scan. However, it is nonspecific and cannot differentiate infection, for example, from neoplasm or trauma.[626] The incidence of false-positive and false-negative results is also significant.[615,653] Use of the three-phase scan technique, consisting of a radionuclide angiogram, an immediate postinjection blood pool image, and a delayed (two- to three-hour) image, has improved the specificity, especially in distinguishing osteomyelitis from septic arthritis,[632] cellulitis, and bone infarction. The increased concentration of radioactive gallium (^{67}Ga) citrate at the site of inflammation is believed to be caused by exudation of in vivo labeled serum protein (transferrin, haptoglobulin, and albumin) and the accumulation of in vivo granulocytes, primarily neutrophils.[626] Thus the two agents may complement each other, and sequential ^{99m}Tc and ^{67}Ga imaging has been shown to yield more information than either test alone.[623] The primary usefulness of ^{67}Ga in acute cases is to confirm the presence of cellulitis and determine whether it is complicated by osteomyelitis. In one study,[658] although both agents gave positive results in acute osteomyelitis or septic arthritis, acute cellulitis was more clearly defined by ^{67}Ga than by ^{99m}Tc blood pool images. Inactive osteomyelitis was characterized by normal ^{67}Ga and abnormal ^{99m}Tc images. More recently, the indium-labeled white cell scan has offered potential for greater specificity in the detection of bone infection.[635,663] However, variability of the labeled white cell pool can result in a low percentage of tagged acute phase polymorphonuclear leukocytes and false-negative results in cases of clinically known osteomyelitis secondary to fracture.

Aspiration and Biopsy

Radionuclide imaging is clearly not indicated in every case of osteomyelitis. Its greatest usefulness is probably in suspected deep-seated bone or joint infection.[633] It is most valuable in ruling out multiple foci of involvement. Identification of the offending organism is crucial to a successful outcome in the management of osteomyelitis; the blood culture is positive in about 50% of untreated cases.[580,632] Although S. aureus (or, more rarely, S. epidermidis) is the offending organism in 60% to 90% of cases,[587,633] direct bone aspiration or surgical biopsy should strongly be considered in patients with negative cultures. In the presence of a draining sinus tract, Mackowiak and associates[631] have shown that the isolation of gram-negative organisms from the sinus tract bears no relation and isolation of S. aureus bears little relation to results from cultures obtained during surgery. Thus, bone biopsy and deep aspiration remain the preferred diagnostic procedures in chronic osteomyelitis.[587,633,638]

BACTERIOLOGY

The organism most frequently isolated from the bone of patients with hematogenous osteomyelitis is S. aureus.[648,661] The presence of this organism as a causative agent for osteomyelitis suggests an inordinate virulence in bone. Notwithstanding the recent increase in the incidence of nonhematogenous osteomyelitis in patients who are potentially exposed to many pathogens, S. aureus remains the most common infecting organism. Antimicrobial drugs have not eliminated staphylococci from recent bone infections.[597] However, drug treatment has resulted in a decrease in clinical recurrence of osteomyelitis with such organisms as Streptococcus and Pneumococcus. The staphylococcal organism is different; it is somehow able to survive within con-

Table 5-9. Bacteriological Findings in Osteomyelitis

Organism	No. of Patients
Staphylococcus aureus alone	65
S. aureus and other microorganisms	19
Proteus	5
Staphylococcus albus or *Staphylococcus epidermidis* with mixed gram-negative organisms	5
Pseudomonas	5
No growth	5
S. epidermidis	4
Aerobacter	3
Escherichia coli	2
Salmonella	2
Bacteroides	1
Beta streptococcus	1
Atypical mycobacterium	1

(Clawson, D.K., and Dunn, A.W.: Management of Common Bacterial Infections of Bones and Joints. J. Bone Joint Surg., 49A:165–182, 1967.)

taminated bone for many years.[579,650] The individual, specific features of the *Staphylococcus* providing for prolonged survival are unknown. However, the prevalence of *S. aureus* in osteomyelitis has decreased from 85% to 90% in previous reports to 60% in both hematogenous and nonhematogenous osteomyelitis.[648] More than one organism may cause nonhematogenous osteomyelitis, partly because of the exposure of a traumatic or surgical wound to an increased number of pathogens. The increased incidence of coagulase-negative staphylococcal infections as reported by culture has led some authors to suggest that this organism be considered pathogenic.[578,658] Cultures are reported as sterile or with "no growth" in several case studies. This may be the result of premature or incomplete antibiotic therapy or may reflect the difficulty in isolation of gram-negative bacteria or anaerobic

pathogens. The *S. aureus* organism has become penicillin-resistant in 60% to 70% of cases.[565] Bacteremic states caused by gram-negative bacilli have recently occurred with greater frequency.[561] However, there has not been a parallel increase in the occurrence of osteomyelitis from gram-negative bacilli. Table 5-9 lists the bacteriologic findings in 118 cases of hematogenous osteomyelitis.[577] Kelly and coworkers[619] have listed the organisms cultured from chronic osteomyelitis of the tibia and femur (Table 5-10).

TREATMENT

The successful management of patients with osteomyelitis depends on prompt, accurate clinical and microbiological diagnosis, followed by the institution of specific antibacterial therapy[602] and débridement where indicated. The orthopaedic surgeon must know whether or not the infecting pathogen will be inhibited or killed by the antibiotic selected for use. The degree of susceptibility of various organisms to antibacterial drugs can be determined in vitro in most cases.

The tube-dilution technique to determine the minimal inhibitory concentration and minimal bactericidal concentration is preferred to the disk-diffusion method for the following reasons[566,591,643,647]:

1. There may be great differences in the relative susceptibility of an organism to several drugs that might be considered equally effective on the basis of disk-diffusion results.
2. Tube-dilution studies allow selection of bactericidal over bacteriostatic drugs.
3. Some strains of *S. aureus* were inhibited but not

Table 5-10. Bacteriological Findings in Chronic Osteomyelitis of Tibia or Femur

Years	Staphylococcus aureus Alone		S. aureus and Gram-Negative Rods		Gram-Negative Rods Alone		Total*
	No. of Patients	%	No. of Patients	%	No. of Patients	%	
1967–70†	35	41	18	21	33	38	86
1963–66	52	84	3	5	7	11	62
1959–62	37	74	3	6	10	20	50
1955–58	47	83	3	5	7	12	57

* Two cultures of *Peptococcus* not included.

† *S. aureus* was the predominant organism in all but four during this period.

(Kelly, P.J.; Wilkowske, C.J.; and Washington, J.A., II: Comparison of Gram-negative Bacillary and Staphylococcal Osteomyelitis of the Femur and Tibia. Clin. Orthop., 96:70–75, 1973.)

killed by serum synthetic penicillinase-resistant penicillins, and these would be detected only by tube-dilution studies.[633]

In the treatment of bone and joint infections, a sufficient concentration of antibiotics must reach the actual site of infection.[594,617] The antibiotic must penetrate joint fluid, hematoma, and infected bone.[560,660] Antimicrobial levels can be achieved in joint fluid with penicillin and its analogues. Chloramphenicol and tetracycline also provide satisfactory levels in joint fluid. Controversy exists over the use of intra-articular antibiotic solutions. Because in most cases adequate antibacterial levels are maintained in joint fluids with intravenous administration, routine joint injections are not advised. However, the systemic toxicity of certain antibiotic agents (kanamycin, gentamicin) may be great enough to justify intra-articular injections in special circumstances. Curtis[583] urged surgical drainage of the infected joint to eliminate the purulent exudate as well as the fibrin clots. He questioned the use of joint irrigation with antibiotics.

A study of antibiotic levels in bone showed no significant difference between the antibiotic concentrations in cortical and cancellous bone.[644,654] Also, a constant intravenous infusion of antibiotics demonstrated that bone levels of antibiotics could be maintained as long as serum levels remained constant. Intravenous infusion was the best method of maintaining such serum levels. It was also demonstrated that satisfactory serum and bone antibiotic concentrations could be consistently achieved by the intravenous administration of an antibiotic (on a milligram per kilogram of body weight dosage schedule) 30 minutes before surgery, followed by a continuous intravenous infusion.

Bone and serum concentrations of various antibiotics after parenteral administration are shown in Table 5-11.

Several recent studies in children with acute osteomyelitis[621,655] have shown that results achieved with a short course of intravenous antibiotics followed by oral antibiotics for 6 weeks are as good as those achieved with prolonged intravenous therapy. However, these studies were done under conditions of closely monitored outpatient compliance, and the routine use of only oral antibiotics, especially on an uncontrolled outpatient basis, is not yet established for severe bone and joint infections.

It has been stated that all too often antibiotics are administered indiscriminately, routinely (rather than selectively), or hastily, with an unrealistic sense of urgency.[629] Estimates indicate that up to 50% of all drugs prescribed in the United States are antibiotics, that antibiotics are being prescribed without proper indication up to 90% of the time, and that 50% to 60% of patients receiving antibiotics in hospitals do not have infections.[573] Certain principles of antibacterial therapy have been outlined by McHenry.[629]

Principles of Antibacterial Therapy

1. Select the drug most likely to be effective with the least side effects.
2. Administer the drug by an appropriate route for sufficient time to eradicate or control infection.
3. Monitor the patient closely for a clinical and bacteriologic response and tolerance of the drug.
4. Modify the dosage when the circumstances indicate.
5. Discontinue the drug when infection is eradicated or controlled, when resistance emerges in vitro or in vivo, or when intolerable side effects develop.
6. Use adjunctive therapeutic measures, including incision and drainage or removal of foreign materials, whenever necessary.
7. Obtain follow-up studies, including the appropriate cultures, after therapy is terminated.

Recommended indications for and dosages of antibiotics are listed in Table 5-12.

Specific problems relate to the use of implant devices and biomaterials. Intra-articular infections and subsequent osteomyelitis are disastrous in the patient who has undergone reconstructive surgery of the hip, knee, or other joint in which bone cement for fixation was used. They are equally devastating in the patient who has undergone intramedullary fixation for a long bone fracture. A common cause of pain after use of an endoprosthesis is sepsis.[593] If detected early, infection usually manifests itself as continued pain in the joint, with characteristic wound changes accompanied by toxicity. The elderly patient may not have a significant rise in temperature or other signs of acute infection. It is necessary to aspirate the affected joint, culture the infecting organisms, and begin antibiotic therapy.[593] Usually removal of the implant devices along with meticulous débridement of involved tissues is necessary.

When a patient has sustained an open fracture, steps to prevent further contamination must be instituted. The ends of bone fragments protruding from a wound should be covered with a sterile dressing. Reduction should not be accomplished by allowing the contaminated fracture fragment to be placed into the depths of a wound without previous cleansing. The cleansing and débridement of a contaminated open fracture should be performed in the operating room. It is a laborious, time-consuming process, but when it is completed, all devitalized tissue should be removed from the wound. Once such débridement and cleansing are finished, attention can be turned to reduction and immobilization of the fracture. Occasionally, in selective instances, internal fixation devices are indicated under such circumstances.[625] The sequential application of an external fixator followed later by definitive treatment by intramedullary nailing of the tibia has been associated with an unacceptably high rate of deep sepsis and should be discouraged.[628] The use of suction-irrigation techniques frequently is indicated.[576,582,589,624] Patzakis and coworkers[642] have recommended the use of cephalothin in the management of open fractures caused by direct

Table 5-11. Concentrations of Various Antibiotics in Bone and Serum After Parenteral Administration

Antibiotic	Time After Administration (minutes)	Mean Serum Concentration (μg/mL)	Mean Bone Concentration (μg/g)	Comment
Penicillins				
Penicillin G				
2 million U IV	60 to 30	0.5 to 9.4	Undetectable	Three doses given before biopsy
Methicillin				
250 mg/kg IV	60 to 180	++	12.1	Human infected bone
1 g IV	60	17.1	3.1	
1 g IM				
Oxacillin				
1 g IV	60	18.9	2.1	
2 g IV	<50	86.1	7.66	
Dicloxacillin				
50 mg/kg IM	60 to 180	++	6.4	Human infected bone
Cephalosporins				
Cephalothin				
1 g IV	60	11.9	3.9	
25 mg/kg IV	<50	52.2	1.9	
40 mg/kg IM	$\approx$30	89 to 107	1.4	
Cefazolin				
50 mg/kg/IV	180	$\approx$10	$\approx$4	Human infected bone
1 g IV	50	$\approx$70	$\approx$15	
Cephradine				
1 g IV	50	$\approx$30	$\approx$15	
Lincomycin				
10 mg/kg SQ	60	3.8	0.5	Rabbit; increased concentration infected in bone
10 mg/kg IV	<50	24.2	3.7	
Clindamycin				
600 mg/8 h IM	120	8.51 ± 1.65	3.77 ± 1.6	Three doses given before biopsy
300 mg/6 h IV	240	6.5	1.3	Increased concentration by electrophoretic method
Aminoglycosides				
Gentamicin				
1.7 mg/kg/8 h IM	120–60	3.7 − 6.0	3.66	Three doses given before biopsy
5.0 mg/kg/12 h SQ	60	12.3 ± 1.9	2.7 ± 0.8	Rabbit; increased concentration in infected bone
Sisomicin				
10 mg/kg/12 h SQ	60	14.4 ± 2.0	2.5 ± 0.6	Rabbit; increased concentration in infected bone
Other Antibiotics				
Rifampin				
40 mg/kg/24 h SQ	60	6.5 ± 1.7	0.9 ± 0.4	Rabbit; increased concentration in infected bone
Carbenicillin				
5 g/4 h IV	90	204	24.5	Three doses given before biopsy

(Modified from Waldvogel, F.A., and Vasey, H.: Osteomyelitis: The Past Decade. N. Engl. J. Med., 303(7):360–370, 1980.)

trauma. In a study of 255 open fractures, they showed that the combined use of penicillin and streptomycin did not alter the rate of infection, whereas the rate of infection in the patients treated with cephalothin was 2.3% (statistically significant with a *p* value of <0.05). More recently, owing to the increasing incidence of gram-negative organisms contaminating open fractures, Gustilo and Anderson have recommended the combined use of a first-generation cephalosporin (cefazolin), an aminoglycoside (tobramycin), and penicillin G to provide coverage for gram-positive, gram-negative, and clostridial organisms.[605] Such broad coverage is particularly necessary for barnyard and farm injuries or any other in which the wound is contaminated with organic matter.[634] Antibiotics are empirically administered for three to five days, at which time the clinical appearance of the wound in conjunction with culture results from postdébridement operative specimens is used to determine the need for further antibiotic therapy. Recent

studies suggest no difference in the rate of infection at the fracture site between one and five days of antibiotic administration in the care of open fractures; characteristics of local wounds such as fracture grade, presence of fixation devices, and occurrence in the lower leg were the primary factors influencing risk of infection.[585,586,662]

The first-generation cephalosporins have good activity against most gram-positive cocci.[590] Second-generation and especially third-generation cephalosporins, although increasing the spectrum of coverage, are usually less active and should not be used for infections caused by gram-positive organisms. In general, the less expensive and more active members of the penicillin group should be used. Cross-sensitivity between the cephalosporins and penicillin is low, and cephalosporins may be used in most patients who are allergic to penicillin provided that the penicillin allergic response did not consist of anaphylaxis. Cephalosporins, because of wider coverage (including gram-negative activity)

Table 5-12. Antibiotics: Indications and Dosages

Antibiotic	Organisms	Daily Dosage*
Penicillin G	*Staphylococcus aureus* (non-penicillinase-producing); *Streptococcus pneumoniae*; *Streptococcus pyogenes*; *Streptococcus faecalis* (together with gentamicin); many anaerobic bacteria	25,000 U/kg/4 h
Vancomycin	Resistant to *Staphylococcus* or gram-positive organisms; penicillin-allergic patients	15 mg/kg/12 h; as 1 g IV q 12 h or 500 mg IV q 6 h
Ampicillin	*Hemophilus influenzae* (β-lactamase O); sensitive strains of *Escherichia coli, Proteus mirabilis,* and salmonella; also effective against same organisms as penicillin	25 mg/kg/4 h†
Methicillin, nafcillin, oxacillin‡	*S. aureus* (penicillinase-producing)	25–30 mg/kg/4 h†
Cephalothin, cephapirin	*S. aureus* (penicillinase-producing); *E. coli, P. mirabilis, Klebsiella;* major use is in mixed infections from *S. aureus* infection in penicillin-allergic patients	25–30 mg/kg/4 h†
Cefazolin	Same as cephalothin but may be given intramuscularly	35 mg/kg/6 h
Carbenicillin§	*Pseudomonas aeruginosa*	70 mg/kg/4 h
Clindamycin	Anaerobic bacteria, especially *Bacteroides fragilis; S. aureus, S. pneumoniae; S. pyogenes;* a major use is against *S. aureus* in penicillin-allergic patients	5 mg/kg/6 h
Gentamicin‖,¶ tobramycin	Most gram-negative bacilli	1–2 mg/kg/8 h¶
Amikacin¶	Most gram-negative bacilli, especially those resistant to gentamicin and tobramycin	5–6 mg/kg/8 h¶

* In each case the dosage relates to lean body weight and is given for intravenous usage.
† Slightly higher doses are generally prescribed for children because of shorter half-life.
‡ These drugs are not indicated for organisms that are sensitive to penicillin.
§ Ticarcillin is used for the same indications and has the same antibacterial spectrum: the dose is two thirds that of carbenicillin.
‖ Gentamicin and tobramycin appear to have identical antibacterial spectra; however, in vitro a given concentration of tobramycin is generally twice as effective as gentamicin against *P. aeruginosa* and this drug is therefore preferred for *Pseudomonas* infection.
¶ The half-life of these drugs is shorter in children, and the same dose should probably be given every 6 hours. The dose must be adjusted daily in cases of renal insufficiency.

and lower toxicity, are preferred over clindamycin and vancomycin. However, one of these latter two drugs is indicated for the patient having had previous anaphylactic reaction to penicillin.[612]

The treatment of osteomyelitis is based on the administration of systemic antibiotics in conjunction with surgery to drain abscesses or débride infected necrotic tissue. In early acute hematogenous osteomyelitis, antibiotic therapy without surgical intervention may result in cure, provided the blood supply has not yet been compromised and adequate antibiotic levels in bone can be obtained.[564,568,600,636] However, in subacute or chronic osteomyelitis, both antibiotics and surgery are necessary for adequate treatment.[575,609,618] The surgical procedure often requires extensive débridement of the involved tissues and the removal of bone; the blood supply to bone is such that its compromise frequently prohibits delivery of antibiotic to the affected areas.

Several reports have suggested the efficacy of closed suction-irrigation techniques for the treatment of chronic osteomyelitis.[576,582,589] Carefully planned surgery with débridement of all devitalized and infected tissues, followed by closure of the wound with insertion of a suction-irrigation system, is considered the treatment of choice by some authors. Jackson and Parson[614] have suggested the use of intermittent distention irrigation in the management of septic joints. This form of treatment has added a valuable new dimension to the management of osteomyelitis.

Many other forms of treatment, including the use of regional perfusion,[607] hyperbaric oxygen,[567,584,606] saucerization, immediate skin grafting,[649] distant or local muscle flaps (see Chapter 4),[599] and pulverized bone,[640] have been suggested for the management of chronic osteomyelitis.

A particularly difficult problem is chronic osteomyelitis in conjunction with an ununited fracture, that is, an infected nonunion. Staged procedures may be necessary to débride the involved tissues, provide rigid fracture fixation, and administer systemic antibiotics. Later, addition of bone graft may be required to achieve sound union of the fracture fragments.

Illustrative Case

Following a closed femoral shaft fracture sustained in an automobile accident, a 21-year-old man underwent open reduction and internal fixation with plate application. During the early postoperative period, purulent drainage from the wound and osteomyelitis of the fractured femur developed (Fig.

5-13). Three months postoperatively, the plate and screws were removed and the patient was placed in a spica cast after 2 weeks of closed suction-irrigation treatment. He remained in the spica cast for 17 weeks, but the wound continued to drain and the culture was positive for *Pseudomonas* (Fig. 5-14).

Eight months after the original injury, he was admitted to the hospital and underwent a massive sequestrectomy of the right femur that left a gap of 13 cm; a Küntscher rod was inserted for stabilization and rigid fixation. The infecting organisms were *Proteus mirabilis* and coagulase-negative *Staphylococcus.* Closed suction-irrigation was instituted, and intravenous administration of ampicillin was begun. After 4 weeks, parenteral antibiotics were discontinued and the patient was given oral ampicillin.

The patient underwent autogenous iliac bone grafting of the involved femur. All cultures taken at surgery, of both bone and soft tissues, were sterile. Ampicillin was continued for 6 months.

Subsequently, the femur united, no drainage occurred, and the patient returned to work as a machinist (Fig. 5-15).

In summary, the orthopaedic surgeon must develop an increasing awareness of the management of both acute hematogenous and nonhematogenous osteomyelitis. He or she must be well versed in the complexities of the management of open fractures and postoperative infections and the selection and use of antibiotics appropriate for these conditions.

POST-TRAUMATIC REFLEX SYMPATHETIC DYSTROPHY

For many years certain vague, ill-defined, widespread, painful conditions have been observed after trauma, infection, or thrombophlebitis of the extremities.[676] A variety of terms, such as *minor causalgia, major causalgia,*[693] *causalgia-like states, post-traumatic painful osteoporosis, Sudeck's atrophy,*[733,734] *reflex dystrophy, post-traumatic dystrophy,*[706] and *shoulder-hand syndrome,*[709,736] have been used to designate these conditions. Several theories regarding the pathogenesis of these conditions have been proposed, but no single theory has been proved. In this section, the individual characteristics of reflex sympathetic dystrophy, the shoulder-hand syndrome, and causalgia are considered. The orthopaedic surgeon is expected to manage these problems, which are often caused by fractures and dislocations, with associated soft tissue, nerve, and vascular injury.

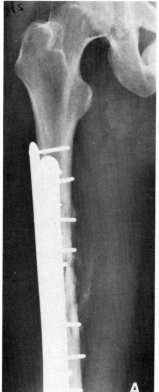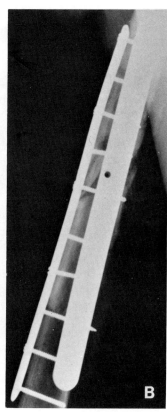

Fig. 5-13. (A) Anteroposterior and **(B)** lateral x-rays of the right femur with dual plates and early osteomyelitis.

More recently, problematic reflex sympathetic dystrophy has been discussed following arthroscopic procedures about the knee, especially when performed in treatment of patellofemoral pain syndromes.[674,698]

PATHOGENESIS

De Takats[676] has suggested a holistic concept under the heading of post-traumatic reflex dystrophy and has characterized this syndrome by chronic sensory stimulus, persistent vasomotor response, motor response, and eventual atrophy of tissue, bone, tendon, and muscle, with joint contractures, chronic edema, and fibrosis. It remains to be demonstrated how a minor injury can cause severe, persistent pain after the injured tissues have healed. A series of reflexes dependent on cross-stimulation between sympathetic efferent and damaged demyelinated sensory fibers may account for the underlying pathophysiology.[678] Livingston[702] proposed that three factors caused a circle of reflexes. He believed that chronic irritation of a peripheral sensory nerve led to an abnormal state of activity in the inter-

nuncial neuron center, which in turn led to a continuum of increased stimulation of efferent motor and sympathetic neurons. Figure 5-16 illustrates the factors that may be involved in a reflex dystrophic state. No single concept of pathogenesis has been proved at this time[673,687,711,738,741]; that there is in fact an abnormal sympathetic reflex is well established.[670,689,716,718,736,737]

REFLEX SYMPATHETIC DYSTROPHY

Pain, hyperesthesia, and tenderness out of proportion to the physical findings are the predominant features in a patient with reflex sympathetic dystrophy.[664,682] The pain may vary in severity and character and may be accompanied by swelling and decreased range of motion in the involved extremity. The skin color, texture, and temperature may vary, depending on the stage of the disease. The diagnosis can be confusing, because these variations may be completely opposite, such as hot or cold, pale or red, sweaty or dry. Early on, increased sweating (hyperhidrosis), redness,[699] warmth, and swelling are more common. In the later stages, pal-

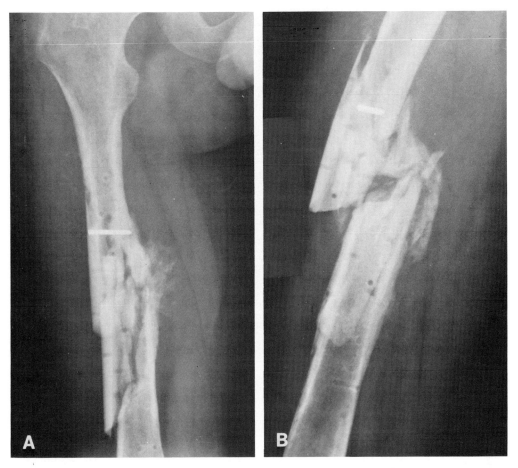

Fig. 5-14. Anteroposterior **(A)** and lateral **(B)** x-rays of the right femur showing chronic osteomyelitis with sequestra formation and nonunion.

lor, with dry and shiny skin, and coolness of the involved part become the predominant features (Fig. 5-17).

Most authors have separated the clinical findings into three stages: early, dystrophic, and atrophic. The first stage is identified by constant burning or aching pain in the extremity. The pain is increased by external stimuli or motion and is out of proportion to the severity of the injury and related physical findings. The stimuli that trigger the pain response may vary from peculiar noises, height, and excitement to emotional upset, vibration, arguments, deep breathing, laughter, or use of certain words.[676,714]

The second stage develops in approximately 3 months. At this stage most patients have significant edema; cold, glossy skin; and a limited range of joint motion. X-ray films often reveal a diffuse osteopenia.

The third, or atrophic, stage is marked by a progressive atrophy of the skin and muscle, joint motion is severely limited by evolving fibrosis, and contractures occur that may be irreversible. Marked, diffuse osteopenia is seen on the x-ray films. The pain may involve the whole limb and approach intractability.

In 1900, Sudeck[733] described acute bony atrophy, relating the onset to "inflammation." Subsequently, Sudeck[734] expanded his concept to include trauma or infection as causes of bone atrophy. He believed that the clinical features of pain, muscle atrophy, cyanosis, and edema developed secondary to the bone atrophy. He also stated that the changes did not occur if a reflex arc was broken, as occurs in such diseases as syringomyelia or poliomyelitis. Lenggenhager[700] has suggested that aseptic inflammation around an involved joint is responsible for the mottled osteodystrophy and has recommended

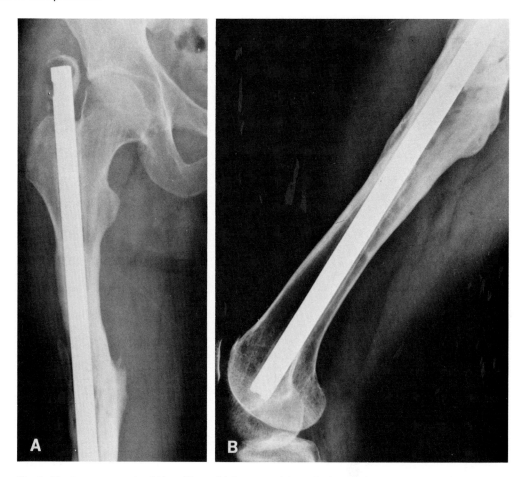

Fig. 5-15. Anteroposterior **(A)** and lateral **(B)** x-rays of the right femur showing union and resolution of osteomyelitis.

forced mobilization, under anesthesia, of the stiffened joints.

The term *Sudeck's atrophy* should not be used if the characteristic radiographic appearance is not present (Fig. 5-18).[715,722] Spotty rarefaction, present in the involved bones, is different from the generalized ground-glass appearance seen with disuse atrophy of bone.[690,691] The radiographic features occur approximately 6 to 8 weeks after the onset of symptoms.[665,669]

Diagnosis

Hartley[688] listed several clinical entities that may cause confusion in the diagnosis of post-traumatic reflex dystrophy; eg, tenosynovitis, disuse atrophy, senile osteoporosis, peripheral neuritis, and peripheral vascular disease states. It is often necessary to distinguish whether the patient's condition is

caused by a major functional overlay in conjunction with a minor organic problem. A local anesthetic block of the appropriate sympathetic ganglia may relieve pain and aid in the diagnosis of reflex sympathetic dystrophy.[704] Scintigraphic patterns characterized by delayed uptake have been useful in the diagnosis and in predicting which patients are likely to respond to therapy.[677,685,697,703,719,725]

Treatment

Prompt immobilization of the injured part may obviate further treatment.[695] Many patients with mild forms of post-traumatic reflex sympathetic dystrophy recover spontaneously following institution of a directed program of functional use of the affected limb. It is important to provide emotional support for the patient with impending or early reflex dystrophy. If conservative measures fail, some form of

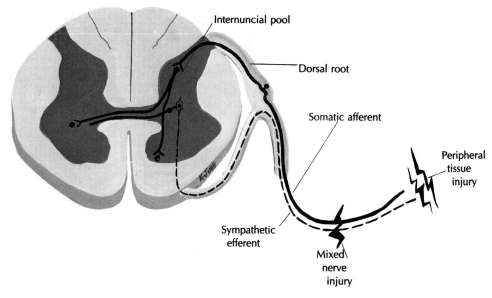

Fig. 5-16. Neural pathways in reflex dystrophy.

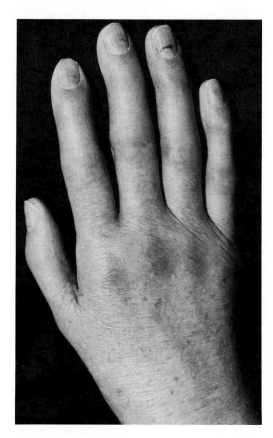

Fig. 5-17. Swollen, pale, stiff fingers in a patient with post-traumatic reflex dystrophy.

sympathetic interruption is used. Interrupting the sympathetic reflex has been attempted by a number of modalities,[674,698] including sympatholytic drugs, given both orally[680,684,726,739] and regionally,[667,671,672,683,686,717] somatic nerve blocks, periodic perineural infusions,[701,712] and stellate ganglion blocks.[724] Infrequently, the abnormal sympathetic reflex may require permanent interruption by surgical sympathectomy.[675,681,682,727,729] Various other medications, including corticosteroids[668,679,731] and calcitonin,[720,742] have been used in the treatment of this problem. Several adjunctive forms of treatment,[740] including transcutaneous nerve stimulation, trigger point injections, and splinting, are helpful and should be considered. A final, imperative note is that all of the preceding often do no more than allow the initiation of a program of functional physical exercise free of pain, which is the real cornerstone of treatment in the recovery of a useful extremity.

SHOULDER-HAND SYNDROME

Steinbrocker and Argyros[730] stated that the shoulder-hand syndrome is a distinctive and severe symptom complex with specific features that allow identification. It may result from external injuries or from internal disorders, such as coronary occlusion or a cerebrovascular accident. It is, however, a syndrome that can be classified as a form of reflex

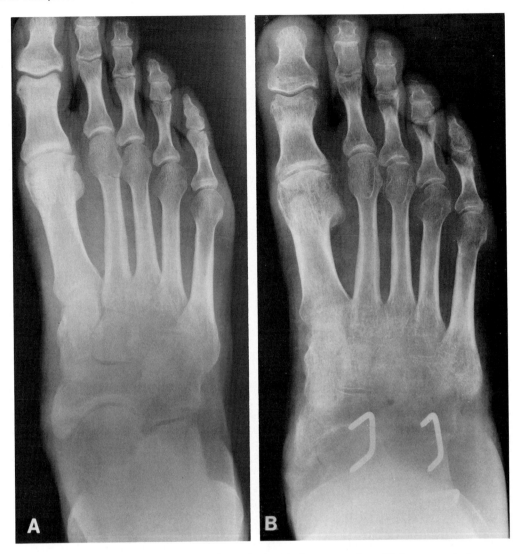

Fig. 5-18. **(A)** Anteroposterior x-ray of the right foot before operation. **(B)** Anteroposterior x-ray of the right foot after operation showing spotty rarefaction, characteristic of Sudeck's atrophy.

dystrophy.[694,710,713,723] The term *shoulder-hand* refers to the chief features of the syndrome—a painful, disabled shoulder associated with painful disability of the hand and fingers. Stiffness is characteristic in both locations.

The syndrome occurs more frequently in older age groups and after cardiac dysfunction.[692,694] It may follow cervical spondylitis, all types of fractures, a cerebrovascular accident, coronary occlusion, or any visceral, musculoskeletal, vascular, or neural process that involves reflex neurovascular responses. The syndrome characteristically evolves through three stages (Table 5-13).

As with other forms of reflex sympathetic dystrophy, the severity of the shoulder-hand syndrome is not proportional to the extent of the underlying disorder. A mild contusion of the shoulder might be followed by severe reflex dystrophy. Some authors believe that prompt recognition leads to more effective treatment.[666,743] No drug is specific for the treatment of the shoulder-hand syndrome; however, it is obvious that the underlying disorders require treatment before any resolution can be expected. Local injections with lidocaine (Xylocaine) and corticosteroids may be both diagnostic and therapeutic.[668,731]

It is inadvisable to manipulate the shoulder under anesthesia. Gentle but progressive active assisted exercises of the shoulder and hand have been most helpful. Contractures are gradually lessened, and pain is decreased. Repeated sympathetic blocks may be effective. The administration of oral corticosteroids is of indefinite value in the management of shoulder-hand syndrome.

The shoulder-hand syndrome may be prevented by early recognition.[730,732] Casts and manipulation should be avoided, and gentle, graduated exercises should be encouraged. Injection of trigger points with lidocaine may prove beneficial.

CAUSALGIA

Causalgia, by definition, means burning pain. In 1864, Mitchell and associates[708] were the first to describe this clinical syndrome. It is associated with a lesion of a peripheral nerve containing sensory fibers and is characterized by extreme pain in the affected extremity. Richards[720] has listed the features of causalgic pain: spontaneous, hot, burning, intense, diffuse, persistent, and intermittent; it is elicited by stimuli that do not necessarily produce physical change. It leads to profound changes in the mental state of the patient. "We consider causalgia to be a clinical syndrome associated with a lesion of a peripheral nerve containing sensory fibers manifested by pain in the affected extremity. This pain is usually of a burning character and is usually located in an area corresponding to the cutaneous distribution of the involved nerve. An integral characteristic of this pain, one whose presence is necessary in order to make the diagnosis, is its accentuation by certain disturbing features of the affected individual's environment."[696]

The incidence of causalgia depends on the criteria accepted for diagnosis. In the Civil War it was estimated to occur in 38% of patients with nerve injuries.[707,728] White and coworkers[741] stated that causalgia occurs in about 5% of wounds of major nerves, especially in those associated with injuries to the median and sciatic nerves. In wartime it was seen most frequently after a high-velocity missile injury with incomplete division of the tibial portion of the sciatic. Incised or lacerated wounds of nerves are rarely complicated by causalgia. It is not a frequent problem in civilian practice.

The exact etiology of causalgia remains uncertain, but it appears crossover effects at the areas of injury permit interaction between efferent sympathetic and afferent sensory fibers.[705,720,735]

The clinical picture is one of excruciating, unbearable pain, with superimposed stabbing, crushing sensations. In about one third of cases the pain begins immediately after injury and in the remaining cases within a week. The duration of pain is extremely variable, reaching maximum intensity 1 or 2 months after injury and, in some cases, persisting for 20 years or more. The pain may regress spontaneously. The area of sensory involvement is usually more than the cutaneous distribution of a single nerve. The extreme guarding of the patient against external stimuli makes motor evaluation of the involved limb difficult, but if the pain is relieved temporarily, the extent of sensory and motor involvement appears to be no greater than that expected from a peripheral nerve lesion without causalgia.[720] Many stimuli aggravate the pain, among them movement, examination, dependence, noise, excitement, touching dry objects, hearing certain words, and laughter. Often the patients are referred for psychological evaluation and are

Table 5-13. Clinical Manifestations of Shoulder-Hand Syndrome

Changes	Shoulder	Hand	Fingers	Vasomotor Changes	Radiographic Changes
Stage I	Pain Limitation of motion Diffuse tenderness	Pain Diffuse marked tenderness Dorsal swelling	Swelling Incomplete painful flexion	Vasodilation Vasospasm (occasionally)	Spotty osteoporosis
Stage II	Pain Early atrophy	Induration of skin	Firm induration Shiny trophic skin	Vasospasm Hyperhidrosis	Progressive diffuse osteoporosis
Stage III	Slight residual pain occurs Limitation of motion	Residual dystrophy and contractures	Diffuse atrophy Residual contractures	Usually absent with dystrophic changes	Generalized osteoporosis

(Modified from Steinbrocker, O., and Argyros, T.G.: The Shoulder–Hand Syndrome; Present Status as a Diagnostic and Therapeutic Entity. Med. Clin. North Am., 42:1533–1553, 1958.)

thought to be emotionally unstable. The image of the patient with severe causalgia holding the involved limb wrapped in a moist towel, anxiously avoiding all contact with external forces, is dramatic and not easily forgotten. Skin changes, such as glossiness, atrophy, moistness, and mottling, reflect the underlying vasomotor instability manifest by either vasoconstriction or dilation.

Operation on the peripheral nerve or its scar has not been effective treatment.[708] Neurolysis does not relieve pain. Alcohol injections have been tried to no avail.[701] Other operations, such as periarterial sympathetic section of the posterior nerve roots and arterial ligation, have not proved helpful in the management of causalgia. In 1930, Spurling[729] described a complete cure of causalgia by cervicothoracic sympathetic ganglionectomy. The World War II experience with this lesion showed that interruption of the appropriate sympathetic nerve fibers is almost always successful in the treatment of causalgia. Sympathetic blocks often provide temporary relief and, in some instances, complete relief following a series of treatments.[720,721] If a sympathetic block is to be done, it should be performed soon after the injury and the onset of symptoms. A satisfactory response to anesthetic sympathetic blockade may be a useful predictor of the anticipated effect of surgical sympathectomy.

In his centennial review of causalgia, Richards[720] stated that certain facts are well established in regard to this syndrome: "(1) True causalgia is rarely seen, except in missile wounds; (2) the nerve injury is usually proximal in the limb and is multiple; (3) the nerve injury is usually incomplete; (4) the anatomic lesions of the nerve are similar to noncausalgic nerve lesions; (5) surgical removal of the involved sympathetic ganglion is an effective mode of treatment."

Although rare, this syndrome represents a challenge in treatment when encountered by the orthopaedic surgeon.

COMPARTMENT SYNDROMES

One of the most devastating complications after a limb injury is ischemic muscle necrosis and subsequent contracture. More than a century ago Richard von Volkmann[784] reported the first account of a post-traumatic muscle contracture of acute onset, with increasing deformity despite splinting and passive exercises. In his classic paper of 1881,[783] he enumerated his reasons for believing that the paralysis and contracture of limbs "too tightly bandaged" resulted from ischemic changes of the muscles. Since that time physicians have become increasingly aware of the many varied circumstances in which increased tissue pressure may compromise the microcirculation. Jepson[759] was the first investigator to prove that paralysis and contracture could be prevented by prompt decompression. He showed in laboratory animals that contracture deformity is caused by a combination of factors, the most important of which are impairment of venous flow, extravasation of blood and serum, and swelling of the tissues, with resulting increased extravascular pressure compromising local tissue perfusion.

The compartment syndrome is a significant clinical problem, causing major functional losses after a wide variety of traumatic, vascular, hematologic, neurologic, surgical, pharmacologic, renal, and iatrogenic conditions.[764] Although it should be familiar to all clinicians, its common characteristics are obscured by the many names and descriptions used to identify it. A compartment syndrome is defined as a condition in which the circulation and function of tissues within a closed space are compromised by an increased pressure within that space. Matsen[769] proposed that there be a unified concept with which to consider all compartment syndromes because the underlying features of all the syndromes are essentially the same, irrespective of etiology or location. The names of some conditions in which compartment syndrome plays a central role are:

1. Volkmann's ischemia[745,751,771,782]
2. Compartment syndrome[746,772,773,775,785]
3. Impending ischemic contractures[779]
4. Rhabdomyolysis[763]
5. Crush syndrome[777]
6. Exercise ischemia[761]
7. Local ischemia[767]
8. Traumatic tension ischemia in muscles[758]
9. Acute ischemic infarction[765]
10. Ischemic necrosis[748]
11. Anterior tibial syndrome[749,768,780]
12. Peroneal nerve palsy[778]
13. Calf hypertension[754]
14. Phlegmasia cerulea dolens[750]

Essentially, any cause of increased compartmental pressure may result in a compartment syndrome. Matsen[769] suggested the following list of etiologies:

I. Decreased compartment size
   A. Closure of fascial defects
   B. Tight dressings
   C. Localized external pressure

II. Increased compartment content
   A. Bleeding
      1. Major vascular injury
      2. Bleeding disorder
   B. Increased capillary permeability
      1. Postischemic swelling
      2. Exercise
         Seizure and eclampsia
      3. Trauma (other than major vascular)
      4. Burns
      5. Intra-arterial drugs
      6. Orthopaedic surgery
   C. Increased capillary pressure
      1. Exercise
      2. Venous obstruction
         Long-leg brace
   D. Muscle hypertrophy
   E. Infiltrated infusion
   F. Nephrotic syndrome

PATHOPHYSIOLOGY

Although the common inciting pathogenic factor in compartment syndromes is increased tissue pressure, three theories have been proposed to explain the development of tissue ischemia found in this pathologic state:

1. Arterial spasm may result from increased intracompartment pressure.[744,751]
2. The theory of critical closing pressure states that because of the small luminal radius and the high mural tension of arterioles, a significant transmural pressure difference (arteriolar pressure minus tissue pressure) is required to maintain their patency. If tissue pressure rises or if arteriolar pressure drops significantly so that this critical pressure difference does not exist (ie, critical closing pressure is reached), the arterioles close.[747]
3. Because of their thin walls, veins will collapse if tissue pressure exceeds venous pressure. If blood continues to flow from capillaries, the venous pressure will rise until it again exceeds tissue pressure and patency is re-established. The augmentation of venous pressure reduces the arteriovenous gradient and, as a result, the tissue blood flow.[762,771]

Ashton[744] studied the effect of increased tissue pressure on regional blood flow and concluded that at least two mechanisms appear to be involved: active closure of small arterioles under the influence of vasomotor tone when transmural pressure is lowered, either by falls in intravascular pressure or rises in tissue pressure, and passive collapse of soft-walled capillaries when tissue pressure rises above the intracapillary pressure. These mechanisms were thought to become particularly important when tissues were surrounded by noncompliant fascial compartments.

The response of skeletal muscle to ischemia or trauma is similar whatever the mechanism of injury.[776] When muscles become anoxic, histamine-like substances are released that dilate the capillary bed and increase the endothelial permeability. Subsequently, intramuscular transudation of plasma occurs with erythrocyte sludging and a decrease of the microcirculatory flow.[757] The muscle gains weight in proportion to the duration of ischemia and has increased as much as 30% to 50% in net weight.[756] The necrosis of muscle is not immediate, because some arterial blood flow often continues, but the intramuscular edema is progressive.[751] It is now known beyond all controversy that after muscle ischemia and direct trauma, muscle has considerable ability to regenerate by the formation of new muscle cells. When only part of the length of a muscle cell succumbs or when some muscle cells disintegrate and others remain viable, marked regeneration can take place. It is therefore extremely important to decompress ischemic muscle as early as possible.[776]

Neural tissues also require a continuous and adequate supply of oxygen. Recent experimental studies on the effects of temporary ischemia, with special reference to intraneural microvascular pathophysiology, have shown that the microvessels of nerves possess an excellent capacity to recover function, even after long periods of ischemia.[766]

DIAGNOSIS

Signs and Symptoms

The clinical presentation of compartment syndromes is often indefinite and confusing, and delays in diagnosis occur even when physicians are aware of the signs and symptoms. The classic signs of impending compartment syndromes are pain, pallor, paresthesias, paralysis, and pulselessness. The prognosis is better if these are *not* always present, since by the time these classic findings have evolved, especially pulselessness, the limb is neither viable nor salvageable. Each sign must be evaluated, separated, and interpreted within the overall clinical picture.

PAIN

Pain is perhaps the earliest and most important and consistent sign. Unfortunately, it is variable, and its presence cannot always be relied on. Compartment syndromes are often associated with inherently painful conditions such as crush injuries and fractures. However, the pain of tissue ischemia is typically described as deep, unremitting, and poorly localized. It is not the type of pain usually associated with a fracture, and it is difficult to control with the usual mild analgesic measures used for fractures. In upper extremity fractures, passive finger extension exacerbates the pain and is an early physical finding of a deep forearm compartment syndrome. In children, one should be alerted if restlessness and pain continue after a fracture reduction.[781]

PALLOR

Pallor may or may not be present. The extremity may appear cyanotic or mottled early in the course of events. Cyanosis is present early, whereas marked pallor in the distal extremity occurs late, after major arterial occlusion has occurred. Neither pallor nor cyanosis should be considered a sign that is necessary for the diagnosis of compartment syndrome.

PARESTHESIA

Paresthesias in the cutaneous distribution of the peripheral nerve coursing through the affected compartment are usually an early sign of impending, but still reversible, compartment syndrome. Sensory disturbance usually precedes motor dysfunction; however, fixed hypoesthesia or anesthesia is a relatively late finding. The presence of true paresthesias, often experienced as a burning or prickling sensation, warrants at least close observation and, in the appropriate clinical context, may dictate a need for definitive treatment of an established compartment syndrome.

PARALYSIS

When a physician waits for obvious motor deficits to occur or for pulses to be obliterated, ischemia has usually been well established for some time and there may well be permanent damage. Motor function is the first nerve function to be lost when a limb is rendered ischemic. Irreversible muscle fiber changes occur as early as 6 hours following the onset of tissue ischemia. Bradley[746] reported that fasciotomy for anterior compartment syndrome resulted in complete recovery in only 13% of those patients who had foot drop at the time of diagnosis.

PULSELESSNESS

The loss of palpable pulses has been shown to occur late, or sometimes not at all, in the course of compartment syndromes.[787] Clinical experience and experimental evidence verify that irreversible tissue damage can occur in a patient with palpable pulses.[770,788]

Intracompartmental Pressures

If one suspects a developing compartment syndrome, constricting casts or circular dressings must be removed immediately. Garfin and associates[753] have presented experimental evidence to substantiate the adverse effects on intracompartmental pressure by the most common offending dressing—the circular cast. With dry Webril cast padding, the average intracompartmental pressure fell 30% after the cast was split on one side, and a 65% reduction in pressure followed spreading of the cast. Splitting of the padding led to only a 10% further reduction in compartment pressure. Complete removal of the cast reduced the pressure by another 15%, for a total decrease of 85% from baseline measurement. With a cast in place it was found that about 40% less fluid, infused into the anterolateral compartment of the leg, was needed to elevate the compartment pressure to levels equivalent to those of limbs not in casts.

Because increased intracompartmental pressure has been incriminated as the primary pathogenic factor in compartment syndromes, and because the diagnosis of these syndromes is often so difficult to make on clinical grounds alone, the measurement of intracompartmental tissue pressures has become a valuable clinical tool. Reneman and Jagenean[774] described a method for determination of total intramuscular pressure, but their technique was rather cumbersome. Whitesides and associates[786,787] advocated the use of a simple pressure-measuring device consisting of a needle and plastic tubing filled with saline solution and air attached to a mercury manometer; they have established tissue pressure measurement criteria as determinants of the need for fasciotomy (Fig. 5-19).

Whitesides and associates' technique requires only a few items that are readily available in most offices and hospitals. Both experimental and clinical experience have demonstrated that normal tissue pressure within closed compartments is approximately 0 mm Hg. This pressure increases markedly in compartment syndromes. There is inadequate perfusion and relative ischemia when the tissue pressure within a closed compartment rises to within 10 to 30 mm Hg of a patient's diastolic blood pressure. Whitesides and coworkers believed that fasciotomy is usually indicated when the tissue pressure rises to 40 to 45 mm Hg in a patient with

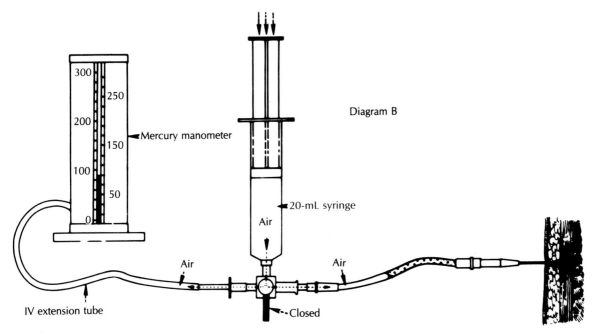

Diagram B

Mercury manometer

20-mL syringe

Air

Air

Air

IV extension tube

Closed

Three-way stopcock open to syringe and both extension tubes

Fig. 5-19. A device for measuring compartment pressures, made up of materials present in most hospitals, has been advocated by Whitesides. *(Reprinted from Whitesides, T. E., Jr.; Haney, T. C.; Morimoto, K.; and Harada, H.: Tissue Pressure Measurements as a Determinant for the Need of Fasciotomy. Clin. Orthop., 113:43, 1975.)*

a diastolic blood pressure of 70 mm Hg and any signs or symptoms of a compartment syndrome. There is no effective tissue perfusion within a closed compartment when the tissue pressure equals or exceeds the patient's diastolic blood pressure. A fasciotomy is definitely indicated in this circumstance, even though distal pulses may still be present. Using their criteria, Whitesides and colleagues had no deficits develop in patients after the physician elected not to perform a fasciotomy on the basis of tissue pressures. Conversely, all patients showed conclusive evidence of a compartment syndrome at operation when Whitesides and associates' suggested tissue pressures were used as an adjunct in making the decision for fasciotomy.[787]

In our institution we have assembled kits for the measurement of intracompartmental pressures. Each kit contains the following items:

1 sterile 20-mL syringe with Luer-Lok tip
1 four-way stopcock
1 18-gauge, 1-¼-inch angiocath intravenous catheter
2 89-cm-long (35-inch) extension tube sets
2 18-gauge needles

1 Telfa adhesive dressing pad
1 set of instructions and diagram, reproduced in Figure 5-20.

Furthermore, commercially available kits now simplify the setup and have transformed the determination of compartment pressures into a quick and easy bedside procedure. However, although pressure measurement is an invaluable adjunct in the evaluation of impending compartment syndrome, especially in the obtunded or comatose patient, careful physical examination remains the cornerstone to early diagnosis and expedient treatment. More recently, diminished tibial venous blood flow, as assessed noninvasively by Doppler identifying loss of normal phasic patterns, accurately predicted the need for surgical fasciotomy.[760]

TREATMENT (FASCIOTOMY)

Jepson's[759] early work proved that the treatment of choice for compartment syndrome is early decompression. Delay in adequately decompressing the offending compartment can result in permanent damage to underlying tissues. Nerves have been

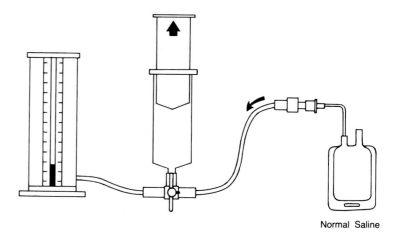

Normal Saline

Fig. 5-20. Instructions for measuring intracompartmental pressure.
1. Clean and prepare the area of the extremity to be evaluated.
2. Assemble your 20-mL syringe with the plunger at the 15-mL mark and connect to an open end of the four-way stopcock (see diagram).
3. Connect sterile plastic IV extension tube and an 18-gauge needle on another end of stopcock and a second IV extension tube to opposite end of stopcock (see diagram) to a blood pressure manometer.
4. Insert the tip of the 18-gauge needle into the saline bag and open the stopcock to allow flow through the needled IV tubing only. Aspirate the saline solution without bubbles into approximately half of the length of the extension tube. Turn the four-way stopcock to close off this tube so that the saline solution is not lost during transfer of the needle.

(continued)

found to demonstrate functional abnormalities (paresthesias and hypoesthesias) within 30 minutes of the onset of ischemia. Irreversible functional loss begins after 12 to 24 hours of total ischemia.[769,771] Muscle shows functional changes after 2 to 4 hours ischemia time, with irreversible functional loss beginning after 4 to 12 hours.[759,786] Ischemia lasting 4 hours gives rise to significant myoglobinuria, which reaches a maximum about 3 hours after the circulation is restored but persists for as long as 12 hours. Contractures are produced after 12 hours of total ischemia.[763,777,779] Capillary endothelium permeability is pathologically altered after 3 hours, resulting in postischemia swelling of 30% to 60%.

Initial decompression should be done by immediate splitting or removal of casts or other compromising circular dressings. If the tissue pressure remains elevated in a patient with any other signs or symptoms of a compartment syndrome, adequate decompressive fasciotomy must be performed as an emergency procedure. (Using Whitesides and associates' criteria, elevation means that the tissue pressure rises to within 10 to 30 mm Hg of the diastolic pressure.)

The technique of fasciotomy is a matter of surgical choice. It may be done either subcutaneously or through limited or extensive skin incisions. However, the surgical goal is salvage of a viable and functional extremity; in no way should the adequacy of decompression be compromised by misdirected concerns over cosmesis and the number or lengths of incisions. It is essential to decompress all tight compartments. The skin must be considered a potentially significant limiting structure.[755]

The classic lower extremity fasciotomy does not provide adequate decompression of all four muscle compartments of the leg. Often the deep posterior compartment has been neglected in discussions or descriptions of fasciotomy, access to which is best obtained behind the posteromedial border of the tibia in the distal third of the leg where the belly of the flexor digitorum longus muscle is exposed. Ernst and Kaufer[752] described fibulectomy-fasciotomy as a way to adequately decompress all four

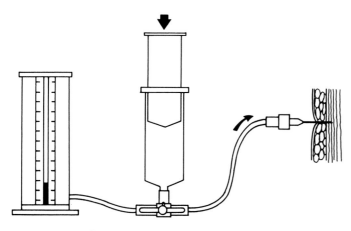

Fig. 5-20 (*continued*)

5. Insert the 18-gauge needle into the muscle of the compartment in which the tissue pressure is to be measured.

6. Turn the stopcock so that the syringe is open to both extension tubes forming a "T" connection as shown in the diagram. This produces a closed system in which the air is free to flow into both extension tubes as the pressure within the system is increased.

7. Increase the pressure in the system gradually by slowly depressing the plunger of the syringe while watching the saline/air meniscus. The mercury manometer will rise as the pressure within the system rises. When the pressure in this system has just surpassed tissue pressure surrounding the needle, a small amount of saline solution will be injected into the tissue and the meniscus will be seen to move. When the column moves, stop the pressure on the syringe plunger and read the level of the manometer. The manometer reading at the time the saline column moves is the tissue pressure in mm Hg.

compartments of the leg. Mubarak and Owen[770] advocated the double-incision fasciotomy, which permits access through two incisions to any or all of the four compartments of the leg when involved with acute or chronic compartment syndromes. The technique of double-incision fasciotomy is as follows.

Anterolateral Incision

The anterolateral incision, used for an approach to the anterior and/or lateral compartment, is 15 to 20 cm long and placed halfway between the fibular shaft and the tibial crest, allowing easy access to both compartments. A smaller incision, or two short incisions, can be adequately used for chronic compartment syndromes. The skin edges are undermined to allow adequate exposure of the fascia. A transverse incision is made just through the fascia in order to identify the intermuscular septum that separates the anterior compartment from the lateral compartment. Identification of the septum is helpful in locating the superficial peroneal nerve that lies in the lateral compartment, adjacent to the septum where it crosses at the junction of the middle and distal thirds of the leg.

With 12-inch Metzenbaum scissors, the *anterior compartment* fascia is opened through the length of the leg. The scissors are gently pushed with the tips opened slightly. Visualization is aided by the use of Army-Navy retractors, and the superficial peroneal nerve is protected in the distal third of the wound. If there is any question of whether the tip of the scissors has strayed from the fascia, the instrument is left in place and a small incision is made over its tip. If the fasciotomy is incomplete, further release can be performed through this small incision.

The *lateral compartment* fasciotomy is made in line with the fibular shaft. The scissors are directed proximally toward the fibular head and distally toward the lateral malleolus such that one is posterior to the superficial peroneal nerve. At the completion of this portion of the procedure, both compartments have been widely decompressed and the superficial peroneal nerve should remain intact and uninjured.

Posteromedial Incision

The posteromedial incision, used for an approach to the superficial and/or deep posterior compartments, is 15 to 20 cm long, slightly distal to the previous incision, and 2 cm posterior to the medial tibial margin. By placing the incision in this location, one avoids injuring the saphenous nerve and vein that course along the posterior margin of the tibia in this locale. Once again, the skin edges are undermined. The saphenous nerve and vein are retracted anteriorly. It is usually easiest to first decompress the *superficial posterior compartment*. Fasciotomy is extended proximally as far as possible and then distally behind the medial malleolus. The Achilles tendon in the superficial posterior compartment and the tendon of the flexor digitorum longus in the deep posterior compartment are identified. The deep posterior compartment is then released distally to proximally under the bridge created by the soleus origin.

The wounds are left open, and delayed primary closure is anticipated in seven to ten days. Skin grafting may be necessary if after a full week there remains sufficient swelling to preclude direct closure of the wound margins.

The authors gratefully acknowledge the assistance of Lori A. Bush in the preparation of this manuscript.

REFERENCES

Hypovolemia (Shock)

1. AIDS and HIV Infection in the United States: 1988 Update. M.M.W.R., 38(Suppl. 4):36, 38, May 12, 1989.
2. Alexander, J.W.; McClellan, M.A.; Ogle, C.K.; and Ogle, J.D.: Consumptive Opsoninopathy: Possible Pathogenesis in Lethal and Opportunistic Infections. Ann. Surg., 184:672–678, 1976.
3. Alexander, M.R.; Ambre, J.J.; Liskow, B.I.; and Trost, D.C.: Therapeutic Use of Albumin. J.A.M.A., 241:2527–2529, 1978.
4. Allen, J.G.: Response to Blood Replacement and Volume Expanders in Acute Hemorrhagic Index Hypovolemia. *In* Mills, L.C., and Moyer, J.H. (eds.): Shock and Hypotension: Pathogenesis and Treatment, pp. 397–400. New York, Grune & Stratton, 1965.
5. Alper, C.A.; Abramson, N.; Block, K.J.; Johnston, R.B.; and Rosen, F.S.: Increased Susceptibility to Infection Associated With Abnormalities of Complement Mediated Functions and of the Third Component (C3). N. Engl. J. Med., 282:349–354, 1970.
6. Altermeier, W.A.; Todd, J.C.; and Inge, W.W.: Gram-neg-

ative Septicemia: A Growing Threat. Ann. Surg., 166:530–542, 1967.
7. American College of Surgeons, Committee on Trauma. Advanced Trauma Life Support Course. Student Manual, 1981.
8. Anderson, R.W.; Simmons, R.L.; Collings, J.A.; Brendenberg, C.E.; James, P.M.; and Levitsky, S.: Plasma Volume and Sulfate Spaces in Acute Combat Casualties. Surg. Gynecol. Obstet., 128:719–724, 1969.
9. Ariel, I.M., and Kremen, A.J.: Compartmental Distribution of Sodium Chloride in Surgical Patients Pre- and Postoperatively. Ann. Surg., 132:1009–1026, 1950.
10. Aronstam, E.M.; Schmidt, C.H.; and Jenkins, E.: Body Fluid Shifts, Sodium and Potassium Metabolism in Patients Undergoing Thoracic Surgical Procedures. Ann. Surg., 137:316–324, 1953.
11. Aviado, D.M.: Pharmacologic Approach to the Treatment of Shock. Ann. Intern. Med., 62:1050–1059, 1965.
12. Baue, A.E.; Tragus, E.T.; Wolfson, S.K., Jr.; Cary, A.L.; and Parkins, W.M.: Hemodynamic and Metabolic Effects of Ringer's Lactate Solution in Hemorrhagic Shock. Ann. Surg., 166:29–38, 1967.
13. Beiting, C.V.; Kozak, K.J.; Kozak, B.A.; Dreffer, R.; Stinnett, J.D.; and Alexander, J.W.: Whole Blood vs. Packed Red Blood Cells for Resuscitation of Hemorrhagic Shock: An Examination of Host Defense Parameters in Dogs. Surgery, 84:194–200, 1978.
14. Blalock, A.: Shock. Further Studies With Particular Reference to the Effects of Hemorrhage. Arch. Surg., 29:837–857, 1934.
15. Blalock, C.V.: Principles of Surgical Care, Shock, and Other Problems, pp. 1–325. St. Louis, C.V. Mosby, 1940.
16. Boba, A., and Converse, J.G.: Ganglionic Blockage and Its Protective Action in Hemorrhage: A Review. Anesthesiology, 18:559–572, 1957.
17. Border, J.R.: Advances and Newer Concepts in Shock. *In* Cooper Surgery Annual, pp. 69–123. New York, Appleton-Century-Crofts, 1969.
18. Border, J.R.; Chenier, R.; McMenamy, R.H.; LaDuca, J.; Seibel, R.; Birkhahn, R.; and Tu, L.: Multiple Systems Organ Failure: Muscle Fuel Deficit With Visceral Protein Malnutrition. Surg. Clin. North Am., 56:1147–1167, 1976.
19. Border, J.R.; LaDuca, J.; and Seibel, R.: Priorities in the Management of the Patient With Polytrauma. Prog. Surg., 14:84–120, 1975.
20. Bove, J.: Transfusion-associated Hepatitis and AIDS. What Is the Risk? N. Engl. J. Med., 317:242–245, 1987.
21. Braunstein, P.: Concealed Hemorrhage Due to Pelvic Fracture. J. Trauma, 4:832, 1963.
22. Byrne, J.J.: Symposium on Shock. Am. J. Surg., 110:293–297, 1965.
23. Cahill, J.M.; Jouasset-Strieder, D.; and Byrne, J.J.: Lung Function in Shock. Am. J. Surg., 110:324–329, 1965.
24. Carey, J.S.; Brown, R.S.; Woodward, N.W.; Yao, S.T.; and Shoemaker, W.C.: Comparison of Hemodynamic Responses to Whole Blood and Plasma Expanders in Clinical Shock. Surg. Gynecol. Obstet., 121:1059–1065, 1965.
25. Chaplin, H.: Packed Red Blood Cells. N. Engl. J. Med., 281:364–367, 1969.

26. Cloutier, C.T.: The Effect of Hemodilutional Resuscitation on Serum Protein Levels in Humans in Hemorrhagic Shock. J. Trauma, 9:514–521, 1969.

27. Cloutier, C.T.; Lowery, B.D.; and Carey, L.C.: Acid-Base Disturbances in Hemorrhagic Shock in 66 Severely Wounded Patients Prior to Treatment. Arch. Surg., 98: 551–557, 1969.

28. Crile, G.W.: Blood Pressure in Surgery: An Experimental and Clinical Research, Philadelphia, J.B. Lippincott, 1903.

29. Dahn, M.S.; Lucas, C.E.; Ledgerwood, A.M.; and Higgins, R.F.: Negative Inotropic Effect of Albumin Resuscitation for Shock. Surgery, 86:235–241, 1978.

30. Doty, D.B.; Hufnagel, H.V.; and Moseley, R.V.: The Distribution of Body Fluids Following Hemorrhage and Resuscitation in Combat Casualties. Surg. Gynecol. Obstet., 130:453–458, 1970.

31. Duff, J.H.; Scott, H.M.; Peretz, D.I.; Mulligan, G.W.; and MacLean, L.D.: The Diagnosis and Treatment of Shock in Man Based on Hemodynamic and Metabolic Measurements. J. Trauma, 6:145–156, 1966.

32. Evarts, C.M.: Low Molecular Weight Dextran. Med. Clin. North Am, 51:1285–1299, 1967.

33. Evers, B.M.; Cryer, H.; and Miller, F.: Pelvic Fracture Hemorrhage. Priorities in Management. Arch. Surg., 124: 422–424, 1989.

34. FDA Drug Bulletin: Use of Blood Components. FDA Drug Bull., 14–15, 1989.

35. Flynn, N.: AIDS: Risk and Treatment, Orthopaedic Audio-Synopsis Foundation. South Pasadena, Calif., 1989.

36. Fortune, J.; Feustel, P.; Saifi, J.; Stratton, H.; Newell, J.; and Shah, D.: Influence of Hematocrit on Cardiopulmonary Function After Acute Hemorrhage. J. Trauma, 27: 243–249, 1987.

37. Friedland, G., and Klein, R.: Transmission of the Human Immunodeficiency Virus. N. Engl. J. Med., 317:1125–1135, 1987.

38. Fulton, R.L., and Jones, C.E.: The Cause of Post-Traumatic Pulmonary Insufficiency in Man. Surg. Gynecol. Obstet., 140:179–185, 1975.

39. Gleckman, R.; Gleckman, R.; and Esposito, A.: Gram-Negative Bacteremic Shock: Pathophysiology, Clinical Features, and Treatment. South. Med. J., 74(3):335–341, 1981.

40. Gollub, S., and Bailey, C.P.: Management of Major Surgical Blood Loss Without Transfusions. J.A.M.A., 198:1171–1174, 1966.

41. Gollub, S.; Svigals, R.; Bailey, C.P.; Hirose, T.; and Shaefer, C.: Electrolyte Solution in Surgical Patients Refusing Transfusion. J.A.M.A., 215:2077–2083, 1971.

42. Gross, S.G.: A System of Surgery: Pathological, Diagnostic, Therapeutique, and Operative, pp. 1–1098. Philadelphia, Lea & Febiger, 1872.

43. Hamit, H.F.: Current Trends of Therapy and Research in Shock. Surg. Gynecol. Obstet., 120:835–854, 1965.

44. Hardaway, R.M., III: Microcoagulation in Shock. Am. J. Surg., 110:298–301, 1965.

45. Hardaway, R.M., III: Intensive Study and Treatment of Shock in Man. Vascular Diseases, 4:53–58, 1967.

46. Hardy, J.D.; Hardy, K.P.; and Turner, M.D.: Massive

47. Hauser, C., and Perry, J.: Massive Hemorrhage From Pelvic Fractures. Minn. Med., 49:285, 1966.

48. Henry, S.B., and Boral, L.I.: The Type and Screen: A Safe Alternative and Supplement in Selected Surgical Procedures. Transfusion, 17:163–168, 1977.

49. Holcroft, J.W.; Trunkey, D.D.; and Lim, R.D.: Further Analysis of Lung Water in Baboons Resuscitated From Hemorrhagic Shock. J. Surg. Res., 20:291–297, 1976.

50. Human Immunodeficiency Virus Infection in the United States: A Review of Current Knowledge. U.S. Department of Health and Human Services. M.M.W.R., 36(Suppl. 6): 1987.

51. Jones, R.C., and Blotchy, M.J.: Initial Management of the Severely Injured Patient. South. Med. J., 62:260–265, 1969.

52. Laks, H.; Pilon, R.; Klovekorn, P.; Anderson, W.; MacCallum, J.; O'Connor, N.: Acute Hemodilution: Effect on Hemodynamics and Oxygen Transport in Anesthetized Man. Ann. Surg., 180:103–109, 1974.

53. Lanser, M., and Saba, R.: Correction of Serum Opsonic Defects After Burn and Sepsis by Opsonic Fibronectin Administration. Arch. Surg., 118:338–342, 1983.

54. Litwin, M.S.: Blood Viscosity in Shock. Am. J. Surg., 110: 313–316, 1965.

55. Lowery, B.D.: Electrolyte Solutions in Resuscitation in Human Hemorrhagic Shock. Surg. Gynecol. Obstet., 133: 273–284, 1971.

56. Lucas, C.E.; Bouwman, D.L.; Ledgerwood, A.M.; and Higgins, R.: Differential Serum Protein Changes Following Supplemental Albumin Resuscitation for Hypovolemic Shock. J. Trauma, 20:47–51, 1980.

57. Lucas, C.E.; Ledgerwood, A.M.; and Higgins, R.F.: Impaired Salt and Water Excretion After Albumin Resuscitation for Hypovolemic Shock. Surgery, 86:544–549, 1978.

58. Lucas, C.E.; Ledgerwood, A.M.; and Higgins, R.F.: Impaired Pulmonary Function After Albumin Resuscitation from Shock. J. Trauma, 20:446–451, 1980.

59. McClellan, M.A., and Alexander, J.W.: The Opsonic Activity of Stored Blood. Transfusion, 17:227–232, 1977.

60. McCullough, J.: Preservation of Opsonic Activity Against *S. aureus* and *E. coli* in Banked Blood. J. Lab. Clin. Med., 79:886–892, 1972.

61. Matsuda, H., and Shoemaker, W.C.: Cardiorespiratory Responses to Dextran 40. Arch. Surg., 110:296–300, 1975.

62. Matsuda, H., and Shoemaker, W.C.: Survivors' and Non-survivors' Response to Dextran 40. Arch. Surg., 110:301–305, 1975.

63. Miller, R.M.; Polakavetz, S.H.; Hornick, R.B.; and Cowley, R.A.: Analysis of Infections Acquired by the Severely Injured Patient. Surg. Gynecol. Obstet., 137:7–10, 1973.

64. Moncrief, J.A.: Shock in the Multiple-Injury Patient. J. Bone Joint Surg., 49A:540–546, 1967.

65. Moore, F.D.: Metabolic Care of the Surgical Patient, pp. 1–1011. Philadelphia, W.B. Saunders, 1959.

66. Moyer, C.A.: Fluid Balance, pp. 1–109. Chicago, Year Book Medical Publishers, 1954.

67. Moyer, C.A.; Margraf, H.W.; and Monago, W.W., Jr.: Burn

Shock and Extravascular Sodium Deficiency Treatment With Ringer's Solution With Lactate. Arch. Surg., 90:799–811, 1965.

68. Munster, A.M.; Hoagland, H.D.; and Pruitt, B.A., Jr.: The Effect of Thermal Injury on Serum Immunoglobulins. Ann. Surg., 172:965–969, 1970.

69. Murray, D.: Complications of Treatment of Fractures and Dislocations: General Considerations. *In* Epps, C. (ed.): Complications in Orthopaedic Surgery, pp. 3–55. Philadelphia, J.B. Lippincott, 1978.

70. Office of Medical Applications of Research, National Institutes of Health: Perioperative Red Cell Transfusion. J.A.M.A., 260:2700–2703, 1988.

71. Olcott, C., IV, and Lim, R.C., Jr.: Specialized Blood Filters and Fresh Whole Blood. J. Am. Coll. Emerg. Phys., 5: 510–511, 1976.

72. Ollodart, R., and Mansberger, A.R.: The Effect of Hypovolemic Shock on Bacterial Defense. Am. J. Surg., 110: 302–307, 1965.

73. Rush, B.F., Jr.; Richardson, J.D.; Bosomworth, P.; and Elseman, B.: Limitations of Blood Replacement With Electrolyte Solutions. Arch. Surg., 98:49–52, 1969.

74. Saba, T.M.; Blumenstock, F.A.; Scovill, W.A.; Bernard, H.: Cryoprecipitate Reversal of Opsonic α-2 Surface Binding Glycoprotein Deficiency in Septic Surgical and Trauma Patients. Science, 201:622–624, 1978.

75. Saba, T.M., and Jaffe, E.: Plasma Fibronectin (Opsonic Glycoprotein): Its Synthesis by Vascular Endothelial Cells and Role in Cardiopulmonary Integrity After Trauma as Related to Reticuloendothelial Function. Am. J. Med., 68:577–594, 1980.

76. Saltz, N.J.: Shock and the Extracellular Fluid Space. Am. J. Surg., 117:603–604, 1969.

77. Schumer, W.; Moss, G.S.; and Nyhus, L.M.: Metabolism of Lactic Acid in the Macacus Rhesus Monkey in Profound Shock. Am. J. Surg., 118:200–205, 1969.

78. Shires, G.T.; Carrico, L.J.; and Canizaro, P.C.: Shock, Major Problems in Clinical Surgery, pp. 1–162. Philadelphia, W.B. Saunders, 1973.

79. Shires, G.T.; Williams, J.; and Brown, F.: Acute Change in Extracellular Fluids Associated With Major Surgical Procedures. Ann. Surg., 154:803–810, 1961.

80. Shires, G.T. (ed.): Care of the Trauma Patient, pp. 3–677. New York, McGraw-Hill, 1966.

81. Shoemaker, W.C.: Sequential Hemodynamic Patterns in Various Etiologies of Shock. Surg. Gynecol. Obstet., 132: 411–423, 1971.

82. Shoemaker, W.C.: Comparison of the Relative Effectiveness of Whole Blood, Transfusions and Various Types of Fluid Therapy in Resuscitation. Crit. Care Med., 4:71, 1976.

83. Shoemaker, W.C., and Brown, R.S.: The Dilemma of Vasopressors and Vasodilators in the Therapy of Shock. Surg. Gynecol. Obstet., 132:51–57, 1971.

84. Shoemaker, W.C.; Elwyn, D.H.; Levine, H.; and Rosen, A.L.: Use of Nonparametric Analysis of Cardiorespiratory Variables as Early Predictors of Death and Survival in Postoperative Patients. J. Surg. Res., 17:301–314, 1974.

85. Shoemaker, W.C.; Montgomery, E.S.; Kaplan, E.; and El-wyn, D.H.: Use of Sequential Physiologic Patterns of Surviving and Nonsurviving Shock Patients for Defining Criteria for Therapeutic Goals and Early Warning of Death. Arch. Surg., 106:630–636, 1973.

86. Shoemaker, W.C., and Munson, D.O.: Effect of Whole Blood and Plasma Expanders on Volume-Flow Relationships in Critically Ill Patients. Surg. Gynecol. Obstet., 137: 453–457, 1973.

87. Simeone, F.A.: Shock. *In* Sabiston, D. (ed.): Davis–Christopher's Textbook of Surgery, pp. 65–94. Philadelphia, W.B. Saunders, 1964.

88. Thal, A.P., and Sardesai, V.M.: Shock and the Circulating Polypeptides. Am. J. Surg., 110:308–312, 1965.

89. Transfusion Alert: Indications for the Use of Red Blood Cells, Platelets, and Fresh Frozen Plasma, Bethesda, Md., U.S. Dept. of Health and Human Services, Public Health Service, National Institutes of Health, 1989.

90. Trudnowski, R.J.: Hydration With Ringer's Lactate Solution. J.A.M.A., 195:545–548, 1966.

91. Valeri, C.R.: Blood Components in the Treatment of Acute Blood Loss: Use of Freeze Preserved Red Cells, Platelets, and Plasma Proteins. Anesth. Analg., 54:1–14, 1975.

92. Villazon, S.A.; Sierra, V.A.; Lopez, S.F.; and Rolando, M.A.: Hemodynamic Patterns in Shock and Critically Ill Patients. Crit. Care Med., 3:215–221, 1975.

93. Weinstein, R.J., and Young, L.S.: Neutrophil Function in Gram-Negative Bacteremia. J. Clin. Invest., 58:190–199, 1976.

94. Wiggers, C.J.: The Present Status of the Shock Problem. Physiol. Rev., 22:74–123, 1942.

95. Wiggers, H.C.; Ingraham, R.C.; Roemhild, F.; and Goldberg, H.: Vasoconstriction and Development of Irreversible Hemorrhagic Shock. Am. J. Physiol., 153:511–520, 1948.

Cardiopulmonary Arrest

96. Briggs, B.A.; and Hayes, H.R.: Cardiopulmonary Resuscitation. *In* Wilkins, E.W., et al. (ed.): MGH Textbook of Emergency Medicine, pp. 27–37. Baltimore, Williams & Wilkins, 1979.

97. Brown, D.L.; Brown, D.L.; and Parmley, C.L.: Second Degree Atrioventricular Block After Methylmethacrylate. Anesthesiology, 56(5):391–392, 1982.

98. The Closed-Chest Method of Cardiopulmonary Resuscitation-Revised Statement. Circulation (Editorial), 31:641–642, 1965.

99. Deyerle, W.; Crossland, S.; and Sullivan, H.: Methylmethacrylate: Uses and Complications. A.O.R.N. J., 29(4):696–697, 700–701, 1979.

100. Drugs of Choice From the Medical Letter, "Cardiac Arrhythmias." Med. Lett. Drugs Ther., 21–23, 1981.

101. Eisenberg, M., et al.: The ACLS Score. J.A.M.A., 246(1): 50–52, 1981.

102. Frank, N., et al.: Circulatory Complications Caused by Bone Cement. Effect of Polymethylmethacrylate on Circulation Parameters of Elderly Patients. M.M.W.R., 121(48):1601–1602, 1979.

103. Gatch, G.: Cardiac Arrest in the O.R. A.O.R.N. J., 32(6): 983–993, 1980.

104. Gross, P.: Drugs to Start the Heart. Emergency Medicine, 11:79–87, 1979.
105. Johnson, J.D.: A Plan of Action in Cardiac Arrest. J.A.M.A., 186:468–472, 1963.
106. Jude, J.R.: Cardiac Arrest and Resuscitation. *In* Management of Surgical Complications, 3rd ed., pp. 108. Philadelphia, W.B. Saunders, 1975.
107. Jude, J.R.: Cardiac Arrest and Resuscitation. *In* Complications in Surgery and Their Management, pp. 114–125. Philadelphia, W.B. Saunders, 1981.
108. Jude, J.R.; Kouwenhoven, W.B.; and Knickerbocker, G.G.: A New Approach to Cardiac Resuscitation. Ann. Surg., 154:311–319, 1961.
109. Kallina, C.: Morbidity and Mortality in Elderly Orthopaedic Patients. Surg. Clin. North Am., 62(2):297–300, 1982.
110. Keret, D., et al: Cardiac Arrest and Death in Hip Replacement. Harefauh, 98(3):119–121, 1980.
111. Kouwenhaven, W.B.; Jude, J.R.; and Knickerbocker, G.G.: Closed Chest Cardiac Massage. J.A.M.A., 173:1064–1067, 1960.
112. Landau, I.: New Legal Risks in Cardiac Arrest. Hospital Physician, 2:80–91, 1966.
113. Levison, M., and Trunkey, D.D.: Initial Assessment and Resuscitation. Surg. Clin. North Am., 62(1):3–8, 1982.
114. Lund, I., and Skulberg, A.: Cardiopulmonary Resuscitation by Lay People. Lancet, 2:702–704, 1976.
115. McIntyre, K.M.; Lewis, A.J.; et al.: Textbook of Advanced Cardiac Life Support. New York American Heart Association, 1981.
116. McIntyre, K.M.; Parker, M.R.; Guildner, C.W.; et al.: Standards and Guidelines for Cardiopulmonary Resuscitation (CPR) and Emergency Cardiac Care. J.A.M.A., 244(5):453–509, 1980.
117. MacKenzie, G.J.; Taylor, S.H.; McDonald, A.H.; and McDonald, K.W.: Haemodynamic Effects of External Cardiac Compression. Lancet, 1:1342–1345, 1964.
118. Messer, J.V.: Cardiac Arrest. N. Engl. J. Med., 275:35–39, 1966.
119. Myerberg, R.J.; Conde, C.A.; Sung, R.J.; Mayorga-Cortes, A.; Mallon, S.M.; Sheps, D.S.; Appel, R.A.; and Castellanos, A.: A Clinical Electrophysiologic and Hemodynamic Profile of Patients Resuscitated From Prehospital Cardiac Arrest. Am. J. Med., 68:568–576, 1980.
120. Myerberg, R.J., et al.: Survivors of Prehospital Cardiac Arrest. J.A.M.A., 244(10):1985–1990, 1982.
121. Newens, A.F., and Volz, R.G.: Severe Hypotension During Prosthetic Hip Surgery With Acrylic Bone Cement. Anesthesiology, 36:298–300, 1972.
122. Powell, J.N.; McGrath, D.J.; Lahiri, S.K.; and Hill, P.: Cardiac Arrest Associated With Bone Cement. Br. Med. J., 3:326, 1970.
123. Safar, P.; Brown, T.C.; Holtey, W.J.; and Wilder, R.J.: Ventilation and Circulation With Closed-Chest Cardiac Massage in Man. J.A.M.A., 176:574–576, 1961.
124. Schuh, F.T.; Schuh, S.M.; Viguera, M.G.; and Terry, R.N.: Circulatory Changes Following Implantation of Methylmethacrylate Bone Cement. Anesthesiology, 39:455–457, 1973.

Fat Embolism Syndrome

125. Aach, R., and Kissane, J. (eds.): Clinicopathologic Conference. Fat Embolism. Am. J. Med., 51:258–268, 1971.
126. Alho, A.; Saikku, K.; Eerola, P.; Koskinen, M.; and Hamaleinen, M.: Corticosteroids in Patients With a High Risk of Fat Embolism Syndrome. Surg. Gynecol. Obstet., 147:358–362, 1978.
127. Allardyce, D.B.: The Adverse Effect of Heparin in Experimental Fat Embolism. Surg. Forum, 22:203–205, 1971.
128. American College of Surgeons: Hospital Trauma Index. Bull. Am. Coll. Surg., 65(a):31–33, 1980.
129. Armin, J., Jr.; and Grant, R.T.: Observations on Gross Pulmonary Fat Embolism in Man and the Rabbit. Clin. Sci., 10:441–469, 1951.
130. Ashbaugh, D.G., and Petty, T.L.: The Use of Corticosteroids in the Treatment of Respiratory Failure Associated With Massive Fat Embolism. Surg. Gynecol. Obstet., 123:493–500, 1966.
131. Bagg, R.J.; Stein, S.; Urban, R.T.; and McKay, D.: Parameters of the Fat Emboli Syndrome (F.E.S.). Orthop. Trans., 3(3):278–278, 1979.
132. Baker, P.L.; Kuenzig, M.C.; and Peltier, L.F.: Experimental Fat Embolism in Dogs. J. Trauma, 9:577–586, 1969.
133. Baker, S.; O'Neill, B.; Haddon, W.; and Long, W.: The Injury Severity Score: A Method for Describing Patients With Multiple Injuries and Evaluating Emergency Care. J. Trauma, 14:187–196, 1974.
134. Barie, P.; Minnear, F.; and Malik, A.: Increased Pulmonary Vascular Permeability After Bone Marrow Injection in Sheep. Am. Rev. Respir. Dis., 123:648–653, 1981.
135. Beck, J.P., and Collins, J.A.: Theoretical and Clinical Aspects of Posttraumatic Fat Embolism Syndrome. Instr. Course Lect. 22:38–87, 1973.
136. Benestad, G.: Falle von Fettembolie mit punktformigen Blutungen in der Haut. Dtsch. Z. Chir., 112:194–205, 1911.
137. Bengston, A.; Larsson, M.; Gammer, W.; and Heideman, M.: Anaphylatoxin Release in Association With Methylmethacrylate Fixation of Hip Prostheses. J. Bone Joint Surg., 69A:46–49, 1987.
138. Benoit, P.R.; Hampson, L.G.; and Burgess, J.H.: Value of Arterial Hypoxemia in the Diagnosis of Pulmonary Fat Embolism. Ann. Surg., 175:128–137, 1972.
139. Bergentz, S.E.: Studies on the Genesis of Posttraumatic Fat Embolism. Acta. Chir. Scand. [Suppl.], 282:1–72, 1961.
140. Bergmann, E.B.: Ein Fall todlicher Fettembolie. Klin. Wocheschr., 10:385–387, 1873.
141. Bivins, B.A.; Madauss, W.C.; and Griffen, W.O., Jr.: Fat Embolism Syndrome: A Clinical Study. South. Med. J., 65:937–940, 1972.
142. Blaisdell, F.W., and Lewis, F.R.: Respiratory Distress Syndrome of Shock and Trauma. *In* Major Problems in Clinical Surgery, Vol. 21. Philadelphia, W.B. Saunders, 1977.
143. Blath, R.A., and Collins, J.A.: The Relationship of Lipuria to Fat Embolism in Rabbits. J. Trauma, 10:901–904, 1970.
144. Bone, L., and Bucholz, R.: Current Concepts Review: The Management of Fractures in the Patient With Multiple Trauma. J. Bone Joint Surg., 68A:945–949, 1986.

145. Bone, L.; Johnson, K.; Weigelt, J.; and Scheinberg, R.: Early Versus Delayed Stabilization of Femoral Fractures. A Prospective Randomized Study. J. Bone Joint Surg. 71A: 336–340, 1989.

146. Bradford, D.S.; Foster, R.R.; and Nossel, H.L.: Coagulation Alterations, Hypoxemia, and Fat Embolism in Fracture Patients. J. Trauma, 10:307–321, 1970.

147. Broder, G., and Ruzumna, L.: Systemic Fat Embolism Following Acute Primary Osteomyelitis. J.A.M.A., 199:1004–1006, 1967.

148. Cahill, J.M.; Daly, B.F.T.; and Byrne, J.J.: Ventilatory and Circulatory Response to Oleic Acid Embolus. J. Trauma, 14:73–76, 1974.

149. Carver, G.M., Jr.: Traumatic Renal Infarction Concurrent With Massive Fat Embolism. J. Urol., 66:331–339, 1951.

150. Cheney, F.; Huang, T.; and Gronka, R.: Effects of Methylprednisolone on Experimental Pulmonary Injury. Ann. Surg., 190:236–242, 1979.

151. Cobb, C.A., Jr., and Hillman, J.W.: Fat Embolism. Instr. Course Lect., 18:122–129, 1961.

152. Collins, J.A.; Gordon, W.C., Jr.; Hudson, T.L.; Irvin, R.W., Jr.; Kelly, T.; and Hardaway, R.M., III: Inapparent Hypoxemia in Casualties With Wounded Limbs: Pulmonary Fat Embolism? Ann. Surg., 167:511–520, 1968.

153. Collins, J.A.; Hudson, T.L.; Hamacher, W.R.; Rokous, J.; Williams, G.; and Hardaway, R.M., III: Systemic Fat Embolism in Four Combat Casualties. Ann. Surg., 167:493–499, 1968.

154. Committee on Medical Aspects of Automotive Safety: Rating the Severity of Tissue Damage. J.A.M.A., 215:277–280, 1971.

155. Crocker, S.H.; Eddy, D.O.; Obenauf, R.N.; Wismar, B.L.; and Lowery, B.D.: Bacteremia: Host-Specific Lung Clearance and Pulmonary Failure. J. Trauma, 21:215–220, 1981.

156. Cuppage, F.E.: Fat Embolism in Diabetes Mellitus. Am. J. Clin. Pathol., 40:270–275, 1963.

157. Czerny, V.: Ueber die klinische Bedeutung der Fettembolie. Klin. Wochenschr., 12:593–595, 604–607, 1875.

158. Derian, P.S.: Fat Embolization—Current Status. J. Trauma, 5:580–586, 1965.

159. Divertie, M.B.: The Adult Respiratory Distress Syndrome. Mayo Clin. Proc., 57:371–378, 1982.

160. Drummond, D.S.; Salter, R.B.; and Boone, J.: Fat Embolism in Children: Its Frequency and Relationships to Collagen Disease. Can. Med. Assoc. J., 101:200–203, 1969.

161. Evarts, C.M.: Emerging Concepts of Fat Embolism. Clin. Orthop., 33:183–193, 1964.

162. Evarts, C.M.: Diagnosis and Treatment of Fat Embolism. J.A.M.A., 194:899–901, 1965.

163. Evarts, C.M.: The Fat Embolism Syndrome: A Review. Surg. Clin. North Am., 50:493–507, 1970.

164. Fabian, T.; Hoots, A.; Stanford, D.; Patterson, C.; and Mangiante, E.: Fat Embolism Syndrome: A Prospective Evaluation in 92 Fracture Patients. J. Trauma, 27:820–820, 1987.

165. Fenger, G., and Salisbury, J.H.: Diffuse Multiple Capillary Fat Embolism of the Lungs and Brain in a Fatal Complication in Common Fractures; Illustrated by a Case. Chicago Medical Journal, 39:587–595, 1879.

166. Field, M.: Fat Embolism From a Chronic Osteomyelitis. J.A.M.A., 59:2065–2066, 1912.

167. Fischer, J.F.; Turner, R.H.; Herndon, J.H.; and Riseborough, E.J.: Massive Steroid Therapy in Severe Fat Embolism. Surg. Gynecol. Obstet., 132:667–672, 1971.

168. Flick, M., and Murray, J.: High Dose Corticosteroid Therapy in the Adult Respiratory Distress Syndrome. J.A.M.A., 251:1054, 1984.

169. Fuschsig, P.; Brucke, P.; Blumel, G.; and Gottlob, R.: A New Clinical and Experimental Concept on Fat Metabolism. N. Engl. J. Med., 276:1192–1193, 1967.

170. Gauss, H.: Studies in Cerebral Fat Embolism: With Reference to the Pathology of Delirium and Coma. Arch. Intern. Med., 18:76–102, 1916.

171. Gauss, H.: The Pathology of Fat Embolism. Arch. Surg., 9:593–605, 1924.

172. Gerbershagen, H.U.: Fettembolie: Therapie mit niedrig viscosem Dextran. Anaesthesist, 21:23–25, 1972.

173. Goris, R.J.A.: The Injury Severity Score. World J. Surg., 7:12–18, 1983.

174. Goris, R.J.A., and Draaisma, J.: Causes of Death After Blunt Trauma. J. Trauma, 22:141, 1982.

175. Goris, R.J.A.; Gimbrere, J.S.F.; Van Niekerk, J.L.M.; Schoots, F.J.; and Body, L.H.D.: Early Osteosynthesis and Prophylactic Mechanical Ventilation in the Multitrauma Patient. J. Trauma, 22:895–903, 1982.

176. Gossling, H.R., and Pellegrini, V.D., Jr.: Fat Embolism Syndrome: A Review of the Pathophysiology and Physiological Basis of Treatment. Clin. Orthop., 165:68–82, 1982.

177. Graber, S.: Fat Embolization Associated With Sickle Cell Crisis. South Med. J., 54:1395–1398, 1961.

178. Gresham, G.A., Kuxzynski, A., and Rosborough, D.: Fatal Fat Embolism Following Replacement Arthroplasty for Transcervical Fractures of Femur. Br. Med. J., 2:617–619, 1971.

179. Grondahl, N.B.: Utersuchungen uber Fettembolie. Dtsch. Z. Chir., 111:56–124, 1911.

180. Gurd, A.R.: Fat Embolism: An Aid to Diagnosis. J. Bone Joint Surg., 52B:732–737, 1970.

181. Hammerschmidt, D.; Weaver, L.; Hudson, L.; Craddock, P.; and Jacob, H.: Association of Complement Activation and Elevated Plasma C5a With Adult Respiratory Distress Syndrome. Lancet, 1:947–949, 1980.

182. Hansen, S., and Winquist, R.: Closed Intramedullary Nailing of the Femur: Kuntscher Technique With Reaming. Clin. Orthop., 138:56–61, 1979.

183. Hausberger, F.X., and Whitenack, S.H.: Effect of Pressure on Intravasation of Fat From the Bone Marrow Cavity. Surg. Gynecol. Obstet., 134:931–936, 1972.

184. Haymaker, W., and Davison, C.: Fatalities Resulting From Exposure to Simulated High Altitudes in Decompression Chambers; Clinico-pathologic Study of 5 Cases. J. Neuropathol. Exp. Neurol., 9:29–59, 1950.

185. Hill, R.B., Jr.: Fatal Fat Embolism From Steroid-induced Fatty Liver. N. Engl. J. Med., 265:318–320, 1961.

186. Immelman, E.J.; Bank, S.; Krige, H.; and Marks, I.N.: Roentgenologic and Clinical Features of Intramedullary Fat Necrosis in Bones in Acute and Chronic Pancreatitis. Am. J. Med., 36:96–105, 1964.

187. Jacobs, R.R.; Wheeler, E.J.; Jelenko, C., III; McDonald, T.F.; and Bliven, F.E.: Fat Embolism: A Microscopic and Ultrastructure Evaluation of Two Animal Models. J. Trauma, 13:980–993, 1973.

188. Johnson, K.; Cadambi, A.; and Seibert, B.: Incidence of Adult Respiratory Distress Syndrome in Patients With Multiple Musculoskeletal Injuries: Effect of Early Operative Stabilization of Fractures. J. Trauma, 25:375–384, 1985.

189. Jones, J.P., Jr.; Engleman, E.P.; and Najarian, J.S.: Systemic Fat Embolism After Renal Homotransplantation and Treatment With Corticosteroids. N. Engl. J. Med., 273:1453–1458, 1965.

190. Kallenbach, J.; Lewis, M.; Zaltzman, M.; Feldman, C.; Orford, A.; and Zwi, S.: "Low-dose" Corticosteroid Prophylaxis Against Fat Embolism. J. Trauma, 27:1173–1176, 1987.

191. Kaplan, J.E., and Saba, T.M.: Humoral Deficiency and Reticuloendothelial Depression After Traumatic Shock. Am. J. Physiol., 230:7–14, 1976.

192. Kearns, T.P.: Fat Embolism of the Retina Demonstrated by Flat Retinal Preparation. Am. J. Ophthalmol., 41:1–2, 1956.

193. Kerstell, J.: Pathogenesis of Posttraumatic Fat Embolism. Am. J. Surg., 121:712–715, 1971.

194. Kerstell, J.; Hallgren, B.; Rudenstam, C.M.; and Svanborg, A.: 1. The Chemical Composition of the Fat Emboli in the Postabsorptive Dog. Acta Med. Scand. [Suppl.], 499:3–18, 1969.

195. King, E.G.; Weily, H.S.; Genton, E.; and Ashbaugh, D.G.: Consumption Coagulopathy in the Canine Oleic Acid Model of Fat Embolism. Surgery, 69:533–541, 1971.

196. Kraus, K.A.: Ueber Fettembolie des Gehirns nach Unfallen. Montasschr. Unfallheilkunde, 58:353–361, 1955.

197. Lachiewicz, P.F., and Ranawat, C.S.: Fat Embolism Syndrome Following Bilateral Total Knee Replacement With Total Condylar Prosthesis: A Report of Two Cases. Clin. Orthop., 160:106–108, 1981.

198. Lehman, E.P., and Moore, R.M.: Fat Embolism Including Experimental Production Without Trauma. Arch. Surg., 14:621–622, 1927.

199. LeQuire, V.S.; Hillman, J.W.; Gray, M.E.; and Snowden, R.T.: Clinical and Pathologic Studies of Fat Embolism. Instr. Course Lect., 19:12–35, 1970.

200. LeQuire, V.S.; Shapiro, J.L.; LeQuire, C.B.; Cobb, C.A., Jr.; and Fleet, W.F., Jr.: A Study of the Pathogenesis of Fat Embolism Based on Human Necropsy Material and Animal Experiments. Am. J. Pathol., 35:999–1016, 1959.

201. Limbird, T.J., and Ruderman, R.J.: Fat Embolism in Children. Clin. Orthop., 136:267–269, 1978.

202. Lindeque, B.; Schoeman, H.; Dommisse, G.; Boeyens, M.; and Vlok, A.: Fat Embolism and the Fat Embolism Syndrome: A Double-Blind Therapeutic Study. J. Bone Joint Surg., 69B:128–131, 1987.

203. Love, J., and Stryker, W.S.: Fat Embolism: A Problem of Increasing Importance to the Orthopedist and the Internist. Ann. Intern. Med., 46:342–351, 1957.

204. Lozman, J.; Deno, C.; Fenstel, P.; Newell, J.; Stratton, H.; Sedransk, N.; Dutton, R.; Fortune, J.; and Shah, D.: Pulmonary and Cardiovascular Consequences of Immediate Fixation or Conservative Management of Long Bone Fractures. Arch. Surg., 121:992–999, 1986.

205. Lynch, M.J.: Nephrosis and Fat Embolism in Acute Hemorrhagic Pancreatitis. Arch. Intern. Med., 94:709–717, 1964.

206. McCarthy, B.; Mammen, E.; Leblanc, L.P.; and Wilson, R.F.: Subclinical Fat Embolism: A Prospective Study of 50 Patients With Extremity Fractures. J. Trauma, 13:9–16, 1973.

207. Manning, J.; Bach, A.; Herman, C.; and Carrico, C.J.: Fat Release After Femur Nailing in the Dog. J. Trauma, 23:322–326, 1983.

208. Maruyama, Y., and Little, J.B.: Roentgen Manifestations of Traumatic Pulmonary Fat Embolism. Radiology, 79:945–952, 1962.

209. Meek, R.N.; Woodruff, B.; and Allardyce, D.B.: Source of Fat Macroglobules in Fractures of the Lower Extremity. J. Trauma, 12:432–434, 1972.

210. Meyers, R., and Taljaard, J.J.F.: Blood Alcohol and Fat Embolism Syndrome. J. Bone Joint Surg., 59A:878–880, 1977.

211. Miller, J.A.; Fonkalsrud, E.W.; Latta, H.L.; and Maloney, J.V., Jr.: Fat Embolism Associated With Extra-corporeal Circulation and Blood Transfusion. Surgery, 51:448–451, 1962.

212. Motamed, H.A.: Fundamental Aspects of Post-multiple Injury Fat Embolism. Clin. Orthop., 82:169–181, 1972.

213. O'Driscoll, M., and Powell, F.J.: Injury, Serum, Lipids, Fat Embolism, and Clofibrinate. Br. Med. J., 4:149–151, 1967.

214. Parker, F.B., Jr.; Wax, S.D.; Kusajima, K.; and Webb, W.R.: Hemodynamic and Pathological Findings in Experimental Fat Embolism. Arch. Surg., 108:70–74, 1974.

215. Pellegrini, V.D. Jr., and Evarts, C.M.: The Fat Embolism Syndrome. In C.M. Evarts (ed.): Surgery of the Musculoskeletal System, 2nd ed., pp. 37–54. New York, Churchill Livingstone, 1989.

216. Pellegrini, V.D., Jr., and Evarts, C.M.: The Fat Embolism Syndrome Revisited: Acute Respiratory Failure Complicating Elective Orthopaedic Surgery, unpublished.

217. Peltier, L.F.: Collective Review: An Appraisal of the Problem of Fat Embolism. Int. Abstr. Surg., 104:313–324, 1957.

218. Peltier, L.F.: The Diagnosis of Fat Embolism. Surg. Gynecol. Obstet., 121:371–379, 1965.

219. Peltier, L.F.: Fat Embolism. A Current Concept. Clin. Orthop., 66:241–253, 1969.

220. Peltier, L.F.: The Diagnosis and Treatment of Fat Embolism. J. Trauma, 11:661–667, 1971.

221. Peltier, L.F.; Adler, F.; and Lai, S.P.: Fat Embolism: The Significance of an Elevated Serum Lipase After Trauma to Bone. Am. J. Surg., 99:821–826, 1960.

222. Pipkin, G.: The Early Diagnosis and Treatment of Fat Embolism. Clin. Orthop., 12:171–182, 1958.

223. Renne, J.; Wurthier, R.; House, E.; Cancro, J.C.; and Hoaglund, F.T.: Fat Macroglobulemia Caused by Fractures or Total Hip Replacement. J. Bone Joint Surg., 60A:613–618, 1978.

224. Rinaldo, J.E., and Rogers, R.M.: Adult Respiratory Distress Syndrome. N. Engl. J. Med., 306(15):900–909, 1982.

225. Riska, E., and Myllynen, P.: Fat Embolism in Patients With Multiple Injuries. J. Trauma, 22:891, 1982.

226. Riska, E.; Von Bonsdorff, H.; Hakkinen, S.; Jaroma, H.; Kiviluoto, O.; and Paavilainen, T.: Prevention of Fat Embolism by Early Internal Fixation of Fractures in Patients With Multiple Injuries. Injury, 8:110, 1976.

227. Riska, E.; Von Bonsdorff, H.; Hakkinen, S.; Jaroma, H.; Kiviluoto, O.; and Paavilainen, T.: Primary Operative Fixation of Long Bone Fractures in Patients With Multiple Injuries. J. Trauma, 17:111–121, 1977.

228. Rokkanen, P.; Alho, A.; Avikainen, V.; Karaharju, E.; Kataja, J.; Lahdensuu, M.; Lepisto, P.; and Tervo, R.: The Efficacy of Corticosteroids in Severe Trauma. Surg. Gynecol. Obstet., 138:69–73, 1974.

229. Rokkanen, P.; Lahdensuu, M.; Kataja, J.; and Julkunen, H.: The Syndrome of Fat Embolism: Analysis of Thirty Consecutive Cases Compared to Trauma Patients With Similar Injuries. J. Trauma, 10:299–306, 1970.

230. Ruedi, T., and Wolff, G.: Vermeidung Postraumatischer Komplikationen Durch Fruhe Definitive Versorgung Von Polytraumatisierten mit Frakturen des Bewegungsapparats. Helv. Chir. Acta, 42:507, 1975.

231. Saldeen, T.: Fat Embolism and Signs of Intravascular Coagulation in a Posttraumatic Autopsy Material. J. Trauma, 10:273–286, 1970.

232. Schnaid, E.; Lamprey, J.; Viljoen, M.; Joffe, B.; and Seftel, H.: The Early Biochemical and Hormonal Profile of Patients With Long Bone Fractures at Risk of Fat Embolism Syndrome. J. Trauma, 27:309–311, 1987.

233. Schonfeld, S.; Ploysongsang, Y.; Dilisio, R.; Crissman, J.; Miller, E.; Hammerschmidt, D.; and Jacob, H.: Fat Embolism Prophylaxis With Corticosteroids: A Prospective Study in High Risk Patients. Ann. Intern. Med. 99:438, 1983.

234. Scriba, J.: Untersuchungen uber die Fettembolie. Leipzig, J.B. Hirschfeld, 1879.

235. Scuderi, C.S.: Fat Embolism: A Clinical and Experimental Study. Surg. Gynecol. Obstet., 72:732–746, 1941.

236. Seibel, R.; Laduca, J.; Hassett, J.; Babikian, G.; Mills, B.; Border, D.; and Border, J.: Blunt Multiple Trauma (ISS 36), Femur Traction, and the Pulmonary Failure-Septic State. Ann. Surg., 202:283–295, 1985.

237. Sevitt, S.: The Significance and Classification of Fat Embolism. Lancet, 2:825–828, 1960.

238. Sevitt, S.: Fat Embolism. London, Butterworth, 1962.

239. Sevitt, S.: Fat Embolism in Patients With Fractured Hips. Br. Med. J., 2:257–262, 1972.

240. Sevitt, S.; Clarke, R.; and Badger, F.G.: Modern Trends in Accident Surgery and Medicine. London, Butterworth, 1959.

241. Shier, M.; Wilson, R.; James, R.; Riddle, J.; Mammen, E.; and Pedersen, H.: Fat Embolism Prophylaxis: A Study of Four Treatment Modalities. J. Trauma, 17:621–629, 1977.

242. Soloway, H.B., and Robinson, E.F.: The Coagulation Mechanism in Experimental Pulmonary Fat Embolism. J. Trauma, 12:630–631, 1972.

243. Sproule, B.J.; Brady, J.L.; and Gilbert, J.A.L.: Studies on the Syndrome of Fat Embolization. Can. Med. Assoc. J., 90:1243–1247, 1964.

244. Stoltenberg, J.J., and Gustilo, R.B.: The Use of Methyl-prednisolone and Hypertonic Glucose in the Prophylaxis of Fat Embolism Syndrome. Clin. Orthop., 143:211–221, 1979.

245. Sutton, G.E.: Pulmonary Fat Embolism and Its Relation to Traumatic Shock. Br. Med. J., 2:368–370, 1918.

246. Talucci, R.; Manning, J.; Lampard, S.; Bach, A.; and Carrico, A.: Early Intramedullary Nailing of Femoral Shaft Fractures: A Cause of Fat Embolism Syndrome. Am. J. Surg., 146:107–111, 1983.

247. Tedeschi, C.G.; Walter, C.E.; Lepore, T.; and Tedeschi, L.G.: An Assessment of the Cerebrospinal Fluid and Choroid Plexus in Relation to Systemic Fat Embolism. Neurology, 19:586–590, 1969.

248. Tedeschi, C.G.; Walter, C.E.; and Tedeschi, L.G.: Shock and Fat Embolism: An Appraisal. Surg. Clin. North Am., 48:431–452, 1968.

249. Ten Duis, H.; Nijsten, M.; Klasen, H.; Binnendijk, B.: Fat Embolism in Patients With an Isolated Fracture of the Femoral Shaft. J. Trauma, 28:383–390, 1988.

250. Tennenberg, S.; Jacobs, M.; and Solomkin, J.: Complement-Mediated Neutrophil Activation in Sepsis- and Trauma-Related Adult Respiratory Distress Syndrome. Arch. Surg., 122:26–32, 1987.

251. Thomas, J.E., and Ayyar, D.R.: Systemic Fat Embolism: A Diagnostic Profile in 24 Patients. Arch. Neurol., 26:517–523, 1972.

252. Trentz, O.; Oesteru, H.J.; Hempelmann, G.; et al.: Kriterien fur die Operabilitat von Polytraumatisierten. Unfallheilkunde, 81:451, 1978.

253. Vance, B.M.: The Significance of Fat Embolism. Arch. Surg., 23:426–465, 1931.

254. Van Der Merwe, C.; Louw, A.; Welthagen, D.; and Schoeman, H.: Adult Respiratory Distress Syndrome in Cases of Severe Trauma—The Prophylactic Value of Methyl-prednisolone Sodium Succinate. South Afr. Med. J., 67:279–284, 1985.

255. Wagner, E.: Die Fettembolie der Lungencapillaren. Arch. Heilk., 6:369–381, 1865.

256. Warner, W.A.: Release of Free Fatty Acids Following Trauma. J. Trauma, 9:692–699, 1969.

257. Warthin, A.S.: Traumatic Lipaemia and Fatty Embolism. Int. Clin., 4:171–227, 1913.

258. Weinberg, H., and Finsterbush, A.: Fat Embolism: Vascular Damage to Bone Due to Blunt Trauma. Intraosseous Phlebography Study. Clin. Orthop., 83:273–278, 1972.

259. Weisz, G.M.: Fat Embolism: Current Problems in Surgery. Chicago, Year Book Medical Publishing, 1974.

260. Weisz, G.M., and Barellai, A.: Nonfulminant Fat Embolism: Review of Concepts on Its Genesis and Orthophysiology. Anesth. Analg., 52:303–309, 1973.

261. Weisz, G.M.; Rang, M.; and Salter, R.B.: Posttraumatic Fat Embolism in Children: Review of the Literature and of Experience in the Hospital for Sick Children, Toronto. J. Trauma, 13:529–534, 1973.

262. Weisz, G.M., and Steiner, E.: The Cause of Death in Fat Embolism. Chest, 59:511–516, 1971.

263. Wilson, J.V., and Salisbury, C.V.: Fat Embolism in War Surgery. Br. J. Surg., 31:384–392, 1944.

264. Wolff, G.; Dittman, M.; Ruedi, Th.; et. al.: Koordination von Chirurgie und Intensivmedizin zur Vermeidung der

Posttraumatischen Respiratorische Insuffizienze. Unfall-hielkunde 81:425, 1978.

265. Zenker, F.A.: Beitrage zur Anatomie und Physiologie der Lunge, Dresden. J. Braunsdorf, 1861.

Hemorrhagic Complications

266. Bachman, F.: Plasminogen Activators. *In* Colman, R.W.; Hirsh, J.; Marder, V.J.; and Salzman, E.W. (eds.): Hemostasis and Thrombosis. Basic Principles and Clinical Practice, 2nd ed., pp. 318–339. Philadelphia, J.B. Lippincott, 1987.

267. Boey, M.L.; Colaco, C.B.; Gharavi, A.E.; Elkon, K.B.; Loizou, E.; and Hughes, G.R.V.: Thrombosis in Systemic Lupus Erythematosus: Striking Association With the Presence of Circulating Lupus Anticoagulant. Br. Med. J., 287:1021–1023, 1983.

268. Bowie, E.J.; and Owen, C.A., Jr.: The Significance of Abnormal Preoperative Hemostatic Tests. *In* Spaet, T.H. (ed.): Progress in Hemostasis and Thrombosis, Vol. 5, pp. 179. New York, Grune & Stratton, 1980.

269. Brettler, D.B.; and Levine, P.H.: Factor Concentrates for Treatment of Hemophilia: Which One to Choose? Blood, 73:2067–2073, 1989.

270. Centers for Disease Control: Update on Acquired Immune Deficiency Syndrome (AIDS) Among Patients With Hemophilia. M.M.W.R., 31:644–652, 1982.

271. Clouse, L.H., and Comp, P.C.: The Regulation of Hemostasis: The Protein C System. N. Engl. J. Med., 314:1298–1304, 1986.

272. Collen, D.: On the Regulation and Control of Fibrinolysis. Thromb. Haemost., 43:77–89, 1980.

273. Colman, R.W.; Hirsh, J.; Marder, V.J.; and Salzman, E.W. (eds.): Hemostasis and Thrombosis: Basic Principles and Clinical Practice, 2nd ed., pp. 1–65. Philadelphia, J.B. Lippincott, 1987.

274. Consensus Development Conference: Platelet Transfusion Therapy. J.A.M.A., 257:1777–1780, 1987.

275. Counts, R.B.; Haisch, C.; Simon, T.L.; Maxwell, N.G.; Heimbach, D.M.; and Carrico, C.J.: Hemostasis in Massively Transfused Trauma Patients. Ann. Surg., 190:91–99, 1979.

276. Francis, C.W., and Marder, V.J.: Physiologic Regulation and Pathologic Disorders of Fibrinolysis. Hum. Pathol., 18:263–274, 1987.

277. Francis, C.W., and Marder, V.J.: Physiologic Regulation and Pathologic Disorders of Fibrinolysis. *In* Colman, R.W.; Hirsh, J.; Marder, V.J.; and Salzman, E.W. (eds.): Hemostasis and Thrombosis. Basic Principles and Clinical Practice, 2nd ed., pp. 358–379. Philadelphia, J.B. Lippincott, 1987.

278. Fuente, (de la) B.; Kasper, C.K.; Rickles, F.R.; and Hoyer, L.W.: Response of Patients With Mild and Moderate Hemophilia A and von Willebrand's Disease to Treatment With Desmopressin. Ann. Intern. Med., 103:6–14, 1985.

279. Harker, L.A., and Slichter, S.J.: The Bleeding Time as a Screening Test for Evaluation of Platelet Function. N. Engl. J. Med., 287:155–159, 1972.

280. Hedner, U., and Kisiel, W.: Use of Human Factor VIIa in the Treatment of Two Hemophilia A Patients With High-Titer Inhibitors. J. Clin. Invest., 71:1836–1841, 1983.

281. Hoyer, L.W.: Review: The Factor VIII Complex: Structure and Function. Blood, 58:1–13, 1981.

282. Levine, P.H.: The Clinical Manifestations and Therapy of Hemophilias A and B. *In* Colman, R.W.; Hirsh, J.; Marder, V.J.; and Salzman, E.W. (eds.): Hemostasis and Thrombosis: Basic Principles and Clinical Practice, 2nd ed., pp. 97–111. Philadelphia, J.B. Lippincott, 1987.

283. Lusher, E.B.: Factor VIII Inhibitors: Etiology, Characterization, Natural History and Management. Ann. N.Y. Acad. Sci., 509:89–102, 1987.

284. Lusher, J.M.; Shapiro, S.S.; Palaszak, J.E.; Rao, A.J.; Levine, P.H.; and Blatt, P.M.: Efficacy of Prothrombin-Complex Concentrates in Hemophiliacs With Antibodies to Factor VIII: A Multicenter Therapeutic Trial. N. Engl. J. Med., 303:421–425, 1980.

285. Marlar, R.A.; Kleiss, A.J.; and Griffin, J.H.: An Alternative Extrinsic Pathway of Human Blood Coagulation. Blood, 60:1353–1358, 1982.

286. Nemerson, Y.: Tissue Factor and Hemostasis. Blood, 71:1–8, 1988.

287. Packham, M.A., and Mustard, J.F.: Platelet Adhesion. Prog. Hemost. Thromb., 7:211–288, 1984.

288. Rapaport, S.: Preoperative Hemostatic Evaluation: Which Tests, If Any? Blood, 61:229–231, 1983.

289. Rapaport, S.I.: Inhibition of Factor VIIa/Tissue Factor-Induced Blood Coagulation: With Particular Emphasis Upon a Factor Xa-Dependent Inhibitory Mechanism. Blood, 73:359–365, 1989.

290. Rosenberg, R.D.: Actions and Interactions of Antithrombin and Heparin. N. Engl. J. Med., 292:146–151, 1975.

291. Ruggeri, Z.M., and Zimmerman, T.S.: von Willebrand Factor and von Willebrand Disease. Blood, 70:895–904, 1987.

292. Shapiro, S.S., and Hultin, M.: Acquired Inhibitors to the Blood Coagulation Factors. Semin. Thromb. Hemost., 1:336–385, 1975.

293. Weiss, H.J.: Platelet Physiology and Abnormalities of Platelet Function. N. Engl. J. Med., 293:531–541, 1975.

Disseminated Intravascular Coagulation

294. Bick, R.: Clinical Relevance of Antithrombin III. Semin. Thromb. Hemost., 8(4), 1982.

295. Bick, R.L.; Bick, M.D.; and Fekete, L.F.: Antithrombin III Patterns in Disseminated Intravascular Coagulation. Am. J. Clin. Pathol., 73:577–583, 1980.

296. Breen, F.A., and Tullis, J.L.: Ethanol Gelatin: A Rapid Screening Test for Intravascular Coagulation. Ann. Intern. Med., 69:1197–1206, 1968.

297. Colman, R.W.; Robboy, S.J.; and Minna, J.D.: Disseminated Intravascular Coagulation: A Reappraisal. Annu. Rev. Med., 30:359–374, 1979.

298. Feinstein, D.I.: Diagnosis and Management of Disseminated Intravascular Coagulation: The Role of Heparin Therapy. Blood, 60:284–287, 1982.

299. Marder, V.J.; Martin, S.E.; Francis, C.W.; and Colman, R.W.: Consumptive Thrombohemorrhagic Disorders. *In* Colman, R.W.; Hirsh, J.; Marder, V.J.; and Salzman, E.W. (eds.): Hemostasis and Thrombosis: Basic Principles and Clinical Practice, 2nd ed., pp. 975–1015. Philadelphia, J.B. Lippincott, 1987.

300. Marder, V.J., and Shulman, N.R.: High Molecular Weight Derivatives of Human Fibrinogen Produced by Plasmin, II. Mechanism of Their Anticoagulant Activity. J. Biol. Chem., 244:2120–2124, 1969.

301. Niewiarowski, S., and Gurewich, V.: Laboratory Identification of Intravascular Coagulation: The Serial Dilution Protamine Sulfate Test for the Detection of Fibrin Monomer and Fibrin Degradation Products. J. Lab. Clin. Med., 77:665–676, 1971.

302. Rickles, F.R., and Edwards, R.L.: Activation of Blood Coagulation in Cancer: Trousseau's Syndrome Revisited. Blood, 62:14–31, 1983.

303. Rubenberg, M.L.; Regoeczi, E.; Bull, B.S.; Dacie, J.V.; and Brain, M.C.: Microangiopathic Haemolytic Anaemia: The Experimental Production of Haemolysis and Red-cell Fragmentation by Defibrination in Vivo. Br. J. Haematol., 14:627–642, 1968.

304. Sack, G.H.; Levin, J.; and Bell, W.R.: Trousseau's Syndrome and Other Manifestations of Chronic Disseminated Coagulopathy in Patients With Neoplasms: Clinical, Pathologic and Therapeutic Features. Medicine (Baltimore), 56:1–37, 1977.

305. Siegal, T.; Seligsohn, U.; Aghai, E.; and Modan, M.: Clinical and Laboratory Aspects of Disseminated Intravascular Coagulation (DIC). A Study of 118 Cases. Thromb. Haemost., 39:122–134, 1978.

306. Spero, J.A.; Lewis, J.H.; and Hasiba, U.: Disseminated Intravascular Coagulation. Findings in 346 Patients. Thromb. Haemost., 43:28–33, 1980.

Thromboembolism

307. Amstutz, H.; Friscia, D.; Dorey, F.; and Carney, B.: Warfarin Prophylaxis to Prevent Mortality From Pulmonary Embolism After Total Hip Replacement. J. Bone Joint Surg., 71A:321–326, 1989.

308. Arfors, K.E.; Hint, H.C.; Dhall, D.P.; and Matheson, N.A.: Counteraction of Platelet Activity at Sites of Laser-Induced Endothelial Trauma. Br. Med. J., 4:430–431, 1968.

309. Atkins, P., and Hawkins, L.A.: The Diagnosis of Deep-vein Thrombosis in the Leg Using 125I-Fibrinogen. Br. J. Surg., 55:825–830, 1968.

310. Barber, F.A.; Burton, W.; and Guyer, R.: The Heparin-Induced Thrombocytopenia and Thrombosis Syndrome. Report of a Case. J. Bone Joint Surg., 69A:935–937, 1987.

311. The Behavior of Thrombi. Arch. Surg., 105:681–682, 1972.

312. Beisaw, N.; Comerota, A.; Groth, H.; Merli, G.; Weitz, H.; Zimmerman, R.; Diseria, F.; and Sasahara, A.: Dihydroergotamine/Heparin in the Prevention of Deep Vein Thrombosis After Total Hip Replacement. A Controlled Prospective Randomized Multicenter Trial. J. Bone Joint Surg., 70A:2–10, 1988.

313. Bergentz, S.E.: Dextran in the Prophylaxis of Pulmonary Embolism. World J. Surg., 2:19–25, 1978.

314. Bergentz, S.E.; Gelin, L.E.; and Rudenstam, C.M.: Fats and Thrombus Formation. An Experimental Study. Thromb. Diath. Haemorrh., 5:474–479, 1961.

315. Bergqvist, D.; Efsing, H.L.; Hallbook, T.; and Hendlund, T.: Thromboembolism After Elective and Post-Traumatic Hip Surgery—A Controlled Prophylactic Trial With Dextran 70 and Low Dose Heparin. Acta Chir. Scand., 145:213–218, 1979.

316. Bergqvist, D.: Dextran in the Prophylaxis of Deep-Vein Thrombosis. J.A.M.A., 258:324–324, 1987.

317. Berman, H.J.: Anticoagulant-induced Alterations in Hemostasis, Platelet Thrombosis, and Vascular Fragility in the Peripheral Vessels of the Hamster Cheek Pouch. In Macmillan, R.L., and Mustard, J.F. (eds.): International Symposium: Anticoagulants and Fibrinolysins, pp. 95–107. Philadelphia, Lea & Febiger, 1961.

318. Bloom, W.L.: Present Status of Plasma Volume Expanders in the Treatment of Shock. Clinical Laboratory Studies. Arch. Surg., 63:739–741, 1951.

319. Bookstein, J.J.: Segmental Arteriography in Pulmonary Embolism. Radiology, 93:1007–1012, 1969.

320. Borgstrom, S.; Gelin, L.; and Zederfeldt, B.: The Formation of Vein Thrombi Following Tissue Injury: An Experimental Study in Rabbits. Acta Chir. Scand. [Suppl.], 247:1–36, 1959.

321. Borow, M., and Goldson, H.: Postoperative Venous Thrombosis. Am. J. Surg., 141:245–251, 1981.

322. Browse, N.L.: The 125I-Fibrinogen Uptake Test. Arch. Surg., 104:160–163, 1972.

323. Bull, J.P.; Ricketts, D.; Squire, J.R.; Maycock, W. d'A.; Spooner, S.J.L.; Mollison, P.L.; and Paterson, J.C.S.: Dextran as a Plasma Substitute. Lancet, 1:134–143, 1949.

324. Bydgeman, S., and Eliasson, R.: Effect of Dextrans on Platelet Adhesiveness and Aggregation. Scand. J. Clin. Lab. Invest., 20:17–23, 1967.

325. Bydgeman, S.; Eliasson, R.; and Gullbring, B.: Effect of Dextran Infusion on the Adenosine Diphosphate Induced Adhesiveness and the Spreading Capacity of Human Blood Platelets. Thromb. Diath. Haemorrh., 15:451–456, 1966.

326. Bydgeman, S.; Eliasson, R.; and Johnson, S.R.: Relationship Between Postoperative Changes in Adenosine Diphosphate Induced Platelet Adhesiveness and Venous Thrombosis. Lancet, 1:1301–1302, 1966.

327. Cheely, R.; McCartney, W.H.; Perry, J.R.; Delany, D.J.; Bustad, L.; Wynia, V.H.; and Griggs, T.R.: The Role of Noninvasive Tests Versus Pulmonary Angiography in the Diagnosis of Pulmonary Embolism. Am. J. Med., 70:17–22, 1981.

328. Collins, R.; Scrimgeour, A.; Yusuf, S.; and Peto, R.: Reduction in Fatal Pulmonary Embolism and Venous Thrombosis by Perioperative Administration of Subcutaneous Heparin. Overview of Results of Randomized Trials in General, Orthopaedic, and Urologic Surgery. N. Engl. J. Med., 318:1162–1173, 1988.

329. Coon, W.W., and Coller, F.A.: Some Epidemiologic Considerations of Thromboembolism. Surg. Gynecol. Obstet., 109:487–501, 1959.

330. Coon, W.W., and Willis, P.W., III: Deep Venous Thrombosis and Pulmonary Embolism. Prediction, Prevention and Treatment. Am. J. Cardiol., 4:611–621, 1959.

331. Couch, N.P.: Guest Editor's Introduction. A.M.A. Archives Symposium on Diagnostic Techniques in Phlebothrombosis. Arch. Surg., 104:132–133, 1972.

332. Crandon, A.J.; Peel, V.R.; Anderson, J.A.; Thompson, V.; and McNicol, G.P.: Postoperative Deep Vein Thrombosis.

Identifying High Risk Patients. Br. Med. J., 281:343–344, 1980.

333. Cronan, J.; Dorfman, G.; and Grusmark, J.: Lower Extremity Deep Venous Thrombosis: Further Experience With and Refinements of Ultrasound Assessment. Radiology, 168:101–107, 1988.

334. Culver, D.; Crawford, J.S.; Gardiner, J.H.; and Wiley, A.M.: Venous Thrombosis After Fractures of the Upper End of the Femur. A Study of Incidence and Site. J. Bone Joint Surg., 52B:61–69, 1970.

335. Davis, F.M., and Qunice, M.: Deep Vein Thrombosis and Anaesthetic Technique in Emergency Hip Surgery. Br. Med. J., 281:1528–1529, 1980.

336. DeLee, J.C., and Rockwood, C.A., Jr.: Current Concepts Review. The Use of Aspirin in Thromboembolic Disease. J. Bone Joint Surg., 62A:149–152, 1980.

337. DeWeese, J.A., and Rogoff, S.M.: Clinical Uses of Functional Ascending Phlebography of the Lower Extremity. Angiology, 9:268–278, 1958.

338. Deykin, D.: Thrombogenesis. N. Engl. J. Med., 276:622–628, 1967.

339. Deykin, D.: Emerging Concepts of Platelet Function. N. Engl. J. Med., 290:144–151, 1974.

340. Dorfman, G.; Cronan, J.; Tupper, T.; Messersmith, R.; Denny, D.; and Lee, C.: Occult Pulmonary Embolism: A Common Occurrence in Deep Venous Thrombosis. Am. J. Radiol., 148:263–266, 1987.

341. Effect of Aspirin on Postoperative Venous Thrombosis. Lancet, 2:441–444, 1972.

342. Ernst, C.B.; Fry, W.J.; Fraft, R.O.; and DeWeese, M.S.: The Role of Low Molecular Weight Dextran in the Management of Venous Thrombosis. Surg. Gynecol. Obstet., 119:1243–1247, 1964.

343. Eskeland, G.; Solheim, K.; and Skjorten, F.: Anticoagulant Prophylaxis, Thromboembolism and Mortality in Elderly Patients With Hip Fractures. Acta Chir. Scand., 131:16–29, 1966.

344. Evans, G., and Mustard, J.F.: Platelet-surface Reaction and Thrombosis. Surgery, 64:273–280, 1968.

345. Evarts, C.M.: Low Molecular Weight Dextran. Med. Clin. North Am., 51:1285–1299, 1967.

346. Evarts, C.M.: Thromboembolic Disease. Instr. Course Lect., 28:67–71, 1979.

347. Evarts, C.M., and Alfidi, R.J.: Thromboembolism After Total Hip Reconstruction. Failure of Low Doses of Heparin in Prevention. J.A.M.A., 225:515–516, 1973.

348. Evarts, C.M., and Feil, E.I.: Prevention of Thromboembolic Disease After Elective Surgery of the Hip. J. Bone Joint Surg., 53A:1271–1280, 1971.

349. Fagan, D.G.: Prevention of Thromboembolic Phenomena Following Operations on the Neck of the Femur. Lancet, 1:846–848, 1964.

350. Fahmy, N., and Patel, D.: Hemostatic Changes and Postoperative Deep Vein Thrombosis Associated With Use of a Pneumatic Tourniquet. J. Bone Joint Surg., 63A:461–465, 1981.

351. Fitts, W.T., Jr.; Lehr, H.B.; Bitner, R.L.; and Spelman, J.W.: An Analysis of 950 Fatal Injuries. Surgery, 56:663–668, 1964.

352. Flanc, C.; Kakkar, V.V.; and Clarke, M.B.: The Detection of Venous Thrombosis of the Legs Using ^{125}I-labeled Fibrinogen. Br. J. Surg., 55:742–747, 1968.

353. Flinn, W.; Sandager, G.; Cerullo, L.; Havey, R.; and Yao, R.: Duplex Venous Scanning for the Prospective Surveillance of Perioperative Venous Thrombosis. Arch. Surg., 124:901–905, 1989.

354. Francis, C.W.; Pellegrini, V.D., Jr.; Harris, C.; and Marder, V.: Antithrombin III Prophylaxis of Venous Thromboembolic Disease After Total Hip or Knee Replacement. Am. J. Med., 87(3B):615–665, 1989.

355. Francis, C.W.; Pellegrini, V.; Marder, V.; Harris, C.; Totterman, S.; Gabriel, K.; Baughman, D.; Roemer, S.; Burke, J.; Goodman, J.; and Evarts, C.: Prevention of Venous Thrombosis After Total Hip Arthroplasty. Antithrombin III and Low-Dose Heparin Compared With Dextran 40. J. Bone Joint Surg., 71A:327–335, 1989.

356. Francis, C.W.; Marder, V.J.; Evarts, C.M.; and Yaukoolbodi, S.: Two Step Warfarin Therapy. Prevention of Postoperative Venous Thrombosis Without Excessive Bleeding. J.A.M.A., 249(3):374–378, 1983.

357. Freeark, R.J.; Bostwick, J.; and Fardin, R.: Posttraumatic Venous Thrombosis. Arch. Surg., 95:567–575, 1967.

358. Froehlich, J.; Dorfman, G.; Cronan, J.; Urbanek, P.; Herndon, J.; and Aaron, R.: Compression Ultrasonography for the Detection of Deep Venous Thrombosis in Patients Who Have a Fracture of the Hip. A Prospective Study. J. Bone Joint Surg., 71A:249–256, 1989.

359. Fulton, G.P.; Akers, R.P.; and Lutz, B.R.: White Thromboembolism and Vascular Fragility in the Hamster Cheek Pouch After Anticoagulants. Blood, 8:140–152, 1953.

360. Gallus, A.S., and Hirsh, J.: Prevention and Treatment of Venous Thromboembolism. Semin. Thromb. Hemost., 11(4):291–331, 1976.

361. Gallus, A.S.; Hirsh, J.; Tuttle, R.J.; Trebilcock, R.; O'Brine, S.E.; Carroll, J.J.; Minden, J.H.; and Hudecki, S.M.: Small Subcutaneous Doses of Heparin in Prevention of Venous Thrombosis. N. Engl. J. Med., 288:545–551, 1973.

362. Genton, E.: Management of Venous Thromboembolism. Adv. Cardiol., 27:305–312, 1980.

363. Gitel, S.N.; Salvati, E.A.; Wessler, S.; Robinson, H.J., Jr.; and Worth, M.N.: The Effect of Total Hip Replacement and General Surgery on Antithrombin III in Relation to Venous Thrombosis. J. Bone Joint Surg., 61A:653–656, 1979.

364. Golodner, H.; Morse, L.J.; and Angrist, A.: Pulmonary Embolism in Fractures of the Hip. Surgery, 18:418–423, 1945.

365. Gronwall, A., and Ingleman, B.: Dextran as a Volume Expander. Acta Physiol. Scand., 7:97–107, 1944.

366. Hamilton, H.W.; Crawford, J.S.; Gardiner, J.H.; and Wiley, A.M.: Venous Thrombosis in Patients With Fracture of the Upper End of the Femur. A Phlebographic Study of the Effect of Prophylactic Anticoagulation. J. Bone Joint Surg., 52B:268–289, 1970.

367. Hampson, W.G.J.; Lucas, H.K.; Harris, F.C.; Roberts, P.H.; McCall, I.W.; Jackson, P.C.; Powell, N.L.; and Staddon, G.E.: Failure of Low-dose Heparin to Prevent Deep-vein Thrombosis After Hip Replacement Arthroplasty. Lancet, 2:795–797, 1974.

368. Harris, W.H.; Athanasoulis, C.; Waltman, A.; and Salzman,

E.: High and Low Dose Aspirin Prophylaxis Against Venous Thromboembolic Disease in Total Hip Replacement. J. Bone Joint Surg., 64A:63–66, 1982.

369. Harris, W.H.; Salzman, E.W.; Athanasoulis, C.A.; Waltman, A.C.; and DeSanctis, R.W.: Aspirin Prophylaxis of Venous Thromboembolism. N. Engl. J. Med., 297:1246–1248, 1977.

370. Harris, W.H.; Salzman, E.W.; and DeSanctis, R.W.: The Prevention of Thromboembolic Disease by Prophylactic Anticoagulation. A Controlled Study in Elective Hip Surgery. J. Bone Joint Surg., 49:81–89, 1967.

371. Harris, W.H.; Saltzman, E.W.; DeSanctis, R.W.; and Coutts, R.D.: Prevention of Venous Thromboembolism Following Total Hip Replacement. J.A.M.A., 220:1319–1322, 1972.

372. Hartman, J.T.; Pugh, J.; Smith, R.; Robertson, W.; Yost, R.; and Janssen, H.: Cyclic Sequential Compression of the Lower Limb in Prevention of Deep Venous Thrombosis. J. Bone Joint Surg., 64A:1059–1062, 1982.

373. Hildner, F.J., and Ormand, R.S.: Accuracy of the Clinical Diagnosis of Pulmonary Embolism. J.A.M.A., 202:567–570, 1967.

374. Hirsh, J.: The Clinical Role of Antiplatelet Agents. Drug Ther., 6:63–74, 1981.

375. Hirsh, J.: Therapeutic Range for the Control of Oral Anticoagulant Therapy. Arch. Intern. Med., 145:1187–1188, 1985.

376. Hirsh, J.: The Optimal Intensity of Oral Anticoagulant Therapy. J.A.M.A., 258:2723–2726, 1987.

377. Hirsh, J., and McBride, J.A.: Increased Platelet Adhesiveness in Recurrent Venous Thrombosis and Pulmonary Embolism. Br. Med. J., 2:797–799, 1965.

378. Huisman, M.; Buller, H.; Ten Cate, J.; and Vreeken, J.: Serial Impedance Plethysmography for Suspected Deep Venous Thrombosis in Outpatients. The Amsterdam General Practitioner Study. N. Engl. J. Med., 314:823–828, 1986.

379. Hull, R.; Hirsch, J.; Jay, R.; Carter, C.; England, C.; Gent, M.; Turpie, A.; McLoughlin, D.; Dogg, P.; Thomas, M.; Raskob, G.; and Okelford, P.: Different Intensities of Oral Anticoagulant Therapy in the Treatment of Proximal Vein Thrombosis. N. Engl. J. Med., 307:1676–1681, 1982.

380. Hull, R.D., and Raskob, G.E.: Current Concepts Review. Prophylaxis of Venous Thromboembolic Disease Following Hip and Knee Surgery. J. Bone Joint Surg., 68A:146–150, 1986.

381. Hull, R.; Raskob, G.; Hirsh, J.; Jay, R.; Leclerc, J.; Geerts, W.; Rosenbloom, D.; Sackett, D.; Anderson, C.; Harrison, L.; and Gent, M.: Continuous Intravenous Heparin Compared With Intermittent Subcutaneous Heparin in the Initial Treatment of Proximal Vein Thrombosis. N. Engl. J. Med., 315:1109–1114, 1986.

382. Hume, M.; Sevitt, S.; and Thomas, D.P.: Venous Thrombosis and Pulmonary Embolism, pp. 1–447. Cambridge, Mass., Harvard University Press, 1970.

383. Jennings, J.J., and Harris, W.H.: A Clinical Evaluation of Aspirin Prophylaxis of Thromboembolic Disease After Total Hip Arthroplasty. J. Bone Joint Surg., 58A:926–927, 1976.

384. Just-Viera, J.O., and Yeager, G.H.: Protection From

Thrombosis in Large Veins. Surg. Gynecol. Obstet., 118:354–360, 1964.

385. Kakkar, V.: The Diagnosis of Deep Vein Thrombosis Using the ^{125}I-Fibrinogen Test. Arch. Surg., 104:152–159, 1972.

386. Kakkar, V.; Fok, P.; Murray, W.; Paes, T.; Merenstein, D.; Dodds, R.; Farrell, R.; Crellin, R.; Thomas, E.; Morley, T.; and Price, A.: Heparin and Dihydroergotamine Prophylaxis Against Thromboembolism After Hip Arthroplasty. J. Bone Joint Surg., 67B:538–542, 1985.

387. Kakkar, V.V.; Howe, C.T.; Flanc, C.; and Clarke, M.B.: Natural History of Postoperative Deep Vein Thrombosis. Lancet, 2:230–232, 1969.

388. Kakkar, V.V.; Spindler, J.; Flute, P.T.; Corrigan, T.; Fossard, D.P.; Crellin, R.Q.; Wessler, S.; and Yin, E.T.: Efficacy of Low Doses of Heparin in Prevention of Deep Vein Thrombosis After Major Surgery. Lancet, 2:101–106, 1972.

389. Kim, Y.H., and Suh, J-S.: Low Incidence of Deep Vein Thrombosis After Cementless Total Hip Replacement. J. Bone Joint Surg., 70A:878–882, 1988.

390. Koekenberg, L.J.L.: Experimental Use of Macrodex as a Prophylaxis Against Postoperative Thromboembolism. Bull. Soc. Int. Chir., 21:501–512, 1962.

391. Landefeld, C.S., and Goldman, L.: Major Bleeding in Outpatients Treated With Warfarin: Incidence and Prediction by Factors Known at the Start of Outpatient Therapy. Am. J. Med., 87:144–152, 1989.

392. Landefeld, C.S.; Rosenblatt, M.; and Goldman, L.: Bleeding in Outpatients Treated With Warfarin: Relation to Prothrombin Time and Important Remediable Lesions. Am. J. Med., 87:153–159, 1989.

393. Langsjoen, P., and Murray, R.A.: Treatment of Postsurgical Thromboembolic Complications. J.A.M.A., 218:855–860, 1971.

394. Laufman, H.: Deep Vein Thrombophlebitis. Current Status of Etiology and Treatment. Arch. Surg., 99:489–493, 1969.

395. Lensing, A.; Prandoni, P.; Brandjes, D.; Huisman, P.; Vigo, M.; Tomasella, G.; Krekt, J.; Ten Cate, J.; Huisman, M.; and Buller, H.: Detection of Deep Vein Thrombosis by Real Time B-mode Ultrasonography. N. Engl. J. Med., 320:342–345, 1989.

396. Leyvraz, P.; Richard, J.; Bachmann, F.; Van Melle, G.; Treyvaud, J.; Livio, J.; and Candarjis, G.: Adjusted Versus Fixed Dose Subcutaneous Heparin in the Prevention of Deep Vein Thrombosis After Total Hip Replacement. N. Engl. J. Med., 309:954–958, 1983.

397. Lotke, P.; Ecker, M.; Alavi, A.; and Berkowitz, H.: Indications for the Treatment of Deep Venous Thrombosis Following Total Knee Replacement. J. Bone Joint Surg., 66A:202–208, 1984.

398. Lowe, L.L.: Venous Thrombosis and Embolism. J. Bone Joint Surg., 63B:155–167, 1981.

399. Lynch, A.; Bourne, R.; Rorabeck, C.; Rankin, R.; and Donald, A.: Deep Vein Thrombosis and Continuous Passive Motion After Total Knee Arthroplasty. J. Bone Joint Surg., 70A:11–14, 1988.

400. McBride, K.; LaMorte, W.; and Menzoian, J.: Can Ventilation-Perfusion Scans Accurately Diagnose Acute Pulmonary Embolism? Arch. Surg., 121:754–757, 1986.

401. MacLean, L.D.; Shibara, H.R.; McLean, A.P.H.; Skinner, G.B.; and Gutelius, J.R.: Pulmonary Embolism; the Value of Bedside Scanning, Angiography and Pulmonary Embolectomy. Can. Med. Assoc. J., 97:991–1000, 1967.

402. Mansfield, A.O.: Alteration in Fibrinolysis Associated With Surgery and Venous Thrombosis. Br. J. Surg., 59:754–757, 1972.

403. Marks, J.; Truscott, B.M.; and Withycombe, J.F.R.: Treatment of Venous Thrombosis With Anticoagulants. Review of 1135 Cases. Lancet, 2:787–791, 1954.

404. Matsuda, M.; Sugo, T.; Sakata, Y.; Murayama, H.; Mimuro, J.; Tanabe, S.; and Yoshitake, S.: A Thrombotic State Due to an Abnormal Protein C. N. Engl. J. Med., 319:1265–1268, 1988.

405. Mavor, G.E., and Galloway, J.M.: Iliofemoral Venous Thrombosis. Pathological Considerations and Surgical Management. Br. J. Surg., 56:45–49, 1969.

406. Medical Letter, The: Dihydroergotamine-Heparin to Prevent Postoperative Deep Vein Thrombosis. Med. Lett. Drugs Ther., 27(688):45–46, 1985.

407. Miletich, J.; Sherman, L.; and Broze, G.: Absence of Thrombosis in Subjects With Heterozygous Protein C Deficiency. N. Engl. J. Med., 317:991–996, 1987.

408. Miller, G.A.H.: The Diagnosis and Management of Massive Pulmonary Embolism. Br. J. Surg., 59:837–839, 1972.

409. Mishkin, F.: Lung Scanning: Its Use in Diagnosis of Disorders of the Pulmonary Circulation. Arch. Intern. Med., 118:65–69, 1966.

410. Mobin-Uddin, K.; McLean, R.; Bolloki, H.; and Jude, J.R.: Caval Interruption for Prevention of Pulmonary Embolism. Arch. Surg., 99:711–715, 1969.

411. Mohr, D.; Ryu, J.; Litin, S.; and Rosenow, E.: Recent Advances in the Management of Venous Thromboembolism. Mayo Clin. Proc., 63:281–290, 1988.

412. Monreal, M.; LaFoz, E.; Navarro, A.; Granero, X.; Caja, V.; Caceres, E.; Salvador, R.; and Ruiz, J.: A Prospective Double-Blind Trial of a Low Molecular Weight Heparin Once Daily Compared With Conventional Low-Dose Heparin Three Times Daily to Prevent Pulmonary Embolism and Venous Thrombosis in Patients With Hip Fracture. J. Trauma, 29:873–875, 1989.

413. Morrell, M.T., and Dunnill, M.S.: The Post Mortem Incidence of Pulmonary Embolism in a Hospital Population. Br. J. Surg., 55:347–352, 1968.

414. Morrell, M.T.; Truelove, S.C.; and Barr, A.: Pulmonary Embolism. Br. Med. J., 2:830–835, 1963.

415. Moser, K., and LeMoine, J.: Is Embolic Risk Conditioned by Location of Deep Venous Thrombosis? Ann. Intern. Med., 94:439–444, 1987.

416. Murphy, E.A.; Mustard, J.F.; Rowsell, H.C.; and Downie, H.G.: Quantitative Studies on the Effect of Dicumarol on Experimental Thrombosis. J. Lab. Clin. Med., 61:935–943, 1963.

417. Negus, D.; Pinto, D.J.; LeQuesne, L.P.; Brown, N.; and Chapman, M.: ^{125}I-labelled Fibrinogen in the Diagnosis of Deep Vein Thrombosis and Its Correlation With Phlebography. Br. J. Surg., 55:835–839, 1968.

418. Neu, L.T., Jr.; Waterfield, J.R.; and Ash, C.J.: Prophylactic Anticoagulant Therapy in the Orthopaedic Patient. Ann. Intern. Med., 62:463–467, 1965.

419. Nicolaides, A.N.; Desai, S.; Douglas, J.N.; Fourides, G.; Dupont, P.A.; Lewis, J.D.; Dodsworth, H.; Luck, R.J.; and Jamieson, C.W.: Small Doses of Subcutaneous Sodium Heparin in Preventing Deep Venous Thrombosis After Major Surgery. Lancet, 2:890–893, 1972.

420. NIH Consensus Conference: Prevention of Venous Thrombosis and Pulmonary Embolism. J.A.M.A., 256:744–749, 1986.

421. Nylander, G.: Phlebographic Diagnosis of Acute Deep Leg Thrombosis. Acta. Chir. Scand. [Suppl.] 387:30–34, 1968.

422. O'Brien, J.R.: Effects of Salicylates on Human Platelets. Lancet, 1:779–783, 1968.

423. O'Brien, J.R.: Detection of Thrombosis With Iodine[125] Fibrinogen. Data Reassessed. Lancet, 2:396–398, 1970.

424. Oster, G.; Tuden, R.; and Colditz, G.; A Cost-Effectiveness Analysis of Prophylaxis Against Deep Vein Thrombosis in Major Orthopaedic Surgery. J.A.M.A., 257:203–208, 1987.

425. Paiement, G.; Wessinger, S.; and Harris, W.: Survey of Prophylaxis Against Venous Thromboembolism in Adults Undergoing Hip Surgery. Clin. Orthop., 223:188–193, 1987.

426. Paiement, G.; Wessinger, S.; Waltman, A.; and Harris, W.: Low-Dose Warfarin Versus External Pneumatic Compression for Prophylaxis Against Venous Thromboembolism Following Total Hip Replacement. J. Arthroplasty, 2:23–26, 1987.

427. Paiement, G.; Wessinger, S.; Waltman, A.; and Harris, W.: Surveillance of Deep Vein Thrombosis in Asymptomatic Total Hip Replacement Patients. Impedance Plebography and Fibrinogen Scanning versus Roentgenographic Phlebography. Am. J. Surg., 155:400–404, 1988.

428. Parker, B.M., and Smith, J.R.: Pulmonary Embolism and Infarction. A Review of the Physiologic Consequences of Pulmonary Arterial Obstruction. Am. J. Med., 24:402–427, 1958.

429. Persson, A.; Jones, C.; Zide, R.; and Jewell, E.: Use of the Triplex Scanner in Diagnosis of Deep Venous Thrombosis. Arch. Surg., 124:593–596, 1989.

430. Pollak, E.W.; Sparks, F.C.; and Barker, W.F.: Pulmonary Embolism. An Appraisal of Therapy in 516 Cases. Arch. Surg., 107:66–68, 1973.

431. Rabinov, K., and Paulin, S.: Roentgen Diagnosis of Venous Thrombosis in the Leg. Arch. Surg., 104:134–144, 1972.

432. Rosenow, E.C., III; Osmundson, P.J.; and Brown, M.L.: Pulmonary Embolism. Mayo Clin. Proc., 56:161–178, 1981.

433. Rothman, R.H., and Booth, R.E.: Prevention of Pulmonary Embolism: A Comparison of ASA and Low Dose Coumadin Regimens. Clin. Orthop., 154:309, 1981.

434. Russell, H.E., Jr.; Bradham, R.R.; and Lee, W.H., Jr.: An Evaluation of Infusion Therapy (Including Dextran) for Venous Thrombosis. Circulation, 33:839–846, 1966.

435. Sabiston, D.C., Jr.: Pathophysiology, Diagnosis and Management of Pulmonary Embolism. Am. J. Surg., 138:384–391, 1979.

436. Salzman, E.W.; Harris, W.H.; and DeSanctis, R.W.: Anticoagulation for Prevention of Thromboembolism Following Fractures of the Hip. N. Engl. J. Med., 275:122–130, 1966.

437. Salzman, E.W.; Harris, W.H.; and DeSanctis, R.W.: Reduction in Venous Thromboembolism by Agents Affecting Platelet Function. N. Engl. J. Med., 284:1287–1292, 1971.

438. Sandritter, W.: Die pathologische Anatomie der Thrombose und Lung en Embolie. Son Derdruck aus Behringwerk-Mitteilungen, 4:37–54, 1962.

439. Schondorf, T.H.; Weber, U.; and Lasch, H.G.: Niedrig dosierts heparin und acetylsalicylsaure nach elektiven operationem am huftgelenk. Dtsch. Med. Wochenschr., 102: 1314–1318, 1977.

440. Sevitt, S., and Gallagher, N.G.: Prevention of Venous Thrombosis and Pulmonary Embolism in Injured Patients. A Trial Anticoagulant Prophylaxis With Phenindione in Middle Aged and Elderly Patients With Fractured Necks of Femur. Lancet, 2:981–989, 1959.

441. Sevitt, S., and Gallagher, N.G.: Venous Thrombosis and Pulmonary Embolism: A Clinicopathological Study in Injured and Burned Patients. Br. J. Surg., 48:475–489, 1961.

442. Sigel, B.; Popky, G.L.; Mapp, E.M.; Feigl, P.; Felix, W.R., Jr.; and Ipsen, J.: Evaluation of Doppler Ultrasound Examination. Its Use in Diagnosis of Lower Extremity Venous Disease. Arch. Surg., 100:535–540, 1970.

443. Sigel, B.; Popky, G.L.; Wagner, D.K.; Boland, J.P.; Mapp, E.M.; and Feigl, P.: A Doppler Ultrasound Method for Diagnosing Lower Extremity Venous Disease. Surg. Gynecol. Obstet., 127:339–350, 1968.

444. Sikorski, J.M.; Hampson, W.G.; and Staddon, G.E.: The Natural History and Aetiology of Deep Vein Thrombosis After Total Hip Replacement. J. Bone Joint Surg., 63B: 171–177, 1981.

445. Smith, G.T.; Dammin, G.J.; and Dexter, L.: Postmortem Arteriographic Studies of the Human Lung in Pulmonary Embolization. J.A.M.A., 188:143–151, 1964.

446. Solonen, K.A.: Prophylactic Anticoagulant Therapy in the Treatment of Lower Limb Fractures. Acta. Orthop. Scand., 33:329–341, 1963.

447. Stamatakis, J.D.; Kakkar, V.V.; Lawrence, D.; Bently, P.G.; Naim, D.; and Ward, V.: Failure of Aspirin to Prevent Postoperative Deep Vein Thrombosis in Patients Undergoing Total Hip Replacement. Br. Med. J., 1:1031–1032, 1978.

448. Stulberg, B.; Insall, J.; Williams, G.; and Ghelman, B.: Deep-Vein Thrombosis Following Total Knee Replacement. An Analysis of 638 Arthroplasties. J. Bone Joint Surg., 66A:194–201, 1984.

449. Swierstra, B.; Van Oosterhout, F.; Ausema, B.; Bakker, W.; Van Der Pompe, W.; and Schouten, H.: Oral Anticoagulants and Dextran for Prevention of Venous Thrombosis in Orthopaedics. Acta Orthop. Scand., 55:251–253, 1984.

450. Swierstra, B.; Stibbe, J.; and Schouten, H.: Prevention of Thrombosis After Hip Arthroplasty. A Prospective Study of Preoperative Oral Anticoagulants. Acta. Orthop. Scand., 59:139–143, 1988.

451. Tubiana, R., and Duparc, J.: Prevention of Thromboembolic Complications in Orthopaedic and Accident Surgery. J. Bone Joint Surg., 43B:7–15, 1961.

452. Turpie, A.; Levine, M.; Hirsh, J.; Carter, C.; Jay, R.; Powers, P.; Andrew, M.; Hull, R.; and Gent, M.: A Randomized Controlled Trial of a Low Molecular Weight Heparin (Enoxaparin) to Prevent Deep Vein Thrombosis in Patients Undergoing Elective Hip Surgery. N. Engl. J. Med., 315: 925–929, 1986.

453. Viamonte, M., Jr.; Koolpe, H.; Janowitz, W.; and Hildner, F.: Pulmonary Thromboembolism—Update. J.A.M.A., 243(21):2229–2234, 1980.

454. Vinazzer, H.; Loew, D.; Simma, W.; and Brucke, P.: Prophylaxis of Postoperative Thromboembolism by Low Dose Heparin and by Acetylsalicylic Acid Given Simultaneously. A Double Blind Study. Thromb. Res., 17:177–184, 1980.

455. Virchow, R.: Die verstopfung den lungenarterie und ihre folgen. Beitr. Exper. Path. Physiol., 2:1–12, 1846.

456. Wacker, W.E.C.; Rosenthal, M.; Snodgrass, P.J.; and Amador, E.A.: A Triad for the Diagnosis of Pulmonary Embolism and Infarction. J.A.M.A., 178:8–13, 1961.

457. Weiss, J.H.; Aledort, L.M.; and Kochwa, S.: The Effect of Salicylates on the Hemostatic Properties of Platelets in Man. J. Clin. Invest., 48:2169–2180, 1968.

458. Wessler, S., and Yin, E.T.: Theory and Practice of Minidose Heparin in Surgical Patients. Circulation, 47:671–676, 1973.

459. Wheeler, H.B.; Pearson, D.; O'Connell, D.; and Mullick, S.C.; Impedance Phlebography. Technique, Interpretation and Results. Arch. Surg., 104:164–169, 1972.

460. Wiley, A.M.: Venous Thrombosis in Orthopaedic Patients: An Overview. Orthop. Surg., 2:388–400, 1979.

461. Winfrey, E.W., III; and Foster, J.H.: Low Molecular Weight Dextran in Small Artery Surgery. Antithrombogenic Effect. Arch. Surg., 88:78–82, 1964.

Gas Gangrene

462. Aitken, D.R.; Mackett, M.C.T.; and Smith, L.L.: The Changing Pattern of Hemolytic Streptococcal Gangrene. Arch. Surg., 117(5):561–567, 1982.

463. Altemeier, W.A., and Culbertson, W.R.: Acute Nonclostridial Crepitant Cellulitis. Surg. Gynecol. Obstet., 87:206–212, 1948.

464. Altemeier, W.A., and Fullen, W.D.: Prevention and Treatment of Gas Gangrene. J.A.M.A., 217(6):806–813, 1971.

465. Altemeier, W.A., and Furste, W.L.: Studies in Virulence of *Clostridium welchii*. Surgery, 25:12–19, 1949.

466. Aufranc, O.E.; Jones, W.N.; and Bierbaum, B.E.: Gas Gangrene Complicating Fracture of the Tibia. J.A.M.A., 209(13):2045–2047, 1969.

467. Boerema, I.: An Operating Room With High Atmospheric Pressure. Surgery, 49(3):291–298, 1961.

468. Bornstein, D.L.; Weinberg, N.; Swartz, M.N.; and Kunz, L.J.: Anaerobic Infections—Review of Current Experience. Medicine, 43:207–232, 1964.

469. Bottini, E.: La Gangrena Traumatica Invadente. Contribuzione Sperimentali ed Illustrazioni Cliniche. Giorn. Reale Accad. Med., 10:1121–1138, 1871.

470. Brummelkamp, W.H.; Boerema, I.; and Hoogendyk, L.: Treatment of Clostridial Infections With Hyperbaric Oxygen Drenching: A Report of 26 Cases. Lancet, 1:235–238, 1963.

471. Colwill, M.R., and Maudsley, R.H.: The Management of Gas Gangrene With Hyperbaric Oxygen Therapy. J. Bone Joint Surg., 50B:732–742, 1968.

472. DeHaven, K.E., and Evarts, C.M.: The Continuing Problem of Gas Gangrene: A Review and Report of Illustrative Cases. J. Trauma, 11:983–991, 1971.

473. Eickhoff, T.C.: An Outbreak of Surgical Wound Infections Due to *Clostridium perfringens.* Surg. Gynecol. Obstet., 114:102–108, 1962.

474. Filler, R.M.; Griscom, N.T.; and Pappas, A.: Posttraumatic Crepitation Falsely Suggesting Gas Gangrene. N. Engl. J. Med., 278(14):758–761, 1968.

475. Fisher, A.M., and McKusick, V.A.: Bacteriodes Infections: Clinical, Bacteriological and Therapeutic Features of 14 Cases. Am. J. Med. Sci., 225:253–273, 1953.

476. Giuidi, M.L.; Proietti, R.; Carducci, P.; Magalini, S.I.; and Pelosi, G.: The Combined Use of Hyperbaric Oxygen, Antibiotics and Surgery in the Treatment of Gas Gangrene. Resuscitation, 9:267–273, 1981.

477. Govan, A.D.T.: An Account of the Pathology of Some Cases of *C. welchii* Infection. J. Pathol. Bacteriol., 58:423–430, 1946.

478. Grossman, M., and Silen, W.: Serious Post-Traumatic Infections With Special Reference to Gas Gangrene, Tetanus and Necrotizing Fasciitis. Postgrad. Med., 32:110–118, 1962.

479. Gye, R.; Rountree, P.M.; and Lowenthal, J.: Infection of Surgical Wounds With *Clostridium welchii.* Med. J. Aust., 48:761–764, 1961.

480. Hayward, N.J.: The Rapid Identification of *C. welchii* by Nagler Tests in Plate Cultures. J. Pathol. Bacteriol., 55:285–293, 1943.

481. Hayward, N.J., and Gray, J.A.B.: Haemolysin Tests for the Rapid Identification of *C. oedematiens* and *C. septicum.* J. Pathol. Bacteriol., 58:11–20, 1946.

482. Holland, J.A.; Hill, G.B.; Wolfe, W.G.; Osterhout, S.; Saltzman, H.A.; and Brown, I.W., Jr.: Experimental and Clinical Experience With Hyperbaric Oxygen in the Treatment of Clostridial Myonecrosis. Surgery, 77:75–85, 1975.

483. Hunt, T.; Halliday, B.; Knighton, D.; Gottrup, F.; Price, D.; Mathes, S.; Chang, N.; and Hohn, D.: Impairment of Microbicidal Function in Wounds: Correction With Oxygenation. *In* Hunt, T.K.; Heppenstall, R.B.; Pines, E.; Rovee, D. (eds.): Soft and Hard Tissue Repair, Biological and Clinical Aspects, pp. 455–468. New York, Praeger, 1984.

484. Jeffrey, J.S., and Thomson, S.: Gas Gangrene in Italy: A Study of 33 Cases Treated With Penicillin. Br. J. Surg., 32:159–167, 1944.

485. Kellett, C.E.: The Early History of Gas Gangrene. Ann. Med. Hist., 1:452–459, 1939.

486. Kemp, F.H.: X-rays in Diagnosis and Localization of Gas Gangrene. Lancet, 1:332–336, 1945.

487. Langley, F.H., and Winkelstein, L.B.: Gas Gangrene: A Study of 96 Cases Treated in an Evacuation Hospital. J.A.M.A., 128:783–792, 1945.

488. MacLennan, J.D.: Anaerobic Infections of War Wounds in the Middle East. Lancet, 2:63–66, 1943.

489. MacLennan, J.D.: Streptococcal Infection of Muscle. Lancet, 1:582–584, 1943.

490. MacLennan, J.D.: Histotoxic Clostridial Infections in Man. Bacteriol. Rev., 26:177–276, 1962.

491. MacLennan, J.D., and MacFarlane, R.G.: Toxin and Antitoxin Studies of Gas Gangrene in Man. Lancet, 2:301–305, 1945.

492. Oakley, C.L.: Gas Gangrene. Br. Med. Bull., 10:52–58, 1954.

493. Pappas, A.M.; Filler, R.M.; Eraklis, A.J.; and Bernhard, W.F.: Clostridial Infections (Gas Gangrene). Diagnosis and Early Treatment. Clin. Orthop., 76:177–184, 1971.

494. Parker, M.T.: Postoperative Clostridial Infections in Britain. Br. Med. J., 3:671–676, 1969.

495. Qvist, G.: Anaerobic Cellulitis and Gas Gangrene. Br. Med. J., 2:217–221, 1941.

496. Rifkind, D.: The Diagnosis and Treatment of Gas Gangrene. Surg. Clin. North Am., 43:511–517, 1963.

497. Robb-Smith, A.H.T.: Tissue Changes Induced by *Clostridium welchii* Type A Filtrates. Lancet, 2:362–368, 1945.

498. Roding, B.; Groeneveld, P.H.A.; and Boerema, I.: Ten Years of Experience in the Treatment of Gas Gangrene With Hyperbaric Oxygen. Surg. Gynecol. Obstet., 134:579–585, 1972.

499. Schwartzman, J.D.; Reller, L.B.; and Wang, W.L.: Susceptibility of *Clostridium perfringens* Isolated From Human Infections to Twenty Antibiotics. Antimicrob. Agents Chemother., 11:695–697, 1977.

500. Smith, L., and DeSpain: Clostridia in Gas Gangrene. Bacteriol. Rev., 13:233–254, 1949.

501. Tonjum, S.; Digranes, A.; Alho, A.; Gjengsto, H.; and Eidsvik, S.: Hyperbaric Oxygen Treatment in Gas-Producing Infections. Acta Chir. Scand., 146:235–241, 1980.

502. Trippel, O.H.; Ruggie, A.N.; Staley, C.J.; and Van Elk, J.: Hyperbaric Oxygenation in the Management of Gas Gangrene. Surg. Clin. North Am., 47:17–27, 1967.

503. Van Beek, A.; Zook, E.; Yaw, P.; Gardner, R.; Smith, R.; and Glover, J.L.: Nonclostridial Gas-Forming Infections. A Collective Review and Report of Seven Cases. Arch. Surg., 108:552–557, 1974.

504. Weinstein, L., and Barza, M.A.: Gas Gangrene. N. Engl. J. Med., 289:1129–1131, 1973.

505. Welsh, F.; Matos, L.; and deTreville, R.T.P.: Medical Hyperbaric Oxygen Therapy. 22 Cases. Aviat. Space Environ. Med., 51:611–614, 1980.

506. Willis, A.T., and Gowland, G.: Some Observations on the Mechanism of the Nagler Reaction. J. Pathol. Bacteriol., 83:219–226, 1962.

507. Willis, A.T., and Hobbs, G.: Some New Media for the Isolation and Identification of Clostridia. J. Pathol. Bacteriol., 77:511–521, 1959.

508. Wilson, T.S.: Significance of *Clostridium welchii* Infections and Their Relationship to Gas Gangrene. Can. J. Surg., 4:35–42, 1960.

509. Wolinsky, E.: Clostridial Myonecrosis. *In* Wyngaarden, J.B., and Smith, L.H. (eds.): Textbook of Medicine, 16th ed. Philadelphia, W.B. Saunders, 1982.

Tetanus

510. American College of Surgeons Committee on Trauma. A Guide to Prophylaxis Against Tetanus in Wound Management. Bulletin American College of Surgeons, 57:32–33, 1972.

511. Aretaeus the Cappadocian: On Tetanus. *In* Adams, F. (ed.): The Extant Works. London, 1856.

512. Brooks, V.B.; Curtis, D.R.; and Eccles, J.C.: The Action of Tetanus Toxin on the Inhibition of Motoneurons. J. Physiol., 135:655–672, 1957.

513. Brown, H.: Tetanus. J.A.M.A., 204:614–616, 1968.

514. Carle, A., and Rattone, G.: Studio Experimentale Sull' Eziologia del Tetano. Geordr. Accad. Med. Torino, 32: 174–180, 1884.

515. Centers for Disease Control: Summary of Notifiable Diseases—United States, 1987. M.M.W.R. 37 (Supplement—Part 2 Graphs and Maps): 41, September 16, 1988.

516. Christensen, M.A.: Important Concepts of Tetanus That Form the Basis for Current Treatment. *In* Eckmann, L. (ed.): Principles on Tetanus. 2nd Proceedings of the International Conference on Tetanus, pp. 455–467. Bern, Hans Huber, 1967.

517. Christensen, N.A.: Treatment of the Patient With Severe Tetanus. Surg. Clin. North Am., 49:1183–1193, 1969.

518. Duchen, L.W., and Tonge, D.A.: The Effects of Tetanus Toxin on Neuromuscular Transmission and on the Morphology of Motor End-Plates in Slow and Fast Skeletal Muscle of the Mouse. J. Physiol., 228:157–172, 1973.

519. Eckmann, L. (ed.): Principles on Tetanus. 2nd Proceedings of the International Conference on Tetanus, pp. 1–577, Bern, Hans Huber, 1967.

520. Furste, W.: Third International Conference on Tetanus: A Report. J. Trauma, 11:721–724, 1971.

521. Furste, W.: Four Keys to 100 Per Cent Success in Tetanus Prophylaxis. Am. J. Surg., 128:616–623, 1974.

522. Furste, W., and Wheeler, W.L.: Tetanus: A Team Disease. Curr. Probl. Surg., Oct:1–72, 1972.

523. Glenn, F.: Tetanus—A Preventable Disease: Including an Experience With Civilian Casualties in the Battle for Manila (1945). Ann. Surg., 124:1030–1040, 1946.

524. Gupta, P.S.; Kapoor, R.; Goyal, S.; Batra, V.K.; and Jain, B.K.: Intrathecal Human Tetanus Immunoglobulin in Early Tetanus. Lancet, 2:439–440, 1980.

525. Habermann, E.: Tetanus. *In* Vinkin, P.J., and Bruyn, G.W. (eds.): Handbook of Clinical Neurology, Vol. 33, Part I, pp. 491–547. New York, North Holland Publishing, 1978.

526. Hardegee, M.C.; Palmer, A.E.; and Duffin, N.: Tetanolysin: In Vivo Effects in Animals. J. Infect. Dis., 123:51–60, 1971.

527. Helting, T.B.; Zwisler, O.; and Wiegandt, H.: Structure of Tetanus Toxin II. Toxin Binding to Ganglioside. J. Biol. Chem., 252:194–198, 1977.

528. Hippocrates: With an English Translation by W.H.S. Jones. Vol. 1, pp. 165. Cambridge, Mass., Harvard University Press, 1923.

529. International Comments Guide Lines Regarding Tetanus. J.A.M.A., 198:687–688, 1966.

530. Jacobs, R.L.; Lowe, R.S.; and Lanier, B.Q.: Adverse Reactions to Tetanus Toxoid. J.A.M.A., 247:40–42, 1982.

531. Kaeser, H.E., and Saner, A.: The Effect of Tetanus Toxin on Neuromuscular Transmission. Eur. Neurol., 3:193–205, 1970.

532. Kerr, J.H.; Corbett, J.L.; Prys-Roberts, C.; Smith, A.C.; and Spalding, J.M.K.: Involvement of the Sympathetic Nervous System in Tetanus. Studies on 82 Cases. Lancet, 2:236–241, 1968.

533. Kitasato, S.: Uber den tetanuserreger. Ztschr. Hyg., 7:225–234, 1889.

534. LaForce, F.M.; Young, L.S.; and Bennett, J.V.: Tetanus in the United States (1965–1966). Epidemiologic and Clinical Features. N. Engl. J. Med., 280:569–574, 1969.

535. Levine, L.; McComb, J.A.; Dwyer, R.C.; and Latham, W.C.: Active-passive Tetanus Immunization. Choice of Toxoid, Dose of Tetanus Immune Globulin and Timing of Injections. N. Engl. J. Med., 274:186–190, 1966.

536. Long, A.: The Army Immunization Program, Vol. III. Preventive Medicine in World War II. Washington, D.C.: U.S. Government Printing Office, 1955.

537. McComb, J.A.: The Combined Use of Homologous Tetanus Immune Globulin and Toxoid in Man. *In* Eckmann, L. (ed.): Principles on Tetanus and Proceedings of the International Conference on Tetanus, pp. 359–367. Bern, Hans Huber, 1967.

538. McComb, J.A., and Dwyer, R.C.: Passive-Active Immunization With Tetanus Immune Globulin (Human). N. Engl. J. Med., 268:857–862, 1963.

539. McCracken, G.H., Jr.; Dowell, D.L.; and Marshall, F.N.: Double-Blind Trial of Equine Antitoxin and Human Immune Globulin in Tetanus Neonatorum. Lancet, 1:1146–1149, 1971.

540. Mellanby, J.H.: Presynaptic Effect of Tetanus Toxin at the Neuromuscular Junction. J. Physiol., 218:68P–69P, 1971.

541. Milledge, J.S.: Hyperbaric Oxygen Therapy in Tetanus. J.A.M.A., 203:875–876, 1968.

542. Murphy, K.J.: Fatal Tetanus With Brain-stem Involvement and Myocarditis in an Ex-Serviceman. Med. J. Aust., 2: 542–544, 1970.

543. Nation, N.S.; Pierce, N.F.; Adler, S.J.; Chinnock, R.F.; and Wehrle, P.F.: Tetanus: The Use of Human Hyperimmune Globulin in Treatment. California Med., 98:305–307, 1963.

544. Pessi, T.; Honkola, H.; and Liikala, E.: Results of Treatment of Patients With Severe Tetanus. Ann. Chir. Gynaecol., 70:182–186, 1981.

545. Ramon, G., and Zoeller, C.: l'Anatoxine tetanique et l'Immunisation Active de l'Homme vis-a-vis du Tetanos. Ann. Inst. Pasteur, 41:803–833, 1927.

546. Recommendation of the Immunization Practices Advisory Committee. Diphtheria, Tetanus and Pertussis: Guidelines for Vaccine Prophylaxis and Other Preventive Measures. M.M.W.R., 30:392–396, 401, 407, 1981.

547. Smith, A.: Tetanus. *In* Beeson, P.B., and McDermott, W. (eds.): Textbook of Medicine, 14th ed. Philadelphia, W.B. Saunders, 1975.

548. Smythe, P.M.: Studies on Neonatal Tetanus, and on Pulmonary Compliance of the Totally Relaxed Infant. Br. Med. J., 1:565–571, 1963.

549. Smythe, P.M.: The Problem of Detubating an Infant With a Tracheostomy. J. Pediatr., 65:446–453, 1964.

550. Smythe, P.M.: Treatment of Tetanus in Neonates. Lancet, 1:335, 1967.

551. Spaeth, R.: Therapy of Tetanus. A Study of Two Hundred and Seventy-Six Cases. Arch. Intern. Med., 68:1133–1160, 1941.

552. Trujillo, M.J.; Castillo, A.; Espana, J.V.; Guevara, P.; and Eganez, H.: Tetanus in the Adult: Intensive Care and Management Experience With 233 Cases. Crit. Care Med., 8:419–423, 1980.

553. Tsueda, K.; Oliver, P.B.; and Richter, R.W.: Cardiovascular Manifestations of Tetanus. Anesthesiology, 40:588–592, 1974.

554. Van Heyningen, W.E., and Messanby, J.: Tetanus Toxin. *In* Kadis, S.; Montie, T.C.; and Ajl, S.J. (eds.): Microbial Toxins, Vol. 2A. New York, Academic Press, 1971.

555. Weed, M.R.; Purvis, D.F.; and Warnke, R.D.: D-Tubocurarine in Wax and Oil: For Control of Muscle Spasm in Tetanus. J.A.M.A., 138:1087–1090, 1948.

556. Wessler, S., and Avioli, L.A.: Tetanus. J.A.M.A., 207:123–127, 1969.

557. White, W.G.: Reactions to Tetanus Toxoid. J. Hyg. (Lond.), 17:283–297, 1973.

558. Woolmer, R., and Cates, J.E.: Succinylcholine in the Treatment of Tetanus. Lancet, 2:808–809, 1952.

559. Wright, G.P.: The Neurotoxins of *Clostridum botulinum* and *Clostridium tetani.* Pharmacol. Rev., 7:413–465, 1955.

Osteomyelitis

560. Alexander, J.W.; Sykes, N.S.; Mitchell, M.M.; and Fisher, M.W.: Concentration of Selected Intravenously Administered Antibiotics in Experimental Surgical Wounds. J. Trauma, 13:423–434, 1973.

561. Altemeier, W.A.; Todd, J.C.; and Inge, W.W.: Gram-Negative Septicemia. A Growing Threat. Ann. Surg., 166:530–542, 1969.

562. Altemeier, W.A., and Wadsworth, C.L.: An Evaluation of Penicillin Therapy in Acute Hematogenous Osteomyelitis. J. Bone Joint Surg., 30A(3):657–679, 1948.

563. Anderson, W.A.D.: Pathology, 4th ed. St. Louis, C.V. Mosby, 1961.

564. Bajpai, J.; Chaturvedi, S.N.; and Khanuja, S.P.S.: Chemotherapy of Acute Bone and Joint Infections. Int. Surg., 62:172–174, 1977.

565. Barber, M., and Waterworth, D.M.: Penicillinase-resistant Penicillins and Cephalosporins. Br. Med. J., 2:344–349, 1965.

566. Barry, A.L.; Garcia, F.; and Thrupp, L.D.: An Improved Single-Disk Method for Testing the Antibiotic Susceptibility of Rapidly-Growing Pathogens. Am. J. Clin. Pathol., 53:149–158, 1970.

567. Bernhard, W.F., and Filler, R.M.: Hyperbaric Oxygenation: Current Concepts. Am. J. Surg., 115:661–668, 1968.

568. Blockey, N.J., and McAllister, T.A.: Antibiotics in Acute Osteomyelitis in Children. J. Bone Joint Surg., 54B(2):299–309, 1972.

569. Bowers, W.H.; Wilson, F.C.; and Greene, W.B.: Antibiotic Prophylaxis in Experimental Bone Infections. J. Bone Joint Surg., 55A:795–807, 1973.

570. Boyd, R.J.; Burke, J.F.; and Colton, T.: A Double Blind Clinical Trial of Prophylactic Antibiotics and Hip Fractures. J. Bone Joint Surg., 55A:1251–1259, 1973.

571. Brown, P.W.: The Prevention of Infection in Open Wounds. Clin. Orthop., 96:42–50, 1973.

572. Butt, W.P.: The Radiology of Infection. Clin. Orthop., 96:20–30, 1973.

573. Caldwell, J.R., and Cluff, L.E.: The Real and Present Danger of Antibiotics. Ration. Drug Ther., 7:1–6, 1973.

574. Charnley, J.: Postoperative Infection After Total Hip Replacement With Special Reference to Air Contamination in the Operating Room. Clin. Orthop., 87:167–187, 1972.

575. Clawson, D.K.: Common Bacterial Infections of Bone. G.P., 32:125–133, 1965.

576. Clawson, D.K.; David, F.J.; and Hansen, S.T.: Treatment of Chronic Osteomyelitis With Emphasis on Closed Suction-Irrigation Techniques. Clin. Orthop., 96:88–97, 1973.

577. Clawson, D.K., and Dunn, A.W.: Management of Common Bacterial Infections of Bones and Joints. J. Bone Joint Surg., 49A:164–182, 1967.

578. Cluff, L.E., and Reynolds, R.C.: Management of Staphylococcal Infections. Am. J. Med., 39:812–825, 1965.

579. Cluff, L.E.; Reynolds, R.C.; Page, D.L.; and Breckenridge, J.L.: Staphylococcal Bacteremia and Altered Host Resistance. Ann. Intern. Med., 69:859–873, 1968.

580. Cole, W.G.; Dalziel, R.E.; and Leitl, S.: Treatment of Acute Osteomyelitis in Childhood. J. Bone Joint Surg., 64B:218–223, 1982.

581. Collins, D.H.: *In* Dodge, O.G. (ed.): Pathology of Bone. London, Butterworth, 1966.

582. Compere, E.L.; Metzger, W.I.; and Mitra, R.N.: The Treatment of Pyogenic Bone and Joint Infections by Closed Irrigation (Circulation) With a Non-toxic Detergent and One or More Antibiotics. J. Bone Joint Surg., 49A:614–624, 1967.

583. Curtis, P.: The Pathophysiology of Joint Infections. Clin. Orthop., 96:129–135, 1973.

584. Davis, J.; Heckman, J.; DeLee, J.; and Buckwold, F.: Chronic Non-Hematogenous Osteomyelitis Treated With Adjuvant Hyperbaric Oxygen. J. Bone Joint Surg., 68A:1210–1217, 1986.

585. Dellinger, E.; Caplan, E.; Weaver, L.; Wertz, M.; Droppert, B.; Hoyt, N.; Brumback, R.; Burgess, R.; Poka, A.; Benirschke, S.; Lennard, E.S.; and Lou, Sr. M.A.: Duration of Preventive Antibiotic Administration for Open Extremity Fractures. Arch. Surg., 123:333–339, 1988.

586. Dellinger, E.; Miller, S.; Wertz, M.; Grypma, M.; Droppert, B.; and Anderson, P.: Risk of Infection After Open Fracture of the Arm or Leg. Arch. Surg., 123:1320–1327, 1988.

587. Dich, V.Q.; Nelson, J.D.; and Haltalin, K.C.: Osteomyelitis in Infants and Children. Am. J. Dis. Child., 129:1273–1278, 1975.

588. Dickson, C.D.: The Clinical Diagnosis, Prognosis, and Treatment of Acute Hematogenous Osteomyelitis. J.A.M.A., 127:212–217, 1945.

589. Dombrowski, E.T., and Dunn, A.W.: Treatment of Osteomyelitis by Debridement and Closed Wound Irrigation-Suction. Clin. Orthop., 43:215–231, 1965.

590. Donowitz, G., and Mandell, G.: Beta-Lactam Antibiotics. N. Engl. J. Med., 318:419–426, 490–500, 1988.

591. Drew, W.L.; Barry, A.L.; O'Toole, R.; and Sherris, J.C.: Reliability of the Kirby-Bauer Disc Diffusion Method for Detecting Methicillin-resistant Strains of *Staphylococcus aureus.* Appl. Microbiol., 24:240–247, 1972.

592. Edwards, M.S.; Baker, C.J.; Wagner, K.H.; Taber, L.H.; and Barrett, F.F.: An Etiologic Shift in Infantile Osteo-

myelitis: The Emergence of the Group B Streptococcus. J. Pediatr., 93(4):578–583, 1978.

593. Evarts, C.M.: Endoprosthesis as the Primary Treatment of Femoral Neck Fractures. Clin. Orthop., 92:69–76, 1973.

594. Evaskus, D.S.; Laskin, D.M.; and Kroeger, A.V.: Penetration of Lincomycin, Penicillin, and Tetracycline Into Serum and Bone. Proc. Soc. Exp. Biol. Med., 130:89–91, 1969.

595. Eyre-Brook, A.L.: Septic Arthritis of the Hip and Osteomyelitis of the Upper End of the Femur in Infants. J. Bone Joint Surg., 42B:11–20, 1960.

596. Ferguson, A.B.: Osteomyelitis in Children. Clin. Orthop., 96:51–56, 1973.

597. Finland, M.; Jones, W.F.; and Barnes, M.W.: Occurrence of Serious Bacterial Infections Since Introduction of Antibacterial Agents. J.A.M.A., 170:2188–2197, 1959.

598. Fogelberg, E.V.; Zitzmann, E.K.; and Stinchfield, F.E.: Prophylactic Penicillin in Orthopaedic Surgery. J. Bone Joint Surg., 52A:95–98, 1970.

599. Ger, R.: Muscle Transposition for Treatment and Prevention of Chronic Post-Traumatic Osteomyelitis of the Tibia. J. Bone Joint Surg., 59A:784–791, 1977.

600. Gillespie, W.J., and Mayo, K.M.: The Management of Acute Hematogenous Osteomyelitis in the Antibiotic Era. J. Bone Joint Surg., 63B:126–131, 1981.

601. Gilmour, W.N.: Acute Haematogenous Osteomyelitis. J. Bone Joint Surg., 44B:841–853, 1962.

602. Gledhill, R.B.: Subacute Osteomyelitis in Children. Clin. Orthop., 96:57–69, 1973.

603. Gordon, S.L.; Greer, R.B.; and Craig, C.P.: Recurrent Osteomyelitis. Report of Four Cases Culturing L-form Variants of Staphylococci. J. Bone Joint Surg., 53A:1150–1156, 1971.

604. Green, W.T., and Shannon, J.G.: Osteomyelitis of Infants. A Disease Different From Osteomyelitis of Older Children. Arch. Surg., 32:462–493, 1936.

605. Gustilo, R., and Anderson, J.: Prevention of Infection in the Treatment of One Thousand Twenty Five Open Fractures of Long Bones. Retrospective and Prospective Analyses. J. Bone Joint Surg., 58A:453–458, 1976.

606. Hamblen, D.L.: Hyperbaric Oxygenation: Its Effect on Experimental Staphylococcal Osteomyelitis in Rats. J. Bone Joint Surg., 50A:1129–1141, 1968.

607. Harley, J.D.; Wilson, S.D.; Worman, L.W.; and Carey, L.C.: Chronic Osteomyelitis: Treatment by Regional Perfusion With Antibiotics. Arch. Surg., 92:548–553, 1966.

608. Harris, N.H.: Some Problems in the Diagnosis and Treatment of Acute Osteomyelitis. J. Bone Joint Surg., 42B:535–541, 1960.

609. Harris, N.H., and Kirkaldy-Willis, W.H.: Primary Subacute Pyogenic Osteomyelitis. J. Bone Joint Surg., 47B:526–532, 1965.

610. Harris, W.H.: Sinking Prostheses. Surg. Gynecol. Obstet., 123:1297–1302, 1966.

611. Hart, V.L.: Acute Hematogenous Osteomyelitis in Children. J.A.M.A., 108:524–528, 1937.

612. Hermans, P., and Wilhelm, M.: Vancomycin. Mayo Clin. Proc., 62:901–905, 1987.

613. Hobo, T.: Zur Pathogenese der akuten haematogen Osteomyelitis, mit Berucksichtigung der Vitalfar beng

Shehre. Acta School Medicine Univ. Kioto, 4:1–29, 1921–1922.

614. Jackson, R.W., and Parson, C.J.: Distention-Irrigation Treatment of Major Joint Sepsis. Clin. Orthop., 96:160–164, 1973.

615. Jones, D.C., and Cady, R.B.: "Cold" Bone Scans in Acute Osteomyelitis. J. Bone Joint Surg., 63B:376–378, 1981.

616. Kahn, D.S., and Pritzker, P.H.: The Pathophysiology of Bone Infection. Clin. Orthop., 96:12–19, 1973.

617. Kanyuck, D.O.; Welles, J.S.; Emmerson, J.L.; and Anderson, R.C.: The Penetration of Cephalosporin Antibiotics Into Bone. Proc. Soc. Exp. Biol. Med., 136:997–999, 1971.

618. Kelly, P.J.: Osteomyelitis in the Adult. Orthop. Clin. North Am., 6(4):983–989, 1975.

619. Kelly, P.J.; Wilkowske, C.J.; and Washington, J.A., II: Comparison of Gram-Negative Bacillary and Staphylococcal Osteomyelitis of the Femur and Tibia. Clin. Orthop., 96:70–75, 1973.

620. King, D.M., and Mayo, K.M.: Subacute Hematogenous Osteomyelitis. J. Bone Joint Surg., 51B:458–463, 1969.

621. Kolyvas, E.; Ahronheim, G.; Marks, M.I.; Gledhill, R.; Owen, H.; and Rosenthall, L.: Oral Antibiotics Therapy of Skeletal Infections in Children. Pediatrics, 65:867–871, 1980.

622. Lazarus, G.S.; Brown, R.S.; Daniels, J.R.; and Fullmer, H.M.: Human Granulocyte Collagenase. Science, 159:1483–1485, 1968.

623. Letts, R.M.; Afifi, A.; and Sutherland, J.B.: Technetium Bone Scanning as an Aid in the Diagnosis of Atypical Acute Osteomyelitis in Children. Surg. Gynecol. Obstet., 140:899–902, 1975.

624. Letts, R.M., and Wong, E.: Treatment of Acute Osteomyelitis in Children by Closed-Tube Irrigation: A Reassessment. Can. J. Surg., 18(1):60–63, 1975.

625. Lhowe, D., and Hansen, S.: Immediate Nailing of Open Fractures of the Femoral Shaft. J. Bone Joint Surg., 70A:812–820, 1988.

626. Lisbona, R., and Rosenthall, L.: Observations on the Sequential Use of ^{99m}Tc-phosphate Complex and ^{67}Ga Imaging in Osteomyelitis, Cellulitis, and Septic Arthritis. Radiology, 123(1):123–129, 1977.

627. Lodwick, G.S.: The Bones and Joints. Atlas of Tumour Radiology. Chicago, Year Book Medical Publishers, 1971.

628. McGraw, J., and Lim, E.: Treatment of Open Tibial Shaft Fractures. External Fixation and Secondary Intramedullary Nailing. J. Bone Joint Surg., 70A:900–911, 1988.

629. McHenry, M.C.: Antibacterial Therapy. Cleve. Clin. Q., 37:43–58, 1970.

630. McHenry, M.C.; Alfidi, R.J.; Wilde, A.H.; and Hawk, W.A.: Hematogenous Osteomyelitis: A Changing Disease. Cleve. Clin. Q., 42:125–153, 1975.

631. Mackowiak, P.A.; Jones, S.R.; and Smith, J.W.: Diagnostic Value of Sinus Tract Culture in Chronic Osteomyelitis. J.A.M.A., 239:2722, 1978.

632. Maurer, A.H.; Chen, D.C.P.; Camargo, E.E.; Wong, D.F.; Wagner, H.N.; and Anderson, P.O.: Utility of Three-Phase Skeletal Scintigraphy in Suspected Osteomyelitis: Concise Communication. J. Nucl. Med., 22(11):941–949, 1981.

633. Mayhall, C.G.; Medoff, G.; and Marr, J.J.: Variation in the Susceptibility of Strains of *Staphylococcus aureus* to Ox-

acillin, Cephalothin and Gentamicin. Antimicrob. Agents Chemother., 10:707–712, 1976.

634. Medical Letter, The: Antimicrobial Prophylaxis in Surgery. Med. Lett. Drugs Ther., 29(750):91–94, 1987.

635. Merkel, K.; Brown, M.; Dewanjee, M.; and Fitzgerald, R.: Comparison of Indium-Labelled-Leukocyte Imaging With Sequential Technetium-Gallium Scanning in the Diagnosis of Low-Grade Musculoskeletal Sepsis. J. Bone Joint Surg., 67A:465–476, 1985.

636. Mollan, R.A.B., and Piggott, J.: Acute Osteomyelitis in Children. J. Bone Joint Surg., 59(B):2–7, 1977.

637. Nettles, J.L.; Kelly, P.J.; Martin, W.J.; and Washington, J.A.: Musculoskeletal Infections Due to Bacteroides. A Study of Eleven Cases. J. Bone Joint Surg., 51A:230–238, 1969.

638. Niekerk, J.P., deV.: Hand Infections: Management and Results Based on a New Classification. A Study of More Than 1,000 Cases. S. Afr. Med. J., 40:316–319, 1966.

639. Ogden, J.A.: Pediatric Osteomyelitis and Septic Arthritis: The Pathology of Neonatal Disease. Yale J. Biol. Med., 52:423–448, 1979.

640. Overton, L.M., and Tully, W.P.: Surgical Treatment of Chronic Osteomyelitis in Long Bones. Am. J. Surg., 126: 736–741, 1973.

641. Paterson, D.C.: Suppurative Arthritis in Children. J. Bone Joint Surg., 48B:586, 1966.

642. Patzakis, M.J.; Harvey, J.P., Jr.; and Ivler, D.: The Role of Prophylactic Antibiotics in the Management of Open Fractures. J. Bone Joint Surg., 56A:532–541, 1974.

643. Petersdorf, R.G., and Sherris, J.C.: Methods and Significance of In Vitro Testing of Bacterial Sensitivity to Drugs. Am. J. Med., 39:766–779, 1965.

644. Prober, C.G., and Yeager, A.S.: Use of the Serum Bactericidal Titer to Assess the Adequacy of Oral Antibiotic Therapy in the Treatment of Acute Hematogenous Osteomyelitis. J. Pediatr., 95(1):131–135, 1979.

645. Robertson, D.E.: Acute Hematogenous Osteomyelitis. J. Bone Joint Surg., 9:8–23, 1927.

646. Rosner, R.: Isolation of Protoplasts of *Staphylococcus Aureus* From a Case of Recurrent Acute Osteomyelitis. Tech. Bull. Reg. Med. Tech., 38:205–210, 1968.

647. Septimus, E.J., and Musher, D.M.: Osteomyelitis: Recent Clinical and Laboratory Aspects. Orthop. Clin. North Am., 10(2):347–359, 1979.

648. Shandling, B.: Acute Hematogenous Osteomyelitis: A Review of 300 Cases Treated During 1952–1959. S. Afr. Med. J., 34:520–524, 1960.

649. Shannon, J.B.; Woolhouse, F.M.; and Eisinger, P.J.: The Treatment of Chronic Osteomyelitis by Saucerization and Immediate Skin Grafting. Clin. Orthop., 96:98–107, 1973.

650. Skinner, D., and Keefer, C.S.: Significance of Bacteremia Caused by *Staphylococcus aureus*. Arch. Intern. Med., 68: 851–875, 1941.

651. Starr, C.I.: Acute Hematogenous Osteomyelitis. Arch. Surg., 4:567–587, 1922.

652. Stevens, D.B.: Postoperative Orthopaedic Infections: A Study of Etiological Mechanisms. J. Bone Joint Surg., 46A:96–102, 1964.

653. Subramanian, G., and McAfee, J.G.: A New Complex of ^{99m}Tc for Skeletal Imaging. Radiology, 99:192–196, 1971.

654. Tetzlaff, T.R.; Howard, J.B.; McCracken, G.H.; Calderon, E.; and Larrondo, J.: Antibiotic Concentrations in Pus and Bone of Children With Osteomyelitis. J. Pediatr., 92(1):135–140, 1978.

655. Tetzlaff, T.R.; McCracken, G.H.; and Nelson, J.D.: Oral Antibiotic Therapy for Skeletal Infections of Children. J. Pediatr., 92(3):485–490, 1978.

656. Trueta, J.: The Three Types of Acute Haematogenous Osteomyelitis: A Clinical and Vascular Study. J. Bone Joint Surg., 41B:671–680, 1959.

657. Tuazon, C.U., and Sheagren, J.N.: Teichoic Acid Antibodies in the Diagnosis of Serious Infections With *Staphylococcus aureus*. Ann. Intern. Med., 84:543–546, 1976.

658. Waldvogel, F.A.; Medoff, G.; and Swartz, M.N.: Osteomyelitis. Clinical Features, Therapeutic Considerations, and Unusual Aspects, pp. 1–101. Springfield, Ill., Charles C. Thomas, 1971.

659. Waldvogel, F.A., and Vasey, H.: Osteomyelitis: The Past Decade. N. Engl. J. Med., 303(7):360–370, 1980.

660. Wilson, F.C.; Worcester, J.N.; Coleman, P.D.; and Byrd, W.E.: Antibiotic Penetration of Experimental Bone Hematomas. J. Bone Joint Surg., 53A:1622–1628, 1971.

661. Winters, J.C., and Cahen, I.: Acute Hematogenous Osteomyelitis. A Review of 66 Cases. J. Bone Joint Surg., 42A:691–704, 1960.

662. Worlock, P.; Slack, R.; Harvey, L.; and MaWhinney, R.: The Prevention of Infection in Open Fractures. An Experimental Study of the Effect of Antibiotic Therapy. J. Bone Joint Surg., 70A:1341–1347, 1988.

663. Wukich, D.; Abreu, S.; Callaghan, J.; Van Nostrand, D.; Savory, C.; Eggli, D.; Garcia, J.; and Berrey, B.: Diagnosis of Infection by Preoperative Scintigraphy With Indium-Labelled White Blood Cells. J. Bone Joint Surg., 69A: 1353–1360, 1987.

Post-traumatic Reflex Sympathetic Dystrophy

664. Amadio, P.: Current Concepts Review. Pain Dysfunction Syndromes. J. Bone Joint Surg., 70A:944–949, 1988.

665. Ascherl, R., and Blumel, G.: Clinical Picture in Sudek's Dystrophy. Fortschr. Med., 99(19):712–720, 1981.

666. Bayles, T.B.; Judson, W.E.; and Potter, T.A.: Reflex Sympathetic Dystrophy of the Upper Extremity (Hand-Shoulder Syndrome). J.A.M.A., 144:537–542, 1950.

667. Benzon, H.T.; Chomka, C.M.; and Brunner, E.A.: Treatment of Reflex Sympathetic Dystrophy With Regional Intravenous Reserpine. Anesth. Analg. (Cleve.), 59(7):500–502, 1980.

668. Berger, H.: The Treatment of Postmyocardial Infarction Shoulder-Hand Syndrome With Local Hydrocortisone. Postgrad. Med., 15:508–511, 1954.

669. Birkenfeld, B.: Erfahrungen mit der Echinacin-Therapie beim Sudeckschen Syndrom. Ther. Ggw., 93:425, 1954.

670. Chapman, L.F.; Ramos, A.O.; Goodell, H.; and Wolff, H.G.: Neurohumeral Features of Afferent Fibers in Man. Arch. Neurol., 4:617–650, 1961.

671. Chuinard, R.G.; Dabezies, E.J.; Goud, J.S.; Murphy, G.A.; and Matthews, R.E.: Intravenous Reserpine for Treatment of Reflex Sympathetic Dystrophy. South. Med. J., 74(12): 1481–1484, 1981.

672. Coffman, J.D., and Davies, W.T.: Vasospastic Diseases: A Review. Prog. Cardiovasc. Dis., 18:123–146, 1975.

673. Collins, W.F., and Randt, C.T.: Evoked Central Nervous System Activity to Peripheral Unmyelinated or ''C'' Fibers in Cat. J. Neurophysiol., 21:345–352, 1958.

674. Cooper, D.; DeLee, J.; and Ramamurthy, S.: Reflex Sympathetic Dystrophy of the Knee. Treatment Using Continuous Epidural Anesthesia. J. Bone Joint Surg., 71A: 365–369, 1989.

675. de Takats, G.: The Technic of Lumbar Sympathectomy. Surg. Clin. North Am., 26:56–69, 1946.

676. de Takats, G.: Sympathetic Reflex Dystrophy. Med. Clin. North Am., 49:117–129, 1965.

677. Doury, P.; Grainer, R.; and Pattin, S.: The Use of Bone Scintigraphy With Technetium 99m Pyrophosphates in the Diagnosis of Algodystrophies. A Report of 74 Observations. Ann. Med. Interne (Paris), 130(11):553–557, 1979.

678. Drucker, W.R.; Hubay, C.A.; Holden, W.D.; and Bukovnic, J.A.: Pathogenesis of Posttraumatic Sympathetic Dystrophy. Am. J. Surg., 97:454–465, 1959.

679. Dwyer, A.F.: Sudeck's Atrophy and Cortisone. Med. J. Aust., 2:265–268, 1952.

680. Edmondson, A.S., and Calandruccio, R.A.: Drug Therapy for Causalgia Syndrome. Mississippi Doctor, 34:239–241, 1957.

681. Erdemir, H.; Gelman, S.; and Galbraith, J.G.: Prediction of the Needed Level of Sympathectomy for Posttraumatic Reflex Sympathetic Dystrophy. Surg. Neurol., 17(5):353–354, 1982.

682. Evans, J.A.: Reflex Sympathetic Dystrophy. Surg. Gynecol. Obstet., 82:36–43, 1946.

683. Farcot, J.M.; Mangin, P.; Laugner, B.; Thiebaut, J.B.; and Foucher, G.: Regional Intravenous Guanethidine for Sympathetic Block Algodystrophic Syndromes. Anesth. Analg. (Paris), 38(7–8):383–385, 1981.

684. Fowler, F.D., and Moser, M.: Use of Hexamethonium and Dibenzyline in Diagnosis and Treatment of Causalgia. J.A.M.A., 161:1051–1053, 1956.

685. Gaucher, A.; Columb, J.N.; Naoun, A.; Netter, P.; Faure, G.; Pourel, J.; and Robert, J.: Scintigraphic Characteristics of Coxopathies: Etiologic Importance. Rev. Rhum. Mal. Osteoartic, 45(11):641–648, 1978.

686. Glynn, C.J.; Basedow, R.W.; and Walsh, J.A.: Pain Relief Following Post-ganglionic Sympathetic Blockage With IV Guanethidine. Br. J. Anesth., 53(12):1297–1302, 1981.

687. Granit, R.; Leksell, L.; and Skoglund, C.R.: Fibre Interaction in Injured or Compressed Region of Nerve. Brain, 67:125–140, 1944.

688. Hartley, J.: Reflex Hyperemic Deossification (Sudeck's Atrophy). Journal of Mount Sinai Hospital, 22:268–277, 1955.

689. Helms, C.A.; O'Brien, E.T.; and Katzberg, R.W.: Segmental Reflex Sympathetic Dystrophy Syndrome. Radiology, 135(1):67–68, 1980.

690. Herrmann, L.G., and Caldwell, J.A.: Diagnosis and Treatment of Posttraumatic Osteoporosis. Am. J. Surg., 51: 630–640, 1941.

691. Herrmann, L.G.; Reineke, H.G.; and Caldwell, J.A.: Post-

traumatic Painful Osteoporosis. A Clinical and Roentgenological Entity. A.J.R., 47:353–361, 1942.

692. Hilker, A.W.: The Shoulder-Hand Syndrome. A Complication of Coronary Artery Disease. Ann. Intern. Med., 31:303–311, 1949.

693. Homans, J.: Minor Causalgia: A Hyperesthetic Neurovascular Syndrome. N. Engl. J. Med., 222:870–874, 1940.

694. Johnson, A.C.: Disabling Changes in the Hand Resembling Sclerodactylia Following Myocardial Infarction. Ann. Intern. Med., 19:433–456, 1943.

695. Johnson, E.W., and Pannozzo, A.N.: Management of Shoulder-Hand Syndrome. J.A.M.A., 195:108–110, 1966.

696. Kirklin, J.W.; Chenoweth, A.I.; and Murphey, F.: Causalgia: A Review of Its Characteristics, Diagnosis and Treatment. Surgery, 21:321–342, 1947.

697. Kozin, F.; Soin, J.S.; Ryan, L.M.; Carrera, G.F.; and Wortmann, R.L.: Bone Scintigraphy in the Reflex Sympathetic Dystrophy Syndrome. Radiology, 138(2):437–443, 1981.

698. Ladd, A.L.; DeHaven, K.E.; Thanik, J.; Patt, R.; and Feuerstein, M.A.: Reflex Sympathetic Imbalance: Response to Epidural Blockade. Am. J. Sports Med., 17(5): 660–668, 1989.

699. Lankford, L.L.: Reflex Sympathetic Dystrophy. *In* Omer, G.E., Jr., and Spinner, M. (eds.): Management of Peripheral Nerve Problems, pp. 216–244. Philadelphia, W.B. Saunders, 1980.

700. Lenggenhager, K.: Sudeck's Osteodystrophy: Its Pathogenesis, Prophylaxis, and Therapy. Minn. Med., 54:967–972, 1971.

701. Lewis, D., and Gatewood, W.: Treatment of Causalgia: Results of Intraneural Injection of 60 Per Cent Alcohol. J.A.M.A., 74:1–4, 1920.

702. Livingston, W.K.: Pain Mechanism: A Physiologic Interpretation of Causalagia and Its Related State, pp. 1–248. New York, Macmillan, 1943.

703. MacKinnon, S., and Holder, L.: The Use of Three-Phase Radionuclide Bone Scanning in the Diagnosis of Reflex Sympathetic Dystrophy. J. Hand Surg., 9A:556–563, 1984.

704. Marti, T.: Wesen und Behandlung des Sudeckschen Syndroms. Praxis, 43:742, 1954.

705. Mayfield, F.H., and Devine, J.W.: Causalgia. Surg. Gynecol. Obstet., 80:631–635, 1945.

706. Miller, D.S., and de Takats, G.: Post-Traumatic Dystrophy of the Extremities: Sudeck's Atrophy. Surg. Gynecol. Obstet., 75:558–582, 1942.

707. Mitchell, S.W.: The Medical Department in the Civil War. J.A.M.A., 62:1445–1450, 1914.

708. Mitchell, S.W.; Morehouse, G.R.; and Keen, W.W.: Gunshot Wounds and Other Injuries of Nerves, pp. 1–164. Philadelphia, J.B. Lippincott, 1864.

709. Moberg, E.: The Shoulder-Hand-Finger Syndrome. Acta. Chir. Scand., 109:284–292, 1955.

710. Munch-Peterson, C.U. The So-called Shoulder-Hand Syndrome. Nord. Med., 51:291–293, 1954.

711. Nathan, P.W.: On Pathogenesis of Causalgia in Peripheral Nerve Injuries. Brain, 70:145–170, 1947.

712. Omer, G.E., Jr., and Thomas, S.: Treatment of Causalgia: Review of Cases at Brooke General Hospital. Tex. Med., 67:93–96, 1971.

713. Oppenheimer, A.: The Swollen Atrophic Hand. Surg. Gynecol. Obstet., 67:446–454, 1938.

714. Pak, T.J.; Martin, G.M.; Magness, J.L.; and Kavanaugh, G.J.: Reflex Sympathetic Dystrophy; Review of 140 Cases. Minn. Med., 53:507–512, 1970.

715. Plewes, L.W.: Sudeck's Atrophy in the Hand. J. Bone Joint Surg., 38B:195–203, 1956.

716. Pool, J.L., and Brabson, J.A.: Pain on Stimulating the Distal Segment of Divided Peripheral Nerves. J. Neurosurg., 3:468–473, 1946.

717. Porter, J.M.; Lindell, T.D.; Leung, B.S.; and Reiney, C.G.: Effect of Intra-arterial Injection of Reserpine on Vascular Wall Catecholamine Content. Surg. Forum, 23:183–185, 1972.

718. Procacci, P.; Francini, F.; Maresca, M.; and Zoppi, M.: Skin Potentials and EMG Changes Induced by Cutaneous Electrical Stimulation, II Subjects With Reflex Sympathetic Dystrophies. Appl. Neurophysiol., 42(3):125–134, 1979.

719. Reiner, J.C.; Moreau, R.; Bernat, M.; Basle, M.; Jallet, P.; and Minier, J.F.: Contribution of Dynamic Isotopic Tests in the Study of Algodystrophies. Rev. Rhum. Mal. Osteoartic., 46(4):235–251, 1979.

720. Richards, R.L.: Causalgia: A Centennial Review. Arch. Neurol., 6:339–350, 1967.

721. Roland, O.: Unsere Erfahrungen mit Depot-Padutin. Zentralbl. Chir., 77:1–147, 1942.

722. Rose, T.F.: Sudeck's Post-Traumatic Osteodystrophy of Limbs. Med. J. Aust., 1:185–188, 1953.

723. Rosen, P.S., and Graham, W.: The Shoulder-Hand Syndrome. Can. Med. Assoc. J., 77:86–91, 1957.

724. Schutzer, S., and Gossling, H.: Current Concepts Review. The Treatment of Reflex Sympathetic Dystrophy Syndrome. J. Bone Joint Surg., 66A:625–629, 1984.

725. Simon, H., and Carlson, D.H.: The Use of Bone Scanning in the Diagnosis of Reflex Sympathetic Dystrophy. Clin. Nucl. Med., 5(3):116–121, 1980.

726. Simson, G.: Propranolol for Causalgia and Sudeck Atrophy (Letter). J.A.M.A., 227:327, 1974.

727. Smithwick, R.H.: The Value of Sympathectomy in the Treatment of Vascular Disease. N. Engl. J. Med., 216:141–150, 1937.

728. Speigel, I.J., and Milowsky, J.L.: Causalgia. J.A.M.A., 127:9–15, 1945.

729. Spurling, R.G.: Causalgia of the Upper Extremity: Treatment by Dorsal Sympathetic Ganglionectomy. Arch. Neurol. Psychiatr., 23:784–788, 1930.

730. Steinbrocker, O., and Argyros, T.G.: The Shoulder-Hand Syndrome; Present Status as a Diagnostic and Therapeutic Entity. Med. Clin. North Am., 42:1533–1553, 1958.

731. Steinbrocker, O.; Neustadt, D.; and Lapin, L.: The Shoulder-Hand Syndrome. Sympathetic Block Compared With Corticotropin and Cortisone Therapy. J.A.M.A., 153:788–791, 1953.

732. Steinbrocker, O.; Spitzer, N.; and Friedman, H.H.: The Shoulder-Hand Syndrome in Reflex Dystrophy of the Upper Extremity. Ann. Intern. Med., 29:22–52, 1948.

733. Sudek, P.: Ueber die akute entzundlicke knocken Atrophie. Arch. Klin. Chir., 62:147–156, 1900.

734. Sudek, P.: Ueber die akute (trophoneurotische) Knoch-

735. Sunderland, S.: Pain Mechanisms in Causalgia. J. Neurol. Neurosurg. Psychiatry, 39:471–480, 1976.

736. Swan, D.M.: Shoulder-Hand Syndrome Following Hemiplegia. Neurology, 4:480–482, 1954.

737. Threadgill, F.D.: Afferent Conduction Via the Sympathetic Ganglia Innervating the Extremities. Surgery, 21:569–594, 1947.

738. Toumey, J.W.: Occurrence and Management of Reflex Sympathetic Dystrophy (Causalgia of the Extremities). J. Bone Joint Surg., 30A:883–894, 1948.

739. Visitsunthorn, U., and Prete, P.: Reflex Sympathetic Dystrophy of the Lower Extremity: A Complication of Herpes Zoster With Dramatic Response to Propranolol. West. J. Med., 135(1):62–66, 1981.

740. Walker, A.E., and Nulsen, F.: Electrical Stimulation of the Upper Thoracic Portion of the Sympathetic Chain in Man. Arch. Neurol. Psychiatr., 59:559–560, 1948.

741. White, J.C.; Heroy, W.W.; and Goodman, E.N.: Causalgia Following Gunshot Injuries of Nerves. Ann. Surg., 128:161–183, 1948.

742. William, E.: Treatment of Reflex Sympathetic Dystrophy by Calcitonin. Rev. Med. Brux., 1(7):457–461, 1980.

743. Young, J.H., and Pearson, A.T.: The Shoulder-Hand Syndrome. Med. J. Aust., 1:776–780, 1952.

Compartment Syndromes

744. Ashton, H.: The Effect of Increased Tissue Pressure on Blood Flow. Clin. Orthop., 113:15–26, 1975.

745. Benjamin, A.: The Relief of Inflatable Plastic Splints on Blood Flow. Br. Med. J., 2:1427–1430, 1966.

746. Bradley, E.L.: The Anterior Tibial Compartment Syndrome. Surg. Gynecol. Obstet., 136(1):289–297, 1973.

747. Burton, A.C.: On the Physical Equilibrium of Small Blood Vessels. Am. J. Physiol., 164:319–329, 1951.

748. Caldwell, R.K.: Ischemic Necrosis of the Anterior Tibial Muscle: Case Report With Autopsy Findings and Review of Literature. Ann. Intern. Med., 46:1191–1199, 1957.

749. Carter, A.B.; Richards, R.L.; and Zachary, R.: The Anterior Tibial Syndrome. Lancet, 2:928–934, 1949.

750. Cywes, S., and Louw, J.H.: Phlegmasia Cerula Dolens: Successful Treatment by Relieving Fasciotomy. Surgery, 51:169–176, 1962.

751. Eaton, R.G., and Green, W.T.: Epimysiotomy and Fasciotomy in the Treatment of Volkmann's Ischemic Contracture. Orthop. Clin. North Am., 3:175–186, 1972.

752. Ernst, C.B., and Kaufer, H.: Fibulectomy-fasciotomy: An Important Adjunct in the Management of Lower Extremity Arterial Trauma. J. Trauma, 11:365–380, 1971.

753. Garfin, S.; Mubarak, S.; Evans, K.; Hargens, A.; and Akeson, W.: Quantification of Intracompartmental Pressure and Volume Under Plaster Casts. J. Bone Joint Surg., 63A:449–453, 1981.

754. Gaspard, D.J.; Cohen, S.L.; and Gaspar, M.R.: Decompression Dermotomy: A Limb Salvage Adjunct. J.A.M.A., 220:831–833, 1972.

755. Gaspard, D.J., and Kohl, R.D.: Compartmental Syndromes

in Which the Skin Is the Limiting Boundary. Clin. Orthop., 113:65–68, 1975.

756. Harman, J.W., and Gwinn, R.P.: The Significance of Local Vascular Phenomena in the Production of Ischemic Necrosis in Skeletal Muscle. Am. J. Pathol., 24:625–638, 1948.

757. Harman, J.W., and Gwinn, R.: The Recovery of Skeletal Muscle Fibers From Acute Ischemia as Determined by Histologic and Chemical Methods. Am. J. Pathol., 25:741–755, 1949.

758. Holden, C.E.A.: Traumatic Tension Ischaemia in Muscles. Injury, 5:223–527, 1973.

759. Jepson, P.N.: Ischemic Contracture, Experimental Study. Ann. Surg., 84:785–795, 1926.

760. Jones, W.; Perry, M.; and Bush, H.: Changes in Tibial Venous Blood Flow in the Evolving Compartment Syndrome. Arch. Surg., 124:801–804, 1989.

761. Kirby, N.G.: Exercise Ischaemia in the Fascial Compartment of the Soleus: Case Report. J. Bone Joint Surg., 52B:738–740, 1970.

762. Kjellmer, I.: An Indirect Method for Estimating Tissue Pressure With Special Reference to Tissue Pressure in Muscle During Exercise. Acta Physiol. Scand., 62:31–40, 1964.

763. Klock, J.C., and Sexton, M.J.: Rhabdomyolysis and Acute Myoglobinuric Renal Failure Following Heroin Use. Calif. Med., 119:5–8, 1973.

764. Lewis, T.: Vascular Disorders of the Limbs, 1–107. London, McMillan, 1936.

765. Lowenberg, E.L.: Acute Ischemic Infarction of the Gastrocnemius Muscle Simulating Deep Vein Phlebitis. J. Cardiovasc. Surg., 6:104–110, 1965.

766. Lundborg, G.: Limb Ischemia and Nerve Injury. Arch. Surg., 104:631–632, 1972.

767. McQuillan, W.M., and Nolan, B.: Ischaemia Complicating Injury. J. Bone Joint Surg., 50B:482–492, 1968.

768. Manson, I.W.: Post-Partum Eclampsia Complicated by the Anterior Tibial Syndrome. Br. Med. J., 2:1117–1118, 1964.

769. Matsen, F.A., III: Compartmental Syndrome: A Unified Concept. Clin. Orthop., 113:8–14, 1975.

770. Mubarak, S.J., and Owen, C.A.: Double-Incision Fasciotomy of the Leg for Decompression in Compartment Syndromes. J. Bone Joint Surg., 59A:184–187, 1977.

771. Parkes, A.R.: Traumatic Ischemia of Peripheral Nerves With Some Observations on Volkmann's Ischemic Contracture. Br. J. Surg., 32:403–413, 1944.

772. Reneman, R.S.: The Anterior and the Lateral Compartment Syndrome of the Leg. The Hague, Mouton, 1968.

773. Reneman, R.S.: The Anterior and the Lateral Compartment Syndrome of the Leg Due to Intensive Use of Muscles. Clin. Orthop., 113:69–80, 1975.

774. Reneman, R.S., and Jagenean, A.H.: The Influence of Weighted Exercise on Tissue (Intramuscular) Pressure in Normal Subjects and Patients With Intermittent Claudication. Scand. J. Clin. Lab. Invest. (Suppl.), 128(31):37, 1973.

775. Reszel, P.A.; Jones, J.M.; and Spittell, J.A.: Ischemic Necrosis of the Peroneal Musculature, A Lateral Compartment Syndrome: A Report of a Case. Mayo Clin. Proc., 38:130, 1963.

776. Sanderson, R.A.; Foley, R.K.; McIvor, G.; and Kirkaldy-Willis, W.H.: Histological Response on Skeletal Muscle to Ischemia. Clin. Orthop., 113:27–35, 1975.

777. Schreiber, S.; Liebowitz, M.; and Berstein, L.: Limb Compression and Renal Impairment (Crush Syndrome) Following Narcotic Overdose. J. Bone Joint Surg., 54A:1683–1692, 1972.

778. Schrock, R.D.: Peroneal Nerve Palsy Following Derotation Osteotomies for Tibial Torsion. Clin. Orthop., 62:172–177, 1969.

779. Spinner, M.; Mache, A.; Silver, L.; and Barsky, A.J.: Impending Ischemic Contracture of the Hand. Plast. Reconstr. Surg., 50:341–349, 1972.

780. Sweeney, H.E., and O'Brien, G.F.: Bilateral Anterior Tibial Syndrome in Association With the Nephrotic Syndrome: Report of a Case. Arch. Intern. Med., 116:487–490, 1965.

781. Tachdjian, M.O.: Pediatric Orthopaedics. pp. 1–766. Philadelphia, W.B. Saunders, 1972.

782. Thomson, S.A., and Mahoney, L.J.: Volkmann's Ischaemic Contracture and Its Relationship to Fracture of the Femur. J. Bone Joint Surg., 33B:336–347, 1951.

783. Volkmann, R.: Die ischaemischem Muskellamungen und Kontrakturen. Zentralbl. Chir., 8:801, 1881.

784. Volkmann, R.: Die Krankheiten der Bewegung surgane. In Pitha, R.V., and Billroth, W.M. (eds.): Handbuch der Chirurgie, Vol. 2. Stuttgart, Ferdinand Enke, 1872.

785. Weitz, E.M., and Carson, G.: The Anterior Tibial Compartment Syndrome in a Twenty-Month-Old Infant: A Complication of the Use of a Bow Leg Brace. Bull. Hosp. Jt. Dis. Orthop. Inst., 30:16, 1969.

786. Whitesides, T.E.; Harada, H.; and Morimoto, K.: The Response of Skeletal Muscle to Temporary Ischemia: An Experimental Study. J. Bone Joint Surg., 53A:1027–1028, 1971.

787. Whitesides, T.E., Jr.; Haney, T.C.; Morimoto, K.; and Harada, H.: Tissue Pressure Measurements as a Determinant for the Need of Fasciotomy. Clin. Orthop., 113:43–51, 1975.

788. Willhoite, D.R., and Moll, J.H.: Early Recognition and Treatment of Impending Volkmann's Ischemia in the Lower Extremity. Arch. Surg., 100:11–16, 1970.

6

Pathologic Fractures

Dempsey Springfield
Candace Jennings

A pathologic fracture is a fracture involving abnormal bone. Typically the fracture occurs during normal activity or with minor trauma, and the failure of bone under these circumstances should alert the surgeon to the presence of a predisposing pathologic condition. The orthopaedic surgeon must do more than just treat the broken bone, because successful management of the patient requires recognition, diagnosis, and treatment of the underlying process. The management of the fracture may be dramatically altered by the associated pathologic condition, and failing to adjust the fracture management may lead to additional difficulties depending on the etiology of the abnormality. Osteoporosis is the most common pathologic condition associated with pathologic fracture, but the management of fractured osteoporotic bone is only occasionally different from that of normal bone.[4] This chapter discusses only briefly the management of fractures of osteoporotic bone. What is usually thought of when pathologic fractures are discussed is carcinoma metastatic to bone with a fracture or "impending fracture," and this chapter concentrates on the management of patients with these fractures. We want to remind the reader, however, of other associated conditions: underlying metabolic disorders, primary benign tumors, and primary malignant tumors. The management of patients with pathologic fractures demands more of the orthopaedic surgeon than the management of similar fractures in normal bone. Initial management, well planned and well executed, will dramatically improve a patient's life, whereas treatment that is not planned and done well will condemn the patient to far more difficulty.

INITIAL EVALUATION

HISTORY AND PHYSICAL EXAMINATION

A patient who presents with a fracture occurring spontaneously or following minor trauma, has an unusual fracture pattern, has had several recent fractures, is elderly, or has a history of a primary malignancy should alert the physician to the possibility of an associated pathologic process. A complete history must be obtained from the patient, beginning with the circumstances surrounding the current injury; the degree of trauma may provide information about the strength of the bone. Patients must be asked specifically about previously diagnosed or treated malignancies, because they may consider themselves "cured" and no longer at risk for recurrence or metastases. Standard questions regarding general health, including recent weight loss, fevers, night sweats, and fatigue, are important. Questions about relevant risk factors, such as smoking, dietary habits, and environmental exposures, should be asked, and a careful review of systems is essential.

The physical examination should be thorough, with careful palpation for lymphadenopathy in the neck, supraclavicular fossa, axilla, and inguinal region; thyroid nodules; breast masses; prostate nodules; rectal masses; and rectal tone. A stool guaiac test is always done. Since common things occur commonly, the history and physical examination can be considered a search for the most likely causes of pathologic fractures, ie, metastatic malignancy and osteoporosis.

RADIOGRAPHIC EVALUATION

X-rays of the symptomatic extremity should be obtained and carefully reviewed with attention to specific lesions and overall bone quality. The pathologic lesion may be obvious, and frequently a diagnosis can be made from the initial x-ray films, history, and physical examination. If the diagnosis is not obvious after the initial evaluation, the x-rays should be examined for diagnostic clues, such as generalized osteopenia, periosteal reaction, thinning of the cortices, abnormal radiodensities in the bone or soft tissue, Looser's lines, calcification of the small vessels, and abnormal soft tissue shadows.

Enneking teaches his students to ask and answer four questions about a lesion seen on a plain x-ray film (W. F. Enneking: personal communication, April, 1974) (Table 6-1). This method has proved helpful in interpreting x-rays of patients with bone lesions. The first question is, ''Where is the lesion located?'' The answer should locate the lesion with respect to the epiphysis, metaphysis, or diaphysis; cortex or medullary canal; and long bone or flat bone. The second question is, ''What is the lesion doing to the bone?'' Lesions associated with a pathologic fracture destroy bone, and the pattern of destruction can be helpful in determining the nature of a process. Is the destruction total, with a complete loss of all bone within the involved area; diffuse, with an area of bone undisturbed but surrounded by areas of resorption; or minimal, with just a hint of bone loss localized to an area of the bone? As a general rule, lesions that permeate through bone with minimal destruction seen radiographically are more aggressive than those that resorb all bone in their pathway. The third question is, ''What is the bone doing to the lesion?'' The degree of maturity of the response gives significant information regarding the character of the tumor. A well-defined, mature reactive rim suggests a slow-growing lesion, especially when no acute periosteal reaction is seen. An intact but abundant periosteal reaction is evidence of an aggressive process, whereas a periosteal reaction that cannot keep up with the tumor (ie, Codman's triangle) suggests an extremely rapidly growing malignant lesion. The fourth question is, ''Are there any clues on the plain

Table 6-1. Enneking's Four Questions

1. Where is the lesion located?
2. What is the lesion doing to the bone?
3. What is the bone doing to the lesion?
4. Are there any clues on the plain films that would provide information about the type of tissue within the lesion?

films that would provide information about the type of tissue within the lesion?'' Calcification is diagnostic of either a cartilage lesion or an infarction of bone. Bone production within the lesion suggests an osteosarcoma or osteoblastoma. A ground-glass appearance is consistent with fibrous dysplasia. This method of looking at x-ray films is extremely helpful, particularly when the diagnosis is not immediately recognizable (Table 6-2).

Osteopenia is the term used to indicate either inadequate bone (osteoporosis) or inadequately mineralized bone (osteomalacia). Using only plain x-ray films, the physician usually cannot distinguish between these two disorders, but there are suggestive differential clues. Looser's lines (compression-side radiolucent lines), calcification of small vessels, and phalangeal periosteal reaction are features of osteomalacia or hyperparathyroidism. Thin cortices and loss of the normal trabecular pattern without other abnormalities are most suggestive of osteoporosis.

When there is an identifiable specific lesion with otherwise normal bone, the initial decision is whether the lesion is inactive (most likely benign) or aggressive (most likely malignant). Small radiolucent lesions that are surrounded by a rim of reactive bone without endosteal or periosteal reaction are inactive or minimally active (ie, usually benign) primary bone tumors. Lesions that erode the cortex but are contained by a well-developed periosteal reaction are usually active benign or a low-grade malignant primary bone tumor, but a metastatic deposit can have this appearance. Large lesions that destroy the cortex and are not contained by the periosteum are aggressive lesions and usually malignant,[16,35] either primary or metastatic. A permeative or ''moth-eaten'' pattern of cortical destruction is most suggestive of a malignancy. Most destructive bone lesions in adults are metastatic carcinoma; however, a solitary bone lesion should be initially considered a primary sarcoma until a primary carcinoma is found or a biopsy reveals metastatic carcinoma or myeloma. Primary bone tumors are most common in patients younger than 50 years of age and usually arise in the metaphysis of a long bone. Metastases are found in older patients and are most commonly at the metaphyseal-diaphyseal junction. When a metastasis is suspected, the remainder of the skeleton should be evaluated for other sites of disease. An avulsion fracture of the lesser trochanter is almost always pathologic, and this specific injury should arouse suspicion of occult metastatic disease (Fig. 6-1).[9,69]

The most common sites of carcinoma metastatic to bone are the spine, ribs, pelvis, femur, and humerus; only rarely do they occur distal to the knees or elbows.[2,8,51,66,91] Therefore, plain x-ray films of the bones at most risk should be obtained. Plain x-ray films of any tender bone also should be examined.[91] A whole-body technetium scan is a useful screen for the entire skeleton,[18,32,78] but we recommend plain x-rays of both humeri, the pelvis, and both femurs in addition to the bone scan. These bones are at risk for pathologic fracture, and plain x-ray assessment is important. In a study of patients with breast carcinoma, 24% of the patients with a

Table 6-2. Classic Answers to Enneking's Four Questions

Nonossifying Fibroma
1. Long bone metaphysis; eccentric medullary canal and cortex
2. Geographic pattern; cortical "expansion"
3. Minimal reaction; periosteum contains lesion
4. Radiolucent

Unicameral Bone Cyst
1. Long bone metaphysis; frequently against epiphyseal plate
2. Geographic pattern; loss of metaphyseal remodeling
3. Well-developed reactive rim
4. Radiolucent; "fallen-leaf" sign with fracture

Enchondroma
1. Long bone metaphysis; common in phalanges of hand
2. Geographic pattern; cortical "expansion"
3. Well-developed reactive rim; periosteum contains lesion
4. Radiolucent with radiodense amorphous nodules within the radiolucency

Aneurysmal Bone Cyst
1. Any location; common in flat bones and spine
2. Geographic pattern medullary canal and cortex
3. Thin reactive rim usually containing the lesion
4. Radiolucent

Osteoblastoma
1. Most common in posterior elements of spine
2. Geographic pattern
3. Marked reaction
4. Neoplastic bone within lesion

Chondroblastoma
1. Long bone epiphysis; periacetabular pelvis
2. Geographic pattern
3. Mild reactive rim
4. Punctate radiodense nodules of calcification

Chondromyxofibroma
1. Long bone metaphysis; eccentric medullary canal and cortex
2. Geographic pattern
3. Mild reactive rim
4. Radiolucent

Ossifying Fibroma and Adamantinoma
1. Cortex of tibia
2. "Bubbly" geographic pattern
3. Modest reaction; periosteum contains lesion
4. Radiolucent

Giant Cell Tumor
1. Long bone metaphysis and epiphysis; to subchondral bone
2. Geographic pattern
3. Minimal reaction
4. Radiolucent

Fibrous Dysplasia
1. Any location; commonly multiple lesions, ipsilateral
2. Geographic pattern
3. No reaction
4. Ground-glass appearance

Ewing's Sarcoma
1. Flat bones, ribs, clavicle, fibula
2. Permeative pattern
3. Periosteal reaction; Codman's triangle, tumor not contained by reactive periosteum
4. Large soft tissue mass associated with lesion

Eosinophilic Granuloma
1. Any location
2. Permeative pattern
3. Modest periosteal reaction
4. Radiolucent

Osteosarcoma
1. Long bone metaphysis
2. Any pattern
3. Marked periosteal reaction
4. Neoplastic bone formation

Chondrosarcoma
1. Any location; periacetabular pelvis common
2. Geographic pattern
3. Minimal reaction
4. Radiolucent; may have radiodensities of calcified cartilage, so-called "smoke rings"

Malignant Fibrous Histiocytoma
1. Long bone metaphysis
2. Geographic/permeative pattern
3. Minimal reaction
4. Commonly associated with Paget's disease or bone infarct

Metastatic Carcinoma
1. Long bone diaphysis
2. Geographic pattern
3. Modest periosteal reaction
4. Radiolucent

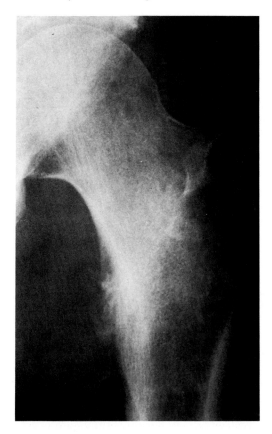

Fig. 6-1. An anteroposterior x-ray of the proximal femur in a patient with known breast cancer. She complained of pain in the groin that worsened with weight-bearing on the extremity. The subtle changes in the lesser trochanter should be diagnostic of a metastasis to the proximal femur. This lesion is easy to miss and if not treated will result in a pathologic fracture. A CT scan is recommended to evaluate the amount of bone destruction, and a bone scan should be done to look for other bone metastases. Prophylactic internal fixation should be considered because of the risk of fracture in this part of the femur.

small primary lesion, otherwise normal results of clinical examination, normal findings from serum chemistries, and normal plain x-ray films had a bone scan that revealed skeletal metastases. The prognostic value of the bone scan was also demonstrated, since 100% of patients with an abnormal bone scan on initial staging had recurrent disease at 5 years, whereas only 26% of those with a normal scan had evidence of disease at the same follow-up interval.[32]

We agree with Steckel and Kagan,[83] who recommend a limited search for the unknown primary

carcinoma. Carcinoma of the breast and carcinoma of the lung account for most metastases to bone; therefore, a chest x-ray film, breast examination, and mammogram are recommended.[1,2,91] Renal, thyroid, and prostate carcinomas are the other three tumors that frequently go to bone, and these organs should be examined. Myeloma should be considered, and skull x-ray films (in addition to immunoelectrophoresis) are recommended. Finally, any organ system implicated by the initial review of systems should be carefully evaluated. More thorough evaluations rarely uncover the primary carcinoma.

LABORATORY EVALUATION

Disturbances in hematologic and/or metabolic parameters can aid in the diagnosis of a primary or secondary disorder associated with pathologic fractures. In all patients in whom a pathologic process is suspected, a baseline laboratory profile should be done, including a complete blood count with a manual differential, peripheral blood smear, and sedimentation rate; serum chemistries and enzymes should include blood urea nitrogen (BUN), serum glucose, liver function tests, albumin, calcium, phosphorus, and alkaline phosphatase. A standard urinalysis is necessary to look for microhematuria, and a 24-hour urine collection is necessary if a complete metabolic evaluation is planned. Serum immunoelectrophoresis is currently the laboratory test of choice as a screen for myeloma.

Patients with osteoporosis have normal values for all the aforementioned laboratory tests, whereas patients with osteomalacia have low serum calcium, low serum phosphorus, high serum alkaline phosphatase, high urinary phosphorus, and high urinary hydroxyproline values. Patients with primary hyperparathyroidism have high serum calcium, alkaline phosphatase, and parathormone; low serum phosphorus; and high urinary calcium, phosphorus, and hydroxyproline. Those patients with renal osteodystrophy have low serum calcium, high serum phosphorus, high serum alkaline phosphatase, and an elevated BUN. When secondary hyperparathyroidism develops in these patients, the serum calcium increases to normal or above normal and the parathormone is also elevated (Table 6-3). Urinary determinations are difficult to assess in patients with secondary hyperparathyroidism owing to the abnormal glomerular filtration. Patients with Paget's disease have normal values for serum calcium and phosphorus but markedly elevated levels of alkaline phosphatase and urinary hydroxyproline. Acid phosphatase is usually elevated in patients with prostatic carcinoma, particularly when the disease has metastasized.

It should be remembered that the serum calcium is a measurement of the unbound calcium in the serum and, therefore, determination of serum protein is important. If the serum protein is lower than normal, the normal range of serum calcium is lowered. Also, patients with a high intake of phosphate have a spuriously low serum calcium.

Hypercalcemia of Malignancy

As many as 75,000 cases of hypercalcemia are diagnosed in the United States each year; most of these patients have primary hyperparathyroidism, but approximately 40% of the patients have a malignancy causing the elevated serum calcium. Rarely, the two causes occur simultaneously. The orthopaedic surgeon managing a patient with metastatic carcinoma to bone must be aware of the risk of hypercalcemia, its symptoms, and management. The malignancies most commonly associated with hypercalcemia are of the lung, breast, kidney, and genitourinary tract. Multiple myeloma and lymphoma may cause hypercalcemia, but they account for fewer than 10% of all cases.[17,33,77] In every patient with metastatic carcinoma to bone, the serum calcium and protein should be measured concurrently. Hypercalcemia can kill a patient and should be diagnosed early and treated.

Although hypercalcemia occurs frequently enough to be a constant concern to any physician treating patients with malignant diseases, it is rarely the presenting clinical feature of a previously undiagnosed malignancy.[17,29] When hypercalcemia occurs in malignancy, it is a poor prognostic sign for the patient; as many as 60% of those patients will not survive longer than 3 months, and only 20% will survive for 1 year. The signs and symptoms are myriad and often vague but classically include nocturia, polydipsia, polyuria, fatigue, irritability, confusion, constipation, urinary tract infections, muscle weakness (especially of proximal muscle groups), joint and bone pain, anorexia, weight loss, nausea, vomiting, abdominal pain, unsteady gait, headache, and blurred vision. Often the signs are of nonspecific deterioration without any focal clues. None of these symptoms is specific, and it is better to diagnose the problem by measuring the serum calcium directly.

There does not appear to be a reliable correlation between the severity of the hypercalcemia and the degree of skeletal involvement.[7,33,79] However, there is some relationship between the type of malignant disease and concurrence of bone metastases and hypercalcemia. For example, lung cancer is likely to cause hypercalcemia without apparent bone metastases, whereas hypercalcemia in multiple myeloma or breast carcinoma and the extent of bone metastases correlate strongly.[79] Histologic evidence suggests that the presence of metastatic disease in bone is not essential for the observation of diffuse osteoclastic activity associated with clinical hypercalcemia.[34]

Once the patient with hypercalcemia is identified, a treatment plan must be established. Outpatient treatment of these patients is unsatisfactory if any long-term effect is expected. The patient with acute hypercalcemia may benefit from vigorous volume repletion; however, this is only a temporizing measure, and the hypercalcemia will recur, often more severely, unless an effort is made to reduce the degree of bone resorption. This reduction can be accomplished in some cases by treating the primary neoplasm directly or by using agents that will reduce osteoclastic activity such as phosphate, mithramycin, calcitonin, indomethacin, or glucocorticoids. A recently developed drug, amino-hydroxy propylidene diphosphonate (APD), has been effective in producing sustained remissions of hyper-

Table 6-3. Disorders Producing Osteopenia

| Disorder | Laboratory Values | | | |
	Serum Calcium	Serum Phosphorous	Serum Alkaline Phosphatase	Urine
Osteoporosis	Normal	Normal	Normal	Normal Ca
Osteomalacia	Normal	Normal	Normal	Low Ca
Hyperparathyroidism	Normal to high	Normal to low	Normal	High Ca
Renal osteodystrophy	Low	High	High	—
Paget's disease	Normal	Normal	Very high	Hydroxyproline
Myeloma*	Normal	Normal	Normal	Protein

* Abnormal serum and/or urine immunoelectrophoresis.

calcemia secondary to malignancy. A recent study[85] reported that in a trial of APD among patients with metastatic breast cancer, hypercalcemia was prevented and there was a significant reduction in bone pain and pathologic fractures. Currently, this drug is available only for investigational use but promises to be a useful clinical tool in the near future.

DIAGNOSIS OF THE PATHOLOGIC PROCESS

The preliminary evaluation may be sufficiently convincing of a diagnosis or at least a category of disease that a biopsy occasionally can be foregone. However, this should be the case only when absolute histologic confirmation of the diagnosis will not alter the clinical management of the patient or in any way affect the successful outcome of the patient's treatment. This is true only for self-healing benign tumors, fibrous dysplasia, and Paget's disease. Categorizing the underlying process into systemic skeletal disease, primary benign disease, primary malignant bone tumor, or metastatic carcinoma will allow selection of the proper treatment plan. If a biopsy is indicated, it should be performed only after careful planning and without interfering with subsequent management of the patient.

INDICATIONS FOR THE METHODS OF BIOPSY

As a general rule, only those lesions suspected of being malignant should be subject to biopsy prior to healing of the fracture. Staging of the tumor prior to a biopsy is best. Staging of the tumor should be completed with accurate anatomic localization and a search for other lesions. Unless the lesion is clearly a metastasis, there is a known primary tumor and a typical x-ray finding, or there are multiple lesions, the lesion should be approached as if it were a primary malignant tumor of bone and the biopsy should not preclude subsequent primary surgical treatment.

STAGING OF TUMORS

There are two primary staging systems for soft tissue tumors but only one for primary bone tumors. Neither system is intended for metastatic carcinoma. The system originally proposed by Enneking and associates can be used for both bone and soft tissue tumors and is probably the most commonly used

system by orthopaedic surgeons.[24] This system separates tumors based on their histologic grade, their anatomic extent, and the presence of metastasis. The histologic grade is either low (I) or high (II). Anatomic extent is either intracompartmental (A) or extracompartmental (B). Those tumors with metastatic sarcoma are placed in a separate stage (III) (Table 6-4). The only other commonly used staging system for musculoskeletal tumors is for soft tissue tumors only and was proposed by a committee commissioned to develop a staging system.[74] This system classifies tumors by their histologic grade, size measured in centimeters, and presence of metastasis. The histologic grades are divided into three groups: low (I), medium (II), and high (III). The size is divided by those less than 5 cm (A) or greater than 5 cm (B). Patients with distant metastasis or invasion of nerves, major vessels, or bone are classified separately in stage IV (Table 6-5).

TECHNIQUE OF BIOPSY

The biopsy must obtain adequate histologic material for diagnosis, contaminate as little local tissue as possible (tissue contaminated by the postbiopsy hematoma must also be considered contaminated by tumor cells), and not adversely affect the treatment of the fracture.[81] Consultation with the pathologist prior to biopsy can be helpful in determining the best area from which to obtain tissue. When possible, the tissue should be obtained from a site unaffected by the fracture, because the bone's reaction to the fracture will produce a confusing histologic picture. (An incisional biopsy obtained from a lesion associated with a pathologic fracture can be exceedingly difficult to interpret because of the fracture callus in-grafted on the underlying tumor.) If a definitive diagnosis can be made on frozen section, the treatment of the tumor and fracture may be completed at the time of the biopsy, but if no diagnosis can be made, it is inappropriate to proceed

Table 6-4. Bone and Soft Tissue Tumor Staging System

Low Histologic Grade	I
Intracompartmental	A
Extracompartmental	B
High Histologic Grade	II
Intracompartmental	A
Extracompartmental	B
Metastatic	III

(Modified from Enneking, W. F.; Spanier, S. S.; and Goodman, M. A.: A System for Surgical Staging of Musculoskeletal Sarcoma. Clin. Orthop., 153:106–120, 1980.)

Table 6-5. Staging of Soft Tissue Sarcoma

Stage I

Ia:	Low histologic grade tumor less than 5 cm in diameter with no regional lymph node or distant metastasis
Ib:	Low histologic grade tumor 5 cm or greater in diameter with no regional lymph node or distant metastasis

Stage II

IIa:	Medium histologic grade tumor less than 5 cm in diameter with no regional lymph node or distant metastasis
IIb:	Medium histologic grade tumor 5 cm or greater in diameter with no regional lymph node or distant metastasis

Stage III

IIIa:	High histologic grade tumor less than 5 cm in diameter with no regional lymph node or distant metastasis
IIIb:	High histologic grade tumor 5 cm or greater in diameter with no regional lymph node or distant metastasis
IIIc:	Tumor of any grade or size with regional lymph node but no distant metastasis

Stage IV

IVa:	Tumor of any grade and any size that grossly invades bone, a major vessel, or a major nerve with or without regional lymph node metastasis but without distant metastasis
IVb:	Tumor with distant metastasis

(Modified from Russell, W. O.; Cohen, J.; Enzinger, S.; Hajdu, S. I.; Heise, H.; Martin, R. G.; Meissner, W.; Miller, W. T.; Schmitz, R. L.; and Suit, H. D.: A Clinical and Pathological Staging System for Soft Tissue Sarcoma. Cancer, 40:1562–1570, 1977.)

with treatment of the tumor or fracture unless this is accomplished without contamination of previously uninvolved tissue. No biopsy procedure is completed until cultures have been obtained.

SPECIFIC TREATMENT

Remembering the rule of common occurrences and assuming a normal distribution of patients, the most common pathologic fracture is due to osteoporosis. Under nearly all circumstances these fractures should be managed as recommended in the accompanying chapters of this text. Adjustments may be necessary because of the weakened bone. Pathologic fractures due to metastatic carcinoma, the second most common cause of pathologic fracture, and the patients in whom they occur demand special considerations (Fig. 6-2).[13,21,39,44,45,48,52,57,63,67,68,76,86,90]

Life expectancy after the diagnosis of metastatic carcinoma continues to increase, and those patients who have skeletal metastases require the most careful considerations. In 1985, 910,000 new cases of primary malignancy were reported in the United States; an estimated 50% of those patients will be alive 5 years later, suggesting a cumulative total number of patients alive with malignant disease to be greater than 2.5 million. Many of these patients will have carcinoma metastatic to bone, especially those with their primary tumor arising from the breast, prostate, lung, kidney, or thyroid. Among those patients, survival with metastatic disease may be several years to a decade.[13,43,88] Because the survival of patients with malignant disease is being improved by advances in early diagnosis and treatment, during the last decade the philosophy of management has changed from one of simply providing comfort in anticipation of an early demise to one of trying to provide pain-free maintenance of normal daily function for a few years. Many routine techniques used to treat nonpathologic fractures are inadequate in the management of pathologic fractures secondary to metastatic carcinoma, and more complex approaches are often necessary.

Most patients with a pathologic fracture from metastatic carcinoma have been treated previously for the primary malignancy, and the diagnosis is only occasionally in question. Patients presenting with a pathologic fracture secondary to metastatic carcinoma but without prior diagnosis should be evaluated so that the primary tumor also may be managed. As outlined in the first section of this chapter, a thorough history and physical examination with attention to lymph nodes, thyroid, breast, rectum, and prostate; chest x-ray film; and baseline laboratory values are requisite in each new patient. Additional studies may include computed tomographic (CT) scan of the lung, renal ultrasound or intravenous pyelogram, ^{99m}Tc bone scan, mammography, and special chemistries as previously outlined. If the primary tumor is not apparent from these tests, it is probably not necessary to continue to search for it.[83] Finding it is unlikely, and if it is found, knowledge of the primary tumor would not lead to a significant difference in the management of the patient. Specifically, it is not necessary to obtain a gastrointestinal series, liver-spleen scan, or CT scans of the head and abdomen unless the patient's history, review of systems, or physical examination suggests an abnormality in one of these locations.

IMPENDING FRACTURES

Many patients who complain of pain are found to have a lesion of bone secondary to metastatic dis-

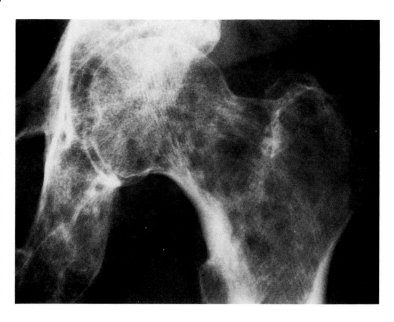

Fig. 6-2. An anteroposterior x-ray of the proximal femur in a patient with known breast cancer. The permeative destruction of the bone is most likely due to metastatic deposits of breast cancer. Disuse osteoporosis may have a similar appearance, and the x-ray diagnosis should be confirmed by a biopsy unless the diagnosis of metastatic disease in the patient has already been confirmed at another site. This permeative destruction of the proximal femur is the most common type of destruction leading to a pathologic fracture. For patients with this type of destruction, we suggest prophylactic internal fixation of the femoral neck and subtrochanteric region.

ease even without a fracture. When the patient is known to have a carcinoma, the principal questions concern whether (1) the patient should be treated with prophylactic surgical stabilization prior to radiation therapy[5,45,75]; (2) he or she should be followed clinically and radiographically; and (3) he or she should be managed by radiation and chemotherapy without prophylactic fixation. Each time a patient with a metastatic deposit in bone is evaluated, these questions must be considered. The term *impending fracture* is used throughout the literature on metastatic disease, but the criteria for what constitutes an impending fracture are arbitrary. Compounding the problem is the fact that patients with lesions classified as impending fractures have been included in many published studies of pathologic fracture treatment, influencing the outcome data of the treatment being tested. Assessing a treatment method for fixation of pathologic fractures and including among the sample numbers many patients with so-called impending fractures may significantly affect the overall results in judging the efficacy of the fixation method and the patient's symptomatic relief. Several studies have formulated guidelines to indicate when prophylactic fixation is necessary, but they are limited by the use of plain, two-dimensional x-ray films, subjective information from the patients, and an inadequate understanding of the biomechanical compromise of the bone by the metastatic carcinoma. Although experienced orthopaedic surgeons may think they have an intuitive sense for which lesions are at risk for frac-

ture, there is considerable controversy about what constitutes an impending fracture and little reliable data to guide us; more definitive guidelines are needed.

Pain is the primary concern of the patient and the major indication for treatment of a bone metastasis, and it has been purported by some authors to be predictive of fracture.[63,67] Although pain is probably not a reliable indicator of impending fracture and is not reason enough for prophylactic fixation, it is the most important reason for some type of treatment, whether it is a surgical stabilization, radiation therapy, chemotherapy, or a combination of modalities.[26,78,84] Not only does pain interfere with a patient's quality of life and indicate a local problem, but it is also cause for prefracture disuse osteopenia, increasing the likelihood of a fracture. Prophylactic internal fixation is a successful method of relieving pain. Fidler assessed preoperative and postoperative pain in patients with impending fractures and found that among patients with 50% to 75% cortical involvement all had moderate to severe pain preoperatively and no or only slight pain after prophylactic internal fixation.[26]

The currently accepted indications for prophylactic internal fixation of impending fractures include loss of 50% or more of the cortex of a long bone, presence of a radiolucent lesion in the femur that measures 2.5 cm or greater in diameter, and increasing pain combined with loss of 50% of the diameter of the bone.[6,25,26,47,71,82] An additional indication for fixation prior to fracture is intractable pain, especially after irradiation has been completed. There are several advantages of prophylactic fixation of an impending fracture. These include decreased morbidity, shorter hospital stay, easier rehabilitation, more immediate pain relief, faster and less complicated surgery, and less blood loss during surgery. In an animal study of prophylactic fixation of bone metastases, Bouma and associates[11] reported a decrease in the incidence of fractures, as well as in lung metastases with prophylactically fixed bone lesions.

All of the currently available studies that use measurements of cortical destruction to predict the risk of fracture due to pathologic lesions have used plain x-ray images. These x-ray films are available, making many retrospective studies possible, but they are limited in several ways: no standardized position or view is used, so x-rays are difficult to compare; permeative lesions probably have the highest fracture risk but cannot be measured by any of the current methods; some bone metastases produce increased density with obscure margins; nearly all metastatic lesions have poorly defined edges, causing considerable error in calculating the percentage of cortical destructions; and the relative risk of different locations in the bone is not considered (Fig. 6-3). Moreover, as Menck and associates[56] pointed out, there are biomechanical factors still to be defined, such as bone strength, the shape of the lesion, and premorbid osteopenia, all contributing to overall fracture risk. In an investigation of bone strength reduction published by McBroom and colleagues,[55] the authors predicted the reduction in flexural strength of their model canine femurs with specifically created defects. Their predictions were based on either of two measurements of defect size: the ratio of hole diameter to bone diameter or the ratio of the defect-reduced cross-sectional area to the intact bone area. They were able to demonstrate variations in the hole-to-bone diameter ratio of up to 10%, using plain radiographs. They suggested that CT scans be used to measure cortical destruction, that CT scans are more accurate than plain x-ray films, and that CT scans are more accurate in predicting the strength reduction caused by metastatic lesions. We are currently participants in a prospective study developing better predictions of impending fractures using special gradient CT scans to assess the size and geometric characteristics of metastatic lesions in human long bones as well as the structural characteristic of the bone immediately adjacent to the metastatic deposit.

The specific methods of surgical treatment for impending fractures are not significantly different

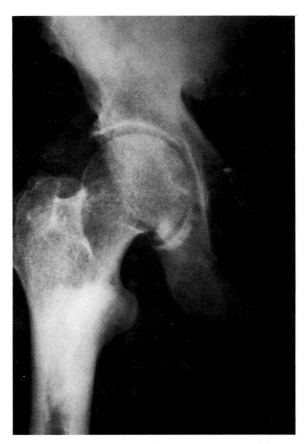

Fig. 6-3. An anteroposterior x-ray of the proximal femur in a patient with known metastatic prostate cancer. Pathologic fractures through lesions with increased density are rare. The lesion should be irradiated if the patient has pain, and internal fixation is indicated only if the pain persists after completion of the irradiation and no other cause is found. Bone metastases that produce increased density are most likely to be due to carcinoma of the prostate; metastatic breast cancer and metastatic lung cancer also have a significant incidence of lesions that produce increased density in the bone. Approximately 90% of prostate metastases cause increased density of the bone, whereas only 60% of breast metastases and 30% of lung metastases produce increased density.

from those for completed pathologic fractures. The operations are easier, surgical and postoperative complications are fewer, and rehabilitation is rapid. One critical caveat when treating patients with impending lesions is that fracture risk is greatest during the surgical positioning, preparation, and draping while the patient is under anesthesia. Patients cannot protect their own extremities and must rely on the surgical team to do this.

GENERAL CONCEPTS IN THE TREATMENT OF PATHOLOGIC FRACTURES

Internal fixation of pathologic fractures is temporary, and the fixation device eventually fails if the bone does not heal. Loss of fixation is the most significant complication of treating pathologic fractures. Healing is slower than it is for fractures through normal bone, particularly when radiation therapy is part of the patient's preoperative or postoperative management,[10,31,78] and all patients with metastatic carcinoma to bone with an impending fracture or completed fracture should receive irradiation as part of their treatment. Poor bone quality is not a contraindication to fixation but demands consideration when selecting the method of fixation. Polymethylmethacrylate (PMMA) can be used to increase the strength of the fixation, but it should *not* be used to replace a segment of bone. PMMA improves the bending strength of a fixation construct and the outcome of fixation in both animal and human studies.[2,4,19,22,36,49,52,59,62,70,80,87] PMMA does not affect the use of therapeutic radiation, nor are the properties of the PMMA affected adversely by the radiation.[22,62] Whether or not PMMA is used in treating a pathologic fracture or stabilizing an impending fracture, PMMA should not be used to replace missing segments of cortical bone permanently. Rather, it is used to improve immobilization of the fracture, increase the strength of the fixation, and reinforce weakened areas of bone while the fracture heals. When PMMA is used, care should be taken to avoid the interposition of cement between fracture fragments that are expected to unite. Autogenous bone graft should be used if necessary, and occasionally an allograft intercalary segment is required. If PMMA is used to replace a segment of bone and the fracture is prevented from healing, the fixation construct will fail. If the patient dies within a few months or makes few demands of the constructed limb, the fixation will be adequate, but otherwise the patient will eventually have an unstable bone.

When the tumor site is exposed in the process of fracture reduction and stabilization, or diagnostic biopsy, all gross tumor should be removed.[2,52] Small defects can be left empty or filled with PMMA if stability is improved, provided bone contact remains. Bone graft, either autograft or allograft, is recommended when fracture union is unlikely without it.

Most patients who present with a pathologic fracture are or will be medically debilitated and require special concern for their general health. In addition to receiving orthopaedic care, each patient should have an internist, medical oncologist, and radiation therapist to assist in the management of the primary tumor as well as metastatic disease. Nutrition is of particular concern; it needs to be assessed by measuring serum albumin, and maintained or improved, even if that requires the addition of enteral or parenteral hyperalimentation perioperatively. Nearly all of these patients will have relative bone marrow suppression and need adequate replacement of blood products. They are likely to suffer larger than usual blood losses at operation because of the hypervascularity of many lesions, thereby demanding greater intraoperative and postoperative replacement. In some circumstances excessive blood loss can be avoided by preoperative angiographic embolization; this is especially useful for metastatic hypernephroma, in which even an open biopsy can lead to life-threatening blood loss (Fig. 6-4**A–C**).[12,14] Other standards of orthopaedic care apply essentially without change,[19] ie, perioperative antibiotic coverage, anticoagulation or other prophylaxis for deep vein thrombosis and pulmonary embolus, aggressive postoperative pulmonary toilet, and early mobilization. Increased weight-bearing and progressive resisted exercises should be delayed until there is evidence of fracture healing; however, joint mobilization and assisted ambulation should not wait, and most patients can be out of bed not later than 2 days postoperatively.

UPPER EXTREMITY FRACTURES

Lesions involving the humeral shaft that have not fractured usually are treated initially with irradiation.[2,15,19,30,58] Prophylactic fixation of an impending humeral fracture is indicated if the patient has persistent pain after irradiation, and when performed for pain or fracture, plate fixation is suggested. While the patient is receiving irradiation, standard splinting techniques are used to reduce the risk of a fracture (Fig. 6-5). Contractures of the shoulder and elbow are common, and these joints should be kept moving. Gentle pendulum exercises can maintain motion in the shoulder and, with appropriate precautions against using torsion, are safe for most humeral shaft, neck, and head defects. Gravity-assisted elbow flexion and extension exercises can be done safely by most patients.

Humeral head fractures and large humeral head lesions should be treated by standard cemented hemiarthroplasty. Replacement of the glenoid surface is not indicated. The goal of humeral head re-

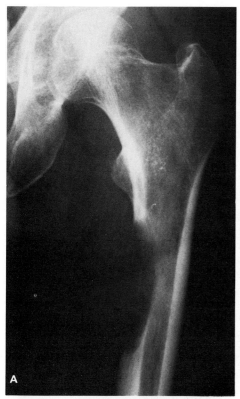

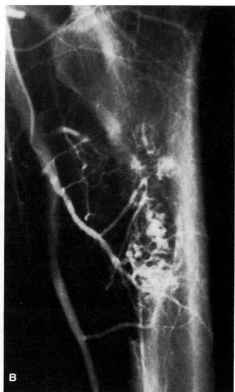

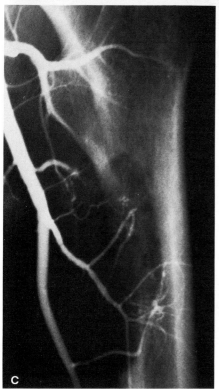

Fig. 6-4. **(A)** An anteroposterior x-ray of the proximal femur in a patient who had carcinoma of the kidney 13 years ago. He complained of groin pain and had been treated for a "pulled muscle" for 6 weeks before this x-ray was taken. This is a typical metastatic lesion. It is in the metaphyseal-diaphyseal junction, has destroyed the cortex, and has an extraosseous soft tissue component. Despite the long time since the original kidney malignancy, this lesion should be suspected of being a metastasis from the hypernephroma. **(B)** On this early phase of the angiogram, the arteriovenous shunting and pooling of dye typical of metastatic hypernephroma can be seen. An operative procedure on this lesion can produce life-threatening hemorrhage. Preoperative embolization is recommended. **(C)** On the postembolization angiogram, marked reduction in vascularity can be seen.

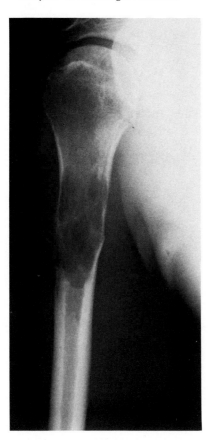

Fig. 6-5. An anteroposterior x-ray of the proximal humerus in a patient with a plasmacytoma of the proximal humerus. He was treated with irradiation without stabilizing the humerus, and a sling and pendulum exercises were used to keep his shoulder moving. If the bone fractures, a resection or stabilization can be done, but if the bone heals without surgery, the patient has better function. Surgery done before irradiation delays and makes the irradiation more difficult.

placement is pain relief and preservation of existing function; range of motion of the joint should not be expected to improve. Postoperative care is routine, with the addition of radiation therapy. When bone destruction or involvement of the glenoid and humeral head is extensive, a resection arthroplasty of the shoulder (Tikoff-Lindberg resection) is suggested (Fig. 6-6).

Although some surgeons recommend prophylactic management of humeral shaft lesions by using flexible rods such as Enders or Rush rods, we prefer to manage impending fractures nonoperatively in the upper extremity. Because this is not ordinarily a weight-bearing extremity, it can be protected appropriately while other treatment, ie, radiotherapy

and chemotherapy is delivered. Occasionally, the patient will require some weight-bearing use of the upper extremities, for example, in crutch or walker-assisted ambulation, and will be treated by prophylactic internal fixation. However, most often nonoperative treatment is continued unless pain persists or until an actual pathologic fracture has occurred. Completed fractures of the humeral shaft should be treated by open reduction and internal fixation with a 4.5-mm compression plate whenever possible. Flexible rods (eg, Enders and Rush rods) provide good alignment but not rigid internal fixation, because they lack adequate rotational control and do not prevent distraction. Although a sling and swathe or functional coaptation brace may provide sufficient alignment of a fractured humerus during radiation treatment, pain relief without rigid immobilization is poor, and a pathologic fracture in the humerus usually does not heal without internal fixation. A 4.5-mm compression plate with a minimum of six cortices in strong or augmented bone above and below the lesion is recommended, and autogenous bone graft should be used if bone destruction is extensive (Fig. 6-7). Rigid fixation may require supplementation with PMMA and/or resection and humeral shortening. New interlocking humeral intramedullary nails are being introduced that may prove as useful in treating the upper extremity as they have been in the lower extremity, but little data are available currently.

Metastases distal to the elbow are unusual, but they pose problems of rotational and angular control similar to those of the proximal lesions of the upper extremity. As with the humeral pathologic fractures, closed treatment is unlikely to succeed, and early internal fixation is recommended. The 3.5-mm compression plate system securing six cortices on each side of the lesion, with or without cement augmentation, provides appropriate fixation in most cases. Fractures of the radial head can be treated by radial head resection. These distal upper extremity lesions are rare, but deserve the same aggressive approach as lesions elsewhere, since the patient's survival does not vary from that of patients with proximal or axial disease.

Metastatic carcinoma to the hand is unusual.[51] Most cases are secondary to lung cancer, although occasionally other primary carcinomas can spread to a bone in the hand. Surgical resection of these metastases is usually the best management.

LOWER EXTREMITY FRACTURES

More than half of all pathologic fractures occur in the proximal part of the femur, and thus they are

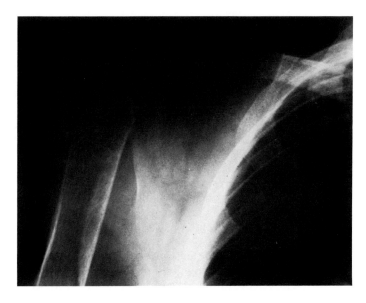

Fig. 6-6. An anteroposterior x-ray of the shoulder in a patient who had a metastasis from a renal cell carcinoma in the humeral head with extension into the shoulder joint. He had no other metastases, and a wide resection was done. He was left with a flail shoulder. This is often called a Tikhoff-Lindberg resection.

the most frequently treated and studied lesions in the literature. Perhaps because of the weight-bearing demands of the extremity, metastatic disease of the femur is the most likely lesion to cause disabling pain. Pathologic fractures of the femur suddenly alter the quality of a patient's life and significantly threaten an individual's level of independence. Without proper surgical attention the patient with a pathologic fracture of the femur will be confined to bed, a situation that is medically and psychologically devastating.

As discussed in other sections, the early diagnosis of primary malignancies, improved treatment of many diseases and their complications, and the improved life expectancy of many patients with metastatic disease create a greater incentive for improved surgical management of metastatic bone disease. In all cases the goal of surgical intervention is to achieve maximum protection of the bone or stabilization of the fracture with the least extensive exposure. There is virtually no place for nonoperative treatment of completed pathologic fractures of the femur. Lesions of the femoral neck, intertrochanteric, and subtrochanteric areas should be prophylactically fixed whenever found because of the high incidence of subsequent fracture and the ease of the operation when done before fracture compared to the difficulties and complications of surgery after a fracture has occurred.

Lesions within the femoral head or neck are successfully treated with replacement arthroplasty, either hemiarthroplasty or total hip replacement.[19,50,52] Total hip replacement is often indicated because there is a high incidence of metastasis within the periacetabular pelvis occurring with lesions of the femoral head and neck.[36,37] The results of treating femoral neck lesions by pinning techniques have been unsatisfactory, with a high rate of nonunion and failure of fixation[58]; this approach is not recommended. As in the upper extremity, we cement endoprosthetic replacements in most cases. When there are adjacent lesions in the subtrochanteric region or proximal shaft, a long femoral stem should be used for prophylactic fixation distally, avoiding a potential postoperative complication and allowing earlier and less protected weight-bearing. All tumor tissue should be curetted from the femoral canal during preparation for implanting the endoprosthesis, and additional cement should be used to enhance the strength of the fixation. Patients with bone metastasis seem to have a greater risk of developing acute pulmonary distress from the use of PMMA,[49] and it is our procedure to thoroughly curet and lavage the involved bone and to be sure that the patient does not have volume depletion when the PMMA is injected.

Solitary intertrochanteric fractures are managed well by the use of a sliding screw and side plate. It is best to obtain bone-to-bone contact, creating a stable configuration. The calcar femorale frequently is affected by metastatic disease; the tumor should be curetted and the medial aspect of the femur stabilized.[41] PMMA is used to improve the fixation of the screws in the bone, not to replace missing bone. The screw and side plate device will fail if healing does not occur. With lesions in the subtrochanteric and diaphyseal regions, both can be stabilized with an intramedullary rod with proximal and/or distal

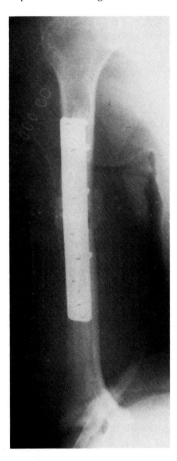

Fig. 6-7. An anteroposterior x-ray of the humerus in a patient with a metastasis to the humeral diaphysis that had been treated with irradiation but fractured. The lesion was exposed and curetted. The humerus was shortened to obtain adequate bone contact. A plate was used to provide immediate, solid stabilization.

screw fixation; PMMA augmentation may be used if necessary. Another alternative is to replace the proximal fragment (femoral head, neck, and trochanter) with an appropriate prosthesis. The bone should not be "built up" with PMMA to fit the femoral prosthesis.

Fractures of the femoral shaft are treated most effectively with an intramedullary device, with or without PMMA.[20,49,59,60] Although compression plates provide excellent rigid internal fixation (experimentally attaining as much as 75% of the normal torsional strength of the bone[3]) their use requires a wide surgical exposure, results in increased blood loss, and provides strength only to the bone under the plate. Intramedullary rod fixation, al-

though not quite as rigid, is technically simple (especially when used as prophylactic fixation of an impending fracture), can be done through a limited exposure, and will strengthen the entire bone. The development of intramedullary nails with proximal and distal interlocking screws has made the use of these devices our preferred method in nearly all patients with impending and pathologic fractures of the femur. When intramedullary rods are used, the canal is overreamed 1.0 to 1.5 mm to avoid high impaction forces during rod placement. The ability to fix the bone both proximally and distally eliminates the complication of telescoping and provides excellent control of length and rotation of the femur. Intramedullary rods are available with the proximal screws directed proximally through the central portion of the femoral neck into the femoral head, thus allowing good fixation for subtrochanteric lesions or the fractured femur with an associated femoral neck lesion, both of which have been difficult to manage in the past. With both proximal and distal interlocking screws, intramedullary rods can be employed to treat lesions and fractures involving most parts of the femur.

When there is a complete fracture and extensive bone destruction, exposure of the fracture, removal of the metastatic tumor, and bone graft may be useful. In this situation PMMA can be used to improve the fixation of the femur but, again, should not be relied on to replace a segment of missing bone. If a gap is present, an intercalary allograft is recommended (Fig. 6-8). If bone contact is minimal, an autogenous bone graft can be used. When there is an impending fracture, an intramedullary rod inserted from the proximal end is sufficient. The rods should be "locked" with fixation screws proximally or distally if the lesion is proximal or distal, or the entire rod can be encased in PMMA. The use of an intramedullary rod and PMMA is most helpful when the patient has multiple lesions or a lesion in the distal metaphysis. When the lesion is in the distal metaphysis, the rod can be introduced from distal to proximal. The technique developed for the retrograde instillation of low-viscosity cement through a fluted intramedullary rod was described by Miller and associates.[59] A small diameter (11-mm), closed-section, fluted intramedullary rod is introduced at the piriform fossa or through the knee. When an intramedullary rod is introduced into the femur from the distal end, a standard knee arthrotomy is used and the femoral canal is opened through the articular surface of the intercondylar notch just anterior to the femoral origin of the anterior cruciate ligament. The femoral canal is

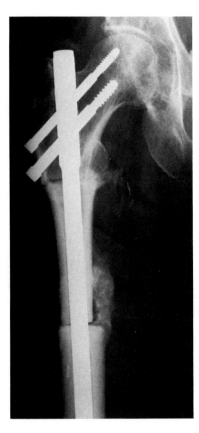

Fig. 6-8. An anteroposterior x-ray of the proximal femur in a patient who has had an intercalary allograft to reconstruct the femur after the resection of a metastatic renal cell carcinoma. This was his first metastasis, 13 years after the initial diagnosis. Metastases first found more than 2 years after the initial tumor has been treated are often best treated by resection. This is especially true of metastases from renal or thyroid carcinomas.

reamed to 15 or 16 mm. The rod is used as a cannula through which the low-viscosity cement is injected, with retrograde filling of the femoral canal (Fig. 6-9A–C). Biomechanical testing of this system and comparison with another rod and cement construct showed a significant improvement in torsional strength. In a clinical trial of this technique, successful results were achieved except in three patients with completed fractures and extensive bone destruction. Although this system can be used in treating completed fractures, we recommend it only for prophylactic fixation.

Supracondylar fractures, like intertrochanteric fractures, are managed well by standard devices such as blade plates, but augmentation with PMMA to improve screw fixation in the weakened metaphyseal bone may be needed.

PELVIC AND ACETABULAR LESIONS

Many metastatic deposits in the bony pelvis do not affect weight-bearing functions and consequently do not need surgical intervention unless an open biopsy is necessary. However, periacetabular lesions, particularly in the medial and superior segments of the acetabulum, present a particularly difficult problem (Fig. 6-10). The loss of function may be gradual and the patient may remain relatively asymptomatic (or the symptoms may be attributed to an adjacent femoral head or neck lesion), and when the patient is seen, extensive destruction has occurred.[39] Surgical reconstruction is difficult and can cause considerable perioperative morbidity, particularly blood loss. Preoperative arteriography is suggested, and if possible, embolization of the tumor should be done.[14] This procedure is safe and can significantly reduce the operative blood loss and risk of intraoperative exsanguination. The periacetabular lesions are best seen on CT scan, on which the extent of tumor destruction can be clearly appreciated.[71] When the lesion is small and the acetabular subchondral bone is intact or has only a small defect, curettage and packing with PMMA is recommended. When a major portion of the acetabular bone is destroyed, a total hip replacement is preferred. Usually a routine acetabular component is adequate, but when the medial and superior acetabulum are destroyed, a protrusion cup is needed. Rarely, a combination of PMMA and Steinmann pins is required to reconstruct the pelvis.[39,46] This demanding surgery is probably best done by someone with extensive experience.

SPINAL FRACTURES

Generally, the symptoms with a compression fracture of a vertebra are minor and can be successfully controlled with temporarily decreased activity or, occasionally, bracing for a short period. Immediate surgical intervention is required only for the patient with actual loss of neurologic function. When documented bone metastases are not present, the major dilemma is whether the underlying pathologic process is osteoporosis or a metastatic deposit.[64] If the patient has had a previous carcinoma or myeloma, if the patient's history and physical examination suggest a carcinoma, if the laboratory results are abnormal (elevated acid phosphatase or abnormal immunoelectrophoresis), or if the plain x-ray films

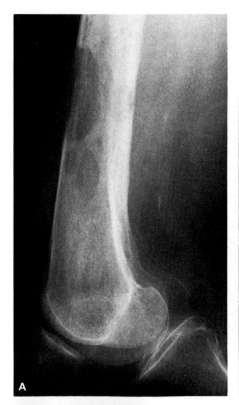

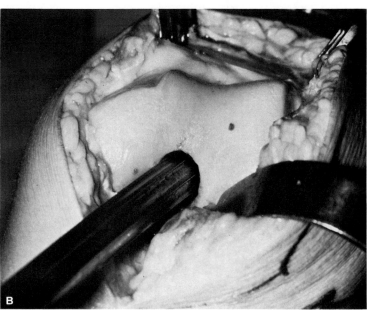

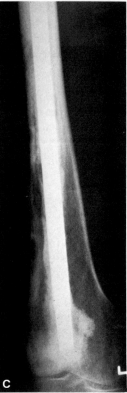

Fig. 6-9. (A) A lateral x-ray of the femur in a woman with known metastatic breast cancer. Metastatic lesions in the distal femur, especially when a large segment of the femur is involved, can be difficult to stabilize. **(B)** In a technique we have used, the intramedullary rod is introduced through the intercondylar notch of the distal femur. An interlocking nail can be used, or methylmethacrylate can be injected through the rod for additional fixation. **(C)** The intramedullary rod is pushed up entirely into the femoral canal before the methylmethacrylate hardens. This method has been successful in stabilizing impending femoral fractures in the distal half of the femur.

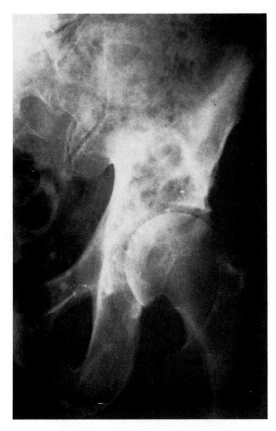

Fig. 6-10. An anteroposterior x-ray of the pelvis in a man with metastatic prostate carcinoma to the ilium just above the acetabulum. Most metastases from prostate carcinoma are "blastic" and do not require stabilization, but this defect in the ilium weakens the acetabulum and should be surgically treated. As long as the subchondral bone is uninvolved or only minimally resorbed, curettage and packing with PMMA is sufficient. Steinmann pins can be used to increase the strength of the reconstruction.

or a bone scan reveal other bone lesions, the patient should be evaluated for a compression fracture due to metastatic disease. If none of the findings are abnormal, the fracture should be assumed to be secondary to osteoporosis. The patient with a suspected malignancy should have a biopsy, but the others should be treated symptomatically. Magnetic resonance imaging (MRI) has been suggested as a means of differentiating an osteoporotic compression fracture from one due to a malignant lesion.[89] When there is complete replacement of the vertebral bone, multiple vertebral body lesions, pedicle involvement, and an intact intervertebral disk, metastatic disease is most likely.

If the patient is treated for an osteoporotic compression fracture but does not respond to the treatment, or if progressive destruction of bone is seen on the follow-up x-ray films, a biopsy should be done. Percutaneous needle biopsy of the lumbar vertebrae can be done under fluoroscopic control and local anesthesia; however, open biopsy through a limited exposure is often better for patient comfort and tolerance, as well as ensuring that diagnostic tissue has been obtained. Biopsy of the thoracic vertebrae can be done through a costotransversectomy or transpedicular approach. We prefer to do biopsies of vertebral body lesions with the transpedicular approach. The patient is positioned prone on the operating table. For thoracic vertebrae, the tip of the transverse process is identified, and for lumbar vertebrae, the superior facet is used as the landmark. The pedicle is just medial to each of these structures. The cortical bone is removed, and the pedicle is found with a small curet and followed into the vertebral body. Then a core biopsy or curet biopsy is taken. A cross-table lateral x-ray film can be taken in the operating room to confirm the position of the instrument.

Skeletal metastases occur most commonly in the spine, affecting the vertebral body more often than the posterior elements. These lesions may remain asymptomatic for months to years and might be appreciated only when a bone scan is done during a routine metastatic work-up. The classic plain x-ray finding is the loss of a pedicle on a plain anteroposterior view of the spine (Fig. 6-11). This sign should be sought carefully in all patients with metastatic disease to bone. As the lesion progresses, the patient will feel moderate to severe pain that can persist for months prior to the onset of focal neurologic deficits. Occasionally the onset of pain is sudden following a pathologic compression fracture. Impingement of the cord or nerve roots may occur either by direct extension of the tumor or secondary to spinal instability and deformity. Early recognition and management by bracing and irradiation will usually result in pain relief, and an operation will be unnecessary. When the patient has compression of the spinal cord, decompression and stabilization are required, and this can usually be accomplished with a laminectomy. A posterior fusion is recommended. When the spine is kyphotic with anterior collapse of the vertebrae and anterior compression of the spinal cord, the patient should be treated by an anterior decompression and stabilization. When the posterior elements are involved and the cord is compressed anteriorly, the patient should have a posterior stabilization and an

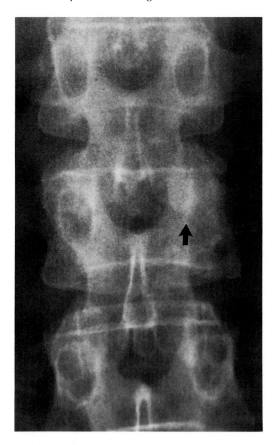

Fig. 6-11. This anteroposterior x-ray of the lumbar spine in a patient who complains of back pain shows a subtle finding that is often called the "winking owl." The cortical bone of the pedicles is seen at the upper outer corners of the vertebral bodies as dense, round structures because we are looking at them in cross section. When metastatic deposits involve the vertebrae, the cortices of the pedicles are usually thinned and therefore cannot be seen on the plain film. This "missing" pedicle *(arrow)* is the closed or "winked" eye and is almost pathognomonic of metastatic disease, but we have also seen it in a patient who had a lymphoma of bone.

anterior decompression (Fig. 6-12). Techniques for anterior and posterior decompression and stabilization, including the use of many instrumentation systems, are described in the literature, and the interested reader is referred there for more detailed information.[27,28,38,40,42,53,54,61,65,76] The literature strongly supports early decompression and stabilization of patients with any neurologic compromise and vertebral collapse, and we agree. When there is minimal or no bone destruction and cord compression is due to the soft tissue extension of

the metastasis, emergent irradiation is recommended. The patient should also be treated with a short course of high-dose corticosteroid to reduce the edema that adds to the compression and neurologic damage.

All patients need a preoperative myelogram or MRI study to verify the level of the lesion and eliminate the possibility of compression at an additional level. Careful correlation of x-ray findings with the clinical neurologic examination will ensure the best management for the patient.

RESECTION AND ALLOGRAFT RECONSTRUCTION

There is an occasional indication for definitive surgical resection of a metastatic focus. A patient with

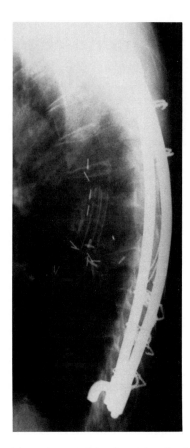

Fig. 6-12. A lateral x-ray of the thoracic spine in a woman with a metastasis to the seventh thoracic vertebra, with extensive destruction of both the posterior elements and the body. She was treated first with posterior decompression and stabilization and then with an anterior decompression, with the rib used as bone graft.

a solitary metastasis from any origin who has been tumor free for more than a couple of years should be considered a candidate for a resection. Renal cell carcinoma and follicular cell thyroid carcinoma are the two tumors most likely to produce isolated bone metastasis years after therapy for the primary tumor.[2] Plasma cell myeloma may present as a solitary lesion. When the patient has a normal serum immunoelectrophoresis and bone marrow aspirate, and despite the 90% risk of diffuse disease developing during the next 10 years, surgical resection of the solitary lesion is an option.

Reconstruction methods are similar to the methods used to reconstruct an extremity after the resection of a primary bone tumor. Because many metastatic deposits are diaphyseal or at the metaphyseal-diaphyseal junction, intercalary allografts are often used to replace the resected segment of bone.

PRIMARY BENIGN DISEASE OF BONE

As a general rule, benign lesions associated with a pathologic fracture eventually require surgical management, although unicameral bone cyst is an exception. Spontaneous healing of a benign tumor after a fracture has been observed, but it does not occur regularly. There is no evidence that the fracture stimulates healing of even the least active lesions. Often the fracture callus temporarily obscures the tumor, but on x-ray films taken after the fracture callus has remodeled, the lesion is usually still present. Nonetheless, surgery is not always required. In a child with a fracture through a unicameral bone cyst, the fracture should be allowed to heal and the patient observed. If the cyst does not heal spontaneously by the time the fracture callus has remodeled, corticosteroid injection is recommended. Curettage is probably best reserved for those unicameral bone cysts that do not heal after three or four corticosteroid injections. A solitary enchondroma in the hand is another example. The fracture will heal, but the lesion will not. If the patient had no symptoms before the fracture occurred and the injury that produced the fracture resulted in a significant force to the bone, then surgery probably is not necessary. If, on the other hand, the patient had symptoms prior to the fracture or if the fracture occurred with minimal or no trauma, it is probably best to use curettage and bone graft for the enchondroma because another fracture is liable to occur in the future. Most other benign tumors should be operated on, but surgery usually is possible and easier if delayed until after the frac-

ture has healed. Closed treatment of the pathologic fracture associated with a benign tumor is usually best and is recommended.

When surgery for a benign bone lesion is necessary, we recommend intralesional excision (simple curettage) for those that usually heal spontaneously (eg, nonossifying fibroma, unicameral bone cyst, enchondroma). Those tumors that do not heal spontaneously (eg, chondroblastoma, osteoblastoma, ossifying fibroma, chondromyxofibroma) should be treated with more aggressive surgery. An en bloc wide surgical excision is the treatment of choice for locally aggressive benign tumors if the resulting function will be normal (ie, fibular head excision). Usually this is not technically possible, and curettage is the initial treatment. If curettage is selected, it should include removal of the reactive bone surrounding the lesion. A wide excision is better if it can be done without excessive permanent sequelae to the skeleton.

Giant cell tumor of bone is a common benign tumor associated with a pathologic fracture in young adults. Our management of this fracture has changed dramatically in the past few years. Until recently, it was believed that those patients who had a pathologic fracture through a giant cell tumor of bone had a particularly aggressive tumor and that they should be treated with a primary resection. The routine management was to allow the fracture, usually grossly displaced, to heal, and then the tumor was widely excised. Although it is recognized that curettage may be inadequate and that the patient has an approximately 50% chance of local recurrence, we recently have elected to treat the patient with a thorough and extended curettage, open reduction of the fracture, packing of the cavity with PMMA, and internal fixation of the reconstructed fracture. Only when the bone has been destroyed beyond reconstruction is it necessary to do a primary excision.

PRIMARY MALIGNANT DISEASE OF BONE

Primary malignant bone tumors include those treated primarily by irradiation (eg, Ewing's sarcoma, myeloma, and non-Hodgkin's lymphoma of bone) and those treated primarily by surgical resection and adjuvant chemotherapy and/or radiation therapy (eg, osteosarcoma, chondrosarcoma, fibrosarcoma, and malignant fibrous histiocytoma). The prognosis for patients presenting with a pathologic fracture through a primary malignant bone tumor is worse than that for patients who do not have a pathologic fracture; however, their management does not differ substantially from that for patients with the same primary sarcoma without a pathologic fracture. Usually it is obvious that the patient has a primary sarcoma, but the clinical presentation and x-ray appearance of chondrosarcoma and malignant fibrous histiocytoma (MFH) of bone are often similar to metastatic carcinoma. When an older adult without a history of a primary carcinoma has a pathologic fracture, chondrosarcoma and MFH of bone should be added to the differential diagnosis.

We recommend whole-lung tomography or CT scan of the lung and ^{99m}Tc bone scan as an initial screening test for possible metastasis from a primary bone sarcoma. Because metastases to the brain, liver, and spleen from sarcoma are rare, it is not necessary to routinely evaluate these organs beyond physical examination and routine laboratory tests. For those patients who have no evidence of neurologic dysfunction on physical examination, no further evaluation is believed needed; however, if the patient has clinical evidence of mental dysfunction (eg, memory abnormalities, seizure, confusion), a CT scan of the brain is indicated. For patients without hepatic or splenic enlargement, and in whom results of the serum liver function tests (ie, SGOT, SGPT, albumin, alkaline phosphatase, total protein, and total bilirubin) and peripheral blood smear are normal, no further investigation is indicated with respect to the liver or spleen. If any of these results are abnormal, a radioisotope liver-spleen scan or abdominal CT scan is required.

Biopsy of a bone sarcoma with an associated pathologic fracture is especially difficult. The healing process will alter the histology and may confuse the pathologist. Whenever possible, the surgeon should perform a biopsy of tissue away from the fracture. When this is not possible, the pathologist should be told. When a soft tissue mass is associated with the tumor, a needle biopsy is usually adequate, but when there is limited extraosseous tissue and the fracture callus has had an opportunity to develop (5 days or more), an open biopsy provides better material and is preferred.

Internal fixation of a pathologic fracture through a primary sarcoma is not appropriate, and when surgical resection of the sarcoma is not required (Ewing's sarcoma, myeloma, lymphoma of bone), the fracture should still be treated closed. If the fracture cannot be treated closed, surgical resection is recommended. Resection without an amputation is more difficult, more likely to be inadequate, and, therefore, is only occasionally recommended.

A radical amputation is the best oncologic treatment of the sarcoma requiring surgical resection (osteosarcoma, chondrosarcoma, fibrosarcoma, MFH) and usually the best treatment for the patient with a primary bone sarcoma and a pathologic fracture.

Those patients with a primary malignancy of bone and pathologic fracture require the carefully coordinated care of an oncology team, including the medical oncologist, radiation therapist, pathologist, radiologist, and orthopaedic surgeon; only with the full complement of care can these patients achieve the best quality of life and maximum life expectancy.

SYSTEMIC SKELETAL DISEASE

When the surgeon is planning the management of patients with a pathologic fracture and a systemic skeletal disease, it is best to separate systemic skeletal diseases into those that can be corrected and those that cannot. The former include renal osteodystrophy, hyperparathyroidism, osteomalacia, and disuse osteoporosis, and examples of the latter include osteogenesis imperfecta, polyostotic fibrous dysplasia, postmenopausal osteoporosis, Paget's disease, and osteopetrosis (Fig. 6-13). As a category, these disorders have in common bones that are weak and predisposed to fracture or plastic deformation. The fracture callus usually does not form normally, and healing occurs slowly. Patients with Paget's disease of bone have an increased incidence of fracture, and delayed union or nonunion are likely to occur when these fractures are treated without internal fixation.

Because the entire skeleton is affected by systemic skeletal disease, the treatment of the fracture must be accomplished without adversely affecting the remainder of the skeleton while the fracture unites. If the underlying process is correctable, treatment should be started and the fracture should then be treated as a nonpathologic fracture. If the underlying process cannot be corrected, the condition of the remainder of the skeleton must be considered when planning treatment of the fracture. Most femoral neck fractures and intertrochanteric fractures are in patients with osteoporosis, and the strength of the bone expected to hold screws or a prosthesis must be considered when planning the surgical fixation technique. Although the bone usually is strong enough to hold the fixation device, occasionally PMMA must be used to hold the screws in the bone. A primary goal in the management of patients with any systemic skeletal disease is to

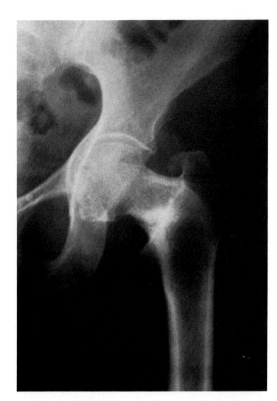

Fig. 6-13. An anteroposterior x-ray of the proximal femur in a woman with osteomalacia. The femoral neck is in varus owing to the bone's inability to withstand the forces of weight-bearing. The bone may need the temporary additional support of an internal fixation device, but more important, the cause of the osteomalacia must be determined and corrected so that the bone can repair itself.

prevent disuse osteoporosis, which may lead to additional pathologic fractures. A secondary goal is to provide long-term mechanical support for the weakened bone. Reduction and internal fixation are indicated so that the patient can remain active. Intramedullary rods provide prolonged support for the bone. PMMA is used if needed for adequate fixation of the device.[4]

SUMMARY

In summary, any abnormality of the bone that reduces the strength of the bone predisposes it to mechanical failure during normal activity or with minimal trauma. The mechanical failure manifests itself as a fracture, and this fracture must be recognized as a pathologic fracture if the patient is to be treated properly. Often, the underlying pathologic process is obvious, but occasionally it is overlooked if not specifically sought. It is the treating physician's responsibility to search for an underlying pathologic process in any patient who sustains a fracture.

REFERENCES

1. Abrams, H.; Spiro, R.; and Goldstein, N.: Metastasis in Carcinoma: Analysis of 1000 Autopsied Cases. Cancer, 3:74–85, 1950.
2. Albright, J.A.; Gillespie, T.E.; and Butaud, T.R.: Treatment of Bone Metastases. Semin. Oncol., 7(4):418–434, 1980.
3. Anderson, J.T.; Erickson, J.M.; Thompson, R.C., Jr.; and Chao, E.Y.: Pathologic Femoral Shaft Fractures Comparing Fixation Techniques Using Cement. Clin. Orthop., 131:273–277, 1978.
4. Bartucci, E.J.; Gonzalez, M.H.; Cooperman, D.R.; Freedberg, H.I.; Barmada, R.; and Laros, G.S.: The Effect of Adjunctive Methylmethacrylate on Failures of Fixation and Function in Patients with Intertrochanteric Fractures and Osteoporosis. J. Bone Joint Surg., 67A:1094–1107, 1985.
5. Beals, R.K.; Lawton, G.D.; and Snell, W.E.: Prophylactic Internal Fixation of the Femur in Metastatic Breast Cancer. Cancer, 28:1350–1354, 1971.
6. Behr, J.T.; Doboz, W.R.; and Badrinath, K.: The Treatment of Pathologic and Impending Pathologic Fractures of the Proximal Femur in the Elderly. Clin. Orthop., 198:173–178, 1985.
7. Bender, R.A., and Hansen, H.: Hypercalcemia in Bronchogenic Carcinoma. A Prospective Study of 200 Patients. Ann. Intern. Med., 80:205–208, 1974.
8. Berretton, B.A., and Carter, J.R.: Current Concepts Review: Mechanisms of Cancer Metastasis to Bone. J. Bone Joint Surg., 68A:308–312, 1986.
9. Bertin, K.C.; Horstman, J.; and Coleman, S.S.: Isolated Fractures of the Lesser Troch in Adults: An Initial Manifestation of Metastatic Malignant Disease. J. Bone Joint Surg., 66A:770–773, 1984.
10. Blake, D.D.: Radiation Treatment of Metastatic Bone Disease. Clin. Orthop., 73:89–100, 1970.
11. Bouma, W.H.; Mulder, J.H.; and Hop, C.J.: The Influence of Intramedullary Nailing upon the Development of Metastasis in the Treatment of an Impending Pathologic Fracture: An Experimental Study. Clin. Exp. Metastasis, 1:205–212, 1983.
12. Bowers, T.A.; Murray, J.A.; Channsangarej, C.; Soo, C.S.; Chuang, V.P.; and Wallace, S.: Bone Metastasis from Renal Carcinoma. J. Bone Joint Surg., 64A:749–754, 1982.
13. Brener, R.A., and Jelliffe, A.M.: The Management of Pathological Fracture of the Major Long Bones from Metastatic Cancer. J. Bone Joint Surg., 40B:652–659, 1958.
14. Carpenter, P.R.; Ewing, J.W.; Cook, A.J.; and Kuster, A.H.: Angiographic Assessment and Control of Potential Operative Hemorrhage with Pathologic Fractures Secondary to Metastases. Clin. Orthop., 123:6–8, 1977.
15. Cheng, D.S.; Seitz, C.B.; and Eyre, H.J.: Nonoperative

Management of Femoral, Humeral, and Acetabular Metastasis in Patients with Breast Carcinoma. Cancer, 45: 1533–1537, 1980.

16. Coerkamp, E.G., and Kroon, H.M.: Cortical Bone Metastasis. Radiology, 169:525–528, 1988.

17. Coggeshall, J.; Merrill, W.; Hande, K.; and DesPrez, R.: Implications of Hypercalcemia with Respect to Diagnosis and Treatment of Lung Cancer. Am. J. Med., 80:325–328, 1986.

18. Coleman, R.E.; Mashiter, G.; Whitaker, K.B.; Moss, D.W.; Rubens, R.D.; and Folgelman, I.: Bone Scan Flare Predicts Successful Systemic Therapy for Bone Metastases. J. Nucl. Med., 29:1354–1359, 1988.

19. Cornell, C.N., and Lane, J.M.: Management of Pathologic Fractures in Patients with Breast Cancer. Surgical Rounds, 9:25–41, 1986.

20. Dobozi, W.R.; Dvonch, V.M.; Saltzman, M.L.; Beigler, D.F.; and Belich, P.: Treatment of Impending Pathological Fractures of the Femur with Flexible Intramedullary Nails. Orthopedics, 7:1682–1688, 1984.

21. Douglass, H.O., Jr.; Shukla, S.K.; and Mindell, E.: Treatment of Pathological Fractures of Long Bones Excluding Those Due to Breast Cancer. J. Bone Joint Surg., 58A:1055–1061, 1976.

22. Eftekhar, N.S., and Thurston, C.W.: Effect of Irradiation on Acrylic Cement with Special Reference to Fixation of Pathological Fractures. J. Biomech., 8:53–56, 1975.

23. Enneking, W.F.: A System of Staging Musculoskeletal Neoplasms. Clin. Orthop., 204:9–24, 1986.

24. Enneking, W.F.; Spanier, S.S.; and Goodman, M.A.: A System for Surgical Staging of Musculoskeletal Sarcoma. Clin. Orthop., 153:106–120, 1980.

25. Fidler, M.: Incidence of Fracture Through Metastasis in Long Bones. Acta Orthop. Scand., 52:623–627, 1981.

26. Fidler, M.: Prophylactic Internal Fixation of Secondary Neoplastic Deposits in Long Bones. Br. Med. J., 1:341–343, 1973.

27. Fidler, M.W.: Anterior Decompression and Stabilization of Metastatic Spinal Fractures. J. Bone Joint Surg., 68B:83–90, 1986.

28. Fidler, M.W.: Pathological Fractures of the Cervical Spine: Palliative Surgical Treatment. J. Bone Joint Surg., 67B: 352–357, 1985.

29. Fisken, R.A.; Heath, D.A.; Somers, S.; and Bold, A.M.: Hypercalcemia in Hospital Patients. Lancet, 1:202–207, 1981.

30. Flemming, J.E., and Beals, R.K.: Pathologic Fracture of the Humerus. Clin. Orthop., 203:258–260, 1986.

31. Gainor, B.J., and Buchert, P.: Fracture Healing in Metastatic Bone Disease. Clin. Orthop., 178:297–302, 1983.

32. Galasko, C.S.B.: Skeletal Metastases. Clin. Orthop., 210: 18–30, 1986.

33. Galasko, C.S.B., and Bunn, J.I.: Hypercalcemia in Patients with Advanced Mammary Cancer. Br. Med. J., 3:573–577, 1971.

34. Graham, W.P., III; Gardner, B.; Thomas, A.N.; Gordon, G.S.; Loken, H.F.; and Goldman, L.: Hypercalcemia in Carcinoma of the Female Breast. Surg. Gynecol. Obstet., 117: 709–714, 1963.

35. Greenspan, A., and Norman, A.: Osteolytic Cortical Destruction: An Unusual Pattern of Skeletal Metastases. Skeletal Radiol. 17:402–406, 1988.

36. Habermann, E.T.: Review of 125 Cases of Pathological Fractures Secondary to Breast Metastases Treated with and Without the Use of Methylmethacrylate. Orthop. Trans., 4:346, 1980.

37. Habermann, E.T.; Sachs, R.; Stern R.E.; Hirsh, D.M.; and Anderson, W.J.: The Pathology and Treatment of Metastatic Disease of the Femur. Clin. Orthop., 169:70–82, 1982.

38. Harrington, K.D.: Anterior Decompression and Stabilization of the Spine as a Treatment for Vertebral Collapse and Spinal Cord Compression from Metastatic Malignancy. Clin. Orthop., 233:177–197, 1988.

39. Harrington, K.D.: The Management of Acetabular Insufficiency Secondary to Metastatic Malignant Disease. J. Bone Joint Surg., 63A:653–664, 1981.

40. Harrington, K.D.: Current Concepts Review: Metastatic Disease of the Spine. J. Bone Joint Surg., 68A:1110–1115, 1986.

41. Harrington, K.D.: Problems of Pathologic Fractures. Complications in Orthopedics, 2(1):4, 1987.

42. Harrington, K.D.: The Use of Methylmethacrylate for Vertebral Body Replacement and Anterior Stabilization of Pathologic Fracture-Dislocation of Spine Due to Metastatic Malignant Disease. J. Bone Joint Surg., 63A:36–46, 1981.

43. Harrington, K.D.; Sim, F.H.; Enis, J.E.; Johnston, J.O.; Dick, H.M.; and Gristina, A.G.: Methylmethacrylate as an Adjunct in Internal Fixation of Pathologic Fractures. J. Bone Joint Surg., 58A:1047–1055, 1976.

44. Heisterberg, L., and Johansen, T.S.: Treatment of Pathologic Fractures. Acta Orthop. Scand., 50:787–790, 1979.

45. Jensen, T.M.; Dillon, W.L.; and Reckling, F.W.: Changing Concepts in the Management of Pathologic and Impending Pathologic Fractures. J. Trauma, 16:496–502, 1976.

46. Johnson, J.T.H.: Reconstruction of Pelvic Ring Following Tumor Resection. J. Bone Joint Surg., 60A:747–751, 1978.

47. Keene, J.S.; Sellinger, D.S.; McBeath, A.A.; and Englser, W.D.: Metastatic Breast Cancer in the Femur: A Search for the Lesion at Risk of Fracture. Clin. Orthop., 203:282–288, 1986.

48. Krebs, H.: Management of Pathologic Fractures of Long Bones in Malignant Disease. Arch. Orthop. Trauma. Surg., 92:133–137, 1978.

49. Kunec, J.R., and Lewis, R.J.: Closed Intramedullary Rodding of Pathologic Fractures with Supplemental Cement. Clin. Orthop., 188:183–186, 1984.

50. Lane, J.M.; Sculco, T.P.; and Zolan, S.: Treatment of Pathological Fractures of the Hip by Endoprosthetic Replacement. J. Bone Joint Surg., 62A:954–959, 1980.

51. Leeson, M.C.; Makley, J.T.; and Carter, J.R.: Metastatic Skeletal Disease Distal to the Elbow and Knee. Clin. Orthop., 206:94–99, 1986.

52. Levy, R.N.; Sherry, H.S.; and Siffert, R.S.: Surgical Management of Metastatic Disease of Bone at the Hip. Clin. Orthop., 169:62–69, 1982.

53. Lord, C.F., and Herndon, J.H.: Spinal Cord Compression Secondary to Kyphosis Associated with Radiation Therapy for Metastatic Disease. Clin. Orthop., 210:120–127, 1986.

54. McAfee, P.C.; Bohlman, H.H.; Ducker, T.; and Eismont, F.S.: Failure of Stabilization of the Spine with Methylmethacrylate. J. Bone Joint Surg., 68A:1145–1157, 1986.

55. McBroom, R.J.; Cheal, E.J.; and Hayes, W.C.: Strength Re-

ductions from Metastatic Cortical Defects in Long Bones. J. Orthop. Res., 6:369–378, 1988.

56. Menck, H.; Schulze, S.; and Larsen, E.: Metastasis Size in Pathologic Femoral Fractures. Acta Orthop. Scand., 59:151–154, 1988.

57. Mikelson, M.R., and Bonfiglio, M.: Pathologic Fractures in the Proximal Part of the Femur Treated by Zickel-Nail Fixation. J. Bone Joint Surg., 58A:1067–1070, 1976.

58. Miller, F., and Whitehill, R.: Carcinoma of the Breast Metastatic to the Skeleton. Clin. Orthop., 184:121–127, 1984.

59. Miller, G.J.; Vander Griend, R.A.; Blake, W.P.; and Springfield, D.S.: Performance Evaluation of a Cement-Augmented Intramedullary Fixation System for Pathologic Lesions of the Femoral Shaft. Clin. Orthop., 221:246–254, 1987.

60. Moehring, H.D.: Closed Flexible Intramedullary Fixation for Pathologic Lesions in Long Bones. Orthopedics, 7:829–834, 1984.

61. Murray, J.A.: Metastasis to Spine (letter). J. Bone Joint Surg., 69A:633–634, 1987.

62. Murray, J.A.; Bruels, M.C.; and Lindberg, R.D.: Irradiation of Polymethylmethacrylate *In Vitro* Gamma Radiation Effect. J. Bone Joint Surg., 56A:311–312, 1974.

63. Murray, J.A., and Parrish, F.F.: Surgical Management of Secondary Neoplastic Fractures About the Hip. Orthop. Clin. North Am., 5:887–901, 1974.

64. Nicholas, J.A.; Wilson, P.D.; and Freiberger, R.: Pathological Fractures of the Spine: Etiology and Diagnosis. J. Bone Joint Surg., 42A:127–137, 1960.

65. Nicholls, P.J., and Jarecky, T.W.: The Value of Posterior Decompression by Laminectomy for Malignant Tumors of the Spine. Clin. Orthop., 201:210–213, 1985.

66. Oni, O.O.A.: Mechanics of Cancer Metastatic to Bone (letter). J. Bone Joint Surg., 69A:309–310, 1987.

67. Parrish, F.F., and Murray, J.A.: Surgical Treatment for Secondary Neoplastic Fractures. J. Bone Joint Surg., 52A:665–686, 1970.

68. Perez, G.A.; Bradfield, J.S.; and Morgan, H.C.: Management of Pathologic Fractures. Cancer, 29:684–693, 1972.

69. Phillips, C.D.; Pope, T.L.; Jones, J.E.; Keats, T.E.; and MacMillan, R.H.: Nontraumatic Avulsion of the Lesser Trochanter: A Pathognomonic Sign of Metastatic Disease? Skeletal Radiol., 17:106–110, 1988.

70. Pugh, J.; Sherry, H.S.; Futterman, B.; and Frankel, V.H.: Biomechanics of Pathologic Fractures. Clin. Orthop., 169:109–114, 1982.

71. Rafii, M.; Firooznia, H.; Kramer, F.; Golimbu, C.; and Sanger, J.: The Role of Computed Tomography in Evaluation of Skeletal Metastasis. CT, 12:19–24, 1988.

72. Ralston, S.; Fogelman, I.; Gardner, M.D.; and Boyle, I.T.: Hypercalcemia and Metastatic Bone Disease: Is There a Causal Link? Lancet, 2:903–905, 1982.

73. Roy-Camille, R.; Saillant, G.; and Mazel, C.: Internal Fixation of the Lumbar Spine with Pedicle Screw Plating. Clin. Orthop., 203:7–17, 1986.

74. Russell, W.O.; Cohen, J.; Enzinger, S.; Hajdu, S.I.; Heise, H.; Martin, R.G.; Meissner, W.; Miller, W.T.; Schmitz, R.L.; and Suit, H.D.: A Clinical and Pathological Staging System for Soft Tissue Sarcoma. Cancer, 40:1562–1570, 1977.

75. Ryan, T.R.; Rowe, D.E.; and Salciccioli, G.G.: Prophylactic Internal Fixation of the Femur for Neoplastic Lesions. J. Bone Joint Surg., 58A:1071–1074, 1976.

76. Santori, F.S.; Ghera, S.; dePalma, F.; and de Chiara, N.: Treatment of Pathological Fractures and Impending Pathological Fractures of the Femur with Ender Nails. Orthopedics, 7:269–274, 1984.

77. Schechter, G.P.; Jaffe, E.S.; Cossman, J.; Horton, J.E.; and Whitcomb, C.C.: Malignant Lymphoma with Hypercalcemia. N. Engl. J. Med., 306:995, 1982.

78. Schocker, J.D., and Brady, L.W.: Radiation Therapy for Bone Metastasis. Clin. Orthop., 169:38–43, 1982.

79. Sherry, M.M.; Greco, F.A.; Johnson, D.H.; and Hainsworth, J.D.: Metastatic Breast Cancer Confined to the Skeletal System: An Indolent Disease. Am. J. Med., 81:381–386, 1986.

80. Sim, F.H.; Daugherty, T.W.; and Ivins, J.C.: The Adjunctive Use of Methylmethacrylate in Fixation of Pathological Fractures. J. Bone Joint Surg., 56A:40–48, 1974.

81. Smith, D.G.; Behr, J.T.; Hall, R.F.; and Dobozi, W.R.: Closed Flexible Intramedullary Biopsy of Metastatic Carcinoma. Clin. Orthop., 229:162–164, 1988.

82. Snell, W., and Beals, R.K.: Femoral Metastases and Fractures from Breast Carcinoma. Surg. Gynecol. Obstet., 119:22–24, 1964.

83. Steckel, R.J., and Kagan, A.R.: Diagnostic Persistence in Working Up Metastatic Cancer with an Unknown Primary Site. Radiology, 134:367–369, 1980.

84. Tong, D.; Gillick, L.; and Hendrickson, F.R.: The Palliation of Symptomatic Osseous Metastases. Cancer, 50:893–899, 1982.

85. van Holten-Verzantvoort, A.Th.; Bijvoet, O.L.M.; Hermans, J.; Harinck, H.I.J.; Elte, J.W.F.; Beex, L.V.A.M.; Cleton, F.J.; Krron, H.M.; Vermey, P.; Neijt, J.P.; and Bligham, G.: Reduced Morbidity from Skeletal Metastases in Breast Cancer Patients During Long-Term Bisphosphonate (ADP) Treatment. Lancet 2:983–985, 1987.

86. Vaughn, P.B., and Brindley, H.H.: Pathologic Fractures of Long Bones. South. Med. J., 72:788–794, 1979.

87. Wang, G.J.; Reger, S.I.; Maffeo, C.; McLaughlin, R.E.; and Stamp, W.G.: The Strength of Metal Reinforced Methylmethacrylate Fixation of Pathologic Fractures. Clin. Orthop., 135:287–290, 1978.

88. Wirth, C.R.: Metastatic Bone Cancer. Curr. Probl. Cancer, 3:1–36, 1979.

89. Yuh, W.T.C.; Zacharck, C.K.; Barloon, T.J.; Satoy, Y.; Sickels, W.J.; and Hawes, O.R.: Vertebral Compression Fractures: Distinction Between Benign and Malignant Causes with MR Imaging. Radiology, 172:215–218, 1989.

90. Zickel, R.E., and Mouradian, W.H.: Intramedullary Fixation of Pathological Fractures and Lesions of the Subtrochanteric Region of the Femur. J. Bone Joint Surg., 58A:1061–1066, 1976.

91. Zimskind, P.D., and Surver, J.M.: Metastasis to Bone from Carcinoma of the Breast. Clin. Orthop., 11:202–215, 1958.

7

Fractures and Dislocations in the Hand

David P. Green
Spencer A. Rowland

Although accurate figures of relative incidence are difficult to derive, fractures of the metacarpals and phalanges are probably the most common fractures in the skeletal system. In 1962, Butt[55] reviewed 200,000 Workers' Compensation injuries and noted that fractures of the hand accounted for 30% of the cases settled and were the most frequently encountered fractures. Emmett and Breck,[93] in their comprehensive review of 11,000 consecutive fractures treated in a busy private practice, found that fractures of the phalanges and metacarpals accounted for 10% of the total.

Perhaps because they are so common, and perhaps because they occur in small bones and are therefore considered minor injuries, these fractures are often relegated for treatment to the more inexperienced members of the medical team. Unfortunately, the results of treatment of fractures in the hand are not universally good,[19] and indeed the incidence of stiffness, malunion, and prolonged functional disability and economic loss is rather striking. As Quigley and Urist[229] pointed out, nowhere else in the body are motion and function more closely related to anatomic structure than in the hand.

GENERAL PRINCIPLES OF MANAGEMENT

INITIAL EVALUATION

The initial evaluation and primary care of an injured hand are critical, for at that time the surgeon has the best opportunity to assess accurately the extent of damage and to restore the altered anatomy. Many authors have observed that the fate of the hand largely depends on the judgment of the physician who first sees the patient.

Maximum functional recovery must be the goal in every hand injury, and this can be achieved only by considering the injury in relation to the patient's needs and life-style. His or her age, hand dominance, and occupation are critical factors, and the opening sentence of the history of any patient with an injured hand should record this information, as in the following example: "A 45-year-old, right-handed electrician. . . ." Knowledge of the patient's avocations or hobbies is important as well, for a clerk or stockbroker may be an accomplished musician or an amateur carpenter.

Precise details about the injury should be obtained. How did it occur (ie, what was the mechanism of injury)? Was it a crushing, tearing, or twisting injury or a clean laceration? A human bite is a notoriously dangerous injury, and a short, curved laceration over a small joint in the hand must be immediately suspected of having been caused by a tooth. Where did the injury occur? Was it in a relatively clean environment, or was it in a stable or a greasy garage? Did it occur on the job or elsewhere? This finding has important financial implications to the patient and may have significant bearing on the outcome. How much time has elapsed since the injury? What has been done in the interim? Has any treatment been given and by whom?

PHYSICAL EXAMINATION

Some fractures and dislocations may be immediately obvious because of local swelling and deformity. Angulation and displacement are often readily apparent, but in fractures of the metacarpals and phalanges it is even more important to recognize rotational malalignment.

One of the greatest pitfalls in treating injuries of the hand is to focus on the obvious fracture and overlook more subtle, but often more significant, damage to soft tissues. One must always determine the precise area of tenderness to accurately assess the damage to soft tissues as well as to bone. For example, if the patient has a swollen proximal interphalangeal (PIP) joint, it is imperative to ascertain whether the maximum tenderness is over the collateral ligaments laterally or over the central slip insertion dorsally. Careful assessment must be made of an open wound with regard to its precise location, its relationship to skin creases, the direction and viability of skin flaps, the extent of actual skin loss, and the degree of contamination of the wound. An open wound should not be probed or handled excessively; gentle inspection with sterile instruments and gloves will give sufficient preliminary information until a thorough exploration can be done in the operating room. Damage to nerves and tendons can usually be determined by careful motor and sensory testing rather than by probing of the wound in the emergency room.

Both open and closed injuries must be examined meticulously for injury to adjacent tendons, nerves, and blood vessels. Precarious circulation may be particularly subtle in closed injuries and must be assessed by noting color and temperature, capillary filling, and patency of collateral circulation by Allen's test[1] at the wrist and in the digit itself.[202]

One always has reason to suspect the presence of foreign bodies in all open or penetrating wounds. X-ray films alone cannot be relied on to uncover foreign bodies, because wood splinters, most types of glass, and many other foreign contaminants are not radiopaque. Xerograms are more likely to show these types of foreign bodies.

Satisfactory physical examination may not be possible without local or regional anesthesia, but the block should be postponed until an initial assessment of nerves and blood vessels has been made in the unanesthetized hand.

RADIOGRAPHIC EXAMINATION

X-rays are essential in virtually all injuries of the hand, even if no bone injury is obvious on clinical examination. Many significant fractures and joint injuries are missed simply because adequate x-rays were not taken on the day of injury. Three views are necessary: posteroanterior (PA), lateral, and oblique. Oblique films are particularly helpful in accurately assessing intra-articular fractures. For injuries involving a finger, a true lateral view of the individual digit is mandatory. Superimposition of the other fingers on a lateral view of the entire hand will obscure significant details that are easily seen on a lateral view of the single digit. Angulation in metacarpal fractures may be difficult to assess accurately on a true lateral film. Added information can be obtained by including a lateral view in 10° supination (for the fourth and fifth metacarpals) or 10° pronation (for the second and third metacarpals).

Again, the temptation is great to concentrate on obvious abnormalities in the x-rays and overlook important but more obscure injuries. For example, one or more carpometacarpal (CMC) joints may be subluxated or dislocated when there is a displaced or angulated fracture of an adjacent metacarpal.

ANESTHESIA FOR HAND INJURIES

Hand injuries cannot be treated properly without adequate anesthesia. In some instances, anesthesia may be necessary to obtain a satisfactory examination, but in virtually all cases, manipulation or reduction requires complete relief of pain. General anesthesia is rarely necessary, unless the patient has concomitant injuries that require it. Axillary or brachial block provides excellent anesthesia, but this is more than is generally required. Intravenous lidocaine (Bier block) provides good muscle relaxation and relief of pain.

We prefer to do most of our fracture manipulations and reductions under regional or digital block. Perhaps the most useful of these is a combined median and radial nerve block at the wrist, which provides excellent anesthesia for the thumb and index and long fingers. We prefer to block the ulnar nerve at the wrist, where it is necessary to add a wheal to block the dorsal sensory branch. If anesthesia of an individual finger is desired, digital block is adequate. It should not be a ring block at the base of the finger because of the greater likelihood of vascular impairment. A metacarpal block at the level of the palmar crease or injection of the nerves in the web space is preferable. Epinephrine should never be used with any local anesthetic agent in the hand because vascular compromise can result. (Moore's[207] book on regional anesthesia is an excellent source of reference for reviewing the aforementioned techniques.)

Small wounds can be adequately anesthetized with local infiltration, but we prefer not to use it to manipulate closed fractures. When local anesthesia is employed, edema of the tissues can be minimized by adding one vial of hyaluronidase (Wydase) to each 30 mL of anesthetic solution.

PROPER USE OF FACILITIES

Closed injuries in the hand are easily treated in the emergency room, plaster room, or office, provided the proper precautions are taken. If any type of intravenous or regional anesthesia is used, one must have immediately available resuscitation equipment such as an airway, Ambu bag, and intravenous drugs. Complications from the use of lidocaine and other local anesthetics are uncommon, but when they do occur, one must be prepared to deal with shock, seizures, and allergic reactions.

All open wounds except the most minor should be treated in an operating room or minor surgery suite. Open fractures and other injuries that require débridement or significant operative dissection should be treated in the operating room.

MASSIVE HAND TRAUMA AND MULTIPLE FRACTURES

Most of the discussions in this chapter deal with the specific management of individual fractures and dislocations in the hand, and little attention is directed toward the severely crushed or otherwise massively injured hand. In dealing with these difficult problems, one can apply the basic guidelines outlined throughout this chapter, but additional principles are pertinent to this type of injury as well.

The ultimate aims must be to return the patient to his or her usual activities as soon as possible and to restore the structure and function of the hand to as near normal as possible. To achieve these goals in the severely injured hand, the surgeon must often manage concomitant injuries that seem to demand diametrically opposed methods of treatment. For example, multiple displaced fractures may create marked instability of the entire hand skeleton, and yet prolonged immobilization can be disastrous. Soft tissue damage accompanying fractures in the hand inevitably evokes a tremendous accumulation of edema fluid. Tendons, ligaments, and intrinsic muscles become bathed in this protein-rich fluid, which rather rapidly becomes transformed into tough, unyielding, fibrous tissue. A bulky com-

pressive dressing properly applied minimizes the initial edema, and early movement helps pump the fluid out of the hand before it can become organized. Prolonged immobilization enhances its conversion into an inelastic encasement of scar.

The experience with massive hand wounds in Vietnam[48] demonstrated rather conclusively that all hand wounds do not require primary closure and that, in fact, some wounds in the hand should *not* be closed at the time of initial débridement. High-velocity missile wounds, severe crush injuries, human bites, and open wounds that have gone untreated for longer than 8 to 12 hours are all contraindications to primary wound closure in the hand. The risk of infection is minimized by careful and adequate débridement, copious irrigation, bulky sterile dressings, and a second look in the operating room three to five days later. At the time of the second operation, delayed primary closure or skin grafting can be done if the wound is surgically clean, or even further débridement with a third look several days hence may be necessary.

Early skeletal alignment is critical in the crushed or otherwise massively injured hand. Peacock[221] has shown how the strategic placement of a few small Kirschner wires at the time of the initial or subsequent operation can often provide enough stability to allow early motion and thereby minimize the stiffness that inevitably results from this type of injury. Finding the ideal compromise between stabilization and mobilization in the massively injured hand will often tax the ingenuity of even the most experienced hand surgeon.

Freeland, Jabaley, and Burkhalter[100,136] have described in detail the concept of delayed primary bone grafting for massive hand trauma. The principle of this method is that all definitive operative repair (which may include a skin flap as well as internal fixation of fractures and bone grafting for segmental defects) is done several days after injury, following thorough débridement on the day of injury and occasionally requiring subsequent débridement(s).

If delayed primary bone grafting is not performed, a useful technique to maintain length in segmental skeletal defects is the "bayonet" spacer, which is easily fabricated from a 0.0625-inch K-wire by the surgeon at the operating table (Fig. 7-1).

GUNSHOT WOUNDS

Clear distinction should be made between high-velocity and low-velocity gunshot wounds. Most civilian gunshot wounds in the hand are caused by

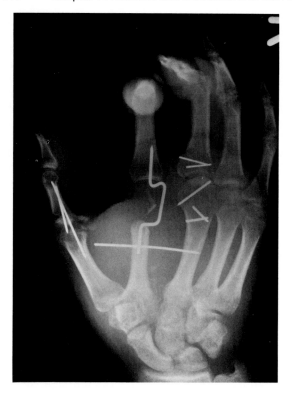

Fig. 7-1. If delayed primary bone grafting is not done, an effective method of maintaining length in segmental skeletal defects is with a "bayonet" spacer, shown here in the index metacarpal. The surgeon can easily fabricate these spacers at the operating table from a 0.0625-inch K-wire by using two pairs of needle-nosed pliers or large needle holders.

low-velocity handguns, and they do not require the extensive débridement required for the massive bone and soft tissue damage resulting from high-velocity wounds seen more frequently in military situations. Several authors[88,109] have pointed out that low-velocity gunshot wounds of the hand are relatively benign injuries. However, Dugas and D'Ambrosia[87] have emphasized the difference between low-velocity, low-caliber (.22) and low-velocity, high-caliber (.45, .357, .38) wounds, noting that the latter require more aggressive débridement.

Fractures and joint damage are common, but nerves and tendons usually seem to escape serious injury in low-velocity gunshot wounds. Nerve injuries are usually neurapraxias and generally recover spontaneously.[87,88]

Treatment should begin with careful assessment of soft tissue damage and appropriate x-ray views to detect bone and joint injury. Minimal superficial débridement (skin edges) of the entrance and exit

wounds, combined with simple cleansing and copious irrigation, is usually sufficient wound management.[243] Exploration of the wound to remove bullet fragments is not necessary unless a large pellet or fragment is superficial and likely to be painful, or possibly if fragments are intra-articular. Lead intoxication (plumbism, saturnism) is a theoretical complication of bullet fragments bathed in synovial fluid,[166,243,279] but probably not from the small joints of the hand. However, lead fragments in a joint can lead to chronic synovitis and eventual joint destruction. Therefore, intra-articular fragments should probably be removed.

The most serious residuals from low-velocity gunshot wounds in the hand are generally those involving the metacarpophalangeal (MP) and PIP joints. Intra-articular fractures with relatively mild comminution may be amenable to the judicious use of Kirschner wires, but more severe comminution with or without bone loss is a prime indication for external fixation[26,152,249] (see p. 488). Major loss of articular surfaces requires bone grafting[100,199] or subsequent arthrodesis.

FRACTURES OF THE DISTAL PHALANX

It is not surprising that fractures of the distal phalanx account for more than half of all hand fractures, because the distal portion of the hand is the most exposed to injury.[193-195] In Butt's[54] series of fractures, the distal phalanx of the long finger was injured more than twice as often as the distal phalanx of the thumb, which was next in frequency.

ANATOMY

The extensor and flexor tendons that insert on the base of the distal phalanx play no role in displacing fractures of the distal phalanx, except for avulsion injuries (which are discussed in the following section). Fibrous septa, which radiate from bone to insert into the skin, form a dense meshwork and probably stabilize the fracture and minimize displacement.[233] Acute swelling and hematoma formation in these closed fibrous compartments undoubtedly account for the severe pain that often accompanies crushing injuries of the distal phalanx.

CLASSIFICATION

Most distal phalangeal fractures are produced by crushing injuries; therefore, extensive soft tissue damage and subungual hematomas are common. Kaplan[148] classified fractures of the distal phalanx

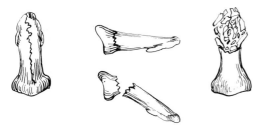

Fig. 7-2. The three general types of fractures of the distal phalanx. (**Left**) Longitudinal fractures rarely show displacement. (**Center**) A transverse fracture may show a marked degree of angulation and may require internal or external splinting. (**Right**) The so-called crushed-eggshell type of comminuted fracture that commonly involves the tuft.

into three general types: longitudinal, comminuted, and transverse (Fig. 7-2). Longitudinal fractures rarely show displacement; however, a transverse fracture close to the base of the phalanx may show a marked degree of angulation. Comminuted fractures usually involve the distal tuft of the phalanx and have been called the "crushed eggshell type."[233] In addition to being the most frequent type, the crushed, comminuted fracture is most commonly associated with soft tissue damage.

TREATMENT

Treatment of nondisplaced fractures should be directed toward the soft tissue damage. Dorsal or volar

splints, which are frequently used for immobilization, may cause severe pain if they are applied too tightly. A hairpin splint or fingertip guard (Fig. 7-3) provides protection without compressing the soft tissues. If such a splint is used for a prolonged period, however, one must be certain that it immobilizes only the distal interphalangeal (DIP) joint and does not block PIP flexion.

Transverse angulated fractures must be reduced and held with either an external splint or a smooth Kirschner wire. No attempt is made to reduce the displaced fragments of the tuft fractures, which resemble a crushed eggshell. The fragments usually are not problematic, but the finger itself can remain painful for many months.

The main reason for splinting fractures of the distal phalanx is to relieve pain. Except in the displaced, transverse variety, these fractures do not require immobilization to hold a reduction. Rather, the splint is provided to protect the tender fingertip from further external trauma.

Most fractures of the distal phalanx rarely require more than 3 to 4 weeks of protective splinting,[56] but these apparently innocuous fractures can result in surprisingly prolonged morbidity, especially if there was concomitant soft tissue crush injury. In an excellent long-term follow-up series, DaCruz and colleagues[80] showed that 31% of tuft fractures had not healed radiographically and 70% of patients had bothersome symptoms at 6 months. These symptoms can be significantly lessened by a home pro-

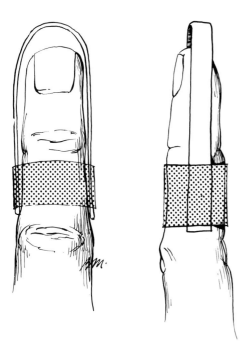

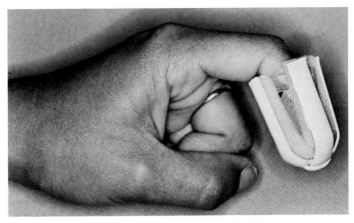

Fig. 7-3. A hairpin splint (**left**) or fingertip guard (**right**) protects the fractured distal phalanx from further injury but allows swelling to occur without tissue compression. Both splints should be fitted so as to not block PIP flexion (**right**).

gram of desensitization modalities supervised by a hand therapist.

NAIL BED INJURIES

Fractures of the distal phalanx are frequently open injuries with significant soft tissue damage. Associated injuries of the nail bed are often more serious and demand more attention than the fracture itself, and yet they are among the most frequently neglected of all injuries.

Evacuation of a subungual hematoma markedly relieves pain. Pressure caused by drilling a hole is unnecessarily painful. The time-honored hot paper clip is a more effective and relatively painless method of draining the hematoma, but a small battery-operated disposable cautery (Accu-Temp, Concept) is even better.

Late nail deformity is often an unavoidable complication following crush injuries of the distal phalanx, but a meticulous repair of the nail bed is the best means of minimizing such deformity.[45,176] Our practice is to attempt to repair the nail bed as carefully as possible with fine (6-0 or 7-0) absorbable sutures, using loupe magnification. If there is loss of nail bed tissue, various types of local and distant nail bed grafts can be considered.[294]

If the nail plate has been avulsed at its base, it is carefully removed, scrubbed with povidone iodine (Betadine), and sutured back into place following repair of the nail bed.[201,295] This not only serves as a protective splint but also minimizes local tenderness. The old nail is pushed off gradually by growth of the new nail. The patient should be told that some deformity of the nail is to be expected, although the full extent of the deformity will not be known until the new nail has fully regrown, a process that usually takes about 4 to 5 months.

When the nail plate has been avulsed or torn and the nail bed laceration is visible, the need for repair of the nail bed is clearly evident. However, when the nail plate is intact, recognition of a significant nail bed laceration is more difficult. Zook[295] has recommended exploration of the nail bed if a subungual hematoma involving greater than 25% of the nail is present. Simon and Wolgin[256] attempted to correlate the association between subungual hematomas and fractures and occult nail bed lacerations. In their series, patients with a subungual hematoma greater than one half the size of the nail had a 60% incidence of nail bed laceration requiring repair, and if there was an associated fracture of the distal phalanx, the incidence was 95%.

Occasionally the base of the nail bed may become entrapped in the fracture site, most commonly seen where the root of the nail has been avulsed from beneath the proximal nail fold. Failure to recognize this complication and extricate the nail bed from the fracture site at the time of the original wound débridement may result in nonunion of the fracture (Fig. 7-4) and a deformed finger.

MALLET FINGER OF TENDON ORIGIN

The term *mallet finger,* by common usage, has come to mean a flexion deformity of the DIP joint resulting from loss of extensor tendon continuity to the distal phalanx.[364] The same clinical picture can be caused by an intra-articular fracture involving one third or more of the dorsal lip of the distal phalanx, but this troublesome fracture is discussed on page 452 under Mallet Finger of Bony Origin.

Mechanism of Injury and Classification

Forcible flexion of the DIP joint is thought to be the mechanism of injury resulting in the "mallet" or "baseball" finger. Bunnell[301] preferred the term *drop finger.* The injury usually occurs when the extensor tendon is taut, as in catching a ball or striking an object with the extended finger. The deformity may result from relatively trivial trauma, and it has been suggested that a familial predisposition[323] or an area of relative avascularity in the tendon[373] may play a role in such patients.

Several patterns of injury may be seen[376]:

1. The extensor tendon fibers over the distal joint may be stretched without completely dividing the tendon. The degree of drop of the distal phalanx is usually not pronounced—a loss of perhaps 5° to 20° extension (Fig. 7-5, **top**)—and the patient retains some weak active extension.

2. The extensor tendon may be ruptured or torn from its insertion into the distal phalanx (Fig. 7-5, **center**).[38,324] In this instance, there is a greater flexion deformity (up to 60°), and the patient has complete loss of active extension at the distal joint.

3. A small fragment of the distal phalanx may be avulsed with the extensor tendon. In this instance, the injury has the same characteristics as the tendon injuries previously mentioned, and the degree of drop depends not on the small fragment, but rather on the amount of loss of continuity of the tendon mechanism. These injuries should be treated as tendon injuries rather than as fractures (Figs. 7-5, **bottom** and

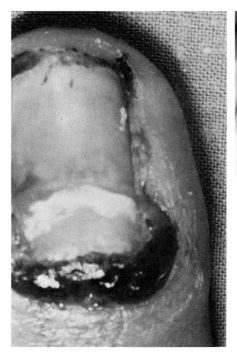
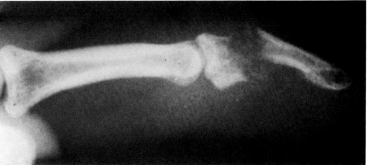

Fig. 7-4. When the root of the nail is avulsed from beneath the cuticle (**left**), one should suspect that the nail bed may be entrapped in the fracture site. The clue to this diagnosis is widening of the fracture line (**right**) and inability to fully reduce the fracture. Failure to extricate the nail bed may result in nonunion of the fracture.

7-6). In the series of Stark and coworkers,[364] 24% of the injuries were associated with small bony avulsion fractures, but this finding had no effect on the final result.

In all of these different types of injuries, if the flexion deformity of the distal joint is severe, a secondary hyperextension deformity of the PIP joint may develop because of imbalance of the extensor mechanism, resulting in a swan-neck deformity (Fig. 7-7).

Methods of Treatment

Considerable controversy has existed as to whether or not the PIP joint need be immobilized in the treatment of mallet finger. Probably in large part because such authorities as Bunnell[301] and Watson-Jones[376] recommended immobilization of the PIP joint in 60° flexion, many authors advised such treatment.[174,178,179,182,183,187,189,193,204,206,210,213,215,218,222]

In 1952, Pratt[349] introduced a method he called an internal splint. A medium-caliber (0.045-inch) smooth Kirschner wire was introduced across the PIP and DIP joints, holding the distal joint in hyperextension and the proximal joint in 60° flexion. The wire was cut off beneath the skin. Casscells and Strange[303,304] modified this technique because some of their patients developed painful and permanent limitation of motion of the PIP joint. They suggested

that only the distal joint be fixed with a Kirschner wire and that the middle joint be maintained in 60° flexion by means of skin plaster. More recently, Evans and Weightman[310] devised a splint that combines static DIP extension with dynamic PIP flexion, which they suggested might reduce tension on the site of tendon rupture and thereby allow a shorter period of splinting.

However, most authors in the current literature believe that *only* the DIP joint need be immobilized.[296,300,306,308,309,318,326,338,340,362,363,366,374] Several types of DIP splints have been described (Fig. 7-8), including at least two modifications of the original Stack splint, one with perforations[326] and another with larger windows,[363] both designed to minimize skin problems. The results of treatment with these various types of splints do not appear to be substantially different,[374] but more minor complications were reported in one series with the dorsal aluminum splint,[366] and in another series patients preferred the Stack splint over the Abouna splint.[374] Regardless of the type of splint used, precise instructions must be given to the patient to achieve optimal results and avoid minor problems[306] (see Authors' Preferred Method subsequently).

Poor results after conservative treatment prompted some surgeons to carry out immediate operative repair of the torn tendon. As early as 1930, Mason[333] had recommended early operative

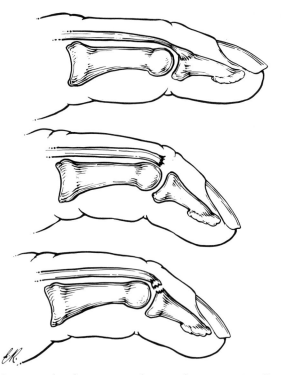

Fig. 7-5. The three types of injury that cause a mallet finger of tendon origin. (**Top**) The extensor tendon fibers over the distal joint are stretched without complete division of the tendon. Although there is some drop of the distal phalanx, the patient retains weak active extension. (**Center**) The extensor tendon is ruptured from its insertion on the distal phalanx. There is usually a 40° to 45° flexion deformity, and the patient has loss of active extension at the distal joint. (**Bottom**) A small fragment of the distal phalanx is avulsed with the extensor tendon. This injury has the same clinical findings as that shown in the center drawing.

repair of the ruptured extensor expansion. Operative treatment is aimed at freshening and approximating the edges of the tear; it is followed by immobilization of the distal and middle joints. An avulsed bone fragment can be reattached with a pull-out wire, but, if small, it may be excised and the tendon reinserted by a pull-out wire through tiny drill holes. The results of operative repair of tendinous mallet fingers are not always satisfactory. Although they may give improved cosmetic results, flexion is often lost, owing to scarring on the dorsal aspect of the joint. The assessment of the late results in Robb's series[354] suggested that early operative repair was unnecessary and even undesirable, a viewpoint shared by most authors.

The imperfect and often harmful results that followed both open and closed treatment led some to believe that the mallet deformity was being overtreated. Stiff PIP joints, pin tract infections, and skin slough were severe penalties to pay for treatment of an injury that rarely caused any functional disability. Some authors[354,356] have stated that in time, practically all mallet deformities of tendinous origin improve gradually to a satisfactory state of recovery without treatment. These authors believed that without treatment, the extensor tendon healed in a lengthened state and that gradual contraction of the fibrous scar tissue took place over the ensuing 6 months, resulting in a satisfactory state of recovery. For this reason, Robb[354] suggested that the only treatment necessary for most patients with mallet finger was the application of an elastic adhesive strapping or a straight spatula splint to relieve the initial discomfort from the injury.

Stark and colleagues[364] analyzed their results with 163 mallet fingers and concluded that not all pa-

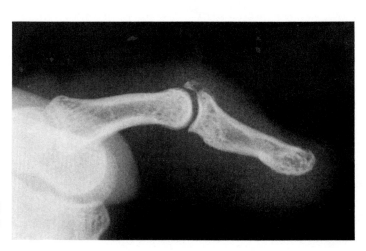

Fig. 7-6. Mallet finger deformities with small fragments such as this should be treated as tendon injuries rather than as fractures.

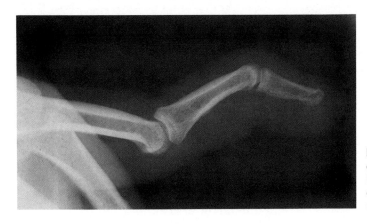

Fig. 7-7. With severe flexion deformity of the distal joint in mallet finger injury, a secondary hyperextension deformity of the PIP joint may occur because of imbalance of the extensor mechanism.

tients with mallet finger should be treated in the same way. Treatment should depend on the elapsed time following injury, the previous treatment, the degree of loss of extension, the degree of functional disability, and the age of the patient. In their series, only four patients were treated surgically and none by Kirschner wire fixation.

The results of treatment of mallet fingers are not universally good by any method. Burke[302] emphasized that assessment at the time of splint removal is valueless because subsequent recurrence of at least some of the extensor lag is likely. Flinchum[311] probably said it best when he noted that "this is a difficult injury to treat without some residual cosmetic or functional loss." Cold weather intolerance has been noted to be the most common late symptom[372] and is not directly related to the amount of residual deformity.[344]

Mikic and Helal[340] reported that although most patients are improved, only about 30% to 40% regain normal function in the DIP joint following treatment. In a very comprehensive study of mallet fingers, Abouna and Brown[296] discovered that the following factors are likely to lead to a poor prognosis: age over 60; delay in treatment more than 4 weeks; an initial active extensor lag greater than 50°; less than 4 weeks of immobilization; and patients with short, stubby fingers. Treatment of patients with associated arthritis (rheumatoid or degenerative) or peripheral vascular disease was particularly unrewarding in their experience.

Authors' Preferred Method of Treatment

ACUTE MALLET FINGER

The authors' preferred treatment for acute mallet finger is *continuous* splinting of *only* the DIP joint for 6 to 10 weeks. We do not immobilize the PIP

joint and have never opted for operative repair of the extensor tendon. Percutaneous Kirschner-wire fixation is used in selected patients. One of us (S.A.R.) uses a simple volar unpadded aluminum splint, which is fashioned to allow three-point pressure (Fig. 7-8**B**). There are two volar points of pressure, one distal and one proximal to the DIP joint. The counterpoint of pressure is applied with adhesive tape over the dorsum of the joint. The other author (D.P.G.) prefers a dorsal padded aluminum splint, which tends to interfere less with the tactile pad of the finger (Fig. 7-8**A**). A Stack[362] plastic mallet finger splint (Fig. 7-8**C**) is frequently used in the first few weeks because it tends to cause less pressure over the sore, swollen dorsum of the DIP joint. The disadvantage of the Stack splint is that it often does not hold the DIP joint in completely full extension. We will also alternate these various types of splints to accommodate and relieve local areas of pressure or tape irritation.

We attempt to position the DIP joint in *slight* hyperextension, but the degree depends on the mobility of the patient's joints and the level of discomfort. The splint should never cause pain, and the amount of hyperextension should never cause blanching of the skin over the DIP joint. (Rayan and Mullins[353] showed that skin blanching occurs in most patients at 50% of total passive hyperextension.) The patient is shown how to take the splint off and reapply it occasionally for skin care, but this requires assistance because two hands are required to hold the joint in extension and properly apply the splint.[306] At no time is the DIP joint allowed to drop into flexion. With the Stack splint, it is important to keep the tip of the finger in contact with the end of the splint, which may require an additional strip of tape placed longitudinally. If the finger does not fit any Stack splint well, Crawford[306]

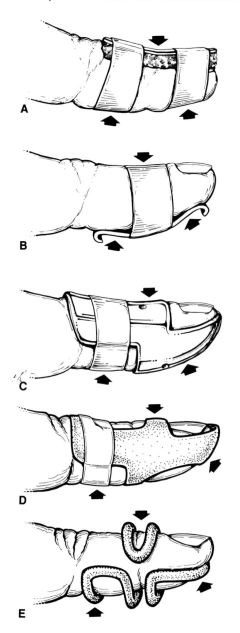

Fig. 7-8. We prefer to immobilize only the DIP joint in treating mallet fingers. This may be done with a dorsal padded aluminum splint (**A**), a volar unpadded aluminum splint (**B**), a Stack splint (**C**), a modified Stack splint (**D**), or an Abouna splint (**E**). Note that each of these splints uses a three-point fixation principle.

suggests using the smaller of the two closest sizes and cutting the splint longitudinally in the midline. To minimize skin irritation with the dorsal aluminum splint, Stern and Kastrup[366] suggested a layer of moleskin or gauze beneath the splint.

This method of treatment is successful only for patients who are reliable and reasonably intelligent, because it requires compliance and cooperation. It is advisable to see these patients after the initial 1 to 2 weeks of treatment to be certain that they understood the instructions and are using the splint properly.

An alternative method of treatment for patients who are unreliable or unable to follow instructions is the finger cast described by Smillie[358] in 1937 (Fig. 7-9), although we rarely use this technique. If it is used, the PIP joint should probably not be immobilized in flexion for more than 3 to 4 weeks.

A minimum of 6 weeks of continuous DIP immobilization is required.[377] Some authors recommend 8 weeks,[306] and one of us (S.A.R.) now routinely splints all mallet fingers for 10 weeks. Some recurrence of the extensor lag is virtually inevitable, and at least 2 to 3 weeks of nighttime splinting of the DIP joint in extension is mandatory after the continuous splint has been discontinued; we prefer a minimum of 4 weeks. Careful follow-up is required, and this treatment must be individualized. Some patients show a greater tendency for recurrence, and in these, the splinting must be applied for more hours each night and for more weeks. If the recurrent extensor lag is severe, Crawford[306] suggests a second course of full-time splinting for 8 weeks. Occasionally, a patient will have difficulty in regaining flexion, and in this situation less part-time splinting is indicated.

Occasionally one sees a patient, such as a dentist or a surgeon, for whom external splinting for a prolonged period would be an economic hardship. In these patients, immobilizing only the distal joint in full extension with a 0.045-inch Kirschner wire is an acceptable method of treatment. The pin is cut off beneath the skin, and the patient can return to his or her usual activities almost immediately. Following removal of the wire at 6 weeks, an additional 4 weeks of external night splinting is recommended. If this technique is used, the patient must be advised of the rare but dreadful complication of osteomyelitis.

LATE MALLET FINGER

A drop finger seen within 3 to 4 weeks should be treated as an acute injury, although the longer the delay, the less successful the result.[296,303,304,364] Mallet deformities that were not seen until 2 to 3 months after injury have been improved with prolonged (at least 8 weeks) splinting of the distal joint.[306,326,347] Auchincloss[297] has suggested that

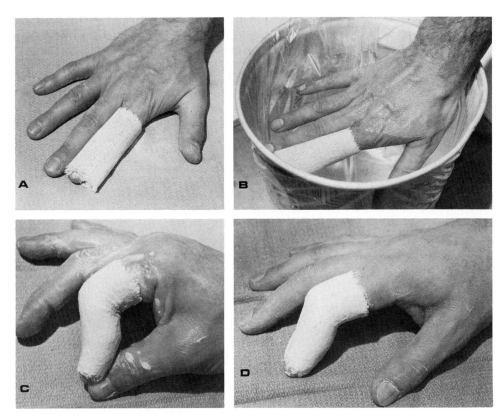

Fig. 7-9. Smillie[358] described a simple method of applying a mallet finger cast. (**A**) An 18-inch strip of 3- or 4-inch dry plaster is rolled into a tube and slipped over the end of the injured finger. No padding is used. (**B**) The patient dips his or her hand into a bucket of water, holding the tube of plaster in place over the finger. (**C**) The patient holds the finger in the correct position of immobilization while the physician smooths out the plaster. (**D**) The completed cast. Removal is facilitated by soaking the plaster. We rarely use this technique.

Kirschner wire splintage may possibly be more effective than external splinting in these patients.

Many patients with late, untreated mallet fingers have no functional problems and require no treatment. For those few patients who do have symptoms, a variety of operative procedures have been proposed, including plication[362] or reefing[303,304,308] of the scarred tendon, tenodermodesis,[322,328,372] arthrodesis[311,364] (more likely to be necessary in the patient with post-traumatic arthritis secondary to a mallet finger of bony origin, discussed subsequently), and even DIP disarticulation[356] (although few, if any, authors endorse Rosenzweig's recommendation for this).

The patients most likely to be symptomatic with late mallet finger are those who develop a swan-neck deformity, with a supple hyperextension posture of the PIP joint that accentuates the DIP extensor lag. Certain carefully selected patients with this problem may be candidates for Fowler's central slip release.[317] However, as Bowers and Hurst[299] have noted, the indications for this procedure are very strict, and the operation must be done with meticulous care to avoid significant potential complications, including weakness of PIP joint extension. Grundberg and Reagan[314] also reported satisfactory results with this procedure but stressed that the swan-neck deformity must be due to a mallet finger and not to pathology at the PIP joint if the operation is to be successful.

Satisfactory correction of such deformities can also be achieved with the spiral oblique retinacular ligament (SORL) reconstruction,[368,327] although this operation is technically more demanding and requires a thorough understanding of the extensor mechanism.

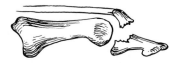

Fig. 7-10. The mallet finger originating from bone injury. The fracture fragment, which involves one third or more of the dorsal articular surface, is often tilted and malrotated, with the remainder of the distal phalanx subluxated volar to the condyles of the middle phalanx.

MALLET THUMB

Disruption of the extensor pollicis longus insertion into the base of distal phalanx can result in a flexion deformity of the thumb similar to that seen in the finger. Both splinting[348,350] and operative repair[307] have been shown to yield satisfactory results, although a review of the cases in these small series suggests that more limited motion in the interphalangeal (IP) joint may follow surgical treatment. In reporting the largest series of mallet thumbs, Miura and coworkers[342] recommended splinting for closed injuries and operative repair for lacerations of the tendon.

MALLET FINGER OF BONY ORIGIN

A fracture involving the dorsal articular surface of the distal phalanx produces a mallet deformity because the extensor tendon is attached to the avulsed fragment. Ordinarily, the fragment includes one third or more of the articular surface (Fig. 7-10). Displacement ranges from minimal separation to a wide gap with tilting and malrotation of the fragment, and the remaining distal phalanx may subluxate volar to the condyles of the middle phalanx (Fig. 7-11). Several authors[305,329] believe that the mallet fracture with volar subluxation is caused by a different mechanism than that causing the usual

hyperflexion injury. They suggest that these fractures, involving 50% or more of the articular surface, are caused by a hyperextension force, and that attempted reduction by extension of the DIP joint will fail. They believe that open reduction and internal fixation (ORIF) is necessary for these fractures.

Management of mallet fractures is controversial. Several authors have cited specific indications for open reduction, including more than 2-mm displacement,[321] 3-mm displacement,[346] more than 30% involvement of the articular surface,[343,346,365] and volar subluxation of the distal phalanx.[296,306,338,343,362,364] However, Schneider[357,377] concluded from a large series of patients with mallet fractures that there is no difference in the results from operative treatment and splinting and that in both groups the fractures heal with a "bump" over the DIP joint. Stern and Kastrup[366] noted a higher complication rate and more limited flexion of the DIP joint in their operated group, and even the staunchest advocates of open reduction[365] concede that "very few had normal motion" in the DIP joint after ORIF.

Operative treatment of a mallet fracture is a deceptively difficult procedure,[377] fraught with many potential problems, including fragmentation of the small dorsal lip fracture, difficulty in exposing and reducing the fragment anatomically, skin slough, loss of fixation postoperatively, and subsequent limited motion in the DIP joint. Stark and colleagues[364,365] emphasized the importance of exact anatomic reduction but noted that one collateral ligament must be divided to provide adequate exposure in order to visualize the articular surface. The technique described by Hamas and associates,[315] in which the extensor tendon is divided 5 mm proximal to the bone (Fig. 7-12), provides good exposure, although at least partial division of one or both collateral ligaments is still necessary to see the articular surface. Our experience with this

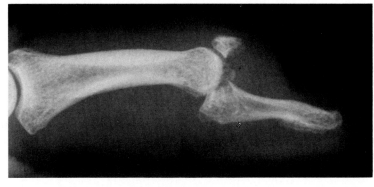

Fig. 7-11. A typical mallet finger of bony origin. Note the displacement of the avulsed fragment and the volar subluxation of the distal phalanx. This is a definite indication for operative treatment. However, open reduction of a mallet fracture is technically difficult, and it is not always possible to achieve precise anatomic reduction.

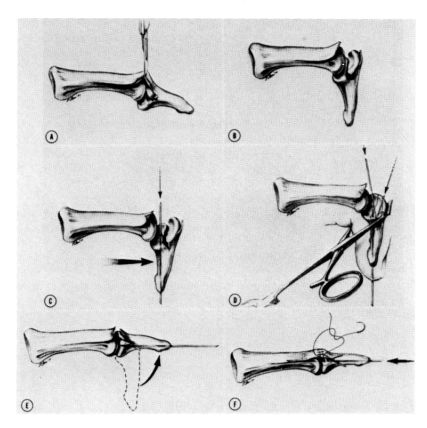

Fig. 7-12. Hamas's technique for open reduction and internal fixation of a mallet fracture in which the extensor tendon is intentionally divided and repaired. Although good exposure and accurate reduction can be achieved with this method, our experience suggests that there may be some increased stiffness of the DIP joint postoperatively because of scarring around the extensor tendon. *(Hamas, R. S.; Horrell, E. D.; and Pierret, G. P.: Treatment of Mallet Finger Due to Intra-articular Fracture of the Distal Phalanx. J. Hand Surg., 3:363, 1978.)*

technique suggests that it may cause more adherence of the extensor tendon and thus limit subsequent DIP motion.

Several methods[315,365,375] have been described for operative fixation of the fracture, each with its advantages and disadvantages. Small Kirschner wires provide better purchase and can usually be left in place longer than a pull-out wire, but even the smallest (0.028-inch) Kirschner wire may shatter the small dorsal fragment.

Authors' Preferred Method of Treatment

Having treated many mallet fractures in the past with open reduction, we have now come to the conclusion that virtually all mallet fractures should be treated with splinting of the DIP joint in much the same fashion as the mallet finger of tendon origin (see p. 449). The reasons for this are that nonoperative treatment avoids all of the potential complications noted previously, and even fractures with rather significant displacement will remodel into a remarkably smooth articular surface (Fig. 7-13). Perhaps most important, in our experience patients treated with splinting tend to regain better range of motion (especially flexion) of the DIP joint than those treated with ORIF.

Our only indication for open reduction is the mallet fracture with volar subluxation of the distal phalanx.

FLEXOR DIGITORUM PROFUNDUS AVULSION

Avulsion of the flexor digitorum profundus tendon from its insertion into the base of the distal phalanx is a relatively uncommon injury, and the diagnosis is frequently missed.[63,163,231] A high index of suspicion and awareness of this injury are imperative, for in most cases early operative treatment is required to achieve a good result.

Mechanism of Injury

Avulsion of the flexor digitorum profundus tendon is caused by forceful hyperextension of the DIP joint while the flexor digitorum profundus is in maximum contraction. It is most commonly seen in athletics, such as when a football player reaches out to tackle the ball carrier and grabs only a handful

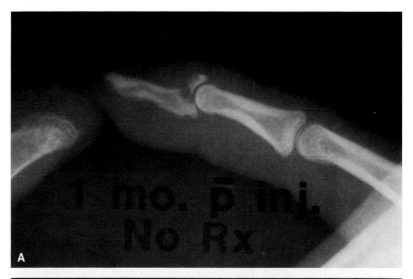

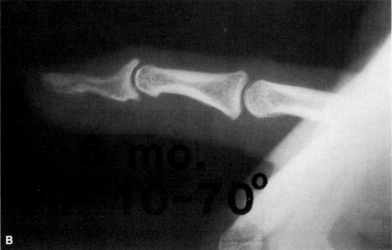

Fig. 7-13. Mallet fractures that are moderately displaced (**A**) usually heal with reasonably good congruity (**B**). This patient had 10° to 70° of active motion in the DIP joint and no pain 6 months after the fracture.

of jersey. The ring finger is involved most frequently, and although the reason for this is not clearly understood, several theories have been suggested.[57,181,288]

The tendon may rupture directly from its insertion into the bone, or it may avulse a fragment of variable size from the base of the distal phalanx. The degree of soft tissue injury and hemorrhage is far greater than that in a simple laceration of the profundus tendon, and this generally results in more extensive scarring within the flexor tendon sheath. As the avulsed tendon end retracts proximally, it may become entrapped at the chiasma of the flexor digitorum superficialis at the level of the PIP joint, and a flexion contracture may subse-

quently develop in that joint. Occasionally, the tendon retracts to the base of the finger or to the level of the lumbrical origin in the palm.

Simultaneous avulsion of both flexor tendons (profundus and superficialis) in the same digit has been described by Culver and associates.[77] They reported a good result in their case by resection of the superficialis and repair of the profundus only.

Classification

The excellent article by Leddy and Packer[164] contributed significantly to our understanding of the different types of pathology seen in this entity. They identified three distinct types of injury that have important implications in treatment:

Type I. The tendon retracts into the palm, severing all blood supply and creating extensive scarring in the tendon sheath. Repair within 7 to 10 days is required.

Type II. The tendon retracts to the level of the PIP joint, and the long vinculum remains intact. Occasionally, a small fleck of bone can be seen on a true lateral x-ray film of the finger (Fig. 7-14**B**). Early treatment is advised, but successful repair can be done as late as 3 months following injury.

Type III. A large bony fragment is avulsed by the tendon and is hung up at the level of the distal (A4) pulley (Fig. 7-14**A**).

Smith[261] and others[52,162] have described a type of injury that cannot be classified in Leddy and Pack-

er's system, and they suggested that this be called type IV. In addition to avulsion of the profundus insertion (with or without a small osseous fragment), there is a separate, concomitant intra-articular fracture at the base of distal phalanx. Early fixation of the intra-articular fracture and reinsertion of the avulsed tendon are both required to restore function.

Diagnosis

If the injury goes unnoticed by the patient, it may not come to the physician's attention for several days or weeks. Even when the patient is seen immediately, the problem may not be obvious, because there is no characteristic deformity. The diagnosis is readily made by demonstrating inability to actively flex the DIP joint.[30,164,224] Pain and local tenderness are usually more marked over the PIP joint, where the retracted end of the tendon has come to rest, than over the point of avulsion at the distal phalanx. If the tendon has retracted into the palm, there will be local tenderness at the level of the A1 pulley.

If a fragment of bone has been torn loose from the distal phalanx by the tendon, lateral and oblique x-rays of the individual finger are mandatory to confirm the diagnosis. The avulsed bone can range in size from a very large fragment[110] to a tiny speck barely visible on x-ray (see Fig. 7-14**B**). In most patients the tendon ruptures directly from the bone and no fragment is seen radiographically; therefore, the diagnosis must be made on the basis of the physical examination.

Treatment

In most cases, early operative reinsertion of the avulsed tendon is mandatory to restore active flexion of the distal joint. The success of repair is directly related to the length of delay following injury, and the most satisfactory results are obtained with immediate operative treatment. As noted, type II injuries can often be treated late, but if the tendon has retracted into the palm (type I), reinsertion will be difficult or impossible after only 7 to 10 days. Although Carroll and Match[61] reported successful repairs as long as 4 weeks after injury, it is usually impossible to bring the contracted tendon back out to its insertion in late cases. Even if it can be accomplished that late, the finger may develop a severe flexion deformity because of muscle contracture and scarring in the sheath.

A frequent technical problem encountered in reinserting the tendon even in early cases is main-

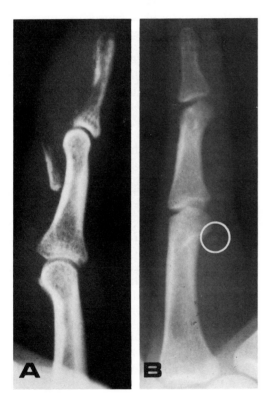

Fig. 7-14. Rupture of the flexor digitorum profundus from its insertion into the distal phalanx may be accompanied by a fragment avulsed from the distal phalanx. (**A**) An unusually large avulsion fragment. (**B**) A very tiny avulsion fragment is seen at the level of condyles of the proximal phalanx. Good-quality x-rays in true lateral and oblique views are necessary to identify the fragment. In most cases, the injury is a pure rupture of the tendon from its insertion, and no fragment is seen. (**A** from Green, D. P.: Commonly Missed Injuries in the Hand. Am. Fam. Physician, 7:114, 1973.)

taining the integrity of the distal (A4) pulley. The avulsed end of the tendon is usually quite broad, and it may be difficult to pass this beneath the intact A4 pulley. It is often necessary to narrow the distal end of the tendon before reinserting it with a pull-out suture into the distal phalanx. Another method of passing the broad end of the tendon beneath the narrow pulley is to split the distal end of the tendon longitudinally and pass each half separately beneath the pulley. In any case, every effort must be made to keep the A4 pulley intact. Failure to do so will seriously impair active flexion of the DIP joint.

Late Treatment

Patients with late, untreated profundus tendon avulsions seek help for one or several of the following reasons: (1) inability to flex the DIP joint, which may result in loss of grip strength; (2) limited motion in the PIP joint, often associated with pain; or (3) a tender fullness in the palm due to flexor tenosynovitis and the retracted stump of the flexor digitorum profundus (FDP). The first priority in these patients is to try to regain full, painless PIP motion with exercise and splinting. Frequently that is all that is needed. If the patient continues to have pain in the PIP joint and/or the palm, excision of the FDP stump from the palm and occasionally a volar scar release of the PIP joint may be indicated. For those people in whom DIP instability in hyperextension with pinch is the main problem, arthrodesis of the DIP joint may be the appropriate treatment. This leaves a small minority of patients who may in fact need active flexion of the DIP joint. FDP tendon grafting through or around an intact superficialis can be done, but not without significant risk of limiting PIP motion. This is an operation that should be done only by a surgeon well versed and experienced in tendon surgery.

The choice of treatment in these patients—therapy alone, arthrodesis of the DIP joint, free tendon grafting, excision of the FDP stump, or doing nothing—demands mature clinical judgment and an understanding of the consequences of each.

FRACTURES OF THE PROXIMAL AND MIDDLE PHALANGES

There is an enormous divergence of opinion regarding the treatment of phalangeal fractures. An understanding of the rationale and principles underlying many different methods of treatment is important, not merely for their historical interest, but because not all fractures in the fingers can or

should be treated in the same manner. Harrison McLaughlin,[190] many of whose tenets are reflected in these pages, used to say that one should not make a fracture fit a favorite treatment. Rather, the method of management should be tailored to the peculiarities of the given fracture and to the needs of the individual patient.

In the section on Methods of Treatment, we describe some of the many techniques that have been advocated, and we attempt to put each in its proper perspective.

ANATOMY

As in other long bone fractures, displacement and angulation in fracture of the phalanges are influenced by two factors: the mechanism of injury and the muscles acting as deforming forces on the fractured bone. The type of injury often determines the nature of the fracture; for example, a direct blow is more likely to cause a transverse or comminuted fracture, whereas a twisting injury will more often result in an oblique or spiral fracture. The direction of angulation seen in fractures of the phalanges primarily depends on the muscles acting on that bone.

Unstable fractures of the proximal phalanx typically present with volar angulation (Fig. 7-15). The proximal fragment is flexed by the bony insertions of the interossei into the base of the proximal phalanx. Although there are no tendons inserting on the distal fragment, it tends to be pulled into hyperextension by the central slip acting on the base of the middle phalanx. Once the stability of the proximal phalanx is lost, there is an accordionlike collapse at the fracture site, aggravated by further pull on the extensor hood by the intrinsic muscles.

The middle phalanx is much less commonly fractured than the proximal phalanx, and muscle forces acting on these fractures are different. The important deforming forces to be considered are the insertion of the central slip into the dorsum of the base of the middle phalanx and the insertion of the flexor digitorum superficialis volarly. The central slip has a well-defined area of insertion, and its action is to extend the middle phalanx. Although the action of the flexor superficialis is to flex the middle phalanx, its insertion is rather complex and is not confined to a short segment of the phalanx. Kaplan[10] has described in detail the decussation of the superficialis tendon to allow the profundus tendon to pass through its two slips, and the reader is referred to Kaplan's textbook for this detailed description. In essence, however, the superficialis di-

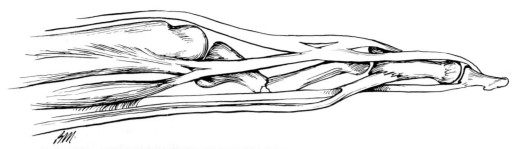

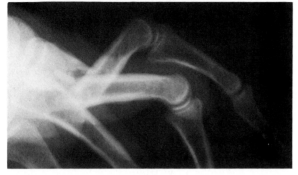

Fig. 7-15. Unstable fractures of the proximal phalanx typically present with volar angulation. (**Top**) The proximal fragment is flexed by the bony insertion of the interossei into the base of the proximal phalanx. Once the stability of the proximal phalanx is lost, there is an accordion-like collapse at the fracture site, aggravated by further pull on the extensor hood by the extrinsic muscles. (**Right**) An x-ray film showing the typical, although somewhat exaggerated, volar angulation. More commonly, the angulation is approximately 30°.

vides into halves, each half turning 90° to allow the profundus to pass through and then completing another 90° rotation to insert into nearly the entire volar surface of the middle phalanx (Fig. 7-16). Careful examination of a disarticulated middle phalanx will reveal that there is a narrow ridge along each side of the middle two thirds of the volar aspect of the bone, into which the superficialis inserts. Many textbooks feature drawings that depict the superficialis insertion as a precise, fixed point on the proximal aspect of the bone. A more accurate representation is illustrated in Figure 7-17, **top,** which shows the very prolonged insertion of the superficialis, extending from a point just distal to the flare of the base to a point only a few millimeters proximal to the neck. A fracture through the neck of the middle phalanx is likely to have volar angulation, as the proximal fragment tends to be flexed by the strong pull of the superficialis (Fig. 7-17, **center**). A fracture through the base of the middle phalanx proximal to the insertion of the superficialis would be more likely to be dorsally angulated owing to the extending force of the central slip on the proximal fragment and a flexing force on the distal fragment by the superficialis (Fig. 7-17, **bottom**). However, fractures through the middle two thirds of the bone may be angulated in either direction or not at all, and the angulation cannot always be predicted with accuracy entirely on the basis of the tendon insertion.[220]

Malrotation at the fracture site is one of the most frequent complications of phalangeal fractures, and one that can be avoided only by careful attention to anatomic detail. When the fingers are flexed, they do not remain parallel, as they are in full extension. Rather, they point toward the region of the scaphoid tubercle, although they do not actually converge on a single fixed point, as is sometimes depicted (Fig. 7-18). Thus, it is relatively easy to detect malrotation when the fingers are in full flexion (Fig. 7-19). With the fingers only semiflexed, it is helpful to use the planes of the fingernails as an additional guide to correct rotation. The opposite hand must be checked for comparison, because often the border fingers lie in a slightly different plane of rotation as seen end-on (Fig. 7-20).

METHODS OF TREATMENT

No Reduction and Early Active Motion (Buddy Taping)

The method that James[140] calls "garter strapping" others refer to as "buddy taping" or "dynamic splinting." The technique is simply to tape the injured finger to an adjacent normal digit and allow and, in fact, encourage the patient to move the finger and to use the hand as normally as possible while the fracture heals. The rationale is that early motion prevents stiffness in the small joints of the finger that almost invariably results from immo-

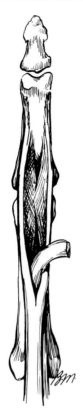

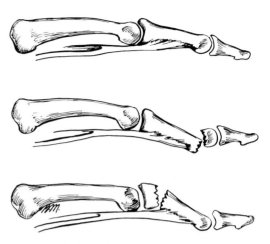

Fig. 7-17. (**Top**) A lateral view showing the prolonged insertion of the superficialis tendon into the middle phalanx. (**Center**) A fracture through the neck of the middle phalanx is likely to have a volar angulation, because the proximal fragment is flexed by the strong pull of the superficialis. (**Bottom**) A fracture through the base of the middle phalanx is more likely to have a dorsal angulation owing to the extension force of the central slip on the proximal fragment and a flexion force on the distal fragment by the superficialis.

Fig. 7-16. The flexor digitorum superficialis has a complicated and extensive insertion into the middle phalanx. Each half of the tendon rotates a full 180° to insert into nearly the entire volar surface of the middle phalanx. Note that fibers from each insertion also cross to the opposite side, forming a broad expanse of tendon beneath the profundus tendon. (*Redrawn from Kaplan, E. B.: Functional and Surgical Anatomy of the Hand, 2nd ed. Philadelphia, J.B. Lippincott, 1965.*)

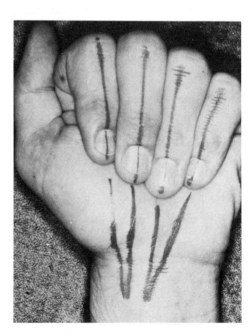

Fig. 7-18. Maintaining correct rotational alignment is one of the most difficult and subtle aspects of treating fractures of the phalanges. When the fingers are flexed, they do not remain parallel as they are in full extension. They point toward the region of the scaphoid, although they do not actually converge on a single fixed point, as is sometimes depicted.

bilization. In a large series of patients with finger fractures, Wright[293] discovered that those treated with early active motion had less stiffness and less economic disability than those treated with immobilization. We basically agree with the idea that stiffness can be minimized and the patient can return to work sooner if the fracture is treated with buddy taping rather than immobilization. However, the method is not suitable for the treatment of all phalangeal fractures. Certain undisplaced fractures and impacted transverse fractures of the phalanges are ideally managed with buddy taping, but only if two basic principles are observed. First, the fracture must truly be stable (ie, undisplaced or impacted) with no angulation in any plane. Coonrad and Pohlman[70] have clearly illustrated the pitfall of misinterpreting an anteroposterior x-ray as showing

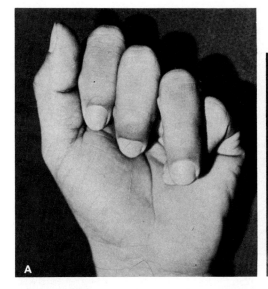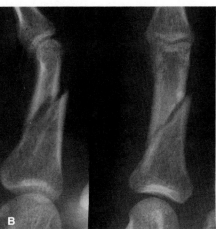

Fig. 7-19. (**A**) Gross malalignment of the ring finger seen in a patient in whom a fracture of the proximal phalanx was allowed to heal with rotational deformity. (**B**) Although subtle malalignment can be evaluated more critically by clinical means, rotational deformity may also be seen radiographically. The wide discrepancy in cross-sectional diameter of the proximal and distal fragments as seen on the lateral view clearly demonstrates a severe rotational deformity. On the anteroposterior view, the deformity is less obvious, although any discrepancy in diameter of the two fragments should alert the physician to the possibility of rotational deformity.

an impacted fracture when in fact the lateral view shows significant volar angulation. Such fractures must be immobilized in flexion and are not amenable to the buddy taping technique. Second, careful clinical and radiographic follow-up of the patient during the healing phase is imperative to immediately recognize displacement or angulation at the fracture site, should it occur.

Closed Reduction and Immobilization

Many fractures of the phalanges can be satisfactorily managed by closed reduction and external immobilization, but several important principles must be followed if this method is to be successful.

1. The closed reduction maneuver must be done before application of the cast or splint, for the splint merely holds the reduction after it has been achieved. The splint must not be relied upon to reduce the fracture.
2. As with fractures of any long bone, the controllable distal fragment must be brought into alignment with the uncontrollable proximal fragment.
3. The fracture must be stable after reduction in order for the splint to maintain the reduction.

Transverse fractures generally fall into this category, but spiral oblique fractures are inherently unstable and it may be impossible to hold them reduced with any sort of splint or cast.

TYPES OF IMMOBILIZATION

A wide variety of splints and casts have been used to immobilize fractures of the phalanges. Since several muscles that act as deforming forces on the fracture originate in the forearm, it is advisable to immobilize the wrist as well as the injured finger. This is generally done with the wrist in approximately 30° of extension.

Circular Cast. A plaster or fiberglass short-arm gauntlet cast that includes the fingers can be used. In small children it is usually necessary to incorporate all four fingers in the cast, but the larger digits in adults may make it possible to immobilize only the fractured finger and a single adjacent finger. This method has the advantage of better stability but the disadvantage of possibly compromising the circulation if the swelling is significant.

Cast With Outrigger. A more commonly used method is to incorporate some sort of outrigger with

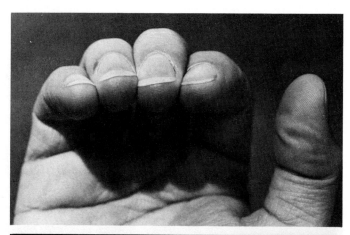

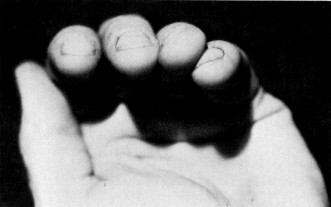

Fig. 7-20. With the fingers only semiflexed, it is helpful to use the planes of the fingernails as an additional guide to correct rotation. The opposite hand must be checked for comparison, because the border fingers frequently lie in a slightly different plane of rotation as seen end-on (**top**). Note the significant rotational malalignment seen in the ring finger (**bottom**).

a short-arm gauntlet cast. Although different types of outriggers can be used, most of these are modifications of the wire finger splint described by Bohler[33] (Fig. 7-21). Because of its rather wide availability, the foam-padded aluminum splint is probably most commonly used in this country, although the stability that it provides leaves something to be desired, and rotational deformity may be more difficult to control. An outrigger made entirely of plaster can be used, but this is more likely to crack or break; reinforcement with a "fin" as described in Chapter 1 and illustrated in Figure 7-22 adds considerable strength without a great deal of additional weight or bulk.

Gutter Splints. Fractures involving the ring or small fingers can be adequately immobilized with an ulnar gutter plaster splint, leaving the radial digits completely free (Fig. 7-23**A**). A similar radial gutter splint, with a hole for the thumb, can be used for fractures in the index and long fingers (Fig. 7-23**B**). These splints are strong and easy to apply;

their major disadvantage is that the plaster tends to "bunch up" in the distal palm, making it more difficult to immobilize the MP joints in flexion.

Anterior and Posterior Splints. Separate, well-padded anterior and posterior plaster splints are more versatile in their application than gutter splints and provide excellent stability. They have the added advantage of allowing the dressing to be split and rewrapped without jeopardizing the reduction if the hand or fingers swell or allowing the wrapping to be tightened if the swelling subsides.

POSITION OF IMMOBILIZATION

Unless there are local factors such as associated injuries that dictate otherwise, the preferred position of immobilization of the hand is the intrinsic plus or so-called J.I.P. James position. James[141] advocated that the MP joints be immobilized in at least 70° of flexion, the PIP joints in no more than 15° to 20° of flexion, and the DIP joints in only 5° to

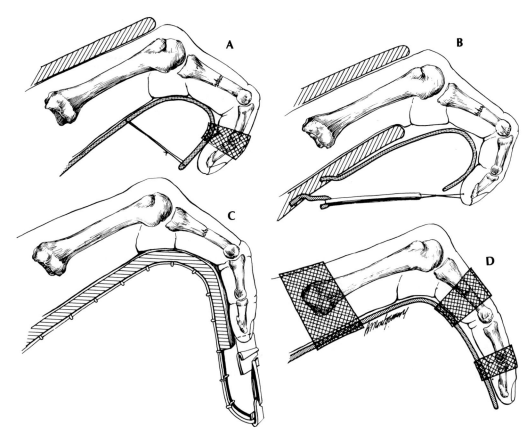

Fig. 7-21. Several types of splinting have been described for treating fractures of the phalanges. (**A**) Böhler described the use of a wire outrigger combined with a dorsal plaster slab that immobilized the wrist. The tip of the outrigger was wired to itself to hold the finger in rather acute flexion. (**B**) Bunnell, and later Boyes, used a modified Böhler splint together with pulp traction, applying just enough tension to maintain the position obtained by manipulation. (**C**) Moberg designed a padded wire ladder that is used widely in Sweden but is not available in the United States. This technique uses a specialized form of nail-pulp traction. (The illustration is slightly inaccurate in that the wire should pass through the periosteum at the tip of the distal phalanx. (**D**) James has advocated that fingers should be immobilized not in the position of function, but rather in a position that more nearly resembles the intrinsic-plus position in which the MP joints are immobilized in at least 70° flexion and the IP joints in minimal flexion (see text).

10° of flexion (see Fig. 7-21**D**). The flexed position of the MP joints is desirable because of the cam effect of the metacarpal head on the collateral ligaments (see p. 516). As James pointed out, the MP joints almost never become stiff in flexion because in that position the collateral ligaments are stretched to their maximum length, whereas stiffness in extension is common because the ligaments will contract if immobilized in their shortened position.

The PIP joints are more likely to become stiff in flexion, but the explanation for this is not so clear-cut. Although the PIP joints can and do occasionally become stiff in extension, the fact that they are more likely to become stiff in flexion lends support to the concept that these joints should preferably be immobilized in minimal flexion. However, this dictum cannot be followed absolutely in treatment of fractures of the phalanges because of the tendency for these fractures to develop volar angulation (see p. 457). It is imperative that the PIP joints be immobilized in sufficient flexion to correct this volar angulation.

Ordinarily it is sufficient to immobilize only the injured finger, but rotational alignment is usually easier to control if an adjacent normal finger is incorporated into the cast or splint.

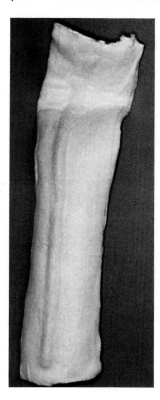

Fig. 7-22. Plaster splints can be strengthened considerably without adding a great deal more weight by using a "fin," which is made by folding several layers of plaster longitudinally.

Closed Reduction and Early Active Motion

Burkhalter and colleagues[49,232] have described a unique method of treating phalangeal fractures that allows early active motion of fractures that require a closed reduction maneuver. This technique is based on the premise that with the MP joints in maximum flexion, the extensor hood is tightened to establish a tension band that provides palmar cortical compression during active flexion (Fig. 7-24**A**). After fracture reduction under digital block anesthesia, a short-arm cast is applied with the wrist in 30° of extension and the MP joints in 90° of flexion (Fig. 7-24**B**). The cast extends dorsally to the level of the PIP joints and is trimmed in the palm to allow full MP and PIP flexion (Fig. 7-24**C**). Simultaneous flexion of the adjacent normal digits is relied on to help control angulation and rotation.

This method is effective in the treatment of transverse fractures of the phalanges with volar angulation referred to previously, but Burkhalter[49] has emphasized that the technique requires great attention to detail on the part of the surgeon and also

"enough maturity to be able to abandon the method if failure is likely."

Traction

Although it is not particularly popular in the current American orthopaedic literature, traction (or extension, as it was often called) frequently has been advocated as the preferred method of treatment for finger fractures throughout the years.[119,198,204,206,210,233] Several types have been described.

SKIN TRACTION

Adhesive tape wrapped circumferentially or diagonally around a finger can provide adequate traction to hold a reduction, but its complications are both bothersome and potentially dangerous. Slipping of the adhesive is a common problem, and even with improved techniques such as that advocated by Schulze,[247] the danger of circulatory compromise is real enough to be of concern. Another disadvantage of skin traction is that it immobilizes the finger in full extension and virtually eliminates active motion of the IP joints while the fracture heals.

The Ellis technique of combined splintage and traction is said by Fitzgerald and Khan[96] to obviate some of these problems. The finger is fixed in extension to the tip of a padded, malleable metal splint and the splint is then flexed, thereby applying isometric traction to the digital skeleton.

PULP TRACTION

The major disadvantage of using a wire passed transversely across the pulp space for traction is the danger of pulp necrosis from squeezing the tip of the finger. Bunnell[47] and Boyes,[40] however, both used pulp traction in conjunction with a Bohler splint (see Fig. 7-21**B**), applying just enough tension to maintain the position obtained by manipulation. Bohler originally used pulp traction[33] but stopped because of complications from improper application.

NAIL TRACTION

Pulling through the nail by means of a wire or silk suture has been advocated, but today it has few supporters as an adjunct to fracture treatment, even though it is frequently used following flexor tendon repair.

NAIL-PULP TRACTION

Moberg[204,205] described extensive experience with a modified type of traction in which a stainless steel

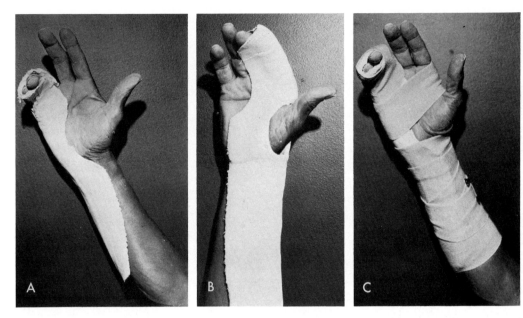

Fig. 7-23. We occasionally use gutter plaster splints in the treatment of phalangeal and metacarpal fractures. (**A**) Fractures involving the ring and small fingers can be adequately immobilized with an ulnar gutter splint, leaving the radial digits completely free. (**B**) A similar splint can be used on the radial side of the hand, cutting out a hole for the thumb. (**C**) The splint is held in place with an elastic bandage, wrapped securely but not tightly.

wire is passed vertically through the nail, the periosteum of the tip of the distal phalanx, and the pulp. He credits his success with this technique and absence of complications to the use of a spreading device, which prevents the wire from squeezing the fingertip (see Fig. 7-21**C**). Since 1948, Moberg has made available throughout Sweden a kit that contains the materials for applying his special nail-pulp traction. Like Boyes, Moberg emphasized that traction is used not to reduce a fracture but only to maintain a reduced fracture in satisfactory position.

SKELETAL TRACTION

Firm traction in the finger can be provided by means of a small Kirschner wire or needle passed transversely through the phalanx and attached to an outrigger by rubber bands in a variety of ways. Specially designed calipers have been used similarly,[60,206] with purchase provided by a tong-type mechanism rather than passage of a wire directly through the entire phalanx. For a fracture of the proximal phalanx, it is desirable to have the wire as close to the fracture as possible, specifically through the distal end of the proximal phalanx. The major disadvantage of this is that it is difficult (several authors say virtually impossible) to insert

a wire transversely through the proximal phalanx without perforating some part of the extensor hood complex. The major disadvantage of traction through the middle or distal phalanx is that it severely restricts or eliminates active motion in the PIP joint during the period of traction. Quigley and Urist[229] concluded that there is only one area in the finger where skin lies directly over fascia and bone, with no underlying tendons or neurovascular bundles; that is a triangular space on the dorsal surface of the middle phalanx, just distal to the insertion of the central slip. They fashioned a traction hook from a Kirschner wire and embedded it into bone in this location.

The banjo type of traction advocated many years ago is now universally condemned. The technique is improper for several reasons: rotation is difficult to control; the fingers are not truly supported; and, most important, stiffness is enhanced by the position of full extension in all joints.

A serious and avoidable complication of traction is pressure necrosis of the volar skin caused by overzealous pull against an unyielding fulcrum. This can be prevented by observing several precautions: (1) padding the wire outrigger with a soft material; (2) never allowing the plaster gauntlet to

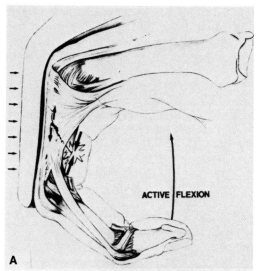

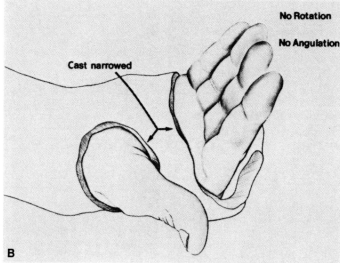

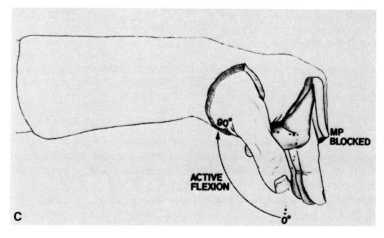

Fig. 7-24. Burkhalter and Reyes's[49,232] method of early mobilization treatment of phalangeal fractures is based on the concept of an intact dorsal soft tissue hinge (**A**). The MP joints are flexed 70 to 90 degrees; the cast extends dorsally beyond the PIP joints (**B**) but is trimmed to allow full PIP flexion (**C**). (*Reyes, F. A., and Latta, L. L.: Conservative Management of Difficult Phalangeal Fractures. Clin. Orthop., 214:24, 1987.*)

extend far enough distally to touch the finger; (3) eliminating acute flexion of the PIP joint; and (4) avoiding excessive traction force.

If traction is used, it should rarely be continued for more than 3 weeks. The most important principle in the use of traction is that its purpose is to maintain a reduction, not to reduce the fracture.

External Fixation

The major indications for external fixation devices in phalangeal fractures are extreme comminution and segmental loss that preclude stabilization by other means,[26,99,234] although occasionally they may be used in conjunction with internal fixation.[99] A more detailed discussion of external fixation devices and techniques is found in the section on Fractures of the Metacarpals (see p. 488).

Closed Reduction and Percutaneous Pin Fixation

The theoretical advantage of closed reduction and percutaneous pinning (CR and PCP) is that an unstable fracture can be rendered sufficiently stable to allow early motion without subjecting the hand to the surgical trauma of open reduction. Excellent results can be achieved with this method, but the procedure is not as easy to perform as one might anticipate.[110] Two knowledgeable surgeons facilitate the technique; one reduces and holds the fracture and the other inserts the pins (Fig. 7-25). A power-driven drill is essential, and although the image intensifier is not absolutely necessary, it certainly makes the procedure easier (except in intra-articular fractures, where the images produced on the monitor are not clear enough to ensure precise

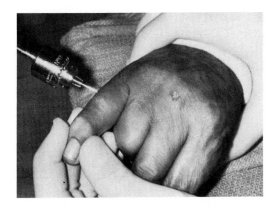

Fig. 7-25. Closed reduction and percutaneous pin fixation of unstable phalangeal fractures is a useful technique but not as easy to perform as one might anticipate. Two knowledgeable surgeons make it easier. One must reduce and hold the fracture while the other simultaneously inserts the pins. (*Green, D. P., and Anderson, J. R.: Closed Reduction and Percutaneous Pin Fixation of Fractured Phalanges. J. Bone Joint Surg., 55A:1652, 1973.*)

anatomic reduction;[176] in such fractures, regular x-ray films are required). Bilos[25] has developed special pins to achieve compression, but we have found smooth Kirschner wires to be entirely satisfactory and simpler to use. Several authors[58,241] have suggested the use of hypodermic needles to serve as guides for more precise pin placement; the surgeon lines up the needle and holds it in position while an assistant inserts the Kirschner wire through the needle. (See Table 7-1 for the proper needle to use with each size Kirschner wire.)

Eaton and colleagues[22] have been staunch advocates of percutaneous pin fixation. They recommend that the procedure be done under wrist block anesthesia because allowing the patient to move the fingers painlessly through a range of motion is the best method of assessing anatomic reduction and stability and of avoiding rotational deformity. They describe quite clearly two distinct methods of CR and PCP. The first is for transverse and short oblique fractures, in which intramedullary pin fixation is used by passing a wire longitudinally to one side of the extensor tendon through the metacarpal head (Fig. 7-26**C**). This technique is particularly well suited for those difficult transverse fractures near the base of the proximal phalanx that tend to develop a recurvatum-type deformity (see p. 457). Reduction is performed by applying longitudinal traction through the middle phalanx while flexing the MP joint to 60° and the PIP joint to at least 45°. A 0.045-inch or 0.035-inch Kirschner

wire is passed across the metacarpal head as noted previously down the medullary canal of the proximal phalanx to the subchondral bone in the condyle. Since the wire crosses the MP joint, a short-arm cast that rigidly immobilizes the MP joints is imperative with this method; both the cast and the Kirschner wire are removed at 3 weeks. A theoretical disadvantage of this method is the transarticular placement of the Kirschner wire,[62] but Cordrey[71] has shown that this will not necessarily result in limitation of motion if the cartilage surfaces are intact.

In the other method, spiral oblique fractures are percutaneously pinned by direct fixation of the fracture,[22,113] although this technique (Fig. 7-26**A**) is considerably more difficult than the intramedullary method used for transverse fractures. There is a narrow margin for error, because a few millimeters' difference in pin placement can easily result in inadequate fixation. Both reduction of the fracture and pin placement are facilitated by the use of a fracture reduction clamp such as the Blalock[29] (Fig. 7-27), AO,[104] or Aesculap (Fig. 7-28). At least two pins (preferably 0.045-inch) must be used, placed as far apart as possible yet providing solid purchase on both fracture fragments. Ideally, the pins should not be parallel to each other, because this may allow the fracture to separate. The pins may be cut off beneath the skin or left to protrude with the tip bent into a small loop or right angle (Fig. 7-29). Although minimal drainage is common from percutaneous pin tracts, it usually resolves with no permanent residual problems after the pins are removed, and the ease of removing pins that have been left protruding through the skin makes this method our preference. With proper pin placement that provides good fracture stability, buddy taping can be instituted immediately and active range of motion encouraged. The pins are removed at 3 weeks, and buddy taping is continued for another 3 weeks.

The main disadvantages of CR and PCP are that it is difficult (especially with spiral oblique frac-

Table 7-1. Hypodermic Needle Guides for Kirschner Wire Placement

Kirschner Wire	Diameter (mm)	Size Needle Required for Guide
0.028-inch	0.712	19-gauge
0.035-inch	0.889	18-gauge
0.045-inch	1.143	16-gauge
0.054-inch	1.372	16-gauge
0.0625-inch	1.588	14-gauge too small

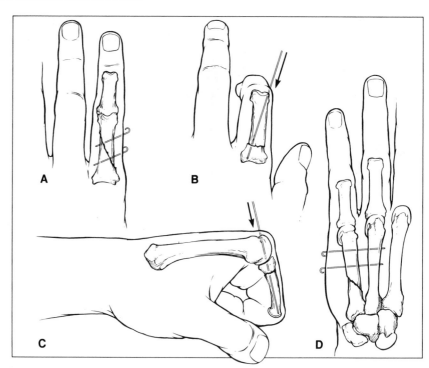

Fig. 7-26. (**A–D**) Four methods of closed reduction and percutaneous pin fixation. See text for details of each.

tures), reduction of the fracture may not be as precise as with open reduction, and parts of the extensor mechanism may be impaled with the Kirschner wires. However, it does avoid the considerable added surgical trauma of open reduction and is therefore an excellent alternative method of treatment for certain fractures. One disadvantage rarely mentioned is that surgeons must expose their own hands to radiation, and Widgerow and colleagues[289] said that they rarely use CR and PCP for precisely this reason.

Open Reduction and Internal Fixation

Unstable fractures that cannot be reduced by closed manipulation and maintained with external splinting require internal fixation. As noted in the preceding section, selected fractures can be reduced by closed manipulation and stabilized with percutaneously placed Kirschner wires, but in some situations open reduction to ensure more precise anatomic reduction is warranted. Specific indications for ORIF vary widely depending on the experience, technical skills, and judgment of the surgeon, but the following would probably be considered appropriate indications by most surgeons:

1. Most intra-articular fractures, although moderate to severe comminution is a relative con-

traindication, again depending on the skills and experience of the surgeon.
2. Multiple fractures.[20,123] The greater the number of fractures, the more necessary it becomes to provide stabilization of the skeleton.
3. Open fractures and associated soft tissue injury. This is a somewhat radical departure from previous concepts, for it was formerly suggested[73] that open fractures were a relative contraindication to open reduction. With wider experience and more precise techniques for open reduction, some authors[123,136] now believe that open injuries with severe soft tissue injury constitute an important indication for open reduction, because providing skeletal stabilization may allow the soft tissue injury to be dealt with more effectively. This does not mean that internal fixation should necessarily be done on the day of injury, and several authors with wide experience have emphasized the importance of delayed primary fixation,[136,197] a concept that has particular application to injuries requiring combined skeletal and soft tissue repair and reconstruction[100] (see the section Gunshot Wounds on p. 443).

Once the decision has been made that internal fixation is indicated, the surgeon has an ever-in-

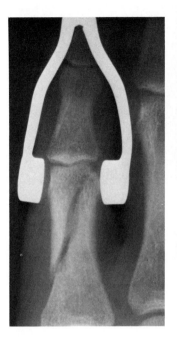
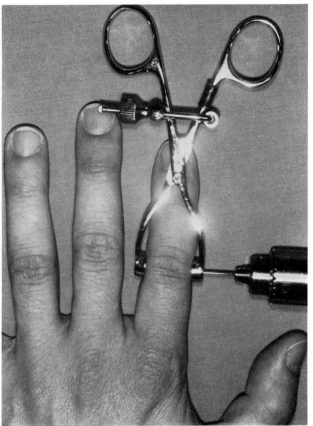

Fig. 7-27. The Blalock clamp is useful in closed reduction and percutaneous pin fixation of fractures of the phalanges. (**Left**) The fracture is reduced, the clamp is applied, and x-ray films confirm the reduction. (**Right**) A hole in the clamp allows exact placement of the pin.

creasing variety of techniques from which to choose, a far cry from the situation in 1924, when Tennant[274] resorted to using a steel phonograph needle for fixation.

KIRSCHNER WIRES

Smooth Kirschner wires remain the most useful and versatile mode of fixation for fractures of the phalanges, despite numerous biomechanical studies that tend to denigrate their efficacy (see p. 473). Placement of the Kirschner wires is largely dependent on the anatomy of the fracture; eg, long spiral fractures are more easily fixed with horizontally or obliquely directed pins, and transverse fractures generally require crossed or longitudinal Kirschner wires. Studies by Namba and colleagues[211] of Kirschner-wire configuration suggest several important technical details:

1. Kirschner wires are best inserted at slow drilling speeds.

2. The diamond-tipped wire (two angled facets) has superior drilling properties but has a greater tendency to "walk" along the cortex before penetrating the bone.

3. The trochar-tipped wire (four angled facets) provides better holding power initially, although at 3 weeks there is no difference in holding power between the trochar and diamond tips.

4. An oblique cutting tip made by the surgeon when a Kirschner wire is shortened in the operating room is clearly inferior in both drilling and holding properties. This implies that for hand surgery the commercially available, double-ended 6-inch Kirschner wires are to be preferred over the standard 9-inch wires.

Ruggeri and colleagues[241] and others[90] have suggested that Kirschner wire placement can be facilitated by using a hypodermic needle as a pin guide, having the surgeon hold the needle while an assis-

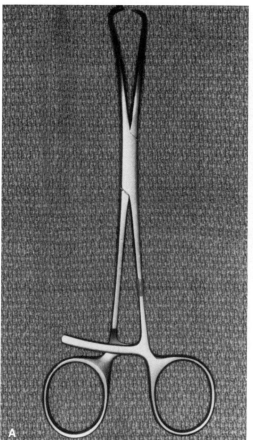

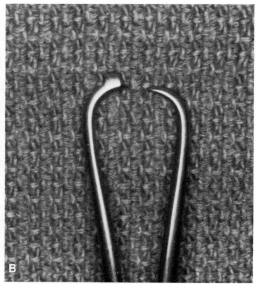

Fig. 7-28. The Aesculap clamp (**A**) is a useful instrument for percutaneous pin fixation. The sharp points hold the reduction achieved, and the small fenestration (**B**) allows precise placement of a K-wire.

tant inserts the Kirschner wire (see Table 7-2 for appropriate-size needles).

Alexander and coworkers[17] noted that slippage at the bone–wire interface is the most common cause of failure of Kirschner wire fixation. This potential problem might theoretically be minimized with the Bilos compression pin, but Noyez and Verstreken[216] have recommended that the Bilos pin be predrilled with a Kirschner wire. Viegas[280] has done laboratory studies to compare the strength of various Kirschner wire configurations.

Some authors have suggested that crossed Kirschner wires may actually distract the fracture site and delay healing.[147] Despite the theoretic disadvantages, however, properly placed crossed Kirschner wires are an excellent, time-proven method of fixation of transverse fractures. O'Brien's description[90,218] of retrograde placement of Kirschner wires is helpful in ensuring proper apposition of the fragments (Fig. 7-30).

INTRAMEDULLARY FIXATION

Intramedullary fixation is an appealing concept, but it has not achieved a high level of popularity in the fixation of hand fractures for a variety of reasons, including difficulty of insertion, impairment of adjacent joint motion, relatively poor control of rotational alignment, and problems with removal. Grundberg[117] described an ingenious technique that obviates some of these disadvantages (Fig. 7-31). A Steinmann pin one size larger than the medullary canal is used to enlarge the proximal and distal canals by drilling first with the sharp end of the pin and then with the blunt end so that it does not penetrate into the adjacent joint. The blunt end is then introduced into the proximal fragment, and the pin is cut off so that it protrudes 1 cm in a phalanx and 1.5 cm in a metacarpal. The fracture is then distracted, and the pin is introduced into the medullary canal of the distal fragment as the fracture is reduced. We have used this method in difficult situations in which other forms of fixation would not suffice; the major problem we encountered was in obtaining adequate purchase on the distal fragment.

Hall[120,121] has described the use of Enders-type flexible intramedullary rods, which he says provides sufficiently rigid fixation to obviate a cast and is but its application to fractures in the hand should be attributed to Lister[171] (Fig. 7-32), who noted that the method is particularly useful in transverse fractures near a joint. Parallel drill holes are made 5 mm distal and proximal to the fracture site with a 0.035-inch Kirschner wire. No. 26–gauge stainless steel monofilament wire is then passed through the holes. Before the wire loop is tied, the 0.035-inch Kirschner wire is driven through the cortex of the distal fragment. With the fracture held reduced under direct vision, the obliquely oriented Kirschner wire is driven back across the fracture site to engage the opposite cortex of the proximal fragment. The wire loop is then tied and its free end buried into a small hole in the adjacent cortex.

Biomechanical studies have shown this to be a consistently rigid method of internal fixation,[102] and Lister[171] has recommended minimal external splinting following its use.

Scheker[245] has suggested that the technique can be facilitated by using a hypodermic needle through which to pass the flexible wire (see Table 7-2 for appropriate-size needles), and additional tips on the technique of intraosseous wiring have been offered by Gingrass and colleagues[103] and Meals.[196] The laboratory studies of Vanik and coworkers[277] concluded that 24-gauge wire is the strongest but is too stiff, and they prefer 26- or 28-gauge wire in the clinical setting. Gingrass and associates[103] recommended 30-gauge wire for comminuted fragments with small fragments, using the straight needle (0.022-inch) that comes swaged on the Ethicon 4-0 pull-out wire for drilling the holes.

TENSION-BAND WIRING

The tension-band concept is a principle of fracture management that has been thoroughly documented by the AO group.[209] In the hand the dorsal surface is generally considered to be the tension side and the palmar surface the compression side.[143] Tension-band wiring applied to the dorsal surface of a phalanx or metacarpal can thus provide good sta-

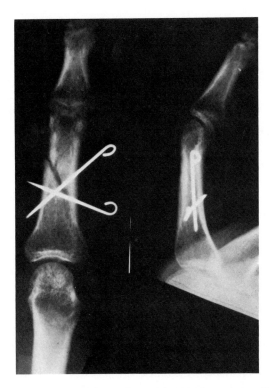

Fig. 7-29. We prefer to leave the K-wires protruding through the skin and bent into a loop to minimize pin migration and facilitate removal later in the office.

therefore a good method to employ in the noncompliant patient. Iselin and Thevenin[133] designed a flexible intramedullary screw that was also reported to allow early motion with no external immobilization. Lewis and colleagues[168,214] have recently reported on an expandable intramedullary device that has been shown in the laboratory to provide good fixation, but long-term follow-up clinical data are lacking at the time of this writing.

INTRAOSSEOUS WIRING

The technique of intraosseous wiring was probably first used by Robertson[237] for arthrodesis of IP joints,

Table 7-2. Needle and Kirschner Wire Sizes for Placing Intraosseous Wiring

Wire Size (No.)	Suture Equivalent	Needle That Will Allow Passage of Wire	Kirschner Wire to Make Hole for Needle
20	5	18-gauge	0.054-inch
22	4	19-gauge	0.045-inch
24	2	19-gauge	0.045-inch
25	1	20-gauge	0.035-inch
26	0	20-gauge	0.035-inch
28	2-0	21-gauge	0.035-inch
30	3-0	21-gauge	0.035-inch
32	4-0	22-gauge	0.035-inch

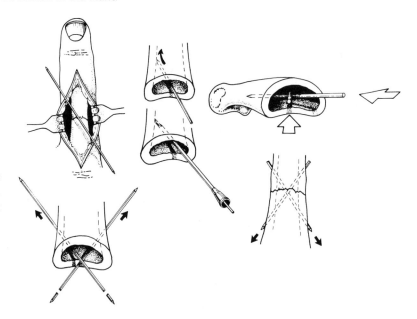

Fig. 7-30. Retrograde placement of crossed K-wires through the fracture site more accurately ensures correct placement than trying to engage both cortices with the fracture reduced. *(O'Brien, E. T.: Fractures of the Metacarpals and Phalanges. In Green, D. P. (ed.): Operative Hand Surgery, p. 615. New York, Churchill-Livingstone, 1982.)*

bility and is the preferred method for fractures requiring internal fixation by Greene and associates.[114] Jupiter and Sheppard[146] use tension-band wiring mainly for avulsion-type fractures such as those seen with mallet and gamekeeper's-type injuries. The preferred wire size for phalangeal fractures is 26 gauge,[114,146] with finer (28 to 30 gauge) used for the smaller intra-articular fractures.[146]

CERCLAGE WIRING

One of the earliest forms of internal fixation in the hand was cerclage wiring, as described by Lambotte in 1928,[159] but it is not widely used today. Gropper and Bowen,[115] however, have found it to be an effective method of fixing oblique and spiral fractures, and Jordan and Grieder[144] have described the use of an angiocath to facilitate passage of the wire around the bone.

ASIF (AO)* TECHNIQUES

With increasing emphasis on rigid internal fixation techniques elsewhere in the skeleton, it is not surprising that these principles have become more popular and widely used in the hand as well. It is important to point out that those most experienced with AO methods[73,123,126,200,267] emphasize that most fractures in the hand can be satisfactorily managed with other techniques. Barton[20] has stated that only

---

* ASIF (Association for the Study of Internal Fixation) is the English translation of AO (Arbeitsgemeinschaft für Osteosynthesefragen).

about 5% of hand fractures require internal fixation; Melone[197] said approximately 10%.

Several biomechanical studies (see p. 473) and clinical experience have shown that properly applied AO minifragment plates and screws provide the most stable form of internal fixation. However, this mechanical superiority must be balanced by individual considerations for each fracture:

1. Is rigid stabilization with plates and screws necessary for mobilization and healing of that fracture?
2. Can rigid fixation of that fracture be achieved, given the fracture configuration and expertise of the surgeon?
3. Do the potential disadvantages—increased soft tissue dissection, increased operative time, and possible subsequent plate removal—outweigh the potential advantages for that fracture?

Virtually all authors with extensive experience using the AO methods stress that the technique is demanding[98,291] and that the margin for error is small.[20,143,197,268] Many have pointed out that the surgeon usually has only one attempt to place a screw in the correct position[79,123,200,268] and that one misplaced screw can compromise the entire operation.[197]

Before using the AO techniques in a patient, the surgeon must prepare himself or herself by reading the excellent books and articles that describe the important principles[46,79,123,126,197,251] and by attending the hands-on instructional courses presented by experienced AO faculty. Beyond that, Hastings[123]

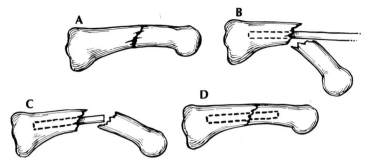

Fig. 7-31. Grundberg has described a method of intramedullary fixation of phalangeal and metacarpal fractures that avoids passing pins through the joints (see text). *(Redrawn from Grundberg, A. B.: Intramedullary Fixation for Fractures of the Hand. J. Hand Surg., 6:572, 1981.)*

has made the excellent suggestion that the surgeon gain experience with these techniques in metacarpal fractures before attempting to fix the more difficult phalangeal fractures.

A detailed and comprehensive description of AO techniques is beyond the scope of this chapter, but it seems appropriate at this point to list the most important and fundamental principles of internal fixation in the hand:

1. Precise preoperative planning is absolutely essential,[46,143,197] using drawings of the fracture fragments superimposed on x-ray films to have a clear idea of what is to be done before entering the operating room. As experience is gained, one should begin to develop the ability to "see" the fracture in three dimensions, which is the hallmark of the true

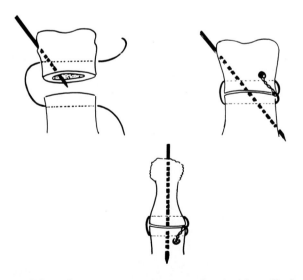

Fig. 7-32. The intraosseous wiring technique described by Lister is good for obtaining stable internal fixation of transverse fractures, especially those adjacent to a joint (see text). *(Lister, G.: Intraosseous Wiring of the Digital Skeleton. J. Hand Surg., 33:428, 1978.)*

AO surgeon. Alternative plans of fixation should be formulated before the operation in the event that it proves impossible to use the AO minifragment implants effectively.

2. The approach should be planned to minimize soft tissue trauma. In the fingers, this usually means a midlateral incision,[74,98,197] preferably on the side of the distal spike, as direct access to this spike facilitates an accurate reduction.[197] At the base of the phalanx, a middorsal, extensor-splitting approach[46] is sometimes required, and more distally in the digit it may be necessary to incise the lateral bands or oblique fibers of the extensor hood. However, the plane between the extensor hood and the periosteum should be disturbed as little as possible, and stripping of the periosteum should be limited to that required only to see the fracture fragments well.[200]

3. After the fracture has been reduced, temporary or "provisional" stabilization should be obtained with small 0.028-inch or 0.035-inch Kirschner wires,[123,183] preferably in positions that will not interfere with subsequent screw placement. Although sometimes difficult to accomplish, this is a most important concept, for it allows the surgeon to direct his or her entire attention to screw and plate placement without having to hold the fracture reduced at the same time.

4. Extreme care must be taken in screw placement, keeping in mind the "one-shot" concept noted previously. Interfragmentary compression should be used by enlarging the screw hole in the proximal cortex.

5. Appropriate hardware must be selected, which usually means 1.5-mm screws in phalanges and 2.0- or 2.7-mm screws (with or without plates) in metacarpals. Plates are rarely indicated in the phalanges,[123,200] although there are several types of specialized implants such as Buchler's condylar plate,[46] which is specif-

ically indicated for fractures close to the MP and PIP joints, and H plates for transverse fractures. Screw fixation alone is usually acceptable in long spiral oblique fractures in which the length of the fracture is greater than two[79,197,267] or two and a half times[143] the diameter of the bone. To avoid splintering of the bone, a fragment should exceed three times the thread diameter of the screw[123] or three to four times the diameter of the drill hole.[136]

6. Use of the correct size drills and taps is imperative, and we find it particularly helpful to have the AO chart depicting such information posted in the operating room in clear view of the surgeon.

7. When using the tap, one must beware of penetrating too deeply, especially when going from dorsal to palmar, where the flexor tendons are intimately contained in the fibro-osseous sheath and are at definite risk.[94] Since there is no calibration on the threads of the tap, the surgeon must first gauge the depth of penetration visually, although with experience he or she will gain the necessary touch to know instinctively when the opposite cortex has been penetrated.

8. Solid bone-to-bone contact must be achieved on the side opposite the plate.[123] If there is a cortical gap, it must be bone grafted to prevent excessive tension on the plate and possible loss of purchase of the screws (Fig. 7-33).

9. X-rays should be taken in the operating room to confirm adequacy of reduction, hardware placement, and depth of screws.

10. Although not always possible, an attempt should be made to close the deep soft tissues, especially to restore the periosteum between the plate and the extensor tendon.

11. The tourniquet should be released and good hemostasis established prior to closure.[200]

12. One of the most important goals of the AO technique is to provide fracture stabilization secure enough to allow early active range of motion, and if this goal is not achieved, the procedure must be considered at least a partial failure. The major cause of less than satisfactory stability is comminution of the fracture, and this brings us back to the first principle: the surgeon must very carefully assess the fracture preoperatively and honestly try to determine if his or her AO skills are capable of providing stable internal fixation.

The most common complication of the AO technique, especially in phalangeal fractures, is an active extensor lag in the PIP joint,[98,136] and the postoperative exercise and splinting program must anticipate this potential problem. The fact that this is a recognized complication of the AO method is implied in the suggestion that plate removal may be combined with extensor tenolysis.[136] Screw removal is generally not necessary,[197] and plate removal is probably not routinely required. Stern and colleagues[268] reported removal of plates in only 25% of their cases, primarily for local tenderness. If the

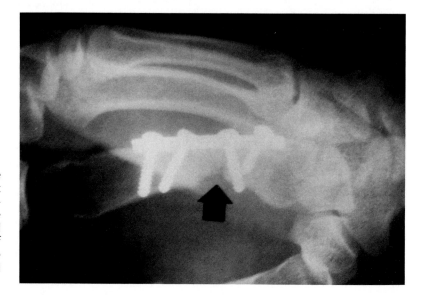

Fig. 7-33. A fundamental principle of internal fixation is that there must be cortical contact on the side opposite the plate. This attempt at plate fixation of a comminuted metacarpal fracture failed because of lack of contact of the volar cortices. A bone graft should have been used to fill the gap *(arrow)*.

plates are removed, however, 4 to 6 months post-operatively is generally given as the appropriate time, followed by protection of the hand for 6 weeks to prevent refracture.[143,197]

Comparison of Internal Fixation Methods

The relative strengths of different types of internal fixation modalities have been studied biomechanically in the laboratory by many investigators.[27,28,108,180,184–186,230,277] Unfortunately, the results of these studies have frequently yielded conclusions that differ from one another, and true comparisons among the various studies are virtually impossible because of the differing testing technique used.[28] However, most have agreed that plates provide the most rigid fixation,[27,28] with tension-band wiring[108] and intraosseous wiring[277] also being superior to Kirschner wires. More study must be done in this area, because the optimum strength and rigidity for fracture healing are unknown.[180] The fundamental question that remains unanswered is, "How strong does internal fixation in the hand *have* to be?"

Amputation

An isolated fracture is, in itself, virtually never an indication for amputation. However, when severe crush injuries have damaged tendons, nerves, and blood vessels as well as bone, it may be the treatment of choice. The decision rests squarely on the judgment of the operating surgeon, although only the most obviously nonviable digits should be amputated as a primary procedure at the initial operation. If there is a reasonable possibility of viability, it is wise to reconstruct the digit as well as possible and allow the natural course of events to help determine the necessity for amputation.

Authors' Preferred Methods of Treatment

EXTRA-ARTICULAR FRACTURES

A few extra-articular fractures of the proximal and middle phalanges do not require reduction; these include undisplaced fractures (Fig. 7-34) and impacted transverse fractures in satisfactory alignment. In the latter group it is particularly important to be certain that neither rotation nor angulation has occurred at the fracture site. Rotation can be more readily appreciated by clinical examination than by x-ray, as noted on p. 459. Angulation can occur in any plane, but in proximal phalangeal fractures, it is almost always with apex volar (recurvatum). Angulation in this plane is easy to over-

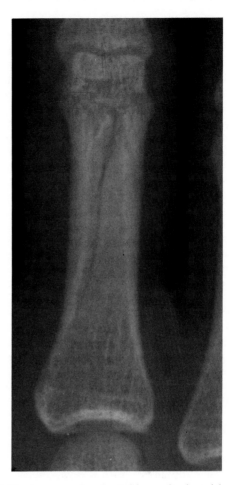

Fig. 7-34. An example of a stable, undisplaced fracture of the proximal phalanx that can be treated by buddy taping to an adjacent normal digit.

look unless true lateral films of good quality are taken. Even a fracture that appears to be in excellent alignment in the posteroanterior view may have 25° to 30° or more recurvatum.[70] The base of the proximal phalanx is often not well visualized in the lateral view, being obscured by superimposition of the other proximal phalanges. Careful interpretation of the x-ray films is essential for accurate initial assessment of the degree of volar angulation in these fractures.

If one can be certain that the fracture is indeed stable and neither angulated nor rotated, then protection, but not immobilization, is required during the period of healing. We prefer buddy taping for these fractures, encouraging active range of motion exercises from the outset. Clinical and x-ray examinations are mandatory after approximately 1

474   Chapter 7. Fractures and Dislocations in the Hand

week of such treatment to be certain that position of the fracture has not changed.

For displaced extra-articular fractures that require reduction, our treatment plan generally follows the algorithm shown in Figure 7-35. Under suitable regional anesthesia (we generally prefer wrist blocks), a closed reduction maneuver is done and x-ray films are taken to evaluate the adequacy of reduction. If acceptable alignment and a stable position have been achieved, external immobilization (splint or cast) is applied. If the fracture can be reduced by closed methods but is unstable, we generally prefer percutaneous pin fixation (CR and PCP). If the fracture cannot be reduced by closed manipulation, then ORIF is indicated. With this general outline as a basis for discussion, we have listed as follows our preferred methods of treatment for the most common types of extra-articular fractures of the phalanges.

Transverse Fracture at the Base of the Proximal Phalanx. As noted previously, the usual angulation in this fracture is recurvatum (apex volar), which we prefer to treat with Burkhalter's method of hyperflexion of the MP joint and immobilization with a dorsal plaster splint (see p. 462 and Fig. 7-24). If the reduction cannot be held with a splint,

we will use Eaton's closed intramedullary pinning technique (see p. 465 and Fig. 7-26**C**). These fractures rarely require open reduction.

Spiral Oblique Fracture of the Proximal Phalanx. This fracture (Fig. 7-36) is inherently unstable and virtually always requires internal fixation, although the choice must be made between CR and PCP and ORIF. If a satisfactory reduction can be obtained with closed manipulation (usually longitudinal traction combined with PIP flexion is sufficient, taking care to correct the rotational alignment), we prefer closed pinning of the fracture site directly with two or three Kirschner wires. As noted on page 465, this may be more difficult than it appears, and a fracture reduction clamp (we prefer the Aesculap) and image intensifier control are of immeasurable help. Sometimes the fracture cannot be reduced satisfactorily by closed manipulation, in which case ORIF is mandatory.

Transverse Fracture at the Neck of the Proximal Phalanx. Although this fracture is more common in children, it can also occur in adults, and it is a classic "booby-trap" fracture.[116] Angulation is usually between 60° and 90° (apex volar); reduction is easy to obtain but difficult to maintain and almost

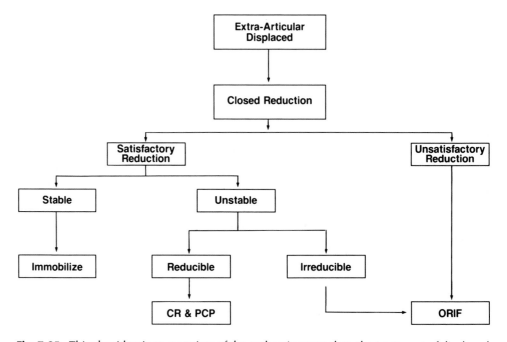

Fig. 7-35. This algorithm is an overview of the authors' approach to the treatment of displaced extra-articular fractures of the phalanges. (CR & PCP = closed reduction and percutaneous pin fixation; ORIF = open reduction and internal fixation)

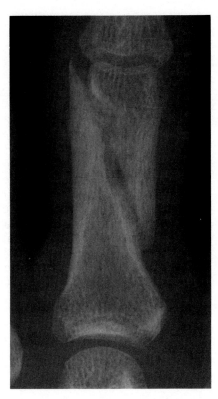

Fig. 7-36. The extra-articular fracture most likely to be unstable after closed reduction is a long oblique fracture of the proximal phalanx. This fracture often requires internal fixation. The surgeon has a choice between closed reduction and percutaneous pinning or open reduction and internal fixation (see text).

impossible to monitor in a cast or splint because superimposition of the other fingers obscures satisfactory x-ray visualization. For this reason we generally prefer CR and PCP, flexing the PIP joint and passing a smooth Kirschner wire either across or to the side of the PIP joint into the medullary canals of the distal and proximal fragments. The pin can be removed at 2 to 3 weeks and motion at the PIP joint safely begun at that point. Occasionally the distal fragment is rotated a full 180°, with the articular surface facing the proximal fracture surface, in which case ORIF is usually required.

Fractures of the Distal Phalanx. Extra-articular fractures of the distal phalanx rarely require internal fixation or even external immobilization. They are frequently associated with significant soft tissue injury, including lacerations of the nail bed, and the most important primary care of these injuries should be directed at the soft tissue damage (see p.

446). The one extra-articular fracture of the distal phalanx that does require operative treatment is a transverse fracture near the base in which the nail bed is trapped in the fracture site and must be extricated (see Fig. 7-4).

Comminuted Fractures of the Proximal and Middle Phalanges. These fractures are most commonly the result of crushing injuries or gunshot wounds and are usually open fractures. Concomitant soft tissue injuries often complicate the treatment, and stable internal fixation is desirable to facilitate treatment of the soft tissues. However, severely comminuted fractures are extremely difficult—sometimes impossible—to restore satisfactorily by open reduction and internal fixation and are best treated with external fixation (see p. 488). Our preference for phalangeal fractures with significant loss of bone is delayed primary bone grafting as described by Freeland and coworkers[100] (see p. 443).

INTRA-ARTICULAR FRACTURES

Truly undisplaced intra-articular fractures are uncommon, but they do occur (Fig. 7-37). They are best treated by carefully guarded and protected early range of motion exercise using the buddy taping system. Immobilization of such fractures often leads to prolonged or even permanent stiffness due to intra-articular adhesions. Again, careful and frequent clinical and radiographic examinations are necessary to check for displacement of the fragments during healing.

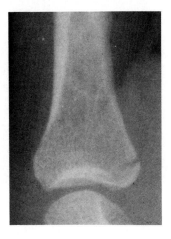

Fig. 7-37. Truly undisplaced intra-articular fractures of the phalanges are uncommon. They can be treated by carefully guarded and protected early range of motion using the buddy taping system.

The goal of treatment in displaced, intra-articular fractures should be anatomic restoration of the joint surface by open reduction and internal fixation.

Condylar Fractures. A fracture that virtually always demands internal fixation is a fracture of one or both condyles of the proximal phalanx, ie, at the level of the PIP joint.[154] A similar fracture occurs at the distal joint, involving the middle phalanx. This fracture most commonly splits off a single condyle (Fig. 7-38), but it may have a Y configuration that displaces both condyles. Failure to stabilize the condylar fracture usually leads to significant displacement, resulting in angulation deformity and incongruity of the articular surface (Fig. 7-39). These fractures can often be treated with percutaneous pin fixation, but only if anatomic alignment can be achieved by closed reduction. If this cannot be accomplished, ORIF is indicated. Adequate operative exposure is the key to success, but it may be difficult to achieve. The surgeon must visualize the articular surface well enough to reduce the fracture anatomically, but at the same time he or she must not excessively strip away the vital soft tissue structures attached to the fragment. We prefer a dorsal approach, splitting the central slip in the midline down to its bony insertion, but extreme care must be taken not to weaken or detach the insertion itself. A midlateral incision avoids the dorsal structures of the extensor aponeurosis, but adequate exposure of the articular surface is often

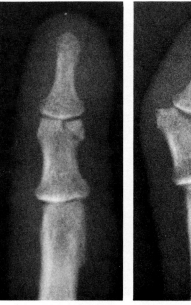
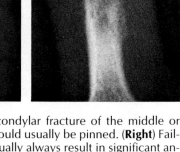

Fig. 7-39. (Left) A condylar fracture of the middle or proximal phalanx should usually be pinned. **(Right)** Failure to do so will virtually always result in significant angular deformity and incongruity of the articular surface.

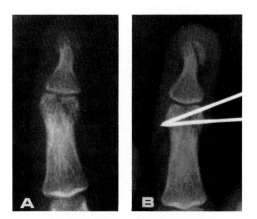

Fig. 7-38. A fracture that virtually always demands internal fixation is a displaced fracture of one or both condyles of the proximal phalanx. **(A)** This fracture most commonly splits off a single condyle, resulting in disruption of the joint and angular deformity of the finger. **(B)** This fracture should be treated with open reduction and exact anatomic restoration of the articular surface.

difficult with this approach and may require cutting the collateral ligament to provide sufficient visualization to effect an anatomic reduction. Some permanent stiffness of the PIP joint is not uncommon following any type of treatment of this injury, but internal fixation stable enough to allow early protected range of motion is the best method of minimizing this.

Avulsion Fractures at the Base of the Proximal Phalanx. Marginal fractures of the base of the proximal phalanx involving the MP joint usually represent avulsion fractures of the collateral ligament. Small or nondisplaced fragments (Fig. 7-40) can be adequately managed by buddy taping. Larger, displaced fractures of this type (Fig. 7-41) will result in incongruity of the articular surface if they are not restored by open reduction and internal fixation. A dorsal approach that splits the extensor hood is generally used, but careful study of the preoperative x-rays is advised to choose the optimal approach. If the large avulsed fragment is seen to be more volar than dorsal, insertion of the small Kirschner wires or AO minifragment screws may be facilitated by a volar approach in which the flexor tendons are retracted and the volar plate reflected.

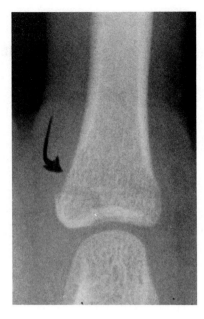

Fig. 7-40. Nondisplaced marginal fractures of the base of the proximal phalanx can be adequately managed by buddy taping.

Avulsion Fractures at the Base of Middle Phalanx. Intra-articular fractures that involve the base of the middle phalanx are usually one of three types: (1) a dorsal chip fracture, which represents an avulsion of bone by the central slip of the extensor tendon, creating a boutonnière deformity; (2) a volar lip fracture, usually combined with a dorsal dislocation or subluxation of the middle phalanx—the so-called fracture-dislocation of the PIP joint (see p. 511); and (3) a lateral chip fracture representing avulsion of bone by the collateral ligament (see p. 502).

Boutonnière Injuries. Boutonnière or buttonhole deformity is caused by disruption of the central slip of the extensor tendon combined with tearing of the triangular ligament on the dorsum of the middle phalanx, which allows the lateral bands to slip below the axis of the PIP joint. Rupture of the central slip causes loss of active extension of the middle phalanx, leading to a flexion deformity of the PIP joint. This is further aggravated by the pull of the lateral bands, which have become flexors of the joint. The PIP deformity is compounded by the limitation of flexion, both passive and active, which develops in the DIP joint. This results from the tenodesis effect of the displaced lateral bands and in time may lead to the fixed hyperextension defor-

mity of the distal joint seen in the classic boutonnière lesion (Fig. 7-42).

Most boutonnière deformities are caused by rupture of the central slip directly from its bony insertion; the diagnosis must be made by clinical examination. The patient with acute injury usually presents not with a typical boutonnière deformity but simply with a swollen, painful PIP joint. Rupture of the central slip is differentiated from the more common injury to the collateral ligament by the location of the maximum area of tenderness on the dorsum rather than the sides of the joint and by the patient's inability to actively extend the PIP joint. If pain prevents active extension, it must be eliminated by digital or metacarpal nerve block so that active motion can be tested. If a patient is suspected of having a ruptured central slip, x-rays of the involved finger should always be made; in some instances, an avulsion fracture will arise from the dorsum of the base of the middle phalanx (Fig. 7-43). Patients with suspected central slip injuries should always be examined seven to ten days after

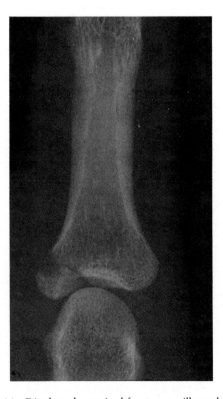

Fig. 7-41. Displaced marginal fractures will result in incongruity of the articular surface if they are not reduced. They usually require open reduction and internal fixation.

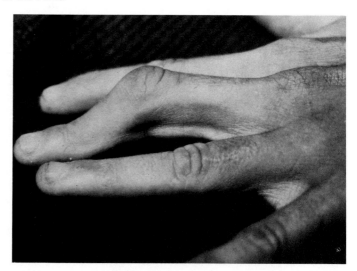

Fig. 7-42. A typical boutonnière deformity with flexion of the PIP joint and hyperextension of the DIP joint. The acute boutonnière injury does not usually present with this typical deformity, but rather with a swollen, painful PIP joint. Early diagnosis is dependent on careful clinical examination (see p. 502).

the injury, when the boutonnière lesion may be more apparent.

A boutonnière lesion without a fracture should be treated closed, by splinting the PIP joint in full extension for 5 to 6 weeks[337,359] (Fig. 7-44). Souter[359] has shown that successful results can be achieved in closed boutonnière lesions in which treatment is delayed up to 6 weeks after injury. It is extremely important that the distal joint not be

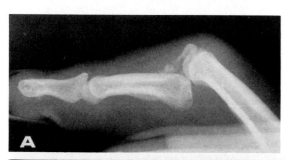

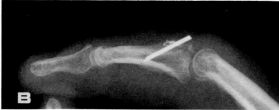

Fig. 7-43. Most boutonnière injuries are purely soft tissue lesions that can be treated by closed methods (see text). **(A)** Occasionally there is a sufficiently large fragment to result in a volar fracture-subluxation of the PIP joint. **(B)** Open reduction and internal fixation of this fracture is sometimes necessary.

immobilized; in fact, it must be actively and passively flexed during treatment. After the initial period of immobilization, a removable splint that holds the PIP joint should be worn at night for at least 4 additional weeks. From the outset of treatment, the patient must be taught to actively and passively bend the distal joint while holding the PIP joint in full extension. Treatment should not be considered complete until active flexion of the distal joint is equal to that in the opposite normal finger.

A boutonnière injury with a displaced avulsion fracture of significant size demands open reduction and internal fixation. At the time of operation, it is important also to repair the triangular ligament to correct the volar subluxation of the lateral bands, although care must be taken not to reef these tendons dorsally under excessive tension because this will limit subsequent flexion of the joint. Postoperative immobilization should be limited to the PIP joint only (in full extension, by means of an external splint or with a smooth Kirschner wire passed obliquely across the joint), and the patient should be carefully instructed in active assisted flexion of the distal joint.

Comminuted Intra-articular Fractures. Severely comminuted intra-articular fractures that involve either the MP joint or the PIP joint are usually not amenable to internal fixation, and attempts to fix such fractures by open reduction are fraught with difficulty and frustration.

In such cases, two options are available: external fixation (see p. 488) and traction (see p. 463). Prior to the use of external fixation or traction, it is often

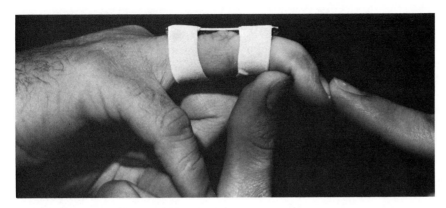

Fig. 7-44. The treatment of closed boutonnière lesions entails two equally important elements: immobilization of the PIP joint in full extension and active and passive flexion of the DIP joint.

helpful to obtain an x-ray with the involved finger suspended in finger traps or distracted manually. If the x-ray shows improvement in the congruity of the articular surface, this gives some assurance that external fixation or traction may be advantageous. On the other hand, if there is no significant improvement in the articular surface, nothing is to be gained from the use of skeletal traction.

For comminuted intra-articular fractures with significant loss of bone, we prefer delayed primary bone grafting as described by Freeland and associates[100] (see p. 443). In these situations, arthrodesis or reconstruction[199] of the involved joint will generally be required.

FOLLOW-UP CARE AND HEALING TIME OF PHALANGEAL FRACTURES

Unfortunately, there is a disturbing tendency to regard fractures of the phalanges as minor injuries and to neglect the important follow-up care they require. Complications often result from finger fractures when an inexperienced surgeon reduces a phalangeal fracture, immobilizes the injured digit, and then tells the patient to return in 3 weeks to have the splint removed. No matter how accurate a reduction is achieved and how carefully the splint is applied, it is imperative that the patient be examined clinically and radiographically from time to time during fracture healing. In particular, patients who are allowed early active motion should be seen periodically, to be instructed and encouraged in the performance of specific exercises to minimize joint stiffness and to regain full active motion.

Immobilization of an injured digit should not be continued until consolidation at the fracture line is visible radiographically. Smith and Rider[260] dem-

onstrated many years ago that the average "roentgenographic" healing time for fractures of the phalanges is 5 months, the range being 1 to 17 months. The important point is that "clinical" healing is evident in 3 to 4 weeks. With the exception of mallet and boutonnière chip fractures, it is rarely necessary to immobilize a closed fracture of a phalanx for longer than 3 weeks; in fact, it is usually detrimental. Some protection should be afforded the digit for 3 more weeks; however, this is easily accomplished by the buddy taping system, which allows the patient to move the joints actively, even in unstable fractures, following the initial 3-week immobilization period.

A final point regarding the period of immobilization is that open fractures do not heal as rapidly as comparable closed fractures in the phalanges. Even in open fractures, however, external immobilization should rarely be continued longer than 4 weeks.

FACTORS INFLUENCING RESULTS

Clearly, the skill of the surgeon is an important element in determining the outcome of fractures in the hand, but there are still many factors over which the surgeon has no control, including: (1) violence of the original injury; (2) associated soft tissue damage; (3) contamination and devascularization of the wound; and (4) age of the patient.[86] Strickland and colleagues[269] reviewed a large series of complicated fractures and concluded that age over 50 and associated tendon injuries (especially extensor) were two of the most important factors that compromised the end result. A somewhat surprising finding in their study was that there was no meaningful difference in the ultimate performance of fractured digits following mobilization during each of the first 4 weeks after fracture, although immobilization for longer than 4 weeks was associated with poorer results.

In a similar study, Huffaker and coworkers[130] found that associated joint injury, more than one fracture in a finger, crush injury, tendon damage, and skin loss were the key factors causing limited range of motion in the injured finger. They further noted that crush injury, tendon damage, and skin loss in the fractured finger frequently caused loss of motion in the unaffected normal fingers.

COMPLICATIONS OF PHALANGEAL FRACTURES

Malunion

Undoubtedly the most common complication of phalangeal fractures is malunion, and this may take several forms.

MALROTATION

Correct rotational alignment is often difficult to maintain in the closed treatment of phalangeal fractures. Immobilizing an adjacent normal digit with the injured finger and carefully monitoring the planes of the fingernails (see p. 460) will help to prevent this complication, but when malrotation does occur, rotational osteotomy is frequently required. Some authors prefer to do the osteotomy directly through the involved phalanx with either a transverse[101,252] or a more complicated step-cut osteotomy.[167,179] In our opinion, however, this is more likely to result in stiffness of the MP or PIP joints, and generally we prefer Weckesser's technique[57,112,287] of doing the osteotomy through the cancellous base of the metacarpal, where rapid healing is ensured.

Weckesser[287] reported that it is possible to correct up to 25° of malrotation with this technique. Studies in cadaver hands by Gross and Gelberman[116] confirmed this for the small finger but suggested that only about 18° to 19° of correction is possible in the index, long, and ring fingers.

In patients with a combined rotation and angulation deformity, the corrective osteotomy must be done at or near the malunion site. Seitz and Froimson[252] have suggested the use of a mini–external fixation device as an aid to correcting the rotational malalignment.

LATERAL DEVIATION

Radial or ulnar deviation following a healed fracture most commonly results from those situations in which there was actual bone loss at the time of injury, eg, in gunshot wounds or crush injuries.

The simplest method of correcting lateral deviation is with a closing wedge osteotomy directly through the site of the malunion.[59] We prefer to do this by removing a small wedge precisely measured on the preoperative x-rays, leaving the soft tissue hinge intact at the apex of the wedge, and using a single, obliquely directed Kirschner wire for fixation.[112] Froimson[101] has described another method for doing this with a series of progressively smaller burs using the Hall drill (Fig. 7-45).

VOLAR (RECURVATUM) ANGULATION

As noted on p. 457, most fractures of the proximal phalanx tend to assume a position of volar angulation at the fracture site. If this is not corrected at the time of reduction, severe residual angulation may occur, which in turn frequently leads to a clawlike deformity of the finger (Fig. 7-46). Froimson[101,252] recommends a dorsal opening wedge osteotomy at the malunion site, but this requires a bone graft, and we generally prefer a volar closing wedge osteotomy.[112] The few millimeters of shortening caused by the closing wedge is compensated for by correcting the angulation.

DISPLACEMENT (SHORTENING)

If a long spiral or short oblique fracture of the proximal phalanx is allowed to heal with shortening, a serious problem may develop. The distal spike of the proximal phalanx may impinge on the base of the middle phalanx, blocking PIP flexion (Fig. 7-

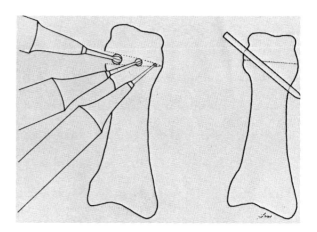

Fig. 7-45. Froimson has described a relatively simple method of performing a closing wedge osteotomy to correct angular deformity of a phalanx by using progressively smaller burs with the Hall drill. *(Froimson, A. I.: Osteotomy for Digital Deformity. J. Hand Surg., 6:585, 1981.)*

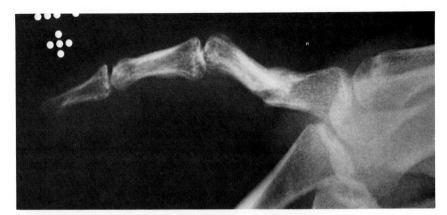

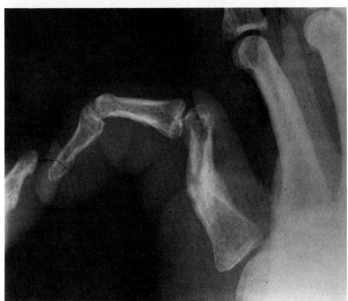

Fig. 7-46. **(Top)** Recurvatum (volar angulation) deformity is a relatively common complication of fractures of the proximal phalanx. It generally results in a compensatory flexion deformity of the PIP joint and limitation of motion in the PIP joint. **(Bottom)** Note that although the PIP joint is in maximum flexion radiographically, apparent (clinical) motion of the finger is limited to about 60°. Osteotomy is often required to correct this deformity.

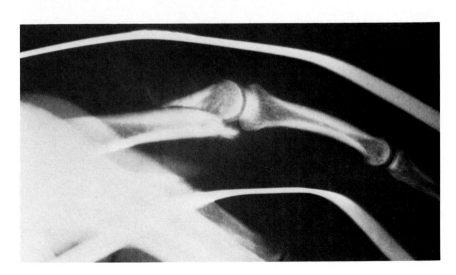

Fig. 7-47. Oblique fractures of the proximal phalanx must be pulled out to length at the time of reduction. Failure to do so, as shown in this inadequate reduction, leaves a protruding volar spike that will significantly limit PIP flexion.

47). If motion is significantly limited, surgical excision of the offending spike can restore good PIP motion[112] (Fig. 7-48).

INTRA-ARTICULAR MALUNION

The most difficult malunion to correct involves a joint surface, a fact that re-emphasizes the importance of anatomic reduction of intra-articular fractures (see p. 476). It is virtually impossible to restore a normal joint in these late situations, but with careful preoperative assessment of the "step-off" (preferably with trispiral tomography) and a precise realignment osteotomy, improved joint congruity can sometimes be accomplished.[169] Joints with significant damage of the articular cartilage are best treated with arthroplasty or arthrodesis.

NONUNION

Nonunion of a phalangeal fracture is a relatively rare complication. It must be kept in mind that radiographic union often requires 4 to 5 months to be complete,[260] and what appears to be delayed union may need only more time (Fig. 7-49). Ohl and Smith[219] described the use of electrical stimulation in the treatment of delayed union of a phalanx, but the efficacy of this modality in phalangeal fractures has not really been established.

Hypertrophic Nonunion.   A true "elephant foot" hypertrophic type of nonunion as described by the AO group[286] is relatively uncommon in the hand.

However, when it does occur, it should be treated by applying a basic AO principle, ie, that the application of a plate without taking down the fracture site will provide sufficiently rigid fixation to allow the fibrous/cartilaginous tissue to undergo metaplasia to bone without the need for a bone graft.[43]

Atrophic Nonunion.   Most nonunions in the hand are of the atrophic variety,[286] and bone grafting is required in the treatment of this type. Atrophic nonunion of the distal phalanx can be successfully stabilized and grafted through the volar midline approach described by Itoh and associates.[135] For infected nonunions, Jupiter and coworkers[147] have emphasized the importance of resecting back to normal bone. Although the treatment of each case must be individualized, we generally prefer a corticocancellous graft, combined with internal fixation to achieve as much stability as possible.

TENDON ADHERENCE

Especially in crush injuries and open fractures, scarring of the flexor or extensor tendons is common. Occasionally, prolonged immobilization may be the cause of tendon adherence. The first step in treatment is an intensive hand rehabilitation program with appropriate exercise and splinting, and surgical treatment should be considered only after maximum passive joint motion has been regained. The diagnosis of flexor tendon adherence is made when the patient has a significant discrepancy be-

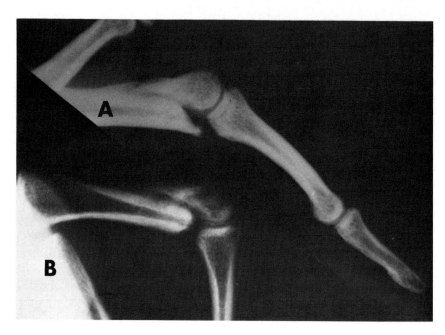

Fig. 7-48. (A) Malunion of a proximal phalangeal fracture with a volar spike limiting flexion of the PIP joint. **(B)** Resection of the spike may improve flexion of the joint.

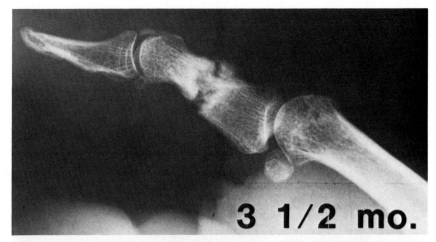

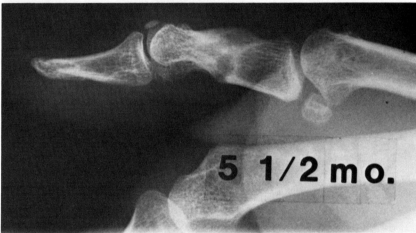

Fig. 7-49. What may appear to be a nonunion of a phalangeal fracture (**top**) often requires only a bit more time (**bottom**). Remember that phalangeal fractures can take up to 5 months to show radiographic healing.

tween active and passive motion (Fig. 7-50). Treatment is tenolysis of the flexor tendons, but such an operation is not to be entered into lightly. It is usually an extensive and technically difficult procedure, preferably done under some type of Neurolept anesthesia that allows active motion on the table to ensure complete correction of the problem. Stark and coworkers[266] have used Silastic sheeting as an interpositional material between tendon and bone in an effort to minimize recurrent adhesions. A highly motivated patient with a reasonably high pain threshold and an intensive postoperative rehabilitation program are also required to maintain the correction achieved at operation.

Because of the broad surface contact between the extensor aponeurosis and proximal phalanx, surgical tenolysis to correct an active extensor lag of the PIP joint is especially difficult and in our experience has been less rewarding than tenolysis of the flexor tendons.

SOFT TISSUE INTERPOSITION

Soft tissue interposition within a fracture site is rarely a problem in the hand except in the distal phalanx, where the nail bed may become entrapped. The two major clues to this complication are (1) avulsion of the root of the nail plate from beneath the proximal nail fold and (2) widening of the fracture site in the lateral x-ray film (see Fig. 7-4). Early recognition is essential, for the nail bed must be surgically extricated from the fracture site and placed back in its normal anatomic position. It is preferred that the nail plate be replaced beneath the proximal nail fold rather than removed.[254]

JOINT STIFFNESS

Limitation of motion in the MP and IP joints following fracture treatment is not uncommon, but a well-supervised rehabilitation program of exercises and splinting will restore full motion in most cases.

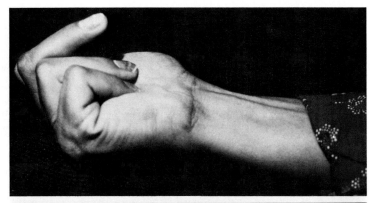

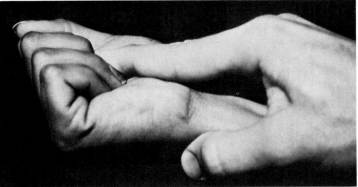

Fig. 7-50. Adherence of the flexor tendons in a patient with a healed fracture of the proximal phalanx. Note the marked discrepancy between active (**top**) and passive (**bottom**) flexion as well as absence of active flexion of the DIP joint with simultaneous PIP flexion (**top**). Full active motion was restored in this finger with an extensive tenolysis of the flexor tendons.

Only after an adequate trial of such therapy should consideration be given to operative treatment.

METACARPAL FRACTURES (EXCLUDING THE THUMB)

ANATOMY

The metacarpals are miniature long bones that are slightly arched in the long axis and concave on the palmar surface.[10,129] Their weakest point is just behind the head.[10]

The proximal ends of the index and long finger metacarpals articulate with the distal carpal row in practically immobile articulations, whereas those of the ring and little fingers have limited anteroposterior motion (see p. 525). The metacarpal shafts radiate like spokes of a wheel, terminating in the bulbous articular heads, which are weakly joined by transverse metacarpal ligaments. The collateral ligaments that join the metacarpal head to the proximal phalanx are relaxed in extension, permitting lateral motion, but become taut when the joint is fully flexed (Fig. 7-51, **left**). This occurs because of the unique shape of the metacarpal head,

which acts as a cam. The distance in extension from the pivot point of the metacarpal to the phalanx is less than the distance in flexion so that the collateral ligament is tightened on flexion of the MP joint (Fig. 7-51, **right**). This anatomic point explains why the MP joints stiffen if the collateral ligaments are allowed to shorten, as they do when the MP joints are immobilized in extension.[140,235,236]

The dorsal and volar interosseous muscles arise from the shafts of the metacarpals and act as flexors at the MP joint. Their deforming force accounts for the dorsal angulation in metacarpal neck and shaft fractures.

Prior to 1932, according to Waugh and Ferrazzano,[285] practically all fractured metacarpals were treated by simple immobilization over a roller bandage, and there was little or no attempt to correct the displacement. Magnuson,[177] in 1928, and McNealy and Lichtenstein,[193] in 1932, advocated treating all metacarpal fractures with a straight dorsal splint, holding the wrist and fingers in extension. The extension method of treatment, either with a straight dorsal splint or with a banjo splint, was recommended by Scudder,[250] Key and Conwell,[153] Cotton,[72] Owen,[220] and others. Neither

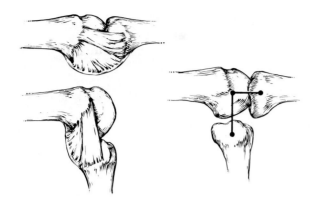

Fig. 7-51. (Left) The collateral ligaments of the MP joints are relaxed in extension, permitting lateral motion, but become taut when the joint is fully flexed. This occurs because of the unique shape of the metacarpal head, which acts as a cam. **(Right)** The distance from the pivot point of the metacarpal to the phalanx in extension is less than the distance in flexion, so that the collateral ligament is tight when the joint is flexed.

method is currently considered acceptable for treating metacarpal fractures.

In 1935, Koch[157] wrote of the disabilities of the hand that resulted from stiffness when the MP joints were immobilized in extension; he advocated immobilizing the hand in the functional position.

CLASSIFICATION

Currently, treatment of a metacarpal fracture is based on its anatomic location, whether it is stable or unstable, and the degree of comminution. Fractures of the metacarpals may be classified according their anatomic location: (1) metacarpal head (ie, distal to the insertion of the collateral ligaments), (2) metacarpal neck, (3) metacarpal shaft, and (4) base of the metacarpal.

FRACTURES OF THE METACARPAL HEAD

McElfresh and Dobyns[188] described a wide variety of fracture patterns in their series of metacarpal head fractures, noting that the second metacarpal was most commonly involved. If possible, these intra-articular fractures should be reduced anatomically and fixed with small Kirschner wires (Fig. 7-52) or AO minifragment screws, although at times the degree of comminution may preclude satisfactory restoration of the articular surface.

Severely comminuted fractures present a difficult challenge. The surgeon must make an honest pre-

operative assessment as to whether he or she possesses the necessary surgical skills to adequately fix the fracture. A distraction view taken with the finger in traction or with manual traction applied (under regional or general anesthesia) often gives a clearer picture of the degree of comminution. If this view reveals comminution that is too severe to allow restoration by open reduction but shows improvement in the articular surface with distraction, an external fixator or traction may be the appropriate treatment for that fracture. If the distraction view shows comminution that precludes open reduction and no improvement in articular alignment, nothing is to be gained from either fixation or prolonged immobilization. In such cases, a short period of splinting is indicated to alleviate pain, followed by early active motion to try to mold the fragments back into some sort of acceptable articular surface. The end result, at best, will be loss of motion without disabling pain.

FRACTURES OF THE METACARPAL NECK

Fractures of the fifth metacarpal neck are one of the most common yet most vexing fractures in the hand. The frequently used appellation *boxer's fracture* is really a misnomer, for professional boxers rarely sustain this injury. However, it is quite common in brawlers and in those whose anger is taken out on a wall or other convenient but unyielding surface; thus the term *fighter's fracture* is a more accurate description.

Virtually all fractures of the metacarpal neck have a typical angulation with apex dorsal and are inherently unstable because of the deforming muscle forces and frequent comminution of the volar cortex (Fig. 7-53). Because of this instability and the difficulties in maintaining reduction, many methods of treatment have been proposed.

It is important to distinguish the treatment of fractures involving the second and third metacarpal necks from that of the fourth and fifth metacarpal necks. As mentioned on p. 525, there is considerably more mobility in the CMC joints of the ring and small fingers, and for this reason significantly less residual angulation can be tolerated in the second and third metacarpals.

Methods of Treatment

NO TREATMENT OR MINIMAL IMMOBILIZATION

Substantial evidence from several countries exists in the literature to suggest that good functional results can be achieved in patients with fractures of

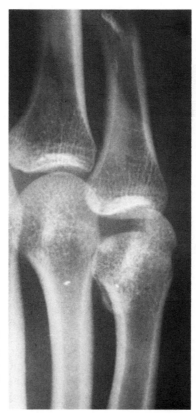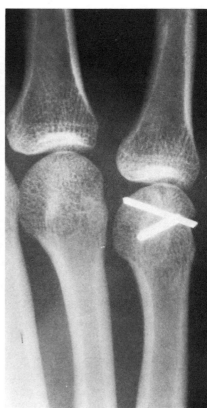

Fig. 7-52. Displaced fractures of the metacarpal head that are not excessively comminuted (**left**) should be treated with anatomic open reduction and internal fixation (**right**).

the fifth metacarpal without any attempt at reduction.[18,91,127,131,189] So long as care is taken to recognize and treat patients with rotational deformity,[18] these authors recommend minimal splinting for pain relief only and gradual resumption of use of the hand. The strongest argument made in defense of this method of treatment is by those who believe that a satisfactory reduction cannot be maintained with cast immobilization,[189] and its major advantage is earlier recovery time. The one drawback is that there will be a cosmetic deformity (loss of prominence of the metacarpal head and a bump on the dorsum of the hand) directly proportional to the degree of angulation, although one cannot assure the patient that a similar deformity will not be present after an attempt at closed reduction and immobilization. McKerrell and colleagues[189] reserved operative treatment for patients demanding a better cosmetic result and willing to accept a longer recovery time but concluded that closed reduction was not indicated because cast or splint immobilization is ineffective in maintaining fracture reduction.

CLOSED REDUCTION AND IMMOBILIZATION WITH PLASTER

One of the earlier and most popular methods of treatment was introduced by Jahss,[139] the so-called 90-90 method or the C-clamp treatment. This method takes advantage of the anatomic fact that the collateral ligaments of the MP joint are tight when the joint is flexed to 90°. With the tight collateral ligaments holding the loose metacarpal head, the PIP joint is flexed and the base of the proximal phalanx is used to push the metacarpal head back into position (Fig. 7-54). Because of the inherent instability of this fracture, Jahss maintained the reduction in plaster with the finger flexed 90° at the MP joint and 90° at the PIP joint, the 90-90 position.

Jahss's method of *reducing* a metacarpal fracture is accepted by most authors, but the use of the 90-90 position to *hold* the reduction has been widely condemned. Even though loss of reduction can be prevented with this position, we strongly advise that it should never be used to immobilize a fracture.

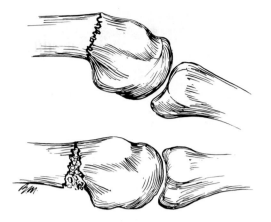

Fig. 7-53. Fractures of the metacarpal neck are basically unstable because of comminution of the volar cortex. For this reason, the reduced fracture tends to settle back to its original angulated position.

The possible complications of permanent stiffness of the PIP joint (Fig. 7-55) and skin slough over the dorsum of the PIP joint far outweigh any loss of function secondary to a malaligned fracture.

Van Demark[276] used Jahss's method of immobilization but avoided the problem of pressure over the PIP joint by holding the finger acutely flexed in the palm with strips of ½-inch adhesive. He reported good results with his method but did not provide any cases with follow-up to support it.

If the 90-90 position should not be used in immobilizing the fracture, then how is the fracture to be held? Herein lies the difficulty, for it is indeed difficult if not impossible to hold a metacarpal fracture reduced with a cast or splint. Theoretically, the MP joint should be immobilized in 70° to 90° of flexion, and Ruby[239] has noted that the key is to avoid too much cast material in the palm. This is difficult to do with an ulnar gutter splint and is best accommodated with anterior and posterior splints.

CLOSED REDUCTION AND FUNCTIONAL BRACING

Several authors[95,105,106,278,281] have advocated that the reduction be maintained with various types of metal and plastic orthoses. The most recent of these is the Galveston brace,[278,281] a commercially available, prefabricated splint that applies the basic concept of three-point fixation of the fracture. This method obviously requires a compliant patient, but even in cooperative patients, it is difficult to maintain precise positioning of the brace for the required 3 to 4 weeks.

CLOSED REDUCTION AND PERCUTANEOUS PIN FIXATION

Because of the difficulty of holding a metacarpal fracture in plaster without using the 90-90 position, many authors have advocated the use of percutaneous Kirschner-wire fixation to hold the fracture after reduction.[23,24,149,208,215,244,272,285] In 1936, Saypol and Slattery[244] introduced a method of transfixing the reduced metacarpal to the adjacent intact metacarpal(s) with smooth Kirschner wires introduced transversely proximal and distal to the fracture site (see Fig. 7-26**D**). They credited Lasher with originating the technique, and it was subsequently popularized in the late 1930s and early 1940s by Bosworth,[36] Waugh and Ferrazzano,[285] Berkman and Miles,[24] and others. More recently, Lamb and associates[158] reported excellent results with this method in a large series of patients.

Vom Saal,[282] Butt,[53] Clifford,[66] and Lord[174] popularized the use of intramedullary pin fixation, and Suman[271] used a combination of intramedullary and transverse pins. Intramedullary fixation has the disadvantage of requiring passage of the pins through the extensor mechanism at the level of the MP joint. Scarring of the extensor hood, with possible joint stiffness and loss of extension, is more likely to occur with this type of treatment if the pins are left in for more than 3 weeks.

The major advantage cited by most advocates of these percutaneous pin fixation techniques is that early motion can be started without external splinting. The pins are generally left in place for 3

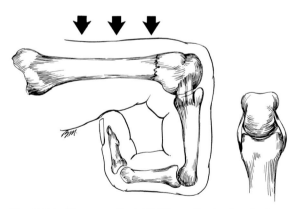

Fig. 7-54. The so-called 90-90 method of reducing a fracture of the metacarpal neck was introduced by Jahss (see text). Although this is the accepted method of *reducing* fractures of the metacarpal neck, it should *never* be used to immobilize a fracture because of possible stiffness of the PIP joint (see Fig. 7-55) or skin slough over the dorsum of the joint.

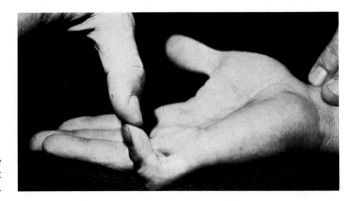

Fig. 7-55. A 90° fixed flexion contracture of the PIP joint in a 26-year-old man following treatment of a metacarpal neck fracture in the 90-90 position.

to 4 weeks, during which time the patient may be allowed to use the hand.

There is a difference of opinion as to whether the pins should be cut off beneath the skin or left to protrude. The likelihood of pin tract infection is minimized by burying the wires, but many authors have reported leaving them out through the skin without serious problems from infection.[36,113,215,221,244,285]

EXTERNAL FIXATION

Makeshift external fixation devices were developed as a logical extension of the transverse pinning method. Dickson[83] suggested that if the ulnar three metacarpals are all fractured, rigidity of fixation can be achieved by leaving the Kirschner wires protruding through the skin and bonding them with acrylic resin (methylmethacrylate) and a longitudinal interconnecting Kirschner-wire strut. Other authors have used similar homemade fixators with cement[75,249] and rigid plastic tubes,[238] and recently there have been several series of cases using commercially available fixators, including the Anderson,[26] AO,[99,263] and mini-Hoffman[99,234,253] devices. Stuchin and Kummer's laboratory comparison[270] of various methods showed that the commercial systems have a clearly superior pin, but greater rigidity was achieved with certain configurations of reinforced bone cement.

The reported complication rate with external fixators is high,[263] and the reader is referred to the articles by Seitz and colleagues[253] and Freeland[99] for details in technique.

External fixation techniques are rarely necessary in fractures of the metacarpal neck. Undoubtedly the most appropriate indication for external fixation in the metacarpals (and phalanges) is to maintain or restore length and alignment in severely comminuted fractures, especially those with segmental bone loss.[26,99,234] This is more likely to occur in fractures of the metacarpal shaft (see p. 491) than in neck fractures.

OPEN REDUCTION AND INTERNAL FIXATION

ORIF is rarely indicated in acute metacarpal neck fractures and is reserved for those unusual instances in which the head has been displaced entirely off the metacarpal shaft (Fig. 7-56).

Authors' Preferred Method of Treatment

As noted, reduction of a metacarpal neck fracture is generally simple, but maintenance of that reduction may be difficult. In fact, it may be impossible to hold an anatomic reduction with any type of external immobilization except perhaps Jahss's 90-90 method. At the same time, it must be re-emphasized that the potential complications of the 90-90 method outweigh the advantages of an anatomic reduction, and we advise against the use of this technique.

Having tried virtually every type of splinting discussed in the preceding section, we have now changed our ideas about fifth metacarpal neck fractures (fighter's fractures), and our indications for reduction are now significantly different than they were in previous editions of this book. We explain to the patient that even if the fracture is reduced and held in a splint or cast for 4 weeks, it is likely that he or she will have some residual angulation at the fracture site (a bump on the dorsum of the hand) and mild loss of prominence of the metacarpal head when making a fist. If the patient understands that the residual deformity will probably be purely cosmetic and that function will probably not be altered, then treatment consists of a removable volar splint that is worn for comfort until the local pain and tenderness subside. If the patient does not wish to accept this, we recommend closed reduction

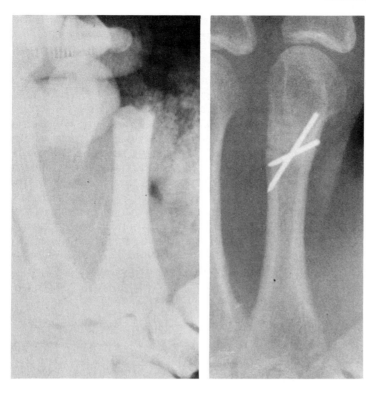

Fig. 7-56. Open reduction and internal fixation is rarely indicated in acute neck fractures and is reserved for those unusual instances in which the metacarpal head and neck have been displaced entirely off the metacarpal shaft, as in this patient.

and percutaneous pin fixation in the operating room (see p. 487).

There is, however, a small group of patients with metacarpal neck fractures who fall into a middle ground between these two extremes. If the angulation is severe, ie, probably 40° or more, a functional deficit ("pseudoclawing") may result (Fig. 7-57). In such patients, one of us (D.P.G.) prefers to do a closed reduction under ulnar-block anesthesia and immobilize the fracture for 4 weeks with an-

terior and posterior splints (see p. 460). I explain to these patients that there will be some mild to moderate residual angulation as noted previously, but the objective of the reduction is to minimize that angulation to eliminate any potential functional deficit. S.A.R. prefers closed reduction and percutaneous pin fixation in these patients.

In making this determination, one must keep in mind that the normal metacarpal neck angle is approximately 15°[16] so that a measured angle of 30°

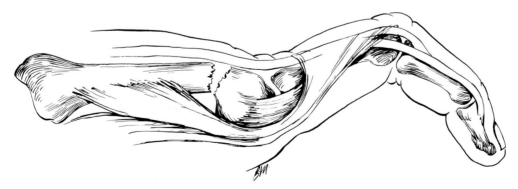

Fig. 7-57. If the angulation in a metacarpal neck fracture is severe, clawing may result when the patient attempts to extend the finger. We have found this to be a good clinical test to supplement the evaluation of the severity of the angulation as seen radiographically.

on the injury films probably represents a true angle of only 15°.

Because of the relative immobility of the second and third CMC joints, less angulation can be accepted in fractures of the metacarpal necks in the index and long fingers. Angulated fractures of these two metacarpal necks should therefore probably be treated with either closed reduction and percutaneous pin fixation or ORIF.

FRACTURES OF THE METACARPAL SHAFT

There are three important potential problems in the management of all metacarpal shaft fractures: shortening, dorsal angulation, and rotational malalignment. Several millimeters of shortening and varying degrees of dorsal angulation are compatible with normal function. However, although dorsal angulation rarely results in functional disability, many patients will be unhappy with the cosmetic appearance of a highly visible bump on the dorsum of the hand. The bump is usually more prominent in a metacarpal shaft fracture than it is in a neck fracture. Malrotation of a metacarpal is a serious complication because it usually interferes with normal flexion of the adjacent fingers.

Fractures of the metacarpal shaft are of three types: transverse, oblique, and comminuted.

Transverse Fractures

Transverse fractures are usually the result of a direct blow, and they generally angulate dorsally because of the interosseous muscles exerting a volar force (Fig. 7-58). Following reduction, these fractures may be immobilized with volar and dorsal splints (or a gutter splint), applying three-point pressure to control the angulation. Rotational alignment is more easily maintained by extending the splints nearly to the tips of the fingers and by including an adjacent normal finger. The same principles that apply to angular deformity of neck fractures apply to shaft fractures. Minimal angulation can be accepted in the second and third metacarpals because there is no compensatory motion at the CMC joints. Some angulation of the fourth and fifth metacarpals may be accepted, although, as noted previously, some patients will find the bump objectionable. The further the fracture is from the MP joint, the more pronounced the dorsal angulation will appear. Therefore, less angulation can be accepted in midshaft fractures than in fractures through the neck (Fig. 7-59).

If reduction is necessary, the same options are available as those discussed for metacarpal neck

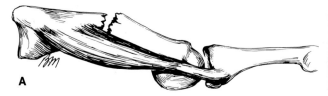

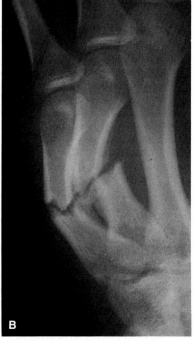

Fig. 7-58. Transverse fractures of the metacarpal are usually the result of a direct blow. (**A**) They generally angulate dorsally because of the interosseous muscles exerting a volar force. (**B**) An x-ray showing the typical dorsal angulation of fractures of the metacarpal shafts.

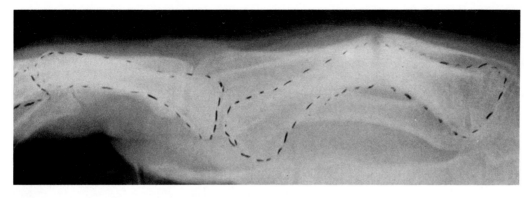

Fig. 7-59. The farther the fracture is from the MP joint, the more pronounced the dorsal angulation will appear and the greater the clawing will be. Therefore, less angulation can be accepted in midshaft fractures than in fractures through the neck of the metacarpal.

fractures (see p. 485). Most transverse metacarpal fractures have a significant amount of soft tissue swelling, and maintenance of reduction may be difficult or impossible with external splinting or casting. If the swelling is not excessive, we prefer separate anterior and posterior plaster splints, although follow-up x-rays at 5 to 7 days are mandatory to detect loss of reduction.

Closed reduction and percutaneous pin fixation is an acceptable method of treatment for some metacarpal shaft fractures, using either transverse or intramedullary pinning, or a combination of the two.[271]

Saypol and Slattery's[244] transverse pinning to an adjacent metacarpal is more applicable to the border metacarpals (second and fifth) but may also be used for the inner metacarpals (third and fourth). Care must be taken to ensure proper rotational alignment and to avoid distraction at the fracture site.

If intramedullary fixation is used, we prefer to insert the pin into the side of the metacarpal head to avoid impaling the extensor hood. A longitudinal pin will control angulation but not rotation and must therefore be supplemented by either a transverse pin, external splinting, or buddy taping.

ORIF is indicated when the fracture cannot be reduced by closed manipulation. Other relative indications include multiple fractures and concomitant soft tissue injury. As noted on p. 443, skeletal stabilization is indicated either primarily or as delayed primary fixation (at 3 to 5 days) in patients who have complex open wounds with significant soft tissue injury. The relative advantages and disadvantages of the various types of internal fixation are discussed on p. 466.

Spiral Oblique Fractures

Spiral oblique fractures of the metacarpal shaft result from a torque force with the finger acting as a long lever.[40] These fractures tend to shorten and rotate rather than angulate. The third and fourth metacarpals tend to shorten less because of the tethering effect of the deep transverse metacarpal ligaments (Figs. 7-60 and 7-61). At least 5 mm of shortening, possibly more, can be accepted without loss of function[31] so long as there is no angulation or rotational malalignment. Such fractures are easily treated with external immobilization (casts or splints). Greater amounts of shortening and rotational deformity are indications for operative treatment, since reduction of these fractures may be difficult to accomplish without direct visualization of the fracture site. Stable internal fixation can usually be achieved with Kirschner wires,[90] AO lag screws,[123] or cerclage wiring.[115]

Another reasonable indication for internal fixation is the subcapital spiral oblique fracture, which, if allowed to heal in the shortened position, may result in impingement at the MP joint level (Fig. 7-62).

Comminuted Fractures

Comminuted fractures of the metacarpal shafts are caused by violent trauma (eg, crush injuries, gunshot wounds) and are frequently associated with a great deal of soft tissue damage. If undisplaced and sufficiently stable to allow early finger motion, these fractures may be treated with external splinting. More commonly, however, they require a combination of internal and external fixation to facilitate

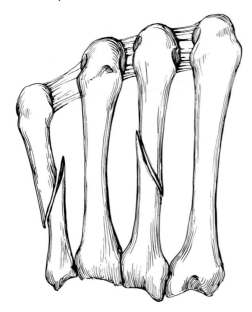

Fig. 7-60. Oblique fractures of the metacarpals tend to shorten and rotate rather than angulate. The third and fourth metacarpals tend to shorten less because of the tethering effect of the deep transverse metacarpal ligament. In the border second and fifth metacarpals, shortening and rotation are likely to be more pronounced.

the treatment of concomitant soft tissue damage and to prevent skeletal collapse (see p. 443). Delayed primary bone grafting may be indicated if there is significant bone loss.[99]

FRACTURES AT THE BASE OF THE METACARPAL

Fractures at the base of the metacarpal are usually stable; however, one should not be complacent about these fractures, because the slightest rotational malalignment will be greatly magnified at the fingertip. The patient's hand in Figure 7-63 demonstrates fractures at the base of the third, fourth, and fifth metacarpals with rotation in all three fingers, leaving a wide gap between the index and long fingers. Since this type of fracture is usually secondary to a crushing injury, the treatment as outlined for comminuted metacarpal shaft fractures should be used. Identification of occult fractures at the base of the metacarpal may be aided by the use of the Brewerton view[150] (see Fig. 7-106). If a fracture at the base of the metacarpal is intra-articular, arthrosis may develop, necessitating an arthrodesis or arthroplasty of the CMC joint later. Fracture-subluxation of the CMC joints is discussed on page 525.

A relatively uncommon injury at the base of the metacarpal is an avulsion fracture attached to the insertion of the extensor carpi radialis longus or brevis. DeLee[82] and Treble and Arif[275] have rec-

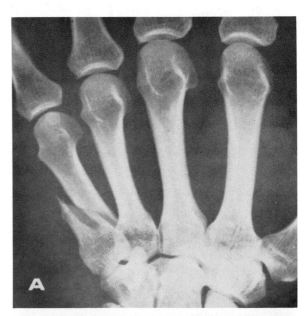

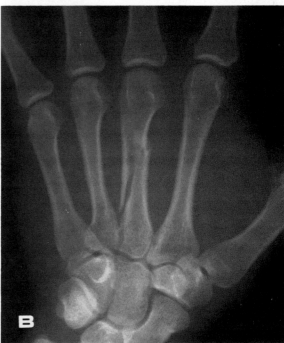

Fig. 7-61. (**A**) An oblique fracture of the proximal shaft of the fifth metacarpal. Note the significant shortening. (**B**) A long oblique fracture of the shaft of the third metacarpal. Note that only minimal shortening has occurred.

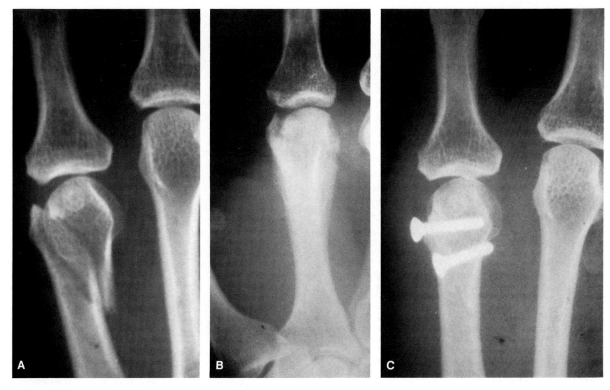

Fig. 7-62. Most spiral oblique fractures of the metacarpals do not displace significantly and can be adequately treated with closed methods. However, if such a fracture involves the neck area (**A**), the fracture may heal such that the proximal spike may impinge on the MP joint (**B**). This fracture is probably best treated with open reduction and internal fixation (**C**).

ommended open reduction, but Crichlow and Hoskinson[74] concluded from their three cases that operative treatment is necessary only if the avulsed fragment causes a bothersome bony prominence. We have treated one patient who avulsed the insertion of his extensor carpi radialis longus without a fragment of bone, in whom persistent symptoms required operative repair at 6 weeks.

COMPLICATIONS OF METACARPAL FRACTURES

The complications seen following metacarpal fractures are related to concomitant soft tissue injury, malunion, overzealous treatment, or pin tract problems.

Fractures involving the shafts and bases of the metacarpals are most commonly due to crushing injuries, and the fractures frequently are open, involving several metacarpals. Frequently, there is soft tissue damage followed by massive edema. Extensor and flexor tendons may be damaged or be-

come adherent to the damaged bone. Interosseous muscles may be damaged, and scarring may result in intrinsic contracture of the hand.

Malunion of the metacarpal neck or shaft virtually always occurs with apex dorsal; the farther it is from the MP joint, the more noticeable the deformity and the more likely it is to disturb the intrinsic and extrinsic muscle balance and cause pseudoclawing and/or a painful grip. Thus, malunion of the shaft is more likely to be symptomatic than that involving the neck. Angulation up to 30° or so is unlikely to cause problems, but if symptoms warrant treatment, we prefer a closing wedge osteotomy.[112] The key to success with this procedure is precise preoperative planning of the osteotomy.

Rotational malalignment is probably the most important complication of metacarpal fractures, and its prevention must be foremost in the mind of the physician managing these injuries. This problem is particularly likely to occur with fractures of the border metacarpals and is much more difficult to control when more than one metacarpal is fractured (see Fig. 7-63). Malunion with rotational deformity may require a rotational osteotomy for correction[67,223,287] (see p. 480).

Stiffness of the proximal and middle finger joints is frequently the result of improper or overzealous treatment. Stiffness of the MP joint is caused by treating the fracture with this joint in extension, allowing the collateral ligaments to shorten. Stiffness of the PIP joint is caused by holding the joint in acute flexion in the 90-90 position or by immobilizing the joint unnecessarily long.

Serious pin tract infection from percutaneously placed Kirschner wires is uncommon, even if the pins are left protruding through the skin. A slight amount of serous drainage is not unusual, but this is rarely a problem if the pins are left in no longer than 4 weeks. Pin tract problems can also be minimized by avoiding skin tension at the time of placement, bending the pins outside the skin to prevent migration, windowing the cast over the pins, and having the patient apply an antiseptic solution (eg, alcohol, Betadine) to the pin-skin interface several times a day.

FRACTURES OF THE THUMB METACARPAL

The thumb is a unique digit, and fractures of the thumb metacarpal are distinctly different from those of other metacarpals. Most thumb metacarpal fractures occur at or near the base, and therefore a thorough knowledge of the anatomy of the CMC joint is essential to understand the mechanism of injury, the pathologic anatomy, and the treatment of these fractures. (See p. 540 for a discussion of the pertinent anatomy.)

CLASSIFICATION

Four distinct fracture patterns may involve the base of the thumb metacarpal,[398,406,407] as illustrated in Figure 7-64. It is particularly important to differentiate intra-articular fractures from the extra-articular types, because management of the two is quite different. Bennett's fracture-dislocation and Rolando's fracture are the intra-articular types, and the extra-articular fracture may have either a transverse or an oblique configuration. The epiphyseal fracture is excluded from this discussion.

BENNETT'S FRACTURE

More properly called a fracture-dislocation, Bennett's fracture was first described by Edward Hal-

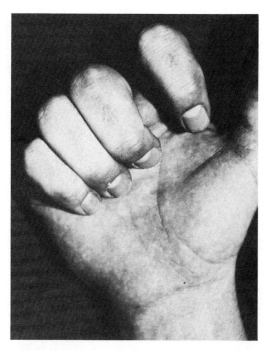

Fig. 7-63. This patient had fractures at the bases of the third, fourth, and fifth metacarpals. All three healed with rotational deformity, leaving a wide gap between the index and long fingers. Correct rotational alignment is particularly difficult to achieve with multiple metacarpal fractures.

loran Bennett[381] in 1882 and has been discussed exhaustively in the world literature since then. The mechanism of injury is an axial blow directed against the partially flexed metacarpal; not surprisingly, many of these injuries are sustained in fistfights. The fracture line characteristically separates the major part of the metacarpal from a small volar lip fragment, producing disruption of the CMC joint (Fig. 7-65). That an avulsion fracture occurs rather than a pure dislocation attests to the strength of the anterior oblique ligament, which anchors the volar lip of the metacarpal to the tubercle of the trapezium. The two primary variables of a Bennett's fracture are the size of the volar lip fragment and the amount of displacement of the shaft. The base of the metacarpal is pulled dorsally and radially by the abductor pollicis longus, while the distal attachment of the adductor further levers the base into abduction (Fig. 7-66).

Methods of Treatment

At least 20 methods of treatment have been advocated for Bennett's fracture since the first large

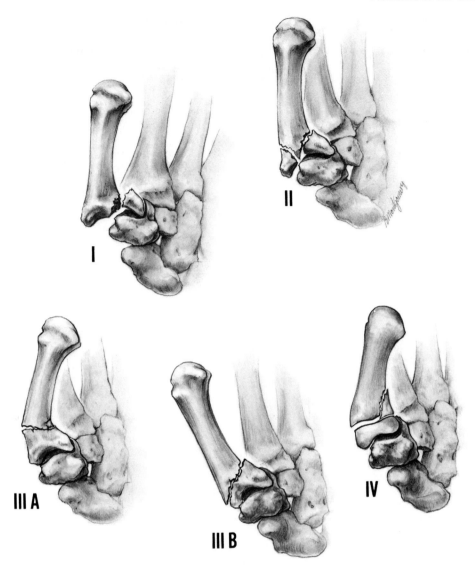

Fig. 7-64. Four distinct fracture patterns may involve the base of the thumb metacarpal. Type I (Bennett's fracture-dislocation) and Type II (Rolando's fracture) are intra-articular. These should be differentiated from the Type III extra-articular fractures, which may be either transverse or oblique. Type IV fractures are epiphyseal injuries seen in children. *(Green, D. P., and O'Brien, E. T.: Fractures of the Thumb Metacarpal. South. Med. J., 65: 807, 1972.)*

clinical series with x-rays in 1904.[408] At one end of the therapeutic spectrum is Blum,[384] who proposed that reduction of the fracture was not necessary and that good results could be achieved with early active motion. Charnley,[387] Roberts and Kelly,[411] Bohler,[33] and Griffiths[399] separately advocated the use of a well-molded plaster cast. Griffiths[399] reported that even in unreduced Bennett's fractures,

the results were not bad, noting that although these patients had some limitation of motion, they were generally free of pain. He concluded that the importance of the joint involvement in this fracture was generally overestimated. Cannon and coworkers[386] further supported this concept with a long-term follow-up study of patients treated nonoperatively, showing that 92% of these patients

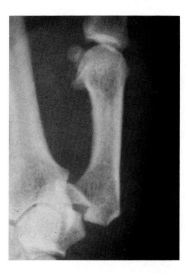

Fig. 7-65. A typical Bennett's fracture-dislocation. The small volar lip fragment remains attached to the anterior oblique ligament that anchors it to the tubercle of the trapezium.

Wagner[420,421] later modified this method further by passing a Kirschner wire from the shaft of the first metacarpal into the trapezium rather than into the second metacarpal, and Salgeback and colleagues[415] used Wagner's technique but with two pins. Wiggins and associates[422] used intramedullary wire fixation following closed reduction because of difficulty in positioning the wires in the manner described by Wagner.

In 1946, Ellis[390] was apparently the first to advocate open reduction, although in his technique the fracture site was not actually exposed. Instead, he reduced the base of the metacarpal and passed small pins into the trapezium, leaving them protruding as a buttress to hold the reduction of the metacarpal. Fisher[391] did a limited open reduction by looping a No. 2 nylon or silk suture around the first metacarpal and passing this out as a pull-out suture in the palm. Badger[380] used a small screw for fixation, obviating plaster immobilization postoperatively.

Gedda and Moberg,[393,394] however, appear to have turned the tide in favor of open reduction with their conclusions that exact anatomic restoration

were asymptomatic at 10 years. They also found in a literature review that only 7 of 456 patients (1.5%) being treated surgically for painful CMC arthritis had a history of a Bennett's fracture.

James and Gibson[403] and Pollen[410] incorporated a felt pad into their casts to prevent the loss of reduction that frequently occurred with plaster alone. Robinson[412] and Watson-Jones[284] each advocated the use of continuous skin traction in addition to a cast, and Bunnell[47] described the method of skeletal traction that at one time was used rather extensively in the treatment of Bennett's fracture. Thoren[418,419] devised a unique method of applying oblique skeletal traction by means of a hook inserted into the base of the first metacarpal. He believed that traction should be applied in the direction of adduction and opposition rather than abduction to bring the displaced shaft back into alignment with the volar lip fragment. Harvey and Bye[401] also suggested adduction as the preferred position of immobilization.

Numerous types of external splints have been advocated, including the Goldthwaite splint[388] and Goldberg's felt pad[396,397] attached to an outrigger. Ross and Sinclair[414] treated a series of patients with the Stader splint, a forerunner of the Roger Anderson device. Closed reduction and percutaneous pin fixation was originally described by Johnson,[405] using Waugh and Ferrazzano's[285] technique of transfixing a fractured metacarpal to an adjacent one.

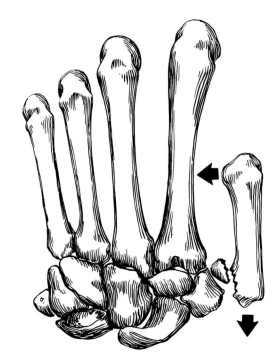

Fig. 7-66. In a Bennett's fracture, the base of the metacarpal is pulled dorsally and radially by the abductor pollicis longus, while the adductor further levers the base into abduction.

of the articular surface would be less likely to lead to post-traumatic arthritis. Despite the absence of any good, long-term studies supporting this concept,[385,409] ORIF has become increasingly popular with surgeons as the treatment of choice. Recommended methods of fixation have included two 0.028-inch K-wires or a 2.0-mm AO screw for smaller fragments[392] and a 2.7-mm AO screw[392,417] or Herbert screw[402] for larger fragments. Foster and Hastings[392] noted that the screw diameter should not exceed 30% of the cortical surface of the volar lip fragment.

Authors' Preferred Method of Treatment

Reports of good results from each of the preceding methods (many in articles with very short-term follow-up) pose a perplexing dilemma for the surgeon choosing a plan of treatment for a patient with a Bennett's fracture. The very fact that so many types of splinting, traction, and other methods of immobilization have been described implies that it is often difficult to achieve and maintain reduction of the articular surface by nonoperative means. We therefore tend to prefer some type of internal fixation in an effort to hold the reduction. Our first choice is closed reduction and percutaneous pin fixation, using 0.045-inch Kirschner wires to hold the shaft of the metacarpal reduced but making no effort to spear the small volar lip fragment with the wires (Fig. 7-67). We used to demand a perfect anatomic reduction, but the results of Cannon and colleagues' previously cited study[386] and the lack of correlation between arthrosis and symptoms[415] suggest that this may not be necessary, and we now accept slight joint incongruity. Only if a reasonable reduction cannot be accomplished with closed reduction (Fig. 7-68) do we resort to ORIF. A small AO cortical screw provides probably the best fixation, but it should be used in this situation only by those familiar with AO principles and techniques (see p. 471). Small Kirschner wires are an acceptable alternative.

Following closed reduction and percutaneous pin fixation, a thumb spica cast is imperative until the Kirschner wires are removed at 4 to 6 weeks. Unprotected motion is allowed sooner following open reduction if secure, rigid fixation has been achieved.

ROLANDO'S FRACTURE

In 1910, Silvio Rolando[413] described a fracture pattern that differed from the classic Bennett's fracture-dislocation. In the fracture he reported, there was, in addition to the volar lip fragment, a large dorsal

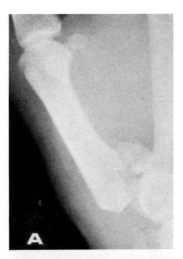

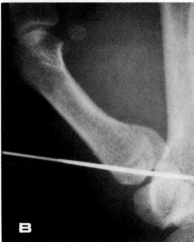

Fig. 7-67. Our preferred method of treatment for Bennett's fracture is an initial attempt at closed reduction and percutaneous pin fixation. (**A**) A typical Bennett's fracture-dislocation. (**B**) Anatomic reduction was achieved by closed reduction and percutaneous pinning. Note that no attempt was made to transfix the small volar fragment; rather the shaft of the metacarpal was held in the reduced position after a reduction had been achieved by closed manipulation.

fragment, resulting in a Y- or T-shaped intra-articular fracture. Although the classic Rolando's fracture is that pictured in Figure 7-64, it should probably more properly be thought of as simply a comminuted Bennett's fracture, because in most instances instead of having the simple Y or T configuration, there is severe comminution. Rolando pointed out that the prognosis was poor following this injury, despite treatment either in a cast or with

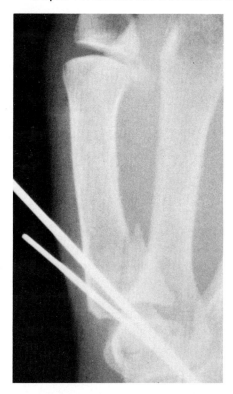

Fig. 7-68. A Bennett's fracture in which a successful reduction was not achieved by the closed method. We believe that inadequate reduction such as this should not be accepted. Either a second attempt at closed reduction or open reduction and internal fixation should be done.

skin traction. More than 75 years later it remains a difficult fracture to treat, but fortunately it is the least common of the adult thumb metacarpal fractures.

Methods of Treatment

The choice of treatment depends primarily on the severity of comminution of the fragments and, to a lesser extent, on the degree of displacement. ORIF should be attempted only if the volar and dorsal components are single large fragments.[392] More commonly, however, the base of the metacarpal is shattered into many fragments and attempts at operative restoration are frustrating, if not impossible (Fig. 7-69). Gelberman and associates[385,395] have reported good results in patients with Rolando's fracture using Thoren's method of oblique traction mentioned on page 497. Longitudinal traction may also be considered in severely comminuted fractures. Before skeletal traction is applied, however,

it is advisable to take an x-ray while a longitudinal traction force is applied to see if the articular surface has improved. If the joint surface has been reasonably restored, a period of traction is justified; if it has not, little will be gained from the use of traction. An external fixator[402] may be the best method of providing that traction force.

For severely comminuted fractures in which the joint surface is not significantly improved on the x-ray taken in traction, we prefer to immobilize the thumb for a minimal period to relieve pain and then begin early active motion in an attempt to remold the badly distorted articular surface. Because of the infrequency of Rolando's fracture, no one has reported a series comparing the results of different forms of treatment. In our experience, the tendency in the past has been to err on the side of overtreatment (ie, to attempt open reduction when it was virtually impossible to restore the articular surface). We repeat that significant comminution is a definite contraindication to operative treatment of this injury.

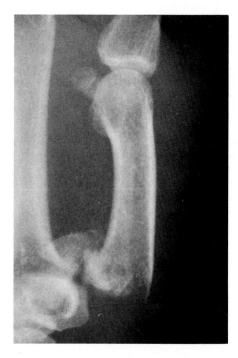

Fig. 7-69. A Rolando's fracture rarely has only the large dorsal and volar fragments. More commonly, it is severely comminuted, as illustrated here. In fractures such as this, open reduction and anatomic restoration of the articular surface are virtually impossible and should not be attempted. (*Green, D. P., and O'Brien, E. T.: Fractures of the Thumb Metacarpal. South. Med. J., 65:807, 1972.*)

EXTRA-ARTICULAR FRACTURES

The extra-articular type is the most frequent fracture in the thumb metacarpal and, fortunately, the simplest to treat. Two basic patterns are seen (Fig. 7-70): a transverse fracture and a less common oblique one. It is particularly important to distinguish these extra-articular fractures from the more serious intra-articular Bennett's and Rolando's fractures because rarely, if ever, is surgery indicated in the management of the extra-articular fractures. This differentiation is usually not difficult on careful study of the x-ray films, although the oblique type may appear at first glance to be a Bennett's fracture. The distinguishing feature is that in the oblique extra-articular type, the fracture line does not enter the joint.

Treatment

One should resist the temptation to overtreat these extra-articular fractures. Anatomic reduction can usually be achieved readily by closed manipulation under regional or local anesthesia; the thumb is immobilized in a short-arm thumb spica cast for 4 weeks. Care must be taken to avoid hyperextension of the MP joint in plaster. Failure to achieve exact alignment of the fracture should not be considered an indication for open reduction. At the worst, the patient with an inadequately reduced transverse fracture is likely to have only a slight prominence at the base of the thumb and possibly some minimal limitation of thumb abduction. Even with 20° to 30° of residual angulation, however, there is usually no detectable limitation of motion.

Occasionally the oblique type of extra-articular fracture may prove somewhat unstable, particularly if there is marked vertical inclination of the fracture line. Even in this type of fracture, however, open reduction is not warranted. If plaster immobilization is unsuccessful in holding the reduction, percutaneous pinning provides a simple method

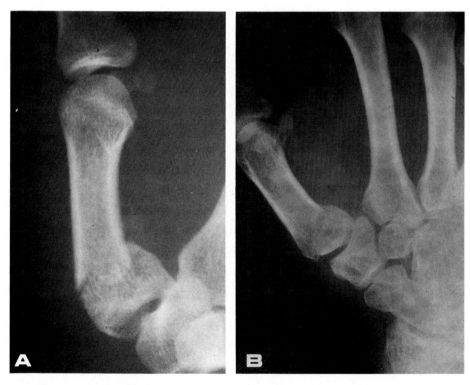

Fig. 7-70. It is particularly important to distinguish these extra-articular thumb metacarpal fractures from the intra-articular varieties. (**A**) The most common fracture of the thumb metacarpal is a transverse extra-articular type. (**B**) Less commonly seen is an oblique extra-articular fracture. This is the fracture that is most frequently confused with a Bennett's fracture. Careful examination of the x-ray film reveals that the fracture line does not enter the joint.

of securing the reduction achieved by closed manipulation.

DISLOCATIONS OF THE DIP JOINT

ACUTE INJURIES

Pure dislocations of the DIP joints of the fingers and the IP joint of the thumb are rare injuries. When they do occur, they are almost always dorsal dislocations and are frequently associated with an open wound. A far more common injury occurring at the DIP joint is a mallet fracture-dislocation, in which the distal phalanx may subluxate volarly (see p. 452). Even the relatively uncommon avulsion of the FDP (see p. 453) is more common than a pure dislocation of this joint. Bowers and Fajgenbaum[432] described volar plate avulsion of the DIP joint that mimics FDP avulsion, even to the point of causing inability to actively flex the DIP joint. They noted that this rare lesion may occur in the absence of actual dislocation of the joint. A similar case was reported by Lineaweaver and Mathes.[475]

SIMULTANEOUS DIP AND PIP DISLOCATIONS

Simultaneous dislocation of both IP joints in the same digit (or the MP and IP joints in the thumb) can occur, most commonly on the ulnar side of the hand in young male athletes.[427] Krishnan[468] has noted that the appearance of such a digit may obscure the clinical diagnosis. Suffice it to say that radiographic examination is mandatory, especially a true lateral view of the individual digit. In all the previously reported cases,[427,450,454,455,466,526,528] closed reduction was easily accomplished, usually under digital block[427,526] or without anesthesia.[466] Good results were reported by all authors except Krebs and Gron,[467] whose patient ultimately required arthrodesis of the PIP joint for severe pain.

IRREDUCIBLE DIP DISLOCATIONS

Irreducible dislocations have been reported in the DIP joint, and there appear to be at least three distinct mechanisms:

1. A pure dorsal dislocation in which the volar plate is avulsed from the neck of the middle phalanx and becomes entrapped in the joint[460,496,499,509,512] similar to a complex dislocation of the MP joint (see p. 521).

2. Entrapment of the long flexor tendon (FDP) in the joint, seen in a dislocation in which there is rupture of one collateral ligament.[267,489,500,504,512] The radiographic key to diagnosis of FDP entrapment is marked lateral displacement of the distal phalanx.[267]

3. Entrapment of an osteochondral fragment[578] or a sesamoid (without attachment to the volar plate)[463] in the joint.

Ifitikhar[453] believed that the volar plate is more likely to be the obstructing element in closed injuries and FDP entrapment the obstructing element in open dislocations of the DIP joint.

Only one case of irreducible palmar dislocation of the DIP joint has been reported.[455]

Treatment

When seen early, DIP dislocations can almost always be easily reduced closed, and they are generally stable after reduction. Hyperextension and mediolateral stress examination should be performed after reduction, and a short period (10 to 12 days) of immobilization of the DIP joint alone is adequate.[521]

The patient with an open DIP dislocation should be afforded all the standard acceptable treatment for any open joint injury (ie, thorough cleansing and débridement) prior to open reduction.

If the dislocation is irreducible, open reduction is required.

CHRONIC (UNREDUCED) DISLOCATIONS

Occasionally a patient presents with an old, unreduced DIP or IP dislocation. If the delay has been as long as 2 to 3 weeks, open reduction will likely be required. This may be somewhat difficult technically because of contracture of the periarticular soft tissues, and the prognosis for joint motion is rather poor.

The joint can be exposed from dorsal, volar, or midlateral incisions. Having tried all of these, we believe that the dorsal approach provides the best exposure, although at least partial transection of the collateral ligament is usually required to see the joint fully and accomplish a reduction from any approach. The longer the joint has been unreduced, the more extensive is the soft tissue dissection required and the more unstable the joint will be postoperatively.

The articular surfaces should be examined carefully at the time of operation. If there is extensive articular damage or erosion, primary arthrodesis is indicated.

DISLOCATIONS AND LIGAMENTOUS INJURIES OF THE PIP JOINT

The PIP joint occupies a position of unique importance in the hand. Loss of motion in this joint severely restricts function. Conversely, if flexion and extension can be maintained in the PIP joint when there is significant damage in the other small joints of the same finger, satisfactory hand function can be preserved. Unfortunately, the propensity for stiffness in the PIP joint is great, not only following injury to the joint itself, but even after prolonged immobilization of an otherwise normal joint. For this reason, the utmost care and concern should be given to injuries involving the PIP joint, and unnecessary immobilization of this joint should be avoided when other injuries in the hand are treated.

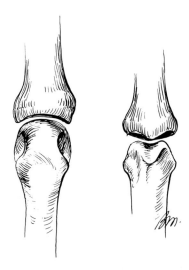

Fig. 7-71. Comparison of the MP and PIP joints as seen in the anteroposterior view. (**Left**) The MP joint is a condyloid joint in which the globular head of the metacarpal articulates with the reciprocally concave base of the proximal phalanx. It allows flexion, extension, abduction, adduction, and a limited amount of circumduction. (**Right**) The PIP joint is essentially a ginglymus or hinge joint, allowing only flexion and extension. It is inherently more stable than the MP joint, by virtue of its bicondylar configuration, which gives it a modified tongue-in-groove appearance.

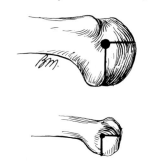

Fig. 7-72. Comparison of the MP (**top**) and PIP (**bottom**) joints as seen in the lateral view. The shape of the head of the proximal phalanx is less eccentric than that of the metacarpal head, and therefore, the cam effect is less significant in the PIP joint.

ANATOMY

The PIP joint, although in some ways similar to the MP joint, has numerous important differences, which have been pointed out by Kuczynski.[11] The PIP joint is essentially a ginglymus or hinge joint, allowing only flexion and extension. It is inherently more stable than the MP joint, by virtue of its bicondylar configuration, which gives it a modified tongue-in-groove appearance (Fig. 7-71). The shape of the head of the proximal phalanx is less eccentric than that of the metacarpal head as seen in the lateral view, and therefore the cam effect is less significant (Fig. 7-72).

The collateral ligaments of the PIP joint are similar to those in the MP joint, with a cordlike collateral ligament proper and a lower accessory ligament (Fig. 7-73). The major difference is that

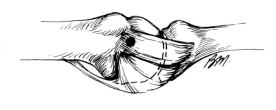

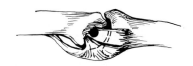

Fig. 7-73. The collateral ligaments of the MP (**top**) and PIP (**bottom**) joints are similar. Both have a cordlike collateral ligament proper and a lower accessory ligament, which attaches directly into the volar plate.

tension in these ligaments is essentially the same in flexion as it is in extension. This is due primarily to two factors: the absence of the cam effect and the parallel alignment of the collateral ligaments, as compared with the divergence of the ligaments in the MP joint. The result of these anatomic peculiarities is that while all parts of the collateral ligaments of the PIP joint are tight in flexion, the volar fibers of the ligament are also tight in extension.[3]

Normal range of motion in the PIP joints is usually at least 0° to 105°, and in many fingers flexion of 120° is easily obtained. As in the MP joint, the volar plate at this level has a firm distal attachment to the base of the middle phalanx and a more flexible proximal attachment to the neck of the proximal phalanx to allow folding with flexion of the joint. Kuczynski[11] has suggested that the volar plate is less mobile in the PIP joint than it is in the MP joint.

Dorsally and dorsolaterally the extensor hood mechanism envelops the joint, while on its volar aspect the volar plate separates the joint from the flexor tendons. (For more detailed descriptions of the ligamentous anatomy around the PIP joint, the reader is referred to the monograph by Milford[13] and the articles by Haines,[9] Landsmeer,[12] and Tubiana and Valentin.[15])

CLASSIFICATION

Injuries of the PIP joints may be classified as collateral ligament injuries, volar plate injuries, dislocations, and fracture-dislocations. In practice, the most important clinical consideration in these injuries is to distinguish between those that are stable and those that are unstable. As a general rule, those that are stable are easy to treat and have the best prognosis.

COLLATERAL LIGAMENT INJURIES (LATERAL DISLOCATIONS)

Collateral ligament injuries are caused by abduction or adduction force applied to the finger, usually in the extended position.[479] Because of the long lever arm, the injury usually involves the PIP joint and is more frequently seen in sports such as football, wrestling, baseball, and basketball. The radial collateral ligament is injured more often than the ulnar collateral ligament.

Collateral ligament injuries may be classified as acute or chronic and further subclassified as stable or unstable. McCue and colleagues[479] defined acute

injuries in their series of patients as those diagnosed within 3 months of injury; most were seen within 3 weeks. We believe that any injury of the lateral ligament diagnosed after 6 weeks should be classified as an old or chronic injury and that the predictable results following collateral ligament repair are uncertain 3 weeks after injury.

Diagnosis

Regardless of the apparent severity or suspected pathology, every injury of the PIP joint should be examined in a systematic and thorough fashion, which must include at least the following major points.

1. Determine the precise area of tenderness. Specifically, the examiner should attempt to ascertain if the maximum tenderness is over the central slip (dorsal), the collateral ligaments (radial and ulnar), or the volar plate (volar).

2. Test for stability of the supporting structures of the joint. The joint should be stressed radially and ulnarly to check the integrity of the collateral ligaments and by passive hyperextension to test the volar plate. Partial tears (sprains) of the collateral ligaments will not allow the joint to open up in excess of physiologic limits. In complete tears (ruptures), there is little or no resistance to lateral deviation stress, and the joint will open on the injured side. Complete tears that are suspected on clinical examination can be documented by stress radiographs, comparing these with stress of the same digit in the uninjured hand.

3. Test both active and passive range of motion, with specific emphasis on the patient's ability to actively extend the PIP joint completely. If he or she is unable to do so because of pain, the examination must be repeated under digital-block anesthesia. Inability to actively extend the PIP joint against resistance is diagnostic of rupture of the central slip, and a boutonnière lesion will result if the patient is not appropriately treated (see p. 477). In the early stages, there will be no limitation of passive flexion of the DIP joint, but within 1 to 2 weeks following injury, this test gains increasing significance. In the patient with a developing boutonnière lesion, passive flexion of the DIP joint will be limited if the PIP joint is held in maximum extension.

4. Obtain at least two (anteroposterior and lateral) x-ray views of the involved finger. Of these, by far the most important is a *true lateral view of*

the individual finger. More errors are made in the diagnosis of PIP joint injuries because of failure to obtain this x-ray than any other single reason. A lateral view of the hand is unacceptable, because important details are obscured by superimposition of the other three fingers. An oblique view, although often helpful in delineating other injuries such as condylar fractures, will often fail to demonstrate the presence or extent of a small chip fracture at the base of the middle phalanx.

In patients with chronic or old collateral ligament injuries, in whom treatment has been ineffective or no primary treatment was instituted, two signs are prominent: instability and swelling.[486] Instability may result from attenuation of the ligament, or there may be total loss of continuity. Swelling at the site of collateral ligament injury is, at times, severe and quite painful, and it may be the patient's main complaint. This may be associated with limitation of joint motion. Swelling is due to excessive reparative connective tissue, which has been described by Moberg[486] as ligamentous callus, at times possibly surrounding tiny avulsion fractures that are too small to be seen radiographically.[461]

Partial tears of the collateral ligament can be difficult to differentiate from complete ruptures on clinical examination alone; therefore, when instability is suspected, stress radiographs (Fig. 7-74) should be compared with those of a finger in the opposite hand. Kiefhaber and colleagues[461] performed extensive laboratory studies on collateral ligament instability and concluded that angulation of greater than 20° is diagnostic of complete rupture. Their studies showed that if the stress x-ray shows angulation of less than 20°, there is a 47% chance of complete rupture, but in these patients the connective tissue layer surrounding the collateral ligament is intact and this will maintain the correct anatomic relationship of the injured structures. They also showed that 94% of PIP collateral ligament ruptures occur at the proximal attachment.

Treatment

ACUTE INJURIES WITH PARTIAL TEARS (SPRAINS)

Most authors agree that incomplete tears of the collateral ligament should be treated with 2 to 5 weeks of buddy taping or immobilization,[480,486] depending on the degree of severity.

Authors' Preferred Method of Treatment. We prefer to treat all partial tears (sprains) of the col-

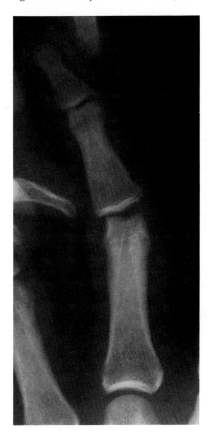

Fig. 7-74. A stress x-ray film of the PIP joint, showing apparent rupture of the radial collateral ligament.

lateral ligaments with buddy taping. The injured finger is taped to a normal adjacent digit, and active motion is encouraged from the outset. The tape is worn continuously for 3 weeks and then only during periods of anticipated stress (eg, participation in sports) for an additional 3 weeks. Usually an athlete is allowed to continue to play during the entire period of treatment.

Regardless of the method of treatment, however, two points must be made clear to the patient from the outset:

1. Full recovery (ie, reaching that point at which there is no residual soreness in the joint) is likely to take what will seem to the patient an inordinately long time (usually several months).
2. There will almost certainly be some permanent residual enlargement of the joint owing to normal healing of the ligament with scar tissue.

ACUTE INJURIES WITH COMPLETE
TEARS (RUPTURES)

Treatment of complete tears of the collateral ligaments of the PIP joints is somewhat controversial.
Some authors advocate simple immobilization of
the finger, although the recommended position and
duration of immobilization vary. Moberg[486] advocated immobilization of the PIP joint in the position
of function for as long as 5 weeks. Eaton and
Littler[440] advised immobilization of the joint in 25°
to 30° of flexion for 2 to 3 weeks, followed by buddy
taping for further protection as active motion is
begun. In discussing McCue's paper,[479] Coonrad
suggested that the finger be immobilized for 3 to 4
weeks and that operative treatment be considered
only if the joint is still unstable after that time. At
one time, Milford[482] suggested splinting the PIP
joint in 60° of flexion for 2 to 3 weeks for complete
ruptures, but he now advocates surgical repair in a
young adult, especially for the radial collateral ligament of the index finger.[483-485] Stern[516] reported
a case in which the collateral ligament became entrapped between the central slip and the lateral
band, preventing closed reduction and therefore
requiring operative treatment.

A few authors[426,457,479,505] have advised surgical
repair of all complete ruptures, but others have recommended more specific indications. Bowers[431]
suggested two indications for operative repair: (1)
inability to achieve a perfectly congruent reduction and (2) "unstressed instability." Wilson and
Liechty[533] advised surgical repair for (1) instability
demonstrated on active range of motion; (2) tissue
interposition preventing joint motion; or (3) lack
of joint congruity on x-ray evaluation.

Authors' Preferred Method of Treatment. We believe that not all complete ruptures of the collateral
ligaments of the PIP joints require operative treatment. One of us (D.P.G.) believes that buddy taping
for 6 weeks is appropriate treatment for most of
these injuries, especially in the long, ring, and small
fingers. Figure 7-75 demonstrates normal stability
of the joint 2 months following injury in a high
school basketball player who had a complete rupture treated with buddy taping while he continued
to play.

The other (S.A.R.) believes that all complete acute
tears of the dominant collateral ligament (radial side
in all fingers except the small finger, in which the

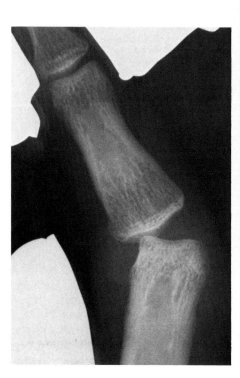
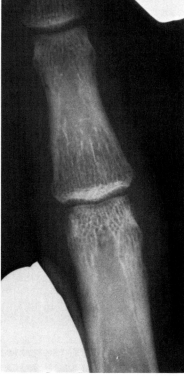

Fig. 7-75. This high school athlete sustained a complete rupture of the collateral ligament of
the PIP joint, easily demonstrated clinically and by stress x-
rays (**left**). Follow-up stress x-
rays taken 2 months later, after
6 weeks of buddy taping,
showed good stability of the
joint (**right**). Most complete
ruptures of the PIP joint collateral ligaments do not require
operative repair (see text).

ulnar collateral ligament is the "dominant" side) should be repaired primarily. It is his experience that in many patients who do not obtain collateral ligament stability following splinting, a large, tender, ligamentous callus develops, which may remain painful and be the patient's major complaint.

The major objection to advocating primary repair for all collateral ligament ruptures is that occasionally the additional operative trauma may result in some limitation of joint motion, which is likely to be more disabling than slight instability, should that result from buddy taping or immobilization alone. As Flatt[444] has pointed out, surgical repair of the collateral ligament is delicate and difficult work. In our experience, it is unusual to obtain full range of motion following any type of operative procedure on the PIP joint. However, we do agree with Milford[483-485] that operative repair should probably be considered for complete rupture of the radial collateral ligament in the index finger of a young adult, where stability is more important than full range of motion.

CHRONIC OR OLD COMPLETE RUPTURES

Patients are occasionally seen with chronic laxity of a collateral ligament because the acute injury was treated either inadequately or not at all. As McCue and coworkers[479] have pointed out, the results of operative treatment in chronic injuries are less satisfactory than those of primary repair. For this reason, reconstruction of chronic ruptures should be considered only if the patient is significantly symptomatic. Moreover, if there is radiographic evidence of articular damage, reconstruction of the ligament is not likely to totally alleviate the patient's symptoms.

In our experience, late reconstruction of a PIP joint collateral ligament is a difficult operation, and the results are somewhat unpredictable, a fact attested to by the paucity of good clinical studies regarding this problem. Noting that the ligament may have healed with lengthening, Redler and Williams[505] merely shortened the ligament and sutured it "under proper tension," a surgical feat that may be somewhat difficult to gauge accurately at operation. In addition to shortening, McCue and associates[479] reinforced the late repair by transferring the radial slip of the superficialis insertion and reattaching it to the proximal end of the ligament with a Bunnell pull-out wire suture. Faithfull[443] reported good results following reconstruction of the lateral ligament with a narrow strip of volar plate detached proximally and sutured into the remnant of collateral ligament on the head of the proximal

phalanx. Since chronic rupture of the collateral ligament is often accompanied by laxity of the volar plate, many of the repairs previously described in the literature employ combined techniques to reconstruct both structures (see p. 508).

DISLOCATIONS OF THE PIP JOINT

There are three types of dislocations of the PIP joint: dorsal, volar, and rotary (Fig. 7-76).

Dorsal PIP Dislocations (Volar Plate Injuries)

Dorsal dislocation is by far the most common type of dislocation in the PIP joint. The physician rarely has an opportunity to see the actual dislocation; reduction is usually accomplished by a coach, a trainer, an observer, or even the patient himself or herself. The mechanism of injury is hyperextension of the joint, but the patient frequently is unable to give a precise history of the mechanism. However, it is important for the examiner to try to ascertain whether the initial displacement of the finger was dorsal or volar, because the treatment implications of these two types of dislocations are radically different.

Although collateral ligament rupture is sometimes a concomitant feature of dorsal dislocation,[486] experimental studies by Benke and Stableforth[430] demonstrated that this is not necessarily so in all cases. What must always occur with dorsal dislocation, however, is rupture of the volar plate. The plate may be torn either at the junction of the membranous and fibrocartilaginous portions of the plate or at its distal attachment into the base of the middle phalanx.[490] The latter may occur with or without a small avulsion chip fracture (Fig. 7-77), and it is important to differentiate this from the far more serious fracture-dislocation of the PIP joint, in which the volar lip fracture involves 20% to 70% of the articular surface and the joint itself is unstable after reduction (Fig. 7-78). The tiny avulsion fracture seen in simple volar plate injuries is rarely displaced and generally heals with only slight spurring of the volar beak of the middle phalanx. Moreover, the presence of the tiny chip provides the physician with clear radiographic evidence of the position of the avulsed volar plate.

Rupture of the volar plate can occur with hyperextension injury of the PIP joint without actual dislocation. Zook and associates[539] pointed out that a transverse skin laceration over the volar aspect of the joint should alert the examiner that the volar plate has probably been torn. Even in the absence of such a laceration, a history of hyperextension

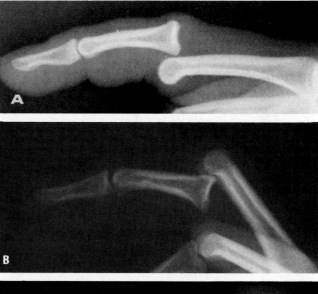

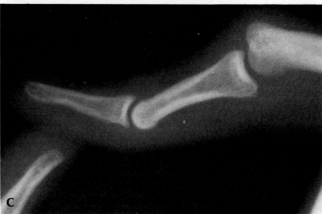

Fig. 7-76. Dislocations of the PIP joints are of three types. Although the common dorsal dislocation (**A**) and the rare volar dislocation (**B**) are easy to reduce, the volar dislocation carries with it a far greater likelihood for permanent impairment because of rupture of the central slip (see text). (**C**) The most uncommon type of dislocation is what we call rotary subluxation. Note that the middle and distal phalanges are seen in true lateral profile and the proximal phalanx has an oblique orientation.

injury of the PIP joint necessitates testing the stability of the volar plate by stressing the joint, under digital-block anesthesia, if necessary.

Stern and Lee[517] studied *open* dislocations of the PIP joint and concluded that the severity of these injuries is generally underestimated. They emphasized the importance of open reduction in the operating room and advocated the use of parenteral antibiotics. Kjeldal[464] emphasized that débridement should precede reduction of the dislocation.

Complex (irreducible) dorsal dislocations of the PIP joint are relatively uncommon but have been reported. The structures blocking reduction have been noted to be the volar plate[449,464,493] and the flexor tendons,[464] and in one case the head of the proximal phalanx was entrapped between the superficialis and profundus tendons.[446]

Patel and associates[497] reported an unusual series of PIP injuries that they called bayonet dislocations because the x-ray films showed displacement in both the anteroposterior and lateral projections. They postulated that *both* collateral ligaments were ruptured in these cases, but seven of their eight cases were treated with closed reduction (the other case was seen late and was treated operatively), and therefore no direct visual confirmation of this assumption was provided.

DIAGNOSIS

If the patient is seen with an unreduced dislocation, x-rays should be taken prior to reduction. More commonly, however, he or she is seen after closed reduction has been done elsewhere, and the clinical appearance is a swollen, painful joint. The

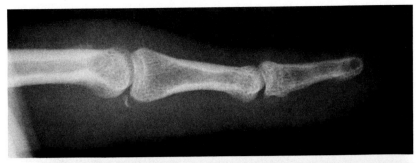

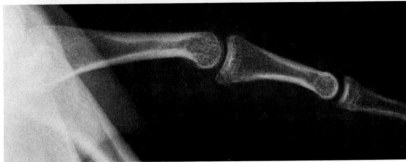

Fig. 7-77. Two types of volar plate avulsion fractures: (**top**) a tiny chip with slight displacement and (**bottom**) a slightly larger fracture with no displacement. These are stable injuries and must be differentiated from the far more serious unstable fracture-dislocation shown in Figure 7-78.

joint must be examined carefully, as described on page 502.

TREATMENT

Acute Injuries.   Most authors advocate immobilization of the PIP joint following dorsal dislocation.[525] Kuczynski's extensive anatomic studies[11] of the PIP joint led him to conclude that if immobilization of that joint cannot be avoided, it should be for as short a period as possible and in no more than 15° of flexion. Sprague[514] suggested 15° to 20° as the appropriate position and 3 weeks the

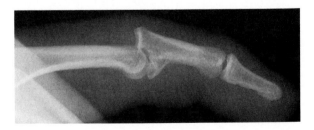

Fig. 7-78. When the volar lip fracture of the middle phalanx involves 20% or more of the articular surface, the remainder of the middle phalanx subluxates dorsally. This unstable injury requires more sophisticated treatment than the small volar plate avulsion fractures shown in Figure 7-77. We generally prefer closed reduction and the dorsal extension block splint method of treatment for this PIP fracture-dislocation.

optimal duration of immobilization. Moller[487] recommended 2 weeks of immobilization for volar plate injuries with proximal tears and 3 to 4 weeks for those with distal avulsions, noting longer morbidity (soreness lasting up to several years) in the latter group. Zook's group[539] suggested that even better results can be achieved with primary surgical repair of the plate.

We prefer to treat all acute volar plate injuries or dorsal dislocations with 3 to 6 weeks of buddy taping. This allows early active motion and prevents hyperextension, which is of course to be avoided in these patients.

Most patients will regain essentially full range of motion, but as noted in the section on collateral ligament injuries, symptoms will usually persist for several months and some permanent swelling of the joint is to be expected, regardless of the method of treatment.

The presence of a tiny avulsion chip fracture does not alter the plan of management, but again we would emphasize that this must be differentiated radiographically from the far more serious fracture-dislocation of the PIP joint, which is discussed on page 511.

For open dislocations, we usually repair the volar plate at the time of joint débridement. Postoperatively, the finger can be immobilized for ten days, followed by active joint exercises. Generally, buddy taping is sufficient to prevent hyperextension of the joint, but if added protection is desired, a dorsal extension block splint can be used for 3 weeks.

Chronic Injuries. Considering the frequency of dorsal dislocations and hyperextension injuries of the PIP joints, relatively few of these patients have chronic symptoms sufficiently troublesome to warrant operative treatment. Recurrent dorsal dislocations of the PIP joint are rare; symptomatic hyperextensibility of the joint secondary to laxity of the volar plate is only a bit more common. In some of these patients a compensatory flexion deformity of the DIP joint may develop, resulting in a typical swan-neck appearance of the finger (Fig. 7-79). Many procedures have been described to correct this problem, all of which have as a common denominator shortening of the attenuated volar plate or creation of some type of checkrein tenodesis to prevent hyperextension of the joint.[423,428,436,465,501,520,530,531] Other types of reconstructive procedures[471,495] have been described for patients with combined chronic laxity of the collateral ligament and volar plate.

A more common problem than symptomatic hyperextensibility or recurrent PIP dislocation is a flexion contracture of the PIP joint. This is generally believed to be due to scarring of the volar plate, with or without an associated chip fracture off the base of the middle phalanx, and has been called a pseudoboutonnière deformity by McCue and associates.[479] The problem can usually be corrected with dynamic splinting and exercise, although occasionally operative treatment may be necessary.[527]

Volar PIP Dislocations

ACUTE INJURIES

Volar dislocations of the PIP joint are relatively rare injuries. They may be pure dislocations (Fig. 7-76**B**) or fracture-dislocations (Fig. 7-80), but the implication of both types is the same: for this type of dislocation to occur, the central slip must be disrupted, and the potential for boutonnière deformity is present. If the dislocation is reduced before the examiner sees the patient and no fracture is present to indicate that it was a volar dislocation, the pitfall is that it will be treated as if it were the much more common dorsal dislocation. Unfortunately, if the finger is treated with splinting in mild to moderate flexion or with buddy taping (both appropriate for a dorsal dislocation), a boutonnière deformity will develop.

Very little is to be found in the literature regarding this uncommon injury. Spinner and Choi[513] reported the largest series (five cases), and their conclusion that open reduction and repair of the central slip is mandatory has been widely quoted since then. However, none of their cases had an adequate trial of primary nonoperative treatment. If the standard treatment for closed boutonnière lesions is nonoperative, why, then, should we consider operative repair of the central slip to be essential in the boutonnière lesion caused by a volar dislocation of the PIP joint? Indeed, Thompson and Eaton[522] advocated splinting of the joint in extension for 3 weeks, followed by dynamic splinting. They advocated primary operative treatment only if the dislocation were irreducible, if the joint surfaces were incongruent after reduction, or if the active extensor lag were in excess of 30°.

Authors' Preferred Method of Treatment. Unless the dislocation is irreducible by closed means, we prefer to treat this injury closed. Following closed reduction of the dislocation, a true lateral radiograph of the finger should be taken to ensure that there is normal congruity of the joint surfaces. The presence of an avulsion fracture at the dorsal base of the middle phalanx (Fig. 7-81) is not an indication for open reduction unless it is displaced and does not reduce adequately with the PIP joint in full extension. If these criteria are met, the treatment is the same as for a closed boutonnière lesion, ie, immobilization of only the PIP joint in full extension with a dorsal splint or an obliquely placed 0.045-inch Kirschner wire, combined with early active and passive flexion exercises of the DIP joint (see p. 477). Continuous splinting is maintained for 4 to 6 weeks, depending on the age of the patient

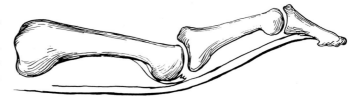

Fig. 7-79. Volar plate injuries of the PIP joint may result in hyperextension deformity of the joint. Some patients may also have a compensatory flexion deformity of the DIP joint secondary to the tenodesing effect of the flexor digitorum profundus tendon.

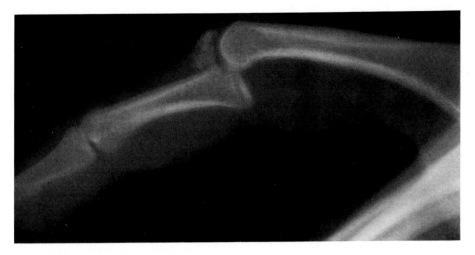

Fig. 7-80. An unstable volar fracture-subluxation of the PIP joint.

(less time in older patients), followed by dynamic extension splinting during the day and static splinting at night (PIP joint in full extension), combined with active range of motion exercises.

If the dislocation cannot be reduced by closed manipulation or if the joint surfaces are not congruent following an attempt at reduction, then primary open reduction is indicated.

CHRONIC INJURIES

Several authors[445,498,502] have discussed the problem of late recognition of volar PIP dislocations and the inevitably poor results in such cases. The key to recognition is, of course, a true lateral x-ray of the involved finger both before and after reduction. Irreducible volar PIP dislocations have been reported, but we believe that the literature on this subject has been unnecessarily confusing because of the failure to differentiate volar dislocation from rotary subluxation. In our opinion, these are two distinct injuries based primarily on the status of the central slip. In volar dislocations, the central slip is ruptured, but in rotary subluxation, it is intact.

Inadequately treated or neglected old volar dislocations will present either as a typical boutonnière deformity or as a flexion contracture of the PIP joint with limited, painful motion. A large series of such patients and the descriptions of operative techniques required to deal with the unusual combination of injuries to the ruptured collateral ligament, volar plate, and extensor mechanism was reported by Peimer and associates.[498]

Rotary PIP Subluxation

Rotary subluxation of the PIP joint is uncommon, but in our opinion, it is clearly a different injury from volar dislocation, even though previous reports in the literature have not always made this distinction.[458,462,488,491,503,512] The mechanism in most cases is a twisting injury,[494] and the resulting pathologic anatomy is buttonholing of one condyle of the head of the proximal phalanx through a longitudinal rent in the extensor hood between the central slip and lateral band, both of which remain intact (Fig. 7-82). The key radiographic feature of rotary subluxation is seen in the lateral view, where

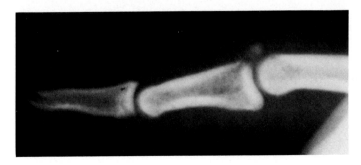

Fig. 7-81. A stable dorsal fracture caused by avulsion by the central slip (analogous to a boutonnière lesion).

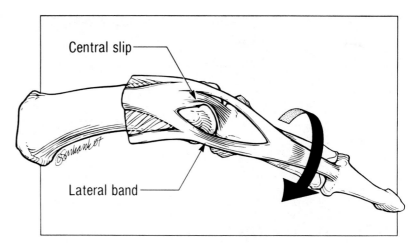

Fig. 7-82. Rotary subluxation of the PIP joint. The condyle of the head of the proximal phalanx is buttonholed between the lateral band and central slip, both of which remain intact.

there is a true lateral profile of the proximal phalanx and an oblique appearance of the middle phalanx (Fig. 7-83), or vice versa.

In the previous edition of this book it was stated that this is always an irreducible dislocation, but one of us (D.P.G.) has subsequently treated two patients successfully with the closed reduction maneuver described by Eaton.[439,522] Under digital-block anesthesia, gentle traction is applied to the finger with both the MP and PIP joints flexed to 90° (Fig. 7-84). This maneuver relaxes the volarly displaced lateral band and allows the band to be disengaged and slip dorsally when a gentle rotary and traction force is applied. Further relaxation of the extensor mechanism can be achieved by dorsiflexion of the wrist. A small pop may be felt as the lateral band reduces to its dorsal position. Successful reduction is followed by full active and passive motion of the PIP joint and must of course be confirmed by post-

reduction x-ray films, especially a true lateral view of the involved digit. If the joint has been successfully reduced, no immobilization is required and early active motion can be started immediately with buddy taping.

Failure of closed reduction is an indication for open reduction. The joint is exposed through a dorsal curved incision, which allows adequate visualization of the entire aponeurosis. A longitudinal rent is found between the intact central slip and one lateral band, with a condyle of the proximal phalanx protruding between these two structures (Fig. 7-85). It is relatively easy to reduce the condyle under direct vision by retracting the lateral band and lifting it from its volarly displaced position beneath the condyle. The collateral ligament should be inspected; if torn, it is repaired. Immediately following reduction, the joint should glide freely through a full range of passive motion. Since the

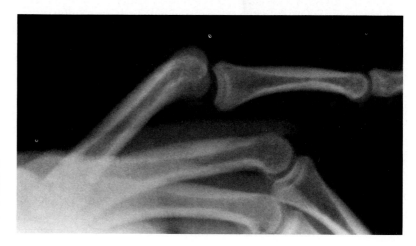

Fig. 7-83. The radiographic key to diagnosis of rotary subluxation of the PIP joint is a true lateral picture of the middle phalanx with a slightly obliqued configuration of the proximal phalanx, or vice versa.

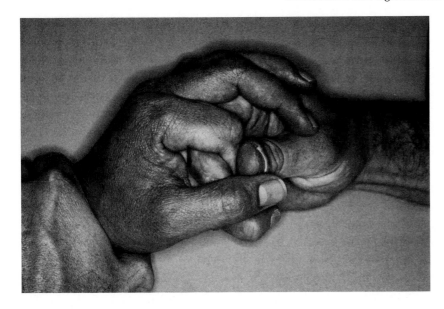

Fig. 7-84. Eaton's[439,522] reduction maneuver for closed reduction of rotary subluxation of the PIP joint. The MP and PIP joints are flexed to relax the lateral bands, and a gentle twisting motion is applied to the middle phalanx.

central slip is intact, minimal postoperative immobilization is required, and we generally prefer to begin active range of motion when the sutures are removed after ten days. If the collateral ligament is repaired, buddy taping for 3 to 4 additional weeks will provide adequate protection.

DORSAL PIP FRACTURE-DISLOCATION

The most potentially disabling injury of the PIP joint is a dorsal fracture-dislocation. Usually as a result of a jamming-type injury, the volar articular surface of the base of the middle phalanx is fractured (usually comminuted and involving up to 75% of the joint surface), and the remaining intact portion of the middle phalanx is subluxated dorsally above the head of the proximal phalanx.

Diagnosis

The clinical picture is usually not dramatic; the PIP joint is simply quite swollen, and range of motion, both active and passive, is severely limited and very

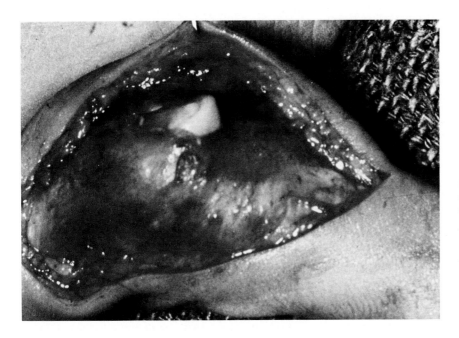

Fig. 7-85. Rotary subluxation of the PIP joint as seen at operation. These uncommon injuries are usually irreducible by closed methods because of buttonholing of the condyle of the proximal phalanx between the central slip and lateral band. However, the joint is usually stable after open reduction (see text).

Fig. 7-86. A classic fracture-dislocation of the PIP joint. There is a volar lip fracture, which is frequently comminuted, as in this patient, and the middle phalanx subluxates dorsally on the proximal phalanx. The injury is frequently missed initially because of the lack of gross clinical deformity and the failure to take an isolated true lateral x-ray film of the involved digit.

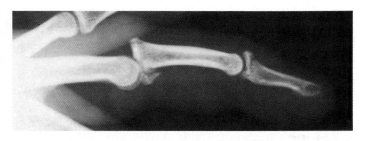

painful. *A true lateral x-ray is mandatory to confirm the diagnosis* (Fig. 7-86). Review of the x-ray reveals dorsal subluxation of the middle phalanx on the proximal phalanx, associated with the fracture of the volar lip of the middle phalanx. The fractured fragment involves at least one third of the volar articular surface of the middle phalanx and, occasionally, up to 75%. However, x-rays fail to reveal the amount of cartilaginous damage; therefore, the size of the fracture cannot be used as the sole criterion for determining the future function of the joint.

Treatment

ACUTE INJURIES

Treatment of the acute injury is rather controversial, and both closed and operative methods have been described. Shulze[511] advocated simple manipulative treatment by placing the joint into extreme flexion while applying traction on the finger. He held the finger in this position with adhesive tape strapping or a malleable aluminum splint, with gradual extension of the finger beginning at seven to ten days; all splinting was discontinued at 3 weeks. Unfortunately, he did not report any cases to demonstrate the effectiveness of his technique. Spray[515] reported two patients treated with taping of the finger in acute flexion with a slightly different technique for 2 and 5 weeks, respectively. Trojan[523] advocated closed reduction and percutaneous pin fixation of the joint with a Kirschner wire for 4 to 6 weeks.

Robertson and coworkers[506] reported seven cases treated with a complicated tridirectional traction device designed to apply longitudinal and volar forces on the middle phalanx and a dorsal force on the proximal phalanx. More recently, Agee[424,425] has described an ingenious force-couple device constructed with Kirschner wires. Schenck[510] has devised a new technique that combines skeletal traction and passive motion, which he has used not only for fracture-dislocations, but also for severely comminuted fractures of the base of the middle

phalanx. Hastings and Carroll[451] have reported the use of a custom-made external fixator that allows immediate active range of motion.

McElfresh and associates[480] first described the extension block splinting method, which is discussed in greater detail subsequently. Strong[519] devised a simpler technique that employs the dorsal extension block principle (Fig. 7-87), and a modification of this method was used by Lange and Engber[472] in three patients who had fracture-dislocations of the PIP joint combined with mallet finger injuries in the same digit.

Wilson and Rowland[532] reported the largest series of patients treated with open reduction and internal fixation. Only one of their patients obtained a full range of motion, but only 4 of their 15 patients had acute injuries (less than 3 weeks old). The major objections to primary open reduction are that (1) the volar lip fragment is almost invariably comminuted and the operation is therefore technically difficult and (2) the 3-week period of postoperative immobilization recommended by the authors further enhances the likelihood of stiffness in an already severely damaged joint. We therefore reserve primary operative treatment for those patients in whom a satisfactory reduction cannot be achieved and maintained by closed reduction and dorsal extension block splinting.

Authors' Preferred Method of Treatment. Our best results with this difficult injury have usually been obtained with the dorsal extension block splinting method described by McElfresh and associates.[480] The method requires careful attention to detail but can result in restoration of a full range of motion if properly applied.

This technique, however, should *not* be used if a satisfactory closed reduction cannot be achieved. Adequacy of reduction must be judged by congruity of the remaining intact articular surface of the middle phalanx with the head of the proximal phalanx (Fig. 7-88). The V sign described by Light[474] (Fig. 7-89) is indicative of an inadequately reduced joint.

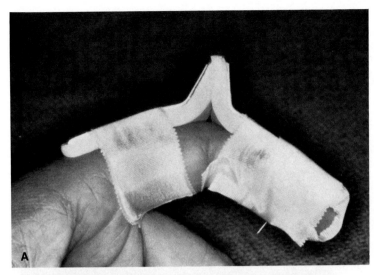

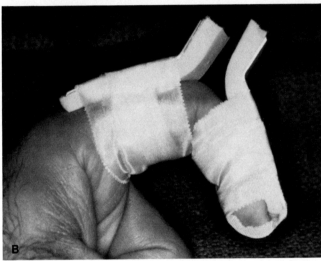

Fig. 7-87. Strong[519] has described a simpler form of dorsal extension block splinting made with two pieces of padded aluminum splint material bent to prevent extension at a predetermined level (**A**) and to allow flexion of the PIP joint (**B**). This method should be used only in very reliable patients who understand the critical importance of not allowing the PIP to extend fully.

It is not necessary for the comminuted volar lip fragment to be anatomically reduced, and usually it remains slightly depressed, but the subluxation of the joint must be reduced anatomically (Fig. 7-90).

If closed reduction cannot be accomplished in an acute injury, the dorsal extension block splinting method should not be used. In such cases, we prefer either ORIF, as described by Wilson and Rowland,[532] or Eaton's volar plate arthroplasty.[441] ORIF is a difficult operation, postoperative stiffness is common, and a long period of passive splinting is needed to restore maximum active range of motion.

Technique of Dorsal Extension Block Splinting. Under digital-block anesthesia, the PIP joint is reduced by longitudinal traction on the digit with simultaneous volarly directed pressure over the subluxated base of the middle phalanx. A lateral radiograph is taken to ensure that the joint can be reduced satisfactorily. This is usually fairly easy to accomplish within a few days of injury but becomes increasingly difficult with time and may be impossible as early as 1 to 2 weeks after injury. If an adequate reduction cannot be documented radiographically, open reduction or volar plate arthroplasty is indicated. McElfresh and coworkers[532] reported success with this method in patients with 30% to 50% of the articular surface involved, and we have been able to use it effectively in some patients with up to 70% involvement.

If the initial test radiograph reveals satisfactory reduction (Fig. 7-90), a short-arm cast is applied, incorporating a 1-inch-wide padded aluminum

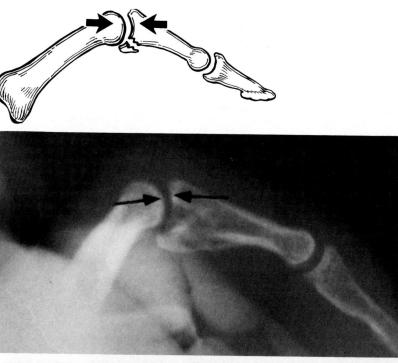

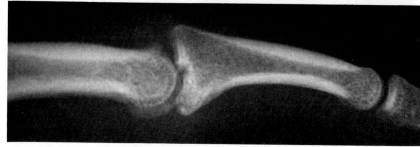

Fig. 7-88. Adequacy of reduction in a PIP fracture-dislocation is judged by congruity between the remaining intact dorsal articular surface of the middle phalanx and the head of the proximal phalanx, as shown **top** and **center.** Compare this with the **bottom** figure, in which there is clearly not an adequate reduction.

splint over the dorsum of the involved finger, extending approximately one-half inch beyond the tip of the digit (Fig. 7-91). The PIP joint is then reduced and the splint bent to conform to the amount of flexion required to maintain the reduction; usually this is about 60°, but occasionally a bit more is necessary. A strip of adhesive tape is applied over the full extent of the aluminum splint and secured to the volar aspect of the cast to prevent inadvertent straightening of the splint (Fig. 7-91**D**). An essential part of the technique is that the proximal segment of the finger must be held firmly to the splint with a strip of half-inch adhesive (Fig. 7-91**A** through **C**); if this is not done, MP joint flexion will cause the proximal phalanx to pull away from the splint, allowing extension of the PIP joint and loss of reduction. Immediately after application of

the splint, another true lateral radiograph is taken to ensure that reduction has been maintained.

Active flexion of the involved finger is allowed and encouraged from the outset, with extension blocked by the splint. The patient is seen at weekly intervals, and if a lateral radiograph shows continued maintenance of reduction, the adhesive tape holding the splint to the cast is cut, the splint is extended to reduce the amount of flexion in the PIP joint, and the tape is reapplied (Fig. 7-92). Usually the flexion can be reduced approximately 15° each week so that full extension is achieved by 4 to 6 weeks (Fig. 7-93). At that time, the splint is removed and buddy taping is applied for an additional 2 to 3 weeks. Most patients regain full active flexion from the beginning and achieve extension gradually over the 4- to 6-week period as the splint

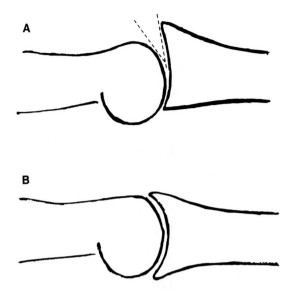

Fig. 7-89. Light[474] has described what he calls the "V" sign of incomplete reduction of a PIP fracture-dislocation. In a satisfactory reduction (**B**) there is parallel congruity between the dorsal base of the middle phalanx and head of the proximal phalanx. In an unsatisfactory reduction (**A**), these two surfaces are neither parallel nor congruent, and the two articular surfaces form a "V." (*Light, T. R.: Buttress Pinning Techniques. Orthop. Rev., 10:49, 1981.*)

is extended. If the patient has not regained full extension of the PIP joint by 6 weeks, dynamic splinting may be used then.

We have limited experience with Strong's[519] simpler type of extension block splint fashioned from two pieces of foam-padded aluminum (see Fig. 7-87), but it does appear to be a reasonable method to use in reliable patients.

CHRONIC INJURIES

Despite the emphasis on the severity of this injury and repeated pleas for early recognition, fracture-dislocations of the PIP joint unfortunately continue to be missed, and these patients turn up with very stiff, painful PIP joints several weeks or even months after the initial injury. As noted, closed reduction is unlikely to be possible beyond 1 to 2 weeks, and other methods of treatment must then be instituted.

Late open reduction using the technique described by Wilson and Rowland[532] may be used in some of these patients. They noted that stripping of the dorsal capsule and division of the collateral ligament and central slip are usually necessary in late cases. They also mentioned that an osteotomy of the united fragment is frequently necessary to improve alignment of the articular surface in old cases, and they used a cortical bone graft from the adjacent proximal phalanx to support the reduced articular fragment. Zemel and associates[536] reported on the use of osteotomy and bone grafting for chronic PIP fracture-dislocations, reporting good results for as long as 10 years postoperatively. McCue and coworkers[479] also used open reduction and osteotomy in late cases, although they did not find the addition of bone graft to be necessary.

Donaldson and Millender[438] were able to do late open reduction without osteotomy by detaching the collateral ligament and performing a dorsal capsulotomy and "minimal freeing" of the extensor mechanism, which allowed reduction of the middle phalanx under direct vision. They pointed out the necessity of restoring the proximal volar pouch, which was consistently obliterated with scarring and adhesions.

For chronic PIP fracture-dislocations, one of us (D.P.G.) prefers the volar plate arthroplasty technique described by Eaton.[439] Eaton has used this procedure as late as 2 years following injury. The operation is technically difficult, but good results can be achieved if the very detailed operative technique described by Eaton and Malerich[441] is followed precisely.

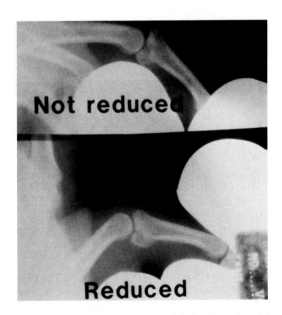

Fig. 7-90. These two x-ray films clearly show the difference between an unsatisfactory reduction of a PIP fracture-dislocation (**A**) and an acceptable reduction (**B**).

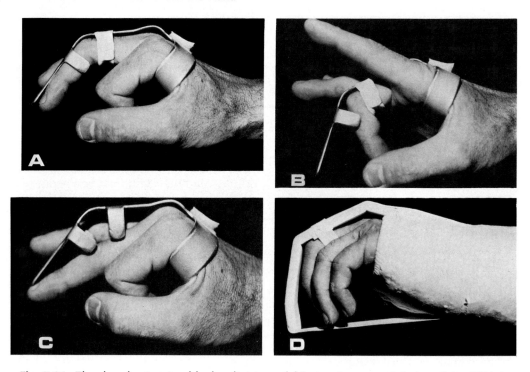

Fig. 7-91. The dorsal extension block splint is useful in treating some injuries of the PIP joint. Extension of the PIP joint can be limited to a predetermined angle (**A**), while at the same time active flexion can be carried out by the patient (**B**). It is particularly important to secure the proximal phalanx to the splint, for if this is not done, flexion of the MP joint allows extension of the PIP joint, thereby negating the function of the splint (**C**). A custom-made orthosis is not necessary. The simplest way to construct the dorsal extension block splint is with a plaster (or fiberglass) gauntlet and a malleable outrigger that is firmly attached to the volar aspect of the cast to prevent bending in extension (**D**).

DISLOCATIONS AND LIGAMENTOUS INJURIES OF THE MP JOINTS (EXCLUDING THE THUMB)

ANATOMY

The MP joint is a condyloid joint that allows flexion, extension, abduction, adduction, and a limited amount of circumduction.[7] The globular head of the metacarpal articulates with the reciprocally concave base of the proximal phalanx, although the surface of the latter has a slightly less acute curve than the metacarpal head. The articular surface of the head is broader on its volar aspect than dorsally, allowing for the recesses in the dorsolateral aspects of both sides of the head to accommodate the collateral ligaments. The stability of the joint depends on the collateral ligaments and volar plate, which together form a snug, boxlike configuration, as noted by Eaton[3] (Fig. 7-94).

Each collateral ligament has essentially two parts: an upper cordlike metacarpophalangeal ligament and a lower accessory, or metacarpoglenoidal, ligament (see Fig. 7-73). The latter, which attaches directly into the volar plate, is less rigid so that it can fold on itself when the joint flexes. Lateral views show that the metacarpal head has an eccentric configuration: the distance from the center of rotation to the articular surface is greater in a volar direction than it is distally (see Fig. 7-72). This produces a camlike effect on the collateral ligaments, making them tight in flexion and lax in extension. One can readily demonstrate this in his or her own hand by noting that passive abduction and adduction are much more restricted with the joint held in maximum flexion than in full extension. This eccentricity of the metacarpal head is the major reason the MP joints are more likely to become stiff in extension than in flexion.

The volar plate of the MP joint is a relatively thick, fibrocartilaginous condensation of the joint

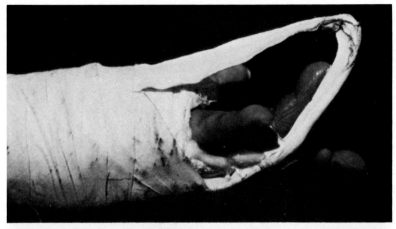

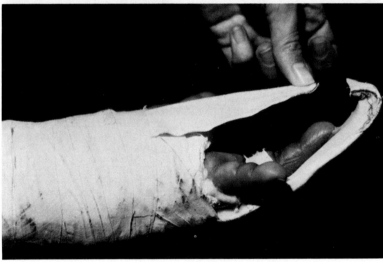

Fig. 7-92. (Top) The outrigger in a dorsal extension block splint must be stabilized with tape to prevent its being inadvertently straightened. **(Bottom)** When the patient is seen at weekly intervals, the tape is cut to allow a measured amount of straightening of the splint and new tape is applied.

capsule forming the anterior wall of the joint. It is firmly attached distally to the base of the phalanx, but its proximal attachment to the neck of the metacarpal is more areolar and flexible, allowing passive hyperextension of the joint and permitting the volar plate to fold on itself in flexion. The volar plates of the four palmar metacarpals are held together firmly by the deep transverse metacarpal ligament, which is, in fact, continuous with the volar plate (Fig. 7-95). Eaton[564] has called this the intervolar plate ligament.

LATERAL MP DISLOCATIONS (COLLATERAL LIGAMENT INJURIES)

Isolated injuries of the collateral ligaments of the finger MP joints are uncommon, presumably because of their relatively protected proximal position within the web space, as well as the protection provided by the adjacent digits. For these same reasons, the diagnosis may be missed early, and the patient may present later with rather vague pain in the region of the MP joint. Most of these injuries appear to involve the radial collateral ligament, and the mechanism of injury is usually an ulnarly directed force on the MP joint.*

Diagnosis

The diagnosis may be suggested by local tenderness and subtle swelling in the valley between the two metacarpal heads directly over the involved collateral ligament. The most specific and significant clinical sign is pain in response to lateral stress with the MP joint held in full extension, with or without

* Murray, J. F. Personal communication, 1982.

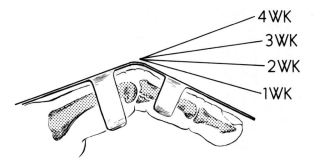

Fig. 7-93. The amount of flexion in the dorsal extension block splint is gradually decreased over several weeks to minimize stiffness in the PIP joint.

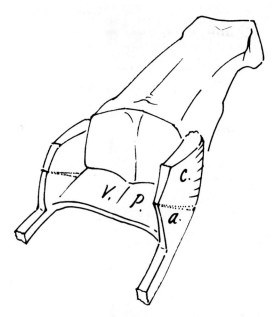

Fig. 7-94. The stability of the MP joint depends, in large part, on the collateral ligaments and volar plate, which together form a snug, boxlike configuration. *(Eaton, R. G.: Joint Injuries of the Hand. Springfield, Ill., Charles C Thomas, 1970.)*

demonstrable instability. Because of the normal laxity of the collateral ligaments with the joint in full extension, stress in this position is usually not painful. Radiographs frequently demonstrate no abnormality, but they may reveal a small avulsion fragment from the metacarpal head (Fig. 7-96). Even relatively large collateral ligament avulsion fractures may be difficult to see on routine x-ray films,[569] and McElfresh and Dobyns[590] have suggested use of the Brewerton view (see Fig. 7-106). Other associated bony injuries include a significant intra-articular corner fracture at the base of the proximal phalanx (Fig. 7-97) in the acute injury or an area of cortical irregularity at the site of attachment of the collateral ligament in chronic injuries (Fig. 7-98).

Ishizuki[583] has reported the largest series of MP joint collateral ligament injuries. All of the 22 patients had arthrograms. The technique of MP joint arthrography is described in detail in his article.

Treatment

ACUTE INJURIES

If the diagnosis is made early (within 10 to 14 days) and if a significant avulsion fracture is not present radiographically, splinting of the joint in 50° flexion for 3 weeks is the recommended treatment,[564] although Ishizuki[583] believes that grossly unstable joints should be repaired surgically. One of us

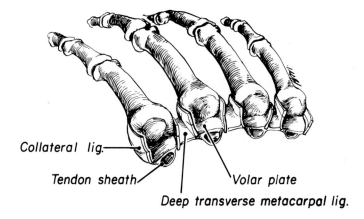

Collateral lig.
Tendon sheath
Volar plate
Deep transverse metacarpal lig.

Fig. 7-95. The volar plates of the four palmar metacarpals are held together firmly by the deep transverse metacarpal ligament, which is, in fact, continuous with the volar plate. Eaton calls this the intervolar plate ligament.

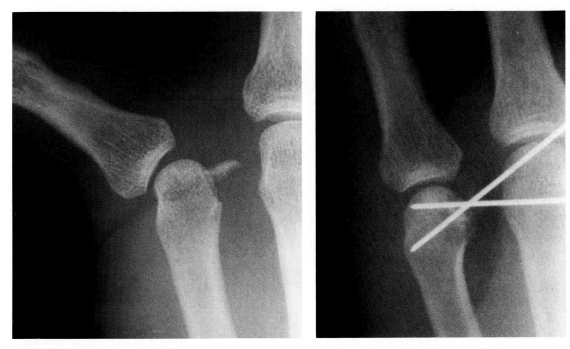

Fig. 7-96. Occasionally, disruption of the collateral ligament of the MP joint is associated with an avulsion fracture off the head of the metacarpal. If such a fracture is displaced (**left**), operative fixation is indicated (**right**).

(S.A.R.) prefers immobilization of the MP joint in full extension to allow the ligament to heal as tightly as possible. If the x-ray film shows wide displacement of a tiny avulsion chip (greater than 2 to 3 mm) or if the fragment involves more than 20% of the articular surface and is displaced or rotated, we believe that primary operative treatment is indicated. Reinsertion of ligament avulsion (with or without a tiny chip fracture) by means of a pull-out suture or internal fixation with small Kirschner wires for corner fractures would be our preferred methods.

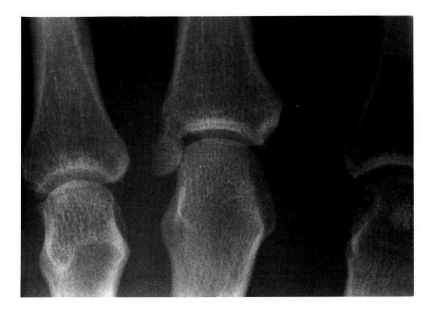

Fig. 7-97. Another indication for open reduction of an MP joint collateral ligament disruption is a large corner fracture of the base of the proximal phalanx.

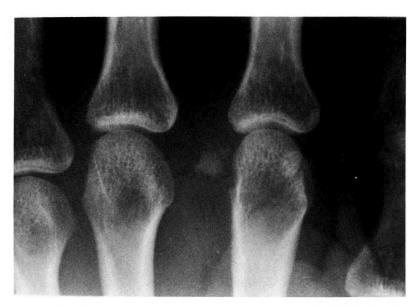

Fig. 7-98. Late, untreated collateral ligament injuries of the MP joint are occasionally (but not always) associated with chronic osseous changes.

CHRONIC INJURIES

As noted in the previous section, finger MP collateral ligament injuries are frequently missed early, and chronic symptoms may result, as suggested in the small series reported by Dray and associates.[562] Although these authors advised against steroid injections, it has been our practice to treat patients presenting with chronic symptoms with a single injection trial and 3 weeks of immobilization, followed by buddy taping to protect the ligament from further injury. Some of these patients continue to have symptoms for many months, but most will become relatively symptom-free in 9 to 12 months.

If symptoms persist beyond this time, operative treatment is indicated, but there is insufficient data in the literature to offer the surgeon clear guidance regarding the best method of surgical treatment. Our limited operative experience with this injury suggests that it may be difficult to identify reparable pathology in chronic cases, and the choices for treatment are reconstruction of the ligament with a free tendon graft as suggested by Dray and associates[562] and Buchler,[558] or excision of the scarred ligament.

DORSAL MP DISLOCATIONS

Two types of dorsal dislocation occur in the MP joint: simple and complex. It is important to differentiate between these two because simple dislocations can be reduced by closed manipulation, whereas complex dislocations are irreducible by closed methods and require open reduction. Both result from hyperextension injuries, and in both the volar plate is torn from its proximal insertion into the neck of the metacarpal. The two can usually be distinguished fairly easily by clinical and radiographic examination, and the surgeon should not have to resort to multiple unsuccessful attempts at closed reduction to conclude that he or she is dealing with an irreducible dislocation.

Simple Dorsal Dislocation (Subluxation)

Eaton[564] correctly refers to simple dorsal dislocation as subluxation of the joint, since the articular surfaces are still in partial contact, but with the proximal phalanx resting in 60° to 90° of hyperextension on the dorsum of the metacarpal head. Closed reduction is relatively simple, although McLaughlin[591] cautioned that it is possible to convert a simple dislocation into a complex dislocation if the reduction is performed by traction alone.

METHOD OF REDUCTION

The proximal phalanx is first hyperextended 90° on the metacarpal, and then the base of the proximal phalanx is *pushed* into flexion, maintaining contact at all times with the head of the metacarpal to prevent entrapment of the volar plate in the joint.

The wrist and the IP joints are flexed during the maneuver to relax the flexor tendons, and the joint usually reduces easily with a palpable and audible "clunk."

Although the reduction can frequently be done without anesthesia, we generally prefer to do it under wrist block, since occasionally pain may preclude a successful reduction and lead the surgeon to the erroneous conclusion that he or she is dealing with a complex dislocation.

Although a short (seven- to ten-day) period of immobilization with the MP joint in 50° to 70° of flexion is acceptable treatment, we generally prefer to allow immediate active motion, preventing hyperextension by buddy taping alone. Recurrent dislocations or chronic symptoms following simple MP dislocations are rare.

Complex (Irreducible) MP Dislocation

Although Farabeuf[565] first coined the term *complex dislocation* in 1876, irreducible dislocation of the MP joints is said to have been described by Malgaigne in his 1855 text.[568,614] Isolated case reports appeared in the early English literature,[548,550,604] but it was not until 1957 that the pathologic anatomy became widely appreciated. In that year, Kaplan[584] published his now classic article in which he described the buttonholing of the metacarpal head into the palm and the anatomy of the constricting factors preventing reduction by closed methods. Although not all authors have agreed with Kaplan about the role of these various structures in preventing reduction, most agree that the most important element preventing reduction is interposition of the volar plate between the base of the proximal phalanx and the head of the metacarpal[549,559,572,574,593] (Fig. 7-99).

Numerous case reports in the earlier literature inferred that this is a rare injury, but more recently reported larger series[542,552,572,579,591,593,596,610] suggest that it is not as uncommon as formerly believed.

Recognition of a complex dislocation should be relatively simple, because there are three clinical and radiographic clues to the diagnosis:

1. The complex dislocation does not present as dramatic an appearance as the simple dislocation (subluxation) described previously. The joint is only slightly hyperextended, with the proximal phalanx lying on the dorsum of the metacarpal head and the finger partially overlapping the adjacent digit. The IP joints are slightly flexed. Radiographically, the proximal phalanx and metacarpal are nearly parallel, with only slight angulation.
2. A consistent finding is puckering of the volar skin. This is more difficult to see when the index finger is involved, since the skin dimple lies within the proximal palmar crease (Fig. 7-100).

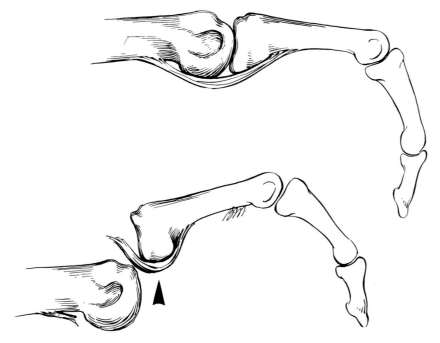

Fig. 7-99. The single most important element preventing reduction in a complex MP dislocation is interposition of the volar plate within the joint space, and it must be extricated surgically.

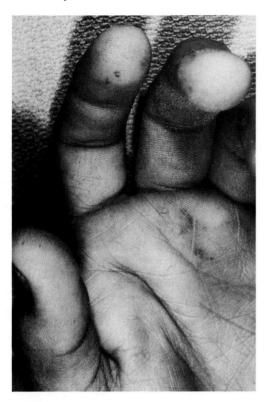

Fig. 7-100. A particularly important clinical sign, which is virtually pathognomonic of a complex dislocation of the index finger, is puckering of the skin in the proximal palmar crease.

It is more readily apparent when the dislocation occurs in the thumb and the dimple is present in the thenar eminence (see Fig. 7-118).

3. A pathognomonic radiographic sign of complex dislocation is the presence of a sesamoid within a widened joint space.[572,599,606,609] Since the sesamoids reside within the volar plate, the presence of a sesamoid within the joint space should be considered an unequivocal sign of a complex dislocation (Fig. 7-101). This finding should not be confused with a chip fracture of the metacarpal head, which may also occur but does not necessarily carry with it the same diagnostic significance. Tsuge and Watari[610] noted that this frequent concomitant injury represents an avulsion fracture of the ulnar tuberosity by the collateral ligament.

Complex dislocations occur most commonly in the index finger, followed in incidence by the thumb and small finger and, rarely, the long and ring fingers. Many other combinations have been described,[543,580,581,613] including simultaneous dislocation of all four MP joints.[616,769]

TREATMENT

An attempt at closed reduction should be made in all dislocations of the MP joint. Even if the pathognomonic signs of a complex dislocation are present, the surgeon is justified in making a single attempt at gentle reduction under adequate anesthesia, but he or she should be prepared to follow this with an immediate open reduction if the manipulation is unsuccessful. The preferred method of closed reduction is that described by McLaughlin[591] (see p. 520). Malerich and associates[589] believe that relaxation of tension on the flexor tendons is critical, suggesting that the closed reduction maneuver should be done with the wrist flexed.

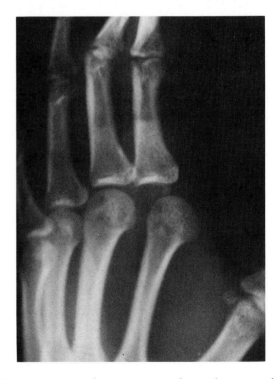

Fig. 7-101. A pathognomonic radiographic sign of a complex dislocation is the presence of a sesamoid within the widened joint space. Since the sesamoids reside in the volar plate, the presence of the sesamoid within the joint space is indicative of interposition of the volar plate within the joint. *(Green, D. P., and Terry, G. C.: Complex Dislocation of the Metacarpophalangeal Joint. Correlative Pathological Anatomy. J. Bone Joint Surg., 55A:1482, 1973.)*

Operative Treatment. The original operative approach to this injury was described by Farabeuf[565] as a dorsal releasing incision. Kaplan[584] presented the logical reasons why a volar approach offers the surgeon more direct visual access to the injury and facilitates the release.

Although most authors favor a volar approach for the open reduction of a complex MP dislocation, Becton and coworkers[551] advocated a dorsal approach, believing that it has the following advantages: (1) better exposure of the volar plate; (2) less likelihood of damage to the digital nerves; and (3) better access for accurate reduction and fixation of an osteochondral fracture of the metacarpal head, if present. Other authors[575,610] have also recommended the dorsal approach for similar reasons, but it has been noted[549,552] that the volar plate has to be split longitudinally from the dorsal approach to effect a reduction; this is not necessary with the volar approach. However, it is easier to excise or fix a concomitant osteochondral fracture of the metacarpal head through the dorsal approach, and we use this when the preoperative x-ray films show such a fracture. Otherwise, we prefer the volar approach.

We believe that the volar approach provides the most direct access to the pathologic anatomy in a complex dislocation, and unless there is a concomitant fracture of the metacarpal head, we use the incision suggested by McLaughlin,[591] which connects the proximal palmar crease with the midradial axis of the index finger. For dislocations in the small finger, an incision in the proximal palmar crease is

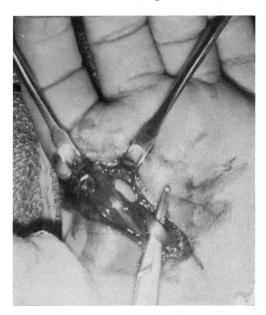

Fig. 7-103. Of extreme importance in the open reduction of a complex MP dislocation is the vulnerable location of the neurovascular bundle caused by displacement of the metacarpal head into the palm. Invariably the digital nerve and artery are tented very tightly and superficially over the prominent metacarpal head and lie immediately beneath the skin.

extended along the mid-ulnar aspect of the finger (Fig. 7-102).

Of extreme importance in the surgical exposure is the vulnerable location of the neurovascular bundle caused by displacement of the metacarpal head into the palm (Fig. 7-103). Invariably, the radial digital nerve and artery in the index finger (the ulnar bundle in the small finger) are tented very tightly and superficially over the prominent metacarpal head, lying immediately beneath the skin. An overly aggressive skin incision can easily injure the neurovascular bundle.

Division of the superficial transverse metacarpal ligaments (transverse fibers of the palmar fascia) facilitates exposure. In the index finger, the metacarpal head is flanked on the radial side by the lumbrical muscle and on the ulnar side by the flexor tendons. In the small finger, the flexor tendons lie on the radial side together with the lumbrical, and the tendon of the abductor digiti quinti lies on the ulnar side. These longitudinal structures must be retracted to provide better exposure of the joint, but releasing them from around the metacarpal neck does nothing to effect a reduction. The most important element preventing reduction is inter-

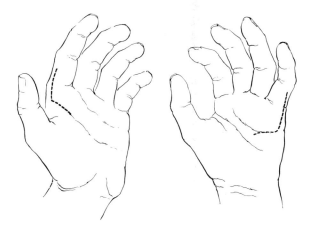

Fig. 7-102. The authors' preferred incisions for open reduction of complex dislocations of the index finger (**left**) and small finger (**right**) MP joints.

position of the volar plate between the base of the proximal phalanx and the head of the metacarpal. The plate has invariably been torn loose from its relatively loose membranous proximal attachment and is found to be wedged in tightly behind (dorsal to) the exposed metacarpal head. The volar plate must be removed manually from the joint before reduction can be accomplished. Avulsion of the volar plate from the neck of the metacarpal is necessarily accompanied by tearing of the plate on both sides from the adjacent deep transverse metacarpal (intervolar plate) ligament, but incompletely so. Extrication of the volar plate with a skin hook is facilitated if the partial tear between the volar plate and the deep transverse metacarpal ligament is completed by a short longitudinal incision (usually on both sides, occasionally on one side).

If care has been taken in removing the volar plate from the joint, it is usually in good condition, with a firm insertion remaining into the base of the proximal phalanx.

It remains a moot and frequently argued point whether or not a true complex dislocation can be reduced by closed manipulation. Our operative experience has led us to believe that it is not possible, but the issue is difficult to resolve because the mere fact of a successful reduction eliminates the opportunity to look and see if the volar plate was in fact entrapped.

Postoperative Care. The joint is invariably stable after reduction, a fact usually confirmed at the operating table by passively moving the joint through a full range of motion. Thus, no immobilization is necessary postoperatively, and early active motion is encouraged, protecting the finger with buddy taping. If the surgeon is concerned about possible instability in hyperextension, a dorsal extension block splint can be used. Hubbard[578] has suggested the use of continuous passive motion postoperatively, but we have not found this necessary.

LATE UNREDUCED COMPLEX MP DISLOCATION

The treatment of a late, untreated, or inadequately treated complex dislocation is considerably more complicated, and the end results are significantly compromised. Murphy and Stark[596] have reported their experience with these difficult injuries, and they note that a second, dorsal incision is necessary to excise the shortened ulnar collateral ligament. None of their six patients with late complex dislocations regained normal range of motion in the finger.

VOLAR MP DISLOCATIONS

Volar dislocation of the MP joint is a rare occurrence.[553,556,595,603,615] Perhaps because it is such an uncommon injury, the pathologic anatomy in volar MP dislocations is not as well understood as in the more common complex dorsal dislocation. The volar plate,[553,595,603] collateral ligament,[553,595] and dorsal capsule[603,615] have all been implicated as a cause of irreducibility. As a result, some authors[553,595] have suggested that both dorsal and volar approaches may be necessary to achieve a reduction.

LOCKING OF THE MP JOINT

Locking of the MP joint in flexion is a relatively uncommon problem. It must be differentiated clinically from the far more common trigger finger caused by stenosis of the flexor tendon sheath in the region of the A1 pulley. In a trigger finger, the "catching" characteristically occurs in the PIP joint, whereas in the condition being considered here, the locking is in the MP joint. The history may implicate a specific traumatic incident in which the finger locks following forcible active flexion of the digit or, more commonly, repeated episodes of catching of the finger following voluntary flexion. The patient may relate that he or she can passively extend the finger with pain, or the pain may have become so severe that he or she cannot extend the finger at all.

On examination, the flexor tendons are intact, and active flexion of the finger may be nearly normal. The key clinical finding is that the MP joint is typically flexed approximately 40° to 50° (Fig. 7-

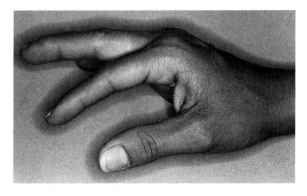

Fig. 7-104. A patient with a "locked" MP joint usually presents with the joint fixed in approximately 40° to 50° flexion (see text).

104), and attempts to straighten the digit are painful or even impossible.

The most frequently recognized cause appears to be the volar plate or collateral ligament catching on an osteophyte on either the side or the volar aspect of the metacarpal head. [541,544,554,561,570, 576,586,605,607] The index finger is most commonly involved,[608] often in older patients with degenerative arthritis, and Goodfellow and Weaver[570] suggested that oblique x-rays of the hand frequently demonstrate these bony projections. Dibbell and Field[561] reported a similar mechanism in a patient with a malunited fracture of the metacarpal head. Other factors mentioned as causes include (1) loose bodies,[588,599] (2) abnormal sesamoids,[566,567] (3) an abnormal fibrous band across the volar aspect of the joint (which may represent a chronic tear of the volar plate),[557,617] and (4) catching of the extensor hood on a dorsal osteophyte.[601]

Treatment

It has been suggested that these patients be observed[608] for at least a month,[576] because spontaneous recovery has been reported in some patients.[544] Forceful manipulation is not recommended, because fracture of the metacarpal head has been reported.[582,586] However, more recent reports[573,600] suggest that *gentle* manipulation may successfully "unlock" the finger, especially if the patient is seen soon after onset. Guly and Azam[573] successfully treated three patients with longitudinal traction combined with alternate medial and lateral rotation under digital-block anesthesia. Posner and coworkers[600] suggested distention of the joint with local anesthetic to aid in reduction. However, if closed reduction is unsuccessful, if spontaneous recovery does not occur, if the condition is extremely painful, or if a fixed contracture of the joint is developing, operative treatment is indicated. The joint is explored through a volar approach,[608] with removal of any offending osteophytes from the metacarpal head or division of the abnormal fibrous bands.

CMC DISLOCATIONS (EXCLUDING THE THUMB)

ANATOMY

The CMC joints of the fingers are arthrodial diarthroses (gliding joints), except the fifth, which is a modified saddle joint.[637] The bases of the metacar-pals articulate with the distal row of the carpal bones and with each other in a complex, interlocking configuration. This is especially true at the base of the second metacarpal, which is forked[652] to receive the convex distal edge of the trapezoid and is also wedged tightly in between the base of the adjacent third metacarpal ulnarly and the trapezium radially. This anatomic arrangement makes precise radiographic visualization of the metacarpotrapezoid joint somewhat difficult.

The joints are strengthened by tough intermetacarpal and CMC ligaments dorsally and volarly; the dorsal ligaments are stronger. Additional reinforcement is provided by the insertions of the wrist flexors and extensors into the bases of the second, third, and fifth metacarpals.

Essentially no movement is possible in the third metacarpocapitate joint, which functions as the stable central post of the hand, as described by Flatt.[635] A very limited amount of anteroposterior gliding is permitted at the base of the second metacarpotrapezoid joint, but the articulations between the bases of the fourth and fifth metacarpals and the hamate are considerably more mobile. Most authors have assumed that up to 20° or 30° of motion is possible in these two joints, but Gunther's cadaver studies[640] revealed only 8° and 15° in the fourth and fifth CMC joints, respectively.

The fifth CMC joint is the most mobile because it is actually a saddle joint similar to the articulation between the thumb metacarpal and the trapezium. A saddle joint is an articulation in which the opposing surfaces are reciprocally concavoconvex. Viewed from the dorsum, the distal surface of the hamate is convex; seen from the ulnar side, it is concave. The bases of both the fourth and fifth metacarpals articulate with the hamate; the distal surface of the hamate is divided into two facets by a faint ridge. The articular surface of the fourth metacarpal is transverse, and that of the fifth metacarpal has an oblique orientation (Fig. 7-105). This sloping articular surface of the fifth CMC joint and the pull of the extensor carpi ulnaris inserting into the base of the fifth metacarpal are the major factors that create instability in fracture-subluxations of this joint.

Two soft tissue relationships of the CMC joints are of extreme importance to the surgeon when operative intervention is required. The deep (motor) branch of the ulnar nerve lies immediately volar to the fifth CMC joint as it winds around the hook of the hamate,[636] and the deep palmar arterial arch lies directly beneath the third metacarpocapitate articulation.

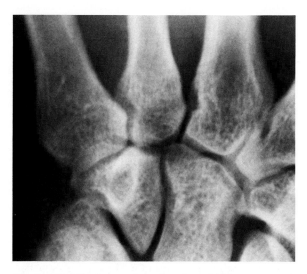

Fig. 7-105. The bases of the fourth and fifth metacarpals both articulate with the hamate. The articular surface of the fourth metacarpal is transverse, and that of the fifth is oblique; the latter is partially responsible for instability of fracture-subluxations of this joint.

MECHANISM OF INJURY

Despite attempts to reproduce CMC dislocations in the laboratory[684] and many hypotheses based on clinical cases, the precise mechanism of these injuries remains somewhat speculative. In general, however, they tend to result either from extreme violence (eg, motorcycle accidents, crush injuries, or blows from heavy falling objects)[642] or from hitting someone or something with the closed fist. Dommisse and Lloyd[632] suggested that the type of fracture or dislocation of the fifth metacarpal is related to the mechanism of injury. They found that direct injury (a crushing blow) tends to produce angulated extra-articular fractures, which do not disrupt the CMC joint and are stable. On the other hand, indirect injury is the cause of unstable intra-articular fracture-dislocations. They postulated that a lever type of strain in which the fifth metacarpal is forced into dorsiflexion causes a bipartite fracture-dislocation, and a direct blow to the metacarpal head produces a longitudinal force that results in a tripartite fracture-dislocation with more proximal migration of the shaft. Their reason for differentiating these two types of fracture-dislocations was that in their experience, closed reduction and percutaneous pin fixation was more likely to be successful in the bipartite fracture than in the tripartite variety. Other authors[621,658] have also suggested that the unstable fracture-dislocation is caused by a force

acting along the longitudinal axis of the fifth metacarpal.

Virtually every combination of CMC dislocations has been reported, in addition to isolated dislocations of each of the four individual joints. Simultaneous dislocation of all four joints generally results from extreme trauma, such as having the hand run over by an automobile,[656] and is likely to be associated with multiple fractures and extensive soft tissue damage.

Most of these dislocations are dorsal, but volar displacement of both the fifth[667,681] and second[675] CMC joints has been reported. Gunther and Bruno[641] described what they called a divergent dislocation, ie, dorsal displacement of the second and third and volar dislocation of the fourth and fifth CMC joints. Concomitant injuries have included dislocation of the fifth MP joint[679] and fractures of the hook of the hamate.[641,667]

DIAGNOSIS

Clinical

The obvious clinical deformity that one might expect to see with this injury is often obscured by marked swelling of the hand. Even when the swelling is severe, however, maximum tenderness can generally be localized to the bases of the metacarpals. In dislocations of the fifth metacarpohamate joint, special attention should be directed to the integrity of the ulnar nerve,[624,636] and in multiple dislocations, a careful assessment of all soft tissues, especially the circulation, must be made. Median nerve injury and avulsion of the wrist extensor tendons[685] have been reported as associated injuries.

Joseph and coworkers[651] have suggested that sprains of the CMC joints are considerably more common than generally believed, and chronic symptoms frequently result. Moreover, the literature still reflects that even frank dislocations are frequently missed when initially seen, and radiographs are mandatory.

Radiographic

Initial radiographic examination should include the three standard views: posteroanterior, lateral, and oblique; the true lateral view is most likely to demonstrate the displacement of the base of the metacarpal.[631,645,680] However, special views may be helpful to determine the exact amount of displacement and the extent of intra-articular comminution. Murless[665] demonstrated that an anteroposterior view (palm up with the forearm in supination) is

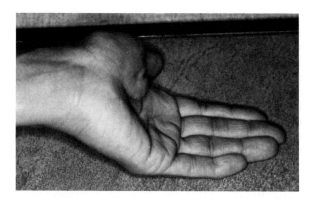

Fig. 7-106. The Brewerton view[623] has been suggested as a method of demonstrating occult fractures at the base of the metacarpals. The x-ray beam is angled 30° from the ulnar side of the hand.

more likely to show small detached fragments than is the standard posteroanterior (palm down) view. Bora and Didizian[621] stated that the most helpful view is with the forearm pronated 30° from a routine anteroposterior view (a 60° supination lateral), and Kaye and Lister[653] suggested the Brewerton view[623] (Fig. 7-106) as a means of demonstrating occult fractures at the base of the metacarpal.

Fisher and colleagues[633,634] have emphasized the principles of parallelism, symmetry, and overlapping articular surfaces in evaluating suspected injuries of the CMC joints. Chmell and coworkers[627] have described what they call the oblique metacarpal line, ie, a straight line drawn on the x-ray film connecting the heads of the ulnar three metacarpals. The amount of shortening of the involved metacarpal can be measured from this line, although comparison with the opposite uninjured hand is advised.

Our own preference, in addition to the standard posteroanterior and lateral views, is to obtain oblique views with the hand pronated and supinated 30° respectively from the true lateral view. Additional oblique views with more or less forearm rotation may be indicated by what is seen in the aforementioned radiographs.

An important point is to be aware of the possible coexistence of dislocation of one CMC joint associated with a displaced fracture of an adjacent metacarpal. Analogous to Monteggia and Galleazi fracture-dislocations in the forearm, the metacarpals are tethered proximally and distally, and if one metacarpal is shortened or significantly angulated, one should always look carefully to rule out dislocation of the base of an adjacent metacarpal[649] (Fig. 7-107). Cain and coworkers[625] reported a series of such patients in whom the fourth metacarpal was fractured and the base of the fifth metacarpal was dislocated dorsally, associated with varying types of fractures of the hamate. Marck and Klasen[660] showed that lateral tomography is the best technique for clearly delineating the nature of these hamate fractures.

TREATMENT

Acute Injuries

CMC dislocations are not rare injuries, but they are sufficiently uncommon that most of the literature regarding them is in the form of case reports or very small series, with many recommendations for treatment based on limited clinical impressions and inadequate data. Because of the conflicting methods of treatment advocated, each with good results reported, we find it difficult to be dogmatic regarding the optimal method of treatment of these injuries.

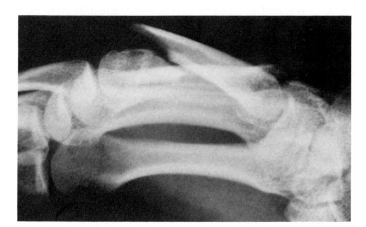

Fig. 7-107. Whenever there is a displaced or angulated fracture of the base or the shaft of a metacarpal, one should be particularly careful to look for dislocation of one or more adjacent CMC joints. In this patient, there is an angulated and shortened fracture of the fifth metacarpal and subluxation of the base of the fourth metacarpal.

METHODS OF TREATMENT

Splinting Without Reduction.   Good evidence suggests that intra-articular fractures of the base of the fifth metacarpal with minimal or no displacement can be adequately treated with a molded cast or splint for 3 to 4 weeks. Disagreement regarding treatment arises, however, in dealing with displaced, intra-articular fracture-subluxations. Several authors, especially in the older literature,[655,673,677,686] have stated or implied that old, unreduced CMC dislocations ultimately become asymptomatic and produce no functional deficit. The validity of these conclusions has to be questioned because of the limited number of cases and extremely short follow-up periods reported. However, in 1974, Petrie and Lamb[670] published what is perhaps the only long-term (average 4 ½ years) follow-up study of a substantial number of patients (23) with essentially untreated fracture-subluxations of the base of the fifth metacarpal. Their rather surprising results, which revealed only one patient with significant symptoms, might tend to dampen one's enthusiasm for open reduction of these injuries. However, even in light of this study, we cannot advocate total neglect for this fracture-dislocation, because our own experience agrees with that of the many authors[642,645,646,650,654] who state that residual subluxation and incongruity of the CMC joints do lead to pain and weakened grip in some patients.

Closed Reduction and Cast Immobilization.   Anatomic or at least acceptable closed reduction is usually not difficult to accomplish if the injury is recognized and treated early. The problem, however, is maintaining that reduction, especially in the presence of significant swelling.[649] If closed reduction and cast immobilization is selected as the method of treatment, careful radiographic monitoring must be done for the subsequent 3 to 4 weeks to detect resubluxation, which is likely.

Closed Reduction and Percutaneous Pin Fixation.   Numerous authors[628,631,638,644,671,682] have demonstrated that the reduction can be maintained with percutaneously placed Kirschner wires after reduction has been achieved by closed manipulation.

Technique.   With the patient under adequate anesthesia with complete muscle relaxation (general anesthesia or brachial block), a strong traction force is applied with finger traps and a counterweight across the upper arm. Uninterrupted traction for five to ten minutes brings the metacarpals out to length, but it does not necessarily reduce the dislocation, and direct pressure must be applied to the bases of the metacarpals to reduce them into their normal anatomic positions (Fig. 7-108). After full reduction has been verified by anteroposterior and lateral radiographs (or with the image intensifier) taken with the hand in traction, two or three 0.045-inch Kirschner wires are passed percutaneously, stabilizing the involved metacarpal to an adjacent intact metacarpal or to the carpus itself, or both. It is imperative to reduce the main shaft of the metacarpal (ie, the subluxation), and it is desirable to anatomically reduce the intra-articular fracture at the base of the metacarpal, although the latter is not always possible. We prefer to bend the pins at a right angle outside the skin to facilitate removal 4 to 6 weeks following reduction. The hand and wrist should be protected in a splint or cast for 6 to 8 weeks.

Open Reduction and Internal Fixation.   Noting the similarity between the fracture-subluxation of the fifth CMC joint and Bennett's fracture in the thumb, numerous authors[621,632,642,646,658,674] have advocated open reduction and internal fixation as the treatment of choice. After discovering that their patients treated with open reduction did not fare as well as those treated with no reduction in the study previously cited, Petrie and Lamb[670] concluded that these two entities are anatomically but not functionally similar, and they argued that the case for open reduction is not strong.

Certainly in some instances open reduction is indicated. Unsuccessful closed manipulation implies some impediment to reduction, including massive swelling,[643,676] interposed fracture fragments,[643,659] interposed soft tissue structures such as the wrist extensor tendons,[643,657] or soft tissue contracture secondary to delay in treatment.[662]

The literature would suggest that open reduction is more likely to be necessary in multiple CMC dislocations,[643,656,663] and open injuries should be treated with open reduction, débridement, appropriate wound care, and, in our opinion, stabilization of the dislocations with multiple Kirschner wires.

Open reduction would also appear to be more frequently necessary in fracture-dislocations of the fifth CMC joint in which the base of the metacarpal is displaced radially across the bases of the other metacarpals[666,673] than it is with the more common pattern of ulnar displacement.

AUTHORS' PREFERRED METHOD

For isolated fracture-subluxation of the CMC joints, including the fifth, we prefer closed reduction and

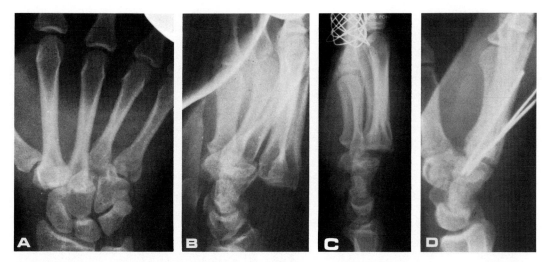

Fig. 7-108. The steps in closed reduction of a CMC dislocation. (**A**) The anteroposterior view shows proximal displacement of the bases of the second and third metacarpals. Note also the fracture of the base of the fifth metacarpal. (**B**) The lateral view dramatically demonstrates dorsal dislocation of the bases of the second and third metacarpals. (**C**) The first step in reduction is to apply a strong traction force, best accomplished by finger traps with countertraction across the upper arm. Traction brings the metacarpals out to length, but it does not necessarily reduce the dislocation. Note that there is still dorsal subluxation of the bases of the metacarpals (**D**) Direct pressure must be applied to the bases of the metacarpals to restore their normal anatomic position. Because of the great propensity for recurrent subluxation following closed reduction alone, we believe that percutaneous pin fixation should routinely be done at the time of closed reduction.

percutaneous pin fixation. Mild to moderate incongruity of the articular surface is accepted (Fig. 7-109), and the major emphasis is on reduction of the subluxation of the metacarpal shaft. This method works equally well when two adjacent joints are dislocated, but we have never attempted to use it with three or four dislocations. Open reduction is more likely to be necessary in the patient with four CMC dislocations. In such situations, Hartwig and Louis[643] noted that reduction and stabilization of the base of the third metacarpal is the key to the reduction of the remaining metacarpals.

Operative treatment is necessary in all open dislocations, and despite the theoretic disadvantage of using internal fixation in an open wound, we believe that it is imperative to use as many Kirschner wires as necessary to restore stability. The massive swelling so often a part of these injuries makes external splinting ineffectual in holding the reduction, and redislocation can be almost guaranteed if internal stabilization is not done.

Chronic Injuries

Unfortunately, CMC dislocations are occasionally missed on initial examination and may present sev-

eral weeks to months following injury. If the subluxation and joint incongruity are mild to moderate, we tend to favor no treatment for those injuries seen more than 3 weeks late. Using Petrie and Lamb's series[670] as the basis for this decision, we would expect some of these patients to become relatively asymptomatic.

If the degree of displacement is marked, or especially if multiple joints are involved, an attempt should probably be made to do a late open reduction. Just how long after injury this can be successfully accomplished is not well documented in the literature, although Imbriglia[650] did so at 3½ months and Bora and Didizian's cases[621] included open reductions done as late as 6 months to 10 years after injury.

For the symptomatic patient with established posttraumatic arthritis, arthrodesis[621,642,643,651,678,683] or arthroplasty is indicated. Clendenin and Smith[630,678] suggested that the fifth CMC joint be fused in 20° to 30° of flexion and also that it is not necessary to fuse the adjacent fourth CMC joint if it is not involved. Surprisingly, none of their patients had any limitation of motion, presumably because of compensatory motion in the triquetro-hamate

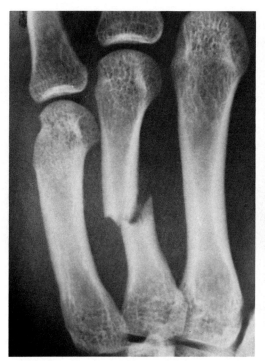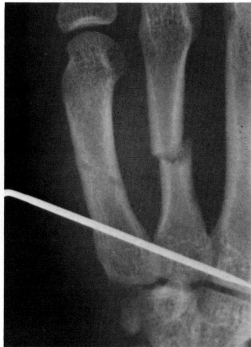

Fig. 7-109. The major goal in closed reduction and percutaneous pin fixation of fracture-subluxations of the fifth CMC joint (**left**) is restoration of length; we will accept mild incongruities of the articular surface as shown on the **right**. Note also the angulated fracture of the shaft of the adjacent fourth metacarpal, a concomitant feature also illustrated in Figure 7-107.

joint.[630] They used a corticocancellous graft carefully fitted into a slot across the joint, with or without Kirschner-wire fixation, similar to the technique described by Joseph and associates.[651]

Arthroplasty of the joint has been advocated by other authors. Black and colleagues[619] prefer simple resection of the impinging osteophytes without any attempt to reduce the subluxated dorsal fragment and shaft. Interposition arthroplasty is favored by others, using either a small Silastic great toe implant[639] or a rolled up tendon ("anchovy").[627]

DISLOCATIONS AND LIGAMENTOUS INJURIES IN THE THUMB

MP JOINT

Anatomy

The MP joint of the thumb is basically a condyloid joint, allowing flexion, extension, abduction, adduction, and a very limited amount of rotation.[708] The range of "normal" motion in the MP joint of the thumb varies widely[698] and appears related to the contour of the metacarpal head.[713] Harris and Joseph[711] noted that motion in joints with flat or "flattish" metacarpal heads tends to be considerably limited. Palmer and Louis[729] recorded that the "normal" arc of MP motion ranges from 5° to 115°. Coonrad and Goldner's studies[698] revealed that the normal range of abduction-adduction varies from 0° to 20°, with an average of 10° (measured with the joint in 15° of flexion). Mediolateral stability is provided mainly by the collateral ligaments.[744]

On the ulnar aspect of the joint, the adductor pollicis muscle is inserted partly through the ulnar sesamoid bone into the volar plate and partly through a powerful tendon directly into the proximal phalanx, with additional fibers fusing with the ulnar expansion of the dorsal aponeurosis.[742,744] This part of the dorsal aponeurosis is called the adductor aponeurosis, and it plays an important role in the pathomechanics of injuries of the ulnar collateral ligament. The adductor aponeurosis directly overlies the ligament and must be divided to provide operative exposure of the ligament. Despite some contradictory studies by Kaplan,[714] most authors now accept Stener's findings that passive stability of the joint is provided by the collateral ligament, with the adductor aponeurosis providing active stabilization against violence tending to abduct the thumb.

Ulnar Collateral Ligament Injury (Gamekeeper's Thumb, Skier's Thumb)

MECHANISM OF INJURY

A sudden valgus (abduction) stress (probably combined with hyperextension[743]) applied to the MP joint of the thumb results in partial or complete disruption of the ulnar collateral ligament and volar plate. In 1955, Campbell[696] reported that chronic laxity of this ligament can develop without a specific incident of acute trauma, and he found this to be an occupational deformity in the hands of British gamekeepers. Their customary method of killing wounded rabbits was such that, over time, attenuation of the ligament resulted in chronic instability of the joint. Through common usage, the term *gamekeeper's thumb* has come to include any injury of the ulnar collateral ligament, although most of these injuries seen currently are acute injuries rather than the chronic stretching of the ligament reported by Campbell.

Several authors[701,707,724] have suggested that acute injuries of the ulnar collateral ligament of the thumb should more properly be called "skier's thumb," since this is probably the most common mechanism of injury and in fact is one of the most common ski injuries.[691,697,703,709] Indeed, this injury was reported in the German literature in 1939 to 1940,[707,746,750] and *skier's thumb* is the preferred appellation in Europe.[707] The ski pole has been implicated as the causative factor, and there has apparently been no decrease in the incidence of this injury with the newer type of strapless poles.[697,701,703,723] Primiano[731] suggested that if a strapless pole is used, injury is less likely to occur if the pole does not block full flexion of the IP joint. A special glove has been designed[704] in an effort to protect the ulnar collateral ligament.

STENER LESION

Stener's important contribution[744] to our understanding of this injury was the recognition that the adductor aponeurosis frequently becomes interposed between the two ends of the torn ligament, thereby preventing adequate healing (Fig. 7-110). The most frequent site of rupture is directly from the distal attachment of the ligament into the proximal phalanx, although interposition may occur

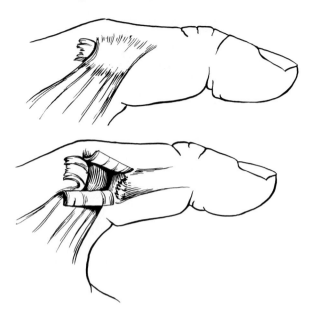

Fig. 7-110. Stener has described how the ruptured end of the ulnar collateral ligament may become displaced and folded back on itself beneath the proximal edge of the adductor aponeurosis. Because of this frequent finding, most authors favor operative repair of complete rupture of the ulnar collateral ligament. *(Redrawn from Stener, B.: Displacement of the Ruptured Ulnar Collateral Ligament of the Metacarpo-phalangeal Joint of the Thumb. J. Bone Joint Surg., 44B:870, 1962.)*

even if the ligament is torn through its substance. Stener found this interposition in 25 of his 39 cases, and other authors[717,725,730,756] have reported an incidence of the Stener lesion ranging from 14% to 83%. Our own impression is that the Stener lesion is present in more than 50% of acute ruptures of the ulnar collateral ligament.

DIAGNOSIS

Clinical. The patient presents with a painful, swollen MP joint of the thumb. Usually the point of maximum tenderness can be localized to the ulnar aspect of the joint. A particularly important point in the evaluation of these patients is to differentiate a sprain (partial tear) from a rupture (complete tear). The obvious way to do this is to determine the amount of radial deviation produced by abduction stress of the MP joint, but this may be more difficult than it sounds. If the joint opens up easily (Fig. 7-111), the diagnosis of rupture is obvious, but pain and muscle spasm may limit passive abduction of the thumb and give a false-negative impression. Unless there is easily demonstra-

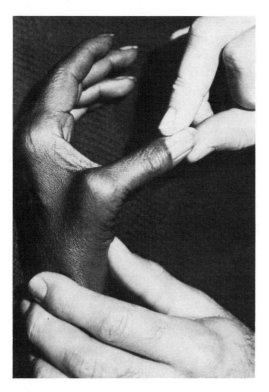

Fig. 7-111. Valgus stress applied to the MP joint of the thumb in a patient with complete rupture of the ulnar collateral ligament (so-called gamekeeper's or skier's thumb).

ble gross instability, we believe that the abduction stress test should be done under some type of anesthesia. Most authors[692,715,716,722,729,730,740,741] advocate local infiltration of the ligament; others prefer a block of the median and radial nerves at the wrist.[705,725,729] Testing should be done with the MP joint in both flexion and extension, and the opposite thumb should be used for comparison. What constitutes an abnormal stress test remains somewhat controversial: Smith[743] said 45°; Frank and Dobyns[705] and Bowers and Hurst[692] said more than 10° greater than the opposite side; and Palmer and Louis[729] said 35° (tested in full flexion). It may be rather difficult to measure the angle of abduction clinically, and Bowers and Hurst[692] noted that clinical estimates consistently were 5° to 15° greater than radiographic measurements in their studies. Therefore, if there is any question about the diagnosis, we believe that the stress test should be measured radiographically.

Radiographic.   Several authors[705,745] have suggested that routine radiographs should be made be-

fore stressing the joint, to prevent possible displacement of an undisplaced fracture. Three types of avulsion fractures may be seen in the initial films; the most common types are a small fragment pulled away from the base of the proximal phalanx (Fig. 7-112**A**) and a large intra-articular fracture involving one fourth or more of the articular surface of the base of the proximal phalanx (Fig. 7-112**B**). Louis and colleagues[721] have identified a third type of avulsion fracture that is attached not to the ulnar collateral ligament but rather to the volar plate. Stothard and Caird's arthrographic studies[747] showed two fractures that probably represented this type of injury, which is not unstable and can be treated with cast immobilization alone.

Stener and Stener[745] have stressed the importance of differentiating avulsion and shear fractures (Fig. 7-113). The latter may originate from the radial side of the head of the metacarpal and are decidedly less common in our experience than the avulsion fractures, which arise from the ulnar aspect of the base of the proximal phalanx.

If no fracture is seen on the initial radiographs and a clear distinction cannot be made on clinical examination between sprain and rupture, or if documentation of the rupture is desired, stress radiographs are indicated. We believe that stress x-rays should be taken, even though Mogan and Davis[724] advised against their use. We agree with Engel, who stated that stress views without anesthesia are of questionable value.[702] Bowers and Hurst[692] believe that the incomplete relief of pain provided by local infiltration anesthesia is a safeguard against further disruption of any of the torn structures, but one of us (D.P.G.) prefers to perform the stress radiographs under median and radial wrist block. Films are taken with the MP joint in full extension, with radial abduction stress applied to the thumb by the surgeon wearing leaded gloves (Fig. 7-114). To our knowledge, no satisfactory method has yet been described to record radiographically the stress test done with the MP joint in flexion.

Arthrography.   Several authors have attempted to evaluate ruptures of the MP collateral ligaments with arthrograms.[692,702,719,734,735,752] This is done by injecting 1 to 2 mL of contrast material (1.2 mL 60% Renografin mixed with 0.8 mL 1% lidocaine) into the joint with a tuberculin syringe in the interval between the extensor pollicis brevis and radial collateral ligament.[692,719] In our opinion, arthrography offers little additional information, unless it can be used to successfully identify the Stener lesion, as Bowers and Hurst[692] attempted to do. We agree with them that this specific use of the

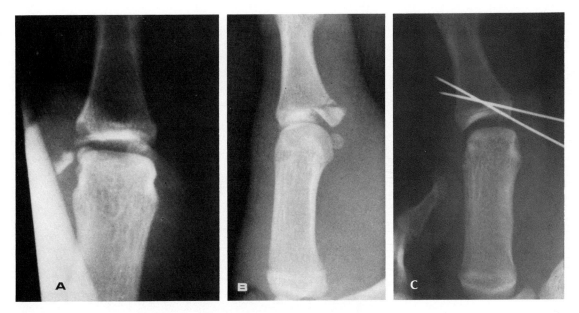

Fig. 7-112. A gamekeeper's thumb may be associated with an avulsion fracture from the base of the proximal phalanx. (**A**) This may be a very small fragment. (**B**) It may be a large fragment involving one fourth or more of the articular surface. Either type, if displaced, requires open reduction. (**C**) A large, displaced fragment avulsed by the ulnar collateral ligament is best treated by open reduction and internal fixation with small, smooth K-wires. Smaller fragments are sometimes more readily fixed with a pull-out suture. (**A** *from Green, D. P.: Am. Fam. Physician, 7:118, 1973.*)

arthrogram has great merit, since it can aid the surgeon in deciding between operative and nonoperative treatment. Mogan and Davis[724] reported that they identified the Stener lesion by arthrography, but they did not correlate their radiographic impressions with operative findings. We agree with other authors[723,747] who believe that it is difficult to identify the Stener lesion by arthrography with any degree of confidence.

Arthroscopy. Arthroscopy does not currently appear to have any value in the diagnosis or treatment of injuries of the MP joint collateral ligament, but Vaupel and Andrews[751] reported its use in one case to treat a chondral defect in the base of the proximal phalanx.

TREATMENT OF ACUTE INJURIES

Partial Tears. There is general agreement that partial tears (sprains) of the ulnar collateral ligament should be treated nonoperatively. We prefer a well-molded thumb spica cast with the MP joint in slight flexion (hyperextension must be avoided) for 3 to 6 weeks, depending on the severity of the injury. Rovere and associates[736] described a fiberglass "mini" thumb spica cast, which they used in hockey players, allowing continued participation

in the sport. Primiano[732] also advocated the use of a modified thumb spica cast that allows full flexion and extension of the wrist.

Complete Tears. Since the publication of Stener's classic article in 1962,[744] there has been increasingly strong support for the operative treatment of all acute ruptures of the ulnar collateral ligament of the thumb[705,715,720,722,728,743] even in the rare case of complete rupture in a child with an open epiphyseal plate.[753] Theoretically, a complete rupture without a Stener lesion can be treated satisfactorily nonoperatively, and Coonrad and Goldner[698] have advocated cast immobilization. However, there are several reasons why we prefer early operative repair of all acute ulnar collateral ligament injuries. (1) The Stener lesion is definitely present in a significant number of cases, and we are not confident that we can differentiate preoperatively the presence or absence of that lesion with any of the currently available modalities. (2) Operative repair of the acute tear is a relatively uncomplicated procedure with minimal morbidity. (3) As is true in ligamentous injuries in other joints, the results of primary repair are better than with any of the late reconstructive operations.[728]

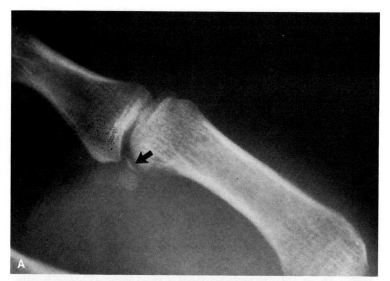

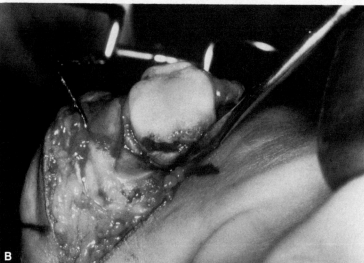

Fig. 7-113. A shear fracture of the metacarpal head (**A**—*arrow*) seen on the x-ray of a patient with a gamekeeper's thumb. These relatively uncommon fractures occur on the radial or volar (**B**) aspect of the metacarpal head and are different from the more typical fracture fragment that is avulsed by the ulnar collateral ligament (see Fig. 7-112).

Associated fractures that are also indications for operative treatment in our opinion are (1) a displaced intra-articular corner fracture involving 25% or more of the articular surface at the base of the proximal phalanx and (2) a small avulsion fracture displaced more than 5 mm. Smith[743] mentioned that volar subluxation of the proximal phalanx is also an indication for surgery.

Operative Technique. The skin incision is centered over the dorsoulnar aspect of the MP joint. Gerber and associates[707] prefer a straight longitudinal incision 1 cm ulnar to the extensor pollicis longus tendon, although this can be gently curved. A dorsal zigzag incision can be used, but the apex of the incision should avoid the transverse skin web to prevent a subsequent scar contracture. Small sensory branches of the radial nerve must be identified and carefully protected throughout the procedure, because a significant incidence of postoperative numbness[712,728,738] and occasional painful neuromas[701] have been reported. The key to the dissection is the adductor aponeurosis, which may be somewhat obscured by the displaced collateral ligament if a Stener lesion is present (see Fig. 7-110). The adductor aponeurosis is carefully divided at its insertion into the dorsal expansion, and both ends are preserved for later repair. The joint capsule is exposed by retracting the dorsal and volar flaps of the hood, and the joint itself is inspected for articular damage; the volar plate and accessory collateral

rotation). The adductor tendon is carefully reattached to the dorsal expansion with 4-0 nonabsorbable sutures. The skin is closed with subcuticular sutures, and a plaster thumb spica splint is applied.

Postoperative Management.   At ten days, the splint and sutures are removed and a thumb spica cast is applied, leaving the IP joint free. The patient must be instructed in active and passive flexion exercises of the distal joint, because stiffness of this joint frequently results from dissection of the extensor hood. At 4 weeks the cast is removed and flexion-extension exercises are instituted for the MP joint; a removable splint is worn to protect the thumb for an

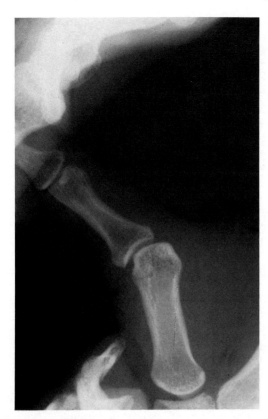

Fig. 7-114. Routine x-rays of the thumb in a patient with a suspected gamekeeper's thumb may show no abnormality. If the slightest amount of instability is found on clinical examination, stress films should be taken to distinguish between a partial and a complete tear. This patient has a complete tear. Note also that the person stressing the thumb is not wearing leaded gloves, an important omission.

ligaments should be inspected as well. If the major (cord) portion of the collateral ligament is torn in its substance, it is repaired with nonabsorbable sutures with the joint in 15° to 20° of flexion. The most common type of pathology is separation of the ligament from the base of the proximal phalanx, with or without a small avulsion fracture. If this is found, the site of attachment of the ligament is roughened with a curette and the ligament is reattached with a pull-out suture over a button on the radial aspect of the thumb (Fig. 7-115). Tiny avulsion fragments are best excised and the ligament advanced into the defect in the proximal phalanx. Large fragments should be anatomically reduced and held with 0.028-inch or 0.035-inch Kirschner wires (two wires are usually necessary to prevent

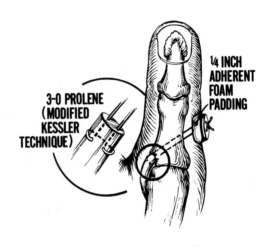

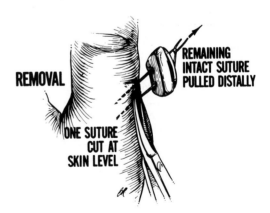

Fig. 7-115. One of us (D.P.G.) prefers this type of pull-out suture over the standard Bunnell pull-out wire. No proximal loop is required, because the suture is pulled distally at the time of removal. Removal of Prolene is considerably less painful for the patient than wire. This type of suture is applicable to any type of situation in which a pull-out suture is required.

additional 2 to 3 weeks. Forceful stress and participation in strenuous athletic activities without splint protection are not allowed until 10 to 12 weeks following the operation, depending on the mobility of the MP joint and the strength of the thumb.

TREATMENT OF CHRONIC INJURIES

If the patient is seen within 2 to 3 weeks of injury, operative repair can usually be accomplished with a reasonable chance of success. Unfortunately, chronic, untreated injuries of the ulnar collateral ligament of the thumb are commonly seen for the first time weeks or months following injury.

Partial Tears.   Untreated sprains of the MP collateral ligaments can produce long-term refractory symptoms, which may be difficult to fully alleviate. If there is no evidence of instability on stress examination, we generally treat these patients with cast immobilization (with or without local steroid injection) for 3 weeks, followed by an intensive course of physical therapy. Perhaps the most important aspect of management of these patients is to make them aware of the chronicity of the problem, emphasizing that it is likely to take several months for their symptoms to subside.

Complete Tears.   The patient with an untreated or inadequately treated rupture of the ulnar collateral ligament with pain and demonstrable instability of the joint is a candidate for reconstruction, since post-traumatic arthritis is likely to develop unless stability is restored. It must be emphasized, however, that no type of soft tissue reconstruction will relieve the patient's pain if post-traumatic arthritis is already established. If preoperative radiographs demonstrate significant arthritic changes, or if significant articular damage is seen at operation, arthrodesis of the MP joint is the treatment of choice.[698,705,710,727]

Several operations have been described for late reconstruction of the ulnar collateral ligament of the thumb. Alldred[689] used a free tendon graft from the fourth toe that was passed through drill holes in the base of the proximal phalanx and head of the metacarpal. Smith[743] advocated a more sophisticated free tendon graft reconstruction, emphasizing the importance of correcting the volar subluxation of the proximal phalanx. He did this by making the transverse drill hole in the proximal phalanx volar to the axis of motion so that the newly created reconstruction of the collateral ligament duplicates the normal ligament by passing distally and volarly from the metacarpal head to

the base of the proximal phalanx. Although Strandell[748] used a free graft in some cases, he also described the use of the extensor pollicis brevis tendon, leaving it attached to its normal insertion and passing the free end through a transverse drill hole in the head of the metacarpal to be reattached to the site of insertion of the original ulnar collateral ligament. Frykman and Johansson[706] employed a slip of the abductor pollicis longus in a similar fashion. Sakellarides and DeWeese[738,740] also used the extensor pollicis brevis, but with a bit more complicated type of reconstruction, and Ahmad and DePalma[688] reported a single case treated with yet another method of using the extensor pollicis brevis. Lamb and Angarita[718] used the palmaris longus tendon left attached at its distal insertion.

Authors' Preferred Method.   We have generally been pleased with the results of the operation described by Neviaser and coworkers,[727] and this is our preference for late reconstruction of the ulnar collateral ligament of the thumb. However, our results with this operation are not as predictable or as uniformly successful as those of primary repair of acute ruptures. Osterman and colleagues[728] reported no functional difference between a free graft and Neviaser's operation but noted slightly less range of motion following the latter.

Operative Technique. The MP joint is exposed through a radially based chevron-type (dorsal zigzag) or gently curved longitudinal incision (see p. 534). The incision must extend far enough volarly to provide good exposure of the adductor tendon, but care must be taken to avoid the transverse skin crease of the web to prevent subsequent scar contracture. Mogensen and Mattsson[725] have noted that the dorsal zigzag incision can be extended across the volar aspect of the joint if necessary. The dorsal sensory nerves are identified and carefully protected throughout the procedure. The tears in the capsule and ligaments are usually bridged by scar, and identification of these structures is more difficult than in the acute repair. Dissection is facilitated by identifying the adductor muscle and tracing its tendon distally to its insertion into the dorsal expansion. The adductor tendon is detached, and care is taken to preserve sufficient tissue to hold a suture. A proximally based U-shaped flap is then created in the scarred, thickened ligament and capsule, leaving it attached to the head of the metacarpal. This flap is advanced distally and sutured into the base of the proximal phalanx with the MP joint in the reduced position (Fig. 7-116). A hole is drilled through the ulnar corner of the proximal phalanx

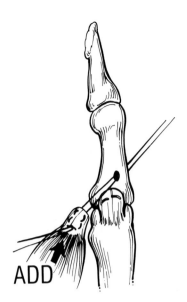

Fig. 7-116. For late reconstruction of ulnar collateral ligament injuries of the MP joint (gamekeeper's thumb), we prefer the technique described by Nevaiser and associates (see text for details). *(Redrawn from Nevaiser, R. I.; Wilson, J. N.; and Lievano, A.: Rupture of the Ulnar Collateral Ligament of the Thumb [Gamekeeper's Thumb]. J. Bone Joint Surg., 53A:1360, 1971.)*

approximately 10 mm distal to the joint, and the adductor tendon is then advanced distally and inserted into this hole with a pull-out suture. Although it is generally not necessary, the MP joint may be stabilized with an obliquely placed 0.045-inch Kirschner wire if the reconstruction seems to be a bit tenuous. One of us (S.A.R.) prefers to use this Kirschner wire in all cases.

Postoperative management is identical to that for acute ligament repair as described on page 535.

Radial Collateral Ligament Injury

Injury of the radial collateral ligament of the MP joint of the thumb is less common than that of the ulnar collateral ligament. Perhaps partly for this reason, the injury is frequently not diagnosed early, and our experience has been that these patients are almost always seen late. Such patients usually present with a tender prominence of the radial aspect of the metacarpal head (Fig. 7-117) and often have pain with activities such as opening a large jar lid or a car door.[695]

Information in the literature is scanty regarding the acute management of such injuries, but anatomically, a situation analogous to the Stener lesion cannot exist on the radial side of the thumb. Theo-

retically, then, nonoperative treatment (cast immobilization) of a complete rupture of the radial collateral ligament is more likely to be successful than similar treatment of an ulnar collateral ligament rupture. However, in one of the few collected series of such patients, Woods and coworkers[755] advised primary repair for complete ruptures.

Authors' Preferred Method of Treatment. For those rare patients in an acute condition with rupture of the radial collateral ligament, we prefer immobilization in a thumb spica cast for 3 to 4 weeks, although one of us (S.A.R.) stabilizes the joint with a percutaneously placed Kirschner wire prior to cast application, and with an additional 2 weeks in the cast following pin removal.

In a few patients seen late with chronic symptomatic joints, we have obtained good results with an operation analogous to the Neviaser reconstruction of the ulnar collateral ligament (see p. 536).

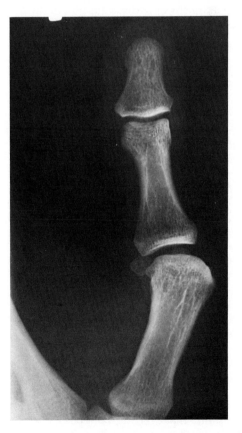

Fig. 7-117. Patients with late, untreated injuries of the *radial* collateral ligament of the MP joint of the thumb usually present with prominence of the radial condyle of the metacarpal.

In this situation, the abductor pollicis brevis is advanced and reinserted approximately 10 mm more distally into the radial aspect of the proximal phalanx. The operation was apparently first suggested by Sutro[749] and more recently advocated by Neviaser and Adams[726] and by Camp and associates.[695] Brewood and Menon[693] have described reconstruction using the extensor pollicis brevis tendon.

Dislocations of the Thumb MP Joint

As in the fingers, dorsal dislocations are more common than volar dislocations in the thumb MP joint. These may be complex (irreducible), usually because of interposition of the volar plate[759] (see p. 521), although entrapment of the flexor pollicis longus has also been reported.[771]

Volar dislocations seem to be almost always associated with collateral ligament ruptures and appear to be more commonly irreducible, owing to interposition of the dorsal capsule and one or both extensor tendons.[761,768,770] Less severe dorsal capsular tears, with or without rupture of the extensor pollicis brevis, have also been reported.[772]

DIAGNOSIS

The most important initial step in management of the dorsal dislocation is to differentiate between a simple and a complex dislocation. As with MP dislocations in the fingers, it is usually possible to make this distinction on the basis of clinical findings rather than to arrive at such a conclusion after repeated successful attempts at closed reduction (see p. 521). The attitude of the finger offers the first clue. In a simple dislocation (subluxation), the phalanx usually rests on the head of the metacarpal in nearly 90° of hyperextension. In the complex dislocation, the proximal phalanx is more nearly parallel to the metacarpal, with only slight hyperextension. The most important diagnostic clinical sign of a complex dislocation is a skin dimple found on the volar aspect of the thenar eminence (Fig. 7-118). Demonstration on x-ray film of a sesamoid within the widened joint space is also pathognomonic of a complex dislocation.

METHODS OF TREATMENT

Simple dislocations of the MP joint can be reduced easily by closed manipulation; complex dislocations cannot. Even in the presence of the pathognomonic skin dimple, however, we believe that a single attempt at closed reduction under adequate anesthesia should be made in all dorsal dislocations of this joint. McLaughlin[591] emphasized the point originally made by Farabeuf[565] that a simple dislocation

can be converted into a complex dislocation by improper reduction. Closed reduction should be performed by first hyperextending the proximal phalanx as far as possible on the metacarpal and then *pushing* against the dorsal surface of the base of the phalanx with the IP joint in flexion. The wrist should be flexed to relax the tension on the flexor tendons. Attempting to reduce the deformity by traction and pulling the phalanx back into position may cause the volar plate to become interposed in the joint, thereby rendering it irreducible.

Following a successful closed reduction, lateral stability of the joint should be carefully tested to check the integrity of the radial and ulnar collateral ligaments. If there is evidence of complete rupture of one of the collateral ligaments, treatment should be directed toward management of this injury, as outlined in the section on injuries of the collateral ligaments on page 533.

Usually the joint will be stable after closed reduction, and protected motion can be started almost immediately. However, 3 to 6 weeks of protection with a removable thumb spica splint may minimize the prolonged MP joint soreness that these patients frequently experience. Few authors advocate immediate repair of the volar plate following a successful closed reduction, since satisfactory healing usually occurs with adequate immobilization. In rare cases, improper healing of the plate may result in chronic pain with either instability in hyperextension or flexion contracture from scarring, necessitating late reconstruction (see Volar Plate Injuries subsequently).

If closed manipulation of the dorsal dislocation fails, the surgeon should be prepared to follow this with an immediate open reduction. The joint is exposed through a volar or dorsal[563] approach, and the entrapped volar plate is extricated from the joint. The tendon of the flexor brevis may also be interposed, and the head of the metacarpal may be found to protrude through the bellies of the thenar intrinsic muscles. In two cases, we have found the tendon of the flexor pollicis longus wrapped around the neck of the metacarpal. Early protected motion should be instituted postoperatively, since stiffness is more common following complex dislocation than it is after a simple dislocation.

Volar Plate Injuries

Relatively little has been written about hyperextension injuries of the MP joint of the thumb.[769] Perhaps the best article is that by Stener[775] in 1963, in which a distinction is made between the passive (volar plate and accessory collateral ligaments) and

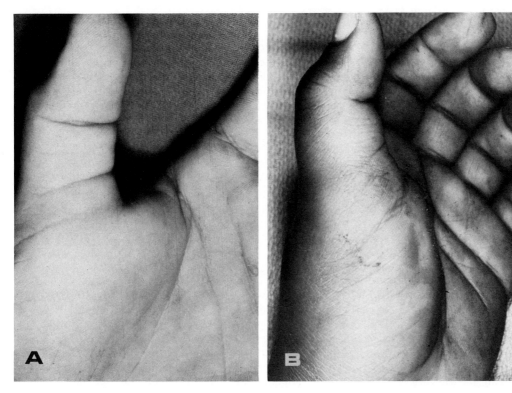

Fig. 7-118. The most important diagnostic clinical sign of a complex dislocation in the thumb is a skin dimple found on the volar aspect of the thenar eminence. (**A**) This patient had a dislocation of the MP joint of the thumb, but no skin dimple was present. This was a simple dislocation that was easily reduced by closed manipulation. (**B**) This patient also had a dislocation of the MP joint of the thumb, but the characteristic skin dimple was present over the thenar eminence. Closed reduction was unsuccessful, and open reduction, which revealed interposition of the volar plate in the joint, confirmed the diagnosis of the complex dislocation.

active (adductor pollicis and flexor pollicis brevis) restraints to hyperextension of the joint. Diagnosis is made by well-localized tenderness over the volar aspect of the joint and excessive hyperextension of the joint. Pain on passive hyperextension is a good diagnostic sign, but if pain limits mobility in the joint, the examination must be performed under anesthesia (local infiltration or, preferably, median plus radial wrist block) to obtain a reliable test. Hyperextension should be compared with the opposite uninjured thumb and tested with the IP joint flexed to relax the flexor pollicis longus.

Stener has suggested that the position of the sesamoids may aid in differentiating between volar plate rupture and tear of the intrinsic muscles; if the sesamoids are displaced distally with the proximal phalanx on hyperextension stress, muscle tear should be suspected. He suggested that muscle rupture should be treated operatively.

Yamanaka and colleagues[779] reported a surprisingly large series of patients with "locking" of the MP joint of the thumb, which they identified as a different entity from the complex MP dislocation. In their 23 patients, the volar plate and radial sesamoid became "hung up" on the more prominent radial condyle of the metacarpal head. In 7 patients, successful reduction was achieved by manipulation, but 16 required open reduction; they advised a radial midlateral approach. Several other reports of locking of the MP joint have appeared, and it is curious that all of these have been by Japanese authors.[763,766,777]

TREATMENT OF ACUTE INJURIES

Despite Stener's studies noted previously, there appears to be little support for his recommendation of primary repair of acute hyperextension injuries of the thumb. Most of these can probably be treated satisfactorily with thumb spica immobilization for 3 to 4 weeks, holding the MP joint in 15° to 20° of flexion.

TREATMENT OF CHRONIC INJURIES

Chronic hyperextension instability of the MP joint of the thumb can cause pain with grasping and pinching. Posner and associates[773] have pointed out that it is important to differentiate a patient who has passive instability due to chronic volar plate injury from a patient who can actively hyperextend the MP joint. The latter individual can stabilize the thumb in flexion when grasping or pinching, but the patient with passive instability cannot.

Although this is a relatively uncommon entity, we have treated several patients in whom this created a painful and functional problem. Operative treatment is required if the patient does not respond to nonoperative modalities (splinting, anti-inflammatory medications, and local injections).

Most of our operative experience has been with volar plate capsulodesis, the idea for which was probably first suggested by Milch[767] in 1929. We have used Zancolli's procedure,[780] although it is technically more difficult in the thumb than in the finger MP joints because of the very large sesamoids in the thumb. If the standard Zancolli technique is used, it is important to suture the proximal end of the volar plate into bone with a pull-out suture. A modification of that technique is to denude the articular cartilage from the sesamoids and create a surgical synostosis between the sesamoids and the metacarpal neck.

Posner and associates[773] have treated this problem with a 1.5-cm advancement of the insertions of the abductor and flexor pollicis brevis, and Kessler[765] has created a crisscross sling across the volar aspect of the MP joint using the full length of the extensor pollicis brevis tendon (left attached at its insertion). Eiken[760] used the palmaris longus tendon left attached at its insertion and passed along the volar aspect of the thumb to the base of the proximal phalanx.

Sesamoid Fractures

Fractures of the sesamoids are uncommon but need to be considered in the differential diagnosis of injuries of the MP joint of the thumb. Most people have five sesamoids in each hand: two at the thumb MP joint, one at the thumb IP joint, and one each at the MP joints of the index and little fingers.[778] Although the latter three may occasionally be absent, the two thumb MP sesamoids are present in virtually 100% of the population,[778] and in this lo-

cation they are found within the volar plate.[572] Bipartite sesamoids have been reported and should be differentiated from fractures.[762,774]

Sesamoids can apparently be fractured by direct trauma[774] or hyperextension injury,[775,757] and Stener[775] has pointed out that the latter mechanism may result in disruption of the volar plate. Arthrography has been used to demonstrate a tear in the volar plate in association with a sesamoid fracture.[757]

Although Stener[775] advocated surgical repair of sesamoid fractures, most of the case reports in the literature have been treated with simple immobilization for 3 to 5 weeks.[757,758,762,764,774,776]

CMC JOINT OF THE THUMB

Anatomy

The CMC joint of the thumb is classically described as a saddle joint, although Eaton and Littler[787] have noted that it is actually formed by two apposing saddles. The base of the first metacarpal is convex in the transverse (radioulnar) plane and concave in the vertical (dorsovolar) plate; the trapezium is concave in the transverse plane and convex in the vertical plane. The volar lip of the metacarpal is somewhat elongated, providing attachment for the volar (anterior oblique) ligament to the tubercle of the trapezium.

Despite a number of scholarly studies,[781,782,789,793,797,799] the ligamentous anatomy of this joint remains somewhat confusing because of differences in terminology and the relative importance relegated to the various ligaments. Eaton and Littler[787] consider the volar (anterior oblique) ligament to be the key structure maintaining thumb stability. Pagalidis and associates[798] and Bojsen-Moller[781] concluded that the most important structure is the first intermetacarpal ligament. It originates from the dorsoradial aspect of the second metacarpal base near the insertion of the extensor carpi radialis longus tendon, and inserts as a broad, fan-shaped bundle into the ulnar aspect of the base of the first metacarpal, usually blending with the anterior and posterior oblique ligaments into the volar-ulnar tubercle of the first metacarpal. They interpreted the function of this ligament as having an important checkrein effect on the base of the first metacarpal to limit radial displacement.

The capsular and ligamentous attachments of the joint are relatively lax, allowing rotation of the thumb metacarpal on the trapezium. Rotation is blocked when the two saddles are tightly apposed

to each other; the ligaments allow sufficient distraction of the two surfaces to permit rotation, while
at the same time becoming taut enough in this
elongated position to guide and limit axial rotation.[793]

A true anteroposterior view (Robert view[794]) is
necessary to show the CMC joint adequately; it
is taken with the hand in maximum pronation
(Fig. 7-119).

Dislocation of the CMC Joint of the Thumb

MECHANISM OF INJURY

Pure dislocations of the CMC joint of the thumb
are uncommon. The mechanism appears to be a
longitudinally directed force with the metacarpal
in slight flexion, allowing the base of the metacarpal
to be levered out in a dorsoradial direction. Because
of the strong attachment of the anterior oblique
ligament (and probably also the first intermetacarpal ligament), this mechanism is more likely to
fracture the volar beak of the metacarpal, resulting
in a Bennett's fracture-subluxation of the joint (see
p. 494). In the less common pure dislocation of the
CMC joint, a tiny fragment of bone may be avulsed
off the base of the metacarpal by the anterior
oblique ligament.[802,803]

TREATMENT OF ACUTE INJURIES

A pure dislocation of the CMC joint of the thumb
without associated fracture (Fig. 7-120) is a deceptively difficult injury to treat. Closed reduction is
simple but may be extremely unstable. Even when
the joint is temporarily stabilized after reduction
with percutaneous pin fixation, the results are not
entirely predictable, and residual subluxation or

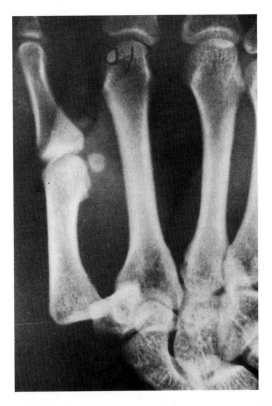

Fig. 7-120. A pure dislocation of the CMC joint of the thumb without associated fracture is an uncommon injury. Closed reduction is easily achieved but extremely unstable.

frank dislocation may recur after removal of
the pins.

The unpredictable and often poor results with
closed reduction led Burkhalter[783] to explore several
of these injuries acutely in an effort to more clearly
understand the pathologic anatomy. Similar to
other authors who have operated on these injuries,[792,800,803] he found that the volar ligament was
intact. Burkhalter further noted that a sleeve of
periosteum was present and that hyperpronation
of the thumb metacarpal reduced the bone into this
periosteal tube. Concluding that supination was an
important element in the mechanism of injury,
Burkhalter treated several subsequent patients with
hyperpronation of the joint combined with percutaneous pin fixation for 6 weeks.

If Burkhalter's observations are correct and the
volar ligament is intact, then open reduction would
not appear to offer any particular advantage, except
perhaps in the rare situation of simultaneous MP
and CMC dislocation as reported by Moore and associates.[796]

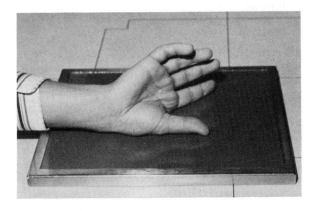

Fig. 7-119. A true anteroposterior view (Robert view) is necessary to adequately show the CMC joint of the thumb. It is taken with the hand in extreme pronation.

In the largest series of these injuries reported (12 patients), Watt and Hooper[802] found that closed reduction and cast immobilization were successful in some cases. However, they pointed out the importance of assessing stability of the joint immediately following reduction and of using a thumb spica cast alone only if the joint is stable. In their series, the best results were achieved in those patients treated on the day of injury.

Authors' Preferred Method of Treatment.   Our experience with this uncommon injury is limited, but on the basis of Burkhalter's observations, our preference is closed reduction with the thumb hyperpronated, supplemented with percutaneously placed Kirschner wires. A thumb spica cast is worn for 4 to 6 weeks, at which time the pins are removed, but the joint is protected for 8 to 10 weeks.

TREATMENT OF CHRONIC INJURIES

In dealing with chronic subluxation of the CMC joint of the thumb, the surgeon should differentiate between post-traumatic and idiopathic subluxation. The latter, seen primarily in women and associated with degenerative arthritis, is far more common than instability of the joint resulting from a single traumatic episode, which is seen predominantly in men.

Chronic post-traumatic instability of the basilar joint of the thumb is so uncommon that virtually everything in the literature regarding treatment is in the form of single case reports. Attempts to stabilize the joint with various forms of free tendon grafts and tenodesis have been reported by Slocum,[801] Eggers,[788] Kestler,[792] Cho,[785] and Jensen.[791] The only technique that has been reported with any reasonably adequate number of patients and follow-up is that described by Eaton and Littler,[787] although even in their series most of the patients had the idiopathic degenerative type of subluxation. Other authors[784,802] have reported successful treatment of chronic CMC dislocations using this method of stabilizing the joint with a strip of flexor carpi radialis tendon, and Magnusson and associates[795] have described a slight modification of the Eaton and Littler procedure.

It must be emphasized that if significant arthritis is present in the CMC joint, this tendon reconstruction procedure is not likely to be successful, and arthroplasty or arthrodesis of the joint should be considered.

REFERENCES

Anatomy

1. Allen, E.V.: Thromboangiitis Obliterans: Methods of Diagnosis of Chronic Occlusive Arterial Lesions Distal to the Wrist With Illustrative Cases. Am. J. Med. Sci., 178: 237–244, 1929.
2. Cleland, J.: On the Cutaneous Ligaments of the Phalanges. J. Anat. Physiol., 12:526, 1878.
3. Eaton, R.G.: Joint Injuries of the Hand. Springfield, Ill., Charles C. Thomas, 1971.
4. Eyler, D.L., and Markee, J.E.: The Anatomy and Function of the Intrinsic Musculature of the Fingers. J. Bone Joint Surg., 36A:1–9; 18–20, 1954.
5. Flatt, A.E.: The Care of Minor Hand Injuries, pp. 15–16. St. Louis, C.V. Mosby, 1959.
6. Gad, P.: The Anatomy of the Volar Part of the Capsules of the Finger Joints. J. Bone Joint Surg., 49B:362–367, 1967.
7. Goss, C.M.: Gray's Anatomy, 26th ed., pp. 322–325, 371–372. Philadelphia, Lea & Febiger, 1954.
8. Grayson, J.: The Cutaneous Ligaments of the Digits. J. Anat., 75:164–165, 1941.
9. Haines, R.W.: The Extensor Apparatus of the Finger. J. Anat., 85:251–259, 1951.
10. Kaplan, E.B.: Functional and Surgical Anatomy of the Hand, 2nd ed. Philadelphia, J.B. Lippincott, 1965.
11. Kuczynski, K.: The Proximal Interphalangeal Joint: Anatomy and Causes of Stiffness in the Fingers. J. Bone Joint Surg., 50B:656–663, 1968.
12. Landsmeer, J.M.F.: Anatomical and Functional Investigations of the Human Finger, and Its Functional Significance. Acta Anat. [Suppl.], 24:1–69, 1955.
13. Milford, L.W.: Retaining Ligaments of the Digits of the Hand. Gross and Microscopic Anatomic Study. Philadelphia, W.B. Saunders, 1968.
14. Smith, R.J.: Non-ischemic Contractures of the Intrinsic Muscles of the Hand. J. Bone Joint Surg., 53A:1313–1331, 1971.
15. Tubiana, R., and Valentin, P.: The Anatomy of the Extensor Apparatus of the Fingers. Surg. Clin. North Am., 44:897–918, 1964.

Fractures of the Phalanges and Metacarpals (Excluding the Thumb)

16. Abdon, P.; Muhlow, A.; Stigsson, L.; Thorngren, K.G.; and Werner, C.O.: Subcapital Fractures of the Fifth Metacarpal Bone. Arch. Orthop. Trauma Surg., 103:231–234, 1984.
17. Alexander, H.; Langrana, N.; Massengill, J.B.; and Weiss, A.B.: Development of New Methods for Phalangeal Fracture Fixation. J. Biomech., 14:377–387, 1981.
18. Arafa, M.; Haines, J.; Noble, J.; and Carden, D.: Immediate Mobilization of Fractures of the Neck of the Fifth Metacarpal. Injury, 17:277–278, 1986.
19. Barton, N.J.: Fractures of the Shafts of the Phalanges of the Hand. Hand, 11:119–133, 1979.
20. Barton, N.J.: Fractures of the Hand (Review Article). J. Bone Joint Surg., 66B:159–167, 1984.

21. Belpomme, C.: External Osteosynthesis of Distal Fractures of the Phalanges by Reposition-fixation of the Fingernail. Int. Surg., 60:219–222, 1975.

22. Belsky, M.R.; Eaton, R.G.; and Lane L.B.: Closed Reduction and Internal Fixation of Proximal Phalangeal Fractures. J. Hand Surg., 9A:725–729, 1984.

23. Belsole, R.: Physiological Fixation of Displaced and Unstable Fractures of the Hand. Orthop. Clin. North Am., 11:393–404, 1980.

24. Berkman, E.F., and Miles, G.H.: Internal Fixation of Metacarpal Fractures Exclusive of the Thumb. J. Bone Joint Surg., 25:816–821, 1943.

25. Bilos, Z.J.: Compression Pin Fixation of Articular Phalangeal Fractures. Orthop. Rev., 12:125–127, 1983.

26. Bilos, Z.J., and Eskestrand, T.: External Fixator Use in Comminuted Gunshot Fractures of the Proximal Phalanx. J. Hand Surg., 4:357–359, 1979.

27. Black, D.M.; Mann, R.J.; Constine, R.; and Daniels, A.U.: Comparison of Internal Fixation Techniques in Metacarpal Fractures. J. Hand. Surg., 10A:466–472, 1985.

28. Black, D.M.; Mann, R.J.; Constine, R.M.; and Daniels, A.U.: The Stability of Internal Fixation in the Proximal Phalanx. J. Hand. Surg., 11A:672–677, 1986.

29. Blalock, H.S.; Pearce, H.L.; Kleinert, H.; and Kutz, J.: An Instrument Designed to Help Reduce and Percutaneously Pin Fractured Phalanges. J. Bone Joint Surg., 57A:792–794, 1975.

30. Blazina, M.E., and Lane, C.: Rupture of the Flexor Digitorum Profundus Tendon in Student Athletes. J. Am. Coll. Health, 14:248–249, 1966.

31. Bloem, J.J.A.M.: The Treatment and Prognosis of Uncomplicated Dislocated Fractures of the Metacarpals and Phalanges. Arch. Chir. Neerl. 23:55–65, 1971.

32. Bohler, L.: The Treatment of Fractures, pp. 98–104. Vienna, Wilhelm Maudrich, 1929.

33. Bohler, L.: The Treatment of Fractures, 5th ed., pp. 898–971. New York, Grune & Stratton, 1956.

34. Borden, J.: Complications of Fractures and Ligamentous Injuries of the Hand. Orthop. Rev., 1:29–38, 1972.

35. Borgeskov, S.: Conservative Therapy for Fractures of the Phalanges and Metacarpals. Acta Chir. Scand., 133:123–130, 1967.

36. Bosworth, D.M.: Internal Splinting of Fractures of the Fifth Metacarpal. J. Bone Joint Surg., 19:826–827, 1937.

37. Botelheiro, J.C.: Overlapping of Fingers due to a Malunion of a Phalanx Corrected by a Metacarpal Rotational Osteotomy—Report of Two Cases. J. Hand Surg., 10B:389–390, 1985.

38. Boyes, J.H.: Bunnell's Surgery of the Hand, 3rd ed. Philadelphia, J.B. Lippincott, 1956.

39. Boyes, J.H.: Bunnell's Surgery of the Hand, 4th ed. Philadelphia, J.B. Lippincott, 1964.

40. Boyes, J.H.: Bunnell's Surgery of the Hand, 5th ed. Philadelphia, J.B. Lippincott, 1970.

41. Boyes, J.H.; Wilson, J.N.; and Smith, J.W.: Flexor Tendon Ruptures in the Forearm and Hand. J. Bone Joint Surg., 42A:637–646, 1960.

42. Brefort, G.; Condamine, J.L.; and Aubriot, J.H.: Functional Results of Seventy-six Cases of Phalangeal and Metacarpal Fractures Studied Using a Hand Emergency Computer Card System. Ann. Chir., 5:25–35, 1986.

43. Brennwald, J.: Bone Healing in the Hand. Clin. Orthop., 214:7–10, 1987.

44. Brown, H.: Closed Crush Injuries of the Hand and Forearm. Orthop. Clin. North Am., 1:253–259, 1970.

45. Brunet, M.E.; and Haddad, R.J.: Fractures and Dislocations of the Metacarpals and Phalanges. Clin. Sports Med., 5:773–781, 1986.

46. Buchler, U.; and Fischer, T.: Use of a Minicondylar Plate for Metacarpal and Phalangeal Periarticular Injuries. Clin. Orthop., 214:53–58, 1987.

47. Bunnell, S.: Surgery of the Hand. Philadelphia, J.B. Lippincott, 1944.

48. Burkhalter, W.E.; Butler, B.; Metz, W.; and Omer, G.: Experiences With Delayed Primary Closure of War Wounds of the Hand in Viet Nam. J. Bone Joint Surg., 50A:945–954, 1968.

49. Burkhalter, W.E.; and Reyes, F.A.: Closed Treatment of Fractures of the Hand. Bull. Hosp. J. Dis. 44:145–162, 1984.

50. Burnham, P.J.: Physiological Treatment for Fractures of the Metacarpals and Phalanges. J.A.M.A., 169:663–666, 1959.

51. Burton, R.I., and Eaton, R.G.: Common Hand Injuries in the Athlete. Orthop. Clin. North Am., 4:809–838, 1973.

52. Buscemi, M.J., and Page, B.J.: Flexor Digitorum Profundus Avulsions With Associated Distal Phalanx Fractures. Am. J. Sports Med., 15:366–370, 1987.

53. Butt, W.D.: Rigid Wire Fixation of Fractures of the Hand. Henry Ford Hosp. Bull., 4:134–143, 1956.

54. Butt, W.D.: Fractures of the Hand: I. Description. Can. Med. Assoc. J., 86:731–735, 1962.

55. Butt, W.D.: Fractures of the Hand: II. Statistical Review. Can. Med. Assoc. J., 86:775–779, 1962.

56. Butt, W.D.: Fractures of the Hand: III. Treatment and Results. Can. Med. Assoc. J., 86:815–822, 1962.

57. Bynum, D.K., and Gilbert, J.A.: Avulsion of the Flexor Digitorum Profundus: Anatomic and Biomechanical Considerations. J. Hand Surg., 13A:222–227, 1988.

58. Caffee, H.H.: Atraumatic Placement of Kirschner Wires. Plast. Reconstr. Surg., 63:433, 1979.

59. Campbell Reid, D.A.: Corrective Osteotomy in the Hand. Hand, 6:50–57, 1974.

60. Carr, R.W.: A Finger Caliper for Reduction of Phalangeal and Metacarpal Fractures by Skeletal Traction. South. Med. J., 32:543–546, 1939.

61. Carroll, R.E., and Match, R.M.: Avulsion of the Flexor Profundus Tendon Insertion. J. Trauma, 10:1109–1118, 1970.

62. Caspi, I.; Engel, J.; and Lin, E.: Intra-articular Bone Formation in Hand Following Wire Fixation. Orthop. Rev., 13:91–92, 1984.

63. Chang, W.H.J.; Thomas, O.J.; and White, W.L.: Avulsion Injury of the Long Flexor Tendons. Plast. Reconstr. Surg., 50:260–264, 1972.

64. Chasmar, L.R.: Metacarpal and Phalangeal Fractures. American Society for Surgery of the Hand, Correspondence Newsletter, 1975.

65. Chuinard, R.G., and D'Ambrosia, R.D.: Tooth Wounds and the Infected Fist. J. Bone Joint Surg., 59A:416–418, 1977.

66. Clifford, R.H.: Intramedullary Wire Fixation of Hand Fractures. Plast. Reconstr. Surg., 11:366–371, 1953.

67. Clinkscales, G.S., Jr.: Complications in the Management of Fractures in Hand Injuries. South. Med. J., 63:704–707, 1970.

68. Conolly, W.B.: The Spontaneous Healing of Hand Wounds. Aust. N.Z. J. Surg., 44:393–395, 1974.

69. Conwell, H.E., and Reynolds, F.C.: Key and Conwell's Management of Fractures, Dislocations, and Sprains, 7th ed. St. Louis, C.V. Mosby, 1961.

70. Coonrad, R.W., and Pohlman, M.H.: Impacted Fractures in the Proximal Portion of the Proximal Phalanx of the Finger. J. Bone Joint Surg., 51A:1291–1296, 1969.

71. Cordrey, L.J.: Intramedullary "Pull-out" Wire Fixation in Surgery of the Hand. Arch. Surg., 8:51–64, 1981.

72. Cotton, F.J.: Dislocations and Joint Fractures, 2nd ed. Philadelphia, W.B. Saunders, 1924.

73. Crawford, G.P.: Screw Fixation for Certain Fractures of the Phalanges and Metacarpals. J. Bone Joint Surg., 58A:487–492, 1976.

74. Crichlow, T.P.K.R., and Hoskinson, J.: Avulsion Fracture of the Index Metacarpal Base: Three Case Reports. J. Hand Surg., 13B:212–214, 1988.

75. Crockett, D.J.: Rigid Fixation of Bones of the Hand Using K-wires Bonded With Acrylic Resin. Hand, 6:106–107, 1974.

76. Culver, J.E.: American Society for Surgery of the Hand, Correspondence Newsletter, 1981.

77. Culver, J.E.; Stanley, E.A.; Amy, E.L.; and Weiker, G.G.: Avulsion of the Profundus and Superficialis Tendons of the Ring Finger. Am. J. Sports Med., 9:184–186, 1981.

78. Curry, G.J.: Treatment of Finger Fractures, Simple and Compound. Finger Amputations. Am. J. Surg., 71:80–83, 1946.

79. Dabezies, E.J., and Schutte, J.P.: Fixation of Metacarpal and Phalangeal Fractures With Miniature Plates and Screws. J. Hand Surg., 11A:283–288, 1986.

80. DaCruz, D.J.; Slade, R.J.; and Malone, W.: Fractures of the Distal Phalanges. J. Hand Surg., 13B:350–352, 1988.

81. Davis, G.D.: A Ball Splint for Hand Fractures. Int. Clin. 1:182–183, 1928.

82. DeLee, J.C.: Avulsion Fracture of the Base of the Second Metacarpal by the Extensor Carpi Radialis Longus. J. Bone Joint Surg., 61A:445–446, 1979.

83. Dickson, R.A.: Rigid Fixation of Unstable Metacarpal Fractures Using Transverse K-wires Bonded With Acrylic Resin. Hand, 7:284–286, 1975.

84. Diwaker, H.N., and Stothard, J.: The Role of Internal Fixation in Closed Fractures of the Proximal Phalanges and Metacarpals in Adults. J. Hand Surg., 11B:103–108, 1986.

85. Dobyns, J.H.: Articular Fractures of the Hand (Abstr.). J. Bone Joint Surg., 48A:610, 1966.

86. Dobyns, J.H.; Linscheid, R.L., and Cooney, W.P.: Fractures and Dislocations of the Wrist and Hand, Then and Now. J. Hand Surg., 8(2):687–690, 1983.

87. Dugas, R., and D'Ambrosia, R.: Civilian Gunshot Wounds. Orthopedics, 8:1121–1125, 1985.

88. Duncan, J., and Kettelkamp, D.B.: Low-velocity Gunshot Wounds of the Hand. Arch. Surg., 109:395–398, 1974.

89. Eaton, R.G.: The Dangerous Chip Fracture in Athletes. Instr. Course Lect., 34:314–322, 1985.

90. Edwards, G.S.; O'Brien, E.T.; and Heckman, M.M.: Retrograde Cross-pinning of Transverse Metacarpal and Phalangeal Fractures. Hand, 14:141–148, 1982.

91. Eichenholtz, S.N.; and Rizzo, P.C.: Fracture of the Neck of the Fifth Metacarpal Bone—Is Overtreatment Justified? J.A.M.A., 178:151–152, 1961.

92. Elton, R.C., and Bouzard, W.C.: Gunshot and Fragment Wounds of the Metacarpus. South. Med. J., 68:833–843, 1975.

93. Emmett, J.E., and Breck, L.W.: A Review of Analysis of 11,000 Fractures Seen in a Private Practice of Orthopaedic Surgery, 1937–1957. J. Bone Joint Surg., 40A:1169–1175, 1958.

94. Fambrough, R.A., and Green, D.P.: Tendon Rupture as a Complication of Screw Fixation in Fractures in the Hand. A Case Report. J. Bone Joint Surg., 61A:781–782, 1979.

95. Ferraro, M.C.; Coppola, A.; Lippman, K.; and Hurst, L.C.: Closed Functional Bracing of Metacarpal Fractures. Orthop. Rev., 12:49–56, 1983.

96. Fitzgerald, J.A.W., and Khan, M.A.: The Conservative Management of Fractures of the Shafts of the Phalanges of the Fingers by Combined Traction-splintage. J. Hand Surg., 9B:303–306, 1984.

97. Flatt, A.E.: Closed and Open Fractures of the Hand. Postgrad. Med. J., 7:17–26, 1966.

98. Ford, D.J.; El-Hadidi, S.; Lunn, P.G.; and Burke, F.D.: Fractures of the Phalanges: Results of Internal Fixation Using 1.5 mm and 2 mm A.O. Screws. J. Hand. Surg., 12B:28–33, 1987.

99. Freeland, A.E.: External Fixation for Skeletal Stabilization of Severe Open Fractures of the Hand. Clin. Orthop., 214:93–100, 1987.

100. Freeland, A.E.; Jabaley, M.E.; Burkhalter, W.E.; and Chaves, A.M.V.: Delayed Primary Bone Grafting in the Hand and Wrist After Traumatic Bone Loss. J. Hand Surg., 9A:22–28, 1984.

101. Froimson, A.I.: Osteotomy for Digital Deformity. J. Hand Surg., 6:585–589, 1981.

102. Fyfe, I.S., and Mason, S.: The Mechanical Stability of Internal Fixation of Fractured Phalanges. Hand, 11:50–54, 1979.

103. Gingrass, R.P.; Fehring, B.; and Matloub, H.: Intraosseous Wiring of Complex Hand Fractures. Plast. Reconst. Surg., 66:383–394, 1980.

104. Glasgow, M., and Lloyd, G.J.: The Use of Modified A.O. Reduction Forceps in Percutaneous Fracture Fixation. Hand, 13:214–216, 1981.

105. Goldberg, D.: Metacarpal Fractures: A New Instrument for the Maintenance of Position After Reduction. Am. J. Surg., 72:758–766, 1945.

106. Goldberg, D.: Closed Functional Bracing of Metacarpal Fractures. Orthop. Rev., 13:139–141, 1984.

107. Gordon, L., and Monsanto, E.H.: Acute Vascular Compromise After Avulsion of the Distal Phalanx With the Flexor Digitorum Profundus Tendon. J. Hand Surg., 12A:259–261, 1987.

108. Gould, W.L.; Belsole, R.J.; and Skelton, W.H.: Tension-band Stabilization of Transverse Fractures: An Experimental Analysis. Plast. Reconst. Surg., 73:111–115, 1984.

109. Granberry, W.M.: Gunshot Wounds of the Hand. Hand, 5:220–228, 1973.

110. Green, D.P.: Non-articular Hand Fractures. The Case for Percutaneous Pinning. In Neviaser, R.J. (ed): Controversies in Hand Surgery. New York, Churchill Livingstone, 1990.

111. Green, D.P.: Commonly Missed Injuries in the Hand. Am. Fam. Physician, 7:111–119, 1973.

112. Green, D.P.: Complications of Phalangeal and Metacarpal Fractures. Hand Clin., 2:307–328, 1986.

113. Green, D.P., and Anderson, J.R.: Closed Reduction and Percutaneous Pin Fixation of Fracture Phalanges. J. Bone Joint Surg., 55A:1651–1654, 1973.

114. Greene, T.L.; Noellert, R.C.; and Belsole, R.J.: Treatment of Unstable Metacarpal and Phalangeal Fractures With Tension Band Wiring Techniques. Clin. Orthop., 214:78–84, 1987.

115. Gropper, P.T., and Bowen, V.: Cerclage Wiring of Metacarpal Fractures. Clin. Orthop., 188:203–207, 1984.

116. Gross, M.S., and Gelberman, R.H.: Metacarpal Rotational Osteotomy. J. Hand Surg., 10A:105–108, 1985.

117. Grundberg, A.B.: Intramedullary Fixation for Fractures of the Hand. J. Hand Surg., 6:568–573, 1981.

118. Gunter, G.S.: Traumatic Avulsion of the Insertion of Flexor Digitorum Profundus. Aust. N.Z. J. Surg., 30:1–8, 1960.

119. Haggart, G.E.: Fractures of the Metacarpal, Metatarsal Bones, and Phalanges Treated by Skeletal Traction. Surg. Clin North Am., 14:1203–1210, 1934.

120. Hall, R.F.: Closed Flexible Intramedullary Rodding of Metacarpal and Phalangeal Fractures. Orthop. Trans., 8:187–188, 1984.

121. Hall, R.F.: Treatment of Metacarpal and Phalangeal Fractures in Noncompliant Patients. Clin. Orthop., 214:31–36, 1987.

122. Hasham, A.I.: Closed Flexor Profundus Injury. J. Trauma, 15:1067–1068, 1975.

123. Hastings, H.: Unstable Metacarpal and Phalangeal Fracture Treatment With Screws and Plates. Clin. Orthop. 214:37–52, 1987.

124. Hawkins, L.G.: Splint Bracing for Unstable Proximal Diaphyseal and Metaphyseal Fractures of the Proximal Phalanx. Correspondence Newsletter, 1982.

125. Hedeboe, J.: Subcapital Fractures of the Fifth Metacarpal. A Classic Method of Treatment Is Abandoned. Ugeskr. Laeger 138:1766–1768, 1976.

126. Heim, U., and Pfeiffer, K.M.: Small Fragment Set Manual. Technique Recommended by the ASIF Group. New York, Springer-Verlag, 1982.

127. Holst-Nielsen, F.: Subcapital Fractures of the Four Ulnar Metacarpal Bones. Hand, 8:290–293, 1976.

128. Howard, L.D., Jr.: The Problem of Metacarpal Fractures of the Hand Due to War Wounds. Instr. Course Lect., 2:196–201, 1944.

129. Howard, L.D., Jr.: Fractures of the Small Bones of the Hand. Plast. Reconstr. Surg., 29:334–334, 1962.

130. Huffaker, W.H.; Wray, R.C.; and Weeks, P.M.: Factors Influencing Final Range of Motion in the Fingers After Fractures of the Hand. Plast. Reconstr. Surg., 63:82–87, 1979.

131. Hunter, J.M., and Cowan, N.J.: Fifth Metacarpal Fractures in a Compensation Clinic Population. A Report on 133 Cases. J. Bone Joint Surg., 52A:1159–1165, 1970.

132. Ikuta, Y., and Tsuge, K.: Micro-bolts and Micro-screws for Fixation of Small Bones in the Hand. Hand, 6:261–265, 1974.

133. Iselin, F., and Thevenin, R.: Fixation of Fractures of the Digits With Intramedullary Flexible Screws. J. Bone Joint Surg., 56A:1096, 1974.

134. Iselin, M.: Avulsion Injuries of the Nail. In Pierre, M. (ed.): The Nail (G.E.M. Monograph), 1st ed. Edinburgh, Churchill Livingstone, 1981.

135. Itoh, Y.; Uchinishi, K.; and Oka, Y.: Treatment of Pseudoarthrosis of the Distal Phalanx With the Palmar Midline Approach. J. Hand Surg., 8:80–84, 1983.

136. Jabaley, M.E., and Freeland, A.E.: Rigid Internal Fixation in the Hand: 104 Cases. Plast. Reconst. Surg., 77:288–298, 1986.

137. Jablon, M.: Articular Fractures and Dislocations in the Hand. Orthop. Rev. 11:61–70, 1982.

138. Jahss, S.A.: Fractures of the Proximal Phalanges: Alignment and Immobilization. J. Bone Joint Surg., 18:726–731, 1936.

139. Jahss, S.A.: Fractures of the Metacarpals: A New Method of Reduction and Immobilization. J. Bone Joint Surg., 20:178–186, 1938.

140. James, J.I.P.: Fractures of the Proximal and Middle Phalanges of the Fingers. Acta Orthop. Scand., 32:401–412, 1962.

141. James, J.I.P.: Common, Single Errors in the Management of Hand Injuries. Proc. R. Soc. Med., 63:69–71, 1970.

142. James, J.I.P., and Wright, T.A.: Fractures of Metacarpals and Proximal and Middle Phalanges of the Finger. J. Bone Joint Surg., 48B:181–182, 1966.

143. Jones, W.W.: Biomechanics of Small Bone Fixation. Clin. Orthop., 214:11–18, 1987.

144. Jordan, S.E., and Greider, J.L.: The Angiocatheter in the Management of Hand Injuries. J. Hand Surg., 11A:446, 1986.

145. Joshi, B.B.: Percutaneous Internal Fixation of Fractures of the Proximal Phalanges. Hand, 8:86–92, 1976.

146. Jupiter, J.B., and Sheppard, J.E.: Tension Wire Fixation of Avulsion Fractures in the Hand. Clin. Orthop., 214:113–120, 1987.

147. Jupiter, J.B.; Koniuch, M.P.; and Smith, R.J.: The Management of Delayed Union and Nonunion of the Metacarpals and Phalanges. J. Hand Surg., 10A:457–466, 1985.

148. Kaplan, L.: The Treatment of Fractures and Dislocations of the Hand and Fingers. Technic of Unpadded Casts for Carpal Metacarpal and Phalangeal Fractures. Surg. Clin. North Am., 20:1695–1720, 1940.

149. Karbelnig, M.J.: Fracture of the Metacarpal Shaft: A Method of Treatment. Calif. Med., 98:269–270, 1963.

150. Kaye, J.J. and Lister, G.D.: Another Use for the Brewerton View (Letter). J. Hand Surg., 3:603, 1978.

151. Kelikian, H.: Osteotomy of the Finger. A Case Report. Bull. Northwestern Univ. Med. School, 21:111–114, 1947.

152. Kessler, I.; Hecht, O.; and Baruch, A.: Distraction-length-

ening of Digital Rays in the Management of the Injured Hand. J. Bone Joint Surg., 61A:83–87, 1979.

153. Key, J.A., and Conwell, H.E.: The Management of Fractures, Dislocations, and Sprains, 5th ed. St. Louis, C.V. Mosby, 1951.

154. Kilbourne, B.C.: Management of Complicated Hand Fractures. Surg. Clin. North Am., 48:201–213, 1968.

155. Kilbourne, B.C., and Paul, E.G.: The Use of Small Bone Screws in the Treatment of Metacarpal, Metatarsal and Phalangeal Fractures. J. Bone Joint Surg., 40A:375–383, 1958.

156. King, T.: Principles in the Treatment of Hand Fractures as Shown in the Technique for a Closed Fracture of the Metacarpal Neck. Med. J. Aust. 1:570–573, 1962.

157. Koch, S.L.: Disabilities of Hand Resulting From Loss of Joint Function. J.A.M.A., 104:30–35, 1935.

158. Lamb, D.W.; Abernethy, P.A.; and Raine, P.A.M.: Unstable Fractures of the Metacarpals: A Method of Treatment by Transverse Wire Fixation to Intact Metacarpals. Hand, 5: 43–48, 1973.

159. Lambotte, A.: Contribution to Conservative Surgery of the Injured Hand. Clin. Orthop., 214:4–6, 1987.

160. Lamphier, T.A.: Improper Reduction of Fractures of the Proximal Phalanges of Fractures. Am. J. Surg., 94:926–930, 1957.

161. Lane, C.S.: Detecting Occult Fracture of the Metacarpal Head: The Brewerton View. J. Hand Surg., 2:131–133, 1977.

162. Langa, V., and Posner, M.A.: Unusual Rupture of a Flexor Profundus Tendon. J. Hand Surg., 11A:227–229, 1986.

163. Leddy, J.P.: Avulsions of the Flexor Digitorum Profundus. Hand Clin., 1:77–83, 1985.

164. Leddy, J.P., and Packer, J.W.: Avulsion of the Profundus Tendon Insertion in Athletes. J. Hand Surg., 2:66–69, 1977.

165. Lee, M.L.H.: Intra-articular and Peri-articular Fractures of the Phalanges. J. Bone Joint Surg., 45B:103–109, 1963.

166. Leonard, M.H.: The Solution of Lead by Synovial Fluid. Clin. Orthop., 64:255–261, 1969.

167. Lewis, R.C., and Hartman, J.T.: Controlled Osteotomy for Correction of Rotation in Proximal Phalanx Fractures. Orthop. Rev., 11:11–15, 1973.

168. Lewis, R.C.; Nordyke, M.; and Duncan, K.: Expandable Intramedullary Device for Treatment of Fractures in the Hand. Clin. Orthop., 214:85–92, 1987.

169. Light, T.R.: Salvage of Intraarticular Malunions of the Hand and Wrist. The Role of Realignment Osteotomy. Clin. Orthop., 214:130–135, 1987.

170. Lipscomb, P.R.: Management of Fractures of the Hand. Am. Surg., 29:277–282, 1963.

171. Lister, G.: Intraosseous Wiring of the Digital Skeleton. J. Hand Surg., 3:427–435, 1978.

172. London, P.S.: Sprains and Fractures Involving the Interphalangeal Joints. Hand, 3:155–158, 1971.

173. Loosli, A., and Garrick, J.G.: The Functional Treatment of a Third Proximal Phalanx Fracture. Am. J. Sports Med., 15:94–96, 1987.

174. Lord, R.D.: Intramedullary Fixation of Metacarpal Fractures. J.A.M.A., 164:1746–1749, 1957.

175. Lowdon, I.M.R.: Fractures of the Metacarpal Neck of the Little Finger. Injury, 17:189–192, 1986.

176. Lucas, G.L.: Internal Fixation in the Hand: A Review of Indications and Methods. Orthopedics, 3:1083–1089, 1980.

177. Magnuson, P.B.: Fractures of Metacarpals and Phalanges. J.A.M.A., 91:1339–1340, 1928.

178. Magnuson, P.B.: Fractures. Philadelphia, J.B. Lippincott, 1942.

179. Manktelow, R.T., and Mahoney, J.L.: Step Osteotomy: A Precise Rotation Osteotomy to Correct Scissoring Deformities of the Fingers. Plast. Recontr. Surg., 68:571–576, 1981.

180. Mann, R.J.; Black, D.; Constine, R.; and Daniels, A.U.: A Quantitative Comparison of Metacarpal Fracture Stability With Five Different Methods of Internal Fixation. J. Hand Surg., 10A:1024–1028, 1985.

181. Manske, P.R., and Lesker, P.A.: Avulsion of the Ring Finger Flexor Digitorum Profundus Tendon: An Experimental Study. The Hand, 10:52–55, 1978.

182. Mansoor, I.A.: Fractures of the Proximal Phalanx of Fingers: A Method of Reduction. J. Bone Joint Surg., 51A: 196–198, 1969.

183. Margles, S.W.: Intra-articular Fractures of the Metacarpophalangeal and Proximal Interphalangeal Joints. Hand Clin., 4:67–74, 1988.

184. Mason, S.M., and Fyfe, I.S.: Comparison of Rigidity of Whole Tubular Bones. J. Biomech., 12:367–372, 1979.

185. Massengill, J.B.; Alexander, H.; Langrana, N.; and Mylod, A.: A Phalangeal Fracture Model—Quantitative Analysis of Rigidity and Failure. J. Hand Surg., 7:264–270, 1982.

186. Massengill, J.B.; Alexander, H.; Parson, J.R.; and Schecter, M.J.: Mechanical Analysis of Kirschner Wire Fixation in a Phalangeal Model. J. Hand Surg., 4:351–356, 1979.

187. Match, R.M.: The Treatment of Fractures of the Hand and the Wrist. Orthop. Rev., 14:35–48, 1985.

188. McElfresh, E.C., and Dobyns, J.H.: Intra-articular Metacarpal Head Fractures. J. Hand Surg., 8:383–393, 1983.

189. McKerrell, J.; Bowen, V.; Johnston, G.; and Zondervan, J.: Boxer's Fractures—Conservative or Operative Management? J. Trauma, 27:486–490, 1987.

190. McLaughlin, H.L.: Trauma. Philadelphia, W.B. Saunders, 1960.

191. McMaster, P.E.: Tendon and Muscle Ruptures: Clinical and Experimental Studies on the Causes and Location of Subcutaneous Ruptures. J. Bone Joint Surg., 15:705–722, 1933.

192. McMaster, W.C.: Intraoperative Reduction of Phalangeal Fractures. Plast. Reconstr. Surg., 56:671–672, 1975.

193. McNealy, R.W., and Lichtenstein, M.E.: Fractures of the Metacarpals and the Phalanges. Surg. Gynecol. Obstet., 60:758–761, 1932.

194. McNealy, R.W., and Lichtenstein, M.E.: Fractures of the Metacarpals and Phalanges. West. J. Surg. Obstet. Gynecol., 43:156–161, 1935.

195. McNealy, R.W., and Lichtenstein, M.E.: Fractures of the Bones of the Hand. Am. J. Surg., 50:563–570, 1940.

196. Meals, R.A.: American Society for Surgery of the Hand, Correspondence Newsletter, 1986.

197. Melone, C.P.: Rigid Fixation of Phalangeal and Metacarpal Fractures. Orthop. Clin. North Am., 17:421–435, 1986.

198. Meltzer, H.: Wire Extension Treatment of Fractures of Fingers and Metacarpal Bones. Surg. Gynecol. Obstet., 55:87–89, 1932.

199. Menon, J.: Reconstruction of the Metacarpophalangeal Joint With Autogenous Metatarsal. J. Hand Surg., 8:443–446, 1983.

200. Meyer, V.E.; Chiu, D.T.; and Beasley, R.W.: The Place of Internal Skeletal Fixation in Surgery of the Hand. Clin. Plast. Surg., 8:51–64, 1981.

201. Michon, J., and Delagoutte, J.P.: Crush Injuries of the Digital Extremities. In Pierre, M. (ed.): The Nail (G.E.M. Monograph), 1st ed. Edinburgh, Churchill Livingstone, 1981.

202. Milford, L.: The Hand. In Crenshaw, A.H. (ed): Campbell's Operative Orthopaedics, 5th ed. St. Louis, C.V. Mosby, 1971.

203. Miller, W.R.: Fractures of the Metacarpals. Am. J. Orthop., 105–108, 1965.

204. Moberg, E.: The Use of Traction Treatment for Fractures of Phalanges and Metacarpals. Acta Chir. Scand., 99:341–352, 1950.

205. Moberg, E.: Emergency Surgery of the Hand. Edinburgh, E.S. Livingstone, 1968.

206. Mock, H.E., and Ellis, J.D.: The Treatment of Fractures of the Fingers and Metacarpals With a Description of the Author's Finger Caliper. Surg. Gynecol. Obstet., 45:551–556, 1927.

207. Moore, D.C.: Regional Block, 4th ed. Springfield, Ill., Charles C. Thomas, 1967.

208. Morton, H.S.: Fractures of the Wrist and Hand. Can. Med. Assoc. J., 51:430–434, 1944.

209. Muller, M.E.; Allgower, M.; Schneider, R.; and Willenegger, H.: Manual of Internal Fixation, 2nd ed., pp. 42–43. New York, Springer-Verlag, 1979.

210. Murray, C.R.: Fractures of the Bones of the Hand. N.Y. State J. Med., 36:1749–1761, 1936.

211. Namba, R.S.; Kabo, J.M.; and Meals, R.A.: Biomechanical Effects of Point Configuration in Kirschner-wire Fixation. Clin. Orthop., 214:19–22, 1987.

212. Nemethi, C.E.: Phalangeal Fractures. Treated by Open Reduction and Kirschner-wire Fixation. Indust. Med. Surg., 23:148–150, 1954.

213. Nichols, H.M.: Manual of Hand Injuries, 2nd ed. Chicago, Year Book Medical Publishers, 1960.

214. Nordyke, M.D.; Lewis, R.C.; Janssen, H.F.; and Duncan, K.H.: Biomechanical and Clinical Evaluation of Expandable Intramedullary Fixation Device. J. Hand Surg., 13A:129–134, 1988.

215. Norman, H.R.C.: Fractures of the Metacarpals Treated by a New Method. Can. Med. Assoc. J., 49:173–175, 1943.

216. Noyez, J., and Verstreken, J.: The Use of the Bilos Compression Pin in Hand Surgery. Acta Orthop. Belg., 53:75–79, 1987.

217. Nunley, J.A.; Goldner, R.D.; and Urbaniak, J.R.: Skeletal Fixation in Digital Replantation. Use of the ''H'' Plate. Clin. Orthop., 214:66–71, 1987.

218. O'Brien, E.T.: Fractures of the Metacarpals and Phalanges. In Green, D.P. (ed.): Operative Hand Surgery, 2nd ed., pp. 709–775. New York, Churchill Livingstone, 1988.

219. Ohl, M.D., and Smith, W.S.: The Treatment of a Phalangeal Delayed Union Using Electrical Stimulation. Orthopedics, 11:585–588, 1988.

220. Owen, H.R.: Fractures of the Bones of the Hand. Surg. Gynecol. Obstet., 66:500–505, 1938.

221. Peacock, E.E.: Management of Conditions of the Hand Requiring Immobilization. Surg. Clin. North Am., 33:1297–1309, 1953.

222. Pedersen, N.T., and Larsen, A.: Incidence of Flexion Contracture Following Fracture of the Fifth Metacarpal Treated by Jahss' Method. Ugeskr. Laeger, 138:1765–1766, 1976.

223. Pieron, A.P.: Correction of Rotational Malunion of a Phalanx by Metacarpal Osteotomy. J. Bone Joint Surg., 54B:516–519, 1972.

224. Posch, J.L.; Walker, P.J.; and Miller, H.: Treatment of Ruptured Tendons of the Hand and Wrist. Am. J. Surg., 91:669–681, 1956.

225. Posner, M.A.: Injuries to the Hand and Wrist in Athletes. Orthop. Clin. North Am., 8:593–618, 1977.

226. Pratt, D.R.: Exposing Fractures of the Proximal Phalanx of the Finger Longitudinally Through the Dorsal Extensor Apparatus. Clin. Orthop., 15:22–26, 1959.

227. Pritsch, M.; Engel, J.; Tsur, H.; and Farin, I.: The Fractured Metacarpal Neck: New Method of Manipulation and External Fixation. Orthop. Rev., 7:122–123, 1978.

228. Pritsch, M.; Engel, J.; and Farin, I.: Manipulation and External Fixation of Metacarpal Fractures. J. Bone Joint Surg., 63A:1289–1291, 1981.

229. Quigley, T.B., and Urist, M.R.: Interphalangeal Joints: A Method of Digital Skeletal Traction Which Permits Active Motion. Am. J. Surg., 73:175–183, 1947.

230. Rayhack, J.M.; Belsole, R.J.; and Skelton, W.H.: A Strain Recording Model: Analysis of Transverse Osteotomy Fixation in Small Bones. J. Hand Surg., 9A:383–387, 1984.

231. Reef, T.C.: Avulsion of the Flexor Digitorum Profundus: An Athletic Injury. Am. J. Sports Med., 5:281–285, 1977.

232. Reyes, F.A., and Latta, L.L.: Conservative Management of Difficult Phalangeal Fractures. Clin. Orthop., 214:23–30, 1987.

233. Rider, D.L.: Fractures of the Metacarpals, Metatarsals, and Phalanges. Am. J. Surg., 38:549–559, 1937.

234. Riggs, S.A., and Cooney, W.P.: External Fixation of Complex Hand and Wrist Fractures. J. Trauma, 23:332–336, 1983.

235. Riordan, D.C.: Fractures About the Hand. South. Med. J., 50:637–640, 1957.

236. Roberts, N.: Fractures of the Phalanges of the Hand and Metacarpals. Proc. R. Soc. Med., 31:793–798, 1938.

237. Robertson, D.C.: The Fusion of Interphalangeal Joints. Can. J. Surg., 7:433–437, 1964.

238. Rosenberg, L., and Kon, M.: An External Fixator in Finger Reconstruction. J. Hand Surg., 11B:147–148, 1986.

239. Ruby, L.K.: American Society for Surgery of the Hand, Correspondence Newsletter, 1982.

240. Ruedi, T.P.; Burri, C.; and Pfeiffer, K.M.: Stable Internal

Fixation of Fractures of the Hand. J. Trauma, 11:381–389, 1971.

241. Ruggeri, S.; Osterman, A.L.; and Bora, F.W.: Stabilization of Metacarpal and Phalangeal Fractures in the Hand. Orthop. Rev., 9:107–110, 1980.

242. Rush, L.V., and Rush, H.L.: Evolution of Medullary Fixation of Fractures by the Longitudinal Pin. Am. J. Surg., 78:324–333, 1949.

243. Russotti, G.M., and Sim, F.H.: Missile Wounds of the Extremities: A Current Concepts Review. Orthopedics, 8:1106–1116, 1985.

244. Saypol, G.M., and Slattery, L.R.: Observations on Displaced Fractures of the Hand. Surg. Gynecol. Obstet., 79:522–525, 1944.

245. Scheker, L.R.: Department of Technique: A Technique to Facilitate Drilling and Passing Intraosseous Wiring in the Hand. J. Hand Surg., 5:629–630, 1982.

246. Schlein, A.P., and Nathan, F.F.: A Dual Finger Fracture. Hand, 4:171–172, 1972.

247. Schulze, H.A.: An Improved Skin-traction Technique for the Fingers. J. Bone Joint Surg., 29:222–224, 1947.

248. Scobie, W.H.: Crush Fracture of Sesamoid Bone of Thumb. Br. Med. J., 2:912, 1941.

249. Scott, M.M., and Mulligan, P.J.: Stabilizing Severe Phalangeal Fractures. Hand, 12:44–50, 1980.

250. Scudder, C.L.: The Treatment of Fractures. Philadelphia, W.B. Saunders, 1926.

251. Segmuller, G.: Surgical Stabilization of the Skeleton of the Hand. Baltimore, Williams & Wilkins, 1977.

252. Seitz, W.H., and Froimson, A.I.: Management of Malunited Fractures of the Metacarpal and Phalangeal Shafts. Hand. Clin., 4:529–536, 1988.

253. Seitz, W.H.; Gomez, W.; Putnam, M.D.; and Rosenwasser, M.P.: Management of Severe Hand Trauma With a Mini External Fixateur. Orthopedics, 10:601–610, 1987.

254. Seymour, N.: Juxta-epiphysial Fracture of the Terminal Phalanx of the Finger. J. Bone Joint Surg., 48A:347–349, 1966.

255. Shapiro, J.S.: Power Staple Fixation in Hand and Wrist Surgery: New Applications of an Old Fixation Device. J. Hand Surg., 12A:218–227, 1987.

256. Simon, R.R., and Wolgin, M.: Subungual Hematoma: Association With Occult Laceration Requiring Repair. Am. J. Emerg. Med., 5:302–304, 1987.

257. Simonetta, C.: The Use of "A.O." Plates in the Hand. Hand, 2:43–45, 1970.

258. Sloan, J.P.; Dove, A.F.; Maheson, M.; Cope, A.N.; and Welsh, K.R.: Antibiotics in Open Fractures of the Distal Phalanx? J. Hand Surg., 12B:123–124, 1987.

259. Smith, C.H.: Compound Fracture of the Fingers. Ann. Surg., 119:266–273, 1944.

260. Smith, F.L., and Rider, D.L.: A Study of the Healing of One Hundred Consecutive Phalangeal Fractures. J. Bone Joint Surg., 17:91–109, 1935.

261. Smith, J.H.: Avulsion of a Profundus Tendon With Simultaneous Intra-articular Fracture of the Distal Phalanx—Case Report. J. Hand Surg., 6:600–601, 1981.

262. Smith, R.J., and Peimer, C.A.: Injuries to the Metacarpal Bones and Joints. Adv. Surg., 2:341–374, 1977.

263. Smith, R.S.; Alonso, J.; and Horowitz, M.: External Fix-ation of Open Comminuted Fractures of the Proximal Phalanx. Orthop. Rev., 16:53–57, 1987.

264. Speed, K.: A Textbook of Fractures and Dislocations. Philadelphia, Lea & Febiger, 1942.

265. Stark, H.H.: Troublesome Fractures and Dislocations of the Hand. Instr. Course Lect., 19:130–149, 1970.

266. Stark, H.H.; Boyes, J.H.; Johnson, L.; and Ashworth, C.R.: The Use of Paratenon, Polyethylene Film, or Silastic Sheeting to Prevent Restricting Adhesions to Tendons in the Hand. J. Bone Joint Surg., 59A:908–913, 1977.

267. Steel, W.M.: The A.O. Small Fragment Set in Hand Fractures. Hand, 10:246–253, 1978.

268. Stern, P.J.; Wieser, M.J.; and Reilly, D.G.: Complications of Plate Fixation in the Hand Skeleton. Clin. Orthop., 214:59–65, 1987.

269. Strickland, J.W.; Steichen, J.B.; Kleinman, W.B.; Hastings, H.; and Flynn, N.: Phalangeal Fractures. Factors Influencing Digital Performance. Orthop. Rev., 11:39–50, 1982.

270. Stuchin, S.A., and Kummer, F.J.: Stiffness of Small-bone External Fixation Methods: An Experimental Study. J. Hand Surg., 9A:718–724, 1984.

271. Suman, R.K.: Rigid Fixation of Metacarpal Fractures. J. R. Coll. Surg. Edinb., 28:51–52, 1983.

272. Sutro, C.J.: Fracture of Metacarpal Bones and Proximal Manual Phalanges: Treatment With Emphasis on the Prevention of Rational Deformities. Am. J. Surg., 81:327–332, 1951.

273. Swanson, A.B.: Fractures Involving the Digits of the Hand. Orthop. Clin. North Am., 1:261–274, 1970.

274. Tennant, C.E.: Use of Steel Phonograph Needle as a Retaining Pin in Certain Irreducible Fractures of the Small Bones. J.A.M.A., 83:193, 1924.

275. Treble, N., and Arif, S.: Avulsion Fracture of the Index Metacarpal. J. Hand Surg., 12B:38–39, 1987.

276. Van Demark, R.: A Simple Method of Treatment of Fractures of the Fifth Metacarpal Neck and Distal Shaft (Boxer's Fracture). South Dakota Medicine, 36:5–7, 1983.

277. Vanik, R.K.; Weber, R.C.; Matloub, H.S.; Sanger, J.R.; and Gingrass, R.P.: The Comparative Strengths of Internal Fixation Techniques. J. Hand Surg., 9A:216–221, 1984.

278. Viegas, S.F.: New Method and Brace for Metacarpal Fractures. Surg. Rounds Orthop., 47–55, 1987.

279. Viegas, S.F., and Calhoun, J.H.: Lead Poisoning From a Gunshot Wound to the Hand. J. Hand Surg., 11A:729–732, 1986.

280. Viegas, S.F.; Ferren, E.L.; Self, J.; and Tencer, A.F.: Comparative Mechanical Properties of Various Kirschner Wire Configurations in Transverse and Oblique Phalangeal Fractures. J. Hand Surg., 13A:246–253, 1988.

281. Viegas, S.F.; Tencer, A.; Woodard, P.; and Williams, C.R.: Functional Bracing of Fractures of the Second Through Fifth Metacarpals. J. Hand Surg., 12A:139–143, 1987.

282. Vom Saal, F.H.: Intramedullary Fixation in Fractures of the Hand and Fingers. J. Bone Joint Surg., 35A:5–16, 1953.

283. Watson-Jones, R.: Fractures and Joint Injuries, 3rd ed. Edinburgh, E.S. Livingstone, 1943.

284. Watson-Jones, R.: Fractures and Joint Injuries, 4th ed. Edinburgh, E.S. Livingstone, 1956.

285. Waugh, R.L., and Ferrazzano, G.P.: Fractures of the Metacarpals Exclusive of the Thumb. A New Method of Treatment. Am. J. Surg., 59:186–194, 1943.

286. Weber, B.G., and Cech, O.: Pseudarthrosis. New York, Grune & Stratton, 1976.

287. Weckesser, E.C.: Rotational Osteotomy of the Metacarpal for Overlapping Fingers. J. Bone Joint Surg., 47A:751–756, 1965.

288. Wenger, D.R.: Avulsion of the Profundus Tendon Insertion in Football Players. Arch. Surg., 106:145–149, 1973.

289. Widgerow, A.D.; Edinburg, M.; and Biddulph, S.L.: An Analysis of Proximal Phalangeal Fractures. J. Hand Surg., 12A:134–139, 1987.

290. Wise, R.A.: An Unusual Fracture of the Terminal Phalanx of the Finger. J. Bone Joint Surg., 21:467–469, 1939.

291. Woods, G.L.: Troublesome Shaft Fractures of the Proximal Phalanx. Early Treatment to Avoid Late Problems at the Metacarpophalangeal and Proximal Phalangeal Joints. Hand Clin., 4:75–85, 1988.

292. Wray, R.C., and Weeks, P.M.: Management of Metacarpal Shaft Fractures. Mo. Med., 72:79–82, 1975.

293. Wright, T.A.: Early Mobilization in Fractures of the Metacarpals and Phalanges. Can. J. Surg., 11:491–498, 1968.

294. Zacher, J.B.: Management of Injuries of the Distal Phalanx. Surg. Clin. North Am., 64:747–760, 1984.

295. Zook, E.G.: Care of Nail Bed Injuries. Surg. Rounds, 44–61, 1985.

Mallet Finger and Boutonniére

296. Abouna, J.M., and Brown, H.: The Treatment of Mallet Finger. The Results in a Series of 148 Consecutive Cases and a Review of the Literature. Br. J. Surg., 55:653–667, 1968.

297. Auchincloss, J.M.: Mallet-finger Injuries: A Prospective, Controlled Trial of Internal and External Splintage. Hand, 2:168–173, 1982.

298. Backdahl, M.: Ruptures of the Extensor Aponeurosis at the Distal Digital Joints. Acta Chir. Scand., 111:151–157, 1956.

299. Bowers, W.H., and Hurst, L.C.: Chronic Mallet Finger: The Use of Fowler's Central Slip Release. J. Hand Surg., 3:373–376, 1978.

300. Brooks, D.: Splint for Mallet Fingers. Br. Med. J., 1:2:1238, 1964.

301. Bunnell, S.: Surgery of the Hand, pp. 490–493. Philadelphia, J.B. Lippincott, 1944.

302. Burke, F.: Editorial: Mallet Finger. J. Hand Surg., 13B:115–117, 1988.

303. Casscells, S.W., and Strange, T.B.: Intramedullary Wire Fixation of Mallet Finger. J. Bone Joint Surg., 39A:521–526, 1957.

304. Casscells, S.W., and Strange, T.B.: Intramedullary Wire Fixation of Mallet Finger. J. Bone Joint Surg., 51A:1018–1019, 1969.

305. Cohn, B.T., and Froimson, A.I.: Case Report of a Rare Mallet Finger Injury. Orthopedics, 9:529–531, 1986.

306. Crawford, G.P.: The Molded Polythene Splint for Mallet Finger Deformities. J. Hand Surg., 9A:231–237, 1984.

307. Din, K.M., and Meggitt, B.F.: Mallet Thumb. J. Bone Joint Surg., 65B:606–607, 1983.

308. Elliott, R.A.: Injuries to the Extensor Mechanism of the Hand. Orthop. Clin. North Am., 1:335–354, 1970.

309. Elliott, R.A.: Splints for Mallet and Boutonniere Deformities. Plast. Reconstr. Surg., 52:282–285, 1973.

310. Evans, D., and Weightman, B.: The Pipflex Splint for Treatment of Mallet Finger. J. Hand Surg., 13B:156–158, 1988.

311. Flinchum, D.: Mallet Finger. J. Med. Assoc. Ga., 48:601–603, 1959.

312. Fowler, F.D.: New Splint for Treatment of Mallet Finger. J.A.M.A., 170:945, 1959.

313. Grundberg, A.B.: Anatomic Repair of Boutonniere Deformity. Clin. Orthop., 153:226–229, 1980.

314. Grundberg, A.B., and Reagan, D.S.: Central Slip Tenotomy for Chronic Mallet Finger Deformity. J. Hand Surg., 12A:545–547, 1987.

315. Hamas, R.S.; Horrell, E.D.; and Pierret, G.P.: Treatment of Mallet Finger Due to Intra-articular Fracture of the Distal Phalanx. J. Hand Surg., 3:361–363, 1978.

316. Harris, C., and Rutledge, G.L.: The Functional Anatomy of the Extensor Mechanism of the Finger. J. Bone Joint Surg., 54A:713–726, 1972.

317. Harris, C., Jr.: The Fowler Operation for Mallet Finger. J. Bone Joint Surg., 48A:613, 1966.

318. Hillman, F.E.: New Technique for Treatment of Mallet Fingers and Fractures of Distal Phalanx. J.A.M.A., 161:1135–1138, 1956.

319. Hovgaard, C., and Klareskov, B.: Alternative Conservative Treatment of Mallet-finger Injuries by Elastic Double-finger Bandage. J. Hand Surg., 13B:154–155, 1988.

320. Howie, H.: The Treatment of Mallet Finger: A Modified Plaster Technique. N.Z. Med. J., 46:513, 1947.

321. Isani, A.: Small Joint Injuries Requiring Surgical Treatment. Orthop. Clin. North Am., 17:407–419, 1986.

322. Iselin, F.; Levame, J.; and Godoy, J.: A Simplified Technique for Treating Mallet Fingers: Tenodermodesis. J. Hand Surg., 2:118–121, 1977.

323. Jones, N.F., and Peterson, J.: Epidemiologic Study of the Mallet Finger Deformity. J. Hand Surg., 13A:334–338, 1988.

324. Kaplan, E.B.: Mallet or Baseball Finger. Surgery, 7:784–791, 1940.

325. Kaplan, E.B.: Anatomy, Injuries and Treatment of the Extensor Apparatus of the Hand and the Digits. Clin. Orthop., 13:24–41, 1959.

326. Kinninmonth, A.W.G., and Holburn, F.: A Comparative Controlled Trial of a New Perforated Splint and a Traditional Splint in the Treatment of Mallet Finger. J. Hand Surg., 11B:261–262, 1986.

327. Kleinman, W.B., and Petersen, D.P.: Oblique Retinacular Ligament Reconstruction for Chronic Mallet Finger Deformity. J. Hand Surg., 9A:399–404, 1984.

328. Kon, M., and Bloem, J.J.A.M.: Treatment of Mallet Fingers by Tenodermodesis. Hand, 14:174–176, 1982.

329. Lange, R.H., and Engber, W.D.: Hyperextension Mallet Finger. Orthopedics, 6:1426–1431, 1983.

330. Lewin, P.: A Simple Splint for Baseball Finger. J.A.M.A., 85:1059, 1925.

331. Littler, J.W.: The Voice of Polite Dissent. A New Method of Treatment for Mallet Finger. Plast. Reconstr. Surg., 58: 499–500, 1976.

332. Littler, J.W., and Eaton, R.G.: Redistribution of Forces in the Correction of the Boutonniere Deformity. J. Bone Joint Surg., 49A:1267–1274, 1967.

333. Mason, M.L.: Rupture of Tendons of the Hand. With a Study of the Extensor Tendon Insertions in the Fingers. Surg. Gynecol. Obstet., 50:611–624, 1930.

334. Mason, M.L.: Mallet Finger. Lancet, 266:1220, 1954.

335. Matev, I.: Transposition of the Lateral Slips of the Aponeurosis in Treatment of Long-standing "Boutonniere Deformity" of the Fingers. Br. J. Plast. Surg., 17:281–286, 1964.

336. Matev, I.: The Boutonniere Deformity. Hand, 1:90–95, 1969.

337. McCue, F.C., and Abbott, J.L.: The Treatment of Mallet Finger and Boutonniere Deformities. Va. Med., 94:623–628, 1967.

338. McFarlane, R.M., and Hampole, M.K.: Treatment of Extensor Tendon Injuries of the Hand. Can. J. Surg., 16: 366–375, 1973.

339. McMinn, D.J.W.: Mallet Finger and Fractures. Injury, 12: 477–479, 1981.

340. Mikic, Z., and Helal, B.: The Treatment of the Mallet Finger by Oakley Splint. Hand, 6:76–81, 1974.

341. Mirza, M.A., and Korber, K.E.: Inverted-U Incision for Exploration of the Distal Phalanx. Ideas and Innovations, 74:548–549, 1984.

342. Miura, T.; Nakamura, R.; and Torii, S.: Conservative Treatment for a Ruptured Extensor Tendon on the Dorsum of the Proximal Phalanges of the Thumb (Mallet Thumb). J. Hand Surg., 11A:229–233, 1986.

343. Mixa, T.M.; Blair, S.J.; and Dvonch, V.M.: Acute and Chronic Management of Mallet Finger. A Case Study. Orthopedics, 8:1044–1046, 1985.

344. Moss, J.G., and Steingold, R.F.: The Long Term Results of Mallet Finger Injury: A Retrospective Study of One Hundred Cases. Hand, 15:151–154, 1983.

345. Nichols, H.M.: Repair of Extensor Tendon Insertion in the Fingers. J. Bone Joint Surg., 33A:836–841, 1951.

346. Niechajev, I.A.: Conservative and Operative Treatment of Mallet Finger. Plast. Reconstr. Surg., 76:580–585, 1985.

347. Patel, M.R.; Desai, S.S.; and Lipson, L.B.: Conservative Management of Chronic Mallet Finger. J. Hand Surg., 11A:570–573, 1986.

348. Patel, M.R.; Lipson, L.B.; and Desai, S.S.: Conservative Treatment of Mallet Thumb. J. Hand Surg., 11A:45–47, 1986.

349. Pratt, D.R.: Internal Splint for Closed and Open Treatment of Injuries of the Extensor Tendon at the Distal Joint of the Finger. J. Bone Joint Surg., 34A:785–788, 1952.

350. Primiano, G.A.: Conservative Treatment of Two Cases of Mallet Thumb. J. Hand Surg., 11A:233–235, 1986.

351. Ramsay, R.A.: Mallet Finger. Lancet, 2:1244, 1968.

352. Ratliff, A.H.C.: Mallet Finger: A Review of Forty-five Cases. Manch. Med. Gaz., 26:4, 1947.

353. Rayan, G.M., and Mullins, P.T.: Skin Necrosis Complicating Mallet Finger Splinting and Vascularity of the Distal Interphalangeal Joint Overlying Skin. J. Hand Surg., 12A: 548–552, 1987.

354. Robb, W.A.T.: The Results of Treatment of Mallet Finger. J. Bone Joint Surg., 41B:546–549, 1959.

355. Roemer, F.J.: Hyperextension Injuries to the Finger Joints. Am. J. Surg., 80:295–302, 1950.

356. Rosenzweig, N.: Management of the Mallet Finger. S. Afr. Med. J., 24:831–832, 1950.

357. Schneider, L.H.: Fractures of the Distal Phalanx. Hand Clin., 4:537–547, 1988.

358. Smillie, I.S.: Mallet Finger. Br. J. Surg., 24:439–445, 1937.

359. Souter, W.A.: The Boutonniere Deformity. A Review of 101 Patients With Division of the Central Slip of the Extensor Expansion of the Fingers. J. Bone Joint Surg., 49B: 710–721, 1967.

360. Souter, W.A.: The Problem of Boutonniere Deformity. Clin. Orthop., 104:116–133, 1974.

361. Spigelman, L.: New Splint for Management of Mallet Finger. J.A.M.A., 153:1362, 1953.

362. Stack, H.G.: Mallet Finger. Hand, 1:83–89, 1969.

363. Stack, H.G.: A Modified Splint for Mallet Finger. J. Hand Surg., 11B:263, 1986.

364. Stark, H.H.; Boyes, J.H.; and Wilson, J.N.: Mallet Finger. J. Bone Joint Surg., 44A:1061–1068, 1962.

365. Stark, H.H.; Gainor, B.J.; Ashworth, C.R.; Zemel, N.P.; and Rickard, T.A.: Operative Treatment of Intra-articular Fractures of the Dorsal Aspect of the Distal Phalanx of Digits. J. Bone Joint Surg., 69A:892–896, 1987.

366. Stern, P.J., and Kastrup, J.J.: Complications and Prognosis of Treatment of Mallet Finger. J. Hand Surg., 13A:329–334, 1988.

367. Stewart, I.M.: Boutonniere Finger. Clin. Orthop., 23:220–226, 1962.

368. Thompson, J.S.; Littler, J.W.; and Upton, J.: The Spiral Oblique Retinacular Ligament (SORL). J. Hand Surg., 3: 482–487, 1978.

369. Urbaniak, J.R., and Hayes, M.G.: Chronic Boutonniere Deformity: An Anatomic Reconstruction. J. Hand Surg., 6:379–383, 1981.

370. Van Demark, R.E.: A Simple Method of Treatment for Recent Mallet Finger. Milit. Surg., 107:385–386, 1950.

371. Van Der Meulen, J.C.: The Treatment of Prolapse and Collapse of the Proximal Interphalangeal Joint. Hand, 4: 154–162, 1972.

372. Warren, R.A.; Kay, N.R.M.; and Ferguson, D.G.: Mallet Finger: Comparison Between Operative and Conservative Management in Those Cases Failing to Be Cured by Splintage. J. Hand Surg., 13B:159–160, 1988.

373. Warren, R.A.; Kay, N.R.M.; and Norris, S.H.: The Microvascular Anatomy of the Distal Digital Extensor Tendon. J. Hand Surg., 13B:161–163, 1988.

374. Warren, R.A.; Norris, S.H.; and Ferguson, D.G.: Mallet Finger: A Trial of Two Splints. J. Hand Surg., 13B:151–153, 1988.

375. Watson, F.M.: American Society for Surgery of the Hand, Correspondence Newsletter, 1983.

376. Watson-Jones, R.: Fractures and Joint Injuries, 4th ed., pp. 645–646. Edinburgh, E & S Livingstone, 1956.

377. Wehbe, M.A., and Schneider, L.H.: Mallet Fractures. J. Bone Joint Surg., 66A:658–669, 1984.

378. Weinberg, H.; Stein, H.C.; and Wexler, M.R.: A New Method of Treatment for Mallet Finger. A Preliminary Report. Plast. Reconstr. Surg., 58:347–349, 1976.

379. Williams, E.G.: Treatment of Mallet Finger. Can. Med. Assoc. J., 57:582, 1947.

Fractures of the Thumb Metacarpal

380. Badger, F.C.: Internal Fixation in the Treatment of Bennett's Fractures. J. Bone Joint Surg., 38B:771, 1956.

381. Bennett, E.H.: Fractures of the Metacarpal Bones. Dublin J. Med. Sci., 73:72–75, 1882.

382. Bennett, E.H.: On Fracture of the Metacarpal Bone of the Thumb. Br. Med. J., 2:12–13, 1886.

383. Billing, L., and Gedda, K.O.: Roentgen Examination of Bennett's Fracture. Acta Radiol., 38:471–476, 1952.

384. Blum, L.: The Treatment of Bennett's Fracture-dislocation of the First Metacarpal Bone. J. Bone Joint Surg., 23:578–580, 1941.

385. Breen, T.F.; Gelberman, R.H.; and Jupiter, J.B.: Intra-articular Fractures of the Basilar Joint of the Thumb. Hand Clin., 4:491–501, 1988.

386. Cannon, S.R.; Dowd, G.S.E.; Williams, D.H.; and Scott, J.M.: A Long-term Study Following Bennett's Fracture. J. Hand Surg., 11B:426–431, 1986.

387. Charnley, J.: The Closed Treatment of Common Fractures. Edinburgh, E & S Livingstone, 1961.

388. Cotton, F.J.: Dislocations and Joint Fractures. Philadelphia, W.B. Saunders, 1910.

389. Dial, W.B., and Berg, E.: Bennett's Fracture. Hand, 4:229–235, 1972.

390. Ellis, V.H.: A Method of Treating Bennett's Fracture. Proc. R. Soc. Med., 39:21, 1946.

391. Fisher, E.: Bennett's Fracture in General Practice. Med. J. Aust., 1:434–438, 1976.

392. Foster, R.J., and Hastings, H.: Treatment of Bennett, Rolando, and Vertical Intraarticular Trapezial Fractures. Clin. Orthop., 214:121–129, 1987.

393. Gedda, K.O.: Studies on Bennett's Fracture: Anatomy, Roentgenology, and Therapy. Acta Chir. Scand. [Suppl.] 193, 1954.

394. Gedda, K.O., and Moberg, E.: Open Reduction and Osteosynthesis of the So-called Bennett's Fracture in the Carpo-metacarpal Joint of the Thumb. Acta Orthop. Scand., 22:249–256, 1953.

395. Gelberman, R.H.; Vance, R.M.; and Zakaib, G.S.: Fractures at the Base of the Thumb: Treatment With Oblique Traction. J. Bone Joint Surg., 61A:260–262, 1979.

396. Goldberg, D.: Thumb Fractures and Dislocations, A New Method of Treatment. Am. J. Surg., 81:227–231, 1951.

397. Goldberg, D.: Metacarpal and Thumb Fractures, A Dynamic Method of Treatment. Orthop. Rev., 7:37–42, 1978.

398. Green, D.P., and O'Brien, E.T.: Fractures of the Thumb Metacarpal. South. Med. J., 65:807–814, 1972.

399. Griffiths, J.C.: Fractures at the Base of the First Metacarpal Bone. J. Bone Joint Surg., 46B:712–719, 1964.

400. Griffiths, J.C.: Bennett's Fracture in Childhood. Br. J. Clin. Pract., 20:582–583, 1966.

401. Harvey, F.J., and Bye, W.D.: Bennett's Fracture. Hand, 8:48–53, 1976.

402. Howard, F.M.: Fractures of the Basal Joint of the Thumb. Clin. Orthop., 220:46–51, 1987.

403. James, E.S., and Gibson, A.: Fractures of the First Metacarpal Bone. Can. Med. Assoc. J., 43:153–155, 1940.

404. James, E.S., and Gibson, A.: Fracture of the First Metacarpal Bone. Can. Med. Assoc. J., 232:153–155, 1940.

405. Johnson, E.C.: Fracture of the Base of the Thumb: A New Method of Fixation. J.A.M.A., 126:27–28, 1944.

406. Macey, H.B., and Murray, R.A.: Fractures About the Base of the First Metacarpal With Special Reference to Bennett's Fracture. South. Med. J., 42:931–935, 1949.

407. McNealy, R.W., and Lichtenstein, M.E.: Bennett's Fracture and Other Fractures of the First Metacarpal. Surg. Gynecol. Obstet., 56:197–201, 1933.

408. Miles, A., and Struthers, J.W.: Original Communications. Bennett's Fracture of the Base of the Metacarpal Bone of the Thumb. Edinburgh Med. J., 15:297–308, 1904.

409. Pellegrini, V.D.: Fractures at the Base of the Thumb. Hand Clin., 4:87–101, 1988.

410. Pollen, A.G.: The Conservative Treatment of Bennett's Fracture-subluxation of the Thumb Metacarpal. J. Bone Joint Surg., 50B:91–101, 1968.

411. Roberts, J.B., and Kelly, J.A.: Treatise on Fractures. Philadelphia, J.B. Lippincott, 1916.

412. Robinson, S.: The Bennett Fracture of the First Metacarpal Bone: Diagnosis and Treatment. Boston Med. Surg. J., 158:275–276, 1908.

413. Rolando, S.: Fracture de la Base du Premier Metacarpien: Et Principalement sur une Variete non Encore Decrite. Presse Med., 18:303–304, 1910.

414. Ross, J.W., and Sinclair, A.B.: The Treatment of Bennett's Fracture With the Stader Splint. J. Can. Med. Serv., 3:507–511, 1946.

415. Salgeback, S.; Eiken, O.; Carstam, N.; and Ohlsson, N.M.: A Study of Bennett's Fracture. Special Reference to Fixation by Percutaneous Pinning. Scand. J. Plast. Reconstr. Surg., 5:142–148, 1971.

416. Spangberg, O., and Thoren, L.: Bennett's Fracture: A Method of Treatment With Oblique Traction. J. Bone Joint Surg., 45B:732–739, 1963.

417. Stromberg, L.: Compression Fixation of Bennett's Fracture. Acta Orthop. Scand., 48:586–591, 1977.

418. Thoren, L.: A New Method of Extension Treatment in Bennett's Fracture. Acta Chir. Scand., 110:485–493, 1956.

419. Thoren, L.: Basal Fractures of the First Metacarpal Bone— A Method of Treatment by Excision. Acta Orthop. Scand., 27:40–48, 1957.

420. Wagner, C.J.: Method of Treatment of Bennett's Fracture Dislocation. Am. J. Surg., 80:230–231, 1950.

421. Wagner, C.J.: Transarticular Fixation of Fracture-dislocations of the First Metacarpal-carpal Joint. West. J. Surg., Obs., and Gyn., 59:362–365, 1951.

422. Wiggins, H.E.; Bundens, W.D., Jr.; and Park, B.J.: A Method of Treatment of Fracture-dislocations of the First

Metacarpal Bone. J. Bone Joint Surg., 36A:810–819, 1954.

Interphalangeal Joints

423. Adams, J.P.: Correction of Chronic Dorsal Subluxation of the Proximal Interphalangeal Joint by Means of a Criss-cross Volar Graft. J. Bone Joint Surg., 41A:111–115, 1959.
424. Agee, J.M.: Unstable Fracture Dislocations of the Proximal Interphalangeal Joint of the Fingers: A Preliminary Report of a New Treatment Technique. J. Hand Surg., 3:386–389, 1978.
425. Agee, J.M.: Unstable Fracture Dislocations of the Proximal Interphalangeal Joint. Treatment With the Force Couple Splint. Clin. Orthop., 214:101–112, 1987.
426. Ali, M.S.: Complete Disruption of Collateral Mechanism of Proximal Interphalangeal Joint of Fingers. J. Hand Surg., 9:191–193, 1984.
427. Ambrosia, J.M., and Linscheid, R.L.: Simultaneous Dorsal Dislocation of the Interphalangeal Joints in a Finger. Case Report and Review of the Literature. Orthopedics, 11:1079–1080, 1988.
428. Bate, J.T.: An Operation for the Correction of Locking of the Proximal Interphalangeal Joint of Finger in Hyperextension. J. Bone Joint Surg., 27:142–144, 1945.
429. Baugher, W.H., and McCue, F.C.: Anterior Fracture Dislocation of the Proximal Interphalangeal Joint. A Case Report. J. Bone Joint Surg., 61A:779–780, 1979.
430. Benke, G.J., and Stableforth, P.G.: Injuries of the Proximal Interphalangeal Joint of the Fingers. Hand, 3:263–268, 1979.
431. Bowers, W.H.: Management of Small Joint Injuries in the Hand. Orthop. Clin. North Am., 14:793–810, 1983.
432. Bowers, W.H., and Fajgenbaum, D.M.: Closed Rupture of the Volar Plate of the Distal Interphalangeal Joint. J. Bone Joint Surg., 61A:146, 1979.
433. Bowers, W.H.; Wolf, J.W.; Nehil, J.L.; and Bittinger, S.: The Proximal Interphalangeal Joint Volar Plate: I. An Anatomical and Biomechanical Study. J. Hand Surg., 5:79–88, 1980.
434. Burton, R.I.: Small Joint Injuries of the Hand. Dynamic and Functional Implications. Hand Clin., 4:11–12, 1988.
435. Cole, I.C.: Principles and Guidelines in Hand Therapy and Rehabilitation During Recovery From Small Joint Injuries. Hand Clin., 4:123–131, 1988.
436. Curtis, R.M.: Treatment of Injuries of the Proximal Interphalangeal Joints of the Fingers. Curr. Pract. Orthop. Surg., 2:125–135, 1964.
437. De Smet, L., and Vercauteren, M.: Palmar Dislocation of the Proximal Interphalangeal Joint Requiring Open Reduction: A Case Report. J. Hand Surg., 9A:717–718, 1984.
438. Donaldson, W.R., and Millender, L.H.: Chronic Fracture-subluxation of the Proximal Interphalangeal Joint. J. Hand Surg., 2:149–153, 1978.
439. Eaton, R.G.: Joint Injuries of the Hand. Springfield, Ill., Charles C. Thomas, 1971.
440. Eaton, R.G., and Littler, J.W.: Joint Injuries and Their Sequelae. Clin. Plast. Surg., 3:85–98, 1976.
441. Eaton, R.G., and Malerich, M.M.: Volar Plate Arthroplasty

of the Proximal Interphalangeal Joint: A Review of Ten Years' Experience. J. Hand Surg., 5:260–268, 1980.
442. Espinosa, R.H., and Renart, I.P.: Simultaneous Dislocation of the Interphalangeal Joints in a Finger. Case Report. J. Hand Surg., 5:617–618, 1980.
443. Faithfull, D.K.: Treatment of Chronic Instability of the Digital Joints Using a Strip of Volar Plate. Hand, 13:36–38, 1981.
444. Flatt, A.E.: The Care of Minor Hand Injuries, pp. 188–189. St. Louis, C.V. Mosby, 1959.
445. Freeman, B.H.; Haskin, J.S., Jr.; and Hay, E.L.: Chronic Anterior Dislocation of the Proximal Interphalangeal Joint. Orthopedics, 8:385–388, 1985.
446. Garroway, R.Y.; Hurst, L.C.; Leppard, J., III; and Dick, H.M.: Complex Dislocations of the Proximal Interphalangeal Joint. A Pathoanatomic Classification of the Injury. Orthop. Rev., 13:21–28, 1984.
447. Green, D.P.: Dislocations and Ligamentous Injuries in the Hand and Wrist. In Evarts, C.M. (ed.): Surgery of the Musculoskeletal System. New York, Churchill Livingstone, 1983.
448. Green, D.P., and Rowland, S.A.: Fractures and Dislocations in the Hand. In Rockwood, C.A., and Green, D.P. (eds.): Fractures. Philadelphia, J.B. Lippincott, 1975.
449. Green, S.M., and Posner, M.A.: Irreducible Dorsal Dislocations of the Proximal Interphalangeal Joint. J. Hand Surg., 10A:85–87, 1985.
450. Hardy, I.; Russell, J.; and McFarlane, I.: Simultaneous Dislocation of the Interphalangeal Joints in a Finger. J. Trauma, 25:450–451, 1985.
451. Hastings, H., and Carroll, C.: Treatment of Closed Articular Fractures of the Metacarpophalangeal and Proximal Interphalangeal Joints. Hand Clin., 4:503–527, 1988.
452. Holtmann, B.; Wray, R.C., Jr.; and Weeks, P.M.: A Frequently Overlooked Injury in the Hand. Mo. Med., 73:477–481, 1976.
453. Iftikhar, T.B.: Long Flexor Tendon Entrapment. Causing Open Irreducible Dorsoradial Dislocation of Distal Interphalangeal Joint of the Finger. A Case Report. Orthop. Rev., 11:117–119, 1982.
454. Ikpeme, J.O.: Dislocation of Both Interphalangeal Joints of One Finger. Injury, 9:68–70, 1977.
455. Inoue, G., and Maeda, N.: Irreducible Palmar Dislocation of the Distal Interphalangeal Joint of the Finger. J. Hand Surg., 12A:1077–1079, 1987.
456. Isani, A.: Small Joint Injuries Requiring Surgical Treatment. Orthop. Clin. North Am., 17:407–419, 1986.
457. Isani, A., and Melone, C.P., Jr.: Ligamentous Injuries of the Hand in Athletes. Clin. Sports Med., 5:757–772, 1986.
458. Johnson, F.G., and Greene, M.H.: Another Cause of Irreducible Dislocation of the Proximal Interphalangeal Joint of a Finger. A Case Report. J. Bone Joint Surg., 48A:542–544, 1966.
459. Jones, N.F., and Jupiter, J.B.: Irreducible Palmar Dislocation of the Proximal Interphalangeal Joint Associated With an Epiphyseal Fracture of the Middle Phalanx. J. Hand Surg., 10A:261–264, 1985.
460. Khuri, S.M.: Irreducible Dorsal Dislocation of the Distal Interphalangeal Joint of the Finger. J. Trauma, 24:456–457, 1984.

461. Kiefhaber, T.R.; Stern, P.J.; and Grood, E.S.: Lateral Stability of the Proximal Interphalangeal Joint. J. Hand Surg., 11A:661–669, 1986.

462. Kilgore, E.S.; Newmeyer, W.L.; and Brown, L.G.: Post-traumatic Trapped Dislocations of the Proximal Interphalangeal Joint. J. Trauma, 16:481–487, 1976.

463. Kitagawa, H., and Kashimoto, T.: Locking of the Thumb at the Interphalangeal Joint by One of the Sesamoid Bones. A Case Report. J. Bone Joint Surg., 66A:1300–1301, 1984.

464. Kjeldal, I.: Irreducible Compound Dorsal Dislocations of the Proximal Interphalangeal Joint of the Finger. J. Hand Surg., 11B:49–50, 1986.

465. Kleinert, H.E., and Kasdan, M.L.: Reconstruction of Chronically Subluxated Proximal Interphalangeal Finger Joint. J. Bone Joint Surg., 47A:958–964, 1965.

466. Konsens, R.M.; Cohn, B.T.; and Froimson, A.I.: Double Dislocation of the Fifth Finger. Orthopedics, 10:1061–1062, 1987.

467. Krebs, B., and Gron, L.K.: Simultaneous Dorsal Dislocation of Both Interphalangeal Joints in a Finger. Br. J. Sports Med., 18:217–219, 1984.

468. Krishnan, S.G.: Double Dislocation of a Finger. A Case Report. Am. J. Sports Med., 7:204–205, 1979.

469. Kuczynski, K.: The Proximal Interphalangeal Joint. Anatomy and Causes of Stiffness in the Fingers. J. Bone Joint Surg., 50B:656–663, 1968.

470. Kuczynski, K.: Less-known Aspects of the Proximal Interphalangeal Joints of the Human Hand. Hand, 7:31–33, 1975.

471. Lane, C.S.: Reconstruction of the Unstable Proximal Interphalangeal Joint: The Double Superficialis Tenodesis. J. Hand Surg., 3:368–369, 1978.

472. Lange, R.H., and Engber, W.D.: Proximal Interphalangeal Joint Fracture-dislocation Associated With Mallet Finger. Orthopedics, 6:571–575, 1983.

473. Levy, I.M., and Liberty, S.: Simultaneous Dislocation of the Interphalangeal and Metacarpophalangeal Joints of the Thumb: A Case Report. J. Hand Surg., 4:489–490, 1979.

474. Light, T.R.: Buttress Pinning Techniques. Orthop. Rev., 10:49–55, 1981.

475. Lineaweaver, W., and Mathes, S.J.: Distal Avulsion of the Palmar Plate of the Interphalangeal Joint of the Thumb. J. Hand Surg., 13A:465–467, 1988.

476. London, P.S.: Sprains and Fractures Involving the Interphalangeal Joints. Hand, 3:155–158, 1971.

477. Lubahn, J.D.: Dorsal Fracture Dislocations of the Proximal Interphalangeal Joint. Hand Clin., 4:15–24, 1988.

478. Lucas, G.L.: Volar Plate Advancement. Orthop. Rev., 4:13–16, 1975.

479. McCue, F.C.; Honner, R.; Johnson, M.C.; and Gieck, J.H.: Athletic Injuries of the Proximal Interphalangeal Joint Requiring Surgical Treatment. J. Bone Joint Surg., 52A:937–956, 1970.

480. McElfresh, E.C.; Dobyns, J.H.; and O'Brien, E.T.: Management of Fracture-dislocation of the Proximal Interphalangeal Joints by Extension-block Splinting. J. Bone Joint Surg., 54A:1705–1711, 1972.

481. Meyn, M.A., Jr.: Irreducible Volar Dislocation of the Proximointerphalangeal Joint. Clin. Orthop., 158:215–218, 1981.

482. Milford, L.: The Hand. *In* Crenshaw, A.H. (ed.): Campbell's Operative Orthopaedics, 4th ed., p. 166. St. Louis, C.V. Mosby, 1963.

483. Milford, L.: The Hand. *In* Crenshaw, A.H. (ed.): Campbell's Operative Orthopaedics, 5th ed., pp. 188–189. St. Louis, C.V. Mosby, 1971.

484. Milford, L.: The Hand. *In* Edmonson, A.S., and Crenshaw, A.H. (eds.): Campbell's Operative Orthopaedics, 6th ed., p. 160. St. Louis, C.V. Mosby, 1980.

485. Milford, L.: Interphalangeal Dislocations. *In* Crenshaw, A.H. (ed.): Campbell's Operative Orthopaedics, 7th ed., pp. 249–253. St. Louis, C.V. Mosby, 1987.

486. Moberg, E.: Fractures and Ligamentous Injuries of the Thumb and Fingers. Surg. Clin. North Am., 40:297–309, 1960.

487. Moller, J.T.: Lesions of the Volar Fibrocartilage in Finger Joints. A 2-year Material. Acta Orthop. Scand., 45:673–682, 1974.

488. Murakami, Y.: Irreducible Volar Dislocation of the Proximal Interphalangeal Joint of the Finger. Hand, 6:87–90, 1974.

489. Murakami, Y.: Irreducible Dislocation of the Distal Interphalangeal Joint. J. Hand Surg., 10B:231–232, 1985.

490. Nance, E.P.; Kaye, J.J.; and Milek, M.A.: Volar Plate Fractures. Radiology, 133:61–64, 1979.

491. Neviaser, R.J., and Wilson, J.N.: Interposition of the Extensor Tendon Resulting in Persistent Subluxation of the Proximal Interphalangeal Joint of the Finger. Clin. Orthop., 83:118–120, 1972.

492. Nichols, H.M.: Manual of Hand Injuries, 2nd ed., p. 310. Chicago, Year Book Medical Publishers 1960.

493. Oni, O.O.A.: Irreducible Buttonhole Dislocation of the Proximal Interphalangeal Joint of the Finger (A Case Report). J. Hand Surg., 10B:100, 1985.

494. Ostrowski, D.M., and Neimkin, R.J.: Irreducible Palmar Dislocation of the Proximal Interphalangeal Joint. A Case Report. Orthopedics, 8:84–86, 1985.

495. Palmer, A.K., and Linscheid, R.L.: Irreducible Dorsal Dislocation of the Distal Interphalangeal Joint of the Finger. J. Hand Surg., 2:406–408, 1977.

496. Palmer, A.K., and Linscheid, R.L.: Chronic Recurrent Dislocation of the Proximal Interphalangeal Joint of the Finger. J. Hand Surg., 3:95–97, 1978.

497. Patel, M.R.; Pearlman, H.S.; Engler, J.; and Lavine, L.S.: Transverse Bayonet Dislocation of the Proximal Interphalangeal Joint. Clin. Orthop., 133:219–226, 1978.

498. Peimer, C.A.; Sullivan, D.J.; and Wild, D.R.: Palmar Dislocation of the Proximal Interphalangeal Joint. J. Hand Surg., 9A:39–48, 1984.

499. Phillips, J.H.: Irreducible Dislocation of a Distal Interphalangeal Joint: Case Report and Review of Literature. Clin. Orthop., 154:188–190, 1981.

500. Pohl, A.L.: Irreducible Dislocation of a Distal Interphalangeal Joint. Br. J. Plast. Surg., 29:227–229, 1976.

501. Portis, R.B.: Hyperextensibility of the Proximal Interphalangeal Joint of the Finger Following Trauma. J. Bone Joint Surg., 36A:1141–1146, 1954.

502. Posner, M.A., and Kapila, D.: Chronic Palmar Dislocation

of Proximal Interphalangeal Joints. J. Hand Surg., 11A: 253–258, 1986.

503. Posner, M.A., and Wilenski, M.: Irreducible Volar Dislocation of the Proximal Interphalangeal Joint of a Finger Caused by Interposition of an Intact Central Slip. A Case Report. J. Bone Joint Surg., 60A:133–134, 1978.

504. Rayan, G.M., and Elias, L.S.: Irreducible Dislocation of the Distal Interphalangeal Joint Caused by Long Flexor Tendon Entrapment. Orthopedics, 4:35–37, 1981.

505. Redler, I., and Williams, J.T.: Rupture of a Collateral Ligament of the Proximal Interphalangeal Joint of the Fingers. Analysis of Eighteen Cases. J. Bone Joint Surg., 49A: 322–326, 1967.

506. Robertson, R.C.; Cawley, J.J., Jr.; and Faris, A.M.: Treatment of Fracture-dislocation of the Interphalangeal Joints of the Hand. J. Bone Joint Surg., 28:68–70, 1946.

507. Rodriguez, A.L.: Injuries to the Collateral Ligaments of the Proximal Interphalangeal Joints. Hand, 5:55–57, 1973.

508. Ron, D.; Alkalay, D.; and Torok, G.: Simultaneous Closed Dislocation of Both Interphalangeal Joints in One Finger. J. Trauma, 23:66–67, 1982.

509. Salamon, P.B., and Gelberman, R.H.: Irreducible Dislocation of the Interphalangeal Joint of the Thumb. Report of Three Cases. J. Bone Joint Surg., 60A:400–401, 1978.

510. Schenck, R.R.: Dynamic Traction and Early Passive Movement for Fractures of the Proximal Interphalangeal Joint. J. Hand Surg., 11A:850–858, 1986.

511. Schulze, H.A.: Treatment of Fracture-dislocations of the Proximal Interphalangeal Joints of the Fingers. Milit. Surg., 99:190–191, 1946.

512. Selig, S., and Schein, A.: Irreducible Buttonhole Dislocation of the Fingers. J. Bone Joint Surg., 22:436–441, 1940.

513. Spinner, M., and Choi, B.Y.: Anterior Dislocation of the Proximal Interphalangeal Joint. A Cause of Rupture of the Central Slip of the Extensor Mechanism. J. Bone Joint Surg., 52A:1329–1336, 1970.

514. Sprague, B.L.: Proximal Interphalangeal Joint Injuries and Their Initial Treatment. J. Trauma, 15:380–385, 1975.

515. Spray, P.: Finger Fracture-dislocation Proximal at the Interphalangeal Joint. J. Tenn. Med. Assoc., 59:765–766, 1966.

516. Stern, P.J.: Stener Lesion After Lateral Dislocation of the Proximal Interphalangeal Joint—Indication for Open Reduction. J. Hand Surg., 6:602–603, 1981.

517. Stern, P.J., and Lee, A.F.: Open Dorsal Dislocations of the Proximal Interphalangeal Joint. J. Hand Surg., 10A:364–370, 1985.

518. Stripling, W.D.: Displaced Intra-articular Osteochondral Fracture—Cause for Irreducible Dislocation of the Distal Interphalangeal Joint. J. Hand Surg., 7:77–78, 1982.

519. Strong, M.L.: A New Method of Extension-block Splinting for the Proximal Interphalangeal Joint—Preliminary Report. J. Hand Surg., 5:606–607, 1980.

520. Swanson, A.B.: Surgery of the Hand in Cerebral Palsy and Muscle Origin Release Procedures. Surg. Clin. North Am., 48:1129–1137, 1968.

521. Thayer, D.T.: Distal Interphalangeal Joint Injuries. Hand Clin., 4:1–4, 1988.

522. Thompson, J.S., and Eaton, R.G.: Volar Dislocation of the Proximal Interphalangeal Joint (Abstr.). J. Hand Surg., 2:232, 1977.

523. Trojan, E.: Fracture Dislocation of the Bases of the Proximal and Middle Phalanges of the Fingers. Hand, 4:60–61, 1972.

524. Tully, J.G., Jr.; Kaphan, M.L.; and Burack, N.D.: Compound Complex Dislocation of Proximal Interphalangeal Joint. Orthop. Rev., 14:81–84, 1985.

525. Vicar, A.J.: Proximal Interphalangeal Joint Dislocations Without Fractures. Hand Clin., 4:5–13, 1988.

526. Watson, F.M., Jr.: Simultaneous Interphalangeal Dislocation in One Finger. J. Trauma, 23:65, 1982.

527. Watson, H.K.; Light, T.R.; and Johnson, T.R.: Checkrein Resection for Flexion Contractures of the Middle Joint. J. Hand Surg., 4:67–71, 1979.

528. Weseley, M.S.; Barenfeld, P.A.; and Eisenstein, A.L.: Simultaneous Dorsal Dislocation of Both Interphalangeal Joints in a Finger. A Case Report. J. Bone Joint Surg., 60A:1142, 1978.

529. Whipple, T.L.; Evans, J.P.; and Urbaniak, J.R.: Irreducible Dislocation of a Finger Joint in a Child. A Case Report. J. Bone Joint Surg., 62A:832–833, 1980.

530. Wiley, A.M.: Chronic Dislocation of the Proximal Interphalangeal Joint: A Method of Surgical Repair. Can. J. Surg., 8:435–439, 1965.

531. Wiley, A.M.: Instability of the Proximal Interphalangeal Joint Following Dislocation and Fracture Dislocation: Surgical Repair. Hand, 2:185–190, 1970.

532. Wilson, J.N., and Rowland, S.A.: Fracture-dislocation of the Proximal Interphalangeal Joint of the Finger. Treatment by Open Reduction and Internal Fixation. J. Bone Joint Surg., 48A:493–502, 1966.

533. Wilson, R.L., and Liechty, B.W.: Complications Following Small Joint Injuries. Hand Clin., 2:329–345, 1986.

534. Wong, J.T.M.: Extensor Mechanism Preventing Reduction of Finger (Abstr.). Med. J. Aust., 1:101, 1978.

535. Woods, G.L., and Burton, R.I.: Avoiding Pitfalls in the Diagnosis of Acutely Injured Proximal Interphalangeal Joint. Clin. Plast. Surg., 8:95–105, 1981.

536. Zemel, N.P.; Stark, H.H.; Ashworth, C.R.; and Boyes, J.H.: Chronic Fracture Dislocation of the Proximal Interphalangeal Joint—Treatment by Osteotomy and Bone Graft (Abstr.). Orthop. Trans., 4:5–6, 1980.

537. Zielinski, C.J.: Irreducible Fracture-dislocation of the Distal Interphalangeal Joint. J. Bone Joint Surg., 65A:109–110, 1983.

538. Zook, E.G.; Van Beek, A.L.; and Wavak, P.: Transverse Volar Skin Laceration of the Finger: A Sign of Volar Plate Injury. Hand, 11:213–216, 1979.

539. Zook, E.G.; Van Beek, A.L.; and Wavak, P.: Transverse Volar Skin Laceration of the Finger: A Sign of Volar Plate Injury. Hand, 11:213–216, 1979.

Metacarpophalangeal Joints

540. Adler, G.A., and Light, T.R.: Simultaneous Complex Dislocation of the Metacarpophalangeal Joints of the Long and Index Fingers. J. Bone Joint Surg., 63A:1007–1009, 1981.

541. Alldred, A.: A Locked Index Finger. J. Bone Joint Surg., 36B:102–103, 1954.

542. Andersen, J.A., and Gjerloff, C.C.: Complex Dislocation of the Metacarpophalangeal Joint of the Little Finger. J. Hand Surg., 12B:264–266, 1987.

543. Araki, S.; Ohtani, T.; and Tanaka, T.: Open Dorsal Metacarpophalangeal Dislocations of the Index, Long, and Ring Fingers. J. Hand Surg., 12A:458–460, 1987.

544. Aston, J.N.: Locked Middle Finger. J. Bone Joint Surg., 42B:75–79, 1960.

545. Baldwin, L.W.; Miller, D.L.; Lockhart, L.D.; and Evans, E.B.: Metacarpophalangeal-joint Dislocations of the Fingers. A Comparison of the Pathological Anatomy of Index and Little Finger Dislocations. J. Bone Joint Surg., 49A:1587–1590, 1967.

546. Barash, H.L.: An Unusual Case of Dorsal Dislocation of the Metacarpophalangeal Joint of the Index Finger. Clin. Orthop., 83:121–122, 1972.

547. Barenfeld, P.A., and Weseley, M.S.: Dorsal Dislocation of the Metacarpophalangeal Joint of the Index Finger Treated by Late Open Reduction. J. Bone Joint Surg., 54A:1311–1313, 1972.

548. Barnard, H.L.: Dorsal Dislocation of the First Phalanx of the Little Finger. Reduction by Farabeuf's Dorsal Incision. Lancet, 1:88–90, 1901.

549. Barry, K.; McGee, H.; and Curtin, J.: Complex Dislocation of the Metacarpo-phalangeal Joint of the Index Finger: A Comparison of the Surgical Approaches. J. Hand Surg., 13B:466–468, 1988.

550. Battle, W.H.: Backward Dislocation of the Fingers Upon the Metacarpus. Lancet, 1:1223–1224, 1888.

551. Becton, J.L., and Carswell, A.S.: The Natural History of an Unreduced Dislocated Index Finger Metacarpophalangeal Joint in a Child. J. Med. Assoc. Ga., 64:413–415, 1975.

552. Becton, J.L.; Christian J.D., Jr.; Goodwin, H.N.; and Jackson, J.G., III: A Simplified Technique for Treating the Complex Dislocation of the Index Metacarpophalangeal Joint. J. Bone Joint Surg., 57A:698–700, 1975.

553. Betz, R.R.; Browne, E.Z.; Perry, G.B.; and Resnick, E.J.: The Complex Volar Metacarpophalangeal-joint Dislocation. A Case Report and Review of the Literature. J. Bone Joint Surg., 64A:1374–1375, 1982.

554. Bloom, M.H., and Bryan, R.S.: Locked Index Finger Caused by Hyperflexion and Entrapment of Sesamoid Bone. J. Bone Joint Surg., 47A:1383–1385, 1965.

555. Bohart, P.G.; Gelberman, R.H.; Vandell, R.F.; and Salamon, P.B.: Complex Dislocations of the Metacarpophalangeal Joint. Operative Reduction by Farabeuf's Dorsal Incision. Clin. Orthop., 164:208–210, 1982.

556. Boland, D.: Volar Dislocation of the Ring Finger Metacarpophalangeal Joint. Orthop. Rev., 13:69–72, 1984.

557. Bruner, J.M.: Recurrent Locking of the Index Finger Due to Internal Derangement of the Metacarpophalangeal Joint. J. Bone Joint Surg., 43A:450–453, 1961.

558. Buchler, U.: American Society for Surgery of the Hand, Correspondence Newsletter, 1987.

559. Burman, M.: Irreducible Hyperextension Dislocation of the Metacarpophalangeal Joint of a Finger. Bull. Hosp. Joint Dis., 14:290–291, 1953.

560. Cunningham, D.M., and Schwarz, G.: Dorsal Dislocation of the Index Metacarpophalangeal Joint. Plast. Reconstr. Surg., 56:654–659, 1975.

561. Dibbell, D.G., and Field, J.H.: Locking Metacarpal Phalangeal Joint. Plast. Reconstr. Surg., 40:562–564, 1967.

562. Dray, G.; Millender, L.H.; and Nalebuff, E.A.: Rupture of the Radial Collateral Ligament of a Metacarpophalangeal Joint to One of the Ulnar Three Fingers. J. Hand Surg., 4:346–350, 1979.

563. Dutton, R.O., and Meals, R.A.: Complex Dorsal Dislocation of the Thumb Metacarpophalangeal Joint. Clin. Orthop., 164:160–164, 1982.

564. Eaton, R.G.: Joint Injuries of the Hand. Springfield, Ill., Charles C. Thomas, 1971.

565. Farabeuf, L.H.F.: De la luxation du ponce en arriere. Bull. de la Soc de Chirurgie, 11:21–62, 1876.

566. Flatt, A.E.: Recurrent Locking of an Index Finger. J. Bone Joint Surg., 40A:1128–1129, 1958.

567. Flatt, A.E.: A Locking Little Finger. J. Bone Joint Surg., 43A:240–242, 1961.

568. Fultz, C.W., and Buchanan, J.R.: Complex Fracture-dislocation of the Metacarpophalangeal Joint. Case Report. Clin. Orthop., 227:255–260, 1988.

569. Gee, T.C., and Pho, R.W.H.: Avulsion-fracture at the Proximal Attachment of the Radial Collateral Ligament of the Fifth Metacarpophalangeal Joint—A Case Report. J. Hand Surg., 7:526–527, 1982.

570. Goodfellow, J.W., and Weaver, J.P.A.: Locking of the Metacarpophalangeal Joints. J. Bone Joint Surg., 43B:772–777, 1961.

571. Gordon, M.H.: Irreduceable Metacarpophalangeal Dislocations. Bull. Hosp. Joint Dis., 37:164–171, 1976.

572. Green, D.P., and Terry, G.C.: Complex Dislocation of the Metacarpophalangeal Joint. Correlative Pathological Anatomy. J. Bone Joint Surg., 55A:1480–1486, 1973.

573. Guly, H.R., and Azam, M.A.: Locked Finger Treated by Manipulation. A Report of Three Cases. J. Bone Joint Surg., 64A:73–75, 1982.

574. Gustilo, R.B.: Dislocation of the Metacarpophalangeal Joint of the Index Finger. Minn. Med., 1119–1121, 1966.

575. Hall, R.F., Jr.; Gleason, T.F.; and Kasa, R.F.: Simultaneous Closed Dislocations of the Metacarpophalangeal Joints of the Index, Long, and Ring Fingers: A Case Report. J. Hand Surg., 10A:81–85, 1985.

576. Harvey, F.J.: Locking of the Metacarpophalangeal Joints. J. Bone Joint Surg., 56B:156–159, 1974.

577. Honner, R.: Locking of the Metacarpophalangeal Joint From a Loose Body. Report of a Case. J. Bone Joint Surg., 51B:479–481, 1969.

578. Hubbard, L.F.: Metacarpophalangeal Dislocations. Hand Clin., 4:39–44, 1988.

579. Hunt, J.C.; Watts, H.B.; and Glasgow, J.D.: Dorsal Dislocation of the Metacarpophalangeal Joint of the Index Finger With Particular Reference to Open Dislocation. J. Bone Joint Surg., 49A:1572–1578, 1967.

580. Iftikhar, T.B., and Kaminski, R.S.: Simultaneous Dorsal Dislocation of MP Joints of Long and Ring Fingers. A Case Report. Orthop. Rev., 10:71–72, 1981.

581. Imbriglia, J.E., and Sciulli, R.: Open Complex Metacar-

pophalangeal Joint Dislocation. Two Cases: Index Finger and Long Finger. J. Hand Surg., 4:72–75, 1979.

582. Inoue, G.; Nakamura, R.; and Miura, T.: Intra-articular Fracture of the Metacarpal Head of the Locked Index Finger Due to Forced Passive Extension. J. Hand Surg., 13B: 320–322, 1988.

583. Ishizuki, M.: Injury to Collateral Ligament of Metacarpophalangeal Joint of a Finger. J. Hand Surg., 13A:456–460, 1988.

584. Kaplan, E.B.: Dorsal Dislocation of the Metacarpophalangeal Joint of the Index Finger. J. Bone Joint Surg., 39A: 1081–1086, 1957.

585. Koniuch, M.P.; Peimer, C.A.; VanGorder, T.; and Moncada, A.: Closed Crush Injury of the Metacarpophalangeal Joint. J. Hand Surg., 12A:750–757, 1987.

586. Langenskiold, A.: Habitual Locking of a Metacarpophalangeal Joint by a Collateral Ligament, a Rare Cause of Trigger Finger. Acta Chir. Scand., 99:72–78, 1949.

587. Le Clerc, R.: Luxations de lindex sur son metacarpien. Rev. D'Orthop., 2:227–242, 1911.

588. Lutter, L.D.: A New Cause of Locking Fingers. Clin. Orthop., 83:131–134, 1972.

589. Malerich, M.M.; Eaton, R.G.; and Upton, J.: Complete Dislocation of a Little Finger Metacarpal Phalangeal Joint Treated by Closed Technique. J. Trauma, 20:424–425, 1980.

590. McElfresh, E.C., and Dobyns, J.H.: Intra-articular Metacarpal Head Fractures. J. Hand Surg., 8:383–393, 1983.

591. McLaughlin, H.L.: Complex "Locked" Dislocation of the Metacarpophalangeal Joints. J. Trauma, 5:683–688, 1965.

592. Milch, H.: Subluxation of the Index Metacarpophalangeal Joint. Case Report. J. Bone Joint Surg., 47A:522–523, 1965.

593. Miller, P.R.; Evans, B.W.; and Glazer, D.A.: Locked Dislocation of the Metacarpophalangeal Joint of the Index Finger. J.A.M.A., 203:138–139, 1968.

594. Minami, A.; An, Kai-Nan; Cooney, W.P.; Linscheid, R.L.; and Chao, E.Y.S.: Ligament Stability of the Metacarpophalangeal Joint: A Biomechanical Study. J. Hand Surg., 10A:255–260, 1985.

595. Moneim, M.S.: Volar Dislocation of the Metacarpophalangeal Joint. Pathologic Anatomy and Report of Two Cases. Clin. Orthop., 176:186–189, 1983.

596. Murphy, A.F., and Stark, H.H.: Closed Dislocation of the Metacarpophalangeal Joint of the Index Finger. J. Bone Joint Surg., 49A:1579–1586, 1967.

597. Murray, J.F.: Personal communication, 1981.

598. Nussbaum, R., and Sadler, A.H.: An Isolated, Closed, Complex Dislocation of the Metacarpophalangeal Joint of the Long Finger: A Unique Case. J. Hand Surg., 11A: 558–561, 1986.

599. Nutter, P.D.: Interposition of Sesamoids in Metacarpophalangeal Dislocations. J. Bone Joint Surg., 22:730–734, 1940.

600. Posner, M.A.; Langa, V.; and Green, S.M.: The Locked Metacarpophalangeal Joint: Diagnosis and Treatment. J. Hand Surg., 11A:249–253, 1986.

601. Quinton, D.N.: Dorsal Locking of the Metacarpophalangeal Joint. J. Hand Surg., 12B:62–63, 1987.

602. Rankin, E.A.; and Uwagie-Ero, S.: Locking of the Meta-

carpophalangeal Joint. J. Hand Surg., 11A:868–871, 1986.

603. Renshaw, T.S., and Louis, D.S.: Complex Volar Dislocation of the Metacarpophalangeal Joint: A Case Report. J. Trauma, 13:1086–1088, 1971.

604. Ridge, E.M.: Dorsal Dislocation of the First Phalanx of the Little Finger. Lancet, 1:781, 1901.

605. Robins, R.H.C.: Injuries of the Metacarpophalangeal Joints. Hand, 3:159–163, 1971.

606. Silberman, W.W.: Clear View of the Index Sesamoid: A Sign of Irreducible Metacarpophalangeal Joint Dislocation. J. Am. Coll. Emerg. Physic. 8:371–373, 1979.

607. Smith, R.J., and Sturchio, E.A.: The Locked Metacarpophalangeal Joint. Bull. Hosp. Joint Dis., 29:205–211, 1968.

608. Stewart, G.J., and Williams, E.A.: Locking of the Metacarpophalangeal Joints in Degenerative Disease. Hand, 13:147–151, 1981.

609. Sweterlitsch, P.R.; Torg, J.S.; and Pollack, H.: Entrapment of a Sesamoid in the Index Metacarpophalangeal Joint. J. Bone Joint Surg., 51A:995–998, 1969.

610. Tsuge, K., and Watari, S.: Dorsal Dislocation of the Metacarpophalangeal Joint of the Index Finger. Hiroshima J. Med. Sci., 22:65–81, 1973.

611. Umansky, A.L.: The Dislocated Index Metacarpophalangeal Joint. (Abstract) J. Bone Joint Surg., 45A:216, 1963.

612. von Raffler, W.: Irreducible Dislocation of the Metacarpophalangeal Joint of the Finger. Clin. Orthop., 35:171–173, 1964.

613. Wilhelmy, J., and Hay, R.L.: Dual Dislocation of Metacarpophalangeal Joints. Hand, 4:168–170, 1972.

614. Wolov, R.B.: Complex Dislocations of the Metacarpophalangeal Joints. Orthop. Rev., 17:770–775, 1988.

615. Wood, M.B., and Dobyns, J.H.: Chronic, Complex Volar Dislocation of the Metacarpophalangeal Joint. Report of Three Cases. J. Hand Surg., 6:73–76, 1981.

616. Wright, C.S.: Compound Dislocations of Four Metacarpophalangeal Joints. J. Hand Surg., 10B:233–235, 1985.

617. Yancey, H.A., Jr., and Howard, L.D., Jr.: Locking of the Metacarpophalangeal Joint. J. Bone Joint Surg., 44A:380–382, 1962.

CMC Joints (Excluding the Thumb)

618. Berg, E.E., and Murphy, D.F.: Ulnopalmar Dislocation of the Fifth Carpometacarpal Joint—Successful Closed Reduction: Review of the Literature and Anatomic Reevaluation. J. Hand Surg., 11A:521–525, 1986.

619. Black, D.M.; Watson, H.K.; and Vender, M.I.: Arthroplasty of the Ulnar Carpometacarpal Joints. J. Hand Surg., 12A: 1071–1074, 1987.

620. Bloom, M.L., and Stern, P.J.: Carpometacarpal Joints of Fingers. Their Dislocation and Fracture-dislocation. Orthop. Rev., 12:77–82, 1983.

621. Bora, F.W., Jr., and Didizian, N.H.: The Treatment of Injuries to the Carpometacarpal Joint of the Little Finger. J. Bone Joint Surg., 56A:1459–1463, 1974.

622. Breiting, V.: Simultaneous Dislocation of the Bases of the Four Ulnar Metacarpals Upon the Last Row of Carpals. Hand, 15:287–289, 1983.

623. Brewerton, D.A.: A Tangential Radiographic Projection for Demonstrating Involvement of the Metacarpal Head in Rheumatoid Arthritis. Br. J. Radiol., 40:233, 1967.

624. Buzby, B.F.: Palmar Carpo-metacarpal Dislocation of the Fifth Metacarpal. Ann. Surg., 100:555–557, 1934.

625. Cain, J.E.; Shepler, T.R.; and Wilson, M.R.: Hamatometacarpal Fracture-dislocation: Classification and Treatment. J. Hand Surg., 12A:762–767, 1987.

626. Chen, V.T.: Dislocation of Carpometacarpal Joint of the Little Finger. J. Hand Surg., 12B:260–263, 1987.

627. Chmell, S.; Light, T.R.; and Blair, S.J.: Fracture and Fracture Dislocation of Ulnar Carpometacarpal Joint. Orthop. Rev., 11:73–80, 1982.

628. Clement, B.L.: Fracture-dislocation of the Base of the Fifth Metacarpal. A Case Report. J. Bone Joint Surg., 17:498–499, 1945.

629. Clendenin, M.B., and Smith, R.J.: Metacarpo-hamate Arthrodesis for Post-traumatic Arthritis. Orthop. Trans., 6:168, 1982.

630. Clendenin, M.B., and Smith, R.J.: Fifth Metacarpal/Hamate Arthrodesis for Posttraumatic Osteoarthritis. J. Hand Surg., 9A:374–378, 1984.

631. Dennyson, W.G., and Stother, I.G.: Carpometacarpal Dislocation of the Little Finger. Hand, 8:161–164, 1976.

632. Dommisse, I.G., and Lloyd, G.J.: Injuries to the Fifth Carpometacarpal Region. Can. J. Surg., 22:240–244, 1979.

633. Fisher, M.R.; Rogers, L.F.; and Hendrix, R.W.: Systematic Approach to Identifying Fourth and Fifth Carpometacarpal Joint Dislocations. A.J.R., 140:319–324, 1983.

634. Fisher, M.R.; Rogers, L.F.; and Hendrix, R.W.: Carpometacarpal Dislocations. CRC Crit. Rev. Diagn. Imaging, 22:95–126.

635. Flatt, A.E.: The Care of Minor Hand Injuries. St. Louis, C.V. Mosby, 1959.

636. Gore, D.R.: Carpometacarpal Dislocation Producing Compression of the Deep Branch of the Ulnar Nerve. J. Bone Joint Surg., 53A:1387–1390, 1971.

637. Goss, C.M.: Gray's Anatomy, 26th ed., pp. 371–372. Philadelphia, Lea & Febiger, 1954.

638. Green, D.P., and Rowland, S.A.: Carpometacarpal Dislocations (Excluding the Thumb). *In* Rockwood, C.A., and Green, D.P. (eds.): Fractures, pp. 323–327. Philadelphia, J.B. Lippincott, 1975.

639. Green, W.L., and Kilgore, E.S.: Treatment of Fifth Digit Carpometacarpal Arthritis With Silastic Prosthesis. J. Hand Surg., 6:510–514, 1981.

640. Gunther, S.F.: The Carpometacarpal Joints. Orthop. Clin. North Am., 15:259–277, 1984.

641. Gunther, S.F., and Bruno, P.D.: Divergent Dislocation of the Carpometacarpal Joints: A Case Report. J. Hand Surg., 10A:197–201, 1985.

642. Hagstrom, P.: Fracture Dislocation in the Ulnar Carpometacarpal Joints. Open Reduction and Pinning—A Case Report. Scand. J. Plast. Recontr. Surg., 9:249–251, 1975.

643. Hartwig, R.H., and Louis, D.S.: Multiple Carpometacarpal Dislocations. J. Bone Joint Surg., 61A:906–908, 1979.

644. Harwin, S.F.; Fox, J.M.; and Sedlin, E.D.: Volar Dislocation of the Bases of the Second and Third Metacarpals. J. Bone Joint Surg., 57A:849–851, 1975.

645. Hazlett, J.W.: Carpometacarpal Dislocations Other Than the Thumb: A Report of 11 Cases. Can. J. Surg., 11:315–322, 1968.

646. Helal, B., and Kavanagh, T.G.: Unstable Dorsal Fracture-Dislocation of the Fifth Carpometacarpal Joint. Injury, 9:138–142, 1977.

647. Henderson, J.J., and Arafa, M.A.M.: Carpometacarpal Dislocation. An Easily Missed Diagnosis. J. Bone Joint Surg., 69B:212–214, 1987.

648. Ho, P.K.; Choban, S.J.; Eshman, S.J.; and Dupuy, T.E.: Complex Dorsal Dislocation of the Second Carpometacarpal Joint. J. Hand Surg., 12A:1074–1076, 1987.

649. Hsu, J.D., and Curtis, R.M.: Carpometacarpal Dislocations on the Ulnar Side of the Hand. J. Bone Joint Surg., 52A:927–930, 1970.

650. Imbriglia, J.E.: Chronic Dorsal Carpometacarpal Dislocations of the Index, Middle, Ring, and Little Fingers: A Case Report. J. Hand Surg., 4:343–345, 1979.

651. Joseph, R.B.; Linscheid, R.L.; Dobyns, J.H.; and Bryan, R.S.: Chronic Sprains of the Carpometacarpal Joints. J. Hand Surg., 6:172–180, 1981.

652. Kaplan, E.B.: Functional and Surgical Anatomy of the Hand, 2nd ed., pp. 28–35, 134. Philadelphia, J.B. Lippincott, 1965.

653. Kaye, J.J., and Lister, G.D.: Another Use for the Brewerton View (Letter). J. Hand Surg., 3:603, 1978.

654. Ker, H.R.: Dislocation of the Fifth Carpo-metacarpal Joint. J. Bone Joint Surg., 37B:254–256, 1955.

655. Kinnett, J.G., and Lyden, J.P.: Posterior Fracture-dislocation of the IV Metacarpal Hamate Articulation: Case Report. J. Trauma, 19:290–291, 1979.

656. Kleinman, W.B., and Grantham, S.A.: Multiple Volar Carpometacarpal Joint Dislocation. J. Hand Surg., 3:377–382, 1978.

657. Lewis, H.H.: Dislocation of the Second Metacarpal: Report of a Case. Clin. Orthop., 93:253–255, 1973.

658. Lilling, M., and Weinberg, H.: The Mechanism of Dorsal Fracture Dislocation of the Fifth Carpometacarpal Joint. J. Hand Surg., 4:340–342, 1979.

659. Lyman, C.B.: Backward Dislocation of the Second Carpometacarpal Articulation. Ann. Surg., 43:905–906, 1906.

660. Marck, K.W., and Klasen, H.J.: Fracture-dislocation of the Hamatometacarpal Joint: A Case Report. J. Hand Surg., 11A:128–130, 1986.

661. McLean, E.H.: Carpometacarpal Dislocation. J.A.M.A., 79:299–300, 1922.

662. McWhorter, G.I.: Isolated and Complete Dislocation of the Fifth Carpometacarpal Joint: Open Operation. Surg. Clin. Chicago, 2:793–796, 1918.

663. Metz, W.R.: Multiple Carpo-metacarpal Dislocations. With the Report of a Case. New Orleans Med. Surg. J., 79:327–330, 1927.

664. Mueller, J.J.: Carpometacarpal Dislocations: Report of Five Cases and Review of the Literature. J. Hand Surg., 11A:184–188, 1986.

665. Murless, B.C.: Fracture-dislocation of the Base of the Fifth Metacarpal Bone. Br. J. Surg., 31:402–404, 1943.

666. Nalebuff, E.A.: Isolated Anterior Carpometacarpal Dislocation of the Fifth Finger: Classification and Case Report. J. Trauma, 8:1119–1123, 1968.

667. North, E.R., and Eaton, R.G.: Volar Dislocation of the

Fifth Metacarpal. Report of Two Cases. J. Bone Joint Surg., 62A:657–659, 1980.

668. Oni, O.O.A., and Mackenny, R.P.: Multiple Dislocations of the Carpometacarpal Joints. J. Hand Surg., 11B:47–48, 1986.

669. Peterson, P., and Sacks, S.: Fracture-dislocation of the Base of the Fifth Metacarpal Associated With Injury to the Deep Motor Branch of the Ulnar Nerve: A Case Report. J. Hand Surg., 11A:525–528, 1986.

670. Petrie, P.W.R., and Lamb, D.W.: Fracture-subluxation of Base of Fifth Metacarpal. Hand, 6:82–86, 1974.

671. Rawles, J.G.: Dislocations and Fracture-dislocations at the Carpometacarpal Joints of the Fingers. Hand Clin., 4:103–112, 1988.

672. Resnick, S.M.; Greene, T.L.; and Roeser, W.: Simultaneous Dislocation of the Five Carpometacarpal Joints. Clin. Orthop., 192:210–214, 1985.

673. Roberts, N., and Holland, C.T.: Isolated Dislocation of the Base of the Fifth Metacarpal. Br. J. Surg., 23:567–571, 1936.

674. Sandzen, S.C.: Fracture of the Fifth Metacarpal Resembling Bennett's Fracture. Hand, 5:49–51, 1973.

675. Schutt, R.C.; Boswick, J.A.; and Scott, F.A.: Volar Fracture-dislocation of the Carpometacarpal Joint of the Index Finger Treated by Delayed Open Reduction. J. Trauma, 21:986–987, 1981.

676. Shephard, E., and Solomon, D.J.: Carpo-metacarpal Dislocation. A Report of Four Cases. J. Bone Joint Surg., 42B:772–777, 1960.

677. Shorbe, H.B.: Carpometacarpal Dislocations. A Report of a Case. J. Bone Joint Surg., 20:454–457, 1938.

678. Smith, R.J.: Malunion of the Base of the Fifth Metacarpal Fracture and Dislocation. American Society for Surgery of the Hand, Correspondence Newsletter. 1980.

679. Stevanovic, M.V., and Stark, H.H.: Dorsal Dislocation of the Fourth and Fifth Carpometacarpal Joints and Simultaneous Dislocation of the Metacarpophalangeal Joint of the Small Finger: A Case Report. J. Hand Surg., 9A:714–716, 1984.

680. Storm, J.O.: Traumatic Dislocation of the Fourth and Fifth Carpo-metacarpal Joints: A Case Report. J. Hand Surg., 13B:210–211, 1988.

681. Tountas, A.A., and Kwok, J.M.K.: Isolated Volar Dislocation of the Fifth Carpometacarpal Joint. Case Report. Clin. Orthop., 187:172–175, 1984.

682. Wainwright, D.: Fractures of the Metacarpals and Phalanges. Proc. R. Soc. Med., 57:598–599, 1964.

683. Watson-Jones, R.: Fractures and Joint Injuries, 4th ed., pp. 635. Edinburgh, E & S Livingstone, 1956.

684. Waugh, R.L., and Yancey, A.G.: Carpometacarpal Dislocation. With Particular Reference to Simultaneous Dislocation of the Bases of the Fourth and Fifth Metacarpals. J. Bone Joint Surg., 30A:397–404, 1948.

685. Weiland, A.J.; Lister, G.D.; and Villarreal-Rios, A.: Volar Fracture Dislocations of the Second and Third Carpometacarpal Joints Associated With Acute Carpal Tunnel Syndrome. J. Trauma, 16:672–675, 1976.

686. Whitson, R.O.: Carpometacarpal Dislocation. A Case Report. Clin. Orthop., 6:189–195, 1955.

687. Wiley, A.M., and Dommisse, I.: Disabilities Following

Basal Fractures and Dislocations of the Ulnar Border of the Hand. Orthop. Rev., 5:43–47, 1976.

MP Joint of the Thumb–Collateral Ligament Injuries

688. Ahmad, I., and DePalma, A.F.: Treatment of Gamekeeper's Thumb by a New Operation. Clin. Orthop., 103:167–169, 1974.

689. Alldred, A.J.: Rupture of the Collateral Ligament of the Metacarpo-phalangeal Joint of the Thumb. J. Bone Joint Surg., 37B:443–445, 1955.

690. Baily, R.A.J.: Some Closed Injuries of the Metacarpophalangeal Joint of the Thumb. J. Bone Joint Surg., 45B:428–429, 1963.

691. Bezes, P.M.H.: Severe Metacarpophalangeal Sprain of the Thumb in Ski Accidents. Ann. Chir. Main., 3:101–112, 1984.

692. Bowers, W.H., and Hurst, L.C.: Gamekeeper's Thumb. Evaluation by Arthrography and Stress Roentgenography. J. Bone Joint Surg., 59A:519–524, 1977.

693. Brewood, A.F.M., and Menon, T.J.: Combined Reconstruction of Volar and Radial Instability of a Thumb Metacarpo-phalangeal Joint. J. Hand Surg., 9B:333–334, 1984.

694. Browne, E.Z.; Dunn, H.K.; and Snyder, C.C.: Ski Pole Thumb Injury. Plast. Reconstr. Surg., 58:19–23, 1976.

695. Camp, R.A.; Weatherwax, R.J.; and Miller, E.B.: Chronic Posttraumatic Radial Instability of the Thumb Metacarpophalangeal Joint. J. Hand Surg., 5:221–225, 1980.

696. Campbell, C.S.: Gamekeeper's Thumb. J. Bone Joint Surg., 37B:148–149, 1955.

697. Carr, D.; Johnson, R.J.; and Pope, M.H.: Upper Extremity Injuries in Skiing. Am. J. Sports Med., 9:378–383, 1981.

698. Coonrad, R.W., and Goldner, J.L.: A Study of the Pathological Findings and Treatment in Soft-tissue Injury of the Thumb Metacarpophalangeal Joint. J. Bone Joint Surg., 50A:439–451, 1968.

699. Curtis, D.J., and Downey, E.F., Jr.: A Simple First Metacarpophalangeal Stress Test. Radiology, 148:855–856, 1983.

700. Davis, P.H.: Arthrography of the Thumb Metacarpo-phalangeal Joint. American Society for Surgery of the Hand, Correspondence Newsletter, 1975.

701. Derkash, R.S.; Matyas, J.R.; Weaver, J.K.; Oden, R.R.; Kirk, R.E.; Freeman, J.R.; and Cipriano, F.J.: Acute Surgical Repair of the Skier's Thumb. Clin. Orthop., 216:29–33, 1987.

702. Engel, J.; Ganel, A.; Ditzian, R.; and Militeanu, J.: Arthrography as a Method of Diagnosing Tear of the Ulnar Collateral Ligament of the Metacarpophalangeal Joint of the Thumb ("Gamekeeper's Thumb"). J. Trauma, 19:106–109, 1979.

703. Engkvist, O.; Balkfors, B.; Lindsjö, U: Thumb Injuries in Downhill Skiing. Int. J. Sports Med., 3:50–55, 1982.

704. Fairclough, J.A., and Mintowt-Czyz, W.J.: Skier's Thumb—a Method of Prevention. Injury, 17:203–204, 1986.

705. Frank, W.E., and Dobyns, J.: Surgical Pathology of Collateral Ligamentous Injuries of the Thumb. Clin. Orthop., 83:102–114, 1972.

706. Frykman, G., and Johansson, O.: Surgical Repair of Rupture of the Ulnar Collateral Ligament of the Metacarpophalangeal Joint of the Thumb. Acta Chir. Scand., 112: 58–64, 1956.

707. Gerber, C.; Senn, E.; and Matter, P.: Skier's Thumb. Surgical Treatment of Recent Injuries to the Ulnar Collateral Ligament of the Thumb's Metacarpophalangeal Joint. Am. J. Sports Med., 9:171–177, 1981.

708. Goss, C.M.: Gray's Anatomy of the Human Body, 26th ed., pp. 324, 372–373. Philadelphia, Lee & Febiger, 1954.

709. Gutman, J.; Weisbuch, J.; and Wolf, M.: Ski Injuries in 1972–1973. A Repeat Analysis of a Major Health Problem. J.A.M.A., 230:1423–1425, 1974.

710. Hagan, H.J., and Hastings, H.: Fusion of the Thumb Metacarpophalangeal Joint to Treat Posttraumatic Arthritis. J. Hand Surg., 13A:750–753, 1988.

711. Harris, H., and Joseph, J.: Variation in Extension of the Metacarpo-phalangeal and Interphalangeal Joints of the Thumb. J. Bone Joint Surg., 31B:547–559, 1949.

712. Helm, R.H.: Hand Function After Injuries to the Collateral Ligaments of the Metacarpophalangeal Joint of the Thumb. J. Hand Surg., 12B:252–255, 1987.

713. Joseph, J.: Further Studies of the Metacarpophalangeal and Interphalangeal Joints of the Thumb. J. Anat., 85: 221–229, 1951.

714. Kaplan, E.B.: The Pathology and Treatment of Radial Subluxation of the Thumb With Ulnar Displacement of the Head of the First Metacarpal. J. Bone Joint Surg., 43A:541–546, 1961.

715. Kessler, I.: Complex Avulsion of the Ulnar Collateral Ligament of the Metacarpophalangeal Joint of the Thumb. Clin. Orthop., 29:196–200, 1961.

716. Kessler, I., and Heller, J.: Complete Avulsion of the Ligamentous Apparatus of the Metacarpophalangeal Joint of the Thumb. Surg. Gynecol. Obstet., 116:95–98, 1963.

717. Lamb, D.W.; Abernethy, P.J.; and Fragiadakis, E.: Injuries of the Metacarpophalangeal Joint of the Thumb. Hand, 3:164–168, 1971.

718. Lamb, D.W., and Angarita, G.: Ulnar Instability of the Metacarpophalangeal Joint of Thumb. J. Hand Surg., 10B: 113–114, 1985.

719. Linscheid, R.L.: Arthrography of the Metacarpophalangeal Joint. Clin. Orthop., 103:91, 1974.

720. Linscheid, R.L.; Grainger, R.W.; and Johnson, E.W.: The Thumb Metacarpophalangeal Joint. Injuries. Minn. Med., 55:1037–1040, 1972.

721. Louis, D.S.; Huebner, J.J., Jr.; and Hankin, F.M.: Rupture and Displacement of the Ulnar Collateral Ligament of the Metacarpophalangeal Joint of the Thumb. Preoperative Diagnosis. J. Bone Joint Surg., 68A:1320–1326, 1986.

722. McCue, F.C.; Hakala, M.W.; Andrews, J.R.; and Gieck, J.H.: Ulnar Collateral Ligament Injuries of the Thumb in Athletes. J. Sports Med., 2:70–80, 1974.

723. Miller, R.J.: Dislocations and Fracture Dislocations of the Metacarpophalangeal Joint of the Thumb. Hand Clin., 4: 45–65, 1988.

724. Mogan, J.V., and Davis, P.H.: Upper Extremity Injuries in Skiing. Clin. Sports Med., 1:295–308, 1982.

725. Mogensen, B.A., and Mattsson, H.S.: Post-traumatic Instability of the Metacarpophalangeal Joint of the Thumb. Hand, 12:85–90, 1980.

726. Neviaser, R.J., and Adams, J.P.: Complications of Treatment of Injuries to the Hand. In Epps, C.H. (ed.): Complications in Orthopaedic Surgery. Philadelphia, J.B. Lippincott, 1978.

727. Neviaser, R.J.; Wilson, J.N.; and Lievano, A.: Rupture of the Ulnar Collateral Ligament of the Thumb (Gamekeeper's Thumb). J. Bone Joint Surg., 53A:1357–1364, 1971.

728. Osterman, A.L.; Hayken, G.D.; and Bora, F.W.: A Quantitative Evaluation of Thumb Function After Ulnar Collateral Repair and Reconstruction. J. Trauma, 21:854–861, 1981.

729. Palmer, A.K., and Louis, D.S.: Assessing Ulnar Instability of the Metacarpophalangeal Joint of the Thumb. J. Hand Surg., 3:542–546, 1978.

730. Parikh, M.; Nahigian, S.; and Froimson, A.: Gamekeeper's Thumb. Plast. Reconstr. Surg., 58:24–31, 1976.

731. Primiano, G.A.: Skiers' Thumb Injuries Associated With Flared Ski Pole Handles. Am. J. Sports Med., 13:425–427, 1985.

732. Primiano, G.A.: Functional Cast Immobilization of Thumb Metacarpophalangeal Joint Injuries. Am. J. Sports Med., 14:335–339, 1986.

733. Reikeras, O., and Kvarnes, L.: Rupture of the Ulnar Ligament of the Metacarpophalangeal Joint of the Thumb. Arch Orthop. Trauma. Surg., 100:175–177, 1982.

734. Resnick, D., and Danzig, L.A.: Arthrographic Evaluation of Injuries of the First Metacarpophalangeal Joint: Gamekeeper's Thumb. A.J.R., 126:1046–1052, 1976.

735. Rosenthal, D.I.; Murray, W.T.; and Smith, R.J.: Finger Arthrography. Radiology, 137:647–651, 1980.

736. Rovere, G.D.; Gristina, A.G.; Stolzer, W.A.; and Garver, E.M.: Treatment of "Gamekeeper's Thumb" in Hockey Players. J. Sports Med., 3:147–151, 1975.

737. Ruby, L.K.: Common Hand Injuries in the Athlete. Orthop. Clin. North Am., 11:819–839, 1980.

738. Sakellarides, H.T.: Treatment of Recent and Old Injuries of the Ulnar Collateral Ligament of the MP Joint of the Thumb. Am. J. Sports Med., 6:255–262, 1978.

739. Sakellarides, H.T.: The Surgical Treatment of Old Injuries of the Collateral Ligaments of the MP Joint of the Thumb Using the Extensor Pollicis Brevis Tendon (A Long-term Follow-up of 100 Cases). Bull. Hosp. Joint Dis., 44:449–458, 1984.

740. Sakellarides, H.T., and DeWeese, J.W.: Instability of the Metacarpophalangeal Joint of the Thumb. Reconstruction of the Collateral Ligaments Using the Extensor Pollicis Brevis Tendon. J. Bone Joint Surg., 58A:106–112, 1976.

741. Schultz, R.J., and Fox, J.M.: Gamekeeper's Thumb. N.Y. State J. Med., 73:2329–2331, 1973.

742. Smith, M.A.: The Mechanism of Acute Ulnar Instability of the Metacarpophalangeal Joint of the Thumb. Hand, 12:225–230, 1980.

743. Smith, R.J.: Post-traumatic Instability of the Metacarpophalangeal Joint of the Thumb. J. Bone Joint Surg., 59A: 14–21, 1977.

744. Stener, B.: Displacement of the Ruptured Ulnar Collateral Ligament of the Metacarpophalangeal Joint of the Thumb.

A Clinical and Anatomical Study. J. Bone Joint Surg., 44B:869–879, 1962.

745. Stener, B., and Stener, I.: Shearing Fractures Associated With Rupture of Ulnar Collateral Ligament of Metacarpophalangeal Joint of Thumb. Injury, 1:12–16, 1969.

746. Sternbach, G.: C.S. Campbell: Gamekeeper's Thumb. J. Emerg. Med., 1:345–347, 1984.

747. Stothard, J., and Caird, D.M.: Experience With Arthrography of the First Metacarpophalangeal Joint. Hand, 13:257–266, 1981.

748. Strandell, G.: Total Rupture of the Ulnar Collateral Ligament of the Metacarpophalangeal Joint of the Thumb. Results of Surgery in 35 Cases. Acta Chir. Scand., 118:72–80, 1959.

749. Sutro, C.J.: Pollex Valgus (A Bunion-like Deformity of the Thumb Corrected by Surgical Intervention). Bull. Hosp. Joint Dis., 18:135–139, 1957.

750. Van Der Kloot, J.F.V.: Injury to the Ulnar Ligament of the Thumb. Arch. Chir. Neerl., 17:179–185, 1965.

751. Vaupel, G.L., and Andrews, J.R.: Diagnostic and Operative Arthroscopy of the Thumb Metacarpophalangeal Joint. A Case Report. Am. J. Sports Med., 13:139–141, 1985.

752. Weston, W.J.: The Normal Arthrograms of the Metacarpophalangeal, Metatarso-phalangeal and Inter-phalangeal Joints. Aust. Radiol., 13:211–218, 1969.

753. White, G.M.: Ligamentous Avulsion of the Ulnar Collateral Ligament of the Thumb of a Child. J. Hand Surg., 11A:669–672, 1986.

754. Wilppula, E., and Nummi, J.: Surgical Treatment of Ruptured Ulnar Collateral Ligament of the Metacarpophalangeal Joint of the Thumb. Injury, 2:69–72, 1970.

755. Woods, D.W.; Mudge, M.K.; and Wood, V.E.: Radial Instability of the Thumb Metacarpophalangeal Joint: A Clinical and Cadaveric Study. Presented at the Scientific Exhibit, AAOS Annual Meeting, San Francisco, 1987.

756. Zilberman, Z.; Rotschild, E.; and Krauss, L.: Rupture of the Ulnar Collateral Ligament of the Thumb. J. Trauma, 5:447–481, 1965.

MP Joint of the Thumb–Volar Plate Injuries

757. Bell, M.J.; McMurtry, R.Y.; and Rubenstein, J.: Fracture of the Ulnar Sesamoid of the Metacarpophalangeal Joint of the Thumb—An Arthrographic Study. J. Hand Surg., 10B:379–381, 1985.

758. Clarke, P.; Braunstein, E.M.; Weissman, B.N.; and Sosman, J.L.: Case Reports. Sesamoid Fracture of the Thumb. Br. J. Radiol., 56:485, 1983.

759. Dutton, R.O., and Meals, R.A.: Complex Dorsal Dislocation of the Thumb Metacarpophalangeal Joint. Clin. Orthop., 164:160–164, 1982.

760. Eiken, O.: Palmaris Longus-tenodesis for Hyperextension of the Thumb Metacarpophalangeal Joint. Scand. J. Plast. Reconstr. Surg., 15:149–152, 1981.

761. Gunther, S.F., and Zielinski, C.J.: Irreducible Palmar Dislocation of the Proximal Phalanx of the Thumb—Case Report. J. Hand Surg., 7:515–517, 1982.

762. Hansen, C.A., and Peterson, T.H.: Fracture of the Thumb Sesamoid Bones. J. Hand Surg., 12A:269–270, 1987.

763. Inoue, G., and Miura, T.: Locked Metacarpo-phalangeal Joint of the Thumb. J. Hand Surg., 13B:469–473, 1988.

764. Jones, R.P., and Leach, R.E.: Fracture of the Ulnar Sesamoid Bone of the Thumb. Am. J. Sports Med., 8:446–447, 1980.

765. Kessler, I.: A Simplified Technique to Correct Hyperextension Deformity of the Metacarpophalangeal Joint of the Thumb. J. Bone Joint Surg., 61A:903–905, 1979.

766. Kojima, T.; Nagano, T.; and Kohno, T.: Causes of Locking Metacarpophalangeal Joint of the Thumb and Its Nonoperative Treatment. Hand, 11:256–262, 1979.

767. Milch, H.: Recurrent Dislocation of Thumb. Capsulorrhaphy. Am. J. Surg., 6:237–239, 1929.

768. Miyamoto, M.; Hirayama, T.; and Uchida, M.: Volar Dislocation of the Metacarpophalangeal Joint of the Thumb—A Case Report. J. Hand Surg., 11B:51–54, 1986.

769. Moberg, E., and Stener, B.: Injuries to the Ligaments of the Thumb and Fingers. Diagnosis, Treatment and Prognosis. Acta Chir. Scand., 106:166–186, 1953.

770. Moneim, M.S.: Volar Dislocation of the Metacarpophalangeal Joint. Pathological Anatomy and Report of Two Cases. Clin. Orthop., 176:186–189, 1983.

771. Onuba, O., and Essiet, A.: Irreducible Dislocation of the Metacarpophalangeal Joint of the Thumb Due to Tendon Interposition. J. Hand Surg., 12B:60–61, 1987.

772. Palmer, R.E.: Injury to Dorsal MCP Joint of the Thumb. Orthop. Rev., 11:127–129, 1982.

773. Posner, M.A.; Langa, V.; and Ambrose, L.: Intrinsic Muscle Advancement to Treat Chronic Palmar Instability of the Metacarpophalangeal Joint of the Thumb. J. Hand Surg., 13A:110–115, 1988.

774. Sinberg, S.E.: Fracture of a Sesamoid of the Thumb. J. Bone Joint Surg., 22:444–445, 1940.

775. Stener, B.: Hyperextension Injuries to the Metacarpophalangeal Joint of the Thumb—Rupture of Ligaments, Fracture of Sesamoid Bones, Rupture of Flexor Pollicis Brevis. An Anatomical and Clinical Study. Acta Chir. Scand., 125:275–293, 1963.

776. Streatfeild, T., and Griffiths, H.F.: Fracture of a Sesamoid Bone. Lancet, 1:1117, 1934.

777. Tsuge, K., and Watari, S.: Locking Metacarpophalangeal Joint of the Thumb. Hand, 6:255–260, 1974.

778. Wood, V.E.: The Sesamoid Bones of the Hand and Their Pathology. J. Hand Surg., 9B:261–264, 1984.

779. Yamanaka, K.; Yoshida, K.; Inoue, H.; Inoue, A.; and Miyagi, T.: Locking of the Metacarpophalangeal Joint of the Thumb. J. Bone Joint Surg., 67A:782–787, 1985.

780. Zancolli, E.: Structural and Dynamic Bases of Hand Surgery, 2nd ed., pp. 212–213. Philadelphia, J.B. Lippincott, 1979.

CMC Joint of the Thumb

781. Bojsen-Moller, F.: Osteoligamentous Guidance of the Movements of the Human Thumb. Am. J. Anat., 147:71–80, 1976.

782. Bojsen-Moller, F.B.: Osteoligamentous Guidance of the Movements of the Human Thumb. Am. J. Anat., 147:71–80, 1976.

783. Burkhalter, W.E.: American Society for Surgery of the Hand, Correspondence Newsletter, 1981.

784. Chen, V.T.: Dislocation of the Carpometacarpal Joint of the Thumb. J. Hand Surg., 12B:246–251, 1987.

785. Cho, K.O.: Translocation of the Abductor Pollicis Longus

Tendon. A Treatment for Chronic Subluxation of the Thumb Carpometacarpal Joint. J. Bone Joint Surg., 52A: 1166–1170, 1970.

786. Eaton, R.G.: Joint Injuries of the Hand, pp. 66–70. Springfield, Ill., Charles C Thomas, 1971.

787. Eaton, R.G., and Littler, J.W.: Ligament Reconstruction for the Painful Thumb Carpometacarpal Joint. J. Bone Joint Surg., 55A:1655–1666, 1973.

788. Eggers, G.W.N.: Chronic Dislocation of the Base of the Metacarpal of the Thumb. J. Bone Joint Surg., 27:500–501, 1945.

789. Haines, R.W.: The Mechanism of Rotation at the First Carpo-metacarpal Joint. J. Anat., 78:44–46, 1944.

790. Hooper, G.J.: An Unusual Variety of Skier's Thumb. J. Hand Surg., 12A:627–629, 1987.

791. Jensen, J.S.: Operative Treatment of Chronic Subluxation of the First Carpometacarpal Joint. Hand, 7:269–271, 1975.

792. Kestler, O.C.: Recurrent Dislocation of the First Carpo-metacarpal Joint. Repaired by Functional Tenodesis. J. Bone Joint Surg., 28A:858–861, 1946.

793. Kuczynski, K.: Carpometacarpal Joint of the Human Thumb. J. Anat., 118:119–126, 1974.

794. Lasserre, C.; Pauzat, D.; and Derennes, R.: Osteoarthritis of the Trapezio-metacarpal Joint. J. Bone Joint Surg., 31B: 534–536, 1949.

795. Magnusson, A.; Bertheussen, K.; and Weilby, A.: Ligament Reconstruction of the Thumb Carpometacarpal Joint Using a Modified Eaton and Littler Technique. J. Hand Surg., 10B:115–116, 1985.

796. Moore, J.R.; Webb, C.A.; and Thompson, R.C.: A Complete Dislocation of the Thumb Metacarpal. J. Hand Surg., 3: 547–549, 1978.

797. Napier, J.R.: The Form and Function of the Carpometacarpal Joint of the Thumb. J. Anat., 89:362–369, 1955.

798. Pagalidis, T.; Kuczynski, K.; and Lamb, D.W.: Ligmentous Stability of the Base of the Thumb. Hand, 13:29–35, 1981.

799. Pieron, A.P.: The Mechanism of the First Carpometacarpal (CMC) Joint. An Anatomical and Mechanical Analysis. Acta Orthop. Scand., 148:7–104, 1973.

800. Shah, J., and Patel, M.: Dislocation of the Carpometacarpal Joint of the Thumb. A Report of Four Cases. Clin. Orthop., 175:166–169, 1983.

801. Slocum, D.B.: Stabilization of the Articulation of the Greater Multangular and the First Metacarpal. J. Bone Joint Surg., 25A:626–630, 1943.

802. Watt, N., and Hooper, G.: Dislocation of the Trapezio-metacarpal Joint. J. Hand Surg., 12B:242–245, 1987.

803. Wee, J.T.K.; Chandra, D.; and Satku, K.: Simultaneous Dislocations of the Interphalangeal and Carpometacarpal Joints of the Thumb: A Case Report. J. Hand Surg., 13B: 224–226, 1988.

8

Fractures and Dislocations of the Wrist

William P. Cooney III
Ronald L. Linscheid
James H. Dobyns

The wrist is a specialized region of the upper extremity that extends from the carpometacarpal joints to the proximal border of the pronator quadratus. The dictionary definitions of the wrist and carpus may be considered identical, but the wrist (*wraeston,* to "twist") generally covers a larger area of interest than the carpus, which is intended to refer only to the two rows of bones between the distal radius and metacarpals. The wrist is the interconnecting group of joints between the hand and forearm and, in common parlance, includes the midcarpal, radiocarpal, and distal radioulnar joints. The orientation of the wrist is based on skeletal landmarks of the distal radius.[282] Motion is described in terms of radiocarpal flexion–extension and radioulnar deviation, as well as distal radioulnar joint pronation and supination (Fig. 8-1).

The carpus is a complex unit of bony articulations that transfers the force and motion of the hand to the supportive forearm and upper extremity.[171,284,323] Rather than a simple hinge joint such as the elbow, or a ball-socket joint such as the hip, the wrist involves a delicate interaction between eight carpal bones that are divided into two carpal rows, the mechanical equivalent of which is not easily simulated.[118,208,284,462] While the primary motions are flexion–extension and radioulnar deviation, the actual motion of carpal bones is much more complex (Fig. 8-2).[118,282] The primary axis of motion resides within the head of the capitate,[361] which is not a singular point but rather an oblique screw axis for combined motions of wrist exten-sion–radial deviation and wrist flexion–ulnar deviation that are quite normal planes of daily movement (see Fig. 8-2). To produce this natural movement, individual carpal bones not only turn up and down and back and forth, but spin and roll about their own axes. To understand the pathophysiology of wrist fractures and dislocations, these functional components need to be understood (see *Kinematics* in this chapter).

Equally important are the muscles and tendons that move the wrist. Their actions are tightly constrained so that their effect on motion and transmission of force can be carefully controlled.

Undoubtedly the ancients were aware of wrist problems, but not much was written until the beginning of the 19th century. A theme, reflected in the writings of the continental physicians, was that most injuries of this area were dislocations of the wrist. Jeanne and Mouchet,[268] Malgaigne,[344] Desault,[144] and others[145,157] diagnosed by clinical exam or confirmed by autopsy dislocations and luxations of the carpus. Sir Astley Cooper produced the first book, *A Treatise on Dislocations and Fractures of Joints* in 1822. It remained for Colles of Dublin[110] and Pouteau of France[439] to differentiate between fractures of the distal radius and wrist dislocations. In the United States, Barton[34] described the volar and dorsal fracture–dislocations of the radiocarpal joint, and Pilcher[436] identified the difference between intra-articular and extra-articular distal radius fractures by description and illustration. The advent of the x-ray allowed swift progression in understand-

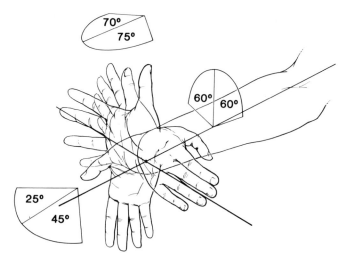

Fig. 8-1. Global motion of the wrist and forearm. The wrist has three degrees of freedom through a complex mechanical arrangement that allows approximately 145° of flexion–extension movement (FEM), 70° of radioulnar deviation (RUD), and 120° of pronosupination through the forearm radioulnar joints. The last provides the torque to accomplish twisting motions.

ing and classifying traumatic injuries of the wrist. Destot[145] produced a remarkable discussion of a variety of wrist injuries in 1926.

Sixteen years ago, when the first version of this chapter on wrist fracture and dislocations was written,[152] the concept of wrist instability had changed only modestly from these earlier writings. It was the work of Lambrinudi,[221,308] Bolton,[221] and later Fisk[183] that recognized that both fracture of the scaphoid and carpal ligament injuries would produce carpal instability. Fisk, in a landmark Hunterian Lecture presentation in 1968,[182] detailed the role of scaphoid instability and carpal collapse. In 1972, Linscheid and coworkers[329] defined traumatic

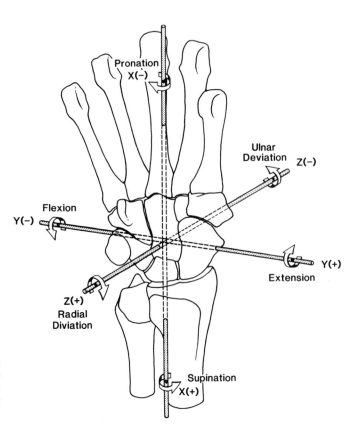

Fig. 8-2. A coordinate system to describe the screw axis of the wrist, which passes through the head of the capitate for flexion Y(−) and extension Y(+); radial deviation Z(+) and ulnar deviation Z(−); and pronation X(−) and supination X(+).

instability of the wrist, bringing forth concepts of dorsal and volar intercalated carpal instability based on the ideas of Landsmeer[309] (DISI and VISI). The term ''sprain'' of the wrist took on new meaning, and the real importance of ligament injuries in producing wrist instability equal to that of wrist fractures became appreciated. The concept of carpal instability has been expanded widely as a result of careful clinical studies and anatomical and biomechanical analyses of the specific pathology involved.[153,327,514] As a result, clear concepts and classifications of the different types of carpal instability have evolved (Table 8-1).

Carpal instability may occur from a variety of different fractures or dislocations with a combination of ligament, bone, capsule, and tendon injury.[118,119,153,356,414] Ligament repair and proper reconstruction of fractured carpal components serve to preserve these support structures for maintenance of normal joint alignment and transmission of forces within this highly tuned and mechanically complex unit.

New information on muscle and tendon physiology,[77] vascularity of the carpal bones,[213,519] the location and function of intrinsic and extrinsic wrist ligaments,[50,210,357] and the three-dimensional motion of individual carpal bones[139,461,490,561] has increased immeasureably our understanding of the surgical anatomy of the wrist. This will assist our efforts toward timely and anatomically accurate reconstruction following acute or delayed trauma.

SURGICAL ANATOMY

GENERAL ANATOMY

From the carpometacarpal joints to the distal border of the pronator quadratus, most of the soft tissues that pass the wrist are bound within rather rigid compartments.[317,318] On the dorsal side the extensor tendons, with the exception of the brachioradialis, pass under an extensor retinaculum that holds them close to bone and maintains their uniform mechanical relationship to the carpus.[518] The six extensor compartments (Fig. 8-3) separate the following tendons: radial wrist abductor (APL) and short thumb extensor (EPB) from the radial wrist extensors (ECRL, ECRB); the long thumb extensor (EPL) in a separate tunnel as it wraps ulnarly around Lister's tubercle; the common finger extensors (EDC) in the fourth or central compartment; the single extensor digiti minimi tendon (EDM) to the fifth digit; and the last or sixth compartment, residing in a groove adjacent to the ulnar styloid, holds the ulnar wrist extensor (ECU).[543]

The volar wrist tendons are tightly constrained within a special compartment, the carpal tunnel (thumb and finger long flexor tendons), except for

Table 8-1. Carpal Instability (Mayo Classification)*

Instability (subluxation)	Dislocation (luxation)	Fracture–dislocation
Perilunate		
Partial or residual	Various stage†	Transosseous
CID‡ type		Transscaphoid perilunate†
Scapholunate dissociation with DISI†		Transradiostyloid perilunate
Lunotriquetral dissociation with VISI		Other combinations
Radiocarpal		
CIND§ type	Dorsal†	Dorsal Barton's
VISI	Volar	Volar Barton's†
DISI	Ulnar	Radial styloid with carpal translation (ulnar, dorsal, radial, volar)
Ulnar translation†		Lunate fossa with carpal translation
Midcarpal		
CIND type	Potential (but	Malunited Colles' fracture (potential, but so rare as
Triquetrohamate (VISI > DISI)†	so rare as to	to be unique)
Scaphotrapeziotrapezoidal (VISI > DISI)	be unique)	With primary MC instability
Capitolunate (DISI > VISI)		With secondary MC instability
Diffuse laxity (DISI > VISI)		

* Instability, dislocations, and fracture–dislocation combined are the most common wrist destabilization pattern.

† The most common instability pattern of the group.

‡ Carpal instability dissociative.

§ Carpal instability nondissociative.

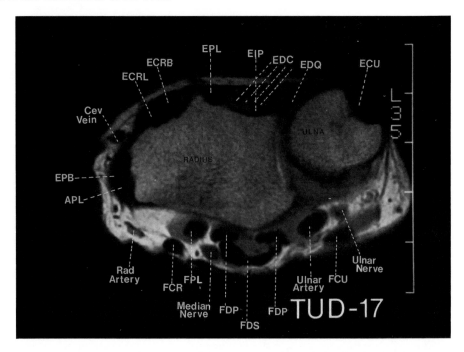

Fig. 8-3. Cross-sectional anatomy of the wrist. MRI through the distal radioulnar joint. Flexor and extensor tendons of the fingers are grouped over the center of rotation so as to impart minimal deviation radially or ulnarly, except for the thumb extrinsic tendons. The wrist motors are distributed peripherally to provide maximum moment arms or establish a wrist position. Dorsal structures, left to right: cephalic vein (*Cev Vein*), extensor carpi radialis longus (*ecrl*), extensor carpi radialis brevis (*ecrb*), extensor pollicis longus (*epl*), extensor indicis proprius, (*eip*), extensor digitorum communis (*edc*), extensor digiti quinti (*edq*), extensor carpi ulnaris (*ecu*). Palmas structures, left to right: extensor pollicis brevis (*epb*), abductor pollicis longus (*apl*), radial artery (*Rad Artery*), flexor carpi radialis (*fcr*), flexor pollicis longus (*fpl*), flexor digitorum profundus (*fdp*), flexor digitorum superficialis (*fds*), flexor carpi ulnaris (*fcu*).

the flexor carpi radialis (FCR) in a separate compartment, the flexor carpi ulnaris (FCU), and palmaris longus (PL). The FCR and FCU control wrist flexion and are uniquely placed to enhance their mechanical advantage through the effect of scaphoid or pisiform motion. The FCU is the most powerful wrist muscle because of its multiple short muscle fibers.[77] The extrinsic tendons of the digits, with the exception of the thumb, are grouped centrally in the frontal plane to afford minimal angulation to the wrist during use, while the wrist motors are grouped peripherally to exert optimum control of the position of the wrist. It is unusual for a muscle belly itself to cross the wrist, because tendons transmit muscle force efficiently with minimal utilization of space. As a consequence, there is little soft tissue protection for the accompanying median and ulnar nerve, and ulnar and radial arteries. These structures are in close proximity to

the wrist dorsal and volar ligaments and underlying bones, rendering them more susceptible to injury with wrist trauma.

TOPOGRAPHIC ANATOMY AND CLINICAL EXAMINATION

Clinical examination of the wrist begins with an appreciation of the topographic anatomy of the wrist (Fig. 8-4).[75,325,349] Dorsally, the wrist extensor tendons can be seen and palpated within each of the six extensor compartments. On the radial side of the wrist, the tendons of the first compartment (EPB and APL) and third compartment (EPL) border the radial and ulnar sides of the anatomic snuff box. One can palpate proximally in the snuff box the radial styloid and, in the mid-third, the waist and distal third of the scaphoid. At the distal end of the snuff box the scaphotrapeziotrapezoidal (STT)

Topographical   anatomy (rt. hand)

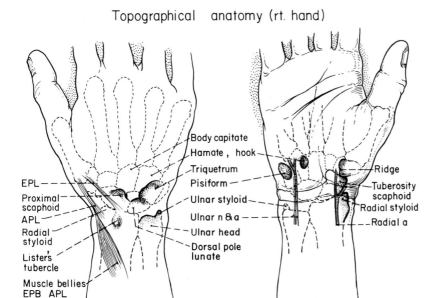

EPL

Proximal scaphoid

APL

Radial styloid

Lister's tubercle

Muscle bellies EPB APL

Body capite
Hamate , hook
Triquetrum
Pisiform
Ulnar styloid
Ulnar n & a
Ulnar head
Dorsal pole lunate

Ridge
Tuberosity scaphoid
Radial styloid
Radial a

Fig. 8-4. Topographical anatomy of the right hand. Bony prominences, readily palpated at the wrist, may be used to locate most major structures, by either palpation or stereotactic approximation. Various movements of the wrist increase the accessibility of certain bony prominences (eg, the dorsal poles of the scaphoid and lunate, the tuberosity of the scaphoid, the body of the scaphoid in the snuffbox, the hamate, the triquetrum, and the pisiform). The ulnar styloid presents in various positions, depending on rotation of the wrist. It is at the ulnar–palmar position in full pronation and the dorso–radial position in full supination.

joint is identified. Moving ulnarly to the EPL is an important landmark, Lister's tubercle, which is the key to identifying both dorsal wrist ganglia and the junction of the scapholunate joint and dorsal scapholunate interosseous ligament. Beneath the extensor tendons the lunate is not easily identified, but the capitate can be felt proximal to the carpometacarpal joint. A prominence in this region is consistent with a *carpe bossu* or carpometacarpal joint arthrosis.[278] On the ulnar side of the wrist, the ulnar head and styloid are identified. Just distal are the ulnar side of the lunate, the triquetrum, and the lunotriquetral joint. The ulnar styloid can be noted to change position volarly with pronation and dorsally with supination. The extensor carpi ulnaris maintains a constant relationship adjacent to the styloid within its own extensor compartment.

An elliptical bony prominence at the base of the thenar muscles, consisting of the trapezial ridge and scaphoid tuberosity, is the most obvious bony landmark on the radial palmar side of the wrist. The radial artery is lateral and the FCR medial to these structures. As one follows the wrist flexion crease ulnarly, the tendon of the palmaris longus (PL) is evident. The position of the median nerve just radial to the PL may be detected by eliciting Tinel's sign. The finger flexor tendons surround the nerve. The lunate, capitate, and body of the triquetrum are deep to these. The ulnar border of the carpal tunnel is formed by the hamate hook and pisiform. The palmar arch pulsates beyond the hook and can be

traced proximally as the ulnar artery. The pisiform is prominent at the base of the hypothenar muscles, articulating dorsally with the triquetrum and held within the FCU, protecting the ulnar side of Guyon's canal.

In the diagnosis of specific injuries, these topographic landmarks are of great value.[325] For example, a scaphoid waist fracture will produce pain and tenderness within the radial snuffbox. Over the dorsal radius, fractures of the radial styloid, radial metaphysis, or lunate fossa of the distal radius can be determined. Scapholunate ligament injuries will demonstrate tenderness just distal to Lister's tubercle, and ballottement of the scaphoid may suggest interosseous ligament damage. Tenderness of the dorsal lunate may suggest Kienböck's disease, while more ulnar tenderness suggests tears of the triangular fibrocartilage or lunotriquetral ligament. Knowing the normal position of the ECU tendon and ulnar styloid helps to differentiate ECU tendinitis from distal radioulnar problems.[91] A number of provocative tests based on the underlying topographic anatomy (see carpal instability) can be performed to confirm or eliminate fracture or ligament injuries. Similar stress testing can assess flexor or extensor tendon damage. Accurate palpation of the cutaneous or deep peripheral nerves and the vascular supply through the radial and ulnar palmar arch arteries can elicit a site of injury. If there are significant fractures or dislocations of the wrist, the normal alignment of the wrist will be displaced, and clinical examination will provide a correct diagnosis before the confirmatory radiologic examinations are completed.

BONES AND JOINTS

The wrist is composed of the distal radius and ulna; the proximal and distal carpal rows, and the base of the metacarpals (Fig. 8-5). The distal carpal row (trapezium, trapezoid, capitate, hamate) forms a

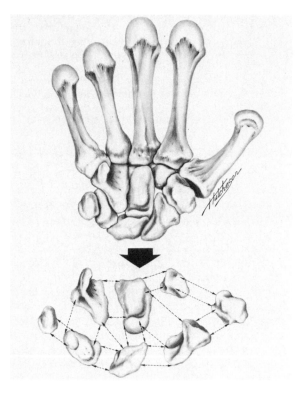

Fig. 8-5. Exploded view of the carpal bones. The wrist is composed of two rows of bones that provide motion and transfer of forces. The distal row (trapezium, trapezoid, capitate, and hamate) is quite stable and moves as a unit. The proximal row (scaphoid, lunate, and triquetrum) is potentially unstable. The carpal bones are supported by extrinsic ligaments attached to roughened areas on dorsal and volar surfaces and intrinsic ligaments attaching intra-articular components, particularly between the scaphoid, lunate, and triquetrum. The radial side of the wrist, exemplified by the scaphoid, provides flexion–extension control over the lunate and distal carpal row. The ulnar side of the wrist exerts rotational control and stability. *(Modified from Taleisnik, J.; and Kelly, P. J.: The Extraosseous and Intraosseous Blood Supply of the Scaphoid Bone. J. Bone Joint Surg. [Am.], 48:1125–1137, 1966.)*

rigid, supportive transverse arch upon which the five metacarpals of the hand are firmly supported. The trapezium, cantilevered radiovolarly from the trapezoid, interfaces the thumb with the proximal row. It provides motion of 10° to 20° at the scaphotrapezial joint and 30° to 42° of rotation/flexion–extension at the metacarpotrapezial joint. Under repetitive stress, the trapezium may shift radially and volarly, increasing compressive stress on the distal scaphoid. The capitate and trapezoid, which shift minimally on each other, are tightly articulated with the second and third metacarpals. The double chevron shape of the second metacarpal on the trapezoid and the third metacarpal styloid on the capitate provide a rigid central strut for the hand. The capitate and hamate slide slightly on each other with wrist motions. Distally they allow moderate motion for the ulnar two metacarpals to enchance the gripping adaptation for the hand. The interlocking of the fifth metacarpal on the ulnar half of the hamate, along with strong volar carpometacarpal ligaments, provides stability.

The proximal carpal row consists of the lunate and triquetrum and, in an anatomic sense, the entire scaphoid. The scaphoid is, however, uniquely positioned to function mechanically as part of both the distal and carpal rows.[341] The short intrinsic ligaments that bind these three bones together around their convex proximal surfaces coordinates their mechanical behavior (Fig. 8-6).

ARTICULAR SURFACES

The articular surfaces of each of the joints that make up the wrist have important roles in subsequent integrated movements of the wrist.[90,317] The eight carpal bones are influenced by the shape of the distal radius, the distal ulna, and triangular fibrocartilage complex. The distal articular surface of the radius is concave and tilted in two planes. In the sagittal plane, there is an average of 14° volar tilt; in the frontal plane, there is an average ulnar inclination of 22°. The triangular fibrocartilage is the ulnar continuation of the distal radius and presents a concave surface for articulation with the lunate and triquetrum. In certain conditions, such as Madelung's deformity or rheumatoid arthritis, the ulnar slope of the radius is accentuated, producing an ulnar shift of the carpus. The variable length of the ulna as a positive or negative variance may influence the carpal position.[130] When it comes into contact with the proximal carpal row it can force a volar tilt to the lunate and triquetrum (VISI deformity).

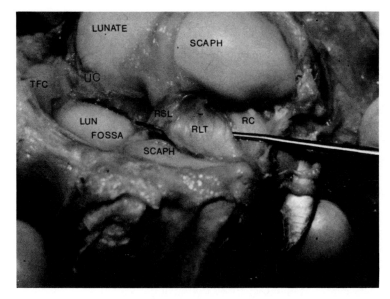

Fig. 8-6. Intra-articular proximal-to-distal view. Intracapsular ligaments of the wrist include the radiocapitate (*RC*), radiolunotriquetral (*RLT*), radioscapholunate (*RSL*), and ulnocarpal (*UC*) ligaments. These ligaments originate from the volar flare of the distal radius (scaphoid and lunate fossae), and insert on the volar aspects of proximal carpal row. The triangular fibrocartilage (*TFC*) extends from ulnar aspect of the distal radius and inserts at the base of the ulnar styloid.

The distal radius also presents two articular surfaces to the scaphoid and lunate, which are important in judging congruent alignment of the wrist after fractures (Colles' type)[76] and in suggesting ligament injuries (dissociation) (Fig. 8-7).[153] A malalignment of the distal radius with loss of volar tilt can also produce a secondary carpal instability.[19,320,521]

The midcarpal joint has an unique articular surface shape, which, as a whole, resembles an acetabulum centered on the lunate. In fact, the midcarpal joint is a combination of three different types of articulation.[118] Laterally, there is a convex distal scaphoid surface articulating with the trapezium and trapezoid (Fig. 8-8). The central part of the midcarpal joint is a concavity of the scaphoid and lunate receiving a convex proximal head of the capitate (Fig. 8-9). Finally, the medial joint of hamate and triquetrum is helicoid in configuration, providing for a sliding movement of the hamate on the triquetrum that influences angulation of the proximal row with wrist movements[552] (see *Kinematics* in this chapter).

The triangular fibrocartilage (TFC) is the main stabilizer of the distal radioulnar joint.[73,290,427,428] It originates from firm attachments on the medial

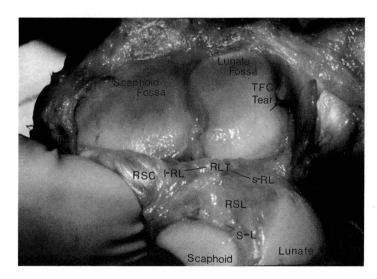

Fig. 8-7. Intra-articular distal-to-proximal view. Volar radioscapholunate (*RSL*) and radiolunotriquetral (*RLT*) blend with the volar aspect of the scapholunate (*SL*) interosseous ligaments (*s-RL*, short radiolunate and *l-RL*, long radiolunate are subdivisions of the radiolunotriquetral ligament, *RLT*).

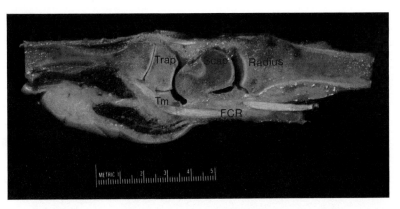

Fig. 8-8. Sagittal view through radius, scaphoid, and trapeziotrapezoidal joints. Note joint configuration, the volar ligaments, the bow-stringing of the *FCR* tendon around the scaphoid tuberosity (*Trap,* trapezoid; *Tz,* trapezium; *Scap,* scaphoid; *FCR,* flexor carpi radialis).

border of the distal radius and inserts into the base of the ulnar styloid.[317] It gives origin to the volar ulnocarpal ligaments and blends imperceptibly into the volar and dorsal radioulnar ligaments,[516] giving the appearance of one discrete structure. The cartilage component is thinnest in the mid-joint contact area, and thickens at the peripheral margins. The TFC blends distally into the ulnar collateral ligament complex (see Fig. 8-9).[424,428] The space between the distal ulna and the TFC is the recessus sacciformis. As a result of phylogenic adaptation of the wrist, a vestigial meniscus of the ulnotriquetral joint merges imperceptibly with the TFC distally.

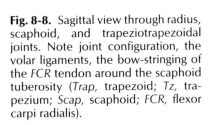

Fig. 8-9. Cross-section anatomy (coronal view) demonstrates the intra-osseous ligaments (*small arrows*) that imperceptibly blend the scaphoid (*Scap*), lunate (*Lun*) and triquetrum (*Triq*) to each other and separate the radiocarpal joint (*RC*) from the midcarpal joint (*MC*). The triangular fibrocartilage (*TFC*) is an ulnar extension of the articular surface of the distal radius, and separates the radiocarpal from the distal radioulnar joint (*DRUJ*). It is the main stabilizer of the distal radioulnar joint.

The wrist is a very congruent structure, with close contact of the articular surfaces during the global motion, combining wrist flexion–extension (FEM) and radioulnar deviation (RUD).[341] Each carpal bone can move three dimensionally in space, rotating, flexing, or extending as well as deviating in response to various wrist positions.[139,461] Conceptually, it resembles a Rubik's cube, in which each component bone's motion will have an effect on adjacent carpal bones.

The wrist must be considered in terms of three-dimensional motion and structure.[171,561] Fractures and dislocations rarely involve only one carpal bone or joint, and radiographic imaging that assists evaluation in three dimensions is needed to understand the pathology that may exist.[394,403]

LIGAMENTS OF THE WRIST

There are two major groups of ligaments of the wrist (Fig. 8-10**A, B**), extrinsic and intrinsic.[48,357,516] The extrinsic ligaments are those that link the carpal bones to the radius, ulna, and metacarpals. The intrinsic ligaments interconnect individual carpal bones.[48,118,133] The transverse carpal ligament or flexor retinaculum connecting the scaphoid tuberosity and trapezial ridge with the hamulus and pisiform provides structural integrity to the proximal carpal arch, as well as constrains the flexor tendons. It connects medially through the pisiform and hypothenar deep fascia with the dorsal retinaculum, completing a circumferential superficial ligament complex.[518]

Extrinsic Ligaments

The deeper extrinsic ligaments[48,50] are condensations within the fibrous capsule and are difficult to distinguish through the superficial adventitia, but are prominent from the intra-articular aspect of the

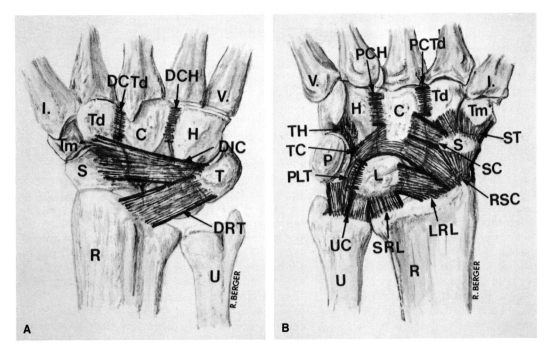

Fig. 8-10. (A) Extrinsic ligaments of the wrist (dorsal): dorsal intercarpal ligament (*DIC*) and dorsal radiotriquetral ligament (*DRT*) [trapezium (*Tm*), trapezoid (*Td*), capitate (*C*), hamate (*H*), scaphoid (*S*), triquetrum (*T*)]. **(B),** Extrinsic ligaments of the wrist (volar): scaphotrapezial (*ST*), radioscaphocapitate (*RSC*), scaphocapitate (*SC*), long radiolunate (*LRL*), short radiolunate (*SRL*), ulnocarpal (*UC*), palmar lunotriquetral (*PLT*), triquetral-capitate (*TC*), triquetral-hamate (*TH*), lunate (*L*), scaphoid (*S*), pisiform (*P*).

joint (see Fig. 8-7). The palmar wrist ligaments originate laterally from a radial-palmar facet of the radial styloid, and are directed in a distal-ulnar direction, where they meet ligaments originating medially from the triangular fibrocartilage and the distal ulna. The stronger and more oblique radial ligaments prevent the carpus from translating ulnarly on the medially angulated slope of the distal radius. The palmar extrinsic ligaments consist of two V-shaped ligamentous bands: one is proximal and connects the forearm to the proximal carpal row; one is distal and connects the forearm to the distal carpal row. The distal limb of the palmar extrinsic ligaments (the arcuate ligaments) consists of the radioscaphocapitate ligament laterally and the ulnocapitate ligament medially (see Fig. 8-10**B**). The proximal limb consists of the radiolunotriquetral and radioscaphoid ligaments laterally and the ulnolunate and ulnotriquetral ligaments medially. The radioscaphoid ligament that inserts onto the tuberosity of the scaphoid is the radial expansion of the radiocapitate ligament, which courses over the palmar concavity of the scaphoid proximal to the tuberosity before inserting on the palmar aspect

of the keel and neck of the capitate. It forms a fulcrum over which the scaphoid rotates (see Fig. 8-8). Between these two rows of ligaments is a thinned area termed the space of Poirier.[437] This area expands when the wrist is dorsiflexed and disappears in palmarflexion. A rent develops during dorsal dislocations, and it is through this interval that the lunate displaces into the carpal canal.[355] The radiocapitate ligament is superficial to the radiolunate, and the former slips over the latter in flexion.

The dorsal ligaments of importance are the radiotriquetral and scaphotriquetral (dorsal intercarpal) ligaments, which describe a V-shape from the dorsal aspect of the distal radius near Lister's tubercle to the triquetrum then back to the dorsal scaphoid rim (see Fig. 8-10**A**).[323,538] The radial capsule is thickened, melding into the radioscaphoid ligament, while the ulnodorsal capsule is augmented by the floors of the fifth and sixth dorsal compartments. There are no true collateral ligaments.

The extrinsic radiolunate ligaments have been subdivided into short and long radiolunate ligaments (see Fig. 8-10**B**). The radioscapholunate ligament of Testut[523] and Kuenz,[304] seen well from the inside of the joint, originates from the palmar aspect of the ridge between the scaphoid and lunate fossae and inserts into the scapholunate interosseous ligament; it acts as a neurovascular supply to the scapholunate interosseous membrane (see Figs. 8-6 and 8-7) and is not a true extrinsic ligament of the wrist. Recent anatomic studies,[50] arthroscopic observations, and ligament testing support these observations.[68]

The final group of extrinsic ligaments support the midcarpal joint and couple the distal carpal bones to each other. On the radial side of the wrist, a V-shaped scaphotrapezial ligament extends from the scaphoid tuberosity to the volar tubercle of the trapezium. Adjacent to it medially are the scaphocapitate and palmar capitotrapezial ligaments and the capitotrapezoidal ligament. On the ulnar side of the wrist, the triquetrocapitate and triquetrohamate ligaments are a continuation of the ulnotriquetral ligament.[10]

Intrinsic Ligaments

The intra-articular intrinsic ligaments of the wrist connect adjacent carpal bones.[329,357,516] They are collections of relatively short fibers that bind the bones of either the proximal or distal carpal rows to each other (see Figs. 8-7 and 8-9).

In the proximal carpal row, the ligaments are intra-articular, connecting the scaphoid to the lunate and the lunate to the triquetrum. There is a contiguous blending of the interosseous ligaments (membranes) with the joint articular cartilage. Laterally, the strong scapholunate interosseous membrane begins volarly and follows the convex arc of the proximal edge of the two bones to the dorsal surface, where there is a thickened collection of more superficial fibers that describe a scapholunate ligament.[333,357,460] This has an important role in carpal stability.[460] The longer fibers of the palmar portion of the scapholunate interosseous membrane allow the scaphoid a greater flexibility than the lunate.

The lunotriquetral interosseous membrane[449,539,540] is similarly formed by stout transverse fibers connecting the proximal edges of triquetrum and lunate. It interdigitates with the dorsal radiotriquetral ligament and palmar ulnotriquetral, ulnolunate, and radiolunotriquetral insertions. Its fibers are more taut, making for a closer lunotriquetral than scapholunate kinematic relationship. The disposition of these ligaments and their strengths are of considerable importance in the ki-

nematics of the joint and the mechanisms of injury.[333,356]

NEUROVASCULAR SUPPLY

The innervation and blood supply of the wrist (Fig. 8-11) come from the regional nerves and vessels.[429] The nerves include the main trunk of the ulnar nerve, running deep to the flexor carpi ulnaris tendon and into Guyon's canal; the main trunk of the median nerve, running between and deep to the flexor carpi radialis and the palmaris longus into the carpal tunnel; the anterior interosseous branch of the median nerve, lying on the interosseous membrane between the ulna and the radius; the posterior interosseous branch of the radial nerve, lying on the posterior surface of the radioulnar interosseous membrane; the superficial sensory branch of the radial nerve, emerging dorsally from beneath the brachioradialis tendon about 5 cm proximal to the radial styloid; and the dorsal cutaneous branch of the ulnar nerve, which branches from the main ulnar trunk and lies subcutaneously across the ulnocarpal sulcus. The palmar cutaneous branch of the median nerve arises from its main trunk, about 4 cm proximal to the wrist crease. These subsidiary branches to the median, ulnar, and radial nerves are readily damaged by lacerations, incisions, and contusions. They are easily visualized just deep to the superficial veins, and should be protected. The potential for a neuralgic pain syndrome is common to all of them.

Circulation of the wrist is obtained through the radial, ulnar, and anterior interosseous arteries and the deep palmar arch. The extraosseous arterial pattern is formed by an anastomotic network of three dorsal and three palmar arches connected longitudinally at their medial and lateral borders by the radial and ulnar arteries.[216,217] The dorsal interosseous does not make a substantial contribution (Fig. 8-11**A**). In addition to transverse and longitudinal anastomoses, there are dorsal to volar interconnections between the dorsal and palmar branches of the anterior interosseous artery.

The palmar transverse archs are the radiocarpal, intercarpal, and deep palmar arch (Fig. 8-11**B**). Two recurrent vessels, one radial and one ulnar, traverse proximally to frequently anastomose with the terminal branches of the anterior division of the anterior interosseous artery. The palmar radiocarpal arch provides the predominant blood supply to the palmar surface of the lunate and triquetrum. The radial and ulnar recurrent arteries supply the distal carpal row. With such a broad collateral circulation present at the wrist, it is rare that damage to one aspect of this extrinsic circulation has a significant effect on the blood supply of the wrist.

The intrinsic blood supply to the carpal bones is an important factor in the incidence of avascular necrosis after trauma.[214,519] Latex injection techniques demonstrate three patterns of interosseous vascularization. The bones in the first group, scaphoid,[440] capitate,[410] (Fig. 8-11**D, E**) and about 20% of lunate (Fig. 8-11**C**), are supplied by a single vessel and thus are at risk for avascular necrosis. The trapezium, triquetrum, pisiform, and 80% of the lunate receive nutrient arteries through two nonarticular surfaces, and have consistent intraosseous anastomoses with a resultant rare occurrence of avascular necrosis. The trapezoid and hamate lack an intraosseous anastamosis and, following fracture, can have avascular fragments.[216] These observations extend previous work, which shows that the blood supply to most carpal bones enters the distal half, leaving the proximal half at risk. There is no interval for example by which the scaphoid can be approached without endangering some of the branches that supply its circulation.[71] With proximal scaphoid fracture the danger of devascularizing the proximal fragment exists. It is important to identify and protect the dorsal and volar radial artery branches to the scaphoid. The lunate blood supply[213] is constantly endangered by common dorsal approaches to the wrist, but the blood supply from the palmar radiocarpal arch is usually sufficient. With fracture–dislocations of the wrist the palmar radiolunate ligament usually remains intact, because the dislocation is distal through the space of Poirier.

MECHANISMS OF INJURY

The usual mechanism of injury (Fig. 8-12) to the wrist is an axial compressive force applied with the wrist in hyperextension, in which the volar ligaments are placed under tension and the dorsal joint surfaces are compressed and subject to shear stresses, especially if the wrist is extended beyond its physiologic limits.[327,328,356,487,542] Depending upon the degree of radial or ulnar deviation, ligament or bony injury or a combination of both will result. The amount of energy absorbed, the direction of the applied force, its point of application, and the strength of the bone and capsule all have a distinct bearing on the pathology and severity of injury (Fig. 8-13).[165,186,367] For example a scaphoid fracture appears to occur when the wrist is dorsi-

flexed past 97° and radially deviated 10°.[553] In this position, the proximal pole of the scaphoid is held viselike by the radius and the proximal radioscaphocapitate ligament, while the distal pole of the bone is carried dorsally by the trapeziocapitate complex. The lunate is unloaded. The radioscaphoid ligament is relaxed by the radial deviation and cannot alleviate the tensile stresses accumulating on the radiovolar aspect of the scaphoid. The tensile fracture then propagates dorsally. The fracture seldom comminutes, because the midcarpal joint attenuates dorsal compression (Fig. 8-14).[553]

Common injuries include a fall from a height, a sports-related collison, or a motor vehicle accident. The injured individual straightens the arm for protection and the body weight and exterior force are concentrated across the wrist. Other mechanisms include palmarflexion, as occurs in an over-the-handle-bars motorcycle accident or twisting injuries in sports where the hand is forcefully rotated against the stationary body. With similar loads, the trained athlete may suffer no significant injury, while the immature individual sustains a physeal separation, and the elderly person suffers a comminuted and displaced fracture.

Mayfield and associates[355,356] and Johnson[272] have pointed out that many injuries of the wrist appear to be sequential variants of perilunate dislocations (Fig. 8-15). Minor injuries such as sprains (stretch or partial tears of carpal ligaments) result from low-energy forces. Ligament tears involve more substantial force to the hand, as when the capitate forcibly distracts the scaphoid and lunate, tearing the interosseous membrane. Higher energy forces result in carpal bone fractures, fracture–dislocations, or ligamentous disruptions of both intrinsic and extrinsic ligaments. The majority of these injuries occur in the perilunate area, and the resulting instability is an important concept in understanding the mechanism of wrist injury.

Following injury, use of the hand potentiates carpal instability, because normal activities generate joint compressive forces that are transmitted across the carpus to the distal radius and to the restraining ligaments.

From the proximal carpal row, the compression loads are transmitted across the radiocarpal joint and, to a lesser degree, across the triangular fibrocartilage to the distal ulna.[165] With the wrist in a neutral position, the loaded carpus will tend to slide down the palmar and ulnarly inclined articular surface of the distal radius. The extrinsic radiocarpal ligaments resist this ulnar translation in order to maintain carpal alignment and stability.

(*text continues on page 577*)

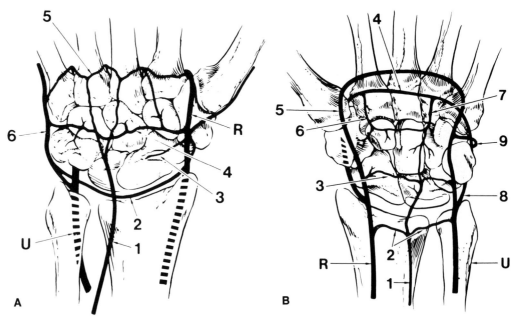

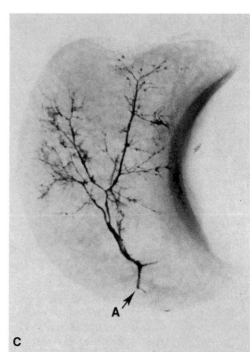

Fig. 8-11. (**A**) Schematic drawing of the arterial supply of the dorsum of the wrist. *R,* Radial artery; *U,* ulnar artery; *1,* dorsal branch, anterior interosseous artery; *2,* dorsal radiocarpal arch; *3,* branch to the dorsal ridge of the scaphoid; *4,* dorsal intercarpal arch; *5,* basal metacarpal arch; *6,* medial branch of the ulnar artery. (**B**) Schematic drawing of the arterial supply of the palmar aspect of the wrist. *R,* Radial artery; *U,* ulnar artery; *1,* palmar branch, anterior interosseous artery; *2,* palmar radiocarpal arch; *3,* palmar intercarpal arch; *4,* deep palmar arch; *5,* superficial palmar arch; *6,* radial recurrent artery; *7,* ulnar recurrent artery; *8,* medial branch, ulnar artery; *9,* branch off ulnar artery contributing to the dorsal intercarpal arch. (**C**) Lunate: lateral view, showing a single large vessel entering the palmar surface and branching within the bone to provide the sole blood supply. This pattern was seen in 20% of the specimens.

(continued)

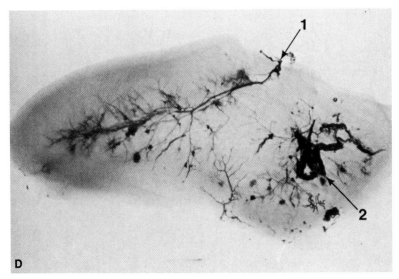

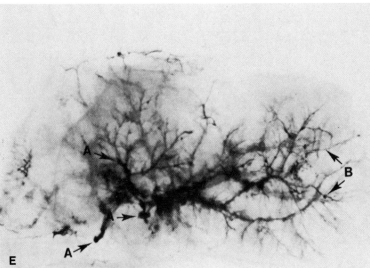

Fig. 8-11 *(continued)*
(**D**) Photograph of a specimen show-ing the internal vascularity of the scaphoid (*1*, dorsal branch of the radial artery; *2*, volar scaphoid branch.) (**E**) Capitate: dorsal view, following clear-ing by Spalteholz technique. Nutrient vessels enter distal third (*A*), with ret-rograde course towards the proximal articular surface and (*B*), terminal ves-sels enter into the head of the capitate. (**A,B**: *Gelberman, R. H.; Panagis, J. S.; Taleisnik, J.; Baumgaertner, M.: The Arterial Anatomy of the Human Carpus. I: The Extraosseous Vascularity. J. Hand Surg., 8(4):367–375, 1983.* **C,E:** *Gel-berman, R. H.; Panagis, J. S.; Taleisnik, J.; Baumgaertner, M.: The Arterial Anatomy of the Human Carpus. II: The Intraosseous Vascularity. J. Hand Surg., 8(4):375–382, 1983.* **D:** *Gelberman, R. H.; Menon, J.: The Vascularity of the Scaphoid Bone. J. Hand Surg., 5(5): 508–513, 1980.*)

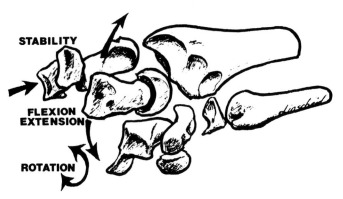

Fig. 8-12. Perilunar dislocation of the wrist occurs in hyperdorsiflexion. Disruption occurs at the scapholunate area and progresses into the space of Poirier and then through the lunotriquetral space. At times, the sequence of injury may be reversed, depending on the orientation at impact. *Forme frustes* are responsible for scapholunate or lunotriquetral dissociations and a variety of wrist sprains.

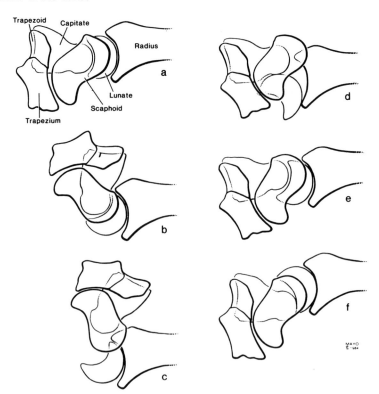

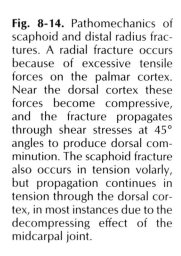

Fig. 8-13. Perilunar dislocation progresses from the neutral position *a*, to extension *b*, to displacement dorsally *c*. As the dislocation rebounds, the carpus may partially displace and flex the lunate. A scapholunate dissociation (*d*) may develop, or with more extensive ligamentous damage, the carpus may settle into a volar dislocation (*e*). This implies more disruption of the ulnar aspect of the proximal row.

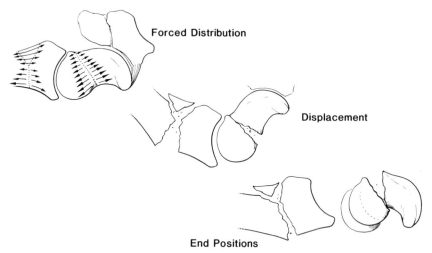

Fig. 8-14. Pathomechanics of scaphoid and distal radius fractures. A radial fracture occurs because of excessive tensile forces on the palmar cortex. Near the dorsal cortex these forces become compressive, and the fracture propagates through shear stresses at 45° angles to produce dorsal comminution. The scaphoid fracture also occurs in tension volarly, but propagation continues in tension through the dorsal cortex, in most instances due to the decompressing effect of the midcarpal joint.

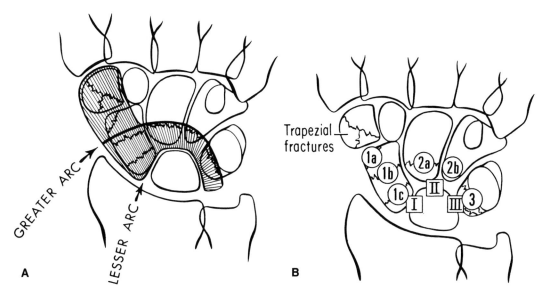

Fig. 8-15. Vulnerable zone of the carpus. (**A**) A lesser arc injury follows a curved path through the radial styloid, midcarpal joint, and lunotriquetral space. A greater arc injury passes through the scaphoid, capitate, and triquetrum. (**B**) Lesser and greater arc injuries can be considered as three stages of perilunate fracture or ligament instabilities. *(Johnson, R. P.: The Acutely Injured Wrist and Its Residuals. Clin. Orthop., 149:33–44, 1980.[272])*

Compressive loads across the triangular fibrocartilage are accepted by the head of the distal ulna, depending upon the relative length of the ulna with respect to the articular surface of the distal radius (± ulnar variance).[544] Redistribution of forces in the forearm are influenced by rotation, ulnar variance, and integrity of the muscles and interosseous membrane.

KINEMATICS

The global motion of the wrist is composed of flexion, extension (FEM), and radioulnar deviation (RUD) (see Fig. 8-1) at the radiocarpal joint, and axial rotation around the distal radioulnar joint (DRUJ).[323,341,471] The radiocarpal articulation acts as a universal joint, allowing a small degree of intercarpal motion around the longitudinal axis related to the rotation of individual carpal bones.[307] The forearm accounts for the most rotation (about 140°) and supplies the hand with the strength necessary to apply vigorous torque. The motion of the radiocarpal joint is flexion–extension of nearly equal proportions (70° each), and radial and ulnar deviation of 20° and 40°, respectively.[86] This amount of motion is possible as a result of complex arrangements between the two carpal rows.[25,171] The wrist motors are attached to the metacarpal bases, but because the carpometacarpal joints are rather rigid, angular deflection is readily transmitted to the distal carpal row and then to the proximal carpal row. The latter, an intercalated segment of connected bones without tendon or muscle attachments,[309,484] is pushed back and forth in response to forces applied distally from the hand. Its stability is dependent on the complex ligament structure described above and the contours of the articular surfaces. During flexion and extension, each carpal row angulates in the same direction with nearly equal amplitude and in a synchronous fashion (Fig. 8-16).[139,171,560,561] During radioulnar deviation, however, the proximal row exhibits a secondary angulation in the sagittal plane to the synchronous motion occuring in the coronal plane. Radial deviation induces flexion of the obliquely situated scaphoid as the trapezium approaches the radius. Through the dorsal aspect of the scapholunate ligament, this motion is transmitted sequentially to the lunate and triquetrum, which flex approximately 25°.[323,333,341,461] As the carpus moves back to full ulnar deviation, the proximal row extends an equal amount. The scaphoid can be observed to extend with ulnar deviation, but it is the proximal

NORMAL CONJUNCT ROTATION

NORMAL SYNCHRONOUS FLEXION/EXTENSION

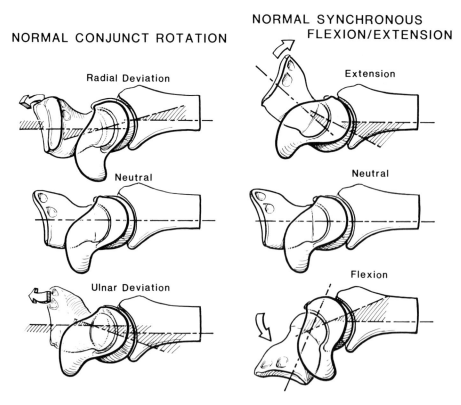

Fig. 8-16. Conjunct rotation of the proximal carpal row occurs in flexion during radial deviation (**upper left**). The axes of the radius and carpal rows are colinear in neutral (**middle left**), and the proximal row extends with ulnar deviation (**lower left**). Angulatory excursions of the proximal and distal rows are essentially equal in amplitude and direction during flexion (**lower right**) and extension (**upper right**). This may be described as synchronous angulation.

migration of the hamate that forces the triquetrum to displace volarly and extend, bringing the lunate with it. This conjunct rotation by varying the length and contour of the proximal carpal row allows for extensive excursion of the wrist while maintaining stability around a longitudinal axis.[323,407] This facility has been described as the "variable geometry" of the proximal carpal row.[281]

When this mechanism is disrupted by fracture or ligamentous injury, the wrist becomes destabilized.[89,329] The usual arcs of motion are no longer synchronous, and the intercarpal contact patterns change. Snapping can be appreciated with motion of the wrist. Symptomatic instability leads, in time, to degenerative changes as a consequence of increased local shear forces and abnormal contact patterns.

Normally, in the coronal plane, the center of rotation of the wrist is located within a small area in the capitate neck (see Fig. 8-2). A line drawn through the axis of rotation parallel with the anatomic axis of the forearm will, with the hand in a neutral position, pass through the head and base of the third metacarpal, the capitate, the radial aspect of the lunate, and the center of the lunate fossa of the radius.[361] The muscle forces in this plane are nearly equally distributed to either side (see Fig. 8-3).

In the sagittal plane with the wrist in neutral flexion–extension, a line passing through the longitudinal axis of the capitate, lunate, and radius will show these to be nearly superimposed or colinear (Fig. 8-17). The scaphoid axis lies 45° to the above and passes between lunate and capitate in a fashion that provides optimal stability to the midcarpal joint. The scaphoid acts as a stabilizing strut or column to support the inherently unstable central column.[329,402] By virtue of its obliquity, the

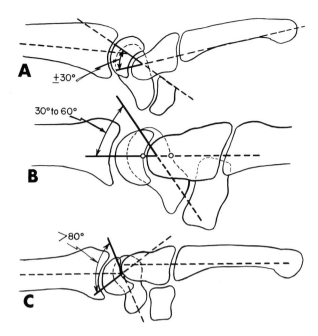

Fig. 8-17. (A) Abnormal volar flexion of the lunate and scaphoid with ±30° volar tilt, diagnostic of a VISI deformity. **(B)** Normal carpal alignment with lunate and capitate colinear and scaphoid angled 45° (normal, 30°–60°), ±15° to the sagittal plane of forearm. **(C)** Abnormal dorsiflexion of the lunate with a vertical scaphoid; scapholunate angle > 80° (normal, 45°–60°), typical DISI deformity.

scaphoid normally is induced to flex when under compressive load, and exerts a similar influence on the lunate. The lunate, however, is also under the influence of the triquetrum, which inherently prefers to extend. For this reason, the lunate may be thought of as being in a state of dynamic balance between two antagonists. It tends to lie in the position of least mechanical potential energy (Fig. 8-18**A**).

When the dynamic balance is interrupted, the lunate will tend to flex with loss of ulnar support from the triquetrum (Fig. 8-18**C**). It will extend when the situation is reversed by loss of radial stability (Fig. 8-18**B**).[460] When the lunate slips into a statically fixed position, arbitrarily considered as greater than 15° of flexion or 10° of extension, a condition defined as volar intercalated segment instability (VISI) or dorsal intercalated segment instability (DISI), respectively, is present (Fig. 8-19).[309] The relative alignment of the scaphoid to the lunate, which approximates 45°, is also important. When this exceeds 70°, the ligamentous linkage with the lunate is usually inoperative. The lunate then gen-

erally adopts an extended position, DISI, and maintains this position even during radial deviation, thus interrupting the normal conjunct rotation and the spatial adaptability of the proximal row. The same is true when the lunate is fixed in flexion, VISI, and will not extend even during ulnar deviation.

The proximal carpal row is also variably unstable in the coronal plane due to the obliquity of the radial articular surface to the plane perpendicular to the longitudinal axis. Joint compressive forces induce the proximal row to slide ulnarly down this inclined plane (Fig. 8-20). This is resisted primarily by the extrinsic radiocarpal ligaments, which run from the radial styloid to the capitate and lunate, and to a lesser extent by the concavity produced by the TFC and underlying ulnar head. Injuries to these structures may allow a partial or complete ulnar translation of the proximal row[323] (see *Carpal Instabilities* in this chapter).

The carpus is also architecturally involved in the transverse and longitudinal archs of the hand that provide structural integrity to withstand extrinsically applied stresses. The faceted, interlocking, rigid second and third carpometacarpal (CMC) joints provide the primary support for the longitudinal arch, while the flattened surfaces of the distal carpal bones supported by short stout intercarpal ligaments do the same for the proximal transverse arch.[278] Even these structures are susceptible to sufficient, applied force, which may weaken or disrupt the arches (see *Axial Collapse Patterns* in this chapter).

The mobility and power of the human thumb place significant stresses along the radial column of the wrist. The thumb tendons are displaced from the center of rotation of the wrist, providing a strong radial moment when they are active. This must be balanced by moments from the ulnar wrist motors. Ordinarily the STT joint plays a minimal role in excursion of the thumb, but a large role in wrist motion. The fourth and fifth CMC joints provide mobility to the ulnar side of the hand, which markedly enhances its ability for spatial adaption.

IMAGING OF THE WRIST

RADIOGRAPHIC EXAMINATION

Radiographic findings are the chief determinant for the specific diagnosis of wrist area fractures and dislocations,[153,222,223,299,325,329,474,514] even though valuable information is available from the history and clinical examination. The two most important views are the posteroanterior and the lateral, each

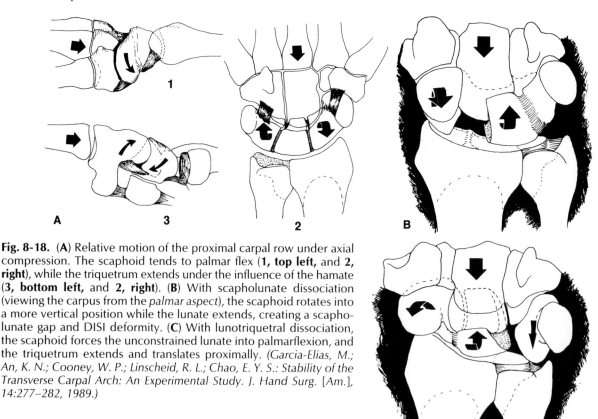

Fig. 8-18. (**A**) Relative motion of the proximal carpal row under axial compression. The scaphoid tends to palmar flex (**1, top left,** and **2, right**), while the triquetrum extends under the influence of the hamate (**3, bottom left,** and **2, right**). (**B**) With scapholunate dissociation (viewing the carpus from the *palmar aspect*), the scaphoid rotates into a more vertical position while the lunate extends, creating a scapholunate gap and DISI deformity. (**C**) With lunotriquetral dissociation, the scaphoid forces the unconstrained lunate into palmarflexion, and the triquetrum extends and translates proximally. (*Garcia-Elias, M.; An, K. N.; Cooney, W. P.; Linscheid, R. L.; Chao, E. Y. S.: Stability of the Transverse Carpal Arch: An Experimental Study. J. Hand Surg. [Am.], 14:277–282, 1989.*)

taken in an exact neutral position. To these two views, we often add four more and consider the entire group of six as a motion study of the wrist. The additional four are posteroanterior views in maximal radial deviation and maximal ulnar deviation, and lateral views in maximal flexion and maximal extension. These six views are adequate in more than 90% of cases in diagnosing fractures and dislocations in this area. The shifting of the carpal bones in the various positions changes the overlap pattern sufficiently, so that most fracture lines can be seen readily on one or more of the views.

In addition, the more subtle changes in the normal relationships of the carpal bones usually can be visualized and measured in one or more of the views. The important angular relationships are probably best visualized in the lateral views. With the normal wrist in neutral position, the longitudinal axes of the long finger metacarpal, the capitate, the lunate, and the radius all fall on the same

line—a line drawn through the center of the head of the third metacarpal, the center of the head of the capitate, the midpoints of the convex proximal and the concave distal joint surfaces of the lunate, and the midpoint of the distal articular surface of the radius (see Fig. 8-17). The longitudinal axis of the scaphoid is drawn through the midpoints of its proximal and distal poles. Using these axes, it is possible to measure angles that define the positions of the carpal bones. For example, the scapholunate angle formed by the intersection of the longitudinal axes of the scaphoid and the lunate averages 47° and ranges from 30° to 60° in normal wrists (see Fig. 8-17). An angle greater than 70° suggests instability, and one greater than 80° is almost certain proof of carpal instability of the dorsiflexion type. A capitolunate angle of more than 20° is also strongly suggestive of carpal instability.

When the lunate lies palmar to the capitate but faces dorsally, the collapse pattern is referred to as dorsiflexion instability (DISI); this pattern is much

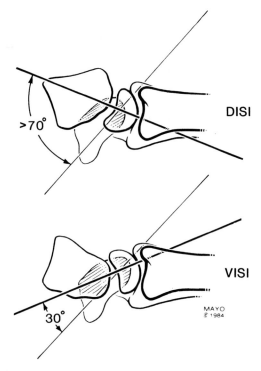

DISI

VISI

MAYO
© 1984

Fig. 8-19. VISI deformity (**bottom**) is usually associated with disruption of the lunotriquetral ligament complex. Neutral position has intact intrinsic ligaments to either side of the lunate. DISI deformity (**top**) is associated with varying degrees of scapholunate disruption.

more common in posttraumatic situations. If the lunate lies dorsal to the capitate and is flexed palmarward, the collapse pattern is called volar flexion instability (VISI) (see Fig. 8-19). Either of these instability patterns may be associated with scapholunate dissociations as well, although there are instances in each category in which scapholunate dissociation cannot be demonstrated, at least on standard x-rays. The palmar (volar) flexion instability pattern is more likely to be associated with triquetrolunate dissociation.

In addition to angular changes, scapholunate dissociation may be marked by more dramatic changes on the posteroanterior view. The normal x-ray shows a fairly constant space between the various carpal bones, which is maintained throughout the range of motion. For instance, the joint width between the scaphoid and the lunate is normally 1 to 2 mm, although it is wider when the scapholunate joint is palmarflexed on the radius. However, with scapholunate dissociation, an increasing gap appears, which may in time be wide

enough to accept proximal migration of the entire capitate head. A spread of more than 3 mm is considered abnormal (Fig. 8-21). In addition, the scaphoid flexes palmarward; this gives the scaphoid less of an elongated profile on the posteroanterior view, and projects the cortical waist of the scaphoid as an overlapping ring of bone inside the scaphoid projection (the "cortical ring sign"), similar to the projection of the hook of the hamate. The lunate also moves into one or the other of the two collapse positions, and this can also be noted on the posteroanterior view by the increasing overlap of the capitate silhouette by a lunate horn (triangular with dorsal horn overlap, wedge shape with volar horn underlap). Another associated deformity that may be seen with either dorsiflexion or palmarflexion instability is that of ulnar translocation of the carpus.[329,447]

SPECIAL IMAGING TECHNIQUES

In addition to these additional views, we have found poly- and trispiral tomography, CT scanning, and magnetic resonance imaging (MRI) to be of particular value in identifying carpal injuries.[51,57,222,430,438] Polytomography should ideally be taken in two planes.[58] Computed tomography with cross-sectional scanning of the carpus[169,468] (see *Carpal Fractures* in this chapter) can be diagnostic for scaphoid malunion and displaced nonunion, capitate fractures, carpal tunnel impingement, and transosseous fracture–dislocations. CT scans are impressive in depicting displacement of distal radius fractures and distal ulna position. MRI[20,57] and ultrasound[188] may provide specific information on stress fractures (scaphoid, capitate, lunate) and avascular necrosis. Bone scans,[40,45,202] while not diagnostic, can assist in confirming a suspected fracture or ligament avulsion injury. Stress x-rays[244] (including traction views) may reveal unsuspected pathology, particularly in fracture–dislocations of the wrist. Arthrography,[49,224,286,315,451] videoradiography,[299,367,474,476] and arthroscopy[68,458] are techniques that can greatly assist in the diagnosis of carpal ligament injuries, as well as both static and dynamic carpal instabilities.

Future imaging techniques will probably include selected use of three-dimensional imaging[394,403,555] in planning reconstructive procedures for malunions and nonunions associated with scaphoid fractures, distal radius fractures, and carpal fracture–dislocations.

At the present time, the ancillary radiographic methods that we use most commonly are the carpal

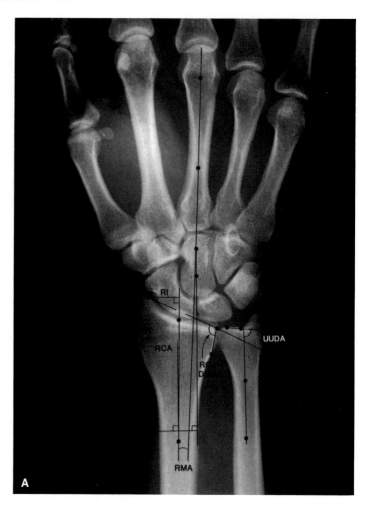

Fig. 8-20. X-ray mapping of the distal radius and ulna. (**A**) Angular measurements of the distal radius and ulna. *RCA,* radius–capitate angle (N = 1° ± 8°). *RI,* radial inclination (N − 24° ± 2.5°). *RCJ–DRUJ,* angle of the radiocarpal joint to the radial margin of the distal radioulnar joint (N = 108 ± 6°). *UUDA,* angle of main axis of ulna to the dome of the ulna (N = 90° ± 8.1°).

(continued)

tunnel view,[313,340,345,559] arthrography, videoradiography[567] with stress loading, polytomography, and cross-section CT scanning. Magnetic resonance imaging has had more frequent application in detecting occult fractures, avascular necrosis, and soft tissue lesions, including triangular fibrocarilage tears. Wrist arthroscopy is an important adjuvant to arthrography, and the techniques currently are quite complementary to each other.[458]

CLASSIFICATION OF WRIST INJURIES AND CARPAL INSTABILITY

The role of instability in carpal injuries has assumed increasing importance since the concept was introduced in the first edition of this book and subsequently was substantially expanded.[324] For a number of years we have been content with a classification system using a combination of the basic diagnostic terms: instability (subluxation), dislocation (luxation), fracture–dislocation, and the types of instability that have been identified (see Table 8-1). Dislocations and fracture–dislocations are always potentially unstable. Fractures and sprains may be stable or unstable and, if the latter, fall into the instability group. The instabilities may be obvious on standard x-rays or may require special imaging techniques or special maneuvers for demonstration.[205,329,332] The most common types of carpal instability (and those initially described) were associated with perilunate dislocations. In identifying this type of instability, one emphasizes the central alignment in a three-link system of rows (radius, proximal carpal row, distal carpal row). Normal balance, as visualized on a lateral x-ray of the carpus, is usually assessed by the near colinear

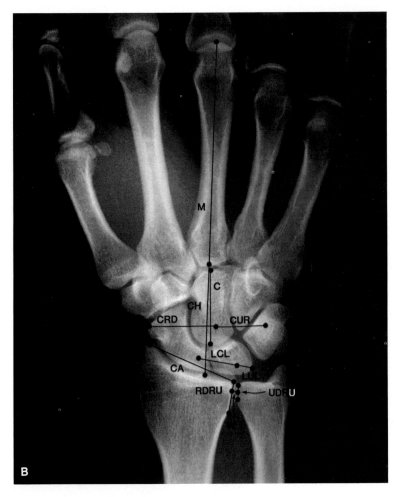

B

Fig. 8-20 *(continued)*
(B) Mean length of articular surface distal radius and ulna. *CRD,* carpal radial distance (N = 20.1 mm ± 1.4) (center of capitate to radial styloid). *CUR,* carpal ulnar distance (N = 18.5 mm ± 3.5) (center of capitate to center of ulnar shaft and base of ulnar styloid); N- 17.1 ± 3.3. *CH,* carpal height (distal capitate to distal radius articular surface) N = 35.6 mm ± 2.4; carpal height ratio (%) 54.3 ± 3.9. *CA,* cord of the arc of the radiocarpal joint; N = 30.9 mm ± 1.7. *RDRU,* length of the radial part of the distal radioulnar joint (sigmoid notch); N = 8.0 mm ± 1.5. *UDRU,* length of the ulnar part of the distal radioulnar joint; N = 6.7 mm ± 1.0. *CUR,* length capitate to axis ulna (carpal–ulnar ratio index CUR/M [%] = 27.1 ± 5). *LCL,* covered length of the lunate (by the radius). *LUL,* uncovered length of lunate (contact with triangular fibrocartilage); N = 6.1 mm ± 2.5. *W,* width distal radioulnar joint (N = 1.7 mm ± 0.5).

alignment of the central column of those rows (radius, lunate, capitate–third metacarpal). Although there is a spectrum of normal on either side of this colinear alignment, a deviation of more than about 15° either way between the links of this chain may be viewed as a lax, diseased, or damaged joint system. The terms for the principal collapse positions remain DISI and VISI.[13,329,330]

Although other types of carpal instability are common and create confusion, one must begin with an understanding of the concepts of perilunate instability.[119,153,355,483,514] Concepts of radial-sided, central, and ulnar-side instabilities of the wrist are helpful in understanding the different types of wrist injuries.[327,355,538] The lateral or radial side of the wrist provides longitudinal stability; the central segment, flexion–extension capability; and the medial or ulnar side, rotational stability (see Fig. 8-5). Carpal instability results from fractures and dislo-

cations of the wrist.[151] On the lateral side of the wrist, fractures involve either the trapezium, scaphoid, and radial styloid (area of ligament origins), or ligament injuries between the scaphoid and lunate or scaphoid and trapezium. Combinations produce wrist fracture–dislocations with variations on the theme of perilunate instability (eg, transscaphoid or transradiostyloid perilunate dislocations).[114] As the disruption propagates centrally, perilunate ligament tears present as dorsal and volar perilunate dislocations, and may culminate in complete lunate dislocation. Eventually, destabilizing injury reaches the medial side of the wrist, and triquetrohamate and triquetrolunate injuries are seen, occasionally with avulsion or chip fractures from either the dorsal or volar surface of the triquetrum as the presenting sign. Although each side of the wrist may be involved eventually (radial and ulnar sides at the radiocarpal level, central segment first

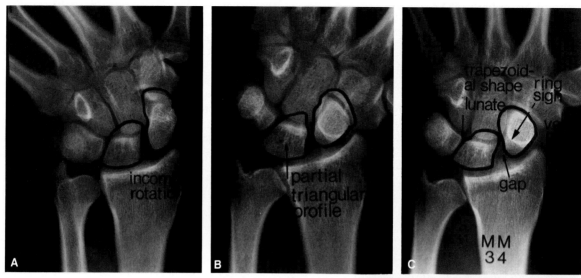

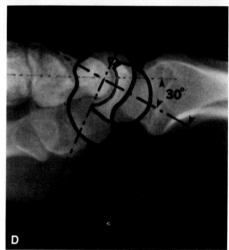

Fig. 8-21. The x-ray findings in scapholunate dissociation. (**A**) Ulnar deviation, increased scapholunate gap with incomplete radial translation of the lunate. (**B**) Radial deviation, scapholunate gap closes, lunate partially rotates; triangular profile of the lunate. (**C**) Gap between scaphoid and lunate exceeds 3 mm; note the trapezoidal shape of the lunate secondary to the volar pole of the lunate rotating under the capitate. Also note foreshortening of the scaphoid due to its flexed position. A ring sign is produced by the cortical outline of the distal pole of the scaphoid. (**D**) Lateral view: the scaphoid is flexed and the lunate extended. The capitate is displaced dorsally relative to the radius. The scapholunate angle exceeds 60°–70°, and the capitolunate angle exceeds 15°–20° (DISI deformity).

at the midcarpal level and perhaps later at the radiocarpal level), the injury pathway can also be viewed as a combination of radiocarpal and midcarpal destabilization.

Another type of wrist instability involves the proximal wrist injuries that present as radiocarpal subluxations or dislocations (ulnar, dorsal, or volar translations). Secondary instability at the radiocarpal or midcarpal joint can result from attenuated volar radiocarpal ligament injuries or from malaligned distal radius fractures (excessive dorsal angulation of the distal radius).

Wrist instability has been recently divided into two broad categories[118]: carpal instability dissociative (CID)[154] and carpal instability nondissociative (CIND).[155] The original concepts of carpal instability

described by Fisk[182] and Linscheid and associates[329] considered carpal instability dissociative (CID) to include perilunate-type collapse patterns that had ligament disruption between bones of the proximal carpal row. The more recent addition of the nondissociative injuries (CIND)[155] includes collapse patterns in which the bones of each carpal row are still strongly attached to each other (ie, the interosseous ligaments are intact). Unfortunately, for peace of mind, dissociative patterns of instability may occur with nondissociative patterns, leading to complexities of both diagnosis and management. We use the acronym CIC to describe this combination or "complex instability of the carpus."

Carpal instabilities lead to abnormal positioning or alignment of the carpal bones by fracture, ligament injury, or both.[13] The most common patterns of carpal malalignment described are (1) DISI, dorsal intercalated segment instability, in which the lunate is dorsiflexed abnormally for any given wrist position; (2) VISI, volar or palmar intercalated segment instability, in which the lunate appears abnormally volar flexed; and (3) ulnar translocation, in which the lunate is abnormally displaced ulnarward from the lunate fossa of the distal radius.

A recent study identified a separate group of axial carpal instabilities[209] characterized by bone and ligament disruptions between the bones of the distal carpal row, with adjacent metacarpals usually included and proximal carpal elements often included. Because they involve intrinsic ligament injuries, they are classified as carpal instability dissociative (CID) injuries.

In applying this classification to acute wrist injuries, the most common types of CID occur between bones of the proximal carpal row, eg, scaphoid fracture or tear of the scapholunate or lunotriquetral ligaments. The transscaphoid perilunate or pure perilunate dislocations provide the highest degree of dissociative carpal instabilities.

Unstable scaphoid fractures[184,252] frequently result in a dissociative radial-side carpal instability. The distal fragment continues to follow the palmarflexion tendency, while the proximal fragment tends to follow the lunate into extension. This results in a DISI type of carpal malalignment. As the distal carpal row migrates proximally, compressive force from the trapezium results in greater mid-scaphoid angulation and additional carpal collapse.

Scapholunate dissociation (SLD), also a radial-side carpal instability, involves a substantial disruption of the ligamentous membrane between the scaphoid and lunate.[329] Lesser degrees of membrane attenuation or partial tear occur, but are not discussed here. The scaphoid, devoid of proximal ligament attachments, rotates around the radiocapitate ligament leading to a dorsal rotary subluxation of the proximal pole. The lunate follows the triquetrum into extension, and a dorsally angulated lunate results (DISI). The primary constraint to scapholunate dissociation is the dorsal half of the scapholunate interosseous membrane, with secondary constraints being the palmar radiocapitate and distal scaphotrapezial ligaments.

Lunotriquetral dissociation (LTD), an ulnar-side carpal instability, involves a substantial disruption of the lunotriquetral and volar radiolunotriquetral ligaments and attenuation or rupture of dorsal radiotriquetral attachments. LTD has been divided into three stages, depending upon involvement of

the above three ligaments. In Stage III, in which lunotriquetral, volar radiolunotriquetral, and dorsal radiotriquetral ligaments are torn, a VISI collapse deformity occurs as the scaphoid induces the lunate into a further flexion stance while the triquetrum extends.[530,538]

Carpal instabilities nondissociative (CIND) can be classified into three groups based on the level of involvement: radiocarpal, midcarpal, and combined radio-midcarpal.[118] The radiocarpal instabilities are commonly associated with complete or partial radiocarpal dislocation or Barton's volar/dorsal fracture–dislocations of the distal radius. The midcarpal instabilities relate to loss of ligament support from the extrinsic scaphotrapezial, scaphocapitate, and triquetrocapitate ligaments. These problems are rarely noted acutely and represent chronic or late presentations of unrecognized sprains of the wrist, often superimposed on a lax ligamentous habitus. Secondary CIND-type midcarpal instabilities that lead to a VISI-type deformity can be seen following malunited distal radius fractures. Combined CID/CIND/CIC are frequent sequellae of the various carpal dislocations (radiocarpal, perilunate, midcarpal), implying severe damage to both the intrinsic and extrinsic radiocarpal ligaments.

The easiest way to differentiate between dissociative and nondissociative instabilities is to perform an arthrogram and note the presence or absence of dye flow between midcarpal and radiocarpal joints. If there is dye flow between compartments, one is probably dealing with a dissociative instability (CID). A lack of communication between the radiocarpal and midcarpal joint favors a nondissociative collapse (CIND). There are multiple reasons for nondissociative proximal carpal row collapse. The proximal carpal row is stabilized both proximally and distally by a complex of capsuloligamentous restraints. Damage to these restraints on *either* side of the proximal carpal row may lead to collapse. The imaging and clinical appearance of the proximal carpal row may be the same whether the destabilization is radiocarpal or midcarpal.

FRACTURES OF THE DISTAL RADIUS

EPONYMS

Modern treatment of fractures of the distal radius requires a clearer definition of the different types of fracture and clarification of the various eponyms associated with this injury. Of all of the fractures that affect the upper extremity, the distal radius fracture is among the most common. Historically, the accurate descriptions of this fracture are ascribed to Pouteau (1783)[439] and Colles (1814),[110] for whom it is classically named. In time, other descriptions of distal radius fractures were credited to Barton (1838),[35] Smith (1854),[494] and Dupuytren (1847).[157] It is more important today to determine the nature of the fracture and to describe the pathology involved than to link diagnosis and treatment to a single name. The type, direction, and amount of displacement are the most important factors[234] relating to treatment and, in this chapter, discussion is directed to the features emphasized as we sort through the preferred methods of treatment for fractures of the distal radius.

ANATOMY

The distal radius and distal radioulnar joints support the carpus with three separate articulations that are of concern in treatment of fractures of the distal radius. The scaphoid fossa and lunate fossa are two concave articular surfaces separated by a dorsal–volar ridge, which define clear articulations for the lunate and scaphoid (see Figs. 8-6 and 8-7). A separate articulation, the sigmoid notch, is present for the head of the ulna. This notch is also concave for contribution to the stability of the distal ulna. The distal articular surface of the radius is aligned to the longitudinal axis of the radius at 14° of volar tilt and 22° of ulnar inclination (see Fig. 8-20). The ulnar side of the wrist is supported in addition by the triangular fibrocartilage (TFC), which articulates with both the lunate and triquetrum. In various degrees of radioulnar deviation, there is greater or lesser contact with the TFC. The length of the ulna varies with pronation and supination, and there are varying degrees of positive or ulnar variance that affect the amount of force transmitted to both the radius and the triangular fibrocartilage.

The dorsal and volar ligaments of the wrist attached to the distal radius, previously described on page 570, are important in the mechanism of fracture and subsequent fragment displacement. These areas include the radial styloid volar facet, where the radiolunate and radiocapitate ligaments originate. The attachments of the dorsal retinaculum are at the first compartment, Lister's tubercle, and the ulnar rim.

The attachments of the dorsal and volar radioulnar ligaments of the TFC ulnarly on the distal radius have importance in lunate fossa fractures (diepunch fractures), disruptions of the TFC, and distal radioulnar joint injuries. The radial border of the TFC is attached along the entire margin of the lunate fossa at its border with the sigmoid notch. The ulnar attachment of the TFC is to the base of the ulnar styloid and distally to the triquetrum with the volar ulnocarpal ligaments.

MECHANISMS OF INJURY

Fractures of the distal radius occur most often from falls on the outstretched hand. The amount of force necessary experimentally to produce these fractures statically varies in the dorsiflexed wrist from 105 kg to 440 kg, with a mean of 195 kg for women and 282 kg for men.[198] Fractures of the distal radius are produced when the dorsiflexion of the wrist varies from 40° to 90°,[553] lesser amounts of force being required at smaller angles. Although the exact mechanism of fracture is not clear, the generally sharp fracture on the palmar aspect of the radial metaphyseal area, compared with the dorsally comminuted fragments, suggests that the radius may first fracture in tension on its palmar surface, with the fracture propagating dorsally where bending moment forces induce compression stresses (see Fig. 8-14). This results in the dorsal cortex comminuting as the fracture proceeds along 45° shear stress lines. Cancellous bone is compacted, further reducing dorsal stability. A high-tensile loading of the palmar radiocarpal ligaments is necessary to transmit the tensile loading to the anterior cortex. Concomitant ligamentous injuries are therefore to be expected.

CLASSIFICATION

The presentation of a classification of fractures of the distal radius must begin with an initial recognition of the different common types of fracture. Colles' fracture is the most common. It involves the distal metaphysis of the radius, which is dorsally displaced and angulated. It occurs within 2 cm of the articular surface, and may extend into the distal radiocarpal or radioulnar joint.[321] Dorsal angulation (silver fork deformity), dorsal displacement, radial angulation, and radial shortening are present. There is often an accompanying fracture of the ulnar styloid, which may signify avulsion of the TFC insertion.

Smith's fracture,[494] or reverse Colles' fracture, is a volar angulated fracture of the distal radius with a "garden spade" deformity.[336] The hand and wrist are displaced forward or volarly with respect to the forearm. The fracture may be extra-articular, intra-articular, or be part of a fracture–dislocation of the wrist (Fig. 8-22).

Barton's fracture is actually a fracture–dislocation or subluxation in which the rim of the distal radius, dorsally or volarly, is displaced with the hand and carpus.[336,432] It is different from a Colles' or Smith's fracture in that the dislocation is the most clinically and radiographically obvious abnormality, with the radial fracture noted secondarily. Some Colles' fractures resemble Barton's fractures when there is significant comminution of the dorsal surface and the fracture location is quite distal on the radius. The volar Barton's fracture is equivalent to a Smith's type III fracture, because both involve volar dislocation of the carpus associated with an intra-articular distal radius component.

Although a number of different classifications have been advanced for fractures of the distal radius, a recent classification that is treatment based and easy to remember will be presented. The Frykman classification[198] was used in the previous edition and has served as a reasonable, although somewhat cumbersome, method of recognition of different fracture types (Table 8-2). The present "universal" classification is modified from Gartland and Werley[211] (Fig. 8-23), and emphasizes the increasing awareness that different treatment modalities are indicated for the variations that exist in distal radius fractures.

Fractures of the distal radius can be broadly classified as extra-articular or intra-articular.[211] The ex-

Table 8-2. Frykman Classification of Colles' Fractures

Fractures	Distal Ulnar Fracture	
	Absent	Present
Extra-articular	I	II
Intra-articular involving radiocarpal joint	III	IV
Intra-articular involving distal radioulnar joint	V	VI
Intra-articular involving both radiocarpal and distal radioulnar joints	VII	VIII

(Data from Frykman, G.: Fracture of the Distal Radius Including Sequelae—Shoulder-Hand-Finger Syndrome, Disturbance in the Distal Radio-ulnar Joint, and Impairment of Nerve Function: A Clinical and Experimental Study. Acta Orthop. Scand., 108[Suppl.]:1–155, 1967.)

tra-articular fractures are generally referred to as Colles' fractures. Extra-articular fractures are either type I, undisplaced and stable, or type II, displaced and unstable. Intra-articular fractures, conversely, are either undisplaced, type III, or displaced, type IV. The displaced type IV has three subcategories: (A) reducible, stable; (B) reducible, unstable; and (C) irreducible (see Fig. 8-23). The treatment decisions are based on the extent of potential instability. The degree of initial displacement provides some criteria for determining instability. In our experience,[120] an unstable fracture is one that presents with greater than 20° of dorsal angulation, has marked dorsal comminution, and radial shortening of 10 mm or more. Secondary instability is present when closed reduction and cast immobilization fails to maintain the initial reduction, and there is residual dorsal angulation of 10° or more and greater than 5 mm of radial shortening. Stable fractures are usually extra-articular with mild to moderate displacement, and when reduced do not redisplace to the original deformity. Unstable fractures are more commonly comminuted, shortened, and have articular fractures that involve not only the radiocarpal joint but also the distal radioulnar joint. These fractures are associated with a higher rate of complications, including loss of reduction, median nerve injury, and instability of the distal radioulnar joint.[115]

Intra-articular fractures of the distal radius have been recognized as having different requirements for treatment than the extra-articular fractures. In addition to the modified Gartland universal classification, several other classifications of intra-articular fractures have been proposed. The Melone[362] classification (Fig. 8-24) recognizes articular fractures as comprising four basic components: the

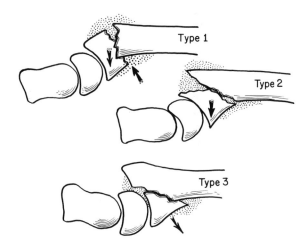

Fig. 8-22. Modified Thomas classification of Smith's fractures. *Type I* is extra-articular, *type II* crosses into the dorsal articular surface, and *type III* enters the radiocarpal joint (and is equivalent to a volar Barton's fracture–dislocation).

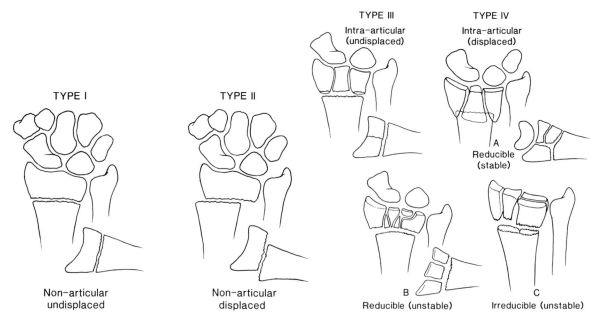

Fig. 8-23. Universal classification of dorsal displaced distal radius fractures. *Type I:* extra-articular, undisplaced; *type II:* extra-articular, displaced; *type III:* intra-articular, undisplaced; *type IV:* intra-articular, displaced: (A) reducible, stable; (B) reducible, unstable; (C) irreducible, unstable. *(Modified from Gartland, J. J. Jr.; Werley, C. W.: Evaluation of Healed Colles' Fractures. J. Bone Joint Surg. [Am.], 33:895–907, 1951; and from Sarmentio, A.; Pratt, G. W.; Berry, N. C.; Sinclair, W. F.: Colles' Fractures: Functional Bracing in Supination. J. Bone Joint Surg. [Am.], 57:311–317, 1975.)*

Fig. 8-24. Melone's intra-articular fracture classification. This classification of articular fractures is based on consistent fracture patterns resulting from the characteristic die-punch mechanism of injury. The fractures generally comprise four basic components. The key medial fragments, owing to their pivotal position, are the cornerstones of both the radiocarpal and distal radioulnar joints, and have been termed the medial complex. Displacement of this complex is the basis for categorization of the articular fracture into specific types. *(Melone, C. P. Jr.: Unstable Fractures of the Distal Radius. In Lichtman, D. M. [ed.]; The Wrist and Its Disorders. Philadelphia, W. B. Saunders, 1987.)*

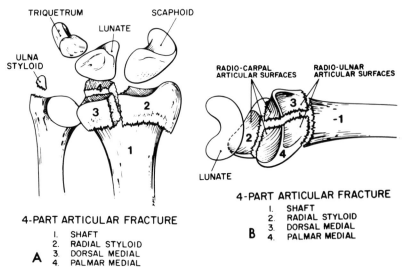

shaft, radial styloid, and dorsal medial and palmar medial components. Variation on the involvement of these fracture fragments results in four different types of intra-articular fractures. Type I is undisplaced and minimally comminuted; type II fractures (die-punch fractures) are unstable with moderate to severe displacement. Comminution of the anterior cortex suggest instability. Type III fractures involve an additional fracture component from the shaft of the radius that can project into the flexor compartment. Type IV fractures involve a transverse split of the articular sufraces with rotational displacement. Unsuccessful reductions are common with Melone types II, III, and IV.

To clearly separate the articular surfaces that may individually be involved with distal radius fractures, we have proposed a modified (Mayo Clinic) classification in which the scaphoid, lunate, and sigmoid notch fossae of the distal radius are considered as separate articulations. Type I fractures are intra-articular but undisplaced; type II fractures are displaced involving the radioscaphoid joint. Type III fractures are displaced involving the radiolunate joint, and type IV fractures are displaced involving both the radioscaphoid and lunate joints and the sigmoid fossa of the distal radius. The radioscaphoid joint fracture (type II) involves more than the radial styloid (the Chauffeur's fracture) and has significant dorsal angulation and radial shortening. The radiolunate fracture (type III) is the die-punch or lunate load fracture, and is often irreducible by traction alone. The radioscaphoid and lunate fracture (type IV) is often a more comminuted fracture involving all of the major joint articular surfaces, and almost always includes a fracture component into the distal radioulnar joint.

The purpose of both the Melone[362] and the above classifications of distal radius fractures is to call attention to the intra-articular fracture, which must be identified as distinct variants of Colles' fracture and which demands more aggressive treatment. Either of these classifications fit well, as further subdivisions of the universal classification of distal radius fractures: type IV—intra-articular.

Throughout the remainder of this chapter, the various types of fracture designations (I, II, III, and IV) refers to the "universal" classification (see Fig. 8-23).

CLINICAL FINDINGS

With the often thinner cortices in the elderly, an extra-articular metaphyseal fracture generally occurs. In younger patients, an intra-articular fracture

with displacement of the joint surfaces is more likely.

On clinical examination, there is obvious deformity of the wrist with dorsal displacement of the hand in the Colles' type fracture (or dorsal Barton's), or volar displacement of the hand and wrist in the Smith's type fracture (volar Barton's).[321] The dorsal aspect of the hand and wrist are usually quite swollen and ecchymosis may be present, especially in the elderly. The wrist should be examined for tenderness not only about the radial fracture site, but also at the distal ulna, elbow, and shoulder. Median nerve function and flexor and extensor tendon action should be tested.[82,104,492,527] Instability of the distal ulna should be assessed, usually after local or regional anesthesia has been obtained.

Associated Injuries and Complications

MEDIAN NERVE INJURY

As a result of the original trauma, distal radius fractures are associated with a number of soft tissue injuries and a variety of potential complications (Table 8-3). The most common associated problem is damage to the median nerve.[115,297,340] With forceful hyperextension, the median nerve is placed under considerable tension. Displacement of fracture fragments can cause direct nerve injury. Inadequate or delayed reduction, hematoma forma-

---

Table 8-3. Complications of Colles' Fractures

Early
  Difficult reduction; unstable reduction maintained only by
    extreme position
  Depressed major articular components
  Distal radioulnar subluxation, dislocation
  Median or ulnar nerve stretch, contusion, or
    compression[532]
  Acute carpal tunnel syndrome
  Postreduction swelling; compartment syndromes[532]
  Errors in external fixation (peripheral nerve injuries)
  Tendon damage
  Pain dysfunction syndromes (early)
  Associated carpal injury
Intermediate and late
  Loss of reduction and secondary deformity
    Malunion and secondary intercarpal collapse deformity
    Radiocarpal arthrosis—inadequate articular surface
      reduction
    Distal radioulnar dissociation and arthrosis
  Stiff hand; shoulder–hand syndrome; arthritic flare
  Pain dysfunction syndrome
  Median nerve compression; carpal tunnel syndrome;
    occasionally ulnar or radial nerve compression
  Tendinous adhesion in the flexor compartment
  Extensor pollicis longus tendon rupture[308,399,492,527]
  Nonunion

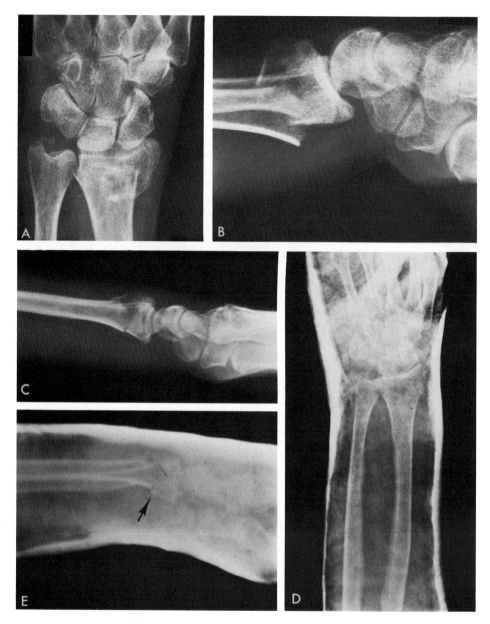

Fig. 8-25. A 54-year-old housewife fell on the palm of her left hand after slipping on ice and sustained a Frykman type VI Colles' fracture. (**A, B**) The fracture line enters the distal radioulnar joint. There is a small avulsion fracture of the ulnar styloid, dorsal angulation of 25°, radial shortening, and dorsal displacement. (**C**) Dorsal angulation was corrected with traction in Chinese finger traps. There is a sharp fracture line on the palmar aspect. The distal fragment lacks approximately 1 mm of complete reduction. There is a comminuted fracture surface dorsally, with evidence of compaction of cancellous bone. (**D**) Postreduction x-rays taken after a circular plaster cast was applied above elbow with the forearm in slight supination, show correction of radial length and radial angulation. (**E**) The lateral view shows that the volar cortex was overcorrected slightly (*arrow*), thus locking its position. Angulation of the articular surface approaches normal palmar flexion of 10° to 15°. The cast is well molded about the forearm, and three-point fixation has been achieved. The cast was split along its ulnar margin to accommodate swelling.

(continued)

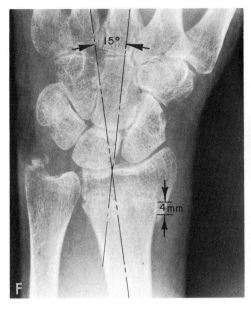
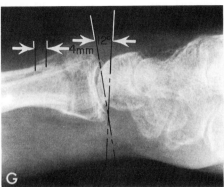

Fig. 8-25 *(continued)*
(F, G) Six weeks later, the fracture shows settling. Radial angulation of 15°, radial shortening of 4 mm, and loss of normal palmar-flexed position of the articular surface to 12° dorsiflexion have occurred in cast. The ulnar styloid appears to be uniting. Clinically, this was an acceptable result. Six months after fracture, there was full range of motion of the fingers, but dorsiflexion was limited to 50°. The woman had slight residual discomfort on supination with active use of the hand.

tion, and increased compartment pressure may produce additional pressure on the nerve. In our review of complications of distal radius fractures, median nerve injury had the most serious sequela.[115]

Prompt reduction of the fracture in the emergency room can help reduce the extent of compression and compromised vascularity. Adequate anesthesia, axillary block, Bier block, or general anesthesia are preferable to hematoma block or intravenous analgesics, except for expedient decompression of the median nerve. Adequate reduction will often relieve paresthesias within a few days. If the symptoms are severe or increasing, carpal tunnel decompression is warranted.[41,352] Open reduction of the fracture or application of external fixation may be applied simultaneously. For mild, chronic median neuropathy, observation may be employed for 3 or 4 months, but should not be ignored.

LOSS OF REDUCTION

Displaced fractures of the radius not uncommonly have a loss of reduction, unless measures are initiated acutely to prevent redisplacement (Fig. 8-25).

Primary percutaneous pin fixation or external fixation should be considered if the original fracture reduction is considered unstable. Fracture stability may be judged at the time of reduction. If there is immediate redisplacement of fracture fragments despite sugar-tong splint or cast support, the fracture is presumed unstable. If the fracture fragments cannot be easily reduced with longitudinal traction, the fracture is probably unstable. Our treatment plan is to obtain as good a closed reduction as possible acutely in the emergency room. If the fracture is unstable, then the patient is scheduled for operating room treatment either the same day or within 48 hours of injury. Even with excellent reduction and adequate casting, there is often gradual shortening at the fracture site as healing occurs.

Late, unrecognized loss of reduction is associated with arthritis of the radiocarpal and distal radioulnar joints,[192] and was the second most common cause of late complications from distal radius fractures in our series. Re-reduction is possible up to 3 weeks from the time of injury, and radiographic re-evaluation of fracture alignment is recommended weekly to prevent loss of reduction, malunion,[270] or the rare nonunion.[246]

DISTAL RADIOULNAR JOINT

Injury to the triangular fibrocartilage is an often unrecognized element of distal radius fractures.[164,261] Although the exact incidence is unknown, we would estimate that approximately 50% of fractures have clinically significant injury to the TFC. These injuries include avulsion of the TFC from the ulnar styloid, in-substance tears of the peripheral rim, and displacement of the lunate fossa with the TFC.[164] It is difficult to test the stability of the distal ulna acutely without incurring redisplacement of the reduced radial fracture. If the ulnar styloid is displaced, it is likely that the TFC will provide diminished support. Placing the forearm in neutral rotation in a long-arm cast situates the TFC in the best alignment for healing. Marked pronation is to be avoided, because this inclines the ulnar head to displace dorsally. By the same token, supination with imperfect radial fragment reduction may result in palmar subluxation of the ulnar head. We would continue long-arm casting for at least 3 weeks, or until forearm rotation is not symptomatic.

To date there have been few advocates for reattachment of the TFC to the ulnar styloid or styloid fixation, but it should be considered when there is gross instability and the ulnar styloid fragment is large, implying total detachment.

OPEN FRACTURES

It is unusual to have an open fracture of the distal radius, but when this occurs it is an indication for emergency operative treatment. Any open injury, even an inside-out puncture wound, should be débrided and the fracture site irrigated using pulsed lavage. If the wound is a result of low-energy trauma, primary closure is acceptable, but if the wound is contaminated, contused, or greater than 2 cm as the result of high-energy trauma, then débridement and delayed wound closure are recommended. External fixation to maintain fracture reduction and allow wound access for dressing changes is preferred. Open reduction and internal fixation with plates or multiple pins is usually contraindicated. The exception would be the small inside-out wound that is primarily closed. Operative quantitative cultures are advisable prior to starting a broad-spectrum antibiotic. Wound closure is performed at 48 to 72 hours.

TREATMENT

Undisplaced Fractures

A large percentage of fractures in the elderly are undisplaced or minimally displaced stable fractures. The goals of treatment in these cases are to protect the area of fracture from further injury and to mobilize the hand and wrist as soon as symptoms allow. Many forms of cast and splints have been described, and the selection can be left to the surgeon's preference.[469,545] Some form of three-point fixation is needed, with a dorsal splint holding the wrist in slight flexion and ulnar deviation. The length of immobilization varies from 3 to 6 weeks. Pain-free motion of the fingers, forearm, and elbow are prerequisites for choosing short-arm cast or splint immobilization.

AUTHORS' PREFERRED METHOD

For stable undisplaced or minimally displaced extra-articular fractures (universal classification types I and II—see Fig. 8-23**A**), we prefer treatment with a light, short-arm fiberglas cast, either at the time of presentation or within 48 hours if a sugar-tong splint was applied in the presence of initial swelling. The cast is applied with the fingers in light traction to help prevent settling (Fig. 8-26).[431] A neutral position of the wrist is desirable. If the fracture was originally slightly displaced, the wrist is placed in no more than slight flexion and ulnar deviation for 3 weeks.

For undisplaced or minimally displaced fractures that are stable but have intra-articular extensions (type III), percutaneous pin fixation may be added where a potential for fracture settling or displacement of the articular fragments is a concern. A short-arm cast is used with percutaneous pins, and the pins are usually removed after 3 to 4 weeks.

Usually by 6 weeks, clinical and radiographic examination demonstrate progression of fracture healing. A custom-designed splint or commercial protective splint is applied. The splint is removed for bathing and exercises, and gradually removed over 2 to 3 weeks when the fracture is solidly healed. Most patients favor the splint for protection, particularly in icy climates. Instructions in active-assisted wrist motion are demonstrated to the patient. These exercises, known as "the six pack" of hand exercises and first described by the senior author (JHD), emphasize complete finger and wrist excursion (see p. 663). Most patients are able to perform these exercises and their rehabilitation on their own, but their progress is rechecked periodically.

Displaced Fractures

In the treatment of displaced fractures of the radius, the fracture type provides an excellent guide to selecting the preferred form of treatment (see Fig. 8-

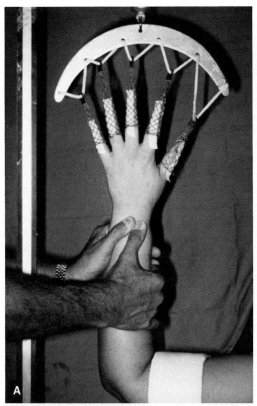

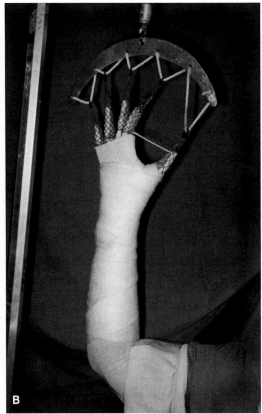

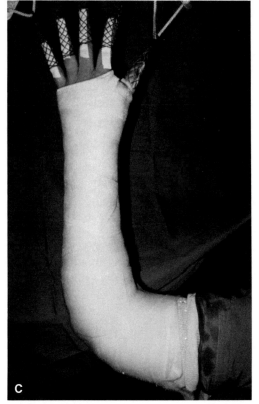

Fig. 8-26. Technique of closed reduction for fractures of the distal radius. Undisplaced fractures are treated in a short-arm cast, while displaced fractures are treated in a long-arm cast. Displaced fractures require (**A**) gentle manipulation and sustained traction, and (**B, C**) application of the long-arm cast while maintaining traction. The finger traps are removed and the cast trimmed to allow for full finger and thumb motion.

23). The principles involve obtaining an anatomic reduction and maintaining that reduction with appropriate methods of immobilization.[63] The importance of anatomic reduction has been demonstrated by clinical studies of the natural history of incompletely reduced fractures, as well as by laboratory assessment of forces and stress loading across the radiocarpal joint. Knirk and Jupiter,[298] Bradway and associates,[76] and others[38,219,362] have correlated the outcome following distal radius fractures with the initial and final fracture displacement. When part of the joint articular surface was displaced more than 2 mm, radial shortening was greater than 5 mm, or dorsal angulation exceeded 20°, less than optimal results were seen. Posttraumatic arthritis was present at the radiocarpal and radioulnar joints in such patients. Wrist motion was decreased, grip strength was less than 50% of normal, and carpal subluxation with wrist instability was evident[19,360] (see *Carpal Instability* in this chapter). These clinical observations have been confirmed by laboratory studies, which show that the effect of loss of radial length creates increased loads across the ulnocarpal joint and decreased force concentration across the radiocarpal joint. Every effort should be made to restore normal length, alignment, and articular surface congruency of the distal radius.[300,431]

CLOSED REDUCTION

An accurate reduction of the fracture is the first step in treatment. Böhler[63] recommended in 1922 that this be performed by longitudinal traction to the hand with countertraction through the forearm. Today, the use of finger-trap traction with proximal brachial countertraction is preferred (Fig. 8-26A). The application of hyperextension and flexion maneuvers to break up the impaction is not recommended. Traction is placed through the thumb, index, and long fingers, and a self-sustained traction holder applies 6 to 12 pounds of countertraction. An axillary block or Bier block is recommended in displaced fractures, because a hematoma block may not provide sufficient anesthesia for distraction reduction. With a dorsally displaced fracture, the reduction is then performed by pushing the distal fragment distally and palmarly while holding the proximal fragment with the fingers around the forearm (Fig. 8-26**A**). When pressure is released, the distal fragment frequently springs back dorsally. Pronation and ulnar deviation of the distal component may also be necessary. Anteroposterior and lateral x-rays are taken to assess the accuracy of the reduction. The goal is to convert the dorsal angulation to neutral or to a slight volar tilt, as well

as to regain radial length. Alignment or slight over-reduction of the volar cortices is essential to prevent redisplacement, because there is little dorsal cortical support in most of these fractures. It should not be necessary to manipulate the wrist in pronation or wrist flexion to obtain or hold the reduction.

For a dorsal Barton's fracture, the reduction is performed in the same manner as a Colles' fracture, but most of these are unstable and pin fixation or open reduction may be needed to maintain reduction. For a Smith's fracture with palmar displacement and palmar angulation of the distal fracture component, traction is used to disimpact the bone surfaces, and dorsal displacement and supination are applied to the distal fragment. Smith's types II and III (see Fig. 8-22) may be unstable, and closed reduction may be insufficient (Fig. 8-27). Image intensification is of immeasurable value in assisting fracture reduction, especially if percutaneous pin fixation is performed. Plain films, however, are essential to assess the final accuracy of the reduction, because fluoroscopic imaging often lacks the clarity required.[399]

Five to ten pounds are used for initial distraction. Occasionally, 15 to 20 pounds (8 to 10 kg) are needed for disimpaction. The wrist should not be maintained with this much distraction during external fixation or pin fixation because the weight of the extremity or 5 pounds countertraction should be sufficient.

If closed reduction of a fracture is unsuccessful, open reduction of the radius may be required, especially to restore joint articular surfaces to normal contour and length, because functional results mirror the radiographic results (Fig. 8-28).

CAST IMMOBILIZATION

After reduction of the fracture is achieved, many methods are available to maintain alignment and prevent redisplacement. The method of immobilization selected depends on the classification status of the fracture (see Fig. 8-23): Is the fracture extra-articular or intra-articular? Is the reduction stable or unstable? How significant is the displacement and amount of comminution present? For most fractures, closed reduction and cast immobilization is preferred. Traction maintained during application allows molding three-point pressure into a long-arm or snugly applied short-arm cast. The volar cortices must be aligned or the distal fragment slightly over-reduced to hold length. Three-point pressure is then applied by molding dorsally over the distal fragment and proximal forearm, and volarly over the distal forearm. A flexed and ulnarly deviated position may actually increase the tendency to redisplacement by displacing the contact area at the radiocarpal joint dorsally; therefore, the wrist is placed in neutral or very slight flexion. The dorsal capsule has no ability to maintain reduction by ligamentotaxis, even when the wrist is fully flexed. Shortening and redisplacement can be minimized when the cast is applied in this fashion, but some subsequent settling is unavoidable.

Excessive wrist flexion also compromises the carpal tunnel and normal flexor tendon function. The forearm should be in neutral rotation in a long-arm cast, so that the ulnar head is fully seated in the sigmoid notch. Restoration of both pronation and supination is more easily achieved from this position.

EXTERNAL FIXATION

In many comminuted and displaced fractures of the distal radius, cast immobilization will not be effective in maintaining the fracture reduction.[26,107,113,120,392,477] Despite increased skills in cast application, there are fractures that are inherently unstable and therefore require immobilization by fixed traction. In the Frykman classification,[198] these fracture types are usually types VII and VIII, in which comminution and displacement are present in addition to intra-articular involvement. Melone has called attention to intra-articular fractures as four-part fractures of increasing severity through four types. Primary external fixation[314,477] should be considered for fracture types II, IVA, and IVB (see Fig. 8-23). Secondary external fixation is indicated when there is loss of reduction following cast immobilization.[113]

Factors that mitigate against adequate reduction include dorsal comminution, interposition of soft tissues volarly, a tendency for dorsal displacement and dorsal angulation of the distal fragment to occur dynamically from soft tissue tension, and greater radial than ulnar instability. To overcome these problems, volar stability must be obtained by adequate locking of the volar cortices and counterforce application to the dorsoradial compressive force. For the latter, the concept of using an external distraction apparatus is appealing. It must be remembered, however, that traction applied in this manner is not well transmitted to the dorsal rim of the radius by ligamentotaxis, because the dorsal ligaments run obliquely and tend to stretch apart rather than exerting equivalent force to the distal fragment from the external fixator.[37]

Our current preference is to accurately reduce the fracture of the distal radius acutely in the emergency room, using traction and adequate anesthesia. If the fracture is considered unstable, we schedule the patient for immediate definitive treatment in the operating room or within 48 hours, as scheduling permits. The specific method of external fixation is less important in treatment of these fractures than adhering to the principle of maintaining reduction with fixed traction (Fig. 8-29).[200,269,405,453,454,458,485] In selecting an external fixator, we prefer a half frame on the radial side of the wrist and forearm for the less comminuted fractures, and a quadrilateral frame centered over the radius for more extensively comminuted fractures. Our experience has included the Hoffman C-series, Orthofix, ASIF half-frame devices, and the Roger Anderson, Mini-Hoffman (Judet), and Ace Colles quadrilateral frame devices.[120]

The fixation frame is assembled and tightened only after the fracture has been completely reduced (see Fig. 8-29). With the exception of one device designed to aid in fracture reduction (Wrist Jack, Hand Biomechanics Laboratory, Sacramento, CA), we believe that the frame and pins should not be used to assist in the reduction. The preferred sequence is longitudinal traction, insertion of half pins, fracture reduction, and assemblage of the external fixation while the wrist is maintained in traction. The external fixation is supplemented with percutaneous pins through the radial styloid for certain intra-articular fractures. A limited open reduction with the external fixation frame in position can also be performed (see below). We have not had experience with external fixation frames that allow early motion through a lateral hinged joint.[106] External fixation with a mini-Hoffman frame in which the pins are placed only into the distal radius and not across the carpus has had limited application in extra-articular distal radius fractures in patients with excellent bone stock, and is an acceptable alternative. Manipulation of intra-articular fragments with percutaneous pins may also be accomplished after the frame is applied. Care must be taken to avoid excessive distraction. The pins-and-plaster technique of external fixation,[107] although appealing in concept,[94] is often difficult in practice.[101,230] Application of the plaster around the pins may prolong the procedure sufficiently to prevent adequate molding of the cast.[101] Subsequent dorsal redisplacement and angulation of the distal fragment has been one factor in our dissatisfaction with the pins-and-plaster technique.

External fixation is maintained for a minimal period of 6 to 8 weeks. After removal of the external fixation frame and pins, removable splint protection

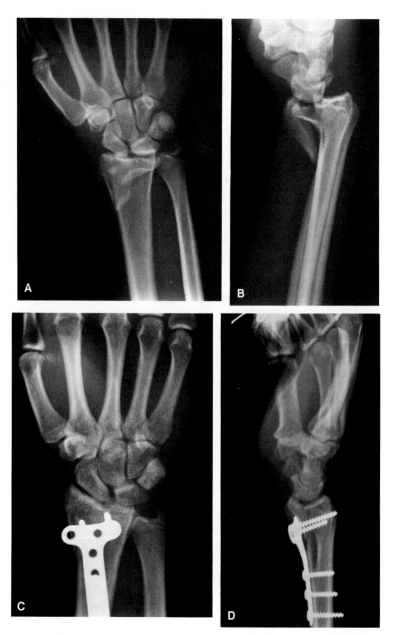

Fig. 8-27. Smith's fracture. Volar displacement of the carpus with a distal radius fracture in a 26-year-old plumber who fell forward from his motorcycle. (**A**) Posteroanterior: oblique fracture through the radius; note the double shadow over the lunate, indicating volar displacement. (**B**) (Lateral) fracture of the distal radial articular surface with volar displacement of the carpus; a comminuted intra-articular fracture (Thomas type III). (**C, D**) Open reduction and volar buttress plate fixation; distal screws were used to hold reduction of the intra-articular fracture components.

(continued)

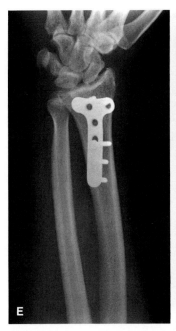
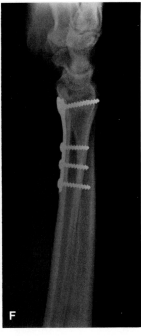

Fig. 8-27 (continued)
(E, F) Reduction well maintained (1 year later) with excellent alignment of joint articular surface and a well-united fracture.

is used for 2 to 3 weeks, because gentle motion is encouraged. Pins can be removed as an outpatient under local anesthesia. Physical therapy should be considered, because distraction across the wrist may delay the return of motion and strength. Pin-tract infection and pin loosening are the major problems with this technique.[554]

PERCUTANEOUS PIN FIXATION

For displaced fractures of the radius, the use of percutaneous pins[105,142,279] has been an accepted practice either alone or to supplement external fixation. Most commonly it is used with a cast or splint. Percutaneous pins are considered for type II, type III, and type IVA fractures. Some surgeons use pins when slippage in the cast is a concern or when the patient is considered unreliable.

A number of techniques have been described. Steinmann pins can be placed down the radial shaft, so that one is inserted through the styloid and the other through the dorsoulnar corner of the distal fragment as intramedullary fixation. The tension produced in the pins as they deflect against the proximal cortices effectively maintains reduction. The ends of the pins are bent at a right angle and are connected with a small metal clamp to prevent rotation.

A second technique involves passing K-wires through the radial styloid with the wrist in traction.

The pins are drilled proximally through the radial styloid until they penetrate the intact cortex of the shaft.[105] K-wires of 0.045 to 0.0625-inch diameter are selected; smaller pins for women and larger pins for men. The pin insertion is performed with a power K-wire driver to allow the surgeon to hold part of the reduction with one hand during the K-wire insertion. Variations include drilling through the ulna until the pin reaches the inner cortex of the styloid[142] or drilling through the radial styloid until it is completely through the ulna (Rayhack technique) (Fig. 8-30). Long-arm cast immobilization must be used if the pins pass between the radius and ulna.

Another method of percutaneous pin fixation is the intrafocal pin technique of Kapandji.[279] In his technique, the K-wires are introduced into the fracture site itself, rather than through the distal fracture fragment. The K-wire can be used to wedge open the fracture reduction and then to prevent the distal fragments from redisplacement. A total of four K-wires are used with this technique (two dorsal and two volar) (Fig. 8-31). Kapandji's original technique involved "feeling for the fracture site" with the tip of the K-wire, followed by manual insertion; however, we prefer image intensification fluoroscopy to assist the insertion. X-rays confirm pin placement. All such procedures are carried out under full sterile preparation and draping. Overhead

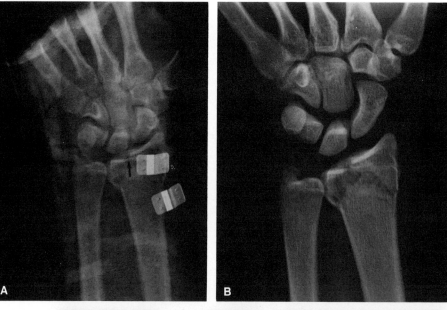

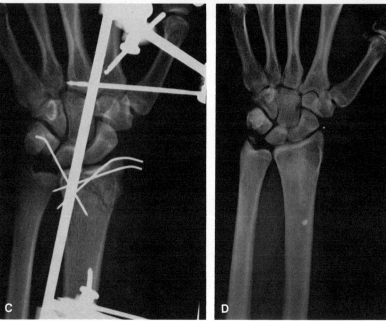

Fig. 8-28. A 32-year-old carpenter fell from a building, fracturing his left distal radius. (**A**) Closed reduction and cast immobilization was performed. A persistent intra-articular step-off involving the lunate fossa of the distal radius was noted (*arrow*). (**B**) After re-reduction with further traction, there was still an intra-articular step-off of greater than 3 mm. (**C**) Limited open reduction and K-wire fixation across the lunate fossa (die-punch) fracture component was performed under sustained traction maintained with an external fixation frame. (**D**) At 4 years follow-up, an anatomic reduction was maintained without evidence of radiocarpal arthrosis. Note complication of a retained fixation pin.

traction is preferred, although some surgeons have devised a lateral traction arm board. After insertion, the K-wires are cut short outside the skin and capped. A sponge padding with an occlusive dressing prevents skin irritation. A short-arm cast is worn for 3 to 6 weeks, depending on the degree of fracture stability. In some cases the cast can be removed at 3 weeks, a splint applied, and radiocarpal motion

started with the pins in place. Some authors recommend windowing the cast and stress-relieving skin incisions if swelling results in pin-site irritation. Careful patient follow-up is needed with all three of these techniques.

Percutaneous pin fixation is an excellent technique, provided the distal radius is not severely comminuted or osteoporotic, because the trabecular bone of the metaphysis provides little inherent stability. It is especially useful for unstable fractures, both extra-articular and intra-articular, in combination with external fixation.

OPEN REDUCTION

One of the recent advances in the treatment of distal radius fractures is the more frequent application of open reduction and internal fixation, especially for intra-articular fractures (Fig. 8-32).[29,32,38,303,362,480] The primary indication is articular fragment[219] displacement, which, if left unreduced, leads to radiocarpal or radioulnar arthritis. While the magnitude of forces across the wrist joint is not known, some have estimated these at 10 to 12 times the grip force. Strenuous activity may require withstanding over 500 pounds of compressive force. Thus, accurate reduction of the intra-articular joint surfaces should be considered along with factors of age, occupation, and activity level during the decision as to whether fracture alignment can best be obtained with closed or open reduction.

The options for open reduction include a longitudinal dorsal approach, a volar approach, a limited transverse dorsal approach, or reduction under arthroscopic control.

Open reduction is preferred when joint incongruity is evident by articular surface displacement of more than 2 mm.[38,76] For a dorsally displaced fracture, a limited dorsal transverse incision is used, distracting the wrist either in traction or with an external fixator. The extensor retinaculum between the third and fourth extensor compartments is reflected, and the wrist capsule is divided in line with the skin incision. A nerve hook, Freer elevator, or percutaneously placed pins can be used to elevate the joint fracture fragments. If there is more than 4 to 5 mm of impaction, a bone graft from the iliac crest or an allograft is recommended to fill the metaphyseal defect.

The choice of fixation depends on the fracture configuration.[314] External fixation supplemented with K-wires that hold the intra-articular fracture components is preferred (see Fig. 8-28). A miniplate (AO/ASIF) is chosen when more proximal comminution is present.[219,265] The dorsal approach for plate fixation involves a longitudinal incision, reflection of the extensor retinaculum, removal of Lister's tubercle, and subperiosteal exposure of the fracture (Fig. 8-33). Temporary K-wire fixation while the defect is packed with a bone graft is usually necessary before application of a mini T-plate. Distal comminution precludes the use of screws in the distal fragment.

A volarly displaced fracture of the Smith's or volar Barton's type is better approached through a volar incision and application of a buttress plate as described by Ellis (see Fig. 8-27).[166] The incision is made through a proximally extended carpal tunnel incision, with reflection of the pronator quadratus from the radius. The plate is contoured to fit the metaphyseal curvature, and distal fragment screws are rarely indicated. This approach may also be necessary to retrieve muscle, tendon,[399] or periosteum that is entrapped and preventing reduction of a dorsally angulated fracture. A displaced volar spike (Melone type III) fracture may also require a volar approach.

During open reduction of the distal radius, the surgeon needs to examine the articular surface reduction of the radioscaphoid, radiolunate, and distal radioulnar joints, and treat each appropriately. There is little indication for primary excision of the distal ulna.[148]

AUTHORS' PREFERRED METHODS

Barton's Fracture. A volar Barton's (Smith's III) is ideally treated by a volar buttress plate.[29,30] A dorsal Barton's (intra-articular Colles') is best treated by closed reduction and external fixation if an adequate reduction can be maintained.[141] Otherwise, open reduction and percutaneous pins, compressive screws, or a dorsal buttress plate can be elected.[432,534]

Chauffeur's Fracture. The radial styloid fracture can usually be treated with closed reduction and percutaneous pin fixation. If, however, the fracture is displaced more than 3 mm, there may be an associated scapholunate[39] dissociation for which we would favor open reduction, repair of the ligament, and anatomic reduction of the radial styloid. Percutaneous pins which, at most, penetrate only two cortices are subject to erosive loosening within the trabecular bone of the metaphysis; therefore, trabecular screws may offer greater security for fixation. Very accurate anatomic alignment is essential to prevent secondary posttraumatic arthrosis.

Smith's Fracture. Open reduction and internal fixation (or external fixation) is the treatment of choice for volar displaced fractures, especially the intra-articular types II and III.[336,524] External fixation for open Smith's fractures is acceptable for wound considerations.[113] Careful reduction with radiographic control and supplemental K-wires may be needed for Smith's type II fractures, to insure anatomic alignment of the radiocarpal joint.[166]

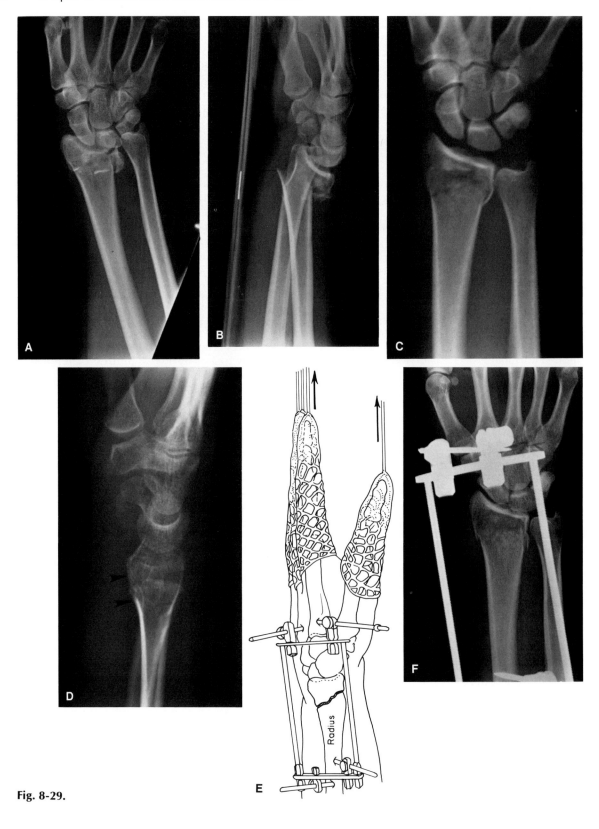

Fig. 8-29.

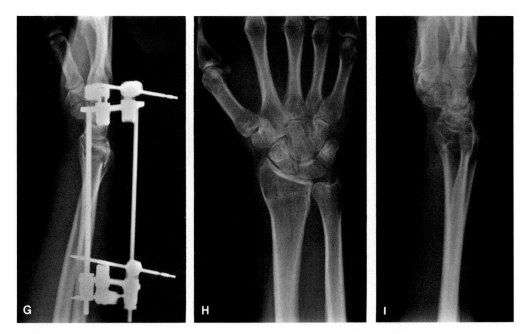

Fig. 8-29. A 32-year-old teacher fell on ice and sustained this intra-articular distal radius fracture (type IV). (**A**) Intra-articular fracture involving the lunate fossa of distal radius. (**B**) Lateral view showing dorsal angulation of 65° with dorsal comminution. (**C**) Traction view, with anatomic reduction achieved. (**D**) Anatomic alignment of the volar cortex (buttress effect). (**E**) External fixation with a quadrilateral frame used to maintain the reduction. (**F, G**) Radiographic appearance (PA and lateral) at 4 weeks; reduction maintained. (**H, I**) End result with nearly normal anatomic alignment of the distal radius 7 months postinjury.

CARPAL INSTABILITIES

Severe wrist injuries with dislocation or fracture–dislocation often develop a wrist instability pattern after spontaneous or manipulative relocation.[272,481] The perilunate dislocation pattern provides a whole spectrum of wrist sprains, fractures, dislocations, and instabilities (Fig. 8-34).[229,272,330,514,478,525] This injury pattern usually begins radially and destabilizes through the body of the scaphoid (scaphoid fracture) or through the scapholunate interval (scapholunate dissociation).[354] Further destabilization passes distal to the lunate, either through the space of Poirier or through the capitate (transcapitate fracture), and then ulnar to the lunate, either through hamate and triquetrum or through the lunotriquetral interval.[354,355,356] This type of perilunate dislocation usually results in a DISI collapse pattern, because the stabilizing influence of the scaphoid is lost first and foremost.

A similar pattern of destabilization can begin ulnarly and propagate radialward around the lunate, such that the lunate is first dissociated from the triquetrum.[449,530,538] The lunate may retain sufficient bonding to the scaphoid that the residual collapse pattern is VISI in nature. Both of these collapse patterns are dissociative (CID) because there is disruption of the ligament bond or the bone structure between the lunate and one or both of the adjacent carpals.[118]

Radiocarpal dislocation is a less common injury, sometimes ligamentous only, but more commonly including a fragment of the radius. It is recognized and traditionally called either a volar or dorsal Barton's fracture-dislocation with a radiocarpal subluxation or dislocation as discussed in the previous section. Either a VISI or DISI instability is possible, and it may be either dissociative or nondissociative, depending upon the degree of damage done to the ligamentous bonds of the proximal carpal row.

There are three other radiocarpal instabilities: ulnar translation of the entire carpus, dorsal translation instabilities, and occasionally volar translation instabilities.[447,470,472] Combinations of these

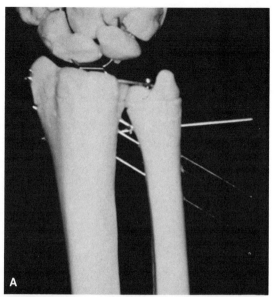

Fig. 8-30. Rayhack technique of percutaneous pin fixation of the distal radius with K-wires (0.45 to 0.625) inserted from the subarticulary region of the distal radius into the stable distal ulna. (**A**) Bone model of percutaneous pin technique. (**B**) Pin fixation of a type II, extra-articular displaced distal radius fracture. (Courtesy of John Rayhack, M.D.)

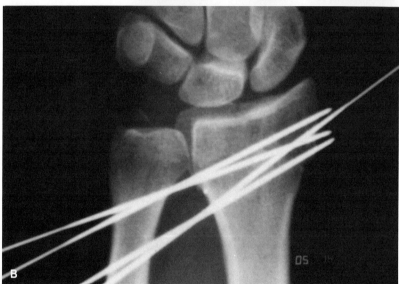

instabilities may occur, although one deformity pattern is usually predominant. The basic patterns are similar in instability, dislocation, and fracture–dislocation, suggesting a spectrum of problems that arise as variations occur in the linkage system within the carpus (see Table 8-1). Using these concepts, it is possible to group all known injuries that result in carpal instability into interrelated categories.

SIGNS AND SYMPTOMS

The most constant and dependable sign of carpal injury is well-localized tenderness. Fractures of the scaphoid, for example, are most tender to pressure in the anatomical snuffbox. Scapholunate and lunate injuries cause tenderness just distal to Lister's tubercle.[238] Triquetral, triquetrolunate, and triquetrohamate ligament injuries result in tenderness over the dorsal margin of the appropriate bone, usually a fingerbreadth distal to the ulnar head. Other clinical findings are highly variable and depend on the extent of carpal disruption. There may be swelling that is severe and generalized or discrete and barely detectable. Changes in shape, attributable to swelling, realignment of the bony architecture, or alterations in soft tissues may occur. Dorsal swelling over the proximal carpal row is suggestive of a ligament avulsion with or without a chip fracture. Marked prominence of the entire carpus dorsally is suggestive of a perilunate dislocation. Compressive stresses applied actively or passively may produce pain at the site of damage.[102] Rather common findings in the wrist area are those of snaps, clicks, shifts, and thuds, which may be palpable and audible.[229]

There are several clinical tests and approaches to diagnosis.[102,222,474] For scapholunate instability, these include the scaphoid lift test, which is a reproduction of pain with dorsal-volar shifting of the scaphoid, and the Watson test,[550] which is painful dorsal scaphoid displacement instability as the wrist moves from ulnar to radial deviation with the tuberosity compressed. For lunotriquetral instability, there is the ballottement test (also called shear or shuck test), in which the triquetrum is displaced dorsally and palmarly on the lunate, demonstrating increased excursion over the normal side and often a painful crepitus. The compression test is a similar displacement of the triquetrum ulnarly during radioulnar deviation, which is also painful. A lax ligamentous habitus is often associated with the ability to subluxate the midcarpal joint by displacing the carpometacarpal unit on the radiocarpal.[509,510] Tendon displacements with audible snaps are easily produced by some people, but are seldom symptomatic.

Distraction can be a good clue to a "lax wrist" or a damaged area, particularly when viewed under fluoroscopic imaging with static traction (approximately 25 pounds) applied. Simple stretching is often revealing when producing pain or subluxation. These and the other movement abnormalities must be correlated with history, clinical findings, and radiologic findings to provide a proper diagnosis.[345]

POSTTRAUMATIC CARPAL INSTABILITY

Carpal instability was used as a category in the initial edition of this text, emphasizing the traumatic etiologies. Subsequent experience has expanded its utility and applicability to the point that most wrist injuries are now involved. First-degree sprains and fractures are usually not associated with instability,[328] but prior trauma, congenital laxity, inflammation, or disease may elevate even these injuries into the instability category. Second- and third-degree sprains, dislocations, and fracture–dislocations are likely to develop carpal instability. The clinical groups to be discussed are radiocarpal, perilunate, midcarpal, and axial injuries. Distal radioulnar joint injuries will be discussed separately.

Radiocarpal Instability

Diagnosis of these injuries is made from a history of appropriate trauma followed by the usual initial findings of swelling, deformity, tenderness, and pain. Swelling and tenderness is most noticeable dorsally at the radiocarpal level and aggravated by wrist motions. Deformity may be an ulnar, dorsal, or volar shift of the carpus. For definitive diagnosis, some deformity should be visible on standard x-rays, although provocative stress may be required to demonstrate the deformity.

The most common injuries at the radiocarpal joint are the well-known fracture–dislocations of the distal radius and carpus[475]; that is, the volar and the dorsal fracture–dislocations (Barton's), styloid fracture dislocations (Chauffeur's) (see *Distal Radial Fractures* in this chapter), and die-punch fracture–dislocations. The pure ligamentous radiocarpal injuries[56] may destabilize the wrist in one of three directions—ulnarward, ulnar translation (UT); dorsally, dorsal translation (DT); or volarly, volar translation (VT).[118,228] True dislocations without fracture of the bony margins are rare and they may sometimes spontaneously reduce, making it even more difficult to demonstrate them. However, they are occasionally seen in unreduced, dramatic fashion with the carpus dorsal to the radius, volar to the radius, or ulnar to the radius.

Ulnar translation is the most frequent radiocarpal instability. It may occur acutely, develop gradually, or be associated with perilunate dislocation residua.[447] It may occur after radiocarpal level injury, when the radiocarpal ligaments are avulsed from their styloidal origins, or after perilunate injury. Clinically the carpus and hand are offset ulnarward. The x-ray appearance is often quite dramatic, with the lunate positioned just distal to the ulna and a large space between the radial styloid and the scaphoid. If the perilunate destabilization is also involved, the lunate and triquetrum slide ulnarly, opening a gap between scaphoid and lunate. In some cases the ulnar shift is subtle, and a decrease in the ulnocarpal index (Chamay[100]) may provide the only clue to diagnosis (see Fig. 8-20). Ulnar translation is also commonly seen in diseases such as rheumatoid arthritis and in developmental deformities such as Madelung's.

Dorsal translation of the carpus and ulnar translation can be seen in two modes: one a true instability secondary to ligament damage, the other an apparent instability due to a carpal shift in response to a change in position of the distal radial articular surface. Ulnar translation may occur with an increase in the radial to ulnar slope of the distal radius.

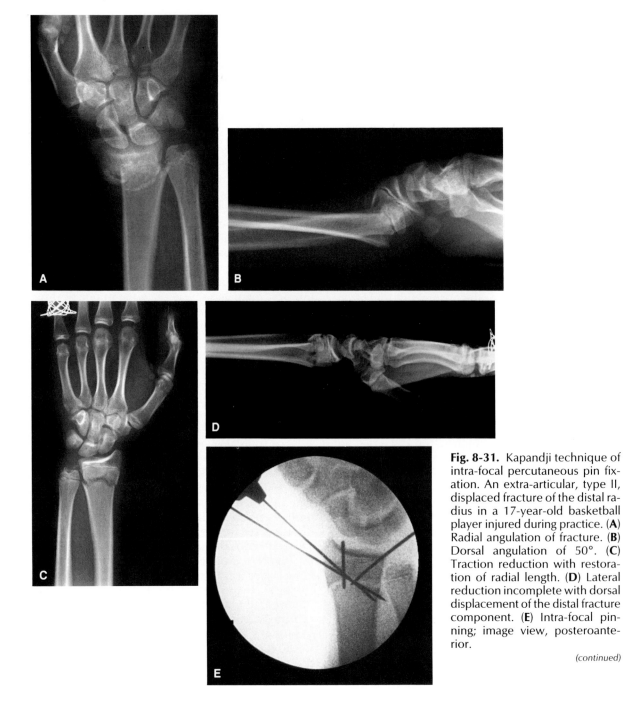

Fig. 8-31. Kapandji technique of intra-focal percutaneous pin fixation. An extra-articular, type II, displaced fracture of the distal radius in a 17-year-old basketball player injured during practice. (**A**) Radial angulation of fracture. (**B**) Dorsal angulation of 50°. (**C**) Traction reduction with restoration of radial length. (**D**) Lateral reduction incomplete with dorsal displacement of the distal fracture component. (**E**) Intra-focal pinning; image view, posteroanterior.

(continued)

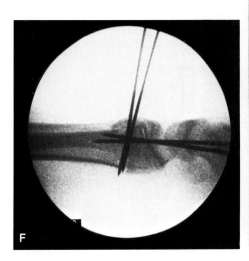
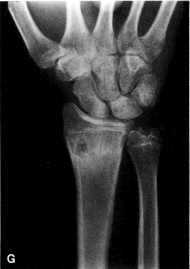
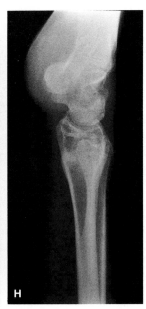

Fig. 8-31 (continued)
(**F**) Intra-focal pinning, lateral; note improved reduction from the wedging effect of the intra-focal (intra-fracture site) K-wires (0.045). (**G, H**) Healed and anatomically aligned distal radius.

Dorsal translation usually occurs following a loss of the normal volar slope of the distal radius from a flexion angle to an extension angle. The latter is a common problem after collapse of a distal radius fracture. The degree of shift of the carpus in response to the new extension slope of the distal radial surface depends to some extent upon laxity of the carpal support ligaments or injury to those ligaments, but even a normal carpus will reposition itself on the changed slope of the distal radius in such a fashion as to maintain the hand parallel to the forearm.

TREATMENT OF RADIOCARPAL INSTABILITY

Unusual dislocations of the radiocarpal joint require immediate reduction, because the deformity of such a dislocation threatens neurovascular structures in the area. While reduction is possible,[556] maintaining or holding the reduction is difficult. We believe that open treatment, both dorsal and volar, should be considered in most carpal dislocations, because residual deformity after these injuries is almost universal. In the acute situation, repair of the damaged extrinsic ligament systems both volarly and dorsally, along with temporary percutaneous wires for 6 to 8 weeks, is appropriate. We also prefer operative ligament repair for those conditions that do not initially manifest as a complete dislocation, but

are diagnosed sometime afterward by an ulnar shift of the carpus (Fig. 8-35 and 8-36). If the carpal shift is the result of the dorsal radial articular surface, the best management is complete reduction and immobilization of the distal radial fracture. One should be certain that the reduction also results in realignment of the carpus, because additional carpal ligament injury is also possible. Late cases of distal radius fracture deformity may require corrective osteotomy and bone graft to restore the position of the radial articular surface (Fig. 8-37). Late identification of ulnar translation deformity or dorsal or volar translation deformity has responded poorly to ligament repairs.[447] The most certain method of controlling possible recurrence of deformity is to carry out a partial or total radiocarpal arthrodesis. Radiolunate fusion has been our preferred technique for this situation, although the variabilities of joint surface damage may suggest radioscaphoid fusion in some cases, and radioscapholunate fusion in others.[326] The latter is usually indicated in the combinations of radiocarpal and perilunate destabilization.

Perilunate Injuries

Perilunate injuries are the most common of the carpal instability patterns.[2,114] These injuries present as pure ligament injuries (scapholunate dissociation
(*text continues on page 609*)

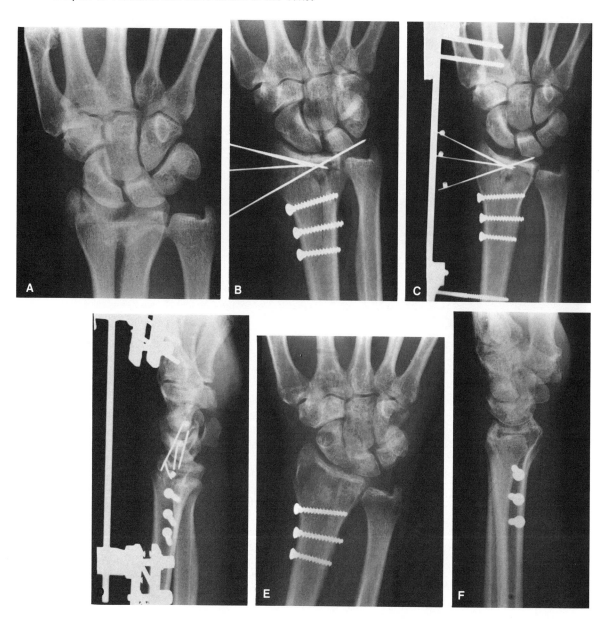

Fig. 8-32. A displaced intra-articular fracture in a 43-year-old motorcyclist was treated with open reduction and internal and external fixation. (**A**) Posteroanterior: intra-articular involvement of the scaphoid and lunate fossae with a longitudinal split component. (**B**) After open reduction, the articular fracture component was fixed with K-wires, and the shaft fracture component was transfixed with cortical bone screws. (**C, D**) An external fixation frame was used for 3 weeks to maintain distraction across the carpus and prevent compression of the articular surface of the distal radius. Motion of the radiocarpal joint was started at 6 weeks. (**E, F**) At follow-up, the articular surface reduction was maintained without evidence of radiocarpal joint abnormality.

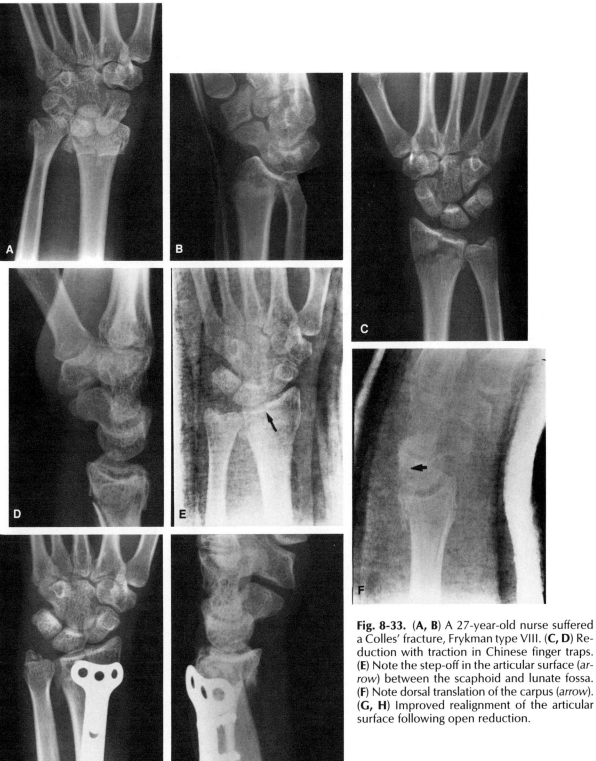

Fig. 8-33. (**A, B**) A 27-year-old nurse suffered a Colles' fracture, Frykman type VIII. (**C, D**) Reduction with traction in Chinese finger traps. (**E**) Note the step-off in the articular surface (*arrow*) between the scaphoid and lunate fossa. (**F**) Note dorsal translation of the carpus (*arrow*). (**G, H**) Improved realignment of the articular surface following open reduction.

607

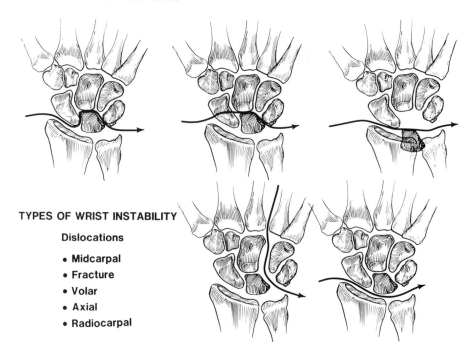

Fig. 8-34. Types of perilunate dislocations. Carpal perilunate dislocations may be purely perilunate ligamentous dislocations (*upper left*); perilunate fracture-dislocations (*upper center*); volar lunate dislocations (*upper right*); axial dislocations (*lower left*); or pure radiocarpal dislocations (*lower right*).

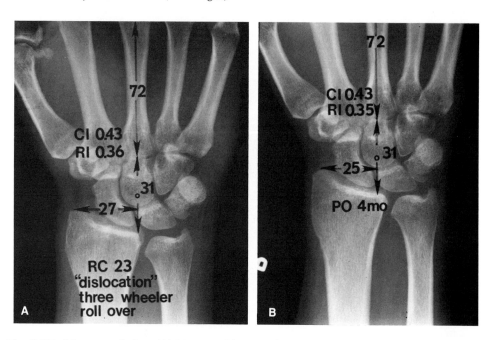

Fig. 8-35. Ulnar translation. (**A**) 23-year-old man who was injured in an all-terrain vehicle rollover. Note lunate displacement and increased radioscaphoid gap. Increased ulnar translation index (radiostyloid capitate head distance/length third metacarpal, Chamay). (**B**) Four months postop there is partial recurrence of the ulnar translation after repair of the radiolunate and radiocapitate ligaments to the radial styloid.

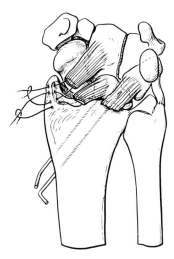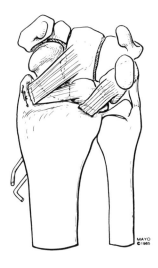

Fig. 8-36. Method of repair of the radiocarpal ligaments to the radial styloid following reduction and K-wire stabilization to the lunate (for ulnar translation).

[SLD] and lunotriquetral dissociation [LTD])[64,66]; as dislocations (perilunate through lunate dislocation spectrum)[6,21,30,55]; and as transosseous, perilunate fracture–dislocations (transcaphoid, perilunate dislocations; transradialstyloid, perilunate dislocations and transscaphoid, transcapitate, perilunate dislocations).[60,114,176] The two subluxations, SLD[338] and LTD,[449] may occur alone, as residua of perilunate dislocations or fracture–dislocations, or in conjunction with other regional injuries such as SLD with fractures of the distal radius, with Kienböck's, with scaphoid fractures, or as LTD with ulnocarpal impingement or triangular fibrocartilage complex (TFCC) tears. Such combinations modify treatment priorities. Here we will consider each entity alone, as if no associations are present.

SCAPHOLUNATE DISSOCIATION

Representing a ligament analogue of the scaphoid fracture, this injury is the most common and most significant ligament injury of the wrist. It is a spectrum of injury ranging from grade I sprains through all gradations of ligament destabilization to scaphoid dislocation.[274,328,412,460] The clinical consequences of the injury depend on the snugness or laxity of the associated and generalized capsuloligamentous system of the wrist. Developmental factors of consequence include an ulna-minus configuration of the wrist,[130] the slope of the radial articular surface, and lunotriquetral coalition. All are probable risk factors.

The mechanism of injury[118] is similar to that of the scaphoid fracture with stress loading of the extended carpus, except it is usually in ulnar (Fig. 8-38) rather than radial deviation. Prior injury, repetitive injury, or the presence of acute or chronic synovitis modify the degree of stress required to the point that the index event may be fairly trivial, such as slamming a car door or catching a basketball.

The diagnosis is made by the appropriate history, complaint localized to the scapholunate area, and physical findings of tenderness, swelling, or deformity in the scapholunate area. The degree of associated stability may be sufficient that only provocative stress[102] (see p. 603) will reveal the classic findings. An easy provocative maneuver is a vigorous grasp that induces pain; another indication is decreasing repetitive grip strength.[131] The patient may also demonstrate pain during flexion–extension or radioulnar deviation. Provocative stress is often accompanied by a click in the region of the proximal scaphoid and sometimes a visible deformity dorsally.[264] The Watson test, producing a painful dorsal protuberance of the proximal pole of the scaphoid, is highly suggestive of SLD (see *Signs and Symptoms*). As the scaphoid flexes to a more vertical orientation with radial deviation, tuberosity compression forces proximal pole subluxation dorsal to the lip of the radius. This test is not absolutely specific for SLD, because it may reposition the entire proximal carpal row if the row, rather than the individual scaphoid, is unstable.

Scapholunate dissociations may be severe enough or old enough to be fixed in malposition with scaphoid flexion and a fixed excessive space between scaphoid and lunate (see Fig. 8-21). A scapholunate gap greater than 2 mm is suspect, and a gap greater than 4 mm is confirmatory.[386] The lateral x-ray appearance of a scapholunate angle greater than 60° is suspect; greater than 80°, con-

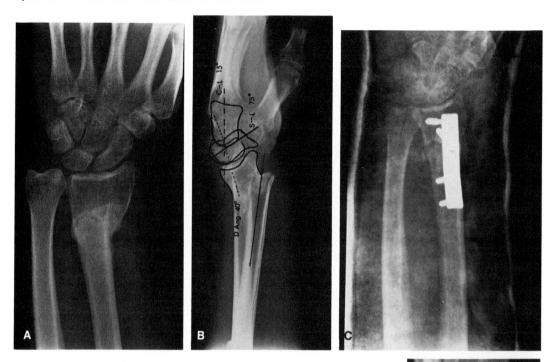

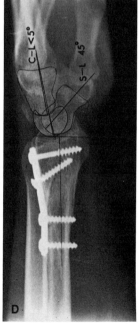

Fig. 8-37. Corrective osteotomy for malunion of the distal radius. (**A**) Shortening and radial deviation of the distal radius (posteroanterior view) and (**B**) dorsal angulation and DRUJ subluxation (lateral view) associated with wrist pain and weakness of grasp. Radiocarpal and midcarpal angulation measurements show radiocarpal (*RC*) angle of 40° from neutral and scapholunate (*SL*) angle of 75°. (**C**) Corrective osteotomy and interposition iliac crest graft restored radial length. (**D**) Lateral x-ray shows slight carpal instability. Note improvement in the radiocarpal and scapholunate angles. The patient's symptoms were significantly improved.

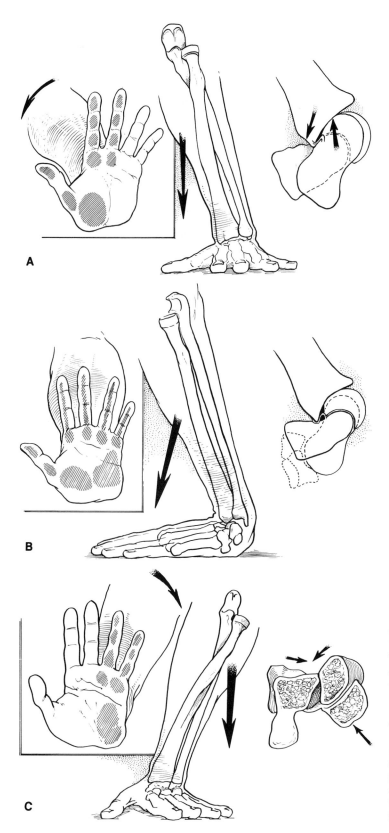

Fig. 8-38. Mechanism of perilunate ligament injuries. (**A**) Dorsiflexion, pronation, and radial deviation load across the radioscaphoid fossa. Torque continues to the ulnar side of wrist. Scaphoid fracture, lunotriquetral ligament tear, or transscaphoid perilunate dislocation may result. (**B**) Dorsiflexion in neutral stresses the midcarpal space. A capitate or lunate fracture may result, or the distal radius will fracture. (**C**) Dorsiflexion in ulnar deviation and supination loads the ulnar side of the wrist and DRUJ. Scapholunate dissociation, triquetrohamate sprain, or perilunate dislocation may result. Tensile stresses of the palmar ligaments may initiate failure at varying locations, depending on the position of the wrist at impact.

firmatory. A capitolunate or radiolunate angle greater than 15° is suspect; greater than 20°, confirmatory. If these findings are not present, the provocative maneuvers discussed above may cause them to appear. If scapholunate instability cannot be seen with grip stress x-rays (Fig. 8-39), then video fluoroscopy using standard and provocative stress motions are observed and recorded. Arthrography[132,315] is then performed to demonstrate dye flow from radiocarpal to midcarpal joint between scaphoid and lunate (Fig. 8-40). It is possible, however, to have an attenuated but still intact scapholunate membrane or a ligament flap that acts as a valve, so that a negative arthrogram does not necessarily rule out the diagnosis. A midcarpal arthrogram may be more diagnostic than a radiocarpal arthrogram, and triple injection arthrograms (radiocarpal, midcarpal, and distal radioulnar) are preferred by some.[315] Arthroscopy can be used to determine the extent of ligament disruption.[68,458]

Treatment. The treatment of scapholunate dissociation has changed significantly over the past ten years,[329] and it is best to consider different op-

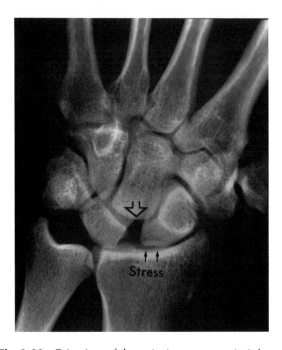

Fig. 8-39. Grip view of the wrist (posteroanterior) demonstrates scapholunate dissociation by forcing the capitate to spread and rotate the scaphoid and lunate apart. Note: (1) increased scapholunate gap, (2) foreshortened scaphoid, and (3) ring sign projection of the vertically oriented scaphoid.

tions for treatment based in part on the duration of injury.[118,119,324,423] There are different treatment plans depending on whether the injury is acute, subacute, or late carpal instability. A current list of treatment alternatives is presented followed by specific recommendations for acute, subacute, and chronic scapholunate instability. For confirmed cases of scapholunate instability, the surgeon should consider one of the following: (1) Protection only in a supportive cast or splint until the natural healing process has concluded. In an acute injury, three-point pressure on the volar scaphoid, dorsal capitate, and dorsal aspect of the distal radius can support and maintain the reduction.[153] (2) Closed reduction and percutaneous pin fixation under image control; a support cast is worn for 8 weeks followed by splint imobilization.[149] (3) Arthroscopic controlled reduction and percutaneous pin fixation. (4) Open reduction and internal ligament repair and fixation.[119,329] (5) Open reduction, ligament repair with soft tissue augmentation, with internal fixation.[61] (6) Intercarpal fusion.[296,548] (7) Proximal row carpectomy[81,277] or wrist fusion.[240,408]

Twenty years ago, reconstruction of the scapholunate ligament was recommended by a technique of tendon graft woven through the scaphoid, lunate, and the volar lip of the distal radius.[153,328,329,423] Although clinical results were often satisfactory (about 75% good or excellent),[225] radiographic correlation was less evident, and these procedures were very difficult to perform.[423] Ligament repair was superceded in many instances by fusion of the distal scaphoid to the trapezium or capitate.[294,295,296] These techniques address only one part of the problem, the unstable scaphoid, and ignore the instability present in the rest of the carpus (ie, lunate and capitate). Difficulty in obtaining congruency of the proximal radioscaphoid articulation[62] at surgery, a significant incidence of nonunion, and late degenerative changes have been noted. The long-term efficacy of intercarpal fusion[294] is now under increasing scrutiny, and the current trend is to look for more reliable ligament and soft tissue repairs for scapholunate dissociation[227,514] presenting early. The controversy between repair and intercarpal fusions will not be resolved soon, but the latter are indicated for late or chronic instability.[550] In the methods of treatment to follow, new concepts in repair or reconstruction of these ligaments will be presented, as well as a review of current techniques for limited intercarpal fusions.

Acute and Subacute Scapholunate Dissociation. Kinematic restoration of the scapholunate complex by ligament repair is a realistic goal when the pa-

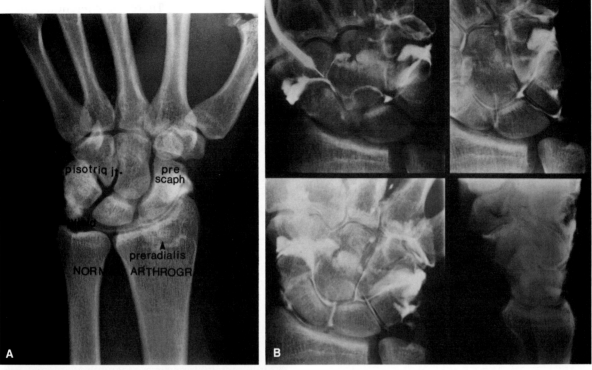

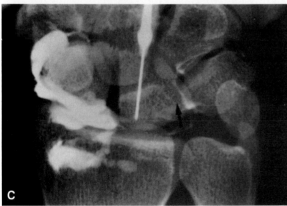

Fig. 8-40. Wrist arthrography. (**A**) Normal radiocarpal arthrogram. Recesses of the prescaphoid, preradialis, prestyloid (ulnar), and pisotriquetral joints have filled. (**B**) Midcarpal arthrogram (serial x-rays) shows gradual presence of dye in the scapholunate and lunotriquetral intervals (**top right**), suggesting a lunotriquetral ligament tear. The radiocarpal joint (**left bottom**) fills, confirming an interosseous ligament tear. (**C**) Abnormal radiocarpal arthrogram with contrast across the lunotriquetral interval (*arrow*).

tient presents early.[149,227] Rapid confirmation of the diagnosis by clinical examination, x-ray studies, arthrography, or magnetic resonance imaging (MRI) is imperative. Arthroscopy of the wrist[68] can assist in confirming the diagnosis and determining the extent of ligamentous damage. The patient who has a mild partial ligament tear may be treated more conservatively than those with significant carpal instability. The patient less than 4 weeks from injury is considered to have an acute tear; if more than 4 but less than 24 weeks, it is a subacute tear. If the time is greater than 6 months from injury,

the tear is chronic and may be reducible or irreducible. Depending on the mechanism of injury and amount of force across the wrist, the scapholunate ligament may be accompanied by injuries to the volar radiocarpal and lunotriquetral ligament or the triangular fibrocartilage.

We believe that ligament repair should be considered in all acute scapholunate injuries, unless the carpus is easily reduced anatomically by closed techniques and remains reduced in sequential x-rays without carpal malalignment by the criteria mentioned above. An increasing scapholunate angle exceeding 60°, a lunocapitate angle exceeding 15°, or an increasing scapholunate gap greater than 3 mm is an indication for operative intervention. There are a number of different reconstruction alternatives, but the most common and direct will be presented.

ACUTE LIGAMENT TEAR—REPAIR TECHNIQUE. The principles for ligament repair (Fig. 8-41) are similar for acute and subacute injuries. The type of repair depends on the quality of the local tissues. Usually, there is sufficient local tissue to perform a direct repair for acute and subacute injuries. The usual technique involves the following: (1) A dorsal incision is centered over Lister's tubercle, reflecting the dorsal wrist capsule in line with the skin incision. The radial capsule is reflected from the scaphoid to its waist. (2) Reduction of the lunate and scaphoid are performed with K-wire "joysticks" inserted in a dorsal to palmar direction. (3) The rim of the scaphoid is freshened to subcortical bone with a small, high-speed burr. (4) When the ligament is attached to the lunate (the usual case), holes are drilled from the waist of the scaphoid in a proximal and medial direction to exit at the scapholunate articulation. (5) Nonabsorbable sutures (2-0 or 3-0 mersilene) are placed in the scapholunate ligament, volar to dorsal. The suture is pulled back through the scaphoid with a second suture on a straight needle. (6) When the sutures for repair are in place, the scaphoid and lunate are reduced with joysticks held in the reduced or slightly overreduced position with pins across the scapholunate and, if needed, radiolunate articulations. (7) The sutures are tied and the capsule repaired. (8) One of us (JHD) reinforces this repair with the radioscaphoid tether (see next section) and a lunate–third metacarpal base tether to restrict DISI malposition.

SUBACUTE LIGAMENT TEAR—REPAIR TECHNIQUE. For subacute scapholunate ligament tears, the addition of local tissue (alone or additionally) may be necessary if the scapholunate ligament has retracted or is deficient. A proximally based dorsal capsule flap[61] (Blatt type) is reflected onto the scapholunate interspace and sutured tautly to the dorsal scaphoid to act as a tether to the proximal pole (Fig. 8-42). Using the techniques described above, it is possible to add this flap to the ligament repair process by placing nonabsorbable sutures from the lunate ligament remnant into the capsular tissue and then out through the scaphoid. A strip of tendon from the radial wrist extensors (ECRL or ECRB) may be substituted, but tendon tissue is not an ideal ligament replacement, and capsular tissue may be preferred.

In both subacute and severe acute scapholunate tears, volar extrinsic ligament attenuation may be found. Use of the arthroscope preoperatively helps to identify these conditions and plan appropriate incisions. A volar approach with direct ligament repair by nonabsorbable sutures can be performed. If there is deficient tissue in the subacute case, part of the flexor carpi radialis can be used to augment the repair process. The radioscaphocapitate (RSC) and radiolunate (RL) ligaments may be advanced into the gap as well. With a large, complete scapholunate ligament tear, a wide scapholunate gap of 5 mm or more, volar ligament repair is usually needed (Fig. 8-43). A carpal tunnel incision extended slightly radially is performed, and the damaged area is identified with a probe inserted from a separate dorsal incision. The interval between the RSC ligament and RL ligament is developed. Sutures may be then placed through the scaphoid proximal pole or remnants of the interosseous membrane, which are then used to pull the radiolunate ligament against the proximal pole to hold the overreduction, which is stabilized by K-wires.

Whether the approach is dorsal or volar or combined, tight repair of the capsular structures is required for acute or subacute dissociation. Internal fixation for a minimal period of 8 weeks is preferred, supplemented with a supportive thumb spica cast. Following cast removal, an orthoplast splint is worn as muscle strength and joint motion are

---

Fig. 8-41. Ligament repair for scapholunate dissociation. (**A**) The scapholunate interosseous membrane (SLIOM) is retained on the lunate. K-wires are introduced into the scaphoid and lunate as toggle arms ("joy sticks"). Both bones are decorticated to the SLIOM attachment. (**B**) Drill holes are made from the proximal scaphoid to the lateral scaphoid sulcus distally (Taleisnik technique). (**C**) Sutures are passed through the SLIOM and are retrieved internally with retrograde straight needles or looped wires. (**D**) Reduction of the lunate by flexion and the scaphoid by extension using toggle wires. (**E**) The sutures are tied after pulling the remnant of the SLIOM tautly against the scaphoid rim. (**F**) SLURPIE procedure. Volar approach with decortication of the contiguous surfaces of the scaphoid and lunate. Fixation is with threaded K-wires after reduction, and the volar ligaments are repaired.

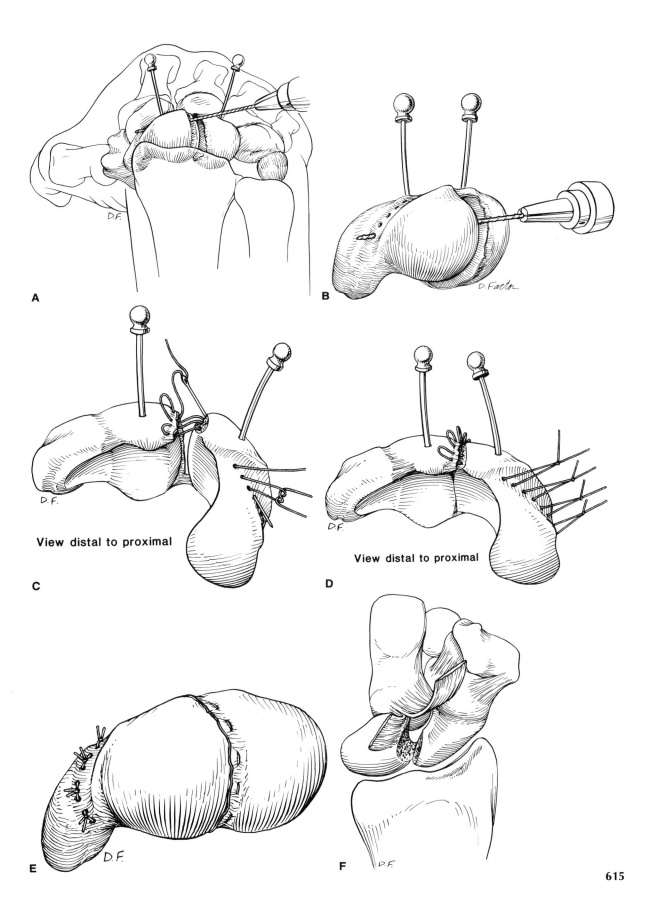

A

B

C

View distal to proximal

D

View distal to proximal

E

F

615

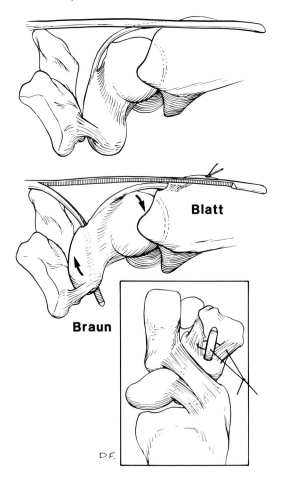

Fig. 8-42. (Top) The scaphoid is flexed and subluxated at the STT joint. **(Middle)** Dorsal capsulodesis as described by Blatt. **(Bottom)** Palmar capsulodesis with a slip of ECRB passed through the scaphoid (Braun).

restored. Return to work or athletic competition is best delayed for a minimum of 6 months, with continued protection during athletic competition.

Chronic Scapholunate Instability—Repair Technique. In cases that present more than 6 months from the time of injury, alternatives for treatment are based on the ability to reduce the carpal instability, the stress demands on the patient's wrist, and the absence of degenerative changes within the carpus. When feasible, restoration of normal carpal anatomy by repair and reconstruction of the support ligaments of the wrist remain the preferred treatment. This requires sufficient local tissue for repair and a correctable carpal instability. When the patient presents with a fixed carpal deformity, local degenerative changes, or work demands that re-

quire heavy lifting or repetitive stress loading, the alternative of partial or complete fusion of the wrist may be preferred.[294,295,296,546,550]

Current techniques for ligament reconstruction include the dorsal capsular flap procedure,[61] a volar ligament reefing procedure,[111] and combined dorsal and volar procedures that add flexor or extensor tendon tissue to the repair site (see Fig. 8-43). The goal of each of these repair techniques involves the addition of local tissue to provide a collagen framework for future stability. Our preferred approach is to start with a dorsal midline incision with access to the wrist between the extensor pollicis longus and the radial wrist extensors laterally and the extensor digitorum communis medially. Because capsular flaps are needed for the reconstruction, they should be anticipated and created during the exposure. For the Blatt type of capsule reconstruction,[61] a long, rectangular flap is made, about 1.5 cm wide, based on the dorsal aspect of the distal radius. For a distal-based flap, one can release the dorsal scaphotriquetral ligament (dorsal intercarpal ligament) from the triquetrum, leaving it attached to the scaphoid rim distally (see Fig. 8-41). The triquetral insertion is brought proximally and sutured to the distal radius. Some surgeons prefer to use part of the extensor carpi radialis brevis left attached distally to be reflected proximally into the scapholunate interval, where it is interwoven into the repair. In the Blatt procedure, the dorsal flap of wrist capsule is sutured in tension distal to the scaphoid center of rotation, so that it tethers the proximal pole in the scaphoid fossa. The flap is sutured to reinforce the local tissue of the scapholunate interval.

Wrist extensor or flexor tendon augmentation procedures require placement of drill holes in bone. This requires precision and technical skill from the surgeon. In this procedure, drill holes are carefully placed in a dorsal-to-volar direction through the scaphoid, and enlarged with an awl (see Fig. 8-43). Part of an extensor or flexor tendon is pulled through a drill hole, after passing to or through the radiolunotriquetral ligament, and then pulled dorsally through the scapholunate interval, where it augments the local ligament repair. A combined dorsal–volar approach is needed to perform this procedure effectively. There is increased risk from placing holes in bone, but it provides a strong static control of the scaphoid as well as the adding local tissue for ligament repair.

The volar approach for scapholunate ligament repair (Conyers technique)[111] is performed through the carpal tunnel incision. A probe or needle passed

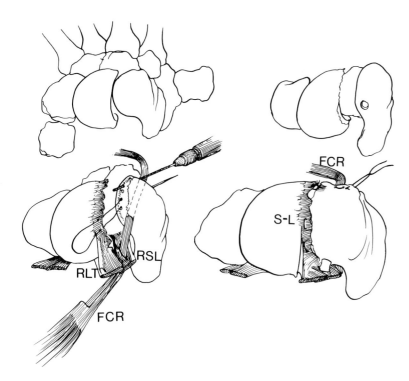

Fig. 8-43. Augmentation of scapholunate ligament repair is demonstrated using half of the flexor carpi radialis (*FCR*) tendon. The scapholunate ligament repair is similar to techniques described in Figure 8-40, with drill holes placed through the scaphoid to the lunate ligament remnant. The dorsal scapholunate ligament is repaired and augmented with a portion of the tendon graft. Radiolunotriquetral (*RLT*), scapholunate ligament (*S-L*), radioscapholunate (*RSL*).

dorsal to volar is helpful in locating the ligament tear. Flaps of radioscaphocapitate and radiolunate ligaments are reflected laterally and medially. The cartilage surfaces that are contiguous to scaphoid and lunate are denuded to subchondral bone to encourage a strong syndesmosis. The scaphoid and lunate are then reduced and pinned with threaded wires that are left in place 8 weeks or more. The volar ligaments are snugly repaired. Motion is delayed 10 to 12 weeks to encourage adequate strength of the syndesmosis.

To correct the malalignment of the carpus, we recommend the following steps in each of these techniques. (1) It is necessary to reduce and pin the lunate to the distal radius or to the distal carpal row to correct lunate dorsal angulation. (2) The scaphoid is reduced to the lunate and the scapholunate interval is pinned. Overreduction of the lunate and scaphoid is preferable. (3) Supplemental fixation of the scaphoid to the capitate or trapezium may be considered. The greater the difficulty in obtaining the reduction or holding the reduction, the more critical strong internal fixation is and the more likely it is that the soft tissue repair will not be successful. For reduction of the scaphoid and lunate, the use of K-wire joysticks is quite helpful. Manual assistance by direct pressure volarly over the tuberosity of the distal (vertical) scaphoid along with

downward pressure on the capitate may be needed. Lateral and posteroanterior x-rays are necessary to confirm that the reduction or overreduction has been obtained prior to final capsule closer.

Following scapholunate ligament reconstruction, immobilization in a thumb spica cast is recommended for 8 to 10 weeks. Splint immobilization for an additional 4 weeks is suggested to allow for collagen tissue healing with gradual stress loading. Supporting splints are best worn intermittently for 6 months to prevent sudden stress to the wrist and allow further collagen maturation.

Scaphotrapeziotrapezoidal (STT) Fusion. The decision regarding intercarpal fusion for scapholunate dissociation is based on the length of time from the original injury, work and strength expectations of the patient, and the ability to reduce and maintain the carpal instability.[435] In addition, findings of radiocarpal and midcarpal arthritis should influence the decision toward intercarpal fusion.[547] Of the partial wrist fusions currently performed for wrist instability, the STT (triscaphe) fusion has had the widest clinical application (Fig. 8-44).[128,159,296,546,548] As described by Watson, the purpose of this procedure is to stabilize the distal scaphoid and thereby hold the proximal pole more securely within the scaphoid fossa of the distal radius. This operation can be performed through a transverse incision

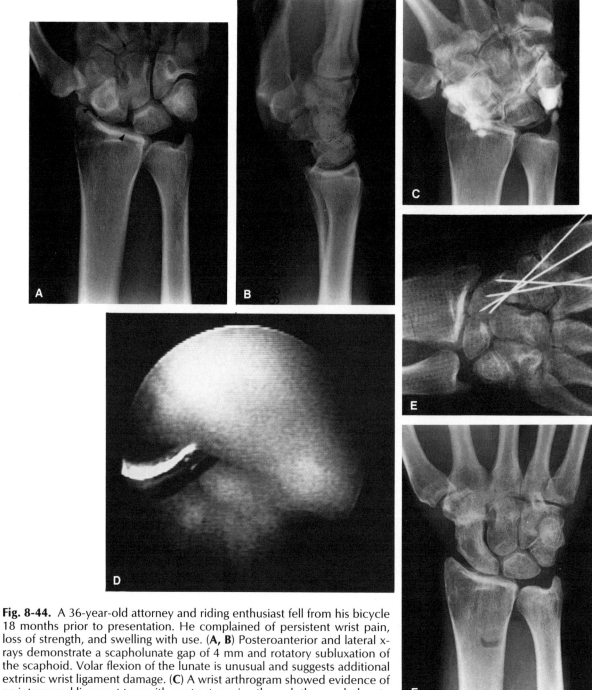

Fig. 8-44. A 36-year-old attorney and riding enthusiast fell from his bicycle 18 months prior to presentation. He complained of persistent wrist pain, loss of strength, and swelling with use. (**A, B**) Posteroanterior and lateral x-rays demonstrate a scapholunate gap of 4 mm and rotatory subluxation of the scaphoid. Volar flexion of the lunate is unusual and suggests additional extrinsic wrist ligament damage. (**C**) A wrist arthrogram showed evidence of an intercarpal ligament tear with contrast passing through the scapholunate interval. (**D**) Arthroscopy was performed to confirm the suspected pathology and to determine the degree of instability. Gross instability between the scaphoid and lunate was noted. (**E**) Fusion of the scaphotrapeziotrapezoidal (STT) joint was performed with a distal radius bone graft and crossed K-wires. (**F**) At 2 years, the fusion was solid with no evidence of radioscaphoid impingement.

(continued)

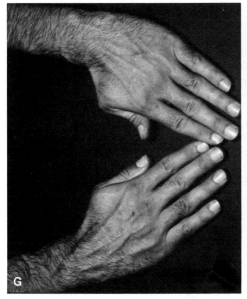

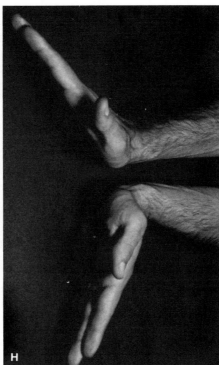

Fig. 8-44 *(continued)*
(G, H) Wrist range of motion after successful
STT fusion.

centered over the STT joint or with the universal longitudinal incision.[159] Arthroscopic examination of both midcarpal and radiocarpal joints may determine the extent of scapholunate ligament and articular cartilage damage, aiding in the choice of preferred treatment.

With either STT fusion[294,295] or the equivalent scaphocapitate (SC) fusion,[208,366] an important component of the procedure is to reduce the vertical scaphoid, close the scapholunate interval, and maintain carpal height.[366,456] Radiographic control is recommended. The ideal flexion angle of the scaphoid is 45°. Fixation of the STT or SC joints is performed with K-wires, screws, or staples. A bone graft from the distal radius or iliac crest is placed between the decorticated distal scaphoid and proximal surface of the trapezium and trapezoid (STT fusion), or between the medial articular surface of the scaphoid and the lateral surface of the capitate (SC fusion). It is essential to realign the scaphoid, correcting its vertical inclination, and to restore carpal height.[546]

Immobilization for intercarpal fusion is usually 8 weeks in a thumb spica cast, followed by a support splint for 4 to 6 weeks. Tomography of the wrist can help determine the degree of consolidation at the fusion site. In our experience, 6 weeks may be too short a time to allow for unprotected wrist motion following an intercarpal fusion. Radiocarpal impingement[197,294] as a complication of STT fusion has led to the recommendation that a concomitant radiostyloidectomy be included.[455]

Authors' Preferred Treatment. We consider localized fusion to be preferable in certain conditions. One of these is the fixed deformity that is difficult to reduce and tends to re-deform unless strong reduction force is maintained. Some carpal deformities are irreducible without extensive soft tissue release, which may cause damage to circulation and joint surfaces; these are better treated with some salvage procedure. This intermediate group between the reducible and salvage groups are probably better treated with intercarpal fusion, eg, STT or SC. Where there is STT joint damage as well as scapholunate dissociation,[243] STT fusion with the scaphoid properly reduced is preferable. In the special situation of scapholunate dissociation and Kienböck's disease, either STT or SC fusion are preferable, plus whatever direct intervention may be desired for the lunate.

Scapholunate dissociation and triquetrolunate

dissociation may be present together. The scapholunate dissociation is usually the most unstable of the two; control of both may be indicated. Joint surface damage of the proximal scaphoid may require other types of localized fusion, such as radioscaphoid or capitolunate fusion, the former retaining and the latter discarding the scaphoid.

There may be an associated instability of the proximal carpal row as well as the dissociative instability between scaphoid and lunate. The ligament–tether augmentations described subsequently will often control such instability. If the tendency for either severe DISI or VISI is marked and it is thought that soft tissue restraint will not control it, a localized fusion may be preferable. If the instability seems to be primarily at the radiocarpal level, radiolunate or radioscapholunate fusion is preferable; if it is primarily at the midcarpal level, scaphocapitate or scapholunocapitate fusion should be satisfactory.

LUNOTRIQUETRAL DISSOCIATION

Lunotriquetral dissociation (LTD) involves a partial or complete tear of interosseous ligaments between the lunate and triquetrum.[449,538] It may present as an isolated injury, as part of the spectrum of perilunate dislocation, or in association with ulnocarpal impingement and triangular fibrocartilage injuries.[350,449] The pathomechanics of lunotriquetral injury that accompany perilunate dislocation are well known,[355,540] but the mechanism of isolated injury requires further study.[530] Because the lunotriquetral joint is more stable than the scapholunate joint, it seems apparent that associated ligament damage, particularly to the dorsal RLTL, must be present before severe, fixed deformities can occur. Diagnosis of lunotriquetral instability involves a history of specific injury with residua of pain and weakness. Tenderness is present dorsally over the lunotriquetral joint, and ballottement of the unstable triquetrum may be possible.[449]

Radiographic diagnosis is more difficult than the diagnosis of SLD because the subtle findings are less pronounced and provocative, stress-induced deformity is less frequent. Subtle angle changes may be demonstrated with special imaging of the wrists,[223] but usually wrist arthrography and/or arthroscopy is needed to demonstrate the loss of membrane continuity between lunate and triquetrum with direct communication between the radiocarpal and midcarpal joints. Fixed deformities are usually VISI,[465,530] because there is dissociation between lunate and triquetrum, and the usual pattern is for the lunate to follow the scaphoid into flexion while the triquetrum extends by sliding distally and volarly on the hamate. Recent studies[538] demonstrate that a tear of the volar lunotriquetral (ulnar portion of volar radiolunotriquetral) and dorsal radiotriquetral ligament are necessary in addition to lunotriquetral ligament tear for the VISI deformity to develop. Isolated interosseous lunotriquetral ligament tears usually will not produce a VISI collapse deformity, unless there is secondary extrinsic carpal ligament attenuation or injury. Lunotriquetral ligament defects are common with ulnocarpal impingement, but these seldom lead to collapse deformities.

Treatment. An acute lunotriquetral dissociation with minimal deformity is ideally treated with a support cast, adding closed reduction and internal fixation of lunate to triquetrum if there is displacement.

A special splint that supports the lunotriquetral joint by maintaining mild, support pressure underneath the pisiform, over the dorsal aspect of the distal ulna, and under the tuberosity of the distal scaphoid with the wrist in extension and ulnar deviation helps to reduce the dissociating stresses.

Lunotriquetral dissociation with angular deformity (Fig. 8-45) or with unsatisfactory results from previous treatment may need open treatment, particularly in the subacute or acute phase. Manual reduction, repair of lax or damaged ligaments, and temporary internal fixation with percutaneous wires across the triquetrum and lunate left in place for 6 to 8 weeks should suffice. The more severely deformed LTDs involve not only a tear of the lunotriquetral interosseous membrane but attenuation of associated extrinsic ligaments. All ligaments that seem to be concerned with lunotriquetral stability should be tightened as necessary, although this is by no means easy to accomplish. The interosseous membrane repair is usually done in a fashion similar to that described for the scapholunate repair, through a dorsal approach in the floor of the fifth dorsal compartment (Fig. 8-46). The ligament is more likely to be stripped from the triquetrum. Capsular flaps are useful for reinforcing the dorsal portion of such a repair or augmenting the dorsal radiotriquetral and dorsal scaphotriquetral ligament system.

If it appears that soft tissue repairs cannot control the tendency to recurrent deformity, lunotriquetral fusion may be indicated. Repair of the dorsal radiotriquetral ligament should also be performed so that a CID-type VISI deformity is not converted to CIND-type VISI following fusion. In most cases, we

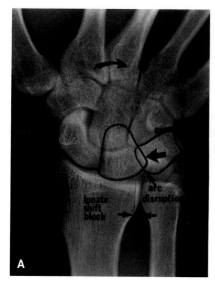

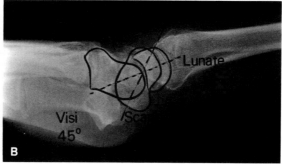

Fig. 8-45. Lunotriquetral dissociation. (**A**) The posteroanterior view demonstrates irregularity of the lunotriquetral arc and a triangular appearance of the lunate. (**B**) The lunate together with the scaphoid is flexed relative to the dissociated triquetrum. *(Reagan, D. S.; Linscheid, R. L.; Dobyns, J. H.: Lunotriquetral Sprains. J. Hand Surg. [Am.], 9(4):502–514, 1984.)*

prefer ligament augmentation procedures that provide satisfactory stabilization; these are preferred over lunotriquetral, radiolunate, or radiolunotriquetral fusion.[528] Lunotriquetral arthrodeses are less reliable than one might think. Nonunions, persistent VISI collapse, symptomatic displacements with RUD, and persistent weakness occur in approximately 35% of patients. Alignment should be accomplished with image intensification at surgery.

PERILUNATE DISLOCATIONS
AND FRACTURE DISLOCATIONS

The common mechanism of perilunate injuries involves a tension disruption of the volar capsuloligamentous apparatus of the wrist, beginning radially and propagating around or through the lunate to the ulnar side of the carpus.[232,355,356,412,414,539,540] A similar pattern begins ulnarward and propagates radially but is not as well documented experimentally. Scapholunate dissociation and lunotriquetral dissociation often remain as residual problems, even after relocation of the perilunate injury. Recurrent collapse tendencies are common whether the injury is the "lesser arc" injury through ligamentous tissue or the "greater arc" injury through bone, or some combination of the two (see Fig. 8-15).[272,356,374] The most common is the transscaphoid perilunate dislocation,[31,114] sometimes given the eponym de Quervain's injury.[143]

Signs and Symptoms. Diagnosis is established by history of a hyperextension injury, and persistent pain, swelling, and deformity.[533] These higher energy injuries produce greater deformity and soft tissue damage. The most common clinical association is median nerve injury, but ulnar neuropathy, arterial injury, and tendon damage may also be seen.[504] The pattern of skeletal deformity is variable.[232,398] The hand and distal carpal row usually remain intact, but the disruption pattern between distal and proximal carpal rows is quite variable.[464] The distal scaphoid dislocates with the distal row, leaving the proximal scaphoid and lunate in near-normal relationship to the forearm. Typically the lunate remains bonded to some degree with the radius and the remainder of the carpus dislocates, usually dorsally, but it may rebound to a volar position.[112] In some instances, the initial dislocation of the majority of the carpus may be volar.[6,228] In the usual situation, the dorsally displaced carpus rebounds to come to rest upon the dorsum of the lunate (see Fig. 8-13).[233,218,367] If the dorsal lunate attachments have been disrupted, the lunate will displace and rotate around its intact volar ligament hinge to present in the carpal tunnel or soft tissues of the forearm.[55] Occasionally, even the volar attachment of lunate is torn, allowing extrusion into the forearm or through the skin.

Radiographic Examination. Diagnosis can be made without x-rays, but the specifics of damage to soft tissue and bone are better appreciated with improved imaging techniques. The basic pattern can be discerned on standard posteroanterior and lateral x-rays, but details of instability, fracture, and fragmentation are much better appreciated with

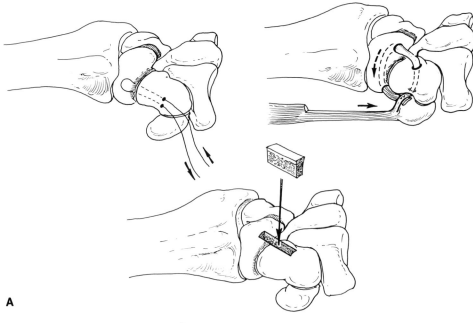

A

Fig. 8-46. Lunotriquetral dissociation. (**A**) Treatment options include direct ligament repair (**top left**), augmentation of repair with half of the flexor carpi ulnaris (**top right**), and lunotriquetral fusion (**bottom**). (**B**) Schematic diagram of the technique to repair the lunotriquetral ligament involves drill holes placed across the waist of the triquetrum into the lunotriquetral interval with a nonabsorbable suture of the lunate remnant. The repair is protected with K-wire fixation for 6 weeks.

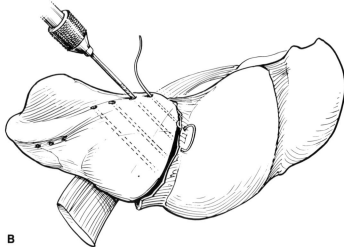

B

traction views obtained with 5 to 10 pounds of finger-trap traction. Approximately 20% of these dislocations are misinterpreted on the initial x-rays. Additional studies of particular value include polytomography, computed tomography, and MRI. Arthrography and arthroscopy may have a useful role in determining the details of injury, if open reduction of the fracture–dislocation is questioned.

Treatment. Acute injuries may be divided into two groups: those which spontaneously reduce or are easily reduced by closed reduction methods, and those that are either open, irreducible, or unstable, once reduced.[2,267] Many of those from the first group will become unstable, rapidly making such distinction hazardous. Nevertheless, there are some spontaneous reductions that are so stable that it is difficult to determine whether a full, perilunate-type dislocation took place; and there are others, which reduce and can be maintained in near-normal alignment in casts and splints. There is no justification for saying that all perilunate injuries require open reduction, although open assessment almost always discloses more damage than anticipated.[114,232] Those injuries that reduce to normal alignment require monitoring on a daily basis for the first week, and on a weekly basis thereafter. These may compare favorably with open treatment on a long-term basis.

The majority of perilunate injuries fall into the open, irreducible, or unstable group, often with neurovascular problems.[112,114,233,414] This group is best treated by open investigation and repair.[2,114,374,387] If there is a neurovascular problem known, a volar approach allows access. Combined with a dorsal approach, this allows both intra-articular and extra-articular damage to be assessed and treated adequately. The surgical access planes are similar to those for treatment of scapholunate and triquetrolunate dissociation, except that it is necessary to release the carpal tunnel.[233] The tearing produced by the injury usually allows sufficient access to damaged areas, but additional incisions may be necessary. The volar capsule may be opened, either along its attachments to the radial rim or through the often torn space of Poirier; the dorsal capsule is usually opened along its origins from the dorsal radial rim, as well as longitudinally in the space between the second and fourth extensor compartments.

For discussion purposes, the perilunate-type injuries will be divided into acute (less than) and chronic (more than) 3 months old. Acute injury will be further subdivided into those that are easily reducible and those open, irreducible, and unstable varieties. The chronic injuries are divided into those

previously untreated and those where previous treatment has failed. Severity of injury must be assessed for both the bone and soft tissues carefully.

Acute (Reduced or Reducible) Perilunate Injury. Some injuries are seen that have probably been dislocated but appear reduced at initial assessment. Ways of confirming this suspicion include stress-test imaging, arthroscopy, and open exploration. Some dislocations reduce with traction or manipulation to a near-normal alignment. Controversy exists as to whether all such injuries should be explored, repaired, and internally fixed, even though some perilunate injuries heal satisfactorily and remain stable with closed management.[114,387,414] Open treatment does not guarantee stability, a good result, or avoidance of complications. Some can be treated by closed methods if patient compliance and management are excellent. Loss of reduction with cast loosening is common. Cast changes with careful maintenance maneuvers may be required during the first 3 to 4 weeks. The basic maintenance maneuver used from the outset is a three-point support system, including pads under the volar aspect of the scaphoid tuberosity and pisiform, plus dorsal pads over the neck of the capitate and over the proximal pole of the scaphoid. The pad under the tuberosity helps to lift and elongate the scaphoid, while the dorsal pad helps control the proximal scaphoid. The pisiform pad transmits a support to the triquetrum, diminishing its tendency to extend (Fig. 8-47). The dorsal pad over the capitate neck depresses the distal row on the proximal row, which

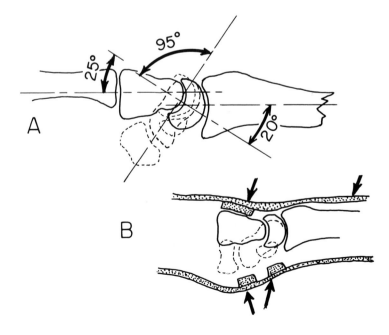

Fig. 8-47. Closed reduction of carpal instability following fracture–dislocations of the wrist can be achieved by three-point fixation. (**A**) Dorsal instability pattern: capitolunate angle 25°, scapholunate angle 95°, radiolunate angle 20°. (**B**) Reduction by pressure applied dorsally over the capitate and distal radius and volarly over the distal pole of the scaphoid and the pisiform.

derotates the extension of the proximal carpal row. There are those who believe that these tendencies are so difficult to maintain that percutaneous fixation is preferable to external support only. The stability characteristics of the specific wrist reveal themselves by the difficulty noted in maintaining reduction with external support only. If reduction is too difficult to either achieve or hold, that be-

comes the indication for open reduction and repair. The success of this method requires adequate imaging with good, standardized posteroanterior and lateral views of the wrist or special imaging techniques.

Acute (Irreducible or Unstable) Perilunate Injury. If the above treatment is unsuccessful or the injury is open, irreducible, unstable, or compromised

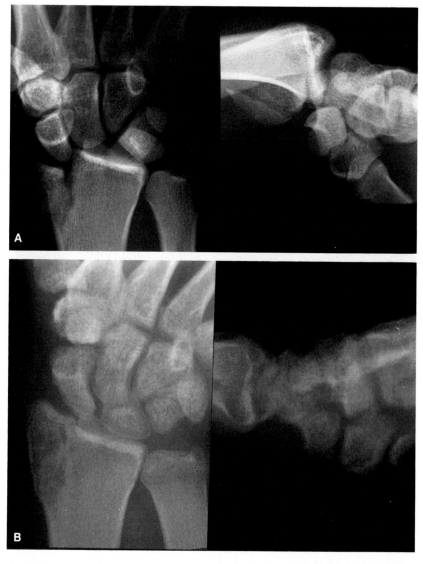

Fig. 8-48. Transradiostyloid perilunate dislocation. (**A**) Proximally displaced radial styloid and scaphoid associated with perilunate dislocation. The lunate is rotated 160° and volarly dislocated. (**B**) Six weeks following closed reduction and percutaneous pinning there is an increased radioscaphoid gap but reasonably good alignment of the carpus.

(continued)

neurovascularly, open reduction, repair, and external or internal fixation are indicated.[174,180,233] There is value in both volar and dorsal approaches. It is easier to examine the cartilage surfaces and intra-articular fragments through the dorsal approach. It is easier to observe and repair volar ligamentous damage through the volar approach, and a volar approach is essential if neurovascular or flexor-tendons are to be assessed. Transscaphoid fractures are often approached from the volar aspect if internal fixation is desired. However, the use of a volar approach only to place a Herbert screw or similar device, ignoring the other widespread requirements of this extensive injury, is inappropriate. It is more important to assess all elements of the injury, restore normal configuration of bony elements, and repair soft tissue damage than to be concerned with the type of fixation device. K-wires that can be inserted swiftly and repetitively are quite adequate for stabilization.

Special Problems.   The two types of perilunate dislocation and fracture–dislocation are the lesser arc or transligamentous injury and the greater arc or transosseous pattern (see Fig. 8-15). Within these major patterns there are many variant patterns.[220] For instance, the scaphoid and lunate may remain partly or totally bonded by ligamentous connections,[21,109,420] and the remainder of the carpus may disrupt around these two bones. In transosseous perilunate fracture–dislocations, a wide spectrum of fracture types is seen, such as transradial styloid, transscaphoid, transcapitate, and transtriquetral in various combinations (Fig. 8-48).[22] Probably the most common distortions are those of the proximal

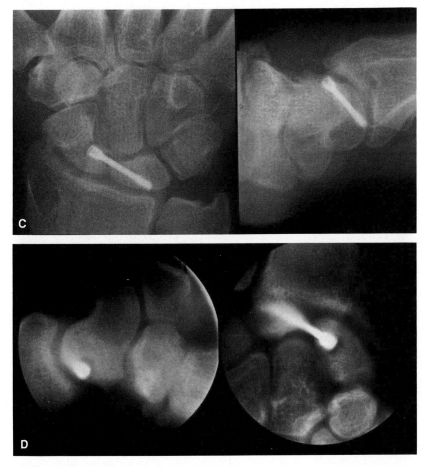

Fig. 8-48 *(continued)*
(C) Eighteen months following attempted scapholunate arthrodesis, with increased scapholunate angle (85°). **(D)** Trispiral tomograms show loosening about the Herbert screw.

capitate and the proximal scaphoid fragment.[348] The capitate fragment is frequently turned 180°, so that its articular surface faces the raw cancellous surface of the major capitate fragment.[348,385,410,503,533] Both capitate and scaphoid fragments (Fig. 8-49) are devascularized by displacement. Any such bony fragment displacement is best anatomically reduced and fixed. Healing is surprisingly good, and restoration of bony architecture is the norm. Autogenous bone graft to restore scaphoid length may be required. Restoration of bony architecture, joint congruency, alignment, and capsular attenuation is probably sufficient in the majority of acute cases of perilunate disruption.

Soft tissue damage is quite common in these high-energy lesions, and it may be obvious that a severe neuropathy or vascular deficiency is present. When these are present, open treatment and evaluation of the structures at risk is essential. Treatment of vascular and nerve injuries should proceed once the fractures are stabilized. Median or ulnar neuropathy, if severe or increasing, is an indication for surgical exploration.

Chronic, Perilunate-Type Injuries. Untreated injuries of this type may be seen months or years after the initial injury.[152,489] The patient is more likely to present because of increasing nerve symptoms or tendon rupture than because of wrist deformity, to which the patient has often become accustomed.

These problems nearly always require some type of salvage operation and will not be discussed further. However, those seen within the first year are still potentially treatable by open reduction, although this will be more difficult because of articular changes and capsular contracture (Fig. 8-50).[489] A good clue to the potential for reduction is distraction of the carpal elements on x-rays obtained with 25 to 30 pounds of traction. An attempt at reduction, repair, and internal fixation should be offered, because even in late cases results can be surprisingly good. Extensive dissection may be required.[218]

Another group of chronic, perilunate-type injuries includes those where prior treatment has not been completely successful. When a bone or bone fragment has been removed, eg, proximal scaphoid or capitate fragment, the alternatives are to rehabilitate the limb and assess the functional level or to consider a salvage procedure such as radiocarpal fusion[147,240] or proximal row carpectomy.[21,126,185,262,408]

MIDCARPAL INSTABILITIES

The difficulties of diagnosing carpal instability of the nondissociative type (CIND) have already been discussed with regard to the radiocarpal instabilities (see Table 8-1).[154,473] The history and the physical findings differ little between radiocarpal and midcarpal types of CIND, unless there are both a

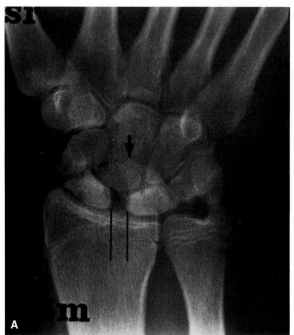

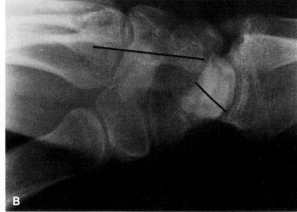

Fig. 8-49. Transscaphoid, transcapitate perilunate dislocation. (**A**) Displaced scaphoid fracture (*small arrows*), increased scapholunate interval, and undisplaced capitate fracture (*large arrow*). Note increased density and bone cysts in the proximal scaphoid and lunate. (**B**) Persistent dorsal subluxation of the capitate and capitolunate instability is present.

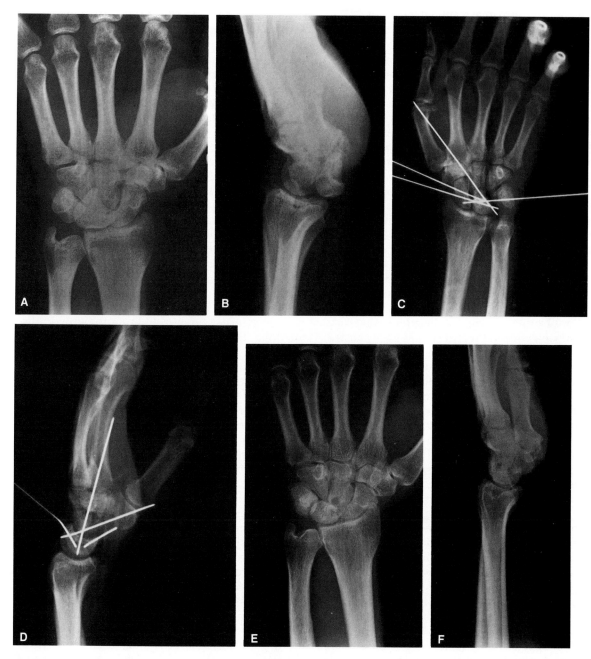

Fig. 8-50. Chronic perilunate dislocation treated by open reduction. **(A)** Posteroanterior and **(B)** lateral x-rays of the nondominant hand of a patient who was seen at our institution 17 weeks after a forced extension injury resulted in perilunate dislocation. The patient was unable to work because of severe, intolerable pain. Grip strength measured 12% of the opposite hand. **(C)** Posteroanterior and **(D)** lateral x-rays at the time of open reduction and temporary K-wire fixation. The scapholunate and lunotriquetral ligaments were also repaired at this time. **(E)** Posteroanterior and **(F)** lateral films 12 months postoperation demonstrate maintenance of reduction. The patient had returned to heavy farm work and reported occasional mild pain after heavy lifting. Grip strength measured 73% of the opposite dominant hand. *(Siegert, J. J.; Frassica, F. J.; Amadio, P. C.: Treatment of Chronic Perilunate Dislocations. J. Hand Surg. [Am.], 13(2):206–012, 1988.)*

recent injury and a localized area of tenderness.[85,155,273,320,335,517] Imaging findings are also almost identical for radiocarpal or midcarpal CIND unless there is evidence of an associated ligament avulsion fracture, significant instability on provocative testing at the midcarpal level, or abnormal articular spacing in either the STT or triquetrohamate joint.[509] Either VISI or DISI deformity or alternating patterns may occur at either level (Fig. 8-51).[154,320,335] In the early stages, these patterns of deformity may be so subtle that they are difficult to detect. Comparison of video motion patterns of the symptomatic wrist to the normal contralateral wrist is often useful. These difficulties are compounded by the fact that ligament insufficiency, either posttraumatic or congenital, may be present at both radiocarpal and midcarpal levels. Visualizing both joints and the intervening proximal carpal row by arthroscopy or surgery gives the final opportunity to decide where the instability is most noticeable. Even then, one may have to judge from subtle deviations from the norm, for the attenuation may not be obvious. Several recent studies have assisted in diagnosis of this condition. Johnson and Carrera[273] described 12 cases in which laxity of or attenuation of the radioscaphocapitate ligament was present. The diagnosis was made by midcarpal stress test in which a pathologic clunk could be reproduced by dorsal–palmar subluxation of the midcarpal joint. A painful snap could be produced with a sudden dorsal subluxation and ulnar shift of the lunate. With good cineradiography, ranging the compressed carpus through the normal range of motion and with subluxation stresses applied during the ranges of motion, one can produce the same catch or click that presented clinically. Differentially testing the midcarpal row and radiocarpal level may help one decide which is the more unstable.

A second clinical test[343] involves dynamic instability through the midcarpal joint produced by extension with radioulnar deviation, producing a "catch-up" clunk as the proximal row snaps from flexion into extension (Fig. 8-52).[558] The clinical literature suggests that triquetrohamate instability, presumed due to damage to the ulnar arm of the volar arcuate ligament, is the most common cause for midcarpal instability.[10,320] Our clinical experience suggests that radiocarpal causes of proximal carpal row instability are as common as midcarpal causes; even at the midcarpal level, STT joint instability and generalized midcarpal instability may be as common as the triquetrohamate variety. Midcarpal instability may be associated with radioscaphocapitate ligament[335] attenuation, leading to loss of radiocarpal wrist stability as well as midcarpal instability.[530] Experience is not yet sufficient to judge how the incidence of midcarpal instability compares to other forms of carpal instability, and therefore treatment alternatives remain limited. Localized fusion placed at the wrong level will not correct the problem, and we have seen instances of satisfactory midcarpal fusion followed by symptomatic radiocarpal instability.

Treatment.   There is no preferred procedure that can be universally applied for midcarpal instability.[343] A solid radius-to-metacarpal (wrist) fusion should solve any instability problem, but the penalties of that treatment are so severe that it should not be applied, unless one is dealing with a fixed deformity and significant arthritis. Many of these wrist problems occur in individuals with congenitally or posttraumatically lax wrists,[509,510] who can control the subluxation tendency to some degree by the sequence of muscle contraction. In such instances external support, limiting the provocative wrist motion, plus musculotendinous training may suffice.

For those with relatively normal joint surfaces but uncontrollable symptoms, the treatment plan is similar to that outlined for radiocarpal CIND. If a specific lesion can be identified, such as damage to radial arcuate ligament (radioscaphocapitate), the ulnar volar arcuate ligament (triquetrocapitate), or the STT capsule, direct repairs are indicated with temporary percutaneous fixation in the corrected alignment. A suitable repair for a midcarpal VISI-CIND is to close the space of Poirier volarly[273] or to construct a dorsal radiocarpal tether between radius and proximal carpal row that limits proximal row excursion. Conversely, for a midcarpal CIND-DISI pattern, one could augment dorsally between proximal carpal row and mid-metacarpal base. If manual reduction is incomplete or recurrence after reduction is rapid at the midcarpal joint, localized fusion across the midcarpal joint is preferable.[85,248,482,528] Radiocarpal fusion is more likely to control the unstable proximal carpal row.[326] Soft tissue augmentation or repair should be protected for 8 weeks with percutaneous pins and external support part-time for another 8 weeks. Proximal row carpectomy is a satisfactory salvage procedure as well.[408,500]

MIDCARPAL INSTABILITY SECONDARY TO MALANGULATION OF THE DISTAL RADIUS

Two occasionally seen conditions can produce a proximal carpal row malalignment that is secondary

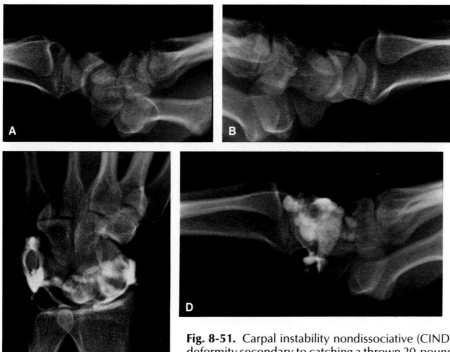

Fig. 8-51. Carpal instability nondissociative (CIND). (**A**) Left wrist shows a VISI deformity secondary to catching a thrown 20-pound weight. The wrist was weak and painful, and a snapping motion could be elicited. (**B**) Right wrist shows normal alignment of the midcarpal joint. (**C, D**) A normal posteroanterior and lateral radiocarpal arthrogram confirms that the VISI deformity is related to extrinsic and not intrinsic carpal ligament injury.

to deformity of the distal radius. The less common is ulnar translation of the carpus from Madelung's deformity. This condition is due to increased radial-to-ulnar slope of the distal radial articular surface. It is developmental (but occasionally posttraumatic)[536] in origin. A much more common problem is posttraumatic deformity of the distal radius related to the attempt of the hand to realign itself with the forearm in the presence of an extension malunion of the distal radius (see Fig. 8-37). In such a circumstance, the carpus has two alternatives, one of which is to translate dorsally on the radial articular surface and articulate with the dorsal half of that radial surface.[52,521] The carpus remains aligned, as does the hand, so that function and appearance remain reasonably good. The carpus is more prominent dorsally and motion is somewhat restricted, particularly flexion, but patients with this realignment pattern infrequently seek additional treatment. More commonly, the proximal carpal row stays aligned normally with the distal radius, but a flexion angulation, DISI, develops at the midcarpal level. Furthermore, the proximal carpal row cannot slide normally in either the radioulnar plane or the

dorsipalmar plane to permit a normal pattern of wrist motion. Over time, this may be accompanied by wrist discomfort, grip weakness, and eventually abnormal wear patterns at both the radiocarpal and midcarpal levels.

Appropriate treatment for distal radius extension malalignment is corrective radial osteotomy with restoration of length and angulation (see Fig. 8-37).[19,179,497] If there are no associated problems, the carpal malalignment usually corrects as the distal radius is corrected. Treatment is relatively simple and results are good. Open-wedge osteotomy of the distal radius, bone graft, and plate fixation is the current preference. If there are associated instabilities of the distal ulna, distal radioulnar joint problems, or fixed deformity of the carpus, then further surgical alternatives, such as ulnar shortening, distal radioulnar joint stabilization, or midcarpal joint fusion, may need to be addressed at the same time.

AXIAL INSTABILITIES

Axial instabilities have recently been separately categorized from other carpal injuries (Fig. 8-53).[93,204,209,396,413,441] These injuries are classically

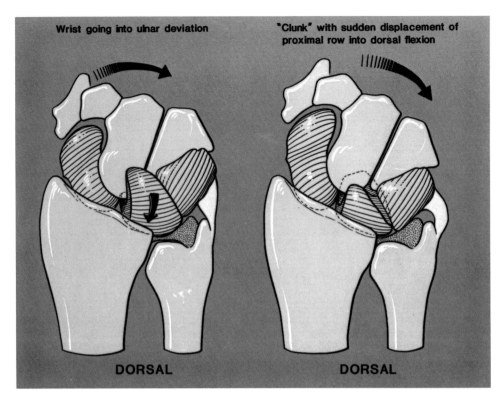

Fig. 8-52. Catch-up clunk. Carpal instability nondissociative is often characterized by sudden displacement of the lunate during radial to ulnar deviation. The palmar-flexed lunate catches as it slides up the radial inclination, then suddenly displaces radially and dorsiflexes with an audible and palpable "clunk." The end positions are normal, but occur as an interrupted rather than a smooth motion transition.

those which present as longitudinal fracture–dislocations of the wrist and, for the most part, have involved high-energy injuries. Traumatic causes have included an exploding truck tire, crushing under heavy objects, and high-pressure machine compression.[204] The basic pathophysiology is collapse of the carpal arch, often with tearing or avulsion of the bony origins of the transverse carpal ligament.[206,207] The focus of this injury is usually in the distal carpus and adjacent metacarpus, occasionally extending either distally into the intermetacarpal area or proximally through the proximal carpal row.[239] The most common pattern is separation of either radial or ulnar components of the carpus with their metacarpal rays from the central carpus.[209] From our review of the more common patterns, a proposed nomenclature is axial-radial, axial-ulnar, or a combination of the two fracture–dislocations (see Fig. 8-53). The carpal elements involved are usually indicated by the term *peri,* if the

discontinuity is primarily ligamentous, as in peritrapezial or peritrapezoidal–trapezial. If the discontinuity is through bone, the term *trans* is employed, as in transtrapezial or transtrapeziotrapezoidal. The accompanying soft tissue disruption is often of more importance than the bone and joint disruption. Neurovascular injury is frequent, sometimes to the point of nonviability of digits.

Diagnosis is established by the history of a force propagating in a sagittal plane (ie, dorsal to palmar crush), often with evidence of severe soft tissue damage, swelling, and open wounds. Standard x-rays should confirm the diagnosis, although the carpal malalignment may be subtle and escape notice. A high index of suspicion is needed. Provocative stress x-rays, tomography, CT, or MRI should be obtained preoperatively and intraoperatively. Evidence of nerve, vascular, musculotendinous, and ligamentous damage is often present—to a severe degree. Instances of median neuropathy are less

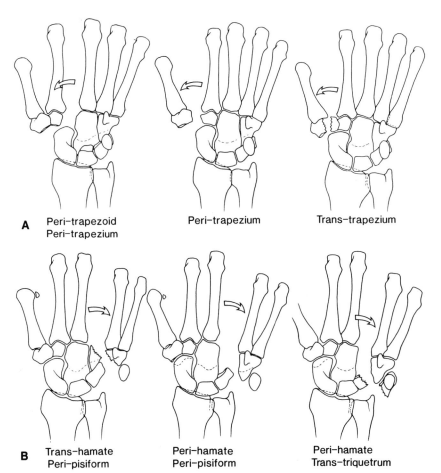

A   Peri-trapezoid   Peri-trapezium   Trans-trapezium
Peri-trapezium

B   Trans-hamate   Peri-hamate   Peri-hamate
Peri-pisiform   Peri-pisiform   Trans-triquetrum

Fig. 8-53. Axial disruptions of the carpus. (**A**) Axial–radial disruption, peritrapezoid and peritrapezial types. (**B**) Axial–ulnar disruptions, transhamate, perihamate, and transtriquetral types. *(Garcia-Elias, M.; Dobyns, J. H.; Cooney, W. P.; Linscheid, R. L.: Traumatic Axial Dislocation of the Carpus. J. Hand Surg. [Am.], 14(3):446–457, 1989.)*

than expected, probably because the carpal tunnel is usually decompressed by the injury.

Treatment.   Initial complete assessment is needed in these injuries for planning of both soft tissue and joint repair. Urgent surgical intervention is often indicated to salvage neurovascular function and restore skeletal alignment[93] (Fig. 8-54). Massive swelling may necessitate decompression of compartments not already decompressed by the injury. Traction can help reduce the axial displacement. Fractures and dislocations, once reduced, can be maintained by K-wires and lag screws. Transcarpal or metacarpal K-wire fixation is usually necessary to prevent redisplacement. Early motion of the hand (flexor and extensor tendons) helps prevent adhesions. Rehabilitation is often prolonged, and prognosis depends upon the severity of soft tissue damage.

FRACTURES OF THE OTHER CARPAL BONES

MECHANISMS OF INJURY

Triquetrum

Fractures of the triquetrum result from a direct blow or from an avulsion injury that may include ligament damage.[36,137,150,203] The triquetrum may be fractured transversely during a perilunate dislocation, but it usually displaces dorsally with the distal carpal row away from the lunate (Fig. 8-55).[87,203] The most common triquetral fracture is probably the impingement shear fracture[69,316] of ulnar styloid against dorsal triquetrum, occurring with the wrist in extension and ulnar deviation, particularly when a long ulnar styloid is present.[203,316] Shear impingement by the hamate against the posteroradial projection of the triquetrum can occur with the wrist in extension and ulnar deviation. A bone avulsion

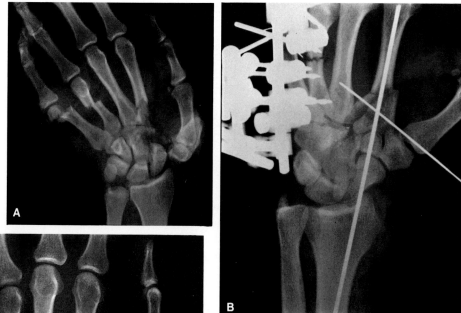

Fig. 8-54. A peritrapezial–trapezoidal axial dissociation in a 19-year-old man who sustained a crush injury of his left wrist. He had associated injuries of intrinsic muscles and extensor tendons, along with fractures of the index, ring, and little metacarpal fractures. (**A**) Radial axial dislocation of the thumb ray through the trapezium and trapezoid articulation with the scaphoid and capitate. Note transverse fractures of the fourth and fifth metacarpals. (**B**) Transverse and axial K-wire fixation of the radial axial fracture–dislocation, and external fixation of the open metacarpal fractures. (**C**) Six years following injury, the skeleton is well aligned. There were residual intrinsic contractures.

with either dorsal or volar ligaments stripped from their triquetral insertions can also occur. The triquetrum is rarely dislocated alone because of the strong ligamentous support dorsally, volarly and ulnarly. Isolated case reports have been described.[54,196]

Trapezium

Fracture through the articular surface of the trapezium is produced by the base of the first metacarpal being driven into the articular surface of the trapezium by the adducted thumb (Fig. 8-56).[17,123,172,275,359] Avulsion fractures caused by the capsular ligaments can occur during forceful deviation, traction, or rotation.[87,271,416] Direct blows to

the palmar arch area or forceful distraction of the proximal palmar arch may result in avulsion of the ridge of the trapezium by the transverse carpal ligament.[123,150,421] Dislocations are occasionally seen.[254,479,486,488,505,512]

Pisiform

The pisiform is generally injured during a fall on the dorsiflexed, outstretched hand.[69,150] A direct blow while the pisiform is held firmly against the triquetrum under tension from the flexor carpi ulnaris leads to either avulsion of its distal portion with a vertical fracture or an osteochondral compression fracture at the pisotriquetral joint (Fig. 8-57). Subluxation or dislocation may occur, usually

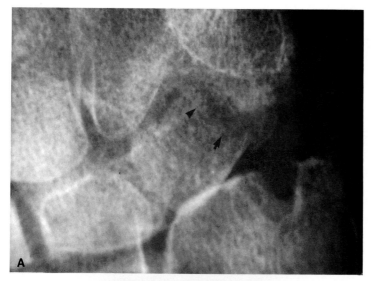

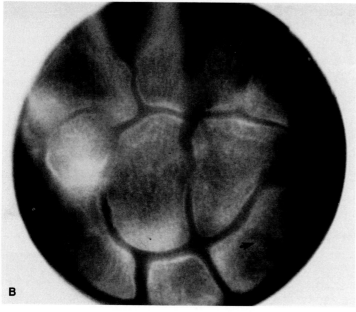

Fig. 8-55. Triquetral fractures. (**A**) An isolated fracture through the body of the triquetrum from an apparent impaction load from the distal ulna. This fracture may also occur from a greater arc injury of the carpus (see Fig. 8-15). (**B**) A tomogram confirms an undisplaced fracture in the body of the triquetrum.

with a combination of wrist extension and flexor carpi ulnaris contraction.[376,535]

Hamate

The hamate may be fractured through its distal articular surface,[347] the other articular surfaces, through the hook (hamulus) of the hamate,[23,59,271] the proximal pole, or the body.[11,69,87,334,373,415,493,502] The hamate also may be dislocated by direct violence.[416] A dorsally displaced articular fracture, the distal portion of the hamate with fifth metacarpal subluxation, occurs when force is applied along the shaft as from a fall or a blow from a fist. Fracture of the hook of the hamate may occur from a fall on the dorsiflexed wrist, with tension exerted through the transverse carpal ligament and piso-hamate ligament (Fig. 8-58).[59,78,97,381] More commonly, sports-related fracture of the hook occurs from the use of clubs, bats, or racquets.[502] Direct force exerted by these objects against the hypothenar eminence or transverse carpal ligament has been implicated. The fracture generally occurs at the base of the hamulus, although avulsion fracture of the tip also may be seen. Osteochondral fracture

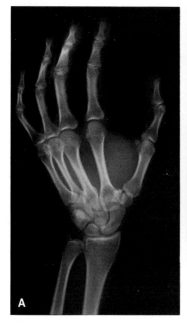

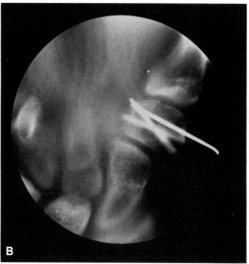

Fig. 8-56. Fracture of the trapezium. (**A**) A comminuted radial fracture of the trapezium with displacement of the first metacarpal base. (**B**) Open reduction and internal fixation with K-wires was performed to realign the joint articular surface.

of the proximal pole probably occurs from impaction injuries against the articular surface of the lunate during dorsiflexion and ulnar deviation. Osteochondral fractures of the triquetral and hamate articular surface may occur in a similar fashion or from a shearing injury, such as that which occurs when a trapped hand is wrenched violently against a steering wheel. Fractures of the body of the hamate[193] and dislocation of the hamate[237] are generally caused by blast injuries or by direct crushing injuries, such as punch-press accidents.

Capitate

Because of its protected position, the body of the capitate is seldom fractured (Fig. 8-59).[3,150,337,338,446,450] Nonunions of the capitate with fracture site erosion and secondary DISI deformity have been recorded.[375] Direct force or crushing blows

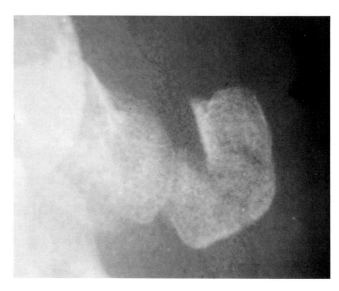

Fig. 8-57. Pisiform fracture. A rather unusual displaced fracture through the body of the pisiform, from a direct blow to the palmar surface of the hand. Treatment was excision of the pisiform.

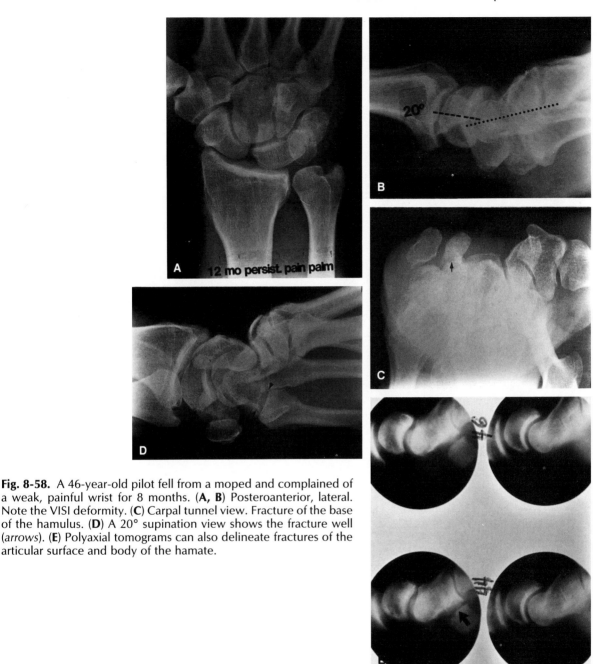

Fig. 8-58. A 46-year-old pilot fell from a moped and complained of a weak, painful wrist for 8 months. (**A, B**) Posteroanterior, lateral. Note the VISI deformity. (**C**) Carpal tunnel view. Fracture of the base of the hamulus. (**D**) A 20° supination view shows the fracture well (*arrows*). (**E**) Polyaxial tomograms can also delineate fractures of the articular surface and body of the hamate.

usually occur with associated injury to the metacarpals and other carpal bones. The capitate, in association with perilunate fracture–dislocation, is more susceptible to fracture through the neck of the bone.[446] A variation of this is the "naviculocapitate syndrome,"[174] in which the capitate and scaphoid are fractured but no dislocation is observed. Because fractures of the scaphoid and the capitate are only stage 1 of the spectrum of injury that culminates in a transscaphoid, transcapitate, perilunate dislocation of the carpus, it is not surprising that the capitate fragment can be frequently rotated 90° to 180° with the articular surface displaced anteriorly or facing the fracture surface of

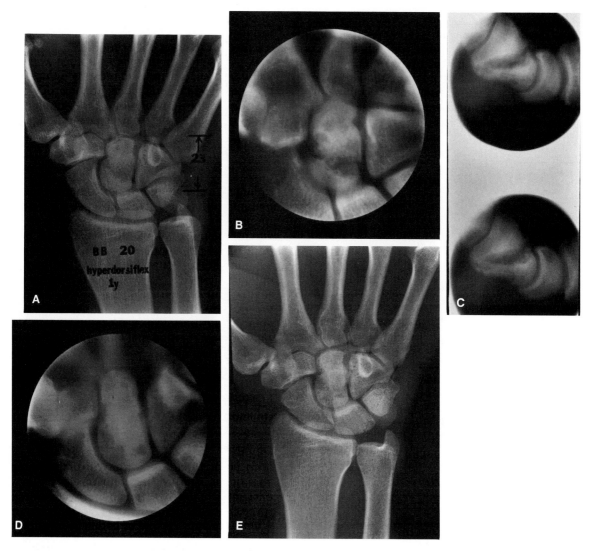

Fig. 8-59. A 20-year-old softball player dorsiflexed his wrist 1 year prior to examination. He had persistent pain in the mid carpus. (**A**) An anteroposterior x-ray was apparently normal except for a suspicious capitate fracture. (**B**) Anteroposterior polyaxial tomograms demonstrated a fracture nonunion through the body of the capitate, with foreshortening. (**C**) Lateral view showed dorsal displacement of the distal fragment. (**D**) The capitate healed 5 months after open reduction, distraction, and fixation with a keyed corticocancellous graft; note sclerosis and mild avascular changes. (**E**) Final radiographic appearance, showing the united capitate.

the capitate neck. Without reduction, avascular necrosis will result. In wrist fracture–dislocations, subtle osteochrondral injuries can be easily overlooked. The mechanism of injury is impingement of the capitate against the dorsal lip of the radius during hyperdorsiflexion, although an opposite mechanism—that of a fall on the hyperflexed wrist—also has been suggested. Nonunion and

ischemia after injury[338,375,444] are rare in the capitate, but they do occur.[445]

Trapezoid

Injury to the trapezoid is generally associated with forces applied through the second metacarpal.[305] Because of it shape and position, the trapezoid is rarely fractured, although axial loading of the second metacarpal can cause dorsal dislocation with rupture of the capsular ligaments.[305,365,452] Palmar dislocation also has been reported. Ligamentous instability produced by similar injury or osteochondral injuries to the trapezoid–second metacarpal, capitate–third metacarpal, or metacarpohamate joints often escape detection. Blast or crush forces can also disrupt the trapezoid sufficient to dislocate or fracture it.

SIGNS AND SYMPTOMS

The signs and symptoms of injuries to the individual carpal bones are pain and tenderness appropriately situated for the injury. Localized swelling, prominence, and limited motion may be present. Stress of muscle–tendon units inserted on or supported by the injured structure may localize symptoms. A knowledge of the deep and topographical anatomy should locate the injury specifically. Neurovascular signs are unusual with these isolated carpal injuries, except for injury of the pisiform and the hook of the hamate, which may affect the ulnar nerve and artery. Tendons on both the flexor and extensor surfaces pass near carpal bone surfaces. Either the fresh raw surface of recent fracture or the roughened exostosis of an old nonunion/malunion may damage any of the flexor or extensor tendons that pass over the carpus.[127]

RADIOGRAPHIC EXAMINATION

Triquetrum

Dorsal chip fractures of the triquetrum are easily overlooked on the anteroposterior view because of the normal superimposition of the dorsal lip on the lunate.[313] Such fractures are usually seen in one of the three lateral views of the recommended motion studies of the wrist; if not, a slightly oblique, pronated lateral view will project the triquetrum even more dorsal to the lunate. Transverse fractures of the triquetral body are usually easily identified on the anteroposterior view.

Trapezium

If fractures of the body of the trapezium cannot be seen on standard views, a true anteroposterior x-ray such as the Robert view (see Chapter 7) to outline the trapezium and first metacarpal base without superimposition may be useful.

Fracture of the trapezial ridge is difficult to identify without carpal tunnel views that silhouette the ridge.

Pisiform

Special views are required to see pisiform injuries. A lateral view of the wrist with the forearm in 20° supination and carpal tunnel views are useful. If subluxation of the pisotriquetral joint is suspected, the diagnosis is made when one or more of the following are present: (1) a joint space more than 4 mm in width, (2) loss of parallelism of the joint surfaces greater than 20°, and (3) proximal or distal overriding of the pisiform amounting to more than 15% of the width of the joint surfaces. The wrist must be in a neutral position during these observations.

Hamate

Fractures and dislocations of the hamate are usually identified on anteroposterior views, particularly when three posteroanterior views are available on the motion studies.[161,334] A dislocation usually results in some rotation that alters the contour of the bone and the normal oval appearance of the hamulus. Fracture of the hook of the hamate is best visualized on the carpal tunnel or 20° supination oblique view.[97,191,430] When there is still doubt, polytomography can confirm the fracture.[161] The hook of the hamate is said to ossify independently and occasionally may fail to fuse with the body of the hamate. This separate bone, known as the os hamulus proprium, can be mistaken for a fracture. Chondral articular injuries are seldom visualized on x-rays.

Capitate

Fractures of the capitate usually can be identified on standard posteroanterior x-rays, although motion studies are recommended to look for displacement. A lucent line through the neck of the capitate may be isolated or may be combined with other fractures or fracture–dislocations.[337,338,533] In such instances, the head of the capitate should be identified on the lateral view to determine if it has been rotated or displaced.

Trapezoid

A trapezoid dislocation or fracture–dislocation is seen on the anteroposterior view as a loss of the normal relationship between the second metacarpal base and the trapezoid. The trapezoid may be superimposed over the trapezium, or the capitate and the second metacarpal may be proximally displaced. Oblique views and tomography may be helpful.

METHODS OF TREATMENT

Isolated injuries of the carpal bones are treated similarly, if undisplaced. Most respond to 6 weeks of support in a short-arm plaster cast. In a few instances, such as the fracture of the neck of the capitate, in which there is instability or vascular deprivation, more complete rest of the upper limb muscles is gained by using a long-arm, full-digit cast, as recommended for some scaphoid fractures.

Dislocations or displaced fractures should be treated in the same fashion. Satisfactory reduction can be accomplished in a finger-trap apparatus with countertraction on the arm and good muscle relaxation. Direct manipulative pressure may be required. If the reduction is unsatisfactory, open reduction and internal fixation[191,193,194] (K-wires, screws, staples) should be used. A fracture of the hook of the hamate may be the sole exception where excision[59,502] is preferred to open reduction and internal fixation.[549] Even some fractures that are satisfactorily reduced by closed methods may be unstable enough to require percutaneous pin fixation. Fractures at the carpometacarpal joint frequently need such fixation. Other indications for open reduction include gross comminution involving an important joint; eg, the trapezium at the thumb carpometacarpal joint will require bone graft to replace bone loss, fusion for irreparable joint damage, or excisional arthroplasty. Revascularization procedures may see increasing use. In a few circumstances in which there is persistent instability, external fixation with slight distraction may be useful.

FRACTURES OF THE SCAPHOID

Fractures of the scaphoid are among the most common fractures of the wrist after fractures of the distal radius, and represent the most common fracture of a carpal bone.[150,393,537] The position of the scaphoid on the radial side of the wrist, as a proximal extension of the thumb ray, makes it vulnerable to injury. Not only does the scaphoid mechanically link the proximal and distal carpal rows, but it is firmly attached at both ends to strong ligament systems that limit and control its motion.[47,357,505,516] It is self evident that the scaphoid flexes with wrist flexion and extends with wrist extension, but it also flexes during radial deviation and extends with ulnar deviation. These factors make immobilization of scaphoid fractures difficult, especially when there

is displacement. This change in position of the scaphoid during different planes of wrist motion confirms the scaphoid's role as the mechanistic key that controls wrist stability and serves as the principal bony support strut. Tensile stresses are generated volarly when excessive hyperextension is applied to the wrist and when tensile forces exceed bone strength, a fracture through the scaphoid will result,[138,245] either alone or in combination with other wrist injury (see *Mechanism of Injury*).

The scaphoid is an irregularly shaped bone, more resembling a deformed peanut than the boat for which it is named. It rests in a plane at 45° to the longitudinal axis of the wrist. Articular cartilage covers 80% of the surface. The proximal pole is constrained to the lunate by an interosseous membrane. The distal pole has a V-shaped scaphotrapezial ligament, a scaphocapitate ligament, and a dorsal capsule. It rests on and is attached along the ulnar aspect of the waist to the radioscaphocapitate ligament. The only other capsular influence is where the dorsal radiocarpal ligament inserts obliquely on a roughened ridge and brings the primary blood supply that enters the scaphoid. Otherwise, the scaphoid has no ligamentous or tendinous attachments and acts with the rest of the proximal carpal row as "intercalated segments" subjected to the forces acting on them.[89,309] Compressive forces, acting across a three-link structure, cause a zig-zag collapse deformity. With a scaphoid fracture, the distal scaphoid tends to flex, and the proximal scaphoid extends with the proximal carpal row. As a consequence, angulation occurs at the fracture site, which gaps open dorsally and gradually assumes the so-called humpback deformity.[18,331,388,491] Studies have recently shown that this deformity may occur at the time of fracture and result in immediate malposition of the scaphoid fragments into radial as well as dorsal angulation.[490] Failure to correct such deformity leads to fracture malalignment, nonunion, or malunion (Fig. 8-60).[322,342]

Despite the lack of direct tendon attachment, joint compressive forces, trapezial–scaphoid shear stress, and capitolunate rotation moments do exert some control on the scaphoid. As a consequence of these biologic and mechanical factors, scaphoid fractures have a high incidence of nonunion (8–10%), frequent malunion, and late sequella of carpal instability and posttraumatic arthritis. We will examine below the diagnosis and treatment of acute scaphoid fractures and address the treatment options available when scaphoid union is either delayed or absent.

ACUTE SCAPHOID FRACTURES

Acute fractures of the scaphoid were first recognized in 1889 by Cousin and Destot[145] before the discovery of x-ray. A clear description was made later, in 1919, by Mouchet and Jeanne.[268] Scaphoid fractures are usually an injury of young male adults occurring after a fall, athletic injury, or motor vehicle accident. Scaphoid fractures in children are uncommon,[7,103,173,235,311,531] because the physis of the distal radius usually fails first.[311] Concomitant fractures of the distal radius and scaphoid[531] have been reported. Similarly, in the elderly, the distal radial metaphysis usually fails with fracture before the scaphoid fractures.

The patient often presents to the emergency room complaining of wrist pain and may be diagnosed as a sprain of the wrist. In sports injuries it is not uncommon for the wrist injury to go unnoticed, with the request for evaluation and treatment delayed.[342]

Signs and Symptoms

The diagnosis of a scaphoid fracture is made on clinical examination where the index of suspicion is raised, and by proper radiographic examination, by which the diagnosis is confirmed.[146] Clinical examination should demonstrate tenderness in the snuffbox region of the wrist, over the tuberosity, or on the proximal pole of the scaphoid just distal to Lister's tubercle. Range of motion will be reduced but not dramatically. There is usually pain at the extremes of motion. Swelling or ecchymosis is not present except in fracture–dislocations. Clearly, these same physical findings may be present with less severe ligament sprains of the wrist, and thus whenever there are any findings suggestive of a scaphoid fracture,[124,146] the emergency physician should treat the patient as a suspected scaphoid fracture.[103]

Radiographic Examination

Radiographic diagnosis of a scaphoid fracture often requires special views and occasionally special tests.[160,173,468] The emergency posteroanterior and lateral radiographs[146] should also include a scaphoid view (anteroposterior with 30° supination and ulnar deviation), which puts the scaphoid in profile. Motion views of the wrist (flexion–extension and radial and ulnar deviation) may demonstrate fracture displacement—an unstable scaphoid fracture (Fig. 8-61). These same x-rays should be repeated at 2 weeks if the initial films were negative. It is imperative for the treating physician to make the diagnosis at this time, because a delay in diagnosis increases the incidence of scaphoid nonunion.[160] If a diagnosis still cannot be confirmed with confidence on routine films, a technetium bone scan,[45,202,411,417] polytomography,[58,223,403] or MRI[51] of the wrist is recommended, in that order of preference.[222,411,417,438] Recently, we have been impressed with the ability of MRI to clearly show a scaphoid fracture when both plain films and even tomography were not diagnostic of a fracture.[57] Some authorities recommend bone scintigraphy as the procedure of choice for a suspected but unconfirmed fracture.[45,202]

When instability of the scaphoid is suspected, careful analysis of the lateral x-ray for intrascaphoid angulation or a dorsally tilted lunate is recommended (see Fig. 8-17). Motion views comparing scaphoid position during radial and ulnar deviation also may demonstrate motion at the fracture site (see Fig.8-61). Polytomography, however, is the best method to determine scaphoid displacement.[51] Lateral tomography or lateral CT (and axial) scanning can be used to measure the exact degree of intrascaphoid angulation or displacement.[332,468] From biplanar trispiral tomography, we have studied the range of normal angulation of the scaphoid in order to detect displacement and instability.[490,491] Measurements appear to be reproducible to within 5° and, when compared with the uninvolved scaphoid, provide information to assess not only the presence of displacement but the accuracy of reduction. Three-dimensional representation of the scaphoid using computed tomography (CT scan) and 3-D imaging provides the ability to describe displacement in all three planes and has promising clinical application.[45,394,403]

Differentiation between an acute scaphoid fracture and a scaphoid nonunion is important for planning treatment, and only proper x-rays can make the difference evident. Not uncommonly, a second injury will draw attention to a minimally symptomatic nonunion aggravated by the recent event. The acute scaphoid fracture is represented by a single line through the bone, occasionally with dorsal–radial comminution and rarely with dorsal angulation. Late presentation of a fracture or established nonunion, conversely, will demonstrate resorption at the fracture site; a space between the fragments; subchondral sclerosis; and displacement on both the posteroanterior and lateral x-rays.[12] A true pseudarthrosis separates delayed acute fracture from established nonunions. The longer the period of time since injury, the greater the cystic resorption, the denser the sclerosis, the more prominent the shortening of the scaphoid, and the greater the loss of carpal height. Secondary degenerative changes are usually present by 10 to 15 years.[322]

Classification

Fractures of the scaphoid may be classified either by the location of the fracture within the bone or by the amount of fracture displacement (stability).

LOCATION

Classification by anatomical location has many proponents, who attempt to correlate fracture union rate with the site of injury (Fig. 8-62). Five different fracture sites have been described: tuberosity, distal third, waist, proximal third, and distal osteochondral fractures.[116,537] All but the tuberosity fractures are intra-articular to a greater or lesser degree.[122,252,443] From a series of scaphoid fractures carefully studied, waist fractures accounted for 80%, proximal pole, 15%; tuberosity, 4%; and distal articular, 1%. The other anatomic classification is based on the direction of the fracture, with horizontal, oblique, avulsion, and comminuted types described.

The healing time for these different fracture types ranges from 4 to 6 weeks for tuberosity fractures, 10 to 12 weeks for distal third and waist fractures, and 12 to 20 weeks for proximal pole fractures.

The blood supply of the scaphoid is critical in regard to fracture location. Gelberman's work[214] confirmed earlier studies,[519] demonstrating that the major blood supply comes from the scaphoid branches of the radial artery, entering the dorsal ridge and supplying 70% to 80% of the bone, including the proximal pole. The second major group of vessels enters the scaphoid tubercle, perfusing only the distal 30% of the bone. With fractures through the waist and proximal third, revascularization will occur only with fracture healing. One can assume that with proper treatment nearly 100% of tuberosity and distal third scaphoid will heal; 80% to 90% of fractures at the waist will heal; and only 60% to 70% of proximal pole fractures will

heal. Similarly, oblique or shear fractures have been shown to have delayed healing in comparison to horizontal fractures. Comminuted or distracted osteochrondral fractures will have the poorest rate of union.

STABILITY

The second major classification of scaphoid fractures subdivides them into either stable or unstable fractures.[116,252] A stable fracture is one that is undisplaced, and it may have an intact cartilage envelope. That is, the fracture may occur within the bony substance of the scaphoid, incompletely separating the two fracture components. X-rays in two planes, as well as motion views, do not show any step-off or displacement of these fractures. The unstable scaphoid fracture, conversely, is by definition displaced with a step-off of 1 mm or more or angulation of the scaphoid in a lateral x-ray (Fig. 8-63). The rate of fracture union and options for treatment change dramatically when one compares unstable and stable scaphoid fractures.

Methods of Treatment

UNDISPLACED FRACTURES

The primary treatment for acute fractures of the scaphoid is cast immobilization.[506] As mentioned earlier, when there is any question regarding the presence of a scaphoid fracture, cast immobilization is recommended for 2 weeks until the diagnosis can be reassessed. The debate between long- and short-arm casts, as well as the position of immobilization, has not been definitely answered, but recent studies should influence our decision.[395] In a recent prospective study, Gellman and coauthors compared short- and long-thumb spica casts and noted decreased time to union and reduced rates of delayed union and nonunion with a long-arm thumb spica cast.[217] This study agrees with earlier reports[84,183,226,537] that noted higher rates of healing with a long-arm cast for 4 to 6 weeks. Conversely, those surgeons who prefer a short-arm thumb spica

Fig. 8-60. A 19-year-old man sustained a scaphoid fracture 1 year ago. (**A**) Anteroposterior: radial displacement and resorption. Note the extended volar pole of the lunate. (**B**) Lateral view showing DISI deformity. (**C, D**) Tomograms. (**C**) The anteroposterior intrascaphoid angle is 70° on the fracture side; (**D**) 45° on the normal side. (**E, F**) The capitolunate angles are (**E**) 19° on the normal side; (**F**) 32° on the fracture side, with dorsal displacement of the capitate. (**G, H**) The intrascaphoid sagittal angles are (**G**) 32° on the normal side; (**H**) 60° on the fracture side, with dorsal displacement of the capitate. (**I, J**) Six weeks postoperation, interpositional bone graft with K-wire fixation of the fracture combined with derotation and pinning of the lunate. (**K**) Three months postoperation, showing healed scaphoid.

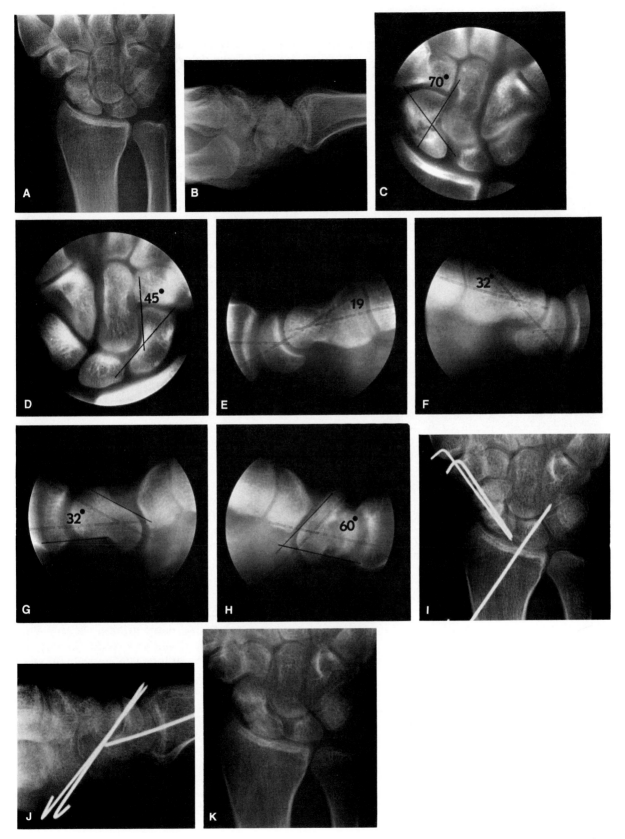

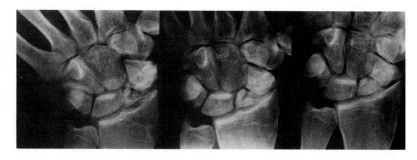

Fig. 8-61. Scaphoid fracture (motion views). (**Left**) With ulnar deviation, a radial gap develops. Neutral deviation (**center**); the fracture line is still obvious. (**Right**) Radial deviation closes the gap. Note the radioscaphoid arthrosis involving the distal pole of scaphoid.

cast point to 95% union rates in their personal series. Tuberosity fractures are undoubtedly suitable for a short-arm cast, while patients with proximal pole fractures are candidates for a long-arm cast.

The recommended position of immobilization for scaphoid fractures varies from full extension to slight flexion, with varying degrees of radial or ulnar deviation. The amount of fracture displacement, alignment in both the posteroanterior and lateral planes, and associated injuries have been analyzed by several biomechanical studies, suggesting that a position of neutral flexion–extension and slight ulnar deviation is the preferred position of undisplaced and minimally displaced scaphoid fractures. To reduce the stress produced by the volar and radiocapitate ligament, Weber and Chao[553] recommended radial deviation and palmar flexion. This

position makes radiographic assessment difficult. From an analysis of simulated displaced fractures,[491] it would appear that slight radial or ulnar deviation is acceptable, along with neutral flexion–extension. If the effect of lunate extension on dorsal gapping of the fracture site is important, then an attempt at flexing the lunate should help control the scaphoid reduction. This can be accomplished by careful molding of the cast. A depression is created over the capitate neck while displacing the carpometacarpal area relative to the forearm. The capitate tends to derotate the lunate and proximal pole, providing better coaptation of the fracture fragments (Fig. 8-64).

For undisplaced stable scaphoid fractures, we recommend a long-arm thumb spica cast, with the wrist in neutral deviation and neutral flexion–extension for 6 weeks, followed by a short-arm thumb spica cast until there is radiographic union confirmed by polytomography.[116] The union rate should exceed 95%. Delay in recognition, delay in initial treatment, and proximal third location of the fracture all negatively influence fracture healing.

DISPLACED FRACTURES

Displaced fractures of the scaphoid require treatment different from that for undisplaced fractures. A displaced fracture, by definition, is one with greater than 1 mm of step-off or more than 60° of scapholunate or 15° of lunocapitate angulation as observed on either plain x-rays or tomography.[117] The degree of instability may vary, and herein lie the different choices for fracture treatment. We believe that there is still a role for a carefully applied long-arm thumb spica cast in the treatment of displaced scaphoid fractures, provided that the fracture can be acceptably reduced and the reduction maintained. To effect the reduction, three-point pressure on the tubercle of the distal scaphoid volarly is combined with dorsal pressure over the capitate and dorsal support at the distal radius, which helps re-

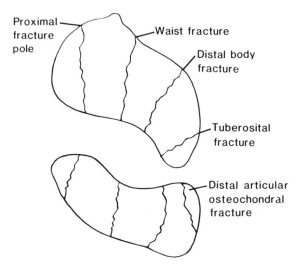

Fig. 8-62. Types of scaphoid fractures. The scaphoid is susceptible to fractures at any level. Approximately 65% occur at the waist, 15% through the proximal pole, 10% through the distal body, 8% through the tuberosity, and 2% in the distal articular surface.

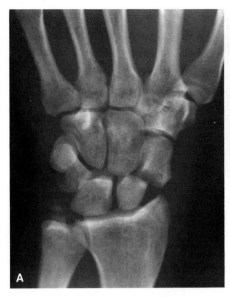

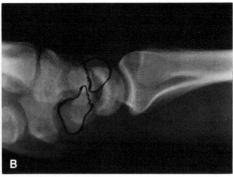

Fig. 8-63. Unstable scaphoid fracture (posteroanterior [**A**] and lateral [**B**] x-rays). Displacement greater than 1 mm is defined as an unstable scaphoid fracture. A displaced scaphoid fracture of this degree is inherently unstable and usually requires open reduction and internal fixation.

duce and maintain the dorsal lunate angulation (see Fig. 8-64). An acceptable reduction includes alignment within 1 mm of displacement and scapholunate angle of not more than 60°. With lateral tomography (or CT scanning), lateral intrascaphoid angulation should not exceed 25° ± 5°, and the posteroanterior angulation not more than 35° ± 5°.

If an accurate fracture reduction cannot be obtained, then other methods of treatment should be considered. These include closed reduction and percutaneous pin fixation, open reduction and pin fixation,[167] and open reduction and compression screw fixation (Fig. 8-65).[88,140,251,253,310] For acute displaced fractures that cannot be easily reduced, we currently recommend open reduction and K-wire fixation of the scaphoid. The technique we prefer is to realign the proximal scaphoid and lunate to the distal radius and secure them with K-wires. The proximal fracture components are stabilized by this procedure. The distal scaphoid can then be

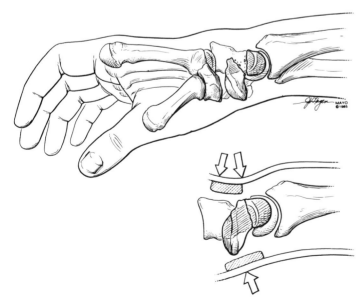

Fig. 8-64. Closed reduction of a displaced scaphoid fracture by three-point pressure. Volar upward pressure is applied on the distal pole of the scaphoid, and dorsal downward pressure is applied on the capitate and lunate. Displacement of the capitate volarly rotates the lunate and proximal pole into flexion and closes the dorsal scaphoid gap.

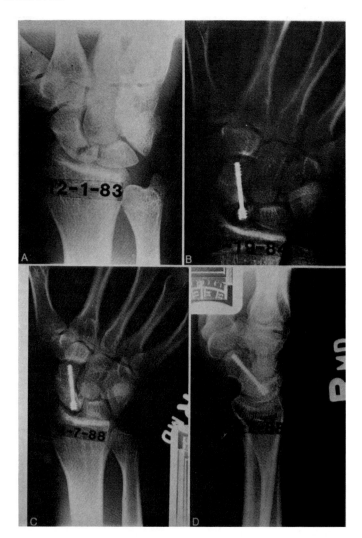

Fig. 8-65. A proximal pole third scaphoid fracture treated with a Herbert screw inserted from the proximal pole. The fracture is reduced from a dorsal approach and the screw inserted into joint cartilage and countersunk. (**A**) Preoperative appearance. (**B**) Immediate postoperative Herbert screw insertion. (**C,D**) Six-year follow-up PA and lateral x-rays. No degenerative changes from proximal screw insertion across scaphoid articular cartilage. (*DeMaagd, R. L.; Engber, W. D.: Retrograde Herbert Screw Fixation for Treatment of Proximal Pole Scaphoid Nonunions. J. Hand Surg. [Am.], 14:996–1003, 1989.*)

reduced onto the proximal fragments and fixed in that position. In addition to K-wire fixation, a long-arm thumb spica cast is maintained for 8 weeks. After K-wire removal, a short-arm cast is applied until fracture healing is confirmed radiographically (preferably with polytomography).

With the advent of new compression screws and staples for the scaphoid, internal fixation has become more popular.[88,253,301,310,346,442] These procedures provide more rigid fixation for the scaphoid and may allow earlier wrist motion. A number of authors have reported their recent experience with such techniques, but clear consensus on the role of screw fixation is lacking.[1,121,187,310,389,397,442] One report[389] includes three acute displaced fractures (Herbert and Fisher type B), all with union but with a 15° decrease in wrist motion. A second report[1]

discussed 9 patients out of a series of 24, in which Herbert screw fixation was used for acute fractures and nonunions. Each of the acute fractures was a significant injury (fracture–dislocations, open or crush injuries). Only 5 of the 9 reported a satisfactory outcome, and union was achieved in only 67%. Problems in correct screw placement were noted in 9 of the 22 cases. Earlier authors[212,353] reported similar experiences with a compression screw of AO design.[353] While providing initial strong fixation, should fracture union not occur, there was eventual loosening of the screw and loss of fixation in all series reported. A recent biomechanical analysis compared the fixation strength of different bone screws and noted less interfragmentary compression with the Herbert screw than was anticipated from its unique design of differential thread-pitch between the distal and proximal screw ends. The correct application of fracture reduction and alignment devices is essential for anatomic screw placement. The development of cannulated screws placed over a K-wire or use of intraoperative imaging will improve the technical factors associated with fracture fixation.[70,187]

The current role for compression screw fixation of scaphoid fractures is limited to displaced fractures displaced proximal pole fractures,[140] and fracture–dislocations.[150] Postfixation cast immobilization is recommended despite proposals for early motion at 2 to 3 weeks.[251] Conclusive studies comparing compression screws with K-wires or cast immobilization of displaced scaphoid fractures are currently lacking,[187] and thus it is inappropriate to recommend their broad application.

SCAPHOID NONUNION

Treatment

STABLE NONUNIONS

In the treatment of nonunion of the scaphoid it is essential to maintain the important principles of fracture healing and at the same time secure correct scaphoid alignment. Four principles to follow include (1) preservation of blood supply, (2) bone apposition by inlay graft, (3) internal fixation for fracture stability, and (4) correction of carpal instability.[117,358,400] Failure of scaphoid bone grafting appears to be associated with inadequate vascularization, unsatisfactory fracture immobilization, insufficient length of immobilization, and instability or displacement. A number of questions are currently being asked regarding the treatment of choice for an undisplaced scaphoid nonunion. What is effect of operative approach on the blood supply? How should avascular necrosis of the scaphoid be confirmed? Is there a role for electrical stimulation of undisplaced scaphoid nonunions? Is internal fixation of the scaphoid nonunion necessary when the nonunion is not displaced?

Russe Bone Graft. From a survey of the literature[24,156,395] and our experience, it appears that a Russe-type inlay bone graft of the scaphoid is the treatment of choice to which other procedures should be compared (Fig. 8-66).[463,501,506] From a review of four different treatment options, the volar Russe[463] type or dorsal–radial Matti[34,351] type had union rates of 86% and 92%, respectively.[117] Studies by others confirm the excellent results associated with the Russe procedure and report union rates of

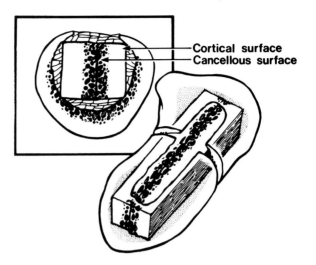

Fig. 8-66. Modified Russe procedure. Two corticocancellous struts are placed in the excavated scaphoid through a volar approach. The remainder of the cavity is packed with cancellous chips. No power equipment is used, to avoid overheating the bone. The curetted interior surfaces of the scaphoid are closely inspected for evidence of vascularity. (*Green, D. P.: The Effect of Avascular Necrosis on Russe Bone Grafting for Scaphoid Nonunion. J. Hand Surg. [Am.], 10:597–605, 1985.*)

85% to 97% for Russe grafting of stable scaphoid nonunions.[24,34,155,395] The need for internal fixation of undisplaced fractures has been questioned by some, but a recent study demonstrated 97% healing rate in combining a Russe procedure with internal fixation.

Our preference and treatment of choice for scaphoid nonunion is volar grafting quite similar to the approach modified by Russe.[112] The bone graft is a combination corticocancellous graft. Russe (as reported by Green)[231] has recommended using a double cortical graft placed side by side (see Fig. 8-66). His technique emphasizes the need to remove the avascular bone and fibrous tissue through a volar bone window, thoroughly excavating both the proximal and distal poles with a curette. We prefer a corticocancellous graft from the iliac crest, which is inset volarly and serves to bridge the fracture gap and correct any displacement or angulation of the scaphoid that has occurred. Supplemental fixation with a K-wire(s) is preferred. Postoperative immobilization in a long-arm thumb spica cast is maintained for 6 weeks. The K-wires are removed and a short-arm thumb spica is worn until fracture union is demonstrated on tomography. A radial styloid or radial metaphysis bone graft can be selected, but the ilium offers a stronger, more compact, trabecular graft that is easier to sculpt for proper fill. Vascularized bone grafts from the distal radius (radial artery)[255,306] or distal ulna (ulnar artery)[236] have been described.

The presence of diminished vascularity of the proximal scaphoid[79] is not a contraindication to a volar inlay bone graft. If fracture union can be achieved, the avascular necrosis will resolve. The time to union is, however, slower and the rate of nonunion is increased. Therefore, it is advantageous to confirm avascular necrosis to determine length and prognosis for successful treatment.[12] Methods of assessing avascular necrosis include bone scan, tomography, and MRI.[175] The latter technique is undoubtedly the most sensitive and specific, but does not provide sequential information on revascularization. Tomography is a better method of assessing fracture union and resolution of avascular changes. The only definitive test for confirming avascular necrosis, however, is a surgical biopsy and the observation at surgery of presence or absence of bleeding from bone. Green[231] reported that when the proximal pole was *completely* avascular (lack of bone bleeding), a definite decrease in the rate of union was noted. If the proximal scaphoid is *completely* avascular, an alternative procedure such as intercarpal fusion,[548] excision of the proximal scaphoid,[158] interposition arthroplasty,[46] or scaphoid allograft[98] should be considered.

Electrical Stimulation. Electrical stimulation (pulsed electromagnetic stimulation—PEMS) has been proposed for undisplaced scaphoid nonunion.[5,43,67,199] Studies suggest that it has a role for fractures 3 to 6 months old. In a study of 44 nonunited fractures that were at least 6 months old, union was achieved in 35, combining electrical stimulation and a thumb spica cast.[199] This study and an unpublished report[43] demonstrated better union with a long-arm cast than a short-arm thumb spica cast. Union rates from these series were 80% and 92%, respectively. The length of stimulation varied from 8 to 10 hours per day. The controversy regarding the use of electrical stimulation in the treatment of scaphoid nonunions, however, remains unsettled, because there have been no controlled patient series comparing cast immobilization alone with electrical stimulation in these studies. Its use in unstable, angulated, displaced nonunions is not indicated. Newer types of pulsed electromagnetic fields with a shorter stimulation period are now available, but there have been no reports on their use in treatment of scaphoid nonunions.

UNSTABLE NONUNIONS

From the work of Fisk[182,183] and later Linscheid and colleagues,[329] instability of the carpus as a result of scaphoid nonunion has had increased recognition. Displaced scaphoid fractures are more difficult to diagnose[168] and treat, and nonunions of the scaphoid with displacement have a lower rate of union with an increased potential for radioscaphoid arthritis.[95,117,307,342,462] Techniques to improve scaphoid alignment by palmar and radiopalmar bone grafting have developed in order to correct scaphoid malalignment[18,184] and to restore normal scaphoid length.[177,178] A number of authors have reported their experience with interposition bone grafting for displaced scaphoid nonunions with internal fixation such as the Herbert screw,[70,121,346] conventional lag screw,[178] or multiple K-wires.[177]

The indications for interposition grafting include gross motion at the nonunion site, scaphoid resorption, and loss of carpal height.[184,331] The operative procedure involves an anterior interposition bone graft, with size based on comparative scaphoid views of the opposite wrist and intraoperative measurements. Using an extended volar Russe approach between the radial artery and flexor carpi radialis, the scaphoid is exposed. A gap is noted as the nonunion is debrided. With the two fragments gently distracted and aligned, reduction is held with a K-wire. The size of the defect is measured in width and depth, and with an oscillating saw the exact dimensions of the graft are removed from the iliac crest. With the graft in place and the scaphoid reduced and held with a K-wire, a Herbert screw is inserted by the technique described by its originator (Fig. 8-67). If there is marked DISI angulation of the lunate, it is best to reduce the lunate and proximal scaphoid by flexing the wrist and pinning the lunate in a reduced position through the radial styloid first.[331,401] An alternative procedure is to use multiple K-wires as described by Fernandez (see Fig. 8-60).[177]

The results of treatment in our series demonstrated a union rate of 81%, although two cases required a secondary interposition graft.[121] Carpal instability as measured by the scapholunate angle was corrected from a preoperative mean of 65° to a postoperative mean of 54°. The capitolunate angle improved from 15° to 3.5°, and the carpal height ratio improved from 0.51 to postoperative 0.54. Complications were related to incorrect placement of the Herbert screw and to resorption of the bone graft. This usually was associated with failure of healing to the proximal pole. Interposition grafting is currently preferred when the volar gap exceeds 3 mm or more. A modification of the Russe procedure using a cross-shaped corticocancellous graft or an extended Russe bicortical graft inserted into the troughs in either pole to prop the scaphoid open for restoration of length may also be used (Fig. 8-68).

A radial approach with partial radial styloidectomy may be indicated in patients with a severe humpback scaphoid deformity, in order to judge the necessary degree of corrective realignment. The dorsal osteophyte of the humpback should be excised to assist in the reduction. This procedure should be chosen with caution, because the traditional Matti–Russe graft has a superior union rate and is capable of correcting mild carpal instability. The Russe technique remains the gold standard to which other scaphoid grafting procedures must be compared.

It may be difficult to completely correct carpal instability in long-standing cases, and these patients may be better served by various salvage procedures.

LUNATE FRACTURES (KIENBÖCK'S DISEASE)

Fractures of the lunate are relatively uncommon[44,99,260,384,522] and often unrecognized, at least until they progress to osteochondrosis of the lunate, at which time they become symptomatic and are diagnosed as Kienböck's disease.[83,287,522] The latter is a condition for which no consistently reliable treatment has been found, and it produces significant disability in a generally young and productive segment of society.[44,368,467] The problem encompasses several aspects of wrist injuries that result in early neglect. First, the injury may be considered a sprain and ignored by the patient. Second, initial x-rays may be negative, because the fracture line remains occult for several weeks, as sometimes seen in the scaphoid. Third, because the lunate is covered by superimposed images of the radius, ulna, and other carpal bones, even lateral x-rays may be read as normal (Fig. 8-69). Fourth, osteonecrosis may be the result of interruption of the vascular supply to the lunate,[216,260,287] which shows no x-ray evidence of injury until sclerosis and osteochondral collapse are seen. Finally, reconstitution of the lunate to its former condition has so far evaded our surgical abilities.[466] There is a recognition that this entity is more prevalent in patients with an ulnar minus variant. Much of the current treatment

methods are based on trying to redistribute the compressive forces across the joint to unload the collapsing part of the lunate. The value of revascularization techniques has so far been unsubstantiated in controlled series.

ANATOMY

The lunate sits like a keystone in the proximal carpal row in the well-protected concavity of the lunate fossa of the radius, anchored on either side by the interosseous ligaments to the scaphoid and triquetrum with which it articulates (see Fig. 8-9). Distally, the convex capitate head fits congruently into the concavity of the lunate. The joint reaction force from the capitate and radius squeezes the lunate ulnarly. The proximal horn of the hamate has a variable articular facet on the distal ulnar surface of the lunate, and ulnar deviation increases the degree of contact of these two bones. The vascular supply of the lunate is primarily through the proximal carpal arcade both dorsally and palmarly.[364] Both Lee[312] and Gelberman and associates[213] have shown the intralunate anastomoses to be of three main types, which can be characterized as I, Y, and X (see *Vascular Anatomy*) (see Fig. 8-11). The degree of cross flow between the two systems probably is subject to considerable variation, and the redundancy available for adequate perfusion of the bone is unknown.

MECHANISMS OF INJURY

Most patients with fractures of the lunate have a history of a dorsiflexion injury, such as a fall on the outstretched hand.[14] Occasionally repetitive use of the hand or a strenuous push will give rise to a "snap" in the wrist. In dorsiflexion, the lunate is displaced onto the volar aspect of the lunate fossa and rotated into extension. The capitate drives against the palmar horn and at the same time pushes the lunate ulnarly. This is resisted by the radiolunate ligament, which exerts tension at its lunate insertion. If there is an ulnar minus variant,[406] the support offered by the TFC and ulnar head will be minimal, and even less when the hand is pronated. The compressive stresses over the proximal convexity of the lunate shift dramatically at the interface between the TFC and radial articular surface. The lack of ulnar support may also allow proximal displacement of the triquetrum, placing further tensile stress on the lunate surface through the lunotriquetral ligament. This appears to provide

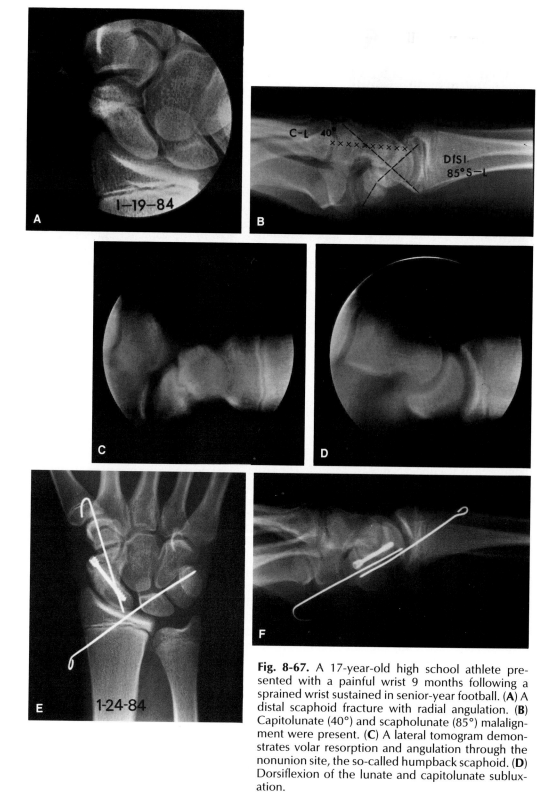

Fig. 8-67. A 17-year-old high school athlete presented with a painful wrist 9 months following a sprained wrist sustained in senior-year football. (**A**) A distal scaphoid fracture with radial angulation. (**B**) Capitolunate (40°) and scapholunate (85°) malalignment were present. (**C**) A lateral tomogram demonstrates volar resorption and angulation through the nonunion site, the so-called humpback scaphoid. (**D**) Dorsiflexion of the lunate and capitolunate subluxation.

(continued)

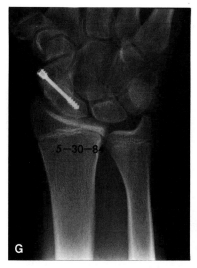

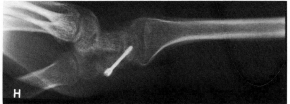

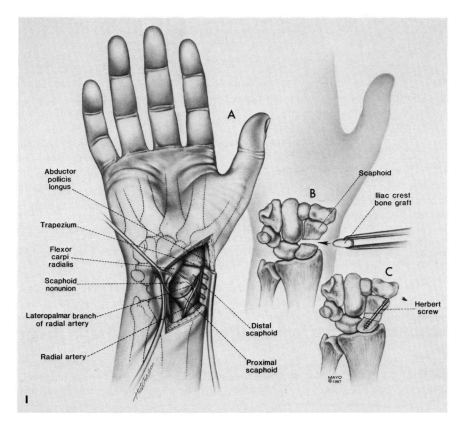

Fig. 8-67. *(continued)*
(E, F) Open reduction, interposition volar wedge bone graft with internal fixation was performed. The proximal scaphoid and lunate were reduced first and pinned; the distal scaphoid was reduced with the interposition bone graft in place and pinned; the Herbert screw was inserted. **(G, H)** Scaphoid union and correction of carpal instability was obtained. **(I)** Operative approach for anterior wedge graft using an extended Russe incision to the scaphotrapezial joint (*A*); interposition iliac crest bone graft (*B*) and internal fixation with Herbert screw (*C*). (**I**: Cooney, W. P.; Linscheid, R. L.; Dobyns, J. H.; and Wood, M. B.: Scaphoid Non-union: Role of Interposition Bone Grafts. J. Hand Surg. [Am.] 13:635–650, 1988.)

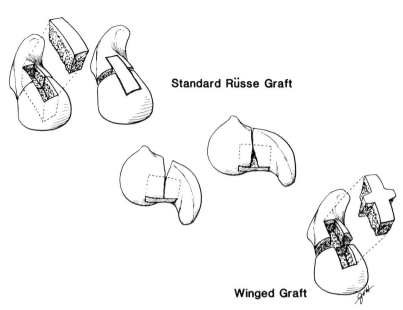

Standard Rüsse Graft

Winged Graft

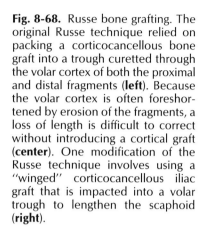

Fig. 8-68. Rüsse bone grafting. The original Rüsse technique relied on packing a corticocancellous bone graft into a trough curetted through the volar cortex of both the proximal and distal fragments (**left**). Because the volar cortex is often foreshortened by erosion of the fragments, a loss of length is difficult to correct without introducing a cortical graft (**center**). One modification of the Rüsse technique involves using a "winged" corticocancellous iliac graft that is impacted into a volar trough to lengthen the scaphoid (**right**).

a reasonable scenario for the transverse fractures that occur in the sagittal plane (see Fig. 8-69). Avulsions of the dorsal pole are more likely due to tension that develops in the scapholunate ligament, because these are frequently seen with SLD. Avulsion fractures of the ulnar aspect of the palmar pole are usually associated with a perilunar dislocation variant. It is also possible that sufficient stress develops where the arteries penetrate the bone to induce devascularization. In this situation, avascularity would precede fracture, rather than vice versa. Indeed, there is considerable evidence that both mechanisms can be responsible for Kienböck's disease.[20,448]

CLASSIFICATION

Fresh fractures of the lunate include dorsal and volar horn avulsion fractures, usually more often from the radial corner than from the ulnar corner.[201] Fractures in the body are most often transverse in the coronal plane. The more common of these is between the mid and volar thirds of the body. A fracture in the sagittal plane suggests that the differential stress across the radioulnar step-off is causative. Collapse of the radial aspect of the lunate is more apparent than on the ulnar side.

Part of the difficulty in describing fractures of the lunate is that the fragmentation that occurs in Kienböck's disease presents confusion between an initiating fracture and the fragmentation due to secondary subcortical collapse patterns.[9] Kienböck's disease is often classified in four or five stages according to the Stahl,[499] DeCoulx,[138] or Lichtman[319] classifications (Table 8-4; Fig. 8-70). This is based on the posteroanterior x-ray appearance, which gives only a partial picture of the condition of the lunate. Ideally, polyaxial or computed tomography should be used for classification purposes.[9,51] Radiodensity changes alone are unreliable criteria for Kienböck's disease, for which the characteristic change is deformity. Not all radiodense lunates deform; if they do not do so, the unique problems associated with Kienböck's disease do not develop.

RADIOGRAPHIC FINDINGS

After the scaphoid, the lunate is the next most fractured carpal bone. As already emphasized, the fracture may be difficult to visualize early, because an undisplaced crack is often hidden by the superimposed structures. The best example is that provided by the palmar cortical line of the radial styloid, which is aligned with the division between the dorsal and palmar thirds of the lunate, where a transverse fracture often occurs. The anteroposterior view of this is in a plane almost perpendicular to the fracture, which is overlapped by the radial rims and, therefore, is not apparent. The palmar horn of the lunate is hidden by the pisiform and scaphoid shadows. For these reasons clinical suspicion must take precedence over the findings on plain films.[378] A Tc[99] bone scan will be positive within 24 hours of injury. Oblique films will help to throw minute

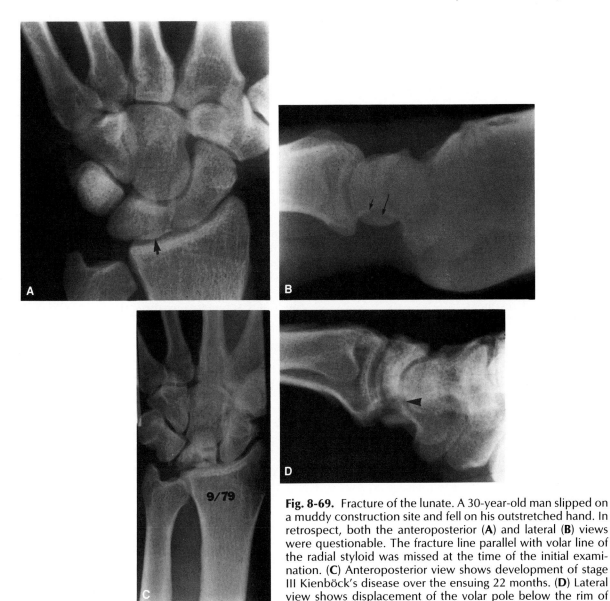

Fig. 8-69. Fracture of the lunate. A 30-year-old man slipped on a muddy construction site and fell on his outstretched hand. In retrospect, both the anteroposterior (**A**) and lateral (**B**) views were questionable. The fracture line parallel with volar line of the radial styloid was missed at the time of the initial examination. (**C**) Anteroposterior view shows development of stage III Kienböck's disease over the ensuing 22 months. (**D**) Lateral view shows displacement of the volar pole below the rim of the radius.

fracture lines into focus on some occasions, but polyaxial tomograms, preferably of the trispiral type, allow the most thorough review (Fig. 8-71). Distraction of a transverse fracture by the intrusion of the capitate, for instance, is easily recognized on tomography but seldom on plain films. Palmar subluxation of the capitate with a palmar horn fracture of the lunate is unlikely to be missed on tomography. When osteonecrotic changes have supervened, they are often apparent in some detail by tomog-

raphy before there is more than a suspicion on regular films. The stage of osteonecrosis is frequently noted to be more advanced than was apparent on standard x-rays. It is also possible to differentiate the primary fracture from the secondary fractures associated with fragmentation. Fragmentation and collapse generally affect the lunate overlying the radial contact area, especially in those wrists with an ulna minus variant.[170,215,302,406] Additional findings that may be of importance in treatment are

Table 8-4. Kienböck's Disease: Classification of Radiographic Stages (Stahl/Lichtman)

Stages

   I: Normal appearance or linear or compression fracture (on tomogram)
  II: Bone density change (sclerosis); slight collapse of radial border.
 III: Fragmentation, collapse, cystic degeneration; loss of carpal height; capitate proximal migration; scaphoid rotation (S-L dissociation).
  IV: Advanced collapse; scaphoid rotation; sclerosis; osteophytes of the radiocarpal joint.

(After Lichtman, D.M.; Alexander, A.H.; Mack, G.R.; and Gunther, S.F.: Kienböck's Disease: Update on Silicone Replacement Arthroplasty. J. Hand Surg., 7:343, 1982.)

the carpal height ratio[361] and the radioscaphoid angle, as a measure of carpal collapse. MRI has also increased our appreciation of the vascular changes that occur within a few days of injury.[20,496] As the cost of this procedure falls, it will assume increasing importance in assessment.

EPONYMS

Kienböck's disease is the well-known eponym for avascular necrosis with deformity of the carpal lunate. It is also described as lunatomalacia, osteonecrosis, and osteochondritis of the lunate.

TREATMENT

Acute Lunate Fractures

The most important factor in treating a fractured lunate is recognition that the fracture may progress to carpal instability, nonunion, or avascular necrosis. Under no circumstances should even a simple fracture of the lunate be treated expectantly in a cast or splint without provision for follow-up studies at close intervals for the first several weeks. Ideally, this should include tomography and, in some instances, MRI. If there is evidence of separation of the lunate fragments by the intrusion of the capi-

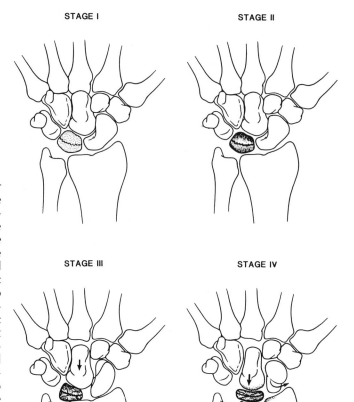

STAGE I   STAGE II

STAGE III   STAGE IV

Fig. 8-70. Staging of Kienböck's disease (after Lichtman). *Stage I:* Routine x-rays (PA, lateral) are normal but tomography may show a linear fracture; usually transverse through the body of the lunate. MRI will confirm avascular changes. *Stage II:* Bone density increase (sclerosis) and a fracture line are usually evident on the PA x-ray. PA and lateral tomograms demonstrate sclerosis, cystic changes, and often a clear fracture. There is no collapse deformity. *Stage III:* Advanced bone density changes are present with fragmentation, cystic resorption, and collapse. The diagnosis is evident from PA x-ray Tomograms (PA, lateral) demonstrate the degree of lunate infractionation and amount of fracture displacement. Proximal migration of the capitate is present and there is mild to moderate rotary alignment of the scaphoid. *Stage IV:* Perilunate arthritic changes are present with complete collapse and fragmentation of the lunate. Carpal instability is evident with scaphoid malalignment and capitate displacement into the lunate space.

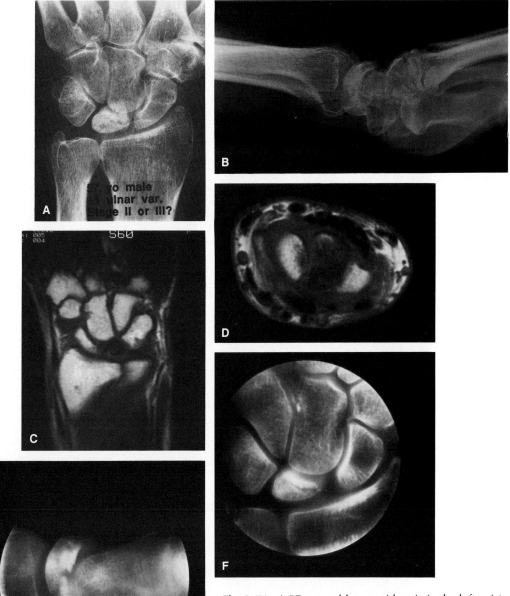

Fig. 8-71. A 57-year-old man with pain in the left wrist after a fall. (**A**) Posteroanterior view shows sclerosis of the lunate, with a +1 ulnar variance. (**B**) Displacement of the volar pole of the lunate. (**C, D**) MRI, showing avascularity of the entire lunate. (**E, F**) Trispiral tomograms. (**E**) Lateral view shows displacement of the volar pole, extrusion of fragments by the capitate, and collapse of the proximal cortical area. (**F**) Sclerosis of the lunate, increased scapholunate space, and intratrabecular collapse.

Fig. 8-72. A 20-year-old garageman injured his wrist when a tire iron slipped. (**A**) Normal left wrist; infractionation and early collapse of the right lunate; ulnar −2 mm. (**B, C**) Anteroposterior and lateral tomograms demonstrate a fracture through the volar pole of the lunate.

(continued)

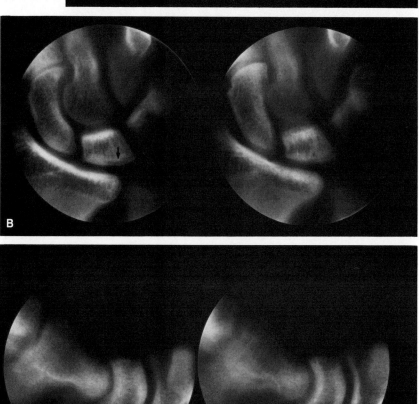

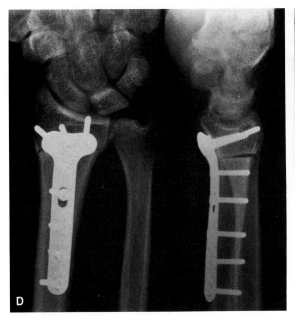

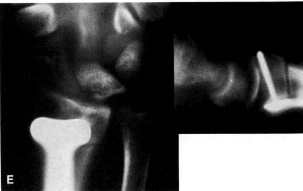

Fig. 8-72 *(continued)*
(D, E) Radial recession to create +1 mm ulnar variance; at 6 weeks. **(D)** healing is apparent on the 12-week tomograms **(E)**.

tate, union will not be possible and the risk of avascular necrosis is sharply increased. The concentration of compressive stresses at the acute angulation of the fracture site prevents the establishment of intraosseous anastomoses.[256] Although the efficacy of internal fixation of the lunate is unproven and the obstacles to successful reduction and fixation are substantial, the consequences of inaction are quite certain. Distraction with an external fixator may allow the lunate fragments to coapt. If there is an ulnar minus variant, a levelling procedure, such as radial recession[15,291] or ulnar lengthening,[27,459,526] can reduce the joint compressive stresses (Fig. 8-72).[15,291,383,404,419,434,508,513,526,529] Immobilization during the expectant period should include a long-arm or Munster-type cast, well molded over the wrist to compress the lunate area.

ESTABLISHED KIENBÖCK'S DISEASE

When Kienböck's disease is established, levelling procedures seem to be the most efficacious approaches to treatment.[467] They do not violate the proximal row, as do the excision replacement procedures,[96,256,285,434,457,511,551,557] and they do relieve forces on the lunate.[433,457,511] Several long-term studies show adequate symptomatic relief and return to work following radial shortening[15,404] or ulnar lengthening.[27] The revascularization procedures[190] have not yet fulfilled their expectations,[16,190] especially without long-term simulta-

neous decompressive procedures.[380,390] Salvage procedures include proximal row carpectomy and arthrodesis. Excision and prosthetic replacements are rarely indicated for acute fractures,[319] and are now seriously questioned for late cases because of silicone synovitis.[96,293,433]

Prognosis

Healing of undisplaced lunate fractures, especially of avulsion injuries at the dorsal or volar horns, is relatively good. A transverse fracture of the body will heal if it remains undisplaced, particularly in adolescents. Nonunion of a lunate body fracture is rare, because most progress to Kienböck's disease. Carpal collapse may occur in advanced Kienböck's disease (stages III, IV). The progressive disintegration of the lunate leads to degenerative changes. Over some years, some of these tend to stabilize and the symptoms may become tolerable at a decreased functional level. Others progress to radiolunate and capitolunate arthritis. Prompt treatment of lunate fractures and early operative intervention, therefore, seems warranted.

COMPLICATIONS OF CARPAL BONE INJURIES

REFRACTURE

The incidence of refracture in the carpal bones is unknown. However, the frequent reinjury of the wrist associated with scaphoid fractures that appear to be healing at 8 or even 12 weeks but are found a few years later to have nonunion suggest that refracture is not infrequent. The use of a protective splint for a considerable time, even after the fracture is thought to be healed, is recommended. Follow-up should be more carefully monitored longer than for other fractures. If clinical findings or routine x-rays are questionable, the status of union should be checked by polytomography, CT scan, or special x-rays, such as giant views.[367]

NERVE INJURY

Nerve injury is relatively uncommon with carpal injuries.[41,297,532] Almost all dislocations and fracture–dislocations of the carpus have at least transient median-nerve symptoms, and many have a sufficient neuropathy to suggest axonotmesis. Those with immediate significant signs of neuropathy are more likely due to direct contusion, hematoma or stretching of the nerve. Those with slowly increasing signs during the first week are more likely due to an incipient carpal tunnel syndrome aggravated by the injury.

Other carpal injuries associated with neuropathy are fractures of the hamate hook[257] and the pisiform, both of which render the juxtaposed ulnar nerve susceptible to injury.[11] Damage to the articular nerve branches may be responsible for chronic wrist sprain pain, eg, the dorsal interosseous nerve at the radiocarpal interval. Damage to the dorsal sensory branches of the radial or ulnar nerves is probably due most often to the pressure of the support apparatus (splint or cast), rather than to direct injury. Vascular injury of significant degree associated with carpal injuries is uncommon.

NONUNION

Nonunion occurs in several of the carpal bones probably because of intermittent forceful compressive stresses, the difficulty of maintaining immobility, and frequent lack of early diagnosis. Scaphoid nonunion[117] is the most common, but similar problems have been observed in the capitate,[195,276,288,375] lunate, pisiform, and hook of hamate.[59,502] Malunion and delayed union also occur for the same reasons.[18] Treatment of nonunion by closed methods may be successful, but malunion must be avoided. Open reduction with bone graft to restore carpal bone configuration and carpal height is often preferable.

PAIN DYSFUNCTION SYNDROME

Dysfunction and dystrophy,[17,28,65,292,418] which combine to be a common serious complication of wrist injuries, can be best introduced by a quotation from John Rhea Barton.

> I do not know of any subject on which I have been more frequently consulted than on deformities, rigid joints, inflexible fingers, loss of the pronating and supinating motions and on neuralgic complaints resulting from injuries of the wrist, and of the carpal extremity of the forearm—one or more of these evils have been left, not merely as a temporary inconvenience, but as a permanent consequence.[35]

The many disabilities that lead to upper limb dysfunction, often referred to as the shoulder–hand syndrome, are common complications of wrist injuries, particularly those that occur in the older age group. The dramatic presentation of the causalgia type[379] has drawn particular attention to the effect of reflex sympathetic dystrophy in such conditions.[379] Nevertheless, the number of cases in which this is the principal factor is relatively small. Shoulder–hand syndrome is a better choice, because the shoulder and hand are the most commonly involved, and hand and wrist involvement more than shoulder involvement.[382] The forearm, elbow, shoulder-girdle, and neck are less commonly involved with pain and limitation of motion.

To cover this spectrum of disabilities, we use the term *pain dysfunction syndrome*.[17] The common denominator of all forms is that of dysfunction, usually precipitated by pain which may be focal, multiple-sited, or even referred.[418]

Other causes of functional inhibition include fear, neurosis, anxiety, and even volition. Sudeck's atrophy or osteoporosis associated with pain and dysfunction is one portion of the spectrum that occurs after carpal injuries and particularly after median nerve irritation.[507] The osteoporosis commonly seen after carpal injury is usually a disuse phenomenon, not the Sudeck type. Treatment consists in identifying and coping with as many of the causes as possible. The most common physiologic pain sources are (1) the injury area generally, (2) autonomic dysfunction, (3) peripheral nerve elements, (4) synovial lined structures, and (5) musculoskeletal trigger areas.[17] Successful treatment of one source alone may allow resolution. More often there are multiple sources that require treatment. Active psychiatric support may be needed. More often evaluation and recommendations are useful with regard to (1) estimates of the degree of neurotic, psychotic, or motivational enhancement of the problem; (2) drug dependency or utility of drugs in management; and (3) suitability of the patient for surgery, for a pain-management center, and so forth. The number of patients with some degree of pain dysfunction syndrome argues for a prophylatic plan that includes (1) control of pain, first by insuring that treatment methods, such as cast or external fixation frames, are not causative; (2) control of dysfunction, beginning with relaxation and rehabilitation techniques for the injured part; and (3) monitoring and graduated retraining to work-level function. Assume that this process will take a year—be happy when it does not.

ISCHEMIC CONTRACTURES

Closed compartment syndromes, both of the forearm or Volkmann type and of the intrinsic compartments of the hand, are not uncommon, particularly if associated with a crush injury.[541] Thus, rigid encasements must be avoided, and careful attention must be paid to all severe and increasing pains that are referred to muscle, nerve, or vascular compartments. If rest, elevation, and resilient bulky dressings are unavailing, measurement of compartment pressures followed by surgical decompression is indicated when positive. Narcotics to control pain following fractures or dislocations are rarely indicated. Dressings (cast, splints) should be first removed and appropriate studies, such as compartment pressure measurements, made. Impending contractures (ischemia) must be promptly treated.

POSTTRAUMATIC CHANGES

Stress fracture has seldom been noted in the carpus.[202,266] However, osteolytic and cystic changes, secondary to episodes of single or repetitive stress, have been reported, especially in certain athletes. In boxers, a condition similar to carpe bossu or os styloideum has been noted, with ridging and exostosis formation, secondary to chondral changes at the carpometacarpal, intercarpal, or intermetacarpal joints of index and mid finger.[87] Similar chondral defects, eburnation, and ridging have been noted at areas of joint impingement where contact occurs during extreme dorsiflexion at the radioscaphoid joint, as in gymnastics. Similar impingement syndromes, usually with considerably more exostosis formation, are seen after dorsal chip fractures of the carpus or Colles' fractures. Associated with these or presenting alone are other posttraumatic residua that include intra-articular menis-

coids, osteochondral fragments, and localized areas of synovitis and ganglion formation.

OTHER COMPLICATIONS

Skin loss, infection, and pathologic fractures are rare and do not warrant discussion. Injuries to neighboring muscles and joints are uncommon from acute carpal injuries, although the secondary arthrosis may, much later, lead to damage of the deep flexors or the extensors. Traumatic arthritis is present to some degree in almost all carpal injuries and may be severe, depending on the degree of chondral-surface damage. Fibrous ankylosis of the carpal joints is associated with the extent of traumatic arthrosis, the degree and persistence of hemorrhage and edema, the length of immobility, and the position during immobilization. The wrist, ankylosed in flexion, makes satisfactory hand function impossible.

INJURIES OF THE DISTAL RADIOULNAR JOINT

Injuries of the distal radioulnar joint (DRUJ) are recognized as integral parts of other fractures including Colles', Smith's, Essex-Lopresti's, and Galeazzi's fractures.[92,108,164,371] They are often relegated to secondary consideration. Until recently, excision of the ulnar head was considered an easy and safe way of dealing with symptoms related to the DRUJ. An increasing awareness of secondary problems after excision has diminished this popularity, and a number of alternatives are now considered preferable. There are a significant number of localized injuries to the DRUJ and ulnar aspect of the wrist.[133,241,250] The diagnosis of many of these problems is difficult because physical and x-ray findings are often subtle or confusing. Interest in the problems of the DRUJ has increased considerably since the first edition of this book.

SURGICAL ANATOMY

The DRUJ provides the distal joint for forearm rotation, the axis of which runs from the center of the radial head proximally to the foveal area of the ulnar head distally (Fig. 8-73).[73,162,280,310,457] The ulnar head has two articular surfaces: the pole, which supports the carpal articulation and is covered by the TFC; and the seat, which articulates with the sigmoid notch of the radius. The TFC is a complex

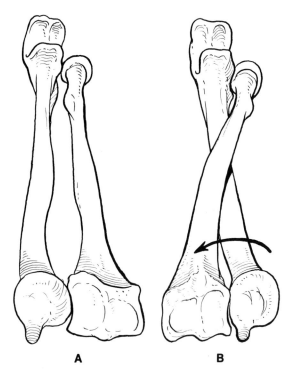

Fig. 8-73. (**A**) In supination, the ulnar head rests against the volar rim of the sigmoid notch. (**B**) In pronation, the ulnar head rests against dorsal lip of the sigmoid notch.

homogenous structure, composed of the dorsal and volar radioulnar ligaments, the articular disc,[108] "meniscus homologue," ulnar collateral ligament, and floor of the sixth dorsal compartment.[317,318,370] The TFC transfers force from the carpus to the ulna, extends the radiocarpal articulation, constrains the ulnocarpal joint, and stabilizes the DRUJ.[290] The radioulnar ligaments arise along the margins of the sigmoid notch of the radius and follow a helical course to converge to an insertion on the base of the ulnar styloid and the fovea of the ulnar pole.[280] On cross section,[289] the ulnar head is slightly elliptical and presents its major axis to the shallow sigmoid notch when in the neutral position. The seat of the ulnar head slides dorsally on the shallow articular crescent of the sigmoid notch during pronation and volarly with supination.[162] This accounts for the greater prominence of the ulnar head clinically with pronation. The dorsal and volar radioulnar ligaments that provide the boundaries of the TFC aid in guiding this motion.[427] The dorsal limb of the TFC becomes taut on pronation and vice versa. Only in the neutral position can the ulnar head be ballotted dorsovolarly to test stability, a

finding more apparent in lax-jointed individuals. There is also a variable amount of longitudinal play in the joint with pronosupination, radioulnar deviation, and forceful grasp. The TFC acts to some extent as a shock absorber between the carpus and the ulnar head.[428]

The relative length of the ulna to the radius is described as ulna variance, which is measured when the forearm is at rest with the elbow and shoulder flexed 90° and the wrist is in neutral flexion–extension and radial–ulnar deviation.[425] Neutral variance is present if the pole of the ulnar head is level with the articular concavity of the lunate fossa in a line perpendicular to the anatomical axis of the forearm. Statically in the ulnar neutral wrist, the relative load across the radioulnar complex is 80% radial and 20% ulnar. With 4 mm of ulna plus, the load changes to approximately 60% radial and 40% ulnar, whereas with an ulna minus the entire load is assumed by the radius.[427] There is increasing evidence to suggest that ulna variance plays a part in a number of symptomatic responses to injury and sustained use.

The final important stabilizer of the DRUJ is provided by the extensor carpi ulnaris (ECU), which lies in a tendon sheath in a groove on the ulnar head radial to the styloid process.[498] It has been suggested that the floor of the sheath and the tendon act as a static and dynamic collateral ligament, respectively.[427] As it is fixed to the ulna, its relative position changes from a dorsoulnar to ulnovolar as the radius moves from full supination to pronation. The dorsal and volar capsules of the DRUJ are lax and provide minimal support.

MECHANISMS OF INJURY

The DRUJ is subjected to a variety of stresses during everyday activity as well as from falls, twisting injuries, and overloads.[369] The joint is particularly vulnerable when in pronation.[92,457,495] The ulnar head lies on the dorsal rim of the sigmoid notch, and is also dorsal to the carpus. With ulnar deviation, the triquetrum compresses the TFC into the palmar aspect of the ulnar head. With hyperpronation the ulnar ligament complex is twisted tautly about the palmarly displaced ulnar styloid, forcing the ulnar head dorsally.[259,495] Both of these mechanisms will force further dorsal subluxation of the ulnar head and disrupt the dorsal capsule and the TFC.[242] Palmar dislocation of the ulnar head invariably occurs with the forearm loaded in supination, where the stretched volar capsule provides little support to resist a pronatory torque applied to the heel of the palm.[125,134,457] The volar radioulnar ligament is capable of providing the dislocating force. Each of these mechanisms may induce chondromalacia of the seat of the ulnar head by shear stress to the cartilage surfaces as they override the rims of the sigmoid notch (Fig. 8-74). The tip of the ulnar styloid may be avulsed or sheared off. A fracture through the base of the ulnar styloid suggests an avulsion of the TFC insertions. The TFC may also be injured by direct compression or shearing stresses between the ulnar head and carpus. An ulna plus variant is often associated with these injuries. Likewise, the radial origins or ulnar insertions may be avulsed by the above mechanisms and can be associated with injury to the tendon sheaths, carpal ligaments, and joints in close proximity.[73,186]

CLASSIFICATION

By convention we speak of dorsal and palmar dislocations of the ulnar head. Chondromalacia or os-

teochondral defects of the ulnar seat may be associated with these injuries or with a lax ligamentous habitus. TFC injuries and ulnolunate impactions are often related to a positive ulna variance. A broad classification follows, recognizing there are often subtleties and interrelations that may occur.[515]

Dislocations/subluxations:[189,377,391,420]
    Ulna dorsal—with or without chondromalacia or osteochondral fracture
    Ulna volar—with or without accompanying radial fracture
Posttraumatic arthrosis:
    Ulnar pole
    Sigmoid notch of radius, with or without intra-articular radial fracture
    Ulnar seat
TFC injuries:[371,409,422]
    Acute tears
        central, radial rim, intralaminar, foveal, styloidal

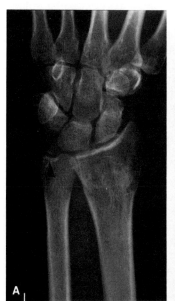
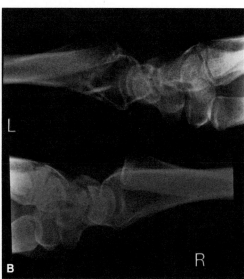
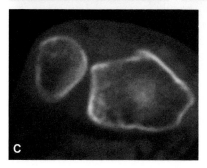

Fig. 8-74. (**A**) Anteroposterior: an ulnar styloid fracture and narrowed distal radioulnar joint of the left wrist. (**B**) Lateral: dorsal subluxation of the left ulnar head (**top**) in comparison to normal right wrist (**bottom**). Note that the ulnar head lies well above the triquetral silhouette. (**C**) CT scan showing dorsal subluxation of the ulnar head.

Chronic tears
  stellate central, ragged radial rim, ulnar surface, styloidal
Styloid fractures:
  Tip, osteochondral
  Mid-styloid
  Base—with or without TFC disruption; radioulnar instability
  Ulnar head—with or without avulsion, floor of sixth compartment, with or without displacement

Impaction injuries:
  Ulnocarpal—functional, ulna plus variance, with or without TFC perforation
  Ulnolunate—chronic, ulnar or lunate cortical sclerosis, cyst formation
  Triquetrostyloid—elongated styloid process, triquetral rim avulsion?
ECU subluxation:[91]
  Lax ligamentous habitus
Associated ulnocarpal injuries or conditions
  Lunatotriquetral tears—with or without ulnocarpal impingement
  Triquetrohamate impaction
  Triquetropisiform chondromalacia
  Osteochondral loose bodies
  Occult carpal fractures
  Carpal instabilities

SIGNS AND SYMPTOMS

Pain on the ulnar aspect of the wrist, usually accentuated with certain movements, and weakness are common complaints.[391,515] Limitation of some motions, snapping, and "giving way" may be included. Dorsal subluxation of the ulna is suggested by ulnar head prominence when the forearm is pronated and by marked limitation of supination.[420] A positive "piano key" sign is a classic sign of instability. Palmar dislocation is evident by apparent narrowing of the forearm, a dimple where the ulnar head should be, and limited pronation. Chondromalacic pain may be elicited with ballottement of the distal ulna in various positions of forearm rotation. TFC tear and ulnocarpal impingement symptoms may be exaggerated by compressing the ulnar head and pisiform between index finger and thumb, followed by ulnar deviation.[409] Tenderness is elicited by pressure at the sulcus below the ulnar styloid. Crepitus is occasionally found during forearm rotation and radioulnar deviation. Disruption of the TFC insertions on the ulna allows an increased passive mobility of the ulnar head on the radius, especially as compared with the opposite wrist. Styloid fractures and loose bodies present with localized tenderness directly over the styloid. ECU subluxation is demonstrated by turning both supinated forearms toward the examiner and forcibly resisting ulnar deviation. This causes the affected tendon to slip out of its groove and bowstring ulnarly. Lunatotriquetral tears are tender directly over the joint, and the symptoms are exaggerated by ballottement dorsovolarly or by triquetral displacement from the ulnar aspect. Triquetrohamate pain is accentuated by extension and ulnar deviation, while pisotriquetral degenerative changes are reproduced by grinding the bones together.

RADIOGRAPHIC FINDINGS

Confirmation of a dorsal ulnar dislocation is often difficult on plain films but usually quite evident on a cross-sectional view with a CAT scan (see Fig. 8-74C).[289,377,420] This will also show fractures and deformity of the sigmoid notch and osteochondral defects. A volar dislocation is easily recognized on a CAT scan but is also usually apparent on plain films, when carefully examined, because the ulnar head is superimposed beneath the edge of the sigmoid notch on the anteroposterior (coronal) view and displaced volar to the radius on the sagittal (lateral) view (Fig. 8-75). An ulna plus variant is often seen on the x-rays of patients with TFC tears, ulnocarpal impingements, lunatotriquetral tears.[425]

Arthrograms can be helpful,[49] but some care may be necessary to prevent a false negative.[451] The prestyloid recess and the pisotriquetral spaces are normal and must not be considered evidence of injury. A two- or three-phase study sequentially injecting the midcarpal, radiocarpal, and distal radioulnar joints is sometimes indicated to be sure that a torn flap of the TFC or lunatotriquetral ligament is not blocking the flow of dye. These studies should be done under the image intensifier and recorded on videotape during wrist motions. Extra-articular disruption of the TFC at the ulnar styloid, for instance, will not be seen on most radiocarpal studies, but would be revealed on a DRUJ study. Fractures may require special views on occasion. Ulnolunate impaction sclerosis and cystic changes are readily identified on tomography. MRI studies will be increasingly valuable, because they show effusions in the DRUJ, chondral lesions, and often the TFC and ligament tears.

TREATMENT

Dorsal subluxation, recognized early, will respond to reduction with the forearm in supination and

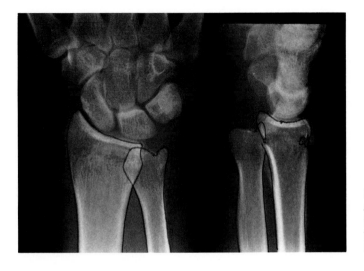

Fig. 8-75. Palmar dislocation of the ulnar head associated with a minimally displaced distal radial fracture. There is narrowing of the anteroposterior silhouette and widening of the lateral silhouette, both clinically and on x-ray.

held in a long-arm cast for 6 weeks.[8] A variety of operations for chronic dislocations have been suggested. These usually employ an augmentation of the ligamentous structures with a strip of tendon.[258] Repair of a peripherally torn TFC should be included. We prefer to include tightening of the ulnocarpal capsule to this repair, because there is often a concomitant carpal supination.

A fresh volar dislocation[133] may reduce with manipulation and pronation, but open reduction is readily justified because the ulnar head is sometimes locked on the under surface of the radius (see Fig. 8-75). Access between the ulnar neurovascular bundle and the flexor profundi tendons will allow the ulna to be pried back into position. An osteochondral indentation may be noted. Immobilization in pronation is usually sufficient to prevent redislocation.

Repair of a torn TFC or ulnar styloid fracture is justified.[409] The same is true when a peripheral injury destabilizes the ulnar TFC by fracturing the styloid or tears the styloid insertion, especially in the athlete or active younger adult. Such repairs can prevent chronic radioulnar instability. A more extensive tearing of the floor of the sixth compartment and ulnocarpal ligaments may be seen. Small ulnar styloid fractures are seldom of significance, but fractures through the base usually imply that the integrity of the TFC is compromised. Immobilization is preferred for 6 weeks, but if there is marked displacement, open reduction with internal fixation should be considered.

Central and radial tears of the TFC may be treated by several methods.[363,426] Arthroscopy enthusiasts have popularized arthroscopic debridement of the central portion of the TFC as the treatment of choice because of the rapid rehabilitation. A "wafer" excision of a few millimeters of the distal ulna, preserving the radioulnar joint, has shown good results. In our hands, there have also been satisfactory results with ulnar recession (Fig. 8-76).[136] This preserves the ulnar head intact, corrects the ulnar plus variance, allows the TFC to heal or be repaired, and provides exposure for concomitant repair of the lunatotriquetral ligament, if indicated. The obvious disadvantage is the presence of an ulnar plate and a longer healing period. Other occasional procedures are pisiformectomy, ulnar styloid excision, triquetral cheilotomy, and loose body removal.

Excision of the ulnar head, the Darrach procedure,[135,148,163] is occasionally indicated when there is irreparable damage in the DRUJ. In some patients the results appear to be quite good,[247] while in others ulnar head excision is disastrous (Fig. 8-77).[53,339,372] Those patients most likely to have a poor result are young women with a loose-jointed habitus. Narrowing of the interosseous space occurs associated with instability of the ulnar stump, impaction of the stump against the radius, and snapping with rotary motions. Later the radius shows scalloping, the ulnar stump remodels into a penciled appearance, and there is persistent weakness.[53] Reconstructive procedures at this stage are unpredictable and often lead to multiple operations. Partial ulnar head excisions with preservation of the styloid and its attachments, with or without soft tissue interposition, may provide better stability but are not free of complications.[74] Preservation of the DRUJ by recession,[72] corrective angulatory osteotomy,[179] or ligamentous stabilizing procedures[80,259]

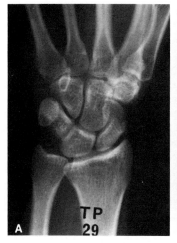
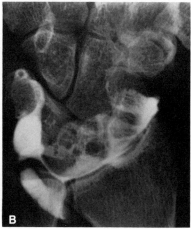
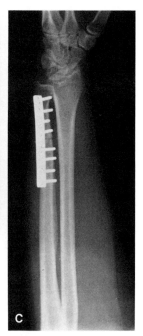

Fig. 8-76. A 29-year-old man with progressive ulnocarpal pain. (**A**) Ulnar plus 2 mm variance. (**B**) Triangular fibrocartilage perforation shown by arthrography. (**C**) Ulnar recession was performed, followed by 8 weeks cast immobilization. The patient was allowed to return to full activities, and he had no pain.

should take precedence, if at all possible. In malunited Colles' fractures, radial corrective osteotomies should be considered.

Dislocation of the ECU has been treated by augmenting the dorsal fascial roof of the sixth compartment with a leaf of the overlying dorsal retinaculum. A slip of flexor carpi ulnaris (FCU) brought through a drill hole to the ulnar side of the ECU groove and carried around the ulnar neck to

be sutured to itself provides a somewhat stronger repair.[91]

PROGNOSIS

Dorsal subluxations of the ulna will recur or worsen without adequate treatment, but are generally quite responsive to treatment as outlined. Palmar dislocations become firmly locked and difficult to reduce

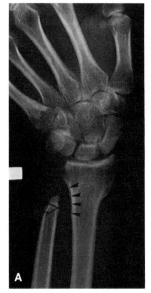
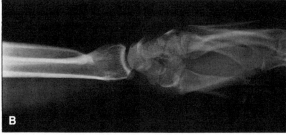

Fig. 8-77. A 28-year-old laborer had a distal radius fracture with moderate dorsal angulation and distal radioulnar joint discomfort. Excision of ulnar head resulted in increased weakness, snapping, and loss of rotation. PA (**A**) and lateral (**B**) x-rays show scalloping of radial metaphysis secondary to lunate stump impingement (*arrows*). A radial corrective osteotomy might have been a better alternative than resection of the distal ulna in this working man.

after 2 or 3 weeks. An osteochondral lesion will worsen with time, as will instabilities of the DRUJ. Symptoms of TFC tears may fluctuate but do not repair themselves spontaneously in most instances. The same is true of ulnar impaction syndromes and lunatotriquetral tears. Surgical treatment of these lesions as outlined is satisfactory.

COMPLICATIONS

Transient sensory symptoms may be the result of irritation of the ulnar nerve in Guyon's canal or at its dorsal sensory branch with the above conditions, although permanent damage is rare. The development of progressive instability is possible with the injuries that affect the TFC. Osteochondral lesions lead to degenerative arthritis, as do the impaction syndromes. Surgical procedures also occasionally develop complications, such as already discussed under the Darrach procedure. Failure of TFC and ligament repairs, as well as nonunion of ulnar osteotomies, occur at times.

PROGNOSIS IN CARPAL INJURIES

In general, the prognosis for recovery from these injuries is excellent, provided diagnosis is made early and appropriate management is carried out swiftly. The time for recovery varies, depending on the type of injury and the treatment requirements, particularly the length of time required for support and healing of damaged tissues. Recovery is practically never complete, if residual deformity involves a joint surface. Severe deformity, such as recurrent or persistent dislocation, collapse deformity or chondral damage, nearly always results in disability sufficient to warrant a reconstructive procedure such as excisional or fibrous arthroplasties, to partial carpal arthrodesis. These procedures, when properly selected, are adequate, but significant disability always results.

POSTTREATMENT CARE AND REHABILITATION OF CARPAL INJURIES

The type of support apparatus used for each condition has been included under the individual topics. Generally, palmar surface splints, combined with resiliant dressings, are used during the immediate posttrauma period of reaction and swelling. After this, the minimal support used should be a short-arm wrist support splint for such entities as dorsal chip fractures, and the maximal support should be a long-arm cast that includes all five digits for certain scaphoid fractures and other precarious carpal body fractures. Some external fixators or internal fixation may be secure enough to minimize external support. Dislocations and fracture–dislocations are treated with supports similar to those used in carpal body fractures, unless there has been associated internal fixation. K-wires, when used percutaneously or for open reduction, are usually left protruding, with the external portion bent at right angles to avoid migration. Antibiotic ointment is applied around the pin site. These cause little trouble (less so in our experience than do buried pins), but must be monitored closely for evidence of looseness or inflammation, or both.

Generally, inflammation is preceded by loosening of a pin. A loose pin should be removed immediately. The first sign of loosening is that the pin can be rotated with manual force alone. In most instances, even snug K-wires are removed in 6 to 8 weeks. The return of a complete range of motion, even in normal joints, can be expected to take about as long as the joint was totally immobilized. The return of comfort and full strength, as judged by the return of grip power and repetitive grip endurance, takes about four times as long as the time that the part was rigidly supported. Nevertheless, the permanently disabling residua associated with pain dysfunction syndrome[17] almost always can be avoided by careful attention to (1) instituting and maintaining shoulder elevation exercises throughout the course of treatment, (2) observing and halting the progression of any neurologic or circulatory deficits, (3) observing and remedying all pain and swelling, (4) avoiding extreme positioning of any joint or part, (5) initiating digit exercises as soon as feasible, and (6) bringing the wrist to a neutral or slightly extended position as soon as this is safe.

Shoulder exercises of the Codman type may be undertaken when some disability of the shoulder restricts elevation. However, the key shoulder exercise to avoid shoulder–hand syndrome is active elevation and rotation. This should be carried out a minimum of 50 times each day if possible. Almost any digit exercise is useful, provided a full range of possible motion is carried out, with the maximal force that is comfortable. Wiggling exercises are inadequate. To ensure that each joint has the maximal chance of being carried through its particular range of motion, we use a set of six exercises (the "six pack hand exercises"): (1) maximal extension of all digits, (2) thumb to each fingertip, (3) the grasp or fist exercise with all fingers flexing to the palmar crease or as near as possible to it, (4) the "claw" exercise with the metacarpophalangeal joints of the fingers kept extended but the interphalangeal joints maximally flexed, (5) the "tabletop" exercise with the metacarpophalangeal joints maximally flexed but the interphalangeal joints extended, and (6) abduction–adduction of all digits in the radioulnar plane.

With these precautions and a gradual increase of function with both duration and force carefully controlled, rehabilitation is seldom a problem. Occasionally, physical therapy modalities, manipulation under anesthesia, articular steroid injection, splinting, and particularly re-education may be required. Re-education with normal patterns of relaxation and integrated contraction are difficult, almost impossible if pain, apprehension, or distraction interfere. The principle resource here is a good, patient therapist, but chemical assistance, blocks, etc., may be needed. Inhibition of some or all of the motors that control the wrist and digits may be so ingrained a pattern that special training may be necessary. The most common instance of this is inhibition of the wrist extensors when pain is associated with wrist extension or when deformity decreases the moment arm distance between the center of wrist motion and the wrist extensor tendon. The patient attempts to extend the wrist with the finger extensors, making it impossible to extend the wrist and make a fist at the same time. The sooner this and other abnormal co-contractions can be identified and corrected, the smoother rehabilitation will be. Recovery from wrist injury is a challenging endeavor but it must be understood and successfully managed because the injury is frequent; loss of time, productivity, and important skills is common.

REFERENCES

1. Adams, B.D.; Blair, W.F.; Reagan, D.S.; and Grundberg, A.B.: Technical Factors Related to Herbert Screw Fixation. J. Hand Surg. [Am.], 13:893–899, 1988.

2. Adkinson, J.W., and Chapman, M.W.: Treatment of Acute Lunate and Perilunate Dislocations. Clin. Orthop., 164: 199–207, 1982.

3. Adler, J.M., and Shaftan, G.W.: Fractures of the Capitate. J. Bone Joint Surg. [Am.], 44:1537–1547, 1962.

4. Agerholm, J.C., and Goodfellow, J.W.: Avascular Necrosis of the Lunate Bone Treated by Excision and Prosthetic Replacement. J. Bone Joint Surg. [Br.], 45:110–116, 1963.

5. Ahl, T.; Andersson, G.; Herberts, P.; and Kalen, R.: Electrical Treatment of Non-United Fractures. Acta Orthop. Scand., 55:585–588, 1984.

6. Aitken, A.P., and Nalebuff, E.A.: Volar Transnavicular Perilunar Dislocation of the Carpus. J. Bone Joint Surg. [Am.], 42:1051–1057, 1960.

7. Albert, M.C., and Barre, P.S.: A Scaphoid Fracture Associated With a Displaced Distal Radial Fracture in a Child. Clin. Orthop., 240:232–235, 1989.

8. Albert, S.M.; Wohl, M.A.; and Rechtman, A.M.: Treatment of the Disrupted Radioulnar Joint. J. Bone Joint Surg. [Am.], 45:1373–1381, 1963.

9. Alexander, A.H., and Lichtman, D.M.: Kienböck's Disease. Orthop. Clin. North Am., 17:461–472, 1986.

10. Alexander, C.E., and Lichtman, D.M.: Ulnar Carpal Instabilities. Orthop. Clin. North Am., 15:307–320, 1984.

11. Ali, M.A.: Fracture of the Body of the Hamate Bone Associated with Compartment Syndrome and Dorsal Decompression of the Carpal Tunnel. J. Hand Surg. [Br.], 11:207–210, 1986.

12. Allen, P.R.: Idiopathic Avascular Necrosis of the Scaphoid: Report of Two Cases. J. Bone Joint Surg. [Br.], 65:333–335, 1983.

13. Allieu, Y.: Carpal Instability Revisited: Ligamentous Instabilities and Intracarpal Malalignments. Ann. Chir. Main, 3:317–321, 1984.

14. Almquist, E.E.: Kienbock's Disease. Clin. Orthop., 202: 68–78, 1986.

15. Almquist, E.E., and Burns, J.F.: Radial Shortening for the Treatment of Kienbock's Disease—A Five to Ten Year Follow-Up. J. Hand Surg., 7:348–352, 1982.

16. Alnot, J.Y.; Badelon, O.; Sommariva, L.; Bocquet, L.; and Grossin, M.: Necrotic Bone Segment Revascularization by the Transfer of a Vascular Bundle. Experimental Study in the Rat. Ann. Chir. Main, 1:274–276, 1982.

17. Amadio, P.C.: Current Concepts Review. Pain Dysfunction Syndromes. J. Bone Joint Surg., 70[Am.]:944–949, 1988.

18. Amadio, P.C.; Berquist, T.H.; Smith, D.K.; Ilstrup, D.M.; Cooney, W.P.; and Linscheid, R.L.: Scaphoid Malunion. J. Hand Surg. [Am.], 14:679–687, 1989.

19. Amadio, P.C., and Botte, M.J.: Treatment of Malunion of the Distal Radius. Hand Clin., 3:541–559, 1987.

20. Amadio, P.C.; Hanssen, A.D.; and Berquist, T.H.: The Genesis of Kienbock's Disease: Evaluation of a Case by Magnetic Resonance Imaging. J. Hand Surg. [Am.], 12: 1044–1049, 1987.

21. Amamilo, S.C.; Uppal, R.; and Samuel, A.W.: Isolated Dislocation of Carpal Scaphoid. J. Hand Surg. [Br.], 10:385–388, 1985.

22. Anderson, W.J.: Simultaneous Fracture of the Scaphoid and Capitate in a Child. J. Hand Surg. [Am.], 12:271–273, 1987.

23. Andress, M.R., and Peckar, V.G.: Fracture of the Hook of the Hamate. Br. J. Radiol., 43:141–143, 1970.

24. Andrews, J.; Miller, G.; and Haddad, R.: Treatment of Scaphoid Nonunion by Volar Inlay Distal Radius Bone Graft. J. Hand Surg. [Br.], 10:214–216, 1985.

25. Andrews, J.G., and Youm, Y.: A Biomechanical Investigation of Wrist Kinematics. J. Biomech., 12:83–83, 1979.

26. Andrianne, Y.; Donkerwolcke, M.; Hinsenkamp, M.; Quintin, J.; Rasquin, C.; El Banna, S.; and Burny, F.: Hoffman External Fixation of Fractures of the Radius and Ulna:

A Prospective Study of Fifty-Three Patients. Orthopedics, 7:845–850, 1984.

27. Armistead, R.B.; Linscheid, R.L.; Dobyns, J.H.; and Beckenbaugh, R.D.: Ulnar Lengthening in the Treatment of Kienböck's Disease. J. Bone Joint Surg. [Am.], 64:170–178, 1982.

28. Atkins, R.M.; Duckworth, T.; and Kanis, J.A.: Algodystrophy Following Colles' Fracture. J. Hand Surg. [Br.], 14: 161–164, 1989.

29. Auffray, Y., and Comtet, J.J.: The Role of Osteosynthesis of the Anterior Surface in Fractures of the Distal End of the Radius (in French). Lyon Med., 219:193–198, 1968.

30. Aufranc, O.E.; Jones, W.N.; and Turner, R.H.: Anterior Marginal Articular Fracture of Distal Radius. J.A.M.A., 196:788–791, 1966.

31. Aufranc, O.E.; Jones, W.N.; and Turner, R.N.: Transnavicular Perilunar Carpal Dislocation. J.A.M.A., 181:130–133, 1962.

32. Axelrod, T.; Paley, D.; Green, J.; and McMurtry, R.Y.: Limited Open Reduction of the Lunate Facet in Comminuted Intra-Articular Fractures of the Distal Radius. J. Hand Surg. [Am.], 13:372–377, 1988.

33. Balfour, G.W.: Diagnosis of Oblique Fractures of the Distal Ulna Using an Extended Pronated View of the Wrist. Case Report. Orthopedics, 13:247–250, 1990.

34. Barnard, L., and Stubbins, S.G.: Styloidectomy of the Radius in the Surgical Treatment of Non-Union of the Carpal Navicular: A Preliminary Report. J. Bone Joint Surg. [Am.], 30:98–102, 1948.

35. Barton, J.R.: Views and Treatment of an Important Injury to the Wrist. Medical Examiner, 1:365, 1838.

36. Bartone, N.F., and Grieco, R.V.: Fractures of the Triquetrum. J. Bone Joint Surg. [Am.], 38:353–356, 1956.

37. Bartosh, R.A., and Saldana, M.J.: Intraarticular Fractures of the Distal Radius: A Cadaveric Study to Determine if Ligamentotaxis Restores Radiopalmar Tilt. J. Hand Surg. [Am.], 15:18–21, 1990.

38. Bassett, R.L.: Displaced Intraarticular Fractures of the Distal Radius. Clin. Orthop., 214:148–152, 1987.

39. Bassett, R.L., and Ray, M.J.: Carpal Instability Associated with Radial Styloid Fracture. Orthopedics, 7:1356–1361, 1984.

40. Bastillas, J.; Vasilas, A.; Pizzi, W.F.; and Gokcebay, T.: Bone Scanning in the Detection of Occult Fractures. J. Trauma, 21:564, 1981.

41. Bauman, T.D.; Gelberman, R.H.; Mubarak, S.J.; and Garfin, S.R.: The Acute Carpal Tunnel Syndrome. Clin. Orthop., 156:151–156, 1981.

42. Baumann, J.U., and Campbell, R.D. Jr.: Significance of Architectural Types of Fractures of the Carpal Scaphoid and Relation to Timing of Treatment. J. Trauma, 2:431–438, 1962.

43. Beckenbaugh, R.D.: Diagnosis and Treatment of Scaphoid Fracture Nonunion. Advances in Orthopaedics, Volume 1, Issue 3, 1985.

44. Beckenbaugh, R.D.; Shives, T.C.; Dobyns, J.H.; and Linscheid, R.L.: Kienbock's Disease: The Natural History of Kienbock's Disease and Consideration of Lunate Fractures. Clin. Orthop., 149:98–106, 1980.

45. Belsole, R.J.; Eikman, E.A.; and Muroff, L.R.: Bone Scintigraphy in Trauma of the Hand and Wrist. J. Trauma, 21:163–166, 1981.

46. Bentzon, P.G.K., and Madsen, A.R.: On Fracture of Carpal Scaphoid Bone. Method for Operative Treatment of Inveterate Fractures. Acta Orthop. Scand., 16:30–39, 1945.

47. Berger, R.A.; Blair, W.F.; Crowninshield, R.D.; and Flatt, A.E.: The Scapholunate Ligament. J. Hand Surg. 7:87–91, 1982.

48. Berger, R.A., and Blair, W.F.: The Radioscapholunate Ligament: A Gross and Histologic Description. Anat. Rec., 210:393–404, 1984.

49. Berger, R.A.; Blair, W.F.; and El-Khoury, G.Y.: Arthrotomography of the Wrist: The Triangular Fibrocartilage Complex. Clin. Orthop., 172:257–264, 1983.

50. Berger, R.A., and Landsmeer, J.M.F.: The Palmar Radiocarpal Ligaments: A Study of Adult and Fetal Human Wrist Joints. Iowa Orthop. J., 5:32–41, 1985.

51. Berquist, T.H. (ed.): Imaging of Orthopedic Trauma and Surgery. Philadelphia, W. B. Saunders, Company, 1986.

52. Bickerstaff, D.R., and Bell, M.J.: Carpal Malalignment in Colles' Fractures. J. Hand Surg. [Br.], 14:155–160, 1989.

53. Bieber, E.J.; Linscheid, R.L.; Dobyns, J.H.; and Beckenbaugh, R.D.: Failed Distal Ulna Resections. J. Hand Surg. [Am.], 13:193–200, 1988.

54. Bieber, E.J., and Weiland, A.J.: Traumatic Dorsal Dislocation of the Triquetrum: A Case Report. J. Hand Surg. [Am.], 9:840–842, 1984.

55. Bilos, J., and Hui, P.W.: Dorsal Dislocation of the Lunate with Carpal Collapse. J. Bone Joint Surg. [Am.], 63:1484–1486, 1981.

56. Bilos, Z.J.; Pankovich, A.M.; and Yelda, S.: Fracture–Dislocation of the Radiocarpal Joint. J. Bone Joint Surg. [Am.], 59:198–203, 1977.

57. Binkovitz, L.A.; Ehman, R.L.; Cahill, D.R.; and Berquist, T.H.: Magnetic Resonance Imaging of the Wrist. Radiographics, 8(6):1171–1202, 1988.

58. Biondelle, P.R.; Vannier, M.W.; Gilula, L.A.; and Knapp, R.: Wrist: Coronal and Transaxial Scanners. Radiology, 163:149–151, 1989.

59. Bishop, A.T., and Beckenbaugh, R.D.: Fracture of the Hamate Hook. J. Hand Surg. [Am.], 13:135–139, 1988.

60. Black, D.M.; Watson, H.K.; and Vender, M.I.: Scapholunate Gap with Scaphoid Nonunion. Clin. Orthop., 224:205–209, 1987.

61. Blatt, G.: Capsulodesis in Reconstructive Hand Surgery: Dorsal Capsulodesis for the Unstable Scaphoid and Volar Capsulodesis Following Excision of the Distal Ulna. Hand Clin., 3:81–102, 1987.

62. Blevens, A.D.; Light, T.R.; Jablonsky, W.S.; Smith, D.G.; Patwardhan, A.G.; Guay, M.E.; and Woo, T.S.: Radiocarpal Articular Contact Characteristics with Scaphoid Instability. J. Hand Surg. [Am.], 14:781–790, 1989.

63. Böhler, L.: The Treatment of Fractures. Translated by Tretter, H.; Luchini, H.B.; Kreuz, K.; Russe, O.A.; and Bjornson, R.G.B., from the 13th German ed. New York, Grune and Stratton, 1956.

64. Bollen, S.R.: Peri-Triquetral-Lunate Dislocation Associated

with Ulnar Nerve Palsy. J. Hand Surg. [Br.], 13:456–457, 1988.

65. Bonica, J.J.: Causalgia and Other Reflex Sympathetic Dystrophies. Postgrad. Med. 53:143, 1973.

66. Bonnel, F., and Allieu, Y.: The Radioulnocarpal and Midcarpal Joints: Anatomical Organisation and Biomechanical Basis. Ann. Chir. Main, 3:287–296, 1984.

67. Bora, F.W.; Osterman, A.L.; and Brighton, C.T.: The Electrical Treatment of Scaphoid Non-Union. Clin. Orthop., 161:33–38, 1981.

68. Botte, M.J.; Cooney, W.P.; and Linscheid, R.L.: Arthroscopy of the Wrist: Anatomy and Technique. J. Hand Surg. [Am.], 14:313–316, 1989.

69. Botte, M.J., and Gelberman, R.H.: Fractures of the Carpus, Excluding the Scaphoid. Hand Clin. 3:149–161, 1987.

70. Botte, M.J., and Gelberman, R.H.: Modified Technique for Herbert Screw Insertion in Fractures of the Scaphoid. J. Hand Surg. [Am.], 12:149–150, 1987.

71. Botte, M.J.; Mortensen, W.W.; Gelberman, R.H.; Rhoades, C.E.; and Gellman, H.: Internal Vascularity of the Scaphoid in Cadavers After Insertion of the Herbert Screw. J. Hand Surg. [Am.], 13:216–222, 1988.

72. Boulas, H.J., and Milek, M.A.: Ulnar Shortening for Tears of the Triangular Fibrocartilaginous Complex. J. Hand Surg. [Am.], 15:415–420, 1990.

73. Bowers, W.H.: Distal Radioulnar Joint. In Green, D.P. (ed.): Operative Hand Surgery, pp. 743–769. Philadelphia, J.B. Lippincott, 1982.

74. Bowers, W.H.: Distal Radioulnar Joint Arthroplasty: The Hemiresection–Interposition Technique. J. Hand Surg. [Am.], 10:169–178, 1985.

75. Boyes, J.H.: Bunnell's Surgery of the Hand, 4th ed., pp. 292–293. Philadelphia, J.B. Lippincott Company, 1964.

76. Bradway, J.K.; Amadio, P.C.; and Cooney, W.P.: Open Reduction and Internal Fixation of Displaced, Comminuted Intra-Articular Fractures of the Distal End of the Radius. J. Bone Joint Surg. [Am.], 71(6):839–847, 1989.

77. Brand, P.; Beach, R.B.; and Thompson, D.E.: Relative Tension and Potential Excursion of Muscles in the Forearm and Hand. J. Hand Surg., 6(3):209–219, 1981.

78. Bray, R.J.; Swafford, A. R.; and Brown, R.L.: Bilateral Fractures of the Hook of the Hamate. J. Trauma, 25:174–175, 1985.

79. Bray, T.J., and McCarroll, H.R. Jr.: Preiser's Disease: A Case Report. J. Hand Surg. [Am.], 9:730–732, 1984.

80. Breen, T.F., and Jupiter, J.B.: Extensor Carpi Ulnaris and Flexor Carpi Ulnaris Tenodesis of the Unstable Distal Ulna. J. Hand Surg. [Am.], 14:612–617, 1989.

81. Briggs, B.T.; Cooney, W.P.; and Linscheid, R.L.: Proximal Row Carpectomy (abstr.). Orthop. Trans., 2:216, 1978.

82. Broder, H.: Rupture of Flexor Tendons, Associated with a Malunited Colles Fracture. J. Bone Joint Surg. [Am.], 36:404–405, 1954.

83. Brolin, I.: Post-Traumatic Lesions of the Lunate Bone. Acta Orthop. Scand., 34:167–182, 1964.

84. Broome, A.; Cedell, C.A.; and Colleen, S.: High Plaster Immobilization for Fracture of the Carpal Scaphoid Bone. Acta Chir. Scand. 128:42–44, 1964.

85. Brown, D.E., and Lichtman, D.M.: Midcarpal Instability. Hand Clin., 3:135–140, 1987.

86. Brumbaugh, R.B.; Crowninschield, R.D.; Blair, W.F.; and Andrews, J.G.: An In-Vivo Study of Normal Wrist Kinematics. J. Biomech. Eng., 104:176–181, 1982.

87. Bryan, R.S., and Dobyns, J.H.: Fractures of the Carpal Bones Other Than Lunate or Navicular. Clin. Orthop., 149:107–111, 1980.

88. Bunker, T.D.; McNamee, P.B.; and Scott, T.D.: The Herbert Screw for Scaphoid Fractures. J. Bone Joint Surg. [Br.], 69:631–634, 1987.

89. Burgess, R.C.: The Effect of a Simulated Scaphoid Malunion on Wrist Motion. J. Hand Surg. [Am.], 12:774–776, 1987.

90. Burgess, R.C.: The Effect of Rotatory Subluxation of the Scaphoid on Radio-Scaphoid Contact. J. Hand Surg. [Am.], 12:771–774, 1987.

91. Burkhart, S.S.; Wood, M.B.; and Linscheid, R.L.: Posttraumatic Recurrent Subluxation of the Extensor Carpi Ulnaris Tendon. J. Hand Surg., 7:1–3, 1982.

92. Buterbaugh, G.A., and Palmer, A.K.: Fractures and Dislocations of the Distal Radioulnar Joint. Hand Clin., 4:361–375, 1988.

93. Cain, J.E. Jr.; Shepler, T.R.; and Wilson, M.R.: Hamatometacarpal Fracture–Dislocation: Classification and Treatment. J. Hand Surg. [Am.], 12:762–767, 1987.

94. Carrozzella, J., and Stern, P.J.: Treatment of Comminuted Distal Radius Fractures with Pins and Plaster. Hand Clin. 4:391–397, 1988.

95. Carrozzella, J.C.; Stern, P.J.; Murdock, P.A.: The Fate of Failed Bone Graft Surgery for Scaphoid Nonunions. J. Hand Surg. [Am.], 14:800–806, 1989.

96. Carter, P.R.; Benton, L.J.; and Dysert, P.A.: Silicone Rubber Carpal Implants: A Study of the Incidence of Late Osseous Complications. J. Hand Surg. [Am.], 11:639–644, 1986.

97. Carter, P.R.; Eaton, R.G.; and Littler, J.W.: Ununited Fracture of the Hook of the Hamate. J. Bone Joint Surg. [Am.], 59:583–588, 1977.

98. Carter, P.R.; Malinin, T.I.; Abbey, P.A.; and Sommerkamp, T.G.: The Scaphoid Allograft: A New Operation for Treatment of the Very Proximal Scaphoid Nonunion or for the Necrotic, Fragmented Scaphoid Proximal Pole. J. Hand Surg. [Am.], 14:1–12, 1989.

99. Cetti, R.; Christensen, S-E.; and Reuther, K.: Fracture of the Lunate Bone. Hand, 14:80–84, 1982.

100. Chamay, A., and Della Santa, D.: Cinematique du Poignet Rheumatoids Apres Resection de la Tete du Culitus. A Propos de 35 Cos. Ann. Chim., 34:711–718,1980.

101. Chapman, D.R.; Bennett, J.B.; Bryan, W.J.; and Tullos, H.S.: Complications of Distal Radial Fractures: Pins and Plaster Treatment. J. Hand Surg., 7:509–512, 1982.

102. Chen, S.C.: The Scaphoid Compression Test. J. Hand Surg. [Br.], 14:323–325, 1989.

103. Christodoulou, A.G., and Colton, C.L.: Scaphoid Fractures in Children. J. Pediatr. Orthop., 6:37–39, 1986.

104. Christophe, K.: Rupture of the Extensor Pollicis Longus Tendon Following Colles' Fracture. J. Bone Joint Surg. [Am.], 35:1003–1005, 1953.

105. Clancy, G.J.: Percutaneous Kirschner Wire Fixation of

Colles Fractures. J. Bone Joint Surg. [Am.], 66A:1008–1014, 1984.

106. Clyburn, T.A.: Dynamic External Fixation for Comminuted Intra-Articular Fractures of the Distal End of the Radius. J. Bone Joint Surg. [Am.], 69:248–254, 1987.

107. Cole, J.M., and Obletz, B.E.: Comminuted Fractures of the Distal End of the Radius Treated by Skeletal Transfixion in Plaster Cast: An End-Result Study of Thirty-Three Cases. J. Bone Joint Surg. [Am.], 48:931–945, 1966.

108. Coleman, H.M.: Injuries of the Articular Disc at the Wrist. J. Bone Joint Surg. [Br.], 42:522–529, 1960.

109. Coll, G.A.: Palmar Dislocation of the Scaphoid and Lunate. J. Hand Surg. [Am.], 12:476–480, 1987.

110. Colles, A.: On the Fracture of the Carpal Extremity of the Radius. Edinb. Med. Surg. J. 10:182–186, 1814.

111. Conyers, D.J.: Scapholunate Intraosseous Reconstruction and Imbrication of the Palmar Carpal Ligaments. J. Hand Surg., 15[Am.]:690–700, 1990.

112. Conway, W.F.; Gilula, L.A.; Manske, P.R.; Kriegshauser, L.A.; Rholl, K.S., Resnik, C.: Translunate, Palmar Perilunate Fracture–Subluxation of the Wrist. J. Hand Surg. [Am.], 14:635–639, 1989.

113. Cooney, W.P.: External Fixation of Distal Radius Fractures. Clin. Orthop., 180:44–49, 1983.

114. Cooney, W.P.; Bussey, R.; Dobyns, J.H.; and Linscheid, R.L.: Difficult Wrist Fractures: Perilunate Fracture–Dislocations of the Wrist. Clin. Orthop., 214:136–147, 1987.

115. Cooney, W.P.; Dobyns, J.H.; and Linscheid, R.L.: Complications of Colles' Fractures. J. Bone Joint Surg. [Am.], 62:613–619, 1980.

116. Cooney, W.P.; Dobyns, J.H.; and Linscheid, R.L.: Fractures of the Scaphoid: A Rational Approach to Management. Clin. Orthop., 149:90–97, 1980.

117. Cooney, W.P.; Dobyns, J.H.; and Linscheid, R.L.: Nonunion of the Scaphoid: Analysis of the Results from Bone Grafting. J. Hand Surg., 5:343–354, 1980.

118. Cooney, W.P.; Garcia-Elias, M.; Dobyns, J.H.; and Linscheid, R.L.: Anatomy and Mechanics of Carpal Instability. Surgical Rounds for Orthopaedics, 1:15–24, 1989.

119. Cooney, W.P.; Linscheid, R.L.; and Dobyns, J.H.: Carpal Instability: Ligament Repair and Reconstruction. *In* Neviaser, R.J. (ed.): Controversies in Hand Surgery, pp. 125–145. New York, Churchill Livingstone, 1990.

120. Cooney, W.P.; Linscheid, R.L.; and Dobyns, J.H.: External Pin Fixation for Unstable Colles' Fractures. J. Bone Joint Surg. [Am.], 61:840–845, 1979.

121. Cooney, W.P.; Linscheid, R.L.; Dobyns, J.H.; and Wood, M.B.: Scaphoid Nonunion: Role of Anterior Interpositional Bone Grafts. J. Hand Surg. [Am.], 13:635–650, 1988.

122. Cooney, W.P.; Ripperger, R.R.; and Linscheid, R.L.: Distal Pole Scaphoid Fractures. Orthop. Trans., 4:18, 1980.

123. Cordrey, L.J., and Ferrer-Torells, M.: Management of Fractures of the Greater Multangular. Report of Five Cases. J. Bone Joint Surg. [Am.], 42:1321–1322, 1963.

124. Corfitsen, M.; Christensen, S.E.; and Cetti, R.: The Anatomical Fat Pad and the Radiological "Scaphoid Fat Stripe." J. Hand Surg. [Br.], 14:326–328, 1989.

125. Cox, F.J.: Anterior Dislocation of the Distal Extremity of the Ulna. Surgery, 12:41–45, 1942.

126. Crabbe, W.A.: Excision of the Proximal Row of the Carpus. J. Bone Joint Surg. [Br.], 46:708–711, 1964.

127. Crosby, E.B., and Linscheid, R.L.: Rupture of the Flexor Profundus Tendon of the Ring Finger Secondary to Ancient Fracture of the Hook of the Hamate: Review of the Literature and Report of Two Cases. J. Bone Joint Surg. [Am.], 56:1076, 1974.

128. Crosby, E.B.; Linscheid, R.L.; and Dobyns, J.H.: Scaphotrapezial Trapezoidal Arthrosis. J. Hand Surg., 3:223–234, 1978.

129. Curtiss, P.H. Jr.: The Hunchback Carpal Bone. J. Bone Joint Surg. [Am.], 43:392–394, 1961.

130. Czitrom, A.A.; Dobyns, J.H.; and Linscheid, R.L.: Ulnar Variance in Carpal Instability. J. Hand Surg. [Am.], 12:205–208, 1987.

131. Czitrom, A.A., and Lister, G.D.: Measurement of Grip Strength in the Diagnosis of Wrist Pain. J. Hand Surg. [Am.], 13:16–19, 1988.

132. Dalinka, M.K.; Turner, M.L.; Osterman, A.L.; and Batra, P.: Wrist Arthrography. Radiol. Clin. North Am., 19:217, 1981.

133. Dameron, T.B. Jr.: Traumatic Dislocation of the Distal Radio-ulnar Joint. Clin. Orthop., 83:55–63, 1972.

134. Darrach, W.: Anterior Dislocation of the Head of the Ulna. Ann. Surg., 56:802–803, 1912.

135. Darrach, W.: Partial Excision of Lower Shaft of Ulna for Deformity Following Colles' Fracture. Ann. Surg., 57:764–765, 1913.

136. Darrow, J.C.; Linscheid, R.L.; Dobyns, J.H.; Mann, J.M.; Wood, M.B.; and Beckenbaugh, R.D.: Distal Ulnar Recession for Disorders of the Distal Radioulnar Joint. J. Hand Surg. [Am.], 10:482–491, 1985.

137. De Beer, J.DeV., and Hudson, D.A.: Fractures of the Triquetrum. J. Hand Surg. [Br.], 12:52–53, 1987.

138. Decoulx, P.; Duquency, A.; and Ammau-Stein, J.: Maladie da Kienboch. Traitment Chirurgical. Lille Chir., 231–250, 1965.

139. Dehne, E.; Deffer, P.A.; and Feighney, R.E.: Patho Mechanics of the Fracture of the Carpal Navicular. J. Trauma, 4:96–113, 1964.

140. DeMaagd, R.L., and Engber, W.D.: Retrograde Herbert Screw Fixation for Treatment of Proximal Pole Scaphoid Nonunions. J. Hand Surg. [Am.], 14:996–1003, 1989.

141. De Oliveira, J.C.: Barton's Fractures. J. Bone Joint Surg. [Am.], 55:586–594, 1973.

142. DePalma, A.F.: Comminuted Fractures of the Distal End of the Radius Treated by Ulnar Pinning. J. Bone Joint Surg. [Am.], 34:651–662, 1952.

143. deQuervain, F.: Clinical Surgical Diagnosis for Students and Practitioners. (Translated from 4th ed. by J. Snowman.) New York, William Wood & Co., 1913.

144. Desault, P.J.: A Treatise on Fractures, Luxations and Other Affections of the Bones (Bichat X. [ed.], and Caldwell C. [trans.]). Philadelphia, Fry & Kammerer, 1805.

145. Destot, E.A.J.: Injuries of the Wrist. A Radiological Study (Atkinson, F.R.B. [trans.]). New York, Paul B. Hoeber, 1926.

146. Dias, J.J.; Thompson, J.; Barton, N.J.; and Gregg, P.J.: Suspected Scaphoid Fractures: The Value of Radiographs. J. Bone Joint Surg. [Br.], 72:98–101, 1990.

147. Dick, H.M.: Wrist Arthrodesis. *In* Green, D.P. (ed.): Operative Hand Surgery, 2nd ed., vol. 1, pp. 155–166. New York, Churchill Livingstone, 1988.

148. Dingman, P.V.C.: Resection of the Distal End of the Ulna (Darrach Operation): An End-Result Study of Twenty-Four Cases. J. Bone Joint Surg. [Am.], 34:893–900, 1952.

149. Dobyns, J.H.: Invited Comment: Ligamentous Reconstruction for Chronic Intercarpal Instability (article by Glickel, S.Z.; and Millender, L.H.). J. Hand Surg. [Am.], 9:526–527, 1984.

150. Dobyns, J.H.; Beckenbaugh, R.D.; Bryan, R.S.; Cooney, W.P.; Linscheid, R.L.; and Wood, M.B.: Fractures of the Hand and Wrist. *In* Flynn, J.E. (ed.): Hand Surgery, 3rd ed., pp. 111–180. Baltimore, Williams & Wilkins, 1982.

151. Dobyns, J.H., and Linscheid, R.L.: Complications of Fractures and Dislocations of the Wrist. *In* Epps, C.H. Jr. (ed.): Complications in Orthopaedic Surgery, vol. 1, pp. 271–352. Philadelphia, J.B. Lippincott, 1978.

152. Dobyns, J.H., and Linscheid, R.L.: Fractures and Dislocations of the Wrist. *In* Rockwood, C.A. Jr., and Green, D.P. (eds.): Fractures, pp. 345–440. Philadelphia, J.B. Lippincott, 1975.

153. Dobyns, J.H.; Linscheid, R.L.; Chao, E.Y.S.; Weber, E.R.; and Swanson, G.E.: Traumatic Instability of the Wrist. A.A.O.S. Instr. Course Lectures, 24:182–199, 1975.

154. Dobyns, J.H.; Linscheid, R.L.; and Cooney, W.P.: Fractures and Dislocations of the Wrist and Hand, Then and Now. J. Hand Surg., 8:687–691, 1983.

155. Dobyns, J.H.; Linscheid, R.L.; and Macksoud, W.S.: Proximal Row Instability Nondissociative. Orthop. Trans., 9:574, 1985.

156. Dooley, B.J.: Inlay Bone Grafting for Non-Union of the Scaphoid Bone by the Anterior Approach. J. Bone Joint Surg. [Br.], 50:102–109, 1968.

157. Dupuytren, B.: On the Injuries and Diseases of Bones (Le Gros Clark, F. [ed., trans.]). London, Sydenham Society, 1847.

158. Dwyer, R.C.: Excision of the Carpal Scaphoid for Ununited Fractures. J. Bone Joint Surg. [Br.], 31:572–577, 1949.

159. Eckenrode, J.F.; Louis, D.S.; and Greene, T.L.: Scaphoid-Trapezium-Trapezoid Fusion in the Treatment of Chronic Scapholunate Instability. J. Hand Surg. [Am.], 11:497–502, 1986.

160. Eddeland, A.; Eiken, O.; Hellgren, E.; and Ohlsson, N.M.: Fractures of the Scaphoid. Scand. J. Plast. Reconstr. Surg., 9:234–239, 1975.

161. Egawa, M., and Asai, T.: Fracture of the Hook of the Hamate. Report of Six Cases and the Suitability of Computerized Tomography. J. Hand Surg., 8:393–398, 1983.

162. Ekenstam, F.W.: The Distal Radio Ulnar Joint. An Anatomical, Experimental and Clinical Study with Special Reference to Malunited Fractures of the Distal Radius [thesis]. Uppsala Universitet, 1984, pp. 1–55.

163. Ekenstam, F.W.; Engkvist, O.; and Wadin, K.: Results From Resection of the Distal End of the Ulna After Fractures of the Lower End of the Radius. Scand. J. Plast. Reconstr. Surg., 16:177–181, 1982.

164. Ekenstam, F.W.; Jakobsson, O.P.; and Wadin, K.: Repair of the Triangular Ligament in Colles' Fracture. No Effect in a Prospective Randomized Study. Acta Orthop. Scand., 60:393–396, 1989.

165. Ekenstam, F.W., Palmer, A.K., and Glisson, R.R.: The Load on the Radius and Ulna in Different Positions of the Wrist and Forearm. Acta Orthop. Scand. 55:363–365, 1984.

166. Ellis, J.: Smith's and Barton's Fractures: A Method of Treatment. J. Bone Joint Surg. [Br.], 47:724–727, 1965.

167. Ender, H.G., and Herbert, T.J.: Treatment of Problem Fractures and Nonunions of the Scaphoid. Orthopedics, 12:195–202, 1989.

168. Engdahl, D.E., and Schacherer, T.G.: A New Method of Evaluating Angulation of Scaphoid Nonunions. J. Hand Surg. [Am.], 14:1033–1034, 1989.

169. Engel, J.; Salai, M.; Yaffe, B.; and Tadmor, R.: The Role of Three Dimension Computerized Imaging in Hand Surgery. J. Hand Surg. [Br.], 12:349–352, 1987.

170. Epner, R.A., and Bowers, W.H.: Ulnar Variance—The Effect of Wrist Positioning and Roentgen Filming Technique. J. Hand Surg., 7:298–305, 1982.

171. Erdman, A.G.; Mayfield, J.K.; Dorman, F.; Wallrich, M.; and Dahlof, W.: Kinematic and Kinetic Analysis of the Human Wrist By Steroscopic Instrumentation. J. Biomech. Eng., 101:124–133, 1979.

172. Failla, J.M., and Amadio, P.C.: Recognition and Treatment of Uncommon Carpal Fractures. Hand Clin., 4:469–476, 1988.

173. Faulkner, D.M.: Bipartite Carpal Scaphoid. J. Bone Joint Surg., 10:284–289, 1928.

174. Fenton, R.L.: The Naviculo-Capitate Fracture Syndrome. J. Bone Joint Surg. [Am.], 38:681–684, 1956.

175. Ferlic, D.C., and Morin, P.: Idiopathic Avascular Necrosis of the Scaphoid: Preiser's Disease? J. Hand Surg. [Am.], 14:13–16, 1989.

176. Fernandes, H.J.A.; Koberle, G.; Ferreira, G.H.S.; and Camargo, J.N. Jr.: Volar Transscaphoid Perilunar Dislocation. Hand 15:276–280, 1983.

177. Fernandez, D.L.: A Technique for Anterior Wedge-Shaped Grafts for Scaphoid Nonunions with Carpal Instability. J. Hand Surg. [Am.], 9:733–737, 1984.

178. Fernandez, D.L.: Anterior Bone Grafting and Conventional Lag Screw Fixation to Treat Scaphoid Nonunions. J. Hand Surg. [Am.], 15:140–147, 1990.

179. Fernandez, D.L.: Correction of Post-Traumatic Wrist Deformity in Adults by Osteotomy, Bone Grafting, and Internal Fixation. J. Bone Joint Surg. [Am.], 64:1164, 1982.

180. Fernandez, D.L., and Ghillani, R.: External Fixation of Complex Carpal Dislocations: A Preliminary Report. J. Hand Surg. [Am.], 12:335–347, 1987.

181. Fick, R.: Handbuch der Anatomie und Mechanik der Gelenke: Unter Berucksichtigung der Bewegenden Muskeln. I. Anatomie der Gelenke. II. Allgemeine Gelenk und Muskelmechanik. III. Spezielle Gelenk und Muskelmechanik. Jena, Gustav Fischer Verlag, 1904–1911.

182. Fisk, G.R.: Carpal Instability and the Fractured Scaphoid. Ann. R. Coll Surg. Edinb., 46:63–76, 1970.

183. Fisk, G.R.: An Overview of Injuries of the Wrist. Clin. Orthop., 149:137–144, 1980.

184. Fisk, G.R.: The Wrist: Review Article. J. Bone Joint Surg. [Br.], 66:396–407, 1984.

185. Fitzgerald, J.P.; Peimer, C.A.; and Smith, R.J.: Distraction Resection Arthroplasty of the Wrist. J. Hand Surg. [Am.], 14:774–781, 1989.

186. Flatt, A.E.: Biomechanics of the Hand and Wrist. *In* Evarts, C.M. (ed.): Surgery of the Musculoskeletal System, 2nd ed., vol. I, pp. 311–329. New York, Churchill Livingstone, 1990.

187. Ford, D.J.; Khoury, G.; El-Hadidi, S.; Lunn, P.G.; and Burke, F.D.: The Herbert Screw for Fractures of the Scaphoid: A Review of Results and Technical Difficulties. J. Bone Joint Surg. [Br.], 69:124–127, 1987.

188. Fornage, B.D.; Schernberg, R.L.; and Rifkin, M.D.: Ultrasound Examination of the Hand. Radiology, 155:785–788, 1985.

189. Foster, R.J., and Hansen, S.T.: Management of Acute Distal Radioulnar Dislocations Associated with Radial Shaft Substance Loss. J. Hand Surg. [Am.], 10:72–75, 1985.

190. Foucher, G., and Saffar, P.L.: Revascularization of the Necrosed Lunate, Stages I and II, with a Dorsal Intermetacarpal Arteriovenous Pedicle. J. Chir. Main., 1:259, 1982.

191. Foucher, G.; Schuind, F.; Merle, M.; and Brunelli, F.: Fractures of the Hook of the Hamate. J. Hand Surg. [Br.], 10:205–210, 1985.

192. Fourrier, P.; Bardy, A.; Roche, G.; Cisterne, J.P.; and Chambon, A.: Approach to a Definition of Mal-Union Callus After Pouteau–Colles Fractures. Int. Orthop. 4:299–305, 1981.

193. Freeland, A.E., and Finley, J.S.: Displaced Dorsal Oblique Fracture of the Hamate Treated with a Cortical Mini Lag Screw. J. Hand Surg. [Am.], 11:656–658, 1986.

194. Freeland, A.E., and Finley, J.S.: Displaced Vertical Fracture of the Trapezium Treated with a Small Cancellous Lag Screw. J. Hand Surg. [Am.], 9:843–845, 1984.

195. Freeman, B.H., and Hay, E.L.: Nonunion of the Capitate: A Case Report. J. Hand Surg. [Am.], 10:187–190, 1985.

196. Frykman, E.: Dislocation of the Triquetrum: Case Report. Scand. J. Plast. Reconstr. Surg., 14:205, 1980.

197. Frykman, E.B.; Ekenstam, F.; and Wadin, K.: Triscaphoid Arthrodesis and Its Complications. J. Hand Surg. [Am.], 13:844–849, 1988.

198. Frykman, G.: Fracture of the Distal Radius Including Sequelae—Shoulder Hand-Finger Syndrome, Disturbance in the Distal Radio-Ulnar Joint, and Impairment of Nerve Function: A Clinical and Experimental Study. Acta Orthop. Scand., 108(suppl.):1–153, 1967.

199. Frykman, G.K.; Taleisnik, J.; Peters, G.; Kaufman, R.; Helal, B.; Wood, V.E.; and Unsell, R.S.: Treatment of Nonunited Scaphoid Fractures by Pulsed Electromagnetic Field and Cast. J. Hand Surg. [Am.], 11:344–349, 1986.

200. Frykman, G.K.; Tooma, G.S.; Boyko, K.; and Henderson, R.: Comparison of Eleven External Fixators for Treatment of Unstable Wrist Fractures. J. Hand Surg. [Am.], 14:247–254, 1989.

201. Fu, F.H., and Imbriglia, J.F.: An Anatomical Study of the Lunate Bone in Kienbock's Disease. Orthopedics, 8:483–487, 1985.

202. Ganel, A.; Engel, J.; Oster, Z.; and Farine, I.: Bone Scanning in the Assessment of Fractures of the Scaphoid. J. Hand Surg., 4:541, 1979.

203. Garcia-Elias, M.: Dorsal Fractures of the Triquetrum: Avulsion or Compression Fractures? J. Hand Surg. [Am.], 12:266–268, 1987.

204. Garcia-Elias, M.; Abanco, J.; Salvador, E.; and Sanchez, R.: Crush Injury of the Carpus. J. Bone Joint Surg. [Br.], 67:286–289, 1985.

205. Garcia-Elias, M.; An, K.N.; Amadio, P.C.; Cooney, W.P.; and Linscheid, R.L.: Reliability of Carpal Angle Determinations. J. Hand Surg. [Am.], 14:1017–1021, 1989.

206. Garcia-Elias, M.; An, K.N.; Cooney, W.P.; Linscheid, R.L.; and Chao, E.Y.S.: Stability of the Transverse Carpal Arch: An Experimental Study. J. Hand Surg. [Am.], 14:277–282, 1989.

207. Garcia-Elias, M.; An, K.N.; Cooney, W.P.; Linscheid, R.L.; and Chao, E.Y.S.: Transverse Stability of the Carpus: An Analytical Study. J. Orthop. Res. 7:738–743, 1989.

208. Garcia-Elias, M.; Cooney, W.P.; An, K.N.; Linscheid, R.L.; and Chao, E.Y.S.: Wrist Kinematics After Limited Intercarpal Arthrodesis. J. Hand Surg. [Am.], 14:791–799, 1989.

209. Garcia-Elias, M.; Dobyns, J.H.; Cooney, W.P.; and Linscheid, R.L.: Traumatic Axial Dislocations of the Carpus. J. Hand Surg. [Am.], 14:446–457, 1989.

210. Garcia-Elias, M.; Vall, A.; Salo, J.M.; and Lluch, A.L.: Carpal Alignment After Different Surgical Approaches to the Scaphoid: A Comparative Study. J. Hand Surg. [Am.], 13:604–612, 1988.

211. Gartland, J.J. Jr., and Werley, C.W.: Evaluation of Healed Colles' Fractures. J. Bone Joint Surg. [Am.], 33:895–907, 1951.

212. Gasser, H.: Delayed Union and Pseudarthrosis of the Carpal Navicular: Treatment by Compression-Screw Osteosynthesis: A Preliminary Report of Twenty Fractures. J. Bone Joint Surg. [Am.], 47:249–266, 1965.

213. Gelberman, R.H.; Bauman, T.D.; Menon, J.; and Akeson, W.H.: The Vascularity of the Lunate Bone and Kienbock's Disease. J. Hand Surg., 5:272–278, 1980.

214. Gelberman, R.H., and Menon, J.: The Vascularity of the Scaphoid Bone. J. Hand Surg., 5:508–513, 1980.

215. Gelberman, R.H.; Salamon, P.B.; Jurist, J.M.; and Posch, J.L.: Ulnar Variance in Kienbock's Disease. J. Bone Joint Surg. [Am.], 57:674–676, 1975.

216. Gelberman, R.H.; Taleisnik, J.; Panagis, J.S.; and Baumgaertner, M.: The Arterial Anatomy of the Human Carpus. Part 1: The Extraosseous Vascularity. Part 2: The Intraosseous. J. Hand Surg., 8:367–375, 1983.

217. Gellman, H.; Caputo, R.J.; Carter, V.; Aboulafia, A.; and McKay, M.: Comparison of Short and Long Thumb-Spica Casts for Non-Displaced Fractures of the Carpal Scaphoid. J. Bone Joint Surg. [Am.], 71:354–357, 1989.

218. Gellman, H.; Schwartz, S.D.; Botte, M.J.; and Feiwell, L.: Late Treatment of a Dorsal Transscaphoid, Transtriquetral Perilunate Wrist Dislocation With Avascular Changes of the Lunate. Clin. Orthop., 237:196–203, 1988.

219. Gessler, W.B., and Fernandez, D.L.: Percutaneous and Open Reduction of the Articular Surface of the Distal Radius. J. Hand Surg. [Am.], in press.

220. Gibson, P.H.: Scaphoid-Trapezium-Trapezoid Dislocation. Hand, 15:267–269, 1983.

221. Gilford, W.W.; Bolton, R.H.; and Lambrinudi, C.: The Mechanism of the Wrist Joint: With Special Reference to Fractures of the Scaphoid. Guy's Hospital Report, 92:52–59, 1943.

222. Gilula, L.A.: Carpal Injuries: Analytic Approach and Case Exercises. A.J.R., 133:503–517, 1979.

223. Gilula, L.A.; Destouet, J.M.; Weeks, P.M.; Young, L.V.; and Wray, R.C.: Roentgenographic Diagnosis of the Painful Wrist. Clin. Orthop., 187:52–64, 1984.

224. Gilula, L.A.; Totty, W.G.; and Weeks, P.M.: Wrist Arthrography: The Value of Fluoroscopic Spot Viewing. Radiology, 146:555–556, 1983.

225. Glickel, S.Z., and Millender, L.H.: Ligamentous Reconstruction for Chronic Intercarpal Instability. J. Hand Surg. [Am.], 9:514–527, 1984.

226. Goldman, S.; Lipscomb, P.R.; and Taylor, W.F.: Immobilization for Acute Carpal Scaphoid Fractures. Surg. Gynecol. Obstet., 129:281–284, 1969.

227. Goldner, J.L.: Treatment of Carpal Instability Without Joint Fusion—Current Assessment. J. Hand Surg., 7:325–326, 1982.

228. Gomez, W., and Grantham, S.A.: Radial Carpal-Volar Lunate Dislocation: A Case Report. Orthopedics, 11:937–940, 1988.

229. Green, D.P.: Dislocations and Ligamentous Injuries of the Wrist. In Surgery of the Musculoskeletal System, 2nd ed., vol. I, pp. 449–515. New York, Churchill Livingstone, 1990.

230. Green, D.P.: Pins and Plaster Treatment of Comminuted Fractures of the Distal End of the Radius. J. Bone Joint Surg. [Am.], 57:304, 1975.

231. Green, D.P.: The Effect of Avascular Necrosis on Russe Bone Grafting for Scaphoid Nonunion. J. Hand Surg. [Am.], 10:597–605, 1985.

232. Green, D.P., and O'Brien, E.T.: Classification and Management of Carpal Dislocations. Clin. Orthop., 149:55–72, 1980.

233. Green, D.P., and O'Brien, E.T.: Open Reduction of Carpal Dislocations: Indications and Operative Techniques. J. Hand Surg., 3:250–265, 1978.

234. Green, J.T., and Gay, F.H.: Colles' Fracture—Residual Disability. Am. J. Surg., 91:636–642, 1956.

235. Greene, M.H.; Hadied, A.M.; and LaMont, R.L.: Scaphoid Fractures in Children. J. Hand Surg. [Am.], 9:536–541, 1984.

236. Guimberteau, J.C., and Panconi, B.: Recalcitrant Non-Union of the Scaphoid Treated with a Vascularized Bone Graft Based on the Ulnar Artery. J. Bone Joint Surg. [Am.], 72:88–97, 1990.

237. Gunn, R.S.: Dislocation of the Hamate Bone. J. Hand Surg. [Br.], 10:107–108, 1985.

238. Gunther, S.F.: Dorsal Wrist Pain and the Occult Scapholunate Ganglion. J. Hand Surg. [Am.], 10:697–703, 1985.

239. Gunther, S.F., and Bruno, P.D.: Divergent Dislocation of the Carpometacarpal Joints: A Case Report. J. Hand Surg. [Am.], 10:197–201, 1985.

240. Haddad, R.J., and Riordan, D.C.: Arthrodesis of the Wrist: A Surgical Technique. J. Bone Joint Surg. [Am.], 49:950–954, 1967.

241. Hamlin, C.: Traumatic Disruption of the Distal Radioulnar Joint. Am. J. Sports Med., 5:93–96, 1977.

242. Hanel, D.P., and Scheid, D.K.: Irreducible Fracture–Dislocation of the Distal Radioulnar Joint Secondary to Entrapment of the Extensor Carpi Ulnaris Tendon. Clin. Orthop., 234:56–60, 1988.

243. Hankin, F.M.; Amadio, P.C.; Wojtys, E.M.; and Braunstein, E.M.: Carpal Instability with Volar Flexion of the Proximal Row Associated with Injury to the Scaphotrapezial Ligament: Report of Two Cases. J. Hand Surg. [Br.], 13:298–302, 1988.

244. Hankin, F.M.; White, S.J.; Braunstein, E.M.; and Louis, D.S.: Dynamic Radiographic Evaluation of Obscure Wrist Pain in the Teenage Patient. J. Hand Surg. [Am.], 11:805–811, 1986.

245. Hanks, G.A.; Kalenak, A.; Bowman, L.S.; and Sebastianelli, W.J.: Stress Fractures of the Carpal Scaphoid. J. Bone Joint Surg. [Am.], 71:938–941, 1989.

246. Harper, W.M., and Jones, J.M.: Non-Union of Colles' Fracture: Report of Two Cases. Br. J. Hand Surg. [Br.], 15(1):121–123, 1990.

247. Hartz, C.R., and Beckenbaugh, R.D.: Long-Term Results of Resection of the Distal Ulna for Post-Traumatic Conditions. J. Trauma, 19:219–226, 1979.

248. Hastings, D.E., and Silver, R.L.: Intercarpal Arthrodesis in the Management of Chronic Carpal Instability After Trauma. J. Hand Surg. [Am.], 9:834–840, 1984.

249. Heim, U.; Pfeiffer, K.M.; and Meuli, H.C.: Small Fragment Set Manual. Technique Recommended by the ASIF Group (Swiss Association for Study of Internal Fixation). New York, Springer-Verlag, 1974.

250. Heiple, K.G.; Freehafer, A.A.; and Van't Hof, A.: Isolate Traumatic Dislocation of the Distal End of the Ulnar or Distal Radioulnar Joint. J. Bone Joint Surg. [Am.], 44:1287–1394, 1962.

251. Herbert, T.J.: Internal Fixation of the Carpus with the Herbert Bone Screw System. J. Hand Surg. [Am.], 14:397–400, 1989.

252. Herbert, T.J.: Scaphoid Fractures and Carpal Instability. Proc. R. Soc. Med., 67:1080, 1974.

253. Herbert, T.J., and Fisher, W.E.: Management of the Fractured Scaphoid Using a New Bone Screw. J. Bone Joint Surg. [Br.], 66:114–123, 1984.

254. Holdsworth, B.J., and Shackleford, I.: Fracture Dislocation of the Trapezio-Scaphoid Joint—The Missing Link? J. Hand Surg. [Br.], 12:40–42, 1987.

255. Hori, Y.; Tamai, S.; Okuda, H.; Sakamoto, H.; Takita, T.; and Masuhara, K.: Blood Vessel Transplantation to Bone. J. Hand Surg., 4:23–33, 1979.

256. Horii, E.; Garcia-Elias, M.; An, K.N.; Bishop, A.T.; Cooney, W.P.; Linscheid, R.L.; and Chao, E.Y.S.: Effect on Force Transmission Across the Carpus in Procedures Used to Treat Kienböck's Disease. J. Hand Surg. [Am.], 15:393–400, 1990.

257. Howard, F.M.: Ulnar-Nerve Palsy in Wrist Fractures. Fracture of the Hamate Bone. J. Bone Joint Surg. [Am.], 43:1197–1201, 1961.

258. Howard, F.M.; Fahey, T.; and Wojcik, E.: Rotatory Subluxation of the Navicular. Clin. Orthop., 104:134–139, 1974.

259. Hui, F.C., and Linscheid, R.L.: Ulnotriquetral Augmentation Tenodesis: A Reconstructive Procedure for Dorsal Subluxation of the Distal Radioulnar Joint. J. Hand Surg., 7:230–236, 1982.

260. Hultén, O.: Uber Anatomische Variationen der Handgelenkknochen. Ein Beitrag zur Kenntnis der Genese zwei verschiedener Mondbeinveranderungen. Acta Radiol., 9:155–168, 1928.

261. Hyman, G., and Martin, F.R.R.: Dislocation of the Inferior Radio-Ulnar Joint as a Complication of Fracture of the Radius. Br. J. Surg. 27:481–491, 1940.

262. Imbriglia, J.E.; Broudy, A.S.; Hagberg, W.C.; and McKernan, D.: Proximal Row Carpectomy: Clinical Evaluation. J. Hand Surg. [Am.], 15:426–430, 1990.

263. Iwegbu, C.G., and Helal, B.: An Unusual Combination of Fractures at the Wrist. Hand, 12:173–175, 1980.

264. Jackson, W.T., and Protas, J.M.: Snapping Scapholunate Subluxation. J. Hand Surg., 6:590–594, 1981.

265. Jakob, R.P., and Fernandez, D.L.: The Treatment of Wrist Fractures with the Small AO External Fixation Device. In Uhthoff, H.K. (ed.): Current Concepts of External Fixation of Fractures, pp. 307–314. Berlin, Springer-Verlag, 1982.

266. James, E.T.R., and Burke, F.D.: Vibration Disease of the Capitate. J. Hand Surg. [Br.], 9:169–170, 1984.

267. Jasmine, M.S.; Packer, J.W.; and Edwards, G.S.: Irreducible Transscaphoid Perilunate Dislocation. J. Hand Surg. [Am.], 13:212–215, 1988.

268. Jeanne, L.A., and Mouchet, A.: Les Lesions Traumatiques Fermees du Poignet, pp.149–165. 28th Congres Francais de Chirurgie, 1919.

269. Jenkins, N.H.; Jones, D.G.; Johnson, S.R.; and Mintowt-Czyz, W.J.: External Fixation of Colles' Fractures: An Anatomical Study. J. Bone Joint Surg. [Br.], 69:207–211, 1987.

270. Jenkins, N.H., and Mintowt-Czyz, W.J.: Mal-Union and Dysfunction in Colles' Fracture. J. Hand Surg. [Br.], 13:291–293, 1988.

271. Jensen, B.V., and Christensen, C.: An Unusual Combination of Simultaneous Fracture of the Tuberosity of the Trapezium and the Hook of the Hamate. J. Hand Surg. [Am.], 15(2):285–287, 1990.

272. Johnson, R.P.: The Acutely Injured Wrist and Its Residuals. Clin. Orthop., 149:33, 1980.

273. Johnson, R.P., and Carrera, G.F.: Chronic Capitolunate Instability. J. Bone Joint Surg. [Am.], 68:1164–1176, 1986.

274. Jones, W.A.: Beware of the Sprained Wrist: The Incidence and Diagnosis of Scapholunate Instability. J. Bone Joint Surg. [Br.], 70:293–297, 1988.

275. Jones, W.A., and Ghorbal, M.S.: Fractures of the Trapezium: A Report on Three Cases. J. Hand Surg. [Br.], 10:227–230, 1985.

276. Jonsson, G.: Aseptic Bone Necrosis of the Os Capitatum. Acta Radiol., 23:562, 1942.

277. Jorgensen, E.C.: Proximal-row Carpectomy: An End-Result Study of Twenty-two Cases. J. Bone Joint Surg. [Am.], 51:1104–1111, 1969.

278. Joseph, R.B.; Linscheid, R.L.; Dobyns, J.H.; and Bryan, R.S.: Chronic Sprains of the Carpometacarpal Joints. J. Hand Surg., 6:172–180, 1981.

279. Kapandji, A.: Intra-Focal Pinning of Fractures of the Lower Extremity of the Radius: Ten Years After (in French). Ann. Chir. Main, 6:57–63, 1987.

280. Kapandji, I.A.: The Inferior Radioulnar Joint and Pronosupination. In Tubiana, R. (ed.): The Hand, pp. 121–129. Philadelphia, W.B. Saunders, 1981.

281. Kapandji, I.A.: Biomécanique du Carpe et du poignet. Ann. Chir. Main, 6:147–169, 1987.

282. Kauer, J.M.G.: Functional Anatomy of the Wrist. Clin. Orthop., 149:9–20, 1980.

283. Kauer, J.M.G.: The Articular Disc of the Hand. Acta Anat. 93:590–605, 1975.

284. Kauer, J.M.G.: The Mechanism of the Carpal Joint. Clin. Orthop., 202:16–26, 1986.

285. Kawai, H.; Yamamoto, K.; Yamamoto, T.; Tadi, K.; and Kaga, K.: Excision of the Lunate in Kienbock's Disease: Results After Long-Term Follow-Up. J. Bone Joint Surg. [Br.], 70:287–292, 1988.

286. Kessler, I., and Silberman, Z.: An Experimental Study of the Radiocarpal Joint by Arthrography. Surg. Gynecol. Obstet., 112:33–40, 1961.

287. Kienböck, R.: Uber tramatische Malazie des Mondbeins und ihre Folgezustände: Entartungsformen und Kompressionsfrakturen. Fortschr. Geb. Roentgenstr. Nuklearmed. Ergangsband, 16:78–103, 1910–1911.

288. Kimmel, R.B., and O'Brien, E.T.: Surgical Treatment of Avascular Necrosis of the Proximal Pole of the Capitate: Case Report. J. Hand Surg., 7:284, 1982.

289. King, G.J.; McMurtry, R.Y.; Rubenstein, J.D.; and Ogston, N.G.: Computerized Tomography of the Distal Radioulnar Joint: Correlation with Ligamentous Pathology in a Cadaveric Model. J. Hand Surg. [Am.], 11:711–717, 1986.

290. King, G.J.; McMurtry, R.Y.; Rubenstein, J.D.; and Gertzbein, S.D.: Kinematics of the Distal Radioulnar Joint. J. Hand Surg. [Am.], 11:798–804, 1986.

291. Kinnard, P.; Tricoire, J.L.; and Basora, J.: Radial Shortening for Kienbock's Disease. Can. J. Surg., 3:261–262, 1983.

292. Kleinert, H.E.: Post-traumatic Sympathetic Dystrophy. Orthop. Clin. North Am., 4:917, 1973.

293. Kleinert, J.M.; Stern, P.J.; Lister, G.D.; and Kleinhans, R.J.: Complications of Scaphoid Silicone Arthroplasty. J. Bone Joint Surg. [Am.], 67:422–427, 1985.

294. Kleinman, W.B.: Long-Term Study of Chronic Scapho-Lunate Instability Treated by Scapho-Trapezio-Trapezoid Arthrodesis. J. Hand Surg. [Am.], 14:429–445, 1989.

295. Kleinman, W.B.: Management of Chronic Rotary Subluxation of the Scaphoid by Scapho-Trapezio-Trapezoid Arthrodesis: Rationale for the Technique, Postoperative Changes in Biomechanics, and Results. Hand Clin., 3:113–133, 1987.

296. Kleinman, W.B.; Steichen, J.B.; and Strickland, J.W.: Management of Chronic Rotary Subluxation of the Scaphoid by Scapho-Trapezio-Trapezoid Arthrodesis. J. Hand Surg., 7:125–136, 1982.

297. Knapp, M.E.: Treatment of Some Complications of Colles' Fracture. J.A.M.A., 148:825–827, 1952.

298. Knirk, J.L., and Jupiter, J.B.: Intra-Articular Fractures of the Distal End of the Radius in Young Adults. J. Bone Joint Surg. [Am.], 68:647–659, 1986.

299. Köhler, A., and Zimmer, E.A.: Borderlands of the Normal and Early Pathologic in Skeletal Rotengenology [Third American ed., based on 11th German ed.]. New York, Grune & Stratton, 1968.

300. Kongsholm, J., and Olerud, C.: Plaster Cast Versus External Fixation for Unstable Intraarticular Colles' Fractures. Clin. Orthop., 241:57–65, 1989.

301. Korkala, O.L., and Antti-Poika, I.U.: Late Treatment of Scaphoid Fractures by Bone Grafting and Compression Staple Osteosynthesis. J. Hand Surg. [Am.], 14:491–495, 1989.

302. Kristensen, S.S.; Thomassen, E.; and Christensen, F.: Ulnar Variance in Kienbock's Disease. J. Hand Surg. [Br.], 11:258–260, 1986.

303. Kristiansen, A., and Gjersoe, E.: Colles' Fracture: Operative Treatment, Indications and Results. Acta Orthop. Scand., 39:33–46, 1968.

304. Kuenz, C.L.: Les geodes du semi-lunaire (thesis). Lyon, 1923.

305. Kuhlmann, J.N.; Fournol, S.; Mimoun, M.; and Baux, S.: Fracture of the Lesser Multangular (Trapezoid) Bone. Ann. Chir. Main, 5:133–134, 1986.

306. Kuhlmann, J.N.; Mimoun, M.; Boabighi, A.; and Baux, S.: Vascularized Bone Graft Pedicled on the Volar Carpal Artery for Non-Union of the Scaphoid. J. Hand Surg. [Br.], 12:203–210, 1987.

307. Kuhlmann, N.; Gallaire, M.; and Pineau, H.: Déplacements du Scaphoide et du Semi-lunaire au Cours des Mouvements du Poignet. Ann. Chir., 32:543–553, 1978.

308. Lambrinudi, C.: Injuries to the Wrist. Guy's Hospital Gazette, 52:107, 1938.

309. Landsmeer, J.M.F.: Studies in the Anatomy of Articulation. I. The Equilibrium of the "Intercalated" Bone. Acta Morphol. Neerl. Scand., 3:287–303, 1961.

310. Lange, R.H.; Engber, W.D.; and Clancy, W.G.: Expanding Applications for the Herbert Scaphoid Screw. Orthopedics, 9:1393–1397, 1986.

311. Larson, B.; Light, T.R.; and Ogden, J.A.: Fracture and Ischemic Necrosis of the Immature Scaphoid. J. Hand Surg. [Am.], 12:122–127, 1987.

312. Lee, M.L.H.: The Intraosseous Arterial Pattern of the Carpal Lunate Bone and Its Relation to Avascular Necrosis. Acta Orthop. Scand., 33:43–55, 1963.

313. Lentino, W.; Lubetsky, H.W.; Jacobson, H.G.; and Poppel, M.H.: The Carpalbridge View: A Position for the Roentgenographic Diagnosis of Abnormalities in the Dorsum of the Wrist. J. Bone Joint Surg. [Am.], 39:88–90, 1957.

314. Leung, K.S.; Shen, W.Y.; Tsang, K.H.; Chiu, K.H.; Leung, P.C.; and Hung, L.K.: An Effective Treatment of Comminuted Fractures of the Distal Radius. J. Hand Surg. [Am.], 15:11–17, 1990.

315. Levinsohn, E.M., and Palmer, A.K.: Arthrography of the Traumatized Wrist. Radiology, 146:647–651, 1983.

316. Levy, M.; Fischel, R.E.; Stern, G.M.; and Goldberg, I.: Chip Fractures of the Os Triquetrum: The Mechanism of Injury. J. Bone Joint Surg. [Br.], 61:355–357, 1979.

317. Lewis, O.J.: The Hominoid Wrist Joint. Am. J. Phys. Anthropol., 30:251–267, 1969.

318. Lewis, O.J.; Hamshere, R.J.; and Bucknill, T.M.: The Anatomy of the Wrist Joint. J. Anat., 106:539–552, 1970.

319. Lichtman, D.M.; Alexander, A.H.; Mack, G.R.; and Gunther, S.F.: Kienbock's Disease—Update on Silicone Replacement Arthroplasty. J. Hand Surg., 7:343–347, 1982.

320. Lichtman, D.M.; Noble, W.H.; and Alexander, C.E.: Dynamic Triquetrolunate Instability: Case Report. J. Hand Surg. [Am.], 9:185–188, 1984.

321. Lidstrom, A.: Fractures of the Distal End of the Radius. A Clinical and Statistical Study of End Results. Acta Orthop. Scand., 41(suppl.):1–118, 1959.

322. Lindström, G., and Nyström, A.: Incidence of Post-traumatic Arthrosis After Primary Healing of Scaphoid Fractures: A Clinical and Radiological Study. [Br.], 15(1):11–13, 1990.

323. Linscheid, R.L.: Kinematic Considerations of the Wrist. Clin. Orthop., 202:27–39, 1986.

324. Linscheid, R.L., and Dobyns, J.H.: Les Types d'Instabilite Anterieure du Carpe. In Razemon, J.-P., and Fisk, G.-R. (eds.): Le Poignet, Monographies du Groupe d'Etude de la Main, pp. 142–146. Paris, Expansion Scientifique Francaise, 1983.

325. Linscheid, R.L., and Dobyns, J.H.: Physical Examination of the Wrist. In Post, M. (ed.): Physical Examination of the Musculoskeletal System, pp. 80–94. Chicago, Year Book Medical Publishers, 1987.

326. Linscheid, R.L., and Dobyns, J.H.: Radiolunate Arthrodesis. J. Hand Surg. [Am.], 10:821–829, 1985.

327. Linscheid, R.L., and Dobyns, J.H.: The Unified Concept of Carpal Injuries. Ann. Chir. Main, 3:35–42, 1984.

328. Linscheid, R.L., and Dobyns, J.H.: Wrist Sprains. In Tubiana, R. (ed.): The Hand, vol. 2, pp. 970–985. Philadelphia, W.B. Saunders, 1985.

329. Linscheid, R.L.; Dobyns, J.H.; Beabout, J.W.; and Bryan, R.S.: Traumatic Instability of the Wrist: Diagnosis, Classification and Pathomechanics. J. Bone Joint Surg. [Am.], 54:1612–1632, 1972.

330. Linscheid, R.L.; Dobyns, J.H.; Beckenbaugh, R.D.; Cooney, W.P.; and Wood, M.B.: Instability Patterns of the Wrist. J. Hand Surg., 8:682–686, 1983.

331. Linscheid, R.L.; Dobyns, J.H.; and Cooney, W.P.: Volar Wedge Grafting of the Carpal Scaphoid. Non-Union Associated with Dorsal Instability Patterns. Orthop. Trans., 6:464, 1982.

332. Linscheid, R.L.; Dobyns, J.H.; and Younge, D.K.: Trispiral

Tomography in the Evaluation of Wrist Injury. Bull. Hosp. Jt. Dis. Orthop. Inst., 44:297–308, 1984.

333. Logan, S.E.; Nowak, M.D.; Gould, P.L.; and Weeks, P.M.: Biomechanical Behavior of the Scapholunate Ligament. Biomed. Sci. Instrum., 22:81–85, 1986.

334. Loth, T.S., and McMillan, M.D.: Coronal Dorsal Hamate Fractures. J. Hand Surg. [Am.], 13:616–18, 1988.

335. Louis, D.S.; Hankin, F.M.; Greene, T.L.; Braunstein, E.M.; and White, S.J.: Central Carpal Instability: Capitate Lunate Instability Pattern: Diagnosis by Dynamic Displacement. Orthopedics, 7:1693–1696, 1984.

336. Louis, D.S.: Barton's and Smith's Fractures. Hand Clin., 4:399–402, 1988.

337. Lowrey, D.G.; Moss, S.H.; and Wollf, T.W.: Volar Dislocation of the Capitate. Report of a Case. J. Bone Joint Surg. [Am.], 66:611–613, 1984.

338. Lowry, W.E., and Cord, S.A.: Traumatic Avascular Necrosis of the Capitate Bone: Case Report. J. Hand Surg., 6:254, 1981.

339. Lugnegard, H.: Resection of the Head of the Ulna in Post-traumatic Dysfunction of the Distal Radio-Ulnar Joint. Scand. J. Plast. Reconstr. Surg., 3:65–69, 1969.

340. Lynch, A.C., and Lipscomb, P.R.: The Carpal Tunnel Syndrome and Colles' Fractures. J.A.M.A., 185:363, 1963.

341. MacConaill, M.A.: The Mechanical Anatomy of the Carpus and Its Bearings on Some Surgical Problems. J. Anat., 75:166–175, 1941.

342. Mack, G.R.; Bosse, M.J.; Gelberman, R.H.; and Yu, E.: The Natural History of Scaphoid Non-Union. J. Bone Joint Surg. [Am.], 66:504–509, 1984.

343. Macksoud, W.S.; Dobyns, J.H.; and Linscheid, R.L.: Non-dissociative Collapse of the Proximal Carpal Row. Presented at 98th Annual Meeting of the American Orthopaedic Association, Coronado, CA, June 10–13, 1985.

344. Malgaigne, J.F.: A Treatise on Fractures (Packard, J.H. [trans.]). Philadelphia, J.B. Lippincott, 1859.

345. Manaster, B.J.; Mann, R.J.; and Rubenstein, S.: Wrist Pain: Correlation of Clinical and Plain Film Findings with Arthrographic Results. J. Hand Surg. [Am.], 14:466–473, 1989.

346. Manske, P.R.; McCarthy, J.A.; and Strecker, W.B.: Use of the Herbert Bone Screw for Scaphoid Nonunions. Orthopedics, 11:1653–1661, 1988.

347. Marck, K.W., and Klasen, H.J.: Fracture–Dislocation of the Hamatometacarpal Joint: A Case Report. J. Hand Surg. [Am.], 11:128–130, 1986.

348. Marsh, A.P., and Lampros, P.J.: The Naviculocapitate Fracture Syndrome. A.J.R., 82:255–256, 1959.

349. Masquelet, A.C.: Clinical Examination of the Wrist. Ann. Chir. Main, 8:159–175, 1989.

350. Mathoulin, C.; Saffar, P.; and Roukoz, S.: Luno-Triquetral Instabilities. Annales de Chirurgie de la Main (Membres Supplement), 9:22–28, 1990.

351. Matti, H.: Uber die Behandlung der Navicularefraktur und der Refractura patellae durch Plombierung mit Spongiosa. Zentrabl. Chir., 64:2353–2359, 1937.

352. Matthews, L.S.: Acute Volar Compartment Syndrome, Secondary to Distal Radius Fracture in Athlete. Am. J. Sports Med., 11:6–7, 1983.

353. Maudsley, R.H., and Chen, S.C.: Screw Fixation in the Management of the Fractured Carpal Scaphoid. J. Bone Joint Surg. [Br.], 54:432–441, 1972.

354. Mayfield, J.K.: Mechanism of Carpal Injuries. Clin. Orthop., 149:45–54, 1980.

355. Mayfield, J.K.; Johnson, R.P.; and Kilcoyne, R.K.: Carpal Dislocations: Pathomechanics and Progressive Perilunar Instability. J. Hand Surg., 5:226–241, 1980.

356. Mayfield, J.K.; Johnson, R.P.; and Kilcoyne, R.K.: Carpal Injuries: An Experimental Approach. Anatomy, Kinematics and Perilunate Injuries. J. Bone Joint Surg. [Am.], 57:725, 1975.

357. Mayfield, J.K.; Johnson, R.P.; and Kilcoyne, R.F.: The Ligaments of the Human Wrist and Their Functional Significance. Anat. Rec., 186:417–428, 1976.

358. Mazet, R. Jr., and Hohl, M.: Fractures of the Carpal Navicular: Analysis of Ninety-One Cases and Review of the Literature. J. Bone Joint Surg. [Am.], 45:82–112, 1963.

359. McClain, E.J., and Boyes, J.H.: Missed Fractures of the Greater Multangular. J. Bone Joint Surg. [Am.], 48:1525–1528, 1966.

360. McMurtry, R.Y.; Axelrod, T.; and Paley, D.: Distal Radial Osteotomy. Orthopedics, 12:149–155, 1989.

361. McMurtry, R.Y.; Youm, Y.; Flatt, A.E.; and Gillespie, T.E.: Kinematics of the Wrist. II. Clinical Applications. J. Bone Joint Surg. [Am.], 60:955–961, 1978.

362. Melone, C.P. Jr.: Open Treatment for Displaced Articular Fractures of the Distal Radius. Clin. Orthop., 202:103–111, 1986.

363. Menon, J.; Wood, V.E.; Schoene, H.R.; Frykman, G.K.; Hohl, J.C.; and Bestard, E.A.: Isolated Tears of the Triangular Fibrocartilage of the Wrist: Results of Partial Excision. J. Hand Surg. [Am.], 9:527–530, 1984.

364. Mestdagh, H.: The Blood Supply of the Lunate. Ann. Chir. Main, 1:246–248, 1982.

365. Meyn, M.A. Jr., and Roth, A.M.: Isolated Dislocation of the Trapezoid Bone. J. Hand Surg., 5:602–604, 1980.

366. Meyerdierks, E.M.; Mosher, J.F.; and Werner, F.W.: Limited Wrist Arthrodesis: A Laboratory Study. J. Hand Surg. [Am.], 12:526–529, 1987.

367. Meyrueis, J.P.; Schernberg, F.; and Gerard, Y.: Radiological Investigation of Instability of the Wrist. In Tubiana, R. (ed.): The Hand, vol. 2, pp. 621–634. Philadelphia, W.B. Saunders, 1985.

368. Michon, J.: Kienbock's Disease and Complications of Injuries to the Lunate Bone. In Tubiana, R. (ed.): The Hand, vol. 2, pp. 1106–1116. Philadelphia, W.B. Saunders, 1985.

369. Mikic, Z.D.: Age Changes in the Triangular Fibrocartilage of the Wrist Joint. J. Anat., 126:367–384, 1978.

370. Mikic, Z.D.: Detailed Anatomy of the Articular Disc of the Distal Radioulnar Joint. Clin. Orthop., 245:123–132, 1989.

371. Mikic, Z.D.: Galeazzi Fracture–Dislocations. J. Bone Joint Surg. [Am.], 57:1071, 1975.

372. Milch, H.: Cuff Resection of the Ulna for Malunited Colles' Fracture. J. Bone Joint Surg., 23:311–313, 1941.

373. Milch, H.: Fracture of the Hamate Bone. J. Bone Joint Surg., 16:459–462, 1934.

374. Minami, A.; Ogino, T.; Ohshio, I.; and Minami, M.: Cor-

relation Between Clinical Results and Carpal Instabilities in Patients After Reduction of Lunate and Perilunar Dislocations. J. Hand Surg. [Br.], 11:213–220, 1986.

375. Minami, M.; Yamazaki, J.; Chisaka, N.; Kato, S.; Ogino, T.; and Minami, A.: Nonunion of the Capitate. J. Hand Surg. [Am.], 12:1089–1091, 1987.

376. Minami, M.; Yamazaki, J.; and Ishii, S.: Isolated Dislocation of the Pisiform: A Case Report and Review of the Literature. J. Hand Surg. [Am.], 9:125–127, 1984.

377. Mino, D.E.; Palmer, A.K.; and Levinsohn, E.M.: The Role of Radiography and Computerized Tomography in the Diagnosis of Subluxation and Dislocation of the Distal Radioulnar Joint. J. Hand Surg. 8:23–31, 1983.

378. Mirabello, S.C.; Rosenthal, D.I.; and Smith, R.J.: Correlation of Clinical and Radiographic Findings in Kienbock's Disease. J. Hand Surg. [Am.], 12:1049–1054, 1987.

379. Mitchell, S.W.: Injuries of Nerves and Their Consequences. Philadelphia, J.B. Lippincott, 1872.

380. Miyaji, N.: Treatment of Lunatomalacia with Vascular Bundle Transplantation (in Japanese). Seikei Geka (Orthopedic Surgery) 31:1591–1594, 1980.

381. Mizuseki, T.; Ikuta, Y.; Murakami, T.; and Watari, S.: Lateral Approach to the Hook of Hamate for Its Fracture. J. Hand Surg. [Br.], 11:109–111, 1986.

382. Moberg, E.: Shoulder-Hand-Finger Syndrome, Reflex Dystrophy, Causalgia. Acta Chir. Scand., 125:523–524, 1963.

383. Moberg, E.: Treatment of Kienbock's Disease by Surgical Correction of the Length of the Radius or Ulna. In Tubiana, R. (ed.): The Hand, vol. 2, pp. 117–1120. Philadelphia, W.B. Saunders, 1985.

384. Mogan, J.V.; Newberg, A.H.; and David, P.H.: Intraosseous Ganglion of the Lunate. J. Hand Surg., 6:61–63, 1981.

385. Monahan, P.R.W., and Galasko, C.S.B.: The Scapho-Capitate Fracture Syndrome: A Mechanism of Injury. J. Bone Joint Surg. [Br.], 54:122–124, 1972.

386. Moneim, M.S.: The Tangential Posteroanterior Radiograph to Demonstrate Scapholunate Dissociation. J. Bone Joint Surg. [Am.], 63:1324–1326, 1981.

387. Moneim, M.S.; Hofammann, K.E.; and Omer, C.E.: Transscaphoid Perilunate Fracture–Dislocation: Result of Open Reduction and Pin Fixation. Clin. Orthop., 190:227, 1984.

388. Monsivais, J.J.; Nitz, P.A.; and Scully, T.J.: The Role of Carpal Instability in Scaphoid Nonunion: Casual or Causal? J. Hand Surg. [Br.], 11:201–206, 1986.

389. Moran, R., and Curtin, J.: Scaphoid Fractures Treated by Herbert Screw Fixation. J. Hand Surg. [Br.], 13:453–455, 1988.

390. Mori, T.; et al: Revitalization of the Osteonecrotic Lunate Bone by Vascular Bundle Transplantation (in Japanese). Seikei Geka (Orthopedic Surgery) 28:1556–1560, 1977.

391. Morrissy, R.T., and Nalebuff, E.A.: Dislocation of the Distal Radioulnar Joint: Anatomy and Clues to Prompt Diagnosis. Clin. Orthop., 144:154–158, 1979.

392. Mortier, J.P.; Baux, S.; Uhl, J.F.; Mimoun, M.; and Mole, B.: The Importance of the Posteromedial Fragment and Its Specific Pinning in Fractures of the Distal Radius. Ann. Chir. Main, 2:219–229, 1983.

393. Mouchet, A.: Fractures Isolees du Scaphoide Carpien. Presse Med., 6:122, 1934.

394. Moutet, F.; Chapel, A.; Cinquin, P.; Rose-Pitet, L.: Three-Dimensional Imaging of the Carpus. Annales de Chirurgíe de la Main (Membres Supplement), 9:32–37, 1990.

395. Mulder, J.D.: The Results of 100 Cases of Pseudarthrosis in the Scaphoid Bone Treated by the Matti–Russe Operation. J. Bone Joint Surg. [Br.], 50:110–115, 1968.

396. Mullan, G.B., and Lloyd, G.J.: Complete Carpal Disruption of the Hand. Hand, 12:39–43, 1980.

397. Müller, M.E.; Algöwer, M.; Schneider, R.; and Willengger, H.: Manual of Internal Fixation, 2nd ed. Berlin, Springer-Verlag, 1979.

398. Murakami, Y.: Dislocation of the Carpal Scaphoid. Hand, 9:79–81, 1977.

399. Murakami, Y., and Todani, K.: Traumatic Entrapment of the Extensor Pollicis Longus Tendon in Smith's Fracture of the Radius: Case Report. J. Hand Surg., 6:238–240, 1981.

400. Murray, G.: End Results of Bone-Grafting for Non-Union of the Carpal Navicular. J. Bone Joint Surg., 28:749–755, 1946.

401. Nakamura, R.; Hori, M.; Horii, E.; and Miura, T.: Reduction of the Scaphoid Fracture with DISI Alignment. J. Hand Surg. [Am.], 12:1000–1005, 1987.

402. Nakamura, R.; Hori, M.; Imamura, T.; Horii, E.; and Miura, T.: Method for Measurement and Evaluation of Carpal Bone Angles. J. Hand Surg. [Am.], 14:412–416, 1989.

403. Nakamura, R.; Horii, E.; Tanaka, Y.; Imaeda, T.; and Hayakawa, N.: Three Dimensional CT Imaging for Wrist Disorders. J. Hand Surg. [Br.], 14:53–58, 1989.

404. Nakamura, R.; Imaeda, T.; and Miura, T.: Radial Shortening for Kienböck's Disease: Factors Affecting the Operative Result. J. Hand Surg. [Br.], 15(1):40–45, 1990.

405. Nakata, R.Y.; Chand, Y.; Matiko, J.D.; Frykman, G.K.; and Wood, V.E.: External Fixators for Wrist Fractures: A Biomechanical and Clinical Study. J. Hand Surg. [Am.], 10:845–851, 1985.

406. Nathan, P.A., and Meadows, K.D.: Ulna-Minus Variance and Kienbock's Disease. J. Hand Surg. [Am.], 12:777–778, 1987.

407. Navarro, A.: In Scaramuzza, R.F. (ed.): El Movimiento de Rotacion en el Carpo y sie Relacion con la Fisio Pathologica de sus Lesiones Traumaticas. Bulletin Trabojos Sociedad Argentina Orthopedia Traumatologia, 34:337–386, 1969.

408. Neviaser, R.J.: Proximal Row Carpectomy for Posttraumatic Disorders of the Carpus. J. Hand Surg., 8:301–305, 1983.

409. Neviaser, R.J., and Palmer, A.K.: Traumatic Perforation of the Articular Disc of the Triangular Fibrocartilage Complex of the Wrist. Bull. Hosp. Jt. Dis. Orthop. Inst., 44:376–380, 1984.

410. Newman, J.H., and Watt, I.: Avascular Necrosis of the Capitate and Dorsal Dorsi-Flexion Instability. Hand, 12:176–178, 1980.

411. Nielsen, P.T.; Hedeboe, J.; and Thommesen, P.: Bone Scintigraphy in the Evaluation of Fracture of the Carpal Scaphoid Bone. Acta Orthop. Scand., 54:303–306, 1983.

412. Nigst, H., and Buck-Gramcko, D.: Luxationen und Subluxationen des Kahnbeines. Handchir. Mikrochir. Plast. Chir., 7:81–90, 1975.

413. Norbeck, D.E.; Larson, B.; Blair, S.J.; and Demos, T.C.: Traumatic Longitudinal Disruption of the Carpus. J. Hand Surg. [Am.], 12:509–514, 1987.

414. O'Brien, E.T.: Acute Fractures and Dislocations of the Carpus. In Lichtman, D.M. (ed.): The Wrist and its Disorders, pp. 129–159. Philadelphia, W.B. Saunders, 1988.

415. Ogunro, O.: Fracture of the Body of the Hamate Bone. J. Hand Surg., 8:353–355, 1983.

416. Ohshio, I.; Ogino, T.; and Miyake, A.: Dislocation of the Hamate Associated with Fracture of the Trapezial Ridge. J. Hand Surg. [Am.], 11:658–660, 1986.

417. Olsen, N.; Schousen, P.; Dirksen, H.; and Christoffersen, J.K.: Regional Scintimetry in Scaphoid Fractures. Acta Orthop. Scand., 54:380–382, 1983.

418. Omer, G.E., Jr., and Thomas, S.R.: The Management of Chronic Pain Syndromes in the Upper Extremity. Clin. Orthop., 104:37, 1974.

419. Ovesen, J.: Shortening of the Radius in the Treatment of Lunatomalacia. J. Bone Joint Surg. [Br.], 63:231–232, 1981.

420. Paley, D.; McMurtry, R.Y.; and Murray, J.F.: Dorsal Dislocation of the Ulnar Styloid and Extensor Carpi Ulnaris Tendon into the Distal Radioulnar Joint: The Empty Sulcus Sign. J. Hand Surg. [Am.], 12:1029–1032, 1987.

421. Palmer, A.K.: Trapezial Ridge Fractures. J. Hand Surg., 6:561–564, 1981.

422. Palmer, A.K.: Triangular Fibrocartilage Complex Lesions: A Classification. J. Hand Surg. [Am.], 14:594–606, 1989.

423. Palmer, A.K.; Dobyns, J.H.; and Linscheid, R.L.: Management of Post-Traumatic Instability of the Wrist Secondary to Ligament Rupture. J. Hand Surg., 3:507–532, 1978.

424. Palmer, A.K.; Glisson, R.R.; and Werner, F.W.: Relationship Between Ulnar Variance and Triangular Fibrocartilage Complex Thickness. J. Hand Surg. [Am.], 9:681–683, 1984.

425. Palmer, A.K.; Glisson, R.R.; and Werner, F.W.: Ulnar Variance Determination. J. Hand Surg., 7:376–379, 1982.

426. Palmer, A.K.; Werner, F.W.; Glisson, R.R.; and Murphy, D.J.: Partial Excision of the Triangular Fibrocartilage Complex. J. Hand Surg. [Am.], 13:391–394, 1988.

427. Palmer, A.K., and Werner, F.W.: Biomechanics of the Distal Radioulnar Joint. Clin. Orthop., 187:26–35, 1984.

428. Palmer, A.K., and Werner, F.W.: The Triangular Fibrocartilage Complex of the Wrist—Anatomy and Function. J. Hand Surg., 6:153–162, 1981.

429. Panagis, J.S.; Gelberman, R.H.; Taleisnik, J.; and Baumgaertner, M.: The Arterial Anatomy of the Human Carpus. Part II. The Intraosseous Vascularity. J. Hand Surg., 8: 375–382, 1983.

430. Papilion, J.D.; DePuy, T.E.; Aulicino, P.L.; Bergfield, T.G.; and Gwathmey, F.W.: Radiographic Evaluation of the Hook of the Hamate: A New Technique. J. Hand Surg. [Am.], 13:437–439, 1988.

431. Parisien, S.: Settling in Colles' Fracture: A Review of the Literature. Bull. Hosp. Jt. Dis. Inst., 34:117–125, 1973.

432. Pattee, G.A., and Thompson, G.H.: Anterior and Posterior Marginal Fracture Dislocations of the Distal Radius: An Analysis of the Results of Treatment. Clin. Orthop., 231: 183–195, 1988.

433. Peimer, C.A.; Medige, J.; Eckert, B.S.; Wright, J.R.; and Howard, C.S.: Reactive Synovitis After Silicone Arthroplasty. J. Hand Surg. [Am.], 11:624–638, 1986.

434. Persson, M.: Causal Treatment of Lunatomalacia: Further Experiences of Operative Ulna Lengthening. Acta Chir. Scand., 100:531–544, 1950.

435. Peyroux, L.M.; Dunaud, J.L.; Caron, M.; Ben Slamia, I.; and Kharrat, M.: The Kapandji Technique and Its Evolution in the Treatment of Fractures of the Distal End of the Radius: Report on a Series of 159 Cases. Ann. Chir. Main, 6:109–122, 1987.

436. Pilcher, L.S.: Fractures of the Lower Extremity or Base of the Radius. Ann. Surg., 65:1, 1917.

437. Poirier, P., and Charpy, A.: Traite d'Anatomie Humaine (Arthrologie). Paris, Masson et Cie, 1897.

438. Posner, M.A., and Greenspan, A.: Trispiral Tomography for the Evaluation of Wrist Problems. J. Hand Surg. [Am.], 13:175–181, 1988.

439. Pouteau, C.: Oeuvres Posthumes de M. Pouteau, vol. 2, p. 251. Paris, P.D. Pierres, 1783.

440. Preiser, G.: Zur Frage der Typischen Traumatischen Ernahrungsstorungen der Kurzen Hand- und Fusswurzelknochen. Fortschr. Geb. Roentgenstr. Nuklearmed. Frgan Zungsband, 17:360–362, 1911.

441. Primiano, G.A., and Reef, T.C.: Disruption of the Proximal Carpal Arch of the Hand. J. Bone Joint Surg. [Am.], 56: 328–332, 1974.

442. Pring, D.J.; Hartley, E.B.; and Williams, D.J.: Scaphoid Osteosynthesis: Early Experience with the Herbert Bone Screw. J. Hand Surg. [Br.], 12:46–49, 1987.

443. Prosser, A.J.; Brenkel, I.J.; and Irvine, G.B.: Articular Fractures of the Distal Scaphoid. J. Hand Surg. [Br.], 13: 87–91, 1988.

444. Rahme, H.: Idiopathic Avascular Necrosis of the Capitate Bone—Case Report. Hand, 15:274–275, 1983.

445. Ralston, E.L.: Handbook of Fractures. St. Louis, C.V. Mosby, 1967.

446. Rand, J.A.; Linscheid, R.L.; and Dobyns, J.H.: Capitate Fractures: A Long-Term Follow-Up. Clin. Orthop., 165: 209–216, 1982.

447. Rayhack, J.M.; Linscheid, R.L.; Dobyns, J.H.; and Smith, J.H.: Posttraumatic Ulnar Translation of the Carpus. J. Hand Surg. [Am.], 12:180–189, 1987.

448. Razemon, J.P.: Pathogenic Study of Kienbock's Disease. Ann. Chir. Main, 1:240–242, 1982.

449. Reagan, D.S.; Linscheid, R.L.; and Dobyns, J.H.: Lunotriquetral Sprains. J. Hand Surg. [Am.], 9:502–514, 1984.

450. Reider, J.J.: Fractures of the Capitate Bone. U.S. Armed Forces Journal, 9:1513–1516, 1958.

451. Reinus, W.R.; Hardy, D.C.; Totty, W.G.; and Gilula, L.A.: Arthrographic Evaluation of the Carpal Triangular Fibrocartilage Complex. J. Hand Surg. [Am.], 12:495–503, 1987.

452. Rhoades, C.E., and Reckling, F.W.: Palmar Dislocation of the Trapezoid: Case Report. J. Hand Surg., 8:85–88, 1983.

453. Riggs, S.A. Jr., and Cooney, W.P.: External Fixation of Complex Hand and Wrist Fractures. J. Trauma, 23:332–336, 1983.

454. Riis, J., and Fruensgaard, S.: Treatment of Unstable Colles' Fractures by External Fixation. J. Hand Surg. [Br.], 14:145–148, 1989.

455. Rogers, W.D., and Watson, H.K.: Radial Styloid Impingement After Triscaphe Arthrodesis. J. Hand Surg. [Am.], 14:297–301, 1989.

456. Rongieres, M.; Mansat, M.; Devallet, P.; Bonnevialle, P.; and Railhac, J.J.: An Experimental Study of Partial Intercarpal Arthrodesis. Ann. Chir. Main, 6:269–275, 1987.

457. Rose-Innes, A.P.: Anterior Dislocation of the Ulna in the Inferior Radio-Ulnar Joint: Case Reports, With a Discussion of the Anatomy of Rotation of the Forearm. J. Bone Joint Surg. [Br.], 42:515–521, 1960.

458. Roth, J., and Haddad, R.G.: Radiocarpal Arthroscopy and Arthrography in the Diagnosis of Ulnar Wrist Pain. J. Arthroscopy, 2:234–243, 1986.

459. Roullet, J., and Walch, G.: Technique of the Elongation of Ulna in the Kienbock's Disease. Results After Ten Years. Ann. Chir. Main, 1:268–272, 1982.

460. Ruby, L.K.; An, K.N.; Linscheid, R.L.; Cooney, W.P.; and Chao, E.Y.S.: The Effect of Scapholunate Ligament Section on Scapholunate Motion. J. Hand Surg. [Am.], 12:767–771, 1987.

461. Ruby, L.K.; Cooney, W.P.; An, K.N.; Linscheid, R.L.; and Chao, E.Y.S.: Relative Motion of Selected Carpal Bones: A Kinematic Analysis of the Normal Wrist. J. Hand Surg. [Am.], 13:1–10, 1988.

462. Ruby, L.K.; Stinson, J.; and Belsky, M.R.: The Natural History of Scaphoid Non-Union. J. Bone Joint Surg. [Am.], 67:428–432, 1985.

463. Rüsse, O.: Fracture of the Carpal Navicular: Diagnosis, Non-Operative Treatment and Operative Treatment. J. Bone Joint Surg. [Am.], 42:759–768, 1960.

464. Russell, T.B.: Inter-Carpal Dislocations and Fracture–Dislocations: A Review of Fifty-Nine Cases. J. Bone Joint Surg. [Br.], 31:524–531, 1949.

465. Saffar, P.: Carpal Dislocations and Sequelar Instability. Ann. Chir. Main, 3:349–352, 1984.

466. Saffar, P.: Replacement of the Lunate by the Pisiform Bone. Ann. Chir. Main, 1:276–279, 1982.

467. Saffar, P., and Gentaz, R.: Comparison Between Surgical and Medical Management of Kienbock's Disease. Ann. Chir. Main, 1:250–252, 1982.

468. Sanders, W.E.: Evaluation of the Humpback Scaphoid by Computed Tomography in the Longitudinal Axial Plane of the Scaphoid. J. Hand Surg. [Am.], 13:182–187, 1988.

469. Sarmiento, A.; Pratt, G.W.; Berry, N.C.; and Sinclair, W.F.: Colles' Fractures: Functional Bracing in Supination. J. Bone Joint Surg. [Am.], 57:311–317, 1975.

470. Sarrafian, S.K., and Breihan, J.H.: Palmar Dislocation of Scaphoid and Lunate as a Unit. J. Hand Surg. [Am.], 15:134–139, 1990.

471. Sarrafian, S.K.; Melamed, J.L.; and Goshgarian, G.M.: Study of Wrist Motion in Flexion and Extension. Clin. Orthop., 126:153–159, 1977.

472. Saunier, J., and Chamay, A.: Volar Perilunar Dislocation of the Wrist. Clin. Orthop., 157:139–142, 1981.

473. Schernberg, F.: Midcarpal Instability. Ann. Chir. Main, 3:344–348, 1984.

474. Schernberg, F.: Static and Dynamic Radioanatomy of the Wrist. Ann. Chir. Main, 3:301–312, 1984.

475. Schoenecker, P.L.; Gilula, L.A.; Shively, R.A.; and Manske, P.R.: Radiocarpal Fracture–Dislocation. Clin. Orthop., 197:237–244, 1985.

476. Schuhl, J.F.; Leroy, B.; and Comtet, J.J.: Biodynamics of the Wrist: Radiologic Approach to Scapholunate Instability. J. Hand Surg. [Am.], 10:1006–1008, 1985.

477. Schuind, F.; Donkerwolcke, M.; Rasquin, C.; and Burny, F.: External Fixation of Fractures of the Distal Radius: A Study of 225 Cases. J. Hand Surg. [Am.], 14:404–407, 1989.

478. Sebald, J.R.; Dobyns, J.H.; and Linscheid, R.L.: The Natural History of Collapse Deformities of the Wrist. Clin. Orthop., 104:140–148, 1974.

479. Seimon, L.P.: Compound Dislocation of the Trapezium: A Case Report. J. Bone Joint Surg. [Am.], 54:1297–1300, 1972.

480. Seitz, W.H. Jr.; Putnam, M.D.; and Dick, H.M.: Limited Open Surgical Approach for External Fixation of Distal Radius Fractures. J. Hand Surg. [Am.], 15(2):288–293, 1990.

481. Sennwald, G.: The Wrist, Anatomical and Pathophysiological Approach to Diagnosis and Treatment. Berlin, Springer-Verlag, 1987.

482. Sennwald, G., and Segmüller, G.: Arthrodèse de la colonne centrale du carpe. Int. Orthop., 13:147–152, 1989.

483. Sennwald, G., and Segmüller, G.: Base anataomique d'un noveau concept de stabilité du carpe. Int. Orthop., 10:25–30, 1986.

484. Seradge, H.; Sterbank, P.T.; Seradge, E.; and Owens, W.: Segmental Motion of the Proximal Carpal Row: Their Global Effect on the Wrist Motion. J. Hand Surg. [Am.], 15(2):236–239, 1990.

485. Seitz, W.H.; Froimson, A.I.; Brooks, D.B.; Postak, P.D.; Parker, R.D.; LaPorte, J.M.; and Greenwald, A.S.: Biomechanical Analysis of Pin Placement and Pin Size for External Fixation of Distal Radius Fractures. Clin. Orthop., 251:207–212, 1990.

486. Sherlock, D.A.: Traumatic Dorsoradial Dislocation of the Trapezium. J. Hand Surg. [Am.], 12:262–265, 1987.

487. Short, W.H.; Palmer, A.K.; Werner, F.W.; and Murphy, D.J.: A Biomechanical Study of Distal Radial Fractures. J. Hand Surg. [Am.], 12:529–534, 1987.

488. Siegel, M.W., and Hertzberg, H.: Complete Dislocation of the Greater Multangular (Trapezium): A Case Report. J. Bone Joint Surg. [Am.], 51:769–772, 1969.

489. Siegert, J.J.; Frassica, F.J.; and Amadio, P.C.: Treatment of Chronic Perilunate Dislocations. J. Hand Surg. [Am.], 13:206–212, 1988.

490. Smith, D.K.; An, K.N.; Cooney, W.P.; Linscheid, R.L.; and Chao, E.Y.S.: Effects of a Scaphoid Waist Osteotomy on Carpal Kinematics. J. Orthop. Res., 7:590–598, 1989.

491. Smith, D.K.; Cooney, W.P.; An, K.N.; Linscheid, R.L.; and Chao, E.Y.S.: The Effects of Simulated Unstable Scaphoid

Fractures on Carpal Motion. J. Hand Surg. [Am.], 14:283–291, 1989.

492. Smith, F.M.: Late Rupture of Extensor Pollicis Longus Tendon Following Colles' Fracture. J. Bone Joint Surg., 28:49–59, 1946.

493. Smith, P.; Wright, T.W.; Wallace, P.F.; and Dell, P.C.: Excision of the Hook of the Hamate: A Retrospective Survey and Review of the Literature. J. Hand Surg. [Am.], 13:612–615, 1988.

494. Smith, R.W.: A Treatise on Fractures in the Vicinity of Joints, and on Certain Forms of Accidental and Congenital Dislocations. Dublin, Hodges & Smith, 1854.

495. Snook, G.A.; Chrisman, O.D.; Wilson, T.C.; and Wietsma, R.D.: Subluxation of the Distal Radio-Ulnar Joint by Hyperpronation. J. Bone Joint Surg. [Am.], 51:1315–1323, 1969.

496. Sowa, D.T.; Holder, L.E.; Patt, P.G.; and Weiland, A.J.: Application of Magnetic Resonance Imaging to Ischemic Necrosis of the Lunate. J. Hand Surg. [Am.], 14:1008–1116, 1989.

497. Speed, J.S., and Knight, R.A.: Treatment of Malunited Colles's Fractures. J. Bone Joint Surg., 27:361–367, 1945.

498. Spinner, M., and Kaplan, E.B.: Extensor Carpi Ulnaris: Its Relationship to the Stability on the Distal Radio-ulnar Joint. Clin. Orthop., 68:124–129, 1970.

499. Stahl, F.: On Lunatomalacia (Kienbock's Disease): A Clinical and Roentgenological Study, Especially on Its Pathogenesis and the Late Results of Immobilization Treatment. Acta Chir. Scand., 45(Suppl. 126):1–133, 1947.

500. Stamm, T.T.: Excision of the Proximal Row of the Carpus. Proc. R. Soc. Med., 38:74–75, 1944.

501. Stark, A.; Brostrom, L.; and Svartengren, G.: Scaphoid Nonunion Treated with the Matti-Russe Technique: Long-Term Results. Clin. Orthop., 214:175–180, 1987.

502. Stark, H.H.; Chao, E.K.; Zemel, N.P.; Rickard, T.A.; and Ashworth, C.R.: Fracture of the Hook of the Hamate. J. Bone Joint Surg. [Am.], 71:1202–1207, 1989.

503. Stein, F., and Siegel, M.W.: Naviculocapitate Fracture Syndrome: A Case Report; New Thoughts on the Mechanism of Injury. J. Bone Joint Surg. [Am.], 51:391–395, 1969.

504. Stern, P.J.: Multiple Flexor Tendon Ruptures Following an Old Anterior Dislocation of the Lunate: A Case Report. J. Bone Joint Surg. [Am.], 63:489–490, 1981.

505. Stevanovic, M.V.; Stark, H.H.; and Filler, B.C.: Scaphotrapezial Dislocation. J. Bone Joint Surg. [Am.], 72(3):449–452, 1990.

506. Stewart, M.J.: Fractures of the Carpal Navicular (Scaphoid): A Report of 436 Cases. J. Bone Joint Surg. [Am.], 36:998–1006, 1954.

507. Sudeck, P.: Uber die akute (reflektorische) Knochenatrophie nach Entzündungen und Verletzungen an den Extremitäten und ihre klinischen Erscheinungen. Fortschr. Geb. Roentgenstr. Nuklearmed. Erganzungsband, 5:277–297, 1901–1902.

508. Sundberg, S.B., and Linscheid, R.L.: Kienbock's Disease: Results of Treatment with Ulnar Lengthening. Clin. Orthop., 187:43–51, 1984.

509. Sutro, C.J.: Bilateral Recurrent Intercarpal Subluxation. Am. J. Surg., 72:110–113, 1946.

510. Sutro, C.J.: Hypermobility of Bones Due to "Over-Lengthened" Capsular and Ligamentous Tissues. Surgery, 21:67, 1947.

511. Swanson, A.B.: Flexible Implant Resection Arthroplasty in the Hand and Extremities. St. Louis, C.V. Mosby, 1973.

512. Tachakra, T.: A Case of Trapezio-scaphoid Subluxation. Br. J. Clin. Pract., 31:162–165, 1977.

513. Tajima, T.: An Investigation of the Treatment of Kienbock's Disease. J. Bone Joint Surg. [Am.], 48:1649–1655, 1966.

514. Taleisnik, J.: Carpal Instability: Current Concepts Review. J. Bone Joint Surg. [Am.], 70:1262–1268, 1988.

515. Taleisnik, J.: Clinical and Technologic Evaluation of Ulnar Wrist Pain. J. Hand Surg. [Am.], 13:801–802, 1988.

516. Taleisnik, J.: The Ligaments of the Wrist. J. Hand Surg., 1:110–118, 1976.

517. Taleisnik, J.: Triquetrohamate and Triquetrolunate Instabilities (Medial Carpal Instability). Ann. Chir. Main, 3:331–343, 1984.

518. Taleisnik, J.; Gelberman, R.H.; Miller, B.W.; and Szabo, R.M.: Extensor Retinaculum of the Wrist. J. Hand Surg. [Am.], 9:459–501, 1984.

519. Taleisnik, J., and Kelly, P.J.: Extraosseous and Intraosseous Blood Supply of the Scaphoid Bone. J. Bone Joint Surg. [Am.], 48:1125–1137, 1966.

520. Taleisnik, J.; Malerich, M.; and Prietto, M.: Palmar Carpal Instability Secondary to Dislocation of Scaphoid and Lunate: Report of a Case and Review of the Literature. J. Hand Surg., 7:606–612, 1982.

521. Taleisnik, J.; Watson, H.K.: Midcarpal Instability Caused by Malunited Fractures of the Distal Radius. J. Hand Surg. [Am.], 9:350–357, 1984.

522. Teisen, H., and Hjarbaek, J.: Classification of Fresh Fractures of the Lunate. J. Hand Surg. [Br.], 13:458–462, 1988.

523. Testut, L., and Latarget, A.: Traite d'Anatomie Humaine. Paris, Doin, 1949.

524. Thomas, F.B.: Reduction of Smith's Fracture. J. Bone Joint Surg. [Br.], 39:463–470, 1957.

525. Thompson, T.C.; Campbell, R.D. Jr.; and Arnold, W.D.: Primary and Secondary Dislocation of the Scaphoid Bone. J. Bone Joint Surg. [Br.], 46:73–82, 1964.

526. Tillberg, B.: Kienbock's Disease Treated with Osteotomy to Lengthen Ulna. Acta Orthop. Scand., 39:359–368, 1968.

527. Trevor, D.: Rupture of the Extensor Pollicis Longus Tendon After Colles' Fracture. J. Bone Joint Surg. [Br.], 32:370, 1950.

528. Trumble, T.; Bour, C.J.; Smith, R.J.; and Edwards, G.S.: Intercarpal Arthrodesis for Static and Dynamic Volar Intercalated Segment Instability. J. Hand Surg. [Am.], 13:384–390, 1988.

529. Trumble, T.; Glisson, R.R.; Seaber, A.V.; and Urbaniak, J.R.: A Biomechanical Comparison of the Methods for Treating Kienbock's Disease. J. Hand Surg. [Am.], 11:88–93, 1986.

530. Trumble, T.E.; Bour, C.J.; Smith, R.J.; and Glisson, R.R.: Kinematics of the Ulnar Carpus Related to the Volar In-

tercalated Segment Instability Pattern. J. Hand Surg. [Am.], 15:384–392, 1990.

531. Vahvanen, V., and Westerlund, M.: Fracture of the Carpal Scaphoid in Children: A Clinical and Roentgenological Study of 108 Cases. Acta Orthop. Scand., 51:909–913, 1980.

532. Vance, R.M., and Gelberman, R.H.: Acute Ulnar Neuropathy with Fractures at the Wrist. J. Bone Joint Surg. [Am.], 60:962, 1978.

533. Vance, R.M.; Gelberman, R.H.; and Evans, E.F.: Scaphocapitate Fractures: Patterns of Dislocation, Mechanism of Injury, and Preliminary Results of Treatment. J. Bone Joint Surg. [Am.], 62:271–276, 1980.

534. Varodompun, N.; Limpivest, P.; and Prinyaroj, P.: Isolated Dorsal Radiocarpal Dislocation: Case Report and Literature Review. J. Hand Surg. [Am.], 10:708–710, 1985.

535. Vasilas, A.; Grieco, R.V.; and Bartone, N.F.: Roentgen Aspects of Injuries to the Pisiform Bone and Pisotriquetral Joint. J. Bone Joint Surg. [Am.], 42:1317–1328, 1960.

536. Vender, M.I., and Watson, H.K.: Acquired Madelung-like Deformity in a Gymnast. J. Hand Surg. [Am.], 13:19–21, 1988.

537. Verdan, C.: Fractures of the Scaphoid. Surg. Clin. North Am., 40:461–464, 1960.

538. Viegas, S.F.; Patterson, R.M.; Peterson, P.D.; Pogue, D.J.; Jenkins, D.K.; Sweo, T.D.; and Hokanson, J.A.: Ulnar-sided Perilunate Instability: An Anatomic and Biomechanic Study. J. Hand Surg. [Am.], 15(2):268–278, 1990.

539. Viegas, S.F.; Tencer, A.F.; Cantrell, J.; Chang, M.; Clegg, P.; Hicks, C.; O'Meara, C.; and Williamson, J.B.: Load Transfer Characteristics of the Wrist: Part I. The Normal Joint. J. Hand Surg. [Am.], 12:971–978, 1987.

540. Viegas, S.F.; Tencer, A.F.; Cantrell, J.; Chang, M.; Clegg, P.; Hicks, C.; O'Meara, C.; and Williamson, J.B.: Load Transfer Characteristics of the Wrist: Part II. Perilunate Instability. J. Hand Surg. [Am.], 12:978–985, 1987.

541. Volkmann, R.: Die ischaemischen Muskellähmungen und Kontrakturen. Zentralbl. Chir., 8:801–805, 1881.

542. Volz, R.G.; Lieb, M.; and Benjamin, J.: Biomechanics of the Wrist. Clin. Orthop., 149:112–117, 1980.

543. Von Lanz, T., and Wachsmuth, W.: Praktische Anatomi: Ein Lehrund Hilfsbuch der anatomischen Grundlagen ärztlichen Handelns, vol. 1, 2nd ed. Berlin, Springer-Verlag, 1938.

544. Voorhees, D.R.; Daffner, R.H.; Nunley, J.A.; and Gilula, L.A.: Carpal Ligamentous Disruptions and Negative Ulnar Variance. Skeletal Radiol., 13:257–262, 1985.

545. Wahlstrom, O.: Treatment of Colles' Fracture. A Prospective Comparison of Three Different Positions of Immobilization. Acta Orthop. Scand., 53:225, 1982.

546. Watson, H.K.: Limited Wrist Arthrodesis. Clin. Orthop., 149:126–136, 1980.

547. Watson, H.K., and Ballet, F.L.: The SLAC Wrist: Scapholunate Advanced Collapse Pattern of Degenerative Arthritis. J. Hand Surg. [Am.], 9:358–365, 1984. Watson, H.K., and Hempton, R.F.: Limited Wrist Arthrodeses. I. The Triscaphoid Joint. J. Hand Surg., 5:320–327, 1980.

548. Watson, H.K.; Goodman, M.L.; and Johnson, T.R.: Limited Wrist Arthrodesis. II. Intercarpal and Radiocarpal Combinations. J. Hand Surg., 6:223–233, 1981.

549. Watson, H.K., and Rogers, W.D.: Nonunion of the Hook of the Hamate: An Argument for Bonegrafting the Nonunion. J. Hand Surg. [Am.], 14:486–490, 1989.

550. Watson, H.K.; Ryu, J.; and Akelman, E.: Limited Triscaphoid Intercarpal Arthrodesis for Rotatory Subluxation of the Scaphoid. J. Bone Joint Surg. [Am.], 68:345–349, 1986.

551. Watson, H.K.; Ryu, J.; and DiBella, A.: An Approach to Kienböck's Disease: Triscaphe Arthrodesis. J. Hand Surg. [Am.], 10:179–187, 1985.

552. Weber, E.R.: Concepts Governing the Rotational Shift of the Intercalated Segment of the Carpus. Orthop. Clin. North Am., 15:193–207, 1984.

553. Weber, E.R., and Chao, E.Y.: An Experimental Approach to the Mechanism of Scaphoid Waist Fractures. J. Hand Surg., 3:142–148, 1978.

554. Weber, S.C., and Szabo, R.M.: Severely Comminuted Distal Radial Fracture as an Unsolved Problem: Complications Associated with External Fixation and Pins and Plaster Techniques. J. Hand Surg. [Am.], 11:157–165, 1986.

555. Weeks, P.M.; Vannier, M.W.; Stevens, W.G.; Gayou, D.; and Gilula, L.A.: Three-Dimensional Imaging of the Wrist. J. Hand Surg. [Am.], 10:32–39, 1985.

556. Weiss, C.; Laskin, R.S.; and Spinner, M.: Irreducible Radiocarpal Dislocation: A Case Report. J. Bone Joint Surg. [Am.], 52:562–564, 1970.

557. Werner, F.W.; Palmer, A.K.; and Glisson, R.R.: Forearm Load Transmission: The Effect of Ulnar Lengthening and Shortening. Transactions of the 28th Annual Meeting of the Orthopaedic Research Society, p. 273. New Orleans, La., January, 1982.

558. White, S.J.; Louis, D.S.; Braunstein, E.M.; Hankin, F.M.; and Green, T.L.: Capitate-Lunate Instability. Recognition by Manipulation under Fluoroscopy. A.J.R., 143:361–364, 1984.

559. Wilson, J.N.: Profiles of the Carpal Canal. J. Bone Joint Surg. [Am.], 36:127–132, 1954.

560. Youm, Y., and Flatt, A.E.: Kinematics of the Wrist. Clin. Orthop., 149:21–32, 1980.

561. Youm, Y.; McMurtry, R.Y.; Flatt, A.E.; and Gillespie, T.E.: Kinematics of the Wrist. I. An Experimental Study of Radial-Ulnar Deviation and Flexion-Extension. J. Bone Joint Surg. [Am.], 60:423–431, 1978.

9

Fractures of the Shafts of the Radius and Ulna

Lewis D. Anderson
Frederick N. Meyer

Chapter 8 includes a discussion of fractures of the distal radius and ulna, and Chapter 10 deals with fractures of the olecranon and radial head. This chapter therefore is confined to fractures of the shaft of both bones of the forearm, single fractures of the radius, and single fractures of the ulna in adults.

We do not know of any eponym associated with fractures of both bones of the forearm. The fracture of the shaft of the ulna with associated dislocation of the radial head was first described by Monteggia[79,95] in 1814 and has been known as the Monteggia fracture since then. The single-bone fracture of the ulna without dislocation of the radial head is often called a nightstick fracture, an obvious reference to one of the mechanisms of injury. The single-bone fracture of the radius in the distal third associated with dislocation of the radioulnar joint has several eponyms. Galeazzi[40,95] of Italy called attention to this treacherous injury in 1934, and since then it has frequently been referred to as Galeazzi's fracture. This combination of injuries is also known as the Piedmont fracture. Hughston[56] of Columbus, Georgia, collected a series of 41 fractures treated by members of the Piedmont Orthopaedic Society and pointed out the difficulties encountered in its treatment. Hughston noted that the French referred to the fracture of the distal radius with dislocation of the ulna as a reverse Monteggia fracture. In Memphis and among graduates of the Campbell Foundation–University of Tennessee Residency Program, one frequently hears this injury called the "fracture of necessity." This description goes back to Dr. Willis C. Campbell's early days,

when he emphasized that this was a fracture in which poor results could be expected with closed treatment. Campbell believed that open reduction was a necessity.

SURGICAL ANATOMY

As has been well described in the literature on the treatment of forearm fractures,[94,100,125] the surgical anatomy of the forearm creates problems in fracture treatment not found in the treatment of diaphyseal fractures of other long bones. The radius and ulna are approximately parallel, but they touch only at the ends. They are bound proximally by the capsule of the elbow joint and the annular ligament and distally by the capsule of the wrist joint, the anterior and posterior radioulnar ligaments, and the fibrocartilaginous articular disk. As Palmer and Werner[87] have shown, the principal stabilizer of the distal radioulnar joint is the triangular fibrocartilage complex. The proximal and distal joints are very complex in both function and structure and are really many joints and not just two. They include the proximal and distal radioulnar joints and the ulnohumeral, radiohumeral, and radiocarpal joints. The ulna is a relatively straight bone, but the radius is much more complex. One frequently hears reference to the ulna moving about the radius when, in fact, the ulna is a relatively fixed strut around which the radius rotates in pronation and supination.[71] In a study of 100 radii from cadavers, Sage[101] pointed out the complexity of the angles and curves

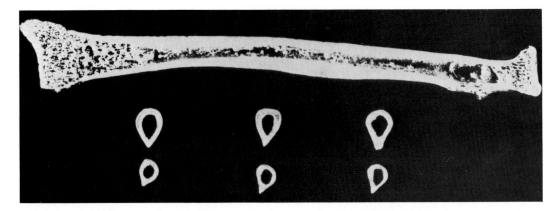

Fig. 9-1. A cross-section contour of the medullary canal of two radii at three points along the diaphysis. *(Sage, F. P.: Medullary Fixation of Fractures of the Forearm. A Study of the Medullary Canal of the Radius and a Report of Fifty Fractures of the Radius Treated with a Prebent Triangular Nail. J. Bone Joint Surg., 41A:1489–1516, 1959.)*

in this bone and the importance of maintaining them, especially the lateral bow of the radius. If this is not done, the patient may not be able to achieve full pronation and supination after fracture (Figs. 9-1 and 9-2).

Between the shafts of the ulna and radius is the interosseous space. The fibers of the interosseous membrane run obliquely across the interosseous space from their distal insertion on the ulna to their proximal origin on the radius. The central portion of the interosseous membrane is thickened and measures about 3.5 cm in width (Fig. 9-3). Exper-

imental studies by Hotchkiss and associates[55] showed that incision of the triangular fibrocartilage complex alone decreased the relative stiffness by 8%. Incision of the triangular fibrocartilage complex and interosseous membrane proximal to the central band decreased the stiffness by only 11%. Incision of the central band, however, decreased stiffness by 71%. The thickened central band of the interosseous membrane is a constant structure and accounts for most of the longitudinal support of the radius if the radial head is resected. If this structure has been injured, proximal migration of the radius may oc-

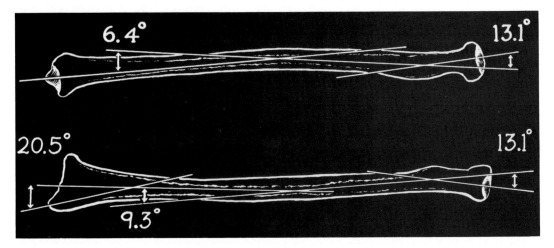

Fig. 9-2. Schematic drawings to show the biplane angulation proximally and distally in the longitudinal axis of the radius. *(Sage, F. P.: Medullary Fixation of Fractures of the Forearm. A Study of the Medullary Canal of the Radius and a Report of Fifty Fractures of the Radius Treated with a Prebent Triangular Nail. J. Bone Joint Surg., 41A:1489–1516, 1959.)*

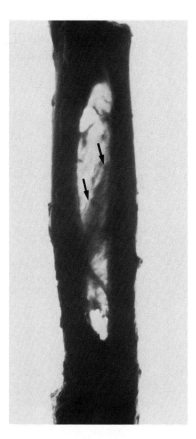

Fig. 9-3. Backlighted photograph of a forearm specimen. The central band is indicated by arrows. *(Hotchkiss, R. N.; An, K.; Sowa, D. T.; Basta, S.; and Weiland, A. J.: An Anatomic and Mechanical Study of the Interosseous Membrane of the Forearm: Pathomechanics of Proximal Migration of the Radius. J. Hand Surg., 14A:256–261, 1989.)*

cur, resulting in painful ulnocarpal impingement. The patient should be warned of this possibility if radial head resection becomes necessary.

Not only are the forearm bones themselves and their associated joints complex, but the muscle groups acting across the forearm cause complex deforming forces when fractures are present. The radius and ulna are joined by three muscles—the supinator, pronator teres, and pronator quadratus—which take origin on one bone and insert on the other. In addition to their named functions, when there is a fracture, these muscles tend to approximate the radius and ulna and decrease the interosseous space.

As Sage[100] has pointed out, the forearm muscles that take origin on the palmar side of the ulna and insert on the radial side of the wrist or hand, such

as the flexor carpi radialis, tend to exert a pronating force. In a similar manner, these muscles, such as the abductor pollicis longus and brevis and the extensor pollicis longus, which have their origins on the ulna and interosseous membrane on the dorsal side and are inserted on the radial side of the dorsum of the wrist, tend to exert a supinating force.

In addition to the supinator muscle itself, the biceps brachii is a powerful supinator of the radius. In fractures of the upper radius below the insertion of the supinator and above the insertion of the pronator teres, two strong muscles (the biceps and the supinator) exert an unopposed force supinating the proximal radial fragment (Fig. 9-4). In fractures of the radius located distal to the pronator teres, the force of the biceps and supinator is somewhat neutralized. In these fractures the proximal fragment of the radius is usually in a slightly supinated or neutral position (Fig. 9-5). In closed treatment of forearm fractures, therefore, the location of the fracture of the radius determines the degree of supination of the distal fragment needed to correct rotational alignment.

If satisfactory functional results are to be achieved in the treatment of fractures of the forearm, it is not sufficient to maintain just the length of each bone. Axial and rotational alignment must be achieved as well, and the radial bow must be maintained. With the complexity of the bones and joints involved, and the many and varied deforming muscle forces, it is extremely difficult to obtain union with sufficient restoration of the anatomy to ensure good functional results by closed treatment (Fig. 9-6). For these reasons, most recent articles in the literature recommend some form of open reduction and internal fixation for displaced diaphyseal fractures of the forearm in adults.

FRACTURES OF BOTH THE RADIUS AND ULNA

MECHANISM OF INJURY

The mechanisms of injury that cause fractures of the radius and ulna are myriad. The most common by far is some form of vehicular accident. Motorcycle accidents have caused an increasing number of these fractures in recent years. Usually the patient does not know exactly what happened because of the sudden nature of the accident. Probably most of these vehicular accidents result in some type of direct blow to the forearm. Other causes of direct blow injuries include fights in which one of the adversaries is struck on the forearm with a stick.

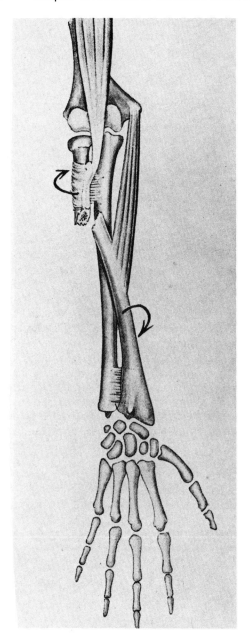

Fig. 9-4. In a fracture of the upper shaft of the radius between the insertion of the supinator and pronator teres, the proximal fragment is supinated and the lower fragment pronated. *(Watson-Jones, R.: Fractures and Joint Injuries, Vol. 2, 4th ed. Edinburgh, E & S Livingstone, 1955.)*

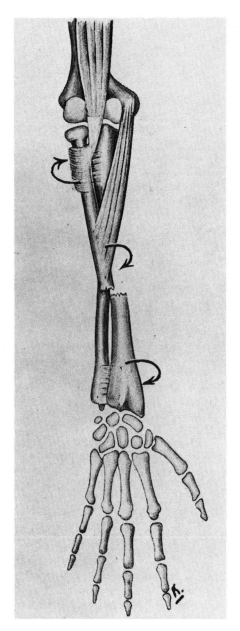

Fig. 9-5. In a fracture of the middle or lower shaft of the radius between the insertions of the pronator teres and the pronator quadratus, the proximal fragment is in midposition. *(Watson-Jones, R.: Fractures and Joint Injuries, Vol. 2, 4th ed. Edinburgh, E & S Livingstone, 1955.)*

Not only do Monteggia and nightstick fractures result from this kind of blow, but fractures of both bones result as well. The person throws the forearm up to protect his or her head, and the forearm is the recipient of the violence.

Pathologic fractures of the forearm bones are not common. If they are excluded, most of the remainder of these fractures result from some type of fall. The force generated is usually much greater than that required to cause a Colles' fracture. Most fore-

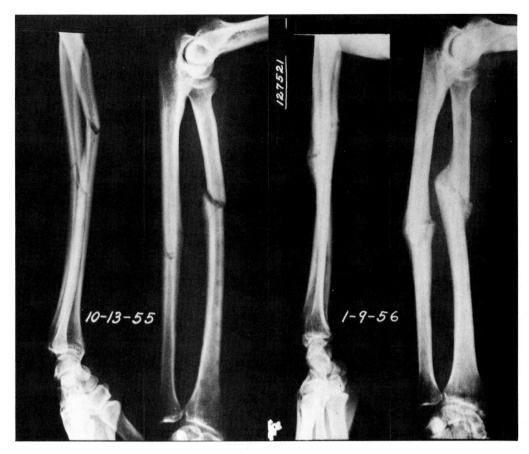

Fig. 9-6. A fracture of the proximal shaft of the radius and midshaft of the ulna treated by closed reduction and cast immobilization. Three months later, the fracture healed with loss of the radial bow and ulnar angulation. Pronation and supination were severely limited.

arm shaft fractures resulting from falls occur in athletics or in falls from heights.

CLASSIFICATION

Fractures of both bones of the forearm are usually classified according to the level of fracture, the degree of displacement and angulation, the presence or absence of comminution, and whether they are open or closed. Each of these factors may have some bearing on the type of treatment to be selected and the ultimate prognosis.

SIGNS AND SYMPTOMS

In adults, undisplaced diaphyseal fractures of the shafts of both bones of the forearm are rare. An injury of sufficient force to break both the radius and the ulna is almost always sufficient to cause displacement. Because shaft fractures of both the

radius and ulna are usually displaced, the signs and symptoms frequently make the diagnosis obvious. They include pain, deformity, and loss of function of the forearm and hand. Palpation along the subcutaneous border of the ulna usually elicits tenderness at the level of the fracture. Some degree of swelling is almost always present and is usually related to both the force causing the injury and the time since the injury. The examiner should not attempt to elicit crepitus, because this may cause additional soft tissue damage. However, it is usually noted when the forearm is aligned for splinting.

The examination should include a careful neurologic evaluation of the motor and sensory functions of the radial, median, and ulnar nerves. Neurologic deficits are not common in closed fractures of the shafts of the radius and ulna, but they do occur. One should also check the vascular status of the forearm as well as the amount of swelling. If the forearm is swollen and tense, compartment pressures should be measured to rule out the possibility of compartment syndrome. Open fractures, especially those caused by gunshot wounds, frequently have associated nerve and major blood vessel involvement. This involvement must be carefully evaluated. In open fractures it is a mistake to probe the wound in the emergency room. This may carry contamination deeper into the wound and increase the risk of infection. The soft tissue damage can be evaluated much better and more safely at the time of formal débridement in the operating room.

RADIOGRAPHIC FINDINGS

Just as the clinical signs and symptoms are usually obvious in shaft fractures of both bones of the forearm, so are the radiologic signs. The configuration of midshaft fractures of the radius and ulna varies depending on the mechanism of injury and the degree of violence involved. Low-energy fractures tend to be transverse or short oblique, whereas high-energy injuries are frequently extensively comminuted or segmented, often with extensive soft tissue injuries.[71]

It is important to note the degree of offset and angulation as well as the amount of shortening and comminution. It is imperative to include the elbow and wrist joints in films to ascertain if there is an associated dislocation or articular fracture.

The nutrient foramen of the radius sometimes is prominent in the anteroposterior views and can be confused with an undisplaced fracture by one not familiar with its location and appearance. It is located at the junction of the proximal and middle thirds of the radius and enters obliquely from distal to proximal. Because it is not usually visualized on the lateral or oblique view, anyone who knows what it looks like should not be confused.

METHODS OF TREATMENT

Undisplaced Fractures

Undisplaced fractures of the shafts of *both* the radius and the ulna are rare in adults. These fractures can usually be treated by immobilization in a well-molded, long-arm cast in neutral pronation-supination with the elbow flexed 90°. The completed cast should extend from the midpalm to the axilla. Angulation of the fractures in the cast can occur. As Patrick[89] has pointed out, angulation occurs because much of the weight of the cast is taken by the collar-and-cuff sling. If the sling is attached to the cast distal to the level of the fractures, as atrophy of the proximal forearm muscles occurs, the cast sags in this area. Distally there is less soft tissue, so the forearm bones are still held firmly by the cast. As a result, angulation occurs (Fig. 9-7). It can be prevented by incorporating a wire or plaster loop on the radial side of the cast proximal to the level of the fractures. Suspending the cast from the patient's neck with a sling through this loop helps prevent angulation of the fractures by keeping the cast firmly against the ulna (Fig. 9-8). The loop should never be placed distal to the fracture, be-

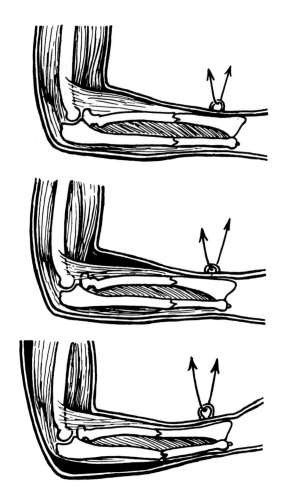

Fig. 9-7. Angulation of the radius and ulna during the period of cast immobilization. (**Top**) Immediately after reduction the cast fits snugly. (**Center**) Swelling has subsided with consequent loosening of the cast in the upper half of the forearm. (**Bottom**) The cast has sagged while still holding the distal fragment firmly, thus causing angulation of the radius and ulna. (*Knight, R. A., and Purvis, G. D.: Fractures of Both Bones of the Forearm in Adults. J. Bone Joint Surg., 31A:755–764, 1949.*)

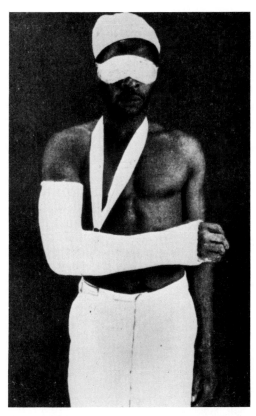

Fig. 9-8. The proper method of suspending a cast by a sling so that the ulnar border of the cast is kept snugly against the forearm to prevent ulnar angulation. *(Knight, R. A., and Purvis, G. D.: Fractures of Both Bones of the Forearm in Adults. J. Bone Joint Surg., 31A:755–764, 1949.)*

cause this increases the chance of angulation. Despite good technique, an initially undisplaced fracture can lose position while immobilized in plaster. For this reason, x-rays should be made in both anteroposterior and lateral planes at weekly intervals. If the fracture does displace, it should be treated as though it were displaced initially.

Plastic Deformation

In 1982, Greene[45] reported a case of a 24-year-old woman with plastic deformation of both bones of the forearm following a conveyor belt injury. Because little or no remodeling occurs in diaphyseal fractures in adults, he recommended closed manipulation under anesthesia, noting that considerable force is required for correction. Scheuer and Pot[106] reported a similar case in 1986 in which the radius and ulna were forcibly fractured by closed manip-

ulation. Their patient required a fasciotomy. They pointed out that the bowing of the bone is often obscure, and if this feature is in doubt, a comparison view of the uninjured arm may be helpful. They believed that incompletely reduced plastic deformities in older children and young adults resulted in significant loss of forearm rotation, and therefore, they recommended closed reduction under general anesthesia with stabilization by intramedullary nailing if necessary.

Displaced Fractures

The treatment of displaced fractures of the shafts of the radius and ulna is difficult. The choice is between closed treatment and open reduction with some form of internal fixation.

CLOSED REDUCTION AND EXTERNAL IMMOBILIZATION

Most series[56,60,89] report a high percentage of unsatisfactory results with closed treatment. However, the report of Sarmiento and associates[103] in 1975 and, more recently, the excellent book by Sarmiento and Latta[104] on the use of early functional bracing for forearm fractures are significant exceptions. Sarmiento reported treatment of 44 fractures of both bones of the forearm. The fractures were initially reduced under anesthesia and the forearms placed in long-arm casts. Reduction was lost in four patients, and open reduction and internal fixation was carried out. The initial long-arm casts were removed after an average of 18 days, and a functional brace was applied that limited pronation and supination but permitted flexion and extension of the elbow. Active exercise of the fingers was encouraged. The results were surprisingly good. In 39 patients the fractures united, and there was only one nonunion. Sarmiento found that 10° malalignment in any plane resulted in only a few degrees' loss of pronation and supination. This finding was supported by the laboratory work of Tarr, Garfinkel, and Sarmiento[117] and Matthews and coworkers.[73] They demonstrated on fresh cadaver specimens that angular and rotatory deformities of 10° or less resulted in minimal limitation of pronation-supination and were readily acceptable to the patient in clinical practice. The healing time averaged 16 weeks for the entire series, including the one nonunion. Some of the patients had less than anatomic reductions, but despite this, good functional results were obtained. Over many years, Sarmiento and his associates have demonstrated considerable skill in the use of functional bracing. Their results have not been duplicated by others to the best of our knowledge. The reader is referred to the book by Sarmiento and Latta[104] for details of treatment by this method.

For the reasons outlined in the discussion of surgical anatomy, it is difficult to reduce and maintain satisfactory position of the fragments by closed methods. Knight and Purvis[60] analyzed 100 adults with shaft fractures of both bones of the forearm treated at the Campbell Clinic, of which approximately half had been treated by closed methods. Of those treated closed, 71% had unsatisfactory results, and the incidence of nonunion and malunion was high. In our hands, closed reduction has been more successful for fractures of both the radius and ulna when the fractures are located in the distal third (Fig. 9-9). If closed treatment is undertaken, the patient must be advised that he or she may require open reduction and internal fixation at any time to ensure solid union in an acceptable position.

As mentioned, both longitudinal and rotational alignment must be correct if good results are to be obtained. The rotational alignment is difficult to determine in ordinary anteroposterior and lateral x-rays. The bicipital tuberosity view recommended by Evans[39] is often helpful (Fig. 9-10). Because the surgeon has no control over the proximal radial fragment with closed methods, he or she must bring the distal radial fragment into correct relationship with the proximal one. Ascertaining the rotation of the proximal fragment from the tuberosity view prior to reduction gives some idea of how much pronation or supination of the distal fragment is needed. The tuberosity view is made with the x-ray tube tilted 20° toward the olecranon, with the subcutaneous border of the ulna flat on the cassette. The x-ray can then be compared with a diagram showing the prominence of the tubercle in various degrees of pronation or supination. As an alterna-

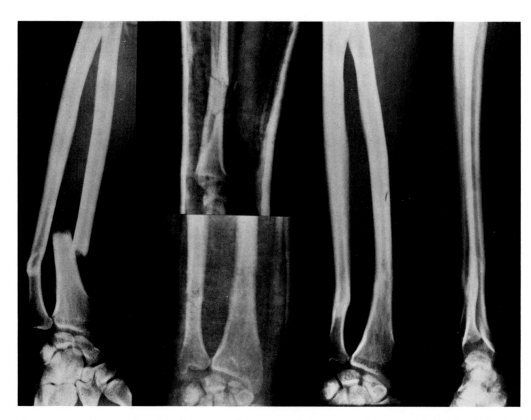

Fig. 9-9. Satisfactory closed reduction and cast immobilization in fractures of the distal third of the radius and ulna. The fractures united with only mild narrowing of the interosseous space. (*Sage, F. P.: Fractures of the Shafts of the Radius and Ulna in the Adult. In Adams, J. P. (ed.): Current Practice in Orthopaedic Surgery, Vol. 1. St. Louis, C.V. Mosby, 1963.*)

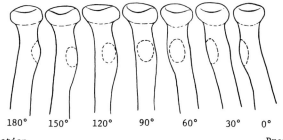

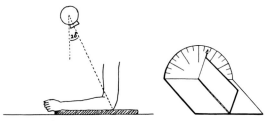

Fig. 9-10. The "tuberosity view." The position of the humeral condyles should be at equal distance from the x-ray film. The appearance of the bicipital tuberosity of the radius is shown at the top in different degrees of pronation and supination. The protractor for measuring rotation is shown at the bottom right. The hand is laid against the vertical plate, and the degree of rotation is read from the calibrated scale. (*Evans, E. M.: Rotational Deformity in the Treatment of Fractures of Both Bones of the Forearm. J. Bone Joint Surg., 27:373–379, 1945.*)

tive, a film of the opposite elbow can be made in a given degree of rotation for comparison.

As a practical matter, we rarely attempt closed treatment for displaced fractures of both bones of the forearm in adults, unless some other condition of the patient prohibits surgery. The results are too uncertain and the period of immobilization too long.

Technique of Closed Reduction. Relaxation of the muscles is mandatory for closed reduction, and general anesthesia is usually best. When the patient is anesthetized, a tuberosity view is obtained if that has not already been done. Finger traps or clove hitches of gauze are then placed on the thumb, index finger, and middle finger to suspend the extremity from an overhead frame or intravenous stand so that the elbow is flexed 90°. Countertraction is applied by means of a loop of muslin, stockinette, or other suitable material that is placed over the distal arm about 3 inches above the elbow. This is tied at a convenient height from the floor so that the surgeon's foot can be placed in it for countertraction. The loop over the distal humerus is padded to prevent excessive pressure. Traction and countertraction are applied while the ulna is palpated, and an attempt is made to reduce it. The radius usually cannot be palpated in the proximal half of the forearm because of swelling and overlying muscles. The forearm is placed in the appropriate amount of supination as determined by the tuberosity view. When the fractures seem reduced and the alignment of the forearm appears good, a single

layer of padding is applied from the midpalm to above the elbow with an extra layer over the bony prominences. A sugar-tong splint is then applied and molded well as it sets. Anteroposterior and lateral x-rays are taken to determine if the reduction is proper. Anything less than near anatomic reduction should not be accepted. If the reduction is not acceptable, the sugar tong is removed and the fractures are remanipulated. Once reduction is acceptable, the muslin loop is removed from the upper arm and the sugar tong is converted into a well-molded, long-arm cast while the extremity is still suspended. As the cast hardens, the plaster is flattened in the area posterior to the distal humerus to prevent the cast from slipping distally. The completed cast should be suspended from the neck by a sling passed through a loop on the radial side of the cast. As mentioned in the discussion of undisplaced fractures, this loop should be at or proximal to the level of the fracture. Once the cast is completed, final x-rays are made.

Aftercare. The circulation and function of the hand must be observed carefully until the swelling begins to decrease. During this period, the arm should be elevated by suspending it from an overhead frame with the fingers uppermost. The elbow should rest on the bed. Active flexion and extension of the fingers should be done at frequent intervals to help reduce edema. If at any time the circulation appears in jeopardy, the cast should be split from the axilla to the hand on both sides. It should be split through the padding to the skin. A loss of reduction is not nearly as bad as gangrene or Volk-mann's ischemic contracture.

Radiographs in two planes should be made at weekly intervals through the cast for the first month and every 2 weeks thereafter until union is solid. Each new set of films should be compared with the *original postreduction films that were accepted.* A common error is to compare the most recent films with the films from the previous visit. If this is done, a gradual loss of reduction goes undetected until it is too late.

The cast should be changed at intervals of 4 to 6 weeks. Each new cast must be applied as carefully as the first one. The fractures can angulate even after some callus is present. There is no margin for error due to a sloppily applied cast.

OPEN REDUCTION AND INTERNAL FIXATION

Over the years many methods of open reduction and internal fixation have been advocated. Open reduction without internal fixation has all the disadvantages of both open and closed treatment and has no place in the modern treatment of fractures of the shaft of the radius and ulna in adults.

In the early 1900s, Lane[11,66,67] of London and Lambotte[11,64,65] of Belgium reported the use of plates on diaphyseal fractures. However, metal reaction led to frequent failures until modern metals for implantation were introduced in 1937 after the work of Venable and associates[123] on electrolysis. Campbell and Boyd[22] used autogenous tibial grafts fixed to the radius and ulna with bone pegs or screws for acute fractures as well as nonunions. Some of these attempts were successful, but unless external immobilization was prolonged, the grafts often developed fatigue fractures before they were revascularized.[60]

Indications for Open Treatment. Mallin[71] recommended the following indications for surgical treatment:

1. All displaced, unstable fractures of radius and ulna in adults
2. All displaced fractures of the radius with greater than 10° angulation or with subluxation of the proximal or distal radioulnar joint
3. Isolated fractures of the ulna with angulation greater than 10°
4. All Monteggia fractures
5. All Galeazzi fractures
6. Open fractures (best treated with internal or external fixation)
7. If compartment syndrome requires fasciotomy, internal or external fixation

Timing of Surgery.   Although we do not necessarily concur with his philosophy of treatment of open fractures, Mallin[71] believes that forearm fractures are best internally fixed as soon after injury as practical, preferably before the onset of swelling. In Hadden's series,[49] 44% of open and 23% of closed fractures were plated during the first 24 hours. His reasons for delaying open treatment included the multiply injured patient in whom other injuries took priority, inexperienced admitting surgeons, and awaiting wound healing in open fractures (early in the series). His current recommendation is primary fixation of open fractures. Chapman and colleagues[24] also recommend fixation of open fractures on the day of injury in most cases unless other injuries preclude fixation.

Fixation With Medullary Nails.   After medullary nailing became popular for fractures of the femur in the late 1940s, various devices for medullary fixation of the radius and ulna were used. In 1957, Smith and Sage[110] reported a series of 555 fractures collected from all over the country in which some form of medullary fixation had been used. The devices included Rush pins, Kirschner wires, Steinmann pins, Lottes nails, and Küntscher V-nails. The results were discouraging (Fig. 9-11). Nonunion resulted in over 20% of the fractures, and malunion and poor function were common in those that did unite. The radial bow was not maintained, and the use of a round pin in a round medullary canal could not control rotation of the fragments (Fig. 9-12). Caden[21] reported a nonunion rate of 16.6% in forearm fractures treated with Rush pins.

In 1959, Sage[101] published his study of the anatomy of the radius and introduced Sage triangular forearm medullary nails. The nail for the ulna is straight and is inserted in a retrograde manner. The nail for the radius is bent to aid in maintaining the radial bow (Fig. 9-13). It is introduced from the radial styloid and driven proximally (Fig. 9-14). The ulnar nail is relatively easy to insert, but the technique for inserting the radial nail is more difficult and exacting. Sage reported good results with his nails (Fig. 9-15). Nonunion occurred in only 6.2% of fractures and delayed union in 4.9%. Other triangular or diamond-shaped nails for the forearm bones were introduced by Ritchey and colleagues[98] and Street.[116] These also grip the cortex well and control rotation but do not preserve the radial bow as well as the Sage nail.

Sage nails are not recommended for fractures of the distal third of the radius beyond the area where the medullary canal has begun to enlarge (Fig. 9-16). Also, one should not attempt to use them if

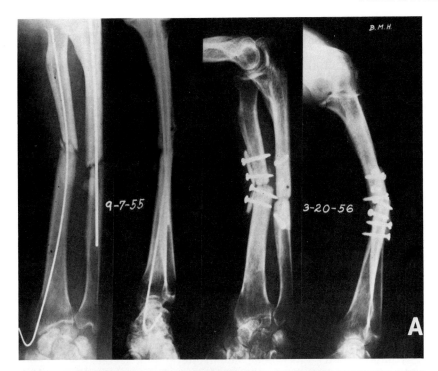

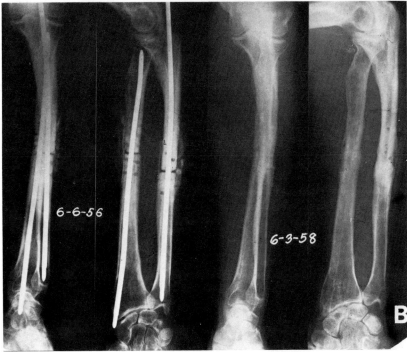

Fig. 9-11. (**A**) Failure of union in fractures of both bones of the forearm resulted from inadequate fixation with Kirschner wires as medullary nails. A second procedure using cortical onlay bone grafts also resulted in failure. (**B**) Eleven months after injury, rigid medullary fixation was achieved with Sage triangular nails. Two years later, the nails have been removed. Union is satisfactory. (Şage, F. P.: Medullary Fixation of Fractures of the Forearm. A Study of the Medullary Canal of the Radius and a Report of Fifty Fractures of the Radius Treated with a Prebent Triangular Nail. J. Bone Joint Surg., 41A:1489–1516, 1959.)

the medullary canal is less than 3 mm in diameter. When his nails are used, Sage[100] recommends routine autogenous iliac bone grafting.

Recently, Street[115] published a report on a series of 137 forearm fractures treated with a square, reamed, intramedullary nail. Nailings were done by either closed or open technique, with the radial nail being introduced distally and the ulnar nail being introduced proximally. Postoperatively, the fractures were immobilized in a long-arm cast for

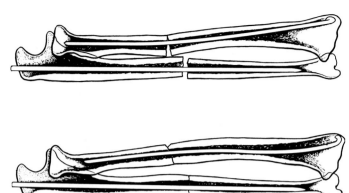

Fig. 9-12. When medullary pins are used in both bones, fixation of the radius must be sufficiently stable to prevent collapse of the radial arch; otherwise, there will be a relative elongation of the radius with distraction of the ulnar fracture, and nonunion may result in either or both bones. *(Smith, H., and Sage, F. P.: Medullary Fixation of Forearm Fractures. J. Bone Joint Surg., 39A:91–98, 1957.)*

4 weeks after which the patient was encouraged to use the arm normally despite the radiographic appearance of the fracture. Street reported a nonunion rate of only 7%. In addition, there were two delayed unions. Street believed that the most likely cause for these failures was either the selection of a nail that was too small or the presence of a butterfly fragment that was devascularized during open reduction. He felt that the technique could be used safely in open fractures but noted that the results were also good for primary débridement and delayed nailing after about 2 weeks. The advantages of this method, especially when done by closed technique, include early union, low incidence of refracture, low infection rate, relatively short operating time, minimal surgical trauma, and less scar than with other methods such as plate fixation.

Technique for Intramedullary Forearm Nails. According to Sisk,[108] when medullary fixation is used for any forearm fracture, errors in selection of the proper length and diameter of the nail, in operative technique, and in aftertreatment contribute to poor results. Disproportion between the size of the nail and the medullary canal often occurs, allowing side-to-side and rotary movements if the nail is too small in diameter. If the diameter is too large, it may explode the shaft of the radius or ulna. Triangular

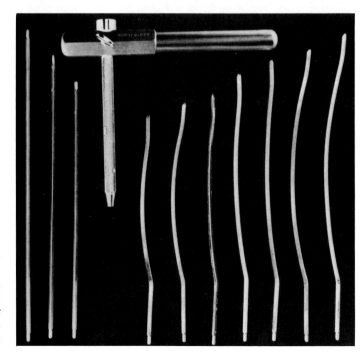

Fig. 9-13. The Sage driver-extractor and full complement of Sage nails for the radius and ulna. *(Sage, F. P.: Medullary Fixation of Fractures of the Forearm. A Study of the Medullary Canal of the Radius and a Report of Fifty Fractures of the Radius Treated with a Prebent Triangular Nail. J. Bone Joint Surg., 41A:1489–1516, 1959.)*

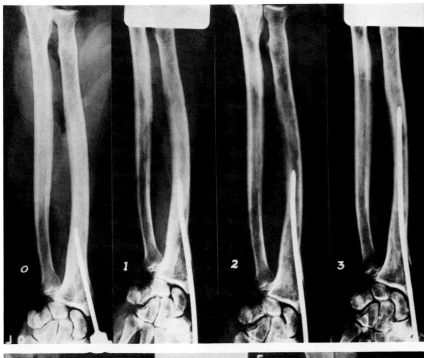

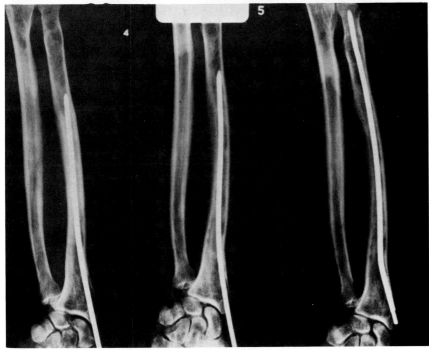

Fig. 9-14. Serial x-rays to show a Sage radial nail being driven up the radius of an amputated specimen. The nail must bend as it traverses the canal and then finally spring back to its original shape. (Sage, F. P.: *Medullary Fixation of Fractures of the Forearm. A Study of the Medullary Canal of the Radius and a Report of Fifty Fractures of the Radius Treated with a Prebent Triangular Nail. J. Bone Joint Surg., 41A:1489–1516, 1959.)*

or diamond-shaped nails are preferred for control of rotation.

Technique for Sage Forearm Nails.[108]   The straight Sage ulnar nail may be used for almost any diaphyseal fracture of the ulna. It may be necessary to

ream the medullary canal, however. The pre-bent Sage radial nail may be used for diaphyseal fractures of the radius unless the fracture is in the proximal one fourth or distal one third of the shaft, where fixation with plates and screws is preferred. The

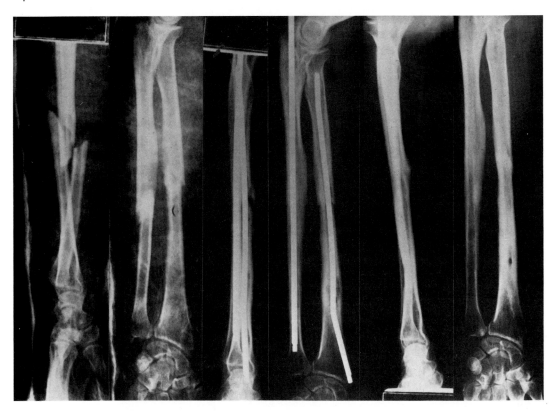

Fig. 9-15. Infection occurred in this radius 6 weeks after nailing. It was believed to be metastatic from an open draining wound present on the knee at the time of nailing. Fortunately, the infection was controlled and union was secured approximately 5 months after nailing. *(Sage, F. P.: Medullary Fixation of Fractures of the Forearm. A Study of the Medullary Canal of the Radius and a Report of Fifty Fractures of the Radius Treated with a Prebent Triangular Nail. J. Bone Joint Surg., 41A:1489–1516, 1959.)*

radial nail should not be used when the medullary canal is less than 3 mm in diameter at its narrowest point. The nail must engage the cortex firmly, and if the cortex is too thin from reaming, the nail will split the shaft.

Prior to beginning the operation, it is imperative that a complete set of Sage nails and insertion equipment be available. This includes a full set of radial and ulnar nails, a combination driver and extractor, a 3-mm drill, and two reamers.

When the ulna alone is to be nailed, the arm is positioned across the chest. When the radius or both bones are to be nailed, the arm is placed on a side table or arm board.

The ulna usually should be nailed first. The fracture is exposed through a short longitudinal incision over the subcutaneous border. Little or no periosteal stripping is required. The fracture is reduced with bone clamps and traction. Special care is taken to obtain exact rotary reduction. To ensure that rotary

reduction is maintained when the nail is driven across the fracture, the surgeon marks opposing points on the proximal and distal fragments with an osteotome. The proximal fragment is delivered into the wound, and an ulnar nail is inserted into the medullary canal to test for fit. If the canal is too small, it is first enlarged with a 3.2-mm drill and then with a reamer. When the reamer passes the smallest diameter of the canal, resistance suddenly ceases. The proximal fragment is reamed until the tip of the reamer is felt beneath the skin at the tip of the olecranon.

After reaming both fragments, the surgeon selects an ulnar nail of correct length by placing it along the ulnar side of the forearm. With the driver threaded on the nail and the elbow flexed to 90°, the nail is driven retrograde up the proximal fragment of the ulna. A small incision is made in the skin over the end of the nail, and the nail is driven farther proximally until its distal end is at the frac-

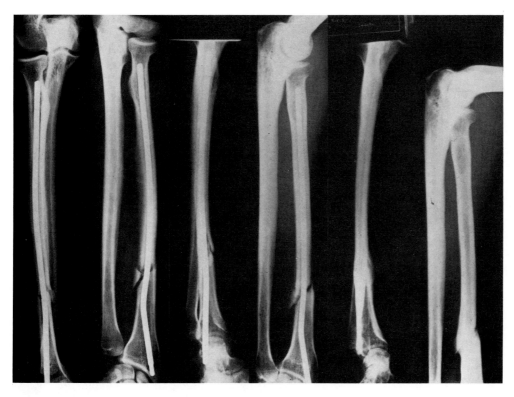

Fig. 9-16. A Sage radial nail was inserted in a fracture that we would now consider too far distal for this form of treatment. Note that telescoping of the nail occurred, resulting in radial shortening and subluxation of the distal radioulnar joint. *(Sage, F. P.: Medullary Fixation of Fractures of the Forearm. A Study of the Medullary Canal of the Radius and a Report of Fifty Fractures of the Radius Treated with a Prebent Triangular Nail. J. Bone Joint Surg., 41A:1489–1516, 1959.)*

ture. The driver is then reversed, reducing the fracture, and the nail is driven down the distal fragment until the driver is within 1.3 cm of the olecranon. Final seating of the nail is delayed until the radius is fixed and radiographs are made confirming the adequacy of reduction.

The radius is then exposed through an appropriate incision. We prefer the volar Henry approach when the fracture is in the distal one half of the shaft and the Thompson dorsal approach when the fracture is in the proximal one half. Once exposed, the fracture is reduced with care to correct any deformity of rotation. The size of the medullary canal is checked with a radial nail, and the proximal and distal segments are reamed if necessary. The fracture is reduced, and the nail is placed along the radial border of the forearm to determine length. The nail should extend from the tip of the radial styloid to within 1.3 cm of the radial head or 3.8 cm of the lateral epicondyle of the humerus.

The wrist is flexed over a folded towel and de-

viated ulnarward so that the radial styloid is accessible. A longitudinal incision 2.5 cm long is made over the radial styloid and carried down to bone at its proximal end but only through the skin distally. Care must be taken to avoid the superficial branch of radial nerve. The periosteum is reflected, and a hole is drilled with a 3.2-mm or 4.8-mm drill through the exposed cortex of the radial styloid. The hole is begun with the drill perpendicular to the cortex, and gradually the handle of the drill is angled distally until the drill is directed toward the lateral epicondyle of the humerus. The drill is advanced 5 or 6 cm, thus producing an oval hole at the point of insertion and a channel that nearly parallels the medullary canal (Fig. 9-17).

The point of the nail is inserted with the nail rotated so that its dorsal or long bow parallels the long arc of the radius. With the wrist in flexion and ulnar deviation, the nail is inserted by hand in a proximal direction as far as possible. If the nail cannot be pushed in for 6 cm, the angle of insertion is

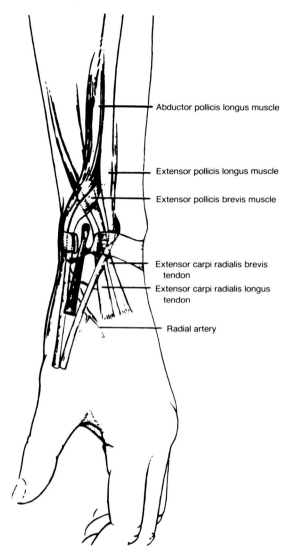

Abductor pollicis longus muscle

Extensor pollicis longus muscle

Extensor pollicis brevis muscle

Extensor carpi radialis brevis tendon

Extensor carpi radialis longus tendon

Radial artery

Fig. 9-17. Medullary nailing of the radius. Nail enters the bone at the radial styloid. Beware of the superficial branch of radial nerve. *(Courtesy of F. P. Sage.) (Sisk, D. T.: Internal Fixation of Forearm Fractures. In Chapman, M. W., and Madison, M. (eds.): Operative Orthopaedics, Vol. 1, pp. 273–285. Philadelphia: J.B. Lippincott, 1988.)*

too acute. The nail is withdrawn and the channel of insertion drilled more obliquely. The driver is threaded on the nail, and while the left hand exerts pressure to depress the nail toward the ulna, the nail is driven in with the right hand. If marked resistance is met, the nail is angled back and forth a few degrees and then driven with moderate blows until it reaches the fracture. When there is an undisplaced butterfly fragment, it is held with a clamp,

the fracture is reduced, and the nail is driven into the proximal fragment leaving 1.3 cm exposed at the radial styloid.

The position of the fracture and the position and length of the nail are checked with anteroposterior and lateral x-rays. If the nails are the correct length, they are then fully seated. The fractures are observed under direct vision to be sure that no distraction occurs. A wire loop is used around a butterfly fragment when it is large and loose. As recommended by Sage, autogenous iliac bone grafts are placed about all fractures of the radius and ulna fixed by medullary nails.

AFTERCARE. A long-arm cast is applied with the elbow at 90° flexion and neutral rotation. The cast is worn for 8 to 12 weeks until enough bridging callus is noted on x-ray. The nails should be removed once union is present but not before 1 year.

COMPLICATIONS. The nail may penetrate the cortex beyond the dorsal curve, or it may split the distal fragment.

Technique for Street Forearm Nails.[115] Proper nail size should be determined prior to surgery, whenever possible. The required length may be determined either by measuring the involved limb or by measuring the radiographs. To avoid the risk of driving the nail through the end of the bone, 1 cm should be subtracted from the measurement. The nail diameter is determined during surgery. As with the Sage nail, a full range of sizes should be available.

In the technique of open nailing, a single skin incision frequently suffices for both bones if the fracture sites are at approximately the same level. Separate subcutaneous approaches are important to avoid continuity of the hematoma of the two fracture sites, with possible synostosis. After the fracture site is exposed, the fragments are mobilized to displace the bone ends sufficiently to ream the canals. It is advisable to expose and ream both bones before nailing either one. The radius is nailed from the distal end. A 1- to 1.5-cm incision is made, extending distally from the dorsal margin of the joint surface at a precise point just lateral to Lister's tubercle; here there is a low ridge on the radius between the extensor carpi radialis longus and brevis tendons. After the skin is incised, the deeper layers are spread gently to avoid damaging the superficial branches of the radial nerve and the dorsal branch of radial artery. The entry portal is directly in line with the medullary canal. At the dorsal margin of the joint, a drill and reamer are introduced at a 45° angle to the joint surface. After the bone is entered 1 to 1.5 cm, with care not to go through the palmar cortex, the angle of the drill is dropped to the axis of the bone and continued another 2 to 4 cm. Before the nail is inserted, it must usually be slightly bent to approximate the bow of the radius, which is mainly lateral but also slightly dorsal. It will be easier to drive the nail if the fracture has been reduced and held with bone-holding forceps. With proper reaming, the nail should drive with some resistance but not require considerable force. When the insertion is almost complete, the driver is removed and reapplied to engage only four turns of the thread. The nail is then driven until the driver abuts the bone.

The nail for the ulna is inserted at the olecranon. A 1-cm longitudinal incision is made over the end of the olecranon, and the insertion of the triceps tendon is split. The reamer is introduced at a point 5 to 8 mm from the dorsal cortex to avoid entering the trochlear notch and 5 mm from the lateral cortex to compensate for the lateral bow. The reamer is then aimed at the fracture site and observed to appear in the canal. The ulna should be reamed all the way to its distal end, because although the canal is wide in this region, the resistance of the cancellous bone may cause distraction of the fracture as the nail is driven home. It may be necessary to withdraw and advance the nail several times while the wrist is held in ulnar deviation to close the gap.

In the technique of closed nailing, an image intensifier is required. It is best to position the arm on an arm board. This allows good visualization with the C-arm. Nail selection and insertion are the same as for open nailing. The nail is inserted into the distal radial and proximal ulnar fragments prior to reduction. Once this has been done, reduction is obtained as described in the discussion of closed reduction. The nail is then driven home. It is important that the nail fit snugly because this proper fit enhances fracture healing and prevents overriding of oblique and comminuted fractures. Since the reduction step can take considerable time, the surgeon must be aware of the amount of radiation exposure he or she is receiving.

Comminuted and segmental fractures are more difficult to treat by closed techniques, but with perseverance treatment can be achieved.

AFTERCARE. X-rays confirming the adequacy of reduction and nail placement are taken before the wounds are closed in the operating room. A long-arm cast is routinely worn for 4 weeks. The position of the forearm in the cast depends on the level of the fracture. Fractures in the proximal third of the forearm are immobilized in supination; fractures in the middle third in neutral; and fractures in the

distal third in pronation. After 4 weeks the cast is removed regardless of the radiographic appearance, and the patient is encouraged to resume normal activities.

COMPLICATIONS. Most complications result from improper selection of nail size. A nail that is too long may be driven through the bone end. One that is too short may not adequately stabilize the fracture. A nail with too great a diameter may split the cortex, and one with a smaller diameter may not adequately control rotation, resulting in delayed union or nonunion of the fracture.

Fixation With Plates and Screws.   Even after better metals became available, many of the early plates used for fractures of the radius and ulna were poorly designed. Failures were common because adequate fixation was not achieved (Fig. 9-18). For a time, the use of plates and screws for the internal fixation of diaphyseal fractures fell into disfavor. Many surgeons treating fractures thought that fixation with a plate and screws held the fracture distracted and caused delayed union and nonunion. This belief was still common in the early 1960s.

Plate-and-screw fixation slowly began regaining favor after Eggers and associates[33-36] introduced the slotted plate (or contact splint, as he preferred to call it). The plate was designed with slots rather than round holes so that, theoretically, the longitudinal muscle pull acting across the fracture would keep the bones in contact and promote union. Whether this actually happens is debatable. After the first few days, fibrous tissue and callus probably grow into the slots so that sliding is no longer possible. In any case, the Eggers plate was a much stronger plate than those used previously, and it provided better fixation. Jinkins and coworkers[59] reported a series of 165 forearm fractures in 1960 in which 145 slotted plates and 20 medullary nails had been used. The overall nonunion rate was only 4.2%. They concluded that the results were best when a slotted plate was used for the ulna and either a slotted plate or a Rush pin was used for the radius.

The idea of using plates through which active compression could be applied began with Danis[26] of Belgium. He published a book in 1949 in which the use of such plates was described. Danis revealed that diaphyseal fractures treated with these plates healed with very little peripheral callus, a phenomenon that he referred to as primary fracture healing. The plate used by Danis had a coapting screw at one end through which compression was applied.

Venable[122] described a similar plate in 1951. Boreau and Hermann[12] introduced a plate with two

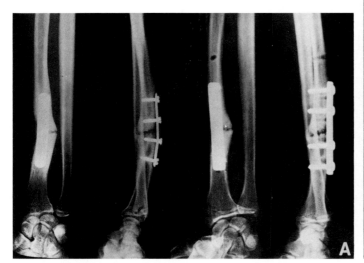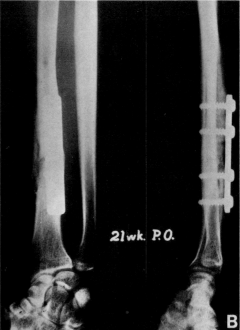

Fig. 9-18. (**A**) An inadequate plate used to treat a fracture at the junction of the middle and distal thirds of the radius. The screws loosened and nonunion resulted. The plate was removed and a compression plate was applied. Note the hole for the compression device. (**B**) Twenty-one weeks after compression plating and bone grafting, satisfactory union is present.

parts in which a cylindrical bolt forced the fragments together. Bagby and Janes[9] modified a Collison plate with oval holes. Compression was achieved by eccentric placement of the screws.

In 1958, Müller, Allgöwer, and Willenegger developed what is now known as the ASIF (AO)* compression plate (Fig. 9-19). The technique for using this plate and other techniques of the Association for the Study of Internal Fixation were published in 1965.[84] The plate is a modification of the plate used by Danis but is much stronger, so more compression can be obtained. Müller visited the Campbell Clinic in about 1959 and introduced the technique of compression plating to us. We first used compression plates in experimental fractures of the femur in dogs (Fig. 9-20).[3] Finding the results to be excellent, we began using the plates in diaphyseal fractures of the radius and ulna in adults in 1960. In the experimental fractures we found that when rigid fixation was achieved with these plates, resorption of the bone at the fracture ends

was not seen radiographically. Resorption was seen radiographically only when infection was present or if the screws had loosened. It appeared that the resorption seen with earlier, less rigid plate fixation and "holding the fracture distracted" was a function of poor fixation with inadequate plates and screws.

In 1972 we reported our clinical experience with the ASIF compression plate for forearm fractures over the 10-year period from 1960 to 1970 at the meeting of the American Academy of Orthopaedic Surgeons in Washington, D.C.[5,6] During this time, 258 adults with displaced fractures of the radius and ulna were treated with compression plate fixation. Fourteen of these patients were lost to follow-up before the outcome was known. The remaining 244 were followed an average of 13.2 months: 112 had fractures of both bones of the forearm, 82 had single fractures of the radius, and 50 had single fractures of the ulna. All 132 patients with single-bone fractures of the radius or ulna were treated with compression plates. Of the 112 patients with both bones fractured, 86 had both fractures fixed with compression plates (Fig. 9-21). Of the remainder, 25 had the fracture of the radius fixed with a compression plate and the fracture of the ulna fixed

---

* ASIF (Association for the Study of Internal Fixation) is the English translation of AO (Arbeitsgemeinschaft für Osteosynthesefragen).

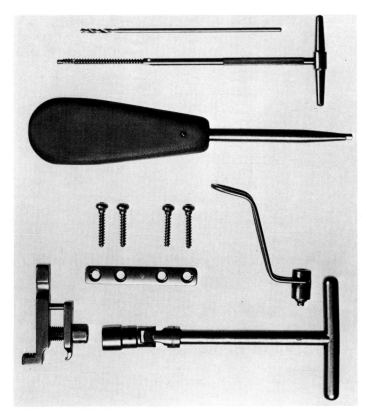

Fig. 9-19. The ASIF (AO) compression instruments. The four-hole plate designed for the human forearm is of heavy construction. The screws have small cores with large threads and are not self-tapping. The drill bit shown at the top has the same diameter as the core of the screws. The tap seen just below the drill bit is used to cut threads in the bone exactly matching those of the screws. The drill guide seen to the right of the screws is used to center the drill exactly so that the heads of the screws countersink accurately into the plate. The compression device (shown at the bottom left with the wrench for tightening this device at the lower right) is rarely used now, having been supplanted by the dynamic compression plate in most cases. *(Anderson, L. D.: Compression Plate Fixation and the Effect of Different Types of Internal Fixation on Fracture Healing. J. Bone Joint Surg., 47A:191, 1965.)*

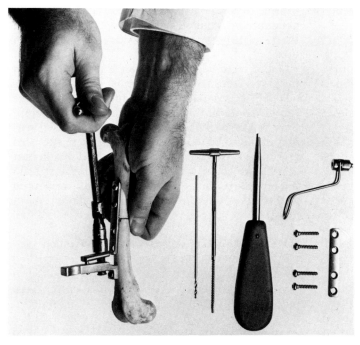

Fig. 9-20. The original ASIF (AO) compression instruments and technique of application with an outboard device. The fracture is reduced and the plate fixed to the upper fragment with two screws. The compression device is hooked into the opposite end of the plate and fixed to the lower fragment with a screw. By tightening of the compression device, the fragments are impacted. A screw is then placed into the second hole from the bottom, the compression device removed, and the final screw placed in the bottom hole. We now tend to favor the dynamic compression plate, which does not require the outboard device. *(Anderson, L. D.: Compression Plate Fixation and the Effect of Different Types of Internal Fixation on Fracture Healing. J. Bone Joint Surg., 47A:191, 1965.)*

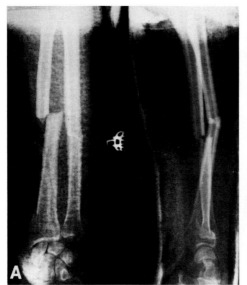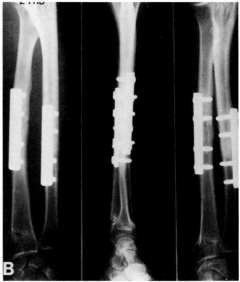

Fig. 9-21. (**A**) Fractures of the radius and ulna in the middle third temporarily immobilized in a cast prior to surgery. Note that there is also a fracture of the distal radius. (**B**) Two years after open reduction and internal fixation with compression plates the radial bow is well maintained and the fractures show good union. The fracture of the distal radius was treated by cast immobilization for 6 weeks.

with some other device (usually a Sage triangular nail). In 1 other patient, the ulna was fixed with a compression plate and the radius with a Sage nail. Thus, 137 fractures of the ulna and 193 fractures of the radius were treated by this method, a total of 330 forearm bones.

Twenty-eight patients (11.4%) had open fractures, and 216 patients (88.6%) had closed fractures. Our policy has been to delay internal fixation in most open fractures until we are sure infection is not present. The period of delay in these 28 patients ranged from 1 to 3 weeks. The average time of delay was 10.6 days.

When we began using the ASIF compression plates, we decided on a policy of using autogenous iliac bone grafts if one third or more of the circumference of the bone was comminuted. Also, in two-bone fractures, if one bone was grafted because of comminution, the other bone was also grafted regardless of its comminution. In accordance with this policy, 63 of the 244 patients (25.9%) had bone grafts applied.

The overall results are shown in Table 9-1 for fractures of the ulna and in Table 9-2 for fractures of the radius. The nonunion rate was 3.7% for the ulna and 2.1% for the radius. The percentage of fractures that united compares favorably with that of other reports in the literature.

The functional results were also very good. Of 223 patients for whom sufficient information was available to determine the degree of function restored, the results were considered excellent in 131, satisfactory in 69, and fair in 16. The results in 7 patients who required additional operations because their fractures failed to unite were considered failures.

There were 28 patients with 38 open fractures in whom internal fixation was delayed. None developed infection. Ninety fractures in 63 patients received bone grafts. The proportion in whom nonunion occurred when bone grafts were used was almost identical to that when grafts were not used (Table 9-3). This fact can be interpreted in different ways. One could conclude that bone grafting did not promote union. However, since grafts were used in the more comminuted fractures, a more reason-

Table 9-1. Results of Compression Plate Fixation for Fractures of the Ulna

	Fractures	Union	Non-union	Rate of Union
Ulna only	50	48	2	96
Ulna and radius	87	84	3	96.5
Total	**137**	**132**	**5**	**96.3**

**Table 9-2. Results of Compression Plate Fixation
for Fractures of the Radius**

	Fractures	Union	Non-union	Rate of Union
Radius only	82	80	2	97.5
Radius and ulna	111	109	2	98.2
Total	**193**	**189**	**4**	**97.9**

able conclusion seems to be that, when bone grafts are used, comminuted fractures heal as well as noncomminuted fractures. Obviously this is not proved; to do so, one would have to treat a series of patients without any bone grafts and then determine whether the rate of nonunion was correlated to the degree of comminution.

The complications in our series of fractures treated with compression plates included nine cases of nonunion (2.7%) and four delayed unions (1.2%) in 330 fractures. Seven of the 244 patients developed significant infection (2.9%) (Fig. 9-22). Four of these infections cleared with antibiotic therapy and caused no further difficulty. The other three failed to unite, and subsequent operations were required. Almost all of the nonunions and delayed unions appeared to have been caused by infection or errors in technique (Fig. 9-23).

Two other complications that we have seen with compression plates have been refracture (if the plate is removed too early) and fracture at the end of the plate from additional trauma. The plate provides very rigid fixation, and the normal stresses acting over the bone beneath the plate are reduced. If the plate is removed early, minor trauma may cause a refracture at or near the site of the original fracture (Fig. 9-24). We do not advocate routine removal of plates. In our experience, the two indications for removal are (1) a prominent plate lying subcutaneously that causes the patient discomfort and (2) the intention of the patient to return to contact sports. Even in these situations, we try to leave the plate in for at least 18 months.

After the plate is removed, the extremity should be protected for about 6 weeks with a right-angle splint with Velcro straps. Since adopting this practice, we have had no further difficulty with refracture. Five such refractures occurred early in the series, when the plates were removed after only a few months. Three fractures were through the screw hole located most distal to the original fracture. In all of these, there was rather violent additional trauma; the forearms were all struck by a baseball bat or similar club. All were minimally displaced

and healed with simple immobilization. (For further discussion of the refracture problem, see p. 718.)

Naiman and coworkers[86] and Dodge and Cody[29] have reported series of diaphyseal fractures of the radius and ulna treated by compression plates. In Naiman and coworkers' series, all 30 fractures united. Dodge and Cody also encountered no nonunions in their 78 patients in whom compression plates were used. However, ten infections occurred; the incidence was 3% in closed fractures and 36% in open fractures.

In 1980, Teipner and Mast[118] published a study comparing double plating with single compression plating for diaphyseal fractures of the forearm. Their double-plating technique was the one described by Jergensen in 1960.[57] The single compression (tension band) was carried out using the recommendations of the ASIF group.[84] Fifty-five patients with 84 fractures were treated using the double-plating technique. In this group there were 82 unions and 2 nonunions. They used a single compression plate in 48 patients with 70 fractures. All 70 of these fractures progressed to union. The authors concluded that both double plating and single compression plating are very effective methods of treating fractures of the diaphysis of the radius and ulna. However, they found that the ASIF compression plating provided a shorter operative time and, at least theoretically, less stress protection of the bone and less devitalization of tissue for exposure. For these reasons, they are now using the single compression plate almost entirely.

In 1981, Rosacker and Kopta[99] reported 54 patients with two-bone fractures of the forearm treated with various fixation devices. Three major types of fixation were used: conventional plates, compression plates, and intramedullary rods. There were 108 fractures in the 54 patients. These workers found that their best results occurred when the fractures were reduced anatomically. The highest percentage of fractures that were anatomically reduced were those treated with compression plates.

**Table 9-3. Results of Compression Plate Fixation
With (c̄) and Without (s̄) Bone Grafting**

	Fractures	Union	Non-union	Rate of Union
Radius s̄ graft	149	146	3	97.3
Radius c̄ graft	44	43	1	97.8
Ulna s̄ graft	91	87	4	95.6
Ulna c̄ graft	46	45	1	97.8
Total	**330**	**321**	**9**	**97.3**

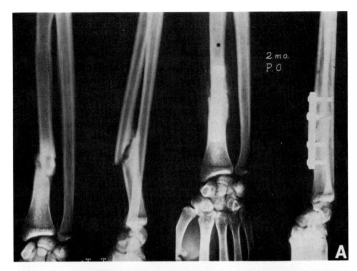

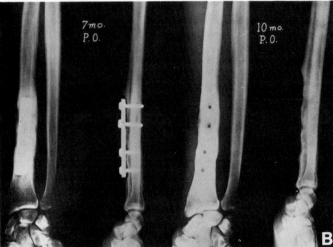

Fig. 9-22. (**A**) A 20-year-old man with an untreated fracture at the junction of the middle and distal thirds of the radius incurred 6 weeks earlier. He was treated with a compression plate applied to the palmar surface of the radius. (**B**) The patient was lost to follow-up but returned at 7 months, at which time he had developed drainage secondary to a *Staphylococcus aureus* infection. Note the periosteal reaction present at the proximal end of the plate and the resorption about the screws in the distal end. The infection resolved when the plate was removed and irrigation-suction treatment was carried out.

The authors suggested that it may be more difficult to apply a compression plate without an anatomic reduction than it is to use a medullary rod or conventional plate. The authors used the criteria of Anderson and coworkers[6] to assess function. Excellent functional results were obtained in 56% of their patients and satisfactory results in 31%. This total of 87% acceptable results is very comparable to the results achieved by Anderson and his group. The one factor most often associated with an excellent result was the adequacy of the reduction. Another factor that Rosacker and Kopta found to be important in obtaining a primary union was delayed surgery. This phenomenon has been observed by others.[62,111] Of Rosacker and Kopta's cases, 19 patients with 38 fractures had their surgery delayed from 1 to 3 weeks for a variety of reasons. All of

these fractures healed primarily. However, the authors pointed out that the economic factors associated with prolonged hospitalization and delayed surgery probably offset the healing benefit of postponing surgery. In contrast to Anderson and associates,[5] Rosacker and Kopta did not advocate primary bone grafting for comminution greater than one third the circumference of the bone. They found that only 11 of their 54 patients required bone grafting for delayed union of their forearm fractures. This is 19%, however, or one in five. Whether to bone graft primarily or not in comminuted fractures is a matter of judgment and opinion. The individual surgeon must decide whether it is better to go ahead and primarily bone graft all fractures that are significantly comminuted while the patient is under an anesthetic and the

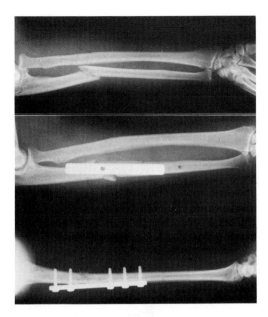

Fig. 9-23. A Monteggia fracture treated by closed reduction of the radial head and compression plate fixation of the ulna. In the bottom films the screws have loosened in the proximal fragment and fixation has been lost. There was an error in technique in that the plate was not centered accurately over the fracture. Nonunion resulted, and a second operation was required.

forearm bones are exposed or else wait to determine if nonunion or delayed union occurs and then perform a second operation for bone grafting. We prefer the former.

Compression plate fixation of forearm fractures is now the preferred technique of most authors.[2,24,49,50,71,108] Sisk[108] pointed out that plates and screws are especially useful for fractures of the distal third or proximal fourth of the radial shaft and of the proximal third of the ulnar shaft. Fractures at these levels are poorly fixed with medullary devices. Chapman and associates[24] suggested that compression plates are indicated in all closed forearm fractures in adults in whom the radius or ulna is angulated greater than 10°. Most of these authors now use the dynamic compression plate rather than the original ASIF plate with an outrigger (Fig. 9-25). This has the advantage of requiring less surgical exposure and has been shown by Anderson and Bacastow[2] to produce results comparable to those with the older-style plate.

Technique of Compression Plating. The technique of compression plating of forearm fractures is discussed in detail in other texts and so is not repeated here.[4,83,84,108] Also, the principles of the AO (ASIF)

techniques are presented in Chapter 1. However, a few important points are emphasized.

Most failures in our and other reported series of fractures of the forearm treated with compression plates have been due to errors in technique or to infection. Before compression plating is undertaken, the surgeon must be thoroughly familiar with the technique and, ideally, should have practiced it in the laboratory. A complete set of equipment must be available, and rigid aseptic technique must be enforced in the operating room.

When the fracture of the radius is located in the distal half of the bone, most authors approach the radius through a volar Henry incision.[6,16,24,25,52] Anderson and associates[6] emphasized that although this is contrary to the principle of placing the plate on the tension side (dorsal radius), the soft tissue coverage on the volar surface is better and the bone contour is flat, making it easier to apply the plate there. Also, there is less soft tissue irritation and thus, presumably, less indication for plate removal. For fractures of the proximal half of the radius, we prefer the dorsal Thompson[6,16,25,119] approach. Some authors, however, recommend using the anterior (Henry) approach for very proximal fractures of the radius. If the fracture is approached dorsally, however, the plate is placed on the dorsal surface of the bone. We believe that there is less hazard to the deep branch of the radial nerve through this approach than through the anterior one. In very high fractures, the nerve can be exposed and retracted. There is, however, greater hazard to the nerve if the plate is subsequently removed through the dorsal approach, when scarring may make visualization of the nerve more difficult. For fractures involving the middle third of the radius, either approach is satisfactory.

For fractures of the ulna, the plate may be placed on either the volar or dorsal surface. The surface to be used is determined by which surface the plate fits better and the location of the comminuted fragments. If there is a butterfly fragment, it is reduced as accurately as possible and the plate is placed over the fragment to hold it in place.

Initially, it was thought that the exposure of the bone should be extraperiosteal. However, following the work of Whiteside and Lesker,[128,129] in which they demonstrated decreased blood flow to damaged muscle and impaired healing of osteotomies following extraperiosteal dissection, most authors[24] now prefer subperiosteal exposure of the fracture, keeping the amount of periosteal stripping to a minimum. Only the fracture site and the surface on which the plate is to be applied should be

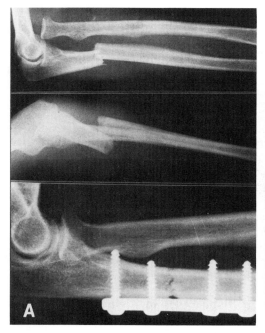
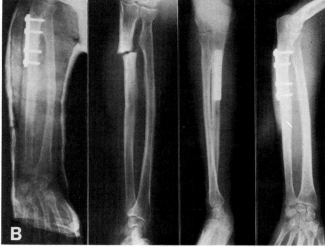

Fig. 9-24. (A) A Monteggia fracture treated by closed reduction of the radial head and compression plate fixation of the ulna. **(B)** The extremity was immobilized in a cast for 6 weeks to allow soft tissue healing about the radial head (**first frame**). At 6 months the plate was removed, and the extremity was not protected. Refracture occurred a month later with minor trauma (**second frame**). A second plate was then applied. Union occurred in 8 weeks with a good functional result (**third and fourth frames**). *(Courtesy of L. D. Anderson and T. D. Sisk.)*

stripped. Anderson, however, still prefers to place the plate on top of the periosteum. This was the technique used in his large series of forearm fractures in which the success rate was 97%.[6]

The ideal length for the plate varies with the size of the plate, the amount of comminution, and the configuration of the fracture. In the last few years, an increasing number of authors[24,49,50] have advocated the use of 3.5-mm plates. Chapman has shown no statistically significant difference in the rates of fracture union between the 4.5-mm dynamic compression plate (DCP) and the 3.5-mm plates. It is important to note, however, that even in a transverse fracture, when the 3.5-mm plates are used, it is usually necessary to use a six-hole plate because the screws must engage a minimum of five cortices on either side of the fracture to obtain adequate fixation. This number is increased to six or seven cortices in very unstable fractures.

If the 3.5-mm DCP is used, the new 3.5-mm cortical screw with 1.25-pitch threads allows the screw to grip the cortex of the bone with additional threads, which improves the pull-out strength. Also, these screws are significantly stronger than the earlier designs of 3.5-mm cortical screws. If the surgeon selects a 4.5-mm DCP, a five- or six-hole plate should be used. It is important to center the plate over the fracture so that no screw will be closer than 1 cm to the fracture line. If screws are placed closer than this, a crack may develop between the screw and the fracture as compression is applied, and fixation will be lost (see Fig. 9-23). It is therefore better to select a longer plate and leave one or two holes empty than to have screws too close to the fracture. In oblique fractures, either an additional lag screw is inserted in a different plane or an interfragmentary lag screw is used through the plate itself. Lag screw fixation across the fracture and any associated fragments increases the strength of the construct up to 40%. Most often, these screws are applied before axial compression of the fracture by the plate (Figs. 9-26 and 9-27).[24]

Whenever possible, comminuted fragments should be secured to the main fragments with lag screws to produce interfragmentary compression. When both the radius and ulna are fractured, both fractures should be exposed and reduced temporarily before a plate is applied to either; otherwise fixation and reduction of one may be lost while an attempt is being made to reduce the other.

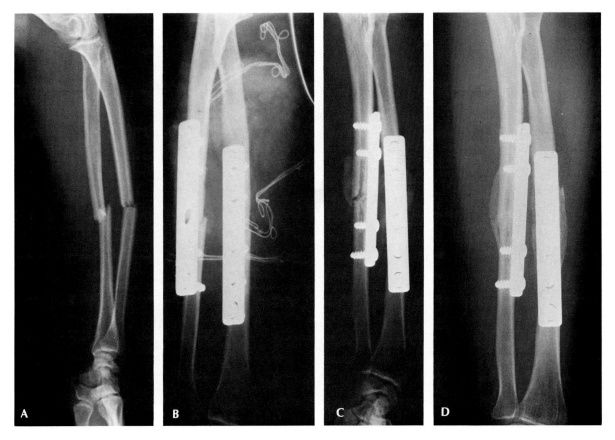

Fig. 9-25. (**A**) Fractures of both bones of the forearm in the middle third. (**B**) X-rays at the time of surgery. Fixation was achieved with two five-hole dynamic compression plates. Because of comminution, one hole in the ulnar plate was left empty and both fractures were bone-grafted. (**C**) At 6 weeks the comminution of the ulna and the iliac bone grafts are easily seen. (**D**) At 1 year the fractures are well united and the bone grafts have been incorporated. The patient had full range of motion in all planes.

Three self-retaining Lane or similar bone-holding forceps are needed for the application of compression plates. After the fracture is reduced and any comminuted fragments are fitted into place, a Lane bone-holding forceps is placed at each end of the plate to secure it temporarily to the bone. The third Lane forceps is placed directly over the fracture at right angles to the other two. Its purpose is to lock the comminuted fragments into place and to prevent shortening of oblique fractures as compression is applied. Some authors report that in unstable fractures, it is technically much easier to fix the plate to one fragment with a single screw before reduction. The fracture is then reduced to the plate bone combination. This technique reportedly necessitates less soft tissue dissection and makes it relatively easy to handle intercalary comminuted bone fragments as well. We have had no experience with this technique, however.

We no longer use the AO tension device routinely in treating forearm fractures, and the reader is referred to the AO Manual of Internal Fixation[83,84] for more information about this technique. We have found the device useful as an adjunct in difficult reductions, however. The external compressor is helpful in reducing shortened and overlapped fragments. In such cases, the plate is applied to one of the major fragments; the articulated tension device is then used to distract the fragments by placing the hook end against the plate. This facilitates reduction. The hook is then reversed to apply tension to the plate (and to compress the fracture)[71] (Figs. 9-28 and 9-29).

Another area where it is helpful is when comminution may make it impossible to achieve perfect alignment and good screw fixation in the comminuted area. The "no touch" technique is used for reduction of the comminuted fragments as follows.

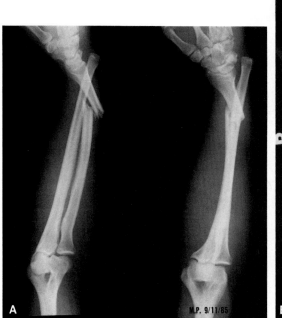
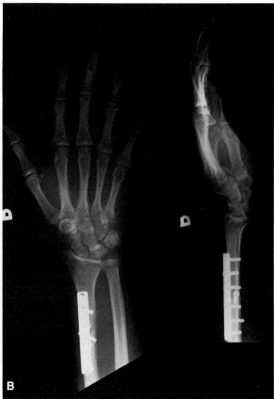

Fig. 9-26. (**A**) Preoperative anteroposterior and lateral x-rays of a 25-year-old man with a closed Galeazzi fracture. (**B**) Postoperative radiographs showing primary fixation with a six-hole, 3.5-mm dynamic compression plate. Note the bicortical screws in the end holes and the separate interfragmentary screw. (*Chapman, M. W.; Gordon, E. J.; and Zissimos, A. G.: Compression-plate Fixation of Acute Fractures of the Diaphyses of the Radius and Ulna. J. Bone Joint Surg., 71A:159–169, 1989.*)

A distractor is applied that pushes against 4.5-mm pins inserted at sites remote from the comminuted or segmental portion. The fragments are distracted sufficiently to obtain good alignment. The comminuted or defect areas are bridged by attaching a well-contoured plate over the intact extreme ends of the fracture. The plate acts as a strut over the comminuted area, which is grafted with bone.

It should be noted that whereas DCPs work well for acute fractures in which the bone is hard, they are not as satisfactory for nonunions and delayed unions as the older compression plates with outboard compression. In nonunions, frequently the bone is softer and the distance available for compression with the DCP is not great enough to allow good compression. Therefore, in nonunions and delayed unions, we prefer to use the older, round-holed ASIF compression plate with outboard compression.

We use autogenous iliac bone grafts if a significant degree of comminution is present. Significant comminution is arbitrarily defined as comminution that involves one third or more of the circumference of the bone.

Finally, it is of utmost importance to close only the subcutaneous tissue and skin. The deep fascia of the forearm is very dense. If it is sutured tightly, edema and hemorrhage may cause increased pressure in the forearm compartments and may lead to a Volkmann's contracture. Obviously, leaving the deep fascia unsutured is important not only with compression plating but also with other forms of internal fixation. We recommend that a closed drainage system be used to decrease the hematoma and resultant swelling. It is removed after 48 hours.

Aftercare. Care after compression plate fixation is tailored to each patient. If the patient is reliable, if the fracture is without significant comminution,

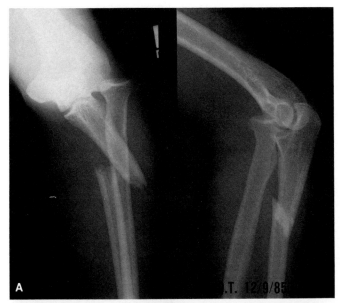

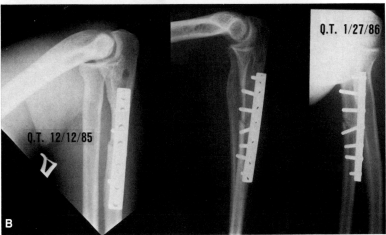

Fig. 9-27. (**A**) Preoperative x-rays of an 18-year-old man with a closed Monteggia fracture. (**B**) Postoperative radiographs showing primary fixation with a seven-hole, 3.5-mm dynamic compression plate, augmented by an olecranon bone graft. Note the unicortical screws on each end of the plate and the use of the center hole as the site for an interfragmentary screw. *(Chapman, M. W.; Gordon, E. J.; and Zissimos, A. G.: Compression-plate Fixation of Acute Fractures of the Diaphyses of the Radius and Ulna. J. Bone Joint Surg., 71A:159–169, 1989.)*

and if stable fixation has been achieved, no external immobilization is necessary (Fig. 9-30). A pressure dressing is applied, and the forearm is elevated from an overhead frame until the swelling begins to subside. As soon as the patient has recovered from the anesthetic, gentle active exercises are begun for the elbow, wrist, and hand. By the end of ten days, such patients have usually regained most of their normal range of motion.

Another category includes the group in which the fracture is not comminuted and stable fixation has been obtained but the patient's reliability is questionable or the fracture is comminuted and stable fixation has not been obtained. One approach is to use a compression dressing with a sugar-tong

splint. After about 10 to 12 days, the sutures are removed and a long-arm cast is applied. The cast is worn until the fracture appears united on x-ray film, usually after about 6 weeks.

Open Fractures of the Radius and Ulna

The ratio of open (compound) fractures to closed fractures is higher for the forearm bones than for any other bone except the tibia.[15] The fact that the ulna has a subcutaneous border throughout its length is the probable reason.

In treating open fractures of both bones of the forearm, we use the classification originally described by Smith[109] and modified by Gustilo and Anderson.[46] Open fractures are classified into three

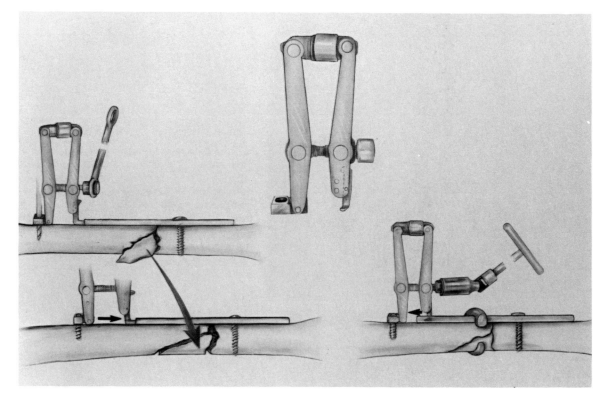

Fig. 9-28. Use of the articulated tension device to assist in initial reduction and provide subsequent stabilization of comminuted fragments. (After Müeller, M. E.; Algöwer, M.; Schneider, P.; and Willenegger, H.: Manual of Internal Fixation, 2nd ed., p. 121. New York, Springer-Verlag, 1979.) (Mallin, B. A.: Principles of Management of Forearm Fractures. In Chapman, M. W. (ed.): Operative Orthopaedics, Vol. 1, pp. 263–271. Philadelphia, J.B. Lippincott, 1988.)

types. Type I is an open fracture with a clean wound less than 1 cm long. Type II is an open fracture with a laceration more than 1 cm long without extensive soft tissue damage, flaps, or avulsions. Type III is either an open segmental fracture, an open fracture with extensive soft tissue damage, or a traumatic amputation. In 1984, Gustilo and colleagues[47,48] further divided type III injuries into A, B, and C. Type III-A injuries are gunshot injuries with adequate coverage of the fractured bone despite extensive soft tissue lacerations, flaps, or high-energy trauma regardless of the size of the wound. Type III-B injuries are farm injuries with extensive soft tissue injury with periosteal stripping and bony exposure, usually associated with massive contamination. Type III-C injuries are open fractures with associated vascular damage requiring repair. Fortunately, the type I and type II wounds are the most common. The usual cause is a sharp spike of bone compounding from within to without. In these fractures we believe that it is safer if the wounds

are débrided and closed either primarily or with a delay of 48 to 72 hours if the wounds are clean. With the patient under anesthesia with good relaxation, an attempt should be made to "hook" at least one of the fractures to prevent excessive shortening. If this cannot be done, shortening can be prevented with pins and plaster while awaiting wound healing. An external fixator may allow better wound management when wounds are extensive. A long-arm cast is applied following the technique described for closed treatment of fractures of both bones of the forearm. When the wounds have healed, usually after 10 to 21 days, one can perform open reduction and internal fixation more safely. As discussed, in our series of forearm fractures treated with compression plates, none of the 28 patients with 38 open fractures developed infections when this policy of delaying open reduction was followed.

An increasing number of authors are recommending primary open reduction and internal fix-

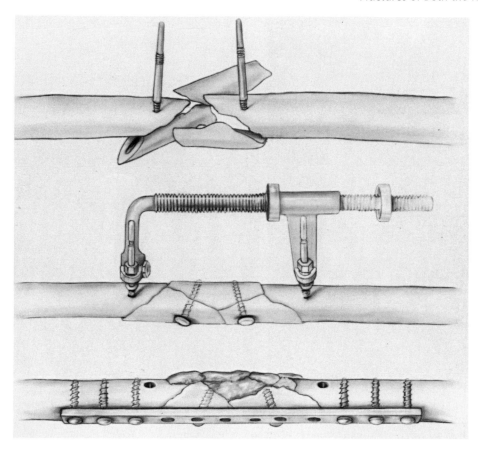

Fig. 9-29. Use of the distracter to assist with reduction and preliminary stabilization of comminuted fractures. *(After Müeller, M. E.; Algöwer, M.; Schneider, P.; and Willenegger, H.: Manual of Internal Fixation, 2nd ed., p. 123. New York, Springer-Verlag, 1979.) (Mallin, B. A.: Principles of Management of Forearm Fractures. In Chapman, M. W. (ed.): Operative Orthopaedics, Vol. 1, pp. 263–271. Philadelphia, J.B. Lippincott, 1988.)*

ation for type I and type II open injuries.[24,32,49,71,77] Chapman even includes some type III-A injuries. If this is to be done, meticulous technique is necessary. After wound cultures have been obtained, cefazolin is administered intravenously in the emergency room. The patient is then taken to the operating room, where the open fracture wound and limb are prepared with povidone soap solution. The wound is copiously irrigated with sterile saline solution using pulsatile lavage. The ends of the bone are exposed using extensile incisions from the open wound. Soft tissue dissection and periosteal stripping are kept to the minimum necessary for adequate exposure. A methodical débridement beginning with the skin and working layer by layer down to the bone is performed. All necrotic tissue is excised. Bone fragments with no soft tissue attach-

ments are usually discarded. The wound is again irrigated with pulsatile saline lavage until a total of 6 to 10 L of saline solution have been used, and 100,000 units of bacitracin is added to the last 2-L bag. Final cultures are taken. Internal fixation is performed as previously described. Although some wounds are closed primarily, most are left open for five to ten days. Antibiotics are given for two to five days postoperatively if there is no evidence of infection and cultures are negative. If the wound is clean without signs of infection, bone grafting is done at the time of closure (Fig. 9-31).

With type III-B and type III-C injuries, management of soft tissue injury is extremely difficult without the use of some form of internal fixation or external fixator. Sisk[108] has used a medullary nail in the ulna to stabilize the forearm while skin graft-

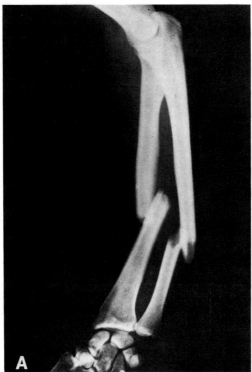
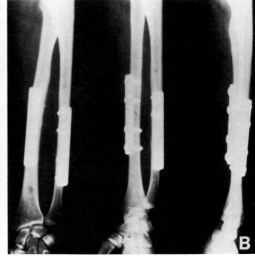

Fig. 9-30. (**A**) Closed fractures of the shafts of the radius and ulna in a cooperative patient. (**B**) Six months after open reduction and compression plate fixation. No external fixation was necessary. Motion was begun early, and functional recovery was complete. Five-hole plates would have been better. (*Anderson, L. D.: Fractures.* In *Crenshaw, A. H. (ed.): Campbell's Operative Orthopaedics, Vol. 1, 5th ed. St. Louis, C.V. Mosby, 1971.*)

ing and similar procedures on the soft tissues are performed. We have found that an external fixator provides good stable fixation of fractures while soft tissue reconstruction is carried out (Fig. 9-32). Godina[44] of Yugoslavia advocated early rather than later soft tissue reconstruction. He reviewed the results of 532 patients who had undergone microsurgical reconstruction following trauma to their extremities. Patients were divided into three groups based on the time from injury to the time of microsurgical reconstruction. Group 1 underwent free flap transfer within 72 hours of injury, group 2 between 72 hours and 3 months, and group 3 between 3 months and 12.6 years. In group 1, the flap failure rate was 0.75%. The infection rate was 1.5%. The average time to fracture healing was 6.8 months with an average hospital stay of 27 days. This was a significant improvement in all categories over patients who had undergone later reconstruction. (See Chapter 4 for a more thorough discussion of soft tissue management of open fractures.)

EXTERNAL FIXATORS

In the past few years, the use of external fixation devices such as the Hoffmann apparatus has grown in popularity as a method of initial management of these severe open fractures of the radius and ulna with soft tissue loss, bone loss, or severe comminution. Their use has been reported by Weiland and associates,[127] DeLee,[27] and Heiser and Jacobs[51] (Figs. 9-33 and 9-34). DeLee noted that there are basically three types of external fixation devices for the forearm bones: the single Hoffmann half-pin frame (Fig. 9-35); the double Hoffmann half-pin frame (Fig. 9-36); and the Hoffmann-Vidal frame with completely transfixing pins (Fig. 9-37). DeLee stated that the indications for the use of complete transfixing pins in the forearm are very limited because of the risk of the pins damaging adjacent neurovascular tissue. Therefore, although the Hoffmann-Vidal frame is the most stable, either the single or the double Hoffmann frame is most often

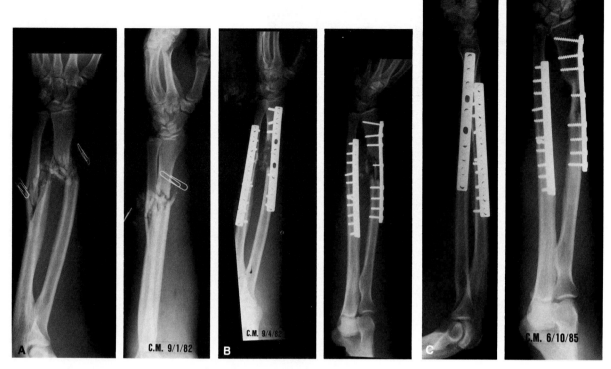

Fig. 9-31. (**A**) Preoperative x-rays in a 32-year-old man with a Type III-A open fracture of the radius and ulna secondary to a high-velocity gunshot wound. (**B**) Postoperative x-rays showing primary fixation with ten-hole, 3.5-mm dynamic compression plates on the radius and ulna. These were augmented by an iliac-crest bone graft at the time of delayed primary closure, 3 days after injury. (**C**) X-rays showing union at 33 months. A normal range of motion was achieved. *(Chapman, M. W.; Gordon, E. J.; and Zissimos, A. G.: Compression-plate Fixation of Acute Fractures of the Diaphyses of the Radius and Ulna. J. Bone Joint Surg., 71A:159–169, 1989.)*

used with half-pins. DeLee suggested the following indications for the use of external fixation in the upper extremity: (1) the presence of severe open wounds with skin and soft tissue loss and a fracture of the radius or ulna; (2) the need to maintain length in cases with bone loss or comminution; (3) open elbow fracture-dislocations with soft tissue loss, in which internal fixation is not advisable; (4) certain unstable distal intra-articular radius fractures; and (5) infected nonunions.

THE CHOICE OF EXTERNAL VERSUS INTERNAL FIXATION IN OPEN FRACTURES

Whether one chooses limited internal fixation or some form of external fixation, the device must be individualized. In most cases, we prefer limited internal fixation as described subsequently because we find the external fixation devices difficult to use on the forearm. If limited internal fixation is chosen, only the minimal amount of metal needed to

stabilize the forearm for wound care should be used. There is no need to fix both bones internally. Medullary nails are better for this purpose than plates and screws. If an infection should develop, screws may pull loose and fixation will be lost. A Sage nail or similar device inserted in the ulna is usually adequate for the immediate purpose. Reconstruction of the radius is left until a later date after there is good soft tissue coverage. Rarely, there may be significant loss of bone from the ulna but not from the radius. In this case the radius is fixed with a medullary nail and the ulna is left for reconstruction later.

As in all open fractures, copious irrigation and meticulous débridement of the wound are extremely important. Antibiotic therapy should be started intravenously in the emergency room after the wound has been cultured and should be continued during and after surgery. Tetanus prophylaxis should be provided.

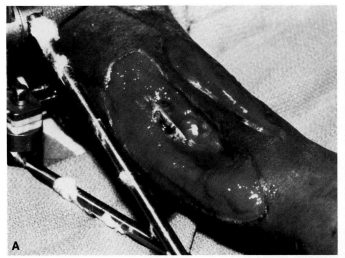

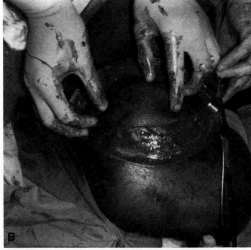

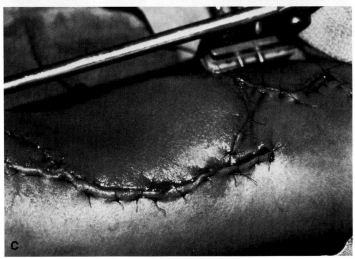

Fig. 9-32. (**A**) A 16-year-old male with extensive bone and soft tissue loss secondary to a gunshot wound of the forearm. After initial stabilization of the forearm with an external fixator, a free scapular flap was used to provide coverage (**B** and **C**).

AUTHORS' PREFERRED METHOD OF TREATMENT

For most displaced fractures of the radius and ulna in adults we prefer ASIF DCP fixation. Closed treatment of these fractures generally yields a high incidence of poor results. On the other hand, the results of compression plate fixation in our 27-year experience have been excellent. The incidence of nonunion has been low (less than 3%), and the functional results have been excellent in most cases. The original ASIF compression plates with outboard compression and the DCPs both give equally good results in acute fractures of the shafts of the radius and ulna. The DCP has the advantage of requiring an incision that is approximately 2.5 cm shorter than that required for the original round-hole plates with outboard compression.

We cannot overemphasize the importance of meticulous attention to the details of operative technique. The need for strict asepsis in the operating room is absolute. Infection and errors in technique are the principal causes of failure. The time of external immobilization with this method is usually less than that with other forms of internal fixation, and in appropriate cases we frequently use no cast at all.

For segmental fractures of the radius we have used one plate on the dorsal surface for the proximal fracture and one on the volar surface for the distal fracture. We have found it difficult to ream and insert Sage nails in segmental fractures of the ra-

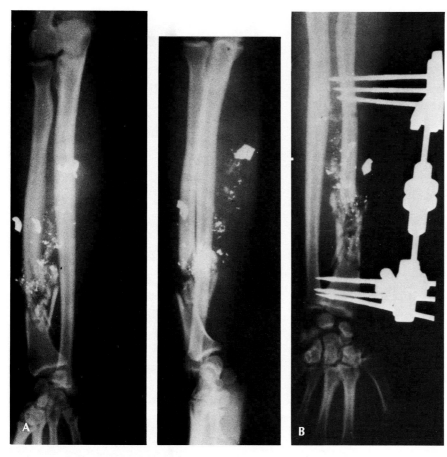

Fig. 9-33. (**A**) A gunshot wound of the distal radius with shortening and disruption of the distal radioulnar joint. (**B**) A single Hoffmann half-pin frame has restored length to the radius and reduced the distal radioulnar joint. *(DeLee, J. C.: External Fixation of the Forearm and Wrist. Orthop. Rev., 10:43–48, 1981.)*

dius. However, they are easier to use for the ulna, and we occasionally will use them for segmental fractures of this bone.

Moderate degrees of comminution can generally be handled with compression plates, but for extensive comminution we prefer a Sage nail for both the radius and the ulna. When the Sage nail is used, comminuted fragments are held in place with circumferential wires, and the fractures are grafted with autogenous iliac bone grafts.

The senior author (L.D.A.) does not like to perform primary internal fixation in open fractures of the shafts of the radius and ulna except in patients with major soft tissue loss, as outlined previously. In most instances, when the wound is relatively small and not too contaminated, the wound is irrigated, débrided, and closed. Antibiotics are used

liberally before, during, and after surgery. The extremity is then immobilized in a cast, and internal fixation is performed as a secondary procedure when the wound is healed. The junior author (F.N.M.) prefers the more aggressive approach, ie, primary internal fixation.

PROGNOSIS

The prognosis for adults with fractures of the radius and ulna depends on many factors. Was the fracture open, and if so, how extensive was the damage and how great was the contamination? Was the fracture displaced or undisplaced, and was there comminution? The surgeon has no control over these and many other factors; they are decided at the time of

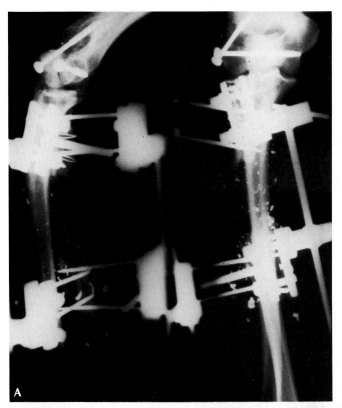

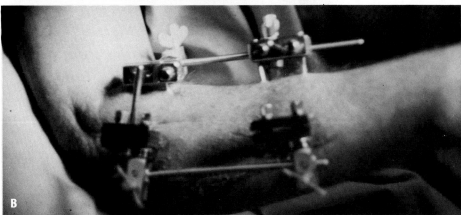

Fig. 9-34. (A) A gunshot wound of the proximal radius in which a 6-cm segment of the proximal radius was blown away with the radial nerve. Fixation was achieved with two single half-pin frames. **(B)** The Hoffmann device in place. Skin coverage was achieved with split-thickness skin grafts.

(continued)

injury. To be sure, the prognosis related to these may be affected by the surgeon's actions and decisions, including early and appropriate treatment.

There are other factors over which the surgeon has more direct control. These include the choice of treatment method (open versus closed reduction), the timing of internal fixation in open fractures, and attention to the details of technique, including gentle soft tissue handling and the prevention of infection.

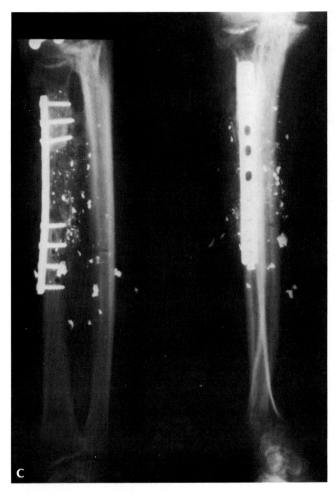

Fig. 9-34 (continued)
(C) After wound healing was achieved, the radius was plated and bone-grafted. Subsequently, tendon transfers for the radial nerve palsy were carried out with good functional results. *(Courtesy of A. J. Weiland.)*

The prognosis for displaced fractures of the radius and ulna in adults treated with closed reduction is generally considered poor in an unacceptably high percentage of patients. For fractures treated with open reduction and rigid internal fixation, the prognosis for achieving union is about 95%. In his series, Sage[101] reported union of 93.8% of the fractures treated with triangular medullary nails, and in our series[4] of forearm fractures treated with compression plates, 97.3% of the fractures united. Approximately 90% had satisfactory or excellent function, and 10% had unsatisfactory or poor function after the first operation. Other articles concerning forearm fractures treated with compression plates report similar results.[2,24,29,49,50,86,102,107,118]

In a group of forearm shaft fractures treated primarily with slotted plates by Jinkins and coworkers,[59] 95.8% united. Caden[21] reported a union rate of 92.5% with slotted plates. Other surgeons have reported similar good results with good rigid fixation both with plates and with medullary nails.[20,98] The important feature common to all these reports in which over 90% of the fractures united was the rigidity of fixation. If medullary nails are used, they must control rotation of the fragments and be sturdy enough to resist angulatory forces. If plates and screws are used, they must be long enough and strong enough to resist loosening and breakage of the fixation. In our experience, the results can be as good for type I, II, or III-A open fractures if open

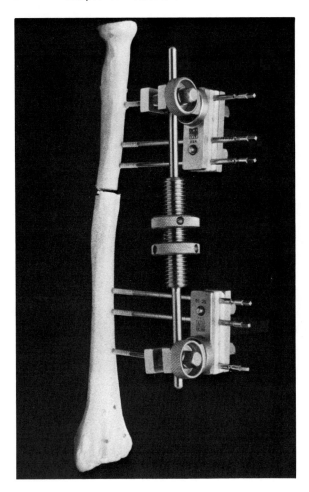

operative procedures are necessary, including the initial débridement and stabilization, skin grafting or pedicle or free flap applications, late reconstruction of the bones, and, frequently, the transfer of tendons. Occasionally, skeletal reconstruction requires creating a one-bone forearm (Fig. 9-38). If infection develops, sequestrectomy and institution of irrigation suction may be necessary. Usually, enough function can be preserved to make all this worthwhile, but the result is generally far from normal. Occasionally, infection and fibrosis of the soft tissues may necessitate amputation.

Fig. 9-35. Single Hoffmann half-pin frame. Three pins above and three pins below the fracture site are connected by a single compression-distraction rod. *(DeLee, J. C.: External Fixation of the Forearm and Wrist. Orthop. Rev., 10:43–48, 1981.)*

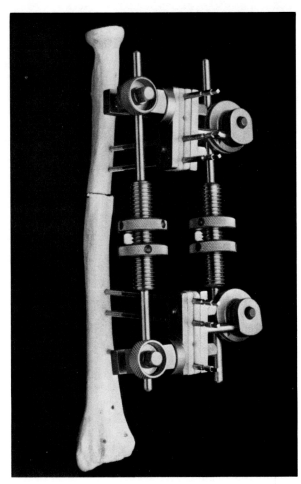

reduction and internal fixation are delayed for 7 to 21 days.

The prognosis for union and good function is much poorer if round medullary nails or inadequate plates are used. Semitubular plates are not recommended. Neither are round medullary nails, which have been reported to lead to nonunion in 14% to 16% of cases.[21,110] Kirschner-wire fixation was reported by Smith and Sage[110] to produce nonunion in 38% of forearm fractures.

For open fractures of the shaft of the radius and ulna with major skin and soft tissue loss, the prognosis must be more guarded. In these cases, several

Fig. 9-36. Double Hoffmann half-pin frame. Three pins above and three pins below the fracture site are connected by two compression-distraction rods. *(DeLee, J. C.: External Fixation of the Forearm and Wrist. Orthop. Rev., 10:43–48, 1981.)*

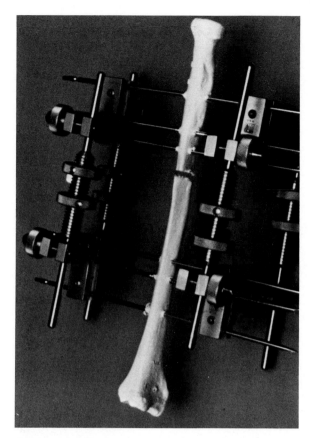

Fig. 9-37. Hoffmann-Vidal frame. Transfixing pins above and below the fracture site are connected by the classic Hoffmann-Vidal frame. This type of external fixation device is rarely indicated in fractures of the radius and ulna. (DeLee, J. C.: External Fixation of the Forearm and Wrist. Orthop. Rev., 10:43–48, 1981.)

COMPLICATIONS

In 1983, Stern and Drury[114] reported on the complications in their series of 87 fractures. A major complication occurred in 18 of 87 patients (28%). These included nonunion in 6 (9.3%). The incidence of nonunion was higher in bones treated with plates in which only four screws were used. Screws loosened in 3 (4.7%). Radioulnar synostosis occurred in 6 (9.4%). Five of the six cases occurred in patients with head injuries. Osteomyelitis occurred in 2 (3.1%) patients with massive crush injuries. One patient (1.6%) had an intraoperative laceration of the radial artery.

Nonunion and Malunion

Nonunion of fractures of the shafts of the radius and ulna is most often seen when infection is pres-

ent, when fixation after open reduction is inadequate, and when adequate reduction was not achieved and maintained following closed treatment. Accurate open reduction and rigid internal fixation will prevent most of these complications. The various methods of treating nonunion are discussed in Chapter 2.

Infection

Despite all attempts to prevent infection, some open fractures and closed fractures treated by open reduction inevitably become infected. With good technique and operating facilities, this group should be small. If infection develops, the wound should be cultured, the sensitivity of the organism should be determined, and appropriate antibiotic therapy should be begun. Superficial infections frequently respond to this treatment alone. If the infection appears to be deep, the wound should be opened to provide drainage, and if the arm is not already immobilized in a cast, a cast should be applied. External support rests the extremity and decreases the chance of the infection causing loss of fixation. If internal fixation is in place and has not loosened, it should not be removed; a fairly high percentage of fractures that have been fixed internally unite in spite of infection if the extremity is held in a cast. After the fracture has healed, the metal can be removed. The residual infection is treated by irrigation-suction (see Fig. 9-22).

We probably should consider treating infections following open reduction more vigorously than we have in the past. Although we have had little experience with early débridement and irrigation-suction in these cases, the results of such management have been good in acute hematogenous osteomyelitis and might have a place here.

In late infections, when fixation has already been lost and nonunion has developed, the metal should be removed along with any sequestra, and irrigation-suction should be instituted. After the infection has cleared, the extremity is maintained in a cast, Orthoplast gauntlet, or leather lacer brace. When the extremity has been free of infection for 6 months, reconstructive procedures can be undertaken with less danger of flaring up the old infection. Appropriate antibiotics should be given before, during, and after the reconstructive surgery.

Nerve Injury

Nerve injuries associated with fractures of both bones of the forearm are uncommon in closed fractures or those with only minor compounding wounds. Prosser and Hooper[92] reported a case in

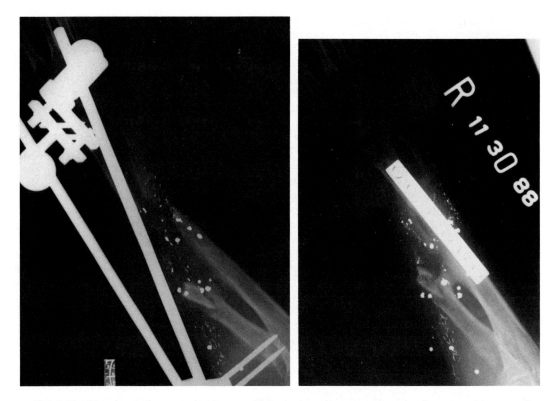

Fig. 9-38. One-bone forearm. A 16-year-old had a gunshot wound to the forearm with extensive skin, muscle, bone, and nerve loss. Following free flap coverage, a one-bone forearm was created for skeletal reconstruction.

which the ulnar nerve was trapped between the bone ends of a greenstick fracture of the ulna. Return of function was complete following removal of the nerve from the bone. Nerve injuries are more common in the major compound wounds with extensive soft tissue loss, such as shotgun injuries. In such an injury, if one of the major nerves is found not to be functioning, it should be explored at the time of débridement to determine whether it is intact or divided. If it is divided, the ends should be tagged together with sutures to prevent retraction and facilitate later repair. If the wound is clean, the nerve cleanly transected, and the soft tissue bed adequate, primary nerve repair at the time of wound closure is probably the appropriate treatment.

Vascular Injury

The collateral circulation of the forearm is good, and if either the radial or the ulnar artery is functioning, the hand and forearm are usually not in jeopardy. When either vessel is patent, the other can simply be ligated. Animal experiments by Gelberman and coworkers[41] and by Trumble and coworkers[120] showed low patency rates if one artery in the forearm is repaired when the other is intact. They thought that this is due to back pressure from the intact vessel and dilation of collateral vessels. It is rare to have both vessels lacerated except in open fractures in which a traumatic near-amputation has occurred. Here the damage to nerves, tendons, and bone is sometimes so severe that amputation may be necessary, although replantation or revascularization using microsurgical techniques is a reasonable alternative in selected cases.

Compartment Syndrome

Relatively little has been written about compartment syndromes in the forearm. Compartment syndromes occur in the forearm both after accidental trauma and after surgery.

In 1975, Eaton and Green[31] reported 19 patients with Volkmann's ischemia, which they considered to be a palmar compartment syndrome of the forearm. The causes of the palmar compartment syndrome included supracondylar fractures, knife wounds of the forearm, and osteotomy of the radius and ulna. They found the most important diagnostic physical finding to be palpable induration of the flexor compartment. Another important early sign is pain on passive extension of the fingers. The radial pulse was absent in only 5 of their 19 patients. This should make us all aware that the presence of a palpable radial pulse does not rule out the presence of a palmar compartment syndrome. Eaton and Green emphasized early decompression not only of the compartment but also of each muscle that shows vascular impairment.

In 1980, Matsen[72] published an excellent book providing a summation of the historical and current knowledge of this subject, including etiology, measurement of compartmental pressures, and treatment. We highly recommend a thorough study of this treatise to all surgeons who treat trauma patients, including those with forearm fractures. (For a more abbreviated discussion of compartment syndromes, see Chapter 5.)

Just as in the leg, it is possible to have a palpable forearm pulse despite increased pressure in the forearm compartments sufficient to obliterate the capillary circulation to the muscles and nerves. This may confuse the picture and delay diagnosis and treatment. In such cases there is decreased sensation in the fingers, little or no function in the forearm muscles, and deep, boring pain in the forearm disproportionate to what one would expect (Fig. 9-39). Pain on passive extension of the fingers is also an important sign of ischemia in the forearm muscles. One should not hesitate to measure compartment pressures. The treatment is early and wide fasciotomy from the elbow to the wrist. At the time of operation, the muscles bulge into the wound. The incision should be allowed to separate, and delayed closure can be done later, sometimes requiring skin grafts.

Closed compartment syndromes that follow surgery on the forearm are usually due to faulty hemostasis and closure of the deep fascia. They can usually be avoided by releasing the tourniquet prior to wound closure to make sure hemostasis is adequate and by closing only the subcutaneous tissue and skin. We know of three patients in whom compartment syndromes developed after open reduction and internal fixation of forearm fractures. In

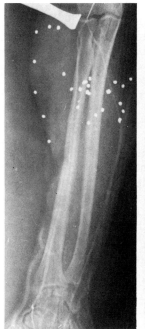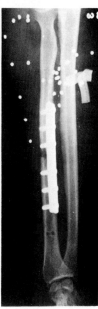

Fig. 9-39. A close-range gunshot wound resulted in a fracture of the radius in the middle third and a closed compartment syndrome. Weak pulses were present at the wrist, but there was decreased sensation in the hand, decreased function of the forearm muscles, and deep, boring pain. The arteriogram showed filling of both radial and ulnar arteries (**first frame**). An immediate anterior and posterior fasciotomy achieved almost immediate return of sensation and motor function. After skin coverage was achieved, the fracture of the radius was treated with a compression plate 5 weeks later.

all three, the deep fascia had been closed. This complication is usually avoidable.

Synostosis

Synostosis of the radius and ulna following fracture is relatively uncommon. In our series of forearm fractures treated with compression plates, 112 patients had fractures of both the radius and ulna and only 3 had a complete synostosis.[5] All three had badly displaced and comminuted fractures of both bones at the same level.

Patients in whom a synostosis develops frequently have a history of either a crushing injury of the forearm or a head injury. If a synostosis develops and the position of the forearm is relatively functional, it is usually best to do nothing. If the position of the forearm is poor, osteotomy to place the hand in a more functional position should be considered. A few cases of successful resection of synostoses have been reported, but usually the heterotopic bone reforms and the synostosis recurs. In 1983, Breit[18] reported good results in a 28-year-old woman who underwent resection of a post-traumatic synostosis, obliteration of the dead space with muscle, prevention of hematoma formation, and early mobilization. Maempel[70] reported two cases of successful excision of a traumatic radioulnar synostosis in which he had used a Silastic sheet interposed between the forearm bones following resection. Vince and Miller[124] reported their results in the treatment of 28 adults with a post-traumatic radioulnar synostosis. They developed a classification system based on the anatomic location of the synostosis. Type 1 involved the distal intra-articular part of the radius and ulna and was the least common in their series. Type 2 involved the nonarticular portion of the distal third and the middle third of the shafts of the radius and ulna. This was the most common. Type 3 involved the proximal third (Fig. 9-40). Seventeen of 28 synostoses were excised. Three of four type 1, none of the ten type 2, and two of three type 3 cross-unions recurred following surgical treatment.

Refracture

In 1988, Deluca and coworkers[28] reported refractures in 7 of 67 patients. Refracture occurred between 42 and 121 days following plate removal. In their series, fracture always occurred through the original fracture site. The average time from original injury to plate removal in refractures was 16

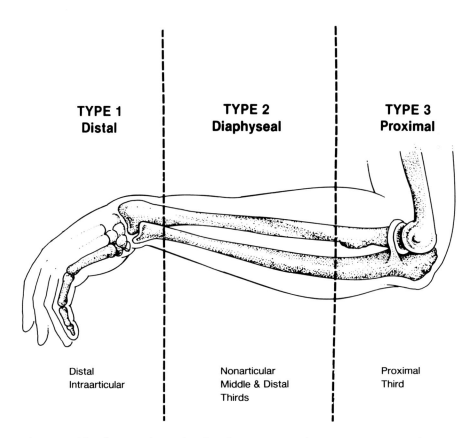

TYPE 1
Distal

TYPE 2
Diaphyseal

TYPE 3
Proximal

Distal
Intraarticular

Nonarticular
Middle & Distal
Thirds

Proximal
Third

Fig. 9-40. This diagram shows the classification system for cross-unions complicating fractures of the forearm. Type 1 (distal) is located in the distal intra-articular part of the forearm. Type 2 (diaphyseal) occurs in the middle and nonarticular distal thirds of the forearm and Type 3 (proximal) in the proximal third, as determined by the length of the ulna. (Vince, K. G., and Miller, J. E.: Cross-union Complicating Fracture of the Forearm: Part 1: Adults. J. Bone Joint Surg., 69A:641, 1987.)

months. No refractures were seen in patients if the plates were removed after 24 months. Of seven refractures, only one had adequate compression. Refracture should be included among the risks of removal. To help identify patients who are at risk, the physician should consider several factors: (1) the nature of the original injury (a disproportionate number of refractures occurred in patients in whom the initial fracture was due to high-energy trauma or a crush injury or was open or associated with other fractures in the extremity); (2) failure to achieve adequate initial compression or reduction in a comminuted fracture; or (3) radiographic determination that the site of the original fracture has remained radiolucent.

Chapman and associates[24] believe that the incidence of refracture can be reduced by the use of 3.5-mm dynamic compression plates. He reported only two refractures in his series and pointed out that both had occurred in fractures in which 4.5-mm plates had been used. In two cases, however, there was early failure of fixation. In one patient a 3.5-mm DCP was used, and in the other, a semitubular plate was used.

Radin and Rose[93] reported a fracture of a semitubular plate within a long-arm cast. The fracture was thought to be due to fatigue caused by the forces generated by the finger flexors. Semitubular plates are not recommended for treatment of forearm fractures except very rarely on the proximal radius or distal ulna.

Muscle and Tendon

Rayan and Hayes[96] reported a case in which the flexor digitorum profundus of the ring finger was trapped between the ends of the ulna in a two-bone forearm fracture. This was not recognized until 2 years later, after the fracture had healed. Release of the entrapped muscle belly resulted in return of full active extension of the ring finger.

FRACTURE OF THE ULNA ALONE (NIGHTSTICK FRACTURE)

UNDISPLACED FRACTURES

Undisplaced or minimally displaced fractures of the shaft of the ulna are fairly common. Most result from a direct blow. Recently, Patel and coworkers[88] and Bell and Hawkins[10] have both reported stress fractures of the ulnar diaphysis in athletes. Fractures in the distal half of the bone usually unite in good

position if they are immobilized in a long-arm cast. The usual time required for union is about 3 months. Loss of position is more common in the proximal half of the bone, where the cast does not provide such good fixation because of greater muscle bulk. If x-rays of these fractures through the cast reveal loss of position, open reduction and internal fixation should be performed.

Just as they reported good results using a functional brace in fractures of both bones of the forearm, Sarmiento and Latta[104] reported excellent results using a functional sleeve in isolated fractures of the ulna. They found that it is not necessary to limit pronation and supination in isolated fractures of the shaft of the ulna. They initially place isolated fractures of the ulna in a long-arm cast with the elbow at 90° flexion and the forearm in a relaxed attitude of supination, with the wrist in neutral or slight dorsiflexion. As soon as the acute symptoms and swelling have subsided, the cast is removed and an adjustable Orthoplast sleeve with Velcro straps is applied. Free motion of the elbow and wrist, as well as pronation and supination, is permitted. As the swelling gradually decreases, the straps on the Orthoplast sleeve are tightened to maintain a firm fit. Sarmiento and Latta reported that they have treated over 250 consecutive isolated fractures of the ulna using this method, with only one nonunion resulting. They do stress that the method is not applicable to Monteggia fractures, in which an anatomic reduction must be obtained and rigid internal fixation of the ulna used to prevent redislocation of the radius. In 1987, Zych and coworkers[130] published a report supporting Sarmiento's results. They concluded that this was an appropriate technique for extra-articlar fractures with angulation in any plane up to 10°. They pointed out that this method should not be used in Monteggia fractures, in unreliable patients, or in patients with a significant neurologic or vascular deficit.

Pollock and coworkers[91] reported excellent results in patients treated with minimal or no immobilization. They compared the fractures of 12 patients treated with a long-arm cast with 42 fractures treated with minimal or no immobilization. In the 12 patients treated with a long-arm cast, the fractures were all in the middle or distal third of the ulnar shaft, and none were displaced greater than one half the diameter of the bone. The average time to union was 10.5 weeks, and the nonunion rate was 8%. The remaining 42 patients were treated one of two ways. Ten patients wore either a short-arm splint or cast for 2 weeks, at which time immobilization was discontinued. In 32 patients, no immobilization was used. An elastic bandage was applied from the palm to the elbow to control swelling. In this group, the average time to union was 6.7 weeks, and no nonunions occurred.

Hoffer and Schobert,[53] however, reported three cases in which they felt that "casual treatment" for nondisplaced ulnar shaft fractures had failed. They recommended the more traditional approach of using a long-arm cast or functional brace.

In our experience, patients have significant pain unless some form of immobilization is used. In the distal third of the ulna, we prefer short-arm cast immobilization,[30] but in fractures of the middle or proximal third of the ulna, we use a long-arm cast.

DISPLACED FRACTURES

We define displaced fractures of the ulna as those with greater than 10° of angulation in any plane or fractures that are displaced greater than 50% of the diameter of the ulna.[30] Displaced fractures of the ulna alone do occur without fracture of the radius or dislocation of the radial head, but if there is much displacement, there is usually some associated injury. One must be sure that the elbow and wrist are well visualized in the x-ray films so that

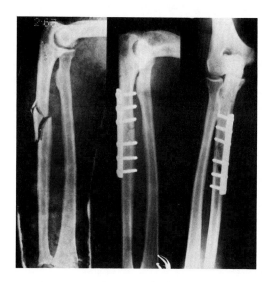

Fig. 9-41. A closed comminuted fracture of the ulna with a large butterfly fragment (**first frame**). Rigid fixation was achieved with a six-hole compression plate and screws. The butterfly fragment was anatomically reduced and held beneath the plate. Films made in the operating room show the fracture lines to be barely visible (**second and third frames**).

these injuries are not missed. In solitary fractures of the ulna, open reduction and internal fixation should be done if there is any significant displacement. For most fractures of the ulna, we prefer a five- or six-hole compression plate. In fractures of the middle or distal third of the ulna, triangular nails work well and may be better than plates if there is extensive comminution over a long area or if the fracture is segmental. Severely comminuted fractures should be bone grafted. In the proximal third of the ulna, the medullary canal is large, and a nail will not provide rigid fixation. Compression plate fixation is better at this level (Fig. 9-41).

MONTEGGIA'S FRACTURE

In 1814, Monteggia[79,95] of Milan published his classic description of the fracture that is associated with his name. Strictly speaking, a Monteggia fracture is a fracture of the proximal third of the ulna with an anterior dislocation of the radial head (Fig. 9-42). As pointed out by Bado[8] and Boyd and Boals,[14] this strict definition accounts for only 60% of ulnar fractures with associated dislocation of the radiohumeral articulation. Bado[8] coined the term *Monteggia lesion* to include the entire spectrum of these injuries. He classified these injuries as follows:

Type I (60% of cases). Anterior dislocation of the radial head. Fracture of the ulnar diaphysis at any level with anterior angulation.

Type II (15% of cases). Posterior or posterolateral dislocation of the radial head. Fracture of the ulnar diaphysis with posterior angulation.

Type III (20% of cases). Lateral or anterolateral dislocation of the radial head. Fracture of the ulnar metaphysis.

Type IV (5% or less of cases). Anterior dislocation of the radial head. Fracture of the proximal third of the radius. Fracture of the ulna at the same level.

Other authors classify these injuries somewhat differently, but it seems clear that the fracture of the proximal third of the ulna with anterior dislocation of the radial head is the most common (type I). In the report of Speed and Boyd[113] in 1940, 83.3% of the radial head dislocations were anterior, 10% were posterior, and 6.7% were lateral. Thus, in their series, Bado's type I lesion was by far the most common, but the type II lesion was more frequently seen than the type III.

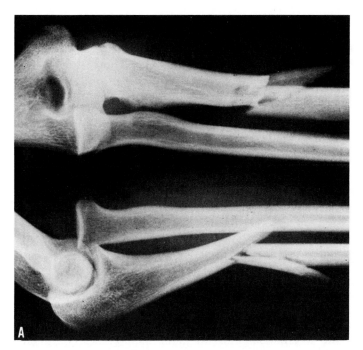

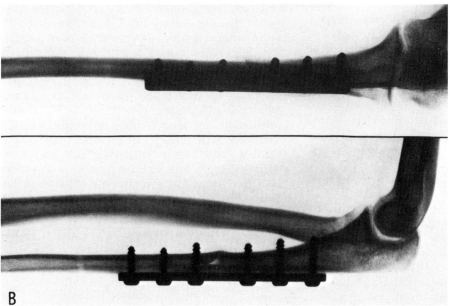

Fig. 9-42. **(A)** Preoperative x-rays of an acute Monteggia lesion in an adult. Note the comminution of the ulna. **(B)** X-rays 3 months postoperatively. *(Boyd, H. B., and Boals, J. C.: The Monteggia Lesion. A Review of 159 Cases. Clin. Orthop., 66:94–100, 1969.)*

MECHANISM OF INJURY

There has been considerable discussion in the literature about the mechanism of injury in Monteggia lesions. The mechanism obviously must vary depending on the type of lesion. The greatest discussion has been about whether the true type I Monteggia fracture is caused by forced pronation of the forearm or by a direct blow over the posterior aspect of the ulna, as when it is struck by a club. Evans[39] reproduced the Monteggia fracture in cadaveric specimens. He placed the humerus in a vise and applied strong pronation to the forearm with a wrench. The shaft of the ulna fractured, and the radial head dislocated anteriorly. Bado[8] agreed with Evans and pointed out that in lateral views of the elbow in type I lesions, the bicipital tuberosity is located posteriorly, indicating full pronation. Evans pointed out that in falls the hand and forearm are usually in full pronation. With the hand planted on the ground, the added weight of the body causes an external rotatory force on the extremity, which produces greater pronation. Evans also cited the lack of hematoma and contusion over the fractured ulna as further evidence that the Monteggia type I fracture is caused by forced pronation in a fall.

On the other hand, we have seen a number of patients with type I lesions who gave no history of a fall but had a definite history of having been struck over the ulna with a baseball bat or similar object. This group of patients did have contusion and hematoma over the ulna, and it seems clear that a direct blow to the ulna was the cause of their injuries. Probably the truth is that the type I Monteggia lesion can be produced either by a fall with forced pronation or by a direct blow over the posterior ulna.

In 1951, Penrose[90] described the mechanism of injury for the type II Monteggia lesion as a variation of posterior dislocation of the elbow. In these type II lesions, the ligamentous attachments of the proximal ulna are stronger than the ulna itself. Thus, the radial head dislocates posteriorly, but the humeroulnar joint remains intact and the ulna fractures.

Bado[8] stated that the mechanism of injury in the type III Monteggia lesion is a direct blow over the inner aspect of the elbow and that this type occurs only in children. However, we have seen at least one such lesion in an adult. In 1976, Germain[42] reported five additional cases of type III Monteggia lesions. He thought that a possible mechanism of injury could be varus stress applied to the elbow with the forearm in a position of hyperpronation.

All five of the type III Monteggia lesions recorded by Germain were in children under the age of 10.

In 1977, Mullick[85] stated that the first type III Monteggia lesion was reported by Weiss in 1941. He noted that from 1941 until 1977 only nine other cases of type III Monteggia lesions were fully reported in the literature and four other cases were briefly mentioned. His bibliography does not include Germain's report. Mullick reported two additional cases and described the nature and mechanism of the injury. In one of his cases the dislocation of the radial head was anterolateral; in the second case, it was posterolateral. He thought that the primary causative force in type III Monteggia lesions is forced adduction. If the primary adduction force is applied while the forearm is in pronation, then the dislocation of the radial head is anterolateral. On the other hand, if the forearm is in midposition or supination when the primary adduction force is applied, the radial head will dislocate posterolaterally. Mullick advised reduction of both anterolateral and posterolateral type III Monteggia lesions under general anesthesia with the elbow in full extension. An abduction force is applied with the forearm in full supination and with pressure applied directly over the dislocated radial head. Supination is used in both anterolateral and posterolateral type III Monteggia lesions because this position puts the fibers of the interosseous membrane on stretch and aids in reduction of the dislocated radial head.

Bado does not describe the mechanism of injury in the type IV Monteggia lesion other than to note that it is a type I lesion with associated fracture of the radial shaft. Possibly a second blow over the radial side of the forearm after the radial head has already dislocated accounts for this injury.

SIGNS AND SYMPTOMS

The signs and symptoms of Monteggia lesions vary with the type. In type I lesions, the radial head can be palpated in the antecubital fossa and there is shortening of the forearm with anterior angulation of the fractured ulna. In type II lesions, the radial head can be palpated posterior to the distal humerus and there is posterior angulation of the ulna. The radial head can be felt laterally in the type III lesions, and there is lateral angulation of the ulnar metaphysis. In the type IV lesions, the radial head is located anteriorly, and there is tenderness and deformity of the radial and ulnar shafts at the level of the fractures.

In all four types of Monteggia lesions there is marked pain and tenderness about the elbow. The patient resists any attempts to move the elbow in flexion-extension as well as pronation-supination.

Associated Nerve Injury

Paralysis of the deep branch of the radial nerve is the most common associated neurologic lesion. Boyd and Boals[14] reported five such cases in their series of 159 patients treated at the Campbell Clinic. These authors noted that spontaneous recovery is the usual course and that exploration is not indicated.

In recent years, an increasing number of articles have pointed to the association of posterior interosseous nerve palsy with Monteggia fractures. Bruce and associates[19] reported a 17% incidence of nerve palsies in their series of Monteggia fractures. All of these involved either the radial nerve or the posterior interosseous nerve. Alvarenga and coworkers[1] also found a significant incidence of radial nerve injury in Monteggia lesions, especially Bado's type II. Mestdagh and colleagues[75] reported four patients with radial nerve palsies in a series of 44 patients. Jessing[58] reported an even higher incidence of radial nerve palsy associated with Monteggia lesions. In his series of 14 patients, radial nerve palsy developed in 6. All of these were confined to the deep branch of the radial nerve. All six of his patients regained full radial nerve function starting 6 to 8 weeks after injury. Therefore, he agreed with Boyd and Boals[14] that exploration of the nerve is not indicated unless function fails to return after the expected time.

Morris[82] and Spar[112] have separately reported irreducible Monteggia lesions with entrapment of the radial nerve. In each of these cases, the posterior interosseus nerve was found to be tightly wrapped around the neck of the radius, thus blocking reduction. The patient described by Morris presented with a complete loss of radial nerve function. In the patient described by Spar, radial nerve motor function was present on admission, but a posterior interosseous nerve palsy developed following unsuccessful closed reduction. In both cases the nerve was extracted surgically from its entrapped position around the neck of the radius and the ulna was internally fixed. Both patients regained full function of the radial nerve.

In 1975, Lichter and Jacobson[69] reported the first known case of tardy palsy of the posterior interosseous nerve secondary to an old Monteggia fracture. This patient was a 46-year-old carpenter in whom weakness had developed in the extensors of the right hand and wrist over the preceding year. The patient related that at the age of 7 he had been struck on the forearm by a golf ball and a mass that had developed over the dorsal aspect of the forearm had persisted. Examination revealed weakness of the muscles innervated by the posterior interosseous nerve and a decreased range of motion in the elbow. Radiographs of the elbow demonstrated dislocation and enlargement of the radial head. Surgery was performed to explore the deep branch of the radial nerve. The enlarged and distorted radial head was found to be attenuating the supinator muscle, and the radial nerve was stretched over the mass. Neurolysis of the posterior interosseous nerve was performed, along with excision of the radial head. The patient made an excellent recovery, although mild weakness of extension of the fingers persisted.

Two years later, in 1977, Austin[7] reported a very similar case in which tardy radial nerve palsy developed 65 years after a Monteggia fracture in a 72-year-old retired laborer. At the time of surgery, a mass of fibrous tissue was found to encase the posterior interosseous nerve, and the nerve was thin and pale. Pronation and supination could be seen to cause pressure on the radial and posterior interosseous nerves in a camlike motion. By the end of 1 month after surgery, strength had begun to return to the extensor muscles of the hand and wrist, and the strength slowly improved over the next 9 months. By that time, the strength of the extensor pollicis longus had returned to grade 4, and that of the finger extensors had returned to grade 3. The extensors of the wrist were also graded at level 4. The residual weakness was not enough to interfere with his part-time employment.

In 1984, Holst-Nielsen and Jensen[54] reported two additional cases of tardy posterior interosseous nerve palsy secondary to old, unreduced radial head dislocations. Both of these cases were treated successfully with decompression of the posterior interosseous nerve only.

Engber and Keene[37] reported a case of anterior interosseous nerve palsy following a type I Monteggia fracture. Two months after injury, the strength of the flexor pollicis longus and the flexor digitorum profundus to the index finger had spontaneously returned to normal. In a cadaveric dissection in which they experimentally created a type I Monteggia fracture, they demonstrated the anterior interosseous nerve to be stretched and tented over the proximal ulnar fragment. The anterior interosseous nerve was noted to have very little mobility at this level and seemed to be tethered just distally.

RADIOGRAPHIC FINDINGS

It would seem that the Monteggia lesions would be obvious on radiographs, but this is not always so. In the 62 patients reported by Speed and Boyd[113] in 1940, 52% of the lesions were not detected until over 4 weeks after the injury. By the 1969 report of Boyd and Boals,[14] which added 97 patients to the series, the proportion of patients with old lesions had decreased to 24%. They concluded that physicians in recent years are doing a better job of recognizing Monteggia fractures. However, it appears we still have some way to go.

The fracture of the ulna is usually obvious and difficult to miss. In the 97 patients reported by Boyd and Boals, the fracture was located in the region of the olecranon or metaphysis in 19, in the proximal third in 69, in the middle third in 8, and in the distal third in only 1. Twelve patients had associated radial head fractures. Six of the 97 patients had Bado type IV lesions with an associated fracture of the shaft of the radius.

There are probably several reasons why the dislocation of the radial head is missed so often. First, the x-ray films may not include the elbow. Second, the x-ray tube may not be centered over the elbow, so that even though the elbow is included in the film, the dislocation may not be obvious. Giustra and associates[43] noted that radiologists also have difficulty with the diagnosis of the Monteggia lesion. They reported that between 1966 and 1972, 400 fractures and dislocations of the wrist and mid- or proximal forearm were seen in their hospital. Five of these injuries proved to be Monteggia lesions, and three of the five were initially misdiagnosed. Giustra stated that a line drawn through the radial shaft and radial head should align with the capitellum in any projection if the radial head is in normal position. This important sign, previously described by McLaughlin,[74] is very helpful in avoiding misdiagnosis of Monteggia lesions. Third, the physician who first sees the patient may be unfamiliar with the lesion and may not realize that dislocation of the radial head is present. He or she may unknowingly reduce the dislocation when aligning the arm to splint it. If such a patient arrives elsewhere for definitive care without the initial x-rays, the new films may appear to be a fracture of the ulna with minimal displacement. A fourth reason for missing the dislocation of the radial head was pointed out by an incident that occurred on

our service at the City of Memphis Hospital. A patient arrived in the emergency room with pain in the forearm after a fall (Fig. 9-43). She came directly to the hospital without referral by another physician. Her x-rays showed a minimally displaced fracture of the proximal third of the ulna, and the radial head was in normal position. The arm was placed in a long-arm cast with the elbow at 90°, and the patient was told to visit the fracture clinic 1 week later. At that time, x-rays through the cast revealed displacement of the fractured ulna and anterior dislocation of the radial head (see Fig. 9-43). On more careful questioning, the patient related that her extremity had been so painful after the fall that she had pulled the arm vigorously and felt a snap in her elbow. After this, the pain was much less severe. Apparently she had reduced her own dislocation and fracture prior to arriving at the emergency room. A more detailed history and careful examination of the lateral elbow for tenderness might have led to the proper diagnosis initially. Fortunately, the diagnosis was picked up after 1 week, the dislocated radial head was reduced, and the ulna was fixed with a compression plate (see Fig. 9-43). The final result was excellent, but if the patient had not returned early for follow-up x-rays, the outcome might not have been a happy one.

The Monteggia fracture remains treacherous, just as Monteggia himself pointed out in 1814.

METHODS OF TREATMENT

There is general agreement that closed treatment is satisfactory for most Monteggia fractures in children,[8,14] but there is considerable controversy as to how these fractures should be treated in adults.

Monteggia[79,95] used closed reduction in his two cases and found it unsatisfactory. The dislocation recurred. Watson-Jones[126] reported that the incidence of myositis ossificans was increased by open reduction of the radial head and reported poor results in 32 of 34 patients initially treated by other surgeons. Bado[8] along with Evans[39] emphasized the importance of reducing the dislocation by supination and maintaining the forearm in that position for 6 to 8 weeks. Bado maintained that conservative treatment is always best for fresh cases of dislocated radial head and usually is best for the fractured ulna.

In their 1940 article, Speed and Boyd[113] found closed treatment unsatisfactory in most acute Monteggia fractures in adults. At that time, they advocated open reduction and internal fixation of the ulna with a Vitallium plate, along with reconstruction of the annular ligament with a fascial loop,

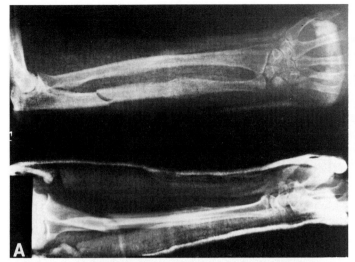

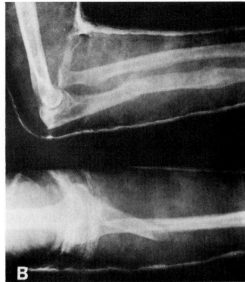

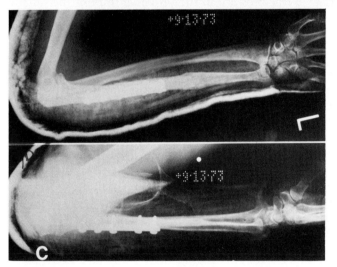

Fig. 9-43. (**A**) X-rays following application of a long-arm cast for what was thought to be a minimally displaced fracture of the ulna. (**B**) Films made 1 week later show dislocation of the radial head and increased angulation of the fracture of the ulna. Careful questioning at that time revealed that the patient probably had reduced her own dislocation of the radial head initially. (**C**) Postoperative films showing a five-hole compression plate applied to the ulna and the elbow maintained 20° above a right angle in a posterior plaster splint.

believing that the loop repair gave added stability and helped prevent redislocation of the radial head. With the relatively inadequate devices available for fixation of the ulnar fracture at that time, the fascial repair may have been helpful.

In the more recent report of 1969, Boyd and Boals[14] recommended rigid internal fixation of the fractured ulna with a compression plate or medullary nail. However, they then stated that open reduction of the dislocated radial head was not indicated unless closed reduction failed. When there is a significant fracture of the head of the radius, Boyd and Boals recommend resection of the radial head at the same time the ulna is internally fixed. Their results were excellent to good in 77% of the acute fractures.

In 1982, Reckling[97] reported on his series of Monteggia lesions and Galeazzi fractures. He found that in children either closed or open treatment yielded good results. In adults, however, he found that the best results were obtained in type I lesions treated with open anatomic reduction, internal stabilization of the ulnar fracture, and closed reduction of the radial head. Factors leading to poor results in type I lesions were failure to obtain anatomic reduction, heterotopic ossification including synostosis of the proximal parts of the radius and ulna, and persistence or recurrence of dislocation of the radial head. In patients in whom the radial head could not be reduced by closed methods, the radial head was usually buttonholed through the intact joint capsule and the annular ligament was displaced but not ruptured. Reckling suggested that reconstruction of the annular ligament is not necessary in these cases. In type II, III, and IV lesions, Reckling found only fair results to be the rule.

Malunion and Nonunion

Untreated or inadequately treated Monteggia fractures that are not seen until 4 to 6 weeks or more after injury present many problems (Fig. 9-44). Usually the ulna has angulated, and the radial head either is unreduced or has dislocated again. Malunion or nonunion of the ulna may be present.

If the patient presents with malunion of the ulna with only a few degrees of angulation and subluxation of the head of the radius, it is best to accept the mild malunion and resect only the head of the radius. If the malunion has occurred with moderate or severe angulation, osteotomy and rigid internal fixation of the ulna along with resection of the radial head are usually indicated.

When there is nonunion of the ulna and subluxation or dislocation of the radial head, realignment of the nonunion, rigid internal fixation, and bone grafting of the ulna should be done. The radial head should usually be resected, except in the rare case in which subluxation is insignificant.

AUTHORS' PREFERRED METHOD OF TREATMENT

We believe that the most important factors in achieving good results in adults with Monteggia lesions are (1) early, accurate diagnosis, (2) rigid internal fixation of the fractured ulna, (3) complete reduction of the dislocated radial head, (4) cast immobilization in the appropriate position (depending on the type of Monteggia lesion) for about 6 weeks, and (5) early open reduction and internal fixation of the fractured radial shaft in Bado's type IV lesions.

The importance of early diagnosis is apparent. If the dislocation is not recognized, the treatment will be inappropriate. Generally, we prefer compression plate fixation for the fractured ulna. Most of these fractures are in the proximal third of the ulna. A medullary nail in this location may not fill the canal and may thus provide less than rigid fixation. For very comminuted fractures in the middle third of the ulna, a triangular medullary nail may be better, but these fractures are not common. Whenever significant comminution is present, we apply autogenous iliac grafts about the fracture.

When the radial head can be reduced completely by closed means, open reduction is unnecessary.

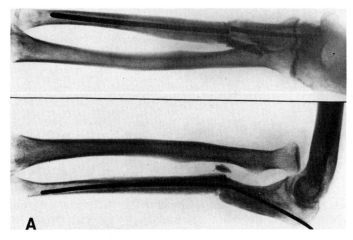
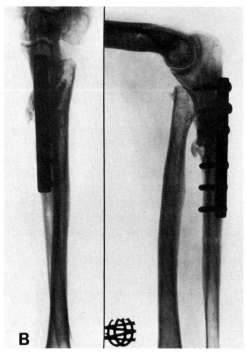

Fig. 9-44. (**A**) Nonunion of the ulna with recurrence of the dislocation of the radial head 4 months after inadequate internal fixation. (**B**) The same patient 4 months after compression plate fixation, bone grafting, and resection of the head of the radius. (*Boyd, H. B., and Boals, J. C.: The Monteggia Lesion. A Review of 159 Cases. Clin. Orthop., 66:94–100, 1969.*)

Open reduction of the radial head is indicated only when an infolded portion of the annular ligament prevents complete reduction or when the radial head is telescoped proximally through an intact annular ligament and hung behind the lateral epicondyle (Fig. 9-45). In the former, the infolded part of the ligament should be removed from the joint to permit reduction of the radial head. In the latter, the ligament must be incised so that the head of the radius can be removed from behind the lateral epicondyle and returned to its proper position. In both, the ligament is repaired after the radial head is reduced. Fascial reconstruction of the annular ligament is very rarely indicated in acute cases of Monteggia fractures. When open reduction of the radial head is required, we prefer the approach recommended by Boyd,[16,17] which uses one incision to expose both the fracture and the dislocation.

In type IV Monteggia lesions, early open reduction and internal fixation of both the fractures of the shaft of the radius and ulna is important. The dislocation can usually be treated closed with postoperative immobilization, as outlined previously.

AFTERCARE

The position in which the elbow and forearm are placed after surgery is of utmost importance. We believe that the type I, III, and IV lesions of the elbow should be held in about 110° of flexion. With rigid fixation of the ulna, we have never seen the radial head redislocate if the elbow is held in this position for 6 weeks after surgery. Supination is probably important when closed treatment is used, but forced supination is unnecessary with good fixation of the ulna if the elbow is maintained in 110° of flexion. The type II lesions with posterior dislocation of the radial head should be maintained in about 70° of elbow flexion for 6 weeks.

Following surgery, radiographs of the forearm and elbow should be made at 2 weeks and again at 6 weeks. After 6 weeks, with the elbow immobilized in plaster as outlined previously, the cast is removed and active exercises are instituted. Passive stretching exercises are contraindicated. Improvement in elbow function generally continues over several months.

COMPLICATIONS

Many complications of Monteggia lesions are the same as those for other fractures of the shafts of the forearm bones. These include infection and nonunion. Redislocation or subluxation of the head of the radius and loss of reduction of the fracture of the ulna are almost always the result of inade-

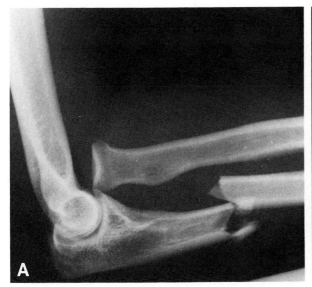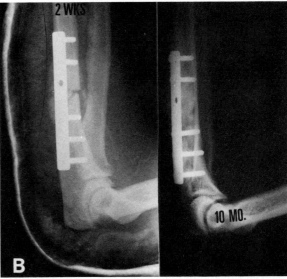

Fig. 9-45. (**A**) A Monteggia fracture in which the intact annular ligament held the radial head dislocated. (**B**) Two weeks after surgery, during which the annular ligament was incised, the radial head was reduced, and the fracture of the ulna was fixed with a compression plate. Iliac grafts were applied because of comminution (**first frame**). Ten months after surgery, function is full except for 10° loss of extension (**second frame**). (*Anderson, L. D.: Fractures. In Crenshaw, A. H. (ed.): Campbell's Operative Orthopaedics, Vol. 1, 5th ed. St. Louis, C.V. Mosby, 1971.*)

quate internal fixation of the fractured ulna or improper positioning of the elbow during the postoperative period. Paralysis of the deep branch of the radial nerve is not uncommon, but function nearly always returns with time, and exploration of the nerve is usually not indicated.

PROGNOSIS

The prognosis for regaining satisfactory or even excellent function following most Monteggia fractures is good, provided the diagnosis is made early and treatment is adequate. In the series reported by Boyd and Boals[14] in 1969, 77% of the results were good or excellent and 23% were fair or poor. This series included all patients treated from 1940 to 1967, and a number of the fair and poor results were from the earlier years, when methods for fixation of the ulnar fracture were not as good as they are now. With rigid fixation of the ulna, the percentage of good and excellent results should be higher, except when infection develops or when there is major soft tissue damage from open wounds.

FRACTURES OF THE RADIUS ALONE

Fractures of the shaft of the radius alone are divided into two distinct groups: fractures in the proximal two thirds of the bone and those at the junction of the middle and distal thirds.

FRACTURES OF THE PROXIMAL RADIUS

Fractures of the upper two thirds of the radial shaft alone are not common in adults. The radial shaft in the proximal two thirds is relatively well padded by the forearm muscles. Most injuries severe enough to fracture the radius at this level will also fracture the ulna. Also, the anatomic position of the radius in most positions of function makes it less likely than the ulna to receive a direct blow.

The rare undisplaced fracture of the shaft of the radius in the proximal two thirds should be immobilized in a long-arm cast with the forearm in mild or full supination, depending on whether the fracture is located above or below the insertion of the pronator teres. The reasons for placing the forearm in supination are outlined in the sections of this chapter dealing with surgical anatomy and fractures of both the radius and ulna.

Undisplaced fractures can become displaced, and frequent x-ray films must be made during the first few weeks. The cast must be maintained until healing has occurred.

Displaced fractures of the proximal one fifth of the radius are probably best treated closed with the forearm in full supination. These fractures are too high for good fixation with plate and screws, and the proximal fragment is too short for a medullary nail to control rotation. If they are completely displaced and cannot be reduced, axial alignment can be achieved and maintained with a medullary nail and rotational alignment maintained with a long-arm cast holding the forearm in full supination. This might also be a rare indication for the use of a semitubular plate. In this location, Chapman and associates[24] recommended an anterior Henry approach. However, in our experience, the posterior Thompson approach allows better visualization of the radial nerve and is therefore safer.

Except for the very high proximal one-fifth fractures, displaced fractures of the radius in the upper two thirds can be treated with plate-and-screw fixation or with an adequate medullary nail as outlined in the section of this chapter on fractures of both the radius and ulna. We usually prefer a compression plate, because it is easier and the results have been good (Fig. 9-46). On the other hand, we have no quarrel with using a medullary nail, provided it controls rotation and maintains the radial bow. The aftertreatment is the same as for fractures of both bones of the forearm treated with open reduction and internal fixation.

FRACTURES OF THE DISTAL SHAFT (GALEAZZI'S FRACTURE)

The solitary fracture of the radius at the junction of the middle and distal thirds has several eponyms. The French, at least as early as 1929, referred to this lesion as a reverse Monteggia fracture.[121] Galeazzi[40,95] described the fracture in 1934 and called attention to the associated dislocation or subluxation of the distal radioulnar joint. He pointed out that subluxation of this joint may be present initially or may occur gradually during treatment. Galeazzi advocated treating the fracture with strong traction through the thumb. Campbell is said to have called this lesion "the fracture of necessity," by which he meant that open reduction and internal fixation was necessary if a good result were to be obtained.

Probably the best description of the fracture of the distal shaft of the radius associated with dislo-

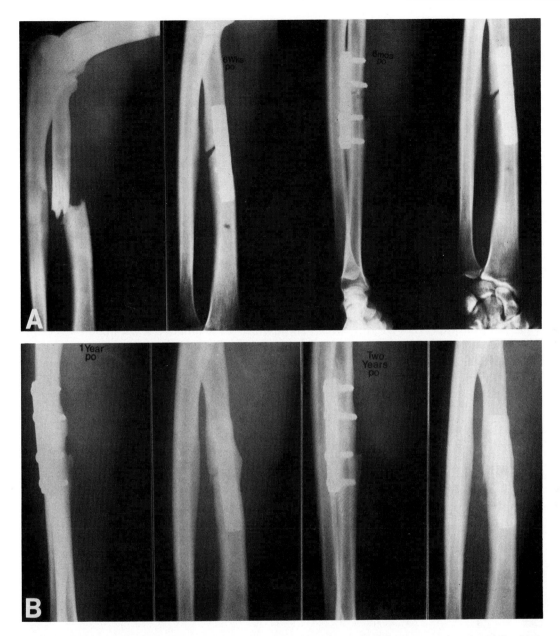

Fig. 9-46. (**A**) A fracture of the shaft of the radius at the junction of the proximal and middle thirds with intact ulna. Open reduction and internal fixation with a four-hole compression plate were performed. Note that the plate was placed on the dorsal aspect of the radius. At 6 months, a portion of the fracture line is still visible. A five-hole plate would have been better, and bone grafts should have been applied. (**B**) Films at 1 year and 2 years showing union. The patient regained full range of motion.

cation of the distal radioulnar joint is that published by Hughston[56] in 1957. He collected 41 cases from members of the Piedmont Orthopaedic Society and called attention to the frequent mistakes in management. His criteria for a satisfactory result were very strict. They included union with perfect alignment, no loss of length, no subluxation of the distal radioulnar joint, and full pronation and supination. Of the 38 fractures treated initially by closed reduction and immobilization, Hughston reported that poor results occurred in 35 (92%). Only three patients had a satisfactory result.

As pointed out by Hughston, four major deforming factors cause loss of reduction. (1) Gravity acting through the weight of the hand, even in a cast, tends to cause subluxation of the distal radioulnar joint and dorsal angulation of the fractured radius. (2) The insertion of the pronator quadratus on the palmar surface of the distal fragment rotates it toward the ulna and pulls it in a proximal and palmar direction. (3) The brachioradialis tends to use the distal radioulnar joint as a pivot point on which to rotate the distal fragment of the radius and at the same time causes shortening. (4) The abductors and extensors of the thumb cause shortening and relaxation of the radial collateral ligament so that one is not able to keep the soft tissue bridge on stretch, even though the wrist is placed in ulnar deviation.

Mechanism of Injury

The two principal causes of Galeazzi's fracture are direct blows on the dorsolateral side of the wrist and falls. Mikic[76] thought that the most probable mechanism of injury in Galeazzi's fracture is a fall on the outstretched hand combined with marked pronation of the forearm. According to Galeazzi,[40,95] this lesion is approximately three times as common as the Monteggia fracture.

Signs and Symptoms

The signs and symptoms vary with the severity of injury and the degree of displacement. In undisplaced or relatively undisplaced fractures, the only deformity may be swelling and tenderness about the fracture. If the displacement is greater, there will be shortening of the radius and posterolateral angulation. Subluxation or dislocation will be evident in the distal radioulnar joint with prominence of the head of the ulna and tenderness over the joint. Most of these are closed fractures. In open fractures, the wound is usually a small puncture wound from within where the distal end of the proximal fragment has protruded through the skin. Nerve and vascular damage is rare.

Radiographic Findings

The fracture at the junction of the middle and distal thirds of the radius usually has a transverse or short oblique configuration (Fig. 9-47). Most do not have significant comminution. If there is much displace-

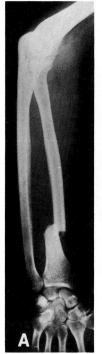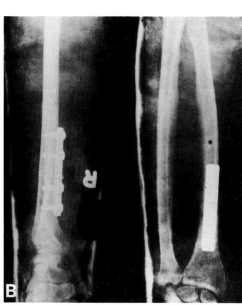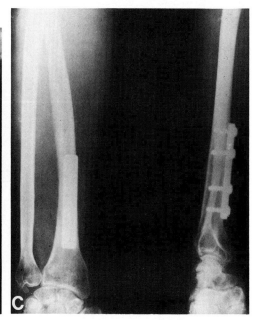

Fig. 9-47. (**A**) A Galeazzi fracture of the distal radial shaft with dislocation of the distal radioulnar joint. (**B**) Successful internal fixation using a four-hole compression plate. Note that the plate was applied on the palmar surface of the radius where the bone is flatter. Compression was applied proximally. (**C**) One year later, union is complete and function is normal.

ment of the fractured radius, the distal radioulnar joint will be dislocated. On the anteroposterior film the radius appears relatively shortened, with an increase in the space between the distal radius and ulna where they articulate. In the lateral view, the fractured radius is usually angulated dorsally and the head of the ulna is prominent dorsally. The injury to the radioulnar joint may be purely ligamentous, or the ligament may remain intact and the ulnar styloid may be avulsed.

Methods of Treatment

From the introductory discussion, it should be apparent that the results of closed treatment are poor.

The deforming forces are so great that even if the fracture is undisplaced initially or if good position is obtained by closed reduction, displacement in the cast is the rule rather than the exception (Fig. 9-48). To obtain good pronation and supination and to avoid derangement and arthritic changes in the distal radioulnar joint, the fracture must unite in an anatomic position. For these reasons, open reduction and internal fixation are almost always the preferred form of treatment.

In their book, Sarmiento and Latta[104] stated that not all isolated fractures of the distal third of the radius have associated distal radioulnar joint pathology or damage to the interosseous membrane.

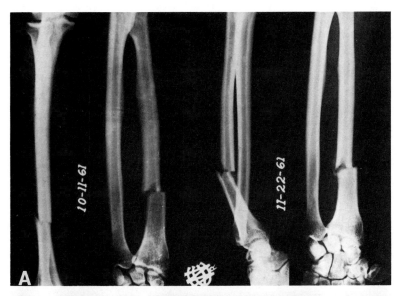

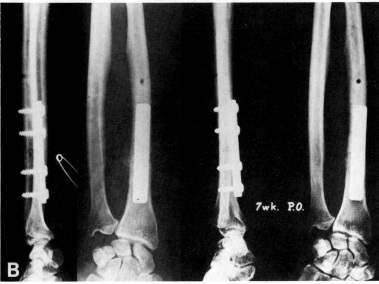

Fig. 9-48. (**A**) Solitary fracture of the distal third of the radial shaft with minimal displacement (**first and second frames**). After 6 weeks' immobilization (by the family physician) in a long-arm cast, the fracture has angulated dorsally and the distal radioulnar joint is seen to be dislocated (**third and fourth frames**). (**B**) Immediate postoperative x-rays showing the fracture fixed with a four-hole compression plate applied to the palmar surface of the radius (**first and second frames**). Seven weeks later, the fracture has united (**third and fourth frames**). (*Anderson, L. D.: Fractures. In Crenshaw, A. H. (ed.): Campbell's Operative Orthopaedics, Vol. 1, 5th ed. St. Louis, C.V. Mosby, 1971.*)

Moore, Lester, and Sarmiento[81] created artificial Galeazzi fractures in cadavers. They found that up to 5 mm of radial shortening occurred after osteotomy alone. Shortening of over 10 mm did not occur unless both the interosseous ligament and the triangular ligament were sectioned. They believe that isolated fractures of the distal third of the radius resulting from axial loading are more likely to be associated with distal radioulnar pathology and injury to the interosseous membrane. Sarmiento suggested that this type of injury requires open reduction and internal fixation. On the other hand, he believes that a similar fracture of the distal third of the radius resulting from a direct blow perpendicular to the bone that displaces the radial fragment ulnarward does not necessarily have associated distal radioulnar joint pathology or injury to the interosseous membrane. He believes that if this latter fracture is transverse and well reduced, it may not require internal fixation and can be treated with good results using his functional bracing method.

Medullary nails do not provide satisfactory fixation for these fractures (see Fig. 9-16). The medullary canal at the level of the fracture is large and continues to enlarge distally. The nail does not prevent medial offset of the distal fragment and shortening of the radius. Also, the medullary canal of the distal fragment is too large for the nail to control rotation.

Small plates and screws also do not provide sufficient fixation to resist the deforming forces. The plates may bend or the screws may pull loose, resulting in loss of position with malunion or nonunion. Plate-and-screw fixation is by far the best method, but if good results are to be expected, the plate must be long enough and the screws must obtain good purchase in both cortices.

In 1975, Mikic[76] of Yugoslavia reported a large series of 125 patients with Galeazzi-type fracture-dislocations of the forearm. Many of his patients in whom the radius alone was internally fixed had a poor result because of failure to maintain reduction of the radioulnar joint. For this reason he advocated pinning the ulna to the radius with one or two percutaneous Kirschner wires. The Kirschner wires are removed after a few weeks. Liang and coworkers[68] also advocated temporary, percutaneous, transradioulnar Kirschner wire fixation for 4 weeks. Mikic advocated the Rush pin as the best method of treatment for fracture of the radius, which in our experience, as outlined previously, has been ineffective because it does not control rotation and allows shortening of the radius. Thus, redislocation of the radioulnar joint is almost in-

evitable with this type of fixation. We have not found redislocation of the distal radioulnar joint to be a problem when rigid fixation of the radius has been achieved using compression plates. However, if for some reason a Rush pin or other medullary nail must be used for the fracture of the radius, then transfixation of the ulna to the radius for a few weeks might be worthwhile. More recently, several other authors[61,78,80,97] have advocated open reduction and plate fixation of the radial fracture. All believed that satisfactory restoration of the radius would adequately treat the distal radioulnar joint disruption.

Authors' Preferred Method of Treatment

We prefer to treat fractures of the junction of the middle and distal thirds of the radius with ASIF compression plates. We have used this method of fixation since 1960, and the results have been excellent. The details of the technique are reported elsewhere,[4,82,84] but a few points about this particular fracture should be emphasized.

At the level of this fracture we prefer the anterior approach of Henry.[16,25,52] The palmar surface of the radius is flat and provides a better bed for the plate.

With the use of a hand table and tourniquet control, a 5- or 6-inch longitudinal incision is made, centered over the fracture in the plane between the flexor carpi radialis and the brachioradialis muscles. The radial artery and veins are identified and retracted to the ulnar side; the brachioradialis and superficial radial nerve are retracted radially. All other structures are retracted ulnarly. The fracture is almost always located just above the proximal border of the pronator quadratus. The insertion of the pronator quadratus is freed from the radius and reflected ulnarward. The palmar surface of the proximal fragment is then exposed for a distance long enough to allow placement of the plate. With the use of self-retaining, bone-holding Lane forceps, the fracture is reduced anatomically. Usually, there is little or no comminution, but if there is, the surgeon should try to fit each fragment anatomically into place. A plate of appropriate length is selected, depending on the obliquity of the fracture and the degree of comminution. In pure transverse fractures, a four-hole 4.5-mm plate or six-hole 3.5-mm plate is adequate, but if there is any comminution or obliquity, a longer plate is necessary. The plate is centered accurately so that at least two 4.5-mm screws or three 3.5-mm screws can be placed in both proximal and distal fragments with no screw closer than 1 cm to the fracture, even if this means leaving a hole in the plate empty.

The plate is clamped to the proximal and distal

fragments with two self-retaining Lane forceps parallel to the plate. A third Lane forceps is placed at right angles to the first two and clamped in place to prevent angulation and shortening when compression is applied. The screws are inserted into the distal fragment first. Cancellous screws with large threads are used if the standard cortical screws do not seat with adequate fixation.

At this point, radiographs are made in anteroposterior and lateral planes to be sure the relationship at the distal radioulnar joint is exactly right. If it is, the screws are inserted into the proximal fragment.

If the procedure is done properly, strong compression can usually be applied to these fractures without disturbing the distal relationship of the radius to the ulna. Occasionally, however, the fracture may be so comminuted or oblique that the radius shortens when compression is applied and the distal relationship is disturbed. If there is significant comminution (there usually is if compression cannot be applied without causing the radius to shorten), autogenous iliac bone grafts are added.

The pronator quadratus is allowed to fall back into position over the plate. The fascia should not be closed, for the reasons discussed previously. The subcutaneous tissue and skin are closed, and a well-molded sugar-tong splint is applied. Final films are made after the cast is in place to confirm that the distal radioulnar joint is reduced anatomically.

Aftercare

After 2 weeks the sutures are removed and a new sugar-tong splint is applied. X-ray films are made. The splint is left in place for a total of 5 or 6 weeks to allow healing of the soft tissues. Then active exercises of the elbow, wrist, and forearm are begun, with emphasis on regaining pronation and supination. Because the plate is well covered with soft tissue, it is seldom necessary to remove it, except in young athletes. If it is removed, the precautions noted previously on p. 718 to prevent refracture should be followed.

Prognosis

Some of the older articles emphasize the poor prognosis for regaining good function after Galeazzi's fracture.[56,126] However, these articles were published before rigid fixation with compression plates was available. The points of Campbell and Hughston are well made. Closed treatment gives poor results, as does inadequate internal fixation. The reduction of both the radial fracture and the distal radioulnar joint must be anatomic, and the fixation must be rigid. Since we began using compression plates for this fracture in 1960, the results have been excellent.

Complications

The complications of Galeazzi's fracture are those incident to all forearm fractures: nonunion, malunion, and infection. The most common complication is angulation of the fracture and subluxation or dislocation of the distal radioulnar joint. In patients with acute fractures, these complications are largely avoidable with skillful surgical technique and rigid fixation.

In 1977, Cetti[23] described an unusual case of blocked reduction of Galeazzi's lesion. He reported two cases in which the extensor carpi ulnaris tendon was caught in the distal radioulnar joint, preventing reduction. In the first case, the fracture of the distal radius was internally fixed with a plate. Two months later, the fracture was healed, but there was marked restriction of pronation and supination. Additional radiographic examination suggested that the inferior radioulnar dislocation was still present or had recurred. At a second operation done 5 months after the first, the distal radioulnar joint was explored. The extensor carpi ulnaris tendon was found to be trapped between the radius and the ulna. The tendon was extracted, and the distal end of the ulna was excised with a good result.

In his second case, attempted closed reduction under general anesthesia was unsuccessful. The lower end of the ulna was then exposed through a dorsal vertical incision, revealing that the distal ulna had erupted dorsally through the capsule of the joint. There was complete separation of the ulnar styloid process, which, with the triangular fibrocartilage, remained in its normal relationship to the distal radius. The tendon of the extensor carpi ulnaris was found trapped between the ulna and the capsule. To reduce the dislocation, the capsule of the distal radioulnar joint had to be incised distally. The tendon could then be displaced and the dislocation of the distal radioulnar joint reduced. These two cases of entrapment of the extensor carpi ulnaris in the distal radioulnar joint associated with Galeazzi's fracture appear to be the only two such cases reported thus far in the literature.

In patients with nonunion and malposition presenting for treatment late (after 6 weeks), it is usually best to realign the radius and apply a bone graft to it. If there has been much resorption of bone at the fracture, a full-thickness iliac graft from the crest can often be used to regain radial length, restore the distal radioulnar relationship, and obtain reasonably good function. Even if the distal ulna must be resected, we believe that it is better to allow the nonunion to heal before doing so. Resecting the distal ulna at the same time that the radius is fixed may lead to problems. Even though the distal relationship may not be satisfactory, the ulna relieves some of the deforming forces on the radius. If it is resected at the same time, the added stress may cause the screws to pull out of the osteoporotic bone. We have seen two patients in whom this complication occurred.

In patients with mild to moderate degrees of malunion of the radius, pronation and supination will be limited and painful. In these, the distal ulna should be resected at the proximal border of the sigmoid notch, but only after the radius is solidly united. When the distal ulna is resected, it should be done subperiosteally, and care should be taken to reconstruct the lateral collateral ligament. (For more details about resection of the distal ulna, see Chapter 8.) Recently, resection of the distal ulna has begun to fall into disfavor, especially in young patients. An alternative to resecting the distal ulna might be to perform a Sauve-Kapandji[105] procedure, an operation in which the distal radioulnar joint is fused and combined with the creation of a pseud-

arthrosis proximal to the fusion (Fig. 9-49). The technique for this procedure is well described elsewhere.[13]

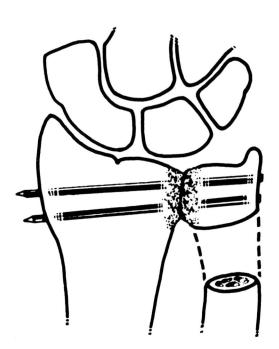

Fig. 9-49. The Sauve-Kapandji procedure as described by Taleisnik *(Bowers, W. H.: The Distal Radioulnar Joint. In Green, D. P. (ed.): Operative Hand Surgery, 2nd ed., pp. 939–989. New York, Churchill Livingstone, 1988.)*

REFERENCES

1. Alvarenga, H.M.; Bonetti, C.L.; Dinhame, K.G.; and Rossi J.D.: Fracture-luxacão de Monteggia. Revta. Paul. Med., 92:108–112, 1978.
2. Anderson, L.D., and Bacastow, D.W.: Treatment of Forearm Shaft Fractures With Compression Plates. Contemp. Orthop., 8(6):17, 1984.
3. Anderson, L.D.: Compression Plate Fixation and the Effect of Different Types of Internal Fixation on Fracture Healing. J. Bone Joint Surg., 47A(1):191–208, 1965.
4. Anderson, L.D.: Fractures. *In* Crenshaw, A.H. (ed): Campbell's Operative Orthopaedics, Vol. 1, 5th ed, pp. 477–691. St. Louis, C.V. Mosby, 1971.
5. Anderson, L.D.; Sisk, T.D.; Park, W.I., III; and Tooms, R.E.: Compression Plate Fixation in Acute Diaphyseal Fractures of the Radius and Ulna (Proceedings). J. Bone Joint Surg., 54A(6):1332–1333, 1972.
6. Anderson, L.D.; Sisk, T.D.; Tooms, R.E.; and Park, W.I., III.: Compression-plate Fixation in Acute Diaphyseal Fractures of the Radius and Ulna. J. Bone Joint Surg., 57A(3):287–297, 1975.
7. Austin, R.: Tardy Palsy of the Radial Nerve From a Monteggia Fracture. Injury, 7:202–204, 1975.
8. Bado, J.L.: The Monteggia Lesion. Clin. Orthop., 50:71–86, 1967.
9. Bagby, G.W., and Janes, J.M.: The Effect of Compression on the Rate of Healing Using a Special Plate. Am. J. Surg., 95:761–771, 1958.
10. Bell, R.H., and Hawkins, R.J.: Stress Fracture of the Distal Ulna: A Case Report. Clin. Orthop., 209:169–171, 1986.
11. Bick, E.M.: Source Book of Orthopaedics, 2nd ed. Baltimore, Wilkins & Wilkins, 1948.
12. Boreau, J., and Hermann, P.: Plague d'osteosynthèse permettant l'impaction des fragments. Presse Med., 60:356, 1952.
13. Bowers, W.H.: The Distal Radioulnar Joint. *In* Green, D.P. (ed.): Operative Hand Surgery, 2nd ed. New York, pp. 939–989. Churchill Livingstone, 1988.
14. Boyd, H.B., and Boals, J.C.: The Monteggia Lesion. A Review of 159 Cases. Clin. Orthop., 66:94–100, 1969.
15. Boyd, H.B.; Lipinski, S.W.; and Wiley, J.H.: Observations on Non-unions of the Shafts of the Long Bones, With a Statistical Analysis of 842 Patients. J. Bone Joint Surg., 43A(1):159–168, 1961.
16. Boyd, H.B.: Surgical Approaches. *In* Crenshaw, A.H. (ed.): Campbell's Operative Orthopaedics, Vol. 1, 5th ed., pp. 58–137. St Louis, C.V. Mosby, 1971.
17. Boyd, H.B.: Surgical Exposure of the Ulna and Proximal Third of the Radius Through One Incision. Surg. Gynecol. Obstet., 71:86–88, 1940.
18. Breit, R.: Post-traumatic Radioulnar Synostosis. Clin. Orthop., 174:149–152, 1983.
19. Bruce, H.E.; Harvey, J.P., Jr.; and Wilson, J.C.: Monteggia Fractures. J. Bone Joint Surg., 56A(8):1563–1576, 1974.

20. Burwell, H.N., and Charnley, A.D.: Treatment of Forearm Fractures in Adults With Particular Reference to Plate Fixation. J. Bone Joint Surg., 46B(3):404–425, 1964.
21. Caden, J.G.: Internal Fixation of Fractures of the Forearm. J. Bone Joint Surg., 43A(8):1115–1121, 1961.
22. Campbell, W.C., and Boyd, H.B.: Fixation of Onlay Bone Grafts by Means of Vitallium Screws in the Treatment of Ununited Fractures. Am. J. Surg., 51:748–756, 1941.
23. Cetti, N.E.: An Unusual Cause of Blocked Reduction of the Galeazzi Injury. Injury, 9:59–61, 1977.
24. Chapman, M.W.; Gordon, J.E.; and Zissimos, A.G.: Compression-plate Fixation of Acute Fractures of the Diaphyses of the Radius and Ulna. J. Bone Joint Surg., 71A:159–169, 1989.
25. Crenshaw, A.H.: Surgical Approaches. In Crenshaw, A.H., (ed.): Campbell's Operative Orthopaedics, Vol. 3, 7th ed., pp. 23–107. St. Louis, C.V. Mosby, 1987.
26. Danis, R.: Uncles theorie et practique de l'osteosynthèse. Paris, Masson & Cie, 1949.
27. DeLee, J.C.: External Fixation of the Forearm and Wrist. Orthop. Rev., 6:43–48, 1981.
28. Deluca, P.A.; Newington, R.W.L.; and Ruwe, P.A.: Refracture of Bones of the Forearm After the Removal of Compression Plates. J. Bone Joint Surg., 70A(9):1372–1376, 1988.
29. Dodge, H.S., and Cody, G.W.: Treatment of Fractures of the Radius and Ulna With Compression Plates: A Retrospective Study of 119 Fractures in 78 Patients. J. Bone Joint Surg., 54A(6):1167–1176, 1972.
30. Dymond, I.W.D.: The Treatment of Isolated Fractures of the Distal Ulna. J. Bone Joint Surg., 66B(3):408–410, 1984.
31. Eaton, R.G., and Green, W.T.: Volkmann's Ischemia: A Volar Compartment Syndrome of the Forearm. Clin. Orthop., 113:58–64, 1975.
32. Edwards, C.C.: Management of Open Fractures in the Multiply Injured Patient. Instr. Course Lect., 37:257–273, 1988.
33. Eggers, G.W.N.; Shindler, T.O.; and Pomerat, C.M.: The Influence of the Contact-compression Factor on Osteogenesis in Surgical Fractures. J. Bone Joint Surg., 31A(4):693–716, 1949.
34. Eggers, G.W.N.; Ainsworth, W.H.; Shindler, T.O.; and Pomerat, C.M.: Clinical Significance of the Contact-compression Factor in Bone Surgery. Arch. Surg., 62:467–474, 1951.
35. Eggers, G.W.N.: Internal Contact Splint. J. Bone Joint Surg., 30A(1):40–52, 1948.
36. Eggers, G.W.N.: The Internal Fixation of Fractures of the Shafts of Long Bones. In Carter, B.N. (ed.): Monographs on Surgery. Baltimore: Williams & Wilkins, 1952.
37. Engber, W.D., and Keene, J.S.: Anterior Interosseous Nerve Palsy Associated With a Monteggia Fracture: A Case Report. Clin. Orthop., 174:133–137, 1983.
38. Evans, E.M.: Pronation Injuries of the Forearm With Special Reference to the Anterior Monteggia Fracture. J. Bone Joint Surg., 31B(4):578–588, 1949.
39. Evans, E.M.: Rotational Deformity in the Treatment of Fractures of Both Bones of the Forearm. J. Bone Joint Surg., 27(3):373–379, 1945.
40. Galeazzi, R.: Uber ein besonderes Syndrom bei Verltzunger im Bereich der Unter armknochen. Arch. Orthop. Unfallchir., 35:557–562, 1934.
41. Gelberman, R.H.; Gould, R.N.; Hargens, A.R.; and Vande Berg, J.S.: Lacerations of the Ulnar Artery: Hemodynamic, Ultrastructural, and Compliance Changes in the Dog. J. Hand Surg., 8:306–309, 1983.
42. Germain, J.P.: Fracture de Monteggia avec luxation laterale de la tête radiale. Union Med. Can., 105(1):56–60, 1976.
43. Giustra, P.E.; Killoran, P.J.; Furman, R.S.; and Root, J.A.: The Missed Monteggia Fracture. Radiology, 110:45–47, 1974.
44. Godina, M.: Early Microsurgical Reconstruction of Complex Trauma of the Extremities. Plast. Reconstr. Surg., 78:285–292, 1986.
45. Greene, W.B.: Traumatic Bowing of the Forearm in an Adult. Clin. Orthop., 168:31–34, 1982.
46. Gustilo, R.B., and Anderson, J.T.: Prevention of Infection in the Treatment of One Thousand and Twenty-five Open Fractures of Long Bones. Retrospective and Prospective Analyses. J. Bone Joint Surg., 58A(4):453–458, 1976.
47. Gustilo, R.B.: Current Concepts in the Management of Open Fractures. Instr. Course Lect., 36:359–366, 1987.
48. Gustilo, R.B.; Mendoza, R.M.; and Williams, D.M.: Problems in Management of Type III Open Fractures: A New Classification of Type III Open Fractures. J. Trauma, 24:742, 1984.
49. Hadden, W.A.; Reschauer, R.; and Seggl, W.: Results of AO Plate Fixation of Forearm Shaft Fractures in Adults. Injury, 15:44–52, 1984.
50. Heim, U., and Pfeiffer, K.M.: Small Fragment Set Manual, 2nd ed., p. 119. New York, Springer-Verlag, 1982.
51. Heiser, T.M., and Jacobs, R.R.: Complicated Extremity Fractures. The Relation Between External Fixation and Non-union. Clin. Orthop., 178:89–95, 1983.
52. Henry, A.K.: Extensile Exposure, 2nd ed. Baltimore, Williams & Wilkins, 1957.
53. Hoffer, M.M., and Schobert, W.: The Failure of Casual Treatment for Nondisplaced Ulna Shaft Fractures. J. Trauma, 24:771–773, 1984.
54. Holst-Nielsen, F., and Jensen, V.: Tardy Posterior Interosseous Nerve Palsy as a Result of an Unreduced Radial Head Dislocation in Monteggia Fractures: A Report of Two Cases. J. Hand Surg., 9A:572–575, 1984.
55. Hotchkiss, R.N.; An, K.; Sowa, D.T.; Basta, S.; and Weiland, A.J.: An Anatomic and Mechanical Study of the Interosseous Membrane of the Forearm: Pathomechanics of Proximal Migration of the Radius. J. Hand Surg., 14A:256–261, 1989.
56. Hughston, J.C.: Fracture of the Distal Radial Shaft: Mistakes in Management. J. Bone Joint Surg., 39A(2):249–264, 402, 1957.
57. Jergensen, F.: Diaphyseal Fractures of the Major Long Bones (Proceedings). J. Bone Joint Surg., 42A(8):1446–1447, 1960.
58. Jessing, P.: Monteggia Lesions and Their Complicating Nerve Damage. Acta Orthop. Scand., 46:601–609, 1975.
59. Jinkins, W.J., Jr.; Lockhart, L.D.; and Eggers, G.W.N.:

Fractures of the Forearm in Adults. South. Med. J., 53: 669–679, 1960.

60. Knight, R.A., and Purvis, G.D.: Fractures of Both Bones of the Forearm in Adults. J. Bone Joint Surg., 31A(4): 755–764, 1949.

61. Kraus, B., and Horne, G.: Galeazzi Fractures. J. Trauma, 25:1093–1095, 1985.

62. Lam, S.J.S.: The Place of Delayed Internal Fixation in the Treatment of Fractures of the Long Bones. J. Bone Joint Surg., 46B(3):393–397, 1964.

63. Lam, S.J.S.: Delayed Internal Fixation for Fractures of the Radial Shaft. Guy's Hosp. Rep., 114:391–400, 1965.

64. Lambotte, A.: Chirgugie operatorie dans les fractures. Paris, Masson & Cie, 1913.

65. Lambotte, A.: L'intervention operatoire dans les fracture de vue de l'osteosynthes avec la description des plusieurs techniques nouvelles. Paris, A. Maloine, 1907.

66. Lane, W.A.: A Lecture on the Operative Treatment of Simple Fractures. Lancet, 1:1489–1493, 1900.

67. Lane, W.A.: The Operative Treatment of Fractures. London, The Medical Publishing Co., 1905.

68. Liang, S.C.; Liang, C.L.; and Liang, C.S.: Galeazzi's Fracture: Report of 22 Cases. Taiwan, Hsueh Hui Tsa Chih, 79:421–426, 1980.

69. Lichter, R.L., and Jacobsen, T.: Tardy Palsy of the Posterior Interosseous Nerve With a Monteggia Fracture. J. Bone Joint Surg., 57A(1):124–125, 1975.

70. Maempel, F.Z.: Post-traumatic Radioulnar Synostosis. A Report of Two Cases. Clin. Orthop., 186:182–185, 1984.

71. Mallin, B.A.: Principles of Management of Forearm Fractures. In Chapman, M.W., and Madison, M. (eds.): Operative Orthopaedics, Vol. 1, pp. 263–271. Philadelphia, J.B. Lippincott, 1988.

72. Matsen, F.A.: Compartmental Syndromes. New York, Grune & Stratton, 1980.

73. Matthews, L.S.; Kaufer, H.; Garver, D.F.; and Sonstegard, D.A.: The Effect on Supination-pronation of Angular Malalignment of Fractures of Both Bones of the Forearm. An Experimental Study. J. Bone Joint Surg., 64A:14–17, 1982.

74. McLaughlin, H.L.: Trauma. Philadelphia, W.B. Saunders, 1959.

75. Mestdagh, H.; Vigier, J.E.; and Mairesse, J.L.: La fracture de Monteggia chez l'adult. Ann Chir., 33(6):417–423, 1979.

76. Mikic, Z.D.: Galeazzi Fracture Dislocations. J. Bone Joint Surg., 57A:1071–1080, 1975.

77. Moed, B.R.; Kellam, J.F.; Foster, R.J.; Tile, M.; and Hansen, S.T., Jr.: Immediate Internal Fixation of Open Fractures of the Diaphysis of the Forearm. J. Bone Joint Surg., 68A(7):1008–1017, 1986.

78. Mohan, K.; Gupta, A.K.; Sharma, J.; Singh, A.K.; and Jain, A.K.: Internal Fixation in 50 Cases of Galeazzi Fracture. Acta Orthop. Scand., 59:318–320, 1988.

79. Monteggia, G.B.: Instituzioni Chirurgiche, Vol. 5. Milan, Maspero, 1814.

80. Moore, T.M.; Klein, J.P.; Patzakis, M.J.; and Harvey, J.P., Jr.: Results of Compression-plating of Closed Galeazzi Fractures. J. Bone Joint Surg., 67A(7):1015–1021, 1985.

81. Moore, T.M.; Lester, D.K.; and Sarmiento, A.: The Sta-

bilizing Effect of Soft-tissue Constraints in Artificial Galeazzi Fractures. Clin. Orthop., 194:189–194, 1985.

82. Morris, A.H.: Irreducible Monteggia Lesion With Radial Nerve Entrapment: A Case Report. J. Bone Joint Surg., 56A(8):1744–1746, 1974.

83. Müller, M.E.; Allgöwer, M.; Schneider, R.; and Willenegger, H.: Manual of Internal Fixation, 2nd ed. Berlin, Springer-Verlag, 1979.

84. Müller, M.E.; Allgöwer, M.; and Willenegger, H.: Technique of Internal Fixation of Fractures. New York, Springer-Verlag, 1965.

85. Mullick, S.: The Lateral Monteggia Fracture. J. Bone Joint Surg., 59A:543–545, 1977.

86. Naiman, P.T.; Schein, A.J.; and Siffert, R.S.: Use of ASIF Compression Plates in Selected Shaft Fractures of the Upper Extremity. Clin. Orthop., 71:208–216, 1970.

87. Palmer, A.K., and Werner, F.W.: The Triangular Fibro-cartilage Complex of the Wrist–Anatomy and Function. J. Hand Surg., 6:153–162, 1981.

88. Patel, M.R.; Irizarry, J.; and Stricevic, M.: Stress Fracture of the Ulnar Diaphysis: Review of the Literature and Report of a Case. J. Hand Surg., 11A:443–445, 1986.

89. Patrick, J.: A Study of Supination and Pronation, With Especial Reference to the Treatment of Forearm Fractures. J. Bone Joint Surg., 28B:737–748, 1946.

90. Penrose, J.H.: The Monteggia Fracture With Posterior Dislocation of the Radial Head. J. Bone Joint Surg., 33B(1): 65–73, 1951.

91. Pollock, F.H.; Pankovich, A.M.; Prieto, J.J.; and Lorenz, M.: The Isolated Fracture of the Ulnar Shaft: Treatment Without Immobilization. J. Bone Joint Surg., 65A(3):339–342, 1983.

92. Prosser, A.J., and Hooper, G.: Entrapment of the Ulnar Nerve in a Greenstick Fracture of the Ulna. J. Hand Surg., 11B:211–212, 1986.

93. Radin, E.L., and Rose, R.R.: Fatigue Fracture of a Forearm Plate Within a Long-arm Cast. Clin. Orthop., 207:142–145, 1986.

94. Ralston, E.L.: Handbook of Fractures. St. Louis, C.V. Mosby, 1967.

95. Rang, M.: Anthology of Orthopaedics. Edinburgh, E & S Livingstone, 1968.

96. Rayan, G.M., and Hayes, M.: Entrapment of the Flexor Digitorum Profundus in the Ulna With Fracture of Both Bones of the Forearm. Report of a Case. J. Bone Joint Surg., 68A(7):1102–1103, 1986.

97. Reckling, F.W.: Unstable Fracture-dislocations of the Forearm (Monteggia and Galeazzi Lesions). J. Bone Joint Surg., 64A(6):857–863, 1982.

98. Ritchey, S.J.; Richardson, J.P.; and Thompson, M.S.: Rigid Medullary Fixation of Forearm Fractures. South. Med. J., 51:852–856, 1958.

99. Rosacker, J.A., and Kopta, J.A.: Both Bone Fractures of the Forearm: A Review of Surgical Variables Associated With Union. Orthopaedics, 4:1353–1356, 1981.

100. Sage, F.P.: Fractures of the Shaft of the Radius and Ulna in the Adult. In Adams, J.P. (ed.): Current Practice in Orthopaedic Surgery. Vol. 1, pp. 152–173. St. Louis, C.V. Mosby, 1963.

101. Sage, F.P.: Medullary Fixation of Fractures of the Forearm:

A Study of the Medullary Canal of the Radius and a Report of Fifty Fractures of the Radius Treated With a Prebent Triangular Nail. J. Bone Joint Surg., 41A(8):1489–1516, 1525, 1959.

102. Sargent, J.P., and Teipner, W.A.: Treatment of Forearm Shaft Fractures by Double Plating. A Preliminary Report. J. Bone Joint Surg., 47A(8):1475–1490, 1965.

103. Sarmiento, A.; Cooper, J.S.; and Sinclair, W.F.: Forearm Fractures: Early Functional Bracing—A Preliminary Report. J. Bone Joint Surg., 57A(3):297–304, 1975.

104. Sarmiento, A., and Latta, L.: Closed Functional Treatment of Fractures. Berlin, Springer-Verlag, 1981.

105. Sauve, L., and Kapandji, M.: Nouvelle technique traitement chirurical des luxations recidivantes isolees de l' extremite inferieure du cubitus. J. Chir. (Paris), 47:589–594, 1936.

106. Scheuer, M., and Pot, J.H.: Acute Traumatic Bowing Fracture of the Forearm. Neth. J. Surg., 38:158–159, 1986.

107. Sisk, D.T.: Fractures of Upper Extremity and Shoulder Girdle. *In* Crenshaw, A.H. (ed.): Campbell's Operative Orthopaedics. Vol. 3, 7th ed., pp. 1557–2118. St. Louis, C.V. Mosby, 1987.

108. Sisk, D.T.: Internal Fixation of Forearm Fractures. *In* Chapman, M.W., and Madison, M. (eds.): Operative Orthopaedics, Vol. 1, pp. 273–285. Philadelphia, J.B. Lippincott, 1988.

109. Smith, H.: Fractures. *In* Speed, J.S., and Smith, H. (eds.): Campbell's Operative Orthopedics, 2nd ed., p. 375. St. Louis, C.V. Mosby, 1949.

110. Smith, H., and Sage, F.P.: Medullary Fixation of Forearm Fractures. J. Bone Joint Surg., 39A(1):91–98, 188, 1957.

111. Smith, J.E.M.: Internal Fixation in the Treatment of Fractures of the Shafts of the Radius and Ulna in Adults. J. Bone Joint Surg., 41B(1):122–131, 1959.

112. Spar, I.: A Neurologic Complication Following Monteggia Fracture. Clin. Orthop., 122:207–209, 1977.

113. Speed, J.S., and Boyd, H.B.: Treatment of Fractures of Ulna With Dislocation of Head of Radius (Monteggia Fracture). JAMA, 115(20):1699–1705, 1940.

114. Stern, P.J., and Drury, W.J.: Complications of Plate Fixation of Forearm Fractures. Clin. Orthop., 175:25–29, 1983.

115. Street, D.M.: Intramedullary Forearm Nailing. Clin. Orthop., 212:219–230, 1986.

116. Street, D.M.: Spectator Letter, 1955.

117. Tarr, R.R.; Garfinkel, A.I.; and Sarmiento, A.: The Effects of Angular and Rotational Deformities of Both Bones of the Forearm. J. Bone Joint Surg., 66A(1):65–70, 1984.

118. Teipner, W.A., and Mast, J.W.: Internal Fixation of Forearm Fractures: Double Plating Versus Single Compression (Tension Band) Plating—A Comparative Study. Orthop. Clin. North Am., 11:381–391, 1980.

119. Thompson, J.E.: Anatomical Methods of Approach in Operations on the Long Bones of the Extremities. Ann. Surg., 68:309–329, 1918.

120. Trumble, T.; Seaber, A.V.; and Urbaniak, J.R.: Patency After Repair of Forearm Arterial Injuries in Animal Models. J. Hand Surg., 12A:47–53, 1987.

121. Valande, M.: Luxation en arrière de cubitus avec fracture de la diaphse radiale. Bull. et Mem. de la Soc. Nat. de Chir., 55:435–437, 1929.

122. Venable, C.S.: An Impacting Bone Plate to Attain Closed Coaptation. Ann. Surg., 133:808–813, 1951.

123. Venable, C.S.; Stuck, W.G.; and Beach, A.: The Effects on Bone of the Presence of Metals; Based Upon Electrolysis: An Experimental Study. Ann. Surg., 105:917–938, 1937.

124. Vince, K.G., and Miller, J.E.: Cross-union Complicating Fracture of the Forearm: Part 1: Adults. J. Bone Joint Surg., 69A:640–653, 1987.

125. Watson-Jones, R.: Fractures and Joint Injuries. Vol. 1, 4th ed. Edinburgh: E & S Livingstone, 1956.

126. Watson-Jones, R.: Fractures and Joint Injuries, Vol. 2, 4th ed. Edinburgh: E & S Livingstone, 1956.

127. Weiland, A.; Robinson, H.; and Futrell, J.W.: External Stabilization of a Replanted Upper Extremity: A Case Report. J. Trauma, 16:239, 1976.

128. Whiteside, L.A., and Lesker, P.A.: The Effects of Extraperiosteal and Subperiosteal Dissection. I. On Blood Flow in Muscle. J. Bone Joint Surg., 60A(1):23–26, 1978.

129. Whiteside, L.A., and Lesker, P.A.: The Effects of Extraperiosteal and Subperiosteal Dissection. II. On Fracture Healing. J. Bone Joint Surg., 60A(1):26–30, 1987.

130. Zych, G.A.; Latta, L.L.; and Zagorski, J.B.: Treatment of Isolated Ulnar Shaft Fractures With Prefabricated Functional Fracture Braces. Clin. Orthop., 219:194–200, 1987.

10

Fractures and Dislocations of the Elbow
Robert N. Hotchkiss
David P. Green

Injuries of the elbow that lead to chronic pain and permanent restriction of motion limit use of the hand in most activities. Positioning of the hand for grip and prehension is dominated by freedom of motion at the elbow. Basic daily activities, from eating to perineal hygiene, require a wide range of positions and movement at the elbow in both flexion and extension and forearm rotation. Any restricted motion of the neck, shoulder, or wrist magnifies impairment of the elbow. More complex tasks, at the workplace or in recreation, require even greater functional demands.

Traditional salvage procedures after trauma, such as arthrodesis and arthroplasty, are especially poor alternatives for the posttraumatic elbow at this time. Except for rare occupational circumstances, there is no ideal position for fusion, and replacement arthroplasty has not yet stood the test of time or durability in the young, active patient. For these reasons, the imperative for diligent and thoughtful management of the injured elbow—to maximize painless, effective motion—becomes more compelling.

Operative procedures for repair and reconstruction of the injured elbow are technically demanding and require careful planning. Because of the proximity of crucial neurovascular structures, a thorough knowledge of the anatomy and extensile exposures is essential. Accurate reduction and stable fixation of bony injuries can often optimize ultimate function and limit long-term disability.

In the literature, the most notable evolution in the management of elbow injuries has been an increasing emphasis on early motion. Irrespective of the specifics of the injury, the importance of early active motion for restoration of effective function cannot be overstated. With this principle in mind, the optimal management of specific fractures and dislocations provides protection, stabilizing those structures damaged, while permitting as much active motion as pain and swelling allow.

ANATOMY

TOPOGRAPHIC ANATOMY

Several bony landmarks of the elbow can be palpated readily. With the elbow in full extension, both epicondyles and the olecranon process lie in the same horizontal plane on the posterior aspect of the elbow. When the elbow is flexed 90°, these points form a nearly equilateral triangle in a plane parallel to the posterior surface of the humerus.[2] In flexion, a fourth bony prominence, the outer border of the capitellum, becomes more evident on the lateral aspect of the humerus. It lies distal and anterior to the lateral epicondyle and should not be confused with it. Just distal to the capitellum the radial head can be palpated; it is most easily found by passively rotating the forearm. A familiarity with the bony prominences of the elbow and their relationships to one another greatly assists the surgeon in perceiving subtle abnormalities during examination of the injured elbow.

When the elbow is flexed, the anconeus muscle lies just distal and posterior to the radiohumeral joint in a triangular area outlined by the radial head, the lateral epicondyle, and the tip of the olecranon. The main portion of the radial collateral ligament extends anteriorly and distally, leaving only the fibrous capsule of the elbow joint underlying this rather small, thin muscle. Any distention of the joint with fluid can best be detected here, and this is the preferred site for aspiration of the joint.

BONES

Lower End of the Humerus

The distal aspect of the humerus divides into medial and lateral columns (Fig. 10-1). Each of these columns is roughly triangular and is bound on its outer border by a supracondylar ridge. The divergence of these two columns increases the diameter of the distal humerus in the medial-lateral plane. From structural and functional standpoints, the distal humerus is divided into separate medial and lateral components, called condyles, each containing an articulating portion and a nonarticulating portion. Included in the nonarticulating portions are the

epicondyles, which are the terminal points of the supracondylar ridges. The lateral epicondyle contains a roughened anterolateral surface from which the superficial forearm extensor muscles arise. The medial epicondyle is larger than its lateral counterpart and serves as the origin of the forearm flexor muscles. The posterior distal portion of the medial epicondyle is smooth and in contact with the ulnar nerve as it crosses the elbow joint. When a condyle loses continuity from its supporting column, as in a fracture, displacement can occur, because no muscles are attached to the condyles to oppose those attached to the epicondyles.

The articulating surface of the lateral condyle is hemispherical and projects anteriorly; it is called the capitellum (capitulum), or "little head." The capitellum is much smaller than the trochlea, and its convex surface articulates with the reciprocally concave head of the radius. These surfaces are in contact throughout only a small portion of the full range of elbow motion.

The articular surface of the medial condyle, the trochlea, is more cylindrical, or spool-like (Fig. 10-

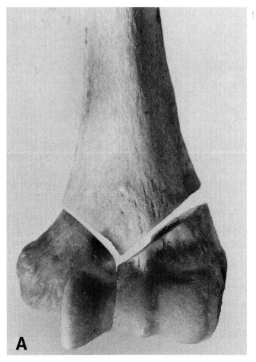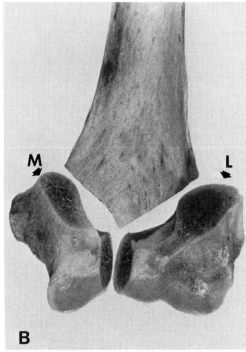

Fig. 10-1. Internal structure of the distal humerus. (**A**) The anterior surface of a normal distal humerus with cuts through the medial and lateral supracondylar columns. (**B**) Rotation of the medial (*M*) and lateral (*L*) supracondylar columns demonstrates their internal structure. The diameter of the medial column (*M*) is smaller than that of the lateral (*L*).

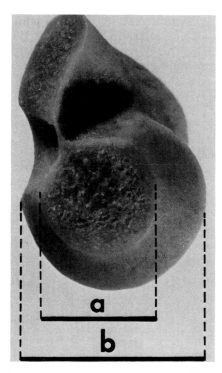

Fig. 10-2. Cross section of the medial condyle through the trochlear groove. The diameter of the bony portion of the center of the groove (*a*) is slightly more than one half that of the medial trochlear ridge (*b*).

2). It has very prominent medial and lateral ridges, which Milch[12] believed are important in maintaining medial and lateral stability of the elbow. Between these ridges is a central groove that articulates with the greater sigmoid (semilunar) notch of the proximal ulna. The diameter of the trochlea at this groove is approximately half that of the medial ridge, and the groove occupies nearly the entire circumference of the trochlea. It originates anteriorly in the coronoid fossa and terminates posteriorly in the olecranon fossa. On the posterior surface of the trochlea the groove is directed slightly laterally. This obliquity of the trochlear groove produces the valgus carrying angle of the forearm when the elbow is extended. Between the lateral ridge of the trochlea and the hemispheric surface of the capitellum, a sulcus separates the medial and lateral condyles. This capitulotrochlear sulcus articulates with the peripheral ridge of the radial head.

Proximal to the condyles on the anterior surface of the humerus lie the coronoid and radial fossae. They receive the coronoid process and radial head, respectively, when the elbow is flexed. Posteriorly, the olecranon fossa is a deep hollow for the recep-

tion of the olecranon, making it possible for the elbow to go into full extension. The bone that separates these anterior and posterior fossae is extremely thin, usually translucent, and occasionally even absent. The presence of extraneous material in the olecranon fossa, such as fracture fragments or an internal fixation device, necessarily impedes full extension of the elbow.

The articular cartilage surface of the capitellum and trochlea projects downward and forward from the end of the humerus at an angle of approximately 30°.[4] The centers of the arcs of rotation of the articular surfaces of each condyle lie on the same horizontal line through the distal humerus. Thus, malalignment of the relationship of one condyle to the other changes their arcs of rotation, limiting flexion and extension[11] (Fig. 10-3).

A bony spine, called the supracondylar process (Fig. 10-4), occasionally projects downward from the anteromedial surface of the humerus. It arises approximately 5 cm superior to the medial epicondyle and is attached to the medial epicondyle by a fibrous band. The process, the shaft of the humerus,

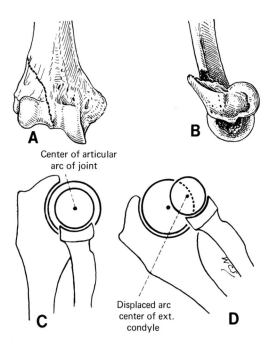

Fig. 10-3. Effects of condylar malalignment. The centers of the articular arc of the separate condyles are located on the same horizontal line through the distal humerus (**A, C**). When there is malalignment of one condyle with another (**B, D**), flexion and extension of the elbow are blocked. *(Magnuson, P.B., and Stack, J.K.: Fractures, 5th ed. Philadelphia, J.B. Lippincott, 1949.)*

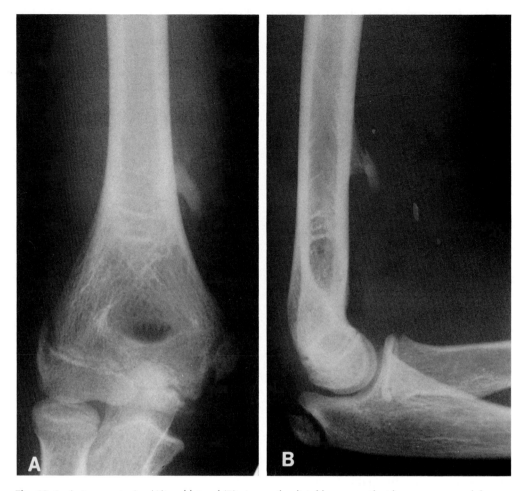

Fig. 10-4. Anteroposterior (**A**) and lateral (**B**) views of a distal humerus that has a supracondylar process.

and the fibrous band form a foramen through which the median nerve and the brachial artery pass. The spur gives origin to a part of the pronator teres muscle and may receive a lower portion of the insertion of the coracobrachialis muscle.

Upper End of the Radius

The proximal end of the radius consists of the disk-shaped head, the neck, and the radial tuberosity; the head and part of the neck lie within the joint. The radial head is not perfectly round; rather, one diameter is consistently 1.5 to 3 cm larger than the other.[24] The shallow concavity of the head articulates with the convex surface of the capitellum, and the border of the head articulates with the lateral side of the coronoid process in the lesser sigmoid (radial) notch. The tuberosity, which is extra-artic-ular, has a rough posterior portion for the insertion of the tendon of the biceps and a smooth anterior surface over which lies a bursa that separates the tuberosity from the tendon.

Upper End of the Ulna

The proximal end of the ulna consists of the olecranon and coronoid processes, which together form the greater sigmoid (semilunar) notch, although their articular surfaces may not always be continuous.[26] The articulation of this notch with the trochlea of the humerus provides inherent bony stability to the hinge joint of the elbow. It is notable that both the medial and lateral collateral ligaments attach to the proximal portion of the ulna.

The triceps inserts by a broad tendinous expansion into the olecranon posteriorly. On the anterior surface, the brachialis muscle inserts into the distal (nonarticular) side of the coronoid process and the tuberosity of the ulna, which lies at the base of the coronoid process.

The head of the radius rests within the lesser sigmoid (radial) notch on the lateral side of the coronoid process. The orbicular (annular) ligament consists of bands of strong fibers, which are intimately and inseparably connected with, but somewhat thicker than, the capsule of the elbow joint. The ligament encircles the head of the radius, retaining it within the radial notch but allowing it enough freedom to rotate easily.

COLLATERAL LIGAMENTS

The collateral ligaments of the elbow supplement the natural stability of the elbow joint.[21] The fan-shaped radial (lateral) collateral ligament originates from the lateral epicondyle and inserts into the orbicular (annular) ligament of the radius. Some posterior fibers go to the ulna just proximal to the posterior origin of the orbicular ligament. The thicker and stronger ulnar (medial) collateral ligament consists of two portions, both arising from the medial epicondyle. The anterior portion attaches to a tubercle (sublime tubercle) on the medial surface of the coronoid. The posterior portion attaches to the medial surface of the olecranon process.

BIOMECHANICS

Unique in the body's collection of diarthrodial joints, the elbow contains two functionally independent articulations that share a synovial compartment but determine motion in two independent axes.[30] The ulnotrochlear articulation directs flexion and extension, and the radiocapitellar joint governs forearm rotation. The ulnohumeral articulation is highly constrained and approximates a hinge with little deviation out of the frontal plane. The instant centers of rotation have been studied and demonstrate little deviation from a true hinge with a single axis.[10,13,14,19,28]

Forearm rotation is centered at the radiocapitellar joint. In forearm rotation, the radius rotates about the ulna, as the ulna is fixed by its articulation at the trochlea. Using these independent axes of motion, the hand can be positioned over a large area in a variety of attitudes. Morrey and colleagues[18] have shown that most activities of daily living require a relatively large range of motion: for flexion and extension 30° to 130° and for pronation and supination 50° each. If a patient loses motion for

any reason, he or she must adapt by using the uninjured extremity or changing shoulder, neck, or body position.

The anteroposterior stability of the elbow results from the static hemicircumferential articulation at the ulnohumeral joint and the dynamic tension provided by the biceps and brachialis anteriorly and the triceps posteriorly. The dynamic stability provided by the flexors and extensors should not be underestimated. The anteromedial ligament and the lateral collateral ligament both provide anteroposterior support in combination with the articular surfaces. A clinical study[494] has shown that up to 50% of the proximal olecranon can be removed without creating instability. In a related biomechanical study,[1] there was a linear decline in stability with each section of the olecranon removed; however, there was no tension in the flexors or triceps. Both authors emphasized the importance of conserving the insertion of the anteromedial collateral ligament.

Most stressful activities such as lifting or throwing exert valgus stress at the elbow. Valgus forces are resisted primarily by a combination of ligaments and joint surfaces and minimally by muscle forces. The anterior portion of the medial collateral ligament is the primary stabilizer to valgus stress in most positions of flexion.[9,15,16,21,22,27] The radial head assists valgus stability by providing a broader base of support and increasing the mechanical advantage of the medial ligament (Fig. 10-5). In full extension, the anterior capsule becomes taut and resists valgus stress. The posterior portion of the medial collateral ligament is thin and contributes little to stability.[9]

Varus stress about the elbow is less problematic. The lateral collateral ligaments and the anconeus muscle confer a combination of static and dynamic stability.[5] The clinical relevance of the varus stabilizers is not yet known. Osborne and Cotterill[390] believed that in cases of recurrent posterior dislocation, the lateral ligaments were paramount and required reconstruction. O'Driscoll and associates have identified a group of patients with posterolateral instability who seem to be deficient of the lateral ulnohumeral collateral ligament.

Joint reaction forces of the elbow have been calculated to reach two to three times body weight during strenuous lifting.[3,14,23] Lifting over the large lever of the forearm magnifies small loads in the hand. Position of the elbow also influences the joint reaction force. As the elbow moves into flexion, the joint reaction force decreases.

When the forearm or hand is loaded in grip or lifting, presumably some load sharing occurs between the ulnohumeral joint and the radiocapitellar joint, but the exact ratio and position dependence are not known. Morrey and coworkers[17] have shown in the cadaver that as the forearm rotates there is a measurable change in the contact at the radiocapitellar joint. The central portion of the interosseous membrane may also play a role in load distribution, since stiffness to longitudinal compression increases from pronation to supination, but the specific relationship *in vivo* is not known[7,8,20] (see Fig. 9-3).

RADIOGRAPHIC ANATOMY

Proper x-rays are vital when evaluating the elbow after trauma. True lateral projections are important when imaging the distal humerus and radiocapitellar joint. Anteroposterior views are also important, but often the elbow is held in the flexed position, causing overlap of the bones. The radial head should be aligned with the capitellum in all views, irrespective of position.

The presence of a so-called fat pad sign can be indicative of trauma[36,37,39] (Fig. 10-6). The radiographic lucency posterior to the distal humerus is the displaced posterior fat from the olecranon fossa, not visible in the normal elbow. If the elbow is extended, the fat pad may be visible simply because of laxity of the triceps. Distention from a hemarthrosis can also displace the anterior fat pad but is less reliable.

FRACTURES OF THE DISTAL HUMERUS

SUPRACONDYLAR FRACTURES

Supracondylar fractures are, by definition, extra-articular. If the joint is involved, they should be classified as intercondylar or transcondylar with proximal extension. Most often the point of fracture is the thin bone between the medial and lateral columns of the distal humerus.[70]

If the distal fragment is displaced posteriorly, it is usually the result of an extension force.[46,51] Anterior displacement reflects a flexion-type injury.[49] Roberts and Kelly[66] credited Kocher with describing four types of fractures, adding adduction and abduction to the flexion and extension types. However, pure displacement in the lateral plane is not seen. We have included these with extension-type fractures.

Extension-Type Supracondylar Fractures

MECHANISM OF INJURY

In Kocher's original classification of supracondylar fractures, the abduction and adduction fractures were thought to be due to pure abduction and adduction forces while the elbow was in extension.[40] Hyperextension (secondary to a fall on the outstretched hand) is often the mechanism.[40] However,

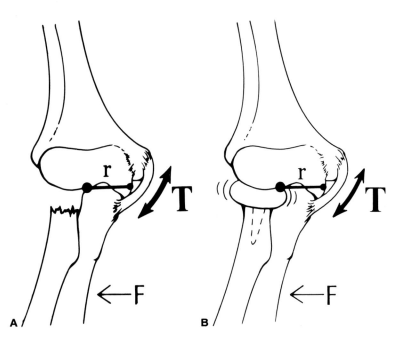

Fig. 10-5. When the radial head is excised, the base of support to valgus stress (*F*) decreases and greater tension (*T*) is experienced by the medial ligaments (**A**). Silicone radial head replacement has not been shown in the laboratory to measurably increase valgus stability (**B**). *(Hotchkiss, R.N., and Weiland, A.J.: Valgus Stability of the Elbow. J. Orthop. Res., 5:372–377, 1987.)*

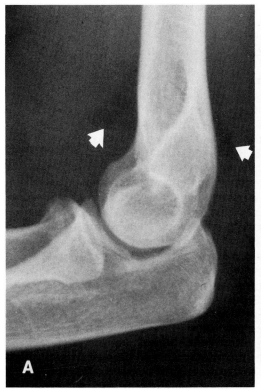
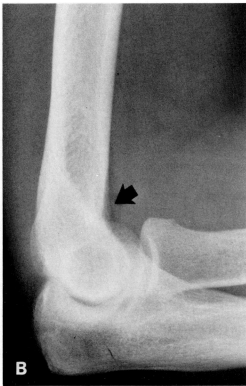

Fig. 10-6. Fat pad sign. (**A**) A lateral view of the elbow joint shows a joint effusion secondary to a minimally displaced fracture of the radial head. There is anterior and superior displacement of the anterior fat pad in the presence of an effusion (*anterior arrow*), and the posterior fat pad is very prominent as well (*posterior arrow*). (**B**) Lateral x-ray of a normal elbow for comparison. The anterior fat pad is barely visualized (*arrow*); the posterior fat pad is not seen.

the authors[66,74] cite direct violence to the elbow as a common cause.

In the lateral view, the fracture usually extends obliquely upward from the anterior distal aspect to posterior proximal aspect. In the extension type, the distal fragment is displaced posteriorly and proximally by the force of the initial injury and by the triceps acting on the proximal ulna. The distal fragment is also usually flexed at the elbow because of the pull of the origins of the forearm muscles on the epicondyles. The sharp, fractured end of the proximal fragment projects forward into the antecubital fossa, where it may contuse or even impale the brachial artery or median nerve.[49] Even if the artery escapes direct injury, vascular impairment may result from massive swelling of the elbow secondary to the frequently severe associated soft tissue injury.[69] Neurovascular complications are an ever-present threat in the management of these difficult injuries.[41,53,69,71]

SIGNS AND SYMPTOMS

The findings in an extension-type supracondylar fracture vary with both the degree of swelling and the displacement of the fracture. Open fractures, although rare, do occur and are usually secondary to direct trauma.[69]

When the patient is seen immediately after the injury, there is little swelling about the elbow, which makes it possible to palpate the bony landmarks.[41] More commonly, however, the patient is seen only after considerable swelling has developed, when the landmarks are not palpable.[69,71] With posterior displacement of the distal fragment, this fracture may be easily confused with a posterior elbow dislocation. Malgaigne's early emphasis on differentiating it from a dislocation[52] leads to the association of the fracture with his name (the Malgaigne fracture).[54] In a supracondylar fracture the three bony landmarks, the medial and lateral epicondyles and the olecranon, maintain their normal spatial relationships.[41] The plane of the equidistant triangle that these points form now lies farther back and not necessarily parallel to the long axis of the humerus.[71] In a posterior dislocation of the elbow the relationship of these three points is disrupted. The tip of the olecranon is posterior to the two epicondyles.

Although Dupuytren[52] pointed out that another pathognomonic sign of this fracture was crepitus, no attempt should be made to elicit it. Uncontrolled manipulation can cause neurovascular damage. The extension-type supracondylar fracture frequently is associated with intense pain and is usually grossly unstable.

Careful initial neurovascular evaluation of the injured arm is essential.[69] Acute injury of the brachial artery and later development of a volar compartment syndrome must be suspected both initially and during the postreduction period.[43,49] Associated injury of all three major nerves has been reported with supracondylar fractures, although apparently the radial nerve is most frequently involved.[43]

RADIOGRAPHIC FINDINGS

The radiographic findings depend on the degree of displacement. In the anteroposterior view, the fracture line is usually transverse in the minimally or displaced or undisplaced fracture, lying just proximal to the articular capsule. In moderately displaced fractures, the distal fragment can lie either medially or laterally in relation to the humeral shaft. In cases of marked displacement there may be either axial rotation of the fragment or angulation in the medial-lateral plane as well. In the lateral view, if the fracture is undisplaced, there may be only a positive fat sign. In those fractures minimally displaced, there may be only a decrease in the angulation of the articular surface with the long axis of the humerus. With marked displacement, the distal fragment is displaced posteriorly and proximally.

METHODS OF TREATMENT

The course of treatment of extension-type supracondylar fractures is influenced greatly by the presence of associated bony and soft tissue injuries (especially neurovascular) in the same limb. In all cases, prompt reduction of the fracture is desirable, but impairment of circulation constitutes a surgical emergency.

Nonoperative Treatment. In nondisplaced or minimally displaced fractures, treatment consists

of posterior plaster splint immobilization for 1 to 2 weeks, after which motion exercise is started.[46,61]

Closed Reduction. In displaced fractures closed reduction is attempted, usually under anesthesia.[70] This relieves tension on the vital neurovascular structures anterior to the elbow joint. First, however, the surgeon must thoroughly examine the x-rays and plan the manipulative maneuvers carefully. The degree of displacement of the distal fragment must be determined, especially the extent of abduction, adduction, medial or lateral displacement, and rotation. Reduction of markedly displaced fractures requires an anesthetic that can give both adequate relaxation and pain relief. This requires, at the minimum, a proximal regional block of the entire extremity or preferably, if the condition of the patient permits, a general anesthetic. An assistant applies countertraction by grasping the upper arm and holds the proximal fragment steady while the surgeon manipulates the distal portion. This is usually best performed by applying traction at the wrist with one hand and guiding the distal fragment during manipulation with the other hand. The proximal pull of the triceps and biceps must first be overcome by longitudinal traction with the elbow extended.[41,59] Smith[71] cautioned against flexion before reduction is obtained, since this may impinge the anteriorly placed neurovascular structures between the sharp ends of the fracture fragments. Once length has been restored by traction—a finding confirmed by a lateral x-ray—the elbow may be hyperextended slightly if extreme care is taken not to overstretch the anterior structures. This tends to unlock the fracture fragments. Once the fragments are free, forward pressure is applied to the distal fragment and backward pressure is applied to the proximal one. At the same time medial or lateral angulation can be corrected.[41,59]

With the fracture fragments now in their proper relationship, the elbow can be flexed gradually.[41] This usually locks the fracture fragment securely in place. The degree of flexion obtainable is usually limited by the amount of swelling about the elbow. The arm must be immobilized in sufficient flexion to maintain fracture reduction. Too much flexion prevents adequate venous return and may even cause occlusion of the brachial artery.[41] The elbow may be flexed just to the point where the radial pulse disappears, and then it should be extended 5° to 10° to accommodate additional swelling. The arm is immobilized in this position with a posterior splint. Patients who have displaced fractures or considerable swelling must be hospitalized after reduction. This allows close observation for the development of any delayed vascular complications.

The decision whether to immobilize the forearm in supination or in pronation is somewhat controversial.[6] Smith[71] pointed out that during reduction the hand must be supinated and directed toward the anterior portion of the shoulder. This helps to obtain adequate rotary alignment. In the past, various authors[66,74] had maintained this position of supination with flexion (the so-called natural splint technique) after reduction had been obtained. Others placed no special emphasis on the position of the forearm,[47,59,68,71,75,78] and DePalma recommended that the forearm be in neutral position.[49] More recent thinking is that the position of the forearm does influence the position of the distal fragment. This is important because the angulation of the distal fragment is responsible for the cubitus valgus or varus deformities.[60,62,72] Böhler[41] believed that the forearm should be in pronation to prevent the more common varus angulation. On the basis of his cadaver and clinical studies, he believed that the varus angulation of the distant fragment resulted from the unopposed pull on the fragment by the pronators of the forearm. Placing the forearm in pronation relaxes these muscles. In full pronation, the rotation of the radius has been exhausted; thus all the forces directed to the forearm are transmitted through the ulna to the humerus. Full pronation tenses the medial collateral ligament, correcting the varus angulation of the distal fragment. Salter,[67] in treating this fracture in children, determines the intact periosteum by the location of the distal fragment in the medial-lateral plane. He then uses this intact periosteum as a hinge to secure the fragments. If there is medial displacement (intact medial periosteum), he recommends that the forearm be pronated. If there is lateral displacement (intact lateral periosteum), the forearm is supinated. Although the periosteum of adults is not as strong as that of children, these general principles can be useful. D'Ambrosia[48] also confirmed with cadaver studies (on the basis of ligament tension) that these fractures were more stable in pronation.

In extension-type fractures with minimal or moderate displacement the principles are essentially the same as for the severely displaced fractures. In many of these there is only loss of the normal condylar angulation.[57] If less than 20° of the condyle-shaft angulation is lost, the position can be accepted.[71] This may result in some decrease of total flexion, but the patient should be able to reach his or her hand to the mouth. In fractures in which the angulation loss is greater than 20°, manipulation should be performed.[46,71]

In cases involving considerable swelling and difficult reduction, the extremity can be placed in

Dunlop's[51] side-arm traction or overhead olecranon pin traction[71,72] until the swelling subsides and a reduction can be attempted with greater ease.

CARE AFTER REDUCTION. X-rays must be taken immediately after reduction. X-rays should then be repeated on about the third and seventh days because occasionally loss of reduction occurs. Special attention must be given to the recognition of varus or valgus angulation of the distal fragments. Varus or valgus angulation can be visualized on a tangential view of the distal humerus through the flexed elbow. The alignment of the distal articular surface with the long axis of the humerus is then measured and compared with that on a similar x-ray of the opposite elbow.

Postoperative immobilization is accomplished by the use of a posterior plaster slab in the proper amount of flexion.[46] This slab can be suspended by a collar-and-cuff arrangement or a sling. A posterior slab probably should be used even in undisplaced fractures, instead of a collar and cuff alone. This provides protection for the tender injured elbow. Circular casts should never be used as the initial method of immobilization. The period of immobilization after reduction lasts from 4 to 6 weeks.[46] Periodic active motion out of the protective splint can be initiated as soon as the fracture is clinically stable. Active motion is facilitated by the application of heat. Passive stretching exercises should never be attempted.

Olecranon Traction. In some fractures, skeletal pin traction through the olecranon may be the treatment of choice (Fig. 10-7).[41] Smith[71] listed four types of severe supracondylar fractures for which Kirschner-wire traction is indicated: (1) when it is impossible to reduce the fracture by other closed methods, (2) when it is possible to reduce the fracture but impossible to maintain the reduction by flexion without compromising the circulation, (3) when swelling is excessive, circulatory impairment is present, or Volkmann's ischemia already threatens, and (4) when associated lesions are present such as compounding of the fracture, additional fractures in the same extremity, or paralysis of a nerve.

The main advantage of this method is that skeletal traction is easier to apply and adjust than skin traction (Fig. 10-8). Either side-arm[61,63,69] or overhead[61,63] skeletal traction can be used. Overhead skeletal traction facilitates edema control, and motion of the elbow can be started early with gravity assisting in flexion. Dressing changes are easily accomplished.[71] Smith[72] suggested that angulation of the distal fragment could be better controlled as well. D'Ambrosia reported no cubitus varus defor-

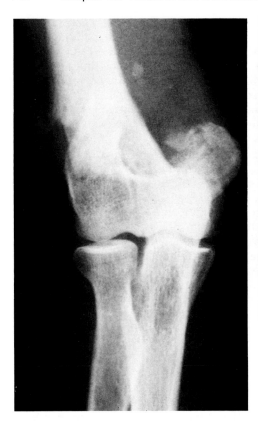
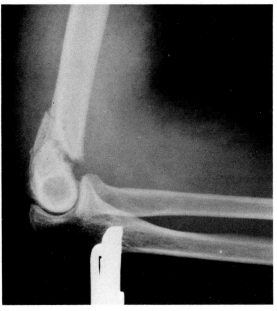

Fig. 10-7. (*Left*) An extension-type supracondylar fracture. (*Right*) Lateral view x-ray demonstrating the fracture line running from posterior-proximal to anterior-distal. Olecranon pin traction resulted in excellent alignment of the fracture.

mities after closed reduction and overhead olecranon pin traction. He believed this was because overhead skeletal traction keeps the forearm in pronation, whereas side-arm traction holds the forearm in the neutral or supinated position, which predisposes to varus deformity.[48] Conn and Wade[46] warned against some of the problems encountered with skeletal pin traction.

Too-early discontinuance of the traction can result in a loss of reduction with poor results.[46] Problems with pin tract infections have been reported.[46,50,63] Although the infection can be easily cleared, marked restriction of motion may result.[46,50,63] Another disadvantage of this method is that it necessitates a lengthy hospitalization.

Operative Methods.   Two operative techniques are available to the surgeon in the treatment of extension-type fractures. One is fixation of the distal fragment with percutaneous Kirschner wires after reduction has been obtained by closed methods. The second is primary open reduction and internal fixation.

Percutaneous Pin Fixation.   Miller[64] first described percutaneous pinning of intercondylar fractures of

the distal humerus in 1939. By directing the wires in a different direction, Swenson[76] adapted its use for supracondylar fractures in children. Although this technique has been used mainly for supracondylar fractures in children and adolescents, Jones reported its use in adults.[58] He modified the technique by allowing the pins to protrude through the skin to facilitate removal. He recommended leaving the pins in 4 to 5 weeks in the adult, followed by 1 to 2 weeks of plaster immobilization. This technique finds application in those fractures that are unstable except in extreme flexion. Stabilization of the fracture by this technique allows the arm to be immobilized in much less flexion. Another indication for this technique is the presence of a fracture of the forearm in the same extremity.[40] In the adult, Kirschner wires may not be strong enough to provide rigid fixation, and small Steinmann pins may be necessary instead.[58] Pin fixation must not be done, of course, unless an adequate reduction can be accomplished. The technique relies heavily on the surgeon's ability to palpate the bony landmarks. Since both reduction and palpation may be difficult or even impossible in the severely swollen elbow, a preliminary period of traction may be necessary

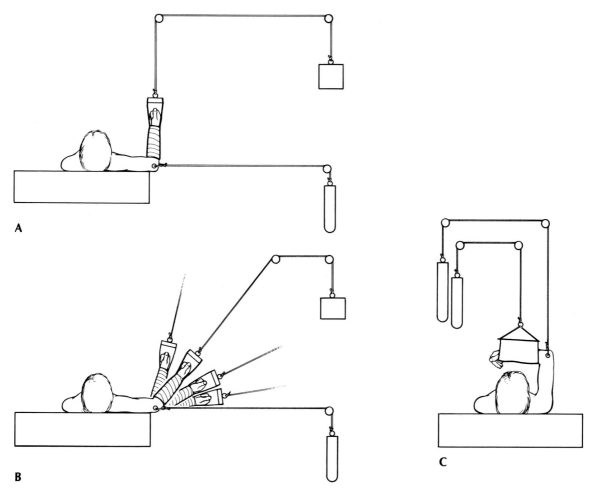

Fig. 10-8. (**A**) Lateral skeletal olecranon pin traction. (**B**) Changing the position of the overhead pulley supporting the forearm (in skin traction) allows early institution of elbow motion. (**C**) Modification of skeletal olecranon pin traction in which the forearm is supported overhead is useful in the early postinjury phase to help decrease swelling.

to allow the swelling to subside. Power equipment for insertion of the pins greatly facilitates the procedure.

In the original descriptions[58,76] the wires were passed medially and laterally through the epicondyles and continued proximally up the respective supracondylar columns. This technique entails some risk to the ulnar nerve during placement of the medial pin. In an effort to avoid this risk, Fowles and colleagues[53] used two pins laterally. One is passed laterally through the lateral epicondyle in the usual manner. A second pin traverses the joint just lateral to the olecranon in the region of the capitulotrochlear sulcus. This pin continues in an axial direction up the humeral shaft. Theoretic disadvantages of this modification include potential

joint contamination by a septic axial pin and inability to extend the elbow fully after pinning because of the axial pin. Childress[45] used a single pin through the olecranon crossing the joint and continuing up the shaft of the humerus.

Open Reduction and Internal Fixation. Primary open reduction is indicated in those fractures in which there is inability to obtain a satisfactory closed reduction, vascular injury, or an associated fracture of the humerus or forearm in the same limb.[40,43,70] In addition, Conn and Wade[46] believed that internal fixation may be the treatment of choice in selected elderly patients to hasten ambulation and joint mobilization.

In those cases in which reduction cannot be obtained, muscle, especially the brachialis, may be interposed between the fracture fragments. In rare instances the proximal humeral fragment may be buttonholed through the brachialis. Attempts at longitudinal traction only tighten the muscle around the protruding fragment. In those patients with vascular injury in whom arterial repair is necessary, the fracture must be stabilized as well. Access to both the antecubital fossa and the distal humerus can be accomplished by the surgical approach of Fiolle and Delmas as described by Henry.[55] In cases without associated vascular injury, the fracture can be approached through combined medial and lateral incisions[44] or through a posterior approach.[61,65] In our experience the posterior approach provides better exposure and better access for internal fixation. After the underlying pathology is corrected, a reduction is obtained by direct visualization. Fracture stabilization can then be achieved by percutaneous pinning[45,53,58,76] or by direct internal fixation.[65] Bryan[43] recommended the use of a special Y-plate for internal fixation of these fractures. Müller and colleagues[65] recommend an AO semitubular or dynamic compression plate on the medial or lateral humeral column with as many screws as possible inserted as lag screws for internal fixation of supracondylar fractures. The surgeon must remember, however, that although simple supracondylar fractures are suitable for internal fixation, conservative treatment has produced better results in patients in whom comminution at the fracture site prevents stable fixation.[56] Unstable internal fixation that necessitates prolonged cast immobilization to maintain the reduction combines the disadvantages of both closed and open treatment and produces the worst clinical results.[61] Early range of motion of the elbow must be possible if open reduction is selected.

Authors' Preferred Method.   The initial evaluation of any serious elbow injury should include a careful assessment for signs of neurovascular injury. Most fractures in the adult distal humerus are intercondylar (not supracondylar), and one should suspect this when first seeing an adult patient with a "supracondylar" fracture.

Undisplaced fractures are immobilized with a long-arm posterior splint for 1 to 2 weeks, and then active motion is begun. It is important to monitor the fracture radiographically for any sign of displacement during the first 2 weeks.

Fractures with displacement are usually unstable, and we seldom use closed manipulation and casting or olecranon pin traction in adults because of the difficulty in maintaining the reduction and pro-

longed immobilization required. If swelling is considerable, immobilization with external splinting is less reliable because adequate flexion is precluded. In certain patients, however, open reduction may be ill advised because of soft tissue injury or other medical problems. In this situation, overhead olecranon pin traction may be a good alternative (see Fig. 10-8).

In most displaced fractures, we prefer open reduction with rigid internal fixation that allows motion in the first few days after injury. Several implants have been designed for use in the distal humerus; however, we believe that double plating offers the most stable configuration.[123] If there is significant comminution or bone loss, then iliac bone graft is added at the time of operation to reduce the likelihood of nonunion. Open reduction and internal fixation of a comminuted fracture of the distal humerus can be an exceedingly difficult procedure, and the surgeon should be experienced in the use of AO techniques before attempting to fix such a fracture.

Open supracondylar fractures should be treated by débridement with the wounds left open and delayed wound closure.[69] These open fractures are usually very unstable because of associated soft tissue stripping at the fracture site. Therefore, primary reduction of the fracture and percutaneous Kirschner-wire or Steinmann-pin stabilization of the fracture should be considered.[58]

Flexion-Type Supracondylar Fractures

This type of injury is quite rare.[47] In Smith's[71] series it occurred in less than 2% and in Siris's[22] series in only 4% of supracondylar fractures. The cause of this fracture is generally believed to be a force directed against the posterior aspect of the flexed elbow.[41,66,71,74] This results in anterior displacement of the distal fragments with the elbow joint. The posterior periosteum is torn, but the anterior periosteum may remain attached, having separated only from the anterior surface of the proximal fragment.[73] Because direct violence is usual in this injury, the fracture is often open, with the sharp proximal fragment piercing the triceps tendon and skin.[43,73] Vascular injuries are rare.

SIGNS AND SYMPTOMS

As in the extension-type fracture, the relationship between the epicondyles and the ulna remains the same, but the plane of their triangle is shifted anterior to the shaft of the humerus. The elbow is flexed, with resistance encountered on attempts at extension. The normal prominence of the posterior aspect of the elbow is absent.

RADIOGRAPHIC FINDINGS

The obliquity of the fracture through the supracondylar region on the lateral view is from proximal anterior to distal posterior (opposite that seen in the extension type). The distal fragment lies anterior to the humerus and is flexed at the elbow. The fracture line, as a rule, is transverse on the anteroposterior projection.

METHODS OF TREATMENT

Nonoperative Treatment.   Flexion-type supracondylar fractures are often difficult to manage.[50,63,73] Closed reduction can be obtained by first applying traction with the forearm flexed.[73] Applying traction with the forearm in extension before reduction is obtained increases the pull of the forearm muscles on the condyles, increasing the flexion of this fragment at the elbow joint. This inhibits reduction and can injure the anterior structures. As the traction is maintained, the distal humeral fragment is pushed posteriorly into position by pressure on its anterior aspect and counterpressure posteriorly on the proximal fragment. Once the fracture is reduced, the fracture fragments can be locked into place by extension of the elbow.

Opinions vary on the best method of immobilization after reduction.[47,49,78] If the anterior periosteum is intact, it can be used as a hinge to hold the distal fragment in place while pressure is applied to the anterior portion of the distal fragment in a posterior direction. This can be achieved by *extension* of the elbow with the posterior force being applied to the distal fragment through the anterior capsule and collateral ligaments. The usual obliquity of the fracture line also helps to buttress the posteriorly applied force on the distal fragment.

In children with an intact, strong, anterior periosteum, this fracture may be stable in extension. However, the thin periosteum present in adults (especially the elderly) offers little resistance and may allow gross displacement of the fracture.[73] In addition, we are opposed to immobilizing the elbow in the extended position for fear of not being able to regain flexion of the elbow after fracture union.[73]

A second method of reducing and holding the distal fragment, based on the fact that the humeral condyles behave as part of the forearm following a supracondylar fracture, was introduced by Soltanpur.[73] The surgeon grasps the humeral condyles in one hand and, with the other hand, maintains the elbow flexed with the forearm in supination. Trac-

tion is applied to the condyles to correct overriding and angulation. An assistant wraps the arm and hand in cast padding, and a circular cast is applied about the upper arm only. When the circular cast dries, the surgeon places one hand under the cast and with the other hand pushes posteriorly to reduce the fracture. The long-arm plaster cast is completed with the arm in this position. The cast is removed in 6 weeks, and elbow motion is instituted. Despite 6 weeks of immobilization, the author reported restoration of nearly complete elbow motion.

Operative Treatment.   For those fractures that cannot be held by closed methods except by extremes of extension, percutaneous pin fixation may be indicated. After the reduction has been accomplished, the pinning should be performed with the elbow flexed.[58] When the elbow is in extension, the bony landmarks may be obscured, making pin placement difficult. Also, flexing the elbow after it has been stabilized in extension can result in loss of reduction.

TRANSCONDYLAR (DICONDYLAR) FRACTURES

There is some controversy whether the transcondylar fracture should be classified as a separate entity. Although most of the earlier fracture texts distinguished it as a separate fracture,[80,83,85,87,89,91–93] others did not.[90] Smith[90] classified transcondylar and supracondylar fractures as a single entity. He believed that for practical purposes the treatment, prognosis, and complications are essentially identical to those of a supracondylar fracture. However, Bryan[81] emphasized that transcondylar fractures are particularly difficult to manage and should therefore be considered separately. He recognized several unique characteristics of these fractures. First, the distal fragment is small with only minimal extra-articular bony area to help control rotation. Second, this small distal fragment, being mainly intra-articular, may allow dislocation of the radiohumeral and ulnohumeral joints during attempted reduction. Third, the amount of bone contact available for union is small even when a perfect reduction is obtained.

Those fractures that pass through both condyles and are within the joint capsule should be classified as transcondylar fractures.[87] Kocher, Ashhurst, and Chutro are credited with distinguishing this fracture from supracondylar fractures.[79,82,88] There appear to be two types, extension and flexion, based on the position of the elbow when fractured.[79] The fracture line is characteristically crescent-shaped or transverse, passing just proximal to the articular surface of the condyles.[88] It also enters the coronoid and olecranon fossae.[79,93] This fracture occurs just proximal to the old epiphyseal line. These fractures may be undisplaced, or the lower fragment may be displaced posteriorly.[79,93] Anterior displacement is distinctly unusual.[79]

The mechanisms of injury and principles of treatment that apply to supracondylar fractures are basically the same in this fracture.[93] There are some differences that merit discussion, however. First, this type of injury is more common in elderly persons with fragile osteoporotic bone. Second, since this fracture lies within the joint cavity, excessive callus production can result in residual loss of motion.[85,87,93] This is especially true if callus develops in the olecranon or coronoid fossae.[81,83,92,93]

Bryan[81] recommended closed reduction (especially of mildly displaced fractures) followed by cast immobilization. If the fracture is not reducible, or if the reduction is unstable, he recommended percutaneous Kirschner-wire fixation. He emphasized the need to restore the normal forward tilt of the distal humerus to preserve a functional arc of elbow motion.

An unusual variation of the transcondylar fracture, recognized by Professor Posadas of Buenos Aires in 1901, is the so-called Posadas's fracture.[79,88,89,91] This injury was described in a monograph on elbow fractures by Chutro in 1904, in which he credits Posadas with the original description.[82] Chutro carefully distinguished between the transcondylar fracture of Kocher and Posadas's fracture. The latter consists of a transcondylar fracture, caused by trauma to the elbow in flexion, in which the distal (dicondylar) fragment is carried anteriorly and there is an associated dislocation of the radius and ulna from the dicondylar fragment. Clinically, the forearm presents in complete extension (and supination), lying along the longitudinal axis of the humerus.[82] The clinical appearance suggests a simple dislocation. The coronoid process appears to become wedged between the anteriorly displaced dicondylar fragment and the proximal supracondylar portion of the humeral diaphysis. Ashhurst[79] emphasized the need to recognize the associated dislocation of the radius and ulna to prevent ankylosis of the elbow. Scudder[89] described how, with improper treatment, the ulna can subsequently develop a pseudarthrosis with the distal portion of the humerus (ie, a type of traumatic arthroplasty). There is no consensus on the preferred

method of treating this fracture. Although Chutro[82] reported the closed treatment of five such injuries, ankylosis in near-complete extension was the result.[79] Ashhurst[79] presented a successful result following closed treatment. However, closed reduction is known to be difficult to obtain and hold.[81,86] Grantham and Tietjen[86] recommended open reduction and internal fixation for this difficult fracture–dislocation.

INTERCONDYLAR T- OR Y-FRACTURES

Intercondylar fractures represent one of the most complicated and challenging fractures in the upper extremity. Watson-Jones[157] wrote "Few fractures are more difficult to treat." The medial and lateral condyles are usually separate fragments, displaced in a T or Y configuration and both unconnected from the humeral shaft and rotated in the axial plane. The goal of treatment is to reestablish the articular congruity and alignment and begin active motion as soon as possible. In most cases, open reduction with rigid internal fixation is preferred.

Mechanism of Injury

The fracture is probably caused by the impact of the ulna in the trochlear groove, forcing the condyles of the distal humerus apart.[96,103] The injury can occur in either flexion or extension.[112,128,161] In the flexion-type injury, Palmer[142] has speculated that the blow against the posterior elbow (olecranon), coupled with contraction of the forearm muscles, produces the fracture with less force than expected. In many instances, however, the forces applied to the posterior flexed elbow are violent, as in motor vehicle injuries. In the flexion-type fracture, the condyles are usually found anterior to the humeral shaft. In the extension-type injury, the ulna is directed anteriorly against the posterior aspect of the trochlea, separating the condyles at the same time as the supracondylar portion is fractured. Another mechanism is that proposed by Wilson and Cochrane,[162] who suggested that the separation of the condyles in this type of fracture may be created by the splitting effect of the humeral shaft as it is forced distally. In the extension-type injury, the condyles are usually found to lie behind the humeral shaft. Whatever the mechanism, there is usually considerable associated soft tissue injury.[96] Some may have open lacerations extending into the fracture site.[96,151] Comminution of the bony fragments is not unusual.[142,151,158] Because of loss of bony continuity, the fracture fragments are displaced by unopposed muscle action.[151] In those with severe displacement, the origins of the forearm muscles pull the epicondyles distally, rotating the condyles so that their articular surfaces face a more proximal direction.[99,142] This converts the trochlear sulcus into a narrow inverted V, making it no longer congruous with the articular surface of the ulna. These actions of the biceps anteriorly and the triceps posteriorly pull the articular surface of the ulna proximally. In an opposing fashion the humeral shaft is forced distally between the rotated condyles.

Signs and Symptoms

Little can be added to points in diagnosis as outlined by Desault[113] in his original description of this injury.

> If the fingers, placed before or behind, press on the limb in the direction of the longitudinal fracture, the two condyles will be separated from each other, the one yielding in an outward, and the other in an inward direction, leaving a fissure or opening between them. The part at the same time expands in breadth. The forearm is almost constantly in a state of pronation. When we take hold of one of the condyles in each hand, and endeavor to make them move in opposite directions, they can be brought alternately forward or backward, and if their surfaces touch, a manifest crepitation is heard.

The key to distinguishing an intercondylar T- or Y-fracture from others is determining the presence of separation of the condyles from each other and from the humeral shaft. With proximal migration of the ulna the arm appears shortened. It is also widened by concomitant condylar separation. The independent mobility of the condyles can be determined by pressing the condyles between the index finger and the thumb. There is crepitus when the condyles are pressed together. Since they are still under the influence of the forearm muscles, the condyles tend to spring back into displacement when the pressure is released. Both the pressure and its release are a source of pain to the patient. The relationship of the epicondyles with the tip of the olecranon process has been disrupted. In those fractures with an extensive degree of displacement there is usually gross instability in all directions.

Radiographic Findings

Good-quality anteroposterior and lateral x-rays are essential in the evaluation of fracture displacement and comminution. Polytomography can also be helpful if the degree of comminution is in doubt. One can usually assume that reality is worse than the x-ray appearance. We have also found computed tomography (CT) scanning to be occasionally helpful in delineating fracture patterns.

In those fractures with considerable displacement of the fragments, the diagnosis is easy. Because of considerable comminution of the fracture fragments, it may be difficult to determine the origin of many small fragments. In those that are undisplaced or minimally displaced, the surgeon must look carefully for the presence of a vertical intercondylar fracture to distinguish this from a simple supracondylar fracture.

Classification

Riseborough and Radin[147] devised a very useful classification of this type of fracture, based on its radiographic appearance (Fig. 10-9). This classification provides some guide to management and prognosis. They defined four types:

I. Undisplaced fracture between the capitellum and trochlea
II. Separation of the capitellum and trochlea without appreciable rotation of the fragments in the frontal plane

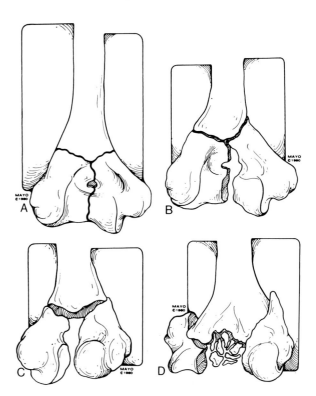

Fig. 10-9. (A) Type I undisplaced condylar fracture of the elbow. (B) Type II displaced but not rotated T-condylar fracture. (C) Type III displaced and rotated T-condylar fracture. (D) Type IV displaced, rotated, and comminuted condylar fracture. *(Bryan, R.S.: Fractures About the Elbow in Adults. Inst. Course Lect. XXX:1981.)*

III. Separation of the fragments with rotary deformity

IV. Severe comminution of the articular surface with wide separation of the humeral condyles

Müller and colleagues[140] have used a somewhat different classification, separating the fractures by the presence of a supracondylar extension or comminution.

We believe that the classification of Riseborough and Radin is more useful for directing treatment and comparison of results. The principal focus of distinction in this classification rests with severity of injury of the articular component of the fracture, a factor that most authors believe determines outcome.[100,117,129,139,142,160]

Methods of Treatment

CLOSED TECHNIQUES

Because of the complexity and technical difficulty of operative treatment, some authors before the 1960s recommended closed treatment for *all* intercondylar fractures. More recently, closed treatment has been recommended for the elderly, for those whose fractures are deemed unsuitable for internal fixation, or for patients whose medical condition prohibits surgery.

Closed methods of treatment can be divided into three categories: (1) cast immobilization; (2) traction (skin, gravity, or skeletal); and (3) early motion, the "bag of bones" technique.

Cast Immobilization. It is difficult to find many advocates[111] of closed manipulation and casting, since this technique usually represents the worst of both worlds—inadequate reduction and prolonged immobilization. Trynin[155] did report a case of closed manipulation and condylar compression in which a carpenter's clamp was used for 4 weeks, but he emphasized the necessity of accurate reduction of the articular surface.

Riseborough and Radin[147] reported five patients treated with manipulation and casting, three with a good outcome and two with a fair result. The degree of displacement in these fractures was minimal (type II). (If casting is used, most recommend starting motion at 3 weeks after injury, using a splint to protect the elbow between exercise sessions.)

Traction. The most popular method of closed treatment is some form of traction[110,112,126,131,135,147,148,153] used either to obtain reduction or to maintain position after manipulation. As late as the 1960s, many authors thought that traction should be used for all intercondylar fractures, but as surgical techniques improved, more authors began recommending its use in type IV injuries or in cases in which open reduction was not feasible. In 1936 Reich[146] perceived the theoretic advantage of open reduction with anatomic restoration but recounted the failures of fixation and believed that traction was a safer alternative. He applied an ice-tong device to the distal humerus and then used traction for 3 weeks or until callus formation was noted.

Olecranon pin traction, reported by many authors, seems to provide the best line of pull to optimize the longitudinal position of the fracture fragments. In the overhead position, swelling rapidly subsides, and the arm and hand are accessible during treatment. In addition, motion of the elbow can begin while in traction as the patient becomes more comfortable. Longitudinal traction alone, however, will not derotate the intercondylar fragments in the axial plane. Skin traction has been reported by some authors,[125,162] but it cannot be applied with more than 5 to 7 pounds because of potential skin slough. Other authors adapted olecranon pin traction to casts or frames that allowed the patient to leave the hospital. Unfortunately, these were often cumbersome or were incorporated into a long-arm cast, which precluded early motion.[143,146,154]

The outcome of displaced fractures treated with traction is difficult to glean from the literature. Riseborough and Radin[147] reported that 8 of their 12 patients with type III injuries had a good result when treated with traction, compared with 4 of 12 with a fair or poor result. Other advocates of traction treatment report somewhat similar results, but the numbers are smaller and reporting methods inconsistent.

In most intra-articular fractures, accurate reduction of the joint surface is usually thought to be one of the most influential factors with respect to outcome. However, with this fracture, some authors have argued otherwise.[98,115,126] In 1932, Hitzrot[126] stated that "anatomic replacement is of secondary importance." Most other authors have disagreed with this position, especially in younger patients.[96,100,107,109,117,125,128,129,130,132,133,140,146,148,156,159,160,163]

Because of the relative rarity of this fracture, a reliable study comparing traction treatment with open reduction and rigid internal fixation has not been possible. Series reporting a comparison of the methods contain patient selection bias or insufficient numbers to allow valid conclusions on a statistical basis.[98,100,147,163] In addition, many of the early series that employed open reduction with internal fixation used a myriad of implants ranging from multiple K-wires to multiple plates and screws, preventing valid comparison with *rigid* fixation and early motion.[125,129] Techniques of exposure have also improved, with more attention given to conservation of the triceps mechanism.[102]

"Bag of Bones" Technique. Eastwood,[115] who popularized this method in England during the 1930s, credited Hugh Owen Thomas as being its originator. It involves simply placing the arm in a collar and cuff initially, in as much flexion as possible. The initial position of flexion is chosen because extension will improve over several months with exercise whereas flexion usually will not.[98,115] The elbow is left hanging free, which is an important point. The effect of gravity on the dependent elbow is thought to enable the fracture fragments to settle into a more natural alignment. Some attempt at initial reduction is made, but the permanent success of this maneuver is questionable.[98] Hand and finger motion are started immediately. Pendulum shoulder motion begins at about seven to ten days. As the swelling and pain subside, the patient is allowed gradually to actively extend the elbow. The fracture is usually united in 6 weeks, at which time the sling is discarded.[98] However, with intensive exercises, the range of motion will improve for 3 to 4 months.[98] In a series reported by Brown and Morgan,[98] the patients achieved an average of 70° of elbow motion. It is significant that in the x-rays presented by both Eastwood[115] and Brown and Morgan,[98] good reductions of the fractures are noted. However, the relationship of fracture reduction to results is not mentioned by either author. One author[156] modified this method by the application of a large padded wooden carpenter's clamp to the condyles, suspending it from the neck. The clamp was tightened as the swelling subsided. In addition to some inherent dangers existing, patients might not accept this modification.

Watson-Jones[157] noted that many of the patients treated with this method had residual loss of extension from excessive anterior tilting of the condyles. Evans believed that although many of his patients treated in this manner had a satisfactory range of motion, a significant number complained of weakness and instability in the elbow.[116] Bickel and Perry[96] also believed that this method does not produce the strong, stable elbow required by a young patient. Therefore, the bag of bones technique appears to be suitable for the elderly patient in whom early ambulation is desired.[112,133] It does

require a good deal of patient motivation and cooperation to achieve a satisfactory result.

OPERATIVE METHODS

The operative methods are (1) pins in plaster, (2) open reduction and internal fixation, (3) distal humeral replacement (prosthetic or allograft), and (4) arthroplasty.

Pins in Plaster. Pins in plaster was originally called blind nailing by Miller.[138] He initially placed the upper extremity in traction with a Kirschner wire in the olecranon. The condyles were then manually reduced and transfixed percutaneously with a second Kirschner wire. A third wire was likewise passed percutaneously through the proximal fragment. While the fracture was maintained in traction, a long-arm cast was applied, incorporating all three wires. Böhler[97] appears to be one of the few other surgeons to have used this technique. Although this method may facilitate maintaining alignment, it contains no provision for elbow motion. The presence of at least two pins penetrating the fracture site greatly enhances the chances of infection and its resultant disability.

Limited Open Reduction and Internal Fixation. In the performance of open reduction and internal fixation, two distinct methods have been reported. Both employ limited surgery to reestablish articular congruity between the humeral condyles. In one method, this is followed by postoperative traction[96,99,116,132] or closed manipulation and casting of the remaining supracondylar component of the fracture.[96,105,116,130,132] In 1953, Evans[116] reported this method in five cases, emphasizing the importance of articular congruity. Once the joint was reconstructed using open reduction and internal fixation between the condyles, the supracondylar portion was managed with splint or cast immobilization. Motion was started after 4 weeks.

Knight[132] reported using olecranon traction once the intercondylar portion was stabilized. Outcome from this technique is difficult to judge. In Evans's[116] series, four of the five patients had flexion contractures of 60° or more.

Open Reduction and Internal Fixation. Open reduction with internal fixation has evolved as the preferred method of treatment for most type II and III fractures.[99–101,104,107,117,122,124,125,128–130,132,140, 148,159,163] Several authors in the 1930s were attracted to the idea of anatomic restoration with early motion, but they were discouraged by the disruptive surgical exposures and the lack of adequate implants.[138,146,160] Since then, improvements in both areas have engendered more confidence in this technique.

Surgical Exposure. To address the problem of exposure, Van Gorder[156] (who credited Campbell with the idea) described a posterior approach to the distal humerus by incising the triceps as a tongue of fascia and folding this distally to the level of the olecranon. Although helpful, this approach still does not permit good exposure of the anterior and distal portions of the joint. In addition, the incision in the triceps mechanism deterred early active motion for fear of rupture.

In 1969, Kelly and Griffin[130] advocated an anterior approach for open reduction. The biceps was retracted medially and the brachialis tendon transected at the level of the coronoid process. No attempt was made to secure the condylar fragments to the shaft of the humerus. There have been no other reports of this approach.

Olecranon osteotomy for exposure of the distal humerus was described for treatment of the ankylosed elbow by MacAusland[134] in 1915. Cassebaum[106,107] subsequently adopted this osteotomy, for distal humeral fracture exposure. Müller[140] later modified the olecranon osteotomy by directing the bone cut so that the joint was not entered. The most recent recommendation of the AO group[122] is a chevron or V-shaped osteotomy (Fig. 10-10), which enters the joint directly opposite the trochlea. The advocates of olecranon osteotomy suggest that better distal exposure is achieved and that there is no requirement for tendon-to-tendon healing. Rigid fixation of the osteotomy allows immediate active motion. Disadvantages, however, are that another "fracture" is created, bearing the risks of technical complication, implant failure, or nonunion.

In 1982, Bryan and Morrey[102] described a triceps-sparing posterior approach to the elbow (Fig. 10-11), initially used for total elbow replacement. The medial border of the triceps and the medial fascia of the forearm are elevated subperiosteally as a single unit in continuity. The ulnar nerve must be identified and protected. Excellent access to the joint is gained without osteotomy or transverse disruption of the triceps mechanism. No studies compare this approach to olecranon osteotomy or have reported its use in trauma, but it has been successfully used in fractures of the distal humerus (see Authors' Preferred Method).

Methods of Fixation. There are two components of the T-type intercondylar fracture that must be secured—the intercondylar and the supracondylar. Because of the interest in articular congruity, more attention initially was given to the intercondylar portion of the fracture.[96,105,116,130,132] As techniques of exposure improved, emphasis on supracondylar fixation increased because of stiffness from immobilization of this portion of the fracture.

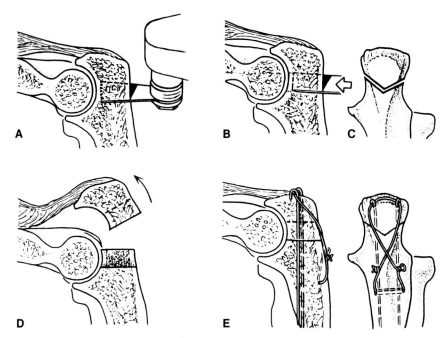

Fig. 10-10. A chevron-shaped olecranon osteotomy can be used for exposure of the distal humerus. *(Heim, U., and Pfeiffer, K.M.: Internal Fixation of Small Fractures, 3rd ed. Berlin, Springer-Verlag, 1988.)*

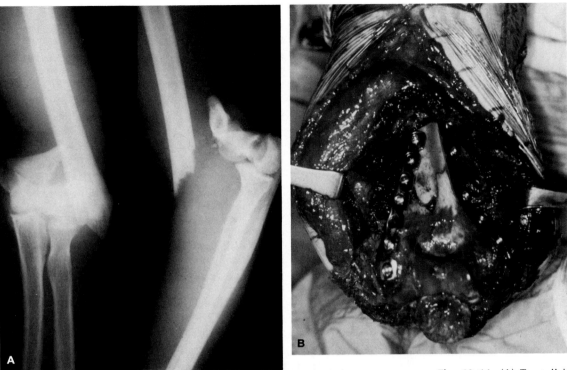

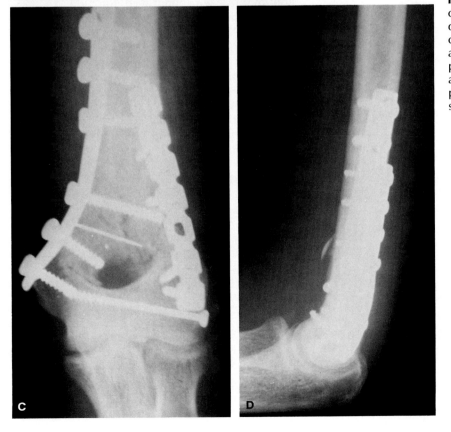

Fig. 10-11. (A) Type II inter-condylar fracture with great displacement of the supra-condylar portion. **(B)** Exposure achieved using the Bryan approach. **(C, D)** Dual-plate fixation using a one-third tubular plate and a 3.5 pelvic reconstruction plate.

The intercondylar portion of the fracture has been secured with multiple K-wires and/or screws. Several authors have stated that secure screw fixation is preferable to multiple K-wire fixation when possible.[122,128,129] Regardless of the implant used, it is important to avoid any impingement in the olecranon fossa or trochlea (Fig. 10-12). If bone is missing, Heim and Pfeiffer[122] and others[117,129] have emphasized the importance of bone grafting any defects in the trochlea, and *not* lagging the fragments.

Because the distal condylar portion of the humerus sits like a barrel on the end of a forked stick, rigid fixation of the supracondylar component without interference with elbow motion has been difficult to achieve. Screws directed from each condyle into the humeral shaft have been used, but the stiffness and fatigue properties of this construct can be low,[123] leading to supracondylar displacement or nonunion.[94,101,123] A posterior Y-shaped plate has also been used for fixation with good results,[100] but it has the disadvantage of single-plane fixation.[123]

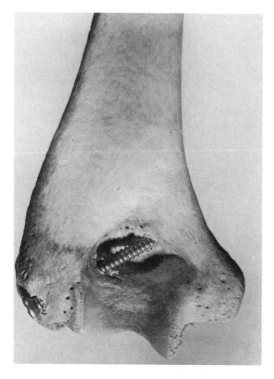

Fig. 10-12. Improper placement of a screw into the lateral supracondylar column can result in its entering the olecranon fossa, which blocks extension of the elbow.

Dual-plate fixation has been used by several authors and seems to provide the most secure fixation. As Gabel and colleagues[117] emphasized in their study of ten patients, no nonunions occurred and active motion was started at the second postoperative day. The recommendations of the AO[122] group are for placement of a semitubular plate medially and a 3.5 reconstruction plate posterolaterally (Fig. 10-13). Helfet and Hotchkiss[123] studied the rigidity and fatigue performance of several methods of fixation in the laboratory, including dual-plate fixation. They concluded that the dual-plate technique, with the plates oriented perpendicularly, offered the most rigid and fatigue-resistant construct, especially in cases of comminution in which interfragmentary compression was precluded. There was no meaningful difference between the use of semitubular plates, reconstruction plates, or a combination of the two as recommended by the AO group.

Distal Humeral Replacement. In 1947, Mellen and Phalen[171] replaced the distal humerus in three patients with a customized acrylic prosthesis. Each patient had an ununited, painful fracture of the distal humerus. They reported follow-up of several months with improved function. In 1954 MacAusland[169] reported good results in four patients with a nylon prosthesis. Venable[176] and others[164,167,174] have used Vitallium with some short-term success. Unfortunately, none of these materials or designs has demonstrated longevity or durability.

Breen and coworkers[165] reported using allograft replacement of the distal humerus in four patients. One allograft became infected and one developed a nonunion; both required removal.

Arthroplasty. Arthroplasty of the elbow using distraction interpositional materials or simple resection is a subject too vast for this chapter.[166,175,177] The primary indication, irrespective of technique, is disabling pain. There is seldom, if ever, a reason to consider these procedures in the setting of an acute fracture. Total elbow replacement should also be considered in the same light. The durability of total elbow replacement in an otherwise healthy and active individual is thus far quite poor,[168,172] exhibiting high rates of loosening and material failure.

AUTHORS' PREFERRED METHOD

Selection of the proper treatment for intercondylar fractures requires careful consideration.[99,147] Each case must be individualized. In the young adult it

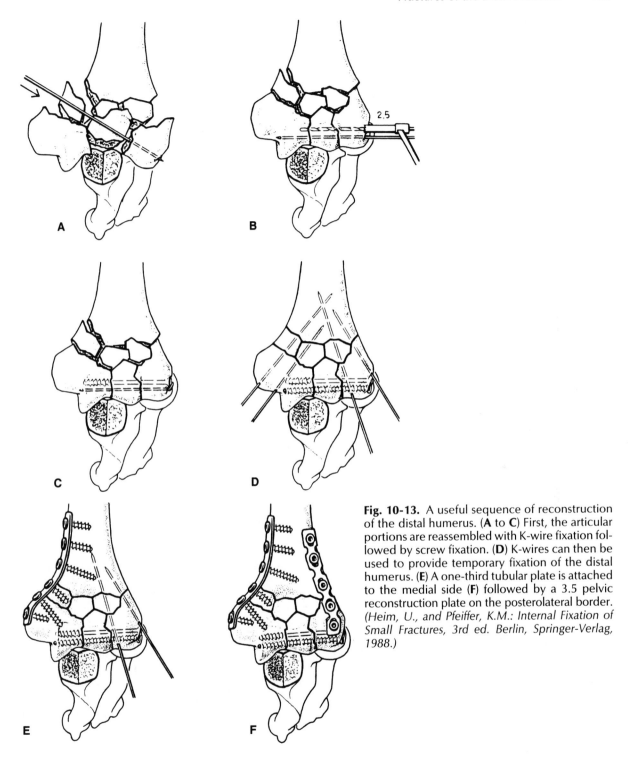

Fig. 10-13. A useful sequence of reconstruction of the distal humerus. (**A** to **C**) First, the articular portions are reassembled with K-wire fixation followed by screw fixation. (**D**) K-wires can then be used to provide temporary fixation of the distal humerus. (**E**) A one-third tubular plate is attached to the medial side (**F**) followed by a 3.5 pelvic reconstruction plate on the posterolateral border. *(Heim, U., and Pfeiffer, K.M.: Internal Fixation of Small Fractures, 3rd ed. Berlin, Springer-Verlag, 1988.)*

is important to obtain as near an anatomic reduction of the articular surface as possible. In the older patient with an excessively comminuted fracture in osteoporotic bone, fixation is often poor[99] or even impossible to achieve. In these patients early restoration of joint motion by nonoperative means is more important than restoration of articular congruity.[99,126,133] It must be emphasized that any method of treatment that requires prolonged immobilization is likely to result in fibrosis or ankylosis of the joint.[151] The final radiographic appearance does not always coincide with the functional result, especially in the elderly.[131]

Type I.   For undisplaced fractures of the distal humerus, we splint the elbow at 90° until swelling subsides. A long-arm cast can be applied, but since active motion is started between the second and third weeks after injury, a bivalved splint or clamshell Orthoplast splint can be used. It is helpful to warn the patient that occasionally displacement can occur. Extension, as with most other injuries of the elbow, is the slowest to return.

Types II and III.   For displaced, unstable fractures, we usually use open reduction with rigid internal fixation. Adequate exposure is essential for accurate reduction and implant placement. Although the transolecranon approach is recommended by the AO group, we prefer the Bryan approach (see Fig. 10-11) for exposure. As Bryan and Morrey[102] have pointed out, it is usually necessary to remove the proximal tip of the olecranon to improve access. Isolation and protection of the ulnar nerve are also important. If the fracture extends more proximally, it may be necessary to expose the radial nerve as well. It is helpful to warn the patient and the family preoperatively that retraction alone can cause temporary palsy of these nerves.

Before surgical reconstruction is done, it is helpful to remember some anatomic points regarding the distal humerus. When transcondylar fixation is obtained, the diameter of the trochlear sulcus is much smaller (approximately one half) than that of the medial trochlear ridge and the lateral condyle. The transfixation device must be centered exactly, or it may enter the articular surface.

The intercondylar fragments are assembled first using a combination of K-wires and small-fragment screws (Fig. 10-14). Loss of articular cartilage can be accepted, but incongruity cannot. As the AO group[122] has taught, lag screws across the condyles can be used only if there is no bone missing or comminution between them. Although a single

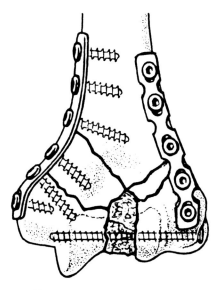

Fig. 10-14. If bone is missing in the intercondylar portion, a corticocancellous bone graft is interposed to reestablish the anatomic proportions. *(Heim, U., and Pfeiffer, K.M.: Internal Fixation of Small Fractures, 3rd ed. Berlin, Springer-Verlag, 1988.)*

screw across the condyles has potential to allow the fragments to rotate, once the condylar portions are securely fixed to the shaft with neutralization plates, this will not happen. The AO cannulated screw system can be especially useful in assembling the distal humerus. Fractures judged by x-ray to be type III without comminution may turn out to be type IV fractures requiring bone graft. We therefore prepare the patient for iliac bone grafting in most cases.

Once the intercondylar portion of the fracture is fixed, the supracondylar component is addressed. If there is adequate bone stock that allows interfragmentary compression of the condylar portion of the fracture to the humeral shaft, multiple lag screws can occasionally be used. The placement of these screws is crucial and must be within the centers of the supracondylar columns, engaging the opposite cortex as a lag screw. Inaccurate placement of these screws will decrease the size of the olecranon fossa, and the olecranon will not fit into the fossa, limiting elbow extension.

In most cases we prefer dual-plate fixation oriented at right angles to one another (see Fig. 10-13). A one-third tubular plate (five or six holes) is fixed to the medial column.[122] The posterolateral column is fixed with a 3.5 pelvic reconstruction plate (five or six holes). If there is any bone gap at the supracondylar junction from comminution, liberal amounts of cancellous bone graft should be added. For fractures with more proximal extension, longer plates can be used.

In reestablishment of condylar-shaft fixation, the epitrochlear ridges, which are often separate fragments, can serve as buttresses to the condyles.[132,158] Their continuity with the humeral metaphysis should be reestablished before the condyles can be stabilized to the shaft.[132,158]

The outcome from this injury greatly depends on postoperative rehabilitation. The elbow is splinted, and active motion is started during the first week after operation. If the gains in extension begin to plateau in the first 6 weeks, it is sometimes useful to add dynamic splinting in the form of a turnbuckle splint, especially if extension is regained slowly.

Type IV. Fractures with excessive comminution in osteopenic bone should be treated with either traction or the bag of bones technique. The older the patient, the less benefit will be achieved from accurate anatomic reduction.

For younger patients, reconstruction of the articular surface can be attempted, as described previously. Bone grafting is usually required to reestablish the anatomic relationship between the condyles. Reconstruction of the type IV fracture requires great patience and skill, but despite the loss of articular cartilage in the trochlear portion, excellent function can be regained. If there is any question about the adequacy of fixation, we will use olecranon pin traction following open reduction.

FRACTURES OF THE HUMERAL CONDYLES

Anatomy and Classification

There appears to be some confusion about the nomenclature of the various anatomic structures of the distal humerus. Some standard anatomy texts[95,119,120] do not differentiate between medial and lateral condyles as separate entities. *Gray's Anatomy*[119] describes the distal end of the humerus as being basically a condyle with articular and nonarticular surfaces. The articular portion is divided into two areas, the capitulum and the trochlea (Fig. 10-15). (We use the term *capitellum* instead of *capitulum* because it is more common in the orthopaedic literature. In our discussion we hope to demonstrate that the terms *capitellum* and *lateral condyle* are not synonymous. The same is true for the terms *trochlea* and *medial condyle*.)

In the discussion of fractures, separation of the distal humerus into medial and lateral condyles is widely accepted.[137,191] The capitulotrochlear sulcus is the terminal dividing point for these condyles.[137] Each condyle contains an articular and a nonarticular portion. The epicondyle is considered part of the nonarticular portion. The articulating portion of the lateral condyle is called the capitellum (capitulu rotuli humeri, eminentia capitata). The articular surface of the medial condyle is called the trochlea. It must be appreciated at this point that fractures of the condyles do not always follow these anatomic boundaries. For example, in a fracture of the lateral condyle or capitellum, a portion of the trochlea is often involved.[191]

During growth there are four separate ossification centers in the distal humerus.[119] The ossification center in the lateral condyle appears during the first year. It forms the bulk of the lateral condyle and a portion of the bone underlying the lateral aspect of the trochlea. The ossification of the medial condyle does not appear until the ninth or tenth year. The epicondyles also have separate ossification centers. The lateral epicondyle center appears at about 12 years and fuses 1 or 2 years later with the main lateral condylar center. The center for the medial epicondyle appears at about 4 to 6 years. Fusion with the main condylar segment does not occur until about the 20th year. In rare instances fusion never occurs.[183] These separate ossification centers have considerable significance in the discussion of fractures of the distal humerus in children. In adults, however, there does not appear to be any residuum in the trabecular pattern within the distal humerus from these separate ossification centers. Thus, it would appear that in adults fractures of the distal humerus depend on the external contour of the bone and the forces applied rather than on intrinsic weakness due to physeal lines.

Distinction between the condyles and their various portions is important in the diagnosis and treatment of these fractures. We shall stipulate that the fracture of the condyle includes separation of both the articular and nonarticular portions, including the epicondyle. There can be isolated fractures of either the articular portion or the epicondylar portion of the condyle. In this instance the remainder of the condyle is still attached to the shaft and to the opposite condyle.

This distinction has practical significance, and some generalities can be made. Fracture of the articular portion alone results in loss of motion, but stability of the elbow by and large remains.[182,183] The fracture fragment is not influenced by muscle

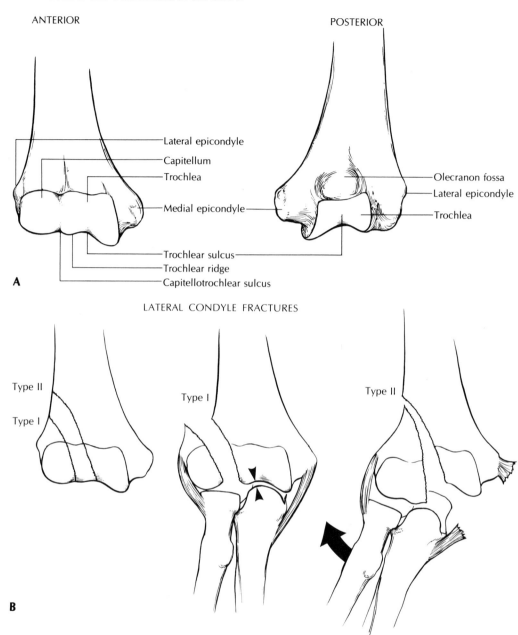

forces. Swelling is minimal because the hematoma is usually restricted by the joint capsule.[191] Fractures of the epicondyles in adults result in local tenderness. There may be some instability. The fracture fragment can also be displaced by muscle forces. Fracture of the entire condyle results in both restriction of motion and instability.[185] There is usually considerable swelling. Fracture of the articular surface alone may be treated by simple excision of the fragment. Fracture of the condyle requires anatomic reduction to restore free motion and fixation to ensure stability.[185,191]

Mechanism of Injury

Several external forces act on the distal humerus.[185] Avulsion forces are usually applied through tension on the collateral ligaments. The tension forces on these collateral ligaments can be increased by lev-

MEDIAL CONDYLE FRACTURES

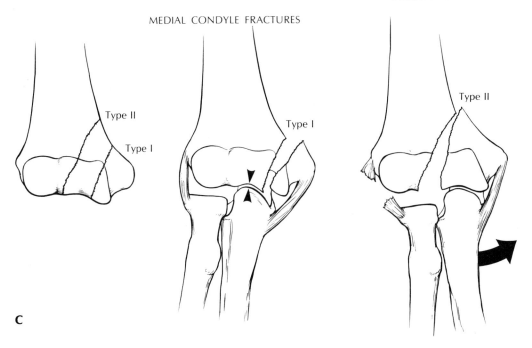

C

Fig. 10-15. Classification of condylar fractures according to Milch[12] and the location of the common fracture lines seen in type I and II fractures of the lateral (**B**) and medial (**C**) condyles. (**A**) Anterior view of the anatomy of the distal articular surface of the humerus. The capitellotrochlear sulcus divides the capitellar and trochlear articular surfaces. The lateral trochlear ridge is the key to analyzing humeral condyle fractures. In type I fractures, the lateral trochlear ridge remains with the intact condyle, providing medial to lateral elbow stability. In type II fractures, the lateral trochlear ridge is a part of the fractured condyle, which may allow the radius and ulna to translocate in a medial to lateral direction with respect to the long axis of the humerus. (**B**) Fractures of the lateral condyle. In type I fractures, the lateral trochlear ridge remains intact, therefore preventing dislocation of the radius and ulna. In type II fractures, the lateral trochlear ridge is a part of the fractured lateral condyle. With capsuloligamentous disruption *medially,* the radius and ulna may dislocate. (**C**) Fractures of the medial condyle. In type I fractures, the lateral trochlear ridge remains intact to provide medial to lateral stability of the radius and ulna. In type II fractures, the lateral trochlear ridge is a part of the fractured medial condyle. With *lateral* capsuloligamentous disruption, the radius and ulna may dislocate medially on the humerus.

erage through the forearm with the elbow in extension. Abduction or adduction of the extended forearm concentrates these forces to one side of the distal humerus. In addition, compressive forces can be applied to the articular surface. These forces may be indirect, being transmitted axially through the radius or ulna from forces applied to the distal portion of the extremity. There are specific areas of the articular surface where greater concentration of force can occur (eg, by the wedge-shaped articular portion of the ulna against the groove of the trochlea or by the rim of the radial head in the capitulotrochlear sulcus). Abduction or adduction of the forearm in extension can further concentrate the force in a given area. Direct forces can be applied

to the elbow as well. This usually occurs on the posterior aspect of the flexed elbow. In this position the lateral condyle is more exposed on the lateral side, while medially the epicondyle is more vulnerable to injury from a direct force. Forces applied directly to the posterior border of the proximal ulna are concentrated in the trochlear groove. If force is applied centrally, both condyles may be wedged apart, producing an intercondylar fracture. If the force is applied eccentrically, fracture of an isolated condyle is produced.[108] Rarely are the forces applied during an injury pure. They are often mixed, resulting in a variety of fracture patterns.

Milch[137] emphasized the importance of differentiating isolated fractures of the humeral condyles from condylar fractures associated with dislocation of the elbow. He pointed out the importance of the lateral trochlear ridge in providing stability of the elbow after fracture of a single condyle. He divided fractures of either condyle into two classes, based on the preservation or loss of the integrity of this ridge. Type I fractures are simple fractures. In this type of fracture the lateral trochlear ridge remains with the intact condyle. Thus, the medial-lateral stability refers to the medial-lateral translocation of the ulna with respect to the distal humerus. Varus or valgus instability secondary to associated contralateral ligament and joint capsule disruption can be present in a type I fracture.[182] Displacement of the fractured condyle can be proximal or distal, depending on the type of injury involved. In the type II fracture the lateral trochlear ridge is a part of the fractured condyle. This allows the radius and ulna to translocate in a medial-lateral direction with respect to the long axis of the humerus if the contralateral collateral ligament and joint capsule are torn.[131,137,191] Therefore, the type II fracture is called a fracture–dislocation. This classification has therapeutic application. Some type I fractures can be treated by closed methods. All type II fractures require open reduction and internal fixation.[137]

Incidence

Fractures of the humeral condyles or their components are uncommon in adults.[148,179,181,183,189] In Knight's series,[186] fractures of a single condyle accounted for only about 5% of fractures of the distal humerus in adults. Fracture of the lateral condyle is more common than fracture of the medial condyle.[181,191] Bryan[179] emphasized the frequent association of humeral condyle fractures with other injuries, such as fractures of both bones of the forearm, which must be considered in planning treatment.

Fractures of the Lateral Condyle

SIGNS AND SYMPTOMS

Fracture of the lateral condyle is recognized by the presence of independent motion of the lateral condyle from the medial condyle and humeral shaft. The condyle may be proximal or distal to the main portion of the humerus, depending on the type of force that created the fracture. As the arm hangs at the side, the carrying angle may be lost.[192] Crepitus usually is present. Radial rotation may accentuate the crepitus.[183] Although intercondylar distance may be widened, the arm does not appear shortened as in intercondylar fractures. Medial el-

bow swelling and tenderness are present in patients with associated medial collateral ligament injury.

RADIOGRAPHIC FINDINGS

The fracture line extends obliquely from either the capitulotrochlear sulcus or the lateral border of the trochlear groove up to the supracondylar ridge. Depending on the type of fracture, there may be lateral translocation of the ulna with respect to the shaft of the humerus. Displacement of the fragment by the action of extensor muscle origin is often present.[179] Lateral condylar fractures must be differentiated from fractures of the capitellum. A fracture of the lateral condyle has both articular and nonarticular components (Fig. 10-16). A fracture of the capitellum involves only the articular surface and its supporting bone. Smith[191] emphasized, however, that in some patients fracture of the lateral condyle is associated with a fracture of the capitellum, the two being separate fragments.

METHODS OF TREATMENT

Nonoperative Treatment. Lateral condyle fractures may be undisplaced or only minimally displaced. These usually can be treated by simple immobilization until stable.[137] Occasionally, percutaneous pinning of such nondisplaced fractures allows earlier institution of elbow motion.[179] Although some authors[192] believe that closed reduction is seldom successful, Conwell and Reynolds[181] described a method of closed reduction for displaced fractures. With the elbow extended and the forearm supinated, manual pressure is applied directly over the fragment for reduction. Adduction of the forearm opens up the lateral aspect of the joint to facilitate the reduction.[178] Anatomic reduction of the condyle is essential, since any displacement interferes with elbow motion.[137] The supinated forearm is then gradually flexed at the elbow. A long-arm cast is applied with lateral molding. There is some question on which position provides maximum stability after reduction. On the basis of the precedents set by Jones, Smith, and Lund, Cotton[182] believed that the best stability was achieved by the splinting effect of the triceps tendon in acute flexion. Milch believed that these fractures are more stable in extension.[137] In extension the olecranon is locked into its opposing fossa of the humerus, which affords medial-lateral stability.[183] Although this position may be tolerated for a brief period by a child, it can result in considerable disability in the adult.[182] We prefer to immobilize these fractures in flexion with the forearm supinated and

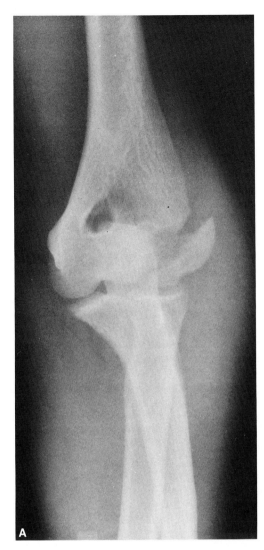

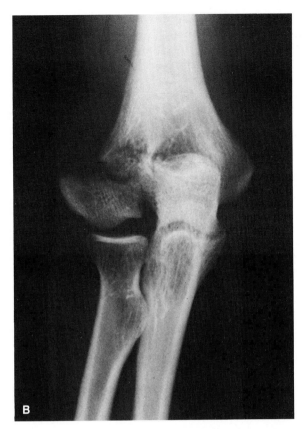

Fig. 10-16. (**A**) This type I fracture of the lateral condyle involves both the articular surface of the capitellum and the nonarticular surface, including the lateral epicondyle. The distal portion of the fracture line emerges just lateral to the capitulotrochlear sulcus. (**B**) Anteroposterior x-ray of a type II fracture of the lateral condyle that involves both the articular surface of the capitellum and the nonarticular surface of the lateral condyle. The distal portion of the fracture line emerges medial to the capitellotrochlear sulcus.

the wrist dorsiflexed slightly to relieve extensor muscle forces on the fragment.

Operative Treatment. The goals of operative intervention appear to be twofold. First, condylar alignment must be reestablished so that the axes of rotation of the condyles are the same.[186] Second, in the type II fracture the integrity of the lateral trochlear wall must be reestablished. Surgery is best performed as soon after the injury as possible.[189] Either the posterior or lateral approach may be used.[178,189] Fixation is usually achieved with screws.[137,180] Care must be taken to preserve the soft tissue attachments to the condylar fragment to protect its vascularity.[137] Smith[191] recommended

repairing the medial collateral ligament, if it is torn, through a separate medial approach. We reserve medial collateral ligament repair for the younger patient engaged in heavy labor when joint stability is not restored by reduction and internal fixation of the lateral condyle.

Complications and Prognosis. The result depends on the degree of comminution of the condyle, accuracy of reduction, and stability of internal fixation. Stable anatomic reduction and early motion help prevent traumatic arthritis and limitation of joint motion.[137,191] Improper reduction or loss of fixation in a type I fracture can lead to cubitus valgus. In a type II fracture this can lead to cubitus valgus and lateral subluxation of the ulna, especially if an associated fracture of the capitellum was removed.[191] This results in a greater deformity because the prominence of the medial condyle is accentuated. No matter what the cause, cubitus valgus may lead to ulnar nerve symptoms, which may require nerve transposition later.[191]

Fractures of the Medial Condyle

Isolated fracture of the medial condyle is a rare injury in the adult.[108,118,178,182,183,191,193] It is noted much less frequently than the lateral condyle fracture, probably because direct blows to the medial side of the elbow more often fracture the prominent medial epicondyle than the deeper medial condyle.[108,144,180,189,191,193]

The mechanism of injury is thought to be either a fall on the outstretched arm with the elbow forced into varus[118] or a fall on the apex of the flexed elbow.[108,181,183,193] The action of the flexor muscles of the forearm tends to displace the fracture distally.[108] Generally, the fracture originates at the depth of the trochlear groove and ascends obliquely to end at the supracondylar ridge. If the primary wedging force on the articular surface is applied by the rim of the head of the radius, then the fracture may originate in the capitulotrochlear sulcus, producing a type II injury. Because it usually involves the trochlear groove, fracture of this condyle may have more disability associated with it.

SIGNS AND SYMPTOMS

Motion of the entire condyle occurs when the medial epicondyle is manipulated. If the radial head is displaced medially with the ulnar and medial condyle fragment, there may be an apparent increased prominence of the lateral condyle and capitellum. Extension of the elbow tends to produce motion of the fragment owing to increased tension on the origin of the forearm flexor muscles.

Signs of ulnar nerve injury or irritation may be present.[137] Lateral joint tenderness and swelling are present in patients with associated injury to the lateral collateral ligament.

METHODS OF TREATMENT

Nonoperative Treatment. In undisplaced fractures, satisfactory treatment can be achieved with a posterior splint. Aspiration of the joint to relieve the hemarthrosis will improve patient comfort.[191] The elbow is flexed and the forearm is pronated with some wrist flexion to relax the muscles that originate on the medial epicondyle.[181,191] Closed reduction of displaced fractures is difficult to achieve

and maintain.[191] X-rays must be taken at frequent intervals to ensure that late displacement of the fragment does not occur.

Operative Treatment. Although some displaced fractures can be reduced closed, it is virtually impossible to maintain a reduction that will prevent a step-off in the articular surface. We prefer anatomic restoration of the articular surface by open reduction and internal fixation (Fig. 10-17). Our goal is to restore joint congruity with stable internal fixation that allows early institution of joint motion.[191] When the fragment is approached, the ulnar nerve must be carefully exposed and protected. Conwell and Reynolds[181] recommended anterior transposition of the nerve if the ulnar groove is involved in the fracture or if the nerve is injured. Firm fixation may be difficult to obtain. The medial supracondylar column is long and narrow. Placement of screws up this column or through the narrow central portion of the trochlear groove may be difficult. Also, it is more difficult to obtain initial purchase of the screws on the pointed medial epicondyle than on the flattened surface of the lateral condyle.

Repair of the lateral collateral ligament is considered only if joint stability is not restored by reduction and fixation of the displaced condyle. Even in this situation, consideration of the patient's age and occupation is critical because repair of the collateral ligament may result in loss of joint motion secondary to scarring. If the fixation is not solid after operation, the extremity should be immobilized as with closed reduction (ie, with the elbow and wrist flexed and the forearm pronated).

COMPLICATIONS AND PROGNOSIS

Because of involvement of the trochlear groove, there is more chance for residual incongruity of critical articular surfaces. This increases the risk of posttraumatic arthritis. In addition, residual displacement of the medial condyle can restrict joint motion.[191] Malunion with the condyle displaced proximally results in cubitus varus.[137] Tardy ulnar nerve symptoms may arise secondary to malunion or excess callus formation.[186]

FRACTURES OF THE ARTICULAR SURFACE OF THE DISTAL HUMERUS

Fractures of the distal humeral articular surface include fractures of the capitellum or trochlea, or both. These fracture lines occur in the coronal plane, parallel to the anterior surface of the hu-

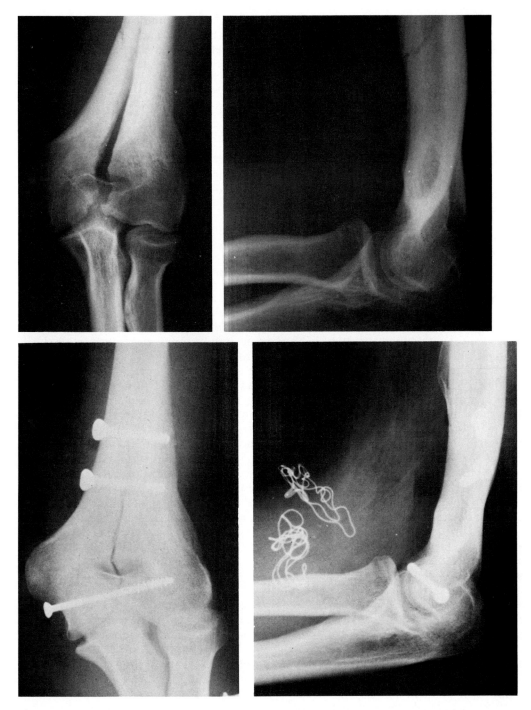

Fig. 10-17. (*Top*) Anteroposterior and lateral x-rays of a fracture of the medial condyle. (*Bottom*) Open reduction and stable internal fixation of the type I medial condyle fracture to allow early range of motion.

merus.[211–213] The fracture fragments therefore consist of the articular surfaces of the capitellum and trochlea with little or no soft tissue attachment.[231]

Compressive wedging or shearing forces are usually involved in producing these fractures. Because of the lack of soft tissue attachment, avulsion forces do not play a role in the production of these fractures.[244] The initial displacement is produced by the causative force. However, further displacement can occur because the fragment has no soft tissue attachments and lies free within the joint cavity.[204,231,244,248]

The fracture fragments consist primarily of articular cartilage with varying amounts of associated subchondral bone.[236,244] Although we will consider fractures of the capitellum and trochlea as separate entities for the purpose of discussion, often both articular surfaces are actually involved.

FRACTURES OF THE CAPITELLUM

Although the first case was described by Hahn in 1853,[224,227] Kocher is credited with calling attention to this fracture in his classic monograph *Fractura Rotuli Humeri*.[203,224,226,231] Thus, fractures of the capitellum are often called Kocher fractures.[241] Fractures of the capitellum are rare. The incidence of this fracture in the numerous series reported in the literature[199,202,209,235,240,248] varies from 0.5% to 1% of all elbow injuries seen.

Both Kocher and Lorenz recognized two types of fractures of the capitellum[224,228] (Fig. 10-18). The type I or Hahn–Steinthal[215,246] type involves a large part of the osseous portion of the capitellum and may contain part of the adjacent lip of the trochlea.[194,196,213,221,225,227,231] The type II or Kocher–Lorenz[224,228] type involves articular cartilage with very little bone attached.[214] Mouchet has described type II fractures as an "uncapping of the condyle."[214,234,236] Type II fractures are reported much less frequently than type I.[212,213,220] Wilson[248] described a third type in which the articular surface is driven proximally and impacted into the osseous portion.

Johansson[219] reported rupture of the ulnar collateral ligament in 8 of 13 cases of capitellar fracture. Collert[201] suggested that restricted mobility following capitellar fracture partly depends on such associated capsular and ligamentous injury.

Emphasis must again be placed on the differentiation between fractures of the capitellum and lateral condyle.[212] A fracture of the capitellum involves only the intra-articular portion of the lateral con-

dyle and does not include the epicondyle or metaphysis. A fracture of the lateral condyle involves the capitellum plus the nonarticular portion, which often includes the epicondyle.[147,212]

ANATOMIC CONSIDERATIONS

The capitellum presents an anterior and inferior articular surface but does not extend posteriorly.[194] The radial head articulates with the anterior surface when the elbow is flexed and with the inferior surface in extension. The radial fossa, a depression on the anterior humerus just above the capitellum, accommodates the margin of the radial head when the elbow is actively flexed. The radial fossa must be cleared of all fracture fragments for the elbow to regain a full range of flexion.

MECHANISM OF INJURY

This fracture is usually produced by the transmission of forces through the radial head, which acts like a piston to shear off the capitellum.[194,221,248] Thus, some authors use the term *anterior shear fracture of the capitellum*.[195,213,224,226,245] This mechanism also helps to explain the occasional association of radial head fractures.[222,226,248]

The mechanism most commonly results when one tries to break a fall and lands on the hand with the elbow in some degree of flexion or falls directly on the elbow in a position of full flexion.[201,214,247]

Bryan[197] suggested that type I fractures result from a force passing from the radius to the humerus in extension, thereby shearing off the capitellum anteriorly, or from a direct lateral blow in flexion. Type II fractures are the result of shearing forces across the joint in varying degrees of flexion.[197]

Milch[233] believed that the location of the fragment gives a clue to the position of the elbow when injured. If the elbow is in extension, the anterior surface of the capitellum is sheared off and the fragment is displaced anteriorly. Injury with the elbow flexed results in the fragment lying in the posterior aspect of the joint. Kocher originally suggested that in the type I fracture the anterior capsule avulsed the fragment when the elbow was forced into hyperextension.[211,226] There are no recent supporters of this mechanism. Because the lateral surface of the capitellum is exposed when the elbow is in a position of semiflexion and semipronation, some authors believe that type I injuries can result from a direct blow to this area.[211,226]

In some instances, especially in the type I fracture, a portion of the lateral trochlear ridge may be

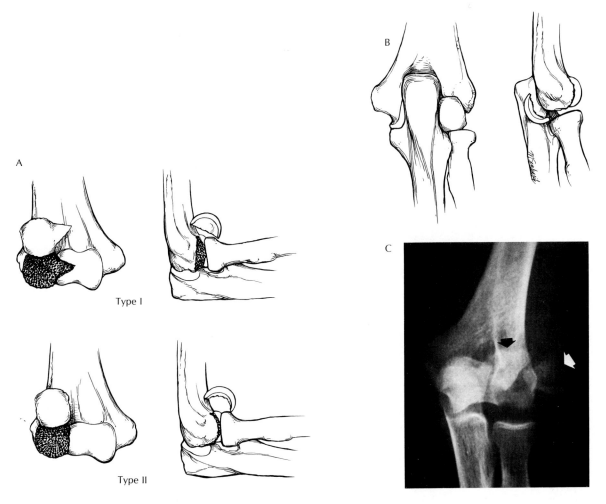

Fig. 10-18. (**A**) The type I (Hahn-Steinthal) capitellar fracture. A portion of the trochlea may be involved in this fracture. The type II (Kocher-Lorenz) capitellar fracture. Very little subchondral bone is attached to the capitellar fragment. There is no fracture through the lateral condyle in the *sagittal* plane in either the type I or II capitellar fracture. (**B**) Although most often the capitellar fragment is displaced anteriorly, occasionally the fracture fragment may be displaced posteriorly. In this instance, an obstruction to extension is noted on physical examination. (**C**) The anteroposterior x-ray is often useful in demonstrating the degree of trochlear involvement. The *arrows* point to two fragments off the capitellotrochlear surface. This may be difficult to recognize on a lateral view.

included. Robertson and Bogart reported a fracture "en masse" of both articular surfaces.[240] This type of fracture may be confused with the Posadas type of transcondylar fracture, which extends through both condyles to their posterior borders. The fracture en masse, however, involves only articular surfaces (Fig. 10-19).

The preponderance of women in most series of capitellar fractures led Grantham and colleagues[214] to suggest a biomechanical-anatomic vulnerability based on the valgus conformation of the female elbow or a metabolic susceptibility because of osteoporosis.

SIGNS AND SYMPTOMS

There is a fair amount of consistency in the reported clinical findings. Since most of the acute symptoms are due to the distention of the joint with blood, there may be a silent interval between the time of

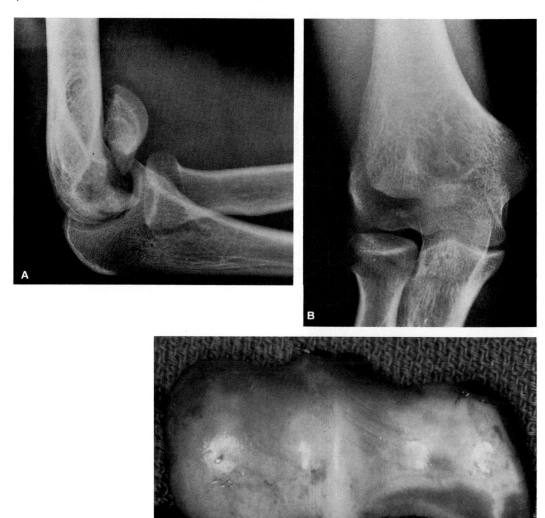

Fig. 10-19. (A to C) A completely displaced and detached intra-articular fracture of the distal humerus of both the capitellum and trochlea.

(continued)

injury and the development of symptoms.[236] Anterior displacement of the fragment results in its impingement on the radial or coronoid fossa, producing a bony block.[205] With posteriorly placed fragments there is no bony block, only pain with flexion as the fragment is forced against the capsule.[203,226]

Range of motion of the elbow is usually limited.[194,212,213,220,224,233] Alvarez and colleagues[194] found that type I fractures result in a mechanical block to flexion, whereas type II fractures usually

demonstrate a block to extension. Pronation and supination are characteristically not limited by this injury.[211,213,220,224,233,247]

Crepitus may be present. Often, the fragments can be palpated anterior to the radial head when the elbow is extended. Since the external bony landmarks maintain their normal relationship, the clinical findings often do not correlate with the acute disability displayed with fracture of the capitellum.[231] Even though concomitant fractures of both the radial head and capitellum are rare, they

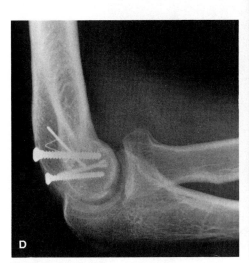
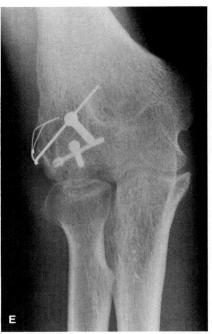

Fig. 10-19 (continued)
(**D, E**) One year after open reduction and internal fixation, there is no sign of ischemic necrosis or collapse.

do occur (Fig. 10-20). Milch[233] emphasized that dual tenderness on the lateral side of the elbow may be an important sign of fractures in both areas.

Tenderness and swelling medially, with or without valgus instability, indicate associated ulnar collateral ligament injury.[201,219,222]

RADIOGRAPHIC FINDINGS

Since the fracture fragments consist largely of cartilage, x-rays do not reveal their true size.[195] The anteroposterior view is often misleading because the outline of the distal humerus is unaffected, and the fracture fragment may not be recognized against the background of the distal humerus.[194] Gejrot[213] and Jopson[220] emphasized, however, that the anteroposterior view is useful in demonstrating the degree of associated trochlear involvement.

Lindem[227] pointed out that the radiographic signs are best appreciated on the lateral x-ray. However, if the lateral x-ray is even slightly oblique, the fragment will be hidden by the humerus and the diagnosis may be missed.[212] The fragment most commonly lies anterior and proximal to the main portion of the capitellum.[231] The articular surface usually faces anteriorly. There may be a lack of the normal cortical margin in the area of the defect on the surface of the capitellum. If the defect is seen

later, there may be union of the fragment with the humerus in the area of the radial fossa. It must be remembered that occasionally the fragment may be displaced posteriorly as reported by Kocher and Lorenz.[215,224,228,231,233] The rare instances of dorsal fractures of both the radial head and the capitellum must always be kept in mind.[233,238] In all fractures of the capitellum the radial head must be carefully evaluated, clinically and radiographically. This is especially important when closed reduction is to be used, with pressure from the radial head to secure the fragment. The opposite is also true; that is, in evaluation of an isolated radial head fracture, the capitellum should be checked carefully for the presence of a fracture as well.[238] In Milch's[233] experience, fracture fragments from a comminuted radial head are rarely displaced in a proximal direction. Thus, if a large fragment is seen in the joint anterior and proximal to the radial head, it should be suspected to have originated from the capitellum rather than from the comminuted radial head.

METHODS OF TREATMENT

There is considerable controversy regarding the appropriate treatment of capitellar fracture. Methods available include nonoperative treatment (with and without closed reduction),[200,213,221,222,231,236,244] open

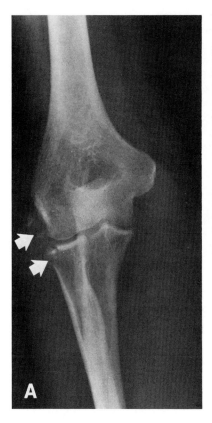

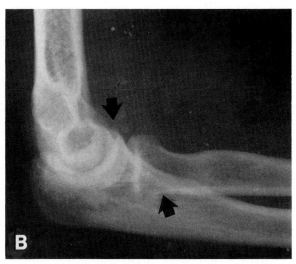

Fig. 10-20. Concomitant fractures of the capitellum and radial head. This injury, sustained by a direct blow, shows fractures of both the capitellum and radial head (*arrows*): (**A**) anteroposterior and (**B**) lateral x-rays. The fragments from the capitellum (*upper arrow*) characteristically lie in the anterior aspect of the joint proximal to the radial head.

reduction (with[206,211,245] and without[213,221] internal fixation), excision,[212,213,220,226,235] and prosthetic arthroplasty.[218] Union of capitellar fractures has been reported following both closed and open reduction even though the capitellar fragment has little soft tissue attachment and vascularity.[230] If reduction (by either closed or open means) is selected, it must be anatomic, since even the slightest displacement is believed to interfere with joint motion.[191,197] Additionally, irrespective of the type of treatment used, supervision of the after-care is essential if a good result is to be expected.

Nonoperative Treatment. Smith[191] recommended nonoperative treatment in a posterior splint for 3 weeks for nondisplaced fractures only. He did not recommend closed reduction of displaced fractures in adults but suggested that such treatment in children and young adults might be efficacious because of more rapid and complete bone healing in these patients.[191] Several authors have emphasized that the lack of soft tissue attachment to the displaced fragment makes closed reduction difficult to achieve and maintain.[194,212,213,244] Because even the slightest

residual displacement will limit the elbow function,[196,212,213] Bryan[197] also believed that the usefulness of closed reduction is limited. Other authors, however, strongly endorse closed reduction.[222] Kleiger and Joseph[222] and Rhodin[236] emphasized that if closed reduction is achieved, excellent results can be anticipated. These authors reserve open reduction for those patients in whom closed reduction fails. The type I injury is most amenable to closed reduction. Reduction must be very accurate, because the smallest amount of displacement can restrict motion of the radiohumeral joint. Most surgeons prefer to manipulate the fracture with the elbow extended.[196,200,203,207,222,236,240] Traction is applied to the forearm with the elbow extended.[200] Pressure is then placed directly over the fracture fragment to effect reduction.[200] Placing a varus stress on the forearm opens the lateral side of the elbow and facilitates replacement of the fracture fragment. Once reduction is accomplished, it is maintained by holding the elbow flexed. The fragment is held in place by the head of the radius. Although Kleiger and Joseph[222] emphasized the need for immobilization in maximum elbow flexion to maintain reduction, Rhodin[236] warned that flexion must be decreased in patients with severe associated swelling to avoid ischemic contracture. Pronation of the forearm seems to secure the radial fixation of the fragment. The ability of the radius to hold the fragment in place has been confirmed at the time of open reduction by Rhodin and Darrach.[206,236] The elbow should be immobilized for 4 to 6 weeks after the reduction.[196,205,222,244]

Operative Treatment.   Open reduction and internal fixation can be very difficult, and unless stable fixation is achieved, excision should be considered.[213] Even with early postoperative motion, partial or complete joint ankylosis may occur despite an anatomic reduction.[198] The surgical approach used for open reduction or excision is posterolateral.[198,220,229,236] In the type I fracture in which an inadequate closed reduction is obtained or there is marked comminution of the fragment, surgical intervention must be performed.

Keon-Cohen[221] found that once an open reduction is obtained, the fragment may be stable and can thus be held in place with the opposing radial head, similar to a closed reduction. Others[198,223,229,245] fix the fragment with a screw. The screw is usually inserted from the posterior aspect of the condyle. The tip engages the bony portion of the fragment, securing it to the condyle. The articular cartilage is therefore not penetrated. Bryan[197] and MacAusland and Wyman[229] suggested fixation with Kirschner wires buried beneath the articular surface. These can be removed later from the posterior aspect of the arm without the joint being reentered.[197] These authors emphasized that early motion (2 to 3 weeks after fracture) is needed and that the radial fossa must be free of all fracture debris to ensure a good result. Collert[201] reported excellent results in 7 of 20 patients treated with internal fixation and open reduction. In the remaining patients, he excised the fragment or simply performed the open reduction without internal fixation. Even when the fracture fragment was devoid of all soft tissue attachment, no avascular necrosis was evident by x-ray.

Simpson and Richards[242] used two Herbert screws in one patient, with a good result. Richards and associates[237] also reported good results using this device in four patients. The advantage of this implant is that the proximal screw head can be countersunk beneath the articular surface.

If the capitellar fragment is comminuted or has little subchondral bone for fixation, excision may be a better alternative.[209,235,244] Smith noted that functional recovery after excision and early motion is superior to that after either closed or open reduction of displaced fractures.[244] He recommended excision early rather than four to five days after injury when hemorrhage and exudate have begun to organize. Splinting is for only 2 to 3 days postoperatively, after which exercise and range of motion are instituted. He specifically noted that proximal migration of the radius with distal radioulnar disconformity is unusual.[244]

Alvarez and colleagues[194] advocated primary excision based on experience with 14 patients. However, only one patient in their series was treated with internal fixation (using K-wires), and only two patients were followed for more than 2 years.

Wilson[248] and MacAusland and Wyman[229] mentioned the association of capitellar fractures with other fractures of the elbow and with dislocation of the joint. In these instances, care should be taken to avoid excision lest the stability of the entire elbow joint be compromised.[229]

A difficult problem in management arises when there are multiple fragments involving both articular surfaces. Additionally, associated fractures of the true lateral condyle may be present.[240,248] Smith[244] believed that the articular fragments (capitellum) should be removed and the associated condylar fractures fixed internally. In his opinion, the lateral instability that is present has not led to ulnar nerve problems or disability. Attempting to replace such multiple fragments necessitates extensive dissection and prolonged postoperative immobilization that may combine to result in ankylosis.[195] On the other hand, simple excision allows early motion and less morbidity.[218,225] Anderson[195] used the epicondyles as the point for deciding on retention or excision of the fragments.

Jakobsson[218] reconstructed the humeral articular surface with an alloy prosthesis in an effort to avoid avascular necrosis of the capitellar fragment and to maintain elbow stability. This approach required two surgical procedures and has not gained popularity.

When both the radial head and capitellum are fractured, MacAusland and Wyman[229] recommended reduction and fixation of the capitellum and excision of the radial head. They warned against fixation of the radial head with excision of the capitellum. They also emphasized that in no instance should both fractures be excised.

In the late diagnosed and unreduced capitellar fracture, the displaced fragment may block flexion. In these cases, excision is the treatment of choice,[195,196,207,221,244] with improvement in flexion noted even when excision is delayed for up to 6 months.[226,227,246]

Avascular Necrosis.   Unlike with the femoral head, complete separation of the capitellum from its blood supply does not usually lead to collapse and arthrosis. Several series have documented healing of the capitellar fragment without collapse, despite its being completely separated from soft tissue at the time of surgery.[201,214,222,225,237,242,245] Even when avascular necrosis is evident on x-ray, the function of the elbow may not be impaired.[222,225]

Presumably, revascularization of the subchondral bone occurs with creeping substitution, but load across the radiocapitellar joint is insufficient during this period to cause collapse and disconformity, as commonly seen in the hip. Therefore, the frightful appearance of the capitellar fragment, completely devoid of soft tissue attachment, should not discourage the surgeon from open reduction with internal fixation.

Authors' Preferred Method.   Fractures of the capitellum usually occur in the same manner as fractures of the radial head. Therefore, it is important to look for associated injuries of the radial head, wrist, and ligaments of the elbow. The lateral condyle of the distal humerus may also be fractured.

Undisplaced fractures of the capitellum are best treated with a posterior splint in approximately 90° of elbow flexion and neutral rotation. Gentle active-motion exercises, avoiding extremes of motion, can be started in as few as ten days. We concentrate first on forearm rotation but avoid full extension and full pronation, since Morrey and colleagues[17] have demonstrated that radiocapitellar force transmission is greatest in this position.

If there is any initial displacement of the fracture, then operative intervention will probably be necessary. In our experience, closed reduction is usually impossible and the reduction, if achieved, is difficult to maintain. In addition, the prolonged immobilization necessary to maintain the reduction may lead to disabling contracture.

For displaced fractures, the goal of operation is anatomic restoration of the articular surface with rigid fixation that permits elbow motion in the immediate postoperative period (see Fig. 10-19). If this cannot be achieved because of comminution or fragment size, then excision should be performed. Before operation, we inform the patient of both possibilities.

Adequate exposure of the fracture is necessary for reduction, since the fragment is often embedded in joint capsule and rotated 90°. Once reduction is achieved, temporary fixation with K-wires is used. Sometimes, the fragment carries a small but sufficient piece of lateral periarticular bone that permits fixation with standard AO (ASIF) screws from the mini-fragment set or the newer cannulated system. The Herbert screw can also be used, with insertion directly into the articular surface. Although insertion using the jig has been described, using the device "freehand" may be simpler. Even with careful technique, fragmentation can occur, necessitating excision.

Whether primary excision or open reduction is performed, active motion is begun within the first week. Even with an appropriately vigorous rehabilitation program, extension often returns slowly. After bony union is achieved, turnbuckle orthoses or dynamic splinting may improve extension.

FRACTURES OF THE TROCHLEA

Isolated fractures of the trochlea are extremely rare.[197,209,244,247] Stimson[247] credited the original description to Laugier in 1853, hence the term *Laugier's fracture*. Very few authors report having seen it as an isolated fracture.[209,216,239,244]

The very structure of the trochlea probably contributes to its rarity as an isolated injury. The capitellum is subject to shear and compressive forces from the head of the radius. It can also be fractured by a direct blow. The trochlea, on the other hand, is deep within the elbow joint and thus protected from direct injury.[197] The transmitted force of the ulna against the trochlea tends to produce more of a wedging action than a tangential shearing force.[197,244] Bryan[197] noted that the shearing forces that may produce a trochlear fracture can be generated in an elbow dislocation; hence, he warned of the association between these two entities.

When the surgeon makes the clinical diagnosis, the signs of effusion, pain, restriction of motion, and crepitus indicate that an intra-articular fracture is probably present. The one finding that should lead the surgeon to suspect a fracture of the trochlea is a fragment lying on the medial side of the joint just distal to the medial epicondyle.[244]

The fracture may extend from the trochlea into the distal portion of the epicondyle.[244] If the fragment is nondisplaced, Smith recommended a posterior splint for 3 weeks followed by exercises and soaks.[244] If the fracture is displaced, the joint should be opened. Large fragments should be replaced and fixed with either a screw or Kirschner wires.[209,244] If internal fixation is used, the elbow should be immobilized only 10 to 14 days before range of motion is begun. If the fragments are too small for fixation, excision and early motion are the treatment of choice.[209,244]

FRACTURES OF THE EPICONDYLES

Each epicondyle has its own ossification center.[258] This has special significance in children, because with tension on the collateral ligaments the point of weakness is at the epiphyseal growth plate rather than the ligaments. Thus, fractures of the epicondyles in children are usually epiphyseal separations most often caused by avulsion.[258,259,266] As primary isolated fractures in adults, they are uncommon.[197,259,266]

Fractures of the Lateral Epicondyle

Fracture of the lateral epicondyle is extremely rare. In fact, many authors have doubted that it even exists as an isolated fracture in adults.[259,267,268] The ossification center of the lateral epicondyle is small and appears in about the 12th year. After it fuses with the main portion of the lateral condyle at puberty, avulsion fractures are even rarer.[258] The lateral epicondyle is almost level with the flattened outer surface of the lateral condyle. Thus, it has only minimal exposure to a direct blow. The treatment involves simple immobilization until the pain subsides, then early motion, similar to the treatment for an undisplaced lateral condyle (Fig. 10-21).

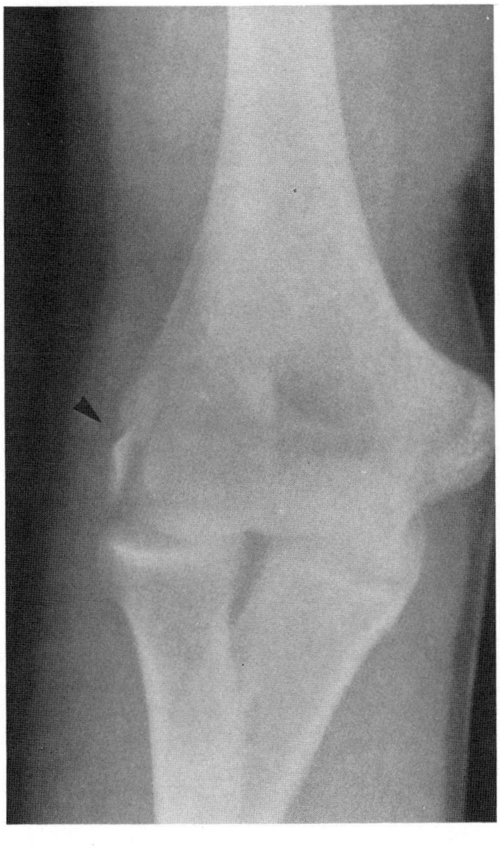

Fig. 10-21. Fracture of the lateral epicondyle (*arrow*) with a small portion of the capitellum as well.

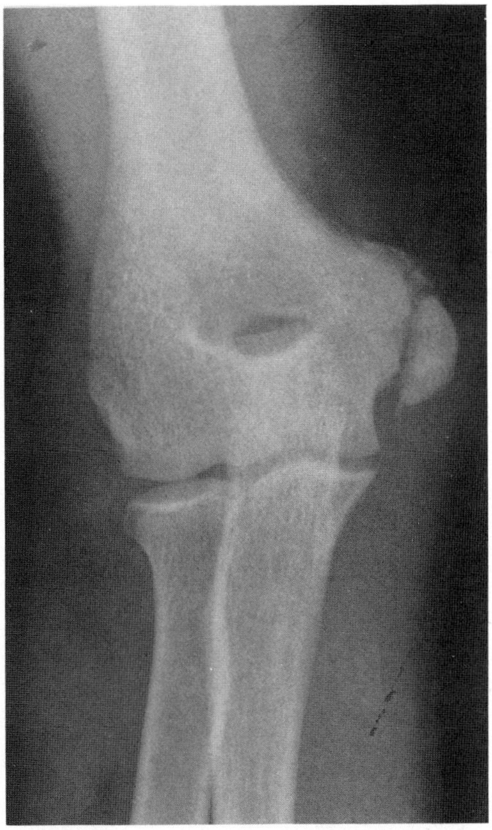

Fig. 10-22. This fracture of the medial epicondyle is relatively undisplaced. There is evidence of periosteal new bone formation proximally along the supracondylar ridge.

Fractures of the Medial Epicondyle

Fracture of the medial epicondyle or epitrochlea (Fig. 10-22) is more common than fracture of the lateral epicondyle.[258,266] Granger first reported fractures of the medial epicondyle in 1818.[253,258,267] In a series of ten cases, he outlined the pertinent anatomy, recognized the difficulty in regaining motion, and noted the favorable results following nonoperative treatment.[253]

Fusion of the ossification center of the medial epicondyle with the distal humerus does not occur until about the 20th year.[257] However, in some adults, fusion may never occur, setting the stage for avulsion fractures of the medial epicondyle in adulthood.[258]

MECHANISM OF INJURY

In the child and adolescent this fragment is commonly avulsed from the humerus during a posterior dislocation of the elbow[258,266] (Fig. 10-23). In many of these fractures associated with dislocations the

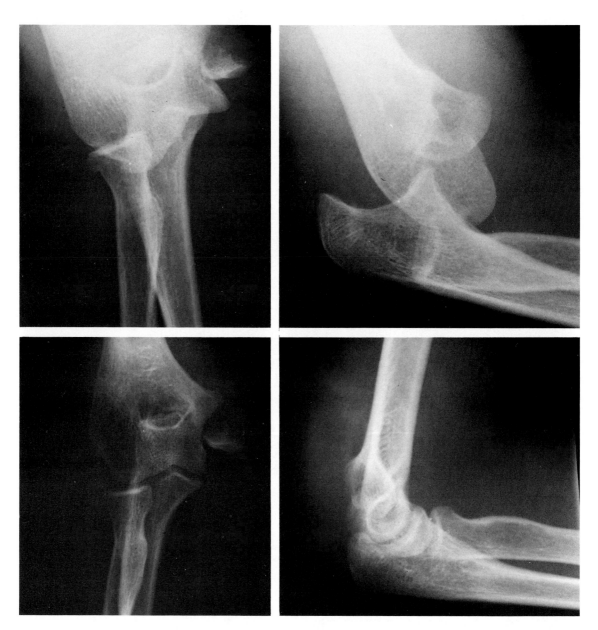

Fig. 10-23. (*Top*) A posterolateral dislocation of the elbow with avulsion of the medial epicondyle. (*Bottom*) Closed reduction of the elbow dislocation was successful, but the position of the medial epicondyle remained unchanged. The patient was managed with simple immobilization for ten days, followed by early range of motion. The patient currently has a full range of motion in the elbow, no ulnar nerve symptoms, and no elbow instability and does not complain of deformity about the joint.

epicondylar fragment may be carried into the joint and remain lodged there when the elbow is reduced[259] (Fig. 10-24). The ulnar nerve can also become trapped with this fragment. After the age of 20 it rarely occurs as a single fracture or associated with a dislocation.[259]

In a series of 143 patients with medial epicondyle fractures, Smith[266] found only two adults in whom the fracture was not associated with other fractures or dislocations of the elbow.

Because there is no residual of the old epiphyseal plate if fusion with the distal humerus occurs, avulsion forces are unlikely to cause this fracture in the adult. Fractures in the adult are not necessarily limited to the area originating from the medial epicondylar ossification center. They can extend into part of the main medial condylar mass as well.[258] These isolated fractures in the adult are most com-monly caused by a direct blow to the epicondyle.[258,259,266] Its prominence on the medial aspect of the elbow makes it especially vulnerable to this type of force.

SIGNS AND SYMPTOMS

In displaced fractures the fragment is usually pulled anterior and distal by the forearm flexor muscles.[253,258] Local tenderness and crepitus over the medial epicondyle are characteristic. Active flexion of the elbow and wrist along with pronation of the forearm will accentuate the pain.[266] Because of the ulnar nerve's proximity to the epicondyle, its function must be evaluated carefully.

RADIOGRAPHIC FINDINGS

There may be a tendency to confuse the normal radiolucent epiphyseal growth plate with an acute

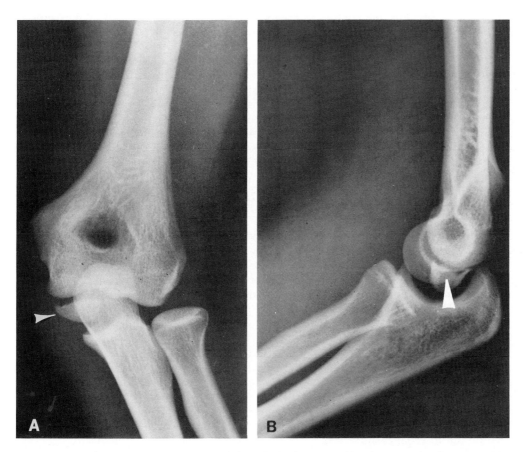

Fig. 10-24. Avulsion of the medial epicondyle with displacement into the joint. (**A**) The epicondyle (*arrow*) is lodged between the medial articular surface of the trochlea and ulna, inhibiting reduction. (**B**) Lateral view of the same patient demonstrating intra-articular location of the medial epicondyle (*arrow*).

fracture of the epicondyle in the adolescent patient. Comparison x-rays of the opposite elbow may be helpful.[253] In those cases in which the epicondylar fragment has been avulsed during a posterolateral dislocation, its presence within the joint must be ruled out.[265] Patrick[261] demonstrated a radiographic clue to its lodgement within the joint. With simple avulsion of the epicondyle, the fragment never migrates distally as far as the joint level. Thus, if the fragment is seen lying at the level of the joint, its intra-articular incarceration must be ruled out.

METHODS OF TREATMENT

General agreement exists on the proper method of treatment of either the minimally displaced fractures or those lodged within the joint.[255,256,259,265] In the minimally displaced fracture, the generally accepted method of treatment is short-term immobilization (seven to ten days) with the elbow and wrist flexed and the forearm pronated.[254] Likewise, those fragments lying within the joint that cannot be extracted by the closed methods advocated by Patrick[261] must be removed operatively.

There is a difference of opinion on the subject of moderately to severely displaced fragments. Three methods of treatment are available to the surgeon: (1) manipulation and short-term immobilization, (2) open reduction with internal fixation, and (3) excision of the fragment.

Smith[266,267] advocated nonoperative treatment with early motion in nearly all cases. In his extensive review of patients with this injury, he was unable to confirm the presence of any previously described disabilities resulting from persistent displacement of the fragment.[266] None of those with fibrous union had pain or disability. Distal displacement of the epicondyle did not result in loss of elbow function or weakness of the flexor-pronator muscles. Only 1 in the 116 patients in his series treated by nonoperative means had any delayed ulnar nerve problems. It was his conclusion that the results with either bony or fibrous union were the same.

Proponents of operative treatment cite the possibility of ulnar nerve symptoms,[254,259,260,266] instability of the elbow with valgus stress testing,[263] wrist flexor weakness, and nonunion of the displaced epicondyle as reason for primary reattachment or excision of the fragment.[259,260,265] Sisk's[265] indication for open reduction and internal fixation was displacement of greater than 1 cm. However, Bernstein and colleagues[253] and Wilson[269] found no patients with ulnar nerve symptoms or wrist flexor weakness when displaced fractures were treated

nonoperatively. In our hands, elbow instability has not been a problem in patients with medial epicondyle fractures associated with elbow dislocation when these injuries are managed nonoperatively. On the contrary, unless early motion is instituted, significant stiffness, not instability, will result.

Additionally, an interesting complication was reported by Roaf,[264] who described a case in which the median nerve had become trapped between the fracture fragments. With healing, two foramina were created through which the median nerve passed. With time and continued motion of the elbow the nerve became frayed at the distal foramen. Total disruption of the nerve resulted.

AUTHORS' PREFERRED METHOD OF TREATMENT

As in other elbow injuries, early resumption of motion is essential to recovery of elbow function. Thus, these fractures are treated by manipulation and immobilization with the forearm pronated and the elbow and wrist flexed in a posterior splint for 10 to 14 days. Active motion is then allowed.

The surgeon must remember that patients with medial epicondyle fractures, especially those associated with an elbow dislocation, may require up to 1 year to regain elbow motion. Should the displaced fragment be unsightly or painful, or if ulnar nerve problems develop, the fragment can be excised later with minimal operative morbidity. Treatment of the entrapped fragment is discussed under dislocation of the elbow (see page 791).

FRACTURES OF THE SUPRACONDYLAR PROCESS

The supracondylar (supracondyloid) process, a congenital variation of the distal end of the humerus, is a bony (or cartilaginous) projection that arises from the anteromedial surface of the humerus approximately 5 cm above the medial epicondyle (Fig. 10-25).[271-275] This process varies greatly in size from a small projection in the middle of a prominent ridge to an actual bony hook.[275] After arising from the anteromedial surface of the humerus, the process is directed downward, forward, and inward toward the medial epicondyle.[271,275] From the tip of the supracondylar process may extend a fibrous arch (which in rare cases may be ossified), the ligament of Struthers, which connects the supracondylar process with the medial epicondyle.[270,273,275] The upper fibers of the pronator teres and some of the lower fibers of the coracobrachialis may arise from the supracondylar process or the ligament of Struthers. Through this small arch formed by the

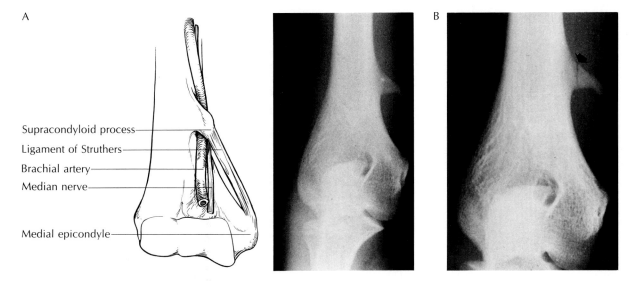

Fig. 10-25. **(A)** The supracondylar process arises from the anteromedial aspect of the distal humerus. It is connected to the medial epicondyle by the ligament of Struthers, which forms a fibro-osseous arch through which pass the median nerve and usually the brachial artery. **(B)** A nondisplaced fracture of a supracondylar process.

supracondylar process, the ligament of Struthers, and the medial epicondyle passes the median nerve and frequently the brachial artery.[270–275]

Fracture of this uncommon process is of clinical significance and bears discussion. The incidence of this process is very low, ranging from 0.6% to 2.7%.[270–274] Because of its long, thin structure and muscle attachments, it is easily fractured.[271] The fracture itself may be quite painful, and the close proximity of the median nerve and brachial artery may result in symptoms of compression of these two structures.[271] One should always suspect its presence in the patient with high median nerve dysfunction.

The mechanism of injury is suspected to be direct trauma to the area, resulting in a fracture through the supracondylar process.[274] The palpation of a painful bony projection on the anteromedial aspect of the distal humerus approximately 5 cm above the elbow should suggest the presence of a fractured supracondylar process.[270] Active extension of the elbow with pronation[270,274] or supination[273] of the forearm may accentuate the pain of the fracture site, median nerve paresthesias, and brachial artery compression.

Although the diagnosis is often made by palpation, radiographic confirmation is essential. Routine anteroposterior and lateral x-rays may fail to demonstrate the bony process because of its origin on the anteromedial humerus.[270,271] Therefore, an oblique x-ray may be required to place the process in sharp profile.[270,271]

Treatment of fractures of the supracondylar process varies.[270,271,273,275] Most heal spontaneously and become asymptomatic with simple immobilization until pain-free; then early elbow motion and muscle-strengthening exercises are instituted.[275] In those that remain painful or produce median nerve dysfunction, surgical excision is indicated.[271,273,275] Kolb and Moore were more cautious in recommending surgical resection.[274] They reported one case of myositis ossificans after removal of the fractured process. Barnard and McCoy[270] emphasized that when surgical excision is elected, removal of the periosteum of the process and the fibers of the pronator teres origin is essential to prevent reformation of the spur.

DISLOCATIONS

The elbow is one of the more highly constrained and stable joints in the body, yet dislocation is not uncommon. Because of this intrinsic stability, re-dislocation is rare in the elbow in contrast to the shoulder. The opposing tension of the triceps and flexors, coupled with the hingelike articulation, confers stability that permits capsular healing even during active motion. The important medial and lateral stabilizing ligaments also seem capable of healing with enough mechanical integrity that repair for acute instability is seldom necessary.

Elbow dislocation has the highest incidence among the 10 to 20-year-old population and is associated with sports injuries.[302] The injury can also occur in the elderly after a fall.

For dislocation to occur without fracture, a combination of levering forces and loading must be applied in a manner that first "unlocks" the olecranon from the trochlea and then translates the articular surfaces out of position. Once dislocation is recognized, prompt reduction with careful attention to the neurovascular status of the arm and hand should be carried out.

CLASSIFICATION

Since most acute elbow dislocations in adults occur at the ulnohumeral joint, most classifications refer to the position of the ulna relative to the humerus following injury. Desault in 1811 described four types of ulnohumeral elbow dislocations.[290] Stimson's classification,[327] which included nearly every possible anatomic position, was adopted by most subsequent authors.[286,326] Unreduced (old) and recurrent dislocations require entirely different treatment and are classified and discussed separately in this section.

Most acute elbow dislocations are posterior (Fig. 10-26) and involve both the radius and ulna.[308,332] The distinction between posterior, posterolateral, and posteromedial is sometimes difficult to determine and seldom influences treatment. The other positions of dislocation—anterior, medial, lateral, and divergent—are rare and require alternative treatment. Pure lateral and medial dislocations are distinct and may require open reduction because of entrapped muscle or nerve. Isolated dislocations of the proximal radius are uncommon in adults, unlike in the pediatric population.

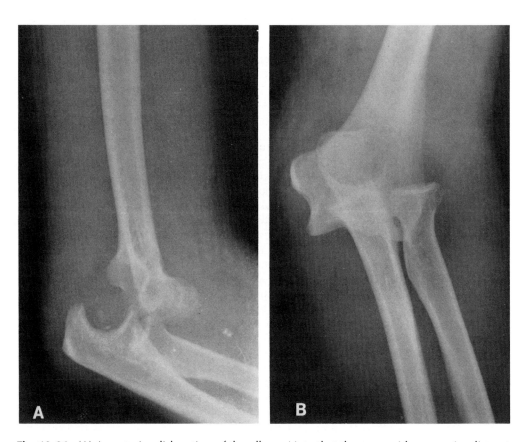

Fig. 10-26. (**A**) A posterior dislocation of the elbow. Note that the coronoid process is adjacent to the olecranon fossa. (**B**) In the anteroposterior view, note the slight lateral displacement of the radius and ulna.

MECHANISM OF INJURY

Posterior dislocations of the elbow are commonly caused by a fall on the hand or wrist. The precise mechanism of dislocation is not known since many patterns of injury share this frequent antecedent. Several authors have speculated that the position of greatest vulnerability is slight hyperextension or at least full extension. As force is transmitted from the fall to the extended elbow, a resultant anterior force is generated that levers the ulna out of the trochlea. As the joint continues to hyperextend, the anterior capsule and collateral ligaments are placed under increasing tension and eventually fail. In addition to hyperextension, a valgus stress usually occurs. In patients who have undergone exploratory surgery immediately after posterior dislocation, nearly all have ruptured the medial collateral ligaments and some even the origin of the flexor mass at the medial epicondyle.[298,329] This valgus stress is not unexpected, given the usual position of the arm away from the body at the time of the fall. In the child, this sudden valgus load can instead cause a fracture of the medial epicondyle through the growth plate.

Anterior dislocations are uncommon and are thought to be caused by impact on the posterior forearm in a slightly flexed position.

INITIAL ASSESSMENT

The first priority of care is to assess the neurovascular status of the hand and forearm *before* manipulation. The physician must attempt to document the status of the brachial artery and median and ulnar nerves because these are most vulnerable and can be entrapped during manipulation. Often, the patient is in great pain and is uncooperative, but nevertheless an attempt should be made. The radiographs must also be scrutinized for associated fractures at the distal humerus, radial head, and coronoid process. One should not hesitate to admit the patient for 24 hours of observation if there is any concern about excessive swelling or the risk of compartment syndrome.

Vascular Injury

Many authors have reported injuries of the brachial artery associated with elbow dislocation.[326,334, 335,342,349,351,354,355,362,365,366,369,370] In 1913 Sherrill[365] repaired the brachial artery "[by] the method described by Carrel and employed by Crile" with good result. In 1937 Eliason and Brown[342] reported ligating the radial and ulnar arteries without repair

and reported good results. Spear and Janes[366] also treated four patients with ligation, but their results were not as satisfying, since one patient demonstrated persistent ischemia in the hand. These authors thought that collateral circulation was adequate in the upper extremity in most cases.

Disputing this, many others have stated strongly that arterial repair with or without reversed saphenous vein grafting should be the standard of care.[331,333–335,343,345,354,355,362,369] Louis and colleagues[354] noted no cold intolerance or claudication in the patients with open and functioning arterial repairs but did find ischemic symptoms in the hand of the patient whose graft clotted. In addition, anatomic studies demonstrated that in dislocation much of the collateral circulation can be disrupted at the time of injury. De Bakey and Simeone's[341] analysis of World War II vascular injuries in the upper extremity also challenged the safety of ligation.

Early recognition of vascular injury is imperative. Loss of pulse does not preclude attempted closed reduction. If, however, arterial flow is not reestablished after reduction and the hand is poorly perfused, the patient should be prepared for immediate arterial reconstruction with saphenous vein grafting. Angiography, if used, should be performed in the operating room, especially if use of the angiography suite delays prompt treatment. If perfusion of the forearm and hand has been poor because of delayed treatment, volar forearm fasciotomy should be performed to reduce the chance of Volkmann's contracture.

A spectrum of arterial injury exists, and vigilance for loss of circulation after reduction due to intimal injury is important. The presence of pulses alone does not ensure adequate circulation to the hand or perfusion of the forearm musculature. It is necessary to examine for signs of increased compartment pressure in the forearm and hand. Pain with gentle passive extension of the digits is the most important early indicator of ischemia. The other clinical features and treatment of compartment syndromes are discussed in Chapter 5 and should be reviewed.

Nerve Injury

The median, ulnar, radial, and anterior interosseous nerves can be injured at the time of elbow dislocation. The relative incidence cannot be derived from the mere volume of case reports, but the radial nerve seems to be the least vulnerable and injury to it the most rarely reported.[371] Injury to the ulnar nerve with entrapment anterior to the joint has also been reported. The valgus displacement that occurs during dislocation can also put the ulnar nerve under stretch.

The median nerve can be injured both at the time of dislocation,[314,346,371] being stretched and attenuated, or during reduction, becoming entrapped in the joint[336,339,340,344,347,352,353,359,360,368] (Fig. 10-27). It is therefore important to examine the patient before and after manipulation for the independent function of each nerve. The most difficult diagnosis is probably the isolated anterior interosseous nerve palsy, since no sensory loss is noted.[338] In cases in which the deficit was present both before and after reduction, it is best for the surgeon to wait and

watch for signs of resolving palsy, counseling the patient that exploration may still be necessary. If there is a decline in function or severe pain in the distribution of the nerve, exploration and decompression are indicated.

After the initial phase of treatment, electromyographic studies demonstrate signs of denervation, but recovery may not be evident. Careful serial clinical examinations are the most helpful. Spontaneous recovery usually occurs, but if none is noted after 3 months, operation should be considered.

POSTERIOR DISLOCATION OF THE ELBOW

Methods of Treatment

CLOSED REDUCTION

After the initial examination of the neurovascular function of the hand and forearm is complete, manipulation and reduction are performed. Many techniques of manipulation have been described[296,305,309,310,312,316] for closed reduction of the posterior dislocation. All the methods employ some form of distraction followed by anterior translation. The principal controversy surrounds the use of hyperextension to "unlock" the olecranon from the distal humerus (Fig. 10-28). Some have advocated this as useful and necessary[310] in certain cases to achieve reduction. There is some danger, however, when full extension or hyperextension is used. Matev[358] and Hallett[347] suggested that hyperextension was responsible for entrapment of the median nerve after elbow dislocation in the cases they reported. Loomis[309] condemned extension and especially hyperextension because of the increased trauma to the brachialis muscle. He recommended reduction in flexion with distal traction on the forearm.

Starkloff positioned the patient prone with the arm hanging over the side of the stretcher, then applied traction with weights hung from the wrist. After 15 to 20 minutes, forward pressure on the olecranon was applied, gently effecting reduction. Parvin[316] also used the prone position (Fig. 10-29), but he used traction applied by the surgeon rather than with weights. Again, after several minutes of traction, the olecranon slipped into reduction with gentle flexion. Meyn and Quigley[312] used a similar technique, except that only the forearm dangles from the edge of the stretcher rather than the whole arm (Fig. 10-30). Lavine used a similar method over the back of a chair. Hankin[296] has more recently described a method of reduction that gently levers

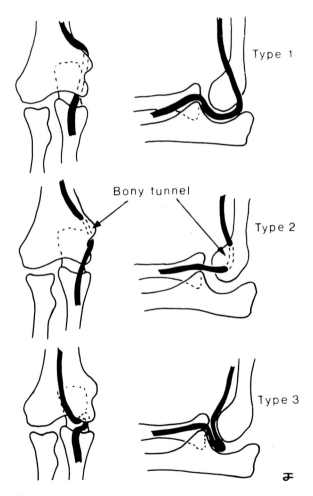

Fig. 10-27. Hallet described three ways in which the median nerve can become entrapped in the elbow. (*Hallet, J.: Entrapment of the Median Nerve After Dislocation of the Elbow. A Case Report. J. Bone Joint Surg., 63B:408–412, 1981.*)

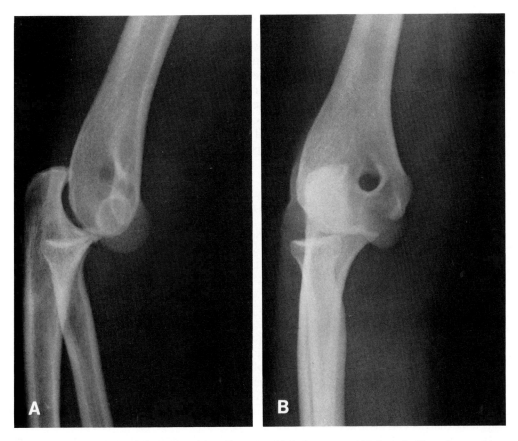

Fig. 10-28. A posterior dislocation of the elbow in which the coronoid is impaled into the trochlea; (**A**) lateral and (**B**) anteroposterior views.

the olecranon over the distal humerus in the flexed position while applying traction. The advantage of these methods is that they require no assistant.

OPEN REDUCTION

The need for open reduction after acute dislocation is rare. Pawlowski and coworkers[318] and Greiss and Messias and colleagues[295] described patients who had irreducible dislocations because soft tissue was entrapped, blocking reduction. Durig[291] recommended that loose intra-articular fragments be removed, but the results of treatment were comparable to those of closed management. Occasionally in the adult (and more often in children), the medial epicondyle can be entrapped, preventing reduction. Purser[320] and Linscheid and Wheeler[308] reported adult patients who required open reduction with extraction of the entrapped medial epicondyle from the joint.

REPAIR OF LIGAMENTS

Some authors have advocated surgical repair of the associated ligamentous injuries.[291,329] However, Josefsson[299] studied 30 patients in a *randomized, prospective* study designed to compare the outcome of surgical versus nonsurgical treatment. They concluded that irrespective of the degree of acute instability when the patients were examined under anesthesia, no benefit was derived from open treatment and repair of the medial ligaments in simple posterior elbow dislocation.

Care After Reduction

There is disagreement in the literature concerning the duration of immobilization after reduction. Loomis[309] and Wadsworth[330] thought that 3 to 4 weeks of immobilization in cast was mandatory to reduce ectopic calcification and allow healing. Protzman[319] and later Mehloff and colleagues[311] as-

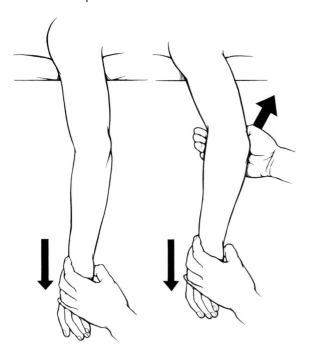

Fig. 10-29. Parvin's method of closed reduction of an elbow dislocation. The patient lies prone on a stretcher, and the physician applies gentle downward traction on the wrist for a few minutes. As the olecranon begins to slip distally, the physician lifts up gently on the arm. No assistant is required, and if the maneuver is done gently, no anesthesia is required. *(Redrawn from Parvin, R.W.: Closed Reduction of Common Shoulder and Elbow Dislocations Without Anesthesia. Arch. Surg., 75:972–975, 1957.)*

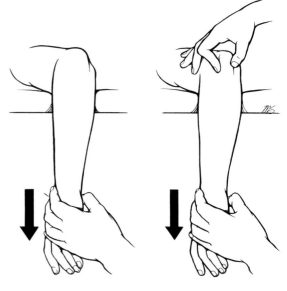

Fig. 10-30. In Meyn and Quigley's method of reduction, only the forearm hangs from the side of the stretcher. As gentle downward traction is applied on the wrist, the physician guides reduction of the olecranon with the opposite hand. *(Redrawn from Meyn, M.A., and Quigley, T.B.: Reduction of Posterior Dislocation of the Elbow by Traction on the Dangling Arm. Clin. Orthop., 103:106–108, 1974.)*

sociated greater contractures and dysfunction with immobilization and recommended motion within the first week after injury. Linscheid also recommended gentle active motion in the first week.[307]

Authors' Preferred Method

As emphasized, the first task of treatment is a careful assessment of any associated neurovascular injuries and concomitant fractures. The vascular status of the hand is paramount. We assess both the radial and ulnar pulses and evaluate the perfusion of the hand. It is important to evaluate capillary refill in the volar fingertips rather than in the nail beds and compare it with that in the uninjured extremity. The median, radial, and ulnar nerves can usually be tested in the hand independently without excessive discomfort to the patient. Both the sensory and motor components of each nerve should be checked.

If the dislocation occurred less than two hours before treatment, closed manipulation with sedation is usually successful. If the dislocation occurred more than four hours before treatment, the task becomes more difficult but still is usually possible without general or axillary block anesthesia. Forceful attempts should be avoided, and if spasm and pain preclude adequate relaxation, general anesthesia can be used. The disadvantage of axillary block is the inability to immediately assess the neurologic function after manipulation and reduction.

The simplest reduction maneuver requires gentle countertraction on the humerus by an assistant while the surgeon applies distal traction on the wrist and proximal forearm. Medial or lateral displacement is corrected first, and then distal traction is continued as the elbow is flexed. Downward pressure by the surgeon on the proximal forearm to disengage the coronoid from the olecranon fossa may be helpful. Hyperextension should be avoided.

When an assistant is unavailable or muscle spasm is more pronounced, Parvin's gravity method[316] (see Fig. 10-29), or that of Meyn and Quigley[312] (see Fig. 10-30), can be used to gradually overcome the spasm. We have no personal experience with Hankin's method,[296] but he reports excellent results with no complications.

After manipulation and reduction, the elbow should be gently ranged passively to test the stability of reduction. Most elbows are stable and do not redislocate at 30° of flexion. Pronation and supination should also be stable. If passive range of motion is not complete or smooth, postmanipulation radiographs should be carefully scrutinized for an associated fracture or entrapment of the medial epicondyle. The presence of valgus laxity is common immediately after reduction, especially if the patient is anesthetized. However, the medial ligaments are extracapsular and probably heal satisfactorily if protected from valgus stress during the healing process.

We usually apply a posterior splint with the elbow in 90° flexion, with loose circumferential wraps. The hand should be accessible for repeated examination for neurovascular dysfunction or compartment syndrome. Most elbows are stable enough after dislocation to permit gentle active motion exercises in both flexion and extension and forearm rotation during the first week after injury. We usually initiate this as soon as the patient will allow it and when swelling has diminished. A removable splint and/or sling between therapy sessions for the first few weeks can be helpful.

If the unanesthetized patient exhibits instability immediately after reduction or redislocates the elbow in the splint, we carefully reexamine the patient in the operating room under fluoroscopy to determine the point of instability. If there are no associated fractures of the coronoid process or radial head, the patient can be fitted with a hinged brace with extension stops set to limit extension before the angle of instability is reached. Active motion can then be commenced. At 3 weeks, the amount of extension allowed in the splint can be increased gradually. Forced passive motion should be avoided, because this can lead to pathologic heterotopic ossification.

The use of formal physical therapy should be determined on an individual basis. Some patients progress with little supervision, whereas others require more comprehensive instruction and surveillance. The shoulder, especially in the elderly, can become quite stiff and painful if not included in the exercise program.

The presence of some heterotopic calcification is not unusual and is seldom of clinical significance.[417,427] Ectopic bone formation is usually seen in the brachialis and the medial or lateral ligaments.

Widespread heterotopic ossification can occur in more severe trauma and is discussed in more detail on page 789.

Outcome

The outcome after simple posterior elbow dislocation has been reported in several series.[278,300,308,311,314,326] Josefsson[300] and coworkers studied 52 patients and found little long-term disability. Most had a slight flexion contracture (10° to 15°) and occasional pain. Recurrent dislocation did not occur; valgus instability was present in few patients but was usually not symptomatic. Full recovery of motion and strength takes 3 to 6 months in most patients. Some patients do not do well, however, especially those with associated fractures or high-velocity trauma.

Recurrent dislocation without associated fracture, congenital deformity, or systemic ligamentous laxity is rare.

UNREDUCED POSTERIOR DISLOCATION OF THE ELBOW

Unreduced posterior dislocations are seen primarily in less developed regions of the world. The precise temporal definition of "old" or "neglected" posterior dislocation is unclear. According to Allende and Freytes,[372] if the joint is unreduced for more than seven days, the chance for closed reduction even after preliminary traction is low.

Several procedures designed to overcome the contracture and shortening of the triceps and release the contracted capsule have been described. We have no personal experience with these methods. Whatever procedure is performed, an extensive understanding of the anatomy is necessary. Open reduction yields better results than leaving the joint dislocated but does not always return the elbow to a functional range of motion.[374,375,377–379]

ANTERIOR DISLOCATION OF THE ELBOW

Anterior dislocation usually occurs after a fall, with a force striking the posterior forearm in the flexed position.[397,398] In 1922 Cohn[397] credited Everts with the original description in 1787. Since then, about 30 cases have been reported in the literature.[396,398–402,404] Because of the blow posteriorly, a fracture of the olecranon can also occur.[397]

Signs and Symptoms

Because brachial artery injury can occur, the same careful assessment for neurovascular injury is recommended. Before reduction, the arm appears shortened, with the forearm held in supination. The distal humerus is prominent posteriorly. The biceps tendon tents the skin anteriorly.

Methods of Treatment

The reduction maneuver is essentially the reverse of the posterior dislocation. Gentle traction is first applied to the forearm to relax the contracted muscles. Posterior and downward pressure is then applied to the forearm with gentle anterior pressure on the distal humerus. Again, after the reduction, a careful examination for neurocirculatory deficit must be done.

The triceps insertion may be stripped and detached in this type of dislocation, and the examiner should test active extension of the elbow.

The elbow is splinted in slightly less than 90° of flexion, depending on the amount of swelling and the status of the triceps. If there is an associated

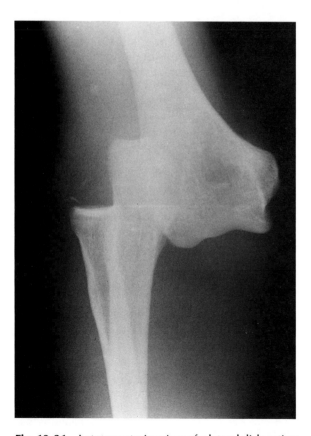

Fig. 10-31. Anteroposterior view of a lateral dislocation in which the olecranon is completely displaced from the trochlea (compare with Fig. 10-32).

olecranon fracture, open reduction with rigid fixation is probably necessary for stability.

MEDIAL AND LATERAL DISLOCATIONS OF THE ELBOW

Medial and lateral dislocations present with a widened appearance of the elbow and normal relative lengths of the arm and forearm. In the anteroposterior x-ray, a pure medial or lateral dislocation shows the greater sigmoid notch of the ulna in the plane of the distal humerus (Fig. 10-31).

In a pure lateral dislocation the greater sigmoid notch may articulate in the capitulotrochlear sulcus (Fig. 10-32), allowing some degree of flexion and extension. This motion may lead the unsuspecting surgeon astray in recognizing the dislocation, especially if there is considerable swelling.

Medial and lateral dislocations are reduced by countertraction on the arm, distal traction on the forearm in mild extension, and then straight medial or lateral pressure. Care should be taken to avoid converting this type into a posterior dislocation, causing further soft tissue damage. The medial dislocation is usually a subluxation rather than a complete dislocation, and soft tissue damage is not as extensive as in the more severe lateral dislocation. Exarchou[294] reported a lateral dislocation that required operative treatment because the anconeus muscle was interposed in the joint, blocking closed reduction.

DIVERGENT DISLOCATION OF THE ELBOW

In divergent dislocation of the elbow, a rare type of dislocation, the radius and ulna dislocate in diverging directions. Two types are seen: anteroposterior and mediolateral (transverse).

The more common anteroposterior type (Fig. 10-33) was first described by Bulley in 1841.[327] It involves a posterior dislocation of the ulna with the coronoid process lodged in the olecranon fossa. The radial head is dislocated anteriorly into the coronoid fossa. Cadaver studies demonstrated that this dislocation could be produced by forced pronation of the forearm after the medial collateral ligament had been cut. Thus, with the forearm in forced pronation and extension, the humerus is forced distally, diverging the radius and ulna.[327] It can be appreciated that, in addition to rupture of the orbicular and collateral ligaments, the interosseous membrane is torn. Clinically, this type of dislocation resembles a posterior dislocation, except that the ra-

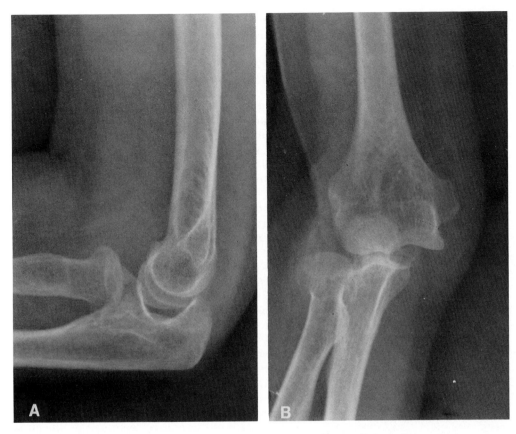

Fig. 10-32. (A) Lateral view of a lateral subluxation of the elbow. The semilunar notch appears to be articulating with the distal humerus. There is no anterior or posterior displacement of the proximal ulna. (B) The anteroposterior view shows that the proximal radius and ulna have shifted laterally as a unit. The semilunar notch of the ulna is articulating in the capitulotrochlear sulcus. This may allow some limited flexion and extension.

dial head is palpable in the antecubital fossa. Reduction is accomplished first by reduction of the ulna in a manner similar to reduction of a posterior dislocation. As the ulnar dislocation is being reduced, simultaneous pressure is applied directly over the radial head to reduce it as well. Smith[325] warned that maintenance of reduction of the radial head may be difficult and may require operative intervention. Most authors recommend that after this injury the elbow should be immobilized in flexion with the forearm supinated.[285,286,325]

The mediolateral (transverse) type is considered by many to be so rare as to be listed as a surgical curiosity.[286,288,325] In Warmont's description of Guersant's original case in 1854, the distal humerus was found to be wedged between the radius laterally and the ulna medially.[401] This lesion should be easily recognized clinically. The elbow appears mark-

edly widened. The articular surface of the trochlea can be palpated readily on the posterior surface of the elbow. Conwell and Reynolds[285] recommended reducing the transverse type by applying traction with the elbow in extension while pressing the proximal radius and ulna together.

DISLOCATION OF THE ULNA ALONE

Isolated dislocation of the ulna can occur in either an anterior or a posterior direction. Stimson[327] described how the ulna can dislocate while the radius remains in position. The radial head serves as the pivot. The medial collateral ligament is torn, whereas the lateral collateral and orbicular ligaments remain intact. The mechanism requires a combination of both angular and axial divergence of the forearm with the humerus. In normal supi-

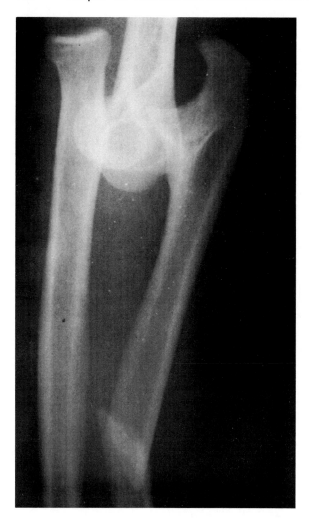

Fig. 10-33. Anteroposterior divergent dislocation of the elbow. The ulna is dislocated posteriorly and the radius anteriorly. This patient also had a fracture of the ulna that required open reduction and internal fixation with an AO (ASIF) plate. The divergent dislocation was reduced closed, and the patient regained nearly full range of painless motion in the elbow.

nation with the proximal ulna secure, only the distal forearm can rotate with the radius. In this injury, proximal fixation of the ulna is lost, allowing the whole forearm, including the proximal ulna, to rotate with the radius. With adduction and posterior rotation of the forearm, the coronoid process becomes displaced posterior to the trochlea. Patients with this injury hold their elbows extended. The forearm loses its normal carrying angle and appears to be in varus. Reduction is achieved by applying

traction in extension to the supinated forearm. The addition of a valgus force to the forearm facilitates the reduction.[325]

The anterior dislocation is much more rare. In this type, the ulna rotates anteriorly and the forearm is abducted. Again, the radius remains as a fixed pivot. The olecranon is carried forward and becomes locked in the coronoid fossa. Patients with this injury are said to keep the elbow flexed.[327] There is also an increase in the carrying angle. Reduction is achieved by direct pressure applied in a posterior direction over the proximal ulna while the forearm is adducted and pronated.

DISLOCATION OF THE RADIAL HEAD ALONE

Isolated dislocation of the proximal radius in an adult is rare, and only ten cases have been reported. In 1974 Wiley and coworkers[412] described two cases but provided no details other than that the direction of the dislocation was lateral. In 1982 Heidt and Stern[407] reported a posterior dislocation, discovered late, treated with radial head excision. In 1984 Burgess and Sprague[403] reported two cases of posterior subluxation following posterior radial head dislocation. In 1984 Ryu and colleagues[409] described closed reduction of an acute posterior dislocation. On the basis of these three reports, it is difficult to ascertain any single mechanism of injury or consistent method of treatment. In two of the reports,[403,407] the radius was reduced and stable in pronation, but in the other, supination was preferred.[409]

Salama[410] reported anterior dislocation after a patient experienced a violent contracture following an electric shock. The dislocation was discovered late, and radial head excision was required.

The diagnosis of radial head dislocation should be made *only after excluding* a Monteggia fracture or congenital dislocation of the radial head. Forced pronation with impact may be the most likely mechanism of injury in isolated posterior radial head dislocation. If the injury occurs, the patient loses some pronation and supination. Dislocation of the radial head is present if a line drawn along the axis of the radial head does not pass through the center of the capitellum in *any* view (Fig. 10-34). It is important to distinguish isolated traumatic radial head dislocation, which is rare, from congenital dislocation of the radial head, which is more common. The adult with congenital radial head dislocation can feel pain after a fall and be reluctant to rotate the forearm as before. In addition, because

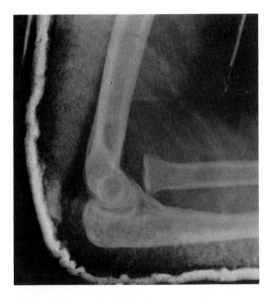

Fig. 10-34. Anterior dislocation of the radial head. The axis of the radial head passes superior to the capitellum. In all dislocations of the radial head, a concomitant fracture of the ulna must be sought.

of growth retardation of the radius, x-rays of the wrist will often demonstrate radioulnar inequality, mimicking acute radioulnar dissociation. However, in congenital radial head dislocation, the radial head is dome-shaped and the capitellum flattened. There is no instability of the wrist and no pain or swelling of the forearm.

RECURRENT DISLOCATION OF THE ELBOW

Chronic instability of the elbow leading to recurrent dislocation is very rare following simple posterior elbow dislocation. Milch[388] in 1936 and Wainwright[394] in 1947 reported cases with recurrent instability caused by bony insufficiency of the proximal ulna, both of which were treated with an anterior bone block procedure. Gosman[382] reported a 15-year-old with recurrent instability with hyperextensible joints, and many of the other reported cases were in children.[390,392] Others reported cases were in the mentally retarded or institutionalized patients.[381,385] No cases of recurrent dislocation have been reported in more recent series following simple posterior dislocation in adults.[300]

The principal pathology that leads to chronic instability and recurrent dislocation is not known (Fig. 10-35). Although anatomic and biomechanical studies have recognized the importance of the an-

terior portion of the medial ligament (Fig. 10-36), Osborne and Cotterill[390] and others[393] have suggested that laxity on the lateral side was the principal deficit. Hassmann and colleagues[384] reported four patients, two of whom were treated with lateral advancement alone and two with both lateral and medial reconstructions. Dryer and associates[380] thought that avulsion of the brachialis and anterior capsule was contributory. Fractures of the coronoid process with displacement may also contribute to instability.

O'Driscoll and coworkers have recently reported deficiency of the lateral *ulnar* collateral ligament leading to posterior-rotary subluxation, which may represent a forme fruste of the lateral laxity identified by Osborne and Cotterill.[390]

In the treatment of recurrent dislocation, it is important to identify which structures are damaged and require reconstruction. In our experience, lateral reconstruction is required in nearly every patient, using the technique as described by Osborne and Cotterill.[390] If the brachialis insertion has been disrupted or the coronoid process displaced, reattachment is helpful, because this restores the anterior tension, seating the olecranon in the distal humerus. Medial ligament reconstruction as described by Jobe and colleagues[455] may also be necessary.

COMPLICATIONS OF ELBOW DISLOCATIONS

Ectopic Calcification and Heterotopic Bone Formation

Calcification of the soft tissue surrounding the elbow is common after trauma.[420,421,423,424,427,428] As Coventry[417] pointed out, however, it is important to distinguish between ectopic calcification, heterotopic bone formation, and myositis ossificans.

Ectopic calcification is mineralization of soft tissue structures "out of place." Calcification of the collateral ligaments and capsule is very common[416] after elbow dislocation and seldom requires treatment.

Heterotopic bone refers to the formation of *trabecular bone* at a location other than where it belongs[413] (Fig. 10-37). Heterotopic bone can form as a result of myositis ossificans (an inflammatory condition that occurs in striated muscle) or bone formation near the joint capsule. Thompson and Garcia[427] noted that myositis will be apparent radiographically within 3 to 4 weeks after injury. Heterotopic bone formation does not always require

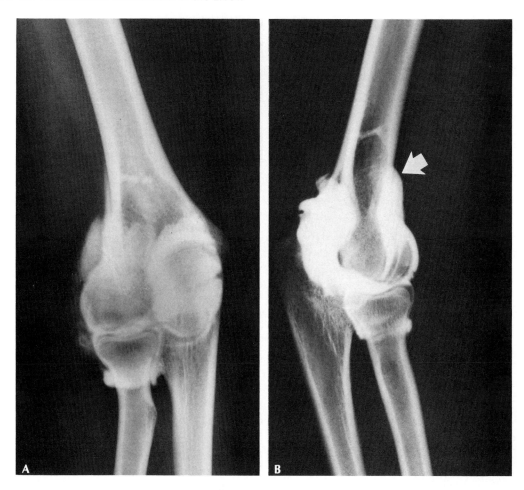

Fig. 10-35. (**A**) Anteroposterior view of a normal elbow indicates the extent of the capsule as demonstrated by an arthrogram. (**B**) On the lateral view, note the superior extension of the joint capsule (*arrow*).

(continued)

treatment, especially if there is no restriction of motion.[428]

Head-injured patients face the greatest risk of disabling heterotopic bone formation about the elbow.[421,426] Another factor that may increase the risk is forced passive (and painful) motion after injury. The combination of fracture with dislocation is also associated with a higher incidence of heterotopic ossification. Long periods of immobilization have also been implicated but not proved.

Prevention or prophylaxis of heterotopic bone formation has been the goal of numerous investigators, especially about the hip after pelvic surgery or total hip replacement.[414,419,422] Coventry and Scanlon[418] reported successful retardation of ectopic

bone around the hip with radiation. Coventry[417] also reported the use of radiation at the elbow in one patient but was reluctant to recommend this uniformly because the radiation ports in the elbow generally include the incision and may delay healing. We have also been reluctant to use this in young people. Diphosphonates have been studied by many but do not seem to reliably inhibit bone induction.[414,419]

Indomethacin probably offers the best choice for prevention at this time. Ritter and Gioe[425] demonstrated a decrease of about 50% in the incidence of heterotopic ossification after total hip replacement. More recently, McLaren[422] also noted a significant decrease of heterotopic bone after pelvic

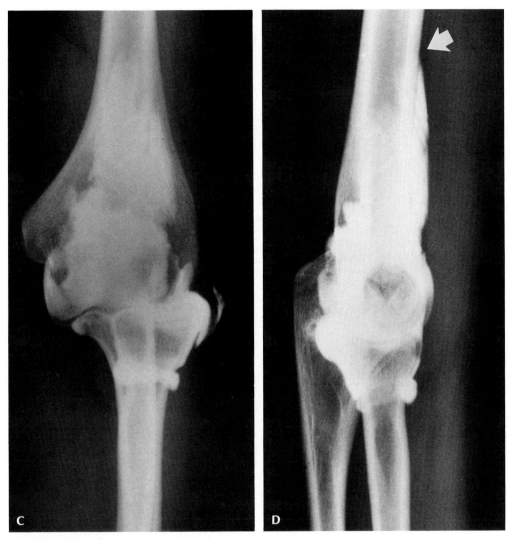

Fig. 10-35 *(continued)*
(**C**) An arthrogram shows the superior excursion of the dye in a recurrent dislocating elbow. (**D**) Lateral view: the dye extends considerably higher than normal *(arrow)*.

surgery. Indomethacin is generally tolerated, but gastrointestinal disturbances or bleeding can occur. We use a dose of 25 mg three times a day, starting as early as possible after injury. A slow-release form of indomethacin is also available.

Associated Fractures

The relative incidence of associated fractures in previously reported series of elbow dislocations has ranged from 12% to 62%.[308,314,322] The most commonly recognized fracture has been that of the medial epicondyle, although these figures do not include osteochondral fractures, which are frequently not recognized but are probably extremely common in elbow dislocations.[291,392]

Fracture–dislocation of the elbow (fracture of the olecranon and anterior dislocation of the radial head) is distinctly different from a pure dislocation, and it is discussed in the section on fractures of the olecranon.

ENTRAPPED MEDIAL EPICONDYLE
A common pitfall of the unwary in the management of posterior dislocation of the elbow is failure to recognize an associated fracture of the medial epicondyle that becomes trapped within the joint after reduction. Immediately after a closed reduction, the elbow should be taken through a full range of motion. If smooth, unrestricted motion is not possible or if there appears to be any type of mechanical

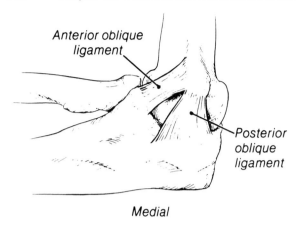

Fig. 10-36. Collateral ligaments of the elbow. Schwab and associates suggested that the medial ligament (especially the anterior portion) is the most important stabilizing ligament in the elbow. *(Schwab, G.H.; Bennett, J.B.; Woods, G.W.; and Tullos, H.S.: Biomechanics of Elbow Instability: The Role of the Medial Collateral Ligament. Clin. Orthop., 146:42–52, 1980.)*

block to motion, entrapment of the medial epicondyle should immediately be suspected as the culprit. If lateral x-rays reveal the avulsed fragment to lie at the level of the joint, it should be assumed that the fragment lies within the joint.[316] Comparison x-rays of the opposite elbow are helpful in making this diagnosis.

Although entrapped medial epicondyle is more common in children and rare in adults, the possibility should be considered with each posterior dislocation. Failure to recognize this complication and to remove the fragment rapidly leads to severe destruction of the articular cartilage.[324]

The entrapped epicondyle can occasionally be extricated by manipulation, either by valgus stress of the forearm accompanied by supination and extension of the wrist and fingers to pull on the flexor muscles or by adduction of the elbow associated with flexion and extension movements of the elbow to express the epicondyle from the joint.[317]

Patrick[317] described a method of attempting to extricate the entrapped epicondyle by simultaneous valgus stress on the elbow and faradic stimulation of the flexor-pronator group of muscles. Usually, however, arthrotomy is necessary to remove the bone, which may then be secured to its normal location with Kirschner wires. Alternatively, the bone can be excised and the common flexor origin reattached directly to bone.

FRACTURES OF THE CORONOID PROCESS

Even though this fracture can occur as an isolated injury, it is most often associated with posterior dislocation of the elbow. The fracture is due to avulsion by the brachialis muscle when the elbow is hyperextended. Conwell and Reynolds[285] treated a patient in whom this occurred when the elbow

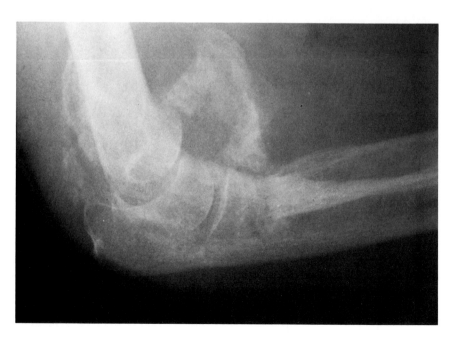

Fig. 10-37. Extensive myositis ossificans of the elbow involving not only the brachialis muscle but also the triceps.

was momentarily subluxated in the hyperextended position. Regan and Morrey[524] reported on 35 patients and established a classification based on the size of the fragment. In patients with large fragments and instability after elbow dislocation, they recommended internal fixation of the fragment to reestablish continuity of the brachialis insertion for stability.

In some cases of associated posterior dislocation, the coronoid process can be more comminuted[324] and a portion of the tip, which is intra-articular, can become loose within the joint.

Displacement of a large fragment of the coronoid has been associated with recurrent dislocation, and some authors recommend that these dislocations be immobilized in as much flexion as obtainable.[289,324,332] The period of immobilization should be 3 to 4 weeks, which is longer than for routine dislocations. Operative intervention appears to be limited to those fractures that interfere with joint motion. This can occur if the fragment is intra-articular or if it unites proximally and forms a significant bony block to flexion. Because of the increased incidence of myositis ossificans with this injury, surgery should be performed either at the time of injury or much later, when the danger of this complication is lessened.

BASEBALL ELBOW (THROWING INJURIES)

Acute fractures and dislocations of the elbow can occur in baseball, but far more prevalent are the chronic maladies associated with repetitive throwing. Throwing injuries of the elbow in the baseball player have been well documented.[441–444, 446,451,453,456,463,465] For many patients, valgus extension overload is a common injury pathway[439,464] (Fig. 10-38). The specific lesions are summarized in Table 10-1. The pitcher is the most common player affected, but others on the team, occasionally infielders, can also be afflicted.

Biomechanics of the throwing motion is a complex topic, and numerous studies in the literature have attempted to describe muscle action and activity during throwing.[462] The throwing motion is commonly divided into five phases: wind up, cocking, acceleration, release/deceleration, and follow-through. During the acceleration phase, the trunk

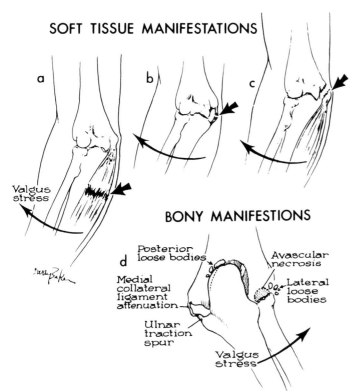

Fig. 10-38. Composite illustration of the types of pathologic conditions seen in the throwing elbow. These are the result of tension on the medial side and compression on the lateral side of the elbow (see also Table 10-1). (Barnes, D.A., and Tullos, H.S.: An Analysis of 100 Symptomatic Baseball Players. Am. J. Sports Med., 6:62–67, 1978.)

Table 10-1. Throwing Injuries of the Elbow (Modified from Slocum[111])

Medial Tension Overload
  Muscular (Flexor-pronator group)
    1. Strain (minor tears)
    2. Rupture
    3. Fascial compartment syndrome (Bennett[101])
    4. Medial epicondylitis
    5. Avulsion of the medial epicondyle
  Ligamentous
    1. Ulnar traction spurs (coronoid process)
    2. Calcium deposits
    3. Medial ligament instability
    4. Loose bodies

Lateral Compression Injuries
    1. Osteochondral fractures of the capitellum
    2. Loose bodies
    3. Posttraumatic arthritis

Extension Overload
    1. Triceps muscle strain
    2. Avulsion fracture tip of olecranon
    3. Olecranon hypertrophy
    4. Loose bodies in the olecranon fossa
    5. Tears of brachialis and anterior capsule
    6. Fixed flexion contractures

and pelvis are positioned forward, and the arm is "catching up" to the rest of the body. The elbow is rapidly extending, and a powerful valgus force is created. This excessive valgus force can cause characteristic injuries to the elbow dependent on the age of the athlete. In younger children, fatigue fractures of the medial epicondyle cause pain and swelling. In the adult, posterolateral osteophytes from valgus overload are seen. There has been concern that throwing a curveball creates more stress on the elbow because of sudden supination of the forearm during release, increasing the chance of injury. High-speed cinematography has shown an increase in the *rate* of extension while throwing a curve but not increased supination during release.[448,459] In a separate study that supported this idea, Sisto and colleagues noted increased electromyographic activity in the extensor carpi radialis longus and brevis (ECRL and ECRB) during acceleration and follow-through when compared to that of the fastball.[462]

Although many sports involve a throwing motion, pitching a baseball is unique because of the position of the trunk and legs, facing the batter and turning on the mound. In other throwing sports, such as the javelin and shot put, more thrust is imparted by the transfer of torsional energy from the legs and trunk.[440,449,459]

As with most injuries due to repetitive trauma, treatment of the baseball elbow begins with pre-

vention and proper technique. Studies have documented that the number of innings pitched is probably the most important factor relating to injury.[446] Throwing the curveball has been cited as causing "Little Leaguer's elbow," and the pitch has been banned in many areas. Others have shown that a *properly* thrown curveball is no more injurious than a traditional fastball.[448,462]

Several simple steps can be taken to prevent or minimize the damage due to pitching.

First, proper conditioning is important. To maintain flexibility and endurance, the pitcher should toss the ball in the off-season without throwing with maximal effort.[466] General conditioning and endurance training allow a more sustained performance. Starting immediately with pitching at maximal velocity leads to early fatigue, poor mechanics, and ultimately extension overload at the elbow.

Second, pain and inflammation should be avoided. Pitching when one is fatigued should be avoided at all costs. An accurate pitch count should be kept during the game with the limit known in advance. If the pitcher begins to show loss of control, this can mean fatigue. Fatigue may cause improper mechanics, leading to injury. The manager and coaches should remain vigilant as the pitch limit is approached.

After throwing, ice applied to the shoulder and elbow seems to decrease the inflammatory response. Ice over the cubital tunnel should be used judiciously, watching for any signs of ulnar nerve dysfunction or injury. After icing, a gentle stretching program to maintain a full range of motion of both the shoulder and elbow should be employed to reduce the potential for contracture and stiffness. On off-days, continued stretching and light tossing are helpful to reduce stiffness. General fitness and conditioning should be maintained and emphasized. Running and bicycling are useful for aerobic conditioning.

Pain in the elbow of the pitcher should raise concern. Overuse injuries can result in permanent dysfunction. The primary cause is usually excessive throwing. Once inflammation and degeneration begin, the process can accelerate, leading to valgus extension overload.

Once the painful elbow develops, treatment to decrease the swelling and inflammation should be started. No competitive throwing is allowed until a full range of motion returns and no pain or tenderness is associated with throwing.

Osteochondritis dissecans of the capitellum can occur in the very young pitcher, but it usually affects those over the age of 10.[458] Changes in the radiocapitellar joint are especially worrisome because of possible permanent loss of function, unlike tendinitis or transient inflammation along the medial elbow. If fragmentation occurs, loose bodies that may require excision can impinge.[458]

Once an athlete is injured, a period of rest with conditioning and stretching is useful until the symptoms of inflammation subside. A defined schedule of rehabilitation is important because it gives the athlete a timetable. If poorly defined exercises of indeterminate duration are prescribed, the athlete is likely to lose confidence and abandon the rehabilitation program. Many graduated rehabilitation programs have been suggested, providing a framework for return.[438]

For pitchers who develop chronic instability of the medial collateral ligament after years of throwing, Jobe and coworkers[455] have described a reconstructive operation that attempts to restore the function of the anterior portion of the medial collateral ligament. This operation is technically demanding. If the tendon graft used in the collateral ligament reconstruction is not precisely placed at the appropriate point of rotation in the humerus, a camlike effect occurs, stretching the newly placed graft. Jobe and associates[455] have reported good results in professional pitchers but only after a carefully monitored program of rehabilitation.

Irrespective of measures taken, pitching a baseball at competitive speeds is an inherently destructive process for most. As Tullos has stated on several occasions, "We do not fix baseball players, we only temporarily improve them. If they continue to pitch, they will continue to have problems."[464]

FRACTURES OF THE OLECRANON

ANATOMY

The olecranon process is a large curved eminence comprising the proximal and posterior portions of the ulna. It lies in a subcutaneous position, which makes it especially vulnerable to direct trauma. Together with the proximal portion of the coronoid process, the olecranon forms the greater sigmoid (semilunar) notch of the ulna, a deep depression that serves as the articulation with the trochlea which allows motion only in the anteroposterior plane and provides stability to the elbow joint. The articular cartilage surface is interrupted by a transverse line of bone, "a bare area," located midway between the tip of the olecranon and the coronoid process. If this is not recognized during reconstruc-

tion of the fractured olecranon, there is a temptation to eliminate any area uncovered by cartilage.

The ossification center for the olecranon appears at 10 years of age and is generally fused to the proximal ulna by the age of 16. There are reports of persistent epiphyseal plates in adults; these are usually bilateral and tend to occur in families.[526] This is not to be confused with patella cubiti, which is a true accessory ossicle located in the triceps tendon at its insertion into the olecranon.[507] Both of these entities may be confused with a fracture, especially when there has been local trauma to the olecranon. They are often bilateral, and comparison x-rays of the uninjured elbow help to differentiate them from fractures.

Posteriorly, the triceps tendon covers the joint capsule before it inserts into the olecranon. The fascia overlying the triceps muscle spreads out medially and laterally like the retinaculum of the quadriceps in the knee. These expansions and the triceps aponeurosis insert into the deep fascia of the forearm and into the periosteum of the olecranon and proximal ulna.

On the posteromedial aspect of the elbow the ulnar nerve passes behind the medial epicondyle to enter the volar surface of the forearm between the two heads of the flexor carpi ulnaris. This relationship must be remembered when a surgical procedure is performed on the olecranon.

MECHANISM OF INJURY

Fractures of the olecranon occur in response to three main types of injury.[540] Direct violence, such as a fall on the point of the elbow or a direct blow to the olecranon, often results in a comminuted fracture.[523] Indirect violence, such as a fall on the outstretched hand with the elbow in flexion, accompanied by a strong contraction of the triceps, can result in a transverse or oblique fracture through the olecranon.[471,483,523,538] Finally, a combination of direct and indirect violence, in which both muscle contraction and direction violence act together, may produce displaced, comminuted fractures.[542]

The transverse or oblique fracture enters the semilunar notch, and the amount of separation of the fragments is influenced by the pull of the triceps muscle (Fig. 10-39). Limited separation of these fragments may be due to the presence of an intact triceps aponeurosis and periosteum of the olecranon, which, in addition to the lateral ligaments and capsule of the elbow joint, resist displacement of the fracture.[538]

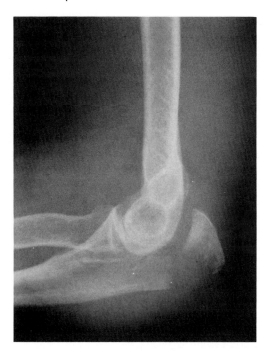

Fig. 10-39. Fracture of the olecranon. Note the comminution and disruption of the articular surface; a true lateral view is necessary to visualize this adequately.

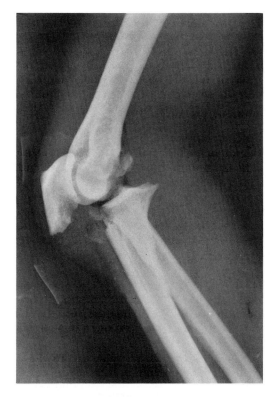

Fig. 10-40. Fracture-dislocation of the elbow (fracture of the olecranon and anterior dislocation of the radius and ulna).

In cases of extreme violence to the elbow, the proximal olecranon fragment often displaces posteriorly, whereas the distal ulnar fragment, together with the head of the radius, may displace anterior to the humerus, resulting in the so-called fracture–dislocation (Fig. 10-40). A fracture–dislocation is far more serious than the isolated olecranon fracture, and persistent or recurrent deformity is likely to occur if the olecranon is not stabilized adequately.

SIGNS AND SYMPTOMS

Because all fractures of the olecranon process have some intra-articular component, there is generally a hemorrhagic effusion of the elbow joint. This results in swelling and pain over the olecranon.[471] There may also be a palpable sulcus at the fracture site, accompanied by a painful and limited range of motion.

Inability to extend the elbow actively against gravity is the most important sign to be elicited; it indicates discontinuity of the triceps mechanism. The presence or absence of this sign often determines the plan of treatment of these fractures.

A careful neurologic evaluation should be done,

since ulnar nerve injuries may accompany fractures of the olecranon, especially in the extensively comminuted fracture that results from direct trauma.[530]

RADIOGRAPHIC FINDINGS

Probably the most common pitfall in the initial evaluation of a fracture of the olecranon is failure to insist on a true lateral x-ray of the elbow. The slightly oblique view, which is frequently obtained in the emergency room, is inadequate to identify precisely the extent of the fracture, the degree of comminution, the amount of disruption of the articular surface in the semilunar notch, and any displacement of the radial head, if present. An anteroposterior x-ray is also important to delineate a fracture line in the sagittal plane.

CLASSIFICATION

No generally accepted classification of olecranon fractures has been presented in the orthopaedic literature.[479,484,500,518] A simple classification of olecranon fractures modified from that of Colton[479] is offered here as a basis for selection of appropriate treatment:

I. Undisplaced fractures
II. Displaced fractures
    A. Avulsion fractures
    B. Oblique and transverse fractures
    C. Comminuted fractures
    D. Fracture–dislocations

To be considered undisplaced, a fracture of the olecranon must meet the following criteria: (1) displacement of less than 2 mm,[488] (2) no increase in this minimal degree of separation with 90° flexion of the elbow, and (3) the patient's ability to extend the elbow actively against gravity.

Displaced fractures include all those that do not meet the preceding criteria, and these usually require open reduction and internal fixation.

Avulsion Fractures

A transverse fracture line separates a small proximal fragment of the olecranon process from the rest of the ulna. This fracture is most common in elderly patients.[523,527,537]

Oblique and Transverse Fractures

The fracture line runs obliquely, starting near the deepest part of the semilunar notch and running dorsally and distally to emerge on the subcutaneous crest of the proximal part of the ulna. This fracture may be a single oblique line, or it may have an element of comminution caused by a fracture in the sagittal plane or a central area of depression in the articular surface.

Comminuted Fractures

This group includes all the severely comminuted fractures of the olecranon, which usually result from direct trauma to the posterior aspect of the elbow. There are multiple fracture planes, often with severe crushing of many fragments. There may be associated fractures of the distal end of the humerus, the shafts of the forearm bones, or the head of the radius.

Fracture–Dislocations

The olecranon fracture is at or near the level of the tip of the coronoid process, so that a plane of instability is located through the fracture site and the radiohumeral joint as well, resulting in an anterior dislocation of the ulna and radius.[475,529,533,543] This fracture is usually secondary to a severe injury, such as a blow to the posterior aspect of the elbow.

METHODS OF TREATMENT

The treatment of fractures of the olecranon has run the gamut from early range of motion of the elbow without regard for the fracture[403,487,523] to precise and open anatomic reduction of the fracture site.[410,484,518,541,542]

Olecranon fractures were mentioned only occasionally in the very early treatises on fracture treatment. Before the era of aseptic surgery, these fractures were splinted in full extension for 4 to 6 weeks.[501] This usually resulted in a stiff elbow with loss of flexion and was the prime reason that early practitioners slowly began to use the position of mid-flexion.[484] This frequently led to nonunion of the olecranon because of separation of fracture fragments, resulting in decreased power of the triceps mechanism.[523]

In 1894, Sachs[487] reported excellent results with rapid restoration of function by dispensing with any form of splinting, allowing the arm to hang in extension, and instituting early massage. After 2 weeks, active movements were started; Sachs reported that full function returned in 6 weeks. This article was written before the discovery of roentgenography, and most of these cases probably represented fibrous union with resultant decreased strength of the olecranon. However, Eliot[487] reported rapid return to relatively normal flexion and extension of the elbow following this treatment regimen, regardless of whether fibrous or bony union resulted. In 1933 Daland[483] presented the first substantial series of olecranon fractures, in which he delineated the signs and symptoms and first recognized the need for accurate reduction of any displaced fracture.

Watson-Jones[538] believed that reduction by closed manipulation could often be achieved with the elbow in full extension with firm pressure over the fragment. He believed that conservative treatment was justified only if the position was accurate. Immobilization was continued for 5 weeks. He noted also that full flexion would be delayed for a year and that the elbow frequently required gentle manipulation at intervals for maximum return.

Undisplaced Fractures

Most authors believe that undisplaced fractures as defined previously are best treated by immobilization in a long-arm cast with the elbow in 45° to 90° of flexion for a short time.[468,471] The elbow should not be placed in full extension for immobilization because stiffness is likely and because, in general, if a fracture is not stable in partial flexion, it will not be stable in full extension.[484]

A follow-up x-ray should be obtained within five to seven days after cast application to make certain that displacement has not occurred. Bony union is usually not complete for 6 to 8 weeks, but generally there is adequate stability at 3 weeks to remove the cast and allow protected range-of-motion exercises, avoiding flexion past 90° until bone healing is complete radiographically. In elderly patients, the period of immobilization should be even less than 3 weeks. A sling can be used for a few days until the patient is comfortable enough to begin active range of motion of the elbow.[527]

Displaced Fractures

Open reduction and internal fixation or primary excision has generally become accepted as the treatment of choice for displaced fractures of the olecranon.[500] There are several disadvantages of nonoperative treatment. (1) Failure to reduce the fracture may allow it to heal in an elongated position by means of a fibrous union; this shortens the distance between the origin and insertion of the triceps muscle, which effectively decreases its power of extension.[523] (2) Articular incongruity secondary to inadequate reduction can lead to post-traumatic arthritis.[488,542] (3) A displaced olecranon fragment can block full extension of the elbow joint.[399,523] (4) Immobilization in full extension for a period sufficient to allow bone healing frequently

results in failure to regain flexion of the elbow. Despite these factors, Perkins[523] and Rowe[527] both suggested conservative treatment of displaced olecranon fractures in elderly patients because the loss of full extension and decreased triceps power are not important in this age group. Rowe[527] stated that simple sling immobilization is all that is needed in these patients.

In an active patient, the aims of treatment of displaced fractures of the olecranon are (1) to maintain power of extension of the elbow, (2) to avoid incongruity of the articular surface, (3) to restore stability of the elbow, and (4) to prevent stiffness of the joint. To achieve this final, and perhaps most important, goal, any mode of internal fixation selected should, ideally, allow the patient to resume protected range of motion reasonably soon after open reduction.[500]

INTERNAL FIXATION

The dilemma of nonunion versus stiffness led Lister in 1884 to choose the fracture of the olecranon to be the first fracture treated by open reduction and internal fixation using his method of antisepsis.[501] Lister provided fixation of the fragment with a wire loop (Fig. 10-41). This method of treatment was modified somewhat as the wire was placed in the form of a ring by Berger in 1902[472] and was later adopted by Böhler in 1929.[473] Modifications of this technique, which was the forerunner of the tension-

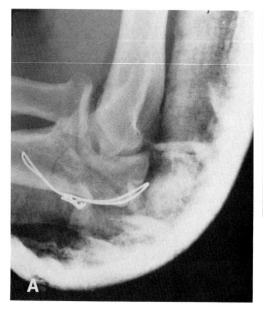

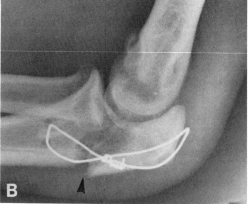

Fig. 10-41. (**A**) Good approximation of a large olecranon fragment by means of a figure-of-eight wire. (**B**) Two months later there is considerable displacement at the fracture site (*arrow*), indicating inadequate fixation by the wire.

band wiring technique advocated by the AO group,[484,518] are now in use.

Multiple methods of internal fixation have been proposed for olecranon fractures. The mechanical advantage that exists in favor of the triceps pull on the small proximal fragment dictates the need for strong internal fixation to prevent displacement of the fracture postoperatively.[525] The surgical principles used in the internal fixation of olecranon fractures include the following[542]:

1. Realignment of the longitudinal axis of the olecranon as accurately as possible and with sufficient stability to allow early controlled motion
2. Preservation of an adequately large coronoid process to form the distal limit of the articular surface
3. Anatomic restoration of the articular surface of the olecranon with the use of cancellous bone grafts to fill in defects in the articular surface

After internal fixation of the fracture, exact surgical repair of the medial and lateral triceps expansion is essential for a good result.

Biomechanics. Two studies[493,520] have attempted to compare the mechanical stability of methods of internal fixation for olecranon fractures. Fyfe and colleagues[493] tested *stiffness* of the configuration. Based on that criterion, the two-knot tension-band technique, as described in the AO technique manual,[518] was optimal. The one-third tubular plate was also quite rigid and optimal in fractures with simulated comminution. Murphy and colleagues[520] used a rapid tension method of testing, measuring *energy-to-failure*, and concluded that the tension-band wiring according to the AO technique[518] and the combination of a 6.5-mm cancellous screw with tension-band wire were essentially equal and optimal. They did not test one-third tubular plate fixation. The method of testing in both of these studies did not include *fatigue analysis*, which is probably the most common mode of failure of the fixation device.

Internal Suture. Rombold[529] was the first to publish a description of the use of the fascial strip suture to repair displaced olecranon fractures. In 1969 Bennett[471] also recommended the use of a fascial strip for internal fixation to avoid the use of metallic internal fixation and its inherent problems. Approximation of the fragments has been attempted with a variety of materials, including fascia, wire, catgut, and nonabsorbable sutures.[471,482,501,504,526,539] In general, these do not provide true internal fixation that is rigid enough to allow early motion, and their use is not recommended.

Intramedullary Fixation. Fixation of displaced olecranon fractures by the use of an intramedullary screw was introduced by W. Russell MacAusland in 1942.[511] Many types of intramedullary devices have also been used, including Rush rods,[529] cancellous (wood) screws,[512,525] large threaded Steinmann pins,[495] and several types of screws designed especially for olecranon fractures[481,495] (Fig. 10-42). The Leinbach screw, which is long enough to gain adequate purchase in the distal fragment, has been known to break at the shank-screw junction.[475,528] Indeed, Rettig and colleagues[525] reported that 50% of patients in whom a malleable screw was used had significant complications. Therefore, if an intramedullary screw is used, these authors recommended that it be long enough to obtain purchase in the medullary canal of the distal ulna and strong enough to resist breakage. They suggested a rigid cancellous compression screw for this purpose.[492] McAtee[481] designed a special compression screw that provides stable internal fixation and permits early range of motion. Johnson and coworkers[503] treated 16 patients with an intramedullary 6.5 cancellous AO (ASIF) screw with good results. He also emphasized the importance of a screw of sufficient length to engage the distal intramedullary canal for adequate fixation.

Bicortical Screw Fixation. In 1969, Taylor and Scham[534] described a modified method of screw fixation for fractures of the olecranon. They advocated its use particularly in transverse and oblique fractures, which occur most frequently at or near the junction of the olecranon and the coronoid processes. Their method uses a posteromedial surgical approach, which allows direct visualization not only of the fracture site but also of the coronoid process. A cortical bone screw is passed from the posterior tip of the olecranon obliquely to engage the anterior cortex of the coronoid process near the sublime tubercle (Fig. 10-43). Wadsworth[536] designed a special screw to obtain this type of bicortical fixation of olecranon fractures. The strong internal fixation achieved with this method allows active range of motion by the patient within 10 to 14 days after operation.

Tension-Band Wiring. Tension-band wiring, a method of internal fixation developed by the AO

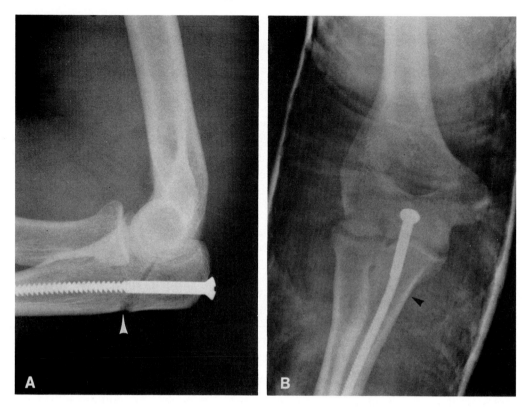

Fig. 10-42. (**A**) Olecranon fracture transfixed with a Leinbach screw. Note the proximity of the fracture site and the junction of the thread and shank of the screw (*arrow*). (**B**) The anteroposterior view shows angulation of the threaded portion of the screw in the medullary canal (*arrow*). Breakage of the screw at the point of angulation and loss of fixation are likely.

group,[496,505,518] differs significantly in technique and principle from conventional cerclage wiring. It is particularly useful in treatment of avulsion fractures. The basic principle is to counteract the tensile forces that act across the fracture site and convert them into compressive forces. To accomplish this, the wire is passed in figure-of-eight fashion around the insertion of the triceps tendon and then distally beyond the fracture site into a transverse drill hole on the posterior (subcutaneous) border of the olecranon (Fig. 10-44). Improved alignment and greater stability can be provided by introducing two parallel Kirschner wires across the fracture site before applying the tension band.[475,476,484,496,514,518] It might seem that this posterior position of the wire would cause the fracture site to gape at the articular surface in the semilunar notch. At the time of operation, this may occur, but the counterpressure of the trochlea under tension by the triceps muscle causes a compression force across the fracture site sufficiently strong to allow immediate active range of motion.[496] As an alternative, Rowland[528] has suggested placing the tension-band wire volar to the long axis and longitudinal pins. A modification of this technique in which both limbs of the figure of eight are twisted has been introduced to allow the wire to be tightened from both sides of the fracture and thereby achieve equal compression.[476,484,496,505]

Several authors have reported problems associated with wire protrusion and pain following tension-band wiring.[502,513,545] Macko and Szabo[513] noted that patients had pain even without proximal migration of the pins. Most authors have emphasized the importance of placing the tension wire deep to the triceps and curling the longitudinal pins so that they are embedded in bone. Even with these measures, many patients require hardware removal.

Murphy and associates[519] reported the use of a 6.5-mm cancellous screw with tension-band wiring in ten patients. In this series, there were fewer complications with prominent hardware as com-

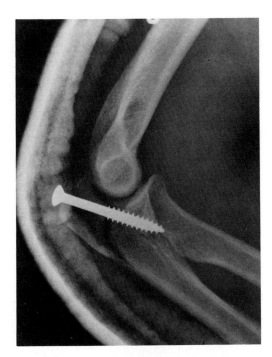

Fig. 10-43. Bicortical fixation of an olecranon fracture. In this case, the threads of the screw cross the fracture site, which is undesirable unless the proximal fragment is overdrilled to give a lag effect.

pared to the use of K-wires at the same institution, though removal was still necessary in some.

Zuelzer Plate. In 1951 Zuelzer first reported the use of a hook plate for fixation of fractures in which one small fragment was separated from the principal part of the bone.[546] This device has since been recommended for fixation of olecranon fractures.[484,541] Weseley and colleagues[541] reported uniformly good results regardless of the degree of comminution, the obliquity of the fracture, or age of the patient. They believed that the advantage of the Zuelzer plate over the tension-band wiring technique was that it did not require supplemental fixation, which is often needed when tension-band wiring is applied to comminuted olecranon fractures.

AO Plate. A one-third tubular plate can be a very useful implant in cases of comminution or oblique longitudinal fractures.[493,496] Where there is comminution with bone loss, the tension-band technique tends to compress and shorten the olecranon. With the use of the plate posteriorly (Fig. 10-45) or on the posterolateral border, adequate rigidity

can usually be achieved with restoration of the anatomy. Bone grafting to compensate for bone loss can also be incorporated with the construct.

Excision. Excision of the proximal fragment and repair of the triceps tendon for a fractured olecranon (Fig. 10-46) was first suggested by Fiolle[491] in 1918. Dunn[486] in 1939 and Wainwright[537] in 1942 each described several cases using this technique; excellent results were reported. Excision of the proximal fragment and triceps repair were popularized in the United States by McKeever and Buck[516] in a classic article in 1947. Their indications for this method of treatment in olecranon fractures were (1) old ununited fractures, (2) extensively comminuted fractures, (3) fractures in elderly people, and (4) any fracture that did not involve the trochlear notch. They were the first to investigate and substantiate the idea that instability of the elbow joint does not result as long as the coronoid process and distal surface of the semilunar notch of the ulna remain intact. They stated that as much as 80% of the olecranon can be removed without danger of producing instability of the elbow joint.[480,516] Lou[510] later reported good results with this technique if the excised fragment was small.

MacAusland and Wyman[512] studied fractures of the olecranon extensively, with particular attention to excising the proximal fragments.[467,468] On the basis of these studies, they made several useful points, as follows, regarding excision of the olecranon.

Much of the olecranon process can be excised as long as the coronoid and anterior soft tissues are intact.

The triceps tendon should be securely reattached to the distal fragment with nonabsorbable sutures; wire is not recommended, since motion of the elbow will cause it to break.[470]

Excision is indicated *only* for isolated fractures of the olecranon. If there is evidence of damage to the anterior structures of the elbow (ie, if there is anterior dislocation of the radial head and shaft of the ulna, ie, a fracture–dislocation of the elbow), primary excision is definitely contraindicated.

Active motion is allowed immediately after operation, but acute flexion is not permitted for several weeks.[470]

MacAusland further pointed out that occasionally during attempted internal fixation, comminution of the olecranon proves more extensive than was initially anticipated, and the surgeon's inability to achieve rigid internal fixation becomes apparent. In such cases, he believes it is better to admit defeat,

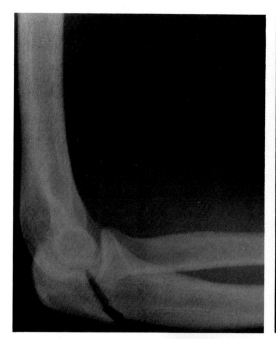
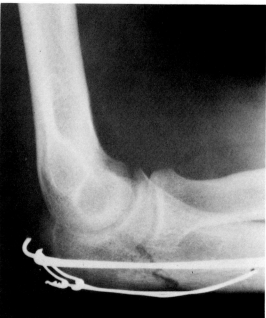
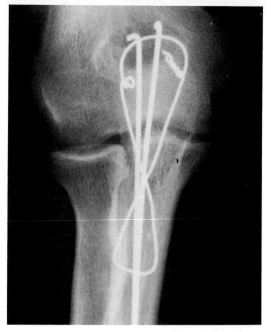
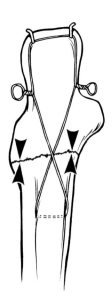

Fig. 10-44. (*Top left*) Oblique fracture of the olecranon. (*Top right*) Open reduction and internal fixation using the AO tension band wiring method of fixation. (*Bottom*) Anteroposterior view demonstrating a modification of the tension band wiring technique in which both limbs of the figure-of-eight wire are twisted. This permits the wire to be tightened on both sides of the fracture to achieve equal compression (note the *arrows*).

as it were, and do a primary excision of the olecranon rather than to persist with a technique that is likely to be unsatisfactory.[470,471,478]

The advantages of excision are that it is an easy and rapid procedure, and it eliminates the possibility of delayed or nonunion and posttraumatic arthritis.[471,478,500,516,535] The disadvantages of excision are said to be triceps weakness, elbow insta-

bility, and loss of elbow motion.[471,498,500,512] However, Rettig and colleagues[525] found elbow motion to be equal following internal fixation or excision. In addition, Gartsman and associates[494] found range of motion, elbow stability, and strength to be equal in patients who underwent open reduction compared with those who underwent excision. However, patients who underwent internal fixation had

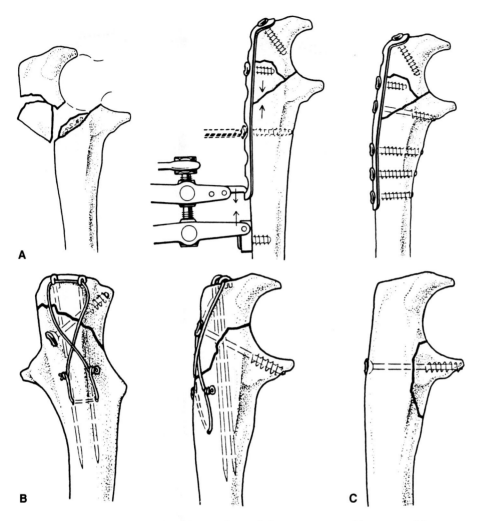

Fig. 10-45. (**A**) Plate fixation can be used to stabilize comminuted fractures of the proximal ulna. (**B**) A combination of screws and wires can also be used. (**C**) Lag screw fixation of the coronoid may be crucial to stability if the fracture is associated with elbow dislocation. *(Heim, U., and Pfeiffer, K.M.: Internal Fixation of Small Fractures, 3rd ed. Berlin, Springer-Verlag, 1988.)*

a much higher incidence of postoperative complications.

During excision, it is important to retain the insertion of the collateral ligaments for stability. The triceps tendon should also be sutured to the remaining bone flush with the articular surface.

AUTHORS' PREFERRED METHOD OF TREATMENT

Undisplaced Fractures

We prefer to treat undisplaced fractures of the olecranon with a short period of immobilization followed by early protected range of motion.

Avulsion Fractures

Generally, the proximal fragment is rather small, and avulsion fractures can be treated adequately either by excision of the fragment and repair of the triceps tendon[537] or by tension-band wiring. Both techniques allow early active range of motion, which is particularly desirable, because most of these fractures occur in older patients.

Transverse Fractures

Transverse fractures are ideally suited to stable internal fixation by tension-band wiring. The modification suggested by Weber provides improved

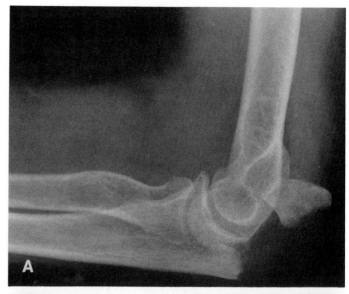

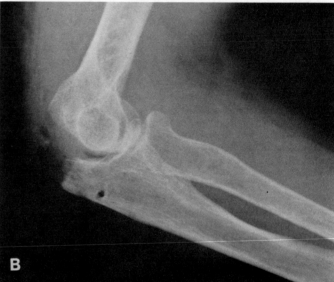

Fig. 10-46. Fracture of the olecranon with rotation of the proximal fragment. (**A**) Lateral view shows wide retraction of the proximal fragment with the elbow in flexion. (**B**) This patient was treated by primary resection of the olecranon fragment and reattachment of the triceps tendon.

fracture rigidity.[484,505] One of us (RNH) prefers the use of a 6.5-mm cancellous screw in combination with the tension-band wiring.

Oblique Fractures

Oblique fractures lend themselves particularly well to bicortical screw fixation.[534] Intramedullary fixation can be quite satisfactory in the simple oblique fracture without comminution. If this method is used, we prefer a large AO cancellous screw that obtains good purchase in the medullary canal of the distal ulna. Stabilization of the oblique fracture with a lag screw before tension-band wiring markedly improves stability.

If there is insufficient obliquity for at least two strong lag screws, a one-third tubular plate can supplement stability. The surgeon should use the technique with which he or she is most familiar.

Comminuted Fractures

Isolated comminuted fractures (ie, those without dislocation of the ulna and radial head and without disruption of the anterior soft tissues) are best treated by excision of the olecranon and secure reattachment of the triceps tendon with nonabsorbable suture to allow early active motion. It is important to retain the collateral ligaments, especially the anteromedial portion for stability.

If the fracture includes part of the ulnar shaft and excision of the olecranon is not possible, AO plate stabilization of the distal fragment combined with tension-band wiring has proved very useful[505] (Fig. 10-47). This technique is also applicable to fracture–dislocations. When comminution or instability precludes a standard approach, a creative combination of lag screws, wires, and plates should be considered. With comminution or bone loss, it is also helpful to have the patient prepared for iliac crest bone grafting if necessary.

Fracture–Dislocations

Fracture–dislocations present a challenging therapeutic problem because of the severe combination of bone and soft tissue damage. Open reduction and internal fixation with restoration of alignment and stability of the ulna is important.[529,543] This can be achieved by the use of some form of intramedullary device or a long screw anchored in the distal medullary canal of the ulna.[543] Primary excision of the olecranon fracture is thought to be contraindicated for fear of anterior translocation of both the radius and ulna.[477,543] Late excision of the olecranon can be considered after healing of the anterior soft tissue structures is complete.

Open Fractures

Many fractures of the olecranon that require open reduction are open because of direct trauma. We do not routinely recommend internal fixation of open fractures, but because these are intra-articular fractures and often result in complete instability of the elbow joint, internal fixation of the fracture after extensive irrigation and débridement is preferred. If the wound is contaminated, it is better to leave the wound open and return in two to three days for a delayed primary closure. Antibiotic coverage should be started preoperatively and continued for 48 to 72 hours postoperatively.

Because most failures of fixation that require reoperation occur in the first postoperative week, x-rays are taken routinely two or three days postoperatively as recommended by Rettig and colleagues.[525]

COMPLICATIONS

Complications of olecranon fractures are mainly decreased range of motion, posttraumatic arthritis,

and nonunion.[475] It is hoped that loss of motion can be minimized by firm internal fixation and early range of motion of the joint.[505] Eriksson and colleagues[488] reported that up to 50% of patients have limited range of motion of the elbow following olecranon fractures, generally with loss of extension. However, in their series, the limitations were not great, and only 3% were aware of it.

Development of posttraumatic arthritis in the elbow is not as common (or perhaps not as noticeable) as in a weight-bearing joint. If reduction to less than 2 mm offset cannot be obtained, the possibility of arthritis developing later is significant. In the event of articular cartilage and bone loss, cancellous grafting in the defect may provide a fibrocartilaginous surface after graft revascularization.[542]

Nonunion of the olecranon has been reported to occur in 5% of olecranon fractures.[488] The treatment of a nonunion should be suited to the patient. In a young, active patient the pseudarthrosis may be taken down and the fracture site reapproximated and held with a tension-band wire or a suitable intramedullary device. Because most of the olecranon is cancellous, bone grafting is seldom needed. If the proximal fragment is large enough, an AO (ASIF) plate may be used with bone grafting (Fig. 10-48).

Excision of the proximal portion of the pseudarthrosis and repair of the triceps tendon is also an acceptable method of management, especially in older patients.

Ulnar nerve symptoms, generally in the form of numbness or paresthesias, have been reported in 10% of patients.[488] These symptoms usually clear spontaneously and require no definitive treatment.

RADIAL HEAD FRACTURES

The proper management of fractures of the radial head is difficult and controversial. The radial head is intra-articular and participates in both flexion and extension as well as forearm rotation; therefore, anatomic restoration of the joint surface and early motion would normally be our guiding principle. Unfortunately, the size, location, and shape of radial head fractures often preclude internal fixation with early motion. Excision, therefore, is the more common operative alternative and remains controversial. The commonly asked questions are: (1) Which fractures should be excised? (2) When should excision be performed, and when should internal fixation be attempted? (3) Should a prosthetic replacement be used?

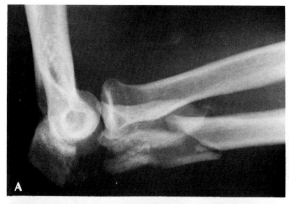
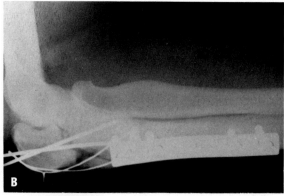

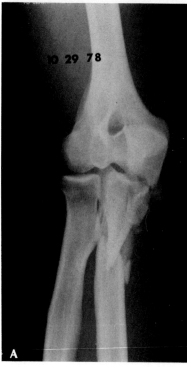
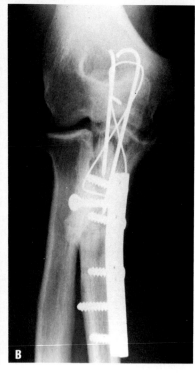

Fig. 10-47. (**A**) Severely comminuted fracture of the olecranon. (**B**) The distal fracture has been stabilized using an AO plate. This essentially converts the comminuted fracture to an oblique fracture of the olecranon, which is then stabilized using the tension-band wiring technique.

(continued)

Ligamentous injury in the elbow and forearm is often associated with radial head fracture. The decision to excise is also influenced by the presence of concomitant injury and its degree of severity. Because of increased recognition of the problems after radial head excision, there is currently more emphasis on preservation of the radial head after fracture.

ANATOMY AND BIOMECHANICS

The radial head is seated in the lesser sigmoid notch and maintains contact with the ulna throughout forearm pronation and supination. Some thought radiocapitellar contact was present only at extremes of flexion, but Morrey and colleagues,[17] using a more dynamic testing model, demonstrated force transmission at all angles, the greatest in full extension. In that same study, pronation also seemed to increase contact and force transmission.

Longitudinal force in grip or lifting activities is transmitted from the wrist to the elbow with load shared by both the radius and ulna. The specific load sharing between the ulna and radius is probably influenced by the position of the forearm in flexion and extension and pronation and supina-

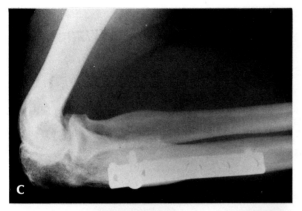

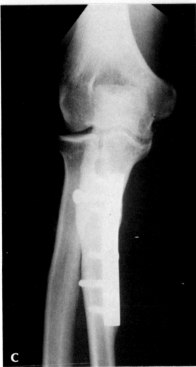

Fig. 10-47 *(continued)*
(C) A follow-up anteroposterior view demonstrates good maintenance of joint congruity.

tion[7,8,17] as well as the relative tension in the biceps. After radial head excision, the central bands of the interosseous membrane help stabilize the radius, resisting proximal translation.[8]

The radial head also contributes to valgus stability when tested in the laboratory,[9,15,17] but the relative contribution *in vivo* is not known (see Fig. 10-5).

Mechanical testing of prosthetic implants has questioned the efficacy of silicone prostheses. Val-gus stability was not enhanced *in vitro* by silicone radial head implants in two independent studies.[592,624] Use of the silicone prosthesis to prevent proximal translation of the radius has also been challenged in the laboratory.[561,591]

MECHANISM OF INJURY

Fractures of the radial head are most frequently caused by direct longitudinal loading—a fall on the outstretched hand (Fig. 10-49). In addition, any injury that causes dislocation of the elbow can also result in fracture of the radial head.

CLASSIFICATION

In 1924 Speed[632] proposed a classification based on two factors—the amount of head involvement, marginal or complete, and the degree of displacement. In 1954 Mason[604] combined these into a single scheme. In 1962, Johnston[594] added elbow dislocation as a type IV fracture.

Type I: Fissure or marginal sector fractures without displacement
Type II: Marginal fractures with displacement
Type III: Comminuted fractures of the whole head
Type IV: Any of the above with elbow dislocation

This classification is useful for treatment of types I and III, but as Mason[604] himself noted, it is not as helpful in directing care for type II fractures. He believed that the existence of a mechanical block was an important factor when considering excision but did not include this factor in his classification. The addition of the type IV classification stressed the increased complexity of the injury when associated with an elbow dislocation. No existing classification accounts for associated injury to the interosseous membrane of the forearm and ligaments of the distal radioulnar joint.

A more useful approach may be to account for the mechanical block and associated injuries in a somewhat different scheme (see Authors' Preferred Method of Treatment).

SIGNS AND SYMPTOMS

Isolated fractures of the radial head usually cause pain on the lateral side of the elbow aggravated by forearm rotation. The examiner must be suspicious and palpate the radial head while passively rotating the forearm. Occasionally, motion elicits painful crepitus. When the fracture is associated with more massive trauma, such as elbow dislocation, the

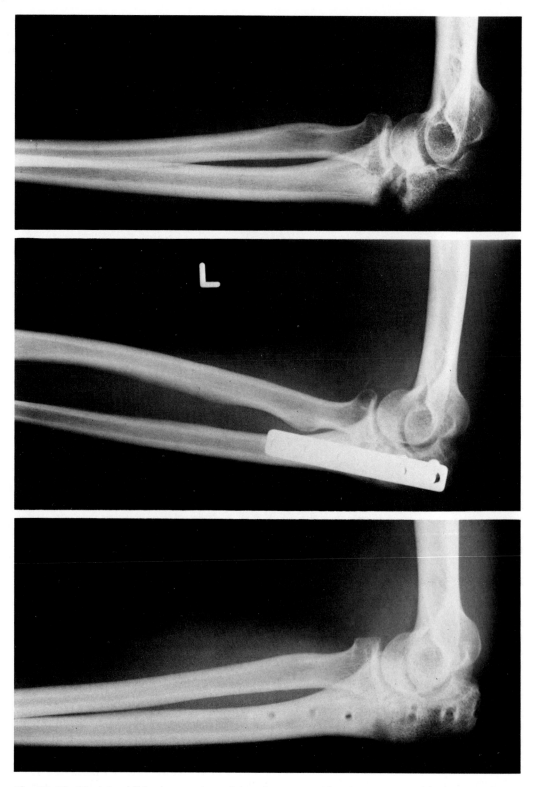

Fig. 10-48. (*Top*) Established nonunion of the olecranon with a large proximal fragment. (*Center*) Articular congruity was reestablished and solid bony union achieved with an AO (ASIF) dynamic compression plate (DCP). (*Bottom*) Follow-up 1 year after plate removal.

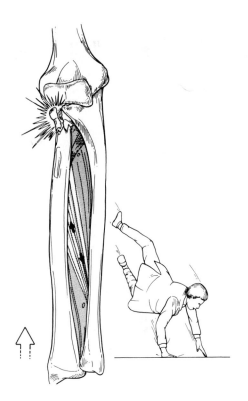

Fig. 10-49. A fall that produces a radial head fracture also can strain or rupture the interosseous membrane (*black arrows*).

swelling and pain can be substantial, precluding adequate palpation or forearm rotation. The forearm and wrist should also be examined for pain and swelling. If wrist pain is present, it is likely that acute radioulnar dissociation occurred and the forearm is unstable.

RADIOGRAPHIC EXAMINATION

X-rays in the anteroposterior and lateral planes of the elbow are usually sufficient to diagnose the fracture. However, if a fat pad sign is present without a noticeable fracture, radiocapitellar views may be helpful. As described by Greenspan and Norman,[31] the radiocapitellar view is taken with the forearm in neutral rotation and the x-ray tube angled 45° cephalad. Posterior elbow dislocation or fracture of the capitellum should also arouse suspicion.[225,627,646] If wrist or forearm pain is present, x-rays of the wrist in the neutral-rotation view should also be taken.

Additional studies may be useful to delineate and quantify the amount of displacement and the size of the fragments. Trispiral polytomography with 2-mm sections in the anteroposterior and lateral planes can be quite helpful. Carefully oriented CT scans using axial cuts may provide additional information.[30] Magnetic resonance imaging (MRI) scans have not yet been widely reported for analysis in acute trauma of the elbow.

METHODS OF TREATMENT

Type I—Nondisplaced Fractures

Retrospective studies of radial head fractures since Thomas in 1905 have concluded that nonoperative treatment of type I fractures (Fig. 10-50) is best.* Some favored immobilization for 2 to 4 weeks in cast.[596,629] In 1939, Eliason and North[595] advocated early motion, but it was Mason and Shutkin's[603] 1943 series with sling immobilization and active motion as early as tolerated that established this as the preferred method of treatment. Since then, few have questioned this practice. Most authors believe that early motion helps to shape and mold slight incongruities without substantial risk of greater displacement.

In addition to early active motion, Postlethwait[622] and others[547,579,589,597,608,621,625] advocated acute aspiration of the hemarthrosis and installation of local anesthetic to reduce pain and assist early active motion. In a prospective study of 80 patients, Holdsworth and colleagues[589] demonstrated that aspiration and injection of local anesthetic increased comfort and improved the initial range of motion but that this practice did not enhance the final outcome.

Most patients with type I fractures can expect good to excellent function after 2 to 3 months of active-motion exercises. Minimal loss of extension is not uncommon and some have occasional pain, aggravated by cold or stress. However, some patients with type I fractures do poorly. Contracture, pain, and inflammation can occur, despite what appears to be a well-aligned, minimally displaced fracture. Radin and Riseborough[626] attributed this to displacement of the fracture, which can occur but is rare.[570] Currey and colleagues[572] reported a patient with an inflammatory condition that histopathologically resembled rheumatoid-like arthritis after an isolated radial head fracture with minimal displacement.

* References 547, 548, 550, 559, 565, 570, 573, 575, 578–580, 584, 588, 593, 594, 596, 598, 603, 604, 608, 616, 617, 623, 626, 629, 632, 640, 643, 645, 647.

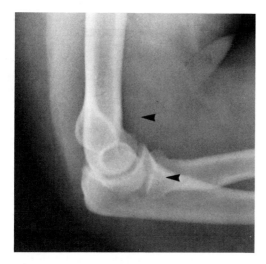

Fig. 10-50. Type I (undisplaced) chisel fracture of the radial head (*lower arrow*). Note the elevation of the anterior fat pad (*upper arrow*), indicating hemarthrosis. The posterior fat pad is small but present.

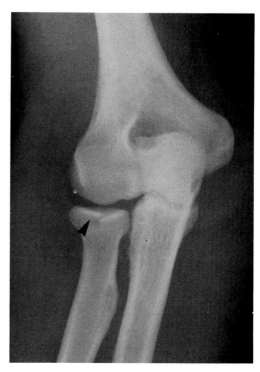

Fig. 10-51. Minimally displaced central depression fracture of the radial head (*arrow*).

In operating on radial head fractures, we have found a high incidence of concomitant osteochondral fractures of the capitellum that were not visible radiographically. This osteocartilaginous impact injury may contribute to a poor result in what otherwise appears to be a simple undisplaced fracture.

Type II—Marginal Fractures With Displacement

The fracture with partial head involvement and displacement (Figs. 10-51 and 10-52) requires careful consideration. The decision to treat with early motion alone or operatively is difficult, and the literature is ambiguous. The principal limitation of the Mason classification is that it provides little guidance for patients with type II fractures. For these fractures, one can find advocates for total excision, partial excision, open reduction with internal fixation, and nonoperative care, each claiming good results. Unfortunately, these series are all retrospective, most affected by drop-out bias and poor specificity of selection criteria.

When Mason[604] examined the results of treatment retrospectively, he concluded that if *any* tilt or displacement was present in fractures involving more than one quarter of the head, excision should be performed. If there was mechanical interference acutely, he recommended immediate excision but did not include this feature in his classification.

Adler and Shaftan and others advocated early motion without excision, even in cases of displacement and comminution.[547,603,645] When pain or a mechanical block was noted later, a delayed excision could then be performed.

The timing of excision has been as controversial as the practice itself. No prospective studies have adequately addressed the question on a comparative basis. Many authors[579,588,626,647] have argued that excision in the first 48 hours was obligatory and that delay would lead to contracture and ectopic calcification. Opposed to this position, Charnley[566] wrote that immediate excision was contraindicated, believing that the physician cannot properly assess the need for excision until 2 weeks after the injury. He recommended that if motion was restricted after 2 weeks, excision should be done at that time. He reported no incidence of ectopic calcification with delayed excision. Adler and Shaftan[547] could find no influence of the timing of excision on outcome. Broberg and Morrey[554] retrospectively evaluated four patients with type II fractures and documented pain relief and some improvement of motion with delayed excision.

Open reduction with internal fixation (Fig. 10-53) has also been recommended for type II fractures by several authors.[558,606,618,619,630] This procedure is

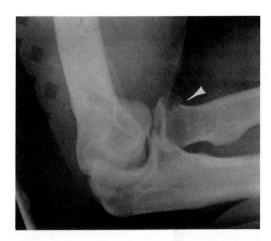

Fig. 10-52. An isolated fracture of the radial head can involve more than 50% of the articular surface (type II) and not require excision if there is no mechanical block.

technically difficult and should be undertaken with care. When concomitant instability exists, either with longitudinal radioulnar dissociation or elbow dislocation, preservation of the radial head can be quite useful and may help to provide needed stability.[619] However, the few, small series in the literature attest to the few fractures that are amenable to open reduction with stable internal fixation.

Small AO (ASIF) screws have been used,[630] and others have employed the Herbert screw for internal fixation of the type II fracture.[558,606] Because the side of the radial head must articulate with the ulna in the lesser sigmoid notch, the Herbert screw is useful because the head of the screw can be countersunk beneath the articular surface. The fragment must be large enough to accommodate the large end of the screw without further fragmentation. One problem with internal fixation is that the location of the fracture may preclude access for insertion of the screw.

Type III—Comminuted Fractures of the Whole Head

Unlike with the type II fracture, there is less disagreement in the literature concerning the proper treatment of comminuted fractures of the radial head (Fig. 10-54). Early excision with immediate motion is nearly universally recommended. A few authors have suggested that early motion after sling immobilization is preferable to early excision, but the number of patients in these series treated in this fashion is small[547,594] and, based on the literature alone, it is difficult to justify this approach. Internal fixation after open reduction is usually precluded because of comminution (Fig. 10-55).

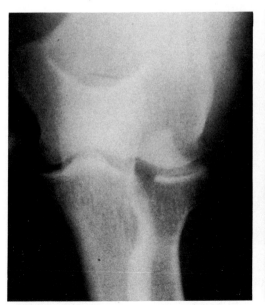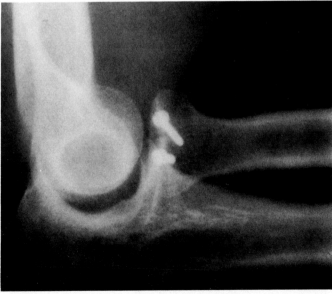

Fig. 10-53. (*Left*) Displaced type II fracture of the radial head with a single fracture line (*right*) treated by open reduction and internal fixation with two AO (ASIF) minifragment screws.

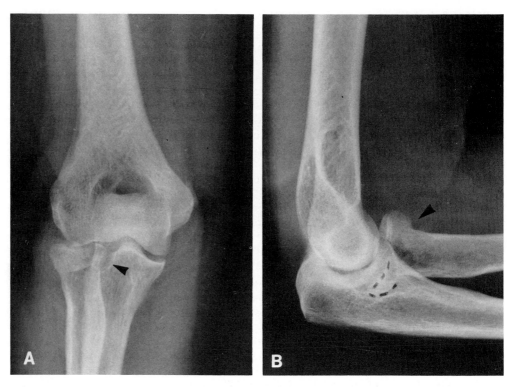

Fig. 10-54. (**A**) Type III (comminuted) fracture of the radial head (*arrow*). (**B**) A lateral view of the same fracture (*arrow*) shows marked displacement not appreciated on the anteroposterior view.

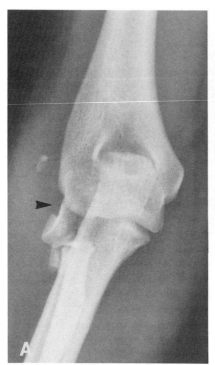

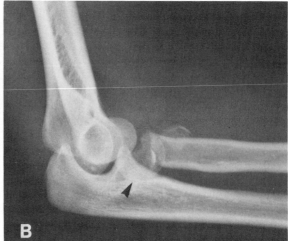

Fig. 10-55. (**A**) Markedly comminuted and displaced fracture of the radial head (*arrow*) and neck. (**B**) The lateral view shows the fracture of the radial neck and rotation of the radial head (*arrow*).

RADIAL HEAD EXCISION AND PROSTHETIC REPLACEMENT

Prosthetic replacement of the radial head was proposed by Speed[633] in 1941 in an attempt to restore radiocapitellar contact and prevent proximal translation of the radius. He implanted ferrule caps over the neck of the radius but found that they displaced and caused inflammation. Others reported the use of metal and acrylic prostheses for radial head replacement, primarily indicated after acute dissociation between the radius and ulna.[551,562,563,567,568] None of these early prostheses seemed to stand the test of time and use.

In the 1970s use of the Swanson silicone rubber prosthesis was reported in several small series with good results.[601,602,644] Interestingly, Mackay and associates[601] noted that despite use of the prosthesis, 4 of the 16 patients demonstrated more than 4 mm of proximal translation of the radius. Sowa and associates[631] also reported several patients with continued proximal translation of the radius, despite use of the prosthesis.

As experience grew with the prosthesis, more reports of material failure and dislocation were published.[552,601,605,612] In addition, particulate synovitis, which had been reported with carpal implants, was also seen in the radial head replacement.[582,648]

The theoretic value of the prosthesis was to improve valgus stability and prevent proximal translation of the radius. However, several independent biomechanical studies have now questioned the mechanical efficacy of the silicone replacement in resisting valgus stress and proximal translation of the radius[561,591,592,624] (Fig. 10-56).

AUTHOR'S PREFERRED METHOD OF TREATMENT

When first examining the patient with a reported radial head fracture, it is important to look for associated injuries of the elbow and forearm. Combination injuries are more common in high-energy trauma but can occur after a simple fall. A more complete examination with less discomfort to the patient can usually be achieved after anesthetizing the elbow joint with aspiration of the hemarthrosis and intra-articular injection of 0.5% Marcaine (Fig. 10-57). The wrist, distal radioulnar joint, and interosseous membrane of the forearm should be examined for tenderness or swelling. If either is present, one should suspect acute radioulnar dissociation.

After examination of the forearm, the medial ligaments of the elbow should be gently palpated for

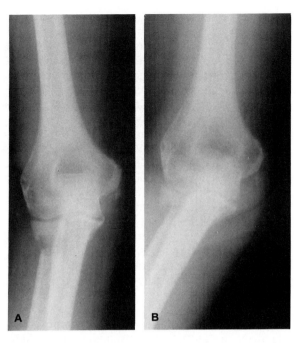

Fig. 10-56. A silicone radial head implant was used in this patient in an attempt to prevent valgus instability (**A**). Six months after injury, stress films (**B**) showed telescoping and compression of the implant, precluding effective capitellar contact. If the prosthesis is used, it is important to excise as little proximal radius as necessary and to use an implant that effectively fills the space.

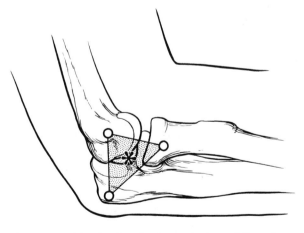

Fig. 10-57. The landmarks for aspiration of the elbow joint are the radial head, lateral epicondyle, and tip of the olecranon. A needle inserted into the center of the triangle (*asterisk*) penetrates only the anconeus muscle and capsule before entering the joint.

swelling or tenderness. If these findings are present, the injury may have been a severe valgus stress causing both a medial ligament tear and radial head fracture. In such patients, there may be greater potential for instability, suggesting greater consideration for radial head preservation.

X-ray interpretation of radial head fractures is quite difficult because of overlapping structures. Positioning of the patient is sometimes difficult because of pain, but a true lateral view is essential. Associated fractures of the capitellum can occur, and the lateral view should be examined for this. It is difficult to judge the degree of comminution and the position of the fragments in many fractures. In these cases, trispiral polytomography can be especially helpful using 2-mm cuts in both the lateral and anteroposterior planes. CT scans can be useful, but the radiologist must orient the gantry carefully to obtain useful information.

Treatment Plan

Mason's[604] classification with a few modifications has been the most frequently quoted and widely adopted scheme since its introduction in 1954. The classification is anatomic and helpful in those patients with uncomplicated undisplaced fractures (type I) and those with severe comminution (type III). In type II fractures, additional emphasis has been placed on degree of displacement, angulation of the fragment, and percentage of head involvement. These are extremely difficult measurements, and no studies to date have prospectively examined the value of subdividing type II fractures with respect to outcome, including Mason's original work. Therefore, even with the modifications and changes suggested, there remains confusion about the treatment of type II fractures. Other authors have also found reason to modify the classification for treatment purposes.[612]

Another drawback is that associated soft tissue injuries of the elbow or forearm do not seem to fit neatly into the otherwise anatomic classification. The radial head can provide stability to the elbow in valgus stress, and in cases in which the anteromedial ligament is disrupted, such as elbow dislocation, preservation of the head may be essential. In cases in which there has been acute dissociation between the radius and ulna (Essex-Lopresti), preservation of the radial head may prevent continued proximal translation of the radius relative to the ulna.

For these reasons, we use a slightly different scheme that attempts to account for more recent information and considers the associated injuries separately.

Factors Influencing Treatment

ANATOMY OF THE FRACTURE
(MASON CLASSIFICATION)

Mason's original classification is used to describe whether or not there is displacement and the degree of comminution. The amount of tilt and the percentage of head involvement are probably important and should be estimated. However, even with polytomography, this is often difficult. In addition to the anatomic description, according to Mason, open reduction with internal fixation may be helpful, dependent on coexistent injuries. It is useful to gauge the suitability for internal fixation, if deemed necessary.

PRESENCE OR ABSENCE OF MECHANICAL BLOCK

The patient can be examined after anesthesia is injected. With the examiner's thumb or fingers over the radial head, gentle passive rotation of the forearm is attempted in several positions of elbow flexion. If there is a definite mechanical block, or severe crepitis, this is noted.

In some cases, the presence of a mechanical block is difficult to judge because of other injuries.

ASSOCIATED INJURIES

Acute Longitudinal Radioulnar Dissociation (ALRUD) (Fig. 10-58).   The forearm should be inspected for signs of acute longitudinal radioulnar dissociation. The wrist must be palpated for tenderness over the distal radioulnar joint and the forearm examined for excessive swelling. X-rays of the wrist in the neutral posteroanterior view can also be helpful. Radiographic comparison with the uninjured side may be necessary (Fig. 10-59).

If there is evidence of injury to the interosseous membrane and distal radioulnar ligaments, radial head preservation becomes more important.

Elbow Dislocation (Medial Ligament Disruption) and/or Fracture of the Coronoid Process.   If there is an associated posterior dislocation (Fig. 10-60), this is usually quite obvious. Injury to the medial collateral ligament with dislocation can be more subtle, and examination for this with gentle palpation, inspecting for swelling and tenderness along the medial elbow, may suggest the diagnosis. It may be helpful to apply valgus stress with anesthesia in an attempt to judge the valgus stability.[21] However,

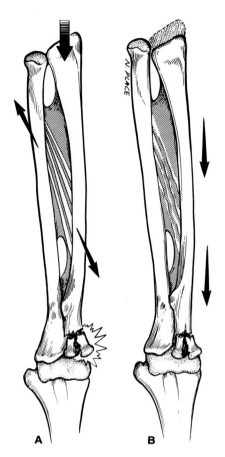

Fig. 10-58. In acute longitudinal radioulnar dissociation (ALRUD), the ligamentous linkage between the radius and ulna may be injured to varying degrees. (**A**) There may be only a sprain without complete disruption. (**B**) Complete dissociation with longitudinal translation and distal radioulnar joint dislocation.

we have found that this is sometimes difficult to interpret under anesthesia with complete loss of tension in the biceps and triceps. Comparison with the uninjured extremity can be helpful and is usually necessary. The combination of medial ligament injury and radial head fracture can lead to gross instability.

A more serious and unstable combination of injuries is the combined radial head fracture, medial ligament disruption, and coronoid process fracture—another "terrible triad." In this situation, there is little to keep the elbow reduced (Fig. 10-61). Open repair and fixation of the coronoid process fracture or reattachment of the brachialis is usually neces-

sary. Direct repair of the medial and lateral ligaments is also usually required. Concomitant excision of the radial head and coronoid process should rarely, if ever, be done, since it may result in marked instability (Fig. 10-62).

Treatment of Specific Fractures

TYPE I FRACTURE (WITH OR WITHOUT ELBOW DISLOCATION)

By definition, type I fractures are not displaced, require no reduction, and should not exhibit any mechanical block to passive forearm rotation. Substantial immediate relief of pain can be provided by aspirating the hematoma and injecting local anesthetic into the joint. The patient is given a sling, or the arm is splinted for a few days. Active forearm rotation is started as soon as tolerated. It is helpful to warn the patient that pain and stiffness can persist for some time and that occasionally the fracture can displace. If weekly gains in range of motion are not occurring, it may be helpful to recommend supervised physical therapy.

Most patients with type I fractures can expect good to excellent function after 2 to 3 months of active-motion exercises. Minimal loss of extension is not uncommon, and some have occasional pain, aggravated by cold or stress. Some patients with type I fractures do poorly. Contracture, pain, and inflammation can occur, despite what appears to be a well-aligned, minimally displaced fracture.

If there was a concomitant posterior elbow dislocation, early motion is still recommended. The healing and rehabilitation process is protracted because of the additional trauma. This injury should be viewed as a posterior elbow dislocation with a radial head fracture, emphasizing care of the dislocation, since the fracture requires no specific intervention, except attention to forearm rotation (see page 782).

TYPE II FRACTURE (WITHOUT ALRUD OR ELBOW DISLOCATION)

Without Mechanical Block. Type II fractures without mechanical block should be treated similarly to type I fractures, as noted previously. Again, the patient should be warned that displacement can occur.

The outcome of fractures of this type is similar to that of the type I fracture, although occasionally the incongruity can result in radiocapitellar ar-

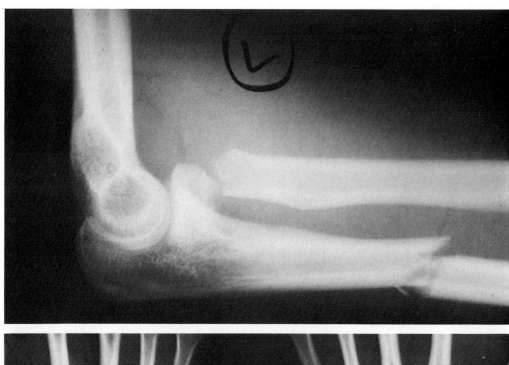

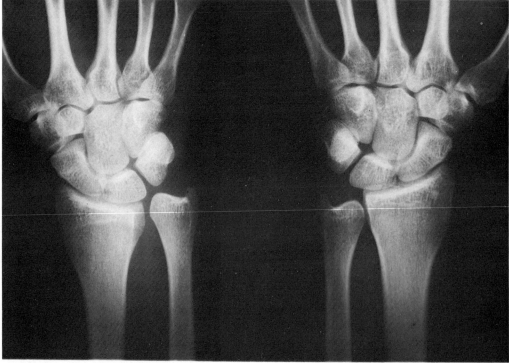

Fig. 10-59. (*Top*) Essex-Lopresti fracture of the radial head (associated with a Monteggia fracture-dislocation in this patient). (*Bottom*) Comparison views of the wrist taken on the day of injury clearly demonstrate proximal migration of the radius and resulting length discrepancy in the radioulnar joint.

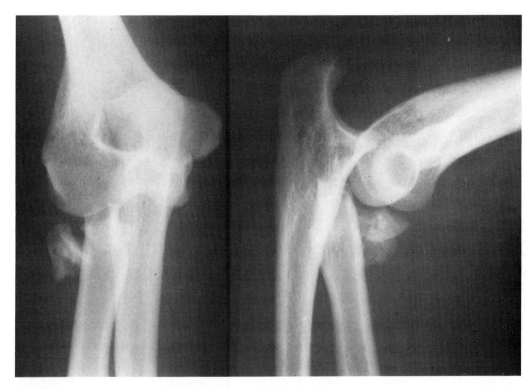

Fig. 10-60. Combination of radial head fracture and elbow dislocation without a coronoid process fracture. In this type of injury, preservation of the radial head should be considered for stability, if technically possible.

throsis and pain. It is helpful to discuss with the patient the possibility of delayed radial head excision.

With Mechanical Block. In the elderly patient, the optimal treatment of the type II fracture with mechanical block is early radial head excision, followed by early active motion. The excision should be performed in the first 24 hours, if possible, to begin immediate range-of-motion therapy.

In younger patients, we consider and evaluate the fracture for internal fixation after open reduction.

When the examination for the presence of a mechanical block is equivocal, it is reasonable to delay excision and follow the patient for several weeks. After the immediate pain and swelling subside, if there is still mechanical limitation, excision can still be performed.

Radial Head Excision. Excision of the radial head is more safely carried out through a posterolateral incision. As Strachan and Ellis[635] noted, the most

vulnerable structure to inadvertent damage is the posterior interosseous nerve. They advised that the incision not extend more than 5 cm distal from the epicondyle. If a more extensile approach is needed, then identification and protection of the nerve should be considered, similar to the posterior (Thompson) approach to the radius.

It is important to remove all fragments and advisable to try to reassemble the excised radial head fragments in order to account for any missing fragments. Intraoperative x-rays can also be helpful if there is any doubt.

Open Reduction and Internal Fixation. Open reduction and internal fixation of the radial head demands patience and careful technique. Before operation, polytomography can be helpful, demonstrating fragmentation and displacement not seen on plain films. We also warn the patient that fixation may not be possible, in which case excision will be necessary. If the reason for attempted internal fixation was to provide stability in the face

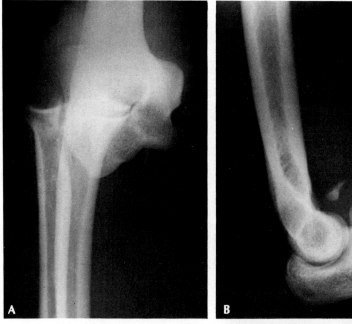

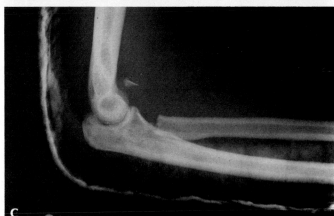

Fig. 10-61. These x-rays illustrate the danger of excising the radial head when there is a concomitant fracture of the coronoid process, even if the coronoid is not removed. (**A**) The initial dislocation film showing a displaced, segmental fracture of the radial head. (**B**) Closed reduction of the elbow. The coronoid process is still markedly displaced. (**C**) The radial head was excised primarily, and the reduced elbow was immobilized in a long-arm splint.

(continued)

of acute dissociation between the radius and ulna or elbow dislocation, but was precluded for technical reasons, insertion of a silicone prosthesis is probably the best alternative. Comminution is often greater than apparent on x-ray or even polytomography, precluding reconstruction. The capitellum may be normal on x-ray but found to be severely damaged on inspection. In these cases, radial head reconstruction may not be indicated.

The size and location of the fragment may also preclude screw fixation with stable, interfragmentary compression. With the use of the Herbert screw, the fragment that accepts the head of the screw must be large enough to not fragment when drilled and tapped. Smaller AO (ASIF) screws can be used for fixation, but the heads of the screws cannot protrude in the zone that articulates with the ulna. Kirschner wires can also be used, but stable fixation is more difficult to achieve with these than with screws.

If internal fixation is precluded for technical reasons and excision performed, proximal translation of the radius can occur despite no apparent injury to the ligaments connecting the radius and ulna.

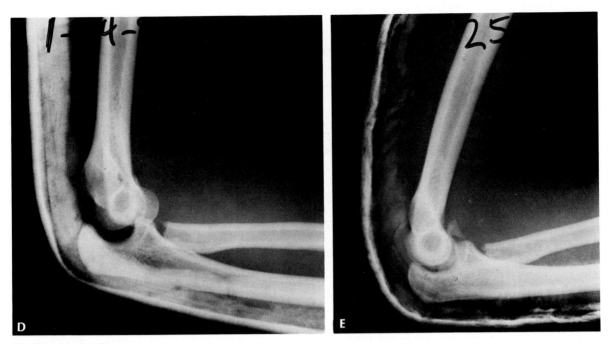

Fig. 10-61 (*continued*)
(**D**) Four days later the elbow resubluxated in the splint. (**E**) On the fifth day the elbow was reduced and held in more flexion.

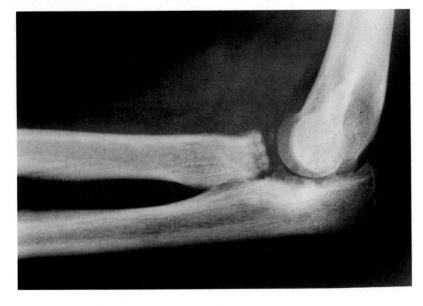

Fig. 10-62. Concomitant excision of the radial head and coronoid process should rarely, if ever, be done, because it may result in severe instability of the elbow joint, as in this patient.

The patient should be warned of this possibility. After excision, early active motion is commenced.

TYPE II FRACTURE WITH ALRUD (ESSEX-LOPRESTI)

Preservation of the radial head is of great importance in these injuries. In most cases, the displaced fragment involves more than 25% of the radial head, and the radius is translated proximally. In these cases, it is helpful to reduce the longitudinal translation first, then to perform open reduction with internal fixation if technically possible. The ulna tends to subluxate dorsally (actually the carpus and radius are volar). Once the fracture of the radial head is fixed, it may be helpful to pin the distal radioulnar joint with the forearm in supination. After 3 weeks, the pins are removed, and gentle forearm rotation is begun, limiting pronation to neutral for 6 weeks.

If the fragment is too small for internal fixation, but displaced and creating mechanical impingement, it would be theoretically better to excise only the fragment, leaving the remaining radial head to protect against proximal migration, although we have had no experience with this procedure, and there are no reports in the literature to document its efficacy.

If the fracture appears to involve less than 25% of the head and there is no mechanical block to motion, we recommend splinting the forearm in full supination for 3 weeks. Then, under supervision, active pronation is allowed to begin from the fully supinated position. It is important to ensure that the distal ulna remains reduced at the distal radioulnar joint during this time. There will likely be some permanent loss of forearm rotation.

TYPE II FRACTURE WITH POSTERIOR ELBOW DISLOCATION

These fractures are generally small fragments off the anterior portion of the radial head. If there is no mechanical block to pronation and supination, we treat this injury as a posterior elbow dislocation.

When the elbow exhibits gross instability and the radial head fracture is large, open reduction with internal fixation should be considered to increase the stability. In these injuries, the coronoid process may also be fractured and the brachialis insertion stripped. In this situation, fixation of the coronoid fracture or reattachment of the brachialis with suture through the ulna can provide critical stability.

If the radial head fracture requires excision, it may be helpful to use the silicone prosthesis for additional support. The use of the prosthesis should be confined to those situations in which, at the time of surgery, the surgeon is convinced that the prosthesis does provide improved stability. To test this during surgery, one should range the elbow with and without the largest acceptable trial prosthesis, applying a valgus stress. During the test, it is important to reestablish tension in the lateral ligamentous complex that was opened (and therefore compromised) to expose the radiocapitellar joint. Using this method, we have found that the prosthesis does not always make a noticeable difference, no matter how theoretically appealing (see Fig. 10-56).

TYPE III FRACTURES WITHOUT ALRUD OR DISLOCATION

For fractures with extensive comminution and displacement without concomitant dislocation or longitudinal dissociation, early excision remains the treatment of choice.

TYPE III FRACTURE WITH ALRUD (ESSEX-LOPRESTI)

As this is written, there is no ideal solution for this combination of injuries. In a type III fracture, the degree of comminution usually requires excision with the subsequent loss of bony support. In rare instances, a two- or three-part fracture can be reconstructed and held with internal fixation. If excision is necessary and performed, continued proximal translation over weeks or months can occur, even with the use of a silicone replacement.[631] The central band of the interosseous membrane has usually been torn and will not likely heal, despite immobilization. It is helpful to warn the patient that the injury is grave and that creation of a radioulnar synostosis with complete loss of forearm rotation may be the only ultimate solution in the months or years ahead.

The decision to excise the radial head in these patients is problematic and should be influenced by the amount of displacement. The radial head, once healed, could provide stability and potentially could prevent symptomatic proximal translation of the radius. Broberg and Morrey[554] have documented that delayed excision of the radial head can provide relief if pain develops, perhaps obviating immediate excision and near-certain chronic instability. However, with most type III fractures, the displacement of the fracture precludes any effective radiocapitellar contact for mechanical stability. In addition, it is necessary to reduce the radius with distal traction and hold it supinated with transfixation pins, to the ulna, preventing any motion and helpful remodeling of the radial head.

The use of the silicone radial head prosthesis is theoretically attractive but is not predictable in preventing proximal translation (Fig. 10-63). With no acceptable alternative currently available, we recommend insertion of the silicone prosthesis with adequate size and firm seating on the proximal radius to act as an effective spacer. Because of the shape of the prosthesis, there is a tendency to use a small size. If the prosthesis is used, the patient should be warned about material failure and continued proximal translation that may ultimately require radioulnar synostosis.

TYPE III FRACTURE WITH ELBOW DISLOCATION

With this combination of injuries, the primary (anteriomedial ligament) and secondary stabilizer (radial head) of the elbow can be compromised leading to gross instability and acute recurrent dislocation (see Fig. 10-61). With excision of the radial head, the base of support against valgus stress is lost (see Fig. 10-5) and "protection" of the healing medial ligament is made more difficult.

To evaluate stability after radial head excision, the surgeon can range the elbow on the operating room table. If it does not dislocate until near 30° of flexion, we do not recommend repair of the medial ligament or use of the silicone prosthesis. All of these elbows will demonstrate valgus instability, but it is the anteroposterior instability that is crucial. Postoperatively, the arm is protected in a hinged orthosis with extension stops. This allows early active motion but protects against valgus stress and recurrent dislocation during capsular healing.

If there is gross anteroposterior instability, it is important to look for injury to the coronoid process or detachment of the brachialis. If this is present, repair of the brachialis insertion or internal fixation of the coronoid should be performed. If the muscle is stripped away without a bony detachment, a Bunnell-type tendon suture can secure the brachialis and be passed through drill holes in the ulna. The medial ligaments can also be repaired with sutures through bone to provide additional stability. In general, we do not repair the medial ligaments after a posterior elbow dislocation (see *Dislocations* on page 782), but we have found that in this setting there is some value in acute repair.

Because the type III radial head fracture is, by definition, comminuted, reduction and internal fixation is usually not an option. It may be helpful to use the silicone prosthesis for additional support, but the use of the prosthesis should be confined to those situations in which, at the time of surgery, the surgeon is convinced that the prosthesis does provide improved stability. To test this during surgery, one should range the elbow with and without the largest acceptable trial prosthesis, applying a mild valgus stress, after repair of the brachialis and medial ligaments. During the test, it is important to hold the lateral capsule of the elbow opposed, giving tension and support to the lateral side of the joint. The lateral ligaments were opened (and therefore compromised) to expose the radiocapitellar joint, and by being open, adds to the instability. Using this method, we have found that the prosthesis does not always make a noticeable difference, no matter how theoretically appealing. If there is a detectable difference, the prosthesis should be of a size that can effectively bear load. It is also necessary to close the lateral capsule snugly around the prosthesis to prevent subluxation.

Frequent postoperative x-rays are mandatory to ensure that the elbow is not dislocating in the splint or cast. Because of the severity of injury, the patient is at high risk for heterotopic bone formation and severe stiffness. During healing and rehabilitation, the orthopaedist is forced to walk a fine line between maximizing early motion and risking recurrent dislocation.

PROXIMAL TRANSLATION OF THE RADIUS—ACUTE AND CHRONIC (RADIOULNAR DISSOCIATION)

Proximal displacement of the radius after radial head fracture or radial head resection has been de-

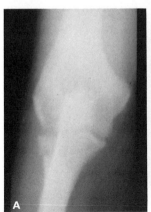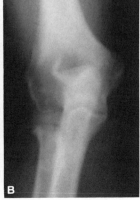

Fig. 10-63. (**A**) A silicone radial head prosthesis was inserted at the time of injury to prevent proximal translation. (**B**) Two years later, symptomatic proximal translation occurred with compression of the prosthesis.

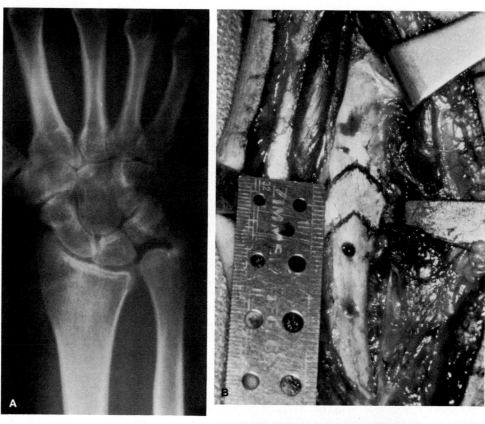

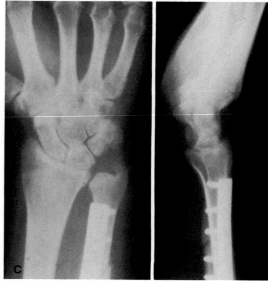

Fig. 10-64. (**A**) Symptomatic proximal translation. (**B,C**) A chevron-type shortening osteotomy was performed with equalization of the radius and ulna at the wrist. (**D**) Several months later, further translation had occurred.

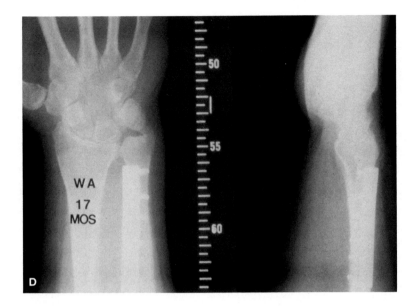

Figure 10-64 (*continued*)

scribed by many investigators over the past 50 years.[549,554,571,574,577,600,601,607,614,626,633,634,638,639] Because of the variable nature of the reports, it is difficult to gauge the incidence of asymptomatic and symptomatic migration, but estimates range from 20% to 90% of patients after radial head resection. Ascertaining the natural history and timing of the proximal translation has not been possible since most reports addressing "proximal migration" did not specify the status of the wrist and forearm ligaments at the time of injury. In addition, it is unclear whether the proximal translation of the radius occurred over the first few weeks, months, or years.

In 1930 Brockman[556] first reported two cases of radioulnar dissociation, the first noted 3 months after injury. Lewis and Thibodeau[600] reported eight patients with proximal translation, but seven of the eight were not skeletally mature at the time of radial head resection and growth retardation may have played a role. In 1941 Speed[633] suggested that radiocapitellar contact was important and attempted to employ the use of a ferrule cap to provide support. Since then, many investigators have attempted to quantify and gauge the clinical significance of the proximal translation.

Despite continued controversy, most series would support the following statement: Proximal translation after radial head fracture and resection occurs in *most* patients to some extent and is *not* always symptomatic, despite disconformity at the distal radioulnar joint.

In 1946 Curr and Coe[571] described a patient with *acute* proximal translation of the radius with disruption of the distal radioulnar joint combined with a radial head fracture. They described the clinical and surgical findings of complete dissociation between the radius and ulna and the difficulty in effectively treating the gross instability. In 1951 Essex-Lopresti[577] reported two cases with similar findings. He suggested preservation of the radial head, if possible, or the use of a rigid prosthesis to maintain a proper longitudinal relationship. In 1988, Khurana and colleagues[597] reported a patient with acute radioulnar dissociation in which the interosseous membrane, visualized in the operating room, was noted to be completely disrupted.

The relationship between *acute* radioulnar dissociation as described by Curr and Coe[571] and the more gradual sounding *proximal migration* of the radius after radial head resection is not known. Most studies of proximal translation of the radius after radial head resection were done after trauma, making it difficult to separate the possible injury itself from the gradual attenuation of the interosseous membrane with longitudinal loading. Rymaszewski[628] did not note proximal translation in a series of 52 patients with rheumatoid arthritis who had undergone radial head resection for radiocapitellar arthrosis. Perhaps lower demand was a factor, though valgus instability of the elbow did develop in many of those patients.

There is probably a continuum of injury, depending on the initial energy and force applied, which causes a partial or complete tear of the in-

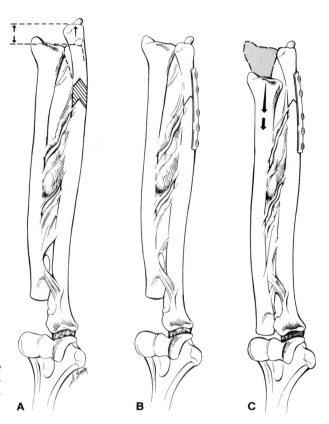

Fig. 10-65. Ulnar shortening usually fails to provide permanent equalization because the ligamentous linkage between the radius and ulna is completely disrupted.

A   **B**   **C**

terosseous membrane and distal wrist ligaments. If these structures are torn completely, then acute displacement can occur at the time of injury. If the ligaments are partially torn, no displacement may be initially present, but with use in grip and lifting activity, the radius can gradually displace.

As of this writing, there is no consistently effective treatment of symptomatic proximal migration of the radius following radial head resection. Some authors have advocated the use of the silicone radial head prosthesis to provide support with radiocapitellar contact.[590,638,644] Others have documented prosthetic failure and the inability of the prosthesis to provide adequate mechanical support[574,601,631] (see Fig. 10-63). Shortening of the ulna is not helpful either (Figs. 10-64 and 10-65). In many cases, as Brockman[556] first suggested in 1930, the creation of a radioulnar synostosis may be the only solution.

OPEN ELBOW INJURIES (SIDESWIPE INJURIES)

Sideswipe injuries[649,650–652] and massive open trauma to the elbow require a comprehensive team approach. Neurovascular injuries must be addressed, along with bony and soft tissue injury. If the hand is not viable and nerve injury is extensive, primary amputation should be considered. An asensate, stiff hand is less useful than a prosthesis. Chapter 4 discusses specific options for coverage of wounds about the elbow. Skeletal stability and soft tissue coverage[651,653,655] are the primary goals of reconstruction. Although rigid internal fixation of all fractures is desirable, external fixation for wound care and soft tissue management is usually mandatory. As soon as feasible, the external fixator should be removed to initiate motion.

REHABILITATION

Proper and timely rehabilitation in the treatment of elbow injuries can reduce disabling contracture and pain. Although the inflammatory response to trauma in the elbow differs little in the initial phases from that in other major joints, one is often struck by the severity of swelling and stiffness from what seemed to be a minor blow or minimal fracture. More severe injuries, such as posterior dislocations or distal humeral fractures, commonly require formal supervised therapy to maximize outcome. The program of mobilization must be individualized to protect injured structures but permit maximal painless motion.

In the acute phase (1 to 6 weeks), the patient with a stable injury should be expected to begin active-motion exercise, both in flexion and extension and pronation and supination. Special attention at this point to sustained position at the extreme in all positions, without excessive pain, is the most effective.

In operative cases, it is helpful to range the elbow in the operating room to determine if there are any limits imposed by the particular fracture or ligamentous repair that would be jeopardized at any one position. One can then rationally design a program of rehabilitation with these constraints in mind. For example, in posterior dislocations, there is usually a safe zone in flexion and extension in which redislocation will not occur. One can then instruct the therapist to remain within that range of motion until healing occurs.

Active-motion exercises with attention to extension are emphasized in the first weeks after injury. If the patient is not showing progress, one can add a dynamic splinting program. *Under no circumstances do we use passive manipulation to increase motion.* This practice carries a very high risk for heterotopic bone formation and subsequent ankylosis.

The use of splints should be coordinated with the therapist and monitored closely. Turnbuckle orthoses, described by Green and McCoy,[431] can be quite effective at reducing flexion contractures. Although these were originally described using leather cuffs, Orthoplast can also be used. Commercially available dynamic splints are available,[433] but we have found that the patients tolerate this form of splinting less well than the turnbuckle orthosis.

Continuous passive motion is attractive and has been recommended by some,[429,435] but there is no evidence to date that the ultimate outcome is influenced by the use of these devices. Extremes of motion are difficult to achieve, and the continuous passive motion devices rarely reach full extension or flexion.

REFERENCES

Anatomy and Biomechanics

1. An, K.N.; Morrey, B.F.; and Chao, E.Y.S.: The Effect of Partial Removal of the Proximal Ulna on Elbow Constraint. Clin. Orthop., 209:270–279, 1986.

2. Anson, B.J., and Maddock, W.G.: Callender's Surgical Anatomy. Philadelphia, W.B. Saunders, 1958.

3. Askew, L.J.; An, K.N.; Morrey, B.F.; and Chao, E.Y.: Isometric Elbow Strength in Normal Individuals. Clin. Orthop., 222:261–266, 1987.

4. Conwell, H.E., and Reynolds, F.C.: Key and Conwell's Management of Fractures. Dislocations, and Sprains, 7th ed. St. Louis, C.V. Mosby, 1961.

5. Funk, D.A.; An, K.N.; Morrey, B.F.; and Daube, J.R.: Electromyographic Analysis of Muscles Across the Elbow Joint. J. Orthop. Res., 5:529–538, 1987.

6. Goss, C.M.: Gray's Anatomy of the Human Body, 36th ed. Philadelphia, Lea & Febiger, 1954.

7. Halls, A.A., and Travill, A.: Transmission of Pressures Across the Elbow Joint. Anat. Rec., 150:243–248, 1960.

8. Hotchkiss, R.N.; An, K.N.; Sowa, D.T.; Basta, S.; and Weiland, A.J.: An Anatomic and Mechanical Study of the Interosseous Membrane of the Forearm: Pathomechanics of Proximal Migration of the Radius. J. Hand Surg., 14A:256–261, 1989.

9. Hotchkiss, R.N., and Weiland, A.J.: Valgus Stability of the Elbow. J. Orthop. Res., 5:372–377, 1987.

10. London, J.T.: Kinematics of the Elbow. J. Bone Joint Surg., 63A:529–0, 1981.

11. MacAusland, W.R.: Arthroplasty of the Elbow. N. Engl. J. Med., 236:97–99, 1947.

12. Milch, H.: Fractures of the External Humeral Condyle. J.A.M.A., 160:529–539, 1956.

13. Morrey, B.F.: Applied Anatomy and Biomechanics of the Elbow Joint. Instr. Course Lect. XXXV: 59–68, 1986.

14. Morrey, B.F.: Biomechanics of the Elbow. *In* Morrey, B.F. (ed.): The Elbow and Its Disorders, vol. 1, pp. 43–61. Philadelphia, W.B. Saunders, 1985.

15. Morrey, B.F., and An, K.N.: Articular and Ligamentous Contributions to the Stability of the Elbow Joint. Am. J. Sports Med., 11:315–319, 1983.

16. Morrey, B.F., and An, K.N.: Functional Anatomy of the Ligaments of the Elbow. Clin. Orthop., 201:84–90, 1985.

17. Morrey, B.F.; An, K.N.; and Stormont, T.J.: Force Transmission Through the Radial Head. J. Bone Joint Surg., 70A:250–256, 1988.

18. Morrey, B.F.; Askew, L.J.; An, K.N.; and Chao, E.Y.: A Biomechanical Study of Normal Elbow Motion. J. Bone Joint Surg., 63A:872–877, 1981.

19. Morrey, B.F., and Chao, E.Y.: Passive Motion of the Elbow Joint. A Biomechanical Analysis. J. Bone Joint Surg., 58A:501–508, 1976.

20. Palmer, A.K., and Werner, F.W.: Biomechanics of the Distal Radioulnar Joint. Clin. Orthop., 187:26–35, 1984.

21. Schwab, G.H.; Bennett, J.B.; Woods, G.W.; and Tullos, H.S.: Biomechanics of Elbow Instability: The Role of the Medial Collateral Ligament. Clin. Orthop., 146:42–52, 1980.

22. Sojbjerg, J.O.; Ovensen, J.; and Nielsen, S.: Experimental Elbow Instability After Transection of the Medial Collateral Ligament. Clin. Orthop., 218:186–190, 1987.

23. Solomonow, M.; Guzzi, A.; Baratta, R.; Shoji, H.; and D'Ambrosia, R.: EMG-force Model of the Elbows Antag-

onistic Muscle Pair. The Effect of Joint Position, Gravity, and Recruitment. Am. J. Phys. Med., 65:223–244, 1986.

24. Stone, C.A.: Subluxation of the Head of the Radius. Report of a Case and Anatomic Experiments. J.A.M.A., 67:28–29, 1916.

25. Strachan, J.C.H., and Ellis, B.W.: Vulnerability of the Posterior Interosseous Nerve During Radial Head Resection. J. Bone Joint Surg., 53B:320–323, 1971.

26. Taylor, T.K.F., and Scham, S.M.: A Posteromedial Approach to the Proximal End of the Ulna for the Internal Fixation of Olecranon Fractures. J. Trauma, 9:594–602, 1969.

27. Tullos, H.S.; Schwab, G.; Bennett, J.B.; and Woods, G.W.: Factors Influencing Elbow Instability. Instruct. Course Lect., VIII:185–199, 1982.

28. Volz, R.B.: Biomechanics Update #2. Basic Biomechanics: Lever Arm, Instant Center of Motion, Moment Force, Joint Reactive Force. Orthop. Rev., 15:677–684, 1986.

29. Youm, Y.; Dryer, R.F.; Thambyrajai, K.; Flatt, A.E.; and Sprague, B.L.: Biomechanical Analysis of Forearm Pronation-Supination and Elbow Flexion-Extension. J. Biomech., 12:245–255, 1979.

Radiology

30. Franklin, P.D.; Dunlop, R.W.; Whitelaw, G.; Jaques, E., Jr.; Blickman, J.G.; and Shapiro, J.H.: Computed Tomography of the Normal and Traumatized Elbow. J. Comput. Assist. Tomogr., 12:817–823, 1988.

31. Greenspan, A., and Norman, A.: Radial Head—Capitellum View: An Expanded Imaging Approach to Elbow Injury. Radiology, 164:272–274, 1987.

32. Grundy, A.; Murphy, G.; Barker, A.; Guest, P.; and Jack, L.: The Value of the Radial Head—Capitellum View in Radial Head Trauma. Br. J. Radiol., 58:965–967, 1985.

33. Hall-Craggs, M.A.; Shorvon, P.J.; and Chapman, M.: Assessment of the Radial Head-Capitellum View and the Dorsal Fat-pad Sign in Acute Elbow Trauma. A.J.R., 145:607–609, 1985.

34. Kohler, A., and Zimmer, E.A.: Borderlands of the Normal and Early Pathologic in Skeletal Roentgenology, 3rd ed. New York, Grune & Stratton, 1968.

35. Koh, A.M.: Soft-Tissue Alterations in Elbow Trauma. A.J.R., 82:867–874, 1959.

36. Murphy, W.A., and Siegel, M.J.: Elbow Fat Pads With New Signs and Extended Differential Diagnosis. Radiology, 124:659–665, 1977.

37. Norell, H.G.: Roentgenologic Visualization of Extracapsular Fat; Its Importance in the Diagnosis of Traumatic Injuries to the Elbow. Acta Radiol., 42:205–210, 1954.

38. Page, A.C.: Critical Evaluation of the Radial Head-Capitellum View in Elbow Trauma. A.J.R., 146:81–82, 1986.

39. Smith, D.N., and Lee, J.R.: The Radiological Diagnosis of Post-traumatic Effusion of the Elbow Joint and Its Clinical Significance: The "Displaced Fat Pad" Sign. Injury, 10:115–119, 1978.

Supracondylar Fractures

40. Anderson, L.: Fractures. *In* Crenshaw, A.H. (ed.): Campbell's Operative Orthopaedics, 5th ed. St. Louis, C.V. Mosby, 1971.

41. Böhler, L.: The Treatment of Fractures, vol. 5. New York, Grune & Stratton, 1956.

42. Browne, A.O.; O'Riordan, M. and Quinlan, W.: Supracondylar Fractures of the Humerus in Adults. Injury, 17:184–186, 1986.

43. Bryan, R.S.: Fractures About the Elbow in Adults. A.A.O.S. Instr. Course Lect. 30:200–223, 1981.

44. Campbell, W.C.: Operative Orthopaedics. St. Louis, C.V. Mosby, 1939.

45. Childress, H.M.: Transarticular Pin Fixation in Supracondylar Fractures of the Elbow in Children. J. Bone Joint Surg., 54A:1548–1552, 1972.

46. Conn, J., and Wade, P.A.: Injuries of the Elbow (A Ten-Year Review). J. Trauma, 1:248–268, 1961.

47. Conwell, H.E., and Reynolds, F.C.: Key and Conwell's Management of Fractures, Dislocations, and Sprains, 7th ed. St. Louis, C.V. Mosby, 1961.

48. D'Ambrosia, R.D.: Supracondylar Fractures of the Humerus—Prevention of Cubitus Varus Deformity. J. Bone Joint Surg., 54A:60–66, 1972.

49. DePalma, A.F.: The Management of Fractures and Dislocations. Philadelphia, W.B. Saunders, 1959.

50. Decoulx, P.; Ducloux, M.; Hespeel, J.; and Coulx, J.: Les Fractures de l'Extremite Inferieure de l'Humerus Chez l'Adulte. Rev. Chir. Orthop., 50:263–273, 1964.

51. Dunlop, J.: Transcondylar Fractures of the Humerus in Childhood. J. Bone Joint Surg., 21:59–73, 1939.

52. Dupuytren, B.G.: On the Injuries and Diseases of Bones. London, Syndenham Society, 1847.

53. Fowles, J.V.; Kassab, M.T.; and Said, K.: Supracondylar Fractures in Children, Stabilization by Two Lateral Percutaneous Pins. Presented at the Canadian Orthopaedic Association Annual Meeting. Winnipeg, Manitoba, 1973.

54. Hamilton, F.H.: A Practical Treatise on Fractures and Dislocations, 8th ed. Philadelphia, Lea Brothers & Co., 1891.

55. Henry, A.K.: Extensile Exposure. Baltimore, Williams & Wilkins, 1945.

56. Horne, G.: Supracondylar Fractures of the Humerus in Adults. J. Trauma, 20:71, 1980.

57. Hoyer, A.: Treatment of Supracondylar Fractures of the Humerus by Skeletal Traction in an Abduction Splint. J. Bone Joint Surg., 34A:623–637, 1952.

58. Jones, K.G.: Percutaneous Pin Fixation of Fractures of the Lower End of the Humerus. Clin. Orthop., 50:53–69, 1967.

59. Keon-Cohen, B.T.: Fractures of the Elbow. J. Bone Joint Surg., 48A:1623–1639, 1966.

60. King, D., and Secor, C.: Bow Elbow (Cubitus Varus). J. Bone Joint Surg., 33A:572–576, 1951.

61. MacAusland, W.R., and Wyman, E.T.: Fractures of the Adult Elbow. A.A.O.S. Instr. Course Lect. XXIV:169–181, 1975.

62. Mann, T.S.: Prognosis in Supracondylar Fractures. J. Bone Joint Surg., 45B:516–522, 1963.

63. Merle D'Aubigne, R.; Meary, R.; and Carlioz, J.: Fractures sus et intercondyliennes recentes de l'adulte. Rev. Chir. Orthop., 50:279–288, 1964.

64. Miller, O.L.: Blind Nailing of the T-Fracture of the Lower End of the Humerus Which Involves the Joint. J. Bone Joint Surg., 21:933–938, 1939.

65. Müller, M.E.; Allgower, M.; Schneider, R.; and Willengger, H.: Manual of Internal Fixation. New York, Springer-Verlag, 1979.

66. Roberts, J.B., and Kelly, J.A.: Treatise on Fractures, 2nd ed. Philadelphia, J.B. Lippincott, 1921.

67. Salter, R.B.: Problem Fractures in Children. A.A.O.S. Instr. Course Lect. Annual Meeting, Dallas, Texas, 1974.

68. Scudder, C.L.: Treatment of Fractures, 9th ed. Philadelphia, W.B. Saunders, 1923.

69. Siris, I.E.: Supracondylar Fractures of the Humerus. Surg. Gynecol. Obstet., 68:201–222, 1939.

70. Sisk, T.D.: Fractures of the Distal End of Humerus. *In* Crenshaw, A.H. (ed.): Campbell's Operative Orthopaedics, 6th ed., pp. 674–683. St. Louis, C.V. Mosby, 1980.

71. Smith, F.M.: Surgery of the Elbow, 2nd ed. Philadelphia, W.B. Saunders, 1972.

72. Smith, L.: Deformity Following Supracondylar Fracture of the Humerus. J. Bone Joint Surg., 42A:235–252, 1960.

73. Soltanpur, A.: Anterior Supracondylar Fracture of the Humerus (Flexion Type). J. Bone Joint Surg., 60B:383–386, 1978.

74. Speed, K.: A Textbook of Fractures and Dislocation. Philadelphia, Lea & Febiger, 1935.

75. Stimson, L.A.: A Treatise on Fractures. Philadelphia, Henry C. Lea's Son & Co., 1890.

76. Swenson, A.L.: Treatment of Supracondylar Fractures of the Humerus by Kirschner-Wire Transfixation. J. Bone Joint Surg., 30A:993–997, 1948.

77. Waddell, J.P.; Hatch, J.; Richards, R.: Supracondylar Fractures of the Humerus—Results of Surgical Treatment. J. Trauma, 28:1615–1621, 1988.

78. Watson-Jones, R.: Fractures and Joint Injuries, vol. 2, 3rd ed. Baltimore, Williams & Wilkins, 1946.

Transcondylar Fractures

79. Ashurst, A.P.C.: An Anatomical and Surgical Study of Fractures of the Lower End of the Humerus. The Samuel D. Gross Prize Essay of the Philadelphia Academy. Philadelphia, Lea & Febiger, 1910.

80. Bohler, L.: The Treatment of Fractures, vol. 1, 5th ed. New York, Grune & Stratton, 1956.

81. Bryan, R.S.: Fractures About the Elbow in Adults. Instr. Course Lect., 30:200–223, 1981.

82. Chutro, P.: Fracturas De La Extremidad Inferior Del Humero En Los Ninos. Buenos Aires, Theses J. Peuser, 1904.

83. Conwell, H.E., and Reynolds, F.C.: Key and Conwell's Management of Fractures, Dislocations, and Sprains, 7th ed. St. Louis, C.V. Mosby, 1961.

84. Cotton, F.J.: Dislocations and Joint Fractures, 2nd ed. Philadelphia, W.B. Saunders, 1924.

85. DePalma, A.F.: The Management of Fractures and Dislocations, vol. 1. Philadelphia, W.B. Saunders, 1959.

86. Grantham, S.A., and Tietjen, R.: Transcondylar Fracture-Dislocation of the Elbow. J. Bone Joint Surg., 58A:1030–1031, 1976.

87. Hamilton, F.H.: A Practical Treatise on Fractures and Dislocations, 8th ed. Philadelphia, Lea Brothers & Co., 1891.

88. Roberts, J.B., and Kelly, J.A.: Treatise on Fractures, 2nd ed. Philadelphia, J.B. Lippincott, 1921.

89. Scudder, C.L.: Treatment of Fractures, 9th ed. Philadelphia, W.B. Saunders, 1923.

90. Smith F.M.: Surgery of the Elbow. Springfield, Ill., Charles C Thomas, 1954.

91. Speed, K.: A Textbook of Fractures and Dislocations, 3rd ed. Philadelphia, Lea & Febiger, 1935.

92. Watson-Jones, R.: Fractures and Joint Injuries, vol. 2, 3rd ed. Baltimore, Williams & Wilkins, 1946.

93. Wilson, P.D., and Cochrane, W.A.: Fractures and Dislocations. Philadelphia, J.B. Lippincott, 1925.

Intercondylar Fractures

94. Ackerman, G.; Jupiter, J.B.: Non-union of Fractures of the Distal End of the Humerus. J. Bone Joint Surg., 70A:75–83, 1988.

95. Anson, B.J., and Maddock, W.B.: Callander's Surgical Anatomy. Philadelphia, W.B. Saunders, 1958.

96. Bickel, W.E., and Perry, R.E.: Comminuted Fractures of the Distal Humerus. J.A.M.A., 184:553–557, 1963.

97. Böhler, L.: The Treatment of Fractures. Vienna, Wilhelm Maudrich, 1929.

98. Brown, R.F., and Morgan, R.G.: Intercondylar T-shaped Fractures of the Humerus. J. Bone Joint Surg., 53B:425–428, 1971.

99. Bryan, R.S.: Fractures About the Elbow in Adults. Instr. Course Lect., 30:200–223, 1981.

100. Bryan, R.S., and Bickel, W.H.: "T" Condylar Fractures of the Distal Humerus. J. Trauma, 11:830–835, 1971.

101. Bryan, R.S., and Morrey, B.F.: Fractures of the Distal Humerus. *In* Morrey, B.F. (ed.): The Elbow and Its Disorders, vol. 1, pp. 302–339. Philadelphia, W.B. Saunders, 1985.

102. Bryan, R.S., and Morrey, B.F.: Extensive Posterior Exposure of the Elbow. Clin. Orthop., 166:188–192, 1982.

103. Burri, C.; Henkemeyer, H.; and Spier, W.: Results of Operative Treatment of Intra-articular Fractures of the Distal Humerus. Acta Orthop. Belg., 41:227–234, 1975.

104. Bush, L.F., and McClain, E.J.: Operative Treatment of Fractures of the Elbow in Adults. Instr. Course Lect., XVI:265–277, 1959.

105. Campbell, W.C.: Operative Orthopaedics. St. Louis, C.V. Mosby, 1939.

106. Cassebaum, W.H.: Operative Treatment of T- and Y-Fractures of the Lower End of the Humerus. Am. J. Surg., 83:265–270, 1952.

107. Cassebaum, W.H.: Open Reduction of T- and Y-Fractures

of the Lower End of the Humerus. J. Trauma, 9:915–925, 1969.

108. Chacha, P.B.: Fracture of the Medial Condyle of the Humerus With Rotational Displacement. Report of Two Cases. J. Bone Joint Surg., 52A:1453–1458, 1970.

109. Conn, J., and Wade, P.A.: Injuries of the Elbow. A Ten Year Review. J. Trauma, 1:248–268, 1961.

110. Conwell, H.E., and Reynolds, F.C.: Key and Conwell's Management of Fractures, Dislocations, and Sprains, 7th ed. St. Louis, C.V. Mosby, 1961.

111. ,Cotton, F.J.: Dislocations and Joint Fractures, 2nd ed. Philadelphia, W.B. Saunders, 1924.

112. DePalma, A.F.: The Management of Fractures and Dislocations. Philadelphia, W.B. Saunders, 1959.

113. Desault, P.J.: A Treatise on Fractures. Luxations and Other Affections of the Bones, 2nd ed. Philadelphia, Kimber & Contrad, 1811.

114. Dunn, A.W.: A Distal Humeral Prosthesis. Clin. Orthop., 77:199–202, 1971.

115. Eastwood, W.J.: The T-Shaped Fracture of the Lower End of the Humerus. J. Bone Joint Surg., 19:364–369, 1937.

116. Evans, E.M.: Supracondylar Y-Fractures of the Humerus. J. Bone Joint Surg., 35B:381–385, 1953.

117. Gabel, G.T.; Hanson, G.; Bennett, J.B.; Noble, P.C.; and Tullos, H.S.: Intraarticular Fractures of the Distal Humerus in the Adult. Clin. Orthop., 216:99–108, 1987.

118. Ghawabi, M.H.: Fracture of the Medial Condyle of the Humerus. J. Bone Joint Surg., 57A:677–680, 1975.

119. Goss, C.M.: Gray's Anatomy of the Human Body, 26th ed. Philadelphia, Lea & Febiger, 1954.

120. Grant, J.C.B.: A Method of Anatomy, 5th ed. Baltimore, Williams & Wilkins, 1952.

121. Hamilton, F.H.: A Practical Treatise on Fractures and Dislocations, 8th ed. Philadelphia, Lea Brothers & Co., 1891.

122. Heim, U., and Pfeiffer, K.M.: Elbow. Internal Fixation of Small Fractures, vol. 3, pp. 107–109.

123. Helfet, D.L., and Hotchkiss, R.N.: Internal Fixation of the Humerus: A Biomechanical Comparison of Methods. J. Orthop. Trauma, 4:260–264, 1990.

124. Henley, M.B.: Intra-articular Distal Humeral Fractures in Adults. Orthop. Clin. North. Am., 18:11–23, 1987.

125. Henley, M.B.; Bone, L.B.; and Parker, B.: Operative Management of Intra-Articular Fractures of the Distal Humerus. J. Orthop. Trauma, 1:24–35, 1987.

126. Hitzrot, J.M.: Fractures at the Lower End of the Humerus in Adults. Surg. Clin. North Am., 12:291–304, 1932.

127. Inglis, A.E., and Pellicci, P.M.: Total Elbow Replacement. J. Bone Joint Surg., 62A:1252–1258, 1980.

128. Johansson, H., and Olerud, S.: Operative Treatment of Intercondylar Fractures of the Humerus. J. Trauma, 11:836–843, 1971.

129. Jupiter, J.B.; Neff, U.; Holzach, P.; and Allgower, M.: Intercondylar Fractures of the Humerus. J. Bone Joint Surg., 67A:226–239, 1985.

130. Kelly, R.P., and Griffin, T.W.: Open Reduction of T-Condylar Fractures of the Humerus Through an Anterior Approach. J. Trauma, 9:901–914, 1969.

131. Keon-Cohen, B.T.: Fractures at the Elbow. J. Bone Joint Surg., 48A:1623–1639, 1966.

132. Knight, R.A.: Fractures of the Humeral Condyles in Adults. South. Med. J., 48:1165–1173, 1955.

133. Knight, R.A.: Management of Fractures About the Elbow in Adults. Instr. Course Lect., XIV:123141, 1957.

134. MacAusland, W.R.: Ankylosis of the Elbow: With Report of Four Cases Treated by Arthroplasty. J.A.M.A., 64:312–318, 1915.

135. Magnuson, P.B., and Stack, J.M.: Fractures. 5th ed. Philadelphia, J.B. Lippincott, 1949.

136. Mellen, R.H., and Phalen, G.S.: Arthroplasty of the Elbow by Replacement of the Distal Portion of the Humerus With an Acrylic Prosthesis. J. Bone Joint Surg., 28:348–353, 1947.

137. Milch, H.: Fractures and Fracture Dislocations of the Humeral Condyles. J. Trauma, 4:592–607, 1964.

138. Miller, O.L.: Blind Nailing of the T Fracture of the Lower End of the Humerus Which Involves the Joint. J. Bone Joint Surg., 21:933–938, 1939.

139. Miller, W.E.: Comminuted Fractures of the Distal End of the Humerus in the Adult. J. Bone Joint Surg., 46A:644–657, 1964.

140. Müller, M.E.; Allgower, M.; Schneider, R.; and Willenegger, H.: Manual of Internal Fixation, 2nd ed. New York, Springer-Verlag, 1979.

141. Niemann, K.M.W.: Condylar Fractures of the Distal Humerus in Adults. South. Med. J., 70:915–918, 1977.

142. Palmer, I.: Open Treatment of Transcondylar T-Fractures of the Humerus. Acta Chir. Scand., 121:486–490, 1961.

143. Patterson, R.F.: A Method of Applying Traction in T and Y Fractures of the Distal Humerus. J. Bone Joint Surg., 17:476–477, 1935.

144. Pollsson, E., and Arnulf, G.: Fracture du Condyle interne-Reposition Sanglante. Lyon Chirurgical, 34:337, 1937.

145. Potter, C.M.C.: Fracture-Dislocation of the Trochlea. J. Bone Joint Surg., 36B:250–253, 1954.

146. Reich, R.S.: Treatment of Intercondylar Fractures of the Elbow by Means of Traction. J. Bone Joint Surg., 18:997–1004, 1936.

147. Riseborough, E.J., and Radin, E.L.: Intercondylar T Fractures of the Humerus in the Adult: A Comparison of Operative and Non-Operative Treatment in Twenty-nine Cases. J. Bone Joint Surg., 51A:130–141, 1969.

148. Scharplatz, D., and Allgower, M.: Fracture Dislocations of the Elbow. Injury, 7:143–159, 1975.

149. Shahriaree, H.; Kooros, S.; Silver, C.M.; and Sheikholeslamzadeh, S.: Excisional Arthroplasty of the Elbow. J. Bone Joint Surg., 61A:922–927, 1979.

150. Sisk, T.D.: Campbell's Operative Orthopaedics, 6th ed. St. Louis, C.V. Mosby, 1980.

151. Smith, F.M.: Surgery of the Elbow, 2nd ed. Philadelphia, W.B. Saunders, 1972.

152. Speed, J.S.: Surgical Treatment of Condylar Fractures of the Humerus. Instr. Course Lect., VII:187–194, 1950.

153. Thomas, T.T.: A Contribution to the Mechanism of Fractures and Dislocations in the Elbow Region. Ann. Surg., 89:108–121, 1929.

154. Thorton, L.: Fractures of the Humerus Treated by Means of the Hoke Plaster Traction Apparatus. J. Bone Joint Surg., 12:911–924, 1930.
155. Trynin, A.H.: Intercondylar T Fracture of Elbow. J. Bone Joint Surg., 23:709–711, 1941.
156. Van Gorder, G.W.: Surgical Approach in Supracondylar "T" Fractures of the Humerus Requiring Open Reduction. J. Bone Joint Surg., 22:278–292, 1940.
157. Watson-Jones, R.: Fractures and Joint Injuries, vol. 2, 3rd ed. Baltimore, Williams & Wilkins, 1946.
158. Wickstrom, J., and Meyer, P.R.: Fractures of the Distal Humerus in Adults. Clin. Orthop., 50:43–51, 1967.
159. Willenegger, H.: Problems and Results in the Treatment of Comminuted Fractures of the Elbow. Reconstr. Surg. Traumatol., 11:118–127, 1969.
160. Wilson, P.D.: Fractures and Dislocations in the Region of the Elbow. Surg. Gynecol. Obstet., 56:335–359, 1933.
161. Wilson, P.D.: Experience in the Management of Fractures and Dislocations. Philadelphia, J.B. Lippincott, 1938.
162. Wilson, P.D., and Cochrane, W.A.: Fractures and Dislocations. Philadelphia, J.B. Lippincott, 1925.
163. Zagorski, J.B.; Jennings, J.J.; Burkhalter, W.E.; and Uribe, J.W.: Comminuted Intraarticular Fractures of the Distal Humeral Condyles. Surgical vs Nonsurgical Treatment. Clin. Orthop., 202:197–204, 1986.

Distal Humeral Fractures—Reconstruction

164. Barr, J.S., and Eaton, R.G.: Elbow Reconstruction With a New Prosthesis to Replace the Distal End of the Humerus. J. Bone Joint Surg., 47A:1408–1413, 1965.
165. Breen, T.; Gelberman, R.H.; Leffert, R.; and Botte, M.: Massive Allograft Replacement of Hemiarticular Traumatic Defects of the Elbow. J. Hand Surg., 13A:900–907, 1988.
166. Deland, J.T.; Garg, A.; and Walker, P.S.: Biomechanical Basis for Elbow Hinge-distractor Design. Clin. Orthop., 215:303–312, 1987.
167. Dunn, A.W.: A Distal Humeral Prosthesis. Clin. Orthop., 77:199–202, 1971.
168. Figgie, H.E.; Inglis, A.E.; Ranawat, C.S.; and Rosenberg, G.M.: Results of Total Elbow Arthroplasty as a Salvage Procedure for Failed Elbow Reconstructive Operations. Clin. Orthop., 219:185–193, 1987.
169. MacAusland, W.R.: Replacement of the Lower End of the Humerus With a Prosthesis. West. J. Surg. Obstet. Gynecol., 62:557–566, 1954.
170. McMaster, W.C.; Tivnon, M.C.; and Waugh, T.R.: Cast Brace for the Upper Extremity. Clin. Orthop., 109:126–129, 1975.
171. Mellen, R.H., and Phalen, G.S.: Arthroplasty of the Elbow by Replacement of the Distal Portion of the Humerus With an Acrylic Prosthesis. J. Bone Joint Surg., 29:348–353, 1947.
172. Morrey, B.F.; Bryan, R.S.; Dobyns, J.H.; and Linscheid, R.L.: Total Elbow Arthroplasty: A Five Year Experience at the Mayo Clinic. J. Bone Joint Surg., 63A:1050–1063, 1981.
173. Nonnenmacher, J., and Schurch, B.: Fractures of the Radial Head and Lesions of the Lower Radius and Ulna in the Adult. The Importance of the Prosthesis in Resection. Ann. Chir. Main., 6:123–130, 1987.
174. Ross, A.C.; Sneath, R.S.; and Scales, J.T.: Endoprosthetic Replacement of the Humerus and Elbow Joint. J. Bone Joint Surg., 69B:652–655, 1987.
175. Shahriaree, H.; Sajadi, K.; Silver, C.; and Sheikholeslamzadeh, S.: Excisional Arthroplasty of the Elbow. J. Bone Joint Surg., 61A:922–927, 1979.
176. Venable, C.S.: An Elbow and an Elbow Prosthesis. Am. J. Surg., 83:271–275, 1952.
177. Volkov, M.V., and Oganesian, O.V.: Restoration of Function in the Knee and Elbow With a Hinge Distractor Apparatus. J. Bone Joint Surg., 57A:591–607, 1975.

Condylar Fractures

178. Böhler, L.: The Treatment of Fractures, vol. 1, 5th ed. New York, Grune & Stratton, 1956.
179. Bryan, R.S.: Fractures About the Elbow in Adults. Instr. Course Lect., vol. 30, pp. 200–223, 1981.
180. Conn, J., and Wade, P.A.: Injuries of the Elbow (A Ten-Year Review). J. Trauma, 1:248–268, 1961.
181. Conwell, H.E., and Reynolds, F.C.: Key and Conwell's Management of Fractures, Dislocations, and Sprains, 7th ed. St. Louis, C.V. Mosby, 1961.
182. Cotton, F.J.: Dislocations and Joint Fractures, 2nd ed. Philadelphia, W.B. Saunders, 1924.
183. Hamilton, F.H.: A Practical Treatise on Fractures and Dislocations, 8th ed. Philadelphia, Lea Brothers & Co., 1891.
184. Kalenak, A.: Ununited Fractures of the Lateral Condyle of the Humerus. A 50 Year Follow-up. Clin. Orthop., 124:181–183, 1977.
185. Keon-Cohen, B.T.: Fractures of the Elbow. J. Bone Joint Surg., 48A:1623–1639, 1966.
186. Knight, R.A.: Fractures of the Humeral Condyles in Adults. South. Med. J., 48:1165–1173, 1955.
187. Masada, K.; Kawai, H.; Kawabata, H.; Masatomi, T.; Tsuyuguchi, Y.; and Yamamoto, K.: Osteosynthesis for Old, Established Non-Union of the Lateral Condyle of the Humerus. 72A:32–40, 1990.
188. Mitsunaga, M.M.; Bryan, R.S.; and Linscheid, R.L.: Condylar Nonunions of the Elbow. J. Trauma, 22:787–791, 1982.
189. Niemann, K.M.W.: Condylar Fractures of the Distal Humerus in Adults. South. Med. J., 70:915–918, 1977.
190. Smith, F.M.: An Eighty-four Year Follow-up on a Patient With Ununited Fracture of the Lateral Condyle of the Humerus. J. Bone Joint Surg., 55A:378–380, 1973.
191. Smith, F.M.: Surgery of the Elbow, 2nd ed. Philadelphia, W.B. Saunders, 1972.
192. Speed, J.S.: Surgical Treatment of Condylar Fractures of the Humerus. Instr. Course Lect., 7:187–194, 1950.
193. Wilson, P.D., and Cochrane, W.A.: Fractures and Dislocations, pp. 175–179. Philadelphia, J.B. Lippincott, 1925.

Capitellar Fractures

194. Alvarez, E.; Patel, M.; Wimburg, G.; and Pearlman, H.S.: Fracture of the Capitellum Humeri. J. Bone Joint Surg., 57A:1093–1096, 1975.

195. Anderson, L.: Fractures. *In* Crenshaw, A.H. (ed.): Campbell's Operative Orthopaedics, 5th ed. St. Louis, C.V. Mosby, 1971.

196. Böhler, L.: The Treatment of Fractures, vol. 1, 5th ed. New York, Grune & Stratton, 1956.

197. Bryan, R.S.: Fractures About the Elbow in Adults. Instr. Course Lect., 30:200–223, 1981.

198. Bush, L.F., and McClain, E.J.: Operative Treatment of Fractures of the Elbow in Adults. Instr. Course Lect., 16:265–277, 1959.

199. Buxton, St J.D.: Fractures of the Head of the Radius and Capitellum Including External Condylar Fractures of Childhood. Br. Med. J., 2:665–666, 1936.

200. Christopher, F., and Bushnell, L.F.: Conservative Treatment of Fracture of the Capitellum. J. Bone Joint Surg., 17:489–492, 1935.

201. Collert, S.: Surgical Management of Fracture of the Capitellum Humeri. Acta Orthop. Scand., 48:603–606, 1977.

202. Conn, J., and Wade, P.A.: Injuries of the Elbow (A Ten-Year Review). J. Trauma, 1:248–268, 1961.

203. Conwell, H.E., and Reynolds, F.C.: Key and Conwell's Management of Fractures, Dislocations, and Sprains, 7th ed. St. Louis, C.V. Mosby, 1961.

204. Cotton, F.J.: Two Unusual Forms of Fracture—Fracture of the Capitellum; Fracture of the Fifth Metatarsal by Inversion. Boston Med. Surg. J., 149:734–736, 1903.

205. Cotton, F.J.: Dislocations and Joint Fractures. Philadelphia, W.B. Saunders, 1924.

206. Darrach, W.: Open Reduction of Fractures of the Capitellum. Ann. Surg., 63:487, 1916.

207. DePalma, A.F.: The Management of Fractures and Dislocations. Philadelphia, W.B. Saunders, 1959.

208. Dushuttle, R.P.; Coyle, M.P.; Zawadsky, J.P.; and Bloom, H.: Fractures of the Capitellum. J. Trauma, 25:317–321, 1985.

209. Eliason, E.L., and North, J.P.: Fractures About the Elbow. Am. J. Surg., 44:88–99, 1939.

210. Flemming, C.W.: Fractures of the Head of the Radius. Proc. R. Soc. Med., 25:1011–1015, 1932.

211. Flint, C.P.: Fractures of the Eminentia Capitata. Surg. Gynecol. Obstet., vol. 7, pp. 343–356, 1908.

212. Fowles, J.V., and Kassab, M.T.: Fracture of the Capitellum Humeri. J. Bone Joint Surg., 56A:794–798, 1974.

213. Gejrot, W.: On Intra-Articular Fractures of the Capitellum and Trochlea of the Humerus With Special Reference to the Treatment. Acta Chir. Scand., 71:253–270, 1932.

214. Grantham, S.A.; Norris, T.R.; and Bush, D.C.: Isolated Fractures of the Humeral Capitellum. Clin. Orthop., 161:262–269, 1981.

215. Hahn, N.F.: Fall von eine besonderes Varietat der Frakturen des Ellenbogens. Zeitschrift Wundarzte und Geburtshelft, 6:185–189, 1853.

216. Hamilton, F.H.: A Practical Treatise on Fractures and Dislocations, 8th ed. Philadelphia, Lea Brothers & Co., 1891.

217. Hendel, D.; Aghasi, M.; and Halperin, N.: Unusual Fracture Dislocation of the Elbow Joint. Arch. Orthop. Trauma Surg., 104:187–188, 1985.

218. Jakobsson, A.: Fracture of the Capitellum of the Humerus in Adults. Treatment With Intra-Articular Chrom-Cobalt-Molybdenum Prosthesis. Acta Orthop. Scand., 26:184–190, 1957.

219. Johansson, O.: Capsular and Ligament Injuries of the Elbow Joint. Acta Chir. Scand. [Suppl.], 287:50–65, 1962.

220. Jopson, J.H.: Fracture of the Capitellum. Int. Clin. Series, 4:232–242, 1913.

221. Keon-Cohen, B.T.: Fractures at the Elbow. J. Bone Joint Surg., 48A:1623–1639, 1966.

222. Kleiger, B., and Joseph, H.: Fracture of the Capitellum Humeri. Bull. Hosp. Joint Dis., 25:64–70, 1964.

223. Knight, R.A.: Fractures of the Humeral Condyles in Adults. South. Med. J., 48:1165–1173, 1955.

224. Kocher, T.: Beitrage zur Kenntniss einiger tisch wichtiger Frakturformen, pp. 585–591. Basel, Sallman, 1896.

225. Lansinger, O., and Mare, K.: Fracture of the Capitellum Humeri. Acta Orthop. Scand., 52:39–44, 1981.

226. Lee, W.E., and Summey, T.J.: Fracture of the Capitellum of the Humerus. Ann. Surg., 99:497–509, 1934.

227. Lindem, M.C.: Fractures of the Capitellum and Trochlea. Ann. Surg., 76:78–82, 1922.

228. Lorenz, H.: Zur Kenntniss der Fractura humeri (eminentiae capitatae). Deutsche Zeitschr. F. Chir., 78:531–545, 1905.

229. MacAusland, W.R., and Wyman, E.T.: Fractures of the Adult Elbow. Instr. Course Lect., 24:169–181, 1975.

230. MacDonald, J.A., and McGoey, P.F.: Fractures of the Articular Portion of the Capitellum of the Humerus in Adults. Canadian Med Assn J 81:634–636, 1959.

231. Mazel, M.S.: Fracture of the Capitellum. J. Bone Joint Surg., 17:483–488, 1935.

232. McManama, G.B., Jr.; Micheli, L.J.; Berry, M.V.; and Sohn, R.S.: The Surgical Treatment of Osteochondritis of the Capitellum. Am. J. Sports Med., 13:11–21, 1985.

233. Milch, H.: Unusual Fractures of the Capitellum Humeri and the Capitellum Radii. J. Bone Joint Surg., 13:882–886, 1931.

234. Mouchet, M.A.: Fractures de L'extremite Inferieure de L'humerus, p. 282. Paris, G. Steinheil, 1898.

235. Patterson, R.F.: Fracture of the Capitellum. J. Tenn. Med. Assoc., 22:277–282, 1929.

236. Rhodin, R.: On the Treatment of Fracture of the Capitellum. Acta Chir. Scand., 86:475–486, 1942.

237. Richards, R.R.; Khoury, G.W.; Burke, F.D.; and Waddell, J.P.: Internal Fixation of Capitellar Fractures Using Herbert Screws: A Report of Four Cases. Can. J. Surg., 30:188–191, 1987.

238. Rieth, P.L.: Fractures of the Radial Head Associated With Chip Fracture of the Capitellum in Adults; Surgical Considerations. South. Surg., 14:154–159, 1948.

239. Roberts, J.B., and Kelly, J.A.: Treatise on Fractures, 2nd ed. Philadelphia, J.B. Lippincott, 1921.

240. Robertson, R.C., and Bogart, F.B.: Fracture of the Capitellum and Trochlea, Combined With Fracture of the Ex-

ternal Humeral Condyle. J. Bone Joint Surg., 15:206–213, 1933.

241. Schultz, R.J.: The Language of Fractures. Baltimore, Williams & Wilkins, 1972.

242. Simpson, L.A., and Richards, R.R.: Internal Fixation of a Capitellar Fracture Using Herbert Screws. Clin. Orthop., 209:166–168, 1986.

243. Sisk, T.D.: Fractures. *In* Crenshaw, A.H. (ed.): Campbell's Operative Orthopaedics, 6th ed. St. Louis, C.V. Mosby, 1980.

244. Smith, F.M.: Surgery of the Elbow, 2nd ed. Philadelphia, W.B. Saunders, 1972.

245. Speed, J.S.: Surgical Treatment of Condylar Fractures of the Humerus. Instr. Course Lect., 7:187–194, 1950.

246. Steinthal, D.: Die isolierte Fraktur der Eminentia capitata in Ellenbogengelenk. Centrallbl. f. Chirurgi 15:17–20, 1898.

247. Stimson, L.A.: A Treatise on Fractures. Philadelphia, Henry C. Lea's Son & Co., 1890.

248. Wilson, P.D.: Fractures and Dislocations in the Region of the Elbow. Surg. Gynecol. Obstet., 56:335–359, 1933.

Trochlear Fractures

249. Bryan, R.S.: Fractures About the Elbow in Adults. Instr. Course Lect., 30:200–223, 1981.

250. Linden, M.C.: Fractures of the Capitellum and Trochlea. Ann. Surg., 76:78–82, 1922.

251. Smith, F.M.: Surgery of the Elbow, 2nd ed. Philadelphia, W.B. Saunders, 1972.

252. Stimson, L.A.: A Treatise on Fractures. Philadelphia, Henry C. Lea's Son & Co., 1890.

Epicondylar Fractures

253. Bernstein, S.M.; King, J.D.; and Sanderson, R.A.: Fractures of the Medial Epicondyles of the Humerus. Contemporary Orthop., 3:637–642, 1981.

254. Conn, J., and Wade, P.A.: Injuries of the Elbow: A Ten-Year Review. J. Trauma, 1:248–268, 1961.

255. Conwell, H.E., and Reynolds, F.C.: Key and Conwell's Management of Fractures, Dislocations, and Sprains, 7th ed. St. Louis, C.V. Mosby, 1961.

256. DePalma, A.F.: The Management of Fractures and Dislocations. Philadelphia, W.B. Saunders, 1959.

257. Goss, C.M.: Gray's Anatomy of the Human Body, 26th ed. Philadelphia, Lea & Febiger, 1954.

258. Hamilton, F.H.: A Practical Treatise on Fractures and Dislocations, 9th ed. Philadelphia, Lea Brothers, & Co., 1891.

259. Keon-Cohen, B.T.: Fractures at the Elbow. J. Bone Joint Surg., 48A:1623–1639, 1966.

260. Knight, R.A.: Fractures of the Humeral Condyles in Adults. South. Med. J., 48:1165–1173, 1955.

261. Patrick, J.: Fracture of the Medial Epicondyle With Displacement Into the Elbow Joint. J. Bone Joint Surg., 28:143–147, 1946.

262. Purser, D.W.: Dislocation of the Elbow and Inclusion of the Medial Epicondyle in the Adult. J. Bone Joint Surg., 36B:247–249, 1954.

263. Rang, M.: Children's Fractures. Philadelphia, J.B. Lippincott, 1974.

264. Roaf, R.: Foramen in the Humerus Caused by the Median Nerve. J. Bone Joint Surg., 39B:748–749, 1957.

265. Sisk, F.D.: Fractures. *In* Crenshaw, A.H. (ed.): Campbell's Operative Orthopaedics. St. Louis, C.V. Mosby, 1980.

266. Smith, F.M.: Medial Epicondyle Injuries. J.A.M.A., 142:396–402, 1950.

267. Stimson, L.A.: A Treatise on Fractures. Philadelphia, Henry C. Lea's Son & Co., 1890.

268. Watson-Jones, R.: Fractures and Joint Injuries, vol. 2, 3rd ed. Baltimore, Williams & Wilkins, 1946.

269. Wilson, J.N.: The Treatment of Fractures of the Medial Epicondyle of the Humerus. J. Bone Joint Surg., 42B:778–781, 1960.

Supracondylar Process Fractures

270. Barnard, L.B., and McCoy, S.M.: The Supracondylar Process of the Humerus. J. Bone Joint Surg., 28:845–850, 1946.

271. Doane, C.P.: Fractures of the Supracondylar Process of the Humerus. J. Bone Joint Surg., 18:757–759, 1936.

272. Genner, B.A.: Fractures of the Supracondyloid Process. J. Bone Joint Surg., 41A:1333–1335, 1959.

273. Hollinshead, W.H.: Anatomy for Surgeons: The Back and Limbs, vol. 3, 2nd ed., p. 354. New York, Harper & Row, 1969.

274. Kolb, L.W., and Moore, R.D.: Fractures of the Supracondylar Process of the Humerus: Report of Two Cases. J. Bone Joint Surg., 49A:532–534, 1967.

275. Lund, H.J.: Fracture of the Supracondyloid Process of the Humerus. J. Bone Joint Surg., 12:925–928, 1930.

Dislocations

276. Aitken, A.P., and Childress, H.M.: Intra-articular Displacement of the Internal Epicondyle Following Dislocation. J. Bone Joint Surg., 20:161, 1938.

277. Biles, J.G., and Grana, W.A.: Ruptured Ulnar Collateral Ligament. Orthopedics, 10:1595–1596, 1987.

278. Borris, L.C.; Lassen, M.R.; and Christensen, C.S.: Elbow Dislocation in Children and Adults. A Long-term Follow-up of Conservatively Treated Patients. Acta Orthop. Scand. 58:649–651, 1987.

279. Broberg, M.A., and Morrey, B.F.: Results of Treatment of Fracture-Dislocations of the Elbow. Clin. Orthop., 216:109–119, 1987.

280. Bush, L.F., and McClain, E.J., Jr.: Operative Treatment of Fractures of the Elbow in Adults. Instr. Course Lect., 16:265–277, 1959.

281. Campbell, W.C.: Malunited Fractures and Unreduced Dislocations About the Elbow. J.A.M.A., 92:122–128, 1929.

282. Caravias, D.E.: Forward Dislocations of the Elbow Without Fracture of the Olecranon. J. Bone Joint Surg., 39B:334, 1957.

283. Carey, R.P.: Simultaneous Dislocation of the Elbow and the Proximal Radio-ulnar Joint. J. Bone Joint Surg., 66B: 254–256, 1984.

284. Conn, J., and Wade, P.A.: Injuries of the Elbow (A Ten-Year Review). J. Trauma, 1:248–268, 1961.

285. Conwell, H.E., and Reynolds, F.C.: Key and Conwell's Management of Fractures, Dislocations, and Sprains, 7th ed. St. Louis, C.V. Mosby, 1961.

286. Cotton, F.J.: Dislocations and Joint Fractures, 2nd ed. Philadelphia, W.B. Saunders, 1924.

287. Cromack, P.I.: The Mechanism and Nature of the Injury in Dislocations of the Elbow and A Method of Treatment. Aust. N.Z. J. Surg., 30:212–216, 1960.

288. DeLee, J.C.: Transverse Divergent Dislocation of the Elbow in a Child. J. Bone Joint Surg., 322–323, 1981.

289. DePalma, A.F.: The Management of Fractures and Dislocations. Philadelphia, W.B. Saunders, 1959.

290. Desault, P.J.: A Treatise on Fractures, Luxations and Other Affections of the Bones. Philadelphia, Kimber & Conrad, 1811.

291. Durig, M.; Mueller, W.; Ruedi, T.P.; and Gauer, E.F.: The Operative Treatment of Elbow Dislocation in the Adult. J. Bone Joint Surg., 61A:239–244, 1979.

292. Edmonson, A.S., and Crenshaw, A.H.: Campbell's Operative Orthopaedics, 6th ed., pp. 499–501. St. Louis, C.V. Mosby, 1980.

293. Ejsted, R.; Christensen, F.A.; and Nielsen, W.B.: Habitual Dislocation of the Elbow. Arch. Orthop. Trauma Surg., 105:187–190, 1986.

294. Exarchou, E.J.: Lateral Dislocation of the Elbow. Acta Orthop. Scand., 48:161–163, 1977.

295. Greiss, M., and Messias, R.: Irreducible Posterolateral Elbow Dislocation. A Case Report. Acta Orthop. Scand., 58: 421–422, 1987.

296. Hankin, F.M.: Posterior Dislocation of the Elbow—A Simplified Method of Closed Reduction. Clin. Orthop., 190:254–256, 1984.

297. Hendel, D.; Aghagi, M.; and Halperin, N.: Unusual Fracture Dislocation of the Elbow Joint. Arch. Orthop. Trauma Surg., 104:187–188, 1985.

298. Josefsson, P.O.; Gentz, C.F.; Johnell, O.; and Wendeberg, B.: Surgical Versus Nonsurgical Treatment of Ligamentous Injuries Following Dislocations of the Elbow Joint. Clin. Orthop., 214:165–169, 1987.

299. Josefsson, P.O.; Gentz, C.F.; Johnell, O.; and Wendeberg, B.: Surgical Versus Non-Surgical Treatment of Ligamentous Injuries following Dislocation of the Elbow Joint. J. Bone Joint Surg., 69A:605–608, 1987.

300. Josefsson, P.O.; Johnell, O.; and Gentz, C.F.: Long-Term Sequelae of Simple Dislocation of the Elbow. J. Bone Joint Surg., 66A:927–930, 1984.

301. Josefsson, P.O.; Johnell, O.; and Wendeberg, B.: Ligamentous Injuries in Dislocations of the Elbow Joint. Clin. Orthop., 214:221–225, 1987.

302. Josefsson, P.O., and Nilsson, B.E.: Incidence of Elbow Dislocation. Acta Orthop. Scand., 57:537–538, 1986.

303. Kuroda, S., and Sakamaki, K.: Ulnar Collateral Ligament Tears of the Elbow Joint. Clin. Orthop., 208:266–271, 1986.

304. Lansinger, O.; Karlsson, J.; Klorner, L.; and Mqare, K.: Dislocation of the Elbow Joint. Arch. Orthop. Trauma Surg., 102:183–186, 1984.

305. Lavine, L.S.: A Simple Method of Reducing Dislocations of the Elbow Joint. J. Bone Joint Surg., 35A:785–786, 1953.

306. Lesin, B.E., and Balfour, G.W.: Acute Rupture of the Medial Collateral Ligament of the Elbow Requiring Reconstruction. Case Report. J. Bone Joint Surg., 68:1278–1280, 1986.

307. Linscheid, R.L.: Elbow Dislocations. In Morrey, B.F. (ed.): The Elbow and Its Disorders, vol. 1, pp. 414–432. Philadelphia, W.B. Saunders, 1985.

308. Linscheid, R.L., and Wheeler, D.K.: Elbow Dislocations. J.A.M.A., 194:1171–1176, 1965.

309. Loomis, L.K.: Reduction and After-Treatment of Posterior Dislocation of the Elbow. Am. J. Surg., 63:56–60, 1944.

310. McLaughlin, H.L.: Trauma, p. 225. Philadelphia, W.B. Saunders, 1959.

311. Mehlhoff, T.L.; Noble, P.C.; Bennett, J.B.; and Tullos, H.S.: Simple Dislocation of the Elbow in the Adult. J. Bone Joint Surg., 70A:244–249, 1988.

312. Meyn, M.A., and Quigley, T.B.: Reduction of Posterior Dislocation of the Elbow by Traction on the Dangling Arm. Clin. Orthop., 103:106–108, 1974.

313. Myers, M.: Dislocations: Diagnosis, Management, and Complications. Surg. Clin. North Am., 48:1391–1402, 1968.

314. Neviaser, J.S., and Wickstrom, J.K.: Dislocation of the Elbow: A Retrospective Study of 115 Patients. South. Med. J., 70:172–173, 1977.

315. Norwood, L.A.; Shook, J.A.; and Andrews, J.R.: Acute Medial Elbow Ruptures. Am. J. Sports Med., 9:16–19, 1981.

316. Parvin, R.W.: Closed Reduction of Common Shoulder and Elbow Dislocations Without Anesthesia. Arch. Surg., 75: 972–975, 1957.

317. Patrick, J.: Fracture of the Medial Epicondyle With Displacement Into the Elbow Joint. J. Bone Joint Surg., 28: 143–147, 1946.

318. Pawlowski, R.F.; Palumbo, F.C.; and Callahan, J.J.: Irreducible Posterolateral Elbow Dislocation: Report of a Rare Case. J. Trauma, 10:260–266, 1970.

319. Protzman, R.R.: Dislocation of the Elbow Joint. J. Bone Joint Surg., 60A:539–541, 1978.

320. Purser, D.W.: Dislocation of the Elbow and Inclusion of the Medial Epicondyle in the Adult. J. Bone Joint Surg., 36B:247–249, 1954.

321. Railton, S.V.: Compound Dislocation of Elbow Joint Without Fracture (Case Report). Can. Med. Assoc. J., 59: 367, 1948.

322. Roberts, P.H.: Dislocation of the Elbow. Br. J. Surg., 56: 806–815, 1969.

323. Schwab, G.H.; Bennett, J.B.; Woods, G.W.; and Tullos, H.S.: Biomechanics of Elbow Instability: The Role of the

Medial Collateral Ligament. Clin. Orthop., 146:42–52, 1980.

324. Smith, F.M.: Displacement of the Medial Epicondyle of the Humerus Into the Elbow Joint. Ann. Surg., 124:410–425, 1946.

325. Smith, F.M.: Surgery of the Elbow. Springfield, Charles C Thomas, 1954.

326. Speed, K.: Fractures and Dislocations. Philadelphia, Lea & Febiger, 1935.

327. Stimson, L.A.: A Treatise on Fractures. Philadelphia, Henry C. Lea's Son & Co., 1890.

328. Thomas, T.T.: A Contribution to the Mechanism of Fractures and Dislocations in the Elbow Region. Ann. Surg., 89:108, 1929.

329. Tullos, H.S.; Bennett, J.; Shepard, D.; Noble, P.C.; and Gabel, G.: Adult Elbow Dislocations: Mechanism of Instability. Instr. Course Lect., XXXV:69–82, 1986.

330. Wadsworth, T.G.: The Elbow, pp. 216–222. New York, Churchill Livingstone, 1982.

331. Wheeler, D.K., and Linscheid, R.L.: Fracture-Dislocations of the Elbow. Clin. Orthop., 50:95–106, 1967.

332. Wilson, P.D.: Fractures and Dislocations in the Region of the Elbow. Surg. Gynecol. Obstet., 56:335–359, 1933.

Neurovascular Injury

333. Amsallem, J.L.; Blankstein, A.; Bass, A.; and Horoszowski, H.: Brachial Artery Injury: A Complication of Posterior Elbow Dislocation. Orthop. Rev., 15:379–382, 1986.

334. Ashbell, T.S.; Kleinert, H.E.; and Kutz, J.E.: Vascular Injuries About the Elbow. Clin. Orthop., 50:107–127, 1967.

335. Aufranc, O.E.; Jones, W.N.; and Turner, R.H.: Dislocation of the Elbow With Brachial Artery Injury. J.A.M.A., 197:719–721, 1966.

336. Ayala, H.; De Pablos, J.; Gonzalez, J.; and Martinez, A.: Entrapment of the Median Nerve After Posterior Dislocation of the Elbow. Microsurgery, 4:215–220, 1983.

337. Banskota, A., and Volz, R.G.: Traumatic Laceration of the Radial Nerve Following Supracondylar Fracture of the Elbow. A Case Report. Clin. Orthop., 184:150–152, 1984.

338. Beverly, M.C., and Fearn, C.B.: Anterior Interosseous Nerve Palsy and Dislocation of the Elbow. Injury, 6:126–128, 1984.

339. Boe, S., and Holst-Nielsen, F.: Intra-articular Entrapment of the Median Nerve After Dislocation of the Elbow. J. Hand Surg., 12B:356–358, 1987.

340. Danielsson, L.G.: Median Nerve Entrapment in Elbow Dislocation. A Case Report. Acta Orthop. Scand., 57:450–452, 1986.

341. DeBakey, M.E., and Simeone, F.A.: Battle Injuries of the Arteries in World War II: An Analysis of 2471 Cases. Ann. Surg., 123:534–579, 1946.

342. Eliason, E.L., and Brown, R.B.: Posterior Dislocation at the Elbow With Rupture of the Radial and Ulnar Arteries. Ann. Surg., 106:1111–1115, 1937.

343. Friedmann, E.: Simple Rupture of the Brachial Artery, Sustained in Elbow Dislocations. J.A.M.A., 177:208–209, 1961.

344. Galbraith, K.A., and McCullough, C.J.: Acute Nerve Injury as a Complication of Closed Fractures or Dislocations of the Elbow. Injury, 11:159–164, 1979.

345. Grimer, R.J., and Brooks, S.: Brachial Artery Damage Accompanying Closed Posterior Dislocation of the Elbow. J. Bone Joint Surg., 67B:378–381, 1985.

346. Gurdjian, E.S., and Smathers, H.M.: Peripheral Nerve Injury in Fractures and Dislocations of Long Bones. J. Neurosurg., 2:202–219, 1945.

347. Hallett, J.: Entrapment of the Median Nerve After Dislocation of the Elbow. J. Bone Joint Surg., 63B:408–412, 1981.

348. Henderson, R.S., and Robertson, I.M.: Open Dislocation of the Elbow With Rupture of the Brachial Artery. J. Bone Joint Surg., 34B:636–637, 1952.

349. Hennig, K., and Franke, D.: Posterior Displacement of Brachial Artery Following Closed Elbow Dislocation. J. Trauma, 20:96–98, 1980.

350. Ho, K.C., and Marmor, L.: Entrapment of the Ulnar Nerve at the Elbow. Am. J. Surg., 121:355–356, 1971.

351. Jackson, J.A.: Simple Anterior Dislocation of the Elbow Joint With Rupture of the Brachial Artery. Am. J. Surg., 47:479–486, 1940.

352. Kerin, R.: Elbow Dislocations and Its Association With Vascular Disruption. J. Bone Joint Surg., 51A:756–758, 1969.

353. Kilburn, P.; Sweeney, J.G.; and Silk, F.F.: Three Cases of Compound Posterior Dislocation of the Elbow With Rupture of the Brachial Artery. J. Bone Joint Surg., 44B:119–121, 1962.

354. Louis, D.S.; Ricciardi, J.E.; and Spengler, D.M.: Arterial Injury: A Complication of Posterior Elbow Dislocation. J. Bone Joint Surg., 56A:1631–1636, 1974.

355. Mains, D.B., and Freeark, R.J.: Report on Compound Dislocation of the Elbow With Entrapment of the Brachial Artery. Clin. Orthop., 106:180–185, 1975.

356. Mannerfelt, L.: Median Nerve Entrapment After Dislocation of Elbow (Report of a Case). J. Bone Joint Surg., 50B:152–155, 1968.

357. Marnham, R.: Dislocation of the Elbow With Rupture of the Brachial Artery. Br. J. Surg., 22:181, 1934.

358. Matev, I.: A Radiological Sign of Entrapment of the Median Nerve in the Elbow Joint after Posterior Dislocation. A Report of Two Cases. J. Bone Joint Surg., 58B:353–355, 1976.

359. Pritchard, D.J.; Linscheid, R.L.; and Svien, H.J.: Intra-articular Median Nerve Entrapment With Dislocation of the Elbow. Clin. Orthop., 90:100–103, 1973.

360. Rana, N.A.; Kenwright, J.; Taylor, R.G.; and Rushworth, G.: Complete Lesion of the Median Nerve Associated With Dislocation of the Elbow Joint. Acta Orthop. Scand., 45:365–369, 1974.

361. Roaf, R.: Foramen in the Humerus Caused by the Median Nerve. J. Bone Joint Surg., 39B:748–749, 1957.

362. Rubens, M.K., and Aulicino, P.L.: Open Elbow Dislocation With Brachial Artery Disruption. Orthopedics, 9:539–542, 1986.

363. Seddon, H.J.: Surgical Disorders of the Peripheral Nerves, 2nd ed. Edinburgh, Churchill Livingstone, 1975.

364. Sharma, R.K., and Covell, N.A.G.: An Unusual Ulnar Nerve Injury Associated With Dislocation of the Elbow. Injury, 8:145–147, 1976.

365. Sherrill, J.G.: Direct Suture of Brachial Artery Following Rupture, Result of Traumatism. Ann. Surg., 58:534–536, 1913.

366. Spear, H.C., and Janes, J.M.: Rupture of the Brachial Artery Accompanying Dislocation of the Elbow or Supracondylar Fracture. J. Bone Joint Surg., 33A:889–894, 1951.

367. Steiger, R.N.; Larrick, R.B.; and Meyer, T.L.: Median-Nerve Entrapment Following Elbow Dislocation in Children (A Report of Two Cases). J. Bone Joint Surg., 51A:381–385, 1969.

368. Strange, F.G., and St, C.: Entrapment of the Median Nerve After Dislocation of the Elbow. J. Bone Joint Surg., 64B:224–225, 1982.

369. Strum, J.T.; Rothenberger, D.A.; and Strate, R.G.: Brachial Artery Disruption Following Closed Elbow Dislocation. J. Trauma, 18:364–366, 1978.

370. Sullivan, M.F.: Rupture of the Brachial Artery From Posterior Dislocation of the Elbow Treated by Veingraft (A Case Report). Br. J. Surg., 58:470–471, 1971.

371. Watson-Jones, R.: Primary Nerve Lesions in Injuries of the Elbow and Wrist. J. Bone Joint Surg., 12:121–171, 1930.

Dislocations—Old

372. Allende, G., and Freytes, M.: Old Dislocation of the Elbow. J. Bone Joint Surg., 24:691–706, 1944.

373. Arafiles, R.P.: Neglected Posterior Dislocation of the Elbow. J. Bone Joint Surg., 69B:199–202, 1987.

374. Billett, D.M.: Unreduced Posterior Dislocation of the Elbow. J. Trauma, 19:186–188, 1979.

375. Kini, M.G.: Dislocations of the Elbow and Its Complications. J. Bone Joint Surg., 22:107–117, 1940.

376. Krishnamoorthy, S.; Bose, K.; and Wong, K.P.: Treatment of Old Unreduced Dislocation of the Elbow. Injury, 8:39–42, 1976.

377. Silva, J.F.: Old Dislocations of the Elbow. Ann. R. Coll. Surg. Engl., 22:363–381, 1953.

378. Speed, J.S.: An Operation for Unreduced Posterior Dislocation of the Elbow. South. Med. J., 18:193–198, 1925.

379. Vangorder, G.W.: Surgical Approach in Old Posterior Dislocation of the Elbow. J. Bone Joint Surg., 14:127–143, 1932.

Dislocations—Recurrent

380. Dryer, R.F.; Buckwalter, J.A.; and Sprague, B.L.: Treatment of Chronic Elbow Instability. Clin. Orthop., 148:254–255, 1980.

381. Ejested, R.; Christensen, F.A.; and Nielsen, W.B.: Habitual Dislocation of the Elbow. Arch. Orthop. Trauma Surg., 105:187–190, 1986.

382. Gosman, J.A.: Recurrent Dislocation of the Ulna at the Elbow. J. Bone Joint Surg., 25:448–449, 1943.

383. Hall, R.M.: Recurrent Posterior Dislocation of the Elbow Joint in a Boy. Report of a Case. J. Bone Joint Surg., 35B:56, 1953.

384. Hassmann, G.C.; Brunn, F.; and Neer, C.S., II: Recurrent Dislocation of the Elbow. J. Bone Joint Surg., 57A:1080–1084, 1975.

385. Jacobs, R.L.: Recurrent Dislocation of the Elbow Joint. Clin. Orthop., 74:151–154, 1971.

386. Kapel, O.: Operation for Habitual Dislocation of the Elbow. J. Bone Joint Surg., 33A:707–714, 1951.

387. King, T.: Recurrent Dislocation of the Elbow. J. Bone Joint Surg., 35B:30–54, 1953.

388. Milch, H.: Bilateral Recurrent Dislocation of the Ulna at the Elbow. J. Bone Joint Surg., 18:777–780, 1936.

389. Mink, J.H.; Eckardt, J.J.; and Grant, T.T.: Arthrography in Recurrent Dislocation of the Elbow. A.J.R., 136:1242–1244, 1981.

390. Osborne, G.; and Cotterill, P.: Recurrent Dislocation of the Elbow. J. Bone Joint Surg., 48B:340–346, 1966.

391. Reichenheim, P.P.: Transplantation of the Biceps Tendon as a Treatment for Recurrent Dislocation of the Elbow. Br. J. Surg., 35:201, 1947.

392. Spring, W.E.: Report of a Case of Recurrent Dislocation of the Elbow. J. Bone Joint Surg., 35B:55, 1953.

393. Symeonides, P.P.; Paschaloglou, C.; Stavrou, Z.; and Pangalides, T.H.: Recurrent Dislocation of the Elbow: Report of Three Cases. J. Bone Joint Surg., 57A:1084–1086, 1975.

394. Wainwright, D.: Recurrent Dislocation of the Elbow Joint. Proc. Rev. Soc. Med. [Biol.], XL:33–34, 1947.

395. Zeier, F.G.: Recurrent Traumatic Elbow Dislocation. Clin. Orthop., 169:211–214, 1982.

Dislocations—Anterior

396. Caravias, D.E.: Forward Dislocation of the Elbow Without Fracture of the Olecranon. J. Bone Joint Surg., 39B:334, 1957.

397. Cohn, I.: Forward Dislocation of Both Bones of the Forearm at the Elbow. Surg. Gynecol. Obstet., 35:776–788, 1922.

398. Oury, J.H.; Roe, R.D.; and Laning, R.C.: A Case of Bilateral Anterior Dislocations of the Elbow. J. Trauma, 12:170–173, 1972.

399. Simon, M.M.: Complete Anterior Dislocation of Both Bones of the Forearm at the Elbow (Review of Recorded Cases and Literature With Report of a Case). Med. J. Rec., 133:333–336, 1931.

400. Staunton, F.W.: Dislocation Forwards of the Forearm Without Fracture of the Olecranon. Br. Med. J., 2:1520, 1905.

401. Tees, F.J., and McKim, L.H.: Case Reports. Anterior Dislocation of the Elbow. Can. Med. Assoc. J., 20:36–38, 1929.

402. Winslow, R.: A Case of Complete Anterior Dislocation of Both Bones of the Forearm at the Elbow. Surg. Gynecol. Obstet., 16:570–571, 1913.

Dislocations—Radial Head

403. Burgess, R.C.; and Sprague, H.H.: Post-traumatic Posterior Radial Head Subluxation—Two Case Reports. Clin. Orthop., 186:192–194, 1984.

404. Evans, E.M.: Pronation Injuries of the Forearm, With Special References to the Anterior Monteggia Fracture. J. Bone Joint Surg., 31B:578–588, 1949.
405. Gleason, T.F., and Goldstein, W.M.: Traumatic Recurrent Posterior Dislocation of the Radial Head. Clin. Orthop., 184:186–189, 1984.
406. Hamilton, W.:
407. Heidt, R.S.; and Stern, P.J.: Isolated Posterior Dislocation of the Radial Head. Clin. Orthop., 168:136–138, 1982.
408. Lancaster, S.; and Horowitz, M.: Lateral Idiopathic Subluxation of the Radial Head. Clin. Orthop., 214:170–174, 1987.
409. Ryu, J.: Pascal, P.E.; and Levine, J.: Posterior Dislocation of the Radial Head Without Fracture of the Ulna. Clin. Orthop., 183:169–172, 1984.
410. Salama, R.: Recurrent Dislocation of the Head of the Radius. Clin. Ortho., 125:156–158, 1977.
411. Southmayd, W.; and Ehrlich, M.G.: Idiopathic Subluxation of the Radial Head. Clin. Orthop., 121:271–274, 1976.
412. Wiley, J.J.; Pegington, J.; and Horwich, J.P.: Traumatic Dislocation of the Radius at the Elbow. J. Bone Joint Surg., 56B:501–507, 1974.

Heterotopic Ossification

413. Ackerman, L.V.: Extra-Osseous Localized Non-Neoplastic Bone and Cartilage Formation (So-Called Myositis Ossificans). J. Bone Joint Surg., 40A:279–298, 1958.
414. Bijvoet, O.L.M.; Nollen, A.J.G.; Slooff, T.J.J.H.; and Feith, R.: Effect of a Diphosphonate on Para-articular Ossification After Total Hip Replacement. Acta Orthop. Scand., 45:926–934, 1974.
415. Bowers, R.F.: Myositis Ossificans Traumatica. J. Bone Joint Surg., 19:215–221, 1937.
416. Buxton, St, J.D.: Ossification in the Ligaments of the Elbow Joint. J. Bone Joint Surg., 20:709–714, 1938.
417. Coventry, M.B.: Ectopic Ossification About the Elbow. *In* Morrey, B.F. (ed.): The Elbow and Its Disorders, vol. 1, pp. 464–471. Philadelphia, W.B. Saunders, 1985.
418. Coventry, M.B.; and Scanlon, P.W.: The Use of Radiation to Discourage Ectopic Bone. A Nine Year Study in Surgery About the Hip. J. Bone Joint Surg., 63A:201–208, 1981.
419. Finerman, G.A.M.; Krengel, W.F.; Lowell, J.D.; Murray, W.R.; and Volz, R.: Role of Diphosphonate (EHDP) in the Prevention of Heterotopic Ossification After Total Hip Arthroplasty: A Preliminary Report. Proceedings of the Fifth Open Scientific Meeting Hip Society, pp. 222–234. St. Louis, C.V. Mosby, 1977.
420. Garland, D.E.; Hanscom, D.A.; Keenan, M.A.; Smith, C.; and Moore, T.: Resection of Heterotopic Ossification in the Adult With Head Trauma. J. Bone Joint Surg., 67A:1261–1269, 1985.
421. Garland, D.E.; and O'Hollaren, R.M.: Fractures and Dislocations About the Elbow in the Head Injured Adult. Clin. Orthop., 168:38–41, 1982.
422. McLaren, A.C.: Prophylaxis With Indomethacin for Heterotopic Bone After Open Reduction of Fracture of the Acetabulum. J. Bone Joint Surg., 72A:245–247, 1990.
423. Mohan, K.: Myositis Ossificans Traumatica of the Elbow. Int. Surg., 57:475–478, 1972.
424. Nollen, A.J.G.; and Slooff, T.J.J.H.: Para-articular Ossifications After Total Hip Replacement. Acta Orthop. Scand., 44:230–241, 1973.
425. Ritter, M.A.; and Gioe, J.J.: The Effect of Indomethacin or Para-Articular Ectopic Ossification Following Total Hip Arthroplasty. Clin. Orthop., 167:113–117, 1982.
426. Roberts, J.B.; and Pankratz, D.G.: The Surgical Treatment of Heterotopic Ossification at the Elbow Following Long-Term Coma. J. Bone Joint Surg., 61A:760–763, 1979.
427. Thompson, H.C., III, and Garcia, A.: Myositis Ossificans: Aftermath of Elbow Injuries. Clin. Orthop., 50:129–134, 1967.
428. Thorndike, A.: Myositis Ossificans Traumatica. J. Bone Joint Surg., 22:315–323, 1940.

Contracture

429. Breen, T.F.; Gelberman, R.H.; and Ackerman, G.N.: Elbow Flexion Contractures: Treatment by Anterior Release and Continuous Passive Motion. J. Hand Surg., 13B:286–287, 1988.
430. Glynn, J.J.; and Niebauer, J.: Flexion and Extension Contractures of the Elbow: Surgical Management. Clin. Orthop., 117:289–291, 1976.
431. Green, D.P.; and McCoy, H.: Turnbuckle Orthotic Correction of Elbow-Flexion Contractures After Acute Injuries. J. Bone Joint Surg., 61A:1092–1095, 1979.
432. Hepburn, G.R.; and Crivelli, K.: Use of Elbow Dynasplint for Reduction of Elbow Flexion Contracture: A Case Study. J. Orthop. Phys. Ther., 5:269–274, 1984.
433. Richard, R.L.: Use of the Dynasplint to Correct Elbow Flexion Burn Contracture: A Case Report. J. Burn Care Rehabil., 7:151–152, 1986.
434. Stern, P.J.; Law, E.J.; Benedict, F.E.; and MacMillan, B.G.: Surgical Treatment of Elbow Contractures in Postburn Children. Plast. Reconstr. Surg., 76:441–446, 1985.
435. Urbaniak, J.F.; Hansen, P.E.; Beissinger, S.F.; and Aitken, M.S.: Correction of Post-traumatic Flexion Contracture of the Elbow by Anterior Capsulotomy. J. Bone Joint Surg., 67A:1160–1164, 1985.
436. Willner, P.: Anterior Capsulectomy for Contractures of the Elbow. J. In. Col. Surg., 11:359–361, 1948.
437. Wilson, P.D.: Capsulectomy for the Relief of Flexion Contractures of the Elbow Following Fractures. J. Bone Joint Surg., 26:71–86, 1944.

Sports Injuries

438. Anderson, T.E.; and Ciocek, J.: Specific Rehabilitation Programs for the Throwing Athlete. Instr. Course Lect. XXXVIII:487–491, 1989.
439. Andrews, J.R.: Bony Injuries About the Elbow in the Throwing Athlete. Instr. Course Lect., XXXIV:323–331, 1985.
440. Ariel, G.B.: Biomechanical Analysis of the Javelin Throw. Track Field Q. Rev., 80:9, 1980.
441. Barnes, D.A.; and Tullos, H.S.: An Analysis of 100 Symp-

tomatic Baseball Players. Am. J. Sports Med., 6:62–67, 1978.

442. Bennett, G.E.: Shoulder and Elbow Lesions of the Professional Baseball Pitcher. J.A.M.A., 117:510–514, 1941.

443. Bennett, G.E.: Shoulder and Elbow Lesions Distinctive of Baseball Players. Ann. Surg., 126:107–110, 1947.

444. Bennett, G.E.: Injuries Characteristic of Particular Sports: Elbow and Shoulder Lesions of Baseball Players. Am. J. Surg., 98:484–492, 1959.

445. Cabrera, J.M.; and McCue, F.C., III: Nonosseous Athletic Injuries of the Elbow, Forearm, and Hand. Clin. Sports. Med., 5:681–700, 1986.

446. DeHaven, K.E.; and Evarts, C.M.: Throwing Injuries of the Elbow in Athletes. Orthop. Clin. North Am., 4:801–808, 1973.

447. Gore, R.M.; Rogers, L.F.; Bowerman, J.; Suker, J.; and Compere, C.L.: Osseous Manifestations of Elbow Stresses Associated With Sports Activities. A.J.R., 134:971–977, 1980.

448. Greene, C.P.: The Curve Ball and the Elbow. *In* Zarins, B.; Andres, J.R.; and Carson, W.G. (eds.): Injuries to the Throwing Arm, pp. 38–39. Philadelphia, W.B. Saunders, 1985.

449. Groppel, J.; and Nirschl, R.P.: A Biomechanical and EMG Analysis of the Effects of Counter-force Braces on the Tennis Player. Am. J. Sports Med., 14:195–200, 1986.

450. Hulkko, A.; Orava, S.; and Nikula, P.: Stress Fractures of the Olecranon in Javelin Throwers. Int. J. Sports Med., 7:210–213, 1986.

451. Indelicato, P.A.; Jobe, F.W.; Kerlan, R.K.; Carter, V.S.; Shields, C.L.; and Lombardo, S.J.: Correctable Elbow Lesions in Professional Baseball Players: A Review of 25 Cases. Am. J. Sports Med., 7:72–75, 1979.

452. Ireland, M.L.; and Andrews, J.R.: Shoulder and Elbow Injuries in the Young Athlete. Clin. Sports Med., 7:473–494, 1988.

453. Jobe, F.W.: Discussion of an Analysis of 100 Symptomatic Baseball Players. Am. J. Sports Med., 6:66–67, 1978.

454. Jobe, F.W.; and Nuber, G.: Throwing Injuries of the Elbow. Clin. Sports Med., 5:621–636, 1986.

455. Jobe, F.W.; Stark, H.; and Lombardo, S.J.: Reconstruction of the Ulnar Collateral Ligament in Athletes. J. Bone Joint Surg., 68A:1158–1163, 1986.

456. King, J.W.; Breslford, H.J.; and Tullos, H.S.: Analysis of the Pitching Arm of the Professional Baseball Pitcher. Clin. Orthop., 67:116–123, 1969.

457. Kovach, J.; Baker, B.E.; and Mosher, J.F.: Fracture Separation of the Olecranon Ossification Center in Adults. Am. J. Sports Med., 13:105–111, 1985.

458. McManama, G.B.; Micheli, L.J.; Berry, M.V.; and Sohn, R.S.: The Surgical Treatment of Osteochondritis of the Capitellum. Am. J. Sports Med., 13:11–21, 1985.

459. Miller, J.E.: Javelin Thrower's Elbow. J. Bone Joint Surg., 42B:788–792, 1960.

460. Morrey, B.F., and An, K.N.: Articular and Ligamentous Contributions to the Stability of the Elbow Joint. Am. J. Sports Med., 11:315–319, 1983.

461. Orava, S., and Hulkko, A.: Delayed Unions and Nonunions

of Stress Fractures in Athletes. Am. J. Sports Med., 16:378–382, 1988.

462. Sisto, D.J.; Jobe, F.W.; Moynes, D.R.; and Antonelli, D.J.: An Electromyographic Analysis of the Elbow in Pitching. Am. J. Sports Med., 15:260–263, 1987.

463. Slocum, D.B.: Classification of Elbow Injuries From Baseball Pitching. Tex. Med., 64:48–53, 1968.

464. Wilson, F.D.; Andrews, J.R.; Blackburn, T.A.; and McCluskey, G.: Valgus Extension Overload in the Pitching Elbow. Am. J. Sports Med., 11:83–88, 1983.

465. Woods, G.W.; Tullos, H.S.; and King, J.E.: The Throwing Arm: Elbow Joint Injuries. J. Sports Med., 1:43–47, 1973.

466. Zarins, B.; Andrews, J.R.; and Carson, W.G.: Injuries to the Throwing Arm. Philadelphia, W.B. Saunders, 1985.

Olecranon Fractures

467. Adler, S.; Fay, G.F.; and MacAusland, W.R.: Olecranon Fractures. J. Bone Joint Surg., 41A:1540, 1959.

468. Adler, S.; Fay, G.F.; and MacAusland, W.R., Jr.: Treatment of Olecranon Fractures. Indications for Excision of the Olecranon Fragment and Repair of the Triceps Tendon. J. Trauma, 2:597–602, 1962.

469. An, K.N.; Morrey, B.F.; and Chao, E.Y.S.: The Effect of Partial Removal of Proximal Ulna on Elbow Constraint. Clin. Orthop., 209:270–279, 1986.

470. Aufranc, O.E., and Jones, W.N.: Open Fracture of the Olecranon. J.A.M.A., 202:427–429, 1967.

471. Bennett, G.S.: Fractures of the Olecranon and Its Repair. Am. J. Orthop. Surg., 11:121–123, 1969.

472. Berger, P.: Le traitement de fractures de l'olecrane et particulierment la sutur de l'olecrane pa un procede (cedarg de l'olecranon). Ga. 2 Hebd. de Med., 2:193–199, 1902.

473. Böhler, L.: The Treatment of Fractures. Vienna, Wilhelm Maudrich, 1929.

474. Böhler, L.: The Treatment of Fractures, vol. 1, 5th ed. New York, Grune & Stratton, 1956.

475. Bryan, R.S.: Fractures About the Elbow in Adults. Instr. Course Lect., XXX:200–203, 1981.

476. Cabanela, M.E.: Fractures of the Proximal Ulna and Olecranon. *In* Morrey, B.F. (ed.): The Elbow and Its Disorders. Philadelphia, W.B. Saunders, 1985.

477. Cave, E.F.: Fractures and Other Injuries. Chicago, Year Book Publishers, 1958.

478. Cave, E.F.: Preoperative and Postoperative Management of Injuries to the Elbow. Clin. Orthop., 38:48–57, 1965.

479. Colton, C.L.: Fractures of the Olecranon in Adults: Classification and Management. Injury, 5:121–129, 1973.

480. Conn, J., and Wade, P.A.: Injuries of the Elbow (A Ten-Year Review). J. Trauma, 1:248–268, 1961.

481. Coughlin, M.J.; Slabaugh, P.B.; and Smith, T.K.: Experience With the McAtee Olecranon Device in Olecranon Fractures. J. Bone Joint Surg., 61A:385–388, 1979.

482. Crenshaw, A.H.: Campbell's Operative Orthopaedics, 5th ed. St. Louis, C.V. Mosby, 1971.

483. Daland, E.M.: Fractures of the Olecranon. J. Bone Joint Surg., 15:601–607, 1933.

484. Deane, M.: Comminuted Fractures of the Olecranon. An Appliance for Internal Fixation. Injury, 2:103–106, 1970.

485. Deliyannis, S.N.: Comminuted Fractures of the Olecranon Treated by Weber-Vasey Technique. Injury, 5:19–24, 1973.

486. Dunn, N.: Operation for Fracture of the Olecranon. Br. Med. J., 1:214–215, 1939.

487. Eliot, E., Jr.: Fracture of the Olecranon. Surg. Clin. North Am., 14:487–492, 1934.

488. Eriksson, E.; Sahlen, O.; and Sandahl, U.: Late Results of Conservative and Surgical Treatment of Fracture of the Olecranon. Acta Chir. Scand., 113:153–166, 1957.

489. Fernandez, G.N.: Pseudarthrosis of the Ulna and Osteoarthritis of the Elbow. A Case Report. J. Bone Joint Surg., 68B:574–576, 1986.

490. Finlayson, D.: Complications of Tension-band Wiring of Olecranon Fractures [Letter]. J. Bone Joint Surg., 68A:951–952, 1986.

491. Fiolle, D.J.: Note sur les fractures de folecrane par projectiles de guerre. Marseille Medical, 55:241–245, 1918.

492. Fitts, W.T., Jr.: Fractures of the Upper Extremity (A Review of Experiences in World War II). Am. J. Surg., 72:393–403, 1946.

493. Fyfe, I.S.; Mossad, M.M.; and Holdsworth, B.J.: Methods of Fixation of Olecranon Fractures: An Experimental Mechanical Study. J. Bone Joint Surg., 67B:367–372, 1985.

494. Gartsman, G.M.; Sculco, T.P.; and Otis, J.C.: Operative Treatment of Olecranon Fractures Excision or Open Reduction With Internal Fixation. J. Bone Joint Surg., 63A:718–721, 1981.

495. Harmon, P.H.: Treatment of Fractures of the Olecranon by Fixation With Stainless-Steel Screws. J. Bone Joint Surg., 27:328–329, 1945.

496. Heim, U., and Pfeiffer, K.M.: Elbow. In Heim, U., and Pfeiffer, K.M. (eds.): Internal Fixation of Small Fractures, 3rd ed., pp. 107–109. Berlin, Springer-Verlag, 1988.

497. Helm, R.H.; Hornby, R.; and Miller, S.W.M.: The Complications of Surgical Treatment of Displaced Fractures of the Olecranon. Injury, 18:48–50, 1987.

498. Hey-Groves, E.W.: Fracture of the Olecranon. Br. Med. J., 1:296, 1939.

499. Holdsworth, B.J., and Mossad, M.M.: Elbow Function Following Tension Band Fixation of Displaced Fractures of the Olecranon. Injury, 16:182–187, 1984.

500. Horne, J.G., and Tanzer, T.L.: Olecranon Fractures: A Review of 100 Cases. J. Trauma, 21:469–472, 1981.

501. Howard, J.L., and Urist, M.R.: Fracture-Dislocation of the Radius and the Ulna at the Elbow Joint. Clin. Orthop., 12:276–284, 1958.

502. Jensen, C.M., and Olsen, B.B.: Drawbacks of Traction-absorbing Wiring (TAW) in Displaced Fractures of the Olecranon. Injury, 17:174–175, 1986.

503. Johnson, R.P.; Roetker, A.; and Schwab, J.P.: Olecranon Fractures Treated With AO Screw and Tension Bands. Orthopedics, 9:66–68, 1986.

504. Keon-Cohen, B.T.: Fractures at the Elbow. J. Bone Joint Surg., 48A:1623–1639, 1966.

505. Kiviluoto, O., and Santavirta, S.: Fractures of the Olecranon. Acta Orthop. Scand., 49:28–31, 1978.

506. Knight, R.A.: Management of Fractures About the Elbow in Adults. Instr. Course Lect., 14:123–141, 1957.

507. Kohler, A., and Zimmer, E.A.: Borderlands of the Normal and Early Pathologic in Skeletal Roentgenology, 3rd ed. New York, Grune & Stratton, 1968.

508. Larsen, E., and Lyndrup, P.: Netz or Kirschner Pins in the Treatment of Olecranon Fractures? J. Trauma, 27:664–666, 1987.

509. Lister, J.: An Address on the Treatment of Fracture of the Patella. Br. Med. J. [Clin. Res.], 2:855–860, 1883.

510. Lou, I.: Olecranon Fractures Treated in the Orthopaedic Hospital, Copenhagen 1936–1947. A Follow-up Examination. Acta Orthop. Scand., 19:166–179, 1949.

511. MacAusland, W.R.: The Treatment of Fractures of the Olecranon by Longitudinal Screw or Nail Fixation. Ann. Surg., 116:293–296, 1942.

512. MacAusland, W.R., and Wyman, E.T.: Fractures of the Adult Elbow. Instr. Course Lect., 24:169–181, 1975.

513. Macko, D., and Szabo, R.M.: Complications of Tension-Band Wiring of Olecranon Fractures. J. Bone Joint Surg., 67A:1369–1401, 1985.

514. Mathewson, M.H., and McCreath, S.W.: Tension Band Wiring in the Treatment of Olecranon Fractures. J. Bone Joint Surg., 57B:399, 1975.

515. McDougall, A.M., and White, J.: Subluxation of the Inferior Radio-ulnar Joint Complicating Fracture of the Radial Head. J. Bone Joint Surg., 39B:278–287, 1957.

516. McKeever, F.M., and Buck, R.M.: Fracture of the Olecranon Process of the Ulna. J.A.M.A., 135:1–5, 1947.

517. Montgomery, R.J.: A Secure Method of Olecranon Fixation: A Modification of Tension-band Wiring Technique. J. R. Coll. Surg. Edinb., 31:179–182, 1986.

518. Muller, M.E.; Allgower, M.; Schneider, R.; and Willenegger, H.: Manual of Internal Fixation, 2nd ed. New York, Springer-Verlag, 1970.

519. Murphy, D.F.; Greene, W.B.; and Dameron, T.B., Jr.: Displaced Olecranon Fractures in Adults. Clinical Evaluation. Clin. Orthop., 224:215–223, 1987.

520. Murphy, D.F.; Greene, W.B.; Gilbert, J.A.; and Dameron, T.B., Jr.: Displaced Olecranon Fractures in Adults. Biomechanical Analysis of Fixation Methods. Clin. Orthop., 224:210–214, 1987.

521. Netz, P., and Stromberg, L.: Non-Sliding Pins in Traction Absorbing Wire of Fractures: A Modified Technique. Acta Orthop. Scand., 53:355–360, 1982.

522. O'Donoghue, D.H., and Sell, L.S.: Persistent Olecranon Epiphysis in Adults. J. Bone Joint Surg., 24:677–680, 1942.

523. Perkins, G.: Fractures of the Olecranon. Br. Med. J. [Clin. Res.], 2:668–669, 1936.

524. Regan, W., and Morrey, B.F.: Fractures of Coronoid Process of the Ulna. J. Bone Joint Surg. 71A:1348–1354, 1989.

525. Rettig, A.C.; Waugh, T.R.; and Evanski, P.M.: Fracture of the Olecranon: A Problem of Management. J. Trauma, 19:23–28, 1979.

526. Rombold, C.: A New Operative Treatment for Fractures of the Olecranon. J. Bone Joint Surg., 16:947–949, 1934.

527. Rowe, C.: The Management of Fractures in Elderly Patients Is Different. J. Bone Joint Surg., 47A:1043–1059, 1965.

528. Rowland, S.A.: Tension Band Wiring of Olecranon Fractures—A Modification of the Technique. Clin. Orthop., in press.

529. Rush, L.V., and Rush, H.L.: A Reconstruction Operation for Comminuted Fractures of Upper Third of the Ulna. Am. J. Surg., 38:332–333, 1937.

530. Scharplatz, D., and Allgower, M.: Fracture Dislocation of the Elbow. Injury, 7:143–159, 1975.

531. Selesnick, F.H.; Dolitsky, B.; and Haskell, S.S.: Fracture of the Coronoid Process Requiring Open Reduction With Internal Fixation. J. Bone Joint Surg., 66A:1304–1305, 1984.

532. Smith, F.M.: Surgery of the Elbow. Philadelphia, W.B. Saunders, 1972.

533. Stug, L.H.: Anterior Dislocation of the Elbow With Fracture of the Olecranon. Am. J. Surg., 85:700–703, 1948.

534. Taylor, T.K.F., and Scham, S.M.: A Posteromedial Approach to the Proximal End of the Ulna for the Internal Fixation of Olecranon Fractures. J. Trauma, 9:594–602, 1969.

535. Van Der Kloot, J.F.V.R.: Results of Treatment of Fractures of the Olecranon. Arch. Chir. Neerlandisum, 16:237–249, 1964.

536. Wadsworth, T.G.: Screw Fixation of the Olecranon After Fracture or Osteotomy. Clin. Orthop., 119:197–201, 1976.

537. Wainwright, D.: Fractures of the Olecranon Process. Br. J. Surg., 29:403–406, 1942.

538. Watson-Jones, R.: Fractures and Joint Injuries, vol. 2, 3rd ed. Baltimore, Williams & Wilkins, 1946.

539. Watson-Jones, R.: Fractures and Joint Injuries, 4th ed. Edinburgh, E.S. Livingstone, 1952.

540. Waxman, A., and Geshelin, H.: Fracture of the Olecranon Process Due to Muscle Pull With the Forearm in Hyperextension. Calif. Med., 66:358–359, 1947.

541. Weseley, M.S.; Barnefeld, P.A.; and Eisenstein, A.L.: The Use of Zuelzer Hook Plate in Fixation of Olecranon Fractures. J. Bone Joint Surg., 58A:859–863, 1976.

542. Willenegger, H.: Problems and Results in the Treatment of Comminuted Fractures of the Elbow. Reconstr. Surg. Traumatol., 11:118–127, 1969.

543. Wilppula, E., and Bakalim, G.: Fractures of the Olecranon. III. Fractures Complicated by Forward Dislocation of the Forearm. Ann. Chir. Gynaecol. Fenn., 60:105–108, 1971.

544. Wilson, P.D.: Fractures and Dislocations in the Region of the Elbow. Surg. Gynecol. Obstet., 56:335–359, 1933.

545. Wolfgang, G.; Burke, F.; Bush, D.; Parenti, J.; Perry, J.; and LaFollette, B.: Surgical Treatment of Displaced Olecranon Fractures by Tension Band Wiring Technique. Clin. Orthop., 224:192–204, 1987.

546. Zuelzer, W.A.: Fixation of Small But Important Bone Fragments With a Hook Plate. J. Bone Joint Surg., 33A:430–436, 1951.

Radial Head Fractures

547. Adler, J.B., and Shaftan, G.W.: Radial Head Fractures, Is Excision Necessary? J. Trauma, 4:115–136, 1964.

548. Arner, O.; Ekengren, K.; and von Schreeb, T.: Fractures of the Head and Neck of the Radius: A Clinical and Roentgenographic Study of 310 Cases. Acta Chir. Scand., 112:115–134, 1957.

549. Aufranc, O.E.; Jones, W.N.; Turner, R.H.; and Thomas, W.H.: Dislocation of the Elbow With Fracture of the Radial Head and Distal Radius. J.A.M.A., 202:131–134, 1967.

550. Bakalim, G.: Fractures of Radial Head and Their Treatment. Acta Orthop. Scand., 41:320–331, 1970.

551. Barrington, T.W.: Radial Head Replacement (Abstract). J. Bone Joint Surg., 51B:778, 1969.

552. Bohl, W.R., and Brightman, E.: Fracture of a Silastic Radial-Head Prosthesis: Diagnosis and Localization of Fragments by Xerography. J. Bone Joint Surg., 63A:1482–1483, 1981.

553. Bohrer, J.V.: Fractures of the Head and Neck of the Radius. Ann. Surg., 97:204–208, 1933.

554. Broberg, M.A., and Morrey, B.F.: Results of Delayed Excision of the Radial Head After Fracture. J. Bone Joint Surg., 68A:669–674, 1986.

555. Broberg, M.A., and Morrey, B.F.: Results of Treatment of Fracture-Dislocations of the Elbow. Clin. Orthop., 216:109–119, 1987.

556. Brockman, E.P.: Two Cases of Disability at the Wrist Joint Following Excision of the Head of the Radius. Proc. R. Soc. Med., 24:904–905, 1930.

557. Buffington, C.B.: The Treatment of Simple and Comminuted Fractures of the Head of the Radius. W. Va. Med. J., 43:198–200, 1947.

558. Bunker, T.D., and Newman, J.H.: The Herbert Differential Pitch Bone Screw in Displaced Radial Head Fractures. Injury, 16:621–624, 1985.

559. Burton, A.E.: Fractures of the Head of the Radius. Proc. R. Soc. Med., 35:764–765, 1942.

560. Buxton St, J.D.: Fractures of the Head of the Radius and Capitellum Including Fractures of Childhood. Br. Med. J. [Clin. Res.], 2:665–666, 1938.

561. Carn, R.M.; Medige, J.; Curtain, D.; and Koneig, A.: Silicone Rubber Replacement of the Severely Fractured Radial Head. Clin. Orthop., 209:259–269, 1986.

562. Carr, C.R.: Metallic Cap Replacement of the Radial Head (Abstract). J. Bone Joint Surg., 53A:1661, 1971.

563. Carr, C.R., and Howard, J.W.: Metallic Cap Replacement of Radial Head Following Fracture. West. J. Surg., 59:539–546, 1951.

564. Carstam, N.N.: Operative Treatment of Fracture of the Head and Neck of the Radius. Acta Chir. Scand., 19:502–526, 1951.

565. Castberg, T., and Thing, E.: Treatment of Fractures of the Upper End of the Radius. Acta Chir. Scand., 105:62–69, 1953.

566. Charnley, J.: The Closed Treatment of Common Fractures. Edinburgh, E & S Livingstone, 1950.

567. Cherry, J.C.: Fracture of the Head of the Radius Treated by Excision and Substitution of an Acrylic Head. J. Bone Joint Surg., 35B:486, 1953.

568. Cherry, J.C.: Use of Acrylic Prosthesis in the Treatment of Fracture of the Head of the Radius. J. Bone Joint Surg., 35B:70–71, 1953.

569. Coleman, D.A.; Blair, W.F.; and Shurr, D.: Resection of the Radial Head for Fracture of the Radial Head. J. Bone Joint Surg., 69A:385–392, 1987.

570. Crawford, G.P.: Late Radial Tunnel Syndrome After Excision of the Radial Head. J. Bone Joint Surg., 70A:1416–1418, 1988.

571. Curr, J.F., and Coe, W.A.: Dislocation of the Inferior Radio-ulnar Joint. Br. J. Surg., 34:74–77, 1946.

572. Currey, J.; Therkildsen, L.H.; and Bywaters, E.G.: Monarticular Rheumatoid-like Arthritis of Seven Years' Duration Following Fracture of the Radial Head. Ann. Rheum. Dis., 45:783–785, 1986.

573. Cutler, C.W.: Fractures of the Head and Neck of the Radius. Ann. Surg., 83:267–278, 1926.

574. Edwards, G.S., and Jupiter, J.B.: Radial Head Fracture With Acute Distal Radioulnar Dislocation—Essex-Lopresti Revisited. Clin. Orthop., 234:61–69, 1988.

575. Eliason, E.L., and North, J.P.: Fractures About the Elbow. Am. J. Surg., 44:88–99, 1939.

576. Epner, R.A.; Bowers, W.H.; and Guilford, W.B.: Ulnar Variance—The Effect of Wrist Positioning and Roentgen Filming Technique. J. Hand Surg., 7:298–305, 1982.

577. Essex-Lopresti, P.: Fractures of the Radial Head With Distal Radial-Ulnar Dislocations. J. Bone Joint Surg., 33B:244–247, 1951.

578. Flemming, C.W.: Fractures of the Head of the Radius. Proc. R. Soc. Med., 25:1011–1015, 1932.

579. Gaston, S.R.; Smith, F.M.; and Baab, O.D.: Adult Injuries of the Radial Head and Neck. Am. J. Surg., 78:631–635, 1949.

580. Gerard, Y.; Schernburg, F.; and Nerot, C.: Anatomical Pathological and Therapeutic Investigation of Fractures of the Radial Head in Adults. J. Bone Joint Surg., 66B:141, 1984.

581. Goldberg, I.; Peylan, J.; and Yosipovitch, Z.: Late Results of Excision of the Radial Head for an Isolated Closed Fracture. J. Bone Joint Surg., 68A:675–679, 1986.

582. Gordon, M., and Bullough, P.G.: Synovial and Osseous Inflammation in Failed Silicone-Rubber Prosthesis. J. Bone Joint Surg., 64A:574–580, 1982.

583. Greenspan, A., and Norman, A.: Radial Head–Capitellum View: An Expanded Imaging Approach to Elbow Injury. Radiology, 164:272–274, 1987.

584. Grossman, J.: Fracture of the Head and Neck of the Radius. New York Med. J., 117:472–475, 1923.

585. Grundy, A.; Murphy, G.; Barker, A.; Guest, P.; and Jack, L.: The Value of the Radial Head–Capitellum View in Radial Head Trauma. Br. J. Radiol., 58:965–967, 1985.

586. Harrington, I.J., and Tountas, A.A.: Replacement of the Radial Head in the Treatment of Unstable Elbow Fractures. Injury, 12:405–412, 1981.

587. Heim, U., and Pfeiffer, K.M.: Elbow. In Heim, U., and Pfeiffer, K.M. (eds.): Internal Fixation of Small Fractures, 3rd ed., pp. 107–109. Berlin, Springer-Verlag, 1988.

588. Hein, B.J.: Fractures of the Head of the Radius. Indust. Med., 6:529–532, 1937.

589. Holdsworth, B.J.; Clement, D.A.; and Rothwell, P.N.: Fractures of the Radial Head—The Benefit of Aspiration: A Prospective Controlled Trial. Injury, 18:44–47, 1987.

590. Horne, G., and Sim, P.: Nonunion of the Radial Head. J. Trauma, 25:452–453, 1985.

591. Hotchkiss, R.N.; An, K.N.; Sowa, D.T.; Basta, S.; and Weiland, A.J.: Pathomechanics of Proximal Migration of the Radius: An Anatomic and Mechanical Study of the Interosseous Membrane of the Forearm. J. Hand Surg., 14A:256–261, 1989.

592. Hotchkiss, R.N., and Weiland, A.J.: Valgus Stability of the Elbow. J. Orthop. Res., 5:372–377, 1987.

593. Jacobs, J.E., and Kernodle, H.B.: Fractures of the Head of the Radius. J. Bone Joint Surg., 28:616–622, 1946.

594. Johnston, G.W.: A Follow-up of One Hundred Cases of Fracture of the Head of the Radius With a Review of the Literature. Ulster Med. J., 31:51–56, 1962.

595. Keon-Cohen, B.T.: Fractures at the Elbow. J. Bone Joint Surg., 48A:1623–1639, 1966.

596. Key, J.A.: Treatment of Fractures of the Head and Neck of the Radius. J.A.M.A., 96:101–104, 1931.

597. Khurana, J.S.; Kattapuram, S.V.; Becker, S.; and Mayo-Smith, W.: Galeazzi Injury With an Associated Fracture of the Radial Head. Clin. Orthop., 234:70–71, 1988.

598. King, B.B.: Resection of the Radial Head and Neck. J. Bone Joint Surg., 21:839–857, 1939.

599. Levin, P.D.: Fracture of the Radial Head With Dislocation of the Distal Radio-Ulnar Joint: Case Report. J. Bone Joint Surg., 55A:837–840, 1973.

600. Lewis, R.W., and Thibodeau, A.A.: Deformity of the Wrist Following Resection of the Radial Head. Surg. Gynecol. Obstet., 64:1079–1085, 1937.

601. Mackay, I.; Fitzgerald, B.; and Miller, J.H.: Silastic Replacement of the Head of the Radius in Trauma. J. Bone Joint Surg., 61B:494–497, 1979.

602. Martinelli, B.: Fractures of the Radial Head Treated by Substitution With the Silastic Prosthesis. Bull. Hosp. Joint Dis., 36:61–65, 1975.

603. Mason, J.A., and Shutkin, N.M.: Immediate Active Motion Treatment of Fractures of the Head and Neck of the Radius. Surg. Gynecol. Obstet., 76:731–737, 1943.

604. Mason, M.L.: Some Observations on Fractures of the Head of the Radius With a Review of One Hundred Cases. Br. J. Surg., 42:123–132, 1954.

605. Mayhall, W.S.T.; Tiley, F.W.; and Paluska, D.J.: Fracture of Silastic Radial-Head Prosthesis. J. Bone Joint Surg., 63A:459–460, 1981.

606. McArthur, R.A.: Herbert Screw Fixation of Fracture of the Head of the Radius. Clin. Orthop., 224:79–87, 1987.

607. McDougall, A., and White, J.: Subluxation of the Inferior Radio-Ulnar Joint Complicating Fracture of the Radial Head. J. Bone Joint Surg., 39B:278–286, 1957.

608. McLaughlin, H.L.: Fracture of the Head of the Radius in Trauma, pp. 221–225. Philadelphia, W.B. Saunders, 1959.
609. Meekison, D.M.: Some Remarks on Three Common Fractures. J. Bone Joint Surg., 27:80–85, 1945.
610. Mikic, Z.D., and Vukadinovic, S.M.: Late Results in Fractures of the Radial Head Treated by Excision. Clin. Orthop., 181:220–227, 1983.
611. Miller, G.K.; Drennan, D.B.; and Maylahn, D.J.: Treatment of Displaced Segmental Radial-Head Fractures. J. Bone Joint Surg., 63A:712–717, 1981.
612. Morrey, B.F.: Radial Head Fracture. *In* Morrey, B.F. (ed.): The Elbow and Its Disorders, vol. 1, p. 378. Philadelphia, W.B. Saunders, 1985.
613. Morrey, B.F.; Askew, L.; and Chao, E.Y.: Silastic Prosthetic Replacement for the Radial Head. J. Bone Joint Surg., 63A:454–458, 1981.
614. Morrey, B.F.; Chao, E.Y.; and Hui, F.C.: Biomechanical Study of the Elbow Following Excision of the Radial Head. J. Bone Joint Surg., 61A:63–68, 1979.
615. Murphy, W.A., and Siegel, M.J.: Elbow Fat Pads With New Signs and Extended Differential Diagnosis. Radiology, 124:659–665, 1977.
616. Murray, R.C.: Fractures of the Head and Neck of the Radius. Br. J. Surg., 28:106–118, 1940.
617. O'Connor, B.T., and Taylor, T.K.F.: The Conservative Approach to Radial Head Fractures (Abstract). J. Bone Joint Surg., 44B:743, 1962.
618. Odenheimer, K., and Harvey, J.P.: Internal Fixation of Fracture of the Head of the Radius. J. Bone Joint Surg., 61A:785–787, 1979.
619. Perry, C.R., and Tessier, J.E.: Open Reduction and Internal Fixation of Radial Head Fractures Associated With Olecranon Fracture or Dislocation. J. Orthop. Trauma, 1:36–42, 1987.
620. Pike, W.: Fracture of the Head of the Radius. (Abstract). J. Bone Joint Surg., 51B:198. 1969.
621. Pinder, J.M.: Fracture of the Head of the Radius in Adults. (Abstract). J. Bone Joint Surg., 51B:386, 1969.
622. Postlethwait, R.W.: Modified Treatment for Fracture of the Head of the Radius. Am. J. Surg., 67:77–80, 1945.
623. Poulsen, J.O., and Tophoj, K.: Fracture of the Head and Neck of the Radius. Acta Orthop. Scand., 45:66–75, 1974.
624. Pribyl, C.R.; Kester, M.A.; Cook, S.D.; Edmunds, J.O.; and Brunet, M.E.: The Effect of the Radial Head and Prosthetic Radial Head Replacement on Resisting Valgus Stress at the Elbow. Orthopedics, 9:723–726, 1986.
625. Quigley, T.B.: Aspiration of the Elbow Joint in the Treatment of Fractures of the Head of the Radius. N. Engl. J. Med., 240:915–916, 1949.
626. Radin, E.L., and Riseborough, E.J.: Fractures of the Radial Head. J. Bone Joint Surg., 48A:1055–1064, 1966.
627. Rieth, P.L.: Fractures of the Radial Head Associated With Chip Fracture of the Capitellum in Adults; Surgical Considerations. South. Surg., 14:154–159, 1948.
628. Rymaszewski, L.A.; Mackay, I.; Amis, A.A.; and Miller, J.H.: Long-term Effects of Excision of the Radial Head in Rheumatoid Arthritis. J. Bone Joint Surg., 66B:109–113, 1984.
629. Sever, J.W.: Fractures of the Head and Neck of the Radius. A Study of End Results. J.A.M.A., 84:1551–1555, 1925.
630. Shumeli, G., and Herold, H.Z.: Compression Screwing of Displaced Fractures of the Head of the Radius. J. Bone Joint Surg., 63B:535–538, 1981.
631. Sowa, D.T.; Hotchkiss, R.N.; and Weiland, A.J.: Symptomatic Proximal Translation of the Radius Following Radial Head Fracture. Submitted, 1990.
632. Speed, K.: Fracture of the Head of the Radius. Am. J. Surg., 38:157–159, 1924.
633. Speed, K.: Ferrule Caps for the Head of the Radius. Surg. Gynecol. Obstet., 73:845–850, 1941.
634. Stephen, I.B.M.: Excision of the Radial Head for Closed Fracture. Acta Orthop. Scand., 52:409–412, 1981.
635. Strachan, J.C.H., and Ellis, B.W.: Vulnerability of the Posterior Interosseous Nerve During Radial Head Resection. J. Bone Joint Surg., 53B:320–323, 1971.
636. Sutro, C.J.: Regrowth of Bone at the Proximal End of the Radius Following Resection of the Radial Head. J. Bone Joint Surg., 17:867–878, 1935.
637. Sutro, C.J., and Sutro, W.H.: Fractures of the Radial Head in Adults With the Complication "Cubitus Valgus." Bull. Hosp. Jt. Dis. Orthop. Inst., 45:65–73, 1985.
638. Swanson, A.B.; Jaeger, S.H.; and La Rochelle, D.: Comminuted Fractures of the Radial Head. J. Bone Joint Surg., 63A:1039–1049, 1981.
639. Taylor, T.K.F., and O'Connor, B.T.: The Effect Upon the Inferior Radio-ulnar Joint of Excision of the Head of the Radius in Adults. J. Bone Joint Surg., 46B:83–88, 1964.
640. Thomas, T.T.: Univ. Penn. Med. Bull., Fractures of the Head of the Radius. An Experimental Study and Report of Cases. 18:184–197, 1905.
641. Vichard, P.; Tropet, Y.; Dreyfus-Schmidt, G.; Besancenot, J.; and Menez, D.: Treatment of Isolated Fractures of the Proximal End of the Radius in Adults: Remarks Concerning 168 Cases. Ann Chir. Main., 6:189–194, 1987.
642. Wadsworth, T.G.: Fractures of the Radial Head and Neck. *In* (ed.): The Elbow, pp. 190–196. Edinburgh, Churchill Livingstone, 1982.
643. Wagner, C.J.: Fractures of the Head of the Radius. Am. J. Surg., 89:911–913, 1955.
644. Weingarden, T.L.: Prosthetic Replacement in the Treatment of Fractures of the Radial Head. J. Am. Osteopath. Assoc., 77:804–807, 1978.
645. Weseley, M.S.; Barenfeld, P.A.; and Eisenstein, A.L.: Closed Treatment of Isolated Radial Head Fractures. J. Trauma, 23:36–39, 1983.
646. Wheeler, D.K., and Linscheid, R.L.: Fracture-Dislocations of the Elbow. Clin. Orthop., 50:95–106, 1967.
647. Wilson, P.D.: Fractures and Dislocations in the Region of the Elbow. Surg. Gynecol. Obstet., 56:335–359, 1933.
648. Worsing, R.A.; Engber, W.D.; and Lange, T.A.: Reactive Synovitis From Particulate Silastic. J. Bone Joint Surg., 64A:581–584, 1982.

Sideswipe Injuries

649. Highsmith, L.S., and Phalen, G.S.: Sideswipe Fractures. Arch. Surg., 52:513–522, 1946.

650. Kuur, E., and Kjaersgaard-Anderson: Side-Swipe Injury
      to the Elbow. J. Trauma, 28:1397–1399, 1988.

651. Meals, R.A.: The Use of a Flexor Carpi Ulnaris Muscle
      Flap in the Treatment of an Infected Nonunion of the
      Proximal Ulna. A Case Report. Clin. Orthop., 240:168–
      172, 1989.

652. Nicholson, J.T.: Compound Comminuted Fractures In-
      volving the Elbow Joint. J. Bone Joint Surg., 28:565–
      575, 1946.

653. Sbitany, U., and Wray, R.C., Jr.: Use of the Rectus Ab-
      dominis Muscle Flap to Reconstruct an Elbow Defect.
      Plast. Reconstr. Surg., 77:988–989, 1986.

654. Shorbe, H.B.: Car Window Elbows. South. Med. J., 34:
      372–376, 1941.

655. Stern, P.J., and Carey, J.P.: The Latissimus Dorsi Flap for
      Reconstruction of the Brachium and Shoulder. J. Bone
      Joint Surg., 70A:526–535, 1988.

656. Wood, C.F.: Traffic Elbow. Kentucky Med. J., 39:78–81,
      1941.

11

Fractures of the Shaft
of the Humerus

Charles H. Epps, Jr.
Richard E. Grant

The shaft of the humerus is capable of a wide range of responses when it is fractured. The surgeon today has many therapeutic options from which to choose. The decision should be based on the type and location of the fracture, the presence of concomitant injuries, and the age and general condition of the patient. Closed methods of treatment are usually successful, although in some fractures union is difficult to obtain. Open methods are sometimes necessary. Work and recreational activities subject this area of the humerus to a diverse array of forces.

ANATOMY

An understanding of the anatomy of the upper arm is essential for proper treatment of fractures of the shaft of the humerus. Anatomically, the shaft may be considered to extend from the upper border of the insertion of the pectoralis major muscle above to the supracondylar ridges below. The upper half of the shaft is cylindrical on cross section; it tends to become flat in the distal portion in an anteroposterior direction. Three borders and three surfaces are described. The anterior border extends from the front of the greater tuberosity above to the coronoid fossa below. The medial border begins with the crest of the lesser tuberosity and ends at the medial supracondylar ridge. The lateral border extends from the back of the greater tuberosity above to the lateral supracondylar ridge. The anterolateral surface presents the deltoid tuberosity, for the insertion of the deltoid, and below this the radial sulcus, which

transmits the radial nerve and profunda artery. The anteromedial surface forms the floor of the intertubercular groove, but it has no outstanding surface markings. The posterior surface is the origin for the triceps and contains the spiral groove.[42]

There are medial and lateral intermuscular septa that divide the arm into anterior and posterior compartments. The biceps brachii, coracobrachialis, and brachialis anticus muscles are contained in the anterior compartment. The neurovascular bundle courses along the medial border of the biceps and includes the brachial artery and vein and the median, musculocutaneous, and ulnar nerves. The posterior compartment contains the triceps brachii muscle and the radial nerve.[49] An interesting variation is the supracondylar process, a projection arising from the anteromedial surface, about 2 inches above the medial epicondyle.[93] When the process is present, the median nerve and the brachial artery take an abnormal course to pass behind it and then forward between a fibrous band connecting the process to the epicondyle.

An analysis of humeral shaft fractures is made possible by an appreciation of the muscle forces that act on the shaft at varying levels (Fig. 11-1). A fracture above the level of the pectoralis major allows the proximal fragment to abduct and rotate internally, owing to action of the rotator cuff (see Fig. 11-1**A**). If the shaft is broken above the deltoid insertion, this muscle pulls the lower fragment outward, while the pectoralis major, latissimus dorsi, and teres major pull the proximal fragments inward (see Fig. 11-1**B**). When the fracture line lies below

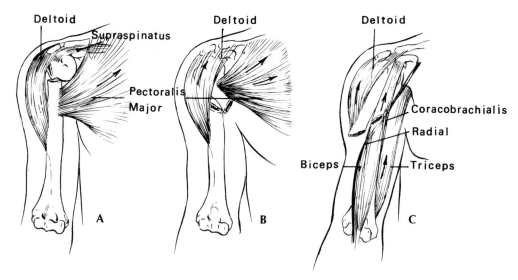

Fig. 11-1. Anatomical factors that influence deformities in typical fractures of the humeral shaft. (**A**) Fracture between rotator cuff and pectoralis major causing abduction and rotation of proximal fragment. (**B**) Fracture between pectoralis major insertion and deltoid producing adduction of proximal fragment. (**C**) Fracture below deltoid insertion causing abduction of proximal fragment.

the deltoid, this muscle and the coracobrachialis draw the upper fragment outward and forward while the lower fragment is drawn upward (see Fig. 11-1**C**). Occasionally, the fracture ends remain in contact with varying degrees of angulation. It is more common for the ends to displace and override. This superior displacement is influenced to a considerable degree by muscle contraction, an observation that was probably responsible for the development of the hanging cast principle.

MECHANISMS OF INJURY

Fractures of the shaft of the humerus occur most frequently as the result of direct violence: falls, direct blows to the arm, automobile injuries, or crushing injuries from machinery.[38] Missiles from firearms or shell fragments may pierce soft tissues and cause fractures. Therefore, many of these fractures are open. Indirect trauma, such as a fall on the elbow or the outstretched hand, or even violent muscle contraction, may cause fracture of the humeral shaft.[2,3] There are reports of fractures incurred when javelins, baseballs, or grenades were thrown violently and usually over-arm.[44] Typically, the injury occurs at the junction of the distal and middle thirds of the shaft.

The common fractures of the adult humerus have been reproduced experimentally by simple me-

chanical means. Fractures at the proximal and distal ends depend on the anatomy of the bone itself, but shaft fractures vary according to the nature and degree of the trauma.[58] Compression forces acting on the humerus may affect either end, but not the shaft. On the other hand, a bending force will produce a transverse fracture of the shaft, and a torsion force will result in a spiral fracture. A combination of bending and torsion will usually produce an oblique fracture, and possibly a butterfly fragment.

The resulting angulation and displacement of the fracture fragments depend on the fracturing forces, the level of fracture, and the influence of muscle pull (see Fig. 11-1).

CLASSIFICATION

Fractures of the shaft of the humerus may be conveniently classified on the basis of various factors. Several categories are used for full descriptive classification of individual fractures.

I. Communication with external environment
   A. Open
   B. Closed
II. Location of fracture
   A. Above pectoralis major insertion
   B. Below pectoralis major insertion but above deltoid insertion
   C. Below deltoid insertion

III. Degree of fracture
  A. Incomplete
  B. Complete
IV. Direction and character of fracture line
  A. Longitudinal
  B. Transverse
  C. Oblique
  D. Spiral
  E. Segmental
  F. Comminuted
V. Associated injury
  A. Nerve
    1. Radial
    2. Median
    3. Ulnar
  B. Blood vessel
    1. Brachial artery
    2. Brachial vein
VI. Intrinsic condition of bone
  A. Normal
  B. Pathologic
    1. Secondary to local bone changes
      a. Bone atrophy
      b. Inflammatory process

      c. Neoplasm
        (1) Benign
        (2) Malignant
    2. Secondary to disorders affecting entire skeleton
      a. Congenital abnormalities
      b. Metabolic bone disease
      c. Disseminated bone disorders of unknown etiology

CLINICAL SIGNS AND SYMPTOMS

When the fracture of the humeral shaft is complete and with displacement, the diagnosis is usually obvious. The extremity is shortened, and there is abnormal mobility or crepitus on gentle manipulation associated with swelling and pain. The diagnosis is more difficult in incomplete fractures or fractures without displacement and is based on disability and point tenderness. The x-ray examination is confirmatory and must include both ends of the bone, the shoulder, and the elbow joint. The examiner must check for possible secondary or associated soft

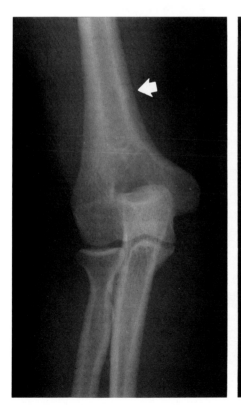 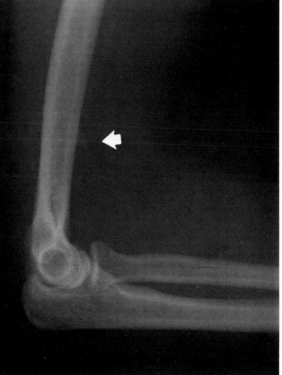

Fig. 11-2. Anteroposterior (**left**) and lateral (**right**) x-rays of the distal humerus demonstrating a supracondylar process. The patient developed transient median nerve symptoms.

tissue injury, carefully examining the entire extremity and the patient in general. The neurovascular status must be evaluated, and the initial examination must establish a baseline for comparison in the event of progressive vascular or neural complications.

RADIOGRAPHIC FINDINGS

Radiographic examination must include not only two views of the entire humerus, but also the shoulder and elbow joints. Anatomical variations in the shaft are uncommon. The supracondylar process, which arises from the anteromedial surface above the medial epicondyle, may be discovered initially on an x-ray film made for trauma (Fig. 11-2). Median nerve symptoms resulting from fracture of the process have been reported by Newman.[74]

METHODS OF TREATMENT

CLOSED METHODS

It was not many years ago that fractures of the shaft of the humerus were high on the list of injuries associated with delayed union and nonunion. Improved methods of closed treatment have reversed this tendency. The numerous methods available today allow considerable individuality in the selection of a technique.[27,47,50,64] The type and level of the fracture, the patient's age and ability to cooperate, the degree of fracture displacement, and the presence of associated injuries are factors that influence the choice of treatment. The nonoperative means most frequently used have been (1) traction by means of a hanging cast, (2) coaptation or U-shaped brachial splint, (3) shoulder spica cast, (4) Velpeau or thoracobrachial casting, (5) abduction humeral splint, and (6) skeletal traction by means of a pin through the olecranon. Functional bracing[83] has been used with increasing frequency in the management of humeral shaft fractures, and occasionally an external fixation device[11] may be indicated.

The Hanging Cast

Caldwell[14,15] introduced the hanging cast technique in 1933, and it has become one of the most widely accepted and successful methods for treatment of humeral shaft fractures. The cast is applied to displaced fractures of the humeral shaft with shortening, and also to oblique and spiral fractures. However, it can be used in most instances, including

comminuted fractures and those involving the distal shaft, when certain principles are carefully observed:[89]

1. The cast must be lightweight and must extend from at least 1 inch proximal to the fracture site to the wrist, with the elbow at a right angle and the forearm in neutral rotation (Fig. 11-3).
2. The arm must always be dependent so as to provide a traction force. The patient should sleep erect or semierect and must avoid supporting the elbow when seated.
3. The sling must be securely fixed at the wrist by a loop made of plaster or other material. To correct lateral angulation, the loop is placed on the dorsum of the wrist; to correct medial angulation, it is placed on the volar side (see Fig. 11-12).
4. Posterior angulation should be corrected by lengthening the sling or suspension apparatus; shortening the sling corrects anterior angulation.

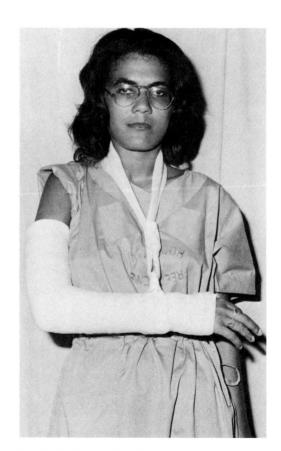

Fig. 11-3. Typical hanging cast.

5. X-ray films of the fracture should be made at weekly intervals, or as frequently as indicated.

6. Exercises should be started immediately. Finger exercises will prevent a stiff hand. If the cast stops at the wrist, this joint is also exercised. As soon as comfort permits, or in a few days, circumduction exercises must be instituted to prevent distraction, shoulder subluxation, and, particularly, adhesive capsulitis (Fig. 11-4). This is accomplished by having the patient bend forward at the waist, allowing the cast to hang free to perform circumduction and pendulum movements.

7. Isometric exercises are also helpful and can be done easily by the patient in the hanging cast or splint. It is believed that isometrics assist in the prevention of distraction and help to pull fragments together.

The requirement that the vertical position be maintained is regarded by some as a disadvantage

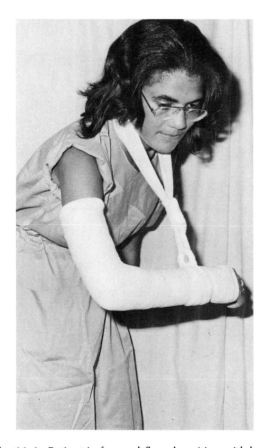

Fig. 11-4. Patient in forward-flexed position with hanging cast swinging free for circumduction and pendulum exercises.

to this method of treatment. However, it can be accomplished easily if the patient is cooperative. Occasionally for an obese person a wedge or pad may be required at the medial aspect of the elbow where angulation occurs from a pendulous breast or redundant tissue. The pad is added if dorsal placement of the wrist loop does not suffice. It is not essential to obtain perfect alignment and apposition. The musculature of the upper arm will accommodate 20° of anterior angulation and 30° of varus angulation without compromising function or appearance.[57] Similarly, bayonet position resulting in shortening up to 1 inch is not noticeable in the upper extremity and requires a minor adjustment in the sleeve lengths of clothing.

Spiral, comminuted, and oblique fractures have the advantage of generous fracture surface areas and tend to heal rapidly (Fig. 11-5). Simple transverse fractures without comminution in some instances fail to unite as promptly and require closer observation to avoid distraction and angulation. Fractures just distal to the insertion of the deltoid muscle are prone to abduction of the proximal fragment and also require special attention.

In the nearly 60 years since its introduction, the hanging cast has enjoyed wide application by a great number of surgeons with outstanding success. Winfield and associates[99] in 1942 reported 136 cases in which the hanging cast was used exclusively. Of these, 103 were available for analysis. There was one case of delayed union and one of nonunion. Stewart and Hundley,[90] in 1955, reported 107 fractures treated in hanging casts; 93.5% of the patients experienced excellent or good results, and 6.5%, fair or poor. In 1959, the Pennsylvania Orthopaedic Society[84] reported a study of 159 fractures of the humeral shaft. The hanging cast was used in 54% of the patients, and of these 96% attained union, in an average of 10 weeks' healing time. Stewart[89] cited a study of Louis Breck and members of the Trauma Committee of the American Academy of Orthopaedic Surgeons in 1961, in which 95.4% of 174 patients with hanging cast treatment obtained good results. The last two reports concern cooperative studies by a number of surgeons and affirm the general applicability of this technique. The current literature[20,52,63,79] and many standard texts[1,18,23,56,65,97] contain reports of success with the hanging cast.

Coaptation Splint

The application of a U-shaped coaptation plaster splint with a collar and cuff is another acceptable method (Fig. 11-6). The prime candidate for this

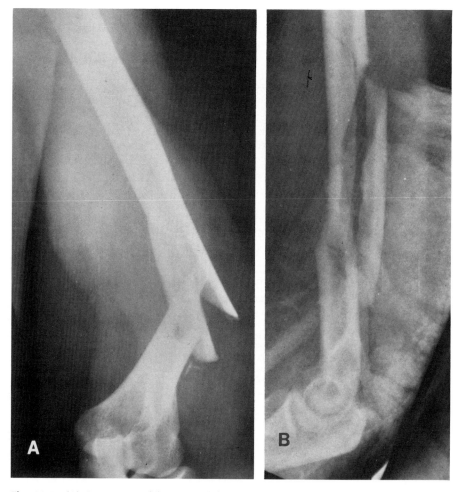

Fig. 11-5. (**A**) Comminuted fracture of the distal humerus. (**B, C**) Fracture in plaster.
(*continued*)

procedure is the patient whose fracture might be distracted by even a light hanging cast. The slab of plaster is placed over thin but adequate layers of padding adhered to wet coatings of benzoin and secured by a Kling bandage to prevent slippage. The slab extends from the axilla around the elbow and over the deltoid. The collar and cuff may be shortened or lengthened to maintain alignment. This technique, sometimes called a "sugar-tong splint," may also be useful as secondary immobilization after a period of time in the hanging cast or other means. It has the distinct advantage of allowing exercises at the elbow, wrist, hand, and shoulder during the entire period of immobilization. Böhler,[7] Charnley,[19] and DePalma[28] expressed a preference for this splint over the hanging cast.

Abduction Humeral Splint

Stewart[89,90] advocated the use of a humeral abduction splint in certain fractures of the shaft. Close and continued observation is required, but increased comfort is cited as an advantage. The splint supports the arm and cast in abduction and maintains the humerus in straight alignment. This method is best used as an adjunct only in the early stages of treatment, because it eliminates the possibility of shoulder exercises.

Shoulder Spica Cast

The shoulder spica has been recommended in the early healing stage of the unstable fracture and where delayed union or nonunion appears immi-

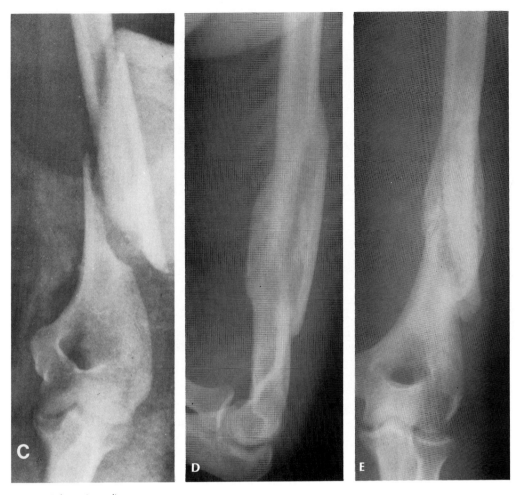

Fig. 11-5 (*continued*).
(**D, E**) The fracture was clinically solid after 2 months and function of the arm was excellent.

nent. It is usually replaced by a simpler form of treatment as soon as the fracture fragments show signs of maintaining reduction. Its drawbacks are the difficulty encountered in applying it, its weight and awkwardness, and patient discomfort in hot, humid climates. Additional problems are encountered if the patient is elderly or obese. From a practical standpoint, it is not clear that the shoulder spica provides better immobilization than other methods.

Open Velpeau-Type Cast

Holm[50] has advocated the open Velpeau-type cast for active and unmanageable children younger than 8 or 10 years and for some older patients unable to cooperate in the use of hanging casts. Axillary and forearm Webril or polyurethane forearm pads are inserted to maintain the desired degree of abduction and flexion of the arm. The elbow is flexed to 90°. Coaptation splints are secured by circumferential turns of plaster, passing around the arm, shoulder, and trunk. The cast is windowed anteromedially to expose the axilla and antecubital fossa and molded carefully about the elbow, axilla, and iliac crest. The cast is cut off around the wrist to allow active wrist and finger exercises. Once healing has progressed enough so that the cast can be removed, a less rigid support is substituted.

Skeletal Traction

Occasionally, in special circumstances when the patient cannot walk, skeletal traction can be used.

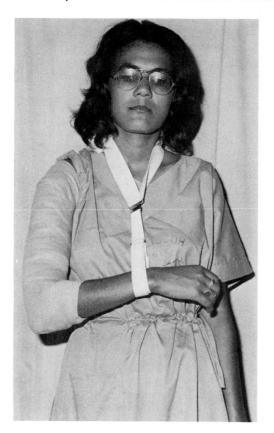

Fig. 11-6. U-shaped coaptation splint and wrist suspension appliance.

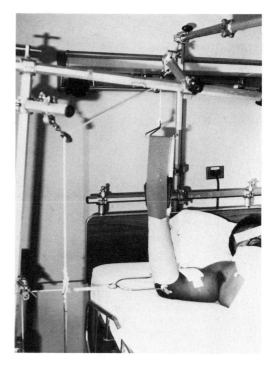

Fig. 11-7. Lateral traction with a Steinmann pin through the olecranon. Note dressing over the compound fracture wound on the anterior aspect of the upper arm. The patient also sustained a posterior dislocation of the right hip in a vehicular accident.

Associated skeletal injuries that require the patient to remain recumbent and extensive open fracture wounds are frequent indications. The method requires the patient's cooperation and close supervision by the surgeon. Traction is provided by a Kirschner wire (0.0625-inch) or a Steinmann pin (3/32- or 7/64-inch), inserted through the olecranon (Fig. 11-7).

The technique of traction is simple, but it should be applied under sterile skin preparation and draping to minimize infection. The procedure may be performed in the emergency room, but the operating room is ideal. The site for insertion is where the olecranon joins the body of the ulna, and a tract down to the periosteum is infiltrated with a local anesthetic. A small nick is made in the skin, and, with a cannulated hand drill, the Kirschner wire or Steinmann pin is inserted in a plane perpendicular to the longitudinal axis of the ulna. If a power drill is used, the pin should be inserted with high torque and low speed to avoid burning the bone.

The ulnar nerve is best avoided by drilling the wire from the medial to the lateral side. If circumstances demand another site, the wire may be inserted in the distal humerus. Soft tissues on the other side of the bone at the point of exit are also infiltrated, thus making the entire procedure relatively painless. The wire is usually drilled until equal lengths protrude from both sides of the elbow, and then sterile dressings are applied. The handle of the Kirschner wire bow should be tightened to minimize the tendency of the wire to bend. The Steinmann pin bow should not be used for a Kirschner wire, nor a Kirschner wire bow for a Steinmann pin. A disposable nylon bow is available that accepts both pins and wires.* The elbow is flexed to 90°, and the forearm is supported by adhesive material or additional skeletal traction.

Active exercises of the hand and wrist are possible and should be encouraged while the arm is in traction.

---

* Salvatore Traction Bow. Wright Manufacturing Co., Memphis, Tenn.

Sling and Swathe

Certain elderly patients may be best managed in a sling and stockinette body swathe.[18] In these cases the reduction is not a critical consideration, but comfort of the patient and disadvantages of other forms of immobilization are major factors. A wedge-shaped axillary pad may be used to obtain a few degrees of abduction in the distal fragment. The apparatus requires frequent adjustment, but this is easy to do. The shoulder is freed for exercises in a week or two, or when comfort permits.

Functional Bracing

The concept of functional bracing has also been applied to fractures of the shaft of the humerus. Sarmiento and colleagues[83] advocated a sleeve or brace firmly compressing the soft tissues surrounding the fractured humerus to maintain alignment of the fragments until healing occurs. The functional sleeve is made of Orthoplast or polypropylene with Velcro straps that permit easy removal and reapplication. The sleeve device may be custom-made or prefabricated. Laterally, the proximal brim approaches the acromion and encircles the arm under the axilla medially. Distally, the sleeve is fashioned to avoid the epicondyles, allowing free elbow motion. A gap in the sleeve permits adjustment by tightening as the swelling subsides (Fig. 11-8). Initially the fracture is treated in a hanging cast, coaptation U-splint, Velpeau bandage, or skeletal traction. After the acute pain and swelling have subsided the functional brace is applied. A standard arm sling is used to maintain the elbow at 90°, and active and passive exercises for the shoulder, elbow, wrist, and hand are begun. As comfort increases, these exercises are permitted with more vigor and excursion. The patient is also allowed to engage in activities of daily living. Sarmiento observed spontaneous correction of angulatory deformities following the initiation of the exercise routine. X-ray examination is easily accomplished through the sleeve. In the initial report 51 cases were treated without nonunion and with consistent restoration of motion of all joints and minimal morbidity.[83]

The use of a similar orthotic device made from two polyethylene splints, a polyethylene hinge, and three elastic webbing straps has been reported by Balfour and colleagues.[4] A shoulder strap of the same elastic webbing is used for suspension of the brace. The time of application is usually between the fourth and seventh days after injury. Rapid fracture union, early restoration of joint mobility, and increased comfort are cited as advantages. A failure rate of 4% (nonunion and delayed union) was reported by these authors.

Naver and Aalberg,[73] adopting the principles of Sarmiento, treated 20 patients with humeral diaphyseal fractures. Prefabricated dynamic bracing was applied for fractures of the humerus within 1 week following the fracture. Ninety percent healed with good anatomical and functional outcome.

Naver's contraindications for dynamic bracing included extremities with major soft tissue defects, unreliable patients, and limbs with excessive angulation or shortening that could increase with functional bracing. Inability to maintain acceptable alignment represented an additional reason for withholding dynamic bracing in a more extensive study of 177 patients reviewed by Zagorski.[100] Minor angulatory deformities associated with dynamic bracing were clinically insignificant; however, residual angulation exceeding 25° or more represented a potential cosmetic problem. Transient inferior subluxation of the shoulder was detected in 5% of patients included in Zagorski's review. Idiopathic inferior glenohumeral subluxation evident at the first follow-up visit resolved within 8 to 10 weeks after injury.

A cast-brace applies the concept of the lower extremity hinged cast brace to the elbow. It can be used for humeral fractures associated with concomitant forearm and distal injuries. This technique, described by McMaster and associates,[66] provides controlled flexion while protecting against varus/valgus stress and translation forces. The cast-brace is constructed from readily available materials and can be applied in an outpatient setting.

External Fixation

External fixation, first used in the treatment of fresh fractures of the lower extremity, has been found to be applicable to the humerus in some cases. The prime indications are markedly comminuted fractures; infected nonunion; bone defect or loss; extensive skin or soft tissue wounds in an open fracture; burn patients with fractures; aged patients in whom immobilization is undesirable; limbs with concomitant fracture in the forearm; or when early mobilization is indicated.

The fixator technique allows the surgeon to adjust the frame components to provide varying degrees of distraction or compression, and neutralization or alignment of humeral fracture fragments. The frame can be adjusted to control rotation and provide easy access to a wound that requires dressing. The frame also facilitates elevation or traction. Half pins are used and should be inserted under general

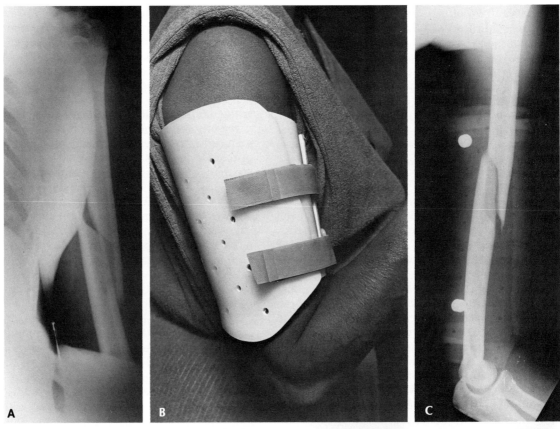

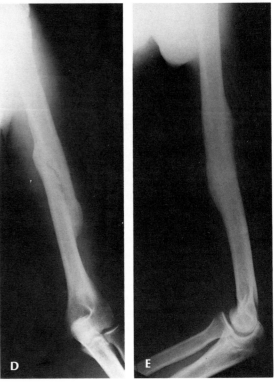

Fig. 11-8. (**A**) Initial x-ray of a spiral fracture of the humerus. (**B**) A functional "sleeve" applied. (**C**) X-ray showing alignment of fragments in the functional sleeve. (**D, E**) Anteroposterior and lateral views of the healed fracture. (*Courtesy of A. Sarmiento, M.D.*)

anesthesia. Two pins are inserted through a drill guide above the fracture and two below the fracture, taking care to engage both cortices. The fracture is manipulated under radiographic control and the external frame is applied with compression where possible. The bony landmarks and zones for pin placement as well as the technique of insertion have been well delineated.[12,43]

Another system that uses polyethylene tubes filled with hardened epoxy resin has also been found to be useful.

It is important that the pins receive daily care and attention. Infected or loose pins should be removed. When union of the fracture has been obtained, the apparatus and the pins are removed without anesthesia.

These methods have two of the advantages of internal fixation: rigid fixation and early mobilization. Kamhin and associates[54] indicated that the risk of injuring the radial nerve during the manipulation for alignment is a real disadvantage. If the location of the fracture threatens the radial nerve, the surgeon may open the fracture site in rare cases. In those injuries associated with an open wound, visualization of the nerve is accomplished more easily.

Humeral fracture stabilization can be achieved by the use of a dynamic axial fixator employing the principles described by Burny.[26] Using a single unilateral bar to connect the specially designed intracortical pins, one can introduce a degree of elasticity to stimulate increased callus formation. A single dynamic external fixator bar and pin system rigid enough to control lateral bending and torque forces facilitates the transmission of controlled distraction, compression, or axial loading across the fracture site once callus formation begins.

DeBastiani[26] applied an external fixator using a single bar with articulating ends and self-tapping screws.

The complications of these techniques include pin tract infection; neurovascular, tendon, and muscle impalement; nonunion; and the bulky frame that can be bothersome in some situations. However, when the technique is applied in the circumstances listed, the surgeon has highly effective methods to supplement conventional treatment of difficult fractures of the humerus (Fig. 11-9).

OPERATIVE METHODS

Open Fractures

The open fracture is an orthopaedic emergency and requires operative treatment. In many cases patients have multiple injuries, and proper consideration must be given to treatment priority. Attention is given first to patency of the airway, hemorrhage, and shock. Tetanus toxoid or antitoxin is given as indicated. A sterile dressing covers the wound, and the limb is splinted until the patient reaches the operating theater.

The wound is cleansed and débrided in the standard orthopaedic manner (see Chapter 3). Care is exercised to avoid injuring blood vessels and nerves. Sterile saline is used in copious amounts, and cultures are taken to identify any pathogens that may be present. Some surgeons elect primary closure for wounds that are seen in the first 6 to 8 hours after injury and are considered "clean." Others routinely leave open all wounds, particularly those seen after 8 to 12 hours, grossly contaminated wounds, and gunshot and combat wounds. Delayed primary closure, after 5 to 7 days, has proved an excellent and safe means of wound care in daily practice as well as under war conditions.[21,35,36,46]

The election of internal fixation, if any, is a matter determined by the experience and judgment of the surgeon. The external fixation devices are excellent in these cases, providing immobilization for the fracture and allowing easy access to the wound. As surgeons gain more experience with the external fixation systems, these devices will probably be used more frequently in the management of difficult open fractures of the humerus.

Closed Fractures

Because closed methods of treatment for humeral shaft fractures have a high rate of success, open reduction is rarely indicated. However, there are situations in which open reduction and internal fixation may be appropriate. First, there are certain segmental fractures in which satisfactory position and alignment cannot be achieved. Second, pathologic fractures secondary to malignancy should be fixed. Some of these also may be treated successfully by coaptation splints. Shaft fractures with associated injuries of the elbow that require early mobilization need internal fixation. Any fracture associated with a vascular injury should be fixed. Last, a spiral fracture of the distal humerus—the type described by Holstein and Lewis,[51] in which a radial nerve palsy may develop after hanging cast treatment or manipulation—may require internal fixation. Similar indications for open reduction and internal fixation have been listed in *Campbell's Operative Orthopaedics.*[25] Another possible indication is Parkinson's disease or another neurologic or systemic disease that would make the hanging cast or its equivalent inappropriate.

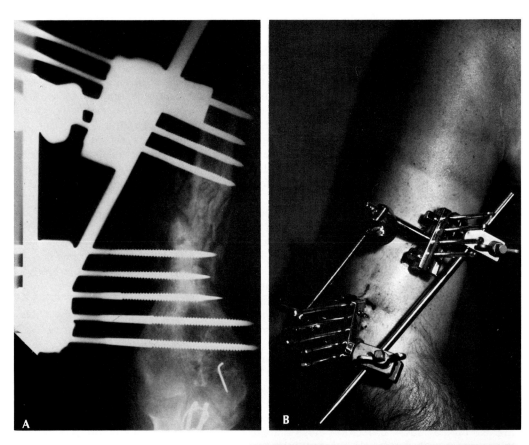

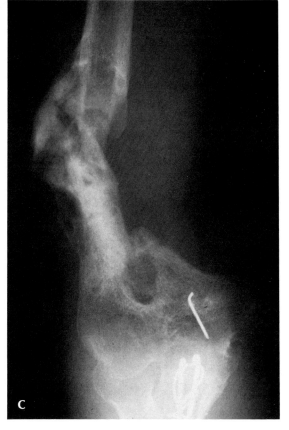

Fig. 11-9. (**A**) Use of an external fixator in the treatment of a complicated open comminuted fracture of the humerus in a multiple trauma patient. (**B**) The external fixator in place. (**C**) The healed fracture with some angulation but a good functional result. *(Courtesy of C.C. Edwards, M.D.)*

The shaft of the humerus is easily approached by medial displacement of the biceps and incision of the brachialis. This exposure avoids the radial nerve, but retraction must be done gently to avoid injury. The proximal shaft may be approached through the deltopectoral groove, and in the distal one third a posterior incision is useful. Excellent descriptions of surgical approaches to this area are available in *Campbell's Operative Orthopaedics,*[25] Banks and Laufman's *Atlas of Surgical Exposures of the Extremities,* and Henry's *Extensile Exposure.*

Once the surgeon has decided that an open reduction is indicated, the techniques and the type of internal fixation must be chosen. Plates provide rigid internal fixation for fresh fractures and nonunions. However, the AO type of plate, developed by Müller and associates,[70,71] is designed to provide not only rigid fixation but also compression (Fig. 11-10). The experience of many surgeons has established this as one of the preferred methods in open reduction.[10,25,72,94] Cancellous bone graft can be added at the time of operation to promote osteosynthesis and minimize the likelihood of nonunion. Postoperatively, there is the advantage that external splinting is not needed, and active mobilization of the whole extremity can be pursued during the entire course of fracture healing. Even if the surgeon wishes to apply external immobilization in the form of a posterior splint for a few weeks or just during wound healing, the early mobility should reduce the tendency for stiffness in all joints.

The external fixation technique is versatile in these circumstances, allowing the surgeon to adjust the frame components to provide varying degrees of distraction, compression, neutralization, or alignment—including rotational alignment of humeral fractures.[43]

Intramedullary rods and nails are used in humeral fractures to maintain alignment and length.[82,92] In general they do not provide as rigid internal fixation as plates. For this reason most rods require supplemental external immobilization, at least during part of the time required for healing.

Intramedullary rods and nails are thought to preserve periosteal blood supply. Successfully treated fractures usually heal by bridging periosteal callus. Micromotion at the fracture site promotes angiogenesis and healing. Radiographs of the humerus stabilized with rigidly reamed rods are characterized by scant and weak callus.[92] Rods of intermediate flexibility promote abundant callus, high strength, and pliability at the fracture site.[89]

Küntscher[60,61] described a technique of intramedullary nailing in which the length and circumference of the nails are carefully determined. This method, applied to properly selected cases, provides the rigid fixation needed for osteosynthesis. Küntscher specifically recommended that external support not be applied. Under these circumstances the patient is allowed active exercise. Multiple intramedullary rods inserted from below by the method of Hackethal[31] have been described as useful. Preliminary reports of a few cases show good results with an elastic plastic pin (of Supramid) inserted in the medullary canal.[75,76]

In a review of 89 fractures treated with intramedullary nailing, Hall[45] noted that the fractures healed within 7.2 weeks, with only one nonunion in a type III open fracture from a shotgun blast. No pain or motion developed at the fracture site despite radiographic evidence of nonunion at 25 months. Range of motion in the elbow varied from 4° to 132°. Average shoulder abduction was 91°, external rotation 54°, and internal rotation 68°. Eight nails backed out, but none in which the eyelets of the nails were tied together with a wire, leading Hall to recommend this step in technique.

Brumback and associates[13] reported immediate closed intramedullary stabilization of humeral diaphyseal fractures in polytrauma patients, with a 94% rate of union and 62% rate of excellent clinical results. Using various portals of entry, intramedullary stabilization was achieved by inserting Rush rods or Enders nails. Retrograde insertion proximal to the olecranon fossa yielded excellent results, in contrast to more flexion contractures and poorer results associated with epicondylar portals. This technique was particularly applicable to patients suffering from multiple trauma, spine fractures, bilateral humeral fractures, and the so called "floating elbow." The authors recommended that antegrade nailing be limited to fractures of the distal third of the humerus and that the portal of entry should avoid the rotator cuff.

In multiply injured patients, the major goals of humeral stabilization are to permit early mobility, maintain pulmonary access, and assure alignment in the supine or noncompliant patient.

The use of Hackethal stacked nailing for humeral shaft fractures was reported by Durbin.[31] Stacked unreamed Hackethal nails were inserted for the fixation of humeral diaphyseal fractures. Minimal blood loss was encountered. Retrograde nail insertion under C-arm control obviated muscle trauma, radial nerve injury, and the extensive exposure required for fixation with plate and screws. The rate of union in 25 patients with adequate follow-up was 92%, with a reoperation rate of 14% for pin adjustment and nonunion.

Seidel[86] has developed a cylindrical unslotted nail.

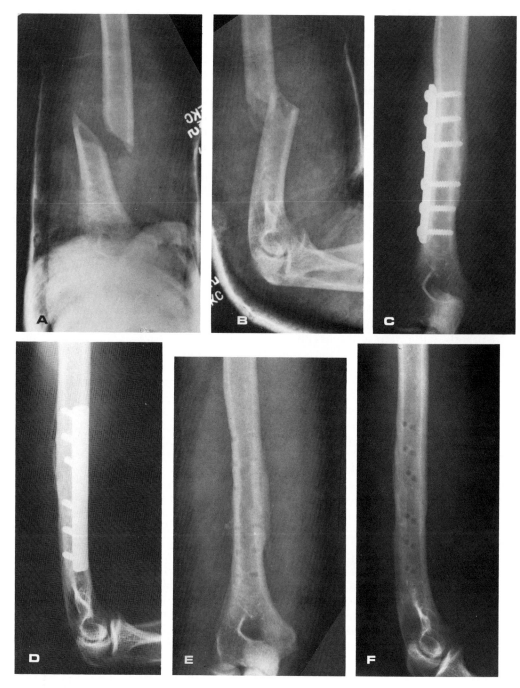

Fig. 11-10. (**A, B**) X-rays of fracture of the junction of the middle and distal thirds of the humerus showing poor position secondary-to soft tissue interposition. (**C, D**) Same fracture after application of an AO compression plate and cancellous bone graft. Union was obtained at 6 weeks. (**E, F**) X-rays of fracture after removal of the plate and screws.

The proximal third of the nail is bent backward at 7.5° from the humeral mid-axis. Stabilization of humeral diaphyseal fractures using the unslotted intramedullary nail may allow early mobilization for polytrauma patients. Distal locking is achieved by intramedullary spreading at the nail tip; proximal locking is performed with two crossed screws.

Stern[88] reviewed intramedullary fixation of humeral shaft fractures. Of 102 fractures operated on, 70 were treated with intramedullary fixation. His indications for this fixation included unsatisfactory alignment after closed treatment, multiple injuries, ipsilateral fracture, retarded healing at 6 to 10 weeks, delayed union at 16 to 30 weeks, and nonunion at more than 32 weeks. The complication rate in the intramedullary rod treatment group was 67%. Forty-five of 70 required additional procedures. Stern's series included complex fractures that failed previous fixation. Several were judged unsuitable for closed treatment.

Vander Griend[95] reported on the use of closed Küntscher nails for humeral diaphyseal fractures. Of 18 fractures treated, 12 were the direct result of trauma, including ten with multiple fractures and two with neurovascular injuries. All were closed fractures. Seventeen of the 18 were treated with antegrade nail placement, and one with retrograde nail placement. Postoperative treatment consisted of a sling only, unless distraction was noted, in which case crutch-walking was initiated to compress the fracture site. Nine of 11 surviving patients had radiographic evidence of union in less than 10 weeks and two had union at 5 to 8 months. All pathologic fractures had pain relief. The Küntscher nail was thought to be useful for the management of closed fractures, polytrauma patients, pathologic fractures, and nonunions. Five centimeters of rod purchase was needed proximal and distal to the fracture site. The most common complication was reduced range of motion, especially shoulder abduction. Limited motion was improved with physical therapy.

Proximal rod impingement may be relieved by the use of a straight nail inserted slightly posterior to the greater tuberosity.

The humeral interlocking intramedullary nail provides a promising alternative for humeral reconstruction and salvage procedures. The implant was introduced to treat complex fractures, nonunions, and pathologic fractures secondary to tumor or severe involutional osteopenia. When comminution, bone loss, or nonunion is present, interlocked intramedullary nailing coupled with appropriate autografting may lead to union and early resumption of function (Fig. 11-11). Ward[96] treated eight fractures using interlocked intramedullary nailing of the humerus—one for delayed union, five for nonunions, and two for pathologic fractures. Intramedullary nailing without interlocking provides poor rotatory control, in his opinion, contributing to an increased rate of nonunion. He recommended a minimum of 2 cm (preferably 4 cm) contact of the rod within the diaphyseal intramedullary canal.

The choice of a technique for intramedullary nailing depends on the training and experience of the surgeon. Infection is particularly unfortunate when it develops after intramedullary nailing or any open procedure that uses internal fixation.

Screw fixation inserted across a long spiral fracture has been used, but the internal fixation is less secure than with other methods. Circumferential wire loops and Parham bands have been used in

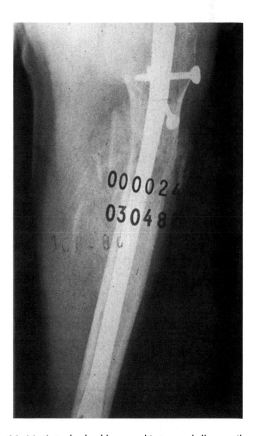

Fig. 11-11. Interlocked humeral intramedullary nail used to reduce a comminuted proximal humeral shaft fracture, with satisfactory reduction and healing. (*Courtesy of Howmedica*)

the past, but alone they seem to have no place in today's armamentarium.

Occasionally, one may wish to use autogenous or homogenous cortical bone grafts for internal fixation. In these circumstances, the plating material provides not only internal fixation but osteosynthesis as well. Such grafts are also useful in bridging defects in the shaft of the humerus.

The level of the fracture may also influence the choice of an internal fixation device. A fracture in the shaft may be suited to either an intramedullary rod or a plate, but fractures at the ends of the humerus demand careful selection of a device. A rod may be better applied proximally, whereas a plate would meet the requirements of a distal fracture.[94]

Interesting and extremely revealing data are available through a comparison of the results obtained by closed treatment as opposed to open reduction in two reported series. Breck's study[89] reported 95.4% good results in 174 fractures treated in hanging casts, while 50 fractures managed by open reduction had 88% good results. In the Pennsylvania Orthopaedic Society study,[84] results were good for 96% of the closed cases treated in a hanging cast and for 88% of the open cases.

AUTHORS' PREFERRED METHODS

Most closed humeral shaft fractures can be appropriately managed by nonoperative methods. We prefer a coaptation splint followed by a functional brace to treat most closed humeral shaft fractures, because this combination has proven simple and effective while minimizing upper extremity joint stiffness associated with other immobilization techniques. However, the functional brace is not recommended for fractures associated with soft tissue injury, in uncooperative patients, or in situations where acceptable alignment cannot be achieved.

Initially we apply a well-molded, U-shaped coaptation splint that is maintained until soft tissue swelling subsides. The patient is encouraged to perform pendulum exercises of the shoulder. Once the fracture site is less mobile and edema recedes, the patient is fitted with a functional brace. Active range of motion exercises of the shoulder, elbow, wrist, and hand are begun early and continued until fracture healing occurs. At each follow-up visit radiographs are taken through the brace to check alignment. The brace is removed when there is clinical and radiographic evidence of bony union. Following removal of the brace, vigorous exercise of the entire extremity is encouraged until full function is restored.

The hanging cast is a viable alternative when functional bracing is not available. Through the years, the hanging cast has been used successfully when applied according to recognized biomechanical principles (Fig. 11-12). Dependency position is essential, and this is maintained in bed by placing an inverted chair under the mattress (Fig. 11-13). Pillows are added to prop the patient in a comfortable position.

For complicated cases that require lateral traction, we prefer using a threaded Steinmann pin (3/32- or 7/64-inch) or a Kirschner wire (0.0625-inch) through the olecranon. This may be used in combination with coaptation humeral splints and a sling, if necessary, to control bowing. When conditions permit, and when the patient is able to walk about, the U-shaped splint or some other means is used.

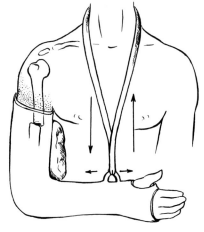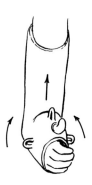

Fig. 11-12. Biomechanical factors of hanging cast technique. Shortening the suspension device corrects anterior bowing, while lengthening corrects posterior bowing. When moved toward the elbow the wrist loop reduces the traction force; when moved toward the wrist, it increases the force. A dorsal position of the loop reduces a varus deformity, and a more volar position reduces a valgus deformity. Note axillary pad to correct varus tendency.

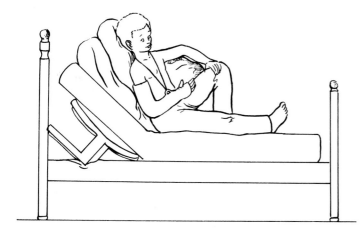

Fig. 11-13. A chair inverted and placed between the mattress and bedspring makes the semi-Fowler's position possible at home.

Very few closed fractures require open reduction. When this is indicated, we prefer to use compression plating in transverse or short oblique fractures. This method provides rigid internal fixation and compression. If open reduction has been postponed for several weeks, we add cancellous bone graft to the primary plating procedure. When alignment is the critical requirement, a Rush rod or a Küntscher nail will suffice; we usually opt for the Rush rod. The indications for open reduction listed above have served us well.

The development of humeral interlocking nails in recent years by Seidel[86] and Ward[96] has added to treatment options under certain circumstances. The interlocking technique allows rotatory stability not provided by the Rush rod or Küntscher nail. The results are preliminary, and future clinical investigations are necessary. However, we have used the Seidel humeral interlocking nail to treat a pathologic fracture secondary to metastatic carcinoma, achieving rigid internal fixation with good palliative relief of pain.

Wound management is a most important consideration in open fractures. Our preference is to perform thorough débridement and irrigation, leaving the wound open. Cultures are taken before treatment and after the final irrigation. The patient is usually given a broad-spectrum antibiotic until a specific organism is cultured, and the best antibiotic is determined by sensitivity studies. Under these circumstances, we usually start intravenous administration of a broad-spectrum antibiotic in the emergency room and continue it for 48 hours postoperatively. If the wound is clinically clean, delayed primary closure is done between the fifth and seventh days. A functional brace, hanging cast, external fixation system, or traction can be used as dictated by other circumstances (Fig. 11-14). The

external fixator frame can be adjusted to provide rigid fixation of the fracture and at the same time allow easy access to a wound that requires dressing.

POSTFRACTURE CARE AND REHABILITATION

It is essential to remember that the rehabilitation of the patient begins immediately after the injury. Immobilization devices should be applied in a manner that will allow maximum active exercise. Early and vigorous movement of the hand is essential if stiffness is to be avoided. The use of functional bracing techniques will minimize stiffness of the adjacent joints. When the hanging cast is used and the wrist is immobilized, the plaster should be trimmed proximal to the metacarpophalangeal joints to allow full flexion of the fingers. The patient is started early on circumduction exercises for the shoulder (see Fig. 11-4). This may not be possible the same day, but it usually can be accomplished by the second or third day after injury. In this manner, adhesive capsulitis of the shoulder can be prevented. The patient in skeletal traction is also instructed to move his fingers and wrist to maintain full mobility of these joints.

Once the cast, splint, or traction has been removed, the patient is started on a well-planned and closely supervised exercise program to regain strength and joint motion in the entire extremity.[29] Stewart[89] made the observation that, barring mechanical interference in any joint—whether from trauma, infection, or other abnormality—the function will return in direct proportion to the strength of the musculature that controls the joint. The elbow merits special attention and should not be passively stretched. Myositis ossificans has been ob-

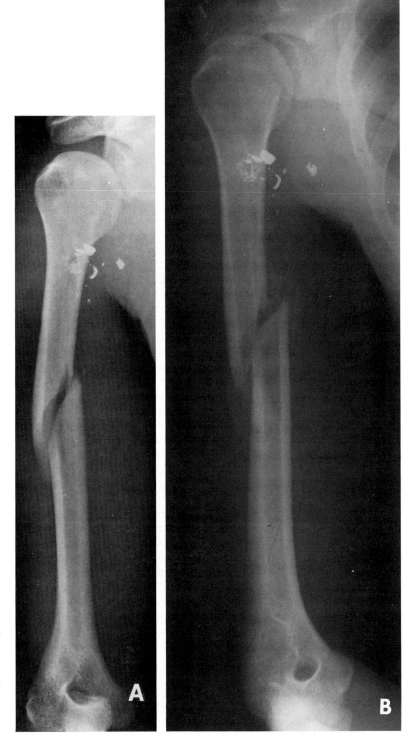

Fig. 11-14. (**A**) An x-ray showing an open fracture of the proximal humerus secondary to gunshot wound, associated with a closed fracture of the mid-shaft. Open fracture wound treated by debridement and left open. (**B**) After 6 weeks in a hanging cast the wound healed without infection and bridging callus was forming satisfactorily. The fracture healed without problems.

served in elbows and is avoided by limiting the exercise to an active routine performed by the patient. The shoulder can be benefited by an assistive and passive program combined with the active routine.

It is vitally important that the surgeon make the patient aware of the importance of the rehabilitation program from the day of injury until maximum recovery has been realized.

PROGNOSIS

Careful consideration of at least eight factors will give the surgeon a fairly accurate prognosis for humeral shaft fractures. The first factor to be weighed is the type of fracture. Spiral and oblique fractures and those that are comminuted tend to heal better than transverse or segmental fractures.

Second, fractures that are in close proximity to either the shoulder or the elbow may have a compromised outcome, depending on the degree of involvement of the soft tissues supporting the joint. Third, an open wound is a significant factor: the open fracture tends to heal more slowly, and there is always the additional risk of infection and osteomyelitis. Fourth, the interposition of soft tissue may make satisfactory reduction impossible by closed means, and open reduction involves entirely different considerations with regard to risk and management. Next, the outcome is affected substantially by the presence of either neural or vascular involvement. Naturally, if both components are injured, the prognosis is more serious. A sixth consideration is the complex situation in which associated fractures in the shoulder, elbow, or forearm may affect the end result. The mode of treatment is a factor. Patients who require thoracobrachial immobilization, instead of the U-type splint or hanging cast, have a greater chance of joint stiffness. Finally, the degree of cooperation by the patient, especially as reflected by willingness to exercise actively, affects the functional result. The surgeon who approaches his patient with an awareness of these prognostic considerations can make enlightened decisions.

COMPLICATIONS

OPEN REDUCTION AND INTERNAL FIXATION

The complications of open reduction and internal fixation of the humerus include infection, nonunion, injury to the radial nerve, prolonged disability, and the potential need for additional procedures to ensure union. Vander Griend[94] reviewed the results of open reduction and internal fixation of humeral diaphyseal fractures using AO plating techniques in 34 patients. Union occurred in 33 of the 34. One fracture failed to unite and required two subsequent operations. The criteria for union included a change in the radiographic appearance of the fracture line. Apparently, there were no correlations among clinical symptoms, function, severity of initial injury, and time to healing. The only complications were two superficial wound infections, one transient postoperative radial nerve palsy, and one surgical division of a radial nerve. Complications were minimized by careful extensile exposure and protection of the radial nerve. Vander Griend's recommendations for open reduction and internal fixation of acute humeral fractures included fractures that were open, those in patients with multiple injuries, those associated with neural or vascular injury, pathologic fractures, and failed closed reductions. He also recommended exploration and internal fixation if a radial nerve palsy develops after closed manipulation, although Shah and Bhatti[87] have shown that this is not always necessary.

Controversy surrounds the use of internal fixation in treating acute fractures of the humeral diaphysis, primarily because of the unacceptable rate of complications reported. Vander Griend's series was unique in that he reviewed all patients treated uniformly using the techniques recommended by the AO group. His complication rate was low and return of function was good in all cases except those with additional major injuries in the fractured limb.[95]

Bell[5] reviewed 34 polytrauma patients treated with AO plating techniques. Thirty-three fractures united. Complications included one nonunion, one failure of fixation, and one infection. No permanent nerve injuries were reported. Bell endorsed AO plating of the humeral diaphysis, finding these techniques useful in multiple trauma patients, preventing fracture disease, and allowing the patient to achieve an early upright position with a pain-free extremity.

Michiels and colleagues[68] reviewed 41 fractures treated surgically. Thirty-two were treated with AO internal fixation and plating, four with external fixation using the Hoffmann external fixation device, and two with intramedullary nailing. Routine removal of AO plates was not carried out. Five patients developed radial nerve palsy postoperatively. One developed a delayed radioulnar synostosis. Intramedullary nailing was subsequently abandoned by Michiels in favor of rigid plate fixation.

Polytrauma patients require rapid recovery of triceps function. Adequate upper extremity function is the primary goal for independent transfer and early ambulation with crutches. Additionally, chest trauma with impaired ventilatory function may be managed more effectively following humeral osteosynthesis and stabilization with internal fixation and plating. However, Michiels[68] encountered a 16% incidence of transient radial nerve palsy after application of AO plates. The plates were not removed routinely because of the vulnerability of the radial nerve at reoperation.

NEURAL COMPLICATIONS

Radial Nerve Palsy

Among complications associated with fractures of the shaft of the humerus, injury to the radial nerve is probably the most common. Fortunately, the wrist drop usually makes this condition easy to recognize. However, in a patient with multiple severe injuries, the examiner may be preoccupied with other matters that are potentially life-threatening, or the patient's unresponsive state may make careful motor examination difficult or impossible. Under these circumstances, radial nerve injury may be overlooked. The examiner must be alert to this possible complication and return, when time and circumstances permit, to make a careful examination of the entire extremity, including its neurovascular status. This practice helps avoid the embarrassment of belated diagnosis of a radial palsy.

It has been estimated that 5% to 10% of patients with humeral shaft fractures demonstrate radial nerve involvement. This is particularly true in spiral fractures in the distal third of the humerus. The displaced fragments may trap the nerve in the fracture site.[32] The anatomical features of this fracture have been analyzed and described by Holstein and Lewis[51] (Fig. 11-15), and Whitson.[98] These authors recommended open reduction through the lateral approach and internal fixation for this particular fracture. However, more recent studies[87,91] have suggested that primary operative intervention is rarely indicated for radial nerve injury associated with fractures of the humerus, even the Holstein-Lewis type.

Most radial nerve injuries are the result of stretching or bruising and are incomplete. Function will return within days or months.[41,55] Where the radial nerve lesion is complete, delayed repair has achieved results as good or better than those of primary repair. Therefore, there is little or no need to explore the nerve unless there is another reason for open intervention.[78] Stewart[89] advised that exploration of the nerve to determine the severity of injury is indicated only in an open fracture. Electromyography and nerve conduction studies are important aids in determining the precise degree of nerve damage and are valuable in monitoring the rate of nerve regeneration. Seddon[85] made the astute clinical observation that the surgeon is justified in waiting until the calendar tells him that the axons regenerating at the rate of 1 mm a day should have reached the most proximal muscle.

Bostman[8] found the incidence of radial nerve

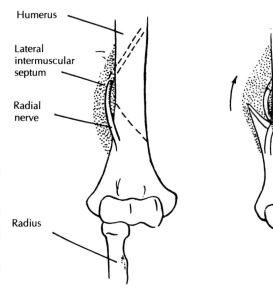

Fig. 11-15. Fractures of the distal third of the humerus may be particularly vulnerable to radial nerve injury. (**Left**) The relationship of the radial nerve to the fracture. (**Right**) Lateral displacement and overriding of the distal fragment. The nerve, fixed to the proximal fragment by the intermuscular septum, is trapped between the fracture surfaces when closed reduction is attempted. (Holstein, A., and Lewis, G.B.: Fractures of the Humerus with Radial Nerve Paralysis. J. Bone Joint Surg., 45A:1382, 1963.)

Humerus

Lateral intermuscular septum

Radial nerve

Radius

palsy to be higher after high-energy accidents. Longitudinal fractures of the distal third of the humeral diaphysis were often associated with laceration or interposition of the radial nerve, whereas transverse fractures of the middle third were more often associated with neurapraxia. Patients with fractures from high-energy injuries are at high risk for nerve damage, and surgical repair and early exploration may be justified, although Bostman suggested that the surgical trauma of nerves in continuity at the time of exploration may contribute to failure of nerve function return.

Bostman's studies suggest that early exploration of the radial nerve and internal fixation of fractures may increase the risk of surgical damage when only neurapraxia is present. The risk of additional nerve injury was demonstrated by several failures of recovery in patients in whom exploration showed an intact or slightly contused nerve. Transverse humeral fractures of the middle third usually manifested neurapraxia only.

Bostman[9] also studied 59 humeral fractures with immediate complete radial nerve palsy: 27 were treated with early (less than 3 weeks) exploration with open reduction and internal fixation using AO plates; 12 underwent surgical exploration after 17 weeks or more in the absence of spontaneous improvement; and 20 were treated with nonoperative management and observation. Five of 27 patients undergoing early exploration were found to have complete nerve transection. Useful recovery was seen in 67% of those patients explored. Twenty-three patients were found to have only bruising of the nerve without discontinuity, and all went on to full recovery.

Pollock[78] evaluated the treatment of radial nerve injury associated with fractures of the humerus. Twenty-four humeral fractures (most in the distal third of the bone) associated with varying degrees of radial nerve palsy were studied. Ostensibly, Pollock agreed with Holstein and Lewis, who believed that humeral fractures at this level most often are at risk for radial nerve injury. However, only 4% of the patients in Pollock's study and 12% of those recorded in the literature had a nerve laceration. The vast majority of patients with humeral fractures and loss of radial nerve function have a lesion-in-continuity. Close follow-up of patients with radial nerve palsy is strongly recommended, especially if impairment persists after fracture healing. Clinical or electromyographic improvement should be apparent at 3½ to 4 months, if the nerve has not been lacerated. Pollock suggested that absence of improvement within this time frame is an indication for nerve exploration. If the nerve has been lacer-

ated or compressed within fracture callus, repair at that time can achieve an excellent result.

Bostman's findings supported "watchful expectancy" as the principle initial policy of management in both immediate and secondary radial nerve palsies. However, he suggested that early exploration of the nerve and rigid internal fixation of the fracture should be considered in fractures showing bayonet apposition, because these have been shown to result in abundant callus formation and radial nerve entrapment. No useful recovery of motor function was seen in 13 of 59 patients with immediate palsy and in two of 16 patients with secondary palsy. In patients with immediate palsy treated by early exploration, eight of 27 did not recover nerve function.

VASCULAR COMPLICATIONS

Humeral shaft fractures can be associated with brachial artery injury. In one series,[40] eleven humeral fractures were associated with brachial artery injuries. One patient developed reflex sympathetic dystrophy, another had a nonunion requiring bone grafting, another osteomyelitis and delayed union, and one developed gangrene secondary to venous insufficiency and infection, requiring amputation.

Arterial defects must be repaired immediately and protected by rigid internal or external fixation. Concomitant prophylactic fasciotomy is encouraged.

The role of arteriography in the evaluation of extremities with long-bone fractures and vascular trauma remains controversial. Some authors have stressed the use of the arteriogram as a diagnostic tool. However, an arteriogram may not always be essential, because the diagnosis can be firmly established clinically in at least 50% of cases, especially with open fractures. The foremost disadvantage of obtaining a preoperative arteriogram is the added delay in definitive treatment. Arteriography does not always contribute to therapeutic decision-making, but may provide additional information when it delineates an ominous absence of collateral circulation. Unnecessary delays for a study of equivocal value are imprudent in the definitive management of a severely ischemic limb. Arterial flow should be reestablished immediately in cases approaching an ischemic time of 6 hours. A temporary intraluminal arterial shunt affords a simple means of reestablishing perfusion.[33,53] A tension-free arterial reconstruction with healthy tissues is critical.

Ligation of the brachial artery above the profunda brachii artery will result in loss of limb in about

50% of cases. However, only 25% of the limbs will require amputation if the level of ligation is below the profunda.[30]

In civilian practice Gainor[40] recommended the following management priorities in a patient with multiple injuries:

1. Resuscitation;
2. Arteriography (not essential in open injuries but helpful in closed trauma);
3. Intraoperative perfusion of the limb with a temporary intraluminal shunt;
4. Rigid bony stabilization with an external fixation device or plates and screws;
5. Wound debridement;
6. Vascular repair with an autogenous vein graft;
7. Neurorrhaphy; and
8. Assessment of the need for fasciotomy.

Fractures complicated by vascular injury constitute severe orthopaedic emergencies and demand prompt restoration of blood supply if the limb is to be saved. Primary control of hemorrhage can be accomplished, usually by direct pressure, while the patient is readied for surgery. If the vascular injury is associated with an open fracture, the vessel should be explored and repaired after the fracture has been stabilized by internal fixation.[80,81] The choice of technique for definitive arterial repair in a particular case is governed by the type and location of the injury. Clean lacerations involving short segments of arterial wall often can be managed by lateral repair. Jagged injuries and gunshot wounds may require excision of segments of artery, after which end-to-end anastomosis is performed, if it can be accomplished without too much tension. If not, a vein graft is required.[22,67]

There are occasions when the artery is sufficiently traumatized to cause vascular spasm. This condition obliterates the vessel without thrombosis or laceration. The effects of spasm may be reversed by periarterial infiltration with Novacaine or Xylocaine. Stellate ganglion blocks may be helpful in some cases. If the spasm persists, the vessel should be explored and the serosal coat, along with its innervation, totally stripped for a distance of at least 3 cm.[89] Most orthopaedic surgeons have not had extensive training or experience in repairing peripheral blood vessels, and in most instances, a vascular surgery consultant should be called.

NONUNION

Delayed union and nonunion of the humeral shaft occur most frequently in transverse fractures, where there is only minimal bone contact between the fragments. Distraction of fractures and the interposition of soft parts are also significant factors. It is paradoxical that open reduction, even though it is performed with good justification, often contributes to nonunion. Treatment should be continued at least 4 months before the surgeon decides that a delayed union is frank nonunion.[89]

Vigorous and definitive treatment is mandatory once the surgeon accepts the diagnosis of nonunion. The skin (especially the extent of any scar tissue) and the circulation of the extremity should be evaluated thoroughly. Essential to success is rigid internal fixation. Today this is perhaps best obtained by compression plating (Fig. 11-16). Intramedullary pinning is also an acceptable means of fixation. The fracture ends are cut back to good bone, and the medullary canal is drilled. If necessary the bone may be shortened an inch or more, and cancellous bone graft is a must, regardless of the means of fixation.[6,16,34] There will be times when wisdom may dictate not disturbing the nonunion site. For example, a transverse fracture with a strong fibrous union being treated with a compression plate would be ideally suited for onlay cancellous bone grafting.[24] Under these circumstances, we prefer not to take down the fibrous union and cut back the ends of the bones. Often, stimulated by the grafts, such a fracture will go on to solid union.

It appears that good results can be predicted with several methods. In 1961 Boyd and others[11] reported 94% union using medullary fixation and autogenous cancellous bone. Campbell[17] reported 93.8% good results in 52 cases of humeral shaft fracture using massive onlay bone grafts. Müller[69] reported the use of rigid fixation by plate or intramedullary nail. Küntscher[60] used the intramedullary nail alone for 786 cases of nonunion, in which nailing was accomplished under x-ray control without direct exposure of the fracture site. The nail was inserted so as to provide rigid fixation, and external support was not used in these cases.

In the larger series of humeral shaft fractures, the incidence of nonunion has ranged from 0% to 13%. Healy[48] found that successful plating of humeral diaphyseal nonunions occurred when the surgeon achieved screw fixation of an average of seven cortices above and seven cortices below the nonunion. Non-reamed intramedullary nails provided no longitudinal or rotational stability, producing unacceptable results. Pulsed electromagnetic field coils supplementing long-arm-cast immobilization failed. Iliac crest cancellous bone grafts are strongly recommended for the surgical manage-

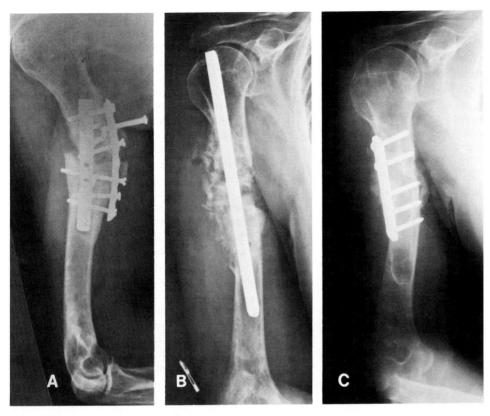

Fig. 11-16. (**A**) An x-ray of a fracture of the humerus with frank nonunion after multiple surgical procedures during a 3-year period. (**B**) An x-ray of the same fracture following removal of plates and intramedullary nailing with bone graft. The fracture did not heal. (**C**) The nonunion finally healed after compression plating and cancellous bone grafts.

ment of specific categories of delayed union or nonunion, such as atrophic nonunions and true synovial pseudarthrosis. Plates are applied to the lateral surface of the humerus through a standard anterolateral approach. Fattah[37] emphasized the need to excise the pseudarthrosis and to provide supplementary autogenous bone graft.

Rigid internal fixation is achieved by open reduction using a broad compression plate.

PATHOLOGIC FRACTURES

The humeral shaft is commonly involved by metastatic disease, and pathologic fractures may result. Parrish[77] observed that displacement and comminution are rare in these neoplastic fractures. The gradual loss of continuity in the cortex of the bone causes some local reaction, including varying degrees of periostitis, osteoblastic activity, hemorrhage, edema, and increased blood supply. These

conditions may lead to sufficient tissue reaction and new bone formation to provide some stability in the region of the neoplastic process before the fracture occurs. In such cases, simple methods of immobilization have been used by Parrish.[77] Approximately 18.5% of breast cancer patients develop evidence of humeral metastatic involvement. Eight pathologic fractures of the humerus were treated conservatively by Fleming[39] with immobilization and application of 2000 to 3000 rads of radiation and chemotherapy.[39] Three of these 8 patients were lost to follow-up; in three the fractures healed; and two developed nonunions.

Although prophylactic internal fixation of humeral metastases was not routinely recommended, operative treatment for pathologic fractures of the humerus was found to be generally superior to nonoperative management.[39] Closed treatment may lead to unsatisfactory results, limited function, incomplete pain relief, and unpredictable healing.

Closed pinning with Rush rods may be useful when multiple tumor foci are present with pathologic humeral diaphyseal fractures. The most noticeable postoperative feature after Rush rod insertion is the almost immediate palliation of the severe pain usually associated with pathologic fractures. With this technique, relief of pain can be achieved without exposing the pathologic fracture and the often-diseased adjacent tissue.

Closed insertion of Rush rods may be supplemented by the injection of polymethylmethacrylate.[59] A 1-inch incision is made over the lateral aspect of the distal humerus and a ¼-inch drill hole is made in the distal lateral cortex. A second proximal drill hole is placed adjacent to the site of the Rush rod insertion. Prior to injection of regular-viscosity cement, the intramedullary rod is visualized within the medullary canal through the ¼-inch drill holes. The polymethylmethacrylate cement is then injected proximal and distal to the fracture site using the ¼-inch lateral cortical portals.

With intramedullary pin fixation, the patient is able to remain mobile if his or her general condition is good. The presence of the nail does not preclude radiation or chemotherapy if either is indicated to treat or control the neoplastic process. Pathologic fractures fixed in this manner go on to solid union in many instances (Fig. 11-17).

LATE COMPLICATIONS

There are other complications of open humeral shaft fractures that present less formidable problems. Once the fracture has proceeded to solid union, refracture has not been observed in our experience or reported to be a significant problem. In cases where there has been healing in the bayonet position or shortening with comminution, the

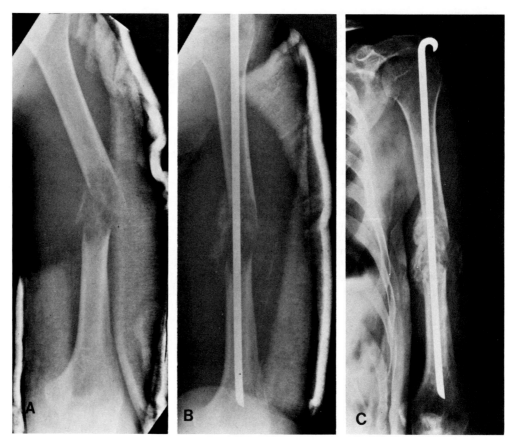

Fig. 11-17. (**A**) An x-ray showing a pathologic fracture through a metastatic lesion resulting from carcinoma of the kidney. (**B**) The same fracture after intramedullary nailing. (**C**) An x-ray after 8 weeks showing healing of fracture.

length descrepancy is not a serious problem. Myositis ossificans seems to be more frequently associated with injuries of the elbow than with those of the humeral shaft. Injuries to neighboring muscles and joints may result in stiffness and loss of function after the fracture has healed. However, regardless of the technique used, when the degree of healing permits a vigorous exercise program, this complication should be minimized.

REFERENCES

1. Adams, J.C.: Outline of Fractures. Edinburgh, E. & S. Livinstone, 1968.
2. American College of Surgeons Committee on Trauma: An Outline of the Treatment of Fracture, 8th ed. Philadelphia, W.B. Saunders, 1965.
3. Baker, D.M.: Fractures of the Humeral Shaft Associated With Ipsilateral Fracture Dislocation of the Shoulder: Report of a Case. J. Trauma, 11:532–534, 1971.
4. Balfour, G.W.; Mooney, V.; and Ashby, M.E.: Diaphyseal Fractures of the Humerus Treated with a Ready-Made Fracture Brace. J. Bone Joint Surg., 64A:11–13, 1982.
5. Bell, M.J.; Beauchamp, C.G.; Kellam, J.K.; and McMurtry, R.Y.: The Results of Plating Humeral Shaft Fractures in Patients with Multiple Injuries: The Sunnybrook Experience. J. Bone Joint Surg., 67B:293–296, 1985.
6. Bennett, G.E.: Fractures of the Humerus With Particular Reference to Nonunion and Its Treatment. Ann. Surg., 103:994–1006, 1936.
7. Bohler, L.: The Treatment of Fractures, Supplementary Volume. New York, Grune & Stratton, 1966.
8. Bostman, O.; Bakalim, G.; Vainionpaa, S.; Wilppula, H.; and Rokkanen, P.: Immediate Radial Nerve Palsy Complicating Fracture of the Shaft of the Humerus: When Is Early Exploration Justified? Injury, 16:499–502, 1985.
9. Bostman, O.; Bakalim, G.; Vainionpää, S.; Wilppula, E.; Patiälä, H.; and Rokkanen, P.: Radial Palsy in Shaft Fracture of the Humerus. Acta. Orthop. Scand., 57:316–319, 1986.
10. Boyd, H.B.; Anderson, L.D.; and Johnston, D.S.: Changing Concepts in the Treatment of Nonunion. Clin. Orthop., 43:37–54, 1965.
11. Boyd, H.B.; Lipinski, S.W.; and Wiley, J.H.: Observations on Nonunion of the Shaft of the Long Bones, With a Statistical Analysis of 842 Patients. J. Bone Joint Surg., 43A:159–168, 1961.
12. Brooker, A.F., and Edwards, C.C. (eds.): External Fixation—The Current State of the Art. Baltimore, Williams & Wilkins, 1979.
13. Brumback, R.H.; Bosse, M.J.; Poka, A.; and Burgess, A.R.: Intramedullary Stabilization of Humeral Shaft Fractures in Patients With Multiple Trauma. J. Bone Joint Surg., 68A:960–970, 1986.
14. Caldwell, J.A.: Treatment of Fractures in the Cincinnati General Hospital. Ann. Surg., 97:161–176, 1933.
15. Caldwell, J.A.: Treatment of Fractures of the Shaft of the Humerus by Hanging Cast. Surg. Gynecol. Obstet., 70: 421–425, 1940.
16. Cameron, B.M.: Shaft Fractures and Pseudarthroses. Springfield, Charles C. Thomas, 1966.
17. Campbell, W.C.: Ununited Fractures of the Shaft of the Humerus. Ann. Surg., 105:135–149, 1937.
18. Cave, E.A.: Fractures and Other Injuries. Chicago, Year Book Publishers, 1958.
19. Charnley, J.: The Closed Treatment of Common Fractures. Baltimore, Williams & Wilkins, 1961.
20. Christensen, S.: Humeral Shaft Fractures: Operative and Conservative Treatment. Acta Chir. Scand., 133:455–460, 1967.
21. Coates, J.B. (ed.): Orthopaedic Surgery in the European Theater of Operations. Washington, D.C., Office of the Surgeon General, Department of the Army, 1956.
22. Connolly, J.: Management of Fractures Associated with Arterial Injuries. Am. J. Surg., 120:331, 1970.
23. Conwell, H.E., and Reynolds, F.C.: Management of Fractures, Dislocations and Sprains, 7th ed. St. Louis, C.V. Mosby, 1961.
24. Coventry, M.B., and Laurnen, E.L.: Ununited Fractures of the Middle and Upper Humerus: Special Problems in Treatment. Clin. Orthop., 69:192–198, 1970.
25. Crenshaw, A.H. (ed.): Campbell's Operative Orthopaedics. St. Louis, C.V. Mosby, 1971.
26. DeBastiani, G.; Aldegheri, R.; and Briviol, R.: The Treatment of Fractures with a Dynamic Axial Fixator. J. Bone Joint Surg., 66B:538–545, 1984.
27. DeGeeter, L.: Treatment of Diaphyseal Humeral Fractures by Percutaneous Pinning. Acta Chir. Belg., 69:198, 1970.
28. DePalma, A.F.: The Management of Fractures and Dislocations. Philadelphia, W.B. Saunders, 1970.
29. Doran, F.S.A.: The Problems and Principles of the Restoration of Limb Function Following Injury as Demonstrated by Humeral Shaft Fractures. Br. J. Surg., 31:351–368, 1944.
30. Doty, D.B.; Treiman, R.L.; Rothschild, P.D.; and Gaspar, M.R.: Prevention of Gangrene due to Fractures. Surg. Gynecol. Obstet., 125:284–288, 1967.
31. Durbin, R.A.; Gottesman, M.J.; and Saunders, K.C.: Hackethal Stacked Nailing of Humeral Shaft Fractures: Experience with 30 Patients. Clin. Orthop., 179:168–174, 1983.
32. Duthie, H.L.: Radial Nerve in Osseous Tunnel at Humeral Fracture Site Diagnosed Radiographically. J. Bone Joint Surg., 39B:746–747, 1957.
33. Eger, M.; Golcman, L.; Goldstein, A.; Hersch, M.: The Use of a Temporary Shunt in the Management of Arterial Vascular Injuries. Surg. Gynecol. Obstet, 132:67–70, 1971.
34. Epps, C.H., Jr.: Nonunion of the Humerus. Instr. Course Lect., XXXVII:161–166, 1988.
35. Epps, C.H., Jr., and Adams, J.P.: Wound Management in Open Fractures. Am. Surg., 27:766–769, 1961.
36. Epps, C.H., Jr., and Cotler, J.M.: Complications of Treatment of Fractures of the Humeral Shaft. In Epps, C.H., Jr. (ed.): Complications in Orthopaedic Surgery, 2nd ed., pp. 231–243. Philadelphia, J.B. Lippincott, 1985.
37. Fattah, H.A.; Halawa, E.E.; and Shaty, T.H.: Nonunion of

the Humeral Shaft: A Report on 25 Cases. Injury, 14: 255–262, 1982.

38. Fenyo, G.: On Fractures of the Shaft of the Humerus. Acta Chir. Scand., 137:221–226, 1971.

39. Flemming, J.E., and Beals, R.K.: Pathologic Fracture of the Humerus. Clin. Orthop., 203:258–260, 1986.

40. Gainor, B.J., and Metzler, M.: Humeral Shaft Fracture with Brachial Artery Injury. Clin. Orthop., 204:154–161, 1986.

41. Garcia, A., Jr., and Maeck, B.H.: Radial Nerve Injuries in Fractures of the Shaft of the Humerus. Am. J. Surg., 99: 625–627, 1960.

42. Goss, C.M. (ed.): Gray's Anatomy, 25th ed. Philadelphia, Lea & Febiger, 1950.

43. Green, S.A.: Complications of External Skeletal Fixation: Causes, Prevention and Treatment. Charles C. Thomas, Springfield, Illinois, 1981.

44. Gregersen, H.N.: Fractures of the Humerus From Muscular Violence. Acta Orthop. Scand., 42:506–512, 1971.

45. Hall, R.F., and Pankovich, A.M.: Ender Nailing of Acute Fractures of the Humerus: A Study of Closed Fixation by Intramedullary Nails Without Reaming. J. Bone Joint Surg., 69A:558–567, 1987.

46. Hampton, O.P., Jr., and Fitts, W.T., Jr.: Open Reduction of Common Fractures. New York, Grune & Stratton, 1959.

47. Harris, W.H.; Jones, W.N.; and Aufranc, O.E.: Fracture Problems. St. Louis, C.V. Mosby, 1965.

48. Healy, W.L.; White, G.M.; Mick, C.A.; Brooker, A.F., Jr.; and Weiland, A.J.: Nonunion of the Humeral Shaft. Clin. Orthop., 219:206–213, 1987.

49. Hollinshead, W.H.: Anatomy for Surgeons, Vol. 3. New York, Hoeber-Harper, 1958.

50. Holm, C.L.: Management of Humeral Shaft Fractures: Fundamentals of Nonoperative Technics. Clin. Orthop., 71:132–139, 1970.

51. Holstein, A., and Lewis, G.B.: Fractures of the Humerus With Radial Nerve Paralysis. J. Bone Joint Surg., 45A: 1382–1388, 1963.

52. Hudson, R.T.: The Use of the Hanging Cast in Treatment of Fractures of the Humerus. South. Surgeon, 10:132–134, 1941.

53. Johansen, K.; Bandyk, D.; Thiele, B.; and Hansen, S.T.: Temporary Intraluminal Shunts: Resolution of a Management Dilemma in Complex Vascular Injuries. J. Trauma, 22:395–402, 1982.

54. Kamhin, M.; Michaelson, M.; and Waisbrod, H.: The Use of External Skeletal Fixation in the Treatment of Fractures of the Humeral Shaft. Injury, 9:245–248, 1977.

55. Kettlekamp, D.B., and Alexander, H.: Clinical Review of Radial Nerve Injury. J. Trauma, 7:424–432, 1967.

56. Key, J.A., and Conwell, H.E.: Fractures, Dislocations and Sprains. St. Louis, C.V. Mosby, 1956.

57. Klenerman, L.: Fractures of the Shaft of the Humerus. J. Bone Joint Surg., 48B:105–111, 1966.

58. Klenerman, L.: Experimental Fractures of the Adult Humerus. Med. Biol. Eng., 7:357–364, 1969.

59. Kuntscher, G.: The Kuntscher Method of Intramedullary Fixation. J. Bone Joint Surg., 40A:17–26, 1958.

60. Kuntscher, G.: Intramedullary Surgical Technique and Its Place in Orthopaedic Surgery: My Present Concept. J. Bone Joint Surg., 47A:809–818, 1965.

61. Kuntscher, G.: Practice of Intramedullary Nailing. Springfield, Charles C. Thomas, 1967.

62. LaFerte, A.D., and Nutter, P.D.: The Treatment of Fractures of the Humerus by Means of Hanging Plaster Cast—"Hanging Cast". Ann. Surg., 114:919–930, 1941.

63. MacAusland, W.R., Jr., and Wyman, E.T.: Management of Metastatic Pathological Fractures. Clin. Orthop., 73: 39–51, 1970.

64. Mann, R., and Neal, E.G.: Fractures of the Shaft of the Humerus in Adults. South. Med. J., 58:264–268, 1965.

65. Mazet, R., Jr.: A Manual of Closed Reduction of Fractures and Dislocations. Springfield, Charles C. Thomas, 1967.

66. McMaster, W.C.; Tivnon, M.C.; and Waugh, T.R.: Cast Brace for the Upper Extremity. Clin. Orthop., 109:126–129, 1975.

67. McNamara, J.J.; Brief, D.K.; Stremple, J.F.; and Wright, J.K.: Management of Fractures With Associated Arterial Injury in Combat Casualties. J. Trauma, 13:17–19, 1973.

68. Michiels, I.; Broos, P.; and Gruwez, J.A.: The Operative Treatment of Humeral Shaft Fractures. Acta Chir. Belg., 86:147–152, 1986.

69. Müller, M.E.: Treatment of Nonunions by Compression. Clin. Orthop., 43:83–92, 1965.

70. Müller, M.E.; Allgower, M.; and Willenegger, H.: Technique of Internal Fixation of Fractures. New York, Springer-Verlag, 1965.

71. Müller, M.E.; Allgower, M.; and Willenegger, H.: Manual of Internal Fixation. New York, Springer-Verlag, 1970.

72. Naiman, P.T.; Schein, A.J.; and Siffert, R.S.: Use of ASIF Compression Plates in Selected Shaft Fractures of the Upper Extremity: A Preliminary Report. Clin. Orthop., 71: 208–216, 1970.

73. Naver, L., and Aalberg, J.R.: Humeral Shaft Fractures Treated With a Ready-Made Fracture Brace. Arch. Orthop. Trauma Surg., 106:20–22, 1986.

74. Newman, A.: The Supracondylar Process and Its Fracture: AJR, 105:844–849, 1969.

75. Nummi, P.: Supramid Pin in Medullary Fixation: A Follow-up Study of Fracture Patients Examined After More Than 10 Years. Acta Chir. Scand., 137:67–70, 1971.

76. Nummi, P.: Intramedullary Fixation with Compression for the Treatment of Fracture in the Shaft of the Humerus: Fixation With Supramid Pin and Two Vitallium Screws. Acta Chir. Scand., 137:71–73, 1971.

77. Parrish, F.F., and Murray, J.A.: Surgical Treatment for Secondary Neoplastic Fractures—A Retrospective Study of 96 Patients. J. Bone Joint Surg., 52A:665–686, 1970.

78. Pollock, F.H.; Drake, D.; Bovill, E.G.; Day, L.; and Trafton, P.: Treatment of Radial Neuropathy Associated With Fractures of the Humerus. J. Bone Joint Surg., 63A:239–243, 1981.

79. Raney, R.B.: The Treatment of Fractures of the Humerus With the Hanging Cast. North Carolina Med. J., 6:88–92, 1945.

80. Rich, N.M.; Baugh, J.H.; and Hughes, C.W.: Acute Arterial Injuries in Vietnam: 1000 Cases. J. Trauma, 10:359–369, 1970.

81. Rich, N.M.; Metz, C.W., Jr.; Hutton, J.E., Jr.; Baugh, J.H.; and Hughes, C.W.: Internal Versus External Fixation of Fractures with Concomitant Vascular Injuries in Vietnam. J. Trauma, 11:463–473, 1971.

82. Rush, L.V., and Rush, H.L.: Intramedullary Fixation of Fractures of the Humerus by the Longitudinal Pin. Surgery, 27:268–275, 1950.

83. Sarmiento, A.; Kinman, P.B.; Calvin, E.G.; Schmitt, R.H.; and Phillips, J.G.: Functional Bracing of Fractures of the Shaft of the Humerus. J. Bone Joint Surg., 59A:596–601, 1977.

84. Scientific Research Committee, Pennsylvania Orthopaedic Society: Fresh Midshaft Fractures of the Humerus in Adults. Penn. Med. J., 62:848–850, 1959.

85. Seddon, H.J.: Nerve Lesions Complicating Certain Closed Bone Injuries. J.A.M.A., 135:691–694, 1947.

86. Seidel, H.: Humeral Locking Nail: A Preliminary Report. Orthopedics, 12:219–226, 1989.

87. Shah, J.J., and Bhatti, N.A.: A Fracture of Humerus and Radial Nerve Paralysis. Orthop. Trans., 6:455, 1982.

88. Stern, P.J.; Mattingly, D.A.; Pomeroy, D.L.; Zenni, E.J.; and Krieg, J.K.: Intramedullary Fixation of Humeral Shaft Fractures. J. Bone Joint Surg., 66A:639–646, 1984.

89. Stewart, M.J.: Fractures of the Humeral Shaft. *In* Adams, J.P. (ed.): Current Practice in Orthopaedic Surgery. St. Louis, C.V. Mosby,.1964.

90. Stewart, M.J., and Hundley, J.M.: Fractures of the Humerus: A Comparative Study in Methods of Treatment. J. Bone Joint Surg., 37A:681–692, 1955.

91. Szaley, E.A., and Rockwood, C.A.: Fractured Humerus With Radial Nerve Palsy. Orthop. Trans., 6:455, 1982.

92. Tarr, R.R., and Wiss, D.A.: The Mechanics and Biology of Intramedullary Fracture Fixation. Clin. Orthop., 212:10–17, 1986.

93. Terry, R.J.: A Study of the Supracondyloid Process in the Living. Am. J. Phys. Anthropol., 4:129–140, 1921.

94. Vander Griend, R.; Tomasin, J.; and Ward, E.F.: Open Reduction and Internal Fixation of Humeral Shaft Fractures. J. Bone Joint Surg., 68A:430–433, 1986.

95. Vander Griend, R.A.; Ward, E.F.; and Tomasin, J.: Closed Kuntscher Nailing of Humeral Shaft Fractures. J. Trauma, 25:1167–1169, 1985.

96. Ward, E.F., and White, J.L.: Interlocked Intramedullary Nailing of the Humerus. Orthopedics, 12:135–141, 1989.

97. Watson-Jones, R.: Fractures and Joint Injuries, 4th ed. Baltimore, Williams & Wilkins, 1960.

98. Whitson, R.O.: Relation of the Radial Nerve to the Shaft of the Humerus. J. Bone Joint Surg., 36A:85–88, 1954.

99. Winfield, J.M.; Miller, H.; and LaFerte, A.D.: Evaluation of the "Hanging Cast" as a Method of Treating Fractures of Humerus. Am. J. Surg., 55:228–249, 1942.

100. Zagorski, J.B.; Latta, L.L.; Zych, G.A.; and Finnieston, A.R.: Diaphyseal Fractures of the Humerus: Treatment With Prefabricated Braces. J. Bone Joint Surg., 70A:607–610, 1988.

12

Fractures of the Shoulder

Louis U. Bigliani
Edward V. Craig
Kenneth P. Butters

Part I: FRACTURES OF THE PROXIMAL HUMERUS

Louis U. Bigliani

The diagnosis and treatment of the proximal humerus fracture are challenging and difficult. Much information has been published in recent decades as new techniques have been developed and old ones rediscovered. Hippocrates[123] is credited with documenting the first fracture of the proximal humerus in 460 B.C. and describing a method of weight traction that aided in bone healing. However, little was written about this subject until the latter part of the 19th century.[26,39,55,109,168,171] These reports discussed treatment of most fractures by immobilization in a sling followed by range-of-motion exercises. This treatment was adequate for undisplaced fractures; however, the more complex fractures were not appreciated or understood, and the results of treatment were poor.

In 1896, Kocher[143] developed an anatomical classification in an attempt to improve diagnosis and treatment, but this simplified scheme was not thorough enough and lacked consistency. Other early attempts at overly simple classifications were confusing and incomplete.[36,39,61,92,95,127,133,136,137,156,177,187,227,241,250,256,275,282,293] Lack of consensus on fracture description and classification made it difficult to evaluate treatment adequately.

In 1934, Codman[48] made a significant contribution when he divided proximal humeral fractures into four basic parts. These parts were divided along the epiphyseal lines and consisted of the head, lesser tuberosity, greater tuberosity, and shaft. The subsequent four-part classification reported by Neer[205] in 1970 is based on this anatomical classification. Neer's classification is a comprehensive system that integrates fracture, anatomy, biomechanics, and displacement, allowing for consistent diagnosis and treatment. It is the most useful and common classification system.

In the early 20th century methods of closed reduction,[4,256] traction,[54,95,136,275] casting,[86,101] and abduction splints[14,53,263,300] were developed to achieve and maintain accurate anatomical alignment of displaced fractures. Often, however, these closed techniques were not sufficient to allow an adequate anatomical reduction. In 1932, Roberts[241] reported that elaborate apparatus and prolonged immobilization were not as beneficial as simpler forms of fixation and early motion. Other authors also stressed the importance of early motion and avoidance of the abduction position.[32,86,127,135,140,302] Howard and Eloesser[127] developed a complex theoretic shoulder model simulating muscle forces and demonstrated that the abduction splint was not beneficial for reduction and control of muscle forces.

Open reduction of severely displaced fracture–dislocations gained popularity during the same period in an effort to provide better anatomical alignment.[19,43,46,61,227,236,250,256,268,281] Roberts[241] and Meyerding[189] suggested the use of open reduction early to improve alignment and avoid malunions that would limit motion. Also, in some instances, internal fixation was performed.[137,177] Suture material, wire, and screws were types of early fixation. In 1949, Widen[307] first reported on intermedullary nailing of a transcervical fracture, and he credited Palmer with the development of the technique. In

1955, Rush[252] described his method of intermedullary nailing for the treatment of displaced fractures, and it became quite popular. In the early 1970s, the ASIF group popularized the use of AO plates and screws for displaced fractures. However, recent reports have stressed a high incidence of complications when this technique is used in more displaced fractures with osteoporotic bone.[148,223,278] Recently refined techniques of internal fixation with wire and nonabsorbable sutures have been successful with a low complication rate.[111,206,213]

In the early 1950s, interest grew in the use of a humeral head prosthesis for the treatment of severely displaced fracture–dislocations of the proximal humerus.[9,75,210,229,239] Closed reduction, open reduction and internal fixation, arthrodesis, and humeral head excision proved generally unsuccessful in the treatment of this problem.[206] In 1955, Neer[203] reported good results with the use of a metal humeral head prosthesis in 27 patients with fracture–dislocations. In 1973, the prosthesis was redesigned to have a more conforming head, and recent technical improvements have led to better results.[212] Currently, there are several types of proximal humeral replacements; the Neer prosthesis is the most common.

Complications of the treatment of proximal humeral fractures are not uncommon and are wide-ranging, including avascular necrosis, malunion, nonunion, infection, and neurovascular injury. This chapter outlines a comprehensive approach to proximal humeral fractures that will aid in diagnosis and treatment.

ANATOMY

It is important to understand the complex anatomy of the shoulder since optimum function of the glenohumeral joint is dependent on proper alignment and interaction of its anatomical structures. Malunion and nonunion of fractures disrupt the balance of forces across the shoulder, interfering with smooth scapula humeral rhythm and causing impingement beneath the subacromial arch.

The shoulder has an almost global range of motion, more than any other major joint in the body. This extent of movement occurs because the glenoid cavity is a shallow socket approximately one third to one fourth the size of the humeral head.[253] Therefore, it depends on capsule, ligaments, and muscle rather than bone for stability. The capsule is quite loose and approximately double the size of the humeral head, allowing for a great deal of motion. The subdeltoid bursa lies on top of the rotator

cuff and greatly facilitates movement of the cuff beneath the coracoacromial arch.

PROXIMAL HUMERUS

The proximal humerus consists of the humeral head, lesser tuberosity, greater tuberosity, bicipital groove, and proximal humeral shaft (Fig. 12-1). It is important to differentiate between the anatomical neck, which is at the junction of the head and the tuberosities, and the surgical neck, which is below the greater and lesser tuberosities. The boundaries of the latter are somewhat variable without a distinct line. Anatomical neck fractures are rare and have a poor prognosis since the blood supply to the

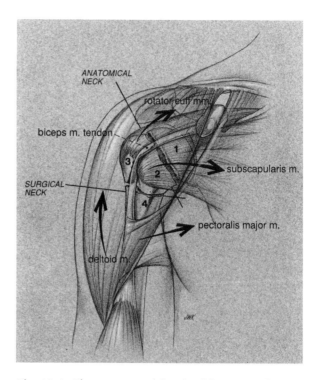

Fig. 12-1. The anatomy of the shoulder is complex and depends on proper alignment and interaction of anatomical structures. Displacement of fracture fragment is due to the pull of muscles attaching to the various bony components. The four anatomical components of the proximal humerus are the head, lesser tuberosity, greater tuberosity, and shaft. The anatomical neck is at the junction of the head and tuberosities, and the surgical neck is below the greater and lesser tuberosities. The subscapularis inserts on the lesser tuberosity, causing medial displacement, whereas the supraspinatus and infraspinatus insert on the greater tuberosity, causing superior and posterior displacement. The pectoralis major inserts on the humeral shaft and displaces it medially.

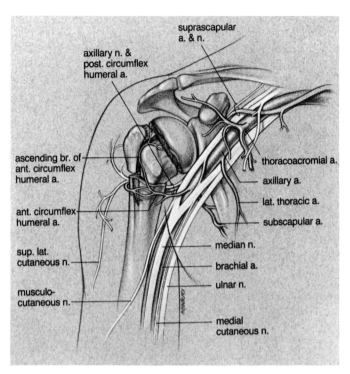

ascending br. of
ant. circumflex
humeral a.

ant. circumflex
humeral a.

sup. lat.
cutaneous n.

musculo-
cutaneous n.

axillary n. &
post. circumflex
humeral a.

suprascapular
a. & n.

thoracoacromial a.

axillary a.

lat. thoracic a.

subscapular a.

median n.

brachial a.

ulnar n.

medial
cutaneous n.

Fig. 12-2. The acromion together with the coracoacromial ligament and the coracoid process form the coracoacromial arch. The brachial plexus and axillary artery are anterior to the coracoid process and can be injured with fractures of the proximal humerus. The major blood supply to the humeral head is through the ascending branch of the anterior humeral circumflex artery, which penetrates the head at the superior aspect of the bicipital groove and becomes the arcuate artery. There are three important nerves about the shoulder: the axillary, suprascapular, and musculocutaneous.

head is completely disrupted (Fig. 12-2). On the other hand, surgical neck fractures are common and the blood supply to the head is preserved. The lesser tuberosity, the area of attachment for the subscapularis muscle, lies on the anterior aspect of the humerus and is smaller than the greater tuberosity. The bicipital or intertubular groove lies between the greater and lesser tuberosities and is on the anterior aspect of the proximal humerus. There are considerable variations in both the height and depth of the groove.[63,124,125] The biceps tendon lies in the bicipital groove and is covered by the transverse humeral ligament. The greater tuberosity lies posterior and superior on the humeral shaft and provides attachment for the supraspinatus, infraspinatus, and teres minor muscles. The greater tuberosity does not protrude above the humeral head. The glenoid is a shallow, convex structure shaped like an inverted comma,[63] approximately one third to one fourth the surface area of the humeral head. It articulates with the humeral head and also provides attachment at its rim for the glenoid labrum and capsule.

ACROMION

The acromion protects the superior aspect of the glenohumeral joint and provides origin and mechanical leverage for the deltoid muscle, which is

a prime mover of the shoulder. It also forms the lateral component of the acromioclavicular joint. The acromion together with the coracoacromial ligament and the coracoid process forms the coracoacromial arch (see Fig. 12-2). This is a rather rigid structure under which the proximal humerus, rotator cuff, and subacromial bursa must pass. Displaced fractures may disrupt the smooth flow of these structures below the coracoacromial arch, which may result in impingement and prevent normal glenohumeral motion. The subacromial (subdeltoid) bursa is a large synovial membrane. The roof is adherent to the undersurface of the coracoacromial ligament, acromion, and deltoid muscle laterally, and the floor is closely adherent to the rotator cuff and greater tuberosity.[125] It also extends anteriorly and posteriorly around the humerus, creating a gliding mechanism facilitating the movement of proximal humerus under the coracoacromial arch. This structure may become injured in even undisplaced fractures, resulting in fibrotic thickening and loss of glenohumeral motion. Early institution of range-of-motion exercises following a fracture limits the formation of bursal adhesions.

ROTATOR CUFF AND MUSCLES

The dynamic interplay of the rotator cuff and deltoid muscles is essential for glenohumeral function.

The stability of the humeral head in the glenoid created by these muscles allows the deltoid muscle to function optimally. The rotator cuff consists of four muscles: the subscapularis, supraspinatus, infraspinatus, and teres minor. The long head of the biceps tendon is another important component of this complex (see Fig. 12-1). The subscapularis is a head depressor and in certain positions an internal rotator. The infraspinatus and teres minor are external rotators. These muscles work as a unit, rather than individually, to maintain dynamic glenohumeral stability.

Since the rotator cuff muscles are attached to the tuberosities, it is important to understand the direction of pull of their fibers because this will facilitate the understanding of displacement of bone fragments. For example, in a fracture of the greater tuberosity, the fragment will be pulled superiorly and posteriorly because of the supraspinatus and teres minor muscles, whereas in a fracture of the lesser tuberosity, the fragment will be pulled anteriorly and medially by the subscapularis muscle. The long head of the biceps attaches to the supraglenoid tubercle of the glenoid and has a stabilizing and depressing action on the humeral head. It is a significant structure to consider in closed reductions since it can act as a tether and block closed reduction. Also, during operative procedures, it is a useful landmark from which the rotator interval can be identified so that bone fragments are properly identified and the rotator cuff muscles are preserved.

Two other important muscles must be considered in relation to the proximal humerus: the deltoid and pectoralis major. The deltoid is a prime mover in the shoulder and originates from the lateral one third of the clavicle, acromion, and spine of the scapula. It inserts at the deltoid tuberosity on the lateral shaft of the humerus and can cause displacement of fractures of the proximal humeral shaft. The pectoralis major is a large fan-shaped muscle that has a broad origin from the clavicle, upper ribs, and sternocostal area. It inserts on the lower portion of the lateral lip of the bicipital groove and can displace the proximal shaft of the humerus medially, as is usually seen in surgical neck fractures.

BLOOD SUPPLY

It is important to consider the blood supply to the proximal humerus, as avascular necrosis is not uncommon following displaced fractures. The major blood supply to the humeral head is from the anterior humeral circumflex artery[145,157,201,236,149] (see Fig. 12-2). Laing[154] was the first to describe the arcuate artery, which is a continuation of the ascending branch of the anterior humeral circumflex as it penetrates the bone. This tortuous artery supplies blood to a large portion of the humeral head. It routinely enters the bone in the area of the intertubicular groove and gives branches to the lesser and greater tuberosities. Also, a small contribution to the humeral head blood supply comes from branches of the posterior circumflex and from the vascular rotator cuff through tendinous osseous anastomosis.

Rothman and Parke[247] have outlined the blood supply to the rotator cuff as routinely derived from six arteries: the anterior humeral circumflex, posterior humeral circumflex, suprascapular, thoracoacromial, suprahumeral, and subscapular. The anterior humeral circumflex is the major supplier to the anterior cuff and the long head of the biceps, while the posterior humeral circumflex and suprascapular anastomosis supply the posterior cuff. The thoracoacromial artery supplies the supraspinatus while the suprahumeral and subscapular arteries supply the anterior inferior aspect of the cuff.

NERVE SUPPLY

Injury to the nerves about the shoulder can occur with fractures. The brachial plexus and axillary arteries are anterior to the coracoid process and can be injured with anterior fracture–dislocations and violent trauma to the proximal humerus (see Fig. 12-2). Isolated injuries to the major nerves innervating the muscles around the shoulder—the axillary, suprascapular, and musculocutaneous—can also occur.

The most commonly injured nerve is the axillary nerve. The axillary nerve is composed of fibers from the fifth and sixth cervical roots, in most cases, and takes its origin from the posterior cord at the level of the axilla. Then it crosses the anterior surface of the subscapularis muscle and dips back posteriorly under its inferior border. It passes along the inferior border of the capsule of the glenohumeral joint and then through the quadrangular space (see Fig. 12-2). After emerging from the quadrangular space, it gives off a branch to the teres minor and divides into anterior and posterior branches. The posterior branch supplies the posterior deltoid and gives off the superolateral brachial cutaneous nerve. The anterior branches supply the middle and anterior deltoid muscles as it winds around the inner surface.

Owing to its relative fixation at the posterior cord and the deltoid, any abnormal downward motion of the proximal humerus can result in traction and injury to this nerve. Also, its close relationship to the inferior capsule makes it susceptible to injury with anterior dislocation and open repairs for anterior fracture–dislocations.

The suprascapular nerve can also be injured, but this is much less common. It is made up of fibers from the fifth and sixth cervical roots and originates from the upper trunk of the brachial plexus. It runs laterally deep to the omohyoid and trapezius, passing through the suprascapular notch (see Fig. 12-2). After giving off two branches to the supraspinatus, it passes around the lateral border of the scapula spine to the infraspinatus. The two points of fixation of the nerve are at its origin from the upper trunk and at the suprascapular notch, where it passes beneath the transverse scapular ligament, making it susceptible to traction injuries.

Injury to the musculocutaneous nerve is rare but does occur. Composed of fibers from C5 to C6 with the occasional addition of C7 fibers, it originates from the lateral cord at the level of the pectoralis minor and passes obliquely distally through the coracobrachialis and between the biceps and brachialis (see Fig. 12-2). In the 93 cadaver shoulders we have dissected, the distance from the coracoid to the point of entrance into the coracobrachialis muscle has been between 3.1 and 8.2 cm with a mean of 5.6 cm.[81] More importantly, 29% entered less than 5 cm from the coracoid. The frequently cited safe zone of 5 to 8 cm is inaccurate. The nerve terminates in the lateral antecubital brachial nerve as it exits the deep fascia at the level of the elbow. Blunt trauma can result in injury to the musculocutaneous nerve as well as traction injuries.

MECHANISM OF INJURY

The most common mechanism of injury for proximal humeral fractures was a fall on outstretched hands from standing height or less.[165] In most instances, severe trauma does not play a significant role. Rather, the trauma need only be minor to moderate in degree because osteoporosis is usually present. The position of the arm and hand during the fall and obesity have also been suggested as factors in young individuals, and the resulting fracture is often more serious. These patients usually have fracture–dislocations with significant soft tissue disruption and multiple trauma. When multiple trauma is treated, the proximal humeral fracture is commonly initially ignored, as attention is focused on more lift-threatening problems. However, as the patient regains consciousness of awareness, complaints of pain in the shoulder may prove secondary to a fracture. Another mechanism of injury, first mentioned by Codman, is excessive rotation of the arm, especially in the abducted position. The humerus locks against the acromion in a pivotal position and a fracture can occur, especially in older patients with osteoporotic bone. Another mechanism of injury is a direct blow to the side of the shoulder. This usually occurs in the lateral position and may result in a greater tuberosity fracture.

An often ignored etiology for fracture–dislocations of the proximal humerus is electrical shock or a convulsive episode.[27,70,109,237,255,265,311] The fracture–dislocation may be anterior or posterior and is often overlooked. Metastatic disease may significantly weaken the bone so that a pathologic fracture may occur with just trivial activity. Whenever a trivial event causes a fracture of the proximal humerus, a pathologic etiology should be considered.

CLASSIFICATION

A workable classification system for fractures of the proximal humerus is necessary for proper management. A classification system must be comprehensive enough to encompass all factors, yet specific enough to allow accurate diagnosis and treatment. Also, it must be flexible enough to accommodate variations and allow logical deductions for treatment. Most proximal humeral fractures are undisplaced and must be differentiated from the more displaced fractures since the treatment is significantly different. Inadequate diagnosis of complex fractures only creates confusion and improper management.

The first steps in any classification system are a thorough knowledge of the anatomy and accurate radiographic views to outline the anatomical structures. The most logical and commonly used classification is the four-part fracture classification developed by Neer[205] in 1970.

NEER CLASSIFICATION

Before the Neer classification, various other methods had been proposed, including anatomical level of location,[32,48,132,136,143] mechanism of injury,[62,276,300] amount of contact by the fracture fragments,[73] degree of displacement,[141] and vascular status of the articular segment.[9,131] Furthermore, others have devised classifications using combinations of the preceding criteria that have resulted in confusion about the diagnosis and treatment of these complex fractures.[21,62,64,74,76,118,141,177,235,241]

In 1896 Kocher was the first to devise a classification of proximal humeral fractures.[143] His classification was based on different anatomical levels for fractures, anatomic neck, epiphyseal region, and surgical neck (Fig. 12-3). The problem with this type of classification is that it does not allow for multiple fractures at two different sites, nor does it differentiate between displaced and undisplaced fractures, which creates confusion because they require different treatment. Classification according to the mechanism of injury can also be misleading, as in the Watson-Jones classification of an abduction or adduction type of fracture.[300] It has since been pointed out that the deformity in these fractures is anterior angulation, and with internal or external rotation of the arm, the fracture can become either an abduction or an adduction fracture.[205,310]

In 1934 Codman[48] made a significant contribution to the understanding of proximal humeral

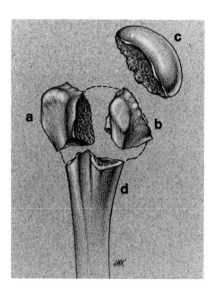

Fig. 12-4. Codman divided the proximal humerus into four distinct fragments that occur roughly along anatomical lines of epiphyseal union. He differentiated the four major fragments as (a) greater tuberosity, (b) lesser tuberosity, (c) head, and (d) shaft. (Adapted from Codman, E.A.: The Shoulder: Rupture of the Supraspinatus Tendon and Other Lesions in or About the Subacromial Bursa. Boston, Thomas Todd, 1934.)

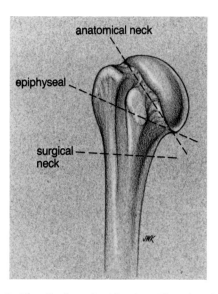

Fig. 12-3. The Kocher classification. This classification is based on three anatomical levels for fractures: anatomical neck, epiphyseal region, and surgical neck. This classification does not allow for differentiation of multiple fractures at two different sites, nor does it differentiate between displaced and undisplaced fractures. (Adapted from Kocher, T.: Beitrage zur Kenntnis einiger praktisch wichtiger Fracturenformen. Basel, Carl Sallman Verlag, 1896.)

fractures by proposing that fractures be separated into four distinct fragments, occurring roughly along the anatomical line of epiphyseal union (Fig. 12-4). He was able to differentiate four major fragments: the anatomical head, the greater tuberosity, the lesser tuberosity, and the shaft. Codman's conclusion was that all fractures were some combination of these different fracture fragments. Furthermore, the musculotendinous cuff attaches to the more proximal fragments and can hold the fractured fragments together.

This was the cornerstone on which Neer,[205] in 1970, based his four-part classification (Fig. 12-5). This was the first truly comprehensive system that considered the anatomy and biomechanical forces resulting in the amount of displacement of fracture fragments and related that to diagnosis and treatment. It is a commonly used classification for proximal humeral fractures and is used extensively in this chapter to identify fracture patterns.

The Neer classification of fractures of the proximal humerus is a system based on the accurate identification of the four major fragments and their relationship to each other. There is nothing to memorize, but an adequate knowledge of the anatomy and the insertions of the tendons of the rotator

Displaced Fractures

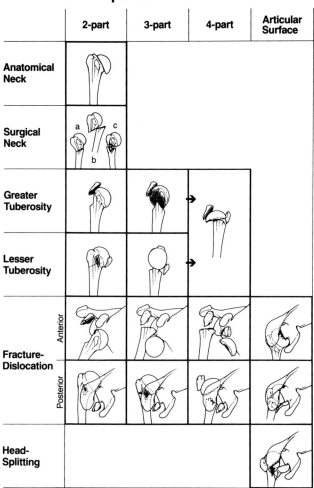

Fig. 12-5. The Neer classification. The most commonly used classification at present is the Neer four-part classification. It is a comprehensive system that encompasses anatomy and biomechanical forces that result in the displacement of fracture fragments. It is based on accurate identification of the four major fragments and their relationship to each other. A displaced fracture is either two-part, three-part, or four-part. In addition, there are fracture–dislocations that can be either two-part, three-part, or four-part. Fissure lines or hairline fractures are not to be considered displaced fragments. A fragment is considered displaced when there is more than 1 cm of separation or a fragment is angulated more than 45° from the other fragments. Impression fractures of the articular surface also occur and are usually associated with an anterior or posterior dislocation. Head-splitting fractures are usually associated with fractures of the tuberosities or surgical neck. *(After Neer, C.S.: Displaced Proximal Humeral Fractures. Part I. Classification and Evaluation. J. Bone Joint Surg., 52A:1077–1089, 1970.)*

cuff are essential to its proper use (see Fig. 12-5). The identification of fragments can be accomplished only with proper x-rays, including the trauma series, which consists of anteroposterior and lateral views in the scapular plane, as well as an axillary view. This fracture system is a concept rather than a numerical classification and sets forth guidelines that are arbitrary and designed to be helpful in recognizing displaced fractures. Emphasis is placed on determining the vascular supply to the humeral head, since avascular necrosis is a common complication of displaced fractures.

Most fractures, over 80%,[213] are minimally displaced, although Rose and associates[243] in 1982 and Horak and Nilsson[126] in 1975 have reported lower incidences, 78% and 61%, respectively. (Minimally displaced fractures must be accurately identified so

that they can be differentiated from the more serious displaced fractures.) In the Neer four-part classification, the four parts are the same as Codman has described: the articular segment or the head, the greater tuberosity, the lesser tuberosity, and the shaft (see Fig. 12-5). When any of the four major segments is displaced over 1 cm, or angulated more than 45°, the fracture is considered displaced. Fissure lines or hairline fractures are not to be considered displaced fragments. A fragment may have several undisplaced components, and these should not be considered separate fragments since they are in continuity and are held together by soft tissue. If the preceding criteria are not met, and there is no displacement of fragments, then the fracture should be considered minimally displaced and there is only one part. In a two-part fracture, one fragment is displaced in reference to the other three fragments. In a three-part fracture, two fragments are displaced in relationship to each other and the other two undisplaced fragments, but the head remains in contact with the glenoid. In a four-part fracture, all four fracture fragments are displaced; the head is out of contact with the glenoid and angulated either laterally, anteriorly, posteriorly, inferiorly, or superiorly. Furthermore, it is detached from both tuberosities as a result of its blood supply. The central focus of this fracture classification is the status of the blood supply to the humeral head and the relationship of the humeral head to the displaced parts and the glenoid.

Neer[205] has also emphasized the term *fracture–dislocation* and the accurate diagnosis of this problem (see Fig. 12-5). A fracture–dislocation exists when the head is displaced outside the joint space rather than subluxated or rotated and there is, in addition, a fracture. Fracture–dislocations can be classified according to direction, usually anterior or posterior, as well as to the number of fracture fragments— that is, two-part, three-part, or four-part. Head-splitting fractures and impression fractures of the articular surface are special fractures (see Fig. 12-5). Impression fractures of the articular surface are graded according to the percentage of the articular surface involved. The general guidelines that have been adopted for these are less than 20%, between 20% and 45%, and greater than 45% of the articular head. Head-splitting fractures can be graded in a similar fashion, but are generally involved with other fractures of the proximal humerus and often are the result of violent trauma.

AO CLASSIFICATION

Recently, on the basis of a review of 730 fractures, Jakob and colleagues[131] and the AO group have modified Neer's classification and have emphasized the vascular supply to the articular segments. The vascular supply to the articular segment plays a pivotal role in the prognosis of a proximal humeral fracture since avascular necrosis is such a common complication. The system is divided into three categories, according to the severity of injury. The least severe is the type A fracture, in which vascular isolation of the articular segment is not present and avascular necrosis is unlikely. It is extracapsular and involves two of the four primary segments. A type B fracture is more severe, and there is partial isolation of the articular segment with a low risk of avascular necrosis. It is partially intracapsular,

and three of the four primary segments are involved. In a type C fracture, the most severe, total vascular isolation of the articular segment occurs with a high risk of avascular necrosis. It is intracapsular, and all four primary segments are involved. In addition, each alphabetic group is subgrouped numerically, with higher numbers generally reflecting greater severity. This more complicated system is supposed to create a framework for more detailed therapeutic and prognostic guidelines; however, long-term results regarding treatment of various fractures have never been presented.

RATING SYSTEM

A consistent method of evaluating results is important. Unless results from different series are reported in a uniform manner, it is difficult to draw valid comparisons. When Hagg and Lundberg[105] reported their series of fractures, they had 52% satisfactory results using Santee's criteria[256] and 35% satisfactory results using Neer's criteria.[206] Confusion persists because authors continue to use their own criteria for evaluation. The most commonly used rating system for fracture has been Neer's, based on 100 units. There are 35 units for pain, 30 units for function, 25 units for range of motion, and 10 units for anatomy. Pain is the most significant factor. An excellent result is over 89 units; satisfactory, over 80 units; unsatisfactory, over 70 units; and failure, under 70 units.

In an effort to standardize results, the American Shoulder and Elbow Surgeons has recently developed a useful rating system for evaluation.[17] The assessment form has five categories: pain, range of motion, strength, stability, and function. It also considers the patient's subjective response to a surgical procedure. Pain is graded from 0 to 5; a score of 0 signifies constant pain and 5 no pain. Both active and passive range of motion are tested in forward flexion, external rotation, and internal rotation. Also, motion should be checked with the patient both sitting and supine. Strength is scored from 0 to 5, from paralysis to normal function. The deltoid, trapezium, biceps, triceps, external rotators, and internal rotators should all be tested. Stability is graded from 0 to 5, from fixed dislocation to a stable joint.

Function is graded from 0 to 4, unable to function to unrestricted activity. Activities of daily living such as cooking, combing hair, as well as throwing and lifting, are tested. Finally, the patient's response is recorded from 0 to 5, worse than before to much improved. It is hoped that this method of evaluation will shortly be widely adopted.

INCIDENCE

Fractures of the proximal humerus are not that uncommon, especially in older age groups. They have previously been reported to account for approximately 4% to 5% of all fractures, but this figure may be low.[165,205,277] A recent epidemiological study reported by Bengner and colleagues[24] from Malmo, Sweden, of more than 2,125 fractures has shown a steady and significant increase in the incidence of proximal humeral fractures. Lind and colleagues[165] noted a similar trend in Denmark and believed that the increased average life span was partially responsible. In two other recent comprehensive studies, one from Rochester, Minnesota,[243] and another also from Malmo, Sweden,[126] the age-adjusted incidence of proximal humeral fractures among adult residents was practically identical—105 and 104 per 100,000 person-years, respectively. Furthermore, it was correlated in the Minnesota study that proximal humeral fractures occur at nearly 70% of the reported rate of proximal femur fractures, all ages considered. A comparison with a previous study concerning proximal femur fractures in the same population was performed.[87] Based on the epidemiological data available, it was concluded that most proximal humeral fractures are primarily osteoporosis-related and an important source of morbidity among the elderly population. Brehr and Cooke[35] also noted a strong similarity in the incidence and pattern of these two fractures.

Proximal humeral fractures were the most common humeral fractures (45%) in Rose and colleagues' study concerning the epidemiological features of humeral fractures in Rochester, Minnesota.[243] In adults more than 40 years of age, the incidence of proximal humeral fractures increases to 76%. The major reason for this is the osteoporosis factor, since the amount of trauma responsible for the fracture was significantly less in the older age group. Shaft and distal humeral fractures are more common in the younger age groups in which more violent trauma is usually associated with the injury. Also, a higher incidence of proximal humeral fractures was noted in women than in men, by a rate of approximately 2 to 1. Horak and Nilsson[126] have also reported increased incidence with age and in females, and the same frequency as fractures of the

proximal end of the femur. The patients with proximal humeral fractures had an increased incidence of alcoholism and prior gastric resection. Furthermore, prevalence of other fractures was about doubled in patients who have had proximal humeral fractures. Rose and colleagues[243] and Horak and Nilsson[126] concluded that osteoporosis was a significant factor in these fractures.

CLINICAL PRESENTATION

Most fractures of the proximal humerus present acutely, and therefore, the most common symptoms are pain, swelling, and tenderness about the shoulder, especially in the area of the greater tuberosity. Palpation of the bony contour of the shoulder may be difficult since the soft tissue covering of the shoulder is generous. Crepitus may be present with motion of the fracture fragments, if they are in contact. However, a fracture of the shoulder is a radiographic diagnosis, and the history and physical signs only corroborate these findings. Ecchymosis generally occurs within 24 to 48 hours of the injury and may spread to the chest wall, flank, and distally down the extremity. It is important to warn the patient that this development may occur, since it may cause alarm that further internal damage has occurred after the initial fracture. In most instances, patients find it difficult to initiate active motion and hold the arm closely against the chest wall. However, history and physical examination are only suggestive of a fracture; the definitive diagnosis is made with the proper x-rays.

A detailed neurovascular evaluation is essential in all fractures of the proximal humerus. The brachial plexus and axillary arteries are just medial to the coracoid process, and injury to these structures is not uncommon. It can occur even in undisplaced fractures.[113,270] It is important to test the peripheral pulses and question the patient about parethesias and loss of sensation in the distal extremity. The easiest way to diagnose a neurovascular complication is to suspect the injury and test for it at the initial examination. The most common nerve that is injured with fractures about the shoulder is the axillary nerve. Sensation should be tested over the deltoid muscle, since testing for deltoid activity or weakness may be very difficult because of pain. Occasionally, in the immediate postfracture or postoperative period, there may be inferior subluxation of the humerus. In most instances, this is secondary to deltoid fatigue or atony, rather than an injury to the axillary nerve.[58,62,79,284,299,309] The arm should be supported in the sling, and gentle isometric exercises will help recover deltoid tone. If the situation is severe and persists for more than 4 weeks, then it must be differentiated from a true axillary nerve palsy.

Examination of the chest should not be ignored, since complications involving the thoracic cavity have been reported after fractures of the proximal humerus. Although rare, they do occur, and several authors have reported intrathoracic penetration by the humeral head associated with fractures.[93,108,226,304] Also, a pneumothorax may occur, especially in patients who have multiple trauma.

Fracture–dislocations of the proximal humerus are difficult to diagnose and often are missed by the initial examiner (Fig. 12-6A).[111,112,122,183,294,295] This is especially true of posterior fracture–dislocations. It is estimated that more than 50% of these injuries are missed by the initial treating physician.[11,112,213] In a fracture–dislocation, there is loss of contour of the shoulder. With an anterior fracture–dislocation, there is an anterior bulge and the posterior aspect of the joint is flattened or hollow. The reverse is true with a posterior fracture–dislocation, where the anterior aspect of the shoulder is flattened, the coracoid is more prominent, and there is a posterior bulge with the axis of the humerus pointing posteriorly. There will always be a loss of external rotation and abduction secondary to pain. However, if there is a surgical neck fracture component to the fracture, rotation and abduction can occur. This diagnosis must be confirmed by proper x-rays, ie, a lateral view in the scapular plane (see Fig. 12-6B), axillary view, or computed tomographic (CT) scan.

When a patient has a convulsive episode or a history of an electrical shock accident and there are pain and swelling about the shoulder, the patient must first be evaluated for a posterior dislocation or fracture–dislocation, as well as an anterior displacement.[13,112,139,265] Although this seems obvious, there was a recent case reported of bilateral posterior fracture–dislocations that were undiagnosed for 14 days after injury.[166] The patient had significant swelling and ecchymosis, as well as a fixed internal rotation contracture. The ecchymosis was attributed to a reaction to a drug prescribed by the initial physician. It cannot be overemphasized that a fixed posterior fracture–dislocation is commonly missed. To avoid this, the examining physician must have a high degree of suspicion so that appropriate radiographs can be ordered.

DIFFERENTIAL DIAGNOSIS

In most instances, the diagnosis of a fracture is readily made when proper and accurate x-rays of

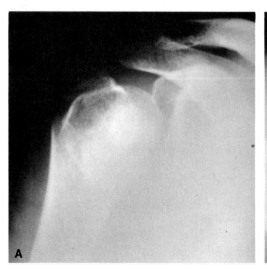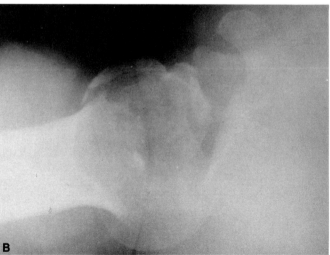

Fig. 12-6. (**A**) An anteroposterior x-ray of an obese female taken in the emergency room was initially read as a minimally displaced fracture. This poor-quality x-ray was the only view taken. The patient was started on early range-of-motion exercises but after 4 weeks had −30° of external rotation, forward elevation to 70°, and no abduction. (**B**) An axillary x-ray taken after 4 weeks reveals a missed posterior fracture–dislocation. An axillary x-ray is essential for diagnosis of posterior fracture–dislocations.

the shoulder are available. However, the patient may have acute pain, after a traumatic incident, with x-rays that rule out a fracture. The differential diagnosis of proximal humeral fractures includes any abnormality that causes acute pain, swelling, and loss of active motion. Acute hemorraghic bursitis, a traumatic rotator cuff tear, a simple dislocation, an acromioclavicular separation, and calcific tendinitis may all present clinically with these symptoms. A fall on an outstretched hand may injure the soft tissues about the shoulder, causing hemorrhage into the subacromial space, leading to inflammation and scarring of the subacromial bursa. If this condition does not resolve several weeks after injury, then one must consider the possibility of a full-thickness rotator cuff tear, especially if the individual is older, if there was a previous anterior dislocation, or both. Greater tuberosity tenderness, weakness of forward elevation and external rotation, an arch of pain, and a positive impingement sign are generally present in these patients. If there is a high degree of suspicion, ultrasonography or an arthrogram may be indicated. Calcific tendinitis may have been a pre-existing problem that was activated by trauma. Patients with an acromioclavicular separation have direct tenderness over the acromioclavicular joint, and in more severe cases the distal clavicle is displaced superiorly. A careful history, in addition to radiographs, will help differentiate a spontaneously reduced dislocation.

Another more important factor to consider is the possibility of an underlying problem that may have contributed to the fracture. Treatment of a pathologic fracture is more complicated, and bone healing is usually compromised. One should suspect that a pathologic fracture may have occurred when a trivial incident is the etiology. Metastatic carcinoma, metabolic bone disease, rheumatoid arthritis, osteonecrosis, and osteoporosis are some of the more common etiologies that may weaken bone and result in a pathologic fracture.

RADIOGRAPHIC EVALUATION

Accurate radiographic evaluation of fractures of the proximal humerus is essential for diagnosis and treatment. Incorrect or oblique x-rays only misrepresent the fracture and create confusion.

TRAUMA SERIES

The trauma series is still the best initial method for diagnosing proximal humeral fractures.[205] This consists of anteroposterior and lateral x-rays in the scapular plane and, if motion and pain permit, an axillary view (Fig. 12-7). The lateral x-ray in the scapular plane is also called the tangential or Y-view of the scapula. This series allows evaluation of the fracture in three separate perpendicular planes so that accurate assessment of fracture displacement can be achieved. The scapula sits obliquely on the chest wall, and the glenoid surface is tilted approximately 35° to 40° anteriorly. Therefore, the glenohumeral joint does not lie in either the sagittal or coronal plane. The anteroposterior and lateral x-rays in this scapular plane can be taken without removing the patient from the sling. They can be done in either a sitting, standing, or prone position. For the anteroposterior x-ray in the scapular plane, the posterior aspect of the affected shoulder is placed up against the x-ray plate and the opposite shoulder is rotated out approximately 40°. This gives a true anteroposterior view of the shoulder joint and avoids any superimposition of other tissues that will obscure bony detail. The lateral x-ray in the scapular plane is accomplished by placing the anterior aspect of the affected shoulder against the x-ray plate and rotating the other shoulder out approximately 40°. The x-ray tube is then placed posteriorly along the scapular spine, and this provides a true lateral view of the shoulder.

The axillary view allows for evaluation in the axial plane and is essential for evaluating the glenoid articular surface and the relationship of anterior and posterior fracture–dislocations (see Fig. 6B). This view is often ignored even though its importance has been stressed for years by several authors.[86,189,206,241,306] An axillary view may also be obtained in either the standing, sitting, or prone position. If possible, the supine position is preferable. The arm can be held by a knowledgeable person in abduction so that further displacement of the fracture does not occur. The x-ray plate is placed above the patient's shoulder, and the arm is gently abducted to 30°. The x-ray tube is placed slightly below the patient, and the beam goes from inferior to superior. It is helpful in these cases to rest the patient's shoulder on a soft cushion so that it is elevated off the table and bony pathology is not obscured. The Velpeau axillary view has also been described, in which the arm is not removed from the sling.[29] The patient is seated and tilted obliquely backward 45°. The plate is below and the x-ray tube above.

In attempting to judge the amount of angular displacement at the surgical neck level, one must

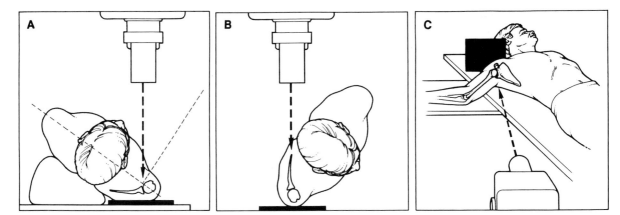

Fig. 12-7. Trauma series. The trauma series consists of anteroposterior and lateral x-rays in the scapular plane as well as an axillary view. These views may be done sitting, standing, or prone. The lateral is called the tangential or Y-view of the scapula. This series allows evaluation of the fracture in three perpendicular planes so that the fracture displacement can be accurately assessed. The scapula sits obliquely on the chest wall, and the glenoid surface is tilted approximately 35° to 40° anteriorly. Therefore, the glenohumeral joint is not in the sagittal or the coronal plane. (**A**) For the anteroposterior x-ray in the scapular plane, the posterior aspect of the affected shoulder is placed up against the x-ray plate and the opposite shoulder is rotated out approximately 40°. (**B**) For the lateral x-ray in the scapular plane, the anterior aspect of the affected shoulder is placed against the x-ray plate and the other shoulder is rotated out approximately 40°. The x-ray tube is then placed posteriorly along the scapular spine. (**C**) The axillary view is performed with the patient supine and the arm supported in abduction. The patient is usually placed on a cushion or foam so that the fracture is not obstructed by the table.

consider the neck shaft angle of the humerus in both the anteroposterior and lateral planes. On the anteroposterior projections, the neck shaft angle is the angle created at the intersection of lines that are perpendicular to the anatomical neck and parallel to the shaft of the humerus. On the lateral radiograph, the neck shaft angle is the angle formed at the intersection of the lines parallel to the anatomic neck and parallel to the shaft of the humerus. Keene and colleagues[138] have demonstrated that the neck shaft angle can vary with humeral rotation. Therefore, it is important to consider the position of the arm when evaluating radiographs and comparing them to the unaffected side, if necessary. In Keene and coworkers' studies of 25 control patients, the average neck shaft angle in the anteroposterior projection was 143°, with a range of 134° to 166°. This angle was less with external rotation and greater with internal rotation. Therefore, it can vary as much as 30° with rotation of the arm. The posterior angulation, which was measured on the lateral x-ray, averaged approximately 25° with a range of −9° to 59°. Supplemental radiographic views, such as transthoracic and various rotational views, can at times be useful to estimate the amount of displacement of specific segments. These can also be useful in malunions, especially with greater tuberosity fractures.

OTHER X-RAY TECHNIQUES

Several other diagnostic tests are helpful, including tomograms and CT. Tomograms can be useful in evaluating a proximal humeral fracture for a non-union or the amount of articular surface (glenoid and humeral head) involvement (Fig. 12-8). However, in most instances, CT has replaced tomography as the initial procedure of choice. Morris and associates have recently reported a series of patients in which CT was helpful in judging the amount of displacement of greater tuberosity fractures.[198] CT is also extremely helpful in evaluating the amount of articular involvement with a head-splitting fracture, impression fractures, chronic fracture–dislocations (Fig. 12-9), and glenoid rim fractures. Magnetic resonance imaging, a relatively new procedure, may hold some promise for evaluating displacement of proximal humeral fractures.

METHODS OF TREATMENT

Many methods of treatment of proximal humeral fractures have been proposed through the years, creating a great deal of controversy and, at times, confusion. Fortunately, most proximal humeral fractures are minimally displaced and can be sat-

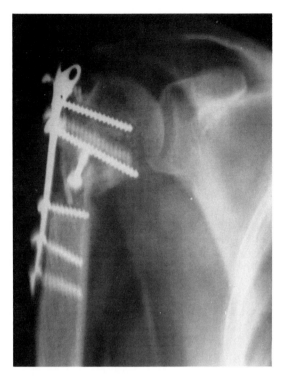

Fig. 12-8. This patient had a nonunion of a comminuted proximal shaft fracture after buttress plate fixation. A tomogram was helpful in establishing a nonunion. Note that the plate is placed extremely high and impinging on the acromion. Also, the plate is distracting the fracture.

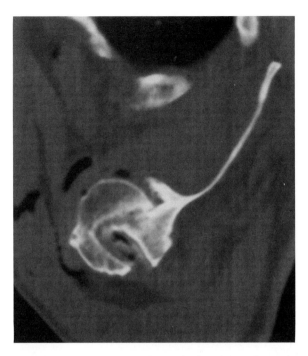

Fig. 12-9. This 64-year-old man had a chronic anterior fracture–dislocation that was missed for approximately 1 year. This CT scan was helpful in evaluating the amount of head and glenoid involvement.

isfactorily treated with a sling and early range-of-motion exercises. The controversy exists when the fractures are significantly displaced. Needless to say, it is imperative to make the appropriate diagnosis initially. Precise x-rays and a reproducible classification system are essential to achieve consistent treatment of displaced fractures. Through the years, various treatment methods have been proposed, including closed reduction, casts, splints, percutaneous pinning, open reduction and internal fixation, and the use of a humeral head prosthesis. However, one method does not fit all cases, and we must discriminate and use sound judgment to determine the appropriate treatment for each fracture.

INITIAL IMMOBILIZATION AND EARLY MOTION

Initial immobilization and early motion has been continually described as having a high degree of success because most proximal humeral fractures are minimally displaced.[76,88,124,197,241,248,302] The

shoulder has a large capsule, allowing a wide range of motion that can compensate for even moderate amounts of displacement. The arm is supported by a sling at the side or in the Velpeau position. A swathe may be needed in the immediate postfracture period to enhance immobilization and comfort. An axillary pad may also be useful. Gentle range-of-motion exercises can be started by 7 to 10 days after a fracture when the pain has diminished and the patient is less apprehensive. It is important to establish that the fracture is clinically stable and moves as a unit before exercises are started. Overly aggressive exercises may distract a minimally displaced fracture and result in a malunion or nonunion (Fig. 12-10). Intermittent x-rays in two perpendicular planes (an anteroposterior–lateral in the scapular plane) are essential to determine if there have been any fractures. Bertoft and colleagues[25] have reported that the greatest amount of improvement in range of movement occurs between 3 and 8 weeks after injury. Therefore, it is very important to have an organized and supervised physiotherapy program in place during this period. The exercises can be performed by the patient at home, but supervision by a physical therapist is beneficial in most instances. The exercises should be performed

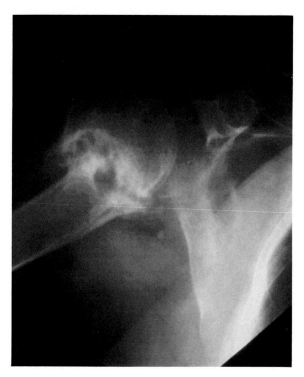

Fig. 12-10. This minimally displaced surgical neck fracture went on to a nonunion. Note the sclerotic margins of the fracture. This patient was started on overly aggressive physiotherapy and was not sufficiently supervised.

at least three to four times a day. The results of this treatment with complex displaced fractures are not as successful.

CLOSED REDUCTION

For years closed reduction has been a popular method of treatment for all types of displaced proximal humeral fractures.[90,101,136,191,241,300,316] However, it is important to differentiate between which fractures are suitable to closed reduction and which are not. Repeated and forcible attempts at closed reduction may complicate a fracture by causing further displacement, fragmentation, or neurovascular injury. Various other types of reduction maneuvers have been used with mixed results.[101,136,191,263,300]

Before a closed reduction is performed, it is important to understand the type of deformity and the forces involved in fracture. Without recognition of pathophysiology of a particular fracture, it is al-

most impossible to perform an adequate closed reduction. Watson-Jones[299] described a classic technique of hyperabduction and traction to achieve a closed reduction. This technique was thought necessary because in the surgical neck "abduction-type fracture" the proximal fragment was pulled into abduction. However, the deformity is anterior angulation and not hyperabduction; therefore, this type of reduction is not necessary. Also, in the displaced two-part surgical neck fracture, the deforming force is created by the pectoralis major muscle and other internal rotators pulling the shaft medially. This force must be neutralized before an adequate reduction can be performed. Adequate relaxation is necessary for a closed reduction. The patient is usually more comfortable supine. An intravenous catheter should be in place in the contralateral arm; a muscle relaxant and narcotic should be given intravenously after a small test dose. Whenever possible, fluoroscopic C-arm visualization should be employed to enhance visualization of the reduction and precise location of the fracture fragments. Also, the stability of the fracture reduction can be tested in different positions. If a fracture after reduction is unstable, further operative stabilization may be necessary.

Two-part Anatomical Neck Fracture

Displaced anatomical neck fractures are difficult to treat by closed reduction. The thickness of the head is quite small and the head may be rotated or angulated in the joint capsule, preventing adequate head and neck alignment. However, several other types of two-part fractures and fracture–dislocations are amenable to closed reduction.

Two-part Surgical Neck Fracture

In the displaced two-part surgical neck fracture, both tuberosities are attached to the head so that it remains in a neutral position. The shaft is usually displaced medially by the pull of the pectoralis major. The hyperabduction overhead technique is not required, nor is significant traction with weight needed. Gentle traction with flexion and some adduction is usually all that is required to get the arm to the pivotal portion so that it can be impacted under the head. If reduction is not possible, there may be interposition of soft tissue, either muscle, capsule, or long head of the biceps muscle. Often, the long head of the biceps is caught in the fracture site, creating a tether that will distract the fracture with repeated attempts at reduction (Fig. 12-11). This situation requires open reduction and internal fixation. An impacted but angulated two-part sur-

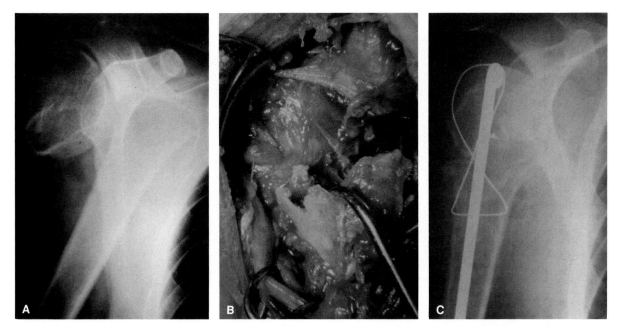

Fig. 12-11. (**A**) An anteroposterior x-ray of a displaced two-part surgical neck fracture. The shaft is displaced medially by the pull of the pectoralis major muscle. Several attempts at closed reduction were performed both in the emergency room and in the operating room under general anesthesia with the use of an image intensifier. However, the fracture could not be reduced. (**B**) Operative photo at the time of surgery showing interposition of the biceps tendon between the proximal fragment and the shaft. The loop retractor is in the biceps tendon, which was tethering the head and wedged between the shaft and the head, preventing reduction. (**C**) A 6-week postoperative x-ray revealing early healing of the fracture, which was fixed with a figure-eight wire. In this instance, a Rush rod was used for longitudinal support because of comminution. The Rush rod was removed to avoid impingement with forward elevation.

gical neck fracture can also be improved with a closed reduction. If the anterior angulation is more than 45°, this will limit forward elevation. The head should be disimpacted from the shaft; then the shaft is reduced and placed underneath the shaft with less anterior angulation. A comminuted fracture can be treated with a closed reduction if it is undisplaced and stable, but displaced and unstable fractures require open reduction and internal fixation to properly align the fragments.[47,49,194,206,251,262,273,279,316]

Two-part Greater Tuberosity Fracture

Greater tuberosity fractures are usually retracted posteriorly and superiorly, and closed reduction is difficult. However, if this fracture is associated with an anterior dislocation, a closed reduction of the glenohumeral dislocation may successfully reduce the greater tuberosity fracture (Fig. 12-12). If the fracture heals in an adequate alignment, the chance of recurrent dislocation is low. However, there is a tendency for the greater tuberosity fragment to dis-

place superiorly and posteriorly after a reduction (Fig. 12-13).[182] If this fragment is not properly reduced, a malunion can occur that will block glenohumeral motion (Fig. 12-14). Oni[221] reported a case in which the greater tuberosity fracture blocked reduction of the anterior glenohumeral dislocation. The literature reports isolated greater tuberosity fractures associated with an anterior dislocation in 5% to 8% of cases.[97,241,260] However, higher rates, between 10% and 15%, have also been reported.[189,191,213,302]

Two-part Lesser Tuberosity Fracture

If the fragment is small and does not block medial rotation, successful treatment by closed reduction of the rare two-part lesser tuberosity fracture has been reported.[131,213,245] Usually, this injury is associated with a posterior dislocation and may also be treated by closed reduction if the articular involvement is minimal and the injury occurred within 2 to 3 weeks (Fig. 12-15). The arm should

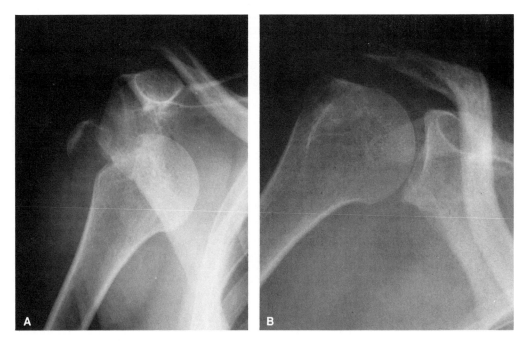

Fig. 12-12. (**A**) An anteroposterior x-ray of a two-part anterior fracture–dislocation with a displaced greater tuberosity fracture. (**B**) After a closed reduction, the greater tuberosity fracture reduced and healed without further displacement. The patient achieved a normal range of motion without any further anterior dislocations.

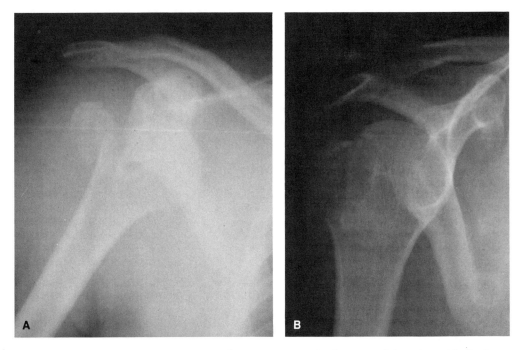

Fig. 12-13. (**A**) An anteroposterior x-ray of a two-part anterior fracture–dislocation with displacement of the greater tuberosity. (**B**) The large greater tuberosity fragment remains displaced and requires open reduction and internal fixation with nonabsorbable sutures.

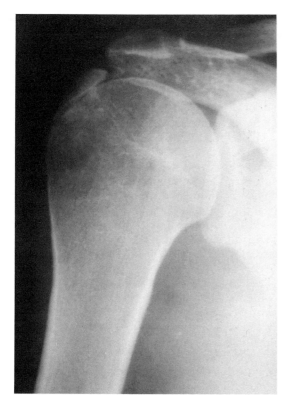

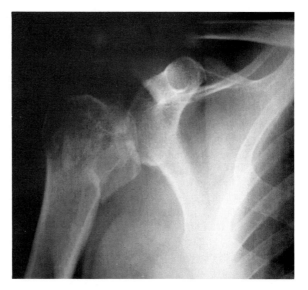

Fig. 12-15. An anteroposterior x-ray of a two-part posterior fracture–dislocation after reduction. The lesser tuberosity fragment was minimally displaced and did not block medial rotation. This injury was treated closed with excellent return of function.

Fig. 12-14. This greater tuberosity malunion resulted from the unopposed pull of the supraspinatus and infraspinatus muscles, which displaced the fragment superiorly and posteriorly. Subacromial attempts at closed reduction were performed both in the emergency room and in the operating room under general anesthesia with the use of an image intensifier. However, the fracture could not be reduced.

be immobilized in neutral or slight external rotation.

Three-part Fractures

Three-part fractures are quite unstable and difficult to treat by closed reduction. They have a tuberosity fragment as well as a surgical neck fragment. In three-part lesser tuberosity fractures, the greater tuberosity is attached to the head, pulling it into external rotation—ie, the articular surface faces anterior. In a greater tuberosity three-part fracture, the lesser tuberosity remains attached to the head, pulling it into internal rotation—ie, the articular surface faces posteriorly. In addition, the shaft is pulled medially by the pectoralis major, adding another component to be considered during the closed reduction. These deforming forces must be consid-

ered when a closed reduction is attempted. The long head of the biceps tendon may also be caught between the fragments, obstructing the reduction. Repeated attempts at a closed reduction in these fractures should not be done because most of them are in elderly people with osteoporotic bone. However, several authors have reported good results with closed reduction of three-part fractures.[76,163,195,316] The better results were in older sedentary individuals with limited goals. The pain relief was adequate, but functional activity was limited. Dingley and Denham[71] have described a modified closed technique for fracture–dislocations. They use a percutaneous pin in the dislocated head to facilitate reduction and then remove the pin. Other literature has reported poor results with closed reduction, a high incidence of pain, malunion, and avascular necrosis.[47,90,105,141,210,279]

Four-part Fractures

Closed reduction of four-part fractures of the proximal humerus generally produces poor results. In various series, there have been extremely high incidences of avascular necrosis, between 13% and 34%.[90,105,141,206,228,259,273,279] Malunion and degenerative arthritis also occur. Lee and Hansen[159] have reported the only series of satisfactory results with closed reduction.

Impression Fractures

If a missed dislocation with an impression fracture is diagnosed within 2 to 3 weeks, and the impression fracture of the head is less than 20%, then an attempt at a closed reduction may be worthwhile. It is important to accurately assess the amount of the head impression fracture with a CT or axillary view to judge whether the reduction will be stable. An adequate result may be obtained with a closed reduction in some displaced fractures, because the shoulder has a great capacity to compensate within a restricted range of motion. Many functional activities involving the shoulder can be done with a restricted range of motion. However, it must be emphasized that an anatomical reduction should be the goal in the treatment of most displaced fractures of the proximal humerus. In older, sedentary individuals, who do not place a great demand on their arm, one may accept a less than perfect closed reduction, especially in the nondominant extremity.

PERCUTANEOUS PINS AND EXTERNAL FIXATION

Percutaneous pinning may be used after a closed reduction if it is unstable.[131,147,150,151] This technique is very useful in the treatment of unimpacted two-part surgical neck fractures. Jacob and coworkers[131] have outlined the technique and reported satisfactory results in 35 of 40 cases. Two distal 2.5 AO threaded tip pins are placed in the proximal shaft just about the deltoid insertion, and then air is drilled into the head fragment using a C-arm image intensifier to visualize the fracture. A pin from the tuberosity into the shaft may enhance fixation. This procedure can be technically difficult, and a power drill is usually required to penetrate the shaft. The pins are removed when there is adequate stability of the fracture, and range of motion can progress without fear of displacement. Kristiansen and Kofoed have recently reported satisfactory results with the use of transcutaneous pin reduction combined with external fixation for three- and four-part fractures.[150,151] In a series of 31 displaced proximal humeral fractures, this technique was compared with closed reduction and the results were better. It is important to place the pins laterally and not medially to avoid injury to neurovascular structures, including the cephalic vein, and to avoid limitation of glenohumeral motion.[147]

PLASTER SPLINTS AND CASTS

Many types of splints and casts have been proposed through the years, with varying success, for the treatment of displaced fractures.[4,14,76,101,130,215,256,] [263,300,302,305,306,312] Currently, a sling and swathe or Velpeau sling is the most commonly used method of immobilization for proximal humeral fractures, and more elaborate devices are generally not required. However, a plaster slab along the humeral shaft and superior aspect of the shoulder can be used for extra support and comfort.

Older literature suggests that reduction in an abducted and flexed position was essential for proper alignment. Milch[191,192] and others[263,300] thought that the abducted and overhead position better neutralized the muscle forces about the shoulder than the anatomical position of Kocher, with the arm at the side. The shoulder spica casts and braces needed to maintain this position were extremely cumbersome and uncomfortable for the patient. These devices began to lose popularity in the 1920s.[241] However, a shoulder spica cast with some degree of abduction (20° to 30°) may be needed to provide extra stability for a severely comminuted fracture of the proximal humerus. Jakob and coworkers[131] recommend the use of an abduction splint for the treatment of selected greater tuberosity fractures.

Good results have been reported with the hanging cast, especially with humeral shaft fractures.[40–42,100,128,130,153,233,306,312] However, a significant amount of patient cooperation is required, and frequent supervision is necessary to avoid angulation and distraction. The weight of a heavy cast may cause distraction of the fracture fragments. This is especially true of comminuted proximal shaft fractures in which there is inferior subluxation.[284] Stewart and Hundley[276] recommended supplementing a hanging cast with an abduction brace for extra support and comfort in the immediate postfracture period. If traction is needed, the weight of the arm should provide sufficient distraction. In general, the use of hanging casts for fractures of the proximal humerus should be avoided, since there is a tendency for distraction of the fracture fragments, leading to nonunion or malunion. The hanging cast technique probably has more application in the treatment of humeral shaft fractures.

SKELETAL TRACTION

The use of traction is not commonly indicated but may be helpful in the management of a comminuted fracture.[140,207,213,215] Traction can be difficult to maintain and restricts patient mobility, especially if the patient has multiple injuries and requires other diagnostic and treatment procedures. However, it can provide temporary benefit until a more definitive procedure can be performed.

The arm should be held in a flexed position and slight adduction to relax the pectoralis major, which is the most important deforming force. The abducted position should be avoided. The shoulder is flexed to 90°, and the elbow is also flexed to 90°. A threaded Kirschner wire, a Steinmann pin, or an AO screw should be placed in the ulna and the forearm and wrist suspended in a sling. This allows some hand and elbow motion to avoid stiffness. The goal is to try to hold the shoulder in a neutral position, since in this fracture both tuberosities are attached to the head and the head is essentially in a neutral position. When there is sufficient callus formation, the traction can be discontinued and the patient's arm placed in a sling or spica cast.

OPEN REDUCTION AND INTERNAL FIXATION

Open reduction of displaced fractures gained popularity in the early part of the 20th century.[19,43,48,97,137,227,241,250,256,281] In many instances, closed reduction and external fixation was unable to correct deformity and maintain reduction sufficiently. Various techniques and devices have been proposed to treat fractures. The choice of technique and devices depends on several factors, including the type of fracture, quality of the bone and soft tissue, and age and reliability of the patient. The goal of internal fixation should be a stable reduction allowing for early motion of the fracture. The current trend is toward limited dissection of the soft tissue about the fracture fragments and a minimal amount of hardware required for stable fixation.[49]

Two-part Anatomical Neck Fracture

Anatomical neck fractures are extremely rare, and very few cases are reported in the literature on which to base a discussion concerning treatment. The prognosis for survival of the head is poor, since it has been completely separated from its blood supply. However, several authors recommend an attempt at open reduction and internal fixation, especially if the patient is young.[64,131,144,213] If the small head cannot be secured to the proximal humerus, then a prosthesis is indicated.

Two-part Surgical Neck Fracture

Two-part displaced surgical neck fractures often require an open reduction and internal fixation because either interposition of soft tissue prevents a closed reduction or the reduction is not stable. Various devices have been proposed for fixation, including intramedullary nails or rods, plates and screws, staples, wire, nonabsorbable suture material, multiple pins, and combinations of these.

The Rush rod technique can be performed through a very limited incision and split in the deltoid and rotator cuff. The rod has been a very popular device, and several authors have reported good results.[162,252,284,303,310] However, the relative lack of fixation of this device to control rotation may be inadequate for some displaced surgical neck fractures. Furthermore, a second procedure may be required to remove the device, since it can impinge against the anterior or inferior acromion during forward elevation and rotation. This technique may be useful in older, debilitated patients in whom minimal surgery is indicated and the functional goals are limited. The use of an AO buttress plate and screw has been associated with good results, especially with two-part surgical neck fractures, but the soft tissue dissection should be limited and the bone quality must be adequate for screw fixation. Yamano[314] has reported a high success rate with a hooked plate. The use of a figure-of-eight tension-band technique with wire or nonabsorbable sutures is also useful and usually provides adequate fixation (see Fig. 12-11; Fig. 12-16). Furthermore, if the quality of the bone is poor, then the wires can be passed through the rotator cuff for proximal fixation, since it may be stronger than the bone. In cases involving comminution, intramedullary fixation with either a Rush rod or Enders nails will improve fixation and maintain length (Fig. 12-17). The Enders rod in Figure 12-18 has been adapted to have a more superior hole for wires and sutures to be passed through. This allows for deeper placement of the nail in the rotator cuff so that it is less prominent, avoiding impingement against the acromion.

Two-part Greater Tuberosity Fracture

Greater tuberosity fractures displaced more than 1 cm may require open reduction and internal fixation because the posterior and superior displacement will cause impingement beneath the acromion[64,182,206] (Fig. 12-19). Screws, wire, and suture material have all been proposed as types of fixation of the greater tuberosity. The rent in the rotator cuff that occurs with displaced greater tuberosity fractures must also be repaired. Screws may not provide adequate fixation in osteoporotic bone (Fig. 12-20). Nonabsorbable sutures are probably a better choice of fixation.

Two-part Lesser Tuberosity Fracture

Displaced isolated fractures of the lesser tuberosity are rare injuries and may require internal fixation with nonabsorbable sutures, especially if the fragment is quite large and blocks medial rotation.[7,103,131,152,181,213,245,266,310] Stangl[274] has described

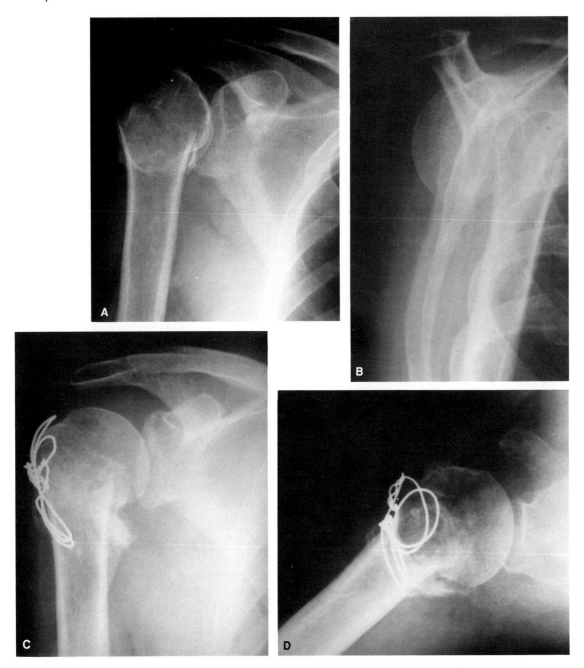

Fig. 12-16. (**A**) Anteroposterior and lateral x-rays of a displaced surgical neck fracture. (**B**) This patient was treated for 3 weeks as an undisplaced fracture on the basis of an anteroposterior x-ray only. The follow-up lateral x-ray in the scapular plane revealed a significant anterior shaft displacement. (**C**) Anteroposterior and lateral x-rays following open reduction and internal fixation with (**D**) two figure-eight wires. The wires are placed through both the cuff and the tuberosities, as well as the proximal shaft.

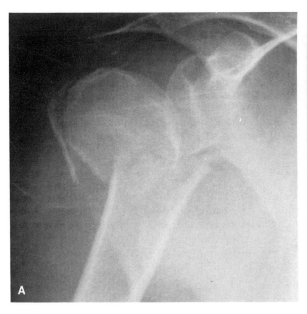
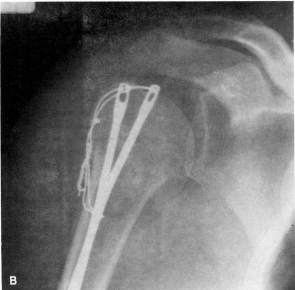

Fig. 12-17. (A) An anteroposterior x-ray of a comminuted displaced surgical neck fracture. (B) Open reduction and internal fixation with two Enders nails as well as a figure-eight wire providing rigid fixation. (*Courtesy of Evan L. Flatow M.D.*)

removal of the bone fragment and suture of the subscapularis tendon to the cortical edge of the fracture site. When the fragment is large, it may involve part of the articular surface.

Three-part Fractures

Open reduction and internal fixation is the treatment of choice of displaced three-part fractures of the proximal humerus.[2,105,111,223,244,257] It is important to avoid extensive exposure and soft tissue dissection of the fragments, which may compromise blood supply. Hagg and Lundberg[105] have reported a high rate of avascular necrosis, between 12% and 25%, in a review of several series of open reduction and internal fixation of three-part fractures.

Regardless of the type of fixation used, it must secure the displaced tuberosity to both the head and shaft. The use of intramedullary nails or rods is usually not adequate fixation to neutralize the deforming forces in this type of fracture and could result in a malunion (Fig. 12-21). Mouradian[200] developed an intramedullary nail with screw fixation for the head and tuberosities. However, the incidence of avascular necrosis was high and follow-up was short. The AO buttress plate technique has been a popular procedure for this fracture, but recent reports from several authors have reflected poor results with the AO plate for both three- and four-part fractures.[148,149,223,278] The complications include avascular necrosis secondary to extensive soft tissue dissection, superior placement of the plate leading to impingement, loss of plate fixation with screw loosening, malunion, and infection. Paavolainen and coworkers[223] reported that the most common technical error was placing the plate too high on the greater tuberosity, which restricted motion and reduced the fracture into a varus deformity (see Fig. 12-8). Kristiansen and Christensen[148] reported 55% unsatisfactory results in a series of 20 patients with two-, three-, and four-part fractures that were managed with plates and screws. Sturzenegger[252] has reported a high incidence (34%) of avascular necrosis.

Neer[206] reported good results with internal fixation of three-part fractures, if the displaced tuberosity is reattached to the shaft and head with either wire or, more recently, nonabsorbable suture. The poor results in his series were due to tuberosity displacement from failure of vertical fixation devices (Rush rods, Kirschner wires, splints) to hold the tuberosities in position. Hawkins and coworkers[111] in 1986 reported, in a series of 15 patients, that good results were obtained in 14 patients with the use of a figure-eight wire for three-part fractures of the proximal humerus. The only early failure in his series occurred in a patient who

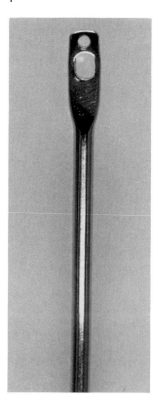

Fig. 12-18. An Enders rod modified with a superior hole for passage of wire or suture. This allows for deeper seating of the rod into the rotator cuff.

had a T plate and screws for fixation. In two patients, avascular necrosis developed, and one patient required a humeral head prosthesis. In osteoporotic bone, the soft tissues of the rotator cuff are stronger than the bone, and these can be used with this technique. The wire is passed through the rotator cuff as well as the bone of the tuberosity, and then attached to the shaft below. This method usually supplies sufficient stability to begin early motion.

Four-part Fractures

Open reduction and internal fixation of four-part fractures generally yields unsatisfactory results, as confirmed by numerous reports.[105,137,148,194,206,223,273,278,280] The complications are essentially the same as with three-part fractures, just more severe and with a higher percentage of avascular necrosis and malunion.

A significant number of four-part fractures occur in the elderly, in whom osteoporosis and poor bone quality are more common. This is not the ideal setting for internal fixation with pins, rods, or plate and screws. Jakob and associates[131] have recently reported that open reduction and internal fixation with multiple pins (minimal fixation techniques) of a subgroup of four-part fractures may be indicated (Fig. 12-22). In this group, the head is impacted on the shaft and the tuberosities are split but in close proximily to the head and shaft. The head is not dislocated or displaced laterally, and some contact with the glenoid is maintained. However, this type of fracture is not a true four-part displacement, according to the Neer classification. The head is elevated, and the tuberosities are placed beneath it. Multiple pins are used to provide fixation and left under the skin subcutaneously. The pins are removed between the fourth and sixth weeks, when early healing and some stability occur. Acceptable function and pain relief may be achieved despite avascular necrosis, because the reasonable position of the head with respect to the glenoid allows adequate glenohumeral congruity. However, long-term follow-up of cases was not reported. As a rule, the results of internal fixation of four-part fractures are generally poor.

Replacement Prosthesis

The use of the humeral head prosthesis for fractures of the proximal humerus was first published in the early 1950s. Several authors reported different designs that were being developed for use in displaced fracture–dislocations of the proximal humerus.[9,75,80,156,210,229,239,291,292] The design that has become the most commonly used was developed by Neer. In 1953, Neer[210] reported the first use of this prosthesis for complex fracture–dislocation of the proximal humerus.

At that time, alternative treatment of this fracture included closed reduction,[86] open reduction and internal fixation,[210,243,258] arthrodesis,[210] and humeral head excision.[133,134] The results were usually unsatisfactory for all these treatments. However, several authors earlier in this century reported satisfactory results with humeral head excision.[190,289] The use of this procedure yields a weakened, short, and painful extremity. In 1955 and 1970 Neer[206,208] reported on a series of patients successfully treated with the proximal humeral prosthesis. The original prosthesis (Fig. 12-23) was revised by Neer in 1973 to a more conforming surface design (Fig. 12-24).

The prosthesis has two head sizes—15 and 22 mm in thickness. The larger gives better leverage and mechanical advantage for forward elevation, but the smaller may be required for coverage by the rotator cuff. There are three stem sizes—7, 9.5, and 12 mm—and two stem lengths—125 and 150

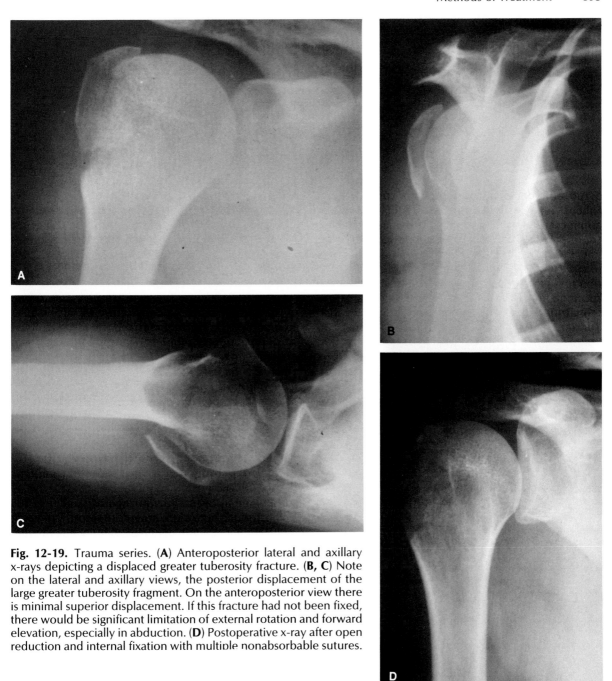

Fig. 12-19. Trauma series. (**A**) Anteroposterior lateral and axillary x-rays depicting a displaced greater tuberosity fracture. (**B, C**) Note on the lateral and axillary views, the posterior displacement of the large greater tuberosity fragment. On the anteroposterior view there is minimal superior displacement. If this fracture had not been fixed, there would be significant limitation of external rotation and forward elevation, especially in abduction. (**D**) Postoperative x-ray after open reduction and internal fixation with multiple nonabsorbable sutures.

mm (see Fig. 12-24). Longer stem lengths are available on special order if needed to bridge a shaft fracture.

The surgical technique has evolved over the past 30 years, and it is reliable for four-part fractures and fracture–dislocations of the proximal humerus. Most recently, Neer and McIlveen[212] have reported better results secondary to technical considerations concerning the anatomical approach, surgical technique, and rehabilitation. Results in 51 of the 61 patients in their series were rated excellent, nine satisfactory, and only one unsatisfactory. The technical considerations are outlined in the next section in the description of the technique. Several other

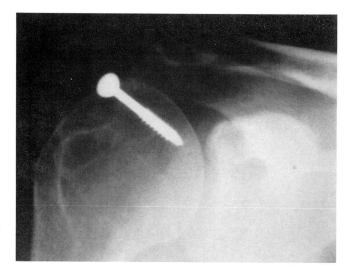

Fig. 12-20. Anteroposterior x-ray of an AO screw that had migrated superiorly with the greater tuberosity fragment. This led to significant impingement and loss of motion. There was loss of fixation of the screw, since it was placed in the soft cancellous bone of the humeral head.

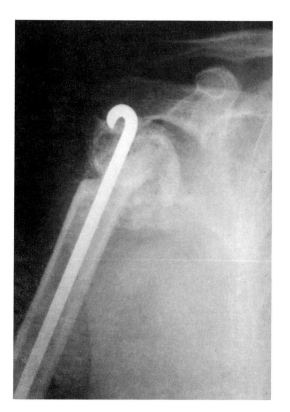

Fig. 12-21. Anteroposterior x-ray of a malunion of a three-part fracture of the proximal humerus. The Rush rod alone was not sufficient to provide adequate fixation of the displaced fragments.

series have reported good results using this prosthesis; pain relief and function were adequate.[65,66,280,288] Others have reported adequate pain relief but a higher incidence of unsatisfactory results secondary to postoperative stiffness and limitation of function.[74,146,176,195,308]

The surgical approach, care of the soft tissue, and postoperative rehabilitation are equally important as the insertion of the prosthesis. A humeral head prosthesis may be required for an anatomical neck fracture if internal fixation is not feasible. Also, in certain comminuted osteoporotic three-part fractures in older individuals, a primary humeral head prosthesis may be a better choice than internal fixation, because the internal fixation does not achieve a stable reduction allowing early motion.[49,213,280] A humeral head prosthesis allows secure tuberosity fixation so that rehabilitation can be started earlier and a more functional result can be achieved. A prosthesis is indicated in head-splitting fractures and also impression fractures in which more than 45% of the articular surface is involved. The results from prostheses in acute fractures are generally better than the results from the use of prostheses in chronic fractures or from revisions of failed internal fixation because of malunion, scar tissue, and muscle contractures.

Fracture–Dislocation

Two- and three-part fracture–dislocations are readily treated by open reduction and internal fixation. In these fracture–dislocations, the vascular supply to the head is maintained by the soft tissue attachments to the intact tuberosity, and therefore, adequate fixation should be attained by the pro-

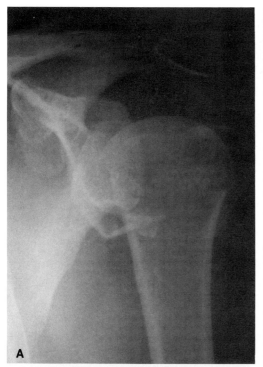

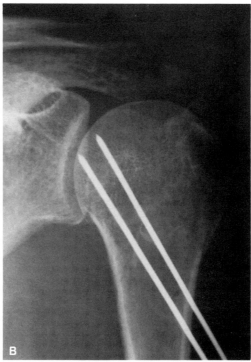

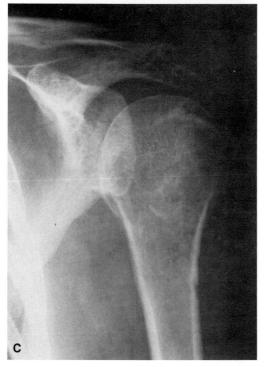

Fig. 12-22. (**A**) An anteroposterior x-ray of a four-part fracture in which there is continuity of the head with the glenoid. (**B**) The head has been elevated and the tuberosities reduced, and two pins are maintaining the reduction. There is minimal internal fixation technique. (**C**) The pins have been removed at 8 weeks, and there is good congruity of the head and the tuberosities. This is early in the fracture period, with a good early result seen. Long-term results with this procedure have not been reported.

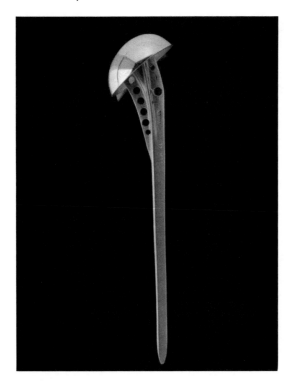

Fig. 12-23. The original Neer I prosthesis, which was designed in 1951.

cedures that have been previously outlined. Redislocation is rare after adequate fracture healing. In two-part fracture–dislocations, a closed reduction may have adequately treated the glenohumeral dislocation, but if there is a persistent tuberosity displacement, this requires open reduction and internal fixation. The results from internal fixation of four-part fracture–dislocations have been poor, and a prosthesis is generally indicated in this type of lesion (Fig. 12-25).

SURGICAL APPROACHES

There are two basic surgical approaches for treatment of the proximal humeral fractures. The first is the superior deltoid approach (Fig. 12-26**A**).[213] The skin incision is made in Langer's lines just lateral to the anterolateral aspect of the acromion. Through this approach the deltoid can be split from the edge of the acromion distally for approximately 4 to 5 cm (Fig. 12-26**B**). The deltoid origin is not removed, allowing exposure of the superior aspect of the proximal humerus. This approach is useful for internal fixation of greater tuberosity fractures

and helpful for the insertion of a proximal intramedullary rod. Rotation, flexion, or extension of the humerus or all three greatly enhance exposure of the underlying structures.

The second approach is a long deltopectoral approach (Fig. 12-27**A**).[214] In this approach both the deltoid origin and insertion are preserved. The skin incision is started just inferior to the clavicle and extends across the coracoid process and down to the area of insertion of the deltoid. The cephalic vein should be preserved and retracted either laterally or medially, depending on which is the easiest direction. The deltopectoral interval is dissected proximally and distally (Fig. 27**B**). If more exposure is needed, the insertion of the deltoid can be partially elevated, and the superior part of the pectoralis major tendon insertion can be divided.

Procedures that split or remove the lateral part of the acromion are unnecessary and may lead to complications. Furthermore, splitting the middle deltoid beyond 5 cm from the edge of the acromion has a high risk of injury to the axillary nerve. Both of these approaches are extremely worthwhile because they preserve deltoid function, which allows a more rapid rehabilitation in the postoperative period. Removal of the deltoid origin is unnecessary because it seriously affects the function of this important muscle and slows the postoperative rehabilitation program. Splitting the middle deltoid beyond 2 inches from the edge of the acromion presents a high risk of injury to the axillary nerve.

AUTHOR'S PREFERRED METHOD OF TREATMENT

Minimally Displaced Fractures

Minimally displaced fractures are treated with a sling and swathe for comfort. The swathe can usually be removed after a few days. On rare occasions, if there is significant swelling and discomfort, I may use a plaster slab on the shaft of the humerus and the superior aspect of the shoulder.

If the fracture is stable, then range-of-motion exercises can be started early—within 10 days when the pain is tolerable. The physician must evaluate the fracture for clinical stability by standing on the side of the patient and supporting the elbow and forearm with one hand and placing the other hand over the proximal humerus. Then one gently rotates the elbow and forearm. If the fracture appears to move as a unit, it is stable, and gentle and passive range-of-motion exercises can be started. Elbow supination, pronation, and flexion can be started while the patient is in the sling. The complete

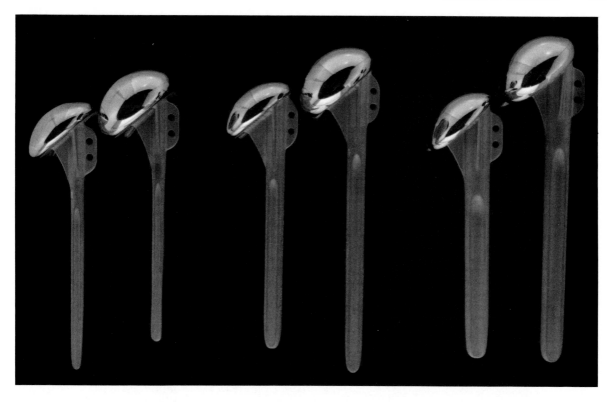

Fig. 12-24. The Neer II prosthesis, which was redesigned in 1973. There are two head sizes (15 and 22 mm) as well as three stem sizes (7, 9.5, and 12 mm) and two stem lengths (125 and 150 mm).

physical therapy regimen is outlined in the rehabilitation section. Frequent radiographic evaluation is needed to check for displacement of fracture fragments.

Two-part Anatomical Neck Fracture

Anatomical neck fractures, as noted, are extremely rare and there are very few reports of treatment.[39,64,131,206] Certainly, no surgeon has treated large numbers of this type of fracture. In young patients, I recommend an attempt at open reduction and internal fixation. If there is some soft tissue attachment to the head and if the quality of the bone is good, it may be possible to achieve fixation to the tuberosities and shaft. In older patients, a primary prosthesis is a better choice, allowing early motion and a more rapid recovery.

Two-part Surgical Neck Fracture

Displaced two-part surgical neck fractures are divided into three distinct types: unimpacted, angulated impacted, and comminuted; most of these can be initially treated by closed reduction. The exception is the severely comminuted surgical neck frac-

ture, in which there is little chance of improved alignment and stability is not possible.

In the displaced surgical neck fracture, the shaft is displaced medially by the pectoralis major and is in close proximity to the brachial plexus and axillary arteries. The head remains within the glenohumeral joint in a neutral position, since both tuberosities are attached. To achieve a closed reduction, gentle traction should be placed on the arm as it is brought out to the side and then gently flexed. Traction should be maintained, and flexion is increased as the arm is gradually adducted to gain reduction of the shaft beneath the head (Fig. 12-28). The adduction neutralizes the pull of the pectoralis major and other internal rotators, which are creating the deformity. Counterpressure by an assistant beneath the armpit or digital pressure on the proximal fragment may be needed to achieve stabilization. An attempt is made to hook the proximal shaft beneath the humeral head, and then the arm is slightly abducted and the shaft is impacted beneath the head. To adequately perform this procedure, it is important to have good relaxation. This may not be possible in an emergency room situation with only

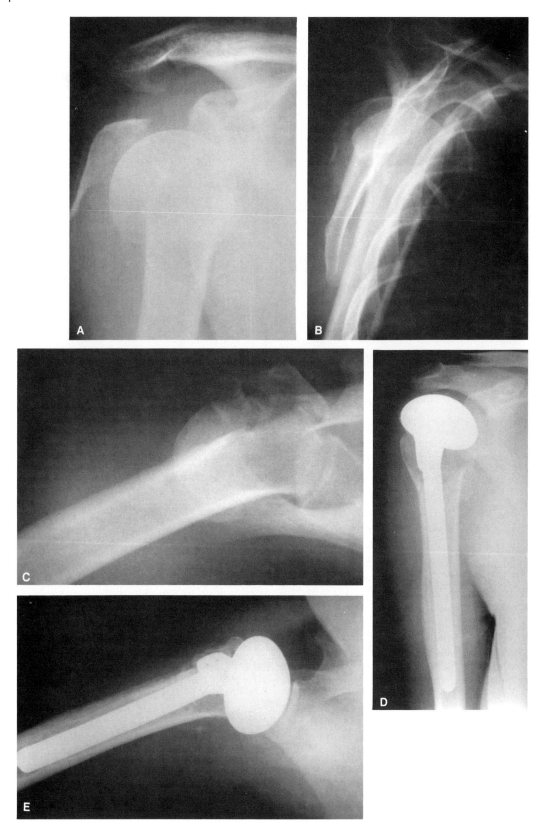

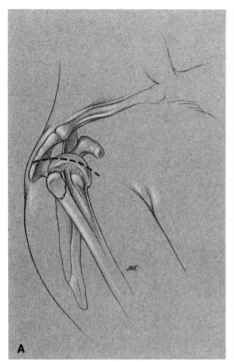 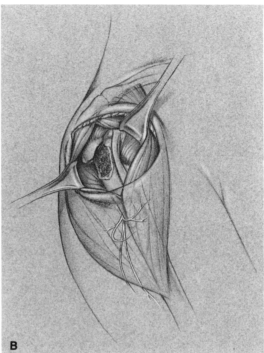

Fig. 12-26. **(A)** Superior anterior approach to the shoulder. The skin incision for the superior anterior approach to the shoulder consists of an oblique incision in Langer's lines beginning on the anterolateral aspect of the acromion and extending down obliquely for approximately 8 to 9 cm. **(B)** Two Richardson retractors are placed in the deltoid as it is split approximately 4 to 5 cm from the tip of the acromion. This gives adequate exposure for greater tuberosity fractures. Great care is made not to extend the slit below 6 cm, since there may be injury to the axillary nerve. Rotation of the humerus allows for improved exposure of the different parts of the proximal humerus.

intramuscular or intravenous analgesics and muscle relaxants. Multiple attempts at closed reduction in the emergency room without adequate relaxation are ill advised.

If the first attempt at closed reduction is unsuccessful, then I prefer to perform the next closed reduction in the operating room under adequate anesthesia and image intensifier control. This monitoring allows precise visualization of the frac-

ture fragments. If a satisfactory reduction is achieved and it is stable, the arm is immobilized in a sling and swathe. However, if the reduction is unstable, then percutaneous pinning should be performed. The patient should be prepared and draped, and intravenous antibiotics should be given. The arm is then reduced and held in a stable position. Two pins are directed proximally, starting above the deltoid insertion through the proximal

←

Fig. 12-25. **(A)** Anteroposterior x-ray in the scapular plane revealing a four-part fracture with the head displaced laterally, the greater tuberosity displaced superior-laterally, and the lesser tuberosity displaced medially. **(B)** Lateral x-ray in the scapular plane revealing the posterior displacement of the greater tuberosity, the head in the center, and the lesser tuberosity medially below the coracoid. **(C)** The axillary view shows the lateral displacement of the head as well as the displacement of lesser and greater tuberosities. **(D)** Anteroposterior and **(E)** axillary x-rays revealing a large humeral head prosthesis in place. In this instance, a press fit was obtained. In most instances, cement is needed to support the prosthesis. Three years postoperatively, the patient has an essentially normal range of motion and activity.

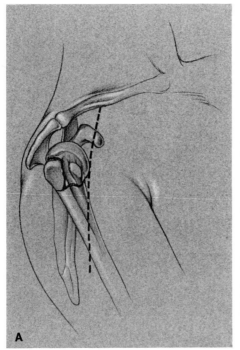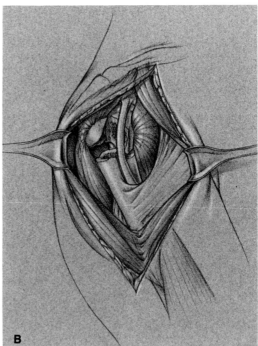

Fig. 12-27. (**A**) A long deltopectoral approach is useful for two-, three-, and four-part fractures. The incision is made from the clavicle medially over the coracoid and extended down to the shaft of the humerus near the deltoid insertion. (**B**) Exposure that can be achieved. The insertion of the pectoralis major also can be released to improve exposure. Care is taken never to remove the deltoid origin from the clavicle. If more exposure is needed, the deltoid insertion can be elevated.

fragment and into the head and tuberosity fragment (Fig. 12-29). These pins should be 2.5-mm terminally threaded AO pins. The use of a power drill is important since it may be difficult to pierce the cortex of the proximal humerus. Each pin should be individually checked with the image intensifier in two perpendicular planes. A third pin is started proximally from above into the greater tuberosity and then into the distal shaft. An additional fourth pin from distal to proximal through the anterior shaft into the head will achieve extra stability, if required. Care must be taken not to enter the articular surface of the head. After this, the arm is rotated and stability is assessed. The pins are cut short beneath the skin and not removed until there is radiographic evidence of fracture stability, usually between 4 and 6 weeks.

If closed reduction is not possible and the percutaneous pinning is unsuccessful, then open reduction and internal fixation is required. There may be soft tissue interposition. The long head of the

biceps can act as a tether in between the fracture fragments and actually prevent reduction by causing distraction (see Fig. 12-11**B**).

The surgical exposure is a long deltopectoral approach in which the origin and insertion of the deltoid are preserved. It provides adequate exposure without injuring the deltoid muscle or axillary nerve. Care should be taken to avoid extensive dissection of the soft tissue from the fracture fragments. I prefer to treat these fractures with a figure-eight wire (18-gauge) technique or No. 5 nonabsorbable nylon suture. Wire provides greater stability but may be an irritant in the subacromial space and may also break or migrate. Therefore, if possible, nonabsorbable sutures or wires should be passed through and under the rotator cuff as well as through the tuberosity. In many instances, the cuff may be better-quality tissue than the bone in the proximal humerus. A large 14- or 16-gauge spinal needle or plastic angiocath is helpful in passing suture or wire through the cuff. A drill hole is made

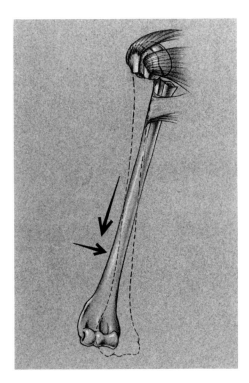

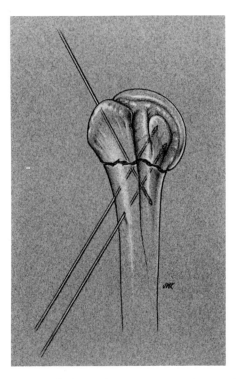

Fig. 12-28. Closed reduction of a surgical neck fracture. To achieve a closed reduction, general traction should be placed on the arm as it is brought out to the side and gently flexed. Traction should be maintained and flexion is increased as the arm is gradually adducted to gain reduction of the shaft beneath the head. Adduction neutralizes the pull of the pectoralis major and other internal rotators that are creating the deformity. Counterpressure by the assistant may be needed beneath the armpit or digital pressure on the proximal fragment to achieve stabilization. The shaft should be beneath the head for a stable reduction.

Fig. 12-29. Technique of percutaneous pinning of surgical neck fractures. The arm is reduced and held in a stable position. Two pins are then directed proximally, starting above the deltoid insertion through the proximal fragment and into the head and tuberosity fragment. These pins should be 2.5-mm terminally threaded AO pins. A power drill must be used because it may be difficult to pierce the cortex. The third pin is started proximally from above into the greater tuberosity and then into the shaft.

in the shaft of the humerus, approximately 1 inch below the fracture site, and the wire or nonabsorbable sutures can be passed through the hole and then looped back in a figure-eight manner. Two separate sutures or wires are used, one through the greater tuberosity and the other through the lesser tuberosity. Then, both sutures or wires are placed through the same drill hole in the proximal humerus. Excellent stability can be achieved, allowing for early range-of-motion exercises. If the longitudinal stability is not sufficient, secondary to comminution or poor bone quality, then intramedullary fixation is necessary to supplement the wire or suture (see Figs. 12-11 and 12-17). The intramedullary fixation may need to be removed at 6 weeks to avoid subacromial impingement.

Impacted surgical neck fractures angulated greater than 45° should be reduced. The deformity is usually in the anterior plane, and malunion will limit forward elevation. Multiple rotational radiographic views, as well as comparison radiographs of the normal shoulder, are important to judge the amount of angulation fully. The reduction maneuver includes abduction and flexion to the pivotal position. This usually distracts the fracture fragments and frees the shaft from under the head, allowing correction of the deformity. A hyperabduction maneuver is not indicated in this fracture because the proximal fragment is not abducted. The head may be reimpacted so that stability can be achieved and early motion started. The arm is immobilized at the side in a sling and swathe.

Initially, comminuted proximal humeral fractures without significant displacement should be

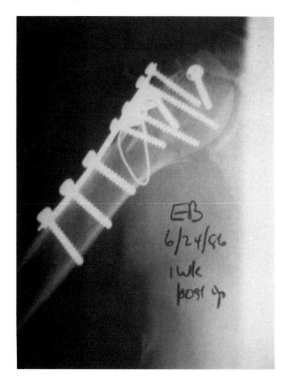

Fig. 12-30. Anteroposterior x-ray of an open reduction and internal fixation with a plate and screws of a comminuted fracture of the proximal humerus. Excellent fixation was achieved, and the patient had excellent union and achieved a good functional result. *(Courtesy of Howard Rosen, M.D.)*

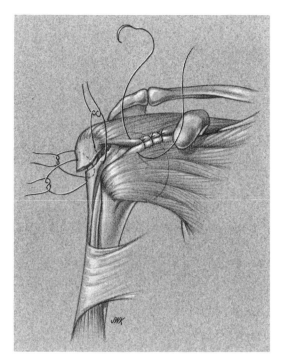

Fig. 12-31. Technique of open reduction and internal fixation of the greater tuberosity fracture. The ideal method of fixation for greater tuberosity fractures is multiple nonabsorbable nylon sutures. The cuff must also be repaired. It is advisable to repair the cuff first, since this reduces tension from the bony sutures and stabilizes the fracture fragment. Several drill holes are placed in the proximal shaft and through the greater tuberosity and then secured.

treated with a sling and swathe and a plaster splint applied along the shaft of the humerus and onto the top of the shoulder. Occasionally, a shoulder spica cast is helpful. Traction is difficult to maintain and tolerate and is a problem in patients with multiple injuries. If closed reduction is not successful, open reduction and internal fixation, with a plate and screws and multiple sutures or wire, if necessary, is indicated (Fig. 12-30). Although this fixation may not be rigid enough to allow early motion, it is adequate to maintain alignment until there is early healing and motion can be started. Addition of a shoulder spica cast can help to enhance fixation.

Two-part Greater Tuberosity Fracture

Two-part greater tuberosity fractures displaced greater than 1 cm require open reduction and internal fixation. A closed reduction is difficult to achieve because there is a tear in the rotator cuff and the fragment is pulled posteriorly and superi-

orly. If left in this position, impingement will develop and the patient will lose motion of the shoulder (see Fig. 12-14). The surgical approach for this type of fracture is a superior approach in Langer's lines (see Fig. 12-26). The deltoid is split a short distance from the acromion for 3 to 4 cm. I prefer to stabilize the bone fragment with multiple nonabsorbable nylon sutures (Fig. 12-31). The rotator cuff must also be repaired. Repairing the rent in the cuff first offers stability and removes tension from the fracture repair. The greater tuberosity is anatomically replaced using several No. 2 nylon sutures (ie, Tevdek) placed through drill holes in the tuberosity and shaft (Fig. 12-32). Bone fragments and hematoma may need to be removed from the fracture surface of the greater tuberosity to improve the reduction. Exercises are started early, on the second or third postoperative day.

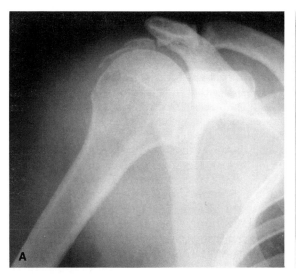
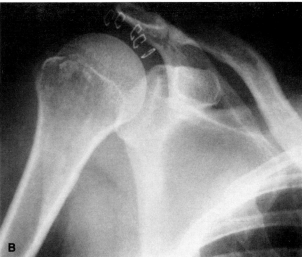

Fig. 12-32. (**A**) Anteroposterior x-ray of the displaced greater tuberosity fracture, which is pulled posteriorly and superiorly by the supraspinatus and the infraspinatus. (**B**) Postoperative x-ray showing stabilization of the fracture with multiple nonabsorbable sutures.

Two-part Lesser Tuberosity Fracture

Displaced isolated fractures of the lesser tuberosity are also extremely rare. If the fragment is small and rotation is not affected, then the arm can be supported in a sling and the patient is instructed about range-of-motion exercises. If the fragment is large and blocks medial rotation, then open reduction and internal fixation with nonabsorbable sutures is needed. The fracture fragment may also be removed and the tendon of the subscapularis repaired back to the proximal humerus.

Three-part Fractures

Most three-part fractures are quite unstable, and closed reduction is difficult. In general, open reduction and internal fixation is the treatment of choice in active patients, since a stable reduction can usually be achieved allowing early motion. Closed reduction is an option only in debilitated patients or patients in whom surgery is contraindicated. The surgical approach to this procedure is also deltopectoral.

Great care must be taken not to denude the fracture fragments of their blood supply, which may lead to avascular necrosis. In most cases, I prefer to use internal fixation of the fragments with No. 5 nonabsorbable sutures or 18-gauge figure-eight wires. The technique is similar to that previously described for two-part surgical neck fractures (Fig.

12-33). The displaced tuberosity should be attached to the head and remaining tuberosity fragment as well as the shaft below (Fig. 12-34). Multiple sutures are necessary for stability. In selected cases, when there is significant osteoporosis and the quality of the bone is poor, not allowing internal fixation, a primary humeral head prosthesis is indicated. This allows earlier mobilization of the shoulder. The patient is usually an older female.

Four-part Fractures

The treatment of choice for four-part fractures of the proximal humerus is a humeral head prosthesis, since other methods of treatment are associated with poor results. Occasionally, in patients less than 40 years of age, without a dislocation, if the head is still in continuity with the glenoid and there appears to be some soft tissue attachment, open reduction may be attempted. Fixation of the head fragment is difficult and best achieved with multiple K-wires that are removed after adequate healing. However, this type of fracture has a high incidence of avascular necrosis.

My preference is use of the Neer humeral head prosthesis. It is available in various sizes. The surgical approach is important because the deltoid must be preserved to allow optimum postoperative shoulder function. The deltoid should not be detached from its origin because this will weaken it.

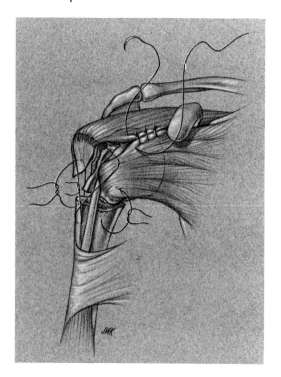

Fig. 12-33. Technique of internal fixation of a three-part fracture. This technique may be done with either absorbable sutures or 18-gauge wire. It is important to secure the displaced tuberosity, in this case the greater tuberosity, to both the head and lesser tuberosity as well as to the shaft below. The lesser tuberosity and head fragment should also be repaired to the shaft below with several sutures. Generally, this gives very stable fixation, allowing for early motion.

A long deltopectoral approach (deltoid on) avoids detachment of the deltoid origin but still allows adequate exposure (see Fig. 12-27). If more exposure is needed, the deltoid insertion should be slightly elevated. Another important aspect is to restore proper length to the humerus, with the prosthesis preserving proper tension in the myofascial sleeve. The tendency is to set the prosthesis against the remaining humeral shaft, which significantly shortens the humerus, creating an unstable situation that leads to inferior subluxation and inability to elevate the extremity. In this situation, the deltoid is shortened and its function is significantly compromised (Fig. 12-35). The addition of cement enhances stability when there is inadequate bony support for the stem, and it allows for adjustment of the prosthesis to the proper length. The prosthesis

has to be set at the proper length and the proper degree of retroversion, which is generally between 30° and 40° (Fig. 12-36). The distal humeral condyles must be palpated to aid in estimating the amount of humeral head retroversion. This is performed with the elbow flexed and the prosthesis in position so that anterior and posterior stability can be assessed. A sponge can be placed into the shaft of the humerus, which allows sufficient support of the prosthesis so that stability can be checked. If part of the biceps groove is intact, then this can be a useful landmark. The lateral fin with holes in it for the prosthesis should sit just at the posterior aspect of the groove (Fig. 12-37).

Secure fixation of the tuberosities is essential to allow early postoperative motion of the shoulder. The tuberosities should be sutured with nonabsorbable suture to each other and to the shaft of the humerus through the fin of the prosthesis (Fig. 12-38). Two or three sutures should be placed from the greater tuberosity to the shaft, and two sutures should be placed from the greater tuberosity through the holes in the fin of the prosthesis to the lesser tuberosity. It is important to close the rent in the rotator cuff. One or two sutures are also passed from the lesser tuberosity to the shaft of the humerus. If possible, the long head of the biceps should be preserved by retracting it anteriorly or posteriorly and then replacing it back into its groove in the humerus. The head of the prosthesis should be positioned above the greater tuberosity to avoid impingement of the greater tuberosity against the acromion (see Fig. 12-25E).

If there is a humeral shaft fracture, it should be stabilized prior to cementing of the prosthesis. This can be done with a cerclage wire and multiple nonabsorbable nylon sutures. The wound is irrigated with saline solution, and two closed-suction irrigation tubes are placed deep in the deltoid muscle. The deltoid is closed with chromic sutures, and if the insertion has been elevated, this should be reattached. The skin is closed with a subcuticular Dexon or nylon suture. Prophylactic antibiotics are given preoperatively, intraoperatively, and postoperatively for 48 hours. The operating physician may start range-of-motion exercises within 48 hours and gently rotate and elevate the arm. Passive-assistive range-of-motion exercises are started on the third postoperative day, and resistive exercises are not performed until there is healing of the tuberosities, generally by 6 weeks. After 6 weeks, the resistance in active exercising is gradually increased and stretching exercises are continued.

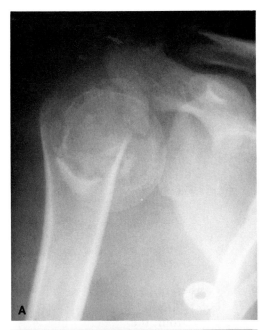

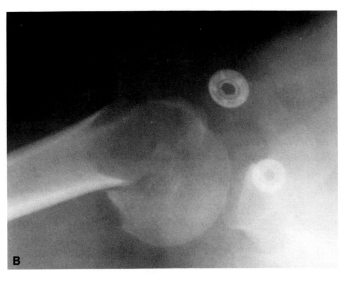

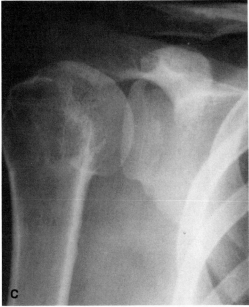

Fig. 12-34. (**A**) Anteroposterior x-ray of a three-part greater tuberosity fracture. (**B**) Axillary x-ray of a three-part greater tuberosity fracture with the shaft and head significantly angulated. (**C**) One-year follow-up anteroposterior x-ray of a three-part greater tuberosity fracture fixed with multiple nonabsorbable sutures. Healing was excellent, and the patient has a full range of motion with normal function.

Fracture–Dislocations

TWO-PART FRACTURE–DISLOCATIONS

Two-part fracture–dislocations should initially be treated by a closed reduction. The head is attached to the shaft and, it is hoped, in most instances, the displaced tuberosity fragment will be reduced to an acceptable position (see Fig. 12-12). Anterior two-part fracture–dislocations are immobilized at the side with a sling and swathe. Posterior fracture–dislocations are immobilized in neutral or slight external rotation with the arm in a cast or brace. There is a tendency for redisplacement of the tuberosity fragment, especially with greater tuberosity fractures. Therefore, frequent follow-up x-rays are

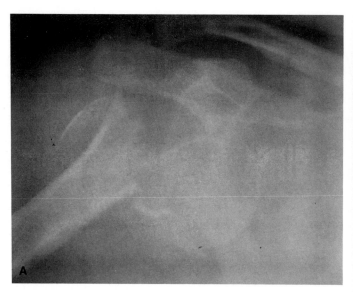

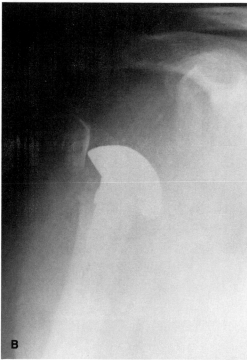

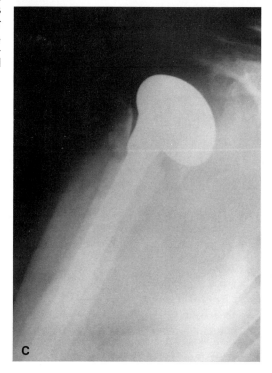

Fig. 12-35. (**A**) Anterior four-part fracture–dislocation with head displaced beneath the coracoid. (**B**) Failed Neer I prosthesis in which the prosthesis was placed up against the proximal shaft, creating an unstable situation leading to inferior subluxation. In addition, both tuberosities became detached as a result of in-adequate fixation. (**C**) Revision of the prosthesis in which cement was used to elevate the prosthesis approximately 4 cm. This was enough to create stability. Enough bone was left on the greater tuberosity to place it beneath the head. This patient, in addition, had a partial axillary nerve palsy. However, he did achieve a pain-free shoulder with approximately 80° of forward elevation and 30° of external rotation.

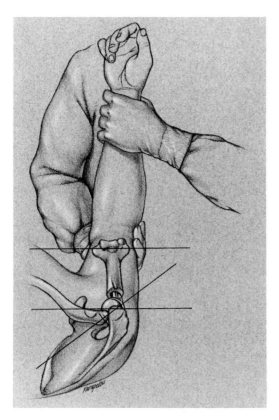

Fig. 12-36. The humeral head prosthesis should be placed in 30° to 40° of retroversion. This can be accomplished by palpating the distal humeral condyles with the elbow flexed and estimating the amount of humeral head retroversion. Anterior and posterior stability should be assessed with the prosthesis in the shaft. A sponge can be stuffed in the shaft of the humerus to allow sufficient support of the prosthesis. If part of the biceps groove is intact, then this can be used as a landmark. The fin of the prosthesis should sit at the anterior aspect of the groove.

essential in the postreduction period. If the tuberosities are displaced, these should be treated the same as two-part fractures.

Usually, with repair of the tuberosity, further glenohumeral dislocations do not occur. Two-part fracture–dislocations involving the anatomical or surgical neck are extremely rare. If an anatomical head fragment is outside, I would use a humeral head prosthesis. With fracture–dislocation involving the surgical neck, I prefer open reduction and internal fixation.

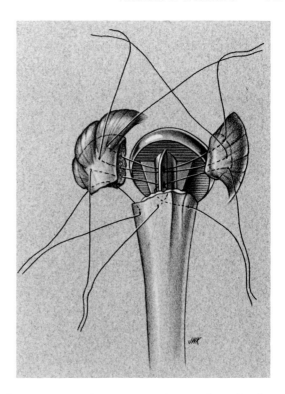

Fig. 12-37. Prosthesis repair. The prosthesis has been cemented into place and is elevated off the shaft. Both tuberosities should be able to fit below the head. The tuberosities should be repaired superior to the head. Drill holes should be placed through both tuberosities and the shaft, and the tuberosities should be attached to each other through the fin of the prosthesis as well as to the shaft below.

THREE-PART FRACTURE–DISLOCATIONS

I prefer open reduction and internal fixation of three-part fracture–dislocations. I might attempt one closed reduction. In anterior fracture–dislocation, it must remembered that the head is very close to the brachial plexus and axillary artery. Therefore, great care must be taken in an open reduction of an anterior three-part fracture–dislocation to gently reduce the head to avoid injury to the neurovascular structures. The glenoid surface should also be inspected for impression fractures. Open reduction and internal fixation using fracture sutures is performed with the same technique as described for three-part fractures.

FOUR-PART FRACTURE–DISLOCATIONS

Four-part fracture–dislocations are treated with a humeral prosthesis. The head is devoid of any soft

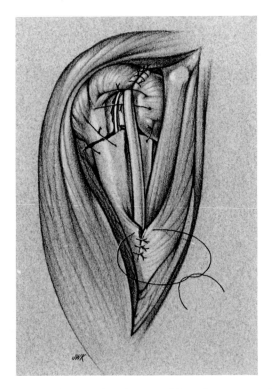

Fig. 12-38. The completed repair of the tuberosities with the rotator cuff interval closed and the biceps preserved. In general, nonabsorbable sutures provide a firm repair, allowing for early motion.

tissue attachment with fracture–dislocations and usually is a free-floating fragment. Once again, great caution should be used in trying to remove the head in an anterior fracture–dislocation (Fig. 12-39), especially if surgery has been delayed for several weeks, since adhesions are usually present. With a posterior fracture–dislocation, there may be excessive posterior instability, and less retroversion may be required for the prosthesis. If the prosthesis is unstable posteriorly, then retroversion may be decreased by 10° to 15°, and this will usually create stability.

Impression and Head-Splitting Fractures

Treatment of impression fractures of the articular surface differs with the size of the defect and the time of the diagnosis. If head involvement is less than 20% and the treatment is within 2 to 3 weeks after injury, closed reduction may be adequate. The arm should be immobilized in external rotation after reduction if the dislocation is posterior. For defects involving 20% to 45% of the anterior head

that are associated with a posterior dislocation, I prefer to use a modification of the McLaughlin procedure as reported by Hughes and Neer[129] involving an anterior approach. The lesser tuberosity, as with the tendon of the subscapularis, is transferred into the defect in the head and fixed with a screw. For head defects greater than 45%, I prefer to use a prosthesis. If the glenoid is fractured, eroded, or worn, it may also require replacement. Generally, impression fractures occur with posterior fracture–dislocations.

Head-splitting fractures also require a prosthesis. These are usually associated with fractures of either tuberosities or the surgical neck (Fig. 12-40). In a young patient, if bone stock is adequate, open reduction and internal fixation may be attempted, but in my experience this is usually a very difficult procedure, associated with a high incidence of failure.

REHABILITATION

Rehabilitation of proximal humeral fractures is essential because adequate motion is needed for optimum function. If a fracture or fracture repair is stable, then therapy should be started early. The most useful rehabilitation protocol is the three-phase system that has been devised by Hughes and Neer[129] (Fig. 12-41). The first phase consists of passive-assistive exercises. In the second phase, active- and early-resistive as well as stretching exercises are started. The third phase is a maintenance program aimed at advanced stretching and strengthening exercises. Application of this system is variable and depends on the type of fracture, the stability of the fracture or fracture repair, and the ability of the patient to comprehend the exercise program. The exercises are performed three to four times per day for 20 to 30 minutes. A hot pack applied 20 minutes before the exercise session is beneficial. Early in the program an analgesic may be needed to control pain, allowing sufficient stretching. Often it is advisable to involve a physical therapist for guidance and management of the exercise program.

Phase I exercises are started early in the post-fracture or postoperative period. If a fracture is minimally displaced or has been treated by closed reduction and is stable, then exercises are generally started between the seventh and tenth days after fracture. The first exercise is usually a pendulum exercise (Codman) in which the arm is rotated both outwardly and inwardly in small circles (see Fig. 41**A** and **B**). The second exercise is supine external rotation with a stick (see Fig. 12-41**C**). It is impor-

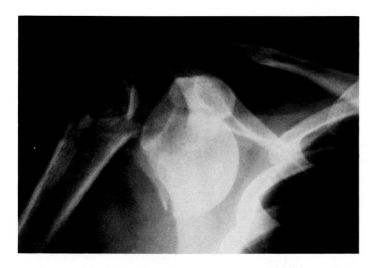

Fig. 12-39. Anteroposterior x-ray of a four-part fracture–dislocation. The head is displaced below the coracoid and is adjacent to the neurovascular bundle.

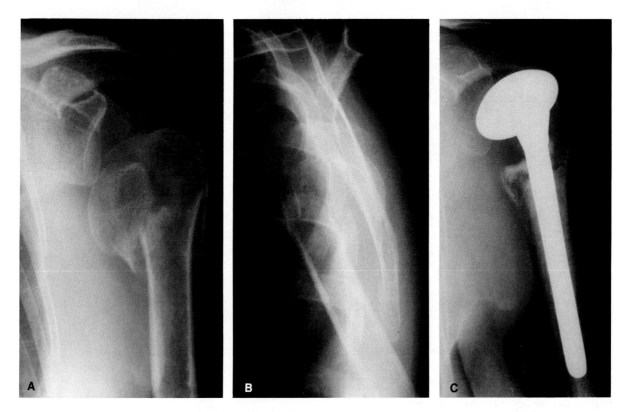

Fig. 12-40. (**A**) Anteroposterior x-ray of a head-splitting fracture in which a significant portion of the articular surface is involved. The superior portion of the head is with the greater tuberosity fragment, and the inferior portion is with the lesser tuberosity fragment. There is also a surgical neck fracture. (**B**) Lateral x-ray in the scapular plane is a head-splitting fracture showing the superior fragment above. The inferior fragment below demonstrates the discontinuity of the articular surface. (**C**) Anteroposterior x-ray of a Neer prosthesis used to repair the head-splitting fracture.

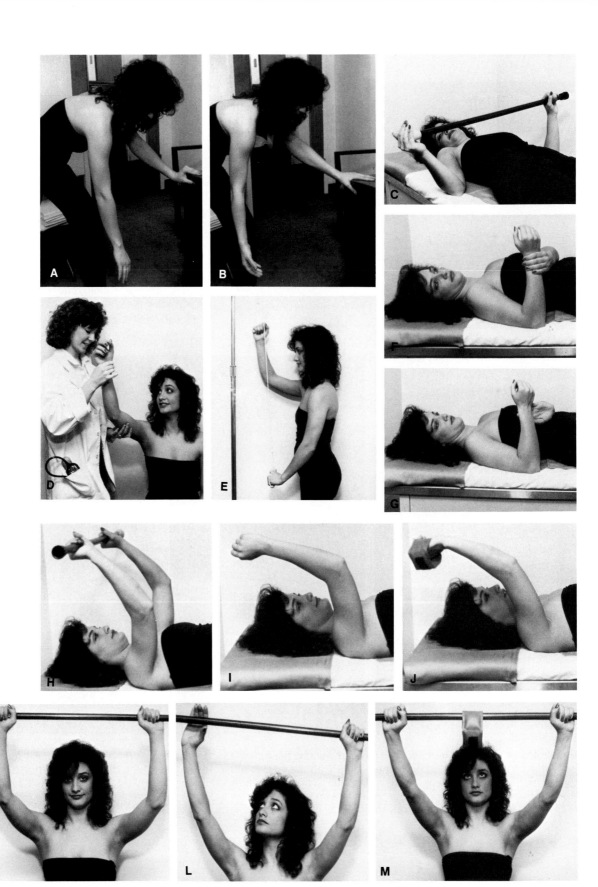

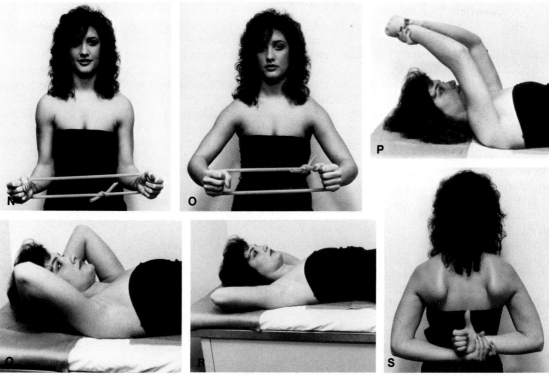

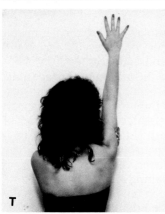

Fig. 12-41. Exercise should be done at least three to four times a day. It is best to warm up first with a hot shower, heating pad, or hot water bottle. The exercise regimen should take between 15 and 20 minutes. (**A, B**) Pendulum exercises are performed with the patient standing and bent over at the waist. Large circles are made with the entire arm with the palm forward and backward. (**C**) External rotation with a stick should be performed supine with the elbow abducted slightly from the side. The noninvolved arm pushes the involved arm out, supplying the power. (**D**) Assisted forward elevation is done by the therapist, with the patient either erect or supine. (**E**) Pulley exercises are performed with the uninvolved arm supplying the power for elevation of the involved arm. (**F, G**) Isometric exercises to strengthen both the external and internal rotators are started with the patient supine. (**H–J**) Active forward elevation with a stick is started supine with the elbow bent. As strength permits, this may be done with the arm un-assisted. Later, a 1- or 2-pound weight can be added for strengthening. (**K–M**) Erect forward elevation can also be performed with a stick using the uninvolved arm to assist the involved arm. As the patient gets stronger, an attempt should be made to release the stick from the involved hand and to lower the arm on its own. Weights can be added for strengthening. (**N**) Strips of rubber sheeting of various strengths or rubber tubing can be used to strengthen the external rotators by placing the tubing around the wrist, keeping the elbows at the side, and externally rotating. (**O**) This can also be used to strengthen the deltoid by abducting the shoulders. In addition, if the rubber tubing is attached to a doorknob and used, the anterior and posterior deltoids can also be strengthened. (**P–R**) As healing permits, the arm is raised overhead with the help of the other arm, and abduction can also be performed. (**S**) Internal rotation is done with the aid of the uninvolved arm or a towel over the shoulder. (**T**) Stretching for a forward elevation can be done against the wall or the end of a door. It is important to try to lean the weight of the body into the wall so as to stretch the shoulder in forward elevation.

tant to support the elbow and the distal humerus with either a folded towel or sheet because this will create a sense of security for the patient. A slight amount of abduction approximately 15° to 20° may also aid in performing this exercise.

Three weeks after fracture, assisted forward elevation (see Fig. 12-41**D**) as well as pulley exercises (see Fig. 12-41**E**) can be added. Extension can be added a little later. Isometric exercises are generally started at 4 weeks (see Figs. 12-41**F** and **G**). After a secure surgical repair, the exercises can be started by the physician within 24 to 48 hours. The physician should start elbow flexion and extension first and then gently assist the patient with pendulum exercises. Supine external rotation and assisted forward elevation, either supine or sitting, are also performed. Between three and five days postoperatively, formal exercises with the therapist are started. These consist of pendulum, pulley supine, external rotation with a stick, supine forward flexion, and extension with a stick. Isometrics can be started after 3 weeks.

Phase II exercises involve early active, resistive, and stretching exercises. The first exercise is supine active forward elevation since gravity is partially eliminated, making elevation easier (see Fig. 12-41**H, I, J**). The forward elevation can then progress to the erect position. The use of a stick in the unaffected arm assists the involved arm in forward elevation (see Fig. 12-41**K, L, M**). As the arm gains strength, active erect elevation can be performed unassisted, but it is important to keep the elbow bent and the arm close to the midline. Strips of rubber sheeting of various strengths (Therabands) are used to strengthen the internal rotators, the external rotators, and anterior, middle, and posterior deltoids (see Figs. 12-41**N** and **O**). Three sets of 10 to 15 repetitions are recommended at each exercise session. Stretching for forward elevation on the top of a door or wall is started, as well as stretching in the door jamb for external rotation (see Fig. 12-41**T**). Also, the arm is raised over the head with hands clasped, and then the hands are placed behind the head and the arms externally rotated and abducted (see Figs. 12-41**P, Q,** and **R**). This exercise is extremely important to achieve abduction and external rotation. Wall climbing is generally not performed because this does not promote stretching. Internal rotation is helped by using the normal arm to pull the involved arm into internal rotation (see Fig. 12-41**S**).

Phase III exercises are generally started at 3 months. Rubber tubing is substituted for the rubber strips to increase resistance. The arm is stretched higher on the wall by leaning the torso into the wall. Also, stretching on the end of the door and prone stretching for forward elevation are extremely useful. A hot shower before stretching promotes relaxation. Light weights could be used after 3 months. These should be started at 1 pound and increased at 1-pound increments, with the limit being 5 pounds. If there is persistent pain after exercises with weights, then the weights should be decreased or eliminated. Strength can be achieved with functional activity. A well-supervised rehabilitation regimen is essential for successful fracture treatment. Even a perfect fracture reduction or surgical repair will not achieve a good result without proper exercises.

COMPLICATIONS

Displaced fractures of the proximal humerus are difficult to manage, and a rather large spectrum of complications has been reported after both closed and open treatment. Some of these include avascular necrosis, nonunion, malunion, hardware failure, frozen shoulder, infection, neurovascular injury, and pneumothorax or pneumohemothorax.

Vascular Injury

Vascular complications following proximal humeral fractures are infrequent, but they do occur and can have profound consequences.[113,117,146,167,206,240,259,270,273,283] Injury to the axillary artery accounts for approximately 6% of all arterial trauma, secondary to fractures of the proximal humerus, and is the most common vascular injury. In a series of 81 fractures, Stableforth[273] reported a 4.9% incidence of arterial damage in displaced fractures. The injury is usually associated with penetrating or violent blunt trauma, resulting in a displaced fracture. However, it has also been reported with minimally displaced fractures. In addition, the risk is increased in older patients with arterial sclerosis because the vessel walls have lost elasticity and cannot stretch in response to the trauma. Therefore, in the elderly, a trivial trauma can result in an arterial injury.

The most common site of injury to the axillary artery is proximal to the takeoff of the anterior circumflex artery. Recent reports have stressed the need to suspect vascular injury whenever there is a fracture near a major vessel because the key to successful treatment is early diagnosis and repair.[113,259,318] The physical examination of the axillary artery may be difficult when pain and muscle spasm prevent abduction. It is important to check the radial pulse in the injured extremity; however, the presence of peripheral pulses may be secondary to collateral circulation. Therefore, an intact radial pulse is not a guarantee that significant arterial injury has not occurred. Doppler ultrasonography can be helpful in detecting a pulse but can also be misleading because collateral circulation can create a pulse detectable by Doppler examination. Other signs include an expanding hematoma, pallor, and parethesias. Paresthesias are probably the most reliable sign of inadequate distal circulation and should raise suspicion of a vascular injury.

If an arterial injury is not recognized, the complication could be catastrophic, including gas gangrene, amputation, and compressive neuropathies of the brachial plexus leading to permanent deficits unless there is early evacuation of the hematoma. Angiography should be performed to confirm the diagnosis and to establish the exact location and nature of the injury. Arterial repair should be performed without delay and, if necessary, coordinated with appropriate orthopaedic fracture repair.

Brachial Plexus Injury

Brachial plexus injuries also occur after fractures of the proximal humerus. Stableforth[273] reported an incidence of 6.1% after fractures of the proximal humerus. Any or all components of the brachial plexus may be involved. Isolated injury to the axillary nerve is not uncommon and has been reported.[28] This is especially true of anterior fracture–dislocations because the nerve courses on the inferior surface of the capsule and is susceptible to injury. Injury to the suprascapular and musculocutaneous nerve is less common. It is thus important to establish, at the time of initial evaluation, if there are any nerve injuries. This can be done clinically by testing skin sensation and motor power. If nerve injury is suspected, it should be explained to the patient and carefully followed. Electromyographic and nerve conduction studies should be used to follow the progress of the injury. In complete axillary nerve injuries that do not show any signs of improvement within 2 to 3 months of injury, early exploration may be indicated.

Chest Injury

Injury to the thorax can also occur after fractures of the proximal humerus.[205,273] There have been several reports of intrathoracic dislocation of the head with surgical neck fractures of the humerus.[93,108,226] In addition, a pneumothorax or a hemopneumothorax can occur after fractures of the proximal humerus.

Myositis Ossificans

Myositis ossificans, especially after fracture–dislocations, has been reported by several authors.[64,206,230] It is unusual for this to occur with uncomplicated fractures, but especially when there is a chronic unreduced fracture–dislocation.

Frozen Shoulder

A frozen shoulder may result if there is inadequate rehabilitation after a fracture or operative repair. It is essential to have a well-organized and monitored physiotherapy program. In general, the first step with a stiff shoulder is to start the patient on a progressive exercise program. In cases of minimally displaced fracture in which there is adequate anatomical congruity, the next step may be a manipulation under anesthesia and arthroscopic débridement of both the joint and subacromial space. The arthroscopic examination creates a brisement and distention of the joint space as well as the subacromial space. Scar tissue and adhesions may also be resected using the arthroscope. If there is painful hardware or impingement of hardware and the patient does have a union, then an open release and removal of hardware may be required.

Avascular Necrosis

Avascular necrosis is not uncommon after both three- and four-part fractures and has also been reported after some two-part fractures.[21,82,90,105,131,141,148,159,200,205,223,259,278,279] In reviewing several large series, Hagg and Lundberg[105] have recently reported an avascular necrosis rate of 3% to 14% after closed reduction of displaced three-part fractures, and a rate of 13% to 34% after four-part fractures. The result is usually a stiff, painful joint. In addition to the avascular necrosis, malunion and glenohumeral arthritis may be present, resulting in significant pain and loss of glenohumeral motion. The example seen in Figure 12-42 is that of an active 72-year-old woman who had a painful stiff shoulder, secondary to avascular necrosis, and a malunion of a four-part fracture, treated by closed reduction and early motion. Degenerative arthritis of the glenohumeral joint developed, and a total shoulder replacement was required for pain relief and improved function. This was an especially difficult procedure to perform since there was joint incongruity and capsular, bursal, and tendon scarring with contracture and loss of bone. However, some reports have described adequate function if there is reasonable congruity of the glenohumeral joint.[199,200]

Besides the severity of the fracture, extensive exposure of soft tissue has been identified as a major

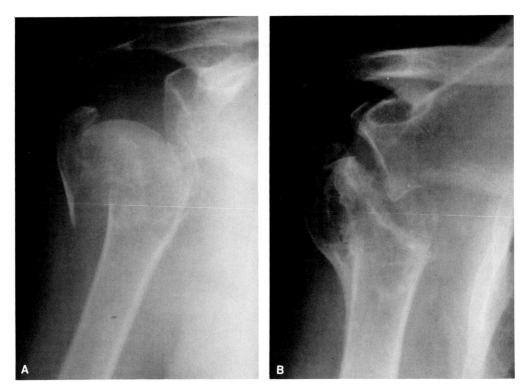

Fig. 12-42. (A) An anteroposterior x-ray of a four-part fracture in an active 72-year-old woman. Her physician believed that there was sufficient congruity of the glenoid and head that early motion could be started and that the patient was too old for an operative procedure. **(B)** Ten months after the fracture, the patient has avascular necrosis and degenerative arthritis. She had significant pain and disability and could not use the upper extremity for even simple activities of daily living. The patient required a total shoulder replacement for pain relief and improved function.

contributing factor. Sturzenegger and associates[278] reported a 34% incidence of avascular necrosis in a series of 17 patients treated with a T-plate. The extensive soft tissue exposure needed for plate fixation was thought to be a factor in this series (Fig. 12-43). The treatment of choice for avascular necrosis is a humeral head prosthesis or total shoulder replacement if the glenoid is involved.

Nonunion

Nonunions of the proximal humerus are not that common[59,73,157,178,206,242,258,272] and usually are associated with displaced fractures, but they can also occur after minimally displaced fractures (see Fig. 12-10). Unfortunately, treatment may be difficult because they often occur in older, debilitated patients with soft, osteoporotic bone. Also, loss of bone stock can occur. The literature on this subject is scarce. In 1964 Sorensen[272] reported on only seven cases, five found in the literature and two of

his own. Neer[205,206] reported 16 cases of nonunions in his paper on displaced proximal humeral fractures in 1970. Eight of the nonunions were secondary to a hanging cast or excessive overhead traction. Other causes after closed treatment include severe displacement; comminution; soft tissue interposition such as capsule, deltoid muscle, or the long head of the biceps; systemic disease; a preexisting stiff glenohumeral joint; an uncooperative patient; and overly aggressive physiotherapy. Nonunion can also occur after open treatment secondary to poor bone quality, inadequate fixation, or infection (Fig. 12-44).

Neer has described a pathologic condition in nonunion of surgical neck fractures in which there is significant resorption of bone beneath the head and a characteristic cavitation of the head fragment, which is produced by the upper end of the shaft (Fig. 12-45). In this situation, there is constant motion because of the unopposed pull of the pectoralis

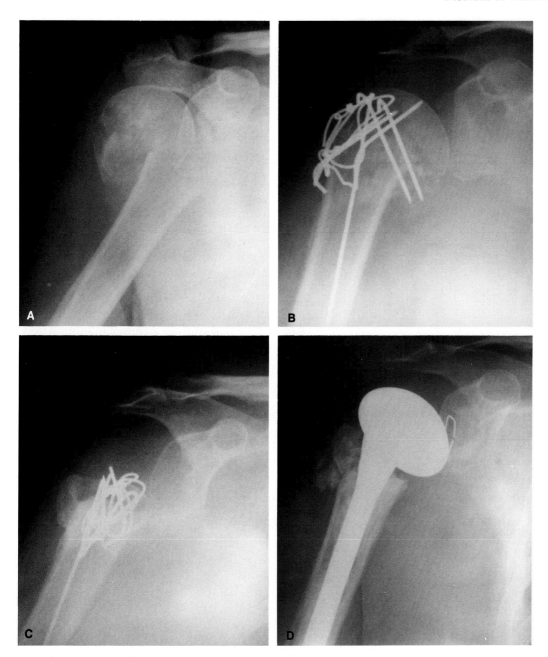

Fig. 12-43. (**A**) Three-part fracture with avascular necrosis. Anteroposterior x-ray of a three-part greater tuberosity fracture. There is displacement of the shaft medially, and the greater tuberosity is rotated and separated from the head. (**B**) Open reduction and internal fixation achieved with numerous pins and wires. Extensive soft tissue dissection was needed for this repair. (**C**) Eight months postoperatively the head has disappeared because there is significant avascular necrosis. (**D**) This failed fracture repair was salvaged with a total shoulder replacement, since the glenoid was also involved with degenerative disease.

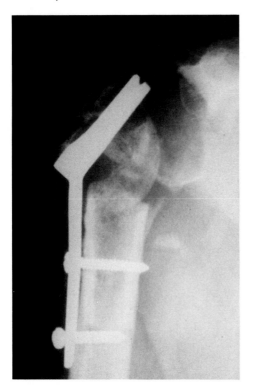

Fig. 12-44. This patient had an open reduction and internal fixation of a four-part fracture with a baby Jewett nail. This hip device was not appropriate for the shoulder, and the patient went on to have a nonunion as well as an infection after this procedure.

major muscle. A pseudarthrosis with a synovial lining occurs because of the communication with the joint and flow of joint fluid into this area. Internal fixation with heavy metal, such as screw and plate fixation, is impossible in this situation because of the poor quality of the remaining humeral head.

The indications for surgical treatment are pain, loss of function, and deformity. Pain may not be severe if the arm is not being used. Open reduction and internal fixation with the addition of autogenous iliac crest bone graft is the preferred treatment. However, a humeral head prosthesis may be necessary if there is articular damage or inadequate bone in the humeral head. Humeral head excision and arthrodesis should be avoided and are strictly salvage procedures. Conservative treatment may be an option in older patients who are pain-free, especially those in whom the nondominant extremity is involved.

The choice of hardware should be either Enders rods and figure-eight wire or suture or a plate and screws. Rods and wire are preferred in surgical neck nonunions and when the bone is soft. A plate is more suited for proximal shaft nonunions with good bone stock so that the screws can hold the cortex. In most cases a spica cast is necessary for 6 to 8 weeks because of poor-quality bone. Electrical stimulation may be a helpful adjunct to promote healing. After the cast is removed, range-of-motion exercises are started and progressed if healing is sufficient. A second procedure may be needed to

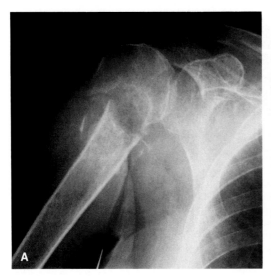
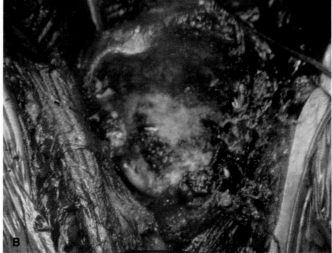

Fig. 12-45. (**A**) Anteroposterior x-ray of a nonunion of the minimally displaced fracture of the proximal humerus. Note the lucent line and the osteoporosis in the subtuberous region. (**B**) Operative photo showing the cavitation beneath the head with significant loss of bone stock.

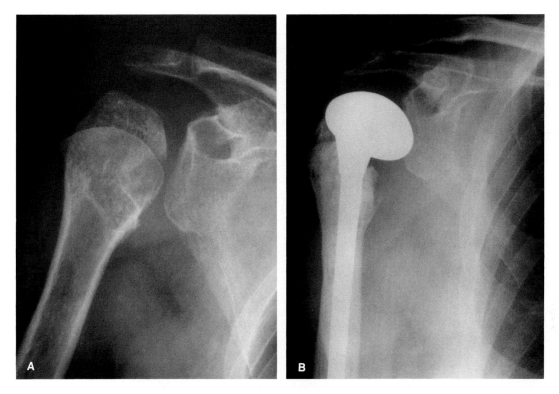

Fig. 12-46. (**A**) Anteroposterior x-ray of a malunion of a four-part fracture in which the greater tuberosity has healed above the head. The patient's surgery was delayed for 8 months because of neurologic complications. (**B**) A prosthesis was eventually inserted, and the repair was quite difficult because of the malunion and scarring of the soft tissues. The patient eventually achieved 130° of forward elevation with 30° of external rotation. There is some discomfort and weatherache, but the patient does have a functional shoulder.

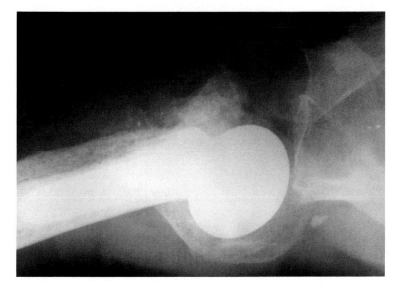

Fig. 12-47. The patient had a posterior fracture–dislocation that was treated with a Neer prosthesis that also dislocated posteriorly. There was extensive myositis ossificans in the soft tissues.

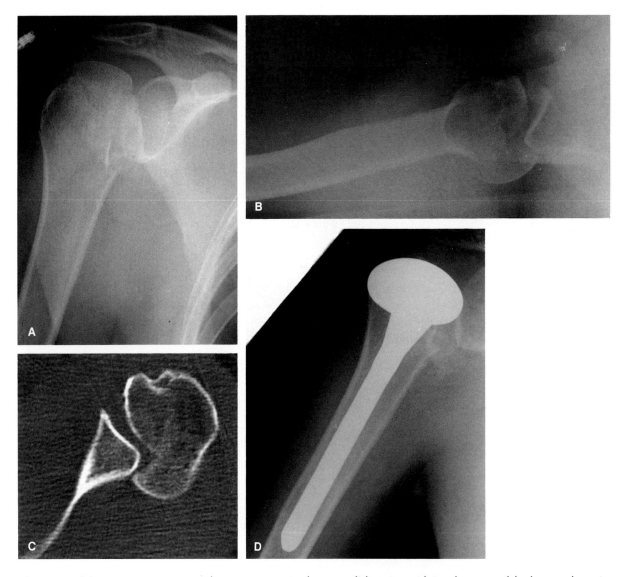

Fig. 12-48. (**A**) Anteroposterior x-ray showing a posterior fracture–dislocation with involvement of the lesser tuberosity as well as a component of the articular surface. (**B**) Axillary x-ray shows significant involvement of the humeral head with a fracture of the lesser tuberosity. (**C**) A CT scan of the head showing a greater than 50% involvement of the articular surface of the head. (**D**) A humeral head prosthesis that was put in excessive retroversion and dislocated posteriorly. The patient had significant pain for approximately 8 months after surgery and had a fixed internal rotation contraction of approximately 30°.

(continued)

release adhesions and remove hardware, especially a prominent rod.

Malunion

Malunion occurs after an inadequate closed reduction or a failed open reduction and internal fixation. This problem is especially difficult to treat because there is excessive scar tissue with retraction of the tuberosities, displacement of the shaft, or both. In addition, neurologic and soft tissue deficits may compromise surgical repair. Greater tuberosity malunions lead to impingement against the acromion[284] (see Fig. 12-14). They are best managed through a superior approach in which the fragment is completely mobilized and all of the scar tissue is lysed. It is important to also mobilize the rotator

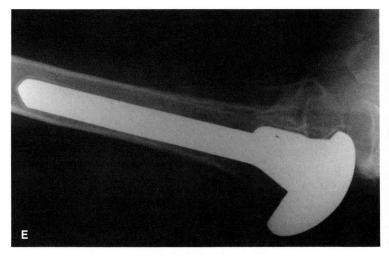

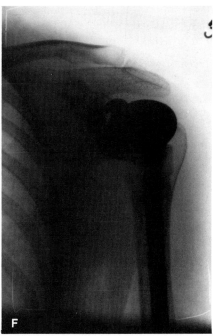

Fig. 12-48 (*continued*)

(**E**) Anteroposterior x-ray shows the prosthesis dislocated posteriorly. (**F**) Anteroposterior x-ray showing a total shoulder replacement that was used to revise the failed humeral head prosthesis. The glenoid was also significantly degenerated. The humeral head was placed in less retroversion, approximately 20°, and this achieved satisfactory stability. In the postoperative period, the patient was held in a neutral position for approximately 2 weeks, and forward elevation was done in the neutral position.

cuff and bring this tissue out to length. These malunions are generally treated the same way as acute greater tuberosity fractures. If there is excessive scarring and there seems to be residual impingement, then an anterior acromioplasty and removal of coracoacromial ligament may be helpful.

Malunions of three-part fractures are more difficult since more components are involved. If avascular necrosis or post-traumatic degenerative arthritis is not present, then osteotomy of the displaced fracture components and internal fixation should be attempted. A prosthesis is generally indicated for avascular necrosis and joint incongruity. A glenoid component may be required if there is arthritis of the glenoid surface. Dissection is quite difficult, and it is important to always be aware of the position of the axillary, suprascapular, and musculocutaneous nerves. A malunion of a surgical neck fracture with increased anterior angulation limits forward elevation. Surgical treatment involves osteotomy to correct the anterior angulation and the rotational deformities.[271]

Malunion and avascular necrosis of a four-part fracture require a prosthesis. The head is usually quite distorted, and often there is significant displacement of the tuberosities (Fig. 12-46). A tuberosity osteotomy must often be performed to allow adequate placement of the humeral head prosthesis. Unless the head is centered and proper length of the humerus is maintained, function will be impaired. The results of these procedures are not as good as those of a primary prosthesis, since the scarring and retraction of the tuberosities and soft tissues often limit the range of motion and restrict overhead function. However, the pain relief is usually satisfactory.

Malunion of a fracture–dislocation is extremely difficult to treat because the head component may be totally out of the glenohumeral joint area and wedged up against the anterior or posterior aspect of the glenoid. Mobilizing the head from the anterior subcoracoid area is especially dangerous because the neurovascular bundle may be attached to the scar tissue surrounding the head. A very careful dissection should be performed. Furthermore, there is an increased incidence of myositis ossificans with fracture–dislocations (Fig. 12-47).

Revision of Failed Prosthesis

Revision of a failed prosthesis is especially difficult. There may be associated soft tissue deficits and bone loss as well as nerve paralysis, which may complicate revision surgery. An electromyogram is helpful in the evaluation before any reconstruction. Revision of a prosthesis is indicated for pain relief since it may be difficult to significantly improve function because of nerve and muscle damage (Fig. 12-48).

Portions of the text and selected illustrations have been used with permission from THE SHOULDER, edited by Charles Rockwood and Frederick Matsen, published by W. B. Saunders Company, Philadelphia, 1990.

REFERENCES

1. Ahlgren, O., and Appel, H.: Proximal Humeral Fractures. Acta Orthop. Scand., 44:124–125, 1973.
2. Ahovuo, J.; Paavolainen, P.; and Bjorkenheim, J.: Fractures of the Proximal Humerus Involving the Intertubercular Groove. Acta Radiol., 30:373–375, 1989.
3. Aitken, A.P.: End Results of Fractures of the Proximal Humeral Epiphysis. J. Bone Joint Surg., 18:1036–1041, 1936.
4. Albee, F.H.: Juxta-epiphyseal Fracture of the Upper End of the Humerus. Med. Rec., 81:847–851, 1912.
5. Albee, F.H.: Restoration of Shoulder Function in Cases of Loss of Head and Upper Portion of the Humerus. Surgery, 32:11–19, 1921.
6. Alberts, K.A., and Engstrom, C.F.: Fractures of the Proximal Humerus. Opuscula Medica, 24(4)121–123, 1979.
7. Andreasen, A.T.: Avulsion Fracture of the Lesser Tuberosity of the Humerus. Lancet, 1:750, 1941.
8. Aldredge, R.H., and Knight, M.P.: Fractures of the Upper End of the Humerus Treated by Early Relaxed Motion and Massage. New Orleans Med. Surg. J., 92:519–524, 1940.
9. De Anquin, C.L., and De Anquin, A.: Prosthetic Replacement in the Treatment of Serious Fractures of the Proximal Humerus. *In* Bayley, I., and Kessel, I. (eds.): Shoulder Surgery. New York, Springer-Verlag, 1965.
10. Ansorge, D.: Fracture Dislocation as a Result of a High Voltage Current Accident. Zentralbl. Chir., 105:465–467, 1980.
11. Arndt, J.H., and Sears, A.D.: Posterior Dislocation of the Shoulder. A.J.R., 94:639–645, 1965.
12. Aufranc, O.E.: Nonunion of Humerus. J.A.M.A., 175:1092–1095, 1961.
13. Aufranc, O.E.; Jones, W. N.; and Turner, R.H.: Bilateral Shoulder Fracture-dislocations. J.A.M.A., 195:1140–1143, 1966.
14. Austin, M.D.: Fractures Hazards, Reporting 3 Uncommon Fracture Cases, With Use of Original Crucifixion Splint in Fracture of Surgical Neck of Humerus. Indiana Med., 16:129, 1923.
15. Autin, A.: Traitement des fractures de l'ESH. These Medicine no. 840. Paris, 1960.
16. Baker, D.M., and Leach, R.E.: Fracture-dislocation of the Shoulder. Report of Three Unusual Cases With Rotator Cuff Avulsion. J. Trauma, 5:659–664, 1965.
17. Bandi, W.: Zur operativen Therapie der Humeruskopfundhalsfrakturen. Unfallheilkunde, 196:38–45, 1976.
18. Bandmann, F.: Beitrag fur Behandlung der Oberarmkopffrakturen. Zentralbl. Chir., 76:97–102, 1951.
19. Bardenheuer, F.H., cited by Hans Lorenz: Die Isolirte Fractur des Tuberculum Minus Humeri. Deut. Zeit. Chir., 58:593, 1900–1901, 1949.
20. Barrett, W.P.; Franklin, H.; Jackins, S.E.; Wyss, C.R.; and Matsen, F.A.: Total Shoulder Arthroplasty. J. Bone Joint Surg., 69A:865–872, 1987.
21. Baudin, P.: Intramedullary Nailing of Fractures of the Proximal Humerus. These Medecine. Bordeaux, 1977.
22. Baxter, M.P., and Wiley, J.J.: Fractures of the Proximal Humeral Epiphysis. Their Influence on Humeral Growth. J. Bone Joint Surg., 68B:570–573, 1986.
23. Bell, H.M.: Posterior Fracture-dislocation of the Shoulder. A Method of Closed Reduction. A Case Report. J. Bone Joint Surg., 47A:1521–1524, 1965.
24. Bengner, U., Johnell, O., Redlund-Johnell, I.: Changes in the Incidence of Fracture of the Upper End of the Humerus During a 3-Year Period. A Study of 2125 Fractures. Clin. Orthop., 231:179–182, 1988.
25. Bertoft, E.S.; Lundh, I., and Ringqvist, I.: Physiotherapy After Fracture of the Proximal End of the Humerus. Scand. J. Rehabil. Med., 16:11–16, 1984.
26. Bigelow, H.J.: A Memoir of Henry Jacob Bigelow. Boston, Little, Brown, 1900.
27. Blasier, R.B., and Burkus, J.K.: Management of Posterior Fracture Dislocations of the Shoulder. Clin. Orthop., 232:199–204, 1988.
28. Blom, S., and Dahlback, L.O.: Nerve Injuries in Dislocations of the Shoulder Joint and Fractures of the Neck of the Humerus. A Clinical and Electromyographical Study. Acta Chir. Scand., 136:461–466, 1970.
29. Bloom, M.H., and Obata, W.: Diagnosis of Posterior Dislocation of the Shoulder With Use of Velpeau Axillary and Angle-up Roentgenographic Views. J. Bone Joint Surg., 49A:943–949, 1967.
30. Boehler, J.: Les fractures recentes de l'epaule. Acta Orthop. Belg., 30:235–242, 1964.
31. Bohler, L.: The Treatment of Fractures, 5th ed. New York, Grune & Stratton, 1956.
32. Bohler, L.: The Treatment of Fractures, 4th English ed. Baltimore, Williams Wood & Co., 1935.
33. Bohler, L.: Die Behandlung von Verrenkungsbruchen der Schulter. Dtsch. Z. Chir., 219:238–245, 1929.
34. Bosworth, D.M.: Blade Plate Fixation. J.A.M.A., 141:1111–1113, 1949.
35. Brehr, A.J., and Cooke, A.M.: Fracture Patterns. Lancet, 1:531–535, 1959.
36. Brickner, W.M.: Certain Afflictions of the Shoulder and

Their Management. International Clinics, 2:191–211, 1924.

37. Brighton, C.T.; Friedenberg, Z.B.; Zemsky, L.M.; and Pollis, R.R.: Direct-current Stimulation on Non-union and Congenital Pseudarthrosis. J. Bone Joint Surg., 57A:368–377, 1975.

38. Brostrom, F.: Early Mobilization of Fractures of the Upper End of the Humerus. Arch. Surg., 46:614–615, 1943.

39. Buchanan, J.J.: Fracture Through the Anatomical Neck of the Humerus With Dislocation of the Head. Ann. Surg., 47:659–671, 1908.

40. Caldwell, G.A.: The Treatment of Fractures of the Upper End of the Humerus. Rocky Mountain Med. J., 40:33, 1943.

41. Caldwell, J.A.: Treatment of Fractures in the Cincinnati General Hospital. Ann. Surg., 97:174–177, 1933.

42. Caldwell, J.A., and Smith, J.: Treatment of Unimpacted Fractures of the Surgical Neck of the Humerus. Am. J. Surg., 31:141–144, 1936.

43. Callahan, D.J.: Anatomic Considerations. Closed Reduction of Proximal Humeral Fractures. Orthop. Rev., 13:79–85, 1984.

44. Carew-McColl, M.: Bilateral Shoulder Dislocations Caused by Electric Shock. Br. J. Clin. Pract., 34:251–254, 1980.

45. Cathcart, C.S.: Movements of the Shoulder Girdle Involved in Those of the Arm on the Trunk. J. Anat. Physiol., 18:211–218, 1884.

46. Chalier, A.: Fracture de l'epaule avec luxation de la tete humerale et avec section tendineuse du long biceps. Repo. Lyon Chir., 29:226, 1932.

47. Clifford, P.C.: Fractures of the Neck of the Humerus. A Review of the Late Results. Injury, 12:91–95, 1980.

48. Codman, E.A.: The Shoulder: Rupture of the Supraspinatus Tendon and Other Lesions in or About the Subacromial Bursa, pp. 262–293. Boston, Thomas Todd, 1934.

49. Cofield, R.H.: Comminuted Fractures of the Proximal Humerus. Clin. Orthop., 230:49–57, 1988.

50. Collin, I.: Brug og misbrug af massage hos ulykkesforsikrede patienter. In Kiaer, S. (ed.): Ulykkesforsikringsbogen. Copenhagen, Nordisk Forog, 1931.

51. Conforty, B.: The Results of the Boytchev Procedure for Treatment of Recurrent Dislocation of the Shoulder. Int. Orthop., 4:127–132, 1980.

52. Conforty, B.: Boytchev's Procedure for Recurrent Dislocation of the Shoulder (Proceedings). J. Bone Joint Surg., 56B:386, 1974.

53. Coonse, G.K.: An Improved Humerus Splint for Hospital Use. J. Bone Joint Surg., 13:374–375, 1931.

54. Coonse, G.K., and Moore, H.: Treatment of Fractures of the Humerus by Mobilization and Traction. N. Engl. J. Med., 203:829–832, 1930.

55. Cooper, A.: A Treatise in Dislocations and Fractures of the Joints. Philadelphia, H.C. Carey & I. Lea, 1825.

56. Cooper, A.: On the Dislocation of the Os Humeri Upon the Dorsum Scapulae and Upon Fractures Near the Shoulder Joint. Guy Hosp. Rep., 4:265–284, 1839.

57. Cotton, F.J.: Dislocations and Joint Fractures. Philadelphia, W.B. Saunders, 1910.

58. Cotton, F.J.: Subluxation of the Shoulder Downward. Boston Med. Surg. J., 185:405–407, 1921.

59. Coventry, M.B., and Laurnen, E.L.: Ununited Fractures of the Middle and Upper Humerus. Special Problems in Treatment. Clin. Orthop., 69:192–198, 1970.

60. Dameron, T.B.: Complications of Treatment of Injuries to the Shoulder. In Epps, C.H. (ed.): Complications in Orthopaedic Surgery, 2nd ed., pp. 247–275. Philadelphia, J.B. Lippincott, 1986.

61. DeBernardi, L.: Sul trattamento della dussazione con frattura dell'estremita superiore dell'omero. Boll. Mem. Soc. Piemontese Chir., 11:193, 1932.

62. Dehne, E.: Fractures at the Upper End of the Humerus. Surg. Clin. North Am., 25:28–47, 1945.

63. DePalma, A.F.: Surgery of the Shoulder, 3rd ed., pp. 372–403. Philadelphia, J.B. Lippincott, 1983.

64. DePalma, A.F., and Cautilli, R.A.: Fractures of the Upper End of the Humerus. Clin. Orthop., 20:73–93, 1961.

65. Des Marchais, J.E., and Benazet, J.P.: Evaluation de l'hemiarthroplastie de Neer dans le traitement des fractures de l'humerus. Can. J. Surg., 26:469–471, 1983.

66. Des Marchais, J.E., and Morais, G.: Treatment of Complex Fractures of the Proximal Humerus by Neer Hemiarthroplasty. In Bateman, J.E., and Welsh, R.P. (eds.): Surgery of the Shoulder. Philadelphia, B.C. Decker, 1984.

67. Destree, C., and Safary, A.: Le traitement des fractures hyumerales, col et diaphyse, par l'enclouage fascicule de Hackethal. Acta Orthop. Belg., 45:666–677, 1979.

68. Dewar, F.P., and Yabsley, R.H.: Fracture-dislocation of the Shoulder. Report of a Case. J. Bone Joint Surg., 49B:540–543, 1967.

69. Dimon, J.H.: Posterior Dislocation and Posterior Fracture Dislocation of the Shoulder. A Report of 25 Cases. South. Med. J., 60:661–666, 1967.

70. Din, K.M., and Meggitt, B.F.: Bilateral Four-part Fractures With Posterior Dislocation of the Shoulder. A Case Report. J. Bone Joint Surg., 65B:176–178, 1983.

71. Dingley, A., and Denham, R.: Fracture-dislocation of the Humeral Head. A Method of Reduction. J. Bone Joint Surg., 55A:1299–1300, 1973.

72. Drapanas, T.; Hewitt, R.L.; Weichert, R.F.; and Smith, A.D.: Civilian Vascular Injuries. A Critical Appraisal of Three Decades of Management. Ann. Surg., 172:351–360, 1970.

73. Drapanas, T.; McDonald, J.; and Hale, H.W.: A Rational Approach to Classification and Treatment of Fractures of the Surgical Neck of the Humerus. Am. J. Surg., 99:617–624, 1960.

74. Duparc, J., and Largier, A.: Les luxations-fractures de l'extremitie superieure de l'humerus. Rev. Chir. Orthop., 62:91–110, 1976.

75. Edelman, G.: Immediate Therapy of Complex Fractures of the Upper End of the Humerus by Means of Acrylic Prosthesis. Presse Med., 59:1777–1778, 1951.

76. Einarsson, F.: Fracture of the Upper End of the Humerus. Acta Orthop. Scand. [Suppl.], 3:10–209, 1958.

77. Ekstrom, T.; Lagergren, C.; and von Schreeb, T.: Procaine Injections and Early Mobilization for Fractures of the Neck of the Humerus. Acta Chir. Scand., 130:18–24, 1965.

78. Elliot, J.A.: Acute Arterial Occlusion. An Unusual Cause. Surgery, 39:825–826, 1956.

79. Fairbank, T.J.: Fracture-subluxations of the Shoulder. J. Bone Joint Surg., 30B:454–460, 1948.

80. Fellander, M.: Fracture-dislocations of the Shoulder Joint. Acta Chir. Scand., 107:138–145, 1954.

81. Flatow, E.L.; Bigliani, L.U.; and April, E.W.: An Anatomic Study of the Musculocutaneous Nerve and Its Relationship to the Coracoid Process. Clin. Orthop., 244:166–171, 1989.

82. Fourrier, P., and Martini, M.: Post-traumatic Avascular Necrosis of the Humeral Head. Int. Orthop., 1:187–190, 1977.

83. Frankau, C.: A Manipulative Method for the Reduction of Fractures of the Surgical Neck of the Humerus. Lancet, 2:755, 1933.

84. Freg, E.K.: Zur operation de bruche am oberen ende des oberarmes. Zentralbl. Chir., 61:851, 1934.

85. Frey, F.: Die Knocherne Heilung von Schienbeinschaftbruchen. Arch. Orthop. Unfallchir., 46:482–484, 1954.

86. Funsten, R.V., and Kinser, P.: Fractures and Dislocations About the Shoulder. J. Bone Joint Surg., 18:191–198, 1936.

87. Gallagher, J.C.; Melton, L.J.; Riggs, B.L.; and Bergstrath, E.: Epidemiology of Fractures of the Proximal Femur in Rochester, Minnesota. Clin. Orthop., 150:163–171, 1980.

88. Garceau, G.J., and Cogland, S.: Early Physical Therapy in the Treatment of Fractures of the Surgical Neck of the Humerus. Indiana Med., 34:293–295, 1941.

89. Garraway, W.M.; Stauffer, R.N.; Kurland, L.T.; and O'Fallon, W.M.: Limb Fractures in a Defined Population. I. Frequency and Distribution. Mayo Clin. Proc., 54:701–707, 1979.

90. Geneste, R., et al.: Closed Treatment of Fracture-dislocations of the Shoulder Joint. Rev. Chir. Orthop., 66:383–386, 1980.

91. Gerard-Marchant, P.: Diagnostic et traitement des luxations de l'epaule compliques de fracture de l'humerus. J. Chir., 31:659–670, 1928.

92. Gibbons, A.P.: Fracture of the Tuberculum Majus by Muscular Violence. Br. Med. J. [Clin. Res.], 2:1674, 1909.

93. Glessner, J.R.: Intrathoracic Dislocation of the Humeral Head. J. Bone Joint Surg., 43A:428–430, 1961.

94. Gold, A.M.: Fractured Neck of the Humerus With Separation and Dislocation of the Humeral Head. Bull. Hosp. Jt. Dis. Orthop. Inst., 32:87–99, 1971.

95. Gordon, D.: Fractures of the Upper End of the Humerus. J.A.M.A., 96:332–336, 1931.

96. Graham, J., and Wood, S.: Aseptic Necrosis of Bone Following Trauma. In Davidson, J.K. (ed.): Aseptic Necrosis of Bone, pp. 113–117, 136–137. Amsterdam, Excerpta Medica, 1976.

97. Greeley, P.W., and Magnuson, P.B.: Dislocation of the Shoulder Accompanied by Fracture of the Greater Tuberosity and Complicated by Spinatus Tendon Injury. J.A.M.A., 102:1835–1838, 1934.

98. Greenhill, B.J.: Persistent Posterior Shoulder Dislocation. Its Diagnosis and Its Treatment by Posterior Putti-Platt Repair. J. Bone Joint Surg., 54B:763, 1972.

99. Grimes, D.W.: The Use of Rush Pin Fixation in Unstable Upper Humeral Fracture. A Method of Blind Insertion. Orthop. Rev., 9:75–79, 1980.

100. Griswold, R.A.; Hucherson, D.C.; and Strode, E.C.: Fractures of the Humerus Treated With Hanging Cast. South. Med. J., 34:777–778, 1941.

101. Gurd, F.B.: A Simple Effective Method for the Treatment of Fractures of the Upper Part of the Humerus. Am. J. Surg., 47:433–453, 1940.

102. Haas, K.: Displaced Proximal Humeral Fractures Operated by Rush Pin Technique. Opuscula Medica, 23:100–102, 1978.

103. Haas, S.L.: Fracture of the Lesser Tuberosity of the Humerus. Am. J. Surg., 63:253–256, 1944.

104. Hackaethal, K.H.: Die Bundelnagelung. Berlin, Springer-Verlag, 1961.

105. Hagg, O., and Lundberg, B.: Aspects of Prognostic Factors in Comminuted and Dislocated Proximal Humeral Fractures. In Bateman, J.E., and Welsh, R.P. (eds.): Surgery of the Shoulder, pp. 51–59. Philadelphia, B.C. Decker, 1984.

106. Hall, M.C., and Rosser, M.: The Structure of the Upper End of the Humerus, With Reference to Osteoporotic Changes in Senescence Leading to Fractures. Can. Med. Assoc. J., 88:290–294, 1963.

107. Hall, R.H.; Isaac, F.; and Booth, C.R.: Dislocations of the Shoulder With Special Reference to Accompanying Small Fractures. J. Bone Joint Surg., 41A:489–494, 1959.

108. Hardcastle, P.H., and Fisher, T.R.: Intrathoracic Displacement of the Humeral Head With Fracture of the Surgical Neck. Injury, 12:313–315, 1981.

109. Hartigan, J.W.: Separation of the Lesser Tuberosity of the Head of the Humerus. N.Y. Med. J., 61:276, 1895.

110. Hawkins, R.J.: Unrecognized Dislocations of the Shoulder. A.A.O.S. Instr. Course Lect., 34:258–263, 1985.

111. Hawkins, R.J.; Bell, R.H.; and Gurr, K.: The Three-part Fracture of the Proximal Part of the Humerus. Operative Treatment. J. Bone Joint Surg., 68A:1410–1414, 1986.

112. Hawkins, R.J.; Neer, C.S.; Pianta, R.M.; and Mendoza, F.X.: Locked Posterior Dislocation of the Shoulder. J. Bone Joint Surg., 69A:9–18, 1987.

113. Hayes, M.J., and Van Winkle, N.: Axillary Artery Injury With Minimally Displaced Fracture of the Neck of the Humerus. J. Trauma, 23:431–433, 1983.

114. Hendenach, J.C.R.: Recurrent Posterior Dislocation of the Shoulder. J. Bone Joint Surg., 23:582–586, 1947.

115. Henderson, M.S.: The Massive Bone Graft in Ununited Fractures. J.A.M.A., 107:1104–1107, 1916.

116. Henderson, R.S.: Fracture-dislocation of the Shoulder With Interposition of Long Head of the Biceps. Report of a Case. J. Bone Joint Surg., 34B:240–241, 1952.

117. Henson, G.F.: Vascular Complications of Shoulder Injuries. A Report of Two Cases. J. Bone Joint Surg., 38B:528–531, 1956.

118. Heppenstall, R.B.: Fractures of the Proximal Humerus. Orthop. Clin. North Am., 6:467–475, 1975.

119. Herbert, J.J., and Paillot, J.: Treatment of Complicated Fractures of the Upper End of the Humerus. Epiphysio-diaphysial Pegging. Rev. Chir. Orthop., 46:739–747, 1960.

120. Hermann, O.J.: Fractures of the Shoulder Joint With Special Reference to Correction of Defects. A.A.O.S. Instr. Course Lect., 2:359–370, 1944.

121. Heuget, L., LaLaude, J.; and Vielpeau, C.: Bone Cement in the Treatment of Certain Fractures of the Proximal Humerus. Ann. Chir., 27:311–313, 1973.

122. Hill, N.A., and McLaughlin, H.L.: Locked Posterior Dislocation Simulating a 'Frozen Shoulder.' J. Trauma, 3:225–234, 1963.

123. Hippocrates: The Genuine Works of Hippocrates. Baltimore, Williams & Wilkins, 1939.

124. Hitchcock, H.H., and Bechtol, C.O.: Painful Shoulder. Observations on the Role of the Tendon of the Long Head of the Biceps Brachii in Its Causation. J. Bone Joint Surg., 30A:263–273, 1948.

125. Hollingshead, W.H.: Anatomy for Surgeons, Vol. 3. *In* The Back and Limbs, 3rd ed. Philadelphia, Harper & Row, 1982.

126. Horak, J., and Nilsson, B.: Epidemiology of Fractures of the Upper End of the Humerus. Clin. Orthop., 112:250–253, 1975.

127. Howard, N.J., and Eloesser, L.: Treatment of Fractures of the Upper End of the Humerus. An Experimental and Clinical Study. J. Bone Joint Surg., 16:1–29, 1934.

128. Hudson, R.T.: The Use of the Hanging Cast in Treatment of Fractures of the Humerus. South. Surgeon, 10:132–134, 1941.

129. Hughes, M., and Neer, C.S.: Glenohumeral Joint Replacement and Postoperative Rehabilitation. Phys. Ther., 55:850–858, 1975.

130. Hundley, J.M., and Stewart, M.J.: Fractures of the Humerus. A Comparative Study in Methods of Treatment. J. Bone Joint Surg., 37A:681–692, 1955.

131. Jakob, R.P.; Kristiansen, T.; Mayo, K.; Ganz, R.; and Müller, M.E.: Classification and Aspects of Treatment of Fractures of the Proximal Humerus. *In* Batemen, J.E., and Welsh, R.P. (eds.): Surgery of the Shoulder. Philadelphia, B.C. Decker, 1984.

132. Johansson, O.: Complications and Failures of Surgery in Various Fractures of the Humerus. Acta Chir. Scand., 120:469–478, 1961.

133. Jones, L.: Reconstructive Operation for Non-reducible Fractures of the Head of the Humerus. Ann. Surg., 97:217–225, 1933.

134. Jones, L.: The Shoulder Joint. Observations on the Anatomy and Physiology With Analysis of Reconstructive Operation Following Extensive Injury. Surg. Gynecol. Obstet., 75:433–444, 1942.

135. Jones, R.: On Certain Fractures About the Shoulder. Ir. J. Med. Sci., 78:282–291, 1932.

136. Jones, R.: Certain Injuries Commonly Associated With Displacement of the Head of the Humerus. Br. Med. J., 1:1385–1386, 1906.

137. Keen, W.W.: Fractures of the Tuberculum Majus. Ann. Surg., 45:938–949, 1907.

138. Keene, J.S.; Huizenga, R.E.; Engber, W.D.; and Rogers, S.C.: Proximal Humeral Fractures. A Correction of Residual Deformity With Long-term Function. Orthopedics, 6:173–178, 1983.

139. Kelly, J.P.: Fractures Complicating Electroconvulsive Therapy and Chronic Epilepsy. J. Bone Joint Surg., 36B:70–79, 1954.

140. Key, J.A., and Conwell, H.E.: Fractures, Dislocations, and Sprains, 7th ed., pp. 348–431. St. Louis, C.V. Mosby, 1961.

141. Knight, R.A., and Mayne, J.A.: Comminuted Fractures and Fracture-dislocations Involving the Articular Surface of the Humeral Head. J. Bone Joint Surg., 39A:1343–1355, 1957.

142. Knowleden, J.; Buhr, A.J.; and Dunbar, O.: Incidence of Fractures in Persons Over 35 Years of Age. A Report to the M.R.C. Working Party on Fractures in the Elderly. Br. J. Prev. Soc. Med., 18:130–141, 1964.

143. Kocher, T.: Beitrage zur Kenntnis einiger praktisch wichtiger Fracturenformen. Basel, Carl Sallman Verlag, 1896.

144. Kofoed, H.: Revascularization of the Humeral Head. Clin. Orthop., 179:175–178, 1983.

145. Krakovic, M., et al.: Indications and Results of Operation in Proximal Humeral Fractures. Mschr. Unfallheilk., 78:326–332, 1975.

146. Kraulis, J., and Hunter, G.: The Results of Prosthetic Replacement in Fracture-dislocations of the Upper End of the Humerus. Injury, 8:129–131, 1976.

147. Kristiansen, B.: External Fixation of Proximal Humerus Fracture. Acta Orthop. Scand., 58:645–648, 1987.

148. Kristiansen, B., and Christensen, S.W.: Plate Fixation of Proximal Humeral Fractures. Acta Orthop. Scand., 57:320–323, 1986.

149. Kristiansen, B., and Christensen, S.W.: Proximal Humeral Fractures. Acta Orthop. Scand., 58:124–127, 1987.

150. Kristiansen, B., and Kofoed, H.: External Fixation of Displaced Fractures of the Proximal Humerus. J. Bone Joint Surg., 69B:643–646, 1987.

151. Kristiansen, B., and Kofoed, H.: Transcutaneous Reduction and External Fixation of Displaced Fractures of the Proximal Humerus. J. Bone Joint Surg., 70B:821–824, 1988.

152. LaBriola, J.H., and Mohaghegh, H.A.: Isolated Avulsion Fracture of the Lesser Tuberosity of the Humerus. A Case Report and Review of the Literature. J. Bone Joint Surg., 57A:1011, 1975.

153. LaFerte, A.D., and Nutter, P.D.: The Treatment of Fractures of the Humerus by Means of Hanging Plaster Cast. "Hanging cast." Ann. Surg., 114:919–930, 1955.

154. Laing, P.G.: The Arterial Supply of the Adult Humerus. J. Bone Joint Surg., 38A:1105–1116, 1956.

155. Lane, L.B.; Villacin, A.; and Bullough, P.G.: The Vascularity and Remodelling of Subchondral Bone and Calcified Cartilage in Adult Human Femoral and Humeral Heads. An Age- and Stress-related Phenomenon. J. Bone Joint Surg., 59B:272–278, 1977.

156. Lasher, W.W.: Fracture Dislocation of the Head of the Humerus. J.A.M.A., 84:356–358, 1925.

157. Leach, R.E., and Premer, R.F.: Nonunion of the Surgical Neck of the Humerus. Method of Internal Fixation. Minn. Med., 48:318–322, 1965.

158. LeBorgne, J.; LeNeel, J.C.; and Mitland, D.: Les lesions de l'artere axillaire et de ses branches consecutives a un traumatisme ferme de l'epaule. Ann. Chir., 27:587–594, 1973.

159. Lee, C.K., and Hansen, H.R.: Post-traumatic Avascular Necrosis of the Humeral Head in Displaced Proximal Humeral Fractures. J. Trauma, 21:788–791, 1981.

160. Lee, C.K.; Hansen, H.T.; and Weiss, A.B.: Surgical Treatment of the Difficult Humeral Neck Fracture. Acromial Shortening Anterolateral Approach. J. Trauma, 20:67–70, 1980.

161. Leikkonen, O.: Osteosynthesis With Special Modified Plate in Fractures of the Proximal End of the Humerus. Ann. Clin. Gynaecol. Fenn., 49:309–314, 1960.

162. Lentz, W., and Meuser, P.: The Treatment of Fractures of the Proximal Humerus. Arch. Orthop. Trauma Surg., 96:283–285, 1980.

163. Leyshon, R.L.: Closed Treatment of Fractures of the Proximal Humerus. Acta Orthop. Scand. 55:48–51, 1984.

164. Lim, T.E.; Ochsner, P.E.; Marti, R.K.; and Holscher, A.A.: The Results of Treatment of Comminuted Fractures and Fracture Dislocations of the Proximal Humerus. Neth. J. Surg., 35:139–143, 1983.

165. Lind, T.; Kroner, T.K.; and Jensen, J.: The Epidemiology of Fractures of the Proximal Humerus. Arch. Orthop. Trauma Surg., 108:285–287, 1989.

166. Lindholm, T.S., and Elmstedt, E.: Bilateral Posterior Dislocation of the Shoulder Combined With Fracture of the Proximal Humerus. A Case Report. Acta Orthop. Scand., 51:485–488, 1980.

167. Linson, M.A.: Axillary Artery Thrombosis After Fracture of the Humerus. A Case Report. J. Bone Joint Surg., 62A:1214–1215, 1980.

168. Lorenz, H.: Die isolirte Fractur des Tuberculum minus humeri. Dtsch. Zeitschr. Chir., 58:593, 1900–1901.

169. Lorenzo, F.T.: Osteosynthesis With Blount Staples in Fracture of the Proximal End of the Humerus. A Preliminary Report. J. Bone Joint Surg., 37A:45–48, 1955.

170. Lovett, R.W.: The Diagnosis and Treatment of Some Common Injuries of the Shoulder Joint. Surg. Gynecol. Obstet., 34:437–444, 1922.

171. Lucas-Championniere, J.: Traitement des fractures par le massage et la mobilisation. Paris, Rueff, 1895.

172. Lundberg, B.J.; Svenungson-Hartwig, E.; and Vikmark, R.: Independent Exercises Versus Physiotherapy in Nondisplaced Proximal Humeral Fractures. Scand. J. Rehabil. Med., 11:133–136, 1979.

173. Luppino, D.; Santangelo, G.; Vicenzi, G.; Innao, V.; and Capelli, A.: Le fratture dell'estremita prossimale dell'omero de interesse chirurgico (studio de 40 casi). Chir. Organi Mov., 67:373–381, 1982.

174. MacDonald, F.R.: Intra-articular Fractures in Recurrent Dislocations of the Shoulder. Surg. Clin. North Am., 43:1635–1645, 1963.

175. Machmull, G., and Weeder, S.D.: Bilateral Fracture of the Anatomical and Surgical Necks of the Humeral Heads. Cases With Bilateral Fracture of the Anatomical and Surgical Necks of the Humeri Due to Convulsion. Radiology, 55:735–739, 1950.

176. Marotte, J.H.; Lord, G.; and Bancel, P.: L'arthroplastie de Neer dans les fractures et fractures-lexatons complexes de l'epaule. A propos de 12 cas. Chirurgie, 104:816–821, 1978.

177. Mason, J.M.: The Treatment of Dislocation of the Shoulder Joint Complicated by Fracture of the Upper Extremity of the Humerus. Ann. Surg., 47:672–705, 1908.

178. Mauclaire, M.: Bull. Mem. Soc. Chir. Paris, 46:572, 1920.

179. Mazet, R.: Intramedullary Fixation in the Arm and the Forearm. Clin. Orthop., 2:75–92, 1953.

180. McBurney, C., and Dowd, C.N.: Dislocation of the Humerus Complicated by Fracture at or Near the Surgical Neck With a New Method of Reduction. Ann. Surg., 19:399–415, 1894.

181. McGuinness, J.P.: Isolated Avulsion Fracture of the Lesser Tuberosity of the Humerus. Lancet, 1:508, 1939.

182. McLaughlin, H.L.: Dislocation of the Shoulder With Tuberosity Fracture. Surg. Clin. North Am., 43:1615–1620, 1963.

183. McLaughlin, H.L.: Locked Posterior Subluxation of the Shoulder. Diagnosis and Treatment. Surg. Clin. North Am., 43:1621–1622, 1963.

184. McLaughlin, H.L.: Posterior Dislocation of the Shoulder. J. Bone Joint Surg., 34A:584–590, 1952.

185. McLaughlin, H.L.: Treatment of Shoulder Injuries. In American Academy of Orthopaedic Surgeons: Regional Orthopaedic Surgery and Fundamental Orthopaedic Problems. Ann Arbor, Mich.: Edwards, 1947.

186. McQuillan, W.M., and Nolan, B.: Ischemia Complicating Injury. A Report of Thirty-seven Cases. J. Bone Joint Surg., 50B:482–492, 1968.

187. McWhorter, G.L.: Fractures of the Greater Tuberosity of the Humerus With Displacement. Surg. Clin. North Am., 5:1005–1017, 1925.

188. Mestdagh, H.; Butruille, Y.; Tillie, B.; and Bocquet, F.: Resultats du traitement des fractures de l'extremite superieure de l'humerus par embrochage percutane. A propos de cent quarantedeux cas. Ann. Chir., 38:5–13, 1984.

189. Meyerding, H.W.: Fracture-dislocation of the Shoulder. Minn. Med., 20:717–726, 1937.

190. Michaelis, L.S.: Comminuted Fracture-dislocation of the Shoulder. J. Bone Joint Surg., 26:363–365, 1944.

191. Milch, H.: The Treatment of Recent Dislocations and Fracture-dislocations of the Shoulder. J. Bone Joint Surg., 31A:173–180, 1949.

192. Milch, H.: Treatment of Dislocation of the Shoulder. Surgery, 3:732–740, 1938.

193. Miller, S.R.: Practical Points in the Diagnosis and Treatment of Fractures of the Upper Fourth of the Humerus. Indust. Med., 9:458–460, 1940.

194. Mills, H.J., and Horne, G.: Fractures of the Proximal Humerus in Adults. J. Trauma, 25:801–805, 1985.

195. Mills, K.L.G.: Severe Injuries of the Upper End of the Humerus. Injury, 6:13–21, 1974.

196. Mills, K.L.G.: Simultaneous Bilateral Posterior Fracture-dislocation of the Shoulder. Injury, 6:39–41, 1974.

197. Moriber, I.A., and Patterson, R.I.: Fractures of the Proximal End of the Humerus. J. Bone Joint Surg., 49A:1018, 1967.

198. Morris, M.F.; Kilcoyne, R.F.; and Shuman, W.: Humeral Tuberosity Fractures: Evaluation by CT Scan and Management of Malunion. Orthop. Trans., 11:242, 1987.

199. Moseley, H.F.: The Arterial Pattern of the Rotator Cuff of the Shoulder. J. Bone Joint Surg., 45B:780–789, 1963.

200. Mouradian, W.H.: Displaced Proximal Humeral Fractures. Seven Years' Experience With a Modified Zickel Supracondylar Device. Clin. Orthop., 212:209–218, 1986.

201. de Mourgues, G.; Razemon, J.-P.; Leclair, H.P.; Comtet, J.J.; and Suares, H.: Fracture-dislocations of the Shoulder Joint. Rev. Chir. Orthop., 51:151–156, 1965.

202. Murphy, J.B.: Nailing of Fracture of Surgical Neck of Humerus After an Unsuccessful Attempt to Secure Union by Bone Transplantation. Surg. Clin. Chicago, 3:531–536, 1914.

203. Neer, C.S.: Articular Replacement for the Humeral Head. J. Bone Joint Surg., 37A:215–228, 1955.

204. Neer, C.S.: Degenerative Lesions of the Proximal Humeral Articular Surface. Clin. Orthop., 20:116–125, 1961.

205. Neer, C.S.: Displaced Proximal Humeral Fractures. Part I. Classification and Evaluation. J. Bone Joint Surg., 52A:1077–1089, 1970.

206. Neer, c.S.: Displaced Proximal Humeral Fractures. Part II. Treatment of Three-part and Four-part Displacement. J. Bone Joint Surg., 52A:1090–1103, 1970.

207. Neer, C.S.: Four-segment Classification of Displaced Proximal Humeral Fractures. A.A.O.S. Instr. Course Lect. 24:160–168, 1975.

208. Neer, C.S.: Indications for Replacement of the Proximal Humeral Articulation. Am. J. Surg., 89:901–907, 1955.

209. Neer, C.S.: Prosthetic Replacement of the Humeral Head. Indications and Operative Technique. Surg. Clin. North Am., 43:1581–1597, 1963.

210. Neer, C.S.; Borwn, T.H.; and McLaughlin, H.L.: Fracture of the Neck of the Humerus With Dislocation of the Head Fragment. Am. J. Surg., 85:252–258, 1953.

211. Neer, C.S.; McCann, P.D.; Macfarlane, E.A.; and Padilla, N.: Earlier Passive Motion Following Shoulder Arthroplasty and Rotator Cuff Repair. A Prospective Study. Orthop. Trans., 11:231, 1987.

212. Neer, C.S., and McIlveen, S.J.: Recent Results and Technique of Prosthetic Replacement for 4-part Proximal Humeral Fractures. Orthop. Trans., 10:475, 1986.

213. Neer, C.S., and Rockwood, C.A., Jr.: Fractures and Dislocations of the Shoulder. In Rockwood, C.A., and Green, D.P. (eds.): Fractures, 2nd ed., pp. 675–707, Philadelphia, J.B. Lippincott, 1984.

214. Neer, C.S.; Watson, K.C.; and Stanton, F.J.: Recent Experience in Total Shoulder Replacement. J. Bone Joint Surg., 64A:319–337, 1982.

215. Neviaser, J.S.: Complicated Fractures and Dislocations About the Shoulder Joint. J. Bone Joint Surg., 44A:984–998, 1962.

216. Newton-John, H.F., and Morgan, D.B.: The Loss of Bone With Age, Osteoporosis, and Fractures. Clin. Orthop., 71:229–252, 1970.

217. Nicola, F.G.; Ellman, H.; Eckardt, J.; and Finerman, G.: Bilateral Posterior Fracture-dislocation of the Shoulder Treated With a Modification of the McLaughlin Procedure. J. Bone Joint Surg., 63A:1175–1177, 1981.

218. Nissen-Lie, H.S.: Pseudarthroses of Humerus. Acta Orthop. Scand., 21:22–30, 1951.

219. North, J.P.: The Conservative Treatment of Fractures of the Humerus. Surg. Clin. North Am., 20:1633–1643, 1940.

220. O'Flanagan, P.H.: Fracture Due to Shock From Domestic Electricity Supply. Injury, 6:244–245, 1975.

221. Oni, O.O.A.: Irreducible Acute Anterior Dislocation of the Shoulder Due to a Loose Fragment From an Associated Fracture of the Greater Tuberosity. Injury, 15:138, 1983.

222. Ostapowicz, G., and Rahn-Myrach, A.: The Functional Treatment of Fractures of the Head of the Humerus. Bruns. Butr. Klin. Chir., 202:96–114, 1961.

223. Paavolainen, P.; Bjorkenheim, J.-M.; Slatis, P.; and Paukku, P.: Operative Treatment of Severe Proximal Humeral Fractures. Acta Orthop. Scand., 54:374–379, 1983.

224. Palmer, I.A.: A Dualistic Method of Treatment Pseudoarthrosis. Acta Chir. Scand., 107:261–268, 1954.

225. Palmer, I.: On the Complications and Technical Problems of Medullary Nailing. Acta Chir. Scand., 101:491–492, 1951.

226. Patel, M.R.; Pardee, M.L.; and Singerman, R.C.: Intrathoracic Dislocation of the Head of the Humerus. J. Bone Joint Surg., 45A:1712–1714, 1963.

227. Phemister, D.B.: Fractures of the Greater Tuberosity of the Humerus. Ann. Surg., 37:440–449, 1912.

228. Pilgaard, S., and Och Oster, A.: Four-segment Fractures of the Humeral Neck. Acta Orthop. Scand., 44:124, 1973.

229. Poilleux, F., and Courtois-Suffit, M.: Des fractures du col chirurgical de l'humerus. Rev. Chir., 133–158, 1954.

230. Post, M.: Fractures of the Upper Humerus. Orthop. Clin. North Am., 11:239–252, 1980.

231. Prillaman, H.A., and Thompson, R.C.: Bilateral Posterior Fracture-dislocation of the Shoulder. A Case Report. J. Bone Joint Surg., 51A:1627–1630, 1969.

232. Proximal Humeral Fractures. What Price History? Editorial. Injury, 12:89–90, 1981.

233. Raney, R.B.: The Treatment of Fractures of the Humerus With the Hanging Cast. North Carolina Med. J., 6:88–92, 1945.

234. Rathbun, J.B., and Macnab, I.: The Microvascular Pattern of the Rotator Cuff. J. Bone Joint Surg., 52B:540–553, 1970.

235. Razemon, J.P., and Baux, S.: Fractures and Fracture-dislocations of the Proximal Humerus. Rev. Chir. Orthop., 55:387–396, 1965.

236. Rechtman, A.M.: Open Reduction of Fracture Dislocation of the Humerus. J.A.M.A., 94:1656–1657, 1930.

237. Reckling, F.W.: Posterior Fracture-dislocation of the Shoulder Treated by a Neer Hemiarthroplasty With a Posterior Surgical Approach. Clin. Orthop., 207:133–137, 1986.

238. Rendlich, R.A., and Poppel, M.H.: Roentgen Diagnosis of Posterior Dislocation of the Shoulder. Radiology, 36:42–45, 1941.

239. Richard, A.; Judet, R.; and Rene, L.: Reconstruction prothetique acrylique de l'extremite superieure de l'humerus specialement au cours des fratures-luxations. J. Chir., 68:537–547, 1952.

240. Rob, C.G., and Standeven, A.: Closed Traumatic Lesions

of the Axillary and Brachial Arteries. Lancet, I:597–599, 1956.

241. Roberts, S.M.: Fractures of the Upper End of the Humerus. An End-result Study Which Shows the Advantage of Early Active Motion. J.A.M.A., 98:367–373, 1932.

242. Rooney, P.J., and Cockshott, W.P.: Pseudarthrosis Following Proximal Humeral Fractures. A Possible Mechanism. Skeletal Radiol., 15:21–24, 1986.

243. Rose, S.H.; Melton, L.J.; Morrey, B.F.; Ilstrup, D.M.; and Riggs, L.B.: Epidemiologic Features of Humeral Fractures. Clin. Orthop., 168:24–30, 1982.

244. Rosen, H.: Tension Band Wiring for Fracture Dislocation of the Shoulder. *In* Proceedings of the 12th Congress of the International Society of Orthopaedic Surgery and Traumatolgie, pp. 939–941. Tel Aviv, October 9–12, 1972.

245. Ross, J., and Lov, J.B.: Isolated Evulsion Fracture of the Lesser Tuberosity of the Humerus: Report of Two Cases. Radiology, 172:833–834, 1989.

246. Rothman, R.H.; Marvel, J.P.; and Heppenstall, R.B.: Anatomic Considerations in the Glenohumeral Joint. Orthop. Clin. North Am., 6:341–352, 1975.

247. Rothman, R.H., and Parke, W.W.: The Vascular Anatomy of the Rotator Cuff. Clin. Orthop., 41:176–186, 1965.

248. Rowe, C.R., and Colville, M.: The Glenohumeral Joint. *In* Rowe, C.R. (ed.): The Shoulder, pp. 331–358. New York, Churchill Livingstone, 1988.

249. Rowe, C.R., and Marble, H.: Shoulder Girdle Injuries. *In* Cave, E.F. (ed.): Fractures and Other Injuries, pp. 250–289. Chicago: Year Book Medical Publishers, 1958.

250. Royster, H.A.: Management of Dislocations of the Humerus Complicated by Fracture of the Neck of the Humerus. J.A.M.A., 49:487–491, 1907.

251. Ruedi, T.: Treatment of Displaced Metaphyseal Fractures With Screw and Wiring Systems. Orthopaedics, 12:55–59, 1989.

252. Rush, L.V.: Atlas of Rush Pin Techniques. Meridian, Mich., Beviron Co., 1959.

253. Saha, A.K.: The Zero Position of the Glenohumeral Joint: Its Recognition and Clinical Importance. Ann. R. Coll. Surg. Engl., 22:223, 1958.

254. Sakai, K.; Hattori, S.; Kawai, S.; Saiki, K.; et al.: One Case of the Fracture at the Attachment of the Subscapularis Muscle. Shoulder Joint, 7:58, 1981.

255. Salem, M.I.: Bilateral Anterior Fracture-dislocation of the Shoulder Joints Due to Severe Electric Shock. Injury, 14:361–363, 1983.

256. Santee, H.E.: Fractures About the Upper End of the Humerus. Ann. Surg., 80:103–114, 1924.

257. Savoie, F.H.; Geissler, W.B.; and Vander Griend, R.A.: Open Reduction and Internal Fixation of Three-part Fractures of the Proximal Humerus. Orthopaedics, 12:65–70, 1989.

258. Scheck, M.: Surgical Treatment of Nonunions of the Surgical Neck of the Humerus. Clin. Orthop., 167:255–259, 1982.

259. Schubl, J.F.: Fracture-dislocations of the Proximal Humerus. These Medecine. Lyon, 1973.

260. Schweiger, G., and Ludolph, E.: Fractures of the Shoulder Joint. Unfallchir 6, 1980.

261. Scudder, C.L.: The Treatment of Fractures, 11th ed., pp. 564–603. Philadelphia, W.B. Saunders, 1939.

262. Sehr, J.R., and Sazabo, R.M.: Semitubular Blade Plate for Fixation of the Proximal Humerus. Journal of Orthopaedic Trauma, 2:327–332, 1989.

263. Sever, J.W.: Fracture of the Head of the Humerus. Treatment and Results. N. Engl. J. Med., 216:1100–1107, 1937.

264. Sever, J.W.: Nonunion in Fracture of the Shaft of the Humerus. Report of Five Cases. J.A.M.A., 104:382–386, 1935.

265. Shaw, J.L.: Bilateral Posterior Fracture-dislocation of the Shoulder and Other Trauma Caused by Convulsive Seizures. J. Bone Joint Surg., 53A:1437–1440, 1971.

266. Shibuya, S., and Ogawa, K.: Isolated Avulsion Fracture of the Lesser Tuberosity of the Humerus. A Case Report. Clin. Orthop., 211:215–218, 1986.

267. Shuck, J.M.; Omer, G.E.; and Lewis, C.E.: Arterial Obstruction Due to Intimal Disruption in Extremity Fractures. J. Trauma, 12:481–489, 1972.

268. Silverskoild, N.: On the Treatment of Fracture-dislocations of the Shoulder-joint. With Special Reference to the Capability of the Head-fragment, Disconnected From Capsule and Periosteum to Enter Into Bony Union. Acta Chir. Scand., 64:227–293, 1928.

269. Sjovall, H.: A Case of Spontaneous Backward Subluxation of the Shoulder Treated by the Clairmont-Ehrlich Operation. Nord. Med. (Hygeia), 21:474–476, 1944.

270. Smyth, E.H.J.: Major Arterial Injury in Closed Fracture of the Neck of the Humerus. Report of a Case. J. Bone Joint Surg., 51B:508–510, 1969.

271. Solonen, K.A., and Vastamaki, M.: Osteotomy of the Neck of the Humerus for Traumatic Varus Deformity. Acta Orthop. Scand., 56:79–80, 1985.

272. Sorensen, K.H.: Pseudarthrosis of the Surgical Neck of the Humerus. Two Cases. One Bilateral. Acta Orthop. Scand., 34:132–138, 1964.

273. Stableforth, P.G.: Four-part Fractures of the Neck of the Humerus. J. Bone Joint Surg., 66B:104–108, 1984.

274. Stangl, F.H.: Isolated Fracture of the Lesser Tuberosity of the Humerus. Minn. Med., 16:435–437, 1933.

275. Stevens, J.H.: Fracture of the Upper End of the Humerus. Ann. Surg., 69:147–160, 1919.

276. Stewart, M.J., and Hundley, J.M.: Fractures of the Humerus. A Comparative Study in Methods of Treatment. J. Bone Joint Surg., 37A:681–692, 1955.

277. Stimson, B.B.: A Manual of Fractures and Dislocations, 2nd ed., pp. 241–260. Philadelphia, Lea & Febiger, 1947.

278. Sturzenegger, M.; Fornaro, E.; and Jakob, R.P.: Results of Surgical Treatment of Multifragmented Fractures of the Humeral Head. Arch. Orthop. Trauma Surg., 100:249–259, 1982.

279. Svend-Hansen, H.: Displaced Proximal Humeral Fractures. A Review of 49 Patients. Acta Orthop. Scand., 45:359–364, 1974.

280. Tanner, M.W., and Cofield, R.H.: Prosthetic Arthroplasty for Fractures and Fracture-dislocation of the Proximal Humerus. Clin. Orthop., 179:116–128, 1983.

281. Tanton, J.: Fractures de l'extremite superiere de l'hu-

merus. *In* LeDentu, A., and Delbet, P. (eds.): Noveau Traite de Chirurgie, Fase 4. Paris, Bailliere et Fils, 1915.

282. Taylor, H.L.: Isolated Fracture of the Greater Tuberosity of the Humerus. Ann. Surg., 54:10–12, 1908.

283. Theodorides, T., and Dekeizer, G.: Injuries of the Axillary Artery Caused by Fractures of the Neck of the Humerus. Injury, 8:120–123, 1976.

284. Thompson, F.E., and Winant, E.M.: Comminuted Fracture of the Humeral Head With Subluxation. Clin. Orthop., 20:94–97, 1961.

285. Thompson, F.R., and Winant, E.M.: Unusual Fracture Subluxations of the Shoulder Joint. J. Bone Joint Surg., 32A:575–582, 1950.

286. Thompson, J.E.: Anatomical Methods of Approach in Operations on the Long Bones of the Extremities. Ann. Surg., 68:309–329, 1918.

287. Tondeur, G.: Les fractures recentes de l'epaule. Acta Orthop. Belg., 30:1–144, 1964.

288. Tonino, A.J., and van de Werf, G.J.I.M.: Hemiarthroplasty of the Shoulder. Acta Orthop. Belg., 51:625–631, 1985.

289. Trotter, E.: Apropos d'un cas de resection de la tete de l'humerus. J. l'Hotel-dieu Montreal, 11:368, 1933.

290. Vainio, S.: Observation on Serious Fractures of the Proximal End of the Humerus. Ann. Clin. Gynaecol. Fenn., 49:302–308, 1960.

291. Valls, J.: Acrylic Prosthesis in a Case With Fracture of the Head of the Humerus. Bal. Soc. Orthop. Trauma, 17:61, 1952.

292. Vander-Ghirst, M., and Houssa, R.: Acrylic Prosthesis in Fractures of the Head of the Humerus. Acta Chir. Belg., 50:31–40, 1951.

293. Van Hook, W.: Fracture Dislocations of the Humeral Head. Boston Medical and Surgical Journal, 187:960–962, 1922.

294. Vastamaki, M., and Solonen, K.A.: Posterior Dislocation and Fracture-dislocation of the Shoulder. Acta Orthop. Scand., 51:479–484, 1980.

295. Vastamaki, M., and Solonen, K.A.: Posterior Dislocation and Posterior Fracture-dislocation of the Shoulder. Acta Orthop. Scand., 50:124, 1979.

296. Veseley, D.G.: Use of the Split Diamond Nail for Fractures of the Humerus, 1958–1961. Clin. Orthop., 41:145–156, 1965.

297. Vichard, P.H., and Bellanger, P.: Ascending Bipolar Nailing Using Elastic Nails in the Treatment of Fractures of the Upper End of the Humerus. Nouv. Presse Med., 7:4041–4043, 1978.

298. Wallace, W.A.: The Dynamic Study of Shoulder Movement. *In* Bayley, I., and Kessel, L. (eds.): Shoulder Surgery, pp. 139–143. New York, Springer-Verlag, 1982.

299. Watson-Jones, R.: Fractures and Joint Injuries, 4th ed., pp. 473–476. Baltimore, Williams & Wilkins, 1955.

300. Watson-Jones, R.: Fractures and Joint Injuries, 3rd ed., pp. 460–461. Baltimore, Williams & Wilkins, 1943.

301. Weise, K.; Meeder, P.J.; and Wentzensen, A.: Indications and Operative Technique in Osteosynthesis of Fracture-dislocations of the Shoulder Joint in Adults. Langenbecks Arch. Chir., 351:91–98, 1980.

302. Wentworth, E.T.: Fractures Involving the Shoulder Joint. N.Y. State J. Med., 40:1282–1288, 1940.

303. Weseley, M.S.; Barenfeld, P.A.; and Eisenstein, A.I.: Rush Pin Intramedullary Fixation for Fractures of the Proximal Humerus. J. Trauma, 17:29–37, 1977.

304. West, E.F.: Intrathoracic Dislocation of the Humerus. J. Bone Joint Surg., 31B:61–62, 1949.

305. Whitman, R.: A Treatment of Epiphyseal Displacements and Fractures of the Upper Extremity of the Humerus Designed to Assure Definite Adjustment and Fixation of Fragments. Ann. Surg., 47:706–708, 1908.

306. Whiston, T.B.: Fractures of the Surgical Neck of the Humerus. A Study in Reduction. J. Bone Joint Surg., 36B:423–427, 1954.

307. Widen, A.: Fractures of the Upper End of Humerus With Great Displacement Treated by Marrow Nailing. Acta Chir. Scand., 97:439–441, 1949.

308. Willems, W.J., and Lim, T.E.A.: Neer Arthroplasty for Humeral Fracture. Acta Orthop. Scand., 56:394–395, 1985.

309. Wilson, G.E.: Fractures and Their Complications. New York, Macmillan, 1931.

310. Wilson, J.N. (ed.): Watson-Jones Fractures and Joint Injuries, 6th ed., pp. 533–545. New York, Churchill Livingstone, 1982.

311. Wilson, J.C., and McKeever, F.M.: Traumatic Posterior (Retroglenoid) Dislocation of the Humerus. J. Bone Joint Surg., 31A:160–172, 180, 1949.

312. Winfield, J.M.; Miller, H.; and LaFerte, A.D.: Evaluation of the "Hanging Cast" as a Method of Treating Fractures of the Humerus. Am. J. Surg., 55:228–249, 1942.

313. Wood, J.P.: Posterior Dislocation of the Head of the Humerus and Diagnostic Value of Lateral and Vertical Views. U.S. Naval Med. Bull., 39:532–535, 1941.

314. Yamano, Y.: Comminuted Fractures of the Proximal Humerus Treated With Hook Plate. Arch. Orthop. Trauma Surg., 105:359–363, 1986.

315. Yano, S.; Takamura, S.; and Kobayshi, I.: Use of the Spiral Pin for Fractures of the Humeral Neck. J. Jpn. Orthop. Assn., 55:1607, 1981.

316. Young, T.B., and Wallace, W.A.: Conservative Treatment of Fractures and Fracture-dislocations of the Upper End of the Humerus. J. Bone Joint Surg., 67B:373–377, 1985.

317. Zadik, F.R.: Recurrent Posterior Dislocation of the Shoulder. J. Bone Joint Surg., 30B:531–532, 1948.

318. Zuckerman, J.D.; Flugstad, D.L.; Teitz, C.C.; and King, H.A.: Axillary Artery Injury as a Complication of Proximal Humeral Fractures. Two Case Reports and a Review of the Literature. Clin. Orthop., 189:234–237, 1984.

Part II: FRACTURES OF THE CLAVICLE
Edward V. Craig

Although clavicular fractures are usually readily recognizable and unite uneventfully with treatment, they occur frequently and can be associated with difficult early and late complications. The fact that the clavicle is the most commonly fractured bone in childhood,[44,255] and that it has been estimated that one of every 20 fractures involves the clavicle,[172] underscores the clinical relevance of these injuries. In fact, fractures of the clavicle may comprise up to 44% of all shoulder girdle injuries.[222]

HISTORICAL REVIEW

The clavicle is entirely subcutaneous, and thus easily accessible to inspection and palpation. This may account for its inclusion in some of the earliest descriptions of injuries of the human skeleton and their treatment. As early as 400 B.C., Hippocrates recorded a number of observations about clavicular fractures:

1. With a fractured clavicle, the distal fragment and arm sag, while the proximal fragment— held securely by the sternoclavicular joint attachments—points upward.
2. It is difficult to reduce and maintain the reduction. Hippocrates noted, "They act imprudently who think to depress the projecting end of the bone. But it is clear that the underpart ought to be brought to the upper, for the former is the moveable part, and that which has been displaced from its natural position."
3. Union usually occurs rapidly and produces prominent callus; and, despite the deformity, healing usually proceeds uneventfully.

Hippocrates also noted:

> A fractured clavicle like all other spongy bone, gets speedily united; for all such bone forms callus in a short time. When, then, a fracture has recently taken place, the patients attach much importance to it, as supposing the mischief greater than it really is . . .; but, in a little time, the patients having no pain, nor finding any impediment to their walking or eating, become negligent, and the physicians, finding they cannot make the parts look well, take themselves off, and are not sorry at the neglect of the patients, and in the mean time the callus is quickly formed.[2]

The Edwin Smith Papyrus provides what is probably the earliest description of the now-accepted method of fracture reduction, indicating that an unknown Egyptian surgeon in 3000 B.C. recommended treating fractures of the clavicle thus:

> Thou shouldst place him prostrate on his back with something folded between his shoulder-blades, thou shouldst spread out with his two shoulders in order to stretch apart his collarbone until that break falls into place.[44,77,172]

Paul of Aegina, a 17th-century Byzantine, reported all that could ever be written about fractures of the clavicle had been written; he noted that treatment options included supine positioning as well as the application of potions of olive oil, pigeon dung, snake oil, and other essences.[158]

Some of the earliest documented cases resulted from reports of riding accidents. In 1702, William III died from a fracture of the clavicle 3 days after his horse shied at a mole hill. Sir Benjamin Brodi described a "diffuse false venous aneurysm" complicating a fracture of the clavicle in Sir Robert Peel, who fell from his horse in 1850 on the way to Parliament. As he lapsed into an unconsciousness, a pulsatile swelling rapidly developed behind the fracture and his arm was paralyzed. The *Lancet* defended the physicians' handling of the case when many skeptics doubted that death could occur from a clavicular fracture.[51,135,283]

Dupuytren, a keen though controversial anatomist and observer, noted in 1839 that the cumbersome devices used to maintain reductions of the clavicle were often unnecessary, and he advocated simply placing the arm on a pillow until union occurred. He observed that some of the devices in use appeared to aggravate the fractures or create new problems. He described one case on which he consulted where bleeding could not be arrested: "When I was summoned I merely removed the apparatus (the pressure of which was the cause of the mischief) and placed the arm on a pillow. The bleeding immediately ceased."[54,283] He railed against cumbersome and painful treatment methods.

Malgaigne, in 1859, concluded that most treatment methods led to healing with residual clavicular deformity,

> . . . but while for a century and a half we see the most celebrated surgeons striving to prefer, or perhaps more strictly

to complicate, the contrivances for treating fractured clavicle we may follow parallel to them another series of no lest estimable surgeons, who disbelieving in these so-called improvements, return to the simplest means, as to Hippocrates before them. If now we seek to judge of all these contrivances by their results we see that most of them are extolled as producing cures without deformity; but we see also that subsequent experience has always falsified these promises. I therefore, regard the thing (absence of deformity) as not impossible, although for my own part I have never seen such an instance.[151]

This well summarizes the results of most conservative treatments for fractured clavicles. That is, most of the fractures unite uneventfully with one of several treatment methods, many of the patients have residual deformity (ie, some shortening and a lump), yet interference with function, cosmesis, activity level, and satisfaction appears to be minimal. In the late 1860s, the present-day ambulatory treatment was described by Lucas-Championniere, who advocated use of a figure-of-eight dressing and suggested that recumbency, popular in his day, be abandoned in favor of early mobilization of the patient.[84] In 1891, Sayer, recognizing the difficulty of maintaining the reduction, advocated an ambulatory treatment that involved a rigid dressing to maintain the reduction and support the extremity. This method was echoed and taught in the textbooks of his time, and still has many advocates today.[229]

Ambulatory treatment with support of the arm, while maintaining satisfactory and acceptable alignment of the fracture fragments, remains the mainstay of care for clavicular fractures.

ANATOMY

The embryology of the clavicle is unique in that it is the first bone in the body to ossify (fifth week of fetal life), and the only long bone to ossify by intramembranous ossification without going through a cartilaginous stage.[80,165,166] The ossification center begins in the central portion of the clavicle, and this area is responsible for growth of the clavicle up to about 5 years of age.[44,69] Although epiphyseal growth plates develop at both the medial and lateral ends of the clavicle, only the sternal ossification center is evident radiographically.[44,262] This medial growth plate is responsible for most of the longitudinal growth of the clavicle—contributing up to 80% of its length.[185] The appearance and fusion of the sternal ossification center occur relatively late, with ossification occurring between 12 and 19 years

of age and fusion to the clavicle occurring between 22 and 25 years.[113,271] Thus, many so-called sternoclavicular dislocations in young adults are, in fact, epiphyseal fractures; this is a potential source of confusion, unless the late sternoclavicular epiphyseal closure is remembered.

Because the clavicle is subcutaneous along its entire length, the only structures that cross it are the supraclavicular nerves.[11] In most people it is possible to grasp the bone and manipulate it, which can be helpful in producing crepitus if an acute fracture is suspected, or movement in the case of a suspected nonunion.

The clavicle is the sole bony strut connecting the trunk to the shoulder girdle and arm, and it is the only bone of the shoulder girdle that forms a synovial joint with the trunk.[143] Its name is derived from the Latin word for "key"—*clavis*—the diminutive of which is *clavicula*, referring to the musical symbol of similar shape.[165]

The shape and configuration of the clavicle are important to its function. They also help explain the pattern of fractures encountered in this bone. Although the clavicle appears nearly straight when viewed from the front, from above it appears as an S-shaped double curve, concave ventrally on its outer half and convex ventrally on its medial half (Fig. 12-49). Though some authors have noted differences in the shape and size of the clavicle between males and females and between dominant and nondominant arms, others have not found this to be so, or have discounted its clinical significance.[50,70,143,185] DePalma found the outer third of the clavicle exhibited varying degrees of anterior torsion, and suggested that changes in torsion might alter stresses and lead to primary degenerative disease in the acromioclavicular joint.[50] The cross section of the clavicle differs in shape along its length, varying from flat along the outer third to prismatic along the inner third. The exact curvature of the clavicle and, to a high degree, its thickness, vary according to the attachments of the muscles and ligaments.[143] The flat outer third is most compatible with pull from muscles and ligaments, whereas the tubular medial third is compatible with axial pressure or pull. The junction between the two cross sections varies in its precise location with the middle third of the clavicle. This junction is a weak spot, particularly to axial loading.[143] This may be one reason why fractures occur so commonly in the middle third. Another may be that the area is not reinforced by muscles and ligaments and is just distal to the subclavius insertion.[102,108,172] It is curious that nature has strengthened, through ligaments or

Right clavicle

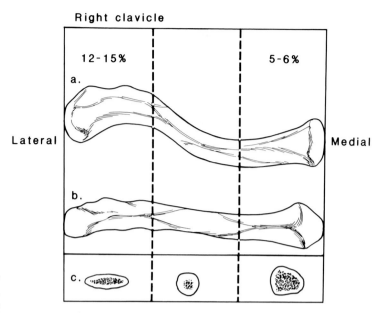

a. Superior view
b. Frontal view
c. Cross sections

Fig. 12-49. The clavicle appears nearly straight when viewed from the front, whereas when viewed from above it appears as an S-shaped double curve. The lateral end of the clavicle is flat in cross section, while the medial aspect is more tubular.

muscular reinforcement, every part of the clavicle except the end of the outer part of the middle third—which in fact is the thinnest part of the bone.[16]

The clavicle articulates with the sternum through the sternoclavicular joint; this joint has little actual articular contact, but surprisingly strong ligamentous attachments. The medial end of the clavicle is moored firmly against the first rib by the intra-articular sternoclavicular joint cartilage (which functions as a ligament), the oblique fibers of the costoclavicular ligaments, and, to a lesser degree, the subclavius muscle.[50] The scapula and clavicle are bound securely through both the acromioclavicular and coracoclavicular ligaments; the mechanism and function behind this have been extensively reported, and contribute significantly to the movement and stability of the entire upper extremity (Fig. 12-50).[78,268] The clavicle in the adult is dense, honeycombed, and lacks a well-defined medullary cavity. The bone of the clavicle has been described as "thick compacta,"[79] and its main nutrient vessel enters just medial to the attachment of the coracoclavicular ligaments.[185]

The tubular third of the clavicle, thicker in cross section, offers protection for the important neurovascular structures that pass beneath the medial third of the clavicle. The intimate relationship be-

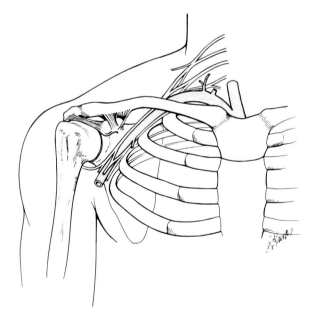

Fig. 12-50. The clavicle is bound securely by ligaments at both sternoclavicular and acromioclavicular joints. It is the only bony strut from the torso to the extremity. The brachial plexus and greater vessels are seen posterior to the medial third of the clavicle between the clavicle and first rib.

tween these structures and the clavicle assumes great importance both in acute fractures, in which direct injury may occur, and in the unusual fracture sequelae of malunion, nonunion, or excessive callus, in which compression may lead to late symptoms. The brachial plexus, at the level that it crosses beneath the clavicle, comprises three main branches. (See Fig. 12-50.) Of these, two are anterior. The lateral anterior branch originates from the fifth, sixth, and seventh cervical roots and forms the musculocutaneous and a branch of the median nerve; the medial anterior branch originates from the eighth cervical and first thoracic roots and forms another branch of the median nerve, the entire ulnar nerve, and the medial cutaneous nerve. The single posterior branch of the plexus forms the axillary and radial nerves. The cord of the brachial plexus, which contains the first components of the ulnar nerve, crosses the first rib directly under the medial third of the clavicle. The other two cords are situated farther to the lateral side and more posteriorly. Therefore, the ulnar nerve is more frequently involved in complications arising from fractures of the medial third of the clavicle.

The space between the clavicle and the first rib has been called the "costoclavicular space." This space has been measured in gross anatomical studies, and often appears quite adequate. However, the costoclavicular space is not as large in living subjects as in cadavers, possibly because the vessels are distended in living subjects and the dimensions of the cords of the brachial plexus are larger than in the cadaver. In addition, the space is diminished in living subjects as the first rib elevates owing to contraction of the scalenus anticus. Hence, when the inner end of the outer fragment of the fractured clavicle is depressed, there is much less space between the first rib and the clavicle, the result being that the vessels (especially the subclavian and axillary vessels) and the nerves (especially the ulnar nerve) may be subjected to injury, pressure, or irritation.[16] The internal jugular, adjacent to the sternoclavicular joint (see Fig. 12-50), usually is not injured with middle-third fractures, but has the potential for injury in more medial trauma involving the sternum and sternoclavicular joint.

SURGICAL ANATOMY

The surgical anatomy relative to the fascial arrangements about the clavicle has been extensively detailed by Abbott and Lucas.[1] Knowledge of these structures will decrease the risk of damage to the neurovascular structures during surgical dissec-

tion.[220] It is useful to divide the fascia into the areas above, below, and behind the clavicle.

Superior to the Clavicle

At the sternal notch a layer of cervical fascia splits into two layers: a superficial layer attached to the front and a deep layer attached to back of the manubrium. The space between these layers contains lymphatics and a communicating vessel between the two anterior jugular veins. The two layers of fascia proceed laterally to enclose the sternocleidomastoid before passing down to the clavicle. For an inch above the clavicle, they are separated by some loose fat. The superficial layer is ill defined and is continuous with the fascia covering the undersurface of the trapezius muscle. A prolongation from the deep layer forms an inverted sling for the posterior belly of the omohyoid muscle; this layer continues to blend with the fascia enclosing the subclavius muscle. Medially, the omohyoid fascia covers the sternohyoid muscle.

Inferior to the Clavicle

Two layers, consisting of muscle and fascia, form the anterior wall of the axilla. The pectoralis major and pectoral fascia form the superficial layer, while the pectoralis minor and clavipectoral fascia form the deep layer. The pectoral fascia closely envelops the pectoralis major. Above, it is attached to the clavicle, and laterally, it forms the roof of the superficial infraclavicular triangle (formed by the pectoralis major, a portion of anterior deltoid, and the clavicle). The deep layer, the clavipectoral fascia, extends from the clavicle above to the axillary fascia below. At the point where it attaches to the clavicle, it consists of two layers, which enclose the subclavius muscle. The subclavius muscle arises from the manubrium and first rib and inserts at the inferior surface of the clavicle. At the lower border of the subclavius, the two fascial layers join to form the costocoracoid membrane. This membrane fills a space between the subclavius above and the pectoralis minor below. This membrane is attached medially to the first costal cartilage and laterally to the coracoid process. Below, it splits into two layers, which ensheathe the pectoralis minor. The costocoracoid membrane is pierced by the cephalic vein, the lateral pectoral nerve, and the thoracoacromial artery and vein.

Deep to the Clavicle

A continuous myofascial layer, which has not been commonly appreciated in surgical anatomy, lies in front of the large vessels and nerves as they pass from the root of the neck to the axilla. From above to below this layer consists of: (1) the omohyoid fascia enclosing the omohyoid muscle, and (2) the clavipectoral fascia, which encloses the pectoralis minor and subclavius muscles.[1] Behind the medial clavicle and the sternoclavicular joint, the internal jugular and subclavian veins join to form the innominate vein. These veins are covered by the omohyoid fascia and by its extension medially over the sternohyoid and sternal thyroid muscle. Behind the clavicle, at the junction between the middle and medial thirds, the junction of the subclavian and axillary veins lies very close to the clavicle and is protected by this myofascial layer.

Between the omohyoid fascia posteriorly and the investing layer of cervical fascia anteriorly is a space, described by Grant, in which the external jugular vein usually joins the subclavian vein at its confluence with the internal jugular vein.[90] Before this junction, the external jugular is joined on its lateral aspect by the transverse cervical and scapular veins, and on its medial aspect by the anterior jugular vein. This anastomosis usually lies just behind the fascial envelope and the angle formed by the posterior border of the sternomastoid muscle and clavicle.[1]

FUNCTION OF THE CLAVICLE

The function of the clavicle may be inferred, in part, by some study of comparative anatomy. Codman has stated, "We are proud that our brains are more developed than the animals: we might also boast of our clavicles. It seems to me that the clavicle is one of man's greatest skeletal inheritances, for he depends to a greater extent than most animals except the apes and monkeys on the use of his hands and arms."[31] Mammals that depend on swimming, running, or grazing have no clavicles, whereas those species that have clavicles appear to be predominantly flyers or climbers. Codman theorized that animals with strong clavicles need to use their arms more in adduction and abduction. The long clavicle may facilitate the placement of the shoulder in a more lateral position, so the hand can be more effectively positioned to deal with the three-dimensional environment.[191] The teleologic role of the clavicle has been disputed, however, because there have been reports of entirely normal function of the upper limb following complete excision of the clavicle.[36,97,106] These reports, combined with observations in patients with congenital absence of the clavicle (cleidocranial dysostosis) who appear

not to show any impairment of limb function, probably are responsible for the often-stated belief that this bone is a surplus part that can be excised without disturbance of function. However, others have noted drooping of the shoulder, weakness, and loss of motion following clavicular excision and have used these observations to attribute to the clavicle its important role in normal extremity function (Fig. 12-51).[218,244]

The clavicle does have several important functions, each of which can be expected to alter not only by excision of the bone, but also by fracture, nonunion, or malunion.

POWER AND STABILITY OF THE ARM

The clavicle, by serving as a bony link from the thorax to the shoulder girdle, provides a stable linkage in the arm–trunk mechanism, and contributes significantly to power and stability of the arm and shoulder girdle, especially in movement above shoulder level.[166] Through the coracoclavicular ligaments, the clavicle transmits the support and force of the trapezius muscle to the scapula and arm.

Although patients with cleidocranial dysostosis and absence of the clavicle do not appear to have significantly decreased motion, and in fact may have increased protraction and retraction of the scapula, they may exhibit some weakness in supporting a load overhead; this further suggests that the clavicle adds stability to the extremity under load in extreme ranges of motion.[106]

The clavicle is predominantly supported and stabilized by passive structures,[143] particularly the sternoclavicular ligaments.[13,14] Though it has been reported that there is EMG evidence of trapezius muscle activity at rest, suggesting a role for that muscle in support of the clavicle,[1] others have not been able to demonstrate that such activity plays any role in clavicular support.

MOTION OF THE SHOULDER GIRDLE

When the arm is elevated 180°, the clavicle angles upward 30° and backward 35° at the sternoclavicular joint. It also rotates upward on its longitudinal axis approximately 50°. During combined glenohumeral, acromioclavicular, and sternoclavicular movement, the humerus moves approximately 120° at the glenohumeral joint and the scapula moves along the chest wall approximately 60°. These complex and combined movements of the joints and their articulating bony structures (ie, scapula, humerus, clavicle) simultaneously seem to

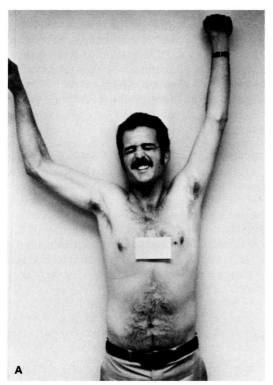
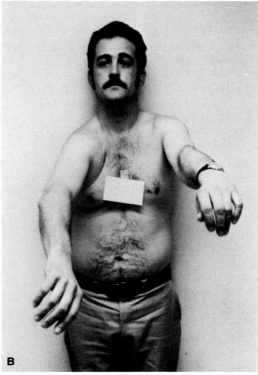

Fig. 12-51. (**A**) A patient who had his right clavicle excised. Eight years following resection, the patient has a painful and limited range of shoulder motion. (**B**) During flexion, the shoulder collapses medially. The patient has no strength in abduction or flexion. He has significant drooping of the upper extremity, which has produced a traction brachial plexitis. (*Courtesy of C. Rockwood, M.D.*)

imply an important role for the clavicle in range of motion of the arm. There is some debate about this, however. It has been observed by some that loss of the clavicle does not in fact impair abduction of the arm[1,282] and may allow full range of motion. However, Rockwood observed loss of the clavicle to result in disabling loss of function, weakness, drooping of the arm, and pain secondary to brachial plexus irritation.[218] (See Fig. 12-51.)

It has been stated that contribution to motion may be the most important function of the clavicle, and that this is related to its curvature—especially the lateral curvature. The 50° rotation of the clavicle on its axis appears to be important for free elevation of the extremity. In fact, direct relationships have been found among the line of attachment of the coracoclavicular ligaments, the amount of clavicular rotation, the extent and relative lengthening of the ligaments, and scapular rotation. Of the total 60° of scapular rotation, the first 30° are related to

elevation of the clavicle as a whole by movement of the sternoclavicular joint, while the next 30° are permitted through the acromioclavicular joint by clavicular rotation and elongation of the coracoclavicular ligaments. Thus, the lateral curvature of the clavicle permits the clavicle to act as crank shaft, effectively allowing half of scapular movement.[142]

The smooth, rhythmic, movement of the shoulder girdle is a complex interaction of muscle groups acting on joints, and both subacromial and scapulothoracic spaces. While it is difficult to break down all of the contributions of the clavicle to the total motion, it appears that its geometric and kinematic design, by permitting rotation, maximizes the stability of the upper limb against the trunk while permitting mobility, particularly of the scapula along the chest wall. The practical result of this is that the glenoid fossa continually moves, facing and contacting the humeral head as the arm is used overhead.[106]

MUSCLE ATTACHMENTS

The clavicle also acts as a bony framework for muscle origins and insertions. The upper third of the trapezius inserts on the superior surface of the outer third of the clavicle, opposite the origin of the clavicular head of the deltoid along its anterior edge. The clavicular head of the sternocleidomastoid muscle arises from the posterior edge of the inner third of the clavicle. The clavicular head of the pectoralis major muscle arises from the anterior edge of the clavicle. During active elevation of the arm these muscles contract simultaneously. It has been suggested, in theory, that the muscles above the clavicle may be directly attached to those below the clavicle as a continuous muscular layer without an interposed bony attachment,[1] but the stable bony framework clearly provides the advantage of a solid foundation for muscle attachment.

The subclavius muscle is the other muscle that inserts on the clavicle. After it arises from the first rib anteriorly at the costochondral junction, it proceeds obliquely and posteriorly into a groove on the undersurface of the clavicle. It appears to aid in depressing the middle third of the clavicle. Fractures of the clavicle often occur at the distal portion of its insertion. In midclavicular fractures, this muscle may offer some protection to the neurovascular structures beneath.

PROTECTION OF THE NEUROVASCULAR STRUCTURES

The clavicle also acts as a skeletal protection for adjacent neurovascular structures and for the superior aspect of the lung. The subclavian and axillary vessels, the brachial plexus, and the lung are directly behind the medial third of the clavicle. As noted earlier, the tubular cross section of the medial third of the clavicle increases its strength and adds to its protective function at this level. The anterior curve of the medial two thirds of the clavicle provides a rigid arch beneath which the great vessels pass as they move from the mediastinum and thoracic outlet to the axilla. It has been shown that during elevation of the arm, the clavicle, as it rotates upward, also moves backward, the curvature providing increased clearance for the vessels.[259] Loss of the clavicle eliminates this bony protection from external trauma.[1]

RESPIRATORY FUNCTION

Elevation of the lateral part of the clavicle results in increased pull on the costoclavicular ligament and subclavius muscle. Owing to the connections between the clavicle and first rib and between the first rib and the sternum, elevation of the shoulder girdle brings about a cephalad motion of the thorax, corresponding to an inspiration. This relationship is made use of in some breathing exercises and in some forms of artificial respiration.[1]

COSMESIS

By providing a graceful curve to the base of the neck, a cosmetic function is served by the smooth subcutaneous bony clavicle. In some patients, after surgical excision the upper limb may fall downward and forward, giving a foreshortened appearance to this area. In addition, the cosmetic function of the clavicle is noted by many concerned patients after excessive formation of callus following clavicular fracture or with deformity secondary to clavicular malunion.[1]

CLASSIFICATION

Although clavicular fractures have been classified by fracture configuration (ie, greenstick, oblique, transverse, comminuted)[236] the usual classification is by location of the fracture. This appears to better compartmentalize our understanding of the fracture anatomy, mechanism of injury, clinical presentation, and alternative methods of treatment.[5,59,67,174,194]

A useful classification is as follows:

Group I—middle-third fractures
Group II—distal-third fractures
  Type I—minimal displacement (interligamentous)
  Type II—displacement secondary to fracture medial to the coracoclavicular ligaments
    A. Conoid and trapezoid attached
    B. Conoid torn, trapezoid attached
  Type III—articular surface fractures
  Type IV—ligaments intact to periosteum (children), with displacement of the proximal fragment
  Type V—comminuted, with ligaments not attached proximally nor distally, but to an inferior, comminuted fragment
Group III—proximal-third fractures
  Type I—minimal displacement
  Type II—significant displacement (ligaments ruptured)
  Type III—intra-articular

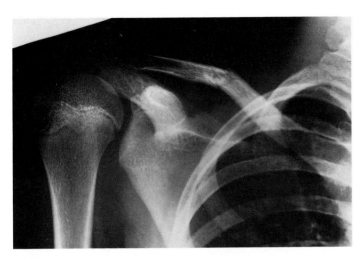

Fig. 12-52. Typical location for a nondisplaced group I fracture of the clavicle.

Type IV—epiphyseal separation (children and young adults)
Type V—comminuted[39]

Group I fractures (middle third) are the most common in both adults and children. The middle third of the clavicle is the point at which the bone changes from a prismatic cross section to a flattened cross section. The force of the traumatic impact follows the curve of the clavicle and disperses upon reaching the lateral curve.[179-181,243] In addition, the proximal and distal segments of the clavicle are mechanically secured by ligamentous structures and muscular attachments, while the central segment is relatively free. Group I fractures account for 80% of all clavicular fractures (Figs. 12-52 to 12-54).[172,222]

Group II fractures account for 12% to 15% of clavicular fractures and are subclassified according to the location of the coracoclavicular ligaments relative to the fracture fragments.[100] Neer first pointed out the importance of these fractures, and subdivided them into three types. The type I fracture is the most common distal fracture, by a ratio of four to one. In this fracture, the ligaments remain intact to hold the fragments together and prevent rotation, tilting, or significant displacement. This is an interligamentous fracture occurring between the conoid and trapezoid or the coracoclavicular and acromioclavicular ligaments (Figs. 12-55 and 12-56).[175]

In type II distal clavicular fractures, the coracoclavicular ligaments are detached from the medial segment. Both the conoid and the trapezoid may be on the distal fragment (type IIA) (Fig. 12-57), or the conoid ligament may be ruptured while the

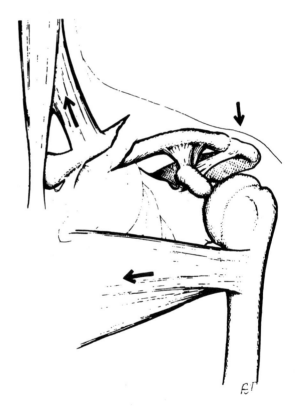

Fig. 12-53. When displacement occurs, the proximal fragment is pulled superiorly and posteriorly by the pull of the sternocleidomastoid, while the distal segment droops forward owing to gravity and the pull of the pectoralis.

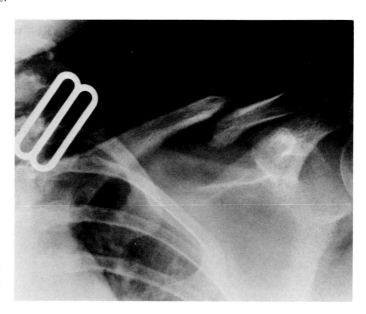

Fig. 12-54. Radiographic appearance of the displacement in a typical group I fracture of the clavicle.

trapezoid ligament remains attached to the distal segment (type IIB)[44] (Fig. 12-58). Four forces act on this fracture; these may impair healing and may contribute to the high incidence of nonunion. These forces are: (1) Weight of the arm—When the patient is erect, the outer fragment, retaining the attachment of the trapezoid ligament to the scapula through the intact acromioclavicular ligaments, is

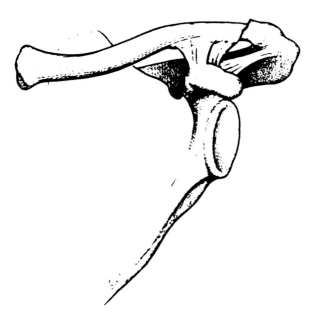

Fig. 12-55. A type I fracture of the distal clavicle (group II). The intact ligaments hold the fragments in place.

pulled downward and forward. (2) Pectoralis major, pectoralis minor, and latissimus dorsi—these structures draw the distal segment downward and medially, causing overriding. (3) Scapular rotation—the scapula may rotate the distal segment as the arm is moved. (4) Trapezius and sternocleidomastoid muscles—the trapezius muscle attaches on the entire outer two thirds of the clavicle, whereas the sternocleidomastoid attaches to the medial third. Thus, these muscles draw the clavicular segment superior and posterior, often into the substance of the trapezius muscle.[174]

Type III distal clavicular fractures involve the articular surface of the acromioclavicular joint alone (Fig. 12-59). Although type II fractures may have intra-articular extension (Fig. 12-60), in type III fractures there is a break in the articular surface without a ligamentous injury. The type III injury may be subtle, may be confused with a first-degree acromioclavicular separation, and may require special views to visualize. It may, in fact, present as late degenerative arthrosis of the acromioclavicular joint. In addition, it has been suggested that "weight-lifters clavicle"—resorption of the distal end of the clavicle—may occur from increased vascularity secondary to microtrauma or microfractures.[26,172,210]

It appears logical to add two more types of distal clavicular fractures, because in some cases bone displacement occurs secondary to deforming muscle forces, yet the coracoclavicular ligaments remain attached to bone or periosteum. Type IV fractures

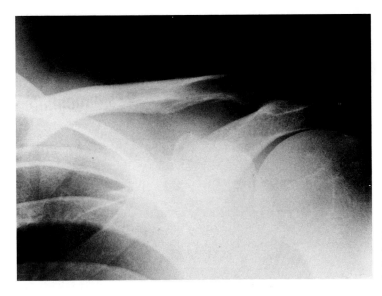

Fig. 12-56. A type I fracture of the distal clavicle seen radiographically. The fragments are held in place securely by intact coraclavicular and acromioclavicular ligaments.

occur in children and may be confused with complete acromioclavicular separation. Called "pseudodislocation" of the acromioclavicular joint, these injuries typically occur in children younger than 16 years.[220] The distal clavicle fractures, but the acromioclavicular joint remains intact. In children and young adults, there is a relatively loose attachment between bone and periosteum. The proximal fragment ruptures through the thin periosteum, and may be displaced upward by muscular forces. The coracoclavicular ligaments remain attached to the periosteum or are avulsed with a small piece of bone.[59,67,220] Clinically and radiographically, it may be impossible to distinguish between grade III ac-

romioclavicular separations, type II fractures of the distal clavicle, and the type IV fracture with rupture of the periosteum.[172,174,175]

In type V fractures, occurring in adults, neither of the main fracture fragments has functional coracoclavicular ligaments. These fragments are displaced by the deforming muscles, as in type I distal clavicular fractures, but the coracoclavicular ligaments are intact and remain attached to a small, third, comminuted intermediary segment.[194] This fracture is thought to be more unstable than the type II distal clavicular fracture (See Fig. 12-60).

Group III fractures, or fractures of the inner third of the clavicle, comprise 5% to 6% of clavicular fractures. As with distal clavicular fractures, these

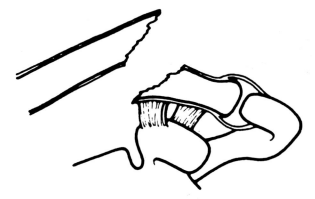

Fig. 12-57. A type IIA distal clavicle fracture. In type IIA, both conoid and trapezoid ligaments are on the distal segment, while the proximal segment, without ligamentous attachments, is displaced. *(Courtesy of C. Rockwood, M.D.)*

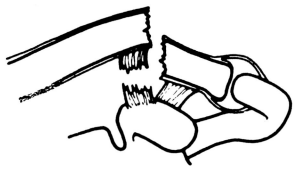

Fig. 12-58. A type IIB fracture of the distal clavicle. The conoid ligament is ruptured, while the trapezoid ligament remains attached to the distal segment. The proximal fragment is displaced. *(Courtesy of C. Rockwood, M.D.)*

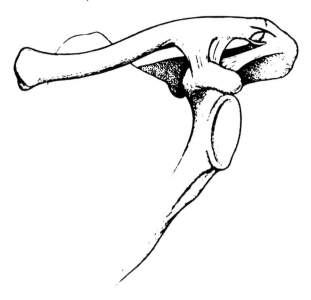

Fig. 12-59. A type III distal clavicle fracture, involving only the articular surface of the acromioclavicular joint. There is no ligamentous disruption or displacement. These fractures present as late degenerative changes of the joint.

can be subdivided according to the integrity of the ligamentous structures. If the costoclavicular ligaments remain intact and attached to the outer fragment, there is little or no displacement.[5,125,203] Satisfactory x-rays are crucial, because these fractures often are overlooked because of bony overlap. When these lesions occur in children, they usually are epiphyseal fractures (Fig. 12-61).[44] In adults, articular surface injuries can also lead to degenerative changes.[172,281]

One additional injury to consider is the panclavicular dislocation ("traumatic floating clavicle").[15,81,111,202] This is not actually classified as a clavicular fracture, but neither is it an isolated sternoclavicular or acromioclavicular separation. In this injury, both sternoclavicular ligaments and coracoclavicular ligamentous structures are disrupted.

MECHANISMS OF INJURY

Because the clavicle is the most frequently fractured bone, a great many mechanisms of injury—both traumatic and nontraumatic—have been reported.[60]

TRAUMA IN INFANTS AND CHILDREN

Fractures of the clavicle in children share many of the same mechanisms of injury as in adults, and may occur either by a direct blow to the clavicle or point of the shoulder or an indirect blow, such as a fall on an outstretched hand. However, some fractures are unique to children, including obstetrical clavicular fractures and plastic bowing injuries.

Birth Fractures

In 15,000 deliveries, between 1954 and 1959, Rubin found clavicular fractures to be the most common birth injury.[223] Although it has been stated that intrapartum traumatic injuries are decreasing

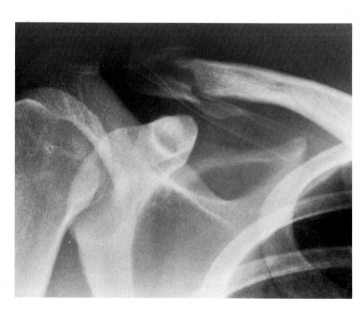

Fig. 12-60. Although there is an intra-articular component to this fracture, it is not a type III fracture, but a type II with intra-articular extension.

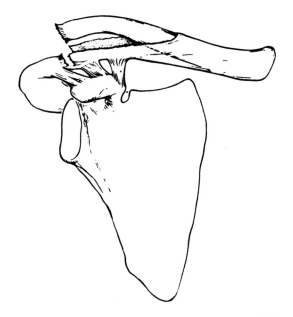

Fig. 12-61. A type IV fracture, which occurs in children and has been called a "pseudodislocation" of the acromioclavicular joint. The coracoclavicular ligaments remain attached to the bone or the periosteum while the proximal fragment ruptures through the thin superior periosteum and may be displaced upward by muscle forces. *(Dameron, T. B., Jr., and Rockwood, C. A., Jr.: Fractures and Dislocations of the Shoulder. In Rockwood C. A., Jr.; Wilkins, K. E.; and King, R. E. (eds.): Fractures in Children, p. 635. Philadelphia, J.B. Lippincott, 1984.)*

owing to improved obstetrical care,[91,269] the incidence of birth-related clavicular fractures remains quite high, and may actually be increasing.[8] Moir found an incidence of clavicular fractures of 5 per 1000 vertex births, increasing to 160 per 1000 in breech presentations.[163] The mechanism of injury in the full-term newborn infant delivered vaginally, when the baby is in a cephalic presentation, is compression of the leading clavicle against the maternal symphysis pubis.[149,256] In a breech delivery, direct traction may occur as the obstetrician, trying to depress the shoulders and free the arm to deliver the head, may produce the same bony injury.[121,186,254]

An overall incidence of approximately 2.8 to 7.2 per 1000 births exists, and several factors appear to be involved (in addition to type of delivery and presentation).

BIRTH WEIGHT

Birth weight clearly plays a role: the incidence of clavicular fractures increases with increasing birth weight and larger children.[29,87] In one study, fewer mothers of infants with clavicular fractures had prenatal care, making the predelivery identification of increased birth weight problematic.[186] Children weighing 3800 to 4000 g and those larger than 52 cm seem to be at more risk for fracture.

SHOULDER DYSTOCIA

In one study no birth fractures occurred in infants with biclavicular diameters of less than 12 cm. The study also suggested that the McRoberts position, as compared with the lithotomy position, decreased the extraction force, the force on the brachial plexus, and the incidence of clavicular fracture.[89]

PHYSICIAN EXPERIENCE

The experience of the physician is probably related to the rate of clavicular birth fractures. Cohen and Otto reported an increased incidence of clavicular fractures when babies were delivered by less experienced residents, with a decreased incidence for each year of obstetrical experience.[30] This certainly is a statistic that merits consideration in obstetrical house staff training.

METHOD OF DELIVERY

The method of delivery also is important. There is an increased risk of fracture with midforceps deliveries, calling into question the wisdom of this obstetrical maneuver. On the other hand, Balata and colleagues noted no fractures in babies delivered by cesarean section.[8]

CONTROL AND TRAUMA OF LABOR

In addition to birth weight and gestational age, Gilbert and Tchabo showed an increased predisposition for clavicular fractures with a prolonged second stage of labor and a primiparous patient.[86] Others have shown that the incidence of severely traumatic delivery and clavicular fractures can be decreased by observing certain procedures to decrease fetal distress at the end of the expulsion phase.[232]

Others have shown no relationship between clavicular fractures and the type of anesthesia, the length of active labor, the length of second stage, Apgar score, or parity of the mother.

The exact type of fracture that occurs during delivery varies, with incomplete, greenstick, and bicortical disruption—with or without displacement—all having been reported.[255]

In one study, males were more commonly affected than females. Also, the right clavicle was fractured more frequently than the left;[8] this is explained by the fact that the presentation of the fetus usually is as the left occiput anterior (LOA), and thus most of the pressure is placed on the right shoulder by the symphysis pubis.[186]

Other Fractures in Infants and Children

Fractures of the clavicle are particularly common in childhood, with nearly half of all clavicular fractures occurring before 7 years of age.[11]

These fractures commonly result from a fall on the point of the shoulder or on an outstretched hand. In younger children, the fall commonly is from a high chair, bed, or a changing table. The fracture may occasionally be caused by a direct violent force applied from the front of the clavicle; as with other fractures of long bones, clavicular fractures may occur in physically abused children.[40]

Direct or indirect trauma to the child's clavicle may result in incomplete or greenstick fractures, rather than displaced fractures.[179] In addition, trauma to the child's clavicle may result in plastic bowing alone, without evidence of cortical disruption. This injury must be differentiated from other causes of bowing (ie, metabolic disorders).[189,203] Such fractures, despite presenting with only bowing, on later examination usually show gross healing of complete fractures with obvious callus on x-ray films.[20,242]

TRAUMA IN ADULTS

The incidence of clavicular fractures in adults appears to be increasing owing to a number of factors, including the rise in high-velocity vehicular injuries and the increased popularity of contact sports for adults.[50,76] The mechanisms of injury of clavicular fractures in adults have been widely reported to consist of either direct or indirect forces. It has generally been assumed that the most common mechanism is a fall on an outstretched hand.[50] However, Allman, when dividing clavicular fractures into three groups, proposed different mechanisms of injuries for each fracture group.[5] He felt that in group I (middle-third) fractures, the most common mechanism was a fall on an outstretched hand, with the force being transmitted up the arm and across the glenohumeral joint and dispersing along the clavicle. He found the group II (distal) fracture most likely to result from a fall on the lateral shoulder, driving the shoulder and scapular downward. In the group III (proximal) fracture, he cited indirect force applied from the lateral side as the most likely mechanism.[203]

Fowler[73] pointed out that almost all clavicular injuries follow a fall or a blow on the point of the shoulder, whereas a blow to the bone itself rarely is the cause (except in athletics, particularly stick sports such as lacrosse or hockey).[239] In a large series of clavicular fractures (342 patients) studied by San Sarankutsy and Turner, 91% had a fall or sustained a blow to the point of the shoulder, while only 1% had a fall on the outstretched hand.[228]

More recently, Stanley and associates studied 150 consecutive patients with clavicular fractures, with 81% of the patients presenting detailed information about the mechanism of injury.[246] These investigators found 94% had fractured the clavicle from a direct blow on the shoulder, while only 6% had fallen on an outstretched hand. Further biomechanical analysis revealed that a direct injury produces a critical buckling load, which is exceeded at a compression force equilavent to the body weight, resulting in fracture of the bone. When the force is applied along the axis of the arm, the buckling force is rarely reached in the clavicle. These investigators recorded fractures at every site along the clavicle with a direct injury to the point of the shoulder, and found that little support could be produced for Allman's concept that fractures at different anatomic sites had different mechanisms of injury. In addition, they theorized that a direct blow to the shoulder might even be the mechanism of injury in those who described a fall on the outstretched hand, for as the hand makes contact with the ground, the patient's body weight and falling velocity are such that movement does not stop, but the fall continues, with the shoulder becoming the upper limb's next contact point with the ground.

Another indirect mechanism of middle-third clavicular fractures occurs from a direct force on the top of the shoulder, which forces the clavicle against the first rib and often produces a spiral fracture of the middle third.[50]

Traumatic fractures of the clavicle have also been reported in association with seizures.[71]

NONTRAUMATIC FRACTURES

It is well recognized that the clavicle can be the site of neoplastic or infectious destruction of bone. Fracture also may occur from relatively minor trauma or following radiation to a neoplastic area (Fig. 12-62). Certainly, lack of a traumatic episode should cause the clinician to consider the possibility of a pathologic bone. In addition to both malignant and benign lesions,[17] pathologic fractures of the clavicle also have been described in association with arteriovenous malformation, an entity that may mimic neoplasm.[162]

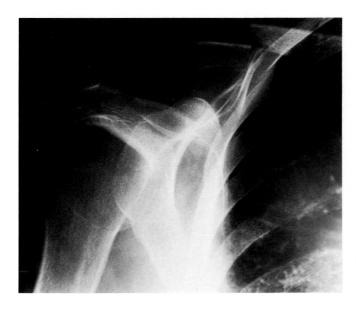

Fig. 12-62. A pathologic fracture of the clavicle from metastatic thyroid carcinoma. The patient presented without a traumatic episode.

Atraumatic stress fractures have also been reported in the clavicle.[124] In addition, spontaneous fractures of the medial end of the clavicle have been reported as "pseudotumors" following radical neck dissection.[41,72,187,253]

Synthetic material used for coracoclavicular disruption has also been reported to produce stress fractures in the clavicle, with subsequent nonunion.[55]

CLINICAL PRESENTATION

BIRTH FRACTURES

There are two clinical presentations of birth fractures—those that are clinically inapparent and those that are clinically apparent (pseudoparalysis).

Clinically inapparent clavicular birth fractures can be very difficult to diagnose, because there are few clinical symptoms. A crack heard during the delivery may be the only clue to the fracture.[11] Although it is uncertain whether these lesions are truly asymptomatic, Farkas emphasized that many clinically inapparent birth fractures are missed in the initial neonatal examination. Of the five cases of clavicular fractures in 300 newborns in his series, none were suspected following routine physical examination in the delivery room and newborn nursery.[68] However, on re-examination, crepitus could usually be demonstrated at the fracture site (Fig. 12-63). In a large study, Joseph and Rosenfeld screened 626 consecutive infants delivered vagi-

nally for fractures, and identified 18 clavicular fractures; of these, 17 were not noted until discharge examinations or follow-up visits, underscoring the need for repeat examinations.[115]

Although these fractures may be easily overlooked, there are some signs that can be helpful. First, clavicular birth fractures usually are unilateral, so close examination may reveal asymmetry of the clavicular contour or shortening of the neck line. Usually it is difficult to feeling the margins of the affected clavicle when compared to the normal side.[115] Often the fracture is first recognized when the swelling caused by fracture callus is recognized by the mother, typically 7 to 11 days after birth.[37]

In *clinically apparent* clavicular birth fractures (Fig. 12-64), the infant's clinical appearance is one of having a "pseudoparalysis" of the extremity, that is, the infant is disinclined or unwilling to use the extremity, and there is a unilateral lack of movement of the entire upper limb, either spontaneously or during elicitation of the Moro reflex.[74,227] Again, because these often are complete fractures, local swelling, tenderness, and crepitus may suggest the diagnosis. Clavicular birth fractures must be distinguished from other conditions that may make the infant disinclined or unable to use the extremity, such as brachial plexus injury, separation of the proximal humeral epiphysis, and acute osteomyelitis of the clavicle or proximal humerus. It is important to remember both a fractured clavicle and a brachial plexus injury may be present.[255] In one study, one of 19 clavicular fractures resulted in brachial plexus injury.[186]

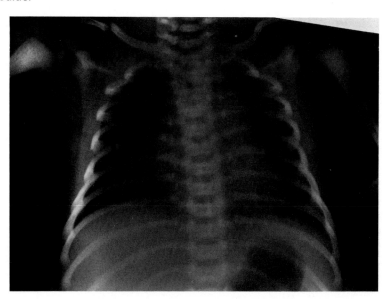

Fig. 12-63. An obstetric fracture in a 1-day-old infant. The fracture is complete and presented with crepitus demonstrable at the fracture site.

OTHER FRACTURES IN INFANTS AND CHILDREN

More than half of clavicular fractures in children occur before the age of 7. Because these fractures may be incomplete or of the greenstick variety, they may not be obvious and thus may be overlooked. The mother may notice that the baby cries after being picked up and appears to be hurt.[11] The baby does not seem to use the arm naturally and cries when it is used for any activities or moved during dressing. On palpation, there may be a tender, uneven, upper border of the clavicle, which is asymmetric when compared to the contralateral side. As with a newborn, the mother may take the baby to the pediatrician because of the "sudden" appearance of a lump (Fig. 12-65).[44]

However, with a complete fracture in a child who is ambulatory and verbal, the diagnosis is usually obvious. In addition to the child's complaints of pain localized to the clavicle, fracture displacement, and the resulting muscle displacement, produces a typical deformity. The shoulder on the affected side may appear lower and droop forward and inward. The child splints the involved extremity against the body and supports the affected elbow with the con-

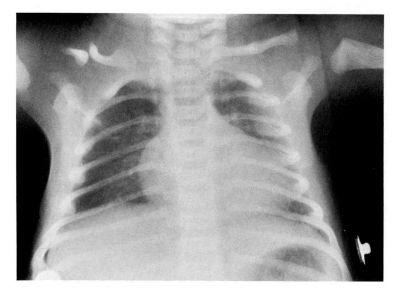

Fig. 12-64. In a newborn with multiple fractures at birth, this clavicular fracture was overlooked until it became evident that the infant had a disinclination to use the extremity. The fracture causes pain, and the infant presents clinically with a "pseudoparalysis" of the extremity (ie, unwillingness to move the upper extremity).

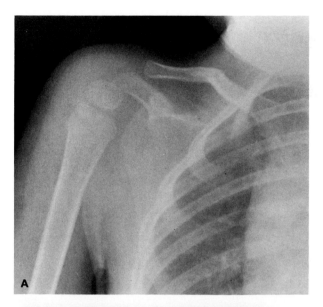

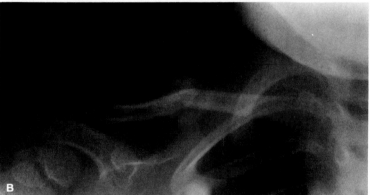

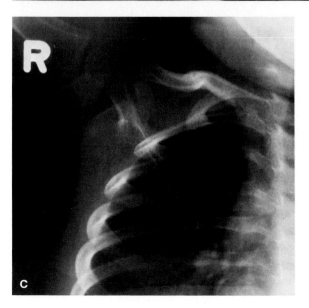

Fig. 12-65. (**A**) A greenstick clavicular fracture in a 2-year-old child. The patient did not use the arm and cried whenever it was elevated. (**B**) Two and a half weeks later, there is prominent callus formation manifest clinically as a bump. (**C**) Five months later the fracture is healed with little residual bump evident.

tralateral hand. Because of the pull of the sterno-cleidomastoid on the proximal fragment, the child tilts the head toward and the chin away from the side of the fracture to relax the pull of this muscle (Fig. 12-66).[255] Physical examination reveals tenderness, crepitus, and swelling typical for this fracture at any age.

Remember that up to 16 years of age, complete acromioclavicular separations are very unusual. What may present clinically as a high-riding clavicle through the acromioclavicular joint and an apparent acromioclavicular separation, often is either a transperiosteal distal clavicular fracture or, more commonly, a rupture through the periosteum with a distal clavicular fracture, in which the coracoclavicular ligaments remain attached to the peri-

osteum. This lesion often is not recognized for what it is in the child younger than 16 years.[59]

Likewise, because the sternal epiphysis is the last long-bone epiphysis to fuse with the metaphysis (usually between 22 and 25 years of age), an epiphyseal injury may occur in the adult patient. Many misdiagnosed sternoclavicular dislocations are, in fact, separations through the medial clavicular epiphysis. Occasionally, sternoclavicular separations occur with adjacent clavicular fractures in children.[23,137]

Atlantoaxial rotatory fixation has recently been emphasized as a traumatic injury accompanying fractures of the clavicle in children. Early diagnosis is important, requiring a high index of suspicion and usually requiring CT scan or fluoroscopy with spot films for diagnosis.[88]

FRACTURES IN ADULTS

Because of the characteristic clinical presentation in adults, displaced fractures of the clavicle present little difficulty with diagnosis if the patient is seen soon after injury. There is usually a clear history of some form of either direct or indirect injury to the shoulder. Clinical deformity is obvious and may be out of proportion to the amount of discomfort the patient experiences.[11] The proximal fragment is displaced upward and backward and may tent the skin. Although compounding of this fracture is unusual, it can occur (Fig. 12-67).[213] The patient usually presents splinting the involved extremity at the side, because any movement elicits pain. The involved arm droops forward and downward (Fig. 12-68). Although the initial deformity may be obvious later, with acute swelling of soft tissue and hemorrhage, the deformity may be obscured. With a fracture near the ligamentous structures (ie, acromioclavicular, sternoclavicular joints), the deformity may mimic a purely ligamentous injury.

Examination reveals tenderness directly over the fracture site, and any movement of the arm is painful. There may be ecchymosis over the fracture site, especially if severe displacement of the bony fragments has produced associated tearing of soft tissue. The patient may angle his head toward the injury, attempting to relax the pull of the trapezius on the fragment. As in children, the patient may be more comfortable with the chin tilted to the opposite side. Gentle palpation and manipulation usually will produce crepitus and motion, and the site of the fracture is easily palpable owing to the subcutaneous position of the bone. The skin over the clavicle, the scapula, or the chest wall may give a clue

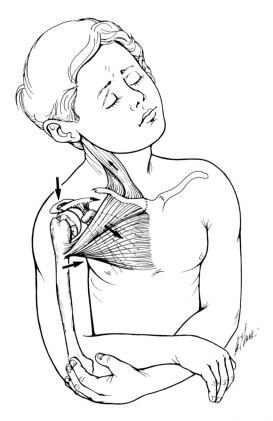

Fig. 12-66. Clinical presentation of a displaced clavicle fracture in a child. The shoulder on the affected side appears lower, and droops forward and inward. The child splints the involved extremity against the body and supports the affected elbow with the contralateral hand. The child tilts the head toward and the chin away from the site of the fracture to relax the pull of the sternocleidomastoid.

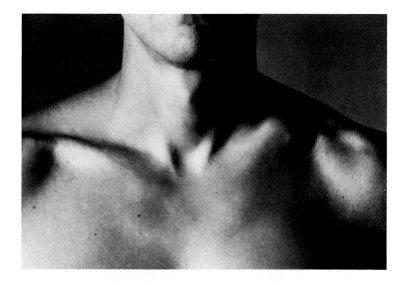

Fig. 12-67. An adult clavicle fracture showing prominence of the proximal fragment, which is displaced upward and backward. This may tent the skin, although compounding is unusual.

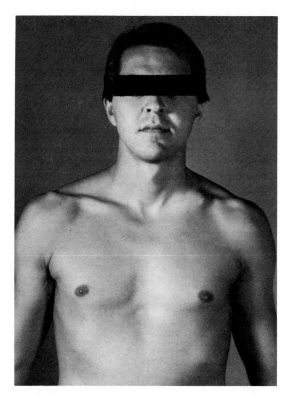

Fig. 12-68. With an adult clavicle fracture, the arm may droop forward and downward to varying degrees.

to the mechanism of injury and may indicate other areas to be evaluated for associated injuries. The lungs must be examined for the presence of symmetric breath sounds, and the whole extremity must be carefully examined.

Undisplaced fractures or isolated fractures of the articular surfaces may not cause deformity, and these may be overlooked unless they are specifically sought for radiographically. If the diagnosis is in doubt, special x-ray views or a repeat x-ray film of the clavicle in 7 to 10 days may be indicated.

The panclavicular dislocation is typically produced by extreme and forceful protraction of the shoulder. This injury usually is the result of a major traumatic episode—such as a high-speed traffic accident, a fall from a height, or a very heavy object falling on the shoulder[81]—although it has been reported following a minor fall at home.[111] Clinically, there is usually bruising over the spine of the scapula, and swelling and tenderness at both ends of the clavicle. This injury is associated with antero-superior sternoclavicular dislocation and either posterosuperior or subjacent displacement of the clavicle. The whole clavicle may be freely mobile and may feel as if it is floating. X-rays usually confirm this injury.

ASSOCIATED INJURIES

In 1830 Gross reported that, "Fractures of the clavicle usually assume a mild aspect, being seldom accompanied by any serious accident."[92] Although statistically most clavicular fractures are relatively innocuous, serious associated injuries may occur. A delay in treating these injuries may be life-threatening.[53] Therefore, it is critical in a patient with a clavicular fracture that a careful examination of the entire upper extremity be performed, with particular emphasis on the neurovascular status, and, as mentioned, a careful examination of the lungs.[53]

Associated injuries accompanying acute fractures of the clavicle may be divided into (1) associated skeletal injuries, (2) injuries to the lungs and pleura, (3) brachial plexus injuries, and (4) vascular injuries.

ASSOCIATED SKELETAL INJURIES

Associated skeletal injuries include separations or fracture–dislocations of the sternoclavicular or acromioclavicular joints (Fig. 12-69).[25,118,137,260] As might be anticipated with ipsilateral sternoclavicular or acromioclavicular joint injuries, closed reduction of the ligamentous injury is usually impossible because of the accompanying clavicular fracture.[118]

Head and neck injuries may be present,[280] especially with displaced distal clavicular fractures; in one series, 10% of patients were comatose.[175]

Fractures of the first rib are frequent, but are easily overlooked.[3,277] These rib fractures may be directly responsible for accompanying lung, brachial plexus, or subclavian vein injuries. Underrecognition of rib fractures may be related to the fact that they are not easily seen on standard chest x-rays. Weiner and O'Dell recommended an anteroposterior view of either the cervical spine or the thoracic spine, plus a lateral view of the thoracic spine to detect rib fractures.[277] The location of first rib fracture may be either the ipsilateral or contralateral rib to the clavicular fracture. Weiner outlined how

a number of these rib fractures occur. The scalenus anticus muscle attaches on a tubercle of the first rib. On either side of this tubercle lies a groove for the subclavian vein anteriorly and the subclavian artery posteriorly. Posterior to the groove for the subclavian artery lies a roughened area for the attachment of the scalene medius muscle. These two muscles elevate the rib during inspiration. The serratus anterior arises from the outer surfaces of the upper eight ribs and fixes the rib posteriorly during inspiration. These structures may interact to contribute to fractures of the first rib as the clavicle is fractured. Three mechanisms have been theorized to be responsible for this combination of injuries: (1) indirect forces transmitted through the manubrium; (2) avulsion fracture at the weakest portion of the rib by the scalene anticus; and (3) injury to the lateral clavicle, which causes an acromioclavicular separation that produces indirect force from the subclavius muscle on the costal cartilage and anterior aspect of the first rib.[204,277]

Fractures of the clavicle may also be associated with scapulothoracic dissociation—disruption of the scapulothoracic articulation presenting with swelling of the shoulder, lateral displacement of the clavicle, severe neurovascular injury, and fracture of the clavicle or the acromioclavicular or sternoclavicular joint.[56]

INJURIES TO THE LUNGS AND PLEURA

A number of authors have commented on the potentially serious complication of pneumothorax or hemothorax associated with fractures of the clavicle. This is a concern because the apical pleura and upper lung lobes lie adjacent to the clavicle (Fig. 12-70). Rowe reported a 3% incidence of pneumothorax in a series of 690 clavicular fractures,

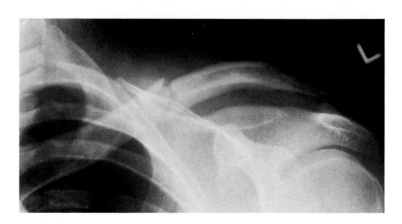

Fig. 12-69. An unusual clavicular fracture associated with a complete acromioclavicular separation. The associated clavicular fracture makes treatment of the ligamentous injury very difficult.

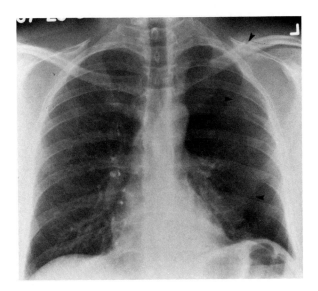

Fig. 12-70. A fracture of the left clavicle associated with a left pneumothorax. The lung markings are absent on the left side. There is also a fracture of the second rib.

although he did not comment on how many had associated rib or scapular fractures.[222] Although it is easy to see how a severely displaced fracture can puncture the pleura with a sharp shard of bone, the x-ray appearance may be misleadingly benign, with little evidence to suggest what might have been significant fragment displacement at the time of injury.[53] Careful physical examination of the lung at the time of the initial presentation is essential, searching for the presence and symmetry of breath sounds. In addition, an upright chest film appears to be important in the assessment of all patients with clavicular fractures who have decreased breath sounds or other physical findings suggestive of a pneumothorax; particularly attention should be paid to the lung outline on the chest film.[150] This is especially true in the multiply traumatized or unconscious patient who has neither obvious blunt chest trauma nor any external signs of trauma to the chest that might yield a clue to lung or pleural complications.[53,109,150,247,250,283]

Tears of the trachea or main bronchi from blunt chest trauma have also been associated with fractures of the clavicle. These usually present either as abnormalities in the appearance of the endotracheal tube (cuff over distention or extraluminal position of tip) or the radiographic appearance of lung collapse toward the lateral chest wall and away from the midline.[267]

BRACHIAL PLEXUS INJURIES

Although nerve injuries with clavicular fractures are rare, acute injuries to the brachial plexus do occur. The neurovascular bundle emerges from the thoracic outlet under the clavicle on top of the first rib.[214,276] As it passes under the clavicle, the neurovascular bundle is protected to a certain extent by the thick, medial clavicular bone. Thus, considerable trauma usually is necessary to damage the brachial plexus and break the clavicle at the same time. When the force is severe enough to do this, a subclavian vascular injury often occurs concomitantly (Fig. 12-71). Forces resulting in nerve injury usually comes from above to downward or from the front to downward. As the force is applied, the nerves may be stretched, with the fulcrum of maximum tension being the transverse process of the cervical vertebra.[156] The roots also can be torn above the clavicle or avulsed from their attachment to the spinal cord.[12] Although the posterior periosteum, subclavius muscles, and bone offer some protection to the underlying plexus, the plexus may be injured directly by bone fragments. This is especially important to emphasize, for manipulation of clavicular fragments should not be done without adequate x-ray studies of the position of these fracture fragments.[270]

If the brachial plexus is directly injured, the ulnar nerve usually is involved, because this portion of the plexus lies adjacent to the middle third of the clavicle.

VASCULAR INJURIES

Acute vascular injuries are unusual, owing to many of the same local anatomic factors that protect the nerves from direct injury. The subclavius muscle and thick deep cervical fascia also act as barriers to direct injury to the vessels. After initial displacement of the fracture fragment occurs, if the adjacent vessels are intact, they are unlikely to be further injured, because the distal fragment is pulled downward and forward by the weight of the limb, while the proximal fragment is pulled upward and backward by the pull of the trapezius. Thus, as with acute nerve injury, a major trauma is usually required to produce an acute vascular insult.[196] Nevertheless, injuries have been reported, even with a greenstick fracture.[161] In addition, acute vascular compression resulting from fracture angulation has been described.[47]

Potential vascular injuries include laceration, occlusion, spasm, or acute compression. The ves-

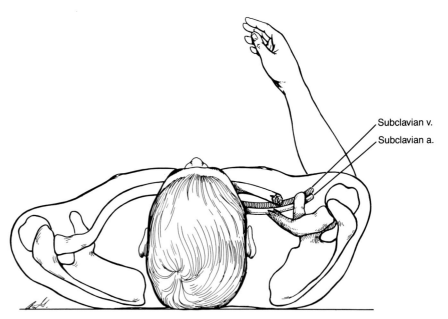

Subclavian v.
Subclavian a.

Fig. 12-71. As the clavicle fractures and displaces, the subclavian vessels immediately posterior to the clavicle may be injured by sharp shards of bone.

sels most commonly injured are the subclavian artery, subclavian vein, and internal jugular vein.[112,129,141,155] The subclavian vein is particularly vulnerable to tearing, because it is fixed to the clavicle by fascial aponeurosis.[93,249] Injuries to the suprascapular artery and axillary artery have also been reported.[107,265] Laceration may result in life-threatening hemorrhage, whereas arterial thrombus and occlusion may lead to distal ischemia. Damage to the arterial wall may lead to aneurysm formation and late embolic phenomena. Venous thrombosis also may be problematic, in that while its clinical presentation is not typically life- or limb-threatening, there is a potential for pulmonary embolism, which certainly may be.[230] Clinical recognition of an acute vascular injury may be difficult, particularly in a patient who is unconscious or in shock. Although a complete laceration certainly may present with a life-threatening hemorrhage or an extremity that is cold, pulseless, and pale, a partial laceration is more likely to present with uncontrolled, life-threatening bleeding. The color and temperature of the extremity may be normal, but the absence of a pulse, the presence of a bruit, or a pulsatile hematoma (as the hematoma is walled off or produces a false aneurysm) should make the clinician strongly suspicious of a major vascular injury.[265] If there is a significant obstruction to blood flow, the injured limb is usually colder than the uninjured limb, and there also may be a difference in blood pressure between the two limbs.[283] Vascular contusion or spasm may result in thrombotic and later thromboembolic phenomena.[278] It is

sometimes difficult to recognize the difference between arterial spasm and interruption or occlusion. It may be reasonable to consider a sympathetic block to help distinguish a spasm from more serious injury.

Although penetrating trauma often focuses attention on the clinical diagnosis of vascular injury, blunt trauma may produce as many as 9% of subclavian artery injuries. In one series, all patients with distal subclavian artery involvement from blunt trauma had fractures of the clavicle and all had absent radial pulses. Eight of 15 had critical ischemia of the hand.[38]

If major injury to a vessel is suspected, an arteriogram should be performed.[283] In the rare event of a torn large vessel, surgical exploration is mandatory. To gain adequate exposure, as much of the clavicle should be excised as needed to isolate and repair the injured major vessel. Although in some instances the vessel may be ligated, ligation of a major vessel in the elderly patient may well be dangerous because of inadequate remaining circulation to the extremity. In any event, a surgeon skilled in the decision-making and techniques regarding vascular repair is essential if a major injury has occurred.

RADIOGRAPHIC EVALUATION

SHAFT FRACTURES

In most instances of clavicular shaft fractures, because of the clinical deformity, the diagnosis is not in doubt, and x-rays are confirmatory. Nevertheless, to get an accurate evaluation of the fragment position, two projections of the clavicle are typically used—an anteroposterior and a 45° cephalic tilt view. In the anteroposterior view, the proximal fragment is typically displaced upward and the distal fragment downward (Fig. 12-72). In the 45° cephalic tilt view, the tube is directed from below upward and more accurately assesses the anteroposterior relationship of the two fragments (Fig. 12-73).[278] Quesana recommended two views at right angles to each other, a 45° angle superiorly and a 45° angle inferiorly, to assess the extent and displacement of clavicular fractures.[207]

Rowe suggested that when ordering an anteroposterior study, the film should include the upper third of the humerus, the shoulder girdle, and the upper lung fields, so other shoulder girdle fractures and pneumothorax can be identified more quickly.[222] The configuration of the fracture is also important, because it may give a clue to associated injuries. While the usual clavicular shaft fracture in the adult is slightly oblique, if more comminuted, and especially if the middle spike is projecting from superior to inferior, this usually results from a greater force, and may alert the surgeon to the potential for associated neurovascular or pulmonary injuries.

Children's fractures may be greenstick, nondisplaced, or present only as bony bowing, and thus the diagnosis of shaft fractures may be more difficult (Fig. 12-74). This is especially true in newborns or infants, where the clinical presentation may be dif-

ficult to assess. Movement by the child or bony overlap may obscure radiographic detail, and an incomplete fracture may not be noted. However, the surrounding soft tissues of the clavicle are normally and frequently displayed as parallel shadows above the body of the clavicle. Although this "accompanying shadow" may not be seen along the proximal third of the clavicle medial to the crossing of the first rib, it is invariably present on most x-rays. Suspicion for clavicular fractures should be aroused by loss of the "accompanying shadow" unilaterally.[242] If there is any doubt about the presence of a fracture in the child, a repeat x-ray taken 5 to 10 days postinjury will usually reveal callus formation.

Recently, use of ultrasound has been described for evaluation of clavicular birth fractures.[121] These fractures may easily be overlooked and may be confused clinically with birth palsy. Katz and associates noted no difference in diagnostic accuracy between ultrasound and plain x-ray studies. In addition, a medial clavicular fracture not seen on plain film was picked up with ultrasonography. In fact, the authors noted that with real-time ultrasound, the individual fracture fragments were seen to move up and down with respiration.

With either plain x-rays or ultrasound, it may be difficult to differentiate congenital pseudoarthrosis from an acute fracture. But the radiographic features, the lack of trauma, and the absence of callus usually help distinguish an atraumatic condition from a birth fracture.

It has been reported that a false-positive Indium-

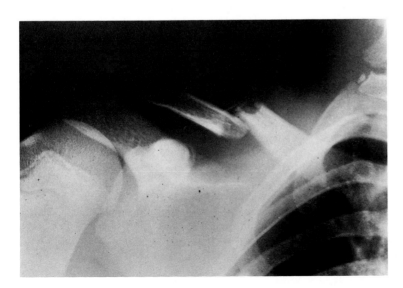

Fig. 12-72. An anteroposterior view of right clavicle fracture, showing the typical deformity with a proximal fragment displaced superiorly.

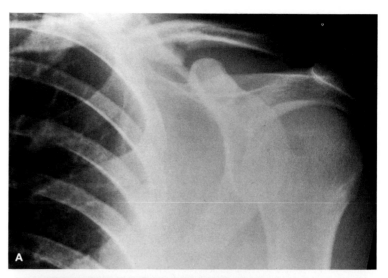

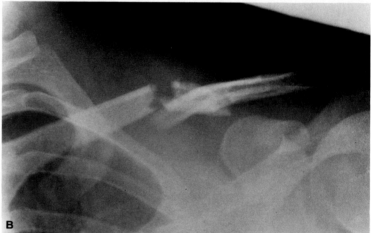

Fig. 12-73. (**A**) An anteroposterior view of a left comminuted clavicular fracture poorly defines and identifies the fracture fragments, owing to overlying bone in the area of the fragments. (**B**) However, when a 20° to 45° cephalic tilt view is obtained, the fracture anatomy is more clearly delineated.

111 white blood cell scan, most useful in identifying infection, can be produced by a fracture of the clavicle. This is a potential source of confusion in the child being evaluated for a febrile episode.[75]

FRACTURES OF THE DISTAL THIRD

In both children and adults, the usual radiographic views obtained for shaft fractures are inadequate to completely assess distal clavicular fractures. The standard exposure for evaluation of shoulder or shaft fractures overexposes the distal clavicle. The usual exposure for the distal clavicle should be approximately one third that used for the shoulder joint. This is especially true if it is important to determine articular surface involvement.

Type II distal clavicular fractures may be particularly difficult to diagnose, because the usual anteroposterior and 40° cephalic tilt views typically do not reveal the extent of injury.[175] If the exposure is appropriate, a distal clavicular fracture may be identified on the anteroposterior and lateral views of the trauma series (Figs. 12-75 and 12-76), but to accurately assess the extent of injury and the presence or absence of associated ligamentous damage, Neer recommended three views: (1) the posteroanterior view of *both* shoulders should be obtained on one plate, with the patient erect and with a 10-pound weight strapped to each wrist (Fig. 12-77). If the distance between the coracoid and medial fragment is increased compared to the normal side, ligamentous detachment from the medial fragment

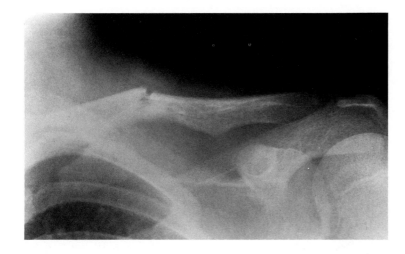

Fig. 12-74. A greenstick fracture of the left clavicle in a 14-year-old patient. In these patients, in whom the fracture line is not complete, the diagnosis may be more difficult to ascertain.

can be assumed to be present. However, because much of the fracture displacement is in the antero-posterior plane, Neer suggested two additional views. (2) An anterior 45° oblique view, with the patient erect and the injured shoulder against the plate gives a lateral view of the scapula and shows the medial fragment posteriorly with the outer fragment displaced anteriorly. (3) A posterior 45° oblique view with the patient erect and the injured shoulder against the plate, also demonstrates the extent of separation of the two fragments.

In a type II distal clavicular fracture, if x-ray views at right angles and with cephalic tilt show good bony overlap and proximity of the fragments, and if crepitation confirms contact between the fragments, stress radiographic views with weights are

probably not necessary; in fact, the use of weights may further displace otherwise minimally displaced fracture fragments (Figs. 12-78 to 12-80).

Articular surface fractures of the distal clavicle are easily overlooked unless high-quality x-rays are obtained. If the fracture is not seen on a plain x-ray view and the clinical suspicion is strong, tomography or CT scan may reveal the presence and extent of an articular surface injury (Fig. 12-81).

FRACTURES OF THE MEDIAL THIRD

Fractures of the medial third may be particularly difficult to detect on routine x-rays owing to the overlap of ribs, vertebrae, and mediastinal shadows. However, a cephalic tilt view of 40° to 45° often

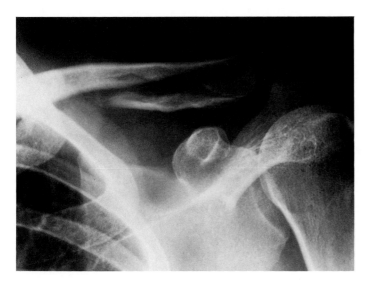

Fig. 12-75. An anteroposterior view of a distal clavicle fracture. This cephalic tilt view (approximately 15°) brings the clavicle and acromioclavicular joint away from the overlying bony anatomy.

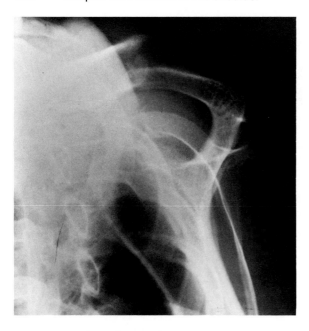

Fig. 12-76. A lateral view of a distal clavicular fracture. The displacement of the proximal segment is identified, but the fracture detail may be obscured by bony and soft tissue anatomy.

reveals the fracture, whether in a child or an adult. In children, particularly, fractures of the medial end of the clavicle are often misdiagnosed as sternoclavicular dislocations, when in fact they are usually epiphyseal injuries. As with distal clavicular injuries, tomography or CT scan may be useful to demonstrate the intra-articular or epiphyseal nature of injuries in this location.

DIFFERENTIAL DIAGNOSIS

ADULTS

In adults, fractures of the shaft of the clavicle usually are not confused with other diagnoses, although pathologic fractures are occasionally difficult to recognize. However, fractures of the distal or medial end of the clavicle may appear clinically to be complete acromioclavicular or sternoclavicular separations, although these rarely present confusion once proper radiographic studies are performed.

CHILDREN

In children, it may easy to confuse injuries to the clavicle with other entities, including congenital and other traumatic conditions.

Congenital Pseudarthrosis

When recognized at birth or shortly thereafter, congenital pseudarthrosis may be confused with either cleidocranial dysostosis or a birth fracture, especially if there is a history of some trauma associated with the delivery. However, birth fractures unite rapidly and leave no disability. The deformity of congenital pseudarthrosis may become more conspicuous as the child grows.[85] Clinically the lump is painless, and there is usually no history of injury, pain, or disability with this lesion.[128,209] It is invariably in the lateral portion of the middle third of the clavicle, and it usually affects the right clavicle, unless there is dextrocardia, when it may occur on the left side.[144,272] Bilateral congenital pseudarthrosis has been reported, particularly when there are bilateral cervical ribs.[44]

The etiology of this entity is unclear. Though a family history is not typical, in some reported cases there has been a familial incidence, raising the question of genetic transmission.[85]

Although there may be a history of trauma with the birth, this is probably incidental and most investigators now agree that congenital pseudarthrosis does not represent a nonunion of normal bone following trauma.[190] Abnormal intrauterine development probably plays the primary role in its appearance, and it has been suggested that pressure from the subclavian artery as it arches over the first rib and under the clavicle may be a primary factor in its development.[144,145] Cervical ribs may also displace the subclavian artery and cause pressure in the same area of the clavicle.[44]

Radiographically there are characteristic changes. The sternal fragment, consisting of the medial third of the clavicle, is larger and protrudes forward and upward, while the lateral half is situated below, pointing upward and backward, ending in a bulbous mass at the pseudarthrosis site. Other identifying features are an increase in the deformity with age, the proximity of the bone ends to one another, and a large, clinically palpable lump. This contrasts quite markedly with cleidocranial dysostosis.

Cleidocranial Dysostosis

Cleidocranial dysostosis is a hereditary abnormality of membranous bone, with the clavicle involved most frequently. The abnormality varies from a central defect to complete absence of the clavicle. The most common presentation is absence of the distal portion of the clavicle.[44,153] Radiographically, it is distinguished from congenital pseudarthrosis by the larger gap between the bone ends, and tapered ends of the clavicle, rather than larger, bul-

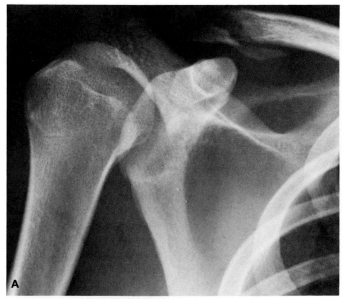

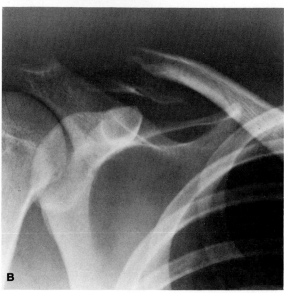

Fig. 12-77. (**A**) A fracture of the right distal clavicle. In an anteroposterior view, the fracture location is suggestive of ligamentous involvement, with the ligaments attached to the distal fragment. (**B**) The extent of ligamentous involvement is confirmed on a weighted view, where there is a widening of the coracoclavicular distance. The coracoclavicular ligaments are attached to the distal clavicular segment.

bous ends.[85] The bone is more clearly aplastic. In addition, multiple membranous bones are involved, and each of these may have its own clinical manifestations. Some children suffer from bossing or other skull defects, smallness of facial bones, scoliosis, abnormal epiphyses of hands or feet, and deficiencies of the pelvic ring. Usually there is a familial history of bone disorders.[4,65]

Sternoclavicular Dislocation

Epiphyseal fractures of the medial end of the clavicle may mimic sternoclavicular separations in children owing to the late closure of the sternal epiphysis. If it is important to distinguish these two entities, tomography or CT scanning may be indicated.

Acromioclavicular Separation

Fracture of the lateral clavicle in children may also appear identical—clinically and radiographically—to a complete acromioclavicular separation. If plain radiography does not identify the small fracture fragment, tomography or CT scanning may. However, because the coracoclavicular ligaments remain

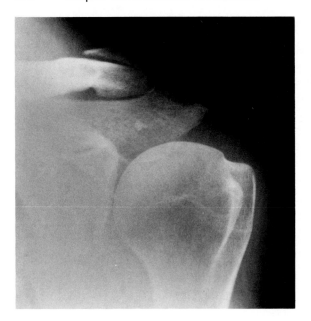

Fig. 12-78. A distal clavicular fracture. The proximal fragment has all the coracoclavicular ligaments attached to it, but there is good bony contact between the two segments.

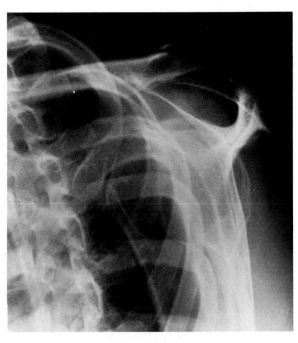

Fig. 12-79. With good bony contact in perpendicular views, weighted views usually are not necessary, and may, in fact, cause distraction of the fragments.

attached to the periosteal tube in children, and healing is uneventful, it is difficult to justify these more elaborate diagnostic modalities.[220,235]

Plastic Bowing

Plastic bowing may occur in young children without complete fracture of the clavicle. This must be differentiated from other causes of clavicular bowing and angulation.[189]

COMPLICATIONS

NONUNION

Despite the frequency of clavicular fractures, nonunion of unoperated shaft fractures is rare, with a reported incidence of 0.9% to 4%.[7,63,114,130,154,173,222,231,258,271] Although there is some debate in the literature as to the definition of clavicular non-

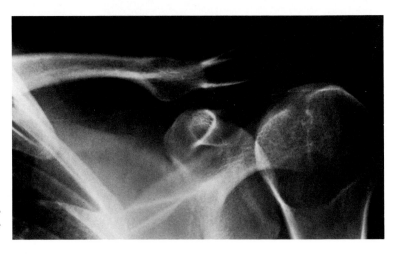

Fig. 12-80. This distal clavicle fracture healed uneventfully with nonoperative treatment.

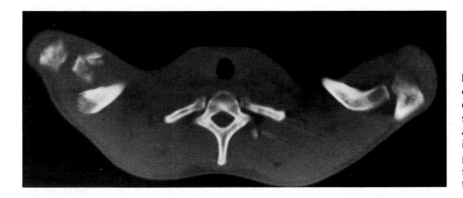

Fig. 12-81. CT scan of a right clavicular fracture. Not only does this image confirm the site of the clavicular fracture as the distal clavicle, but it identifies a previously unsuspected intra-articular extension of the distal clavicle fracture.

union, most authors consider it to be defined as failure to show clinical or radiographic progression of healing at 4 to 6 months;[116,142,206,225,279] there are some temporal differences between atrophic and hypertrophic nonunions. Manske and Szabo reported that tapered, sclerotic, atrophic bone ends at 16 weeks were unlikely to unite, and thus could be assumed to be a nonunion, but classified other fractures as delayed unions after 16 weeks as long as there were some signs of healing.[152] Bilateral post-traumatic pseudarthrosis also has been reported in an adult.[99]

While nonunion of the clavicle occurs predominantly in adults, it has also been described in children.[183] However, when nonunion is seen in a child, it is likely to be a congenital pseudarthrosis.

Predisposing Factors

There appear to be several factors predisposing to nonunion of the clavicle:

1. Inadequate immobilization
2. Severity of trauma
3. Refracture
4. Distal-third fracture
5. Marked displacement
6. Primary open reduction.

INADEQUATE IMMOBILIZATION

It has long been recognized that the clavicle is one of the most difficult bones to immobilize properly and completely following fracture while providing the patient with the simplicity and comfort that are ideal and practical in fracture treatment. Immobilization, by whatever means, should be continued until union is complete, though it may be difficult to determine this time with certainty. Rowe suggested the usual healing period of fractures of the middle third of the clavicle to be: infants—2 weeks;

children—3 weeks; young adults—4 to 6 weeks; adults—6 weeks or more.[222] It has been recognized, moreover, that radiographic union may progress more slowly than clinical union, with x-ray evidence of union not appearing for 12 weeks or more.[222] When in doubt, immobilization should probably be continued. It has been suggested that once a fracture is clinically united, with no motion or tenderness at the fracture site, a gradual increase in activity may safely be permitted, even if radiographic union is incomplete.[222]

SEVERITY OF TRAUMA

Up to half of clavicular fractures resulting in nonunion follow severe trauma.[117] In their series, Wilkins and Johnston reviewed 33 nonunited clavicle fractures.[279] Many of these patients had severe trauma—manifest by the degree of displacement of the fracture fragments, the amount of soft tissue damage, and associated injuries (eg, multiple long-bone, spine, pelvic, and rib fractures). The authors pointed out the similarities between the clavicle and the tibia, another subcutaneous long bone prone to nonunion, and emphasized that the subcutaneous position of the clavicle predisposes it to more severe trauma, more severe soft tissue damage, and thus, to nonunion.[279] As with other bones, open fractures have been implicated as a factor in nonunion of the clavicle.[142] Late perforation of the skin with a free compounding fragment has also been reported.[213]

It should be noted that many factors associated with clavicular nonunion—such as the degree of displacement, compounding, operative management, poor immobilization, and soft tissue interposition—may simply reflect cases associated with more severe trauma to the clavicle; thus, the independent statistical importance of some these associations with nonunion may be questioned.

REFRACTURE

Some authors have identified refracture of previously healed clavicular fractures as contributing to nonunion.[117,154] In Wilkins and Johnston's series, 7 of 31 nonunions were in such patients.[279] There appears to be no relationship between nonunion following refracture and the length of time between injuries, the age of the patient, the duration of immobilization of the original fracture, or the severity of the initial or subsequent traumatic injuries. It has been theorized that because the vascular anatomy of fractured bone remains altered for a long period, even after fracture union,[215] reinjury might in some way prevent this altered blood supply from reacting to the new fracture.[279]

DISTAL-THIRD FRACTURE

Approximately 85% of nonunions of the clavicle occur in the middle third of the bone.[211] Despite this, it appears that distal-third clavicle fractures are much more prone to nonunion than shaft fractures. In his series on clavicular nonunions, Neer noted that distal clavicle fractures accounted for over half of nonunited clavicles following closed treatment.[173] He found several reasons for this: (1) Distal clavicular fractures are very unstable, and the muscle forces and weight of the arm tend to displace the fracture fragments.[241] (2) Because distal clavicular injuries often result from severe trauma, there is extensive local soft tissue injury, and other associated injuries may affect generalized biologic and specific fracture healing.[175] (3) Distal fractures are difficult to secure adequately with external immobilization.

Even in fractures where union might occur with closed methods, the union time for distal clavicular fractures is often lengthy, and this long healing time, combined with soft tissue trauma, may lead to stiffness and prolonged disability from disuse. For these reasons, Neer advocates early open reduction and internal fixation for this injury.[174,175]

MARKED DISPLACEMENT

In a large series reported by Jupiter and Leffert, the degree of displacement was the most significant factor in producing a nonunion.[117] However, in many clavicular fractures, marked displacement is often associated with other factors that delay fracture healing, such as severe trauma, soft tissue damage, open fractures, and soft tissue interposition. Manske and Szabo felt soft tissue interposition alone was a major contributing factor in fractures that failed to heal, and at surgery they frequently found a fracture fragment impaled in the trapezius muscle.[152] They particularly implicated soft tissue interposition in the development of atrophic nonunions. However, others have reported that muscle interposition is uncommon.[117]

PRIMARY OPEN REDUCTION

Some authors have associated primary open reduction of acute clavicular shaft fractures with an increased incidence of nonunion, while others have reported nonunion following osteotomy of the clavicle or radiation therapy.[131,214] Rowe reported an incidence of 0.8% nonunion in fractures treated nonoperatively, which rose to 3.7% in those treated operatively.[222] Neer had a similar experience, with a nonunion rate of 0.1% in fractures treated nonoperatively, versus 4.6% when the initial fracture was treated surgically.[173] Schwartz reported a nonunion rate of 13% in patients with primary open reduction of clavicular fractures, although he suggested inadequate internal fixation may have played a prominent role in this high incidence.[234] Poigenfurst reported a complication rate of 10%, with four nonunions in 60 fresh clavicular fractures treated with internal plate fixation.[200]

Poor internal fixation, rather than the surgery itself, may play the primary role in the increased incidence of nonunion in clavicular fractures treated with primary surgery (Fig. 12-82). Zenni reported a series of 25 acute clavicular fractures treated with primary open reduction, using an open intramedullary pin or cerclage suture and bone grafting; all of these healed without complications.[286] In some reports of an increased incidence of nonunions with open reduction, it is probable that the operative fractures included difficult cases—those with severe trauma, soft tissue damage, and associated injuries—thus contributing to the poor results. Nevertheless, the excellent results obtained with nonoperative treatment are undeniable, and primary open reduction of clavicular fractures is rarely indicated.

Radiographic Evaluation

Although nonunion often may be demonstrated clinically by motion at the fracture site, radiographic confirmation is obtained on anteroposterior and 45° cephalic tilt views. The radiographic signs of nonunion may not always be clear. If there is minimal displacement of the fracture fragments and no gross motion, tomography (or even a bone scan) may be useful to demonstrate the presence of a nonunion in a symptomatic patient (Figs. 12-83 and 12-84). As with other fractures, nonunions of the

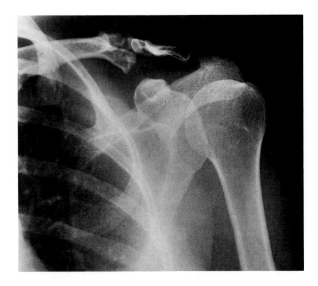

Fig. 12-82. An x-ray view of a nonunited distal clavicular fracture following primary open reduction and internal fixation using an intramedullary pin. *Inadequate* internal fixation may be a contributing factor in nonunion of surgically treated acute fractures.

clavicle may present with hypertrophic or atrophic bone ends. There may be real or apparent bone loss, particularly if there has been comminution. It is particularly helpful in evaluating nonunions to obtain an anteroposterior film of both clavicles on a single large cassette. In this way the distance from sternum to acromion can be measured on the normal side and compared with the symptomatic side. This may help in deciding whether primary osteosynthesis with bone grafting will be adequate, or whether an intercalary segment of bone will be needed to span the area of segmental bone loss.

Symptoms

Approximately 75% of patients with nonunited clavicular fractures are symptomatic, with moderate to severe pain.[117,152] However, there is some evidence that patients with atrophic nonunions, although symptomatic initially, may become less so with time.[279] Nonunion pain may radiate to the neck, down into the forearm, or even into the hand—especially if there is nerve irritation.[225] Patients may complain of grating or crepitation, which is often palpable. The shoulder may appear to sag forward, inward, and medially, and the apex of the medial fragment may be observed angling upward underneath the trapezius. Twenty five percent or more of patients may be affected by neurologic symptoms, often owing to compromise of the bra-

chial plexus by overabundant callus.[117,225] Likewise, chronic vascular symptoms may result from pressure on the subclavian vein, producing symptoms of thoracic outlet syndrome.[9,33,117,198]

It must be emphasized that when considering nonunion as the cause of a patient's painful symptoms, nonunion may be an incidental finding. A careful history and physical examination must be obtained, because many soft tissue and bony abnormalities around the shoulder, including posttraumatic arthrosis of either the sternoclavicular or acromioclavicular joints, may mimic the symptoms of a nonunion; these degenerative changes in the joint may appear several years after the injury.[279]

Physical Examination

Physical examination may reveal motion as the clavicle is manipulated, or pain upon pressure at a nonunion site. Prominent bone of comminuted fragments may be palpable. Occasionally there may be limited range of motion at the shoulder joint, but this often is associated with soft tissue, subacromial, or glenohumeral joint disease rather than as a direct result of the clavicular nonunion. If there are neurologic symptoms, often these are referred to the ulnar nerve distribution, and instrinsic weakness may occur.[83,225]

MALUNION

In children with clavicular fractures, foreshortening is frequent but has not been reported to be a problem, and the angular deformity will often remodel. However, in adults, there is no remodeling potential, and shortening or angulation may occur. This has been described by some as being purely a cosmetic deformity with little interference with function.[11] However, Eskola and associates reported that patients with shortening of the clavicular segments of greater than 15 mm at follow-up examination had statistically significantly more pain than those without these findings, and these authors recommended taking care to avoid the acceptance of a shortened clavicle.[62]

If the malunited fracture is a significant cosmetic or functional problem, simply shaving down the bone may be inadequate.[172] Several authors have recommended osteotomy, internal fixation, and bone graft.[11] The patient must be made aware, however, that nonunion may be a sequela, and that the cosmetic appearance of the surgical scar may be more troublesome than the bump from the malunited bone.

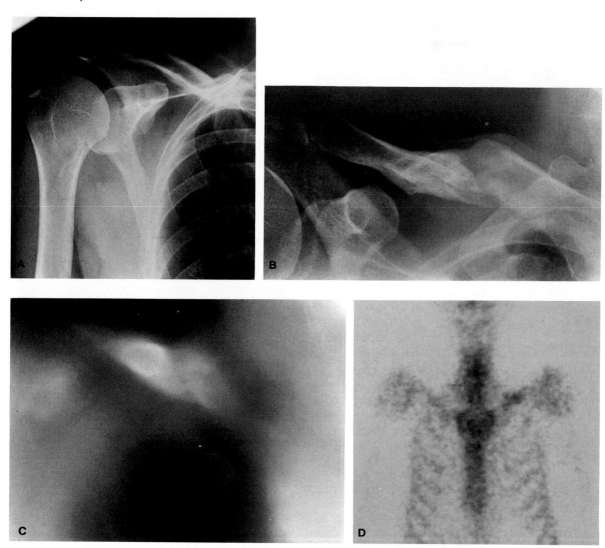

Fig. 12-83. (A) An anteroposterior view of the right shoulder in a patient who has pain following a clavicle fracture. The fracture area is poorly seen on this view. **(B)** A 45° cephalic tilt view shows the clavicle much more clearly, but it is still uncertain whether there is clear bridging of the fracture site. **(C)** Tomography suggests a lucent line in the area of the fracture that occurred 4 years earlier. **(D)** A bone scan shows increased activity in the right clavicle, which confirms the presence of a clavicular nonunion.

NEUROVASCULAR COMPLICATIONS

The large amount of callus that follows healing of a clavicular fracture in a child rarely causes compression of the costoclavicular space, and usually the callus mass decreases with time.[44] In adults, however, late neurovascular sequelae can follow both united and ununited fractures.[27,82,167,235,252,262]

Normally, the sternoclavicular angle and anterior bow of the clavicle provide abundant room for the brachial plexus and subclavian vessels in the costoclavicular space. Although there is some normal variability in the width and space between the clavicle and first rib, this room is usually adequate.[104] Occasionally a congenital anomaly—such as a bifid clavicle or a straight clavicle with no medial or anterior angulation (Fig. 12-85)—may narrow the costoclavicular space and cause neurovascular compression.[221] Thus, it is not surprising that abundant callus or significant fracture deformity in

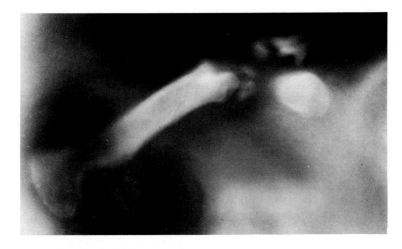

Fig. 12-84. A tomogram showing bone fragmentation in a clear-cut nonunion of the clavicle.

some patients may narrow this space enough to cause symptoms, which most frequently involve the subclavian vessels, the carotid artery, or the brachial plexus.[34,45,105,120] Although these compression phenomena are infrequent, they are important, because their clinical presentation may be confusing to the clinician and problematic for the patient until definitive treatment is instituted. Several vascular structures have been reported to be involved in compression syndromes.

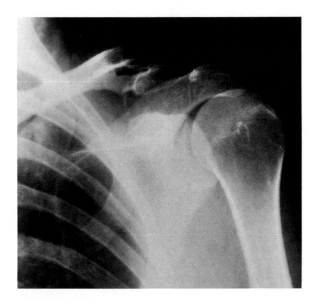

Fig. 12-85. A partial or complete bifid clavicle may narrow the normal space between the clavicle and the first rib, leading to neurovascular compression syndromes.

Carotid Artery

Obstruction of the carotid artery may lead to symptoms of syncope. This would be expected to be associated with fracture deformity or callus at the medial end of the clavicle.

Subclavian Vein

Compression of the subclavian vein between the clavicle and first rib, with subsequent obstruction, is probably the most common late vascular complication, and it may be accompanied by plexus and subclavian artery involvement.[132] The point of this obstruction has been shown by Lusskin to be the site where the vein crosses the first rib and passes beneath the subclavius muscle and costoclavicular ligament.[148] Some authors have emphasized the role of the subclavius muscle and the condensation of the clavipectoral fascia known as the costocoracoid ligament in producing venous obstruction and subsequent thrombosis.[148] The syndrome is characterized by dilitation of the veins of the upper extremity and anterior chest on the affected side, produced by congestion of the collateral venous network. This compression is relieved by a downward thrust of the shoulder.[66,146,226,251] Lusskin reported that this costoclavicular syndrome could be distinguished from the typical anterior scalene, cervical rib, and thoracic outlet compression syndromes, which may also produce arterial and neurologic symptoms, but are typically reproduced by the Adson maneuver. The other syndromes are not typically accentuated by shoulder girdle extension.[47,95,104,238] The treatment depends on the offending structure. If it is overabundant callus, addressing the surgery to the clavicle may be indicated. However, if the clavicle is more normal, it might make more sense to resect the first rib.

Subclavian Artery

Subclavian artery compression was reported by Guilfoil, who described a case of thrombosis secondary to a clavicular nonunion.[95] Although injury to this artery is well recognized in acute clavicular injuries,[93,170] it is unusual as a late complication secondary to overabundant clavicular callus or nonunion. However, Yates recorded a case of death from embolus to the basilar artery, which originated from a thrombosis in the subclavian artery following nonunited clavicular fracture.[284]

Aneurysm

Both traumatic aneurysms[28,49,176] and pseudo-aneurysms[236] have been reported following clavicular fractures. These may present as pulsatile masses or soft tissue densities in the area of the clavicular fracture or nonunion, and may also be the source of thrombi.

Brachial Plexus

Several neurologic symptoms have been described relating to late complications of clavicular fractures.[94] Because the onset of symptoms varies from the time of fracture to the establishment of nonunion, the late sequelae can be confused with nerve injuries occurring at the time of acute injury. Thus, it is particularly important to do a careful neurologic examination of the patient with an acute fracture. While an early nerve injury is usually a traction neuropraxia, involves the lateral cord, and has a guarded prognosis, late compression neuropathies typically affect the medial cord, produce ulnar nerve symptoms, and have more benign prognoses. Typically associated with middle-third fractures, the proximal tip of the distal nonunion fragment is pulled downward and posteriorly, bringing it into contact with the neurovascular bundle, which is squeezed by the nonunion site above and the first and second ribs below. As one would expect, this problem is more common with hypertrophic than atrophic nonunions (Fig. 12-86).

The diagnosis of late compression syndrome is usually made by a careful history, physical examination, and electrical studies such as EMG and nerve conduction velocities.[16,61,104,123,148,160,181,225] MRI may be helpful to outline the relationship between the brachial plexus and hypertrophic callus or clavicular fragments (Fig. 12-87).

POST-TRAUMATIC ARTHRITIS

Post-traumatic arthritis may follow intra-articular injuries of both sternoclavicular and acromioclavicular joints, although degenerative disease of the distal clavicle is much more common. Often, this is the result of a unrecognized intra-articular (type III) fracture. The patient may present with symptoms specifically related to pain at the acromioclavicular joint, or symptoms of impingement owing to an inferior protruding osteophyte of the acromioclavicular joint, causing extrinsic pressure on the subacromial bursa and rotator cuff.[171] Radiographically, there may be cystic changes, spur formation, or narrowing of the acromioclavicular joint, or there may be resorption of the distal clavicle.[110] Further radiology studies may be needed to define the lesion, especially in the area of the sternoclavicular joint, and additional tomograms or CT scan may be indicated. The symptoms often decrease following a diagnostic injection of 1% Xylocaine into the affected joint. If appropriate nonoperative treatment, including nonsteroidal medications or a steroid injection, do not provide lasting relief, surgical excision of the joint may be indicated. If the outer clavicle is to be resected, the distal 2 cm of bone are removed, lateral to the coracoclavicular ligaments, and the deltoid is repaired to the trapezius fascia. If resection of the sternoclavicular joint is indicated, the clavicular head of the sternocleidomastoid muscle may be used to fill in the area of resection.[172]

TREATMENT

As early as the late 1920s, more than 200 treatment methods had already been described for fractures of the clavicle (Fig. 12-88).[133,139] In general, excellent results have been reported with nonoperative treatment of these fractures.

The exact method of treatment of the fractured clavicle depends on several factors, including the age and medical condition of the patient, the location of the fracture, and associated injuries.

CHILDREN

Because of the excellent healing potential in children and the tremendous remodeling that goes on with growth, there is little role for any form of treatment other than nonoperative in children. In fact, it has been stated that operative treatment is

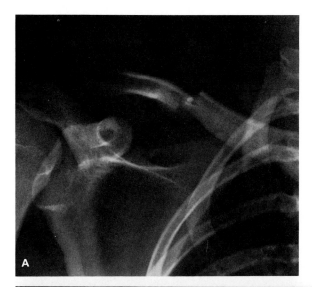

Fig. 12-86. (**A**) A mid-clavicular fracture in an adult, with a mild degree of displacement. This was treated with a figure-of-eight splint, which was discontinued early so motion could be started. (**B**) An anteroposterior view showing abundant callus formation. It is unclear whether the fracture has united. (**C**) A cephalic tilt view confirms the presence of a nonunion with hypertrophic callus. The patient had symptomatic paresthesias, suggestive of irritation of the brachial plexus.

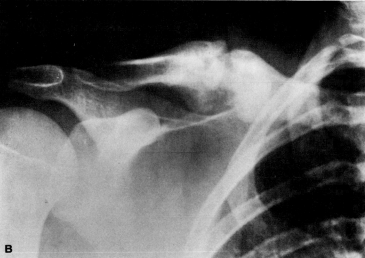

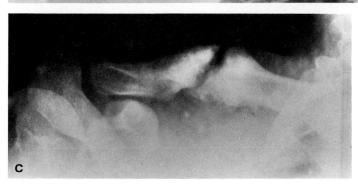

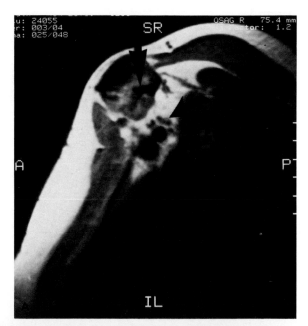

Fig. 12-87. (A) An MRI scan showing the location of a hypertrophic callus (*large arrow*) and brachial plexus (*small arrow*). MRI can image actual encroachment on the brachial plexus, which was minimal in this case. (B) The patient was treated with a DCP and bone grafting for this symptomatic, hypertrophic nonunion, with debulking of the callus.

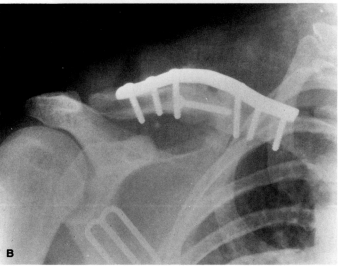

contraindicated in children.[255] Occasionally, however, operative management may be indicated, such as for débridement of an open fracture, for neurovascular compromise that does not resolve with closed reduction, for severe, irreducible displacement of the fragments, or for mediastinal compression associated with posteriorly displaced medial clavicular fractures.[19,42,108,140,161] While it is generally agreed that closed methods are usually successful, the exact method may vary, because children differ in comprehension levels and ability to cooperate with nonoperative treatment regimens.

In the newborn with a birth fracture, little treatment is needed other than to keep the baby comfortable. Healing is usually rapid, occurring within the first 2 weeks with no untoward effects. However, the nurse and mother must be instructed in methods of careful, safe, and gentle turning of the infant to minimize discomfort. The arm may be gently bound to the child for a few days to increase the comfort level.[44] Direct pressure over the clavicle while dressing the child is avoided.

In children, for a greenstick or nondisplaced fracture, treatment often involves wearing a sling

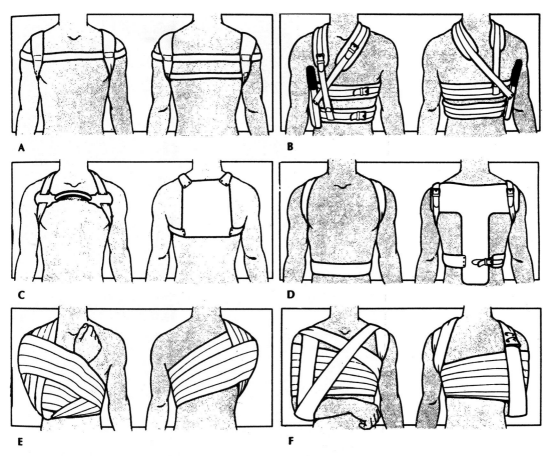

Fig. 12-88. A variety of closed treatment methods have been used for fractures of the clavicle. A number of these are illustrated: (**A**) the Parham support; (**B**) the Bohler brace; (**C**) the Taylor clavicle support; (**D**) unidentified support; (**E**) a Velpeau wrap; and (**F**) a modified Velpeau wrap. *(Dameron, T. B., Jr., and Rockwood, C. A., Jr.: Fractures and Dislocations of the Shoulder. In Rockwood C. A., Jr.; Wilkins, K. E.; and King, R. E. (eds.): Fractures in Children, p. 609. Philadelphia, J.B. Lippincott, 1984.)*

until the symptoms have subsided.[216] In displaced fractures or those requiring reduction, most treatment methods use some form of a figure-of-eight bandage or splint, either alone or reinforced with plaster, to hold the shoulder upward and backward to reduce the degree of displacement. Fortunately, in children, these fractures heal rapidly without much morbidity (Fig. 12-89).[201] Treatment of older children and teenagers may be more troublesome, frequently requiring plaster reinforcement because of high activity levels.

Frequent adjustment is often needed by the physician or parent to treat young patients with figure-of-eight methods; this can prove frustrating for both the patient and the surgeon. There is a real question as to whether there is any significant long-term advantage to aggressive attempts to maintain the reduction with these treatment methods.

ADULTS

In adults with clavicular fractures, as with other fractures, the goal of treatment is to achieve bone healing with minimum morbidity, minimal loss of function, and minimal residual deformity. Keeping this in mind, some traditional, cumbersome, methods of immobilization of clavicular might best be reevaluated. The main principles of nonoperative treatment historically have included several points: (1) to brace the shoulder girdle to raise the outer fragment upward, outward, and backward; (2) to depress the inner fragment; (3) to maintain reduction; and (4) to enable the ipsilateral elbow and hand to be used so that associated problems with immobilization can be avoided.

An extensive review of the literature would lead one to conclude that immobilization is nearly im-

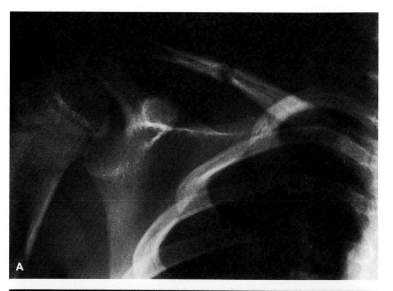

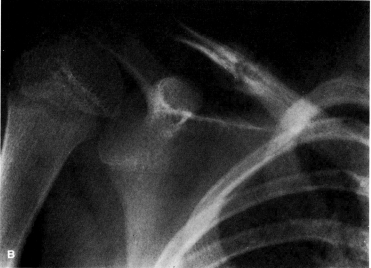

Fig. 12-89. Fractures in children heal quickly with minimum morbidity, using simple immobilization. (**A**) An x-ray view of a clavicular fracture in a 5-year-old. (**B**) After 14 days, there is no pain, with significant callus formation.

possible to achieve, that deformity and shortening are usual, and that even if some shortening occurs, it generally does not interfere with function. The literature is replete with methods of various complexity to immobilize the clavicle, and treatment has been described ranging from long-term recumbency alone[11,208] to ambulatory treatment[34] to internal fixation methods.[21,108,122,136,138,164,169,177,193,197,224,286]

METHODS

Simple Support

The simplest form of treatment is to provide support for the arm (Fig. 12-90). This might include a sling alone, a sling and swathe, a Sayer bandage, or a Velpeau bandage.[139] No attempt is made to maintain

a clavicular reduction, provided that satisfactory positioning of the bone appears to be present and union might be anticipated.[199] Although sling treatment is certainly the simplest way to treat the fractured clavicular shaft, it is often unsettling to the orthopaedic surgeon who wishes to effect realignment of the fracture fragments. This probably explains the popularity of the many methods to effect and maintain closed reduction.

Closed Reduction

A closed reduction is followed by an attempt to maintain reduction by bringing the distal fragment up and back. This may involve use of a bandage alone (including the figure-of-eight),[18,208] a bandage with plaster reinforcement,[35,285] or full immobilization of the shoulder in a spica cast (Figs. 12-91

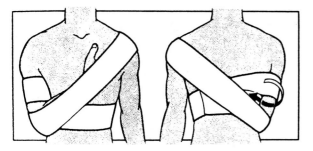

Fig. 12-90. Modification of a Sayer bandage, which is intended not to reduce the fracture, but simply to support the arm. *(Dameron, T. B., Jr., and Rockwood, C. A., Jr.: Fractures and Dislocations of the Shoulder. In Rockwood C. A., Jr.; Wilkins, K. E.; and King, R. E. (eds.): Fractures in Children, p. 617. Philadelphia, J.B. Lippincott, 1984.)*

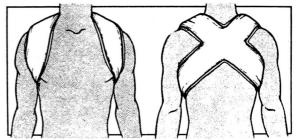

Fig. 12-91. A Billington yoke, used to maintain a reduction, consists of a plaster figure-of-eight. *(Dameron, T. B., Jr., and Rockwood, C. A., Jr.: Fractures and Dislocations of the Shoulder. In Rockwood C. A., Jr.; Wilkins, K. E.; and King, R. E. (eds.): Fractures in Children, p. 617. Philadelphia, J.B. Lippincott, 1984.)*

and 12-92).[127,172,192,222,264] A variety of materials have been described to maintain the closed reduction including metal, leather, plastic, plaster, and muslin.[172] The position required to reduce the fracture and maintain reduction (upward, lateral, and backward) is difficult to achieve, is often uncomfortable to the patient, and occasionally has been reported to cause symptoms of either neurovascular compression or even displacement of the fragment[222] if careful attention is not paid to placing the external immobilization precisely. Few studies have attempted, in a controlled fashion, to evaluate whether vigorous efforts to effect and maintain reduction provide greater chance for a better outcome than simple arm support. In two studies directly comparing figure-of-eight dressings to sling support, it was noted that figure-of-eight dressings were time consuming, required frequent adjustments, might contribute to other problems, and had more complications than simple sling treatment. The authors concluded that functional and cosmetic sequelae of the two methods were identical, with alignment of the healed fracture unchanged from the initial displacement.[6,159] Another group studied the recovery time following conservative treatment of clavicular fractures in 140 patients. There was no difference in the speed of recovery between the sling and the figure-of-eight, although patient age at the time of fracture did affect the recovery, with 33% of patients older than 20 years still having symptoms 3 months after injury.[245]

Open or Closed Reduction With Internal Fixation

A number of devices have been described for treatment of clavicular fractures with internal fixation.[98,188,240] These devices have included circlage sutures,[264] intramedullary devices (Stein-

mann pin, Kirschner wire, Knowles, Perry, Rush pins),[21,24,138,164,169,177,193,197,224,237,286] or plate fixation.[130,168]

Open or Closed Reduction With External Fixation

In some instances, such as open fractures or septic nonunions, external fixation can be considered. In one study using the Hoffman device, the average time for the external fixator to be left on was 51 days, there were no pleural or vascular complications, and all fractures united.[233] However, this is not a technique with which there is extensive experience, and there is a potential for complications with this procedure.[43]

Primary Excision of Fracture Fragment

In rare instances, primary excision of both ends of the fracture with skin closure and intentional formation of a pseudarthrosis has been advocated.[195]

Although distal clavicular fractures may heal quite well without surgical treatment,[219,220] the deforming forces and high incidence of nonunion have led many authors to recommend primary open reduction and internal fixation,[64] using either an intramedullary pin[174,175] or some method of dynamic fixation to bring the proximal clavicle segment to the distal segment (Figs. 12-93 and 12-94).[122] Others have used a coracoclavicular screw.[266]

Complications have been reported with each of these methods, including migration of intramedullary wires. In addition, musculocutaneous nerve injuries have been reported with coracoid process transfers to the proximal clavicular segment.[28] Plate fixation is often impractical because of the small distal segment. Some type of intramedullary device not prone to migration might offer the safest method of treatment for distal clavicular fractures.

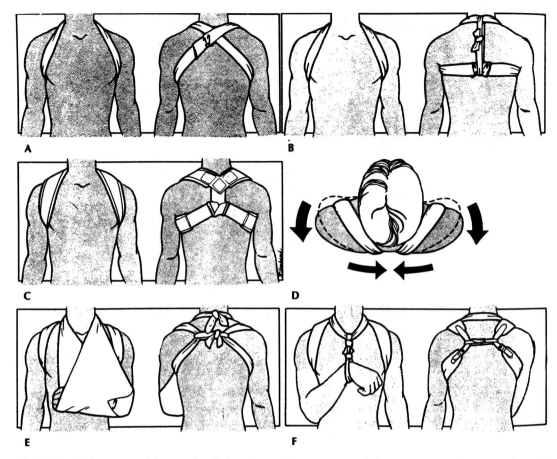

Fig. 12-92. Other types of figure-of-eight bandages. These are intended to maintain reductions achieved by closed means. (**A**) Stockinette padded with three layers of sheet wadding and held in place with safety pins. (**B**) Padded stockinette with the upper and lower borders tied to one another; this knot is tightened daily, increasing tension to maintain the reduction. (**C**) A commercial figure-of-eight support. (**D**) Superior view of the patient, showing how the figure-of-eight support pulls the shoulder up and backward. (**E**) A modified figure-of-eight bandage with a sling. (**F**) A figure-of-eight support used with a collar and cuff. (*Dameron, T. B., Jr., and Rockwood, C. A., Jr.: Fractures and Dislocations of the Shoulder. In Rockwood C. A., Jr.; Wilkins, K. E.; and King, R. E. (eds.): Fractures in Children, p. 618. Philadelphia, J.B. Lippincott, 1984.*)

Treatment of Nonunion

Asymptomatic clavicular nonunions need not be treated. In addition, nonunions in the elderly should probably be considered for nonoperative treatment. Nonoperative methods to obtain union have been reported, in particular, use of electrical stimulation; however, there have been only a few documented cases of healing of clavicular nonunions by pulsed electromagnetic fields,[22,48] and most authors share the view that there is little role for electrical stimulation in the treatment of clavicular nonunions. This especially true because operative methods have shown such high degrees of success.[10,32]

Indications for surgical treatment are: (1) pain or aching clearly attributable to the nonunion; (2) shoulder girdle dysfunction, weakness, or fatigue; and (3) neurovascular compromise.[193] While bone drilling has been suggested as a means of stimulating a delayed union to progress,[205] there is little role for this in established nonunion.

Partial claviculectomy, with excision of the nonunion site, has been reported as a means of treating ununited clavicular fractures. Certainly, in the short term, this may alleviate the crepitus and often will eliminate the pain.[152] However, many patients treated in this way remain mildly to moderately symptomatic,[117,279] the stabilizing function of the clavicle is lost, and neurogenic symptoms may be

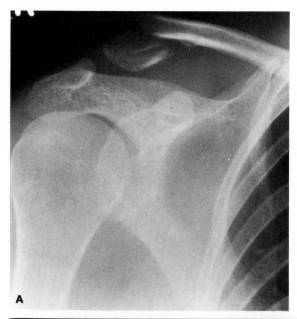

Fig. 12-93. (A) A distal clavicular fracture. The ligaments are attached to the distal clavicular piece, and there is high-riding and instability of the proximal fragment. Open reduction with internal fixation was elected as the treatment method because of the potential for nonunion in this fracture. (B) Intramedullary fixation was accomplished with a heavy Kirschner wire, bent to prevent migration. (C) Fracture healing occurred uneventfully. Once the fracture heals, the shoulder and clavicle are stable because the ligaments are attached to the distal fragment.

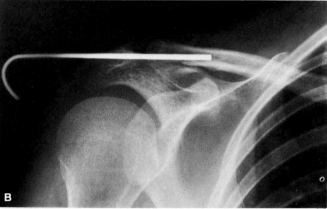

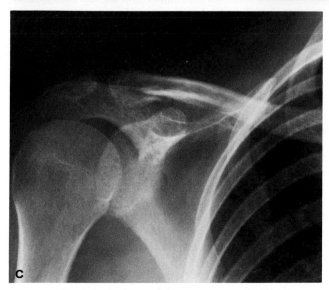

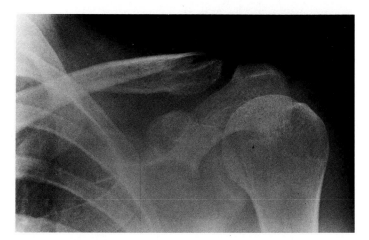

Fig. 12-94. Distal clavicular fractures may heal quite well without surgical treatment in some instances, as evidenced by this x-ray. The view is in an adult who had an oblique distal clavicular fracture treated nonoperatively. Clinical and radiographic union have occurred.

a problem.[142,279] However, resection of the nonunion, and filling the defect with cancellous bone chips may stimulate regeneration of the clavicle, and, in addition, may decompress the neurovascular structures if nonunion is accompanied by symptoms of thoracic outlet syndrome.[33] Surgical treatment most commonly consists of an attempt to gain union through some means of internal fixation with bone grafting. The techniques for surgical treatment of nonunions have evolved, as have internal fixation techniques for other long-bone fractures and nonunions.

Several open treatment methods have been detailed. Some authors have used wire sutures through the ends of either clavicular fragment and through iliac crest graft.[11,83,173] Sutures of other materials—including catgut, braided suture, and even loops of kangaroo tendon—have also been used.[172] Simple intrafragmentary screw fixation has been advocated, with fixation of the iliac bone as onlay graft and cancellous bone grafting at either junction.[157,225] However, because the clavicle exhibits so much movement in multiple planes, and because these methods control rotation poorly, neither suture nor screw fixation is secure enough to be reliable without additional protection. External cast or brace support is necessary to prevent screw or wire breakage and possible wire fragment migration, which can produce disastrous results.[134,158,184]

Open reduction with intramedullary fixation is popular. Fixation is achieved with Kirschner wires[147,154,172,182,234,258,263,273] (with or without screws), Steinmann pins,[126,174,222] Knowles pins,[177] or modified Hagie pins.[217] Although reports have been encouraging with these methods, rotation is

poorly controlled under most circumstances, the intramedullary fixation can be difficult to insert if there are atrophic bone ends (especially with the flat, curved clavicle), and external plaster support often is required. In addition, distraction of the fracture at the nonunion site with threaded pins may occur.[126] The intramedullary device may bend or break, and a number of complications have been reported with pin migration (Fig. 12-95).[134,158,184] Despite reports of success,[261] the complication rate can be high with intramedullary fixation—as high as 75% in one series.[279]

The application of rigid internal fixation in acute fractures has facilitated management of many traditionally difficult fractures, and this concept of rigidly immobilizing fragment ends has had natural applications to the treatment of nonunions as well. Although rigid internal fixation techniques using AO plates without bone grafting have been reported to be successful in clavicular nonunions,[101,206,248] the addition of supplemental bone graft to rigid plating has been the most popular treatment of clavicular nonunions. With this method of treatment, union rates have approached 100%.[57,58,119,206,212,261,275] Manske and Szabo reported an incidence of 100% union by 10 weeks postoperatively without complications, using open reduction and internal fixation with compression plating and bone grafting.[152] Jupiter and Leffert reported on 23 clavicular nonunions, including two resulting from clavicular osteotomies for surgical access, with an overall success rate of 89% in achieving union. However, 93.7% of those treated with grafting and dynamic compression plating achieved union.[117] Eskola and associates reported 20 of 22 clavicular nonunions healing with rigid

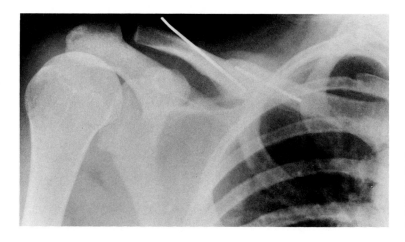

Fig. 12-95. A complication of intramedullary fixation with a Kirschner wire or Steinmann pin. Insufficient bone purchase combined with motion can lead to hardware failure and migration of pins, with potentially catastrophic results.

plate fixation and bone grafting, but warned against shortening of the clavicle to achieve union.[63] For this reason, if resection of the sclerotic edges of the atrophic margin to achieve primary osteosynthesis would result in significant clavicular shortening, many authors recommend intercalary bone grafting along with plate fixation (Fig. 12-96).[16,142] Plate fixation with bone grafting is reliable, safe, and has few complications; in addition, the internal fixation usually is so secure that no postoperative external cast immobilization is needed, and a sling alone is usually adequate. The plate does have the disadvantage of requiring a second operation to remove the hardware if it irritates the skin.[52] In addition, screw holes weaken the bone, and protection is needed after hardware removal.

There is one instance in which intramedullary fixation is probably the treatment of choice. In nonunion of the distal third of the clavicle, particularly type II distal clavicular fractures, the distal fragment usually is too small for adequate plate and screw fixation; there has been excellent success using intramedullary fixation with bone grafting for this specific nonunion.[175]

Medial clavicular nonunions, although rare, are particularly troublesome to treat (Fig. 12-97). The proximity to the sternoclavicular joint and vital structures make intramedullary fixation worrisome, and often there is little proximal bone with which to secure a standard DCP. Thinner plates are often prone to breakage. A postoperative spica cast may be required.

Treatment of Neurovascular Complications

The treatment for late neurovascular lesions depends on the cause of the compromised structures. Following a fracture of the middle third of the clav-icle, if there is neurovascular compromise secondary to massive callus formation and callus debulking is risky, if internal fixation with bone grafting of pseudarthrosis is impractical because of comminution, or if there is a malunion with a severe deformity and realignment osteotomy cannot be achieved, then resection of the middle third of the clavicle may be the best choice. Abbott and Lucas outlined the areas of the clavicle that can be resected without untoward sequelae, as well as the areas that do less well with resection.[1] Though some authors advocate total claviculectomy, it is probably wiser to do careful subtotal resections when possible.

If there is excessive callus build-up or malunion of the clavicle, and the lesion is amenable to bone grafting and plate fixation, then removal of the hypertrophic callus build-up and realignment osteotomy (with or without segmental interposition of bone graft and cancellous bone grafting), will often relieve the neurovascular symptoms.

If the clavicle has a satisfactory appearance and is stable, enlargement of the costoclavicular space, and thus neurovascular decompression, can be accomplished by resecting the first rib and partially excising the scalene muscle or subclavius muscle.[47,235]

POSTOPERATIVE CARE

Following operating treatment of a nonunion or an acute fracture, the patient is placed in a sling and swathe in the operating room. The postoperative x-ray should include not only the fracture site and internal fixation, to verify fracture alignment and hardware placement, but also enough of the lung to ensure that no injury has occurred during

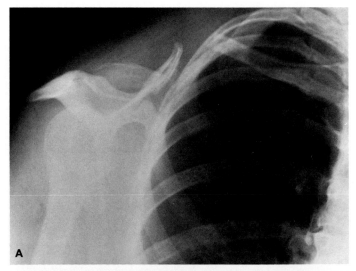

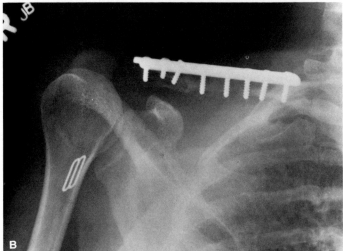

Fig. 12-96. (A) Radiograph in a 26-year-old woman who fractured her clavicle 5 years previously. A painful nonunion was present, with an intermediate gap and atrophic ends. **(B)** Rigid internal fixation was accomplished using a DCP with an intercalary bone graft. Clinical and radiographic union occurred.

surgery. When comfortable, the patient is discharged and wound care is the same as for any shoulder surgery.

If the glenohumeral joint and the subacromial bursa have not been surgically violated and are otherwise not diseased, there appears to be no need for early range of motion exercises, because shoulder range of motion, if normal preoperatively, will usually remain so. Thus, the patient may be kept safely supported in a sling or immobilizer until radiographic signs of union occur without fear of producing a frozen shoulder.

Early postoperative, isometric exercises for the rotator cuff may be begun, although isometric strengthening of trapezius and deltoid are delayed until their suture junction is healed securely (3 to 4 weeks). Range of motion following surgery is not permitted past 45° flexion in the plane of the scapula until there are clinical signs of union, usually at 4 to 6 weeks.

When clinical or radiographic union is present, the patient may begin full range of motion, particularly forward elevation (using an overhead pulley) and external rotation (using a cane or stick); hyperextension–internal rotation may also be added. Resistive exercises of the deltoid, trapezius, cuff, and scapular muscles are gradually added to the rehabilitation program. When radiographic union is present, full active use of the arm is permitted.

The patient is not permitted to return to full, strenuous work or athletic activities until there is a nearly full range of shoulder motion, strength

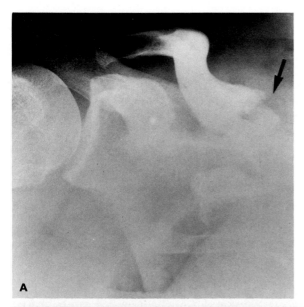

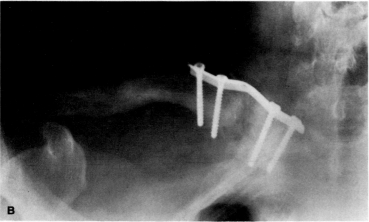

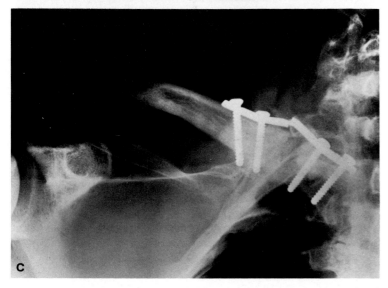

Fig. 12-97. (**A**) A medial clavicular nonunion (*arrow*) may be difficult to treat with internal fixation. It is a dangerous area for intramedullary fixation, and often it is difficult to obtain six cortices with plate fixation. (**B**) This medial clavicular nonunion was treated with plate fixation. Only four cortices could be obtained for purchase on the medial fragment, a semitubular plate was used. (**C**) A small plate with inadequate rigidity, when combined with poor postoperative protection, can lead to hardware failure in a medial clavicular fracture.

has returned to near normal, and bone healing is presumed solid. In adults, this is usually 4 to 6 months postoperatively.

AUTHOR'S PREFERRED METHODS

Newborns and Infants

Despite some information that clavicular fractures in newborns may be asymptomatic, I prefer to ensure comfort by treating clavicular birth fractures for a few days. The newborn is supine for many hours a day, often on his back, and a newborn who is not particularly active may be treated simply by avoiding pressure on the clavicle during dressing, taking care to handle the infant gently, and avoiding movement of the affected arm during feeding, diapering, and dressing. When the newborn is prone, soft padding may be placed under the anterior aspect of the shoulder to use the weight of the body to help keep the lateral clavicle back. Avoiding handling of a newborn is neither practical nor desirable. If "pseudoparalysis" is present (ie, the infant avoids use of the arm because of pain), I prefer to place a thick cotton pad (ABD) in the axillae, flex the elbow fully to 90°, and gently strap the arm to the chest with a padded elastic, Kling, or Kerlex bandage. A sling is difficult to apply and maintain and is not necessary. The parents may be taught to reapply the bandage for skin care and after bathing. Usually within 7 to 10 days, the patient is asymptomatic. Healing is usually complete by 2 weeks. The infant will use the arm normally once symptoms subside. Unrestricted use of the arm is permitted once the wrap is off, and the parents may be reassured that deformity and exuberant callus will remodel in time. After adequate healing, the infant is retested with the Moro reflex to ensure that the disinclination to move the arm was, in fact, a pseudoparalysis and did not constitute inability to move the arm secondary to an injury to the brachial plexus.[255]

Children

AGES 2 TO 12 YEARS

Young children are treated symptomatically. Before the age of 6 years, no attempt is made to reduce a clavicular fracture, because it will remodel and the large lump will be gone in 6 to 9 months.[255] The child is made more comfortable with a figure-of-eight bandage. Commercial figure-of-eight bandages usually are too large, and the simplest way to construct one is to use 2-inch stockinette filled with cotton wadding, cast padding, or felt. The child

is seated and the figure-of-eight dressing is applied as follows: The surgeon, standing behind the patient, passes the stockinette across the front of the uninjured clavicle, through the uninjured axilla and across the back, through the axilla on the fracture site, across the front of the anterior shoulder and clavicle on the fracture site, and across the back behind the neck. To help keep the shoulder up and back, tension is placed on the stockinette, and a safety pin binds both ends of the stockinette together as the tension is maintained. An elastic bandage or 2-inch tape securing the bandage can be placed from one posterior strap to the other, maintaining the tension and securing the position. Alternatively, the figure-of-eight stockinette may be criss-crossed behind the patient before being applied to the fracture side, then subsequently pinned and tightened. If the 2-inch stockinette appears to irritate the skin, an ABD cotton pad can be placed beneath the anterior straps. Parents should be instructed to tighten the figure-of-eight bandage to maintain this tension, by reapplying the anchoring safety pin. This should be done without taking the stockinette off. The stockinettes have a tendency to loosen quickly and should be retightened 2 or 3 days after the initial application and then weekly thereafter. I prefer to see the child weekly to assure that the bandage is secure, that there are no skin problems, neurovascular irritation, or any other problems with treatment. Parents should be made aware of potential circulatory difficulties or skin problems if the bandage is too tight. I ask them to practice tightening the bandage with my supervision to minimize their anxiety at handling the bandage adjustment. In young children, 3 weeks of immobilization is usually adequate, but in the older ambulatory child, clinical signs of union such as absence of tenderness to pressure over the fracture site or movement of the arm can help the physician decide when immobilization may be discontinued. Although union typically occurs in 3 to 6 weeks, symptoms often are dramatically diminished within the first 2 to 3 weeks (Fig. 12-98).

Nondisplaced fractures, incomplete fractures, or plastic bone bowing need not be treated with figure-of-eight bandages; the position is unlikely to change with ambulatory treatment if activity can be curtailed and reinjury avoided, and a simple sling for comfort until clinical union takes place is sufficient.

The child should avoid unusually vigorous activities such as gym class until the bone is solid, typically at about 3 months.

Repeat x-ray evaluation is not necessary at each return visit. I typically order an x-ray of the involved

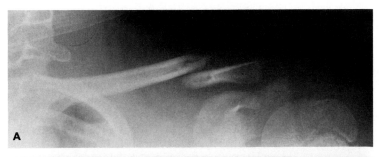

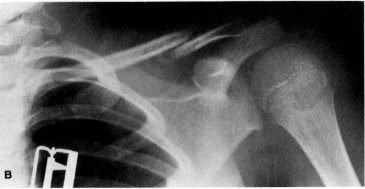

Fig. 12-98. (**A**) A 9-year-old boy with a fracture of the lateral portion of the middle third of the clavicle. (**B**) Two and a half weeks postoperatively, periosteal reaction and early callus formation can be seen. Clinically, the shoulder was not tender. Because union progresses rapidly in childhood fractures of the clavicle, little effort is made to produce and maintain a reduction.

shoulder with the immobilization in place, one more x-ray to check the progress of healing and the amount of callus, and then one final x-ray when union is definite (between 6 and 12 weeks). A final x-ray showing healing is helpful, in case of reinjury.

AGES 12 TO 16 YEARS

Children 12 to 16 years old may be difficult to treat, because their activity level often frustrates the most aggressive attempts to maintain reduction and immobilization. While in very young children little or no attempt is made to reduce clavicular fractures, teenagers have limited remodeling potential and reduction should be attempted before immobilization. Teenagers are often self-conscious about the deformity and bump that may remain after the fracture is healed; this is another reason to attempt closed reduction. With meticulously sterile technique and careful preparation of the area, the hematoma is infiltrated with 6 to 10 cc of 1% Xylocaine or Marcaine, and the resulting anesthesia usually permits reduction and molding of the fracture into satisfactory position. With the fracture reduced, a 4-inch stockinette with cast padding may be passed in the figure-of-eight fashion described for young children. To reduce the fracture, the teenager sits on a stool, and the physician's knee is placed in the patient's midback between both scapulae; both shoulders are brought upward and

backward and the fracture may be molded into place. In more active children, a plaster yoke should be considered, fashioned in the same way as the figure-of-eight bandage. However, the skin should be well protected with cast padding, felt, or cotton wadding in stockinette, with the soft padding extending past the sharp edges of the plaster. The cast may be trimmed in any area where the edges are sharp. Treatment for 6 weeks is usually adequate in the older child and adolescent. In cooperative older children and young adults, a commercial figure-of-eight clavicular splint, which usually is an elastic bandage with well-padded areas for the axillae, may be applied. The commercial splint has several advantages, including easy removal for bathing and more resistance to "stretching out" as days go by than the fashioned stockinette. The figure-of-eight bandage does not reduce or rigidly immobilize the fracture, but may serve as a reminder to hold the shoulders "back" when the child wants to slump forward.[44]

Despite some suggestions that there may not be long-term differences between the use of the sling and the figure-of-eight bandage, my preference is still to apply the figure-of-eight wrap, after an attempt to reduce the fracture, maintaining alignment of the clavicle. The figure-of-eight bandage has one advantage that the sling does not: it leaves both hands and elbows free for activities of daily living.

In addition, the sling, in its usual position, holds the arm forward and inward, and the distal clavicular segment is not in a position to be lined up with the proximal segment.

In older children, the fractures usually heal within 6 weeks. However, I generally maintain the clavicular immobilizer for 4 weeks after healing to serve as a reminder to restrict activities. Vigorous athletic activities should be avoided until union is solid, which in the teenager should be at 12 to 16 weeks.[44,47]

In the multiply traumatized child the clavicular fracture can be treated by recumbency. A small pillow is placed between the scapulae, allowing the weight of the arm to reduce the fracture (Fig. 12-99). If recumbent treatment is to be instituted, a sling may make the arm more comfortable.

MEDIAL AND DISTAL FRACTURES

I prefer to treat both medial and distal clavicular fractures in children with a sling for support and an ace wrap for comfort. Medial clavicular fractures

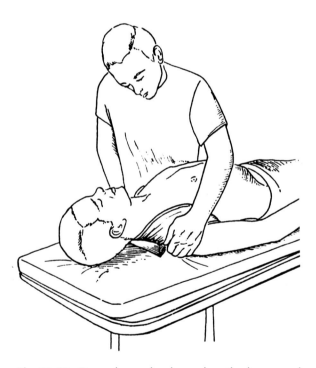

Fig. 12-99. Recumbency has been described as one of the treatment methods for clavicular fractures, especially in the mutiply traumatized person. A bump or pillow is placed between the scapulae, allowing the weight of the arm to reduce the fracture. A multiply traumatized patient may well be managed by reduction and rigid internal fixation.

are rare problems and rarely produce significant displacement. Lateral clavicular fractures, although clinically dramatic (appearing as a high-grade acromioclavicular separation), are stable, because the coracoclavicular and acromioclavicular ligaments remain attached to the periosteal tube and both sides of the joint respectively. Despite the degree of displacement, the bone will remodel in time (Fig. 12-100). For lateral clavicular fractures, I find a figure-of-eight bandage difficult to maintain over the most lateral aspect of the shoulder; the sling and swathe is more practical and quite comfortable. The healing potential in children negates the need for precise maintenance of reduction.

Adults

Fractures of the adult clavicle are much more difficult to treat, as the quality of the bone and periosteum is different from children, and associated soft tissue or bony injury is often greater. In addition, the potential for healing is less in adults than in children.

SHAFT FRACTURES

Despite the broad range of treatment methods for clavicular shaft fractures, in adults I prefer a commercially available figure-of-eight splint following closed reduction. To reduce the clavicle, the patient is seated on a stool with the surgeon behind, and after meticulous preparation, the fracture area and fracture hematoma are infiltrated with 8 to 12 cc of 1% Xylocaine. The physician's knee is placed between the scapulae, both outer edges of the shoulder are held securely, and the shoulders are pulled upward, outward, and backward (Fig. 12-101). The fracture may then be manipulated into place. The commercially available figure-of-eight bandage, usually with ABD to pad the area of the axilla, is preferred because it is more comfortable, less cumbersome, and more cosmetic than options such as a plaster spica; also, with the figure-of-eight bandage, immobilization of the fracture is as adequately achieved as in more drastic and bulky forms of external fixation. The figure-of-eight has the added advantage of keeping both hands and elbows free. If some patients feel more comfortable, a sling may be added to provide additional support for the arm; this also may make sleeping more comfortable. Because adults usually have more trouble healing the fracture than children, immobilization must be maintained for 6 to 8 weeks. Although I permit rotation of the arm at the side in any direction and to any extent, I limit active use of the arm until clinical union takes place. If refracture occurs dur-

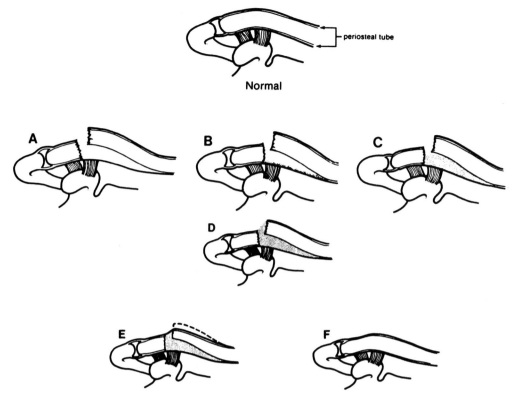

Fig. 12-100. The sequence of events in a typical type IV distal clavicular fracture in a child. (**A**) The ligaments remain attached to the periosteal tube, as the medial clavicular fragment ruptures through the superior thin periosteum. This may mimic an acromioclavicular separation. (**B**) Early filling of the area between the periosteum and the bone. (**C**) Further filling in of the bone. (**D**) Bridging callus reaches the top of the medial clavicular segment. (**E**) Early remodeling begins, with further consolidation of the fracture. (**F**) Remodeling leads to complete union. Such fractures are best treated nonoperatively, and excellent results can be expected. *(Dameron, T. B., Jr., and Rockwood, C. A., Jr.: Fractures and Dislocations of the Shoulder. In Rockwood C. A., Jr.; Wilkins, K. E.; and King, R. E. (eds.): Fractures in Children, p. 628. Philadelphia, J.B. Lippincott, 1984.)*

ing treatment, continued immobilization is appropriate. Athletics are not permitted for at least 6 weeks following clinical and radiographic union. At 6 to 8 weeks, the patient is taken out of the figure-of-eight bandage and placed in a sling for an additional 3 to 4 weeks for added protection, while gentle isometric and mobilization exercises are begun.

INDICATIONS FOR PRIMARY OPEN FIXATION

My indications for operative treatment of acute clavicular fractures are:

1. Neurovascular injury or compromise that is progressive or fails to reverse with closed reduction of the fracture
2. Severe displacement caused by comminution with resulting severe angulation and tenting of the skin—enough to threaten its integrity— which fails to respond to closed reduction
3. An open fracture that requires operative debridement
4. Multiple trauma, where patient mobility is desirable and closed methods of immobilization are impractical or impossible
5. A "floating" shoulder, with a displaced clavicular fracture and an unstable scapular fracture
6. Many type II distal clavicle fractures (see below)
7. Inability of the patient to tolerate closed immobilization (eg, neurologic problems of Parkinsonism, seizure disorders, or other neurovascular disorders)[257]
8. In the very rare patient where the cosmetic lump over the healed clavicle is intolerable, and the patient is willing to exchange this for a po-

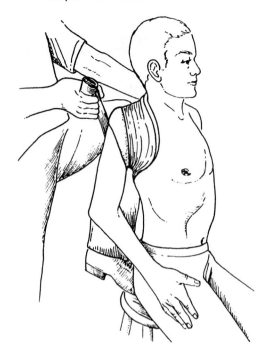

Fig. 12-101. A method of reducing the clavicle and applying a figure-of-eight bandage. The physician's knee is placed between the scapulae, both outer edges of the shoulder are held securely, and the shoulders are pulled upward, outward, and backward.

tentially equally noncosmetic surgical scar and the possibility of a nonunion.

Although there are quite a number of relative or absolute indications for surgery, it must be emphasized that very few fractures of the shaft need to be treated with primary open reduction and internal fixation.[172,181]

If surgery for a fractured clavicle is to be undertaken, historically the choices have been between plate fixation (AO) and intramedullary fixation.[158,167] I prefer intramedullary fixation for acute fractures for the following reasons: (1) Less exposure of the fracture is required, and therefore there is a smaller skin incision; (2) Because little periosteal stripping is needed, there is less interference with the healing potential of the fracture. (3) Removal of hardware is less problematic and can usually be done with a local anesthetic. (4) No screw holes remain to act as potential areas of weakness of the bone.

Although use of a threaded Steinmann pin, bent at the lateral end to avoid migration, has been well described, my preference is for use of a Knowles

pin, a method described by Neviaser. The Knowles pin has a hub that is large enough to prevent pin migration and is easily palpable beneath the skin for removal. The threaded distal end of the pin also helps prevent migration. To insert this pin, the patient sits in a beach-chair position, and a small, horizontal incision is made at the level of the fracture, which is then exposed. The fracture is reduced and held with towel clips. The Knowles pin is drilled from lateral to medial, entering the clavicle at the posterior lateral aspect of the acromion (avoiding the acromioclavicular joint, if possible). It is then directed toward the medial fragment of the clavicle and down the intramedullary portion of the medial fragment.

Alternatively, a 4-mm Steinmann pin may be drilled retrograde from medial to lateral after the fracture is exposed, entering the lateral fragment at the fracture site and emerging at the posterolateral aspect of the acromion. At the point of egress of the pin, a Knowles pin is drilled antegrade through the acromion, following the Steinmann pin as the pin is withdrawn. At the fracture site, the fracture is reduced and held with towel clips, and the Knowles pin is drilled into the medullary canal. If the Knowles pin penetrates the anterior cortex, and the tip of the pin is excessively prominent, it may be cut even with the anterior edge of the clavicle to avoid prominence under the skin. In addition, the subacromial space must be palpated to ensure the intramedullary pin is not in the subacromial space, but is, in fact, transacromial.

I also prefer to add bone graft acutely, along with internal fixation, when any acute shaft fracture is treated with open reduction and internal fixation.

DISTAL CLAVICLE FRACTURES

In type I distal clavicular fractures, the ligaments are intact, displacement is minimal, and the patient may be treated with a sling for comfort, early isometric exercises, and discontinuation of the immobilization as symptoms permit.

Type II distal clavicular fractures, as discussed previously, are difficult to treat nonoperatively. Immobilization is difficult, the fragments are distracted by muscle forces and the weight of the arm, the proximal fragment is unstable and has no ligamentous attachment, and nonunion occurs all too frequently. The usual sling does not reduce the deformity, and the use of a figure-of-eight bandage can actually increase the deformity by holding the proximal fragment posteriorly. Although closed treatment has been successful,[220] union often is delayed and shoulder stiffness may increase morbidity.

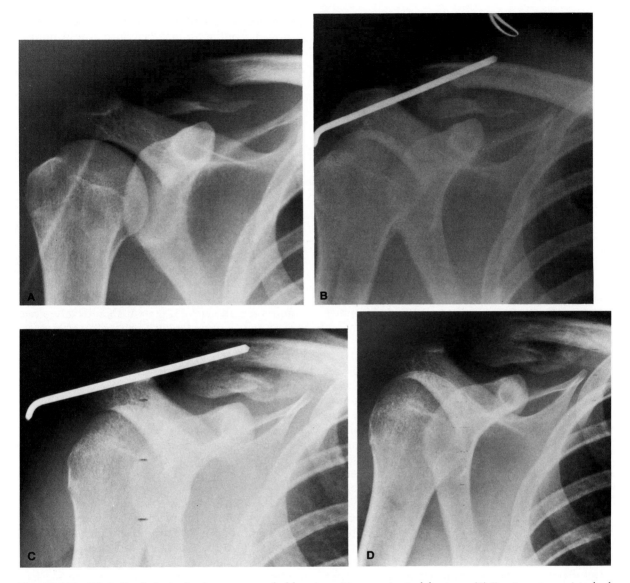

Fig. 12-102. (A) A distal clavicular fracture—probably a type V, comminuted fracture. (B) Treatment consisted of intramedullary fixation using a heavy Steinmann pin. (C) Early healing. (D) Internal fixation is removed, and radiographic union has occurred.

However, if there is obvious bony contact, as manifested by crepitus and a radiographic bone wedge, nonoperative treatment may logically be considered. Patients with type II distal fractures are probably best treated with open reduction and internal fixation acutely if the fragments are displaced and the fracture is unstable. The operative treatment depends on the size of the lateral fragment and the position and integrity of the coracoclavicular ligaments relative to the fragments.

Although a variety of encircling wires,[179,181] pins

(Fig. 12-102), and sutures[175] binding the proximal fragment to the coracoid process have been described, I prefer open intramedullary fixation with a Knowles pin (Fig. 12-103). Remember that, because of the fracture anatomy, the coracoclavicular ligaments usually are attached to the distal fragment, with the proximal fragment pulled upward by contraction of the trapezius muscle. Therefore, if fracture union can be achieved, the acromioclavicular joint and clavicle are stable.

With the patient in the beach-chair position and

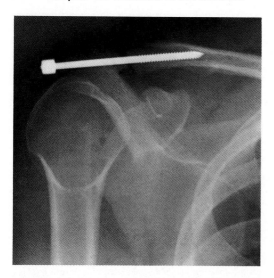

Fig. 12-103. A Knowles pin is often a preferable method of internal fixation, because the hub prevents migration and is easily palpable for later removal. It can be buried underneath the skin.

the head turned away from the side of the fracture, a small vertical incision is made at the fracture site. The deltoid–trapezius interval is split horizontally, and the fracture site is exposed. I often place a very heavy nonabsorbable suture or tape around the coracoid process and proximal clavicular segment to secure the reduction. This is passed prior to reduction of the fracture. In addition, prior to reduction, a Knowles pin is drilled from the posterolateral aspect of the acromion to emerge from the medullary canal of the distal clavicular segment. Once the pin is seen and the subacromial space is palpated to make certain that the pin has not violated it, the fracture is reduced. Reduction may be maintained with towel clips, and the Knowles pin is advanced through the intramedullary canal of the proximal clavicular fragment. If the pin penetrates the anterior cortex, this is usually not a problem, and any excessive pin length can be cut flush with the anterior clavicle. The nonabsorbable suture or tape from the coracoid to the clavicle is then securely tied for added fixation. Although both conoid and trapezoid ligaments may be attached to the distal clavicular segment, not infrequently the conoid ligament is torn with the trapezoid alone attached to the distal segment. If this is the case, the conoid ligament may be sutured into the clavicular periosteum or into the clavicular insertion of the trapezoid ligament. With adequate internal fixation of an acute fracture of the lateral clavicle, I typically

do not add bone graft because union usually ensues; however, bone graft may be added. The patient is then placed in a sling and swathe postoperatively, and isometric exercises are begun in the early postoperative period. The Knowles pin is removed after radiographic signs of early fracture healing (6 weeks); because the coracoclavicular sutures contribute to security, early healing has generally occurred by this time, and removal is especially helpful if the hub of the Knowles pin is irritating the skin.

Type III fractures of the distal clavicle are not often recognized acutely. When they are seen acutely, if unstable, or when they appear as an extension of a type II injury into the joint, they should be treated as type II injuries. If they lead to symptomatic late degeneration of the acromioclavicular joint, the distal 2 cm of clavicle may be excised with little morbidity and excellent results. When a type III distal fracture is treated surgically in the acute stage, the distal fragment should be retained because of its attachment to the coracoclavicular ligaments, unless there is hopeless damage of the articular surface or severe comminution. In extremely rare instances, if it is necessary to excise the distal segment, the proximal clavicular segment must be stabilized, usually with an intramedullary pin, and the ligaments transferred from the distal fragment to the proximal fragment. Occasionally the coracoacromial ligament may be secured to the proximal fragment acutely.[274]

MEDIAL CLAVICLE FRACTURES

Fractures of the medial clavicle require symptomatic support only, unless there is severe neurovascular compromise or injury. If this occurs, and the fracture must be operated on, open reduction should be considered. However, even if this fracture is openly reduced, I prefer to avoid intramedullary fixation because of the difficulty of securing and positioning the fragment and the danger of pin migration, which has the potential for catastrophic results.

NONUNION

Fortunately, clavicular nonunions are rare. When they do occur, 75% are in the shaft (30% atrophic, 70% hypertrophic) and 25% are in the distal third.[117,152] An asymptomatic nonunion need.

My preference for treatment of a symptomatic clavicular shaft nonunion is to use a compression plate and bone graft; ideally, I use a six- or seven-hole DCP (3.5-mm) with at least six cortices secured on each clavicular segment. I prefer a DCP plate

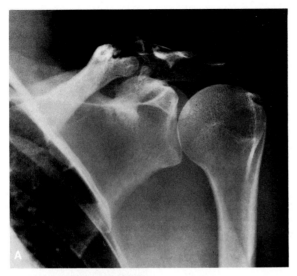

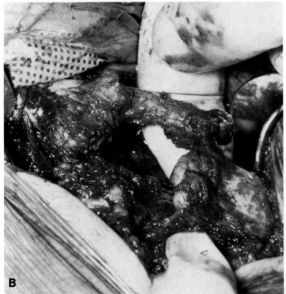

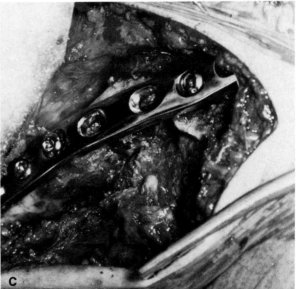

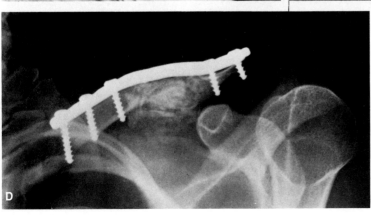

Fig. 12-104. (A) Three years after a clavicle fracture, this patient has a symptomatic left clavicular nonunion. The ideal treatment is bone grafting and rigid internal fixation, preferably with a DCP. **(B)** Intraoperative photograph showing small, thin, tapered sclerotic edges of the nonunion. **(C)** A seven-hole DCP was used with massive cortical cancellous grafting. Only two screws could be placed in the small lateral segment. **(D)** Healing has occurred. A disadvantage of plate fixation for nonunion is that the plate may need to be removed if it causes subcutaneous irritation.

because it uses small fragment screws, as compared with the 4.5-mm screws for the semitubular plate. In addition, compression appears to be less difficult to achieve (Fig. 12-104).

The surgical technique requires the patient to be in a semiseated or beach chair position with the head turned to the opposite shoulder. A horizontal incision is made parallel to the medial clavicular segment along its superior border. The interval between the deltoid and the trapezius is found, and a horizontal incision is made in this interval. The ends of the clavicle are exposed subperiosteally and any interposed soft tissue is removed (Figs. 12-105 and 12-106). In a hypertrophic nonunion, the excessive callus buildup and excessively hypertrophic bone may be shaved down to a more normal clavicular size to facilitate fitting of the plate. With an atrophic nonunion, if the sclerotic ends need to be resected, an intercalary segment of iliac crest graft is fashioned to fit between the two clavicular segments. If it is anticipated in an atrophic nonunion that an intercalary bone graft will be needed, it is useful to be able to palpate the distance from the acromial tip to the midsternum both on the injured and uninjured sides (Figs. 12-107 and 12-108). In addition, preoperatively the distance between the acromion and the sternum on each side can be measured on

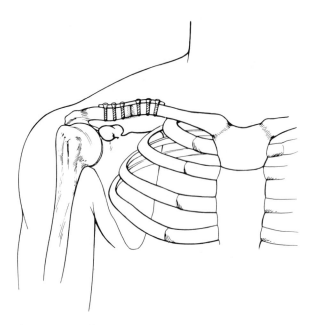

Fig. 12-106. Illustration of internal fixation and bone grafting of a nonunited middle-third clavicular fracture. At least six cortices should be incorporated into the DCP. Care must be taken so the screws do not project too far inferiorly. The bone graft should be packed in the nonunion site and inferiorly, but *not* in the retroclavicular space.

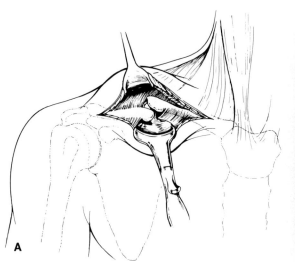
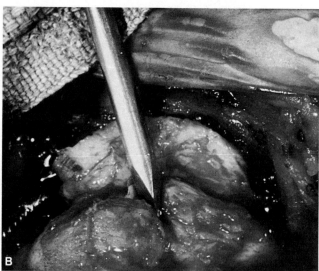

Fig. 12-105. Surgical treatment of symptomatic nonunion. (**A**) Operative approach. A horizontal incision is made. The trapezius and deltoid are elevated off of the clavicle and the nonunion is exposed. Blunt retractors protect the retroclavicular vital structures. (**B**) The nonunion is exposed. Sclerotic edges are trimmed and fibrous tissue is removed. Usually the fragments are large enough to take six cortices on either side of the fracture.

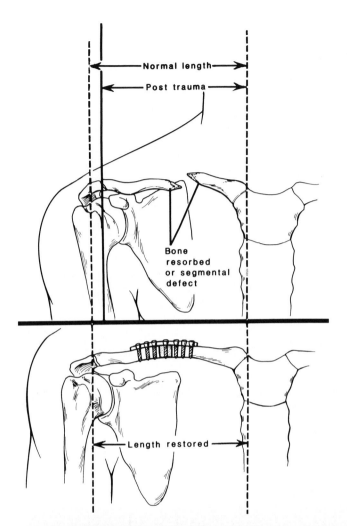

Fig. 12-107. In an atrophic clavicular nonunion, there are often tapered sclerotic edges, and an intercalary bone graft may be needed between the two ends of the nonunion. The normal manubrial acromial length is demonstrated. The post-traumatic manubrial acromial length decreased due to bone resorption or a segmental defect. To restore the normal length of the clavicle, an intercalary bone graft can be placed between the two sides of the nonunion. It is often helpful to internally fix the intercalary segment (fibula or iliac crest) with a cortical screw.

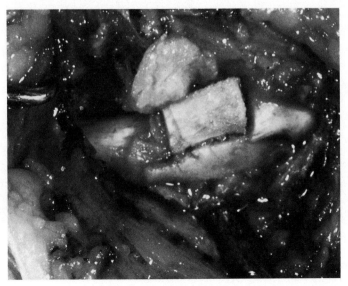

Fig. 12-108. Operative photograph of intercalary bone graft segment placed between the two sides of a nonunion.

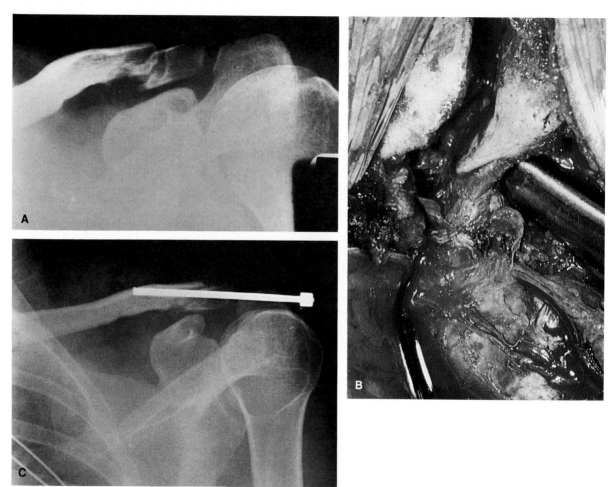

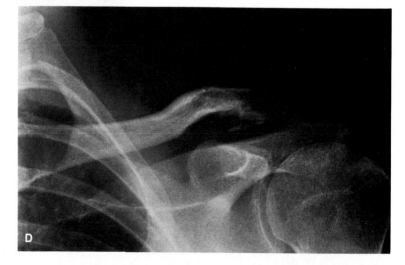

Fig. 12-109. (**A**) Two years after a type II distal clavicle fracture, a painful nonunion has occurred. (**B**) Exposure of the nonunion reveals the ligaments on the small distal segment and fibrous tissue between the bone ends. (**C**) Internal fixation with a Knowles pin (which has been cut off where it protruded past the anterior cortex) and bone grafting of the nonunion site were performed. Ligament reconstruction is not ordinarily needed, because the ligaments remain attached to the distal fragment. (**D**) Clinical and radiographic union have occurred.

an x-ray taken on a large cassette. This helps judge how much clavicular length will need to be made up by intercalary graft.

Blunt retractors (ie, Darrach, Bennet) are used to protect the infraclavicular structures during drilling of the plate holes. I prefer to place the plate superiorly and have not found this to be cosmetically or symptomatically a problem. I use a 3.5-mm DCP—six- or seven-hole, depending on the fracture configuration—(Synthes, Wayne, Penna.) and I attempt to get three screws in each clavicular segment as bicortical fixation. Occasionally an interfragmentary screw can be used if the bony anatomy warrants it and the nonunion anatomy is oblique enough (See Fig. 12-87**B**). The plate is contoured to the clavicle and secured to the bone. If an intercalary iliac crest segment is to be used, the middle hole of a seven-hole plate may be used to place a screw from the plate directly into the intercalary segment. Following secure plate fixation, iliac crest bone is placed at the fracture site along the superior and inferior clavicular borders. Excessive bone should not be placed posteriorly and inferiorly, to avoid late irritation or crowding of the neurovascular structures. The trapezius and deltoid fascia are repaired and the patient is placed in a sling and swathe postoperatively.

For lateral clavicular nonunions, I prefer the same method of internal fixation as with acute fractures—that is, use of a Knowles pin. However, iliac crest graft is always added (Fig. 12-109). In addition I usually add, as with an acute fracture, a piece of Mersilene tape or heavy nonabsorbable suture from the coracoid around the proximal fragment of the clavicle. In this type of procedure, the fracture site is exposed as with an acute fracture, the Knowles pin is passed from the posterolateral corner of the clavicle, across the acromioclavicular joint and small distal segment, and, after the nonunion edges are trimmed to satisfactory bone, the Knowles pin is advanced across the nonunion site. Coracoclavicular fixation is then tightened and bone graft is added. As with an acute fracture, the Knowles pin is taken out after 6 to 8 weeks.

For medial clavicular nonunions, my preference is for plate fixation and graft rather than intramedullary devices. However, purchase on the medial fragment may be difficult, compromising the thickness and size of the plate which may be used. If less than six-cortex purchase must be accepted, a supplementary spica cast is recommended.

Remember that the healing time for a nonunion of the adult clavicle is longer than for an acute fracture. This may often require a period of 3 to 6 months, and the patient should be protected until radiographic signs of union are present. A sling is usually enough immobilization for at least 6 to 8 weeks, and gentle range of motion may be begun once immobilization is discontinued. Removal of the plate is optional after healing of the fracture, while the intramedullary Knowles pin is removed after approximately 6 weeks.

In the rare instance where the surgeon is confronted with a previously excised lateral clavicular segment and an unstable proximal segment following a type II distal clavicle fracture, I use Mersilene tape around the proximal segment to secure the segment to the coracoid, then transfix the proximal segment with an intramedullary Knowles pin after reduction, and transfer the coracoacromial ligament into the end of the clavicle.[178,274]

Portions of the text and selected illustrations have been used with permission from THE SHOULDER, edited by Charles Rockwood and Frederick Matsen, published by W. B. Saunders Company, Philadelphia, 1990.

REFERENCES

1. Abbott, L.C., and Lucas, D.B.: The Function of the Clavicle: Its Surgical Significance. Ann. Surg., 140:583–599, 1954.
2. Adams, C.F.: The Genuine Works of Hippocrates. Baltimore, Williams & Wilkins, 1939.
3. Aitken, A.D., and Lincoln, R.E.: Fractures of the First Rib Due to Muscle Pull: Report of Case. N. Engl. J. Med., 220:1063–1064, 1939.
4. Alldred, A.J.: Congenital Pseudoarthrosis of the Clavicle. J. Bone Joint Surg., 45B:312–319, 1963.
5. Allman, F.L.: Fractures and Ligamentous Injuries of the Clavicle and Its Articulation. J. Bone Joint Surg., 49A:774–784, 1967.
6. Anderson, K.; Jensen, P.O.; and Lauritzen, J.: Treatment of Clavicular Fractures: Figure-of-Eight Bandage Vs. a Simple Sling. Acta Orthop. Scand., 57:71–74, 1987.
7. Apeli, L., and Burch, H.B.: Study on the Pseudoarthrosis of the Clavicle. *In* Chapcal, G. (ed.): Pseudarthroses and Their Treatment. Eighth International Symposium on Topical Problems in Orthopaedic Surgery, pp. 188–189. Stuttgart, Thieme, 1979.
8. Balata, A.; Olzai, M.G.; Porcu, A.; Spano, B.; Ganau, R.; and Corchia, C.: Fractures of the Clavicle in the Newborn. Ital. Ped., 6(1):125–129, 1984.
9. Bargar, W.L.; Marcus, R.E.; and Ittleman, F.P.: Late Thoracic Outlet Syndrome Secondary to Pseudoarthrosis of the Clavicle. J. Trauma, 24:857–859, 1984.
10. Basom, W.C.; Breck, L.W.; and Herz, J.R.: Dual Grafts for Nonunion of the Clavicle. S. Med. J., 40:898–899, 1987.
11. Bateman, J.E.: The Shoulder and Neck. Philadelphia, W.B. Saunders, 1978.

12. Bateman, J.E.: Nerve Injuries About the Shoulder in Sports. J. Bone Joint Surg., 49A:785–792, 1967.

13. Bearn, J.G.: An Electromyographic Study of the Trapezius, Deltoid, Pectoralis Major, Biceps, Triceps, Muscles During Static Loading of the Upper Limb. J. Anat., 140:103–108, 1961.

14. Bearn, J.G.: Direct Observation in the Function of the Capsule to the Sternoclavicular Joint in Clavicular Support. J. Anat., 10:159–170, 1967.

15. Beckman, T.: A Case of Simultaneous Luxation of Both Ends of the Clavicle. Acta Chir. Scand., 56:156–163, 1934.

16. Berkheiser, E.J.: Old Ununited Clavicular Fractures in the Adult. Surg. Gynecol. Obstet., 64:1064–1072, 1937.

17. Bernard, T.N., and Haddad, R.J.: Enchrondroma of the Proximal Clavicle: An Unusual Cause of Pathologic Fracture Dislocation of the Sternoclavicular Joint. Clin. Orthop., 167:239–241, 1982.

18. Billington, R.W.: A New (Plaster Yoke) Dressing for Fracture of the Clavicle. South. Med. J., 24:667, 1931.

19. Bonnett, J.: Fracture of the Clavicle. Arch. Chir. Neerlandicum, 27:143–151, 1975.

20. Bowen, A.D.: Plastic Bowing of the Clavicle in Children: A Report of Two Cases. J. Bone Joint Surg., 65A:403–405, 1983.

21. Breck, L.: Partially Threaded Round Pins With Oversized Threads for Intramedullary Fixation of the Clavicle and the Forearm Bones. Clin. Orthop., 11:227–229, 1958.

22. Brighton, C.T., and Pollick, S.R.: Treatment of Recalcitrant Nonunion With a Capacatively Coupled Electrical Field. A Preliminary Report. J. Bone Joint Surg., 67A:577–585, 1985.

23. Brooks, A.L., and Henning, G.D.: Injuries to the Proximal Clavicular Epiphysis. J. Bone Joint Surg., 54A:1347, 1972.

24. Bronz, G.; Heim, D.; and Posterla, C.: Die stabile Clavicula Osteosynthese. Unfallheilkunde, 84:319–325, 1981.

25. Butterworth, R.D., and Kirk, A.A.: Virginia Med., 79:98, 1952.

26. Cahill, B.R.: Osteolysis of the Distal Part of the Clavicle in Male Athletes. J. Bone Joint Surg., 64A:1053–1058, 1982.

27. Campbell, E.; Howard, W.B.; and Breklund, C.W.: Delayed Brachial Plexus Palsy Due to Ununited Fracture of the Clavicle. J.A.M.A., 139:91–92, 1949.

28. Caspi, I.; Ezra, E.; Nerubay, J.; and Horoszovski, H.: Musculocutaneous Nerve Injury After Coracoid Process Transfer for Clavicle Instability. Acta Orthop. Scand., 58:294–295, 1987.

29. Cayford, E.H., and Tees, F.J.: Traumatic Aneurysm of the Subclavian Artery as a Late Complication of Fractured Clavicle. Can. Med. Assoc. J., 25:450–452, 1931.

30. Cohen, A.W., and Otto, S.R.: Obstetric Clavicular Fractures. J. Reprod. Med., 25:119–122, 1980.

31. Codman, E.A.: The Shoulder—Rupture of the Supraspinatus Tendon and Other Lesions in or About the Subacromial Bursa. Boston, T. Todd Co., 1934.

32. Connolly, J.F.: Electrical Treatment of Nonunion: Its Use and Abuse in 100 Consecutive Fractures. Orthop. Clin., 15:89–106, 1984.

33. Connolly, J.F., and Dehne, R.: Delayed Thoracic Outlet Syndrome From Clavicular Non-Union: Management by Morseling. Nebr. Med. J., 71:303–306, 1986.

34. Connolly, J.F., and Dehne, R.: Nonunion of the Clavicle and Thoracic Outlet Syndrome. J. Trauma, 29:1127–1132, 1989.

35. Conwell, H.E.: Fractures of the Clavicle. J.A.M.A., 90:838–839, 1928.

36. Cook, T.: Reduction and External Fixation of Fractures of the Clavicle in Recumbency. J. Bone Joint Surg., 36A:878–880, 1954.

37. Copeland, S.M.: Total Resection of the Clavicle. Am. J. Surg., 72:280–281, 1946.

38. Costa, M.C., and Robbs, J.V.: Nonpenetrating Subclavian Artery Trauma. J. Vasc. Surg., 8:71–75, 1988.

39. Craig, E.V.: Fractures of the Clavicle. In Rockwood, C.A. Jr., and Matsen, F.A., III (eds.): The Shoulder, pp. 367–412. Philadelphia, W.B. Saunders, 1990.

40. Cumming, W.A.: Neonatal Skeletal Fractures: Birth Trauma, or Child Abuse? J. Canad. Assoc. Rad., 30:30–33, 1979.

41. Cummings, C.W., and First, R.: Stress Fracture of the Clavicle After a Radical Neck Dissection. Case Report. Plast. Reconstr. Surg., 55:366–367, 1975.

42. Curtis, R.J., Jr.: Operative Treatment of Children's Fractures of the Shoulder Region. Orthop. Clin. North Am., 21:315–324, 1990.

43. Dameron, T.B., Jr.: External Fixation of the Clavicle for Fracture or Nonunion in Adults (letter). J. Bone Joint Surg., 71A:1272, 1989.

44. Dameron, T.B., Jr., and Rockwood, C.A., Jr.: Fractures of the Shaft of the Clavicle. In Rockwood, C.A., Jr.; Wilkins, K.E.; and King, R.E. (eds.): Fractures in Children, pp. 608–624. Philadelphia, J.B. Lippincott, 1984.

45. Dannohl, C.; Meeder, P.J.; and Weller, S.: Costoclavicular Syndrome: a Rare Complication of Clavicular Fracture. Aktuelle Taumatologie, 18:149–151, 1988.

46. Das, N.K., and Deb, H.K.: Synovioma of the Clavicle. Report of a Case. J. Int. Coll. Surg., 35:776–780, 1961.

47. Dash, U.N., and Handler, D.: A Case of Compression of Subclavian Vessels by a Fractured Clavicle Treated by Excision of the First Rib. J. Bone Joint Surg., 42A:798–801, 1960.

48. Day, L.: Electrical Stimulation in the Treatment of Ununited Fractures. Clin. Orthop., 161:54–57, 1981.

49. De Bakey, E.; Beall, C., Jr.; and Ukkasch, D.C.: Recent Developments in Vascular Surgery With Particular Reference to Orthopaedics. Am. J. Surg., 109:134–142, 1965.

50. DePalma, A.: Surgery of the Shoulder, 3rd ed., pp. 348–362. Philadelphia, J.B. Lippincott, 1983.

51. Dickson, J.W.: Death Following Fractured Clavicle. Br. Med. J. 2:666, 1952.

52. Dolin, M.: The Operative Treatment of Midshaft Clavicular Nonunions (letter). J. Bone Joint Surg., 68A:634, 1986.

53. Dugdale, T.W., and Fulkerson, J.B.: Pneumothorax Complicating a Closed Fracture of the Clavicle: A Case Report. Clin. Orthop., 221:212–214, 1987.

54. Dupuytren, Le Baron: On the Injuries and Diseases of Bone (Clark, L., trans.). London, Sydenham Society, 1847.

55. Dust, W.N., and Lenczner, A.M.: Stress Fracture of the

Clavicle Leading to Nonunion Secondary to Coracoclavicular Reconstruction With Bacron. Am. J. Sports Med., 17:128–129, 1989.

56. Ebraheim, N.A.; An, H.S.; Jackson, W.T.; Pearlstein, S.R.; Burgess, A.; Tscherne, H.; Hass, N.; Kellam, J.; and Wipperman, B.U.: Scapulothoracic Dissociation. J. Bone Joint Surg., 70:428–432, 1988.

57. Echtermeyer, V.; Zwipp, H.; and Oestern, H.J.: Fehler und Gefahren in der Behandlung der Fracturen und Pseudarthrosen des Schlusselbeins. Langenbecks Arch. Chir., 364: 351–354, 1984.

58. Edvardsen, P., and Odegard, O.: Treatment of Posttraumatic Clavicular Pseudoarthrosis. Acta Orthop. Scand. 48: 456–457, 1977.

59. Eidman, D.K.; Siff, S.J.; and Tullos, H.S.: Acromioclavicular Lesions in Children. Am. J. Sports Med., 9:150–154, 1981.

60. Elliott, A.C.: Tripartite Injury of the Clavicle: A Case Report. S. Afr. Med. J., 70:115, 1986.

61. Enker, S.H., and Murthy, K.K.: Brachial Plexus Compression by Excessive Callus Formation Secondary to a Fractured Clavicle: A Case Report. Mt. Sinai J. Med., 37:678–682, 1970.

62. Eskola, A.; Vainionpaa, S.; Myllynen, P.; Patiala, H.; and Rokkanen, P.: Outcome of Clavicular Fracture in 89 Patients. Arch. Orthop. Trauma Surg., 105:337–338, 1986.

63. Eskola, A.; Vainionpaa, S.; and Myllyen, P.: Surgery for Ununited Clavicular Fracture. Acta Orthop. Scand., 57: 366–367, 1986.

64. Eskola, A.; Vainionpaa, S.; Patiala, H.; et al: Outcome of Operative Treatment in Fresh Lateral Clavicle Fracture. Ann. Chir. Gynaecol., 76:167–168, 1987.

65. Fairbank, H.: Cranio-Cleido-Dystostosis. J. Bone Joint Surg., 31B:608, 1949.

66. Falconer, M.A., and Weddell, G.: Costoclavicular Compression of the Subclavian Artery and Vein. Lancet, 2:539, 1943.

67. Falstie-Jensen, S.: Psuedodislocation of the Acromioclavicular Joint. J. Bone Joint Surg., 64B:368–369, 1982.

68. Farkas, R., and Levine, S.: X-Ray Incidence of Fractured Clavicle in Vertex Presentation. Am. J. Obstet. Gynecol., 59:204–206, 1950.

69. Fawcett, J.: The Development and Ossification of the Human Clavicle. J. Anat., 47:225–234, 1913.

70. Fich, R.: Handbuch der Anatomie und Mechanic der Galanke. *In* Bvdeleben, V. (ed.): Handbuch der Anatomie des Menschen, Vol. 2, Section 1, pp. 163–187. Jema, Gustava Discher, 1910.

71. Finelli, P.F., and Cardi, J.K.: Seizure as a Cause of Fracture. Neurology, 39:858–860, 1989.

72. Fini-Storchi, O.; LoRusso, D.; and Agostini, V.: "Pseudotumors" of the Clavicle Subsequent to Radical Neck Dissection. J. Laryngol. Otol., 99:73–83, 1985.

73. Fowler, A.W.: Fractures of the Clavicle. J. Bone Joint Surg., 44B:440, 1962.

74. Freedman, M.; Gamble, J.; and Lewis, C.: Intrauterine Fracture Simulating a Unilateral Clavicular Pseudarthrosis. J. Assoc. Radiol., 33:37–38, 1982.

75. Friedman, R.J., and Gordon, L.: False Positive Indium-111 White Blood Cell Scan in Enclosed Clavicle Fracture. J. Orthop. Trauma, 2:151–153, 1988.

76. Frobenius, H., and Betzel, A.: Injuries and Their Causes in Bicycle Accidents. Unfallchirurgie (Munchen), 13:135–141, 1987.

77. Fry, J.: Photo of the "Edwin Smith Surgical Papyrus." *In* Rockwood, C.A.; Wilkins, K.E.; and King, R.E. (eds.): Fractures in Children, Philadelphia, J.B. Lippincott, p. 679. 1984.

78. Fukuda, K.; Craig, E.V.; An, K.N.; Cofield, R.H.; and Chao, E.Y.: Biomechanical Study of the Ligamentous System of the Acromioclavicular Joint. J. Bone Joint Surg., 68A: 434–440, 1986.

79. Gardner, E.D.; Grey, D.J.; and Orahilly, R.: Anatomy, p. 108. Philadelphia, W.B. Saunders, 1960.

80. Gardner, E.: The Embryology of the Clavicle. Clin. Orthop., 58:9–16, 1968.

81. Gearen, P.F., and Petty, W.: PanClavicular Dislocation: Report of a Case. J. Bone Joint Surg., 64A:454–455, 1982.

82. Gebuhr, P.: Brachial Plexus Involvement After Fractures of the Clavicle. Ugeske-Laeger, 150:105–106, 1988.

83. Ghormley, R.K.; Black, J.R.; and Cherry, J.H.: Ununited Fractures of the Clavicle. Am. J. Surg., 51:343–349, 1941.

84. Gibbon, J.H.: Lucas-Championnierer and Mobilization in the Treatment of Fractures. Surg. Gynecol. Obstet., 43: 271–278, 1926.

85. Gibson, D.A., and Carroll, N.: Congenital Pseudoarthrosis of the Clavicle. J. Bone Joint Surg., 52B:629–643, 1970.

86. Gilbert, W.M., and Tchabo, J.G.: Fractured Clavicle in Newborns. Int. Surg., 73:123–125, 1988.

87. Gitsch, V.G., and Schatten, C.: Frequenz und potentielle Faktoren in der Genese der geburtstraumatisch bedingten Klavicula fraktur. Zent. Gynakol., 109:909–912, 1987.

88. Goddard, N.J.; Stabler, J.; and Albert, J.S.: Atlanto-Axial Rotatory Fixation in Fracture of the Clavicle: An Association and a Classification. J. Bone Joint Surg., 72B:72–75, 1990.

89. Gonik, B.; Allen, R.; and Sorab, J.: Objective Evaluation of the Shoulder Dystocia Phenomenon: Effect of Maternal Pelvic Orientation on Bone Reduction. Obstet. Gynecol., 74:44–48, 1989.

90. Grant, J.C.B.: A Method of Anatomy, 5th ed. Baltimore, Williams & Wilkins, 1952.

91. Gresham, E.L.: Birth Trauma. Ped. Clin. North Am., 22: 317, 1975.

92. Gross, S.D.: The Anatomy, Physiology, and Diseases of the Bones and Joints, p. 67. Philadelphia, John Grigg, 1830.

93. Gryska, P.F.: Major Vascular Injuries. N. Engl. J. Med., 266:381–385, 1982.

94. Guattieri, G., and Frassi, G.: Late Truncal Paralysis of the Brachial Plexus in Sequela of Fracture of the Clavicle. Arch Ortopedia., 74:840–848, 1961.

95. Guilfoil, P.H., and Christiansen, T.: An Unusual Vascular Complication of Fractured Clavicle. J.A.M.A., 200:72–73, 1967.

96. Guillemin, A.: Dechrune de la Vein Sous-Claviere par Fracture Fermie de la Clavicule. Bull. Mem. Soc. Nat. Chir., 56:302–304, 1930.

97. Gurd, F.B.: The Treatment of Complete Dislocation of the Outer End of Clavicle: A Hitherto Undescribed Operation. Ann. Surg., 113:1094–1097, 1941.

98. Hackstock, H., and Hackstock, H.: Surgical Treatment of Clavicular Fracture. Unfallchrurg, 91:64–69, 1988.

99. Hargan, B., and Macafee, A.L.: Bilateral Pseudoarthrosis of the Clavicles. Injury, 12:316–318, 1981.

100. Heppenstall, R.B.: Fractures and Dislocations of the Distal Clavicle. Orthop. Clin. North Am., 6(2):447–486, 1975.

101. Hicks, J.H.: Rigid Fixation as a Treatment for Hypertrophic Nonunion. Injury, 8:199–205, 1976.

102. Hoyer, H.E.; Kindt, R.; and Lippert, H.: Zur Biomechanik der menschlichen Clavcula. Z. Orthop., 118:915–922, 1980.

103. Houston, H.E.: An Unusual Complication of Clavicular Fracture. J. Ky. Med. Assoc., 75:170–171, 1977.

104. Howard, F.M., and Schafer, S.J.: Injuries to the Clavicle With Neurovascular Complications: A Study of Fourteen Cases. J. Bone Joint Surg., 47A:1335–1346, 1965.

105. Hughes, A.W., and Sherlock, D.A.: Bilateral Thoracic Outlet Syndrome Following Nonunion of Clavicles Associated With Radio-osteodystrophy Injury. J. Bone Joint Surg., 19:40–41, 1988.

106. Inman, V.T., and Saunders, J.B.: Observation on the Function of the Clavicle. Calif. Med., 65:158–165, 1946.

107. Iqbal, O.: Axillary Artery Thrombosis Associated With Fracture of the Clavicle. Med. J. Malaysia, 26:68–70, 1971.

108. Jablon, M.; Sutker, A.; and Post, M.: Irreducible Fractures of the Middle Third of the Clavicle. J. Bone Joint Surg., 61A:296–298, 1979.

109. Jackson, W.J.: Clavicle Fractures: Therapy is Dictated by the Patient's Age. Consultant, October, p. 177, 1982.

110. Jacobs, P.: Post-traumatic Osteolysis of the Outer End of the Clavicle. J. Bone Joint Surg., 46B:705–707, 1964.

111. Jain, A.S.: Traumatic Floating Clavicle: A Case Report. J. Bone Joint Surg., 66B:560–561, 1984.

112. Javid, H.: Vascular Injuries of the Neck. Clin. Orthop., 28:70–78, 1963.

113. Jit, I., and Kulkrani, M.: Times of Appearance and Fusion of Epiphysis at the Medial End of the Clavicle. Indian J. Med. Res., 64:773–792, 1976.

114. Johnson, E.W., Jr., and Collins, H.R.: Nonunion of the Clavicle. Arch. Surg., 87:963–966, 1963.

115. Joseph, P.R., and Rosenfeld, W.: Clavicular Fractures in Neonates. Am. J. Dis. Child., 144:165–167, 1990.

116. Joukainen, J., and Karaharju, E.: Pseudoarthrosis of the Clavicle. Acta Orthop. Scand., 48:550, 1977.

117. Jupiter, J.B., and Leffert, R.D.: Nonunion of the Clavicle. J. Bone Joint Surg., 69A:753–760, 1987.

118. Kanoksikarin, S., and Wearne, W.N.: Fracture and Retrosternal Dislocation of the Clavicle. Aust. N. Z. J. Surg., 48:95–96, 1978.

119. Kabaharjve, E.; Joukainen, J.; and Peltonen, J.: Treatment of Pseudoarthrosis of the Clavicle. Injury, 13:400–403, 1982.

120. Karwasz, R.R.; Kutzner, M.; and Krammer, W.G.: Late Brachial Plexus Lesion Following Clavicular Fracture. Unfallchurg., 91:45–47, 1988.

121. Katz, R.; Landman, J.; Dulitzky, F.; and Bar-Ziv, J.: Fracture of the Clavicle in the Newborn: An Ultrasound Diagnosis. J. Ultrasound Med., 7:21–23, 1988.

122. Katznelson, A.; Nerubay, J.; and Oliver, S.: Dynamic Fixation of the Avulsed Clavicle. J. Trauma, 16:841–844, 1976.

123. Kay, S.P., and Eckardt, J.J.: Brachial Plexus Palsy Secondary to Clavicular Nonunion: A Case Report and Literature Survey. Clin. Orthop., 206:219–222, 1986.

124. Kaye, J.J.; Nance, E.P., Jr.; and Green, N.E.: Fatigue Fracture of the Medial Aspect of the Clavicle: An Academic Rather Than Athletic Injury. Radiology, 144:89–90, 1982.

125. Key, J.A., and Conwell, E.H.: The Management of Fractures, Dislocations, and Sprains, 2nd ed., p. 437. St. Louis, C.V. Mosby, 1937.

126. Khan, M.A.A., and Lucas, H.K.: Plating of Fractures of the Middle Third of the Clavicle. Injury, 9:263–267, 1978.

127. Kini, M.G.: A Simple Method of Ambulatory Treatment of Fractures of the Clavicle. J. Bone Joint Surg., 23:795–798, 1941.

128. Kite, J.H.: Congenital Pseudoarthrosis of the Clavicle. South. Med. J., 761:703–710, 1968.

129. Klier, I., and Mayor, P.B.: Laceration of the Innominate Internal Jugular Venous Junction: Rare Complication of Fracture of the Clavicle. Orthop. Rev., 10:81–82, 1981.

130. Koch, F.; Papadimitriou, G.; and Groher, W.: Die Clavicula pseudoarthroseihse Entstehung und Behandlung. Unfallheilkunde. 74:330–337, 1971.

131. Koelliker, F., and Ganz, R.: Results of the Treatment of Clavicular Pseudarthrosis. Unfallchirurg (Berlin), 92:164–168, 1989.

132. Koss, S.D.; Giotz, H.T.; Redler, N.R.; et al: Nonunion of a Midshaft Clavicle Fracture Associated With Subclavian Vein Compression: A Case Report. Orthopedic Rev., 18:431–434, 1989.

133. Kreisinger, V.: Sur le Traitement des Fractures de le Clavicule. Rev. Chir., 43:376, 1927.

134. Kremens, V., and Glauser, F.: Unusual Sequelae Following Pinning of Medial Clavicular Fracture. Am. J. Roentgenol., 74:1066–1069, 1956.

135. Lancet (editorial): Sir Robert Peel's Death. Lancet, 2:19, 1850.

136. Lee, H.G.: Treatment of Fracture of the Clavicle by Internal Nail Fixation. N. Engl. J. Med., 234:222–224, 1946.

137. Lemire, L., and Rosman, M.: Sternoclavicular Epiphyseal Separation With Adjacent Clavicular Fracture. J. Pediatr. Orthop., 4:118–120, 1984.

138. Lengua, F.; Nuss, J.; Lechner, R.; Baruthio, J.; and Veillon, F.: The Treatment of Fracture of the Clavicle by Closed Medio-Lateral Pinning. Rev. Chir. Orthop., 73:377–380, 1987.

139. Lester, C.W.: The Treatment of Fractures of the Clavicle. Ann. Surg., 89:600–606, 1929.

140. Liechtl, R.: Fracture of the Clavicle and Scapula. In Webber, B.G.; Brunner, C.; and Freuler, F. (eds.): Treatment of Fractures in Children and Adolescents, pp. 88–95. New York, Springer-Verlag, 1988.

141. Lim, E., and Day, L.J.: Subclavian Vein Thrombosis Fol-

lowing Fracture of the Clavicle: A Case Report. Orthopedics, 10:349–351, 1987.

142. Lipton, H.A., and Jupiter, J.B.: Nonunion of Clavicular Fractures: Characteristics and Surgical Management. Surg. Rounds Orthop., July, 1988.

143. Ljunggren, A.E.: Clavicular Function. Acta Orthop. Scand., 50:261–268, 1979.

144. Lloyd-Roberts, G.C.; Apley, A.G.; and Owen, R.: Reflections Upon the Etiology of Congenital Pseudoarthrosis of the Clavicle. J. Bone Joint Surg., 57B:24–29, 1975.

145. Lombard, J.J.: Pseudoarthrosis of the Clavicle: A Case Report. S. Afr. Med. J., 66:151–153, 1984.

146. Lord, J.W., and Rosati, J.M.: Neurovascular Compression Syndromes of the Upper Extremity. CIBA Clinical Symposia, 10(2), 1958.

147. Lukin, A.V., and Grishken, V.A.: Two Cases of Successful Treatment of Fracture Dislocation of the Clavicle. Ortop. Travmatol. Protez., 11:35, 1987.

148. Lusskin, R.; Weiss, C.A.; and Winer, J.: The Role of the Subclavius Muscle in the Subclavian Vein Syndrome (Costoclavicular Syndrome) Following Fracture of the Clavicle. Clin. Orthop., 54:75–84, 1967.

149. Madsen, E.T.: Fractures of the Extremities in the Newborn. Acta Obstet. Gynecol. Scand., 34:41–74, 1955.

150. Malcolm, B.W.; Ameli, F.N.; and Simmons, E.H.: Pneumothorax Complicating a Fracture of the Clavicle. Can. J. Surg., 22:84, 1979.

151. Malgaigne, J.F.: A Treatise on Fractures, pp. 374–401. (Transl. by Packard, J.H.) Philadelphia, J.B. Lippincott, 1859.

152. Manske, D.J., and Szabo, R.M.: The Operative Treatment of Mid-Shaft Clavicular Non-Unions. J. Bone Joint. Surg., 67A:1367–1371, 1985.

153. Marie, P., and Sainton, P.: On Hereditary Cleidocranial Dysostosis. Clin. Orthop., 58:5–7, 1968.

154. Marsh, H.O., and Hazarian, E.: Pseudoarthrosis of the Clavicle (abstract). J. Bone Joint Surg., 52B:793–970, 1970.

155. Matry, C.: Fracture de la Clavicule Gauche au Tiers Interne: Blessure de la Vein Sous-Claviere. Osteosynthese Bull. Mem. Soc. Nat. Chir., 58:75–78, 1932.

156. Matz, S.O.; Welliver, P.S.; and Welliver, D.I.: Brachial Plexus Neuropraxia Complicating a Comminuted Clavicle Fracture in a College Football Player: Case Report and Review of the Literature. Am. J. Sports Med., 17:581–583, 1989.

157. Mayer, J.H.: Nonunion of Fractured Clavicle. Proc. Roy. Soc. Med., 58:182, 1965.

158. Mazet, R.: Migration of a Kirschner Wire From the Shoulder Region Into the Lung: Report of Two Cases. J. Bone Joint Surg., 25:477–483, 1943.

159. McCandless, D.N., and Mowbray, M.: Treatment of Displaced Fractures of the Clavicle. Sling Vs. Figure-of-Eight Bandage. Practitioner, 223:266–267, 1979.

160. Miller, D.S., and Boswick, J.A.: Lesions of the Brachial Plexus Associated With Fractures of the Clavicle. Clin. Orthop., 64:144–149, 1969.

161. Mital, M.A., and Aufranc, O.E.: Venous Occlusion Following Greenstick Fracture Clavicle. J.A.M.A., 206:1301–1302, 1968.

162. Mnaymneh, W.; Vargas, A.; and Kaplan, J.: Fractures of the Clavicle Caused by Arteriovenous Malformation. Clin. Orthop., 148:256–258, 1980.

163. Moir, J.C., and Myerscough, P.R.: Operative Obstetrics, 7th ed., Baltimore, Williams & Wilkins, 1964.

164. Moore, T.O.: Internal Pin Fixation for Fracture of the Clavicle. Am. Surg., 17:580–583, 1951.

165. Moseley, H.F.: The Clavicle: Its Anatomy and Function. Clin. Orthop., 58:17–27, 1968.

166. Moseley, H.F.: Shoulder Lesions, pp. 207–235. New York, Churchill Livingstone, 1972.

167. Mulder, D.S.; Greenwood, F.A.; and Brooks, C.E.: Post-Traumatic Thoracic Outlet Syndrome. J. Trauma, 13:706–713, 1973.

168. Mueller, M.E.; Allgower, N.; and Willenegger, H.: Manual of Internal Fixation. New York, Springer-Verlag, 1970.

169. Murray, G.: A Method of Fixation for Fracture of the Clavicle. J. Bone Joint Surg., 22:616–620, 1940.

170. Natali, J.; Maraval, M.; Kieffer, E.; and Petrovic, P.: Fractures of the Clavicle and Injuries of the Subclavian Artery: Report of 10 Cases. J. Cardiovasc. Surg., 16:541–547, 1975.

171. Neer, C.S., II: Impingement Lesions. Clin. Orthop., 173:70–77, 1983.

172. Neer, Charles S., II: Fractures of the Clavicle. In Rockwood, C.A., Jr., and Green, D.P. (eds.): Fractures in Adults, pp. 707–713. Philadelphia, J.B. Lippincott, 1984.

173. Neer, C.S., II: Nonunion of the Clavicle. J.A.M.A., 172:1006–1011, 1960.

174. Neer, C.S., II: Fractures of the Distal Third of the Clavicle. Clin. Orthop., 58:43–50, 1968.

175. Neer, C.S., II: Fracture of the Distal Clavicle With Detachment of Coracoclavicular Ligaments in Adults. J. Trauma, 3:99–110, 1963.

176. Nelson, H.P.: Subclavian Aneurysm Following Fracture of the Clavicle. St. Bartholomew (Hospital Report), 65:219–229, 1932.

177. Neviaser, R.J.; Neviaser, J.S.; and Neviaser, T.J.: A Simple Technique for Internal Fixation of the Clavicle. Clin. Orthop., 109:103–107, 1975.

178. Neviaser, J.S.: Acromioclavicular Dislocations Treated by Transference of the Coracoacromial Ligament. Bull. Hosp. Joint. Dis., 12:46–54, 1951.

179. Neviaser, J.S.: Injuries of the Clavicle and Its Articulations. Orthop. Clin. North Am., 11:233–237, 1980.

180. Neviaser, J.S.: Injuries in and about the Shoulder Joint. Instr. Course Lect., XIII:187–216, 1956.

181. Neviaser, J.S.: The Treatment of Fractures of the Clavicle. Surg. Clin. North Am., 43:1555–1563, 1963.

182. Neviaser, R.J.: Injuries to the Clavicle and Acromioclavicular Joint. Orthop. Clin. North Am., 18:433–438, 1987.

183. Nogi, J.; Heckman, J.D.; Hakala, M.; and Sweet, D.E.: Nonunion of the Clavicle in the Child: A Case Report. Clin. Orthop., 110:19–21, 1975.

184. Noriell, H.; and Llewelleyn, R.C.: Migration of a Threaded Steinmann Pin From an Acromioclavicular Joint Into the Spinal Canal: A Case Report. J. Bone Joint Surg., 47A:1024, 1965.

185. Ogden, J.A.; Conologue, G.J.; and Bronson, N.L.: Ra-

diology of Postnatal Skeletal Development: The clavicle. Skeletal Radiol., 4:196–203, 1979.

186. Oppenheimer, W.L.; David, A.; Growdon, W.A.; Dorey, F. J.; and Davlin, L.B.: Clavicle Fractures in the Newborn. Clin. Orthop., 250:176, 1990.

187. Ord, R.A., and Langon, J.D.: Stress Fracture of the Clavicle: A Rare Late Complication of Radical Neck Dissection. J. Maxillofac. Surg., 14:281–284, 1986.

188. O'Rourke, I.C., and Middleton, R.W.: The Place and Efficacy of Operative Management of Fractured Clavicle. Injury, 6:236–240, 1975.

189. Ostreich, A.E.: The Lateral Clavicle Hook—An Acquired as Well as a Congenital Anomaly. Pediatr. Radiol., 11: 147, 1981.

190. Owen, R.: Congenital Pseudoarthrosis of the Clavicle. J. Bone Joint Surg., 52B:642–652, 1970.

191. Oxnard, C.E.: The Architecture of the Shoulder in Some Mammals. J. Morphol., 126:249–290, 1968.

192. Packer, B.D.: Conservative Treatment of Fracture of the Clavicle. J. Bone Joint Surg., 26:770–774, 1944.

193. Paffen, P.J., and Jansen, E.W.: Surgical Treatment of Clavicular Fractures With Kirschner Wires: A Comparative Study. Arch. Chir. Neerl., 30:43–53, 1978.

194. Parkes, J.C., and Deland, J.D.: A Three-Part Distal Clavicle Fracture. J. Trauma, 23:437–438, 1983.

195. Patel, C.V., and Audenwalla, H.S.: Treatment of Fractured Clavicle by Immediate Partial Subperiosteal Resection. J. Postgrad. Med., 18:32–34, 1972.

196. Penn, I.: The Vascular Complications of Fractures of the Clavicle. J. Trauma, 4:819–831, 1964.

197. Perry, B.: An Improved Clavicular Pin. Am. J. Surg., 112: 142–144, 1966.

198. Pipkin, G.: Tardy Shoulder Hand Syndrome Following Ununited Fracture of Clavicle: A Case Report. J. Missouri Med. Assoc., 643–646, August, 1951.

199. Piterman, L.: "The Fractured Clavicle." Aust. Fam. Phys., 11:614, 1982.

200. Poigenfurst, J.; Reiler, T.; and Fischer, W.: Plating of Fresh Clavicular Fractures: Experience With 60 Operations. Unfallchirurgie, 14:26–37, 1988.

201. Pollen, A.G.: Fractures and Dislocations in Children. Baltimore, Williams & Wilkins, 1973.

202. Porral, A.: Observation d'une Double Luxation de la Clavicule Droite Juniva. Hibd. Med. Chir. Part., 2:78–82, 1831.

203. Post, M.: Current Concepts in the Treatment of Fractures of the Clavicle. Clin. Orthop., 245:89–101, 1989.

204. Post, M.: Injury to the Shoulder Girdle. In Post, M. (ed.): The Shoulder: Surgical and Non-Surgical Management, pp. 432–447. Philadelphia, Lea & Febiger, 1988.

205. Pusitz, M.E., and Davis, E.V.: Bone-Drilling in Delayed Union of Fractures. J. Bone Joint Surg., 26A:560–565, 1944.

206. Pyper, J.B.: Nonunion of Fractures of the Clavicle. Injury, 9:268–270, 1978.

207. Quesana, F.: Technique for the Roentgen Diagnosis of Fractures of the Clavicle. Surg. Gynecol. Obstet., 42:4261–4281, 1926.

208. Quigley, T.B.: The Management of Simple Fracture of the Clavicle in Adults. N. Engl. J. Med., 243:386–290, 1950.

209. Quinlan, W.R.; Brady, P.G.; and Regan, B.F.: Congenital Pseudoarthrosis of the Clavicle. Acta Orthop. Scand., 51: 489–492, 1980.

210. Quinn, S.F., and Glass, T.A.: Post Traumatic Osteolysis of the Clavicle. South. Med. J., 76:307–308, 1983.

211. Rabenseifner, L.: Zur Atiologie und Therapie bei Schlusselbeinpsuedarthosen. Acta Traumatol., 11:130–132, 1981.

212. Raymakers, E., and Marti, R.: Nonunion of the Clavicle. In Pseudarthroses and Their Treatment. Eighth International Symposium on Topical Problems in Orthopaedic Surgery. Thieme, 1979.

213. Redmond, A.D.: A Complication of Fracture of the Clavicle (letter). Injury, 13:352, 1982.

214. Reid, J., and Kenned, J.: Direct Fracture of the Clavicle With Symptoms Simulating a Cervical Rib. Brit. Med. J. 2:608–609, 1925.

215. Rhinelander, F.W.: Tibial Blood Supply in Relation to Fracture Healing. Clin. Orthop., 105:34–81, 1974.

216. Ring, M.: Clavicle. In Ring, M. (ed.): Children's Fractures, 2nd ed. Philadelphia, J.B. Lippincott, 1983.

217. Rockwood, C.A.: Fractures of the Outer Clavicle in Children and Adults. J. Bone Joint Surg., 64B:642, 1982.

218. Rockwood, C.A.: Personal Communication.

219. Rockwood, C.A.: Management of Fracture of the Clavicle and Injuries of the SC Joints. Orthop. Trans., 6:422, 1982.

220. Rockwood, C.A.: Treatment of the Outer Clavicle in Children and Adults. Orthop. Trans., 6:472, 1982.

221. Rosati, L.M., and Lord, J.W., Jr.: Neurovascular Compression Syndromes of the Shoulder Girdle. New York, Grune and Stratton, 1961.

222. Rowe, C.R.: An Atlas of Anatomy and Treatment of Mid-Clavicular Fractures. Clin. Orthop., 58:29–42, 1968.

223. Rubin, A.: Birth Injuries: Incidence, Mechanisms and End Result. Obstet. Gynecol., 23:218–221, 1964.

224. Rush, L.V., and Rush, H.L.: Technique of Longitudinal Pin Fixation in Fractures of the Clavicle and Jaw. Miss. Doctor, 27:332, 1949.

225. Sakellarides, H.: Pseudoarthrosis of the Clavicle. J. Bone Joint Surg., 43A:130–138, 1961.

226. Sampson, J.J.; Saunders, J.B.; and Capp, C.S.: Compression of the Subclavian Vein by the First Rib and Clavicle With Reference to Prominence of the Chest Veins as a Sign of Collaterals. Am. Heart J., 19:292–315, 1940.

227. Sandford, H.N.: The Moro Reflex as a Diagnostic Aid in Fracture of the Clavicle and the Newborn Infant. Am. J. Dis. Child., 41:1304–1306, 1931.

228. Sankarankuty, M., and Turner, B.W.: Fractures of the Clavicle. Injury, 7:101–106, 1975.

229. Sayer, L.: A Simple Dressing for Fractures of the Clavicle. Am. Pract., 4:1, 1871.

230. Scarpa, F.J., and Levy, R.M.: Pulmonary Embolism Complicating Clavicle Fracture. Conn. Med., 43:771–773, 1979.

231. Schewior, T.: Die Durckpallenostesynthese bei Schlusselpein pseudarthrosen. Acta Traumatol., 4:113–125, 1974.

232. Schrocksnadel, H.; Heim, K.; and Dapunt, O.: The Clavicular Fracture—A Questionable Achievement in Modern

Obstetrics. Geburtshilfe Und Frauenheilkunde, 49:481–484, 1989.

233. Schuind, F.; Pay-Pay, E.; Andrianne, Y.; Donkerwolcke, M.; Rasquin, C.; and Burny, F.: External Fixation of the Clavicle for Fracture or Nonunion in Adults. J. Bone Joint Surg., 70A:692–695, 1988.

234. Schwartz, V.N., and Leixnering, M.: Technik und Ergebieniesse der Klavikula-markdrahtung. Zentralbl-Chir., 111:640–647, 1986.

235. Shauffer, I.A., and Collins, W.V.: The Deep Clavicular Rhomboid Fossa. J.A.M.A., 195:778–779, 1966.

236. Shih, J.; Chao, E.; and Chang, C.: Subclavian Pseudoaneurysm After Clavicle Fracture: A Case Report. J. Formosan Med. Assoc., 82:332–335, 1983.

237. Siebermann, R.P.; Spieler, U.; and Arquint, A.: Rush Pin Osteosynthesis of the Clavicle as an Alternative to Conservative Treatment. Unfallchirurgie, 13:303–307, 1987.

238. Siffrey, and Aulong: Thrombose Post-Traumatique de l'Artere Sous-Claviere Gauche. Lyon Chir., 51:479–481, 1956.

239. Silloway, K.A.; Mclaughlin, R.E.; Edlich, R.C.; and Edlich, R.F.: Clavicular Fractures and Acromioclavicular Joint Injuries in Lacrosse: Preventable Injuries. J. Emerg. Med., 3:117–121, 1985.

240. Simpson, L.A., and Kellam, J.: Surgical Management of Fractures of the Clavicle, Scapula, and Proximal Humerus. Orthop. Update Series, 4:1–8, 1985.

241. Smith, R.W.: A Treatus on Fractures in the Vicinity of Joints, pp. 209–224. Dublin, Hodges & Smith, 1847.

242. Snyder, L.A.: Loss of the Accompanying Soft Tissue Shadow of Clavicle With Occult Fracture. South Med. J., 72:243, 1979.

243. Sorrells, R.B.: Fracture of the Clavicle. J. Arkansas Med. Soc., 71:253–256, 1975.

244. Spar, I.: Total Claviculectomy for Pathological Fractures. Clin. Orthop., 129:236–237, 1977.

245. Stanley, D., and Norris, S.H.: Recovery Following Fractures of the Clavicle Treated Conservatively. Injury, 19:162–164, 1988.

246. Stanley, D.; Trowbridge, E.A.; and Norris, S.H.: The Mechanism of Clavicular Fracture. J. Bone Joint Surg., 70B:461–464, 1988.

247. Steenburg, R.W., and Ravitch, M.M.: Cervico-Thoracic Approach for Subclavian Vessel Injury From Compound Fracture of the Clavicle: Considerations of Subclavian Axillary Exposures. Ann. Surg., 1:839, 1963.

248. Steffelaar, H., and Heim, V.: Sekundare Plattenosteosynthesen an der Clavicula. Arth. Orthop. Unfallchir., 79:75, 1974.

249. Steinberg, I.: Subclavian-Vein Thrombosis Associated With Fractures of the Clavicle. Report of Two Cases. N. Engl. J. Med., 264:686–688, 1961.

250. Stimson, L.A.: A Treatise on Fractures, p. 332. Philadelphia, Henry A. Lea's Son, 1883.

251. Stone, P.W., and Lord, J.W.: The Clavicle and its Relation to Trauma to the Subclavian Artery and Vein. Am. J. Surg., 98:834–839, 1955.

252. Storen, H.: Old Clavicular Pseudoarthrosis With Late Appearing Neuralgias and Vasomotor Disturbances Cured by Operation. Acta Chir. Scand., 94:187, 1946.

253. Strauss, M.; Bushey, M.J.; Chung, C.; and Baum, S.: Fractures of the Clavicle Following Radical Neck Dissection or Postoperative Radiotherapy: A Case Report and Review of the Literature. Laryngoscope, 92:1304–1307, 1982.

254. Swischuk, L.E.: Radiology of Newborn and Young Infants, 2nd ed., p. 630. Baltimore, Williams & Wilkins, 1981.

255. Tachdjian, M.O.: Pediatric Orthopaedics. Philadelphia, W.B. Saunders, 1972.

256. Tanchev, S., Kolishev, K.; Tanchev, P.; Gramcheva, O.; and Asparukhov, A.: Etiology of a Clavicle Fracture Due to the Birth Process. Akus-Ginecol., 24:39–43, 1985.

257. Taylor, A.R.: Nonunion of Fractures of the Clavicle: A Review of 31 Cases. J. Bone Joint Surg., 51B:568–569, 1969.

258. Taylor, A.R.: Some Observations on Fractures of the Clavicle. Proc. Roy. Soc. Med., 62:1037–1038, 1969.

259. Telford, E.D., and Mottershead, S.: Pressure at the Cervicobrachial Junction: An Operative and an Anatomical Study. J. Bone Joint Surg., 30B:249, 1948.

260. Thomas, C.B., Jr., and Friedman, R.J.: Ipsilateral Sternoclavicular Dislocation and Clavicular Fracture. J. Orthop. Trauma, 3:355–357, 1989.

261. Thompson, A.G., and Batten, R.C.: The Application of Rigid Internal Fixation to the Treatment of Nonunion and Delayed Union Using AO Technique. Injury, 8:88, 1977.

262. Todd, T.W., and D'Errico, J., Jr.: The Clavicular Epiphysis. Am. J. Anat., 41:25–50, 1928.

263. Tregonning, G., and Macnab, I.: Post-Traumatic Pseudoarthrosis of the Clavicle. J. Bone Joint Surg., 58B:264, 1976.

264. Trynin, A.H.: The Bohler Clavicular Splint in the Treatment of Clavicular Injuries. J. Bone Joint Surg., 19:417–424, 1937.

265. Tse, D.H.W.; Slabaugh, P.B.; and Carlson, P.A.: Injury to the Axillary Artery by a Closed Fracture of the Clavicle. J. Bone Joint Surg., 62A:1372–1373, 1980.

266. Tsou, P.N.: Percutaneous Cannulated Screw Coracoclavicular Fixation for Acute Acromioclavicular Dislocations. Clin. Orthop., 243:112–121, 1989.

267. Unger, J.M.; Schuchmann, G.G.; Grossman, J.E.; and Pellett, J.R.: Tears of the Trachea and Main Bronchi Caused by Blunt Trauma: Radiologic Findings. Am. J. Roentgenol., 153:1175–1180, 1989.

268. Urist, M.R.: Complete Dislocation of the Acromioclavicular Joint. J. Bone Joint Surg., 28:813–837, 1946.

269. Valdes-Dopena, M.A., and Arey, J.B.: The Causes of Neonatal Mortality: An Analysis of 501 Autopsies on Newborn Infants. J. Ped., 77:366, 1970.

270. Van Vlack, H.G.: Comminuted Fracture of the Clavicle With Pressure on Brachial Plexus: Report of Case. J. Bone Joint Surg., 22A:446–447, 1940.

271. Wachsmudh, W.: Allgemiene und specielle Operadion slettie, pp. 375. Berlin, Springer-Verlag, 1956.

272. Wall, J.J.: Congenital Pseudoarthrosis of the Clavicle. J. Bone Joint Surg., 52A:1003–1009, 1970.

273. Watson-Jones, R.: Fractures and Other Bone and Joint Injuries, pp. 90–91. Edinburgh, E. & S. Livingstone, 1940.

274. Weaver, J.K., and Dunn, H.K.: Treatment of Acromioclavicular Injuries Especially Acromioclavicular Separation. J. Bone Joint Surg., 54A:1187–1198, 1972.

275. Weber, B.G.: Pseudoarthrosis of the Clavicle. In Pseudoarthrosis: Pathophysiology, Biomechanics, Therapy, Results, pp. 104–107. New York, Grune and Stratton, 1976.

276. Weh, L., and Torklus, D.Z.: Fracture of the Clavicle With Consecutive Costoclavicular Compression Syndrome. Z. Orthop., 118:140–142, 1980.

277. Weiner, D.S., and O'Dell, H.W.: Fractures of the First Rib Associated With Injuries to the Clavicle. J. Trauma, 9:412–422, 1969.

278. Widner, L.A., and Riddewold, H.O.: The Value of the Lordotic View in Diagnosis of Fractured Clavicle. Rev. Int. Radiol., 5:69–70, 1980.

279. Wilkins, R.M., and Johnston, R.M.: Ununited Fractures of the Clavicle. J. Bone Joint Surg., 65A:773–778, 1983.

280. Wilkes, J.A., and Hoffer, M.: Clavicle Fractures in Head-Injured Children. J. Orthop. Trauma, 1:55–58, 1987.

281. Worcester, J.N., and Green, D.P.: Osteoarthritis of the Acromioclavicular Joint. Clin. Orthop., 58:69–73, 1968.

282. Wood, V.E.: The Results of Total Claviculectomy. Clin. Orthop., 207:186–190, 1986.

283. Yates, D.W.: Complications of Fractures of the Clavicle. Injury, 7:189–193, 1976.

284. Yates, A.G., and Guest, D.: Cerebral Embolus Due to Ununited Fracture of the Clavicle and Subclavian Thrombosis. Lancet, 2:225–226, 1928.

285. Young, C.S.: The Mechanics of Ambulatory Treatment of Fractures of the Clavicle. J. Bone Joint Surg., 13:299–310, 1931.

286. Zenni, E.J., Jr.; Krieg, J.K.; and Rosen, M.J.: Open Reduction and Internal Fixation of Clavicular Fractures. J. Bone Joint Surg., 63A:147–151, 1981.

Part III: FRACTURES AND DISLOCATIONS OF THE SCAPULA

Kenneth P. Butters

The scapula has an important role in arm function. It sits congruently against the ribs and stabilizes the upper extremity against the thorax. It also links the upper extremity and the axial skeleton through the glenoid, acromioclavicular, clavicle, and sternoclavicular joints. The scapula is subject to indirect injury through axial loading on the outstretched arm (scapular neck), through direct trauma—often high energy, from a blow or fall (body)—and through direct trauma to the point of the shoulder (acromion, coracoid). Shoulder dislocation may cause glenoid fracture. Traction by muscles or ligaments may cause avulsion fractures. Scapular fracture patterns have been identified and are discussed.

Fracture of the scapula occurs infrequently,[70] the incidence being 3% to 5% of shoulder girdle injuries[39,104] and 0.4% to 1% of all fractures.[86,122] This low incidence may be due to its thickened edges, its great mobility with recoil, and its position between layers of muscle. The mean age of patients with scapular fractures is 35 to 45.[3,69,119]

Associated injuries to other points in the shoulder girdle, the thoracic cage, and soft tissues are common and may lead to delayed diagnosis of the scapular fracture. Such problems as cervical spine fracture or vascular injury often require immediate attention. Operative surgical indications for scapular fracture are rare. Significant trauma is required to fracture the scapula, as evidenced by the cause of injury—motor vehicle accidents in about 50% of cases[49,69] and motorcycle accidents in 11% to 25%.

ANATOMY

The practice of orthopaedics is applied anatomy. Bony contour, muscle attachments, and the location of adjacent neurovascular structures should be understood in the evaluation of scapular fractures and certainly should be studied before surgery.

The anterior scapular surface is covered with the attachment of the subscapularis muscle, and the serratus anterior muscle attaches to the anterior medial border of the scapula (Figs. 12-110 and 12-111). The posterior scapula has on its surface the

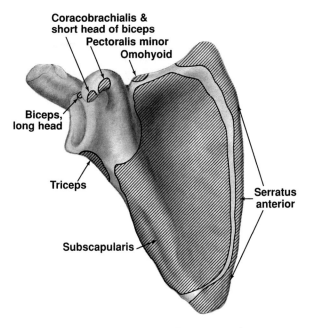

Fig. 12-110. The muscle attachments to the anterior surface of the scapula.

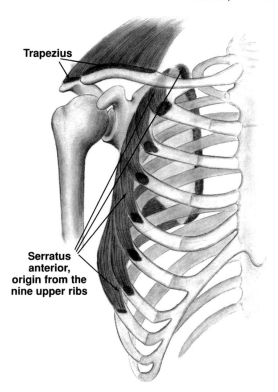

Fig. 12-111. A schematic showing the primary scapular stabilizing muscles. The serratus anterior passes deep to the scapula, attaching to the medial border holding the scapula against the chest wall.

supraspinatus and infraspinatus muscles, and the trapezius muscle overlies the supraspinatus and attaches to the spine and clavicle (Fig. 12-112). The deltoid overlies a portion of the infraspinatus posteriorly and the lateral subscapularis anteriorly; its origin is from the scapular spine, acromion, and anterior clavicle. Many other muscles attach to the scapular margin—the levator scapulae and rhomboids to the medial border, the teres minor and teres major from the lateral border, and an inconsistent latissimus attachment to the inferior tip of the scapula. The pectoralis minor, the short head of the biceps, and the coracobrachialis attach to the coracoid; the long head of the biceps attaches to the superior glenoid; and the triceps attaches to the inferior glenoid (Figs. 12-110 and 12-113).

The coracoid process projects upward, forward, and lateral from the superior border of the scapula. The brachial plexus and axillary artery run posterior to the pectoralis minor tendon, which inserts on the medial aspect of the base of the coracoid. Just medial to the coracoid base is the scapular notch, bridged by the transverse scapular ligament. The suprascapular nerve passes through the notch under the ligament, and the suprascapular artery passes over the ligament. The acromion continues laterally from the spine; a gap between it and the neck of

the scapula constitutes the spinoglenoid notch, transmitting the suprascapular nerve and vessels to the infraspinatus. Figure 12-113B shows this relationship and the proximity of the axillary and suprascapular nerves and the brachial plexus to the scapula.

The dorsal scapular and accessory nerves travel with the deep and superficial branches of the transverse cervical artery, respectively, parallel to and medial to the vertebral border of the scapula.

Most shoulder function involves simultaneous humeral and scapular movements with a definite rhythm. The scapula is a platform for the upper extremity. It rotates into abduction to assist the arm with forward elevation and undergoes adduction, elevation, or depression to help position the extremity. With all these movements, the scapula is in its bed against the chest wall. Scapular fracture malunion, soft tissue scarring, and muscle and nerve injury can all affect rhythm and limit scapular excursion, decreasing shoulder motion.

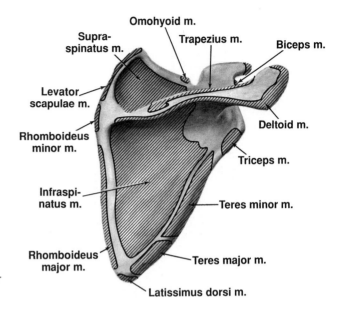

Fig. 12-112. The muscle attachments to the posterior surface of the scapula.

CLASSIFICATION OF FRACTURES OF THE SCAPULA

Certain fracture patterns are seen in the scapula. They are described by anatomic area for ease of discussion (ie, body and spine, glenoid neck, intra-articular, glenoid, coracoid, and acromion). Several areas of the scapula are often involved, but the neck (10% to 60%) and body (49% to 89%) are most common.[3,49,69,121] Zdravkovic and Damholt[125] divided scapular fractures into three types: I—fractures of the body; II—fractures of the apophysis, including the coracoid and acromion; and III—fractures of the superior lateral angle, including the neck and glenoid. This classification was devised to separate the type III fracture, which is generally considered the most difficult to treat. Displaced or comminuted

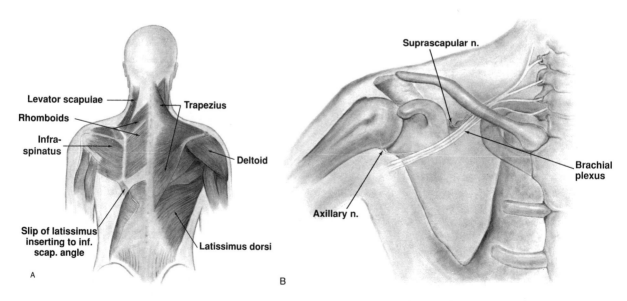

Fig. 12-113. **(A)** The posterior torso musculature, superficial (**right**) and deep (**left**). **(B)** A schematic diagram showing the positions of the brachial plexus relative to the scapula.

type III (neck and glenoid) fractures constituted only 6% of this entire series of scapular fractures.

Thompson and colleagues,[119] in their trauma center series of wide-impact blunt trauma, classified scapular fractures into class I—the coracoid and acromion and small fractures of the body; class II—the glenoid and neck; and class III—major scapular body fractures. Class II and III fractures were much more likely to have associated injuries. Ideberg[48] has proposed a classification of five types of intra-articular glenoid fractures (described later in this chapter).

CLINICAL PRESENTATION

Throughout the literature, a classic clinical description of scapular fracture, that of the scapular glenoid neck, is noted. According to Hitzrot and Bolling,[45] Sir Astley Cooper described flattening of the shoulder and prominence of the acromion. When the deformity was reduced by supporting the elbow, the movement was associated with bony crepitus. Interestingly, two of his three cases proved to be humeral neck fractures. Some authors have tried to make a clinical diagnosis by measuring arm length or midline-to-coracoid distance[45] without finding that this offers consistent, accurate help in diagnosis.

The typical presentation is that the arm is held adducted and protected from all movements, with abduction especially painful. Local tenderness is present. The shoulder may appear flattened with a displaced neck or acromion fracture. Ecchymosis is less than expected from the degree of bony injury present, as opposed to fracture of the upper humerus. Pain with deep inspiration may be present with coracoid fracture (pectoralis minor) or body fracture (serratus anterior). One should always be aware of the possibility of associated pneumothorax, either immediate or delayed. With body fractures especially, deep swelling may be quite painful, producing "pseudorupture of the rotator cuff."[85] Neviaser[85] described the syndrome of weak cuff function and loss of active arm elevation, which is probably only inhibition of muscle contractions from intramuscular hemorrhage and which usually resolves within a few weeks. This syndrome can be differentiated from rotator cuff tear, since the fracture is seen on x-ray and the swelling present with fracture and pseudorupture syndrome exceeds that normally seen with a cuff tear. As noted, a scapular fracture often presents with associated injuries needing more urgent treatment.

ASSOCIATED INJURIES AND COMPLICATIONS

Significant associated injuries occur in 35% to 98% of scapular fractures. The higher incidence is attributed to admissions to trauma units for serious injuries.[3,30,49,69,119,121] This figure reflects the degree of trauma necessary to fracture the scapula.

Fischer[30] and Thompson[119] and their associates have stated that direct scapular trauma and resultant scapular body fracture from wide-impact trauma have a particularly high incidence of associated ipsilateral upper torso injuries, so these fractures should be regarded as warnings. Similarly, the diagnosis of scapular fracture is often delayed while more urgent care is provided.[3]

Pneumothorax was found in 16 of 30 patients in a prospective study of fractured scapulae.[71] Interestingly, 10 of the 16 pneumothoraces were delayed in onset from one to three days. A follow-up chest x-ray, physical examination, and blood gas determinations should therefore be considered in patients with scapular fractures. Other series have reported a lower overall incidence of pneumothorax (11% to 38%).[3,30,119]

Ipsilateral fractured ribs are present in 27% to 54% of cases.[119] Correlation with pneumothorax is probably strong enough to warrant a prophylactic chest tube before early surgery is done for other injuries.[30] Armstrong and Vanderspuy found a fracture of the scapula with an underlying first rib fracture a particularly severe injury.[3]

Pulmonary contusion, which can be a life-threatening associated injury, is present in 11% to 54% of scapular fractures.[30,119] This injury may result in marked oxygen desaturation requiring tracheal intubation and positive end-expiratory pressure ventilation. Figure 12-114 illustrates several common associated injuries. Fracture of the clavicle frequently (23% to 39%) is associated with a fracture of the glenoid or glenoid neck. This may represent a continuation of an impaction force. Brachial plexus injury (5% to 13%) is usually a supraclavicular type with a poor prognosis.[3,30,49,69,119] In their series, McGahan and colleagues noted the association of brachial plexus injury with injuries about the acromion. They postulated that this may be due to depression of the shoulder and contralateral neck flexion as a mechanism of injury.[67,82] However, in Fischer and coworkers' series of badly injured patients in the trauma unit, 70% of the brachial plexus injuries seen occurred with major body fracture caused by wide, blunt trauma. Also, 57% of those patients with scapular fracture and a brachial plexus

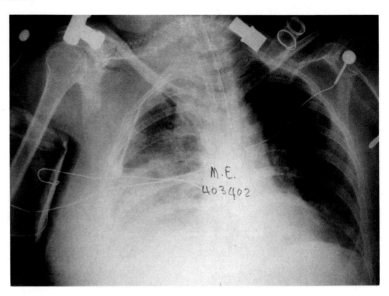

Fig. 12-114. X-ray of a multiple trauma patient with a fractured neck of the scapula and associated upper extremity fractures and pulmonary contusion.

injury also had arterial injury of the ipsilateral upper torso. A scapular fracture alone had an 11% incidence of arterial injury.[30] Case reports in the literature of nerve and arterial injuries[69,89,114] with scapular fracture supplement the trauma studies and reinforce the importance of a complete neurovascular examination. Skull fractures, which occur in 24% of patients with scapular fractures, and closed head injuries, which occur in 20%, generate concern, especially with a history of loss of consciousness.[69]

Distal extremity and spinal injury, blunt abdominal trauma, and pelvic fracture are all reported to increase in occurrence with major scapular body fracture.

Associated injuries were responsible for the 15% mortality that occurred with scapular fracture in the patients reported by Fischer and colleagues[30] and in 10% of the patients reported by Armstrong and Vanderspuy.[3] Half of these deaths were from pulmonary contusion with sepsis.

In summary, then, the presence of scapular fracture on initial anteroposterior chest x-ray is an indication for a good work-up for additional torso and extremity trauma on the injured side. In McGahan's and Armstrong's series, 50% of the fractures had grave associated injuries and no scapular surgery could even be carried out, indicating simple immobilization treatment followed by range of motion exercises.[3,69]

DIFFERENTIAL DIAGNOSIS

X-RAY EVALUATION

Fracture of the scapula requires x-ray diagnosis, but visualization is not always easy. Superimposition of the thorax may cloud the structural details of the scapula; however, most scapular fractures can be adequately evaluated by multiple plane views. A single view cannot provide all the information. A true anteroposterior view of the shoulder and an axillary and true scapular lateral view (trauma series) show glenoid (Fig. 12-115), neck, body (Fig. 12-116), and acromion (Fig. 12-117) fractures. The axillary lateral view is helpful for acromial and glenoid rim fractures, and the cephalic tilt or Stryker notch view is useful for coracoid fractures (Fig. 12-118). Tomograms have not been very helpful in the overall evaluation of scapular fractures; they can be used in carefully chosen planes to evaluate union or displacement of the fracture.

The oblique position of the scapula on the chest wall and its narrow width make tomographic evaluation difficult to interpret. A computed tomographic (CT) scan in the standard transverse plane again may not allow a three-dimensional concept of the fracture. The CT scan can be used in evaluating a glenoid fracture to confirm the reduced position of the humeral head. A three-dimensional reconstruction can be used to evaluate the shoulder girdle complex.[87]

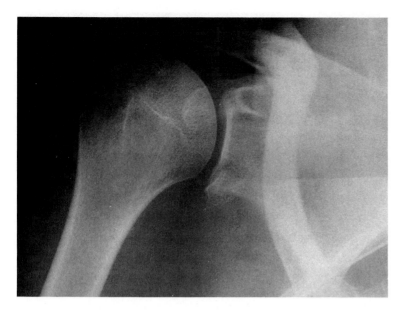

Fig. 12-115. A true anteroposterior view of the glenoid showing an anteroinferior glenoid fracture.

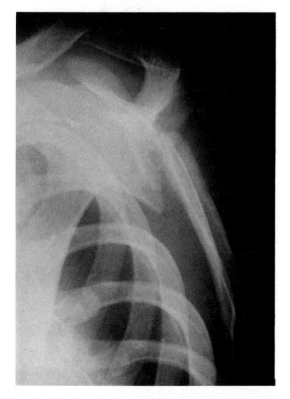

Fig. 12-116. A true (tangential) scapular lateral view (trauma series lateral view) showing a displaced scapular body fracture with a bayonet position.

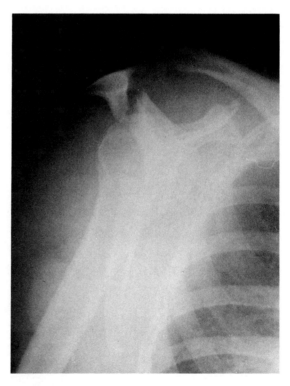

Fig. 12-117. The fractured base of the acromion is well seen on a true (tangential) scapular lateral view.

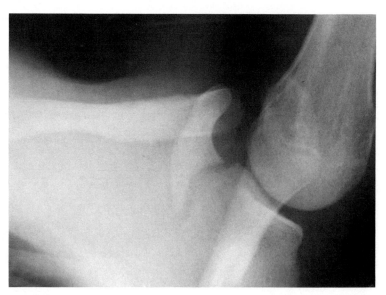

Fig. 12-118. A fracture of the base of the coracoid is best seen on a Stryker notch view.

EPIPHYSEAL LINES

Most important in the discussion of differential diagnosis is understanding the development of the scapula and its ossification pattern.[67,90,117] At birth the body and spine form one ossified mass, and the coracoid, acromion, glenoid, and inferior angle are all cartilaginous. At 3 to 18 months of age, a center of ossification, which may be bipolar, appears at the midcoracoid. At 7 to 10 years of age, the coracoid base, including the upper third of the glenoid, ap-

pears. Sometimes called a subcoracoid bone, it joins the rest of the coracoid at 14 to 16 years of age (adolescence). An ossification center at the tip and a shell-like center at the medial apex of the coracoid may appear at the same time and go on to fusion at ages 18 to 25 (Figs. 12-119 and 12-120).

Two or three acromial centers form at ages 14 to 16, coalesce at age 19, and fuse to the spine at ages 20 to 25. Failure of this to occur, with persistence of one ossification center past age 25, is known as *os acromiale.*

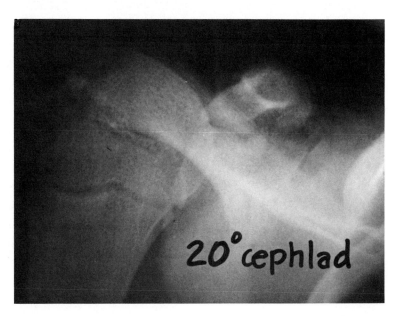

Fig. 12-119. A normal ossification pattern at the base of the coracoid. A crescent-shaped center is seen at the apex of the coracoid.

The glenoid fossa ossifies from four sources: (1) the coracoid base (including the upper third of the glenoid); (2) the deep portion of the coracoid process; (3) the body; and (4) the lower pole (joining the body at ages 20 to 25 and deepening the glenoid cavity). At ages 8 to 13 the glenoid border may be dentate from irregular ossification.[54]

At the inferior angle of the scapula, an ossification center appears at age 15 and fuses at age 20; the vertebral border center appears at ages 16 to 18 and fuses by the 25th year. The ossification centers may be asymmetrical, and comparison films may not be helpful.

OS ACROMIALE

Clinically, os acromiale is the best-known separate bone, resulting from failure of coalescence of the adjacent ossification centers. It stimulates acromial fracture. The open epiphyseal line occurs at the level of the acromioclavicular joint (Fig. 12-121).[9] (Interestingly, Liberson's classic 1937 study was stimulated by a worker's compensation claim.[61]) The unfused apophysis is present in 2.7% of random patients and when present is bilateral in 60%.[61] Four ossification centers are present in the acromion, as seen in Figure 12-122. The most common site of nonunion is between the meso-acromion and the meta-acromion at the mid-acromioclavicular joint. An axillary lateral x-ray is essential for an accurate description. Factors favoring the diagnosis of os acromiale over fracture are bilateral-occurrence rounded borders with uniform space and the position of the bony ossification center even with or above the posterior acromion on the anteroposterior view. Norris[88] has reported that the unfused physis has been mistaken for fracture and that there is an association between os acromiale and rotator cuff tear. Fracture separation, or at least some movement at this site, has been seen during acromioplasty, and surgical fixation with pins or screws at the time of cuff repair has been necessary.[82,83]

GLENOID DYSPLASIA

Scapular neck dysplasia (hypoplasia of the glenoid) resembling an impaction of the glenoid may have an associated acromial or humeral head abnormality. It usually has a benign course; many cases are found inadvertently, first being evaluated in the sixth or seventh decade of life.[95,99] Rockwood has seen glenoid dysplasia present in individuals of college age and become symptomatic with increased athletic use of the shoulder.[100] One might suspect

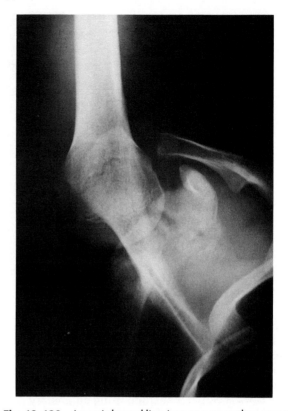

Fig. 12-120. An epiphyseal line is seen across the upper third of the glenoid. It serves as a common growth plate for the upper portion of the glenoid and for the base of the coracoid process. This may be confused with a fracture and is the precise location of most type III glenoid fractures.

an increased incidence of impingement with medial head position and less rotator cuff lever arm. Figure 12-123 is a radiograph of a 60-year-old with mild shoulder pain and stiffness.

NORMAL SCAPULAR FORAMINA

Scapular foramina[99] from disrupted ossification of the body and neck are common. They appear benign and are well circumscribed.

TYPES OF FRACTURES AND METHODS OF TREATMENT
GLENOID NECK (EXTRA-ARTICULAR) FRACTURE

The literature of the early 20th century interestingly parallels that of today. A fractured scapula was thought to be produced by trauma, usually of great

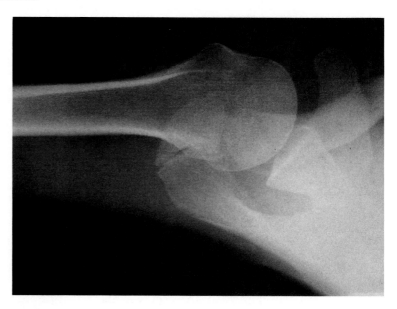

Fig. 12-121. Os acromiale.

violence, with associated injuries. The treatment was usually conservative. The published work focused on displaced scapular neck fractures. Scudder[112] believed that traction with abduction of the arm was helpful. Cotton and Brickley[18] in 1921 described a closed reduction, using an axillary pad and three weeks of bed rest with "hypnotics" and a pillow placed between the scapulae. Hitzrot and Bolling[45] in 1916 believed that manipulation and traction had no effect, and even with displace fractures the results were satisfactory enough that reduction attempts were unnecessary. The posterior approach was used if surgery was done on intra-articular fractures. Findlay[29] in 1931 kept even his patients with scapular body fractures flat in bed for ten days. Most authors agreed that "early motion" was important.

A fracture of the neck of the scapula is probably the second most common scapular fracture, occurring from direct trauma, a fall on the point of the shoulder, or a fall on the outstretched arm from impaction. True anteroposterior, tangential scapular lateral, and axillary lateral x-ray films and often CT are necessary to confirm the extra-articular nature of the fracture and the reduced position of the humeral head.

With neck fracture, the glenoid articular surface is intact and the fracture pattern extends from the suprascapular notch area across the neck to the lateral border of the scapula. The glenoid and coracoid may be comminuted or remain as an intact unit. The glenoid neck fracture is often displaced, but an intact clavicle and acromioclavicular joint will limit this displacement and enhance stability as opposed

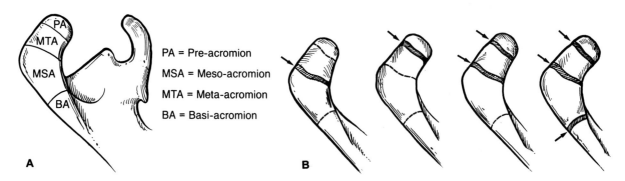

Fig. 12-122. (A) The diagram represents the ossification centers of the acromion. **(B)** The most common site of failure of ossification is between the meso-acromion and the meta-acromion.

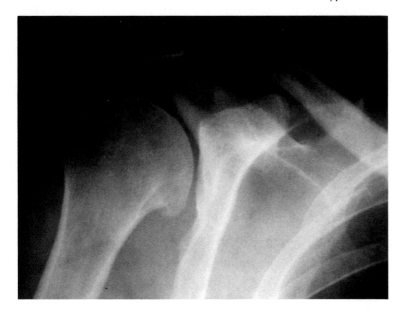

Fig. 12-123. Scapular dysplasia.

to what occurs with the clavicle fracture seen in Figure 12-124.

Reduction of the scapular neck fracture and restoration of the glenoid to its anatomic position are not necessary. Sling immobilization for comfort is probably enough. Further displacement is rare. In a study of neck and body fractures, Lindblom and Leven found that, if untreated, all healed in the position displayed at the time of the primary examination.[62]

For displaced fracture, DePalma[21] recommends closed reduction and olecranon pin traction for 3 weeks, followed by use of a sling. Bateman[6] favored closed reduction in a shoulder spica for 6 to 8 weeks in those cases in which "shortening of the neck is sufficient to favor subluxation or interfere with abduction." McLaughlin[70] believed that most neck fractures were impacted, making attempts at correction difficult.

Most series report good range of motion and function in follow-up of neck and body fractures (Fig. 12-125).[48,62,121] Armstrong and Vanderspuy[3] reported that some residual stiffness was present in six of seven neck fractures, but their patients had

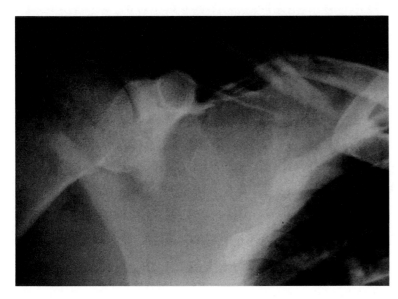

Fig. 12-124. A scapular neck fracture with an associated body and clavicle fracture.

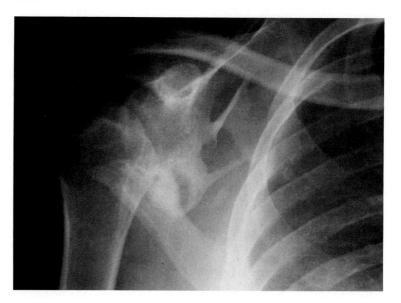

Fig. 12-125. A healed glenoid neck fracture with marked medial displacement. The patient had a full range of shoulder motion.

no functional disability. Zdravkovic and Damholt[125] came to the same conclusion in a study with an average follow-up of 9 years. Gagney and colleagues,[34] in a French article, found a good result in only 1 of 12 displaced fractures. They thought that the injury would "disorganize the coracoacromial arch" and recommended open reduction. A fractured surgical neck may be significantly displaced. Hardegger and coworkers believed that the amount of displacement and stability depends on the presence of an associated fracture of the clavicle or a coracoclavicular ligament tear. The altered gle-

nohumeral-acromial relationship results in "functional imbalance."[39] They recommended open reduction and scapular fixation of this fracture. Figure 12-126 is an x-ray of such a scapular neck fracture with an associated fractured clavicle, and Figure 12-127 shows the importance of an intact clavicle in glenoid fracture stability.

GLENOID (INTRA-ARTICULAR) FRACTURE

Intra-articular glenoid fractures may lure the orthopaedist into choosing surgical treatment. True

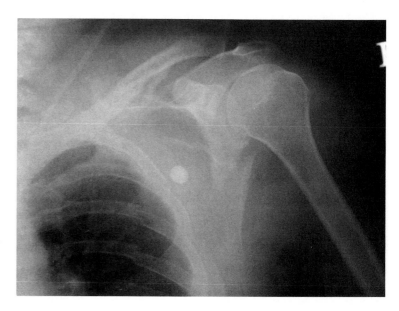

Fig. 12-126. Surgical stabilization should be utilized for this unstable glenoid neck fracture associated with a fractured clavicle. Hardegger recommends a scapular plate; the author has used clavicular plate fixation.

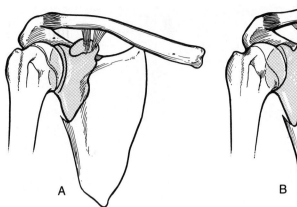
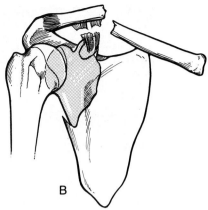

Fig. 12-127. This diagram shows the distinction between stable (**A**) and unstable (**B**) scapular neck fractures. The association of a scapular neck fracture with either a fractured clavicle or disruption of the coracoclavicular ligament creates an unstable fracture.

anteroposterior, axillary lateral, and West Point views and often CT scans are needed to assess these fractures. A direct force on the lateral shoulder or indirect axial compression of the extremity may cause a stellate glenoid fracture. Most of these require no reduction since the head remains centered (Figs. 12-128 and 12-129).

Ideberg[47,48] classified glenoid fractures into five types (Fig. 12-130), based on 300 cases: type I—avulsion of the anterior margin; type II—transverse fracture through the glenoid fossa, with an inferior triangular fragment displaced with the humeral head; type III—oblique fracture through the glenoid exiting at the midsuperior border of the scapula,

often associated with acromioclavicular fracture or acromioclavicular dislocation; type IV—horizontal, exiting through the medial border of the blade; and type V—which combines type IV with a fracture separating the inferior half of the glenoid.

Type I

A type I fracture is an anterior avulsion fracture occurring most probably from dislocations and subluxations but in some cases from direct injury. These fractures, if displaced, may predispose to instability. Usually, continuity is maintained between the capsule, labrum, and fracture fragment. Interestingly, however, a history of recurrent dislocation

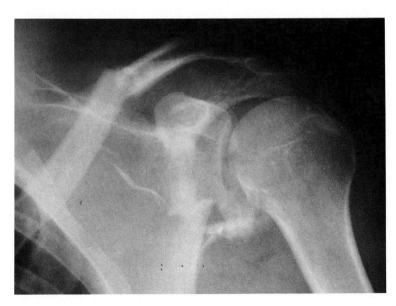

Fig. 12-128. A comminuted glenoid articular surface fracture with satisfactory position.

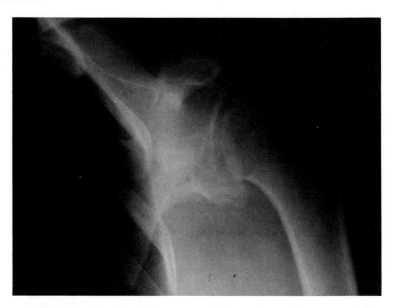

Fig. 12-129. The fracture in Figure 12-128 healed well without problems and with good preservation of the joint surface.

may precede the episode, causing a fracture of the anterior glenoid margin. Figure 12-131 shows such a fracture repaired with open reduction and AO screw fixation.

Ideberg believed that the size of the fragment is not prognostic for further instability.[48] DePalma thought that displacements greater than 10 mm, particularly if the size of the fragment is one fourth that of the glenoid, would indicate an open reduction.[21] Late open reduction of the displaced fragment or reconstruction of the anterior glenoid is difficult, often requiring a bone graft or coracoid bone block. In their Bankart study, Rowe and colleagues found that those fractures involving one fourth or even one third of the glenoid had equal success with repair compared with those in which one sixth or less of the glenoid was involved.[107]

According to Rockwood, a fracture involving one fourth of the glenoid fossa that is associated with shoulder instability is an indication for open reduction of the fragment with screw fixation.[100] A CT scan is helpful in determining fragment size and humeral head position (Fig. 12-132).

Ideberg's indication for operation is persisting subluxation or an unstable reduction (recurrent instability soon after reduction). No details were given, but 125 to 130 cases of glenoid avulsion in Ideberg's report had a satisfactory outcome. Of the 68 patients with associated dislocations, 11 had surgery, 5 with satisfactory results.

A distinction must be made between a glenoid avulsion fracture and a small glenoid rim or labrum avulsion fracture, which is commonly seen with traumatic anterior shoulder instability. These latter lesions are evidence of injury from traumatic anterior instability, not an indication for acute repair or reconstruction. Posterior rim fractures are much less common, and similar judgment is applied.

When the decision is made to treat a large anterior glenoid fracture nonsurgically, a follow-up x-ray must be taken and a physical examination done. A chronic dislocation may occur, especially in older patients, and postreduction resubluxation may go unnoticed.[57]

Type II

A type II fracture involves a transverse or oblique fracture through the glenoid with the inferior glenoid as a free fragment. The humeral head may subluxate inferiorly, with the fragment leading the surgeon to consider open reduction (Figs. 12-133 to 12-135).

Type III

A type III fracture involves the upper third of the glenoid and includes the coracoid; it may occur along the old epiphyseal line separating ossification centers. This fracture is often accompanied by a

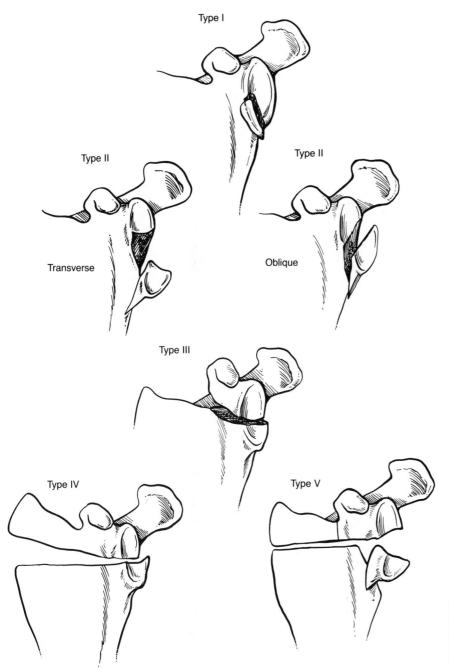

Type I

Type II

Transverse

Type II

Oblique

Type III

Type IV

Type V

Fig. 12-130. Ideberg's classification of intra-articular fracture of the glenoid into five types based on fracture patterns.

fractured acromion or clavicle or by acromioclavicular separation (Figs. 12-136 to 12-138).

Intact glenohumeral ligaments may keep the incongruity slight, and early motion may spontaneously improve fracture position. Open reduction is difficult, as it is in type II fractures. One technique uses an anterior arthrotomy (deltopectoral approach) as used for anterior reconstruction, plus superior exposure for a superior-to-inferior glenoid screw. Partial-thickness clavicle removal or even resection of the distal clavicle may need to be done to clear a path for the screw. Five of Ideberg's 17

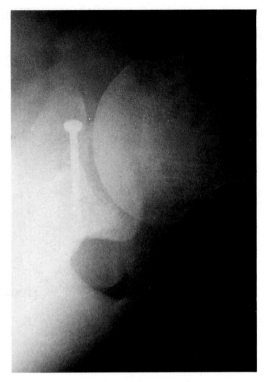

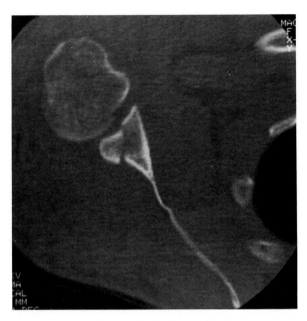

Fig. 12-132. A CT scan showing a large glenoid fracture with residual humeral head subluxation.

Fig. 12-131. An anterior glenoid fracture seen on an axillary view after open reduction and internal fixation.

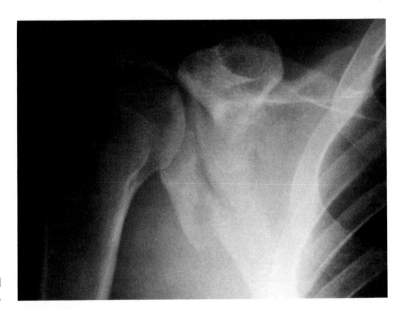

Fig. 12-133. A type II (oblique) glenoid fracture treated with early rehabilitation.

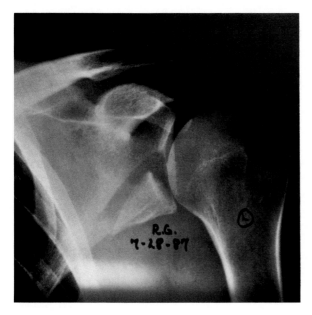

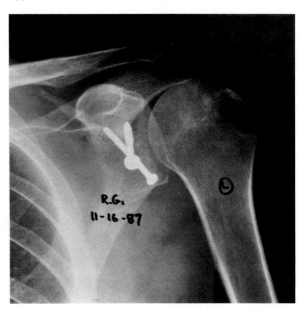

Fig. 12-134. An anterior glenoid fracture associated with anterior shoulder instability.

Fig. 12-135. Anterior glenoid rim fracture fixed with open reduction and fixation with two screws.

cases of type III fractures had a poor result, usually with associated injuries. Only one of the 17 had open reduction.

Type IV

A type IV fracture is a horizontal glenoid fracture extending all the way through the body to the axillary border. Four of Ideberg's 23 patients had poor

results from an extra-articular origin, and 3 of the 23 from glenoid irregularity. Again, open reduction was difficult.

Type V

Type V fractures combine types II and IV. Direct violent trauma was the cause in most cases, often delaying scapular treatment and probably influ-

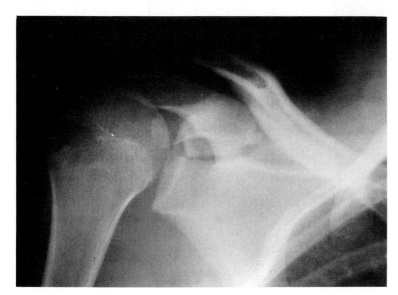

Fig. 12-136. A type III glenoid fracture near the original epiphyseal line.

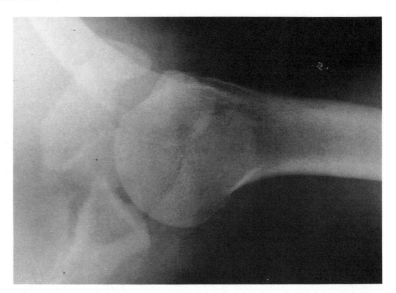

Fig. 12-137. A type III glenoid fracture including the base of the coracoid and the upper third of the glenoid, seen on an axillary view.

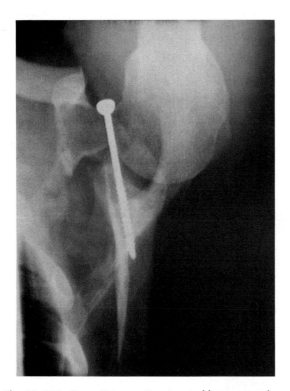

Fig. 12-138. Type III nonunion, treated by open reduction through the anterior and superior approaches with resection of the distal clavicle.

encing the results. Interestingly, of the 7 patients out of 20 who had poor results, all 7 had surgery, whereas only 1 of 13 with good results had open reduction (Figs. 12-139 and 12-140).

Ideberg's experiences with fractures of types II through V, which represent 40% of the total series, are summarized as follows. Closed reduction under anesthesia was always unsuccessful in improving fracture position at the time, but some late improvement in displacement was seen in most of the conservatively treated fractures. This improvement in fracture position may come from molding by muscle forces across the joint. A good result occurred in 75% of the cases of types II to V and was obtained mainly by early mobilization. Open reduction, however, can also produce a good result. Associated problems, such as other fractures about the shoulder, nerve, or muscle lesions, may worsen the outcome.

Some European literature suggests a more aggressive surgical indication to treatment of scapular fractures. Basing their evaluation on true anteroposterior, tangential scapular lateral, and axillary lateral x-rays, Hardegger and coworkers[39] described eight varieties of fracture with some surgical indication: (1) fracture of the body with a lateral spike entering the joint; (2) fracture of the glenoid rim with instability after reduction of dislocation; (3) fracture of the glenoid fossa, displaced; (4) extra-articular fracture of the glenoid neck with lateral and distal displacement; (5) similar displaced neck fractures with a displaced clavicle fracture or cor-

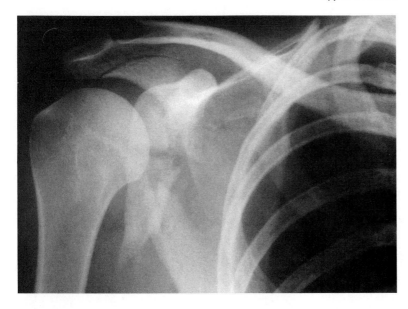

Fig. 12-139. Type V glenoid fracture.

acoclavicular ligament rupture (they thought that these extra-articular fractures resulted in functional imbalance and altered the glenohumeral-acromial relationship); (6) fracture of the acromion (if significant displacement is present, nonunion may develop or the deltoid may tilt the acromion fragment inferiorly, interfering with rotator cuff function); (7) fracture of the coracoid, displaced with neurovascular compression or with coracoclavicular ligament rupture; and (8) avulsion of the coracoid tip in an athlete.

The surgical approach is anterior for anterior glenoid rim and coracoid fractures. The posterior approach is employed for neck and glenoid fossa fractures, detaching the infraspinatus and using a lag screw or inferior buttress plate fixation.

SCAPULAR BODY FRACTURE

Direct violence and sudden contraction of divergent muscles may cause fractures of the body of the scapula. Other reported causes include electrical

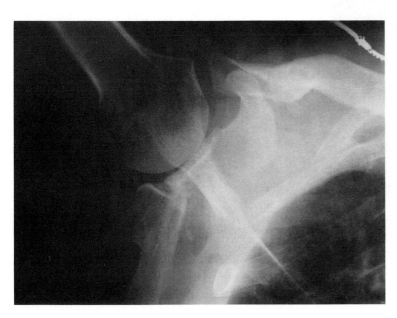

Fig. 12-140. Type V glenoid fracture, well healed, with good functional motion without pain.

shock treatments and accidental electrical shock causing seizures.[10,43,66,118] Of all scapular fractures, body fractures have the highest incidence of associated injury. Scapular fractures may be quite comminuted and displaced. True anteroposterior and trauma lateral (tangential scapular lateral) x-rays of the shoulder will show the scapular body fracture (Figs. 12-141 and 12-142). Axillary and cephalic tilt views may also be helpful in looking for other fractures, since injury often is not isolated to the body. CT is not usually helpful in treatment (Fig. 12-143). In the immediate treatment of these fractures, no reduction is attempted. The patient is given local ice and immobilization for comfort. Cross-strapping with adhesive moleskin to immobilize the scapula in a nonambulatory patient was described by Bateman and Neer.[6,83] Such immobilization may produce a stiff shoulder.[70] Pendulum exercises, use of overhead pulleys, and a further passive or active assisted range-of-motion program are begun within a week after injury. Multiple muscle attachments form an excellent environment for healing, and nonunion is rare. Pain may persist until the fracture is solid, but a full range of motion

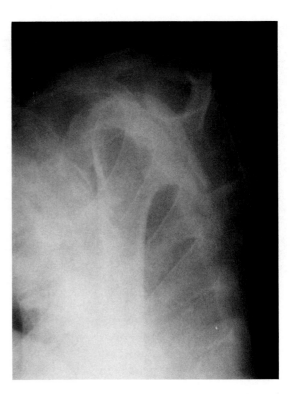

Fig. 12-142. A true (tangential) scapulolateral view showing a comminuted body fracture.

should be the goal in rehabilitation to mobilize the scapula, and progressive-resistance exercises to the rotator cuff and deltoid are essential.

Normal bony anatomy is not necessary for good function in a healed scapular body fracture. Perceived malunion with scapulothoracic irritation rarely restricts shoulder function, although when accompanied by associated scarring, it may impair scapular motion.

The literature includes mention of operative treatments of body fractures. These include an acute excision of a displaced inferolateral fragment[40] and an open reduction for body fracture, which "interferes in unity of the scapula in performing function as adjunct to arm elevation."[31]

ACROMION FRACTURE

The acromion commonly absorbs direct superior blows, and acromioclavicular separation is a much more common sequela than acromion fracture. Most acromial fractures have very little displacement. Commonly the fracture line is lateral to the acromioclavicular joint, causing confusion with os acromiale. In addition to the standard views, x-ray

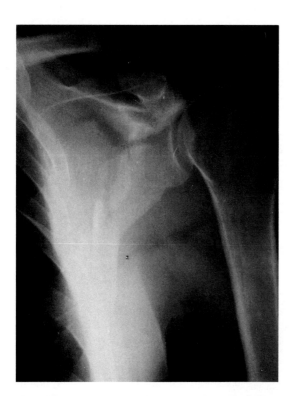

Fig. 12-141. A comminuted fracture of the body of the scapula.

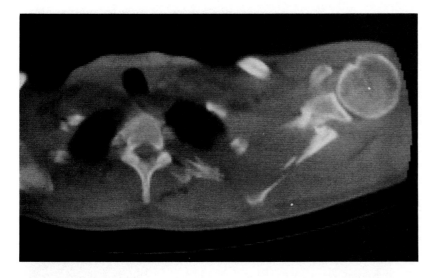

Fig. 12-143. A CT scan showing fracture of the body with an intact glenohumeral joint.

evaluation must include axillary and 30° caudal tilt views. A supraspinatus outlet view may be helpful, as well as x-rays of the contralateral shoulder to look for os acromiale (bilateral in 60% of patients) and to compare acromial configuration.

Another mechanism of acromial fracture is traumatic or superior displacement of the humeral head. This often causes an associated extensive rotator cuff tear. If the humeral head is displaced upward in the subacromial space (acromiohumeral distance is reduced), a rotator cuff tear should be suspected and an arthrogram obtained. A stress fracture can occur in association with the superior migration of the humeral head, as is seen with long-standing cuff disease (Fig. 12-144). Cuff repair and open reduction of the end of the acromion probably should be done. Acromionectomy should, as always, be avoided. An acromial avulsion by deltoid force has been reported.[58]

A nondisplaced fracture of the acromion should respond well to initial symptomatic treatment and the use of a sling for 3 weeks. Rehabilitation is begun immediately with range-of-motion exercises—passive initially—progressing to isometrics and an active program of rotator cuff and deltoid progressive-resistance exercises after fracture healing.

Results of simple acromial fracture treatment are

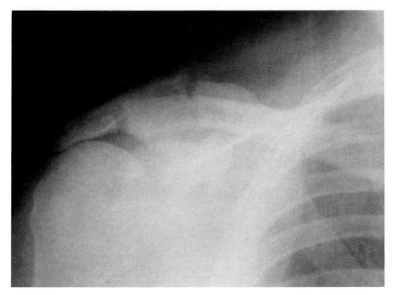

Fig. 12-144. A stress fracture of the acromion in a patient with cuff arthropathy.

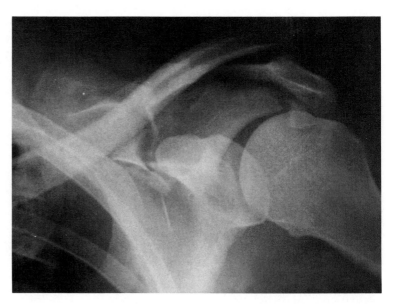

Fig. 12-145. A patient with a displaced acromion fracture is a candidate for open reduction.

generally good. Loss of motion, however, was noted by Wilbur and Evans,[121] who recommended cast immobilization in 60° of abduction, 25° of forward flexion, and 25° of external rotation for 6 weeks. Displaced fractures occasionally require elevation and Kirschner-wire or screw fixation to eliminate impingement or to reduce the acromioclavicular joint (Fig. 12-145).[83] Acromial nonunion is reported in isolated cases. I have experience with two cases of symptomatic nonunions of fracture of the acromion. One case became asymptomatic with pro-

longed protection, and the other healed after open reduction and fixation with Kirschner-wire–tension band fixation and bone graft. Darrach[20] recommended open reduction, fixation, and immobilization. Ruther[110] used a bone graft and cast. Wong-Pack and associates used a plate across the clavicle to the acromion.[124] Mick and Weiland employed a lag screw and plate along the scapular spine.[75] Neer reminds us that no more than a small fragment of acromion should ever be excised.[83]

A fracture of the base of the acromion near the

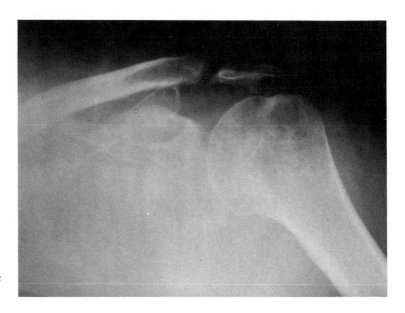

Fig. 12-146. A nonunion of a fracture of the acromion.

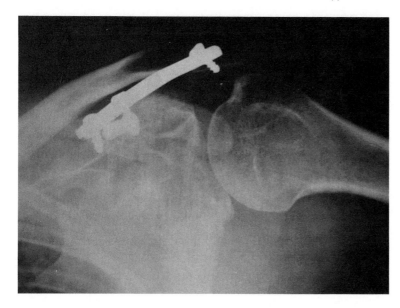

Fig. 12-147. Nonunion of the acromion, fixed with an intercalary graft and AO plate anchored along the spine of the scapula.

spine, if displaced, may progress to nonunion, and acute open reduction fixation is a good option (Figs. 12-146 to 12-148). As always, when early surgery for the scapular fracture is contemplated, the clinical picture, age, and occupation of the patient must be carefully considered. With the small cross section of contact area in acromion fractures, postoperative protection is necessary.

CORACOID FRACTURE

The coracoid is an important part of the attachment of the limb flexion muscles and ligaments, especially those stabilizing the clavicle. The coracoid is not readily visualized by an anteroposterior x-ray film; an axillary view and an anteroposterior cephalic tilt view of 35° to 60° are needed (Fig. 12-149). A Stryker notch view[124] and Goldberg[37] posterior oblique 20° cephalic tilt views are also helpful. Weight-hanging films may also be helpful if an associated acromioclavicular separation is present. Fractures of the coracoid may be isolated, occurring from a direct blow to the coracoid or to the point of the shoulder. Coracoid fracture may also occur along with acromioclavicular dislocation, with the coracoclavicular ligaments remaining intact.[9,50,126]

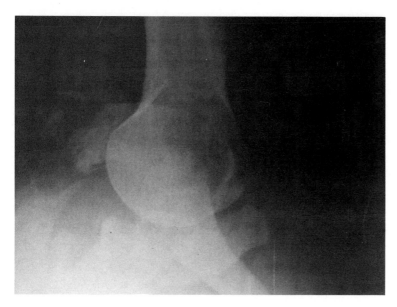

Fig. 12-148. Nonunion of the acromion after a comminuted scapular fracture, well seen on an axillary view.

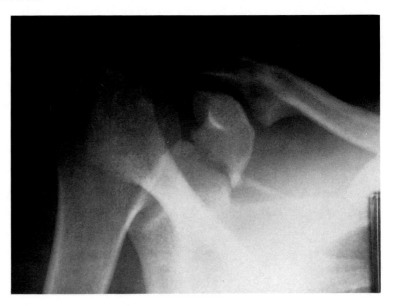

Fig. 12-149. A 35° cephalic tilt view showing a fracture of the base of the coracoid.

This occurs with traction exerted on the intact ligaments, avulsing the coracoid at its base or through an epiphyseal line. A radiographic clue to diagnosis is a normal and symmetrical coracoclavicular distance on x-ray and clinical evidence of third-degree acromioclavicular separation with a high-riding clavicle (Fig. 12-150). A cephalic tilt view, especially taken to evaluate the clavicle, may reveal the fracture. I believe the best view is the Stryker notch view. This coracoid fracture may be overlooked when attention is restricted to the obvious acro-

mioclavicular separation. The coracoid tip may be avulsed by muscle pull of the biceps and coracobrachialis[103] or from direct contact from a dislocating humeral head.[35,70] Garcia-Elias and Salo pointed out that this association is easily missed and that follow-up postreduction axillary lateral x-ray evaluation is necessary if pain continues in the shoulder (Fig. 12-151).[35] Fatigue fractures, such as trapshooter's shoulder,[11] have been reported. There are case reports of coracoid fractures with complications from surgical use of the coracoclavicular

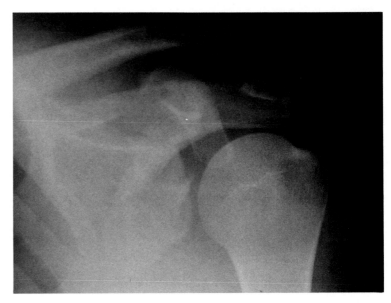

Fig. 12-150. A third-degree acromioclavicular separation with fractured base of the coracoid and a comminuted glenoid fracture. Note the normal coracoclavicular distance, indicating intact ligaments.

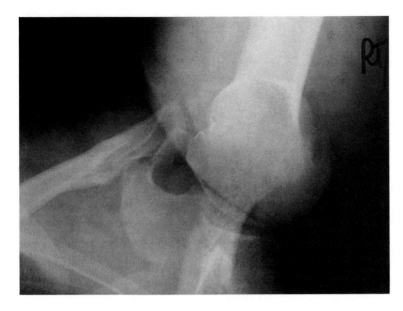

Fig. 12-151. Fracture of the coracoid tip from a direct blow, seen on Stryker notch, cephalic tilt view.

tape fixation[78] and from medial migration of the humeral head from cuff arthropathy (Fig. 12-152).

The fracture occurs most commonly through the base and is minimally displaced unless significant acromioclavicular separation occurs. A fracture line may extend across the suprascapular notch to the superior surface of the scapula or into the upper third of the glenoid. Confusion may exist concerning a normal accessory ossification center; such a center may be present at the ligament insertion at the site of an avulsion. (See the section on epiphyseal lines.)

In the coracoid fracture with acromioclavicular separation, surgical and nonsurgical treatment appear to offer equally favorable results. The literature is unclear about the time required for union, but no nonunions are reported. Some authors believe that open reduction is indicated but only for treatment of the acromioclavicular separation. Stability of the fractured coracoid is supplied by the coracoacromial and coracoclavicular ligaments superiorly and by the pectoralis minor and conjoined tendon inferiorly. For the isolated coracoid fracture, therefore, most authors believe that no specific

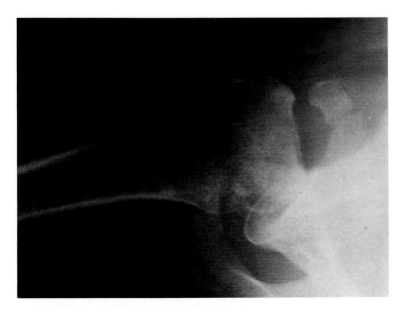

Fig. 12-152. A stress fracture of the coracoid from medial humeral head migration in cuff arthropathy.

treatment is needed since an anatomic alignment is not essential for adequate function or healing. For a displaced fracture, especially with associated acromioclavicular separation, Bateman recommended shoulder spica or acromioclavicular fixation.[6] Other authors' indications for surgery include "marked displacement,"[106] associated acromioclavicular separation,[59,64,83,113,121] and compression of the brachial plexus.[83] Neer also described suprascapular nerve paralysis with fracture in the area of the suprascapular notch. Electromyography is essential in the diagnosis, and early exploration is usually indicated.[83]

McLaughlin believed that fibrous union is not uncommon but is rarely symptomatic.[70] Garcia-Elias and Salo reported a painful coracoid nonunion, discovered late after shoulder dislocation, which did well after excision of the fragment.[35] Both Steindler[115] and Benton and Nelson[8] have reported that the tip of the coracoid can be excised and the conjoined tendons reattached to the remaining coracoid process.

AVULSION FRACTURES OF THE SCAPULA

Some of these injuries have been discussed within the anatomic groups, but they are mentioned here for completeness owing to a common mechanism. Scapular fracture due to avulsion of its many muscular and ligament attachments is uncommon. Four mechanisms may be involved[44]: (1) uncoordinated muscle contraction due to electrical shock, electroconvulsive therapy, or seizures; (2) muscle pull as the result of trauma or unusual exertion; (3) ligamentous avulsion; and (4) stress fracture near a muscle attachment.

A coracoid fracture may occur by means of a coracoclavicular ligament avulsion associated with acromioclavicular separation,[50,83,113] resisted muscle force (coracobrachialis, short head of the biceps) with direct blow,[22,103] and stress fracture of the tip.[8,11] An electroshock treatment caused an avulsion fracture.[52,97] A superior scapular border avulsion is seen as an extension of the fractured coracoid, created by the coracoclavicular ligament or possibly by avulsion of the omohyoid muscle.[50] Deltoid avulsion of the acromion is seen in case reports[44,58,98] and can be easily confused with os acromiale.

RESULTS OF TREATMENT

Results of treatment of scapular fractures have been reported generally across the spectrum of injuries,

and functional results have been satisfactory with conservative treatment. McGahan and coworkers,[69] Lindblom and Leven,[62] McLaughlin,[70] Zdravkovic and Damholt,[125] and Armstrong and Vanderspuy[3] all had series of patients with fractures of the scapula treated nonsurgically. Few patients had long-term disability of the shoulder. Steindler[125] in 1946 reported insignificant disability associated with nonsurgical treatment and found occasional limitation of abduction in neck fractures with grating and limitation of motion due to surrounding scar in body fractures. He thought that intra-articular glenoid fracture, however, could lead to painful post-traumatic arthritis. Armstrong and Vanderspuy[3] found 6 of 11 extra-articular neck fractures to have residual stiffness but no functional disability. Three of their six patients with glenoid fractures, however, had restricted painful movement on follow-up. Wilbur and Evans[121] grouped acromion, glenoid, and coracoid fractures and found 10 of 11 to have a decreased range of motion, with poor results in only 2. Zdravkovic and Damholt[125] found 23 of 28 patients to have moderately severe deformity on x-ray in follow-up, but only 2 had restricted elevation (both cases were intra-articular glenoid fractures). Only two patients changed occupation, and only one had severe osteoarthritis after 9 years. Again, published results support conservative management of most scapular fractures.

AUTHOR'S PREFERRED TREATMENT

GLENOID NECK FRACTURE

Reduction of displaced extra-articular scapular neck fractures is not necessary to obtain a good clinical result. Early experience with traction did not improve the position of the fracture and necessitated prolonged recumbency and hospital stay. Symptomatic local care, followed in a few days by passive exercises, allows satisfactory motion and does not interfere with fracture healing. When a displaced clavicle fracture accompanies a medially displaced glenoid neck fracture, an unstable segment that includes the glenoid, acromion, and lateral clavicle is created. Stabilization by plate fixation of the clavicle allows for much faster rehabilitation.

BODY AND SPINE

Patients are examined for associated injuries, which are very common with body fractures. Symptomatic treatment is indicated. Ice and sling immobilization are followed by stretching exercises and later, after fracture healing, by scapular mobilization and shoulder girdle strengthening.

GLENOID

X-ray evaluation is important. Axillary and West Point views as well as CT are used to diagnose significant glenoid fractures involving 25% or more of the joint surface. One must separate these from a small avulsion fracture. If these larger fragments are displaced, open reduction and small AO screw fixation are indicated, possibly using the new AO small cannulated 3.5-mm screws. The chance for recurrent instability if these fractures are left untreated, especially in the younger age group, approaches 100%. The operative approach, although difficult, is easier than later reconstruction with fragment fixation, iliac bone graft, coracoid bone block, or Bankart repair. I start gentle motion at seven days in these patients.

The other types of glenoid fractures described by Ideberg (types II through V) have less clear indications for operative treatment. If the humeral head is centered on the major portion of the glenoid and the shoulder joint is stable, then nonsurgical treatment is indicated as the head remains intracapsular. When the humeral head appears to be subluxated along with a major fragment, surgical treatment with capsular repair is indicated. Again, a work-up with carefully positioned tomograms and CT gives the surgeon a three-dimensional view of the fracture. I usually prefer the anterior approach to re-

duce the fracture, combined with superior visualization to pass the screw. The path of the screw is cleared by partial-thickness clavicle removal or even by resection of the distal clavicle. It is critical to understand the obliquity of the fracture before this can be planned. This surgery is most difficult, and the fixation often is not pleasing.

ACROMION

As stated, most fractures of the acromion are without significant displacement. They should be protected in a supervised passive and active assisted exercise program with no resisted deltoid function until union occurs. If there has been upward movement of the humeral head, fracturing the acromion, then the rotator cuff must be investigated and repaired. The presence of os acromiale must be remembered as part of the differential diagnosis for fracture; its presence alone is associated with an increased incidence of cuff disease.[83] The use of a dorsal tension band wire is a good technique for fixation of acromial fractures.

CORACOID

The Stryker notch or the 35° cephalic tilt view provides the information needed to assess the displacement of the coracoid fracture. Complete third-degree acromioclavicular separation combined with the significantly displaced coracoid fracture is an indication for open reduction of both injuries with trans-acromioclavicular Steinmann pin fixation (Fig. 12-153). I have experience with two late ex-

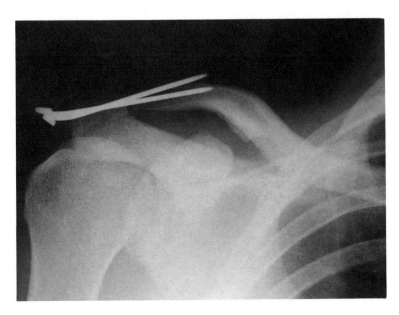

Fig. 12-153. Open reduction of the acromioclavicular joint with transacromion clavicular joint pins.

plorations of suprascapular nerve injury in association with coracoid and body fractures and agree with Neer, who favors early exploration of the nerve.

OTHER DISORDERS

DISLOCATION OF THE SCAPULA

Dislocation of the scapula between the ribs and into the thoracic cage is very rare. Ainscow describes one type with little violence and a pre-existing factor such as generalized laxity or locking osteochondroma.[1] The medial border is lodged between the third and fourth ribs or in the fourth to fifth intercostal space.[84] A second type is associated with more violent trauma involving chest injury. This is a rare variation of the injury and usually causes fracture of the scapula and ribs. The rhomboid muscles must be stretched or torn.[53] The diagnosis is suspected on examination of the upper extremity and inspection of the posterior chest wall but may be missed owing to associated injuries or may not be appreciated on anteroposterior views of the chest.

Nettrour and colleagues' series had a case in which the displaced scapula was thought to be a chest wall hematoma on plain chest films.[84] The Nettrour anterior oblique or tangential scapular lateral (trauma lateral) view or CT scan will confirm the diagnosis. Reduction under general anesthesia is accomplished by hyperabducting the arm and manually manipulating the axillary border, rotating the scapula forward and at the same time pushing

it back, as described by DePalma.[21] Acute reduction is usually stable, but adhesive strapping plus collar and cuff is recommended by Key and Conwell.[53] Late discovery may require open reduction and soft tissue reattachment to maintain reduction.[83]

SCAPULOTHORACIC DISSOCIATION

A new term, *scapulothoracic dissociation,* describes violent lateral displacement of the scapula with clavicle disruption and severe soft tissue injury (ie, to the brachial plexus and with or without vascular disruption) with intact skin.[24,25] It has been described by Ebraheim and coworkers[25] as "closed, traumatic forequarter amputation" and has been infrequently reported, since most patients have died. Soft tissue injury includes complete or partial tears of the deltoid, pectoralis, and posterior scapular muscles. Vascular disruption occurs most frequently at the level of the subclavian artery. Most often there is complete avulsion of the brachial plexus, but incomplete neuropraxia is possible. Bony injury may appear as acromioclavicular or sternoclavicular separation or clavicle fracture. Ipsilateral upper extremity fractures are often also present. Associated injuries are usually discovered early, without full appreciation of the magnitude of the injury. The diagnosis is made when a nonrotated chest x-ray shows significant lateral displacement of the scapula as measured by the distance from the sternal notch to the coracoid, glenoid margin, or medial scapular border. Kelbel and associates[51] found the ratio of the medial border to spine distances to be 1.5 or greater. Figure 12-154 shows this measurement.

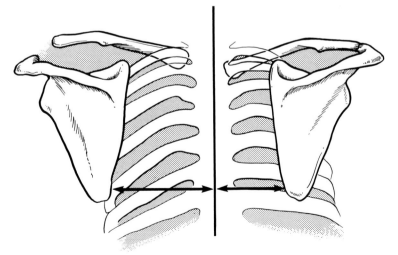

Fig. 12-154. A diagram of scapulothoracic dissociation, demonstrating a lateral displacement of the scapula on the injured side (**left**) compared with the normal side (**right**) on a nonrotated chest x-ray.

The primary mode of injury is direct trauma occurring, for example, during a motorcycle, mill wheel, hay baler, or motor vehicle accident.[91] Extremities are flail and pulseless, but swelling from dissecting hematoma may be the only external signs. A more distal vascular injury may divert attention from the more severe proximal injury. Following resuscitation of the patient, the chest x-ray should be carefully inspected and arteriography performed to delineate the vascular lesion. Exploration to restore vascular integrity and diagnose the level and severity of the brachial plexus injury is next. On the basis of this information and on assessment of scapular muscle damage, early above-elbow amputation and shoulder fusion are considered.[24,25] Rorabeck found no advantage to shoulder arthrodesis in this setting.[102] If parts of the brachial plexus remain intact, vascular and neurologic repair for limb salvage is indicated.

Portions of the text and selected illustrations have been used with permission from THE SHOULDER, edited by Charles Rockwood and Frederick Matsen, published by W. B. Saunders Company, Philadelphia, 1990.

REFERENCES

1. Ainscow, D.A.: Dislocation of the Scapula. J. Coll. Surg. Edinb., 27:56–57, 1982.
2. Anderson, L.D.: Fractures. *In* Crenshaw, A.H. (ed.): Campbell's Operative Orthopaedics, 6th ed., p. 662. St. Louis, C.V. Mosby, 1971.
3. Armstrong, C.P., and Vanderspuy, J.: The Fractured Scapula: Importance in Management Based on a Series of 62 Patients. Injury, 15:324–329, 1984.
4. Aston, J.W., and Gregory, C.F.: Dislocation of the Shoulder With Significant Fracture of the Glenoid. J. Bone Joint Surg., 55A:1531–1533, 1973.
5. Banerjee, A.K., and Field, S.: An Unusual Scapular Fracture Caused by a Water Skiing Accident. Br. J. Radiol., 58:465–467, 1985.
6. Bateman, J.E.: The Shoulder and Neck, 2nd ed. Philadelphia, W.B. Saunders, 1978.
7. Benchetrit, E., and Friedman, B.: Fracture of the Coracoid Process Associated With Subglenoid Dislocation of the Shoulder. J. Bone and Joint Surg., 61A:295–296, 1979.
8. Benton, J., and Nelson, C.: Avulsion of the Coracoid Process in an Athlete. J. Bone Joint Surg., 53A:356–358, 1971.
9. Bernard, T.N.; Brunet, M.E.; and Haddad, R.J., Jr.: Fractured Coracoid Process in Acromioclavicular Dislocations. Clin. Orthop., 175:227–231, 1983.
10. Beswick, D.R.; Morse, S.D.; and Barnes, A.U.: Bilateral Scapular Fractures From Low Voltage Electrical Injury—A Case Report. Ann. Emerg. Med., 11:12–13, 1982.
11. Boyer, D.W.: Trap Shooter's Shoulder: Stress Fracture of the Coracoid Process. J. Bone Joint Surg., 57A:862, 1975.
12. Caffey, J. (ed.): Pediatric X-ray Diagnosis, 7th ed., pp. 320–321. Chicago, Year Book Medical Publishers, 1978.
13. Cameron, H.U.: Snapping Scapula: A Report of Three Cases. Eur. J. Rheumatol. Inflamm., 7:66–67, 1984.
14. Charlton, M.R.: Fracture, Neck of the Scapula. N.W. Med., 37:18–21, 1938.
15. Cigtay, O.S., and Mascatello, V.J.: Scapular Defects: A Normal Variation. A.J.R., 132:239–241, 1979.
16. Cockshott, W.P.: The Coracoclavicular Joint. Radiology, 132:313–316, 1979.
17. Cooley, L.H., and Torg, J.S.: "Pseudo-winging" of the Scapula Secondary to Subscapular Osteochondroma. Clin. Orthop., 162:119–124, 1982.
18. Cotton, F.J., and Brickley, W.J.: Treatment of Fracture at the Neck of the Scapula. Boston Med. Surg. J., 185:326–329, 1921.
19. Coues, W.P.: Fracture of the Coracoid Process of the Scapula. N. Engl. J. Med., 212:727–728, 1935.
20. Darrach, W.: Fractures of the Acromion Process of the Scapula. Ann. Surg., 59:455–456, 1914.
21. DePalma, A.F.: Surgery of the Shoulder, 3rd ed., pp. 366–367. Philadelphia, J.B. Lippincott, 1983.
22. De Rosa, G.P., and Kettelkamp, D.B.: Fracture of the Coracoid Process of the Scapula: A Case Report. J. Bone Joint Surg., 59A:696–697, 1977.
23. Dzioba, R.B., and Quinlan, W.J.: Avascular Necrosis of the Glenoid. J. Trauma, 24:448–451, 1984.
24. Ebraheim, N.A.; An, S.; Jackson, W.T.; Perlstein, S.R.; Burgess, A.; Tscherne, H.; Hass, N.; Kellam, J.; and Wipperman, B.U.: Scapulothoracic Dissociation. J. Bone Joint Surg., 70A:428–432, 1988.
25. Ebraheim, N.A.; Pearlstein, S.R.; Savolaine, E.R.; et al: Scapulothoracic Dissociation (Avulsion of the Scapula, Subclavian Artery, and Brachial Plexus): An Early Recognized Variant, A New Classification, and a Review of the Literature and Treatment Options. J. Orthop. Trauma, 1:18–23, 1987.
26. Edeland, H.G., and Zachrisson, H.E.: Fracture of the Scapular Notch Associated With Lesion of the Suprascapular Nerve. Acta Orthop. Scand., 46:758–763, 1975.
27. Fery, A., and Sommelet, J.: Fractures de l'apophyse coracoide. Rev. Chir. Orthop., 65:403–407, 1979.
28. Findlay, R.T.: Fractures of the Scapula and Ribs. Am. J. Surg., 38:489–494, 1937.
29. Findlay, R.T.: Fractures of the Scapula. Ann. Surg., 93:1001–1008, 1931.
30. Fischer, R.P.; Flynn, T.C.; Miller, P.W.; and Thompson, D.A.: Scapular Fractures and Associated Major Ipsilateral Upper-torso Injuries. Curr. Concepts Trauma Care, 1:14–16, 1985.
31. Fischer, W.R.: Fracture of the Scapula Requiring Open Reduction: Report of a Case. J. Bone Joint Surg., 21:459–461, 1939.
32. Friedrich, B., and Winter, G.: Zur Operativen Therapie von Frakturen der Scapula. Chirurg, 44:37–39, 1973.
33. Froimson, A.I.: Fracture of the Coracoid Process of the Scapula. J. Bone Joint Surg., 60A:710–711, 1978.
34. Gagney, O.; Carey, J.P.; and Mazas, F.: Les fractures recentes de l'omoplate a propos de 43 cas. Rev. Chir. Orthop., 70:443–447, 1984.

35. Garcia-Elias, M., and Salo, J.M.: Nonunion of a Fractured Coracoid Process After Dislocation of the Shoulder. J. Bone Joint Surg., 67B:722–723, 1985.

36. Gleich, J.J.: The Fractured Scapula, A Significance in Prognosis. Missouri Med., 77:24–26, 1980.

37. Goldberg, R.P., and Vicks, B.: Oblique Angle to View for Coracoid Fractures. Skeletal Radiol., 9:195–197, 1983.

38. Halpern, A.A.; Joseph, R.; Page, J.; and Nagel, D.A.: Subclavian Artery Injury and Fracture of the Scapula. J. Am. Coll. Emerg. Physicians, 8:19–20, 1979.

39. Hardegger, F.H.; Simpson, L.A.; and Weber, B.G.: The Operative Treatment of Scapular Fractures. J. Bone Joint Surg., 66B:725–731, 1984.

40. Harmon, P.H., and Baker, D.R.: Fracture of the Scapula With Displacement. J. Bone Joint Surg., 25:834–838, 1943.

41. Hayes, J., and Zehr, D.: Traumatic Muscle Avulsion Causing Winging of the Scapula. J. Bone Joint Surg., 68A:495–497, 1981.

42. Heatly, M.D.; Breck, L.W.; and Higinbotham, N.L.: Bilateral Fracture of the Scapula. Am. J. Surg., 71:256–259, 1946.

43. Henneking, K.; Hofmann, D.; and Kunze, K.: Skapulafrakturen nach electrounfall. Unfallchirurgie, 10:149–151, 1984.

44. Heyse-Moore, G.H., and Stoker, D.J.: Avulsion Fractures of the Scapula. Skeletal Radiol., 9:27–32, 1982.

45. Hitzrot, T., and Bolling, R.W.: Fracture of the Neck of the Scapula. Ann. Surg., 63:215–234, 1916.

46. Hollinshead, R., and James, K.W.: Scapulothoracic Dislocation (Locked Scapula). J. Bone Joint Surg., 61A:1102–1103, 1979.

47. Ideberg, R.: Unusual Glenoid Fractures: A Report on 92 Cases. Acta Orthop. Scand., 58:191–192, 1987.

48. Ideberg, R.: Fractures of the Scapula Involving the Glenoid Fossa. In Bateman, J.E., and Welsh, R.P.: Surgery of the Shoulder, pp. 63–66. Toronto, B.C. Decker, 1984.

49. Imatani, R.J.: Fractures of the Scapula. A Review of 53 Fractures. J. Trauma, 15:473–478, 1975.

50. Ishizuki, M.; Yamaura, I.; Isobe, Y.; Furuya, K.; Tanabe, K.; and Nagatsuka, Y.: Avulsion Fracture of the Superior Border of the Scapula. A Report of Five Cases. J. Bone Joint Surg., 63A:820–822, 1981.

51. Kelbel, J.M.; Hardon, O.M.; and Huurman, W.W.: Scapulothoracic Dissociation—A Case Report. Clin. Orthop., 209:210–214, 1986.

52. Kelly, J.P.: Fractures Complicating Electroconvulsive Therapy in Chronic Epilepsy. J. Bone Joint Surg., 36B:70–79, 1954.

53. Key, J.A., and Conwell, H.E.: The Management of Fractures. Dislocations and Sprains. St. Louis, C.V. Mosby, 1964.

54. Kohler, A., and Zimmer, E.A.: Borderlands of the Normal and Early Pathologic Skeletal Roentgenogram. New York, Grune & Stratton, 1968.

55. Kopecky, K.K.; Bies, J.R.; and Ellis, J.H.: CT Diagnosis of Fracture of the Coracoid Process of the Scapula. Comput. Radiol., 8:325–327, 1984.

56. Kozlowski, K.; Colavita, N.; Morris, L.; and Little, K.E.T.: Bilateral Glenoid Dysplasia (Report of Eight Cases). Aust. Radiol., 29:174–177, 1985.

57. Kummel, B.M.: Fractures of the Glenoid Causing Chronic Dislocation of the Shoulder. Clin. Orthop., 69:189–191, 1970.

58. Laing, R., and Dee, R.: Fracture Symposium. Orthop. Rev., 13:717–720, 1984.

59. Lasda, N.A., and Murray, D.G.: Fracture Separation of the Coracoid Process Associated With Acromioclavicular Dislocation. Clin. Orthop., 134:222–224, 1978.

60. Leffmann, R.: A Case of "Rattling Shoulder Blade." Acta Med. Orientalia, 6:292–295, 1947.

61. Liberson, F.: Os Acromiale—A Contested Anomaly. J. Bone Joint Surg., 19:683–689, 1937.

62. Lindblom, A., and Leven, H.: Prognosis in Fractures of the Body and Neck of the Scapula. Acta Chir. Scand., 140:33–47, 1974.

63. Longabaugh, R.I.: Fracture Simple, Right Scapula. U.S. Naval Med. Bull., 27:341–343, 1924.

64. Mariani, P.P.: Isolated Fracture of the Coracoid Process in an Athlete. Am. J. Sports Med., 8:129–130, 1980.

65. Mathews, R.E.; Cocke, T.B.; and D'Ambrosia, R.D.: Scapular Fractures Secondary to Seizures in Patients Without Osteodystrophy. J. Bone Joint Surg., 65:850–853, 1983.

66. McCally, W.C., and Kelly, D.A.: Treatment of Fractures of the Clavicle, Ribs and Scapula. Am. J. Surg., 50:558–562, 1940.

67. McClure, J.G., and Raney, R.B.: Anomalies of the Scapula. Clin. Orthop., 110:22–31, 1975.

68. McGahan, J.P., and Rab, G.T.: Fracture of the Acromion Associated With Axillary Nerve Deficit. Clin. Orthop., 147:216–218, 1980.

69. McGahan, J.P.; Rab, G.T.; and Dublin, A.: Fractures of the Scapula. J. Trauma, 20:880–883, 1980.

70. McLaughlin, H.L.: Trauma, pp. 236–237. Philadelphia, W.B. Saunders, 1959.

71. McLennen, J.G., and Ungersma, J.: Pneumothorax Complicating Fractures of the Scapula. J. Bone Joint Surg., 64A:598–599, 1982.

72. McWilliams, C.A.: Subscapular Exostosis With Adventitious Bursa. J.A.M.A., 63:1473–1474, 1914.

73. Mencke, J.B.: The Frequency and Significance of Injuries to the Acromion Process. Ann. Surg., 59:233–238, 1914.

74. Michele, A.A., and Davies, J.J.: Scapulocostal Syndrome (Fatigue-Postural Paradox). N.Y. State J. Med., 50:1353–1356, 1950.

75. Mick, C.A., and Weiland, A.J.: Pseudo-arthrosis of a Fracture of the Acromion. J. Trauma, 23:248–249, 1983.

76. Milch, H.: Snapping Scapula. Clin. Orthop., 20:139–150, 1961.

77. Milch, H.: Partial Scapulectomy for Snapping in the Scapula. J. Bone Joint Surg., 32A:561–566, 1950.

78. Milch, H., and Burman, M.S.: Snapping Scapula and Humerus Varus. Arch. Surg., 26:570–588, 1933.

79. Moneim, M.S., and Balduini, F.C.: Coracoid Fractures—A Complication of Surgical Treatment by Coraclavicular Tape Fixation. A Case Report. Clin. Orthop., 168:133–135, 1982.

80. Montgomery, S.P., and Loyd, R.D.: Avulsion Fracture of the Coracoid Epiphysis With Acromioclavicular Separation. J. Bone Joint Surg., 59:963–965, 1977.

81. Moseley, H.F.: Shoulder Lesions, 2nd ed., pp. 171–175. New York, Paul Hoeber, 1953.

82. Mudge, M.K.; Wood, V.E.; and Frykman, G.K.: Rotator Cuff Tears Associated With Os Acromiale. J. Bone Joint Surg., 66A:427–429, 1984.

83. Neer, C.S., II: Fractures About the Shoulder. In Rockwood, C.A., and Green, D.P. (eds.): Fractures, pp. 713–721. Philadelphia, J.B. Lippincott, 1984.

84. Nettrour, L.F.; Krufty, L.E.; Mueller, R.E.; and Raycroft, J.F.: Locked Scapula: Intrathoracic Dislocation of the Inferior Angle. J. Bone Joint Surg., 54A:413–416, 1972.

85. Neviaser, J.: Traumatic Lesions: Injuries in and About the Shoulder Joint. Instr. Course Lect., XIII:187–216, 1956.

86. Newell, E.D.: Review of Over 2,000 Fractures in the Past Seven Years. South. Med. J., 20:644–648, 1927.

87. Norris, T.: Fractures and Dislocations of the Glenohumeral Complex. In Chapman, M. (ed.): Operative Orthopedics, pp. 205–210. Philadelphia, J.B. Lippincott, 1984.

88. Norris, T.R.: Unfused Epiphysis Mistaken for Acromion Fracture. Orthopedics Today, 3:12–13, 1983.

89. Nunley, R.L., and Bedini, S.J.: Paralysis of the Shoulder Subsequent to Comminuted Fracture of the Scapula: Rationale and Treatment Methods. Phys. Ther. Rev., 40:442–447, 1960.

90. Ogden, J.A., and Phillips, S.B.: Radiology of Postnatal Skeletal Development. Skeletal Radiol., 9:157–169, 1983.

91. Oreck, S.L.; Burgess, A.; and Levine, A.M.: Traumatic Lateral Displacement of the Scapula: A Radiologic Sign of Neurovascular Disruption. J. Bone Joint Surg., 66A:758–763, 1984.

92. Orthopedic Knowledge Update, 1985, Scapular Fractures.

93. Parsons, T.A.: The Snapping Scapula and Subscapularis Exostosis. J. Bone Joint Surg., 55B:345–349, 1973.

94. Pate, D.; Kursunoglu, S.; Resnick, D.; and Resnick, C.S.: Scapula Foramina. Skeletal Radiol., 14:270–275, 1985.

95. Pettersson, H.: Bilateral Dysplasia of the Neck of the Scapula and Associated Anomalies. Acta Radiol. [Diagn.] (Stockh.), 22:81–84, 1981.

96. Protiss, J.J.; Stampfli, F.W.; and Osmer, J.C.: Coracoid Process Fracture Diagnosis in Acromioclavicular Separation. Radiology, 116:61–64, 1975.

97. Ramin, J.E., and Veit, H.: Fracture of the Scapula During Electroshock Therapy. Am. J. Psychiatry, 110:153–154, 1953.

98. Rask, M.R., and Steinberg, L.H.: Fracture of the Acromion Caused by Muscle Forces. J. Bone Joint Surg., 60A:1146–1147, 1978.

99. Resnick, D.; Walter, R.D.; and Crudale, A.S.: Bilateral Dysplasia of the Scapular Neck. AJR, 139:387–390, 1982.

100. Rockwood, C.A.: Personal communication, 1989.

101. Rockwood, C.A.: Management of Fractures of the Scapula. Orthopaedic Transactions, 10:219, 1986.

102. Rorabeck, C.H.: The Management of the Flail Upper Extremity in Brachial Plexus Injuries. J. Trauma, 20:491–493, 1980.

103. Rounds, R.C.: Isolated Fracture of the Coracoid Process. J. Bone Joint Surg., 31A:662–663, 1949.

104. Rowe, C.R.: Fractures of the Scapula. Surg. Clin. North Am., 43:1565–1571, 1963.

105. Rowe, C.R.: The Bankart Procedure. A Study of Late Results (Proceedings). J. Bone Joint Surg., 59B:122, 1977.

106. Rowe, C.R.: The Shoulder, pp. 373–381. New York, Churchill Livingstone, 1987.

107. Rowe, C.R.; Patel, D.; and Southmayd, W.W.: The Bankart Procedure—A Long-term End-result Study. J. Bone Joint Surg., 60A:1–16, 1978.

108. Rubenstein, J.D.; Abraheim, N.A.; and Kellam, J.F.: Traumatic Scapulothoracic Dissociation. Radiology, 157:297–298, 1985.

109. Rush, L.V.: Fracture of the Coracoid Process of the Scapula. Ann. Surg., 90:1113–1114, 1929.

110. Ruther, H.: Therapy of Pseudoarthroses of the Scaphoid, Internal Malleollus, and Acromion. Ztschr. Orthop., 79:485–499, 1950.

111. Sandrock, A.R.: Another Sports Fatigue Fracture: Stress Fracture of the Coracoid Process of the Scapula. Radiology, 117:274, 1975.

112. Scudder, C.L. (ed.): The Treatment of Fractures, 4th ed., pp. 201–212. Philadelphia, W.B. Saunders, 1904.

113. Smith, D.M.: Coracoid Fracture Associated With Acromioclavicular Dislocation. A Case Report. Clin. Orthop., 108:165–167, 1975.

114. Stein, R.E.; Bono, J.; Korn, J.; and Wolff, W.I.: Axillary Artery Injury in Closed Fracture of the Neck of the Scapula—A Case Report. J. Trauma, 11:528–531, 1971.

115. Steindler, A.: Traumatic Deformities and Disabilities of the Upper Extremity, pp. 112–118. Springfield, Ill., Charles C Thomas, 1946.

116. Strizak, A.M., and Cowen, M.H.: The Snapping Scapula Syndrome. J. Bone Joint Surg., 64A:941–942, 1982.

117. Tachdjian, M.O.: Pediatric Orthopedics, pp. 1553–1555. Philadelphia, W.B. Saunders, 1972.

118. Tarquinio, T.; Weinstein, M.E.; and Virgilio, R.W.: Bilateral Scapular Fractures From Accidental Electric Shock. J. Trauma, 19:132–133, 1979.

119. Thompson, D.A.; Flynn, T.C.; Miller, P.W.; and Fischer, R.P.: The Significance of Scapular Fractures. J. Trauma, 25:974–977, 1985.

120. Varriale, P.L., and Adler, M.L.: Occult Fracture of the Glenoid Without Dislocation. J. Bone Joint Surg., 65A:688–689, 1983.

121. Wilbur, M.C., and Evans, E.B.: Fractures of the Scapula—An Analysis of Forty Cases and Review of Literature. J. Bone Joint Surg., 59A:358–362, 1977.

122. Wilson, P.D. (ed.): Experience in the Management of Fractures and Dislocations (Based on an Analysis of 4390 Cases) by the Staff of the Fracture Service MGH, Boston. Philadelphia, J.B. Lippincott, 1938.

123. Wolfe, A.W.; Shoji, H.; and Chuinard, R.G.: Unusual Fracture of the Coracoid Process. Case Report and Review of the Literature. J. Bone Joint Surg., 58A:423–424, 1976.

124. Wong-Pack, W.K.; Bobechko, P.E.; and Becker, E.J.: Fractured Coracoid With Anterior Shoulder Dislocation. J. Can. Assoc. Radiol., 31:278–279, 1980.

125. Zdravkovic, D., and Damholt, V.V.: Comminuted and Severely Displaced Fractures of the Scapula. Acta Orthop. Scand., 45:60–65, 1974.

126. Zettas, J.P., and Muchnic, P.D.: Fracture of the Coracoid Process Base and Acute Acromioclavicular Separation. Orthop. Rev., 5:77–79, 1976.

127. Zilberman, Z., and Rejovitzky, R.: Fracture of the Coracoid Process of the Scapula. Injury, 13:203–206, 1982.

13

Subluxations and Dislocations About the Glenohumeral Joint

Charles A. Rockwood, Jr.
Steven C. Thomas
Frederick A. Matsen III

HISTORICAL REVIEW

EARLY DESCRIPTIONS

The first report of a shoulder dislocation is found in humankind's oldest book, the Edwin Smith Papyrus (3000–2500 B.C.).[1425] Hussein[569] reported that in 1200 B.C. in the tomb of Upuy, an artist and sculptor to Ramses II, there was a drawing of a scene that was strikingly similar to Kocher's method of reduction (Fig. 13-1).

The most detailed early description of anterior dislocations came from the father of medicine, Hippocrates, who was born in 460 B.C. on the island of Cos.[5] Hippocrates described the anatomy of the shoulder, the types of dislocations, and the first surgical procedure. In one of his classic procedures for reduction, he stressed the need for suitably sized leather-covered balls to be placed in the axilla, for without them the heel could not reach the head of the humerus in his reduction maneuver. Other hippocratic techniques are described by Brockbank and Griffiths (Fig. 13-2).[161]

Hippocrates wrote,

It deserves to be known how a shoulder which is subject to frequent dislocations should be treated. For many persons owing to this accident have been obliged to abandon gymnastic exercises, though otherwise well qualified for them; and from the same misfortune have become inept in warlike practices, and have thus perished. And this subject deserves to be noticed, because I have never known any physician [to] treat the case properly; some abandon the attempt altogether, and others hold opinions and practice the very reverse of what is proper.

Hippocrates criticized his contemporaries for improper burning of the shoulder, a treatment popular at the time. In this first description of a surgical procedure for recurrent dislocation of the shoulder, he described how physicians had burned the top, anterior, and posterior aspects of the shoulder, which only caused scarring in those areas and promoted the downward dislocation. He advocated the use of cautery in which an oblong, red-hot iron was inserted through the axilla to make eschars, but only in the lower part of the joint. Hippocrates displayed considerable knowledge of the anatomy of the shoulder, and he warned the surgeon not to let the iron come in contact with the major vessels and nerves because this would cause great harm. Following the burnings, he bound the arm to the side day and night, for a long time, "for thus more especially will cicatrization take place, and the wide space into which the humerus used to escape will become contracted."

In the centuries that followed, more refined descriptions of shoulder conditions and their management were published. The text by H. F. Moseley[872] has a particularly good section on the historical aspects of management of shoulder instability.

HUMERAL HEAD DEFECT

The defect created by the anterior margin of the glenoid in the posterolateral aspect of the humeral head has long been recognized. In 1861, Flower[390] described the anatomic and pathologic changes

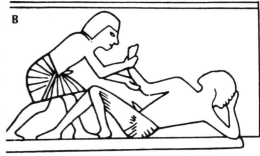

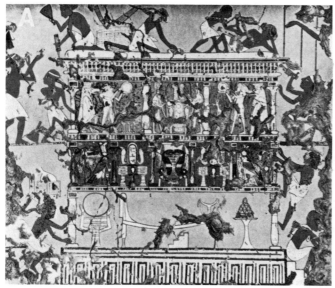

Fig. 13-1. The Kocher technique is 3000 years old. (**A**) Drawing from the tomb of Upuy in 1200 B.C. (From The Metropolitan Museum of Art.) (**B**) Schematic drawing of the picture in the upper right corner of the tomb painting depicting a patient on the ground while a man—possibly a physician—is manipulating a dislocated shoulder in the technique of Kocher. *(Hussein M.K.: Kocher's Method Is 3,000 Years Old. J. Bone Joint Surg., 50B:669–671, 1968).*

found in 41 traumatically dislocated shoulders from specimens in London museums. He wrote that "where the head of the humerus rests upon the edge of the glenoid fossa absorption occurs, and a groove is evacuated, usually between the articular head and the greater tuberosity." In 1880, Eve[360] reported an autopsy on a patient who died 12 hours after an acute anterior dislocation in which he found the deep groove in the posterolateral aspect of the head. Joessel[606] also observed the defect. According to Hill and Sachs,[530] beginning in 1882, publications appeared by Kuster,[679] Cramer,[258] Löbker,[743] Schúller,[1193] Staffel,[1252] and Francke[258] that described the finding of a posterolateral defect in humeral heads resected for relief of chronic or recurrent dislocation.

In 1887, Caird[179] of Edinburgh concluded that in the true subcoracoid dislocation there must be an indentation fracture of the humeral head produced by the dense, hard anterior lip of the glenoid fossa. In cadaver experiments, he was able to produce the head defect. He said that the hard, dense glenoid lip would cut into the soft cancellous bone like a knife.

Hermodsson's text[522] on radiographic studies of anterior dislocations of the shoulder offers the best review of the changes detectable by radiography.

Largely through the efforts of Moseley of Montreal, the text was translated from German to English in 1963. Hermodsson's work has shown that the posterolateral humeral head defect is the result of a compression fracture caused by the anterior glenoid rim following the exit of the humeral head from the glenoid fossa. He also made several observations about fresh, acute traumatic anterior dislocations: (1) the defect is seen in the majority of cases; (2) the longer the head is dislocated, the larger the defect will be; (3) the defect generally is larger with an anteroinferior dislocation than with an anterior dislocation; and (4) the defect generally is larger in recurrent anterior dislocations of the shoulder.

Hermodsson reported that in 1898 Franke made the first mention of radiographic changes in the humeral head associated with recurrent dislocation of the shoulder. In 1925, Pilz[1024] reported the first detailed radiographic examination of recurrent dislocation of the shoulder and stated that routine radiographs were of little help. He stressed the need for an angled-beam projection to observe the defect. Currently, all the special views that demonstrate the posterolateral humeral head defect involve an angled projection of the x-ray beam.

In 1940 Hill and Sachs[530] published a very clear and concise review of the available information on

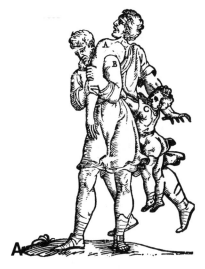

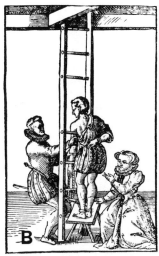

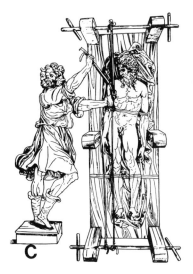

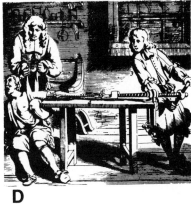

Fig. 13-2. Modified techniques of Hippocrates to reduce dislocations of the shoulder. (**A**) Reduction over the operator's shoulder (from the Venice edition of Galen in 1625). (**B**) Reduction over the rung of a ladder. When the step stool on which the patient is standing is withdrawn, the weight of the patient's body produces a reduction of the dislocation (from deCruce in 1607). (**C**) The use of a rack to reduce the shoulder dislocation (Vidius). (**D**) Reduction of the dislocation by a medieval type of screw traction (from Scultetus in 1693). (*Brockbank, W., and Griffiths, D. L.: Orthopaedic Surgery in the 16th and 17th Centuries. J. Bone Joint Surg., 30B:365–375, 1948*).

the humeral head compression fracture defect that now carries their names.

ANTERIOR CAPSULE DEFECTS

According to the Hunterian Lecture given by Reeves in 1967, Roger of Palermo in the 13th century taught that the lesion in an acute dislocation was a capsular rupture. This concept was later challenged by Hunter, Flower,[390] Caird,[179] Broca and Hartmann,[160] Perthes,[1018] and Bankart,[75,76] who noted that the lesion in traumatic anterior instability was caused by the shearing of the anterior soft tissue structures from the glenoid, secondary to forward translation of the humeral head.

ROTATOR CUFF INJURIES

In 1880, Joessel[606] reported on his careful postmortem studies of four cases of known recurrent dislocations of the shoulder. In all cases he found a rupture of the posterolateral portion of the rotator cuff from the greater tuberosity and a greatly increased shoulder joint capsule volume. He also noted fractures of the humeral head and the anterior glenoid rim. He concluded that cuff disruptions that did not heal predisposed to recurrence of the problem; that recurrences were facilitated by the enlarged capsule; and that fractures of the glenoid or head of the humerus resulted in a smaller articular surface, which may tend to produce recurrent dislocation. However, his four patients were elderly and may have had the degenerative cuff changes so common in older people.

THE "ESSENTIAL LESION" OF RECURRING DISLOCATIONS: BONE DEFECTS VERSUS SOFT TISSUE DEFECTS AND OTHERS

Roentgen's discovery of x-ray in 1895 ushered in new evaluations and studies on the anatomy of the anterior glenoid and on humeral head defects. These studies gave further impetus to the theory that the posterolateral defect of the humeral head was the essential lesion that produced recurrent anterior dislocations. Bankart,[75] following the concepts of Broca and Hartmann[160] and Perthes,[1018] continued to claim that the essential lesion was the detached labrum and capsule from the anterior glenoid (referred to by subsequent authors as the Bankart lesion) (Fig. 13-3). Later experimental and clinical work by Reeves[1074] and Townley[1309] suggested that other lesions can be responsible for recurrent dislocation, such as lack of bleeding at the time of the initial traumatic dislocation, detachment of the subscapularis tendon, and variance in the attachment of the inferior glenohumeral ligament.

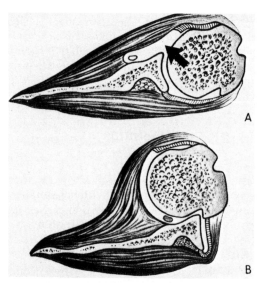

Fig. 13-3. (A) Perthes' concept of the detached anterior capsule and labrum with formation of a subscapular pouch (**arrow**).[1018] Note the loose body anterior to the neck of the glenoid. **(B)** Diagram of the anatomic relations during anterior dislocation. Note the posterolateral notch in the humeral head.

Moseley and Overgaard[869] found laxity in 25 consecutive cases, and DePalma and associates[285] reported subscapularis laxity, ruptures, and decreased muscle tone in 38 consecutive cases. Several of their cases, like those of Hauser,[487] revealed a definite defect along the anterior or inferior aspect of the subscapularis tendon, as if the tendon had been partially torn from its bone attachment, along with separation of those muscle fibers that insert into the humerus directly below the lesser tuberosity. McLaughlin,[822] DePalma and associates,[285] Jens,[598] and Reeves[1072] noted at the time of surgery (but before arthrotomy), that with abduction and external rotation the humeral head would dislocate under the lower edge of the subscapularis tendon. Symeonides[1281] biopsied the subscapularis muscle tendon unit at the time of surgery and found microscopic evidence of "healed post-traumatic lesions." He identified lengthening of the subscapularis muscle, which leads to a decrease in power, as the prime factor producing instability of the shoulder.

EARLY TREATMENT OF ACUTE TRAUMATIC INTERIOR DISLOCATIONS

Hippocrates[538] discussed in detail at least six different techniques to reduce the dislocated shoulder. From century to century the literature has included woodcuts, drawings, and redrawings illustrating modifications of Hippocrates' teachings by such investigators as Paré, de Cruce, Vidius, and Scultetus. Some of Hippocrates' techniques are still in use today.

In 1870 Theodore Kocher,[656] a Nobel Prize winner for medicine in 1909, gave a somewhat confusing report of his technique for levering in the anteriorly dislocated shoulder. Had Kocher not been so famous as a thyroid surgeon, his article might have received only scant attention.

EARLY OPERATIVE RECONSTRUCTIONS FOR ANTERIOR INSTABILITY

Most of the published literature on shoulder dislocations is concerned with the problem of recurrent anterior dislocations. As mentioned previously, Hippocrates[538] described the use of a white-hot poker to scar the anteroinferior capsule. Since then more than 100 different operative procedures have been developed to manage the recurrent anterior dislocation. The reader who has a yearning for the detailed history should read the classic texts by Moseley[872] and Hermodsson.[522]

Various operative techniques have been based on the posterolateral defect and the soft tissue disruptions on the front of the shoulder. Bardenheuer[80] in 1886 and Thomas[1291,1292] from 1909 to 1921 discussed capsular plication or shrinking; in 1888, Albert[16] performed arthrodesis; and in 1901, Hildebrand[529] deepened the glenoid socket.

In 1906, Perthes[1018] wrote a classic paper on the operative treatment of recurrent dislocations. He stated that the operation should be directed to a repair of the underlying lesion (ie, repair of the capsule, the glenoid labrum detachment from the anterior bony rim, and the rotator cuff tear). He repaired the capsule with suture to the anterior glenoid rim through drill holes and in several cases used staples to repair the anterior capsular structures (Fig. 13-4). This report gave the first description of repair of the anterior labrum and capsule to the anterior glenoid rim. Two patients were followed for 17 years, one for 12 years, two for 3 years, and one for 1 year and 9 months. All had excellent function with no recurrences.

The muscle-sling myoplasty operation was used in 1913 by Clairmont and Ehrlich.[211] The posterior

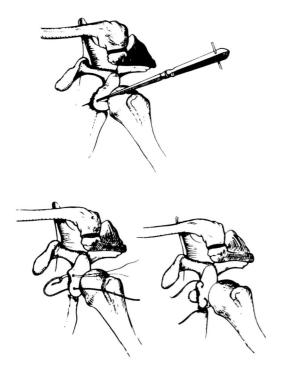

Fig. 13.-4. Method of repair used by Perthes in 1906.[1018] The labrum and anterior capsule were reattached using either suture, as shown, or small staples in the anterior rim of the glenoid.

third of the deltoid, with its innervation left intact, was removed from its insertion on the humerus, passed through the quadrilateral space, and sutured to the coracoid process. When the arm was abducted the deltoid contracted, which held up the humeral head. Finsterer,[383] in a similar but reversed procedure, used the coracobrachialis and the short head of the biceps from the coracoid and transferred them posteriorly. Both operations failed because of high recurrence rates.

In 1923 Bankart[75] first published his operative technique, noting that only two classes of operations were used at that time for recurrent dislocations of the shoulder: (1) those designed to diminish the size of the capsule by plication or pleating,[1291,1292] and (2) those designed to give inferior support to the capsule.[211] Bankart condemned both in preference to his procedure. He said the essential lesion was the detachment or rupture of the capsule from the glenoid ligament. He recommended repair using interrupted sutures of silkworm gut passed between the free edge of the capsule and the glenoid ligament. At that time he did not repair the lateral capsule to the bone of the anterior glenoid rim. In his 1939 article, Bankart[76] described the essential lesion as a "detachment of the glenoid ligament from the anterior margin of the glenoid cavity" and stated that "the only rational treatment is to reattach the glenoid ligament (or the capsule) to the bone from which it has been torn." He further wrote that "the glenoid ligament may be found lying loose either on the head of the humerus or the margin of the glenoid cavity" and that "in every case the anterior margin of the glenoid cavity will be found to be smooth, rounded, and free of any attachments, and a blunt instrument can be passed freely inwards over the bone on the front of the neck of the scapula." He recommended the repair of the lateral capsule down to the raw bone of the anterior glenoid and held it in place with suture through drill holes made in the anterior glenoid rim with sharp, pointed forceps. Although no references were listed in either article, Bankart must have been greatly influenced by the previously published work of Broca and Hartmann[160] and particularly of Perthes,[1018] which described virtually identical pathology and repair.

Beginning in 1929, Nicola[919–923] published a series of articles on management of recurrent dislocations of the shoulder. He used the long head of the biceps tendon and the coracohumeral ligament as a suspension checkrein to the front of the shoulder (Fig. 13-5). Because of technical difficulties and the high rate of recurrences, this procedure has

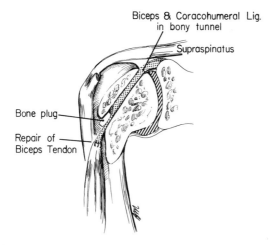

Fig. 13-5. In the Nicola operation, the long head of the biceps and the coracohumeral ligament are passed through a bony tunnel in the head of the humerus to act as a ''checkrein'' ligament.[921]

been abandoned. Henderson[512,513] described another checkrein operation that looped half of the peroneus longus tendon through drill holes in the acromion and the greater tuberosity. The Henderson tenosuspension operation also has been abandoned. Gallie and LeMesurier[411] described the use of autogenous fascia lata suture in the treatment of recurrent dislocations of the shoulder in 1927. This procedure has been modified and used by Bateman.[88]

POSTERIOR GLENOHUMERAL INSTABILITY

In 1839, in a Guy's Hospital report, Sir Astley Cooper[246] described in detail a dislocation of the os humeri upon the dorsum scapulae. This report is a classic, for Cooper presented most of the characteristics associated with posterior dislocations: the dislocation occurred during an epileptic seizure; pain was greater than with the usual anterior dislocation; external rotation of the arm was entirely impeded, and the patient could not elevate his arm from his side; the shoulder had an anterior void or flatness and a posterior fullness; and the patient was ''unable to use or move his arm to any extent.'' In this report of a case in which Cooper had acted as a consultant, a reduction could not be accomplished and the patient never recovered the use of his shoulder. A postmortem examination of the shoulder, performed 7 years later, revealed that the subscapularis tendon was detached and the infra-

spinatus muscles were stretched posteriorly about the head of the humerus. The report suggested that the detached subscapularis was ''the cause of the symptoms.'' Cooper[246] further described a resorption of the anterior aspect of the humeral head where it was in contact with the posterior glenoid—probably the first description of the so-called reversed Hill-Sachs lesion.

Another classic article on the subject was published in 1855 by Malgaigne,[779] who reported 37 cases of posterior dislocations of the shoulder. Three cases were his own and 34 were from literature. This series of cases was collected 40 years before the discovery of x-rays, and it points out that with adequate physical examination the correct diagnosis can be made.

ANATOMY OF THE GLENOHUMERAL JOINT

SURGICAL ANATOMY

The Skin

Shoulder stabilization surgery usually can be accomplished through cosmetically acceptable incisions in the lines of the skin. Anteriorly the surgeon can identify the prominent anterior axillary crease by adducting the shoulder. An incision placed in the lower part of this crease provides excellent access to the shoulder for anterior repair, yet heals nicely with a subcuticular closure (Fig. 13-6 to 13-8). When cosmesis is a concern, the incision can be made more into the axilla as described by Leslie and Ryan (Fig. 13-9 and 13-10).[715]

Posteriorly, an analogous vertical incision in line with the extended posterior axillary crease (best visualized by extending the shoulder backwards) also heals well (Fig. 13-11). Fortuitously, these creases lie directly over the joint to which the surgeon needs access.

The First Muscle Layer

The shoulder is covered by the deltoid muscle arising from the clavicle, acromion, and scapular spine. The anterior deltoid extends to a line running approximately from the midclavicle to the midlateral humerus. This line passes over the cephalic vein, the anterior venous drainage of the deltoid, and the coracoid process. The deltoid is innervated by the axillary nerve, whose branches swoop upward as they extend anteriorly. The commonly described ''safe zone'' 5 cm distal to the acromion does not

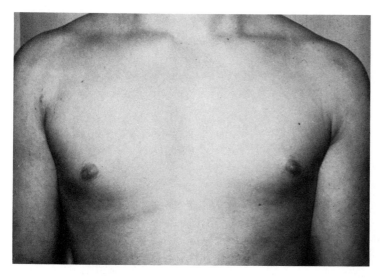

Fig. 13-6. Cosmetic anterior approach on patient's right shoulder. The incision is made in the skin crease. *(Matsen, F. A., III; Thomas, S. C.; and Rockwood, C.A., Jr.: Anterior Glenohumeral Instability. In Rockwood, C. A., and Matsen, F. A., III (eds.): The Shoulder, Fig. 14-4. Philadelphia, W. B. Saunders, 1990.)*

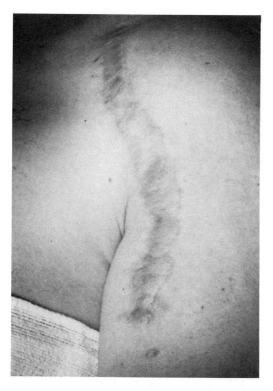

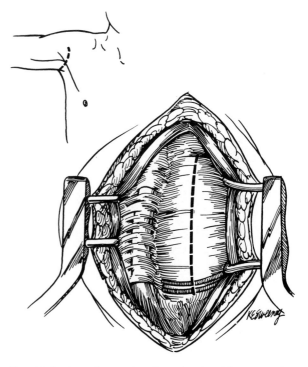

Fig. 13-7. A noncosmetic approach across the front of the shoulder. *(Matsen, F. A., III; Thomas, S. C.; and Rockwood, C. A., Jr.: Anterior Glenohumeral Instability. In Rockwood, C. A., and Matsen, F. A., III (eds.): The Shoulder, Fig. 14-5. Philadelphia, W. B. Saunders, 1990.)*

Fig. 13-8. Anterior approach to the shoulder. Note the skin incision in the axillary line (**inset**). Also note the position of the subscapularis incision 1 cm medial to its insertion. *(Matsen, F. A., and Thomas, S. C.: Glenohumeral Instability. In Evarts, C. M. (ed.): Surgery of the Musculoskeletal System, Vol. 2, 2nd ed. p. 1454. New York, Churchill Livingstone, 1989.)*

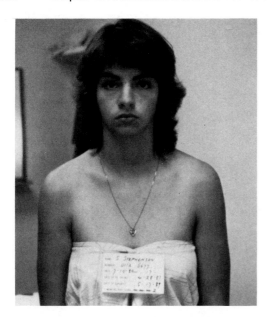

Fig. 13-9. The cosmetic axillary incision. With the arm at the patient's side, the axilliary incision used to perform an anterior capsular shift reconstruction is not visible.

take into account these anterior branches, which may come as close as 2 cm to the acromion. The deltoid abuts against the pectoralis major muscle, the clavicular head of which assists the anterior deltoid in forward flexion. Its medial and lateral

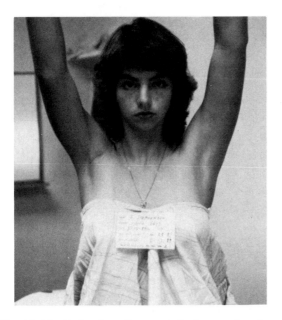

Fig. 13-10. Only when the arm is in the overhead position is the axillary incision noticeable.

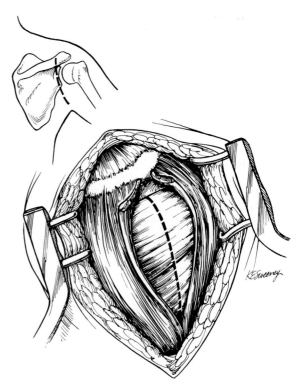

Fig. 13-11. Posterior approach for treatment of posterior glenohumeral instability. The skin incision is centered over the posterior glenoid rim (**inset**). Note the deltoid-splitting approach to minimize the amount of deltoid origin that must be released. Also note the incision in the infraspinatus and teres minor tendons. *(Matsen, F. A., and Thomas, S. C.: Glenohumeral Instability. In Evarts, C. M. (ed.): Surgery of the Musculoskeletal System, Vol. 2, 2nd ed. p. 1465. New York, Churchill Livingstone, 1989.)*

pectoral nerves are not in the surgical field of shoulder stabilization. Splitting the deltopectoral interval just medial to the cephalic vein preserves the deltoid's venous drainage and takes the surgeon to the next layer. It is important to note that extension of the shoulder tightens the pectoralis major and the anterior deltoid as well as the coracoid muscles, compromising the exposure. Thus assistants must be reminded to hold the shoulder in slight flexion to relax these muscles and facilitate exposure.

Posteriorly, the medial edge of the deltoid is too medial to provide useful access to the glenohumeral joint. Access must be achieved by splitting the deltoid, which is most conveniently done at the junction of its middle and posterior thirds. This junction is marked by the posterior corner of the acromion.

The site is favorable for a split because it overlies the joint and also because the axillary nerve exiting the quadrangular space divides into two trunks (its anterior and posterior branches) in an inferior location.

The Coracoacromial Arch and the Clavipectoral Fascia

The coracoid process is the "lighthouse" of the anterior shoulder, providing a palpable guide to the deltopectoral groove, a locator for the coracoacromial arch, and an anchor for the coracoid muscles (the coracobrachialis and short head of the biceps) that separate the lateral "safe side" from the medial "suicide" where the brachial plexus and major vessels lie. The surgeon fully appreciates the value of such a lighthouse when it is lacking—for example, when reexploring a shoulder for complications of a coracoid transfer procedure. The clavipectoral fascia covers the floor of the deltopectoral groove and can be easily identified by rotating the humerus. This permits the surgeon to observe the moving subscapularis beneath the fascial layer. Incising the fascia up to but not through the coracoacromial ligament preserves the stabilizing function of the coracoacromial arch. The bursa separates the structures that do not move on humeral rotation (the deltoid, coracoid muscles, acromion, and coracoacromial ligament) from those that do (the rotator cuff, long head of the biceps tendon, and humeral tuberosities). Posteriorly a similar plane exists between the nonrotating and the rotating structures. Anteriorly or posteriorly, this plane provides a convenient place for medial and lateral retractors.

The Zone of the Nerves

The axillary nerve runs between the deltoid and the coracoid muscles on one side and the rotator cuff on the other. Sweeping a finger from superior to inferior along the anterior aspect of the subscapularis muscle catches the axillary nerve, hanging like a chain passing beneath the shoulder joint. Tracing this nerve proximal and medial leads the finger to the bulk of the brachial plexus. Tracing it laterally and posteriorly leads the finger beneath the shoulder capsule toward the quadrangular space. From a posterior vantage the axillary nerve is felt exiting the quadrangular space beneath the teres minor and extending laterally, where it is applied to the deep surface of the deltoid muscle. By virtue of its prominent location in close proximity to the shoulder joint anteriorly, inferiorly, and posteriorly, the axillary nerve is the most frequently injured structure in shoulder surgery (Fig. 13-12). The musculocutaneous nerve lies on the deep surface of the coracoid muscles and penetrates the coracobrachialis with one or more branches lying a variable distance distal to the coracoid. (Again, the

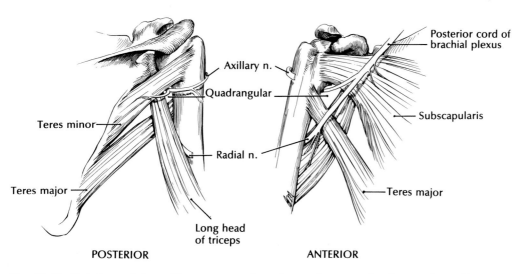

Fig. 13-12. Relations of the axillary nerve to the subscapularis muscle, the quadrangular space, and the neck of the humerus. With anterior dislocations the subscapularis is displaced forward, which creates a traction injury to the axillary nerve. The nerve cannot move out of the way because it is held above by the brachial plexus and below where it wraps around behind the neck of the humerus.

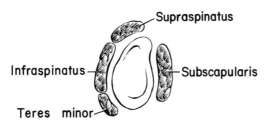

Fig. 13-13. A cross section through the glenohumeral joint shows the muscles that make up the rotator cuff. The subscapularis is the muscle most commonly used in anterior reconstructions of the shoulder, whereas the infraspinatus is the muscle most commonly used to perform posterior soft tissue reconstructions.

often-described 5-cm "safe zone" for the nerve beneath the process refers only to the average position of the main trunk and not to an area that can be entered recklessly.) The musculocutaneous nerve is vulnerable to injury from retractors placed under the coracoid muscles and to traction injury in coracoid transfer. Knowledge of the position of these nerves can make the shoulder surgeon both more comfortable and more effective.

The Rotator Cuff

The next layer of the shoulder is the rotator cuff (Fig. 13-13). The tendons of the muscles in the rotator cuff blend in with the capsule as they insert to the humeral tuberosities. Thus, in reconstructions that require splitting of these muscles from the capsule, the splitting is more easily accomplished medially, before the blending becomes complete. The nerves to these muscles run on their

deep surfaces: the upper and lower subscapular to the subscapularis and the suprascapular to the supraspinatus and infraspinatus (Fig. 13-14). Medial dissection on the deep surface of these muscles may jeopardize their nerve supply.

The cuff is relatively thin between the supraspinatus and the subscapularis (the "rotator interval"). This allows the cuff to pass around the coracoid process as the arm is elevated and lowered. Splitting this interval toward the glenoid may be helpful when mobilization of the subscapularis is needed.

The tendon of the long head of the biceps originates from the supraglenoid tubercle. It runs beneath the cuff in the area of the rotator interval and exits the shoulder beneath the transverse humeral ligament and between the greater and lesser tuberosities. In the bicipital groove of the humerus this tendon is endangered by procedures that involve lateral transfer of the scapularis tendon across the groove.

The Scapulohumeral Ligaments

Usually there are five scapulohumeral ligaments: the coracohumeral and the superior, middle, anteroinferior, and posteroinferior glenohumeral ligaments. As will be discussed in greater detail, these ligaments are important static stabilizers of the shoulder when they are under tension. Considerable variations have been noted in the size of these ligaments and in their attachment to the scapula. These variations may explain why certain shoulders appear more prone to instability. The anteromedial and anteroinferior glenohumeral ligaments often are avulsed from the glenoid or glenoid labrum in traumatic anterior instability. Secure repair of these

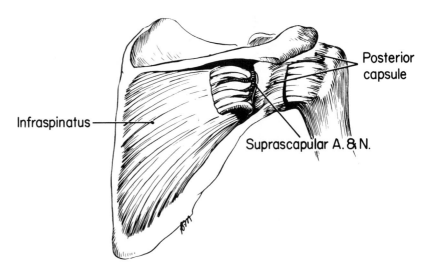

Fig. 13-14. A posterior view of the shoulder joint. Note that the suprascapular artery and nerve enter the infraspinatus muscle. In performing soft tissue reconstructions, care should be taken to avoid excessive medial traction on the muscle, which could damage these structures.

avulsions is an important aspect of management of recurrent traumatic glenohumeral instability (Figs. 13-15 and 13-16).

FACTORS IN GLENOHUMERAL STABILITY

The glenohumeral joint is suited for mobility. The large spherical head of the humerus articulates with the small, shallow glenoid fossa of the scapula. The glenoid provides little coverage of the head, particularly when the shoulder is (1) adducted, flexed and internally rotated, (2) abducted and elevated, or (3) adducted at the side with the scapula rotated downward.[275,777,1163,1322] Despite this lack of coverage, the normal shoulder precisely constrains the humeral head to within 1 mm of the center of the glenoid cavity throughout most of the arc of movement.[562,1035,1036] It is amazing that this seemingly unstable joint is able to provide this precise centering, resist the gravitational pull on the arm hanging at the side for long periods, allow for the lifting of large loads, permit throwing a baseball at speeds approaching 100 miles an hour, and hold together during the application of an almost infinite variety of forces of differing magnitude, direction, duration, and abruptness. Rather than asking why the shoulder dislocates in some patients, perhaps we should ask how it can be so stable in most individuals. We suggest that glenohumeral stability results from a hierarchy of mechanisms, including those that do not require the expenditure of energy by muscles ("passive" mechanisms) and those that do ("active" mechanisms). In this way, nature conserves energy while reserving the ability to call up muscular reinforcement as needed.

Passive Mechanisms

It is apparent that muscle activity is not required to hold the shoulder together. The intact shoulder of a fresh anatomical specimen is quite stable. The anesthetized and paralyzed shoulder does not fall apart in the operating room. Basmajian and Bazant[86] used electromyography of the deltoid, supraspinatus, infraspinatus, biceps, and triceps in a series of young men to show that *none* of these muscles is active when the arm hangs quietly at the side. In cadaver studies Kumar and Balasubramaniam[673] found the position of the humeral head was maintained without muscle activity (with the entire arm hanging down) in 18 of 24 cadaver shoulders. Thus, it is appropriate to discuss "passive" stabilizing mechanisms of the glenohumeral joint, which include joint conformity, finite joint volume, adhesion/cohesion, ligamentous and capsular restraints, and the glenoid labrum.

JOINT CONFORMITY

Saha[1163] demonstrated that there is considerable variation in the radii of the curvature of the glenoid fossa. The contour may be almost flat or slightly curved or may have a definite socket-like appearance. The stability of the glenohumeral joint is affected by the size, shape, and tilt of the glenoid fossa.

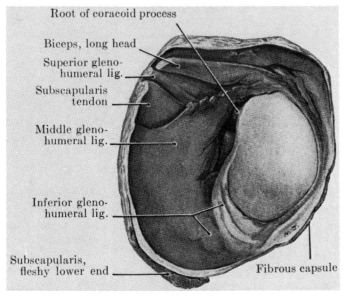

Fig. 13-15. Anterior glenohumeral ligaments. This drawing shows the anterosuperior, anteromedial, and anteroinferior glenohumeral ligaments. The anteromedial and anteroinferior glenohumeral ligaments are often avulsed from the glenoid or glenoid labrum in traumatic anterior instability. (*Grant's Atlas of Anatomy*, 4th ed. Baltimore; Williams & Wilkins, 1956.)

Root of coracoid process

Biceps, long head

Superior gleno-humeral lig.

Subscapularis tendon

Middle gleno-humeral lig.

Inferior gleno-humeral lig.

Subscapularis, fleshy lower end

Fibrous capsule

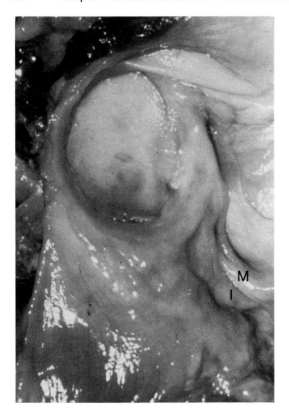

Fig. 13-16. Cadaver dissection of the glenoid and associated glenohumeral ligaments. This dissection demonstrates the anterior glenohumeral ligaments. Note the relationship of the anteroinferior (**I**) and the anteromedial (**M**) glenohumeral ligaments to the anterior rim of the glenoid. *(Matsen, F. A., III; Thomas, S. C.; and Rockwood, C. A., Jr.: Anterior Glenohumeral Instability. In Rockwood, C. A., and Matsen, F. A., III (eds.): The Shoulder, Fig. 14-10. Philadelphia, W. B. Saunders, 1990.)*

Cyprien and co-workers[265] studied the humeral retrotorsion and glenohumeral[265] relationship in normal patients and in patients with recurrent anterior dislocation and found essentially no difference. However, when they studied the affected and unaffected shoulders in the group of patients with recurrent dislocation, they found that the diameter of the glenoid and the contact index were smaller in the dislocated shoulders than in the normal shoulders. Whether these changes were the cause or the effect of the instability is unclear. Brewer and associates[157] measured the "retroversion" of the glenoid in ten adolescents with 17 posteriorly unstable shoulders. They concluded that "excessive retroversion is a developmental deformity and is considered the primary etiology of posterior insta-

bility of the shoulder." However, their data are also consistent with the hypothesis that the deformity is a result (rather than a cause) of the instability: a major right–left difference in glenoid tilt (>10°) was found only when one shoulder had experienced numerous dislocations and the other none. Perhaps even more important is the fact that the apparent tilt of the glenoid surface on the axillary view varies with the angle at which the radiograph is obtained (Fig. 13-17).

Randelli and Gambrioli[1059] used computed tomography (CT) to perform glenohumeral osteometry. They found no significant developmental differences in glenohumeral index, glenoid anteroposterior orientation, and humeral retrotorsion between 50 normal subjects and 40 patients with recurrent anterior dislocations. They concluded that erosions and fractures may affect the apparent orientation and anteroposterior diameter of the glenoid.

The depth of the bony glenoid is enhanced by the contributions of the articular cartilage and the glenoid labrum, which, by virtue of their relative compliance, provide an element of plasticity that can enhance the quality of the glenohumeral fit (similar to the "feathered" edge of a contact lens) (Fig. 13-18). The concavity and the fit of the glenoid to the humeral head provide stability to the joint, which is enhanced by forces pressing the ball into the socket (see Active Mechanisms).

FINITE JOINT VOLUME

When one pulls on the plunger of a plugged syringe, a relative vacuum is created that resists displacement of the plunger. Anatomical studies, surgical findings, attempts at aspiration, and magnetic resonance images all confirm that there is minimal (<1 cc) free fluid in the normal shoulder joint. The normal shoulder is sealed by the capsule so that outside fluid cannot enter it. Thus, like the syringe, the shoulder joint is stabilized by its limited joint volume. As long as the joint is a closed space containing minimal free fluid, the joint surfaces cannot be easily distracted or subluxated. Small translations of the humerus on the glenoid can be balanced by fluid flow in the opposite direction, allowing a nonuniform gap to open in the joint space. This gap can increase until all available fluid has been mobilized, at which point further motion of the joint is resisted by negative fluid pressure in the joint. This negative pressure pulls the capsule inward toward the joint space, putting its fibers "on the stretch." Individuals with more stretchy capsules (see the discussion of the AMBRI syndrome) will

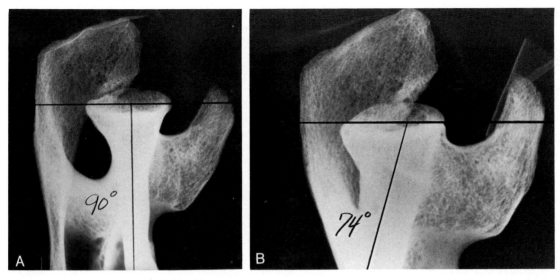

Fig. 13-17. Two radiographs of the same cadaver scapula showing the variation in apparent glenoid retroversion depending on the radiographic projection. *(Matsen, F. A., III; Thomas, S. C.; and Rockwood, C. A., Jr.: Anterior Glenohumeral Instability. In Rockwood, C. A., and Matsen, F. A., III (eds.): The Shoulder, Fig. 14-11. Philadelphia, W. B. Saunders, 1990.)*

allow greater translation than those with stiff joint capsules.

This mechanism is aided by the fact that intra-articular pressure is normally slightly negative.[718,882,1227] This negative intra-articular pressure is likely to be the result of the high osmotic pressure in interstitial tissues, which draws water from the joint. For example, if the colloid osmotic pressure of normal synovial fluid is 10 mm Hg and that of the synovial interstitium is 14 mm Hg, the equilibrium pressure in the joint fluid will be −4 mm Hg.[1227] This negative intra-articular pressure adds a small amount of resistance to distraction (about one ounce per square inch) to the limited joint volume effect. The greater importance of these osmotic effects lies in the fact that they provide a mechanism by which free fluid is scavenged from the joint space.

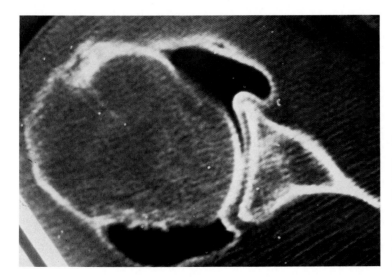

Fig. 13-18. CT arthrogram of glenohumeral joint. The depth of the bony glenoid is enhanced by contributions of the articular cartilage and the glenoid labrum. This further increases the stability of the glenohumeral joint. *(Matsen, F. A., III; Thomas, S. C.; and Rockwood, C. A., Jr.: Anterior Glenohumeral Instability. In Rockwood, C. A., and Matsen, F. A., III (eds.): The Shoulder, Fig. 14-12. Philadelphia, W. B. Saunders, 1990.)*

ADHESION/COHESION

The stabilization mechanism changes when the gap between the articular surfaces becomes very small. Viscous and intermolecular forces begin to dominate, preventing ready fluid motion and providing a cohesive bond between the glenoid and humerus. We term this the "adhesion/cohesion mechanism." A familiar example is provided by two wet microscope slides pressed together. Water is held to their surfaces by *adhesion*. They can readily slide on each other but cannot be pulled apart easily by forces applied at right angles to their flat surfaces—the water holds them together by *cohesion*. Joint surfaces also are wet with joint fluid that holds them together by adhesion/cohesion. This joint fluid interface has the highly desirable properties of (1) having high tensile strength (difficult to pull apart), and (2) having little shear strength (allows sliding of the two joint surfaces on each other with low resistance).[1227] An important distinction is that the adhesion/cohesion mechanism does not put the capsular fibers on the stretch, because viscous forces suffice to prevent fluid from entering the joint space. Thus, stability is provided entirely by forces exerted by and on the articular surfaces. It is also noteworthy that adhesion/cohesion forces do not stabilize a prosthetic shoulder replacement, because metal and polyethylene are insufficiently compliant to provide the necessary near-perfect congruence and because water does not adhere to their surfaces.

Both the limited joint volume effect and the effect of adhesion/cohesion would be reduced or eliminated by the addition of excess fluid (gas or liquid) to the joint. This phenomenon was well described by Humphry in 1858.[566]

> In many joints—the ball and socket joints for instance—though the ligaments assist, as just mentioned, in preventing dislocation, it is quite clear that the articular surfaces cannot, under ordinary circumstances, be directly held in apposition by them, inasmuch as they must be loose in the whole circumference to permit the movements of the joint in every direction. If the ligament were sufficiently tight at any one part to hold the bones together, it must of necessity prevent the movement in one direction, which we know is not the case. The experiments of Weber upon the hip-joint were, I believe, the first to prove the fact that atmospheric pressure is the real power by which the head of the femur is held in the acetabulum when the muscles are at rest. One convincing experiment is easily repeated; hold up a side of the pelvis, with its appended lower extremity, the joint not having been opened, and then bore a hole through the acetabulum, so as to admit air into the hip-joint. The weight of the limb causes it to drop from half an inch to an inch, the head of the thigh-bone is pulled out of the acetabulum, as soon as the air is

permitted to pass between the articular surfaces. In the unopened state of the joint, therefore, the weight of the limb is entirely borne by atmospheric pressure, so that both ligaments and muscles, the latter especially, are relieved in a corresponding manner. The same fact may be shown with regard to the shoulder and other joints, in a greater or less degree, though obviously the illustration is easiest in the hip and shoulder. The advantages of this construction, and the facilities it affords for easy movement by leaving all the muscles free to act upon the joint, need no demonstration. We have only to remember that this power is in continual operation to appreciate the amount of animal force that is economized by it.

The contribution of atmospheric pressure to shoulder stability is also described in *Gray's Anatomy* (second edition, 1963): "The looseness of the capsule is so great that the arm will fall about an inch from the scapula when the muscles are dissected and a hole made in it to remove the atmospheric pressure." Kumar and Balasubramaniam again demonstrated this effect in cadaver shoulders.[673] They fixed the scapula to a frame in the vertical position while the arm hung free. Radiographs were taken to determine the presence of glenohumeral subluxation. The results of these studies are so striking that they are quoted here:

> In none of the shoulders was any subluxation of the joint demonstrable radiographically after dividing the muscles; but, when the capsule was then punctured [with an 18 gauge needle], marked inferior subluxation of the humeral head was seen. This occurred regardless of where the capsule was punctured. Provided atmospheric air was able to gain access into the glenohumeral joint, subluxation was always noted. As soon as the capsule was punctured percutaneously a hissing sound was heard as air rushed into the joint and it subluxated: the subluxation was confirmed radiographically. The point of puncture of the capsule did not affect these findings. No further subluxation beyond the position reached after percutaneous puncture of the capsule occurred when the overlying muscles were subsequently divided.

They found that once air had been admitted, the intact shoulder could be subluxated manually into any position with minimal force. Before air had been admitted, "a fair amount of force" was necessary to produce subluxation. It seems likely that the air admitted into the joint eliminated the stabilizing effect of the limited joint volume and also interrupted the continuity of the fluid cohesion holding the wet joint surfaces together. The change in shoulder stability with admission of air has been quantitated by Sidles and co-workers.[1224] The addition of blood to the joint in an intracapsular fracture may produce inferior subluxation by similar mechanisms.[250,368,900,971,972,1295,1296] It is of note that finite volume and adhesion/cohesion also operate in the subacromial bursa, providing additional resistance to inferior displacement of the humerus.

These stabilizing mechanisms may be overwhelmed by the application of traction, as in the cracking of the metacarpophalangeal joint. A "crack" is produced as the joint cavitates: subatmospheric pressure within the joint releases gas (>80% carbon dioxide) from solution in the joint fluid. This is accompanied by a sudden jump in the joint separation. Once a joint has cracked it cannot be cracked again until about 20 minutes later when all the gas has been reabsorbed.[1125,1329] (We are indebted to Peter Simkin of the University of Washington, Division of Rheumatology, who pointed us to the important literature on joint volume and adhesion/cohesion effects in joint stability.)

LIGAMENTOUS AND CAPSULAR RESTRAINTS

Ligamentous and capsular restraints are a fourth passive mechanism of joint stability. The joint capsule is large, loose, and redundant. The capacity of the glenohumeral joint capsule is larger than that of the humeral head to allow for the full and free range of motion of the shoulder. By virtue of their mandatory redundancy, the capsule and its ligaments cannot prevent glenohumeral translation when the joint is in most of its range. This is because the capsular ligaments must be under tension to exert an effect, and this occurs only when the joint approaches the end of its range of motion. Kaltsas[627] studied some of the material properties of the shoulder capsule and found it to be more elastic and stronger than the capsule of the elbow.

The three anterior glenohumeral ligaments were first described by Schlemm.[1187] Whereas Codman[220] believed that the ligaments are only a variable thickening of the capsule, Fick,[380] Weitbrecht,[1387] Delorme,[301] Moseley and Overgaard,[869] Reeves,[1075] Turkel and associates,[1322] DePalma,[294] and McLaughlin[822] agreed that the superior, middle, and inferior glenohumeral ligaments are distinguishable and important for joint stability (See Fig. 13-15.)

The constant yet diminutive *superior glenohumeral ligament* extends from the anterosuperior edge of the glenoid (near the origin of the tendon of the long head of the biceps) to the top of the lesser tuberosity of the humerus (with a portion of the coracohumeral ligament).

The dense but variable *middle glenohumeral ligament* originates from the supraglenoid tubercle, the superior labrum, or the scapular neck. It attaches to the base of the lesser tuberosity of the humerus with the posterior aspect of the subscapularis muscle. Its distal half is fused with the tendon of the subscapularis. It is usually 1 to 2 cm wide and 4 mm thick. It is poorly defined or absent in 30% of shoulders.[292] In four cases of recurrent dislocation, Moseley and Overgaard found the middle glenohumeral ligament either was not discernible or was attached to the neck of the scapula rather than the labrum.[869]

The *inferior glenohumeral ligament* extends from the anteroinferior labrum and glenoid lip to the lesser tuberosity of the humerus just inferior to the middle glenohumeral ligament. The inferior glenohumeral ligament reinforces the capsular area between the subscapularis and the origin of the long head of the triceps. The experimental work on primates that was reported by Reeves[1072,1074] demonstrated the importance of the inferior glenohumeral ligament in preventing anterior dislocation of the shoulder. He further pointed out that in most instances the anteroinferior glenohumeral ligament inserted primarily into the inferior labrum and only partially into bone. Turkel and associates[1322] pointed out three parts of this ligament: the superior band, the anterior axillary pouch, and the posterior axillary pouch. They proposed that the superior band of the inferior glenohumeral ligament was a major stabilizer of the joint.

Delorme,[301] DePalma,[293] and Moseley and Overgaard[869] documented variability in the glenohumeral ligaments, which sometimes were very poorly defined. (See Fig. 13-15.) They also demonstrated great variation in the size and number of synovial recesses that form in the anterior capsule above, below, and between the glenohumeral ligaments. They have shown from dissections that if the capsule arises at the labrum, there are few if any synovial recesses (in this situation there is a generalized blending of all three ligaments, which leaves no room for synovial recesses or weaknesses, and hence the anterior glenohumeral capsule is stronger). However, the more medially the capsule arises from the glenoid (ie, from the anterior scapular neck), the larger and more numerous are the synovial recesses. The end result can be a thin, weak anterior capsule. Uhthoff and Piscopo[1325] demonstrated in an embryological study that in 52 specimens the anterior capsule inserted into the glenoid labrum in 77% and into the medial neck of the scapula in 23%. These congenital variations may play a major role in the relative frequency of bilateral glenohumeral instability. (See Bilateral Shoulder Instability, p. 19.)

Ovesen and co-workers,[971–978] Turkel and colleagues,[1322] and Warren and associates[1362] have demonstrated the role of the anterior and posterior capsule and capsular ligaments in limiting the translation and rotation of the humerus. We emphasize that glenohumeral ligaments can exert an effect only if they are under tension. Thus, these ligaments provide a checkrein function that is the last guardian of shoulder stability after all other passive and dynamic mechanisms have been overwhelmed. Examples of restraint provided by capsular ligaments have been demonstrated in cadaver studies as follows:

1. The anteroinferior capsule restrains anterior subluxation of the abducted arm.[972]
2. The middle glenohumeral ligament limits external rotation at 45° of abduction.[1322]
3. The inferior glenohumeral ligament limits external rotation at 45° to 90° of abduction.[1322]
4. The posterior capsule and the teres minor restrain internal rotation.[974,978]
5. The lower two thirds of the anterior capsule and the lower subscapularis restrain abduction and external rotation.[974,975]

Schwartz and co-workers[1198] performed selective arthroscopic cutting experiments on cadaver shoulders to quantitate the contribution of the capsular structures to glenohumeral stability. They pointed out that clinically, instability usually was accompanied by both anterior and posterior lesions. They concluded:

1. The inferior glenohumeral ligament in concert with the posteroinferior capsule provided the primary restraint to anterior translation.
2. The middle glenohumeral ligament (when present) provided a secondary restraint to anterior dislocation.
3. The posteroinferior capsule provided the primary posterior restraint to posterior dislocation.
4. The posterosuperior capsule and superior glenohumeral ligament provided secondary restraint to posterior dislocation.

Howell and associates[562] used axillary roentgenograms to document the anteroposterior position of the humeral head on the glenoid. They found that posterior translation of the humeral head occurs in normal subjects with the arm in extension and external rotation. This posterior translation is absent in shoulders with anterior instability. These authors suggest that this posterior translation is the result of the tension in the intact anterior capsule and ligaments.

The *coracohumeral ligament* extends from the lateral border of the horizontal arm of the coracoid process, below the coracoacromial ligament, to the transverse humeral ligament bridging the greater and lesser tuberosities between the supraspinatus and subscapularis tendon insertions.[457] Basmajian and Bazant[86] have carried out cadaver dissections demonstrating that the coracohumeral ligament and the superior capsule became quite taut when the arm was in adduction, and suggested that this tension helped to stabilize the humeral head in the glenoid. In contrast, when the shoulder was abducted to the mid-range, the superior capsule became more lax and the humeral head became more unstable. They proposed that the coracohumeral ligament held the humeral head on the slope of the glenoid, providing substantial stability that was further enhanced by upward rotation (abduction) of the scapula and by supraspinatus contraction. Ovesen and Nielsen[971] demonstrated that cutting the coracohumeral ligament gave rise to distal subluxation of the humerus in the vertically mounted shoulder. The authors concluded that the superior capsuloligamentous structures are the most important structures preventing distal subluxation of the humeral head. However, they did not consider that cutting the superior capsuloligamentous structures must have admitted air to the joint—an action that in itself can produce downward subluxation (see under Finite Joint Volume and Adhesion/Cohesion). Thus, although the coracohumeral ligament provides stability to the adducted shoulder, it is probably insufficient by itself, as was demonstrated in the 24 shoulders studied by Kumar and Balasubramaniam[673] that became downwardly unstable with only the admission of air into the joint.

GLENOID LABRUM

The glenoid labrum is a fibrous rim that serves to deepen the glenoid fossa and allow attachment of the glenohumeral ligaments and the biceps tendon to the glenoid. It is the interconnection of the periosteum of the glenoid, the glenoid bone, the glenoid articular cartilage, the synovium, and the capsule. At the posterosuperior section the labrum is continuous with the long head tendon of the biceps. Anteriorly it is continuous with the inferior glenohumeral ligament. (See Figs. 13-15 and 13-16.)[457,874,874a,1313] Bankart deemed its detachment from the glenoid the essential lesion responsible for the high incidence of recurrent anterior dislocations. The labrum is detached in most cases of traumatic anterior instability (Fig. 13-19).[75,76]

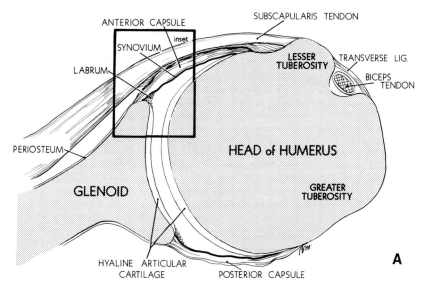

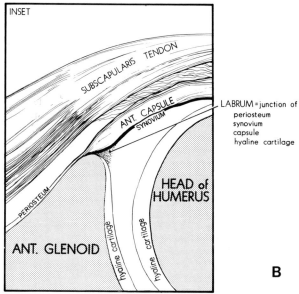

Fig. 13-19. Normal shoulder anatomy. (**A**) A horizontal section through the middle of the glenohumeral joint demonstrating normal anatomic relationships. Note the close relation of the subscapularis tendon to the anterior capsule. (**B**) A close-up view in the area of the labrum. The labrum is essentially devoid of fibrocartilage and is composed of tissues from the nearby hyaline cartilage, capsule, synovium, and periosteum.

DePalma[293] and Olsson[959] have shown that the incidence of severe recurrent dislocations is low in elderly patients, in whom labral degeneration is more common. Townley[1309] and Reeves[1072-1074] removed the anterior glenoid labrum through a posterior approach and found that as long as the anterior capsular mechanism remained a strong structural unit, anterior displacement of the humeral head was prevented. Thus, the integrity of the labrum itself may not be as important as the security of the attachment of glenohumeral ligaments to the glenoid.

Microscopic studies by Moseley and Overgaard,[869] Townley,[1309] and Gardner[420] have shown that a small amount of fibrocartilage exists at the junction of the hyaline cartilage of the glenoid and fibrous capsule. The vast majority of the labrum consists of dense fibrous tissue with a few elastic fibers. A defect in the glenoid labrum lessens the effective depth of the fossa and thus can be expected to diminish the constraint of the head and facilitate the translation of the head in the direction of the defect. In fresh cadavers, Sidles and co-workers[1224] showed that excision of the labrum reduced by just over

50% the stabilization provided by glenoid geometry against distal subluxation.

BONY RESTRAINTS

The glenoid prevents the humerus from moving medially. It faces anteriorly at an angle of about 45 degrees with the coronal plane, which places it behind the humeral head for most forward uses of the arm. The acromion, coracoid, and coracoacromial ligament limit the extent of posterosuperior, superior, and anterosuperior motion of the humeral head, "backstopping" the other stabilizing mechanisms (Fig. 13-20).

Active Mechanisms

The role of dynamic stability can easily be demonstrated in the normal subject. When the subject is completely relaxed, the humerus can be pushed forward and backward with respect to the scapula. If the subject contracts the muscles (for example, by slightly abducting the shoulder), the anteroposterior excursion is virtually eliminated.

Dynamic glenohumeral stability is provided by the long head of the biceps and the muscles of the rotator cuff: the subscapularis, the supraspinatus, the infraspinatus, and the teres minor. The cuff muscles serve several stabilizing functions. First, by virtue of the blending of their tendons with the glenohumeral capsule and ligaments, selective contraction of the cuff muscles can adjust the tension in these structures, producing "dynamic" ligaments, as proposed by Cleland in 1866.[218] Second,

by contracting together, they press the humeral head into the glenoid fossa, locking it into position and thus providing a secure scapulohumeral link for upper extremity function.[1035] Sidles and associates[1224] demonstrated that the resistance of the shoulder to distal subluxation is proportionally increased by 67% of the applied compressive load. Thus, a 3-kg increase in the forces pushing the head into the glenoid increases the resistance to distal subluxation by 2 kg. Third, by contracting selectively, the rotator cuff muscles can resist displacing forces resulting from contraction of the principal shoulder motors.[869,1281] For example, when the pectoralis major and anterior deltoid muscles elevate and flex the shoulder, they tend to push the humeral head out the back of the glenoid fossa; this displacement is resisted by contraction of the subscapularis, infraspinatus, and teres minor muscles. Similarly, when the lateral deltoid initiates shoulder abduction, the supraspinatus and the long head of the biceps actively resist upward displacement of the humeral head relative to the glenoid fossa. Patients who can consciously relax these stabilizing muscles can achieve voluntary glenohumeral subluxation and dislocation. Conversely, patients with capsular instability can increase the security of their glenohumeral joints by strengthening the rotator muscles. Dynamic stability is most effective if the contractions of all shoulder muscles are coordinated with one another; strength alone is insufficient. Thus, repetitive coordination exercises such as swimming are an important tool for enhancing dynamic stability.[605]

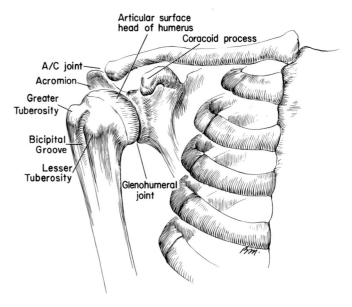

Fig. 13-20. Normal bony architecture of the shoulder joint.

Conclusion

We conclude that the shoulder has a hierarchy of supporting mechanisms. Minimal loads, such as gravitational pull on the arm, are resisted by passive mechanisms such as the concavity of the joint surface provided by the glenoid and its labrum, the finite joint volume, and the adhesion/cohesion of joint fluid. Larger loads, such as those encountered in serving a tennis ball, washing a car, or picking up a child, are resisted by the action of cuff muscles whose contraction is coordinated with that of the prime movers to balance displacing forces. These mechanisms cost the body some energy but do not threaten its integrity. Finally, the ability of the shoulder to resist massive loads depends on the ligaments, the capsule, and the bony support of the joint. For example, the severe abduction–external rotation forces of a fall in skiing or a "clothesline" tackle in football challenge the anteroinferior glenohumeral ligaments. If these ligaments do not hold, a subluxation or dislocation occurs.

The function, movements, and biomechanics of the shoulder joint are further detailed in articles by Inman and colleagues,[578] Lucas,[750] Saha,[1163,1169] Bechtol,[96] Colachis and Strohm,[231] Dvir and Berme,[329] Engin,[349] Poppen and Walker,[1036] Turkel and co-workers,[1322] Jobe and associates,[603] and Gainor and colleagues.[405]

BILATERAL SHOULDER INSTABILITY

Some of the factors contributing to joint stability are congenitally determined, such as the particular collagen makeup of the patient's ligaments, the arrangement of the glenohumeral ligaments and their method of attachment to the glenoid, the tilt of the glenoid face, the size and depth of the glenoid, the thickness of the glenoid labrum, the torsion of the humerus, and the variations in cuff muscle anat-

omy. These factors are likely to affect both shoulders similarly. Thus, variations in these factors among individuals could have a major effect on the propensity of both shoulders to be unstable. Other factors affecting both shoulders include the patient's age, predilection for trauma, and presence of seizures. In light of these considerations, it is not surprising that the incidence of bilateral glenohumeral instability is higher than would be expected if instability were distributed randomly among shoulders. Hovelius and co-workers[557] found that 17% of their patients aged 23 to 29 years with shoulder instability had this problem in both shoulders. In further support of a genetic predisposition, they found that the incidence of dislocation in other family members was 5% as compared with the population-wide incidence of 1.7%. O'Driscoll and Evans[949] reviewed 257 patients having DuToit capsulorrhaphy for recurrent instability; 13% developed contralateral instability within 15 years (Fig. 13-21).

MOVEMENTS OF THE SHOULDER

Specific Joint Movements

Older literature states that the motion of the shoulder was quite simple, inferring that the first 90° of abduction was in the glenohumeral joint and the remaining 90° came from scapular elevation and rotation. However, in 1944, in a classic article on shoulder function, Inman and co-workers[578] demonstrated that motion was a complex action.

Motion of the upper extremity involves motion of four separate joints about the shoulder complex: (1) the glenohumeral joint, (2) the acromioclavicular joint, (3) the sternoclavicular joint, and (4) the so-called scapulothoracic joint, which effects movement between the scapula and the thoracic cage. Complete elevation of the arm, in either flex-

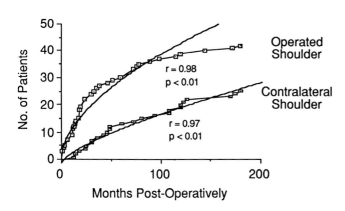

Fig. 13-21. Incidence of contralateral shoulder instability from the data of O'Driscoll and Evans.[949] Thirteen percent of the patients with normal contralateral shoulders at the time of surgery developed contralateral instability within 15 years. *(Matsen, F. A., III; Thomas, S. C.; and Rockwood, C. A., Jr.: Anterior Glenohumeral Instability. In Rockwood, C. A., and Matsen, F. A., III (eds.): The Shoulder, Fig. 14-14. Philadelphia, W. B. Saunders, 1990.)*

ion or abduction, depends on the free motion in all of the joints of the shoulder complex.

GLENOHUMERAL MOTION

Between the humerus and the glenoid fossa, 120° of passive motion is possible without moving the scapula. Beyond this point motion is blocked by the neck of the humerus against the acromion process. The glenohumeral joint is capable of only 90° of active abduction. If the arm is in full internal rotation, only 60° of glenohumeral motion is possible, because the greater tuberosity impinges on the acromion process. In external rotation, the greater tuberosity is rotated behind the acromion.

SCAPULOTHORACIC MOTION

In full abduction or flexion, the scapula rotates outward 60° (Fig. 13-22). The rotation begins after the first 30° of abduction or 60° of glenohumeral flexion and then moves smoothly and synchronously with the movement of the glenohumeral joint.

CLAVICLE AND STERNOCLAVICULAR MOTION

The clavicle is a very freely moveable and frequently moved joint. During full overhead motion the clavicle elevates 35° and rotates on its long axis 45° to 50°. With protraction and retraction of the arm the clavicle motion totals 35°. Downward displacement of the clavicle is prevented by the sternoclavicular ligaments.

ACROMIOCLAVICULAR MOTION

A total range of motion of 20° was reported by Inman and colleagues[578] and by others, but we have only been able to detect 5° to 8° of motion (refer to the section on Injuries to the Acromioclavicular Joint).

Interaction of the Deltoid and Short Rotators During Arm Motion

The deltoid is the primary muscle for flexion, abduction, and extension of the arm. However, the muscles of the rotator cuff serve a very important role in shoulder motion. Saha[1162,1164,1169] has confirmed the work of Inman and colleagues[578] and has shown that the short rotators function as horizontal stabilizers and steering muscles: they help to hold the humeral head in the glenoid during abduction. During abduction the power of the subscapularis is primarily between 120° and 150° and acts to glide and roll the head posterior in the glenoid, to counteract the tendency toward anterior subluxation. The large infraspinatus and the smaller teres minor act to prevent anterior displacement of the head and to pull the head down and backward, while the deltoid abducts the arm. Saha has shown by electromyography that the latissimus dorsi helps to hold the head back during shoulder motion and is most active from 60° to 180°.[1161,1163]

Other Abduction Mechanisms

LONG HEAD OF THE BICEPS TENDON

In the anatomic position, the long head of the biceps tendon is ineffective to flex or abduct the arm, because it is anterior and medial to the center of the head of the humerus. However, when the arm is externally rotated and during abduction and flexion, the long head of the biceps tendon serves as a secondary head depressor. This mechanism is a weak

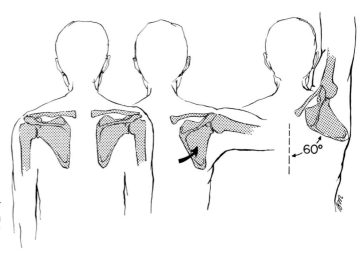

Fig. 13-22. During full elevation of the upper extremity, the scapula rotates outward 60°. In general, the scapula rotates on the thorax 1° for every 2° of glenohumeral elevation.

one and may be used to help abduct the arm of a patient who has paralysis of the deltoid muscle.

SUPRASPINATUS MECHANISM

Lucas[750] pointed out that the supraspinatus mechanism is similar to the biceps mechanism, except that the muscle motor is on the scapula and the insertion is on the greater tuberosity of the humerus. In addition, the tendon in the anatomic position is more nearly over the center of the head. Electromyographic studies reveal that the supraspinatus acts with the deltoid muscle throughout the entire range of motion of arm elevation.

SUMMARY OF SHOULDER MOTION

In summary, then, motion of the shoulder is complex.[1162,1164,1169] All four joints of the shoulder (ie, glenohumeral, scapulothoracic, acromioclavicular, and sternoclavicular) must be freely moveable.[578] There is keen interaction between the deltoid and the rotator cuffs (ie, supraspinatus, subscapularis, infraspinatus, and teres minor). The short rotators guide, steer, and maintain the humeral head in the glenoid fossa. They depress or hold down the humeral head, so that although the deltoid elevates the arm primarily, the subscapularis, along with the infraspinatus and teres minor, prevent anterior subluxation of the head. The infraspinatus and the teres minor externally rotate the humerus to prevent impingement of the greater tuberosity into the acromion during abduction.

Full elevation of the arm is accomplished by a 2:1 ratio of glenohumeral to scapulothoracic motion; scapular rotation of 60°; and clavicular upward rotation of 40° to 50° and elevation of 30° to 40°. Rotation and upward displacement occur in the sternoclavicular joint, and some motion occurs at the acromioclavicular joint.

For more detailed information on the function, movements, and biomechanics of the shoulder joint, see the articles by Inman and colleagues,[578] Lucas,[750] Saha,[1163,1169] Bechtol,[96] Colachis and Strohm,[231] Dvir and Berme,[329] Engin,[349] Poppen and Walker,[1036] Turkel and co-workers,[1322] Jobe and associates,[603] and Gainor and co-workers.[405]

CLASSIFICATION OF GLENOHUMERAL INSTABILITY

Glenohumeral instability may be classified according to the degree of instability, the chronology of instability, whether substantial force initiated the process (ie, traumatic or atraumatic), whether the patient intentionally contributes to the shoulder's instability (ie, voluntary or involuntary), and the direction in which the humeral head translates in relation to the glenoid fossa.

DEGREE OF INSTABILITY

Dislocation of the glenohumeral joint is the complete separation of the articular surfaces; immediate, spontaneous relocation does not occur. Glenohumeral *subluxation* is defined as symptomatic translation of the humeral head on the glenoid without complete separation of the articular surfaces. This is in contrast to the small amount of glenohumeral translation that occurs in normal shoulder function.[562,1035] Subluxation of the glenohumeral joint is transient and often momentary: the humeral head quickly and spontaneously returns to its normal position in the glenoid fossa. In a series of patients with anterior shoulder subluxation reported by Rowe and Zarins,[1135] 87% were traumatic and more than 50% were not aware that their shoulders were unstable. Like dislocations, subluxations may be traumatic or atraumatic, anterior, posterior, or inferior, acute or recurrent, or they may occur after surgical repairs that did not achieve complete shoulder stability. Recurrent subluxations may coexist with or be initiated by glenohumeral dislocation. Rowe and Zarins[1134,1144] reported Hill-Sachs compression fractures in 40% of the patients in their series on subluxation of the shoulder, an observation indicating that at some time these shoulders had been completely dislocated. *Apprehension* refers to the fear that the shoulder will subluxate or dislocate. This fear may be more functionally limiting than the instability itself.

CHRONOLOGY OF INSTABILITY

Congenital instability may result from absence or abnormalities of the proximal humerus or glenoid, such as excessive retroversion of the head of the humerus or malformation of the glenoid. A glenohumeral dislocation is *acute* if seen within the first day or so after its occurrence; otherwise, it is *chronic*. A dislocation is *locked* (or *fixed*) if the humeral head has been impaled on an edge of the glenoid, making reduction difficult. If a glenohumeral joint has been unstable on multiple occasions, the instability is *recurrent*. Recurrent instability may consist of repeated glenohumeral dislocations, subluxations, or both.

CONTRIBUTING FACTORS

Rowe[1144] carefully analyzed 500 dislocations of the glenohumeral joint and determined that 96% were *traumatic* (caused by a major injury) and the remaining 4% were *atraumatic*. DePalma,[292] Rockwood,[1113] and Collins and Wilde[233] also recognized the importance of distinguishing between traumatic and atraumatic instability of the shoulder. This distinction is critical in the selection of treatment. Patients with *traumatic* shoulder instability usually have a *unilateral* problem, usually have a *Bankart* lesion, and *surgery* is usually required to manage the problem—thus, the acronym "TUBS." Patients with *atraumatic* shoulder instability usually have an *atraumatic* initial injury, may have *multidirectional* instability, usually have *bilateral* shoulder instability, and usually respond to a *rehabilitation* program. However, should surgery be performed, the surgeon must pay particular attention to performing an *inferior* capsular shift—thus, the acronym "AMBRI." If a patient intentionally subluxates or dislocates his or her shoulder, instability is described as *voluntary.* If the instability occurs unintentionally, it is *involuntary.* Voluntary and involuntary instability may coexist. Voluntary anterior dislocation may occur with the arm at the side or in abduction/external rotation. Voluntary posterior dislocation may occur with the arm in flexion, adduction, and internal rotation, or with the arm at the side. The relatively frequent association of voluntary dislocations of the shoulder with emotional instability and psychiatric problems has been noted by several authors.[188,1129] The desire to voluntarily dislocate the shoulder cannot be treated surgically.

Neuromuscular causes of shoulder instability have been reported as well. Percy[1014] described a woman who, following an episode of encephalitis, developed a posterior dislocation. Kretzler and Blue[662] have discussed the management of posterior dislocations of the shoulder in children with cerebral palsy. Sever,[1213] Fairbank,[367] L'Episcopo,[680] Zachary,[1416] and Wickstrom[1394] reported techniques for the management of neurologic dislocation of the shoulder caused by upper brachial plexus birth injuries.

DIRECTION OF INSTABILITY

Anterior Dislocations

Subcoracoid dislocation is the most common type of anterior dislocation. The usual mechanism is a combination of shoulder abduction, extension, and external rotation producing forces that challenge the anterior capsule and ligaments, the glenoid rim, and the rotator cuff mechanism. The head of the humerus is displaced anteriorly with respect to the glenoid and is inferior to the coracoid process (Fig. 13-23). Other types of anterior dislocation include *subglenoid* (the head of the humerus lies anterior and below the glenoid fossa) (Fig. 13-24), *subclavicular* (the head of the humerus lies medial to the coracoid process, just inferior to the lower border of the clavicle) (Fig. 13-25), and *intrathoracic* (the head of the humerus lies between the ribs and the thoracic cavity) (Fig. 13-26).[442,875,1003,1183,1390] These rarer types of dislocation are usually associated with severe trauma. There is a high incidence of fracture of the greater tuberosity of the humerus and rotator cuff avulsion. Neurologic, pulmonary, and vascular complications can occur, as can subcutaneous emphysema. West[1390] reported a case of intrathoracic dislocation in which with reduction the humerus was felt to slip out of the chest cavity with a sensation similar to that of slipping a large cork from a bottle. His patient, who had an avulsion fracture of the greater tuberosity and no neurologic deficit, regained a functional range of motion and returned to his job as a carpenter.

Posterior Dislocations

Posterior dislocations may leave the humeral head in a *subacromial* (head behind the glenoid and beneath the acromion), *subglenoid* (head behind and beneath the glenoid), or *subspinous* (head medial to acromion and beneath the spine of the scapula) location. The subacromial dislocation is the most common by far (Fig. 13-27). Posterior dislocations are frequently locked. Hawkins and co-workers[500] reviewed 41 such cases related to motor vehicle accidents, surgeries, and electroshock therapy.

Inferior Dislocations

Inferior dislocation of the glenohumeral joint was first described by Middeldorpf and Scharm[842] in 1859. Lynn[754] carefully reviewed 34 cases in 1921, and Roca and Ramos-Vertiz[1102] reviewed 50 cases from the world literature in 1962. Laskin and Sedlin[692] reported a case in an infant. Three bilateral cases have been reported by Murrard,[888] Langfritz,[691] and Peiro and co-workers.[1012] Lucas and Peterson[751] also reported a 16-year-old boy who got his arm caught in the power take-off of a tractor and had an open luxatio erecta injury.

Some authors have categorized luxatio erecta as a type of anterior dislocation, but we believe, because of the anatomic relationships, that this type of dislocation belongs in a separate category (ie,

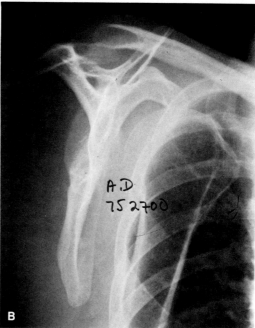

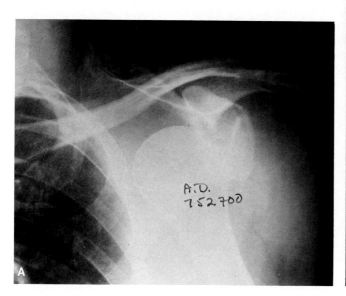

Fig. 13-23. Subcoracoid dislocation. **(A)** Anteroposterior view reveals that the head is medially displaced away from the glenoid fossa. On this view it is impossible to tell whether the head is anteriorly or posteriorly dislocated. **(B)** On the true scapular lateral view the humeral head is completely anterior to the glenoid fossa. *(Matsen, F. A., III; Thomas, S. C.; and Rockwood, C. A., Jr.: Anterior Glenohumeral Instability. In Rockwood, C. A., and Matsen, F. A., III (eds.): The Shoulder, Fig. 14-15. Philadelphia, W. B. Saunders, 1990.)*

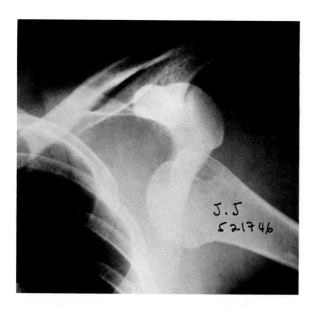

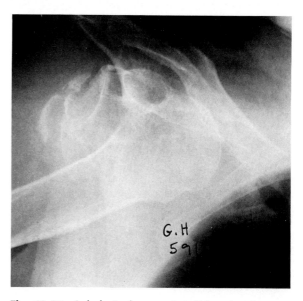

Fig. 13-24. Subglenoid dislocation. Note that the humeral head is completely inferior to the glenoid fossa.

Fig. 13-25. Subclavicular anterior dislocation in a 74-year-old man. Note that the majority of the head is medial to the coracoid and beneath the mid-clavicle. There is an associated fracture of the greater tuberosity secondary to the medial displacement of the head of the humerus.

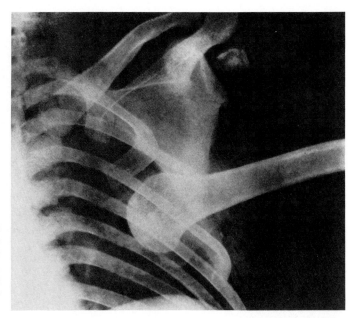

Fig. 13-26. An intrathoracic anterior dislocation of the left shoulder. Note the wide interspace laterally between the third and fourth ribs and the avulsion fracture of the greater tuberosity, which remained in the vicinity of the glenoid fossa. *(West, E. F.: Intrathoracic Dislocation of the Humerus. J. Bone Joint Surg., 31B:61, 1949).*

the humerus is turned upside down, with the entire humeral head below the glenoid fossa). It differs from the anterior and posterior subglenoid dislocations of the glenohumeral joint in that with the luxatio erecta dislocation, the superior aspect of the articular surface of the humeral head is directed inferiorly and is not in contact with the inferior glenoid rim.

Severe soft tissue injury or fractures about the proximal humerus occur with this dislocation (Fig. 13-28). At the time of surgery or autopsy, various authors have found avulsion of the supraspinatus,

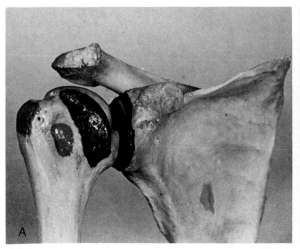
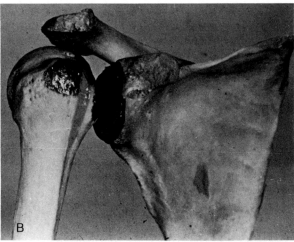

Fig. 13-27. The subacromial posterior dislocation can appear deceptively normal on x-ray films. **(A)** Normal position of the humeral head in the glenoid fossa. **(B)** In the subacromial type of posterior shoulder dislocation, the arm is in full internal rotation and the articular surface of the head is completely posterior, leaving only the lesser tuberosity in the glenoid fossa. This positioning explains why abduction—and particularly external rotation—is blocked in posterior dislocations of the shoulder.

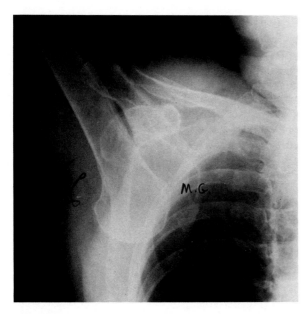

Fig. 13-28. Anteroposterior x-ray film of the inferior dislocation reveals that the entire humeral head and surgical neck of the humerus are inferior to the glenoid fossa.

pectoralis major, or teres minor muscles and fractures of the greater tuberosity.[668,692,754,842,888,1102]

Superior Dislocations

Speed[1248] reported that Langier, in 1834, was the first to record a case of superior dislocation of the glenohumeral joint, and Stimson[1261,1262] reviewed 14 cases that had been reported in the literature prior to 1912. In current literature little is mentioned about this type of dislocation, but undoubtedly occasional cases occur. The usual cause is an extreme forward and upward force on the adducted arm. With displacement of the humerus upward, fractures may occur in the acromion, acromioclavicular joint, clavicle, coracoid process, or humeral tuberosities (Fig. 13-29). Extreme soft tissue damage occurs to the capsule rotator cuff, biceps tendon, and surrounding muscles. Clinically, the head rides above the level of the acromion. The arm is short and adducted to the side. Shoulder movement is restricted and quite painful. Neurovascular complications are usually present. Treatment consists of closed reduction and restoration of the damaged tissues.

INCIDENCE AND MECHANISMS OF INJURY OF SHOULDER INSTABILITY

INCIDENCE

The shoulder is the most commonly dislocated major joint in the body, accounting for 45% of 8056 dislocations at the Central Outpatient Department of the Injured of Budapest.[634] Cave[199] reported a series of 1600 shoulder injuries, of which 394 were dislocations; of these, 84% were anterior glenohumeral dislocations, 12% were acromioclavicular, 2.5% were sternoclavicular, and only 6 of the 394, or 1.5%, were posterior dislocations.

The incidence of posterior dislocations is estimated at 2% but is difficult to ascertain because of

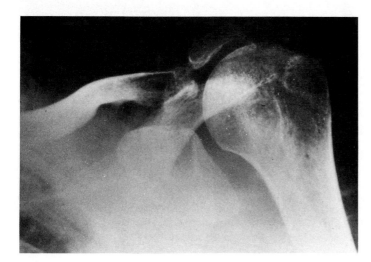

Fig. 13-29. Superior dislocation of the left shoulder. Note that the head of the humerus is displaced superiorly from the glenoid fossa and that the fracture of the acromion process has also been displaced upward.

the frequency with which this diagnosis is missed. Thomas[1289] reported seeing only 4 cases of posterior shoulder dislocation in 6000 x-ray examinations. The literature reflects that the diagnosis of posterior dislocation of the shoulder is missed in over 60% of cases.[348,508,1009,1344] A 1982 article by Rowe and Zarins[1134] indicates that the diagnosis was missed in 79% of cases! McLaughlin[820] stated that posterior shoulder dislocations are sufficiently uncommon that their occurrence creates a "diagnostic trap."

The largest reported and complete series of posterior dislocations of the shoulder (37 cases) was recorded by Malgaigne[779] in 1855, 40 years before the discovery of x-rays. He and his colleagues made the diagnosis by performing a *proper physical examination.* Cooper[246] stated that the physical findings are so classic that he called it "an accident which cannot be mistaken."

MECHANISMS

Atraumatic Instability

In patients with constitutionally lax shoulders, instability can develop with no or minimal injury.[422,1050,1135] If the shoulder muscles become deconditioned, the dynamic stability may be lost, so the joint is launched on a self-perpetuating cycle of more instability → less use → more shoulder dysfunction → more instability. This situation is reminiscent of the interrelationship of patellar instability and quadriceps weakness.

Traumatic Instability

The normal shoulder can become unstable as a result of trauma. Although the shoulder can be dislocated by *direct* trauma such as a blow directed at the proximal humerus, *indirect* force is the most common cause of shoulder sprain, subluxation, or dislocation. The combination of abduction, extension, and external rotation forces applied to the arm may result in an anterior dislocation. Axial loading of the adducted, internally rotated arm may produce a posterior dislocation.[857]

Dislocations may result from violent muscle contraction, by electrical shock or convulsive seizures.[13,188,384,491,734,809,813,960,1050,1206] Although the resulting dislocation may be anterior, it is usually posterior. The combined strength of the internal rotators (latissimus dorsi, pectoralis major, and subscapularis muscles) simply overwhelms the external rotators (infraspinatus and teres minor muscles) (Fig. 13-30).

Other mechanisms for traumatic posterior dislocation of the shoulder include a direct force applied to the anterior shoulder (Fig. 13-31) or an indirect posterior force applied through the arm up to the shoulder (Fig. 13-32).

Inferior dislocation may be produced by a hyperabduction force that causes impingement of the neck of the humerus against the acromion process, which levers the head out inferiorly. The humerus is then locked with the head below the glenoid fossa and the humeral shaft pointing overhead. The force

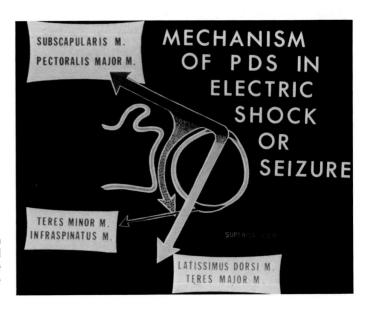

Fig. 13-30. Mechanism of posterior dislocation of the shoulder that is caused by an accidental electrical shock or a convulsive seizure. The strong internal rotators simply overpower the weak external rotators.

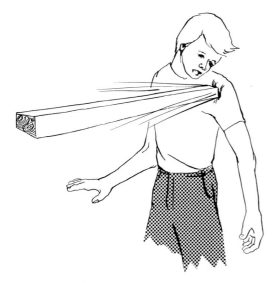

Fig. 13-31. Mechanism of injury for posterior dislocation of the shoulder. A direct force to the anterior shoulder pushes the humeral head out posteriorly.

may be so great as to force the head out through the soft tissues and the skin. As noted earlier, Lucas and Peterson[751] reported a 16-year-old boy who caught his arm in the power take-off of a tractor and suffered an open luxatio erecta injury.

CLINICAL PRESENTATION

DISLOCATIONS

History

Glenohumeral instability presents in many ways, ranging from a vague sense of shoulder dysfunction to an obvious fixed dislocation.[1050,1134,1135] The his-

tory should attempt to define the mechanism of injury, including the position of the arm, the amount of applied force, and the point of force application. Injury with the arm in extension, abduction, and external rotation favors anterior dislocation. Electroshock, seizures, or a fall on the flexed and adducted arm is more consistent with posterior dislocation. It is important to determine the amount of trauma that initiated the instability as well as the force required to produce subsequent episodes. A violent injury from a fall while skiing is associated with a quite different pathologic process and requires different management than a shoulder that becomes unstable without any particular precipitating episode (ie, swinging a badminton racket or throwing a ball). When there is a prior history of instability we inquire how long the shoulder was "out," whether radiographs were taken, and what was done to reduce the shoulder. Previous radiographs and medical records are frequently most helpful in supporting the diagnosis. The history should also solicit evidence of neurologic or rotator cuff problems after previous episodes of shoulder instability. Finally, the previous treatment and its effectiveness needs to be investigated, including rehabilitation and surgery.

Physical Examination

ANTERIOR DISLOCATION

The physical examination of the anteriorly dislocated shoulder should be diagnostic. The acutely dislocated shoulder is very painful. Muscles are in spasm in an attempt to stabilize the joint. The humeral head may be palpable anteriorly. The posterior shoulder shows a hollow beneath the acromion. The arm is held in slight abduction and external rotation. Anterior dislocation usually pro-

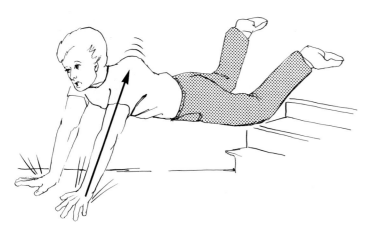

Fig. 13-32. Mechanism of injury of posterior dislocation of the shoulder. An indirect force is applied up through the upper extremity to the shoulder. This is particularly true when the upper extremity is in flexion, adduction, and internal rotation.

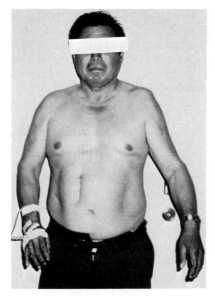
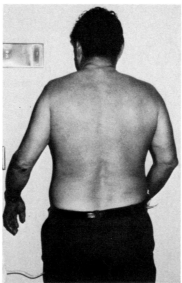
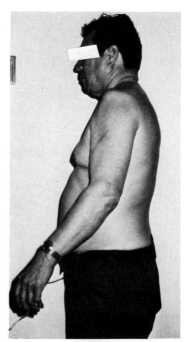

Fig. 13-33. Acute anterior dislocation of the left shoulder. In the frontal (**top left**) and posterior (**top center**) views note that the left arm is held in abduction and slight external rotation. In the frontal view there is some squaring off of the corner of the left shoulder. In the lateral view (**top right**) note the marked prominence of the acromion process. Following reduction (**bottom**) the arm is in normal position. Both shoulders are now rounded.

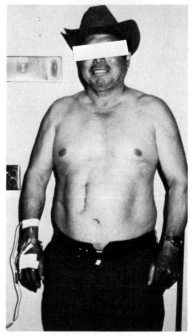

duces a shoulder incapable of complete internal rotation and abduction (Fig. 13-33). Because of the frequent association of nerve injury, particularly the axillary nerve, and, to a lesser extent, vascular injuries,[125] an essential part of the physical examination of the anteriorly dislocated shoulder is the assessment of the neurovascular status of the upper extremity and the charting of the findings prior to reduction.

POSTERIOR DISLOCATION

Recognition of a posterior dislocation may be impaired by the lack of a striking deformity of the shoulder and by the fact that the shoulder is held in the traditional sling position of adduction and internal rotation (Fig. 13-34). However, a directed physical examination will reveal the diagnosis. The classic features of a posterior dislocation include:

1. Limited external rotation of the shoulder (often to less than 0°)

2. Limited elevation of the arm (often to less than 90°)
3. Posterior prominence and rounding of the shoulder compared with normal
4. Flattening of the anterior aspect of the shoulder
5. Prominence of the coracoid process on the dislocated side (Fig. 13-35).

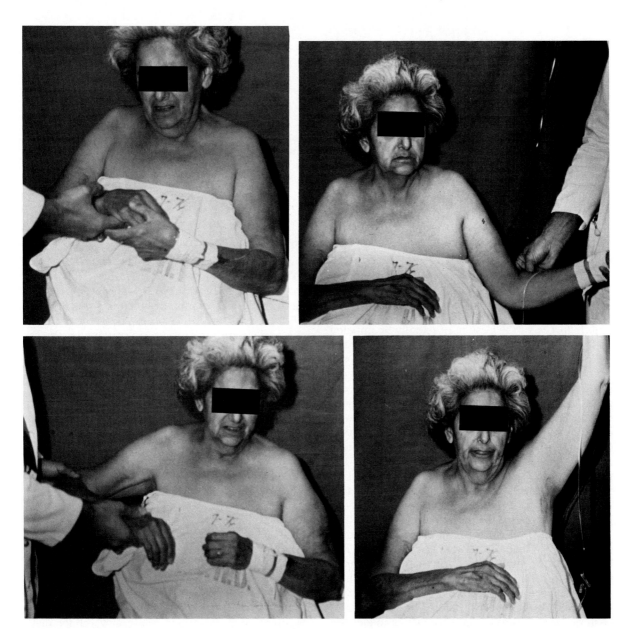

Fig. 13-34. This patient has an acute posterior dislocation of the right shoulder with loss of external rotation and abduction. (**Top left**) Any type of maneuver to externally rotate the right shoulder produces severe pain. (**Top right**) In the normal shoulder, external rotation is free and easy and without pain. (**Bottom left**) Abduction of the dislocated shoulder again produces significant pain. (**Bottom right**) Note presence of full abduction of the normal left shoulder.

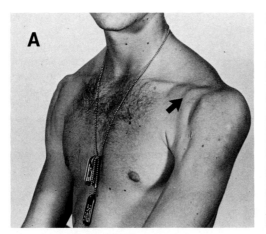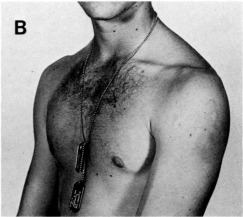

Fig. 13-35. Prominence of the coracoid process in posterior dislocations. (**A**) In this patient with a voluntary posterior dislocation of the left shoulder, note the anterior prominence of the coracoid process and the conjoined tendon (**arrow**). (**B**) With the shoulder in the normal position, the coracoid process is not visible.

Asymmetry of the shoulder contours can often be best visualized by viewing the shoulders from above while standing behind the patient (Fig. 13-36).

The motion is limited because the head of the humerus is fixed on the posterior glenoid rim by muscle forces, or the head may actually be impaled on the glenoid rim. With time, the posterior rim of the glenoid may further impact the fracture of the humeral head and produce a deep hatchet-like defect or V-shaped compression fracture, which engages the head even more securely. Patients with old, unreduced posterior dislocations of the shoulder may have 30° to 40° of glenohumeral abduction and some humeral rotation owing to enlargement of the groove. With long-standing disuse of the muscles about the shoulder, atrophy will be present, which accentuates the flattening of the anterior shoulder, the prominence of the coracoid, and the fullness of the posterior shoulder.

Proper physical examination is essential. Rowe and Zarins[1134] reported 23 cases of unreduced dislocation of the shoulder, of which 14 were posterior. Hill and McLaughlin[533] reported that in their series the average time from injury to diagnosis was 8 months. In the interval before the diagnosis of posterior dislocation of the shoulder is made, the injury may be misdiagnosed as "frozen shoulder,"[533,817,818] for which vigorous therapy may be mistakenly instituted in an attempt to restore the range of motion.

INFERIOR DISLOCATION

In a subglenoid dislocation the arm is abducted about 30°, internally rotated, and shortened. Nobel[930] reported a case of this rare type of dislocation in which the acromion–olecranon distance was shortened by 1.5 inches.

A patient with luxatio erecta usually has the humerus locked in a position somewhere between 110° and 160° of abduction (Fig. 13-37). The head of the humerus may be palpated on the lateral chest wall. Pain is quite severe. The condition is more common among the elderly. The mechanism of injury is a hyperabduction force, impinging the neck of the humerus on the acromion, which levers the head inferiorly out of the glenoid fossa (Fig. 13-38).

SUPERIOR DISLOCATION

Superior dislocations of the shoulder are very rare. The usual mechanism is a severe upward force on the adducted arm up against the acromion (ie, a fall from a great height whereby the weight of the body forces the head superiorly).

BILATERAL DISLOCATIONS

Mynter[889] first described bilateral shoulder dislocations in 1902; according to Honner,[541] only 20 cases were reported prior to 1969. Bilateral dislocations have been reported by McFie,[809] Yadav,[1412] Onabowale and Jaja,[960] Segal and colleagues,[1206]

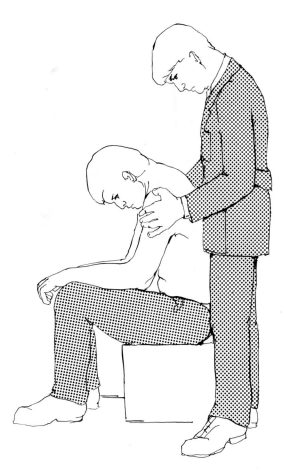

Fig. 13-36. The anterior and posterior aspects of the shoulders can best be visualized by having the patient sit on a low stool, with the examiner standing behind him. Then the injured shoulder can easily be compared with the uninjured one.

Goodfellow and Boldero,[448] and Carew-McColl.[188] Most of these cases were the result of convulsions or violent trauma. Peiro and co-workers[1012] reported bilateral erect dislocation of the shoulders in a man caught in a cement mixer. Bilateral dislocation of the shoulder secondary to accidental electrical shock has been reported by Carew-McColl[188] and Fipp[384] and Rockwood[1104] (Fig. 13-39). Nicola and co-workers[918] reported cases of bilateral posterior fracture–dislocation following a convulsive seizure (Fig. 13-40). Ahlgren and associates[13] reported three cases of bilateral posterior fracture–dislocation associated with a convulsion. Lindholm and Elmstedt[734] reported a case of bilateral posterior fracture–dislocation following an epileptic seizure, which was treated by open reduction and internal fixation with screws. Parrish and Skiendzielewski[995]

reported a patient with bilateral posterior fracture–dislocations after status epilepticus. The diagnosis was missed for more than 12 hours. Pagden and associates[982] reported two cases of posterior shoulder dislocation following seizures related to regional anesthesia.

RECURRENT INSTABILITY

History

The challenge of diagnosis is greater in the shoulder with recurrent instability. Particularly in the shoulder with recurrent subluxation, the condition is much less obvious to the patient and the physician. Yet, the same diagnostic steps—the history, the physical examination, and the roentgenograms—usually will point to the diagnosis. With traumatic instability, the patient usually can describe the initial injury in great detail (ie, a sharp stabbing pain, a closed reduction done by a physician usually with sedation, and a residual aching shoulder for several weeks). In most cases of recurrent traumatic anterior instability, the injury results from a forced abduction and external rotation of the shoulder. A classic example is the defender who tries to make an arm tackle on the ball carrier and ends up having his arm pulled back into extension, abduction, and external rotation. Similarly, a skier may fall on an abducted arm or a kayaker may have the arm pulled back over the head while bracing in white water. This movement is associated with a sharp, stabbing pain in the shoulder. Spontaneous reduction may occur immediately, or the patient may require a manipulative reduction. Records and roentgenograms from the initial episode are most valuable. Subsequently, the shoulder may demonstrate recurrent subluxation,[1113] "dead arm syndrome,"[1134] or frank dislocation when it resumes the extended, abducted, and externally rotated position. Recurrent traumatic posterior instability may begin with a fall on the outstretched arm or a blow on the front of the shoulder.

Recurrent instability may also have an atraumatic onset. Without a major injury, the humeral head starts to slide out of its normal position. This instability may be anterior, posterior, inferior, or multidirectional. Patients with atraumatic instability may describe aggravation of their problem by trauma. Careful questioning usually reveals that the original injury was minor in nature and occurred with such things as taking an overhead swing at a tennis ball, lifting up a garage door, a minor fall on the shoulder, or swinging a baseball bat. Several

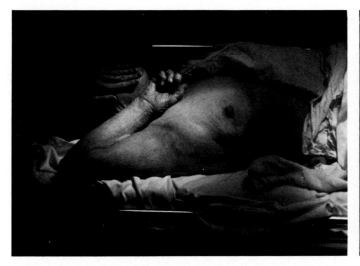
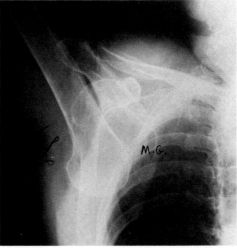

Fig. 13-37. Inferior dislocation (luxatio erecta) of the right shoulder in a 75-year-old woman. (**Left**) Note that the arm is directed upward in relationship to the trunk. The hand of the flexed elbow is lying on the anterior chest. (**Right**) Anteroposterior x-ray film of the inferior dislocation reveals that the entire humeral head and surgical neck of the humerus are inferior to the glenoid fossa.

important clues that suggest the diagnosis of atraumatic subluxation or dislocation can be obtained from the patient: the original injury was a minor one and (usually) was not associated with significant pain; the subluxation or dislocation reduced spontaneously; the patient returned to activities without much pain or problem; and the patient has generalized ligament laxity (ie, the opposite shoulder, the metacarpophalangeal joints, elbows, knees, and so forth). The symptoms include feelings of recur-

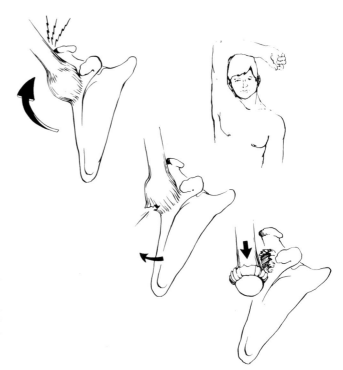

Fig. 13-38. Mechanism of luxatio erecta. With hyperabduction of the humerus, the shaft abuts the acromion process, which stresses and then tears the capsule inferiorly and evers the head out inferiorly. The head and neck may be buttonholed through a rent in the inferior capsule, or the entire capsule may be separated. The rotator cuff muscles are always detached, and there may be an associated fracture of the greater tuberosity.

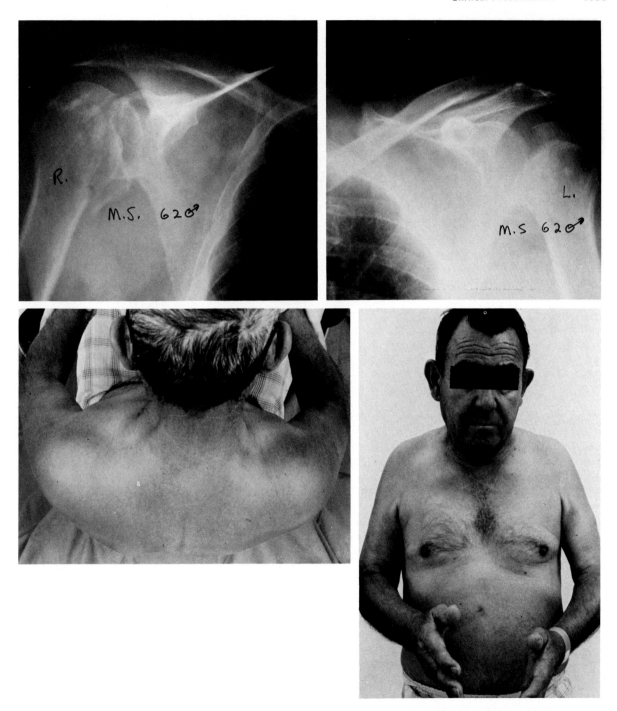

Fig. 13-39. This patient had an accidental electrical shock and has bilateral fracture and posterior dislocation of the shoulders. (**Top left**) Anteroposterior x-ray film of the right shoulder. (**Top right**) Anteroposterior x-ray film of the left shoulder. The patient had severe limitation of external rotation and abduction and the final diagnosis was confirmed by scapular lateral x-ray films. (**Bottom left**) Note the fullness of the posterior aspect of both shoulders when viewed from above the patient. (**Bottom right**) The patient has no abduction and has −30° of external rotation. He is unable to supinate the hand and forearm because of the marked internal rotation of both humeri secondary to the injury.

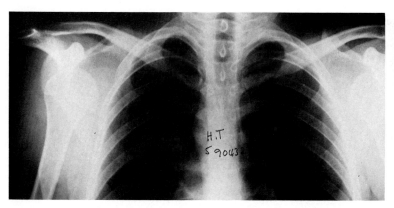
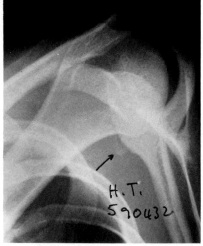

Fig. 13-40. (**Left**) Anteroposterior x-ray film of both shoulders reveals bilateral acute traumatic anterior dislocation of the shoulders as a result of seizures in a 22-year-old patient. Both shoulders were reduced without difficulty. (**Right**) A modified scapular lateral view reveals fracture of the anteroinferior rim of the glenoid.

rent instability, apprehension, or dislocation. A good history of the onset, positions of instability, and past treatment is very helpful in diagnosis.

We routinely ask whether the patient can dislocate the shoulder voluntarily. If the answer is "yes," the surgeon must determine whether voluntary instability is the preponderant problem (in which case surgical stabilization is unlikely to succeed) or just a minor facet of a shoulder that usually goes out involuntarily. The patient with voluntary instability usually has no history of injury, but can remember since childhood the ability to slip one or both shoulders out of place with minimal discomfort. In the late teens or twenties, the patient may note that the shoulder begins to slip out of place when a stress is placed on it (Fig. 13-41).

Physical Examination

Like the history, physical examination of the shoulder with suspected recurrent instability is challenging. We usually start by seeking evidence of generalized ligamentous laxity, such as contralateral shoulder instability, hyperextension of the knees, elbows, and metacarpophalangeal joints, thumb flexibility, and flat feet. The strength of the anterior, middle, and posterior deltoid and the external rotators is next checked; a screening neurologic examination is also performed. Weakness of external rotation suggests the possibility of a rotator cuff tear or a suprascapular nerve injury. Perhaps the most important part of the examination is the performance of stress tests to challenge the stability of the joint in various directions, observing

both the resulting translation and the degree of apprehension demonstrated by the patient with each test. It is particularly helpful if a specific test reproduces the sensation that is problematic for the patient ("That's what that happens!"). In the performance of these tests, it is important that the patient be as relaxed as possible so the examiner is testing static (capsular) and not dynamic (muscular) stability. In interpreting the significance of the degree of translation on a given test, it is helpful to use the contralateral shoulder and previous examinations of other shoulders as a standard of what is normal.

Drawer Test. For the drawer test (Fig. 13-42), the patient is seated with the forearm resting on the lap and the shoulder relaxed. The examiner stands behind the patient. One of the examiner's hands stabilizes the shoulder girdle (scapula and clavicle) while the other grasps the proximal humerus. The humeral head is pressed gently toward the scapula to center it in the glenoid, assuring a neutral starting position. Starting from this neutral position, the humerus is first pushed forward to determine the amount of anterior displacement relative to the scapula. The normal shoulder reaches a firm endpoint with only slight anterior translation, no clunking, and no pain or apprehension. A clunk or snap on anterior subluxation or reduction may suggest a labral tear or Bankart lesion. The humerus is returned to the neutral position and then pulled backward to determine the amount of posterior translation relative to the scapula. The normal

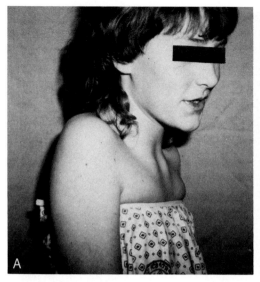
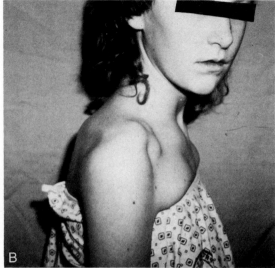

Fig. 13-41. Voluntary instability. This patient had no significant history of injury but could voluntarily dislocate her shoulder with minimal discomfort. Patient with the right shoulder reduced (**A**) can posteriorly dislocate voluntarily (**B**). *(Matsen, F. A., III; Thomas, S. C.; and Rockwood, C. A., Jr.: Anterior Glenohumeral Instability. In Rockwood, C. A., and Matsen, F. A., III (eds.): The Shoulder, Fig. 14-20. Philadelphia, W. B. Saunders, 1990.)*

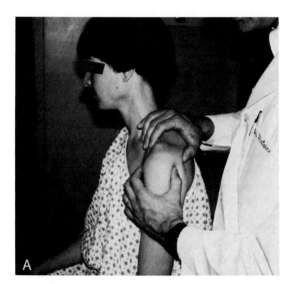
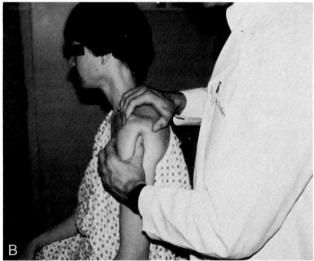

Fig. 13-42. Drawer test. (**A**) With the patient seated and the forearm resting in the lap, the examiner stands behind the patient and stabilizes the shoulder girdle with one hand while grasping the proximal humerus with the other, pressing the humeral head gently toward the scapula to center it in the glenoid. (**B**) The head is then pushed forward to determine the amount of anterior displacement relative to the scapula. It can then be returned to the neutral position and a posterior force applied to determine the amount of posterior translation relative to the scapula. *(Matsen, F. A., III; Thomas, S. C.; and Rockwood, C. A., Jr.: Anterior Glenohumeral Instability. In Rockwood, C. A., and Matsen, F. A., III (eds.): The Shoulder, Fig. 14-21. Philadelphia, W. B. Saunders, 1990.)*

shoulder allows posterior translation up to about one half of the humeral head diameter. Increased anterior and posterior translation suggests multidirectional instability. This test has the advantage of eliciting evidence of capsular laxity without threatening the patient with dislocation—a threat that may lead to a false-negative test from protective muscle contraction.

Sulcus Test.   For the sulcus test (Figs. 13-43 and 13-44), the patient sits with the arm relaxed at the side. The examiner pulls the arm downward. Inferior instability is demonstrated if a sulcus or hollow appears inferior to the acromion. This test is often positive in multidirectional instability.

Fulcrum Test.   For the fulcrum test (Fig. 13-45), the patient lies supine at the edge of the exami-

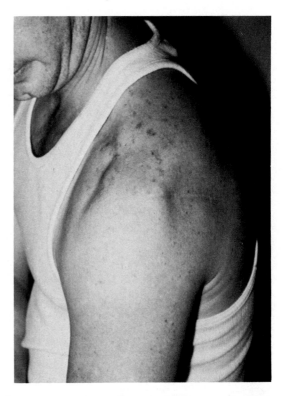

Fig. 13-44. Positive sulcus sign. This patient had a posterior repair for glenohumeral instability. However, he continues to have inferior instability and demonstrates the sulcus (or hollow) just inferior to the anterior acromion during this sulcus test. A capsular shift is indicated. *(Matsen, F. A., III; Thomas, S. C.; and Rockwood, C. A., Jr.: Anterior Glenohumeral Instability. In Rockwood, C. A., and Matsen, F. A., III (eds.): The Shoulder, Fig. 14-23. Philadelphia, W. B. Saunders, 1990.)*

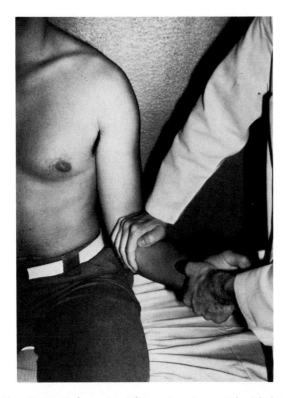

Fig. 13-43. Sulcus test. The patient is seated with his arm relaxed and at the side. The examiner pulls downward on the arm. Inferior instability is demonstrated if a sulcus (or hollow) appears inferior to the acromion. This patient has a negative sulcus test. *(Matsen, F. A., III; Thomas, S. C.; and Rockwood, C. A., Jr.: Anterior Glenohumeral Instability. In Rockwood, C. A., and Matsen, F. A., III (eds.): The Shoulder, Fig. 14-22. Philadelphia, W. B. Saunders, 1990.)*

nation table with the arm abducted to 90°. The examiner places one hand on the table under the glenohumeral joint to act as a fulcrum. The arm is gently and progressively extended and externally rotated over this fulcrum. Maintaining gentle passive external rotation for a minute fatigues the subscapularis, challenging the capsular contribution to the anterior stability of the shoulder. The patient with anterior instability will usually become apprehensive as this maneuver is carried out (watch the eyebrows for a clue that the shoulder is getting ready to dislocate).

Crank or Apprehension Test.   For the crank (or apprehension) test (Fig. 13-46), the patient sits with the back toward the examiner. The arm is held in 90° of abduction and external rotation. The examiner pulls back on the patient's wrist with one

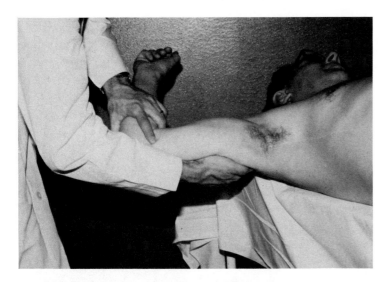

Fig. 13-45. Fulcrum test. With the patient supine and the shoulder at the edge of the examination table, the arm is abducted to 90°. The examiner's right hand is used as a fulcrum while the arm is gently and progressively extended and externally rotated. In the presence of anterior instability, the patient becomes apprehensive or the shoulder translates with this maneuver. *(Matsen, F. A., III; Thomas, S. C.; and Rockwood, C. A., Jr.: Anterior Glenohumeral Instability. In Rockwood, C. A., and Matsen, F. A., III (eds.): The Shoulder, Fig. 14-24. Philadelphia, W. B. Saunders, 1990.)*

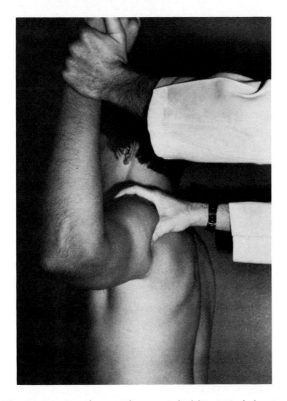

Fig. 13-46. Crank test. The arm is held in 90° abduction and external rotation. The examiner's left hand pulls back on the patient's wrist while his right hand stabilizes the back of the shoulder. The patient with anterior instability becomes apprehensive with this maneuver. *(Matsen, F. A., III; Thomas, S. C.; and Rockwood, C. A., Jr.: Anterior Glenohumeral Instability. In Rockwood, C. A., and Matsen, F. A., III (eds.): The Shoulder, Fig. 14-25. Philadelphia, W. B. Saunders, 1990.)*

hand while stabilizing the back of the shoulder with the other. The patient with anterior instability usually will become apprehensive with this maneuver. Again, we refer to apprehension as a feeling that the shoulder is getting ready to dislocate, rather than just pain (which could come from other conditions such as impingement) (Fig. 13-47).

Jerk Test (Posterior Instability).   For the jerk test (Figs. 13-48 and 13-49), the patient sits with the arm internally rotated and flexed forward to 90°. The examiner grasps the elbow and axially loads the humerus in a proximal direction. While axial loading of the humerus is maintained, the arm is moved horizontally across the body. In many patients with recurrent posterior instability this test will produce a sudden jerk when the humeral head slides off the back of the glenoid. When the arm is returned to the original position of 90° abduction, a second jerk may be observed—that of the humeral head returning to the glenoid.

Push–Pull Test (Posterior Instability).   For the push–pull test (Fig. 13-50), the patient lies supine with the shoulder off the edge of the table. The arm is in 90° of abduction and 30° of flexion. Standing next to the patient's hip, the examiner pulls up on the wrist with one hand while pushing down on the proximal humerus with the other. The shoulders of normal, relaxed patients often will allow 50% posterior translation on this test. Greater degrees of translation, apprehension, or reproduction of the patient's symptoms suggest pathologic pos-

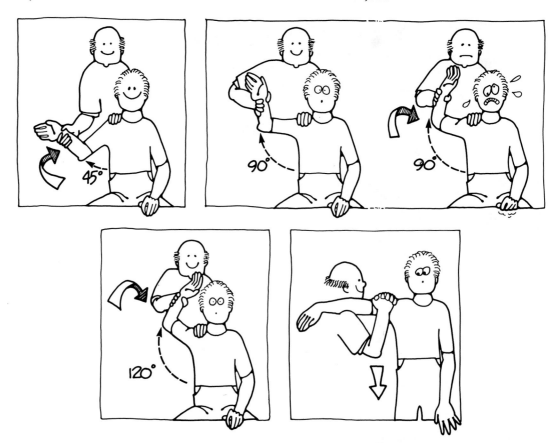

Fig. 13-47. Evaluation of the injured shoulder in varying degrees of abduction. (**Top left**) External rotation force is applied to the arm in 45° of abduction. (**Top right**) The shoulder is abducted 90°. Next, the external rotation force with some extension is applied, which produces pain, usually posteriorly, and marked apprehension in the patient. In my experience it is this position that most commonly produces pain and severe apprehension. (**Bottom left**) The external rotation and extension force is applied to the arm in 120° of abduction. This does cause apprehension in some patients but not as marked with the arm in 90° of abduction. (**Bottom right**) The Feagin test. With the patient's elbow resting on the top of the physician's shoulder, a downward force on the proximal humerus in some instances produces apprehension.

terior instability. This test should be performed on both sides to compare the degrees of translation and the patient's response.

If apprehension on these tests cannot be easily differentiated from painful subacromial impingement, a subacromial injection of lidocaine can help eliminate the symptoms of impingement.[898]

Instability in more than one direction (multidirectional instability) is not uncommon. Thus, all directions of glenohumeral instability are routinely examined, even in the patient with documented recurrent anterior shoulder dislocations.

RADIOGRAPHIC AND LABORATORY EVALUATION

PLAIN RADIOGRAPHY

With a dislocated shoulder, the physician needs to know the following: (1) the direction of the dislocation, (2) the existence of associated fractures (displaced or not), and (3) possible barriers to relocation. If a dislocation is confirmed, reduction and postreduction films can be accomplished on the x-

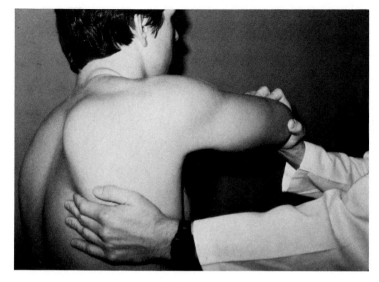

Fig. 13-48. Jerk test. The patient's arm is abducted to 90° and internally rotated. The examiner axially loads the humerus while the arm is moved horizontally across the body. The left hand stabilizes the scapula. Patients with recurrent posterior instability may demonstrate a sudden jerk as the humeral head slides off the back of the glenoid or when it is reduced by moving the arm back to the starting position. *(Matsen, F. A., III; Thomas, S. C.; and Rockwood, C. A., Jr.: Anterior Glenohumeral Instability. In Rockwood, C. A., and Matsen, F. A., III (eds.): The Shoulder, Fig. 14-27. Philadelphia, W. B. Saunders, 1990.)*

ray table. (The patient certainly appreciates not being moved for each of these steps.)

Radiographs in the Plane of the Body

Radiographs of the shoulder are most conveniently identified by the plane of the projection. For many years the standard shoulder films have been taken with the film in the plane of the body.

ANTEROPOSTERIOR VIEW

The anteroposterior view is obtained with the patient's back flat on the cassette and the x-ray beam

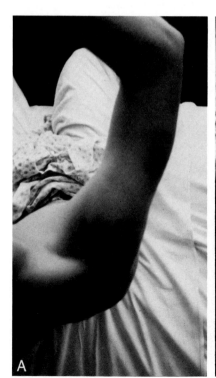
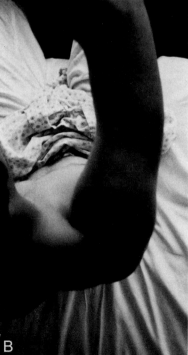

Fig. 13-49. Positive jerk test. **(A)** Normal appearance of the shoulder before the patient performs a jerk test. **(B)** With axial loading and movement of the arm horizontally across the body, the humeral head slides off the back of the glenoid, as demonstrated by the prominence in the posterior aspect of the patient's shoulder. This maneuver resulted in a sudden jerk and some discomfort. *(Matsen, F. A., III; Thomas, S. C.; and Rockwood, C. A., Jr.: Anterior Glenohumeral Instability. In Rockwood, C. A., and Matsen, F. A., III (eds.): The Shoulder, Fig. 14-27. Philadelphia, W. B. Saunders, 1990.)*

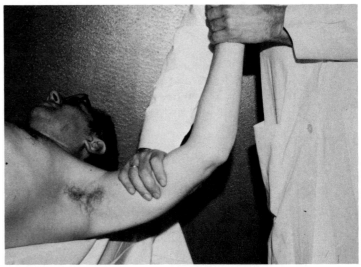

Fig. 13-50. Push–pull test. The patient lies supine and relaxed with the shoulder at the edge of the examination table. The examiner pulls up on the wrist with one hand while pushing down on the proximal humerus with the other. Approximately 50% posterior translation of the humerus on the glenoid is normal in relaxed patients. *(Matsen, F. A., III; Thomas, S. C.; and Rockwood, C. A., Jr.: Anterior Glenohumeral Instability. In Rockwood, C. A., and Matsen, F. A., III (eds.): The Shoulder, Fig. 14-28. Philadelphia, W. B. Saunders, 1990.)*

at right angles to this plane and centered on the shoulder. This may be called the "AP in the plane of the body." However, this is not a true anteroposterior view of the glenohumeral joint, because the scapula lies on the posterolateral chest wall at an angle of 30° to 45° from the frontal plane. Hence, the glenoid is open or faces anteriorly 45°, and the view projects a significant overlap of the humeral head on three fourths to seven eighths of the glenoid (Fig. 13-51).

Although the anteroposterior view in the plane

of the body may provide sufficient information to diagnose the various types of anterior dislocations and the subspinous and subglenoid types of posterior dislocations, it is insufficient to diagnose the most common type of posterior dislocation—the subacromial. Frequently, this dislocation is missed on this view because the displacement is essentially at right angles to the plane of the film. Even posterior dislocations associated with a fracture can appear deceptively normal.

We do not recommend the use of radiographic

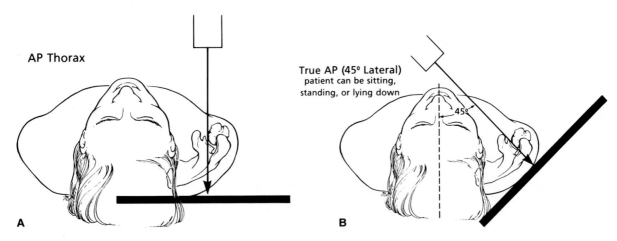

Fig. 13-51. **(A)** Anteroposterior x-ray view of the shoulder taken in the plane of the thorax. Note that the film is actually an oblique view of the glenohumeral joint. **(B)** To obtain a true anteroposterior view of the glenohumeral joint, the beam must be angled 45° or the patient can rotate the body until the scapula is parallel to the x-ray cassette. *(Rockwood, C. A.; Szalay, E. A.; Curtis, R. J.; Young, D. C.; and Kay, S. P.: X-ray Evaluation of Shoulder Problems. In Rockwood, C. A., and Matsen, F. A., III (eds.): The Shoulder, Figs. 5-1, 5-2. Philadelphia, W. B. Saunders, 1990.)*

views in the plane of the body to routinely evaluate the glenohumeral joint. McLaughlin has said that the reliance on anteroposterior radiographs will lead the unwary orthopaedist into a "diagnostic trap."[820] However, a number of radiographic signs that suggest posterior dislocation have been described on the anteroposterior view in the plane of the body. These signs include the following:

1. Absence of the normal elliptical overlap shadow. Normally on the routine anteroposterior view an overlap shadow is created by the head of the humerus superimposed on the glenoid fossa of the scapula. The shadow is a smooth-bordered ellipse. In posterior dislocations, the articular surface of the humeral head is posterior to the glenoid and the elliptical overlap shadow is distorted (Fig. 13-52).

2. Vacant glenoid sign. Normally on the routine anteroposterior view the humeral head fills the majority of the glenoid cavity. However, in posterior dislocations with the head resting behind the glenoid, the glenoid fossa appears to be partially vacant. Arndt and Sears[50] refer to

this as a "positive rim sign" and state that if the space between the anterior rim and the humeral head is greater than 6 mm, it is highly suggestive of a posterior dislocation (Fig. 13-53).

3. The "trough line." Cisternino and colleagues[210] and Demos[302] have reported on the high incidence of a "trough line" on the anteroposterior x-ray film. This is a result of the impaction fracture of the humeral head caused by the posterior rim of the glenoid and is analogous to the Hill-Sachs impaction fracture line seen with anterior dislocation of the shoulder. These authors reported that the trough line on the anteroposterior x-ray films was present in 75% of their 20 cases of posterior dislocation.

4. Loss of profile of the neck of the humerus. In posterior dislocations of the shoulder, the arm is in full internal rotation; thus, a profile of the neck of the humerus is not seen. However, the same is true for the normal shoulder when the radiograph is taken with the arm in internal rotation. If anteroposterior films of an injured shoulder in internal or external rotation do not

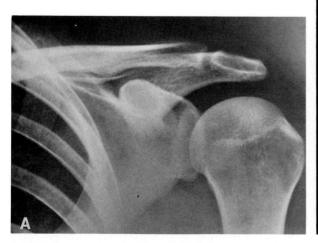
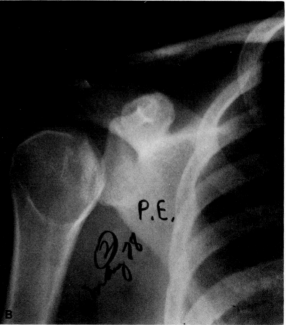

Fig. 13-52. Absence of the normal elliptical shadow in posterior dislocation of the shoulder. (**A**) In the anteroposterior view of a normal left shoulder, note that the humeral head in the glenoid fossa creates an elliptical overlap shadow with the posterior glenoid fossa. The head of the humerus is parallel to the anterior glenoid rim. (**B**) With posterior dislocation of the right shoulder the articular surface does not seem to fit appropriately into the glenoid fossa. The head seems to be laterally and inferiorly displaced from the glenoid.

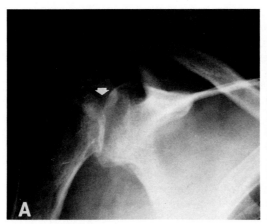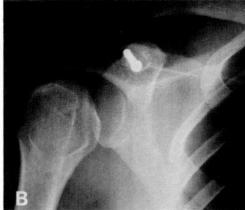

Fig. 13-53. Vacant glenoid sign and "trough line" of posterior dislocation. **(A)** The anterior three fourths of the glenoid is vacant because only the lesser tuberosity is in the glenoid fossa. There is an impaction or indentation fracture of the anterior humeral head caused by the rim of the posterior glenoid **(arrow)**. **(B)** Practically the entire glenoid fossa is vacant. Only a small edge of the lesser tuberosity is visible in the lower posterior fossa.

show the profile of the neck of the humerus on either view, then posterior dislocation of the shoulder is suggested.

5. Void in the inferior or superior glenoid fossa. With posterior dislocation the humeral head is occasionally displaced upward or downward, leaving a void in the inferior or superior third of the glenoid fossa. This is not seen in the normal shoulder.

TRANSTHORACIC LATERAL VIEW

As with the anteroposterior view in the plane of the scapula, we discuss the transthoracic lateral view for the reader's interest but do not recommend it for the analysis of glenohumeral pathology. In this view, the lateral aspect of the involved arm and shoulder is placed against the cassette and the normal arm over the head of the patient. The x-ray beam is directed through the chest.

Dorgan[321] reported that obesity, as well as some technical factors, may prevent accurate identification of the glenohumeral joint in the transthoracic lateral view. He credits Dr. Albert Moloney of Boston with interpreting a "break in the normal scapulohumeral arch" (Moloney's line). Normally in this projection a smooth or rounded dome-type of arch is created by the shaft of the humerus, the head of the humerus, and the lateral or axillary border of the scapula. In posterior dislocations of the shoulder, the head and neck of the humerus are behind and superimposed on the glenoid fossa; hence, the smooth dome shape is obliterated. Con-

sequently, the top of the arch comes to a narrow apex created by the shaft of the humerus, which meets the axillary border of the scapula. In anterior dislocations the opposite is true; that is, the dome of the arch becomes quite wide. This widening occurs (1) because the head is displaced anteriorly, and (2) because the arm is in external rotation and places more of the neck on profile, which widens the arch.

Radiographs in the Plane of the Scapula

Rather than views referred to the plane of the body, we suggest a standard series of radiographs referred to the plane of the scapula for all injured shoulders: an anteroposterior view in the plane of the scapula, a lateral scapular view, and an axillary view.

ANTEROPOSTERIOR VIEW

In 1923 Grashey[459] recognized that to take a true anteroposterior radiograph of the shoulder joint, the direction of the x-ray beam must be perpendicular to the plane of the scapula. This view is most easily accomplished by placing the scapula flat on the cassette (a position the patient can help achieve) and passing the x-ray beam at right angles to this plane, centering it on the coracoid process. We refer to this view as an "AP in the plane of the scapula" (Fig. 13-54). In the normal shoulder the articular surface of the humeral head is separated clearly from the glenoid fossa by a radiographic joint space. This view can be taken with the arm in a sling and

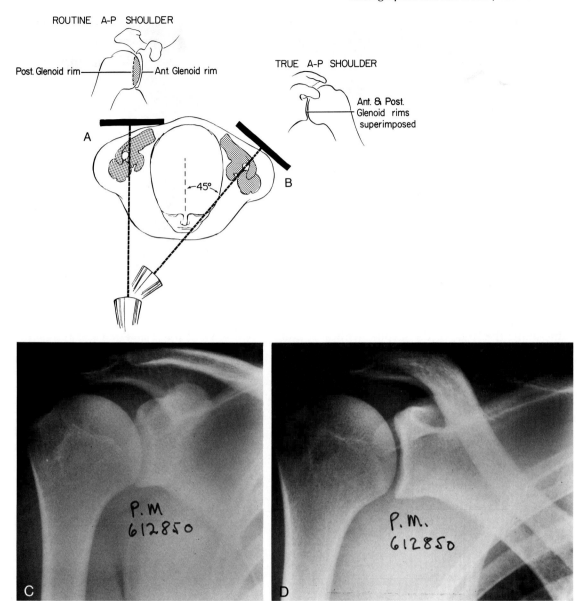

Fig. 13-54. (A, B) Note the great difference between the two angles of the x-ray beam, the placement of the cassettes, and the schematic drawings of the glenohumeral joint. (**C**) An x-ray film of the shoulder in the plane of the thorax. (**D**) An x-ray film of the shoulder taken in the plane of the scapula. *(Rockwood, C. A.; Szalay, E. A.; Curtis, R. J.; Young, D. C.; and Kay, S. P.: X-ray Evaluation of Shoulder Problems. In Rockwood, C. A., and Matsen, F. A., III (eds.): The Shoulder, Fig. 5-4. Philadelphia, W. B. Saunders, 1990.)*

only requires positioning of the entire body rather than the arm (Fig. 13-55).

LATERAL VIEW

The view at right angles to the anteroposterior in the plane of the scapula is the "scapular lateral" view (Fig. 13-56).[817,818,820,901,1104] Like the antero-

posterior view, it can be obtained by positioning the body and not the arm. Here the cassette is placed anterolateral to the deltoid and the scapula is positioned perpendicular to it (Fig. 13-57). Because the posterior aspect of the body of the scapula is easy to palpate, this position can be reliably achieved. The beam is placed parallel to the spine

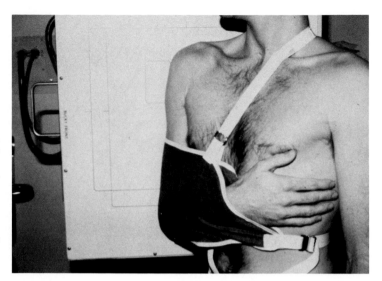

Fig. 13-55. Positioning of the patient in a sling for an anteroposterior x-ray view in the plane of the scapula. The scapula is placed flat on the cassette. The x-ray beam is positioned at right angles to the cassette and centered on the coracoid process. *(Matsen, F. A., III; Thomas, S. C.; and Rockwood, C. A., Jr.: Anterior Glenohumeral Instability. In Rockwood, C. A., and Matsen, F. A., III (eds.): The Shoulder, Fig. 14-31. Philadelphia, W. B. Saunders, 1990.)*

of the scapula and perpendicular to the cassette. To aid the radiological technician, the physician can draw a line along the spine of the scapula with a marking pen. The x-ray cassette is placed anterolateral to the shoulder, which will be perpendicular to the line on the scapula. The x-ray beam is directed down the line on the spine onto the cassette.[1104] In this view, the contour of the scapula projects as the letter Y (Fig. 13-58).[452] The downward stem of the Y is projected by the body of the scapula; the upper forks are projected by the coracoid process anteri-

orly and by the spine and acromion posteriorly. The glenoid is located at the junction of the stem and the two arms of the Y and appears as a dense circle of bone. In obese people the circular density of the glenoid may not be seen, but it is always located at this intersection. In the normal shoulder the humeral head is at the center of the arms of the Y, that is, about the glenoid fossa. In posterior dislocations the head is seen posterior to the glenoid; in anterior dislocations it is anterior to the glenoid.

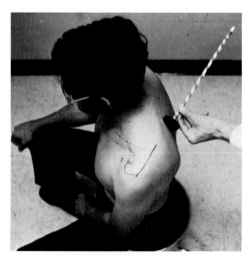
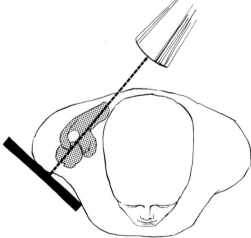

Fig. 13-56. (Left) Demonstration of how a heavy line drawn on the skin over the spine of the scapula with a marking pen helps the technician to visualize the positioning of the patient for a scapular lateral x-ray view. The beam is directed down the spine of the scapula in the line of the pointer. **(Right)** The cassette should be placed on the anterolateral aspect of the shoulder and held perpendicular to the beam of the x-ray.

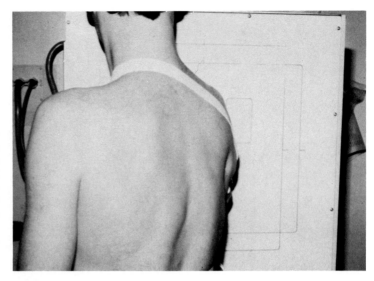

Fig. 13-57. Position of the patient in the sling for a scapular lateral x-ray view. The scapula is positioned perpendicular to the cassette. The beam should be placed parallel to the spine of the scapula and perpendicular to the cassette. (*Matsen, F. A., III; Thomas, S. C.; and Rockwood, C. A., Jr.: Anterior Glenohumeral Instability. In Rockwood, C. A., and Matsen, F. A., III (eds.): The Shoulder, Fig. 14-34. Philadelphia, W. B. Saunders, 1990.*)

Even though the anteroposterior view may suggest a posterior dislocation of the shoulder, the scapulolateral x-ray film will definitely confirm the diagnosis (Fig. 13-59).

AXILLARY VIEW

In the axillary view, first described by Lawrence in 1915,[700,836] the cassette is placed on the superior aspect of the shoulder. The arm is abducted enough to allow the radiographic beam to pass between the chest and the arm in a direction perpendicular to the cassette (Fig. 13-60**A**) from the shoulder. In the presence of shoulder trauma, this view is usually obtained with the patient supine and the beam horizontal, but it may also be obtained with the patient prone or standing. In some situations when the patient cannot abduct the arm more than 30° to 40°, a curved cassette or a rolled cardboard cassette can be placed in the axilla; then the radiographic beam would come from a superior position (Fig. 13-60**B**). An effort should always be made to take the axillary radiograph because it not only is diagnostic of shoulder dislocation but also offers a special premium in that it will often demonstrate the presence and size of head compression fractures, as well as fractures of the glenoid or of the lesser tuberosity of the humerus (Figs. 13-61 through 13-64).

Some modifications of the axillary view have been described. In his text on radiographic positioning, Jordan demonstrated the various techniques for obtaining axillary lateral views.[624]

The trauma axillary lateral view of Tietge and Ciullo can be taken while the patient is in the supine position (Fig. 13-65). Cleaves[216,836] and Teitge and Ciullo[1038] have described variations on this view. Bloom and Obata[126] have modified the axillary technique so the arm does not have to be abducted. They call this the Velpeau axillary lateral view. While wearing a sling or Velpeau dressing, the patient leans backward 30° over the cassette on the table (Fig. 13-66). The x-ray tube is placed above the shoulder and the beam projected vertically down through the shoulder onto the cassette.

SUMMARY

In summary, in the evaluation of a possible dislocation or fracture–dislocation of the shoulder, we recommend the three orthogonal projections of the shoulder (anteroposterior and lateral in the plane of the scapula and axillary view), which provide a sensitive assessment of shoulder dislocation. The use of fewer views or other less interpretable projections may obscure significant pathologic processes. If the three views cannot be taken, or if there is a question regarding the diagnosis, a CT scan will be of great assistance.

RADIOGRAPHIC EVALUATION OF RECURRENT GLENOHUMERAL INSTABILITY

The radiographic evaluation of recurrent glenohumeral instability is more subtle. The approaches may be grouped into stress views and views seeking fixed abnormalities. *Stress views* may document the amount of glenohumeral translation with loading in various directions. Inferior translation may be documented by taking an anteroposterior view in

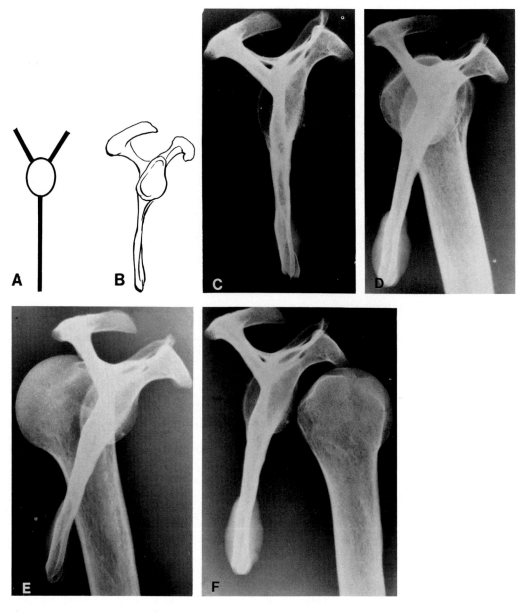

Fig. 13-58. Interpretation of a true lateral x-ray film of the shoulder. (**A**) The schematic drawing illustrates how a lateral view of the scapula projects as the letter Y. (**B**) Drawing of the lateral view of the scapula. (**C**) True lateral x-ray film of the scapula. Note that the glenoid fossa is located at the junction of the base of the spine and the base of the coracoid, with the body of the scapula projecting vertically. (**D**) The true lateral view of the glenohumeral joint shows the humeral head well centered about the glenoid fossa. (**E**) In the subacromial posterior dislocation of the shoulder, as seen on the true lateral view, the articular surface of the head of the humerus is directed posterior to the glenoid fossa. (**F**) In anterior subcoracoid dislocations of the shoulder, as seen on the true lateral view, the humeral head is anterior to the glenoid fossa and below the coracoid process.

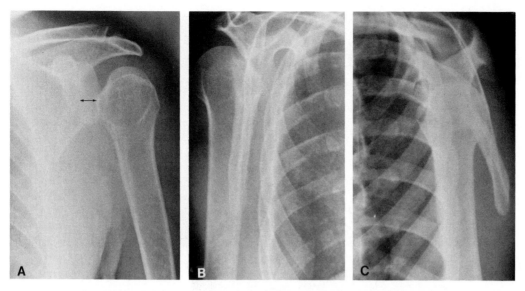

Fig. 13-59. The importance of true lateral x-ray views of the shoulder. (**A**) Subacromial posterior dislocation of the left shoulder is visualized on the anteroposterior view. Note the vacant glenoid sign and anteromedial humeral head defect. (**B**) A true scapular lateral of the posterior dislocation of the left shoulder reveals that the humeral head is displaced posteriorly out of the glenoid fossa. (**C**) The true lateral of the normal and opposite shoulders reveals that the humeral head is centered about the glenoid fossa, which is located at the junction of the base of the coracoid process, the base of the spine, and the acromion process with the vertical body of the scapula.

the plane of the scapula while a sulcus test is performed. Anterior translation is best demonstrated on an axillary view taken while the fulcrum test is performed. Posterior translation is most easily documented on an axillary view taken while the push–pull test is performed. Although these tests may demonstrate translation, they do not confirm that the translation is causing the patient's problem (ie, asymptomatic shoulders may demonstrate substan-

tial posterior translation). Furthermore, the inability to achieve a positive stress view does not necessarily exclude the diagnosis of instability (muscle action or incorrect technique may produce a false-negative test).

Fixed abnormalities may provide valuable clues to the direction of instability and the contributing factors to instability. The anteroposterior view in the plane of the scapula and the axillary view may re-

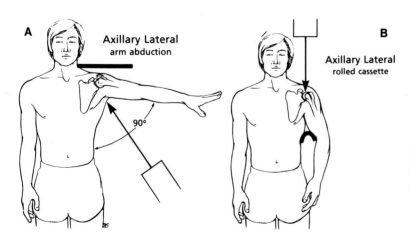

Fig. 13-60. (**A**) The axillary lateral x-ray view. Ideally, the arm is abducted 70° to 90° and the beam is directed superiorly up to the x-ray cassette. (**B**) When the patient cannot fully abduct the arm, a curved cassette can be placed in the axilla and the beam directed inferiorly through the glenohumeral joint onto the cassette. *(Rockwood, C. A.; Szalay, E. A.; Curtis, R. J.; Young, D. C.; and Kay, S. P.: X-ray Evaluation of Shoulder Problems. In Rockwood, C. A., and Matsen, F. A., III (eds.): The Shoulder, Figs. 5-5, 5-6. Philadelphia, W. B. Saunders, 1990.)*

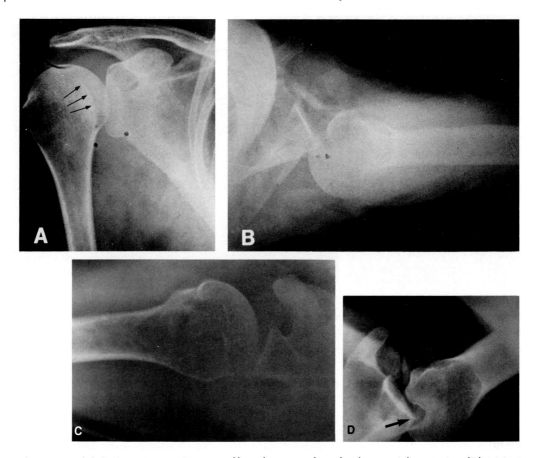

Fig. 13-61. (**A**) An anteroposterior x-ray film of an unreduced subacromial posterior dislocation of the shoulder is deceptively normal in appearance. However, the anterior two thirds of the glenoid fossa is vacant and the dense vertical line lateral to the head of the humerus is suggestive of an impaction fracture (**arrow**). (**B**) An axillary lateral view confirms the anteromedial impaction fracture of the humeral head. Note that the entire articular surface of the head of the humerus is posterior to the glenoid fossa. (**C**) An axillary lateral view of the normal left shoulder shows the normal articulation of the humeral head with the glenoid fossa and normal relations of the humeral head to the coracoid process and the acromion process. (**D**) The axillary lateral x-ray film of the right shoulder shows a subacromial posterior dislocation of the right shoulder with a large antero-medial compression fracture defect of the humeral head, the so-called reverse Hill-Sachs sign (**arrow**).

veal anterior or posterior glenoid lip fractures, new bone formation, or rounding of the glenoid lip in the presence of recurrent instability. Modifications of the axillary view may help identify glenoid rim changes.

THE WEST POINT AXILLARY LATERAL VIEW

Rokous[1118] and colleagues described what has become known as the "West Point axillary view."[1104] For this view the patient is placed prone on the x-

ray table with the involved shoulder on a pad raised 7.5 cm from the top of the table. The head and neck are turned away from the involved side. With the cassette held against the superior aspect of the shoulder, the x-ray beam is centered at the axilla, 25° downward from the horizontal and 25° medial. The resulting x-ray is a tangential view of the anteroinferior rim of the glenoid (Fig. 13-67). Using this view, Rokous and associates demonstrated bony abnormalities of the anterior glenoid rim in 53 of

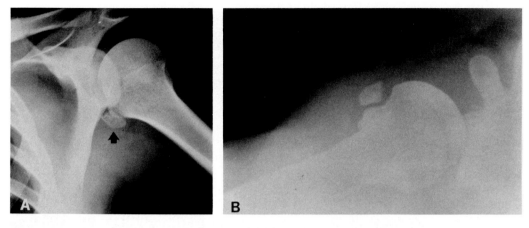

Fig. 13-62. Avulsion fracture of lesser tuberosity associated with posterior dislocation. (**A**) An axillary lateral view of the left shoulder reveals the old smooth-bordered fragment of the lesser tuberosity. (**B**) An anteroposterior view of the left shoulder taken with the arm in 45° of abduction and full internal rotation. Note the avulsion fracture of the lesser tuberosity (**arrow**). The patient had a history of an acute traumatic posterior dislocation that was reduced on the playing field.

63 patients whose histories indicated traumatic subluxation of the shoulder. Cyprien and co-workers[265] demonstrated lessening of the glenoid diameter and shortening of the anterior glenoid rim in shoulders with recurrent anterior dislocation. Blazina and Satzman[124] also reported anteroinferior glenoid rim fractures seen on the axillary view in nine cases.

THE APICAL–OBLIQUE VIEW

Garth and associates[423] described the apical oblique projection of the shoulder. For this view, the patient sits with the scapula flat against the cassette (as for the anteroposterior view in the plane of the scapula). The arm may be in a sling. The x-ray beam is directed perpendicular to the cassette (45° to the

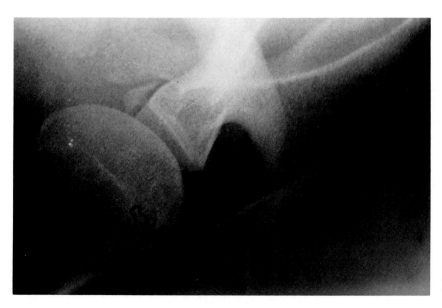

Fig. 13-63. Axillary lateral view demonstrating fracture of the anterior glenoid rim associated with anterior dislocation.

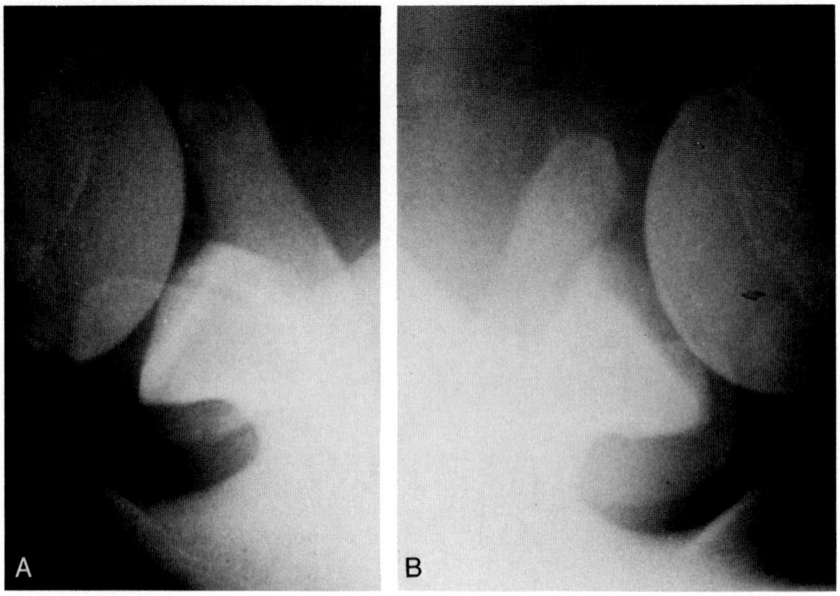

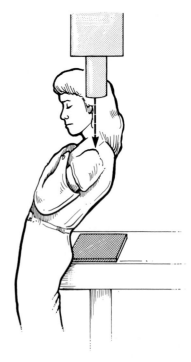

Fig. 13-64. Bilateral axillary views. (**A**) Rounding of the anterior glenoid rim as a result of recurrent anterior glenohumeral dislocation is evident on this axillary view. (**B**) Normal side is shown for comparison. (*Matsen, F. A., III; Thomas, S. C.; and Rockwood, C. A., Jr.: Anterior Glenohumeral Instability. In Rockwood, C. A., and Matsen, F. A., III (eds.): The Shoulder, Fig. 14-42. Philadelphia, W. B. Saunders, 1990.*)

coronal plane) and 45° caudally, and is centered on the coracoid. The beam then passes tangential to the articular surface of the glenohumeral joint and the posterolateral aspect of the humeral head. This view will also reveal both anterior glenoid lip defects and posterolateral impression fractures of the humeral head (Fig. 13-68).

SPECIAL VIEWS FOR HUMERAL HEAD DEFECTS

Humeral head defects may also be seen, confirming previous anterior dislocations in the case of pos-

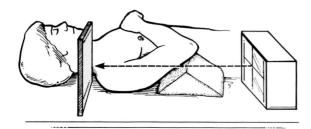

Fig. 13-65. Positioning of the patient for the trauma axillary lateral x-ray view. The patient is supine. The elbow is elevated by a piece of foam rubber, allowing the x-ray beam to pass from inferior up through the glenohumeral joint onto the x-ray cassette, which is superior to the shoulder. (*Modified from Tietge, R. A., and Ciullo, J. V.: The CAM Axillary X-Ray. Orthop. Trans., 6:451, 1982.*)

Fig. 13-66. Positioning of the patient for the Velpeau axillary lateral x-ray view, as described by Bloom and Obata. (*Modified from Bloom, M. R., and Obata, W. G.: Diagnosis of Posterior Dislocation of the Shoulder With Use of the Velpeau Axillary and Angled Up Radiographic Views. J. Bone Joint Surg., 49A:943–949, 1967.*)

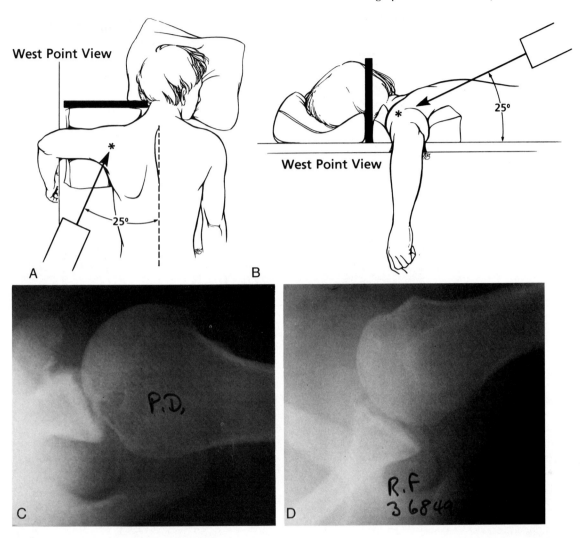

West Point View

West Point View

25°

25°

*

*

A   B

P.D.

R.F
36844

C   D

Fig. 13-67. **(A,B)** Positioning of the patient for the West Point x-ray view to visualize the anteroinferior glenoid rim of the shoulder. *(Modified from Rokous, J. R.; Feagin, J. A.; and Abbott, H. G.: Modified Axillary Roentgenogram. Clin. Orthop., 82:84–86, 1972.)* **(C, D)** Examples of calcification on the anteroinferior glenoid rim as noted on the West Point x-ray view.

terolateral defects and posterior dislocations in the case of anteromedial defects (Fig. 13-69). A number of special views have been described for identifying humeral head defects.

1. Hermodsson's internal rotation technique (anteroposterior radiograph in internal rotation). Hermodsson recommended that the patient be supine with a sandbag placed under the elbow to put the humerus horizontal to the top of the table. The arm is adducted to the side of the patient, the humerus is internally rotated 45°, and the forearm lies across the anterior trunk.

The x-ray beam is tilted 15° toward the feet and centered over the humeral head.[522]

2. Adams' modification of the internal rotation view. Adams' modification[7] is essentially the same view recommended by Hermodsson but with internal rotation increased from 70° to 100°.

3. Hermodsson's tangential view. To obtain marked internal rotation of the humerus, the elbow is flexed 90° and the dorsum of the hand is placed behind the trunk, over the upper lumbar spine. The thumb points upward. The film

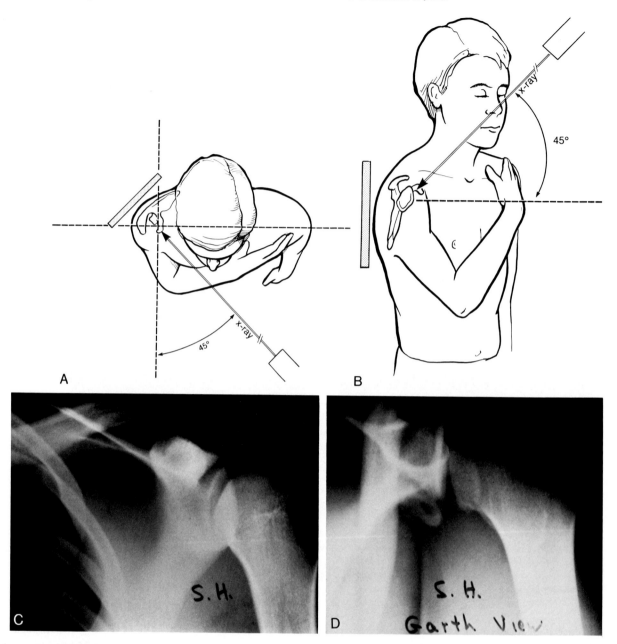

Fig. 13-68. (**A,B**) Positioning of the patient to obtain the apical-oblique x-ray. This is a true anteroposterior view of the glenohumeral joint with a 45° caudal tilt of the x-ray beam. *(Modified from Garth, W. P., Jr.; Slappey, C. E.; and Ochs, C. W.: Radiographic Demonstration of Instability of the Shoulder: The Apical Oblique Projection, A Technical Note. J. Bone Joint Surg., 66A:1450–1455, 1984.)* (**C**) An x-ray film of the left shoulder in the plane of the thorax that does not reveal any significant abnormality. (**D**) In the apical-oblique view, note the calcification on the anteroinferior glenoid rim. (Courtesy of Dr. Garth.)

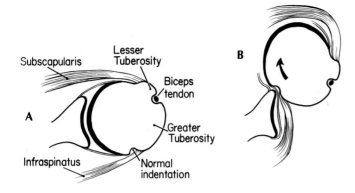

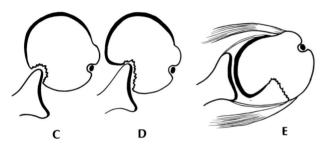

Fig. 13-69. A horizontal section through the gleno-humeral joint shows the formation of a posterolateral humeral head defect. (**A**) Normal anatomic relation-ships. (**B**) Anterior dislocation without a compression fracture defect. (**C**) A small posterolateral defect. (**D**) A large compression fracture defect. (**E**) Following re-duction, the defect is quite evident and has deformed the normal articular surface of the humeral head.

cassette is held superior to the adducted arm, and the x-ray tube is placed posterior, lateral, and inferior to the elbow joint, making a 30° angle with the humeral axis.[872]

4. Hill-Sachs view. An anteroposterior radiograph is made of the shoulder with the arm in marked internal rotation (Fig. 13-70).

5. Stryker notch view. The patient is supine on the table with the cassette placed under the shoulder.[478] The palm of the hand on the side with the affected shoulder is placed on top of the head, with the fingers directed toward the back of the head. The elbow should point straight upward. The x-ray beam tilts 10° to-ward the head, centered over the coracoid pro-cess (Fig. 13-71). This technique was developed by William S. Stryker and reported by Hall and co-workers.[478] They stated they could demon-strate the humeral head defect in 90% of 20 patients with a history of recurring anterior dislocation of the shoulder.

6. Didiee view. For this view, the patient is prone on the table with the cassette under the shoul-der.[315,872,1009] The forearm is behind the trunk, as for the tangential view of Hermodsson. The arm is parallel to the top of the table with a 3-

inch pad placed under the elbow. The dorsum of the hand is on the iliac crest with the thumb directed upward. The x-ray tube is directly lat-eral to the shoulder joint, and the beam is an-gled 45°.

7. Cephaloscapular projection. Oppenheim and co-workers[962] described a view in which the x-ray beam is passed from superior to inferior across the glenoid face to a cassette behind the patient, who is leaning forward.

8. Apical oblique view. As noted above, with this view, posterolateral impression fractures can be noted.[422,423]

In their classic article, Hill and Sachs[531] evaluated the relationship of humeral head defects to shoulder instability. They concluded that more than two thirds of anterior shoulder dislocations are compli-cated by a bony injury of the humerus or scapula. We quote:

> Compression fractures as a result of impingement of the weakest portion of the humeral head, that is, the posterior lateral aspect of the articular surface against the anterior rim of the glenoid fossa are found so frequently in cases of ha-bitual dislocation that they have been described as a typical defect . . . These defects are sustained at the time of the

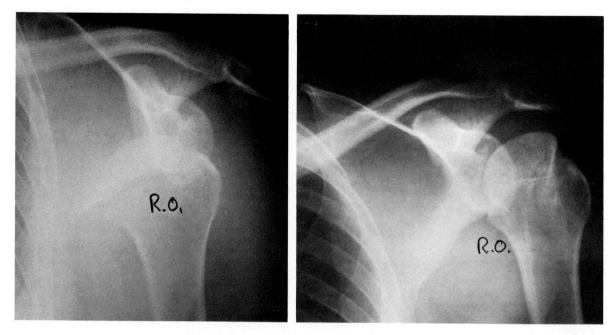

Fig. 13-70. Demonstration of the Hill-Sachs compression fracture. (**Left**) Anteroposterior x-ray film demonstrates subcoracoid anterior dislocation. (**Right**) Appearance postreduction and with the humerus held in internal rotation. Note the posterolateral humeral head defect and the sharp, dense spine of bone impaction running downward from the top of the humeral head toward the center of the humeral head. This is a line of condensation of bone and is the result of an impaction fracture caused by the anterior glenoid rim.

original dislocation . . . A special sign is the sharp, vertical, dense medial border of the groove known as the line of condensation, the length of which is correlated with the size of the defect.

Hill and Sachs reported the defect in only 27% of 119 acute anterior dislocations and in 74% of 15 recurrent anterior dislocations. However, they stated that the incidence of the groove defect was low because it was only in the last 6 months of their 10-year study (1930 to 1940) that they used the special radiographic views. The size of the defect varied in length (cephalocaudal) from 5 mm to 3 cm, in width from 3 mm to 2 cm, and in depth from 10 to 22 mm.[531]

Incidence of Humeral Head Defects

Using the Adams technique, Symeonides[1281] reported humeral head defects in 23 of 45 patients who had recurrent anterior dislocations of the shoulder—an incidence of 50%. However, at the time of surgery he could confirm only 18 of these, bringing the incidence down to 40%. In the remaining five cases he was only able to palpate the groove that is normally located between the greater tuberosity and the humeral head.

Eyre-Brook[363] reported an incidence of the humeral head defects of 64% in 17 recurrent anterior dislocations, and Brav[154] recorded a rate of 67% in 69 recurrent dislocations. Rowe[1127] noted defects in 38% of 125 acute dislocations, and in 57% of 63 recurrent dislocations. Adams[6] noted defects at the time of surgery in 82% of 68 patients. Palmar and Widen[984] found defects at surgery in all of 60 patients.

Danzig and colleagues[272] reported that in cadaveric and clinical studies, no single view consistently revealed humeral head compression fractures. Pavlov and co-workers[1009] found that the Stryker notch view taken in internal rotation best revealed the posterolateral humeral head defect, while the anterior glenoid lip was best evaluated by the Didiee and West Point views. Rozing and associates[1150] found that humeral head defects most often were seen by the Stryker notch view, and that glenoid rim defects were most easily seen on a coronal projection with the beam angled 45° craniocaudal.

The demonstration of a humeral head defect

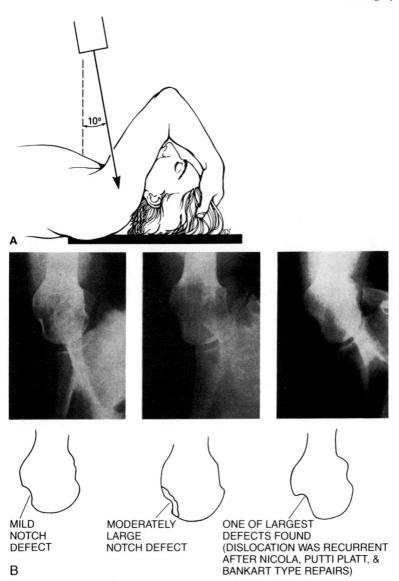

MILD NOTCH DEFECT

MODERATELY LARGE NOTCH DEFECT

ONE OF LARGEST DEFECTS FOUND (DISLOCATION WAS RECURRENT AFTER NICOLA, PUTTI PLATT, & BANKART TYPE REPAIRS)

B

Fig. 13-71. (**A**) The position of the patient for the Stryker notch view. The patient is supine with the cassette posterior to the shoulder. The humerus is flexed approximately 120° so that the hand can be placed on top of the patient's head. Note that the angle of the x-ray tube is 10° superior. (**B**) Defects in the posterolateral aspect of the humeral head are seen in three different patients with recurring anterior dislocations of the shoulder. (*Modified from Hall, R. H.,; Isaac, F.; and Booth, C. R.: Dislocation of the Shoulder with Special Reference to Accompanying Small Fractures. J. Bone Joint Surg., 41:489–494, 1959.*)

confirms that the shoulder has been dislocated, and reveals in which direction. Furthermore, the presence of such a defect usually suggests a traumatic cause of the instability. When these factors are already known—for example, in a 17-year-old whose recurrent anterior dislocations began with a well-documented abduction–external rotation injury in football—we tend not to spend a great deal of effort demonstrating the humeral head defect because (1) it is very likely to be present even if not seen on the radiographs, and (2) the existence of such a lesion does not in itself alter our management of the patient.

SPECIAL RADIOGRAPHIC STUDIES

Arthrography

Single- and double-contrast arthrograms can be used to evaluate previously dislocated shoulders for rotator cuff tears. This is especially important if a patient fails to regain strength of flexion and rotation after a shoulder dislocation.

Computed Tomography

Through the use of computed tomographic (CT) scans, we can study the cross-sectional anatomy of the shoulder in great detail. These scans are helpful

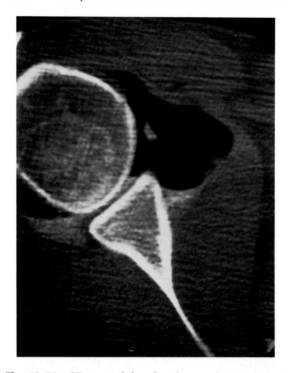

Fig. 13-72. CT scan of the glenohumeral joint with air contrast. This study demonstrates a bony avulsion from the anterior glenoid rim. *(Matsen, F. A., III; Thomas, S. C.; and Rockwood, C. A., Jr.: Anterior Glenohumeral Instability. In Rockwood, C. A., and Matsen, F. A., III (eds.): The Shoulder, Fig. 14-46. Philadelphia, W. B. Saunders, 1990.)*

in revealing the extent of fractures of the glenoid or humeral head compression fractures. Gould and colleagues[454] used CT to demonstrate a loose body blocking reduction of the shoulder. CT offers a method for determining the size and locations of glenoid rim defects.[1209] When previous glenoid bone blocks have been carried out or hardware inserted, CT is useful for examining the possibility of their encroachment on the humeral head.[256,258,273] Injecting small amounts of air and radio-opaque contrast into the joint prior to CT scanning often highlights the glenoid labrum. This imaging technique may permit preoperative identification of attenuation, tears, and displacement of the labrum as well as stripping and stretching of the anterior shoulder joint capsule (Figs. 13-72 through 13-74).[151,256,340,636,654,812,825,1055,1056,1221]

OTHER DIAGNOSTIC TESTS

Fluoroscopy

Norris[936] described a technique for the fluoroscopic evaluation of the shoulder under anesthesia. This examination is performed in the axillary projection while the shoulder is stressed anteriorly or posteriorly. Norris found that any anterior subluxation was likely to be abnormal, but that posterior displacement of up to 50% of the humeral head may be normal. If surgeons recognize this normal posterior laxity, unnecessary posterior tightening can

Fig. 13-73. CT scan of the glenohumeral joint. Note the posterior humeral head defect and the anterior glenoid defect, well demonstrated on this scan. *(Matsen, F. A., III; Thomas, S. C.; and Rockwood, C. A., Jr.: Anterior Glenohumeral Instability. In Rockwood, C. A., and Matsen, F. A., III (eds.): The Shoulder, Fig. 14-47. Philadelphia, W. B. Saunders, 1990.)*

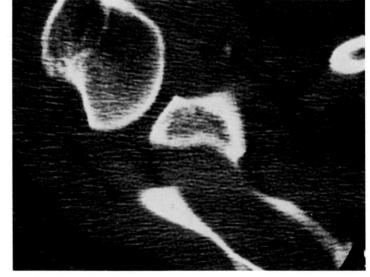

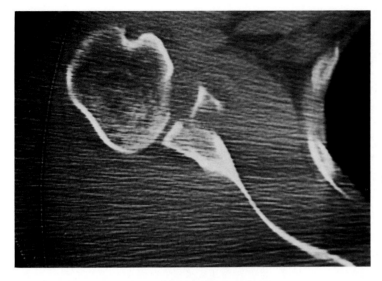

Fig. 13-74. CT scan of the glenohumeral joint. This scan shows a fracture of the anterior glenoid rim secondary to anterior glenohumeral dislocation. *(Matsen, F. A., III; Thomas, S. C.; and Rockwood, C. A., Jr.: Anterior Glenohumeral Instability. In Rockwood, C. A., and Matsen, F. A., III (eds.): The Shoulder, Fig. 14-48. Philadelphia, W. B. Saunders, 1990.)*

be avoided. Other tests may be indicated in the evaluation of the patient with glenohumeral instability, such as electromyography if there is a concern about brachial plexus injury.

Arthroscopy

Shoulder arthroscopy is being used by some to evaluate glenohumeral instability. This technique allows inspection of the humeral head and anteromedial or posterolateral defects. It also allows observation of the anterior glenoid for the scuffing that often accompanies recurrent anterior instability and for labral or ligamentous anomalies and injuries.[35,194,398,422,473,612,726,825,852,957,992,1395,1396,1427] We currently reserve this technique for the rare instances in which substantial question concerning the diagnosis remains even after a thorough history, physical examination, and radiographic studies.

COMPLICATIONS OF INJURY

COMPLICATIONS OF TRAUMATIC ANTERIOR DISLOCATIONS

Ligaments and Capsular Changes

Because the ligament and capsule are stretched or stripped off the rim and neck of the scapula, the most common complication following a traumatic anterior dislocation of the shoulder is a recurrence of the shoulder instability.

Fractures and Bony Changes

Bony injuries have been discussed briefly earlier in this chapter. Essentially they consist of compression fractures of the humeral head (the Hill-Sachs lesion), fractures of the anterior glenoid lip, fractures of the greater tuberosity, and fractures of the acromion or coracoid process associated with the superior dislocation of the shoulder (Figs. 13-75 through 13-77). Benchetrit and Friedman[103] and Wong-Pack and associates[1409] reported on fractures of the coracoid process that may not be recognized on routine anteroposterior x-ray films. Verrina[1344] reported a patient who developed voluminous ossification of the joint following an easily reduced anterior dislocation of the shoulder.

Ferkel and co-workers[376] pointed out the risk of creating displaced fractures at the time of reduction of an anterior shoulder dislocation. Both their patients were in their 50s and had subcoracoid dislocations with greater tuberosity fractures. Each attempted reduction using simple traction created a displaced fracture of the anatomic neck (Fig. 13-78).

Cuff Tears

Rotator cuff tears may accompany anterior and inferior glenohumeral dislocations.[1001,1020,1072,1281] Petterson reported 27 ruptures of the rotator cuff in 47 patients with anterior dislocation.[1020] Tijmes and co-workers[1301] reported cuff rupture in 28% of anterior dislocations. The frequency of this complication increases with age: in patients older than 40 years, the incidence exceeds 30%; after age 60, it exceeds 80%. Rotator cuff tears may present as pain or weakness on external rotation and abduction.[497,1020,1074,1392] Johnson and Bayley,[609] in a se-

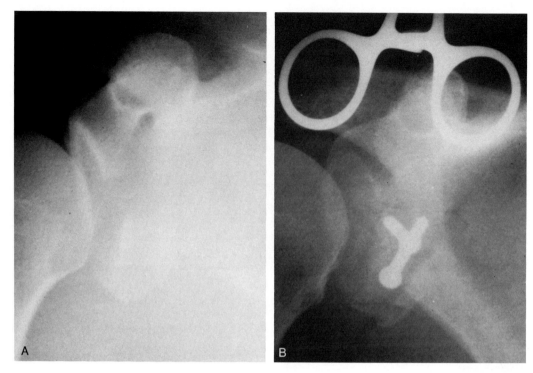

Fig. 13-75. Anterior glenoid rim fracture. (**A**) An anteroposterior x-ray film demonstrates an anterior glenoid rim fracture secondary to traumatic anterior dislocation. (**B**) An intraoperative anteroposterior x-ray film shows reduction and screw fixation of an anterior glenoid rim fracture. *(Matsen, F. A., III; Thomas, S. C.; and Rockwood, C. A., Jr.: Anterior Glenohumeral Instability. In Rockwood, C. A., and Matsen, F. A., III (eds.): The Shoulder, Fig. 14-49. Philadelphia, W. B. Saunders, 1990.)*

ries of 12 complications following acute anterior dislocation, stressed that rotator cuff injury can be obscured by an axillary nerve injury. Shoulder ultrasonography[764] or arthrography is considered in patients older than 40 years, in those with substantial initial displacement of the humeral head (such as in a subglenoid dislocation), and in those demonstrating a slow return of active function after a glenohumeral dislocation (Fig. 13-79). Prompt operative repair of this tendon rupture is usually indicated.

McLaughlin and MacLellan[815] point out that the incidence of recurrence is low when shoulder dislocation occurs by disruption of the posterior structures—the greater tuberosity and cuff. Their series of 90 shoulder dislocations associated with tuberosity fractures showed only one recurrence. In Rowe's series[1129,1144] there were only three recurrences among 75 such cases.

Vascular Injuries

Vascular damage most frequently occurs in elderly patients with stiffer, more fragile vessels. The injury may be to the axillary artery or vein or to the branches of the axillary artery—the thoracoacromial, subscapular, circumflex, and rarely the long thoracic. Approximately 200 cases have been reported in the literature. Injury may occur at the time of either dislocation or reduction (Fig. 13-80).[44,262,467,595]

ANATOMY

The axillary artery is divided into three parts that lie medial to, behind, and lateral to the pectoralis minor muscle (Fig. 13-81). The sites most commonly injured are in the second part, when the thoracoacromial trunk is avulsed, and in the third part, when subscapular and circumflex branches are avulsed or the axillary artery is totally ruptured.

MECHANISM OF INJURY

Damage to the axillary artery can take the form of a complete transection, a linear tear of the artery caused by avulsion of one of its branches, or an intravascular thrombus, perhaps related to an intimal tear. Brown and Navigato[166] observed that

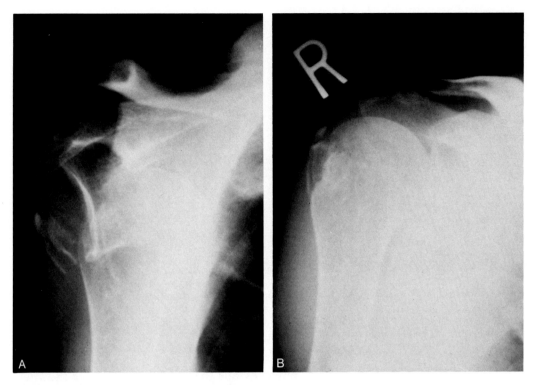

Fig. 13-76. Greater tuberosity fracture. (**A**) An anteroposterior x-ray film prior to reduction showing a fracture of the greater tuberosity. (**B**) A postreduction anteroposterior x-ray film of a greater tuberosity fracture. *(Matsen, F. A., III; Thomas, S. C.; and Rockwood, C. A., Jr.: Anterior Glenohumeral Instability. In Rockwood, C. A., and Matsen, F. A., III (eds.): The Shoulder, Fig. 14-50. Philadelphia, W. B. Saunders, 1990.)*

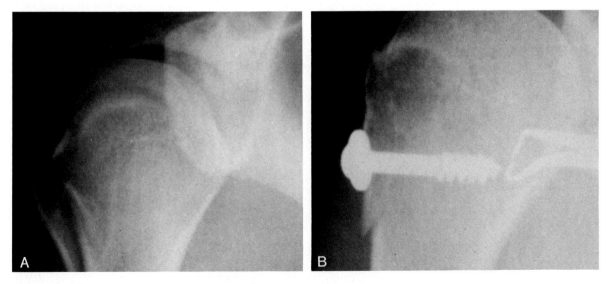

Fig. 13-77. (**A**) An x-ray film showing a displaced greater tuberosity fracture. (**B**) An intraoperative x-ray film showing screw fixation of a greater tuberosity fracture. *(Matsen, F. A., III; Thomas, S. C.; and Rockwood, C. A., Jr.: Anterior Glenohumeral Instability. In Rockwood, C. A., and Matsen, F. A., III (eds.): The Shoulder, Fig. 14-53. Philadelphia, W. B. Saunders, 1990.)*

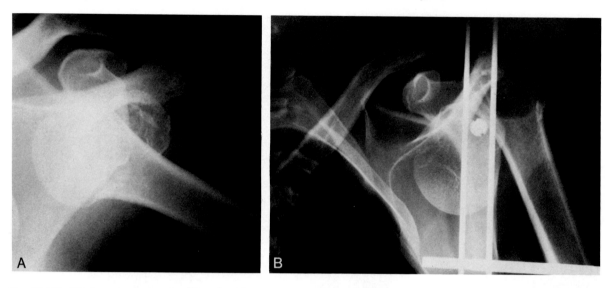

Fig. 13-78. (**A**) An anteroposterior view showing an anteroinferior dislocation with an associated greater tuberosity fracture. (**B**) An anteroposterior view after attempted reduction. *(Matsen, F. A., III; Thomas, S. C.; and Rockwood, C. A., Jr.: Anterior Glenohumeral Instability. In Rockwood, C. A., and Matsen, F. A., III (eds.): The Shoulder, Fig. 14-54. Philadelphia, W. B. Saunders, 1990.)*

the artery is relatively fixed at the lateral margin of the pectoralis minor muscle. With abduction and external rotation, the artery is taut; when the head dislocates, it dislocates the axillary artery forward, and the pectoralis minor acts as a fulcrum over which the artery is deformed and ruptured. Milton[849] proposed that the axillary artery is fixed in its third part by the circumflex and subscapular branches, and that these branches hold the artery in place and prevent it from escaping injury when the humeral head displaces forward. Jardon and coworkers[595] reported two cases in which the axillary artery was fixed by scar to the pericapsular tissues and transected during displacement of the capsule. Watson-Jones[1375] reported the case of a man who had multiple anterior dislocations that

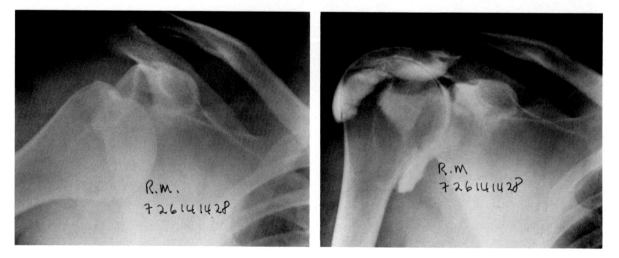

Fig. 13-79. (**Left**) Anteroposterior x-ray film of the right shoulder of a 55-year-old patient with an anterior subcoracoid dislocation. (**Right**) Arthrogram done 4 weeks later revealed rupture of the rotator cuff with dye extending into the subacromial bursa.

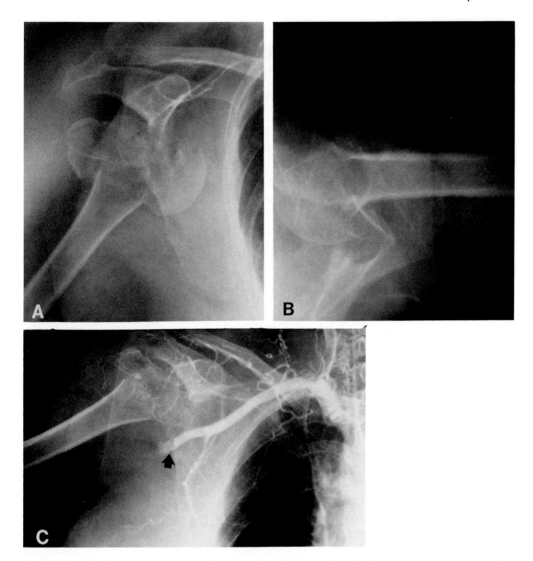

Fig. 13-80. Fracture–dislocation of the right shoulder associated with thrombosis of the axillary artery in a 71-year-old woman. (**A**) An anteroposterior view reveals a 7-day-old fracture–dislocation of the right shoulder. Note the comminution of the proximal end of the humerus and the location of the articular surface of the humerus—anterior in the subcoracoid position. (**B**) An axillary lateral view demonstrates the displacement of the head anterior to the glenoid. Manipulation was unsuccessful in accomplishing reduction, and the surgeon elected to resect the head of the humerus, which was a free fragment. Following excision of the fragment, the right hand was pale and there was no palpable brachial or radial pulse. (**C**) Arteriogram was interpreted as showing a thrombus (**arrow**) 3 cm distal to the subscapular artery. The shoulder was reexplored immediately, and through an arteriotomy an intimal tear approximately 3.8 cm long was identified. Following the removal of the intimal tear there was prompt return of back bleeding. Following closure of the artery and release of the vascular clamps, the radial and ulnar pulses returned and the hand immediately became pink. The postoperative course was uneventful.

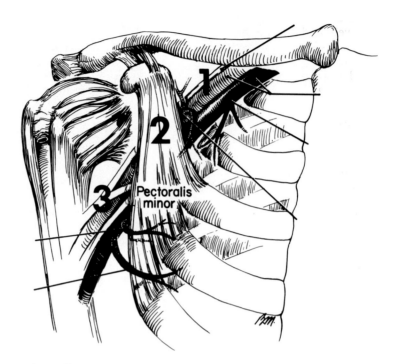

Fig. 13-81. The axillary artery is divided into three parts by the pectoralis minor muscle; the second part is behind the muscle and the third part is lateral to it.

he reduced himself. Finally, when the man was older, the axillary artery ruptured during one of the dislocations and he died.

INJURY AT THE TIME OF DISLOCATION

Vascular injuries are commonly associated with inferior dislocation.[418,716,754,828] Gardham and Scott[418] reported an axillary artery occlusion with an erect dislocation of the shoulder in a 40-year-old patient who had fallen headfirst down an escalator. Although we often consider vascular complications as a phenomenon of older patients, they can occur at any age. Baratta and co-workers[79] reported the case of a 13-year-old boy who ruptured his axillary artery with a subcoracoid dislocation sustained while wrestling. Vascular injuries also have been reported by Drury and Scullion,[325] Fitzgerald and Keates,[385] Sarma and co-workers,[1181] Bertrand and colleagues,[110] Lescher and Andersen,[714] and Stein.[1255]

INJURY AT THE TIME OF REDUCTION

Vascular damage at the time of reduction occurs primarily in the elderly, particularly when an old anterior dislocation is mistaken for an acute injury and a closed reduction is performed. The axillary artery is bound down by the pectoralis minor muscle and frequently by anterior pericapsular scarring; it is brittle and cannot withstand the traction required to reduce an old dislocation. The injury can also occur during any forceful manipulation in younger patients who, because of locked acute dislocation, have excessive forces applied during reduction.

The largest series of vascular complications associated with closed reduction of the shoulder has been reported by Calvet and co-workers,[183] who in 1941 collected 90 cases. This paper, revealing the tragic end results, must have accomplished its purpose because there have been very few reports in the literature since then dealing with the complications that occur during reduction. In their series, in which 64 of 91 reductions were performed many weeks after the initial dislocation, the mortality rate was 50%. The other patients lost either the arm or the function of the arm. Besides the long delay from dislocation to reduction, Guibe[468] stated that excessive forces were commonly used to reduce difficult dislocations of the shoulder. He quotes Delpeche, who observed a case in which the force of 10 men was used to accomplish the shoulder reduction, damaging the axillary vessel. Kirker[649] described a case of rupture of the axillary artery and axillary vein and brachial plexus palsy, but he was uncertain as to when the complication occurred (at the time of dislocation or reduction). Stener[1256] also reported a case of axillary artery damage in which he could not determine when the injury occurred.

SIGNS AND SYMPTOMS

Vascular damage may be obvious or subtle. Findings may include pain, expanding hematoma, pulse deficit, peripheral cyanosis, peripheral coolness and pallor, neurologic dysfunction, and shock. An arteriogram should confirm the diagnosis and locate the site of injury.

TREATMENT AND PROGNOSIS

Patients suspected of having major arterial injury need a large-bore intravenous line, and blood must be sent for type and cross match. Jardon and co-workers[595] reported that the bleeding can be controlled before operation by digital pressure on the axillary artery over the first rib. The patient in severe shock or ischemia should be taken promptly to the operating room, where emergent treatment can be rendered. Jardon and co-workers[595] have recommended that the axillary artery be explored through the subclavicular operative approach, as described by Steenburg and Tavitch.[1254] The results of simple ligation of the vessels in the elderly patient have been disappointing, probably because of poor collateral circulation and the presence of arteriosclerotic vascular disease.[617,649,1335] Even when ligation has been performed in younger patients with good collateral circulation, approximately two thirds of these patients have lost some of the function of the upper extremity—some by developing upper extremity claudication. The treatment of choice is to restore normal circulation to the arm; this can be done by repair of the lesion or by using a graft or prosthesis. We agree that it is most important to resect the damaged artery back to normal intima before the vessel is repaired to prevent late thrombus. Lev-el and associates[716] reported a patient who had an injury to the axillary artery and who subsequently developed a thrombus that required resection and vein graft. Gardham and Scott[418] reported a case in 1980 in which the axillary artery was damaged in its third part and was managed by a bypass graft using the saphenous vein. Excellent results have been reported by Henson,[519] Cranley and Krause,[259] Stevens,[1258] McKenzie and Sinclair,[813] Brown and Navigato,[166] Gibson,[439] Rob and Standeven,[1097] and Jardon and co-workers.[595]

Neural Injuries

The brachial plexus and the axillary artery lie immediately anterior, inferior, and medial to the glenohumeral joint.[457] It is not surprising, therefore, that neurovascular injuries frequently accompany traumatic anterior glenohumeral dislocations.

ANATOMY

The axillary nerve originates off the posterior cord of the brachial plexus. It crosses the anterior surface of the subscapularis muscle and angulates sharply posteriorly to travel along the inferior shoulder joint capsule. It then leaves the axilla to exit through the quadrangular space below the lower border of the teres minor muscle, where it hooks around the posterior and lateral humerus on the deep surface of the deltoid muscle. (See Fig. 13-12.)

MECHANISM OF INJURY

According to Milton,[848,849] McGregor postulated that the nerve is crushed between the head of the humerus and the axillary border of the scapula (Fig. 13-82). Stevens[1258] pointed out that in normal anatomy the path of the axillary nerve is directly across the anterior surface of the subscapularis muscle. In an anterior dislocation the head displaces the subscapularis tendon and muscle forward, creating traction and direct pressure on the nerve. Nerve injuries are divided into three groups:

1. *Neurapraxia*—transient denervation produced by a mild injury to the nerve. Recovery is usually complete in 1 to 2 months.
2. *Axonotmesis*—complete denervation produced by a moderate to severe injury of the nerve, in which the nerve cells die but regeneration can be accomplished through the intact nerve sheaths. The recovery rate is approximately 2.5 cm per month.
3. *Neuronotmesis*—complete denervation that occurs when the axons and the sheaths are transected. Recovery is poor without careful nerve repair. This rarely occurs as a result of anterior dislocation of the shoulder.

INCIDENCE

McLaughlin reported nerve injuries in 2% of recurrent dislocations and in 10% of acute dislocations. Watson-Jones[1374] reported 14% and Rowe[1143] 5.4%. DePalma[287] reported 5%; Mumenthaler and Schliack[885] 15% and Brown[167] 25% of 76 cases. Gariepy[421] stated that the nerve injury is more common than is realized. Tuszynski[1323] has written on two patients with temporary injury to the bra-

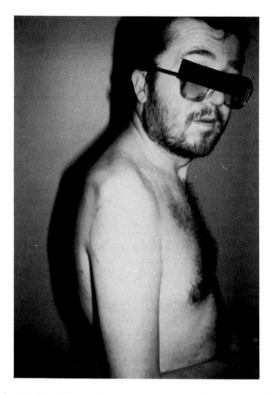

Fig. 13-82. This patient sustained an axillary nerve palsy secondary to glenohumeral dislocation. Note the area of decreased sensation diagrammed on the lateral aspect of the proximal humerus. Also note the presence of significant wasting. *(Matsen, F. A., III; Thomas, S. C.; and Rockwood, C. A., Jr.: Anterior Glenohumeral Instability. In Rockwood, C. A., and Matsen, F. A., III (eds.): The Shoulder, Fig. 14-56. Philadelphia, W. B. Saunders, 1990.)*

chial plexus following anterior dislocation of the shoulder. Pasila and co-workers,[1002] in a review of 226 patients with acute dislocation of the shoulder, found an incidence of complications of 25%. There were 25 brachial plexus injuries and 19 axillary nerve injuries. Parsons and Rowley[998] demonstrated that delayed reduction of a shoulder dislocation could cause deterioration of neurologic function.

The axillary is the most commonly involved nerve: reported incidences of first-time anterior glenohumeral dislocations accompanied by significant axillary nerve injury range from one in three to one in twenty.[125,467,705,1002,1143] The likelihood of an axillary nerve injury increases with the age of the patient, the duration of the dislocation, and the amount of trauma that initiated the dislocation.[125,1001] Other nerves injured are the radial,

musculocutaneous, median, ulnar, and the entire brachial plexus.

Livson[742] presented an extensive electromyographic analysis of 11 cases of shoulder dislocation with nerve injury. The axillary nerve was most commonly injured, but more proximal involvement of the posterior and median cords of the brachial plexus was also observed.

Blom and Dahlback,[125] in a very careful electromyographic study of 73 patients with anterior dislocation or fracture of the humeral neck, showed that the incidence of nerve injury was 35%. Of the 73 patients studied, 26 had nerve damage (17 partial injuries and 9 complete denervations). Of the 26 nerve injuries, 22 were confined to the axillary nerve. In the remaining 4, the breakdown was as follows: axillary and musculocutaneous nerves, 1; axillary and radial nerves, 1; radial nerve, 1; and musculocutaneous and median nerves, 1. In their series, more than half the patients older than 50 years had damage to the axillary nerve. They observed that the transient, partial denervations of the axillary nerve were responsible for the poor recovery following anterior dislocation. They noted that if a patient's recovery is delayed beyond 1 to 3 months, it may well be the result of an unrecognized partial axillary nerve injury.

Blom and Dahback[125] also demonstrated that the usual sensory testing of the axillary nerve (ie, checking the skin sensation just above the deltoid insertion on the lateral shoulder) is completely unreliable (Fig. 13-83). They found that most patients who had axillary nerve damage had no sensory loss, not even three patients who, by electromyography, showed complete denervation of the axillary nerve. In addition, they stated that there were three other patients who had sensory loss but normal electromyographic patterns. They stressed that the patient who has somewhat delayed functional recovery probably has partial damage to the axillary nerve.

DIAGNOSIS

The diagnosis of nerve injury is considered in any patient having neurologic symptoms, or signs such as weakness or numbness. Nerve injury may also present as delayed recovery of active shoulder motion after glenohumeral dislocation. Blom and Dahlback[125] demonstrated that the usual sensory testing of the axillary nerve (ie, checking the skin sensation just above the deltoid insertion on the lateral shoulder) is unreliable. An electromyogram provides objective evaluation of neurologic function, provided that 3 or 4 weeks have passed between the injury and the evaluation.

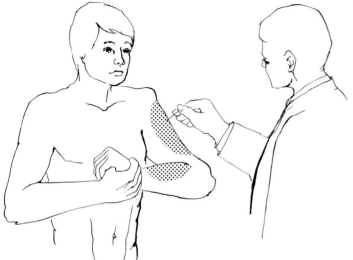

Fig. 13-83. The examiner is testing skin sensation for damage to the axillary nerve before reduction of the anterior dislocation of the left shoulder. The other area to be tested is the dorsal aspect of the forearm, which is supplied by the musculocutaneous nerve. However, testing the skin for abnormalities may be unreliable.[125]

TREATMENT AND PROGNOSIS

It is generally agreed that most axillary nerve injuries resulting from anterior dislocation are traction neurapraxias and will recover completely. Blom and Dahlback[125] reported full functional and electromyographic recovery at 3 to 5 months in 26 cases of partial and complete axillary nerve denervation. Brown[167] reported almost complete recovery in 76 cases. His treatment consisted of "watchful expectancy," without galvanic stimulation or exploration of the nerve. Assmus and Meinel[56] reported that patients with partial axillary nerve palsy frequently recovered in 2 to 6 weeks, and that complete reinnervation could be expected by 1 year. However, a poor prognosis resulted if the axillary nerve did not recover after 10 weeks.

In summary, damage to the axillary nerve is a common complication of anterior dislocations of the shoulder; regardless of whether the damage is partial or complete, the result is usually a normal, functioning shoulder. The incidence of axillary nerve denervation is higher in elderly patients, and the overall incidence is probably in the range of 30%. The classic technique of checking the lateral shoulder for abnormal skin sensation is an unreliable indicator of axillary nerve damage.

Recurrence of Dislocation

Recurrent dislocation is the most common complication following an acute traumatic anterior dislocation of the shoulder. Several factors should be considered in evaluating the risk of recurrence, including patient age, type and duration of immobi-

lization, and presence of fractures at the time of the initial dislocation.

PATIENT AGE

The age of the patient at the time of the initial dislocation has a major effect on the incidence of redislocation.[1131,1144] McLaughlin and MacLellan[815] observed that 95% of 181 primary traumatic dislocations in teenagers recurred. Henry and Genung[517] found an 85% to 90% redislocation rate for acute traumatic anterior dislocations in young patients (average age, 19 years). Before the age of 20, the incidence is reported by Rowe,[1144] McLaughlin and Cavallaro,[814] and others[872] to be between 80% and 92%. After the age of 40, the incidence drops sharply to 10% to 15%. The majority of recurrences occur within 2 years of the first traumatic dislocation.[6,76,293,365,814,874,875,1143,1144,1309]

Simonet and Cofield[1228] found an overall incidence of recurrence in 116 patients followed for more than 4 years to be 33%; 66% in patients younger than 20 years, 17% in patients 20 to 40 years, and zero in patients older than 40 years. However, they did point out that the recurrence rate in athletes younger than 20 years was 80%, but only 30% in nonathletes of a similar age group. Hovelius[557] followed 257 primary shoulder dislocations in 254 patients between the ages of 12 and 40 years. They found two or more recurrences in 55% of patients up to 22 years old, 37% in patients 23 to 29 years old, and 12% in patients 30 to 40 years old.

Kiviluoto and co-workers[651] again emphasized that patients younger than 30 are more prone to recurrent dislocations, whereas those older than 30 are more likely to develop shoulder stiffness. Rowe and Sakellarides[1131] reported 66 patients with an average age of 60 years in which the recurrence rate was 4.5%. McLaughlin and MacLellan reported a recurrence rate of 1.1% in a similar population.[815]

Recurrences are more common in men than in women. Moseley[872] quotes several series in which the ratios range from four to one to six to one. Rowe[1144] reports that recurrent dislocations are neither more nor less common in the dominant shoulder, nor does the weaker shoulder tend to suffer primary or recurrent dislocations more frequently than the stronger, dominant one. Rowe[1131,1144] also has pointed out that the recurrence rate varies inversely with the severity of the original trauma; in other words, the more easily the dislocation occurred initially, the more easily it recurs.

IMMOBILIZATION OF INITIAL DISLOCATION

In many clinical series, the incidence of recurrence seems to be affected very little by the type and length of immobilization of the shoulder following initial dislocation. In their report of a series of 573 dislocations of the shoulder, McLaughlin and Cavallaro[814] concluded that the length of time the shoulder was immobilized after initial anterior dislocation was of little importance. Hovelius and associates[551] compared 112 patients whose shoulders were immobilized for 3 to 4 weeks with 104 patients who used the shoulder as early and as freely as possible and found an equal recurrence rate after 2 years. Ehgartner[337] found the same recurrence rate in patients who were immobilized in plaster-of-paris Velpeau and in patients who used a sling. Rowe and Sakellarides[1131] were unable to document that prolonged immobilization lessened the incidence of redislocation.

By contrast, Stromsoe and co-workers[1271] followed 99 patients and found a 6.4% recurrence rate in shoulders immobilized for 3 weeks, and a 12% recurrence rate in those immobilized for less than 3 weeks. Kazar and Relovszky[634] reported a 10% to 15% incidence of recurrence with a lower incidence for those immobilized longer than 1 week.

Aronen and Regan[51] reported on 20 naval midshipmen with first-time shoulder dislocations who were treated with a specific, aggressive postdislocation program and followed for an average of 35.8 months (age averaged 19.2 years). The shoulders were immobilized in a sling for 3 weeks. Isometric deltoid and internal rotation exercises were started at 2 weeks. The patients were not allowed to return to activity until there was no evidence of weakness or atrophy and no apprehension on abduction and external rotation. Patients required an average of 3 months to reach these goals. These patients had no recurrent dislocations; two had recurrent subluxations. This is comparable to the result of Yoneda,[1414] who found good results in 83% of patients in a program emphasizing postimmobilization exercises.

ASSOCIATED FRACTURES

Hovelius[557] reported on 256 shoulders with primary dislocations in patients 12 to 40 years of age. Although age was the primary factor, as described earlier, the presence of fractures also seemed to have an effect. A moderate humeral head defect was correlated with an increased incidence of recurrence in patients older than 22 years. Of 32 shoulders with fractures of the greater tuberosity, dislocations recurred only in one. These two factors may be related. These fractures were four times as common in patients older than 30 years, 23% of whom has fractures, compared with only 8% among patients younger than 30 years. Other series include fracture of the greater tuberosity with anterior glenohumeral joint dislocations in approximately 15% to 35% of patients.[288,815,1125] The redislocation rates of shoulders with greater tuberosity fractures were low in these series as well.

We conclude that the injuries sustained by young patients in traumatic dislocations are relatively unlikely to heal in a manner yielding a stable shoulder. Probably the most important of these difficult injuries is avulsion of the glenohumeral ligament from the anterior glenoid lip and neck of the scapula. Older patients tend to stretch the capsule or avulse the greater tuberosity, either of which is likely to heal leaving a stable shoulder. In atraumatic instability, there is no lesion and thus a high chance of recurrence. The degree of trauma and the age of the patient seem to be more important than the specifics of past dislocation management in determining the recurrence rate.

COMPLICATIONS OF TRAUMATIC POSTERIOR DISLOCATIONS

Fractures

Fractures of the posterior glenoid rim and of the proximal humerus (upper shaft, tuberosities, and head) are quite common in traumatic posterior dislocations of the shoulder.[946,947,1289,1403] Vichard and Arnould[1348] reported 11 cases of posterior dislocation associated with fractures. The commonly associated compression fracture of the anteromedial portion of the humeral head is produced by the posterior cortical rim of the glenoid. It is best visualized on an axillary view or a CT scan. This lesion, sometimes called a "reversed Hill-Sachs lesion," often occurs at the time of the original posterior dislocation. It becomes larger with multiple posterior dislocations of the shoulder. Large humeral head defects are seen in the patient with an old, unreduced posterior dislocation.

The posterior rim of the glenoid may be fractured and displaced in posterior dislocations (Fig. 13-84). This occurs not only with direct forces from an anterior direction that push the humeral head out posteriorly, but also with indirect types of dislocations such as occur during seizures or accidental electrical shock.

Fracture of the lesser tuberosity of the humerus may accompany posterior dislocations. The subscapularis muscle comes under considerable tension in this dislocation and may avulse the lesser tuberosity onto which it inserts. Although the fracture may be seen on anteroposterior and lateral x-ray films of the glenohumeral joint, it is best seen on the axillary view and on CT scan.

When the x-ray films reveal a comminuted fracture of the proximal humerus, one should be aware that the head fragment may be displaced posteriorly. Because of the distortion of the fragments, it is impossible to determine the exact position of the head without axillary lateral x-ray or CT scan studies. In the series of 16 cases of posterior dislocation of the shoulder reported by O'Connor and Kacknow,[947] 12 had comminuted fractures of the proximal humerus. In 8 of the 12 fractures, the diagnosis of posterior dislocation was initially missed. Kavanaugh[633] reported posterior dislocation of the shoulder associated with a fracture of the shaft of the humerus.

Other Complications

Neurovascular injuries and cuff tears are much less common with posterior dislocations than with anterior dislocations. Recurrence is very common with (1) atraumatic posterior dislocation, and (2) large bony defects of the humerus and/or glenoid resulting from traumatic posterior dislocation.

DIFFERENTIAL DIAGNOSIS

The differential diagnosis of the acute dislocation includes contusion, fracture, and acute rotator cuff tear, all of which may coexist. Radiographs in three planes should resolve the diagnosis of dislocation. The differential diagnosis of recurrent instability is more difficult. It includes all causes of recurrent shoulder dysfunction, such as impingement, cuff tear, loose bodies, glenohumeral joint surface roughness, and snapping scapula. A careful history of the first episode and circumstances of recurrence, plus repeated physical examinations that include stress tests and radiographs to look for clues of instability, should lead to the correct diagnosis.

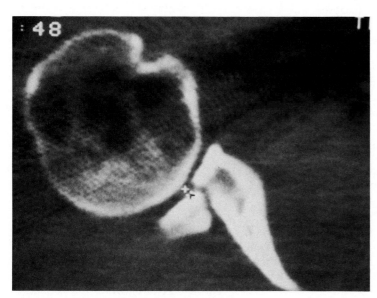

Fig. 13-84. A CT scan of the glenohumeral joint demonstrates a fracture of the posterior glenoid rim as a result of posterior dislocation of the glenohumeral joint. *(Matsen, F. A., III; Thomas, S. C.; and Rockwood, C. A., Jr.: Anterior Glenohumeral Instability. In Rockwood, C. A., and Matsen, F. A., III (eds.): The Shoulder, Fig. 14-57. Philadelphia, W. B. Saunders, 1990.)*

TREATMENT

ANTERIOR AND POSTERIOR DISLOCATIONS

Anterior Dislocations

ACUTE TRAUMATIC ANTERIOR DISLOCATIONS

Acute dislocations of the glenohumeral joint should be reduced as quickly and gently as possible. Whenever possible, a complete set of radiographs should be obtained prior to reduction to rule out associated bony injuries. Early relocation promptly eliminates the stretch and compression of neurovascular structures, minimizes the amount of muscle spasm that must be overcome to effect reduction, and prevents progressive enlargement of the humeral head defect in locked dislocations. The extent of anesthesia required to accomplish a gentle reduction depends on many factors, including the amount of trauma that produced the dislocation, the duration of the dislocation, the number of previous dislocations, whether the dislocation is locked, and to what extent the patient can voluntarily relax the shoulder musculature. When seen acutely, some dislocations can be reduced without medication. At the other extreme, reduction of a long-standing, locked dislocation may require a brachial plexus block or general anesthetic with muscle relaxation. Many practitioners use narcotics and muscle relaxants to aid in the reduction of shoulder dislocations. A potential trap exists: the dosages required to produce muscle relaxation while the shoulder is dislocated may be sufficient to produce respiratory depression once the shoulder is reduced. Our recommendation is that if these medications are to be used, they should be administered through an established intravenous line. This produces a more rapid onset, a short duration of action, and the opportunity to adjust the required dose more appropriately. Furthermore, resuscitation (if necessary) is facilitated by the prospective presence of such a route of access. Airway management tools should be readily available.

Two different principles have been used in the reduction of shoulder dislocation—traction and leverage. Many of the older texts and some of the more current ones prefer the leverage techniques, but more recently, concern has grown over the possibility of damaging the capsule, axillary vessels, and the brachial plexus when applying the great force used during leverage. (See Fig. 13-2.)

Hippocratic Technique. Hippocrates' original technique[5] is still effective when only one person is available to reduce the shoulder. The stockinged foot of the physician is used as countertraction. The heel should not go into the axilla (ie, between the anterior and posterior axillary folds), but should extend across the folds and against the chest wall. Traction should be slow and gentle; as with all traction techniques, the arm may be gently rotated internally and externally to disengage the head (Fig. 13-85).

Stimson's Technique. Although Lewis A. Stimson[1261–1265] of New York City is credited for the method of reduction that bears his name, he attributed it to Dr. Cole, a house-staff physician of the Chambers Street Hospital. It was a variation of Stimson's technique of obtaining muscle relaxation in the prone position to reduce a posterior dislocation of the hip. The patient is placed prone on the edge of the examining table while downward traction is gently applied (Fig. 13-86).[1265] McLaughlin thought the weight of the arm may be sufficient to reduce the shoulder. The use of weights is a subsequent modification of the original technique. Appropriate weights are taped to the wrist of the dislocated shoulder, which hangs free off the edge of the table. Five pounds is usually sufficient, but more or less weight may be used depending on the size of the patient. When using this technique, one should be patient since it may take 15 to 20 minutes for the reduction to occur. However, it is important that patients not be left unattended in this position, particularly if narcotics and muscle relaxants have been administered.

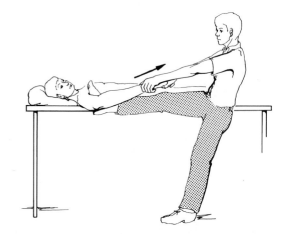

Fig. 13-85. Hippocratic technique of closed reduction. Note that the heel of the physician is not in the axilla and that the foot extends anteriorly and posteriorly across the axillary folds of the axilla.

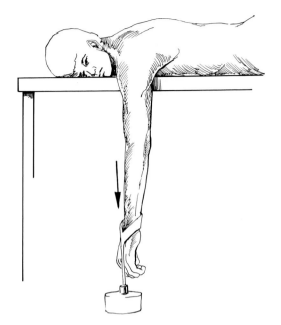

Fig. 13-86. The modified Stimson technique of closed reduction. The amount of weight hung from the hand depends on the size of the patient.

Milch's Technique.   In 1938 Milch[843] described a technique for reduction that employed abduction and external rotation. With the patient supine, the arm is abducted and externally rotated, and the thumb is used to gently push the head of the humerus back in place. Lacey[681] modified the technique by performing the maneuver with the patient prone on an examining table. Russell and associates[1156] reported on the ease and success of this technique.

Kocher's Leverage Technique.   In this maneuver, the humeral head is levered on the anterior glenoid and the shaft is levered against the anterior thoracic wall until the reduction is completed. We do not recommend it for routine use because of the complications that can occur during the leverage and manipulation.[1099] DePalma[293] warned that undue forces used in rotation leverage can damage the soft tissues of the shoulder joint, the vessels, and the brachial plexus. Beattie and co-workers[95] reported a fracture of the humeral neck during a Kocher procedure. Other authors have reported spiral fractures of the upper shaft of the humerus and further damage to the anterior capsular mechanism when the Kocher leverage technique of reduction was used. McMurray[826] reported that of 64

dislocations reduced by the Kocher method, 40% recurred, whereas of 112 dislocations reduced by gently lifting the head in place, only 12% recurred.

Miscellaneous Techniques.   Since 1975, numerous articles have been described dealing with simple techniques to reduce the dislocated shoulder: the forward elevation maneuver by Steel,[1253A] Janecki and Shahcheragh,[593] and Waldron;[1360] the external rotation method by Leidelmeyer[710] and Mirick and co-workers;[850] the scapular manipulation by Anderson and colleagues;[29] the modified gravity method by Lippert;[737] the crutch and chair technique by Parisien[993] and the chair and pillow technique by White.[1392] Manes[783] and Clotteau and colleagues[219] described other modifications.

CHRONIC ANTERIOR TRAUMATIC DISLOCATIONS

A glenohumeral joint that has been dislocated for several days is a chronic dislocation. As the chronicity of the dislocation increases, so do the difficulties and complications of reduction. The old, persistent, unreduced chronic dislocation is usually a very difficult problem to handle. When one encounters an elderly patient with pain in the shoulder whose x-ray films reveal an anterior dislocation, a very careful history is needed to determine whether the initial injury occurred acutely or a week to several months earlier.

The condition is noted most commonly in elderly people and in those whose general mental status may prevent them from seeking help at the time of the injury. Ten of 14 patients presented by Bennett[105] were more than 50 years old. The dislocation may be produced by a trivial injury, because with increasing age there is weakness and degeneration of the soft tissues.[850] In younger patients, the late diagnosis of an old, unreduced anterior dislocation of the shoulder is unusual, but may occur when the patient is unconscious for a period with severe multiple injuries.

McLaughlin[816] describes this type of shoulder dislocation as the most difficult of all. It is difficult to establish criteria for when to attempt closed reduction, when to operate and reduce the shoulder, and when to simply leave it alone. There are no established rules because conditions (ie, age of patient, length of time from dislocation, degree of symptoms, range of motion, radiographic findings, and general stability of the patient) can vary so much. If a closed reduction is to be performed, it should be done with minimal traction, without leverage, and with total muscle relaxation under controlled general anesthesia. Usually within 2 to

3 weeks of the dislocation, the humeral head is firmly impaled on the anterior glenoid, and there is so much soft tissue contraction and interposition that it is impossible to perform a gentle closed reduction. If a gentle closed reduction fails, an open procedure should be considered. This can be very difficult because of the distorted anatomy of the axillary artery and nerves, and because the structures are tight and "scarred down." Some older patients' old dislocations produce minimal symptoms, so nontreatment is selected owing to the hazards of open treatment. Ganel and co-workers[416] reported on four elderly patients with long-standing persistent dislocations of the shoulder who had relatively good functional results.

In performing an open reduction, the subscapularis and anterior capsule are incised near their insertion. External rotation and lateral traction usually will disimpact the humerus from the glenoid. The humerus is then gently internally rotated while lateral traction is applied to reduce the head. Leverage is avoided because the head is usually very soft. If the posterolateral head defect is greater than 40% or if the head collapses during reduction, a humeral head prosthesis is inserted. The subscapularis and capsule are then repaired. The shoulder is carefully inspected for cuff tears and vascular damage.

Schulz and associates[1194] reported that of 61 chronic dislocations in 58 patients, 17 (24%) were posterior and 44 (76%) were anterior. These dislocations occurred primarily among elderly people; more than half the dislocations were associated with fracture of the tuberosities, head or neck of the humerus, glenoid, or coracoid process, and more than one third involved neurologic deficits. Closed reduction was attempted in 40 shoulders and was successful in 20. Of the 20 shoulders successfully reduced (3 posterior and 17 anterior), the duration of dislocation exceeded 4 weeks in only one instance. Open reduction was performed in 20 and humeral head excision in six. Eight patients were not treated, and five shoulders were irreducible.

Perniceni and coworkers[1016] described the reinforcement of the anterior shoulder complex in three patients with old, unreduced anterior dislocations of the shoulder. They used the Gosset[452] technique, which places a rib graft between the coracoid and the glenoid rim. Rowe and Zarins[1134] reported on 24 patients with unreduced dislocations of the shoulder and operated on 14 of them. They concluded the operative treatment gave better results than previously reported.

INDICATIONS FOR EARLY SURGERY

In addition to the need for open reduction for the rare irreducible dislocation, a few other situations exist in which early surgery may be indicated in the early management of shoulder dislocations.

Soft Tissue Interposition. If the rotator cuff, capsule, or biceps tendon prevents reduction, operative reduction will be required. Tietjen[1300] reported a case of avulsion of the supraspinatus, infraspinatus, and teres minor, which at the time of surgery were interposed between the humeral head and the glenoid.

Displaced Fracture of the Greater Tuberosity. Although fractures of the greater tuberosity are not uncommon with anterior shoulder dislocations, the tuberosity usually reduces into an acceptable position when the shoulder is reduced. Occasionally, the greater tuberosity fragment displaces up under the acromion process or is pulled posteriorly by the cuff muscles. If the greater tuberosity remains displaced following reduction of the shoulder joint, consideration should be given to anatomical reduction and internal fixation of the fragment and repair of the attendant split in the tendons of the rotator cuff. It is relatively easy to determine the amount of superior displacement of the tuberosity fragment on the anteroposterior roentgenogram in the plane of the scapula. The scapular lateral radiograph is helpful to determine the amount of posterior displacement. If the tuberosity is allowed to heal with posterior displacement, it may produce not only the functional equivalent of a rotator cuff tear, but also a bony block to external rotation. Norris and co-workers[935] found that CT scans were necessary to define the anteroposterior position of displaced tuberosity fragments in 10 of 18 cases.

Glenoid Rim Fracture. Aston and Gregory[57] reported three cases in which large anterior fractures of the glenoid occurred as a result of a fall on the lateral aspect of the abducted shoulder. A fracture of the anterior glenoid lip may be associated with an anterior dislocation, recurring subluxation, or recurrent anterior dislocation. Open reduction and internal fixation of displaced lip fractures offers the opportunity to anatomically restore the capsule and ligamentous attachments to the glenoid.

SPECIAL PROBLEMS

Occasionally it may be necessary to perform an early surgical reconstruction in a patient who re-

quires absolute and complete shoulder stability before being able to return to his or her occupation
(eg, someone involved in the construction of a high-
rise building who has to walk and balance on steel
beams, or an athlete whose income depends on
having a full, stable range of motion). A surgical
repair done 2 weeks after the initial traumatic injury
will allow the patient to have full function and stability more reliably than the usual treatment of 3
to 4 weeks in a shoulder immobilizer.

MATSEN'S PREFERRED METHOD OF ANTERIOR REDUCTION

I find that reduction of either anterior or posterior
glenohumeral dislocations usually can be effected
by traction on the abducted and flexed arm. The
elbow is also flexed to relax the neurovascular
structures of the arm. This maneuver may be carried
out with the patient in either a prone or supine
position, as long as the body is fixed to resist the
traction force. The only drawback with the prone
position (Stimson's maneuver) is the discomfort the
patient experiences in assuming it. I commonly
place the patient supine with a sheet around the
thorax, with the loose ends on the side opposite
the shoulder dislocation, where they are held by
an assistant (Fig. 13-87). The surgeon stands on the
side of the dislocated shoulder near the patient's
waist. The elbow of the dislocated shoulder is flexed
to 90°. A second sheet, tied loosely around the surgeon's waist, is looped over the patient's forearm
so it lies just distal to the flexed elbow. While the
assistant provides countertraction by pulling on the
sheet around the patient's thorax, the surgeon applies traction to the shoulder by leaning back
against the sheet around his waist and grasping the
forearm. Steady traction along the axis of the arm
will usually effect reduction. Anesthesia, muscle
relaxants, and analgesics are often unnecessary
with this gentle method. To this basic maneuver,
one may add gentle rocking of the humerus from
internal to external rotation, or outward pressure
on the proximal humerus from the axilla. These
additions are particularly useful if prereduction axillary roentgenograms show the humeral head to
be impaled on the glenoid rim. Postreduction
roentgenograms are used to confirm reduction and
to detect fractures. A postreduction neurovascular
check is routine.

ROCKWOOD'S PREFERRED METHOD OF ANTERIOR REDUCTION

I prefer the traction and countertraction method
(Fig. 13-88). I use a combination of narcotics, with

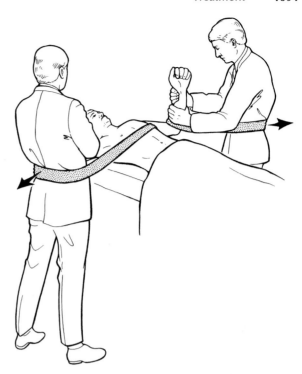

Fig. 13-87. Reduction technique for anterior glenohumeral dislocation. The patient lies supine with a sheet
placed around the thorax, then around the assistant's
waist; this provides countertraction. The surgeon stands
on the side of the dislocated shoulder near the patient's
waist with the elbow of the dislocated shoulder flexed
to 90°. A second sheet is tied loosely around the waist
of the surgeon and looped over the patient's forearm,
thereby providing traction while the surgeon leans back
against the sheet, grasping the forearm. Steady traction
along the axis of the arm will usually cause reduction.
The surgeon's hands are free to gently rock the humerus
from internal to external rotation or to provide gentle
outward pressure on the proximal humerus from the
axilla. (Matsen, F. A., III; Thomas, S. C.; and Rockwood,
C. A., Jr.: Anterior Glenohumeral Instability. In Rockwood,
C. A., and Matsen, F. A., III (eds.): The Shoulder, Fig. 14-
58. Philadelphia, W. B. Saunders, 1990.)

muscle relaxants or tranquilizers, and perform the
reduction in the emergency department. An intravenous line is routinely established in the normal
arm. Half the narcotics are given intramuscularly,
and half are given through the intravenous tubing,
followed by administration of a tranquilizer or
muscle relaxant. A sheet, folded to form a 5-inch
swathe, is used as the countertraction to stabilize
the chest. After 5 to 6 minutes have passed, very
gentle traction is applied to the involved arm in

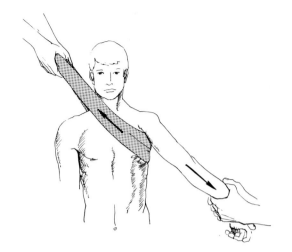

Fig. 13-88. Closed reduction of the left shoulder with traction against countertraction. *(Matsen, F. A., III; Thomas, S. C.; and Rockwood, C. A., Jr.: Anterior Glenohumeral Instability. In Rockwood, C. A., and Matsen, F. A., III (eds.): The Shoulder, Fig. 14-59. Philadelphia, W. B. Saunders, 1990.)*

line with the deformity, and the traction is increased very gradually against the countertraction. Occasionally, gentle internal and external rotation is used to disengage the head from the glenoid rim. With very gentle and gradual traction, the reduction can be accomplished without pain, and sometimes even without any palpable sensation of reduction. In some larger patients, the reduction may be so atraumatic that neither the physician nor the patient feels or sees the reduction. It is only after traction has been discontinued that the patient moves his arm about, stating that everything is all right. If this technique is unsuccessful and there are no other contraindications, I prefer to use general anesthesia, again with traction–countertraction maneuvers, instead of the leverage type of reduction.

POSTREDUCTION MANAGEMENT

After reducing the glenohumeral joint, repeat anteroposterior and lateral x-ray views are obtained in the plane of the scapula to verify the adequacy of the reduction and to provide an additional opportunity to detect fractures of the glenoid and proximal humerus. The patient's neurologic status is checked, including the sensory and motor functions of all five major nerves in the upper extremity. The strength of the pulse is verified and evidence of bruits or an expanding hematoma is sought.[467] The integrity of the rotator cuff is initially evaluated

by observing the strength of isometric external rotation and abduction.

Trimmings[1315] demonstrated that aspiration of the hemarthrosis from the shoulder can be an effective means of reducing discomfort after the shoulder is reduced.

Because recurrent glenohumeral instability is the most common complication of glenohumeral dislocation, postreduction treatment focuses on optimizing shoulder stability. Thus, two potentially important elements in postreduction treatment are protection and muscle rehabilitation. Reeves demonstrated in primates that it took 3 months before normal capsular patterns of collagen bundles were observed, 5 months before the subscapularis tendon was histologically normal, and 4 to 5 months before tensile strength was regained.[1074] It is unknown whether labral tears or ligamentous avulsions from the glenoid heal, or how long this might take. In any event, it is apparent that the shoulder should not be immobilized for the length of time required for complete healing. Traumatic anterior dislocations in young patients are usually managed by 2 to 5 weeks of postreduction immobilization; shorter periods are indicated for patients older than 30 years, owing to their lower predilection for recurrence and greater tendency for shoulder stiffness.[651,814,815,1144,1414] (See under Complications of Injury for further discussion of the relationship between the period of immobilization and the incidence of recurrence.)

The position of immobilization should be one of comfortable adduction and internal rotation. This position relaxes the injured anterior structures. Tight bandaging is not required, and the immobilization need not be absolute. The elbow should be fully extended at least several times a day. Allowing the arm to externally rotate to zero degrees twice a day is helpful in preventing "sling soreness." It is again emphasized that persons older than 30 years tend to develop stiffness of the shoulder, elbow, and hand with immobilization. Thus, in this population, mobilization may be instituted within a week after anterior dislocation. In this approach, external rotation is allowed to 30° and flexion to 90° for the first 3 weeks, then to 40° and 140°, respectively, for the next 3 weeks.

During the period of protection, the patient is instructed in progressive isometric exercises, particularly of the internal and external shoulder rotator muscles. The patient will not be well served by the atrophy of disuse. After the period of immobilization, more vigorous rotator-strengthening exercises using rubber tubing or weights are prescribed. Strong subscapularis and infraspinatus muscles are ideally situated to increase glenohumeral stability.[1163] Range-of-motion exercises are rarely needed after a routine glenohumeral dislocation in a young patient. Swimming is recommended at 6 weeks to enhance endurance and coordination. By 3 months after the dislocation, most patients should have almost full flexion and rotation of the shoulder. The patient is not allowed to use the injured arm in sports or for over-the-head labor until normal rotator strength and nearly full forward elevation are achieved. Any deviation from the expected course of recovery requires careful reevaluation for occult fractures, loose bodies, rotator cuff tears, peripheral nerve injuries, and glenohumeral arthritis. Matsen's management of first dislocations in a 17-year-old and a 38-year-old are contrasted in Table 13-1.

In the very rare situation in which a locked anterior dislocation cannot be managed as described here, open reduction may be accomplished after the subscapularis and anterior capsule are incised from the lesser tuberosity. After open reduction, the subscapularis and capsule are repaired.

Posterior Dislocations

REDUCTION OF ACUTE POSTERIOR DISLOCATIONS

Patients with acute, traumatic posterior dislocations of the shoulder usually have much more pain than those with acute, traumatic anterior dislocations. The use of intravenous narcotics, combined with muscle relaxants or tranquilizers to reduce the dislocation, may be unsuccessful; general anesthesia with muscle relaxation may be required. Closed reduction usually can be accomplished once the muscle spasm has been eliminated. With the patient supine, traction should be applied to the adducted arm in the line of the deformity, along with a gentle lifting of the head back into the glenoid fossa. Care should be taken not to force the arm into external rotation; if the head is locked posteriorly on the glenoid rim, the forced rotation could produce a fracture of the head or shaft of the humerus. If the maneuver is done gently after good muscle relaxation has been achieved, the reduction is atraumatic. If the prereduction radiographs show that the head is locked on the posterior glenoid, distal traction on the arm should be combined with lateral traction on the upper arm. A folded towel or soft roller bandage can be used by an assistant to apply the lateral traction. In locked posterior dislocations, reduction may be facilitated by gently internally rotating the humerus to stretch out the posterior capsule and cuff musculature before reduction is attempted.

If gentle closed reduction of a locked posterior glenohumeral dislocation is not possible, open reduction may be accomplished through an anterior deltopectoral approach.[319,500,608,670,683,818,1121] Be-

Table 13-1. Comparison of Management of First Anterior Dislocation in Patients of Two Ages

	17-Year-Old Patient	38-Year-Old Patient
Pathology anticipated	Inferior glenohumeral ligament avulsion from glenoid	Capsule and/or cuff tear
Neurovascular check	X	X
Three radiographic views relative to plane of scapula	X	X
Radiographic findings	Posterolateral head defect Possible anteroinferior glenoid chip	Possible greater tuberosity fracture —
Reduction by two-sheet method	X	X
Postreduction neurovascular examination	X	X
Postreduction radiographs	X	X
Possible cuff tear	—	X
Possible axillary palsy	X	X
Sling	X	X
Elbow straightening twice daily	X	X
Immediate isometrics for rotator muscles	X	X
Concern about stiffness	—	X
Avoid external rotation beyond 0° and flexion beyond 90° for	6 weeks	2 weeks
Start vigorous range-of-motion exercises	3 months	6 weeks
Start vigorous internal and external strengthening	6 weeks	2 weeks
Start swimming	6 weeks	Earlier if possible
Concern about redislocation	High	Low

cause local anatomy is significantly distorted, the tendon of the long head of the biceps is used as a guide to the lesser tuberosity. The subscapularis is released either by lesser tuberosity osteotomy or by direct incision. With the glenoid thus exposed, open reduction is carried out. After reduction, the humeral head defect may be rendered extra-articular by filling it with the subscapularis tendon[818,819,823] or the lesser tuberosity.[1104] If the humeral head defect involves more than 30% of the articular surface, prosthetic replacement may be indicated.

Moeller[857] reported on a patient who had an open acute posterior dislocation of the left shoulder. The shoulder was totally unstable following reduction with tears of the rotator cuff, biceps tendon, and subscapularis tendons. The patient had associated injury to the axillary and suprascapular nerves.

Hawkins and co-workers[500] reviewed 41 cases of locked posterior shoulder dislocations. The average interval between injury and diagnosis was 1 year! In seven shoulders the deformity was accepted. Closed reduction was successful in only 6 of the 12 cases in which it was attempted.

POSTREDUCTION CARE

If the shoulder is stable after closed reduction, McLaughlin recommended immobilization in a sling-and-swathe position. However, if the shoulder tends to subluxate or redislocate in the sling-and-swathe position, a shoulder spica or some type of modification should be used. The amount of external rotation is determined by applying the cast with the arm in its most stable position. Cautilli and colleagues[196,197] do not recommend the sling-and-swathe position (internal rotation), because it places the injured posterior structures under tension. Their immobilization technique consists of a padded plaster cast around the waist and a padded circle of plaster around the wrist. These two casts are then connected by a wooden bar and held in place with plaster. The shoulder is usually immobilized in neutral to slight external rotation. A sling of stockinette may be used to support the arm.

Wilson and McKeever[1403] stated that many acute traumatic posterior dislocations are unstable and recommended the use of Steinmann pins to maintain reduction. In their technique, after the shoulder has been reduced, two pins are drilled in cruciate fashion down from the acromion process into the reduced humeral head. The pins are removed after 3 weeks and rehabilitation begins. There is a danger of pin breakage when the pins are placed from the acromion into the head or from the head into the glenoid.

A large anteromedial humeral head defect, as is occasionally seen on axillary lateral x-ray views, may predispose to recurrent dislocations. Therefore, the shoulder can best be immobilized with the arm in external rotation to allow posterior capsular healing. Scougall[1202] has shown in monkeys that a surgically detached posterior glenoid labrum and capsule heal soundly without repair. He concluded that the best position of immobilization to allow healing for all posterior structures is in abduction, external rotation, and extension; and that this position should be maintained for 4 weeks.

EARLY SURGERY IN ACUTE TRAUMATIC POSTERIOR DISLOCATIONS

Indications for surgery include a major displacement of an associated lesser tuberosity fragment, a major fragment off the posterior glenoid, an irreducible dislocation, open dislocation, or an unstable reduction.

The specific indication for the McLaughlin operation is the presence of an anteromedial humeral head defect so large that a stable reduction cannot be achieved. Through an anterior approach, the subscapularis is detached from the lesser tuberosity; the shoulder is reduced and the subscapular tendon is transferred into the head defect.[716,820] Neer[1104] modified this operation by transferring the lesser tuberosity with the tendon into the defect. The added fragment of the lesser tuberosity helps fill the space in the defect, and it is simpler to perform, because the lesser tuberosity can be secured into the defect with a bone screw (Fig. 13-89). Nicola and co-workers[923] reported a successful result in a patient who had bilateral posterior fracture–dislocations following a seizure, and who was treated with Neer's modification of the McLaughlin procedure.

In their series of locked posterior dislocations, Hawkins and associates[500] used subscapularis transfer into the defect, lesser tuberosity transfer, hemiarthroplasty, and total shoulder arthroplasty, according to the specific problem.

McLaughlin recommended a sling-and-swathe position following the transfer of the subscapularis muscle for 2 weeks. Rockwood[1104] recommends immobilization of the arm in a position of neutral rotation in a modified shoulder spica cast for 6 weeks (Fig. 13-90). The rehabilitation program following removal of the cast consists of 3 to 4 weeks' gentle use of the shoulder for everyday living activities, followed by gentle stretching exercises, and finally, resistive exercises to gain strength in the internal and external rotators and the deltoid mus-

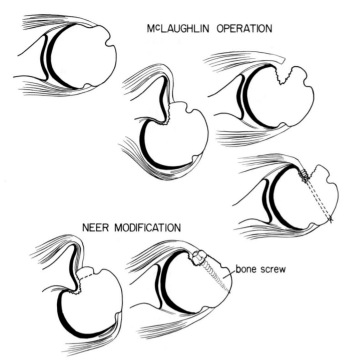

Fig. 13-89. When there is a large anteromedial humeral head defect, McLaughlin recommended that following reduction through an anterior approach the tendon of the subscapularis be transferred into the humeral head defect. Neer has modified the procedure by transferring the lesser tuberosity with the attaching subscapularis tendon into the defect.

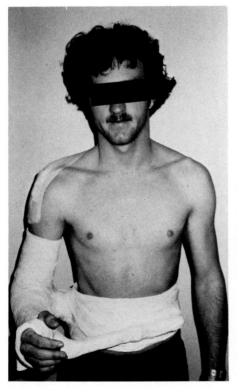
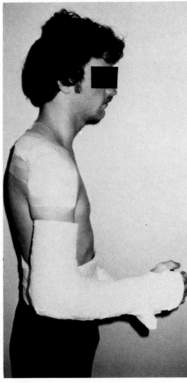

Fig. 13-90. Frontal and side views of the type of cast used following posterior surgical reconstruction and following acute traumatic posterior dislocation of the shoulder. This is a lightweight, long-arm cast connected to a well-padded band of plaster about the waist. The arm is maintained in neutral rotation, in slight extension, and in 15° to 20° of abduction.

cles. The patient should not return to any heavy lifting or heavy work until full range of motion and strength have been regained—usually after 3 to 6 months.

Rowe and Zarins[1134] did not use a postoperative cast or brace following reconstruction of unreduced posterior dislocation. Instead, they positioned the arm at the side of the body, posterior to the coronal plane, and held it with a strip of Elastoplast tape or a canvas restraint.

CHRONIC POSTERIOR DISLOCATIONS

If a patient, especially an older patient, has had a chronic posterior dislocation for months or years, and if there is minimal pain and a functional range of motion, surgery may not be indicated (Fig. 13-91). However, if disability exists and there is good bone stock to the glenohumeral joint, reconstruction should be considered. Rowe and Zarins,[1134] in a review of 23 patients with chronic dislocations that had been unreduced over 3 weeks, found that 14 were posterior and 8 were anterior. Fourteen of these shoulders were operated upon. Seven patients had open reduction with preservation of the humeral head; one had a total shoulder replacement two received humeral head prostheses, and four were treated with humeral head resection.

AUTHORS' PREFERRED METHOD OF TREATMENT

Our management of acute traumatic posterior dislocations begins with a definition of the extent and chronicity of the injury. A complete radiographic evaluation is necessary, including anteroposterior and lateral views in the plane of the scapula and an axillary view. Careful note is made of associated fractures, including the extent of the impression fracture of the anteromedial humeral head. A gentle closed reduction is attempted, using axial traction on the arm. If the head is locked on the glenoid rim, gentle internal rotation may stretch out the posterior capsule to facilitate reduction. Lateral traction on the proximal humerus may unlock the humeral head. Once it is unlocked, the humerus is gently externally rotated. After reduction is achieved and confirmed by postreduction radio-

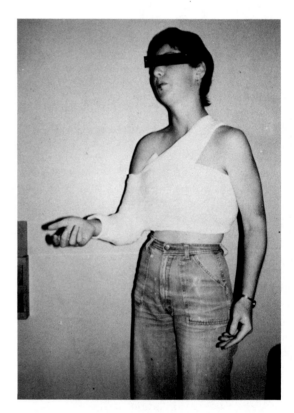

Fig. 13-92. Handshake cast. After closed reduction of an acute traumatic posterior dislocation is confirmed by x-ray films, a cast is applied in neutral rotation and slight extension for 3 weeks. *(Matsen, F. A., III; Thomas, S. C.; and Rockwood, C. A., Jr.: Anterior Glenohumeral Instability. In Rockwood, C. A., and Matsen, F. A., III (eds.): The Shoulder, Fig. 14-60. Philadelphia, W. B. Saunders, 1990.)*

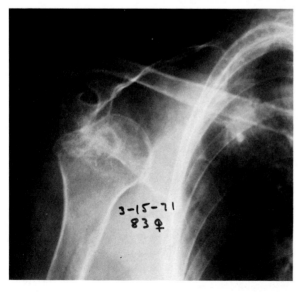

Fig. 13-91. Unreduced anterior dislocation in an 83-year-old patient. Because she had very little pain and 75° of flexion, it was elected to treat this dislocation nonoperatively.

graphs, the reduction is maintained for 3 weeks by a cummerbund "handshake" cast in neutral rotation and slight extension (Fig. 13-92). This position relaxes the injured structures. External rotation and deltoid isometrics are carried out during immobilization. After removal of the cast, a vigorous internal and external rotator-strengthening program is initiated. Range of motion is allowed to return with active use. Vigorous physical activities are not resumed until the shoulder is strong and 3 months have elapsed since reduction. Swimming is encouraged to develop endurance and muscle coordination.

If, on axillary lateral radiographs, the head of the humerus has a large reverse Hill-Sachs compression fracture and is locked on the posterior rim of the glenoid, an anterior approach should be used to reduce the humeral head, and the subscapularis tendons can be used to transfer into the defect in the humeral head (Fig. 13-93).

RECURRENT INSTABILITY

Recurrent Anterior Instability

In the management of recurrent glenohumeral instability, perhaps the greatest challenge is to be sure of what condition is being treated. At the risk of oversimplifying, we have found it useful to recognize that most patients with recurrent instability fall into one of two large groups. The first is characterized by a history of definite *trauma* initiating a problem of *unidirectional* shoulder instability.

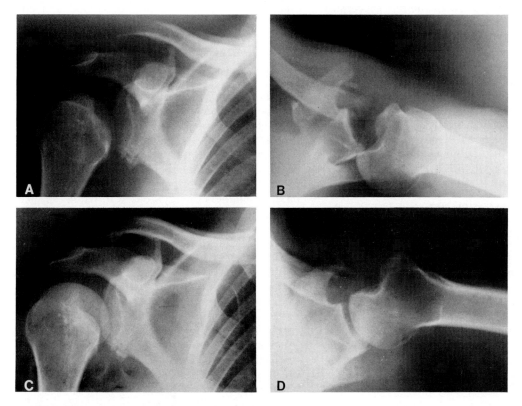

Fig. 13-93. Management of permanent posterior dislocation of the shoulder. (**A**) Subacromial permanent posterior dislocation of the right shoulder reveals a vacant glenoid sign and the appearance that the posterior glenoid rim has created a large defect in the humeral head. (**B**) The axillary lateral view confirms the large anteromedial compression defect in the humeral head. Note the majority of the articular surface of the humeral head is posterior to the glenoid fossa. (**C**) The anteroposterior view shows that following the McLaughlin reconstruction, through an anterior approach, the humeral head is well within the glenoid fossa. (**D**) An axillary lateral x-ray film confirms that the head of the humerus is relocated to the glenoid fossa. The subscapularis tendon has been transferred into the depth of the anteromedial defect, which blocks recurrent dislocations during internal rotation of the shoulder.

These shoulders usually have definite structural damage. When the direction of traumatic instability is anterior, the shoulders commonly have ruptures of the glenohumeral ligaments at their glenoid attachments, referred to as *Bankart* (Perthes) lesions. Finally, these shoulders frequently require *surgery* to achieve stability. To help remember this grouping, we use the acronym TUBS (Table 13-2). A typical patient is a 17-year-old skier whose recurrent anterior instability began with a fall on an abducted, externally rotated arm.

Patients in the second group have no history of significant trauma; thus, instability is *atraumatic*. These patients are much more prone to have *multidirectional* instability that is *bilateral*. *Rehabilitation*, especially rotator cuff–strengthening and coordination exercises, is the first line of treatment. If surgery is performed, laxity of the *inferior* capsule must be managed with an inferior capsular shift. The acronym for this group is AMBRI (Table 13-2). A typical patient is a 15-year-old swimmer whose shoulders are becoming painful, and on examination are found to be loose in all directions.

Although many variants of these basic themes exist, it is essential to differentiate the shoulder that goes out because it has suffered a major injury from one that goes out because it is constitutionally loose. This fundamental distinction can become obscured in some of the very involved classifications that have been proposed.

NONOPERATIVE MANAGEMENT

Coordinated, strong contraction of the muscles of the rotator cuff is one of the important mechanisms of shoulder stability. Sidles and co-workers[1224] have shown that a compressive load applied to the glenohumeral joint is able to resist a translational force two thirds as large as the compressive force. Shoulders with looser capsules, such as those of pitchers, swimmers, and gymnasts, have a greater relative dependence on this dynamic stabilizing mechanism.

Table 13-2. Two Types of Recurrent Instability

Traumatic
Unidirectional
Bankart lesion (avulsion of glenohumeral ligaments from glenoid)
Surgery is often necessary
Atraumatic
Multidirectional
Bilateral
Rehabilitation enhances stability
Inferior capsular shift should be a part of repair if surgery is necessary

Saha and associates[1160–1163,1168,1169] point to deficiencies of the posterior shoulder depressor or steering muscles as a major factor in recurrent instability. Many, if not most, of these deficiencies in muscle strength should respond to vigorous internal and external rotator–strengthening exercises. Both internal and external rotator strength contribute to anterior and posterior stability. Coordinated contractions of the cuff muscles help hold the humerus in the glenoid and resist potentially displacing forces. Rotator-strengthening exercises are most effectively performed by keeping the humerus close to the body and rotating the arm against the resistance of rubber tubing, spring exercises, or weights in the sidelying position. A useful goal is to strive for sufficient strength in both directions to rotate 20 times against a resistance of 20% of the body weight (the "20–20" goal). Rockwood and colleagues[1103] found that 12% of patients with traumatic subluxation, 80% with anterior atraumatic subluxation, and 90% with posterior instability responded to a special rehabilitation program. (See Fig. 13-129.)

Although any form of glenohumeral instability may benefit from this rehabilitation, it is particularly indicated in patients with the AMBRI syndrome. Nonoperative management is desirable for patients with voluntary instability, for those with posterior glenohumeral instability, and for those requiring a supranormal range of motion (such as baseball pitchers and gymnasts) in whom surgical management often does not permit return to a competitive level of function.[497,1129,1163]

Because the coordination of muscle contraction is a key element of dynamic stability, smooth repetitive activities (eg, swimming) play an essential role in this treatment program. In addition to rotator strengthening and coordination exercises, patients with voluntary shoulder instability require a careful explanation of the importance of avoiding intentional glenohumeral subluxation or dislocation. They must understand that each time they let the shoulder go out of joint it makes it looser and more prone to unpredictable instability.

OPERATIVE MANAGEMENT

In contemplating a surgical approach to anterior glenohumeral instability, it is essential to identify any factors that may compromise the surgical results, such as generalized ligamentous laxity, multidirectional instability, or significant bony defects of the humeral head or glenoid. When these conditions exist, it is necessary to tailor the surgical procedure to the specific pathology.

Surgical stabilization of the glenohumeral joint is considered if instability or apprehension repeatedly compromises shoulder comfort or function in spite of a reasonable trial of internal and external rotator strengthening and coordination exercises. A vigorous effort to stabilize the shoulder with exercises is particularly indicated in patients with multidirectional or posterior instability and in athletes requiring a completely normal or supranormal range of motion. Surgical stabilization is not indicated in patients with a refractory desire to voluntarily subluxate or dislocate the glenohumeral joint. Surgery is especially not indicated in patients with atraumatic instability who are emotionally unstable.

Many surgical procedures have been described for the treatment of recurrent anterior glenohumeral instability. Tightening, and to some degree realigning, the subscapularis tendon and partially eliminating external rotation are the goals of the Magnuson-Stack and the Putti-Platt procedures. The Putti-Platt operation also tightens and reinforces the anterior capsule. Reattachment of the capsule and glenoid labrum to the glenoid lip is the goal of the Bankart repair, the DuToit staple capsulorrhaphy, and the Eyre-Brook capsulorrhaphy.[364,365] Augmentation of the bony anterior glenoid lip is the objective of anterior bone block procedures. The Bristow procedure transfers the tip of the coracoid process with its muscle attachments and also creates a musculotendinous sling across the anteroinferior tendon at the front of the glenohumeral joint. An anterior glenoid bone buttress procedure is the objective of the Oudard and Trillat procedure. A large posterolateral humeral head defect may be approached by limiting external rotation, by filling the defect with the infraspinatus tendon, or by performing a rotational osteotomy of the humerus.[196,197,1273,1381]

Capsular Repairs

Bankart Procedure. The Bankart repair was apparently first done by Perthes[1018] in 1906, who recommended the repair of the anterior capsule to the anterior glenoid rim. He was not in doubt about the pathology of traumatic instability: "In every case the anterior margin of the glenoid cavity will be found to be smooth, rounded, and free of any attachments, and a blunt instrument can be passed freely inwards over the bare bone on the front of the neck of the scapula." He reattached the capsule to the glenoid rim by placing drill holes through the bone. Credit for this type of repair should go to

Perthes, but the popularity of the technique stems from the work of Bankart,[75,76] who first performed the operation in 1923 on one of his former house surgeons. The procedure commonly used today is based on Bankart's 1939[75] article, in which he discusses the repair of the capsule to the bone of the anterior glenoid through the use of drill holes and suture. The subscapularis muscle, which is carefully divided to expose the capsule, is reapproximated without any overlap or shortening. Bankart reported 27 consecutive cases with "full movements of the joint and in no case has there been any recurrence of the dislocation."[124,1118,1135,1143]

Hovelius and co-workers[556] found a 2% redislocation rate after the Bankart procedure, compared with 19% after the Putti-Platt operation. More than one third of patients younger than 25 years were dissatisfied with the results of the Putti-Platt procedure. Rowe and Zarins[1135] reported a series of 50 subluxating shoulders with good or excellent results in 94% after a Bankart repair; Bankart lesions were found in 32 of these shoulders.

Rowe and co-workers[1127] reported on 51 shoulders with fractures of the anterior rim of the glenoid. Eighteen shoulders had fractures involving one sixth or less of the glenoid, 26 involved one fourth of the glenoid, and 7 had one third of the anterior glenoid fractured. In this group of patients, who were treated with Bankart repair without particular attention to the fracture, the overall incidence of failure was 2%.

Many shoulder surgeons consider this the procedure of choice for management of traumatic unidirectional instability, which is almost always associated with avulsion of the glenohumeral ligaments from the glenoid.

Staple Capsulorrhaphy. In the DuToit staple capsulorrhaphy, the detached capsule is secured back to the glenoid using staples.[326,1233] Actually, the staple repair had been described 50 years earlier by Perthes. Rao and associates[1067] reported follow-up on 65 patients having DuToit staple repair of the avulsion of the capsule from the glenoid rim. Of these, 94% had separation of the labrum from the rim. Good to excellent results were obtained in 98%; 58% were able to return to athletics. Two patients showed radiographic evidence of loose staples.

O'Driscoll and Evans[949] reviewed 269 consecutive DuToit capsulorrhaphies in 257 patients for a median follow-up of 8.8 years. Eighty-eight percent of the procedures were performed for dislocations and 12% for subluxations. Fifty-three per cent of the patients had postoperative pain. Internal and external rotation were limited. Recurrence was reported in 28% if stapling alone was done and in 8% if a Putti-Platt procedure was added; 11% had staple loosening, migration, or penetration of cartilage. Staple complications contributed to pain, physical restrictions, and osteoarthritis.

The use of staples for surgical repairs may be associated with major complications (Figs. 13-94 and 13-95).[1429]

Subscapularis Muscle Procedures

Putti-Platt Procedure. In 1948 Osmond-Clark[964] described this procedure, which was used by Sir Harry Platt of England and Vittorio Putti of Italy. Platt first used this technique in November 1925. Some years later, Osmond-Clarke saw Putti perform essentially the same operation that had been his standard practice since 1923. Scaglietta,[1184] one of Putti's pupils, revealed that the operation may well have been performed first by Codivilla, Putti's teacher and predecessor. Neither Putti nor Platt ever described the technique in the literature.

In the Putti-Platt procedure, the subscapularis tendon is divided 2.5 cm from its insertion. The anterior shoulder joint capsule, which adheres to the posterior surface of the subscapularis tendon, may be opened in the same plane as the tendon is divided so the joint can be inspected. The lateral stump of the tendon is attached to the "most convenient soft-tissue structure along the anterior rim of the glenoid cavity."[964] If the capsule and labrum have been stripped from the anterior glenoid and the neck of the scapula, the tendon is sutured to the deep surface of the capsule, and "it is advisable to raw the anterior surface of the neck of the scapula, so that the sutured tendo-capsule will adhere to it."[964] After the lateral tendon stump is secured, the medial muscle stump is lapped over the lateral stump, producing a substantial shortening of the capsule and subscapularis muscle.

In those instances when the medial capsule can be separated from the medial muscle tendon unit, the capsule is sutured on top of the secured lateral tendon and the medial muscle tendon unit is then secured over the capsule laterally in the area of the greater tuberosity of the humerus. The exact placement of the lateral stump into the anterior soft tissues and of the medial stump into the greater tuberosity is determined so that after the procedure, the arm should externally rotate to the neutral position.

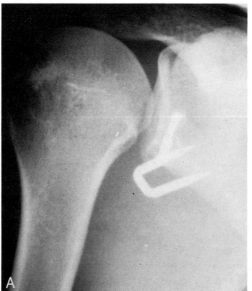
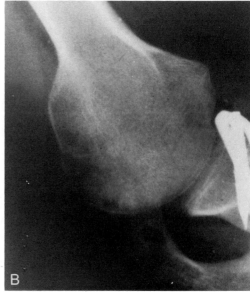

Fig. 13-94. Complications of staple capsulorrhaphy. (**A**) An anteroposterior x-ray film showing a prominent staple on the inferior glenoid rim. (**B**) An axillary view showing staple impingement on the head of the humerus. *(Matsen, F. A., III; Thomas, S. C.; and Rockwood, C. A., Jr.: Anterior Glenohumeral Instability. In Rockwood, C. A., and Matsen, F. A., III (eds.): The Shoulder, Fig. 14-61. Philadelphia, W. B. Saunders, 1990.)*

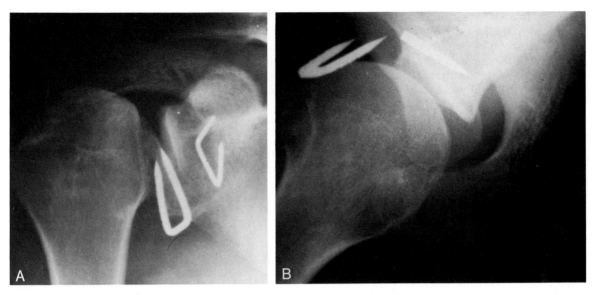

Fig. 13-95. Loose staple after staple capsulorrhaphy. (**A**) An anteroposterior x-ray film showing a loose staple in the glenohumeral joint. (**B**) Axillary view. (*Matsen, F. A., III; Thomas, S. C.; and Rockwood, C. A., Jr.: Anterior Glenohumeral Instability. In Rockwood, C. A., and Matsen, F. A., III (eds.): The Shoulder, Fig. 14-62. Philadelphia, W. B. Saunders, 1990.*)

Blazina and Satzman[124] described the use of the Putti-Platt procedure to manage anterior shoulder subluxation. Watson-Jones[1379] and other authors have recommended that the Bankart and Putti-Platt procedures be combined (ie, following meticulous repair of the capsule to the glenoid, they "double-breast" the subscapularis rather than merely reapproximating it). Weber[1381] reattaches the capsule with screws and then shortens the subscapularis.

Symeonides[1281] reported 33 cases in which the subscapularis and anterior capsule were overlapped without attempting to suture the lateral flap to the glenoid.

Quigley and Freedman[1053] reported the results of 92 Putti-Platt operations; of these patients, 11 had more than a 30% loss of motion. Seven had recurrent instability after surgery.

Leach and coworkers,[702] in 1981 reported a series of 78 patients who had been treated with a modified Putti-Platt procedure. The only failure was in a diabetic who had a recurrence during a seizure following an insulin reaction. Loss of external rotation averaged between 12° and 19°.

Collins and associates[234] reviewed a series of 58 Putti-Platt procedures and 48 Putti-Platt–Bankart procedures. The redislocation rate was 11% (some because of significant trauma); 20% had residual pain, and the average restriction of external rotation was 20°.

Hovelius and colleagues,[556] in a follow-up of 114 patients who underwent either Bankart or Putti-Platt reconstruction, found a recurrence rate of 2% in 46 patients treated with the Bankart procedure and of 19% in 68 patients treated with a Putti-Platt procedure. Follow-up ranged from 1.5 to 10 years.

Since the description of the Putti-Platt technique by Osmond-Clarke[964] in 1948, authors have described the technique as securing the lateral tendon into the "rawed" anterior glenoid rim of the scapula. In effect, this would create a tenodesis of the subscapularis tendon. With only a 2.5-cm lateral stump of the tendon to work with, there is no way one can attach the lateral stump of the subscapularis tendon to the anterior glenoid of the neck of the scapula and have the patient be able to externally rotate the arm beyond the neutral position or flex, extend, abduct, or elevate the upper extremity. Because the radius of the humerus is approximately 2.5 cm, a 2.5-cm stump of subscapularis fused to the anterior glenoid would limit the total humeral rotation to one radian, or 57°. If the lateral stump of the subscapularis tendon is attached to the raw bone of the anterior glenoid, and if the patient develops a functional range of motion, this suggests the tendon was disrupted from the glenoid. This was confirmed by Symeonides,[1281] who performed an autopsy on a patient who had had a Putti-Platt procedure 22 months before his unexpected death.

Angelo and Hawkins[42] presented a series of eight patients who developed osteoarthritis an average of 15 years after Putti-Platt repair. A common feature of these shoulders is that they had never gained more than zero degrees of external rotation after shoulder repair. The authors hypothesized that the excessive tightness of the anterior repair changed the joint mechanics, resulting in increased wear.

The Putti-Platt procedure is contraindicated in multidirectional instability (AMBRI), because tightening the front of the shoulder will only increase the likelihood of posterior instability. In traumatic instability (TUBS), the data suggest that the Putti-Platt procedure, which limits external rotation, is not necessary if the Bankart lesion is solidly repaired.

Magnuson-Stack Procedure.   Transfer of the subscapularis tendon from the lesser tuberosity across the bicipital groove to the greater tuberosity was originally described by Paul Magnuson and James Stack in 1940.[629,773–775,846] In 1955, Magnuson recommended that in some cases the tendon should be transferred not only across the bicipital groove, but also distally into an area between the greater tuberosity and the upper shaft. In this manner, when the arm is abducted, the subscapularis muscle tendon unit acts more effectively as a sling to support the head of the humerus. DePalma[293] also recommended the tendon be transferred to the upper shaft below the greater tuberosity. He interpreted this procedure as being designed to strengthen the anterior muscle barrier to the front of the shoulder and to produce a dynamic force that, on elevation of the arm, forces and holds the head of the humerus in the glenoid fossa. The tendon has been attached to the shaft into a bone trough with sutures, a staple, or a boat nail. Karadimas,[629] in the largest single series of Magnuson-Stack procedures (154 patients), reported a 2% recurrence rate.

Badgley and O'Connor[68] and Bailey[71,72] reported a combination of the Putti-Platt and the Magnuson-Stack operations; they used the upper half of the subscapularis muscle to perform the Putti-Platt procedure and the lower half of the muscle to perform the Magnuson-Stack procedure.

Although the Magnuson-Stack procedure has been successfully applied, it is losing favor to more specific surgical repairs. For example, if isolated laxity of the subscapularis is the cause of recurrent instability, it should be manageable by internal rotation–strengthening exercises. The capsular avulsion common to most cases of traumatic instability can be specifically repaired without loss of rotation. The complications observed with the Magnuson-Stack procedure include excessive anterior tightening with posterior subluxation or dislocation (Fig. 13-96), damage to the biceps (Fig. 13-97), and recurrent instability.

Bone Block

Eden-Hybbinette Procedure.   The Eden-Hybbinette procedure was performed independently by Eden[334] in 1918 and by Hybbinette[571] in 1932. Eden[334] first used tibial grafts, but both authors finally recommended use of iliac grafts. This procedure is supposed to extend the anterior glenoid. It has been used by Palmar and Widen,[984] Lavik,[697] and Hovelius[551] in treating shoulder subluxation and dislocation. Lavik[697] modified the procedure by inserting the graft into the substance of the anterior glenoid rim. Lange[689] inserted the bone graft into an osteotomy on the anterior glenoid. Hehne and Hubner[508] reported a comparison of the Eden-Hybbinette–Lange and the Putti-Platt procedures in 170 patients; their results seemed to favor the latter. Paavolainen and co-workers[981] reported on 41 cases of Eden-Hybbinette procedures; three had recurrent instability, and external rotation was diminished an average of 10%. They found the results similar to their series of Putti-Platt operations. In each group 10% developed degenerative joint disease.

Oudard Procedure.   In 1924, Oudard[969] described a method in which the coracoid process was prolonged with a bone graft from the tibia. The graft (4 × 3 × 1 cm) was inserted between the sawed-off tip and the remainder of the coracoid and was directed laterally and inferiorly. The graft acted as an anterior buttress that served to prevent recurrent dislocations. Oudard[969] also shortened the subscapular tendon. Later, he published another method of obtaining the elongation of the coracoid by performing an oblique osteotomy of the coracoid and displacing the posterolateral portion to serve as a bone block.

Bone blocks rarely seem to be the procedure of choice for increasing shoulder stability. One must be concerned about procedures that may bring the humeral head into contact with bone that is not covered by articular cartilage, because of the high risk of degenerative joint disease. Soft tissue repairs and reconstructions would appear to be safer and more effective for dealing with all but the most unusual situations.

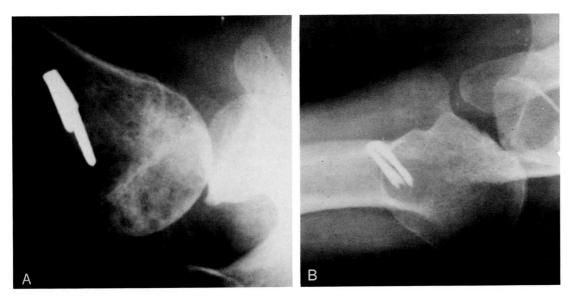

Fig. 13-96. Magnuson-Stack procedure. (**A**) This axillary view shows posterior subluxation of the humeral head on the glenoid as a result of excessive anterior tightening with the Magnuson-Stack procedure. (**B**) Another patient's axillary view shows excessive anterior tightening from the Magnuson-Stack procedure, resulting in posterior glenohumeral displacement of the humeral head. *(Matsen, F. A., III; Thomas, S. C.; and Rockwood, C. A., Jr.: Anterior Glenohumeral Instability. In Rockwood, C. A., and Matsen, F. A., III (eds.): The Shoulder, Fig. 14-63. Philadelphia, W. B. Saunders, 1990.)*

Coracoid Transfer

Trillat Procedure. Trillat[1313,1314] and Leclerc-Chalvet[131,932,1313,1314] performed an osteotomy at the base of the coracoid process and then displaced the coracoid downward and laterally. The displaced coracoid is held in position by a special nail-pin or screw. The pin is passed into the scapula above the inferiorly displaced subscapularis muscle, which effectively shortens the muscle.

Bristow-Helfet Procedure. The Bristow procedure was given its name by the late J. Arthur Helfet[511] of Cape Town, South Africa. He named the operation after his mentor, W. Rowley Bristow, because

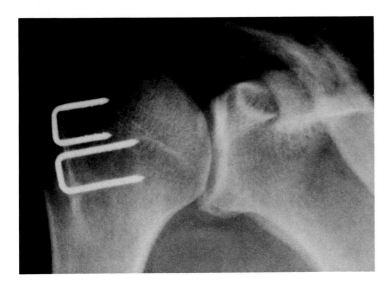

Fig. 13-97. Staple impingement on the long head of the biceps tendon. This anteroposterior x-ray film shows the position of the staple resulting in tendon impingement. Anterior shoulder pain resolved on staple removal. *(Matsen, F. A., III; Thomas, S. C.; and Rockwood, C. A., Jr.: Anterior Glenohumeral Instability. In Rockwood, C. A., and Matsen, F. A., III (eds.): The Shoulder, Fig. 14-64. Philadelphia, W. B. Saunders, 1990.)*

of "Bristow's ability to reduce fussy surgical problems to simple and logical essentials." In the 1958 article, Helfet states, "In his memory I present details of an operation which he showed me nineteen years ago and which I have since used exclusively for recurring dislocation of the shoulder."

Helfet originally described detaching the tip of the coracoid process from the scapula just distal to the insertion of the pectoralis minor muscle, leaving the conjoined tendons (ie, the short head of the biceps and the coracobrachialis) attached. Through a vertical slit in the subscapularis tendon, the joint is exposed and the anterior surface of the neck of the scapula is "rawed up." The coracoid process with its attached tendons is then passed through the slit in the subscapularis and kept in contact with the raw area on the scapula by suturing the conjoined tendon to the cut edges of the scapularis tendon.

In 1958, T. B. McMurray (son of T. P. McMurray of hip osteotomy fame) visited Dr. Newton Mead[827] of Chicago and described modifications of the Bristow operation that were being used in Capetown, Johannesburg, and Pretoria. Mead and Sweeney[827] reported the modifications in more than 100 cases. The modifications consist of splitting the subscapularis muscle and tendon unit in line with its fibers to open the joint and firmly securing the coracoid process to the anterior glenoid rim with a screw. May[803] modified the Bristow procedure further by vertically dividing the entire subscapularis tendon from the lesser tuberosity; after exploring the joint, he attaches the tip of the coracoid process with the conjoined tendon to the anterior glenoid with a screw. The subscapularis tendon is then split horizontally and reattached—half the tendon above and half below the transferred conjoined tendon—to the site of its original insertion.

Helfet[511] reported that the procedure not only "reinforced" the defective part of the joint, but also had a "bone block" effect. Mead,[827] however, does not regard the bone block as being a very important part of the procedure and believes that the transfer adds a muscle reinforcement at the lower anterior aspect of the shoulder joint which prevents the lower portion of the subscapularis muscle from displacing upward as the humerus is abducted. Bonnin[137,138] modified the Bristow procedure in the following way: he does not shorten or split the subscapularis muscle tendon unit, but for exposure he divides the subscapularis muscle at its muscle–tendon junction, and, following the attachment of the coracoid process to the glenoid with a screw, he reattaches the subscapularis on top of the conjoined

tendon. Results with this modification in 81 patients have been reported by Hummel and associates.[565]

Torg and co-workers[1304] reported their experience with 212 cases of the Bristow procedure. In their modification, the coracoid was passed over the superior border rather than through the subscapularis. Their postoperative instability rate was 8.5% (3.8% redislocation and 4.7% subluxation). Ten patients required reoperation for screw-related problems; 34% had residual shoulder pain and 8% were unable to do overhead work. Only 16% of athletes were able to return to their preinjury level of throwing. Carol and associates[190] reported on the results of the Bristow procedure performed for 32 recurrent dislocating shoulders and 15 "spontaneous" shoulder instabilities. At an average follow-up of 3.7 years, only one patient had recurrent instability, and the average limitation of external rotation was 12°. Hovelius and co-workers[551] reported follow-up on 111 shoulders treated with the Bristow procedure. At 2.5 years their postoperative instability rate was 13% (6% dislocation and 7% subluxation). External rotation was limited an average of 20°, and 6% required reoperation because of screw-related complications. Muscle strength was 10% less in the operated shoulder. Chen and colleagues[206] found that after the Bristow procedure, the reduced strength of the short head of the biceps was compensated for by increased activity in the long head.

Lamm and co-workers[685] and Lemmens and de Waal Malefijt[713] have described four special x-ray projections to evaluate the position of the transplanted coracoid process: anteroposterior, lateral, oblique lateral, and modified axial. Lower and co-workers[749] used CT to demonstrate the impingement of a Bristow screw on the head of the humerus. Collins and Wilde[233] and Nielsen and Nielsen[926] reported that while they had minimal problems with recurrence of dislocation, they did encounter problems with screw breakage, migration, and nonunion of coracoid to scapula. Hovelius and colleagues[552,558] reported only a 50% rate of union of the coracoid to the scapula.

Norris and associates[935] evaluated 24 patients with failed Bristow repairs; only two had union of the transferred coracoid. Causes of failure included (1) residual subluxation, and (2) osteoarthritis from screw or bone impingement or overtight repair. They pointed to the difficulty of reconstructing a shoulder after a failed Bristow procedure. In 1988, Ferlic and DiGiovine,[377] reported on 51 patients treated with the Bristow procedure. They had a 10% incidence of redislocation or subluxation and a 14% incidence of complications related to the screw. An additional surgical procedure was required in 14% of the patients.

In 1989, Rockwood and Young[1107] reported on 40 patients who had previously been treated with the Bristow procedure. Thirty-one underwent subsequent reconstructive procedures: 10 had a capsular shift reconstruction; 4 required capsular release; 4 had total shoulder arthroplasty; 1 had an arthrodesis; and 6 had various combined procedures. The authors concluded the Bristow procedure was nonphysiologic and was associated with too many serious complications, and recommended that it not be performed for routine anterior reconstruction of the shoulder.

There also appears to be a significant problem with recurrent subluxation after the Bristow procedure.[558a,767,809] Hill and co-workers[531] and MacKenzie[766] noted failures to manage subluxation with this procedure.

Latarjet Procedure. First described in 1954, the Latarjet procedure[693–696,1000] involves the transfer of a larger portion of the coracoid process than is used with the Bristow procedure, along with the biceps and coracobrachialis tendons, to the antero-inferior aspect of the neck of the scapula. Instead of the raw cut surface of the tip of the coracoid process being attached to the scapula, as in the Bristow-Helfet procedure, the coracoid is laid flat on the neck of the scapula and held in place with

one or two screws. Tagliabue and Esposito[1282] have reported on the Latarjet procedure in 94 athletes. Vittori has modified the procedure by turning the subscapularis tendon downward and holding it displaced downward with the transferred coracoid. Pascoet and associates[1000] reported on the Vittori modification in 36 patients, with only one recurrence.

Although many surgeons use coracoid transfer procedures, the redislocation rates after these operations appear to be no lower than those of other operations for shoulder instability. Yet complications are frequent and can have major consequences (see Complications of Injury) (Figs. 13-98 and 13-99). Coracoid transfer does not address the primary pathology of either traumatic or atraumatic glenohumeral instability, and presents the risks of hardware and bone blocks. Finally, coracoid transfer procedures are extremely difficult and hazardous to revise. The subscapularis and axillary neurovascular structures are scarred in abnormal positions. It is also difficult to regain normal suppleness of the subscapularis muscle. In addition, the axillary and musculocutaneous nerves are at risk in the revision of failed transfers.

Other Open Repairs

Gallie Procedure. Gallie and LeMesurier[411,412] originally described the use of autogenous fascia lata to create new ligaments between the anteroin-

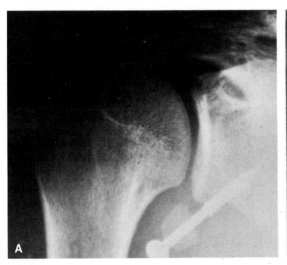
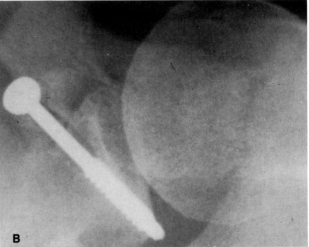

Fig. 13-98. Nonunion of coracoid process after the Bristow procedure. **(A)** An anteroposterior x-ray film shows nonunion of the coracoid process. **(B)** An axillary view of a different patient shows nonunion of the coracoid process after the Bristow procedure. *(Matsen, F. A., III; Thomas, S. C.; and Rockwood, C. A., Jr.: Anterior Glenohumeral Instability. In Rockwood, C. A., and Matsen, F. A., III (eds.): The Shoulder, Fig. 14-66. Philadelphia, W. B. Saunders, 1990.)*

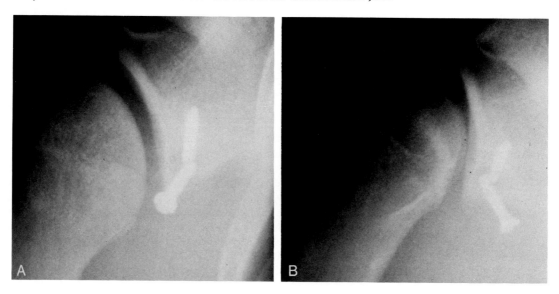

Fig. 13-99. Anteroposterior x-ray films showing broken screws with the humerus in external rotation (**A**) and internal rotation (**B**). *(Matsen, F. A., III; Thomas, S. C.; and Rockwood, C. A., Jr.: Anterior Glenohumeral Instability. In Rockwood, C. A., and Matsen, F. A., III (eds.): The Shoulder, Fig. 14-69. Philadelphia, W. B. Saunders, 1990.)*

ferior aspect of the capsule and the anterior neck of the humerus in 1927. Bateman[88] of Toronto has also used this procedure.

Nicola Procedure. Toufick Nicola's name is usually associated with this operation, but the procedure was first described by Rupp[1155] in 1926 and Heymanowitsch[528] in 1927. In 1929, Nicola[921] published his first article in which he described the use of the long head of the biceps tendon as a checkrein ligament. The procedure has been modified several times.[919–923] Recurrence rates have been reported to be between 30% and 50%.[191,619,1381]

Saha Procedure. A. K. Saha[1159–1169] reported on the transfer of the latissimus dorsi posteriorly into the site of the infraspinatus insertion on the greater tuberosity. He observed that during abduction, the transferred latissimus reinforces the subscapularis muscle and the short posterior steering and depressor muscles by pulling the humeral head backward. He has used the procedure for traumatic and atraumatic dislocations, and in 1969 reported 45 cases with no recurrences.[1166]

Boytchev Procedure. Boytchev first reported an open repair procedure in 1951 in the Italian literature,[146,147] and later modifications were developed by Conforty.[236] The muscles that attach to the cor-

acoid process, along with the tip of the coracoid, are rerouted deep to the subscapularis muscle, between it and the capsule. The tip of the coracoid, with its muscles, is then reattached to its base in the anatomic position. Conforty[236] reported on 17 patients, none of whom had a recurrence of dislocation. Ha'eri[474] reported 26 cases with a minimum of 2-year follow-up.

Connolly Procedure. When the recurrent anterior dislocation is associated with a large posterolateral humeral head defect, Connolly has transferred the tendon insertion of the infraspinatus into the defect.[239,240] This keeps the defect from sliding anteriorly over and onto the glenoid and converts the defect into an extra-articular structure. This operation is essentially a mirror image of the McLaughlin procedure used in posterior dislocations of the shoulder when there is a large anterior bone defect in the humeral head.

Osteotomy of the Proximal Humerus. Debevoise and associates[296] have shown that humeral torsion is abnormal in the repeatedly dislocating shoulder. In 1969, B. G. Weber[1381] of Switzerland reported a rotational osteotomy that increased the retroversion of the humeral head. He also shortened the subscapularis muscle (Fig. 13-100). The indications

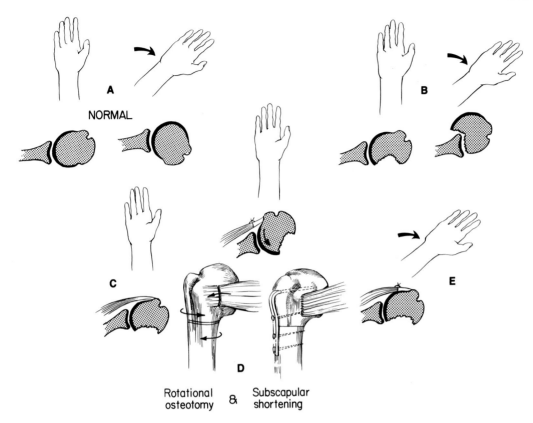

NORMAL

Rotational
osteotomy   &   Subscapular
shortening

Fig. 13-100. Weber osteotomy of the proximal humerus to prevent recurrent anterior dislocation. (**A**) Normally when the arm is externally rotated, the posterior articular surface of the humerus stays in contact with the glenoid fossa. (**B**) However, during external rotation, when there is a large posterolateral humeral head defect, the articular surface of the head is decreased, which causes the recurrent anterior dislocation. The humerus is then held impinged by the anterior glenoid rim. (**C, D, E**) With external rotation, according to Weber, if the normal retroversion of the humeral head is increased by proximal humeral osteotomy and subscapularis shortening, the defect does not come in contact with the anterior glenoid rim, and recurrences are prevented. (*Redrawn from Weber, B. G.: Operative Treatment for Recurrent Dislocation of the Shoulder. Injury, 1:107–109, 1969.*)

were a moderate to severe posterior lateral humeral head defect, which he found in 65% of his patients with recurrent anterior instability. By increasing the retroversion, the posterolateral defect is delivered more posteriorly, and the anterior undisturbed portion of the articular surface of the humeral head articulates against the glenoid. Following this procedure, even with external rotation of the arm, the posterolateral defect no longer engages the glenoid cavity. In 1984, Weber and colleagues[1380] reported a redislocation rate of 5.7%, with good to excellent results in 90%. Most patients required reoperation for plate removal.

This procedure also includes an anterior capsular reefing, making it difficult to determine the effect of the osteotomy itself. Although posterolateral humeral head defects are common in recurrent traumatic instability, we do not usually find these defects to be a significant factor if the capsular pathology is managed appropriately.

Osteotomy of the Neck of the Glenoid. In 1933, Meyer-Burgdorff reported on decreasing the anterior tilt of the glenoid by a posterior closing-wedge osteotomy. Saha[1169] has written about an anterior opening-wedge osteotomy with bone graft into the neck of the glenoid to decrease the tilt.

Caution must be observed in determining the glenoid version from plane roentgenograms. Change in angulation of the beam can change the apparent version substantially. (See Fig. 13-17.) There is little evidence that glenoid version is the primary problem in recurrent glenohumeral instability. Thus, glenoid osteotomy is too hazardous a procedure for use in ordinary situations.

Arthroscopic Repair

Arthroscopic repair of the Bankart lesion using a staple was performed by Johnson as early as 1980.[612] In this procedure, a metal staple is used to reattach the torn labrum or capsule to the roughened edge of the glenoid. Johnson recommends at least 3 weeks of immobilization. Concern about the safety of using staples and the high redislocation rate has given rise to other arthroscopic techniques (Fig. 13-101). Morgan and Bodenstab[863] reported 25 arthroscopic shoulder stabilizations using a transglenoid absorbable suture. In Johnson's[1111a] first series of 106 patients treated with the arthroscopic staple technique, he reported a recurrence of subluxation or dislocation in 21%. Caspari[193,194] reported on his arthroscopic transglenoid technique, and Wolf[1405] reported the use of a screw to reattach the labrum. Currently, arthroscopic repairs with biodegradable materials are being studied by Warren[1365] and Johnson.[613] Andrews[30–40] has extensively reported on the arthroscopic evaluation and treatment of glenoid labral problems. Ellman,[342–344] Hawkins,[488–489] Esch,[355–359] Jobe,[601–605] Gartsman[425–427] and many others are currently studying the use of the arthroscope in the evaluation and management of shoulder instabilities.

Our experience with open repairs leads us to predict that arthroscopic repair of atraumatic multidirectional instability (AMBRI) is too extensive a procedure to be performed under arthroscopic control. However, the traumatic tearing of the glenohumeral ligaments from the glenoid (TUBS) is suited to arthroscopic repair, once a safe technique is developed which yields results comparable with those obtained with an open Bankart repair.

POSTOPERATIVE MANAGEMENT

Postoperatively, the arm is immobilized in adduction and internal rotation. This can be accomplished by supporting the arm in a standard sling and then securing the arm to the trunk with a soft roller bandage, or by using one of the standard shoulder immobilizers that are commercially available. Some authors recommend postoperative immobilization for 4 to 6 weeks, after which a rehabilitation program is begun. This may be too long, in that limitation of external rotation is a problem after shoulder repair, particularly in the older patient or in the throwing athlete. Rowe and associates[1128] recommend immobilization for just 2 to 3 days, after which the arm is completely free. Their patients are instructed to gradually increase the motion and function of the extremity.

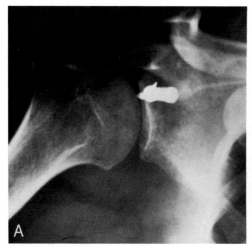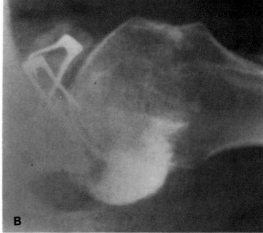

Fig. 13-101. (**A**) An anteroposterior x-ray film shows the position of an arthroscopically placed staple. Impingement on humeral head is suggested by this view. (**B**) An axillary x-ray film with contrast material demonstrates impingement of the staple on the humeral head. *(Matsen, F. A., III; Thomas, S. C.; and Rockwood, C. A., Jr.: Anterior Glenohumeral Instability. In Rockwood, C. A., and Matsen, F. A., III (eds.): The Shoulder, Fig. 14-71. Philadelphia, W. B. Saunders, 1990.)*

RESULTS

Most of the reported series on the various types of reconstructions have yielded "excellent" results. However, it is very difficult to determine how each author graded his results. For example, if the patient has no recurrences after repair, but has loss of 45° of external rotation and cannot throw, is that a fair, good, or excellent result? The simple fact that the shoulder no longer dislocates cannot be considered an excellent result. Although the older literature suggested that the goal of surgery for anterior dislocations of the shoulder was to limit external rotation, more modern literature suggests that a reconstruction can both prevent recurrent dislocation and allow a nearly normal range of motion and comfortable function.

COMPLICATIONS OF SURGICAL PROCEDURES

Complications of surgical repairs for anterior glenohumeral instability may be grouped into several categories the most significant of which are infection, recurrent instability, complications secondary to misdiagnosis, neurovascular injuries, hardware-related complications, and limited motion.

Postoperative Infection.   Thorough skin preparation, adhesive plastic drapes, and prophylactic antibiotics are useful in reducing contamination by axillary bacterial flora. It also is important to prevent the accumulation of a significant hematoma by achieving good hemostasis, obliterating any dead space, and using a suction drain if significant bleeding persists. Finally, it is important to keep the axilla clean and dry postoperatively by using a gauze sponge as long as the arm is held at the side.

Recurrent Instability.   The published incidence of recurrent dislocation after the standard anterior repairs ranges from 0% to 18%. A 1975 review by Rockwood of 1634 reconstructions compiled from the literature revealed that the incidence of recurrence averaged 3%. In a 1983 review of 3187 procedures (Table 13-3), this incidence was unchanged.[1104] This review included 432 Putti-Platt operations, 571 Magnuson-Stack operations or modifications, 513 Bankart operations or modifications, 45 Saha operations, 203 Bankart–Putti-Platt combinations, 750 Bristow operations, 115 Badgley combined procedures, 254 Eden-Hybbinette operations, 277 Gallie operations or modifications, and 27 Weber operations. However, for the most part, the results were based on whether or not the patient's shoulder redislocated after the operative procedure.

Morrey and Jones,[865] in a long-term follow-up study of 176 patients that averaged 10.2 years, found a recurrence rate of 11%. The operative reconstructions were of the Bankart and Putti-Platt types. Among the 20 patients with recurrences, half were related to athletic activities, inadequate immobilization, a history of contralateral dislocation, or a family history of shoulder dislocation. In 7 of the 20 patients, the recurrence occurred 2 years or more after surgery. The need for long-term follow-up was further emphasized in a recent study by O'Driscoll and Evans,[949] who followed 269 consecutive staple capsulorrhaphies for a minimum of 8.8 years. Twenty-one percent experienced recurrent instability; this incidence increased progressively with the length of follow-up.

Rowe and colleagues[1133] reported on the management of 39 patients with recurrence of instability after various surgical repairs. Of 32 who were reoperated upon, 84% had unrepaired avulsions of the capsule and labrum from the anterior glenoid rim. Excessive laxity was thought to be the primary cause of instability in four shoulders. Twenty-two of the 24 shoulders reoperated on with a Bankart repair and followed for at least 2 years had a good or excellent result.

Rockwood and Young[1107] reported on 40 shoulders in 39 patients who had failed Bristow procedures. The complications following the procedure included recurrent anterior instability, recurrent posterior instability, articular cartilage injury, severe irreversible joint damage, failure of the coracoid to unite to the scapula, loosening of the screw, and neurovascular injury.

Following revisions of the failed Bristow procedures, excellent and good results were achieved in only 50% of the patients. Six patients had fair results and 14 had poor results. The poor results were in patients who had so much destruction of the glenohumeral joint that fusion or total shoulder arthroplasty had to be performed.

The surgical management of a failed Bristow operation is complicated and extremely difficult. The extensive scarring, especially about the musculocutaneous and axillary nerves, makes reconstruction tedius and complex. As noted, the authors concluded that the Bristow procedure is nonphysiologic—that is, it does not direct itself to the basic pathology of the problem—and should not be used for routine anterior shoulder instability.

Complications Secondary to Misdiagnosis.   Another major category of complications arises from failure of diagnosis. It is essential to differentiate

**Table 13-3. Incidence of Recurrence Following Various Reconstructions
for Anterior Dislocations of the Shoulder***

Procedure	Authors	Year	No. Cases		Recurrence (%)	
Putti-Platt	Adams[6]	1948	37		5.4	
	Brav[154]	1955	41		7.3	
	Jeffery[596]	1959	34		3.0	
	Osmond-Clarke[965]	1965	140		1.4	
	Truchly[1318]	1968	102		0	
	Leach and associates[702]	1981	78		1.2	
			432	Total	3.0	Average
Magnuson-Stack and modifications	Giannestras[437]	1948	31		6.4	
	Palumbo and Quirin[986]	1950	13		0	
	Vare[1337]	1953	30		0	
	Alldred[19]	1958	10		0	
	DePalma and Silberstein[286]	1963	75		2.7	
	Jens[598]	1964	42		9.0	
	Bryan and associates[170]	1969	53		7.5	
	Magnuson and Stack[773]	1943	6		0	
	MacAusland[759]	1956	21		9.5	
	Gartland and Dowling[424]	1954	14		0	
	Robertson[1100]	1954	14		0	
	Karadimas and associates[629]	1980	154		2.0	
	Aamoth and O'Phelan[1]	1977	40		2.5	
	Hovelius and associates[551]	1979	68		1.9	
			571	Total	4.1	Average
Bankart and modifications	Adams[6]	1948	18		5.5	
	Townley[1309]	1950	26		0	
	Rowe[1144]	1956	75		1.3	
	Du Toit and Roux[326]	1956	150		5.0	
	Dickson and Devas[314]	1957	50		4.0	
	Boyd and Hunt[143]	1965	49		4.1	
	Rowe and associates[1128]	1978	145		2.5	
	Thomas and Matsen[1290]	1989	63		2.6	
			513	Total	3.2	Average
Saha	Saha[1162]	1967	45		0	
			45	Total	0	Average
Bankart–Putti-Platt combination	Watson-Jones[1378]	1948	52		2.0	
	Viek and Bell[1350]	1959	39		2.5	
	Weber[1381]	1969	62		1.6	
	Lambdin and associates[684]	1971	50		5.0	
			203	Total	2.8	Average
Bristow	Helfet[511]	1958	30		3.0	
	McMurray[826]	1961	73		2.7	
	May[803]	1970	16		0	
	Collins and Wilde[233]	1973	50		0	
	Hill and associates[530]	1981	107		2.0	
	Lombardo and associates[746]	1976	51		2.0	
	Nielsen and Nielsen[926]	1982	18		0	
	Barrett and associates[83]	1982	50		4.0	
	Mackenzie[766]	1980	16		0	
	Hummel and associates[565]	1982	81		0	
	Hovelius and associates[552]	1983	111		6.0	
	Allman[22]	1974	50		0	
	Sweeney and associates[1278]	1975	97		3.0	
			750	Total	1.7	Average
Badgley combinations (ie, Putti-Platt, Nicola, and Magnuson-Stack)	Bailey[71]	1967	115		1.7	
			115	Total	1.7	Average

Table 13-3. Incidence of Recurrence Following Various Reconstructions for Anterior Dislocations of the Shoulder* (*continued*)

Procedure	Authors	Year	No. Cases		Recurrence (%)	
Eden-Hybbinette and modifications	Palmar and Widen[984]	1948	128		4.0	
	Oster[966]	1969	78		18.0	
	Said and Medbo[1170]	1970	21		0	
	Bonnin[137]	1973	27		0	
			254	Total	6.0	Average
Gallie	Gallie and LeMesurier[411]	1948	175		4.0	
	Bateman[88]	1963	102		1.9	
			277	Total	2.9	Average
Weber	Weber[1381]	1969	27		0	
			27	Total	0	Average

* Total number of studies: 53; total number of cases: 3187; average % of recurrence: ±3.0%.

traumatic unidirectional instability (TUBS) from atraumatic multidirectional instability (AMBRI) before carrying out any surgical repair. The consequences of mistaking multidirectional instability for pure anterior instability are substantial. In this situation, if only the anterior structures are tightened, limited external rotation and posterior subluxation may lead to the rapid loss of glenohumeral articular cartilage and postsurgical degenerative joint disease. This complication can be prevented *only* by accurate preoperative diagnosis. It also points out the necessity for preserving external rotation during the postoperative period, and reassessing with axillary roentgenograms any shoulder that appears to vary from the expected course.

Neurovascular Injuries. The musculocutaneous nerve runs as a single or multipartite structure obliquely through the coracobrachialis for a variable distance distal to the coracoid process. In this location, it may be injured by (1) dissection to free up the coracoid process, (2) retraction, or (3) inclusion in suture.[1221] Helfet[511] described one case in which the nerve had a high penetration into the coracobrachialis and became impinged where the conjoined tendon entered the slit made in the subscapularis tendon. The axillary nerve may be injured in dissection and suture of the inferior capsule and subscapularis. Rockwood specifically recommends that the axillary nerve be routinely palpated and protected with a retractor during anterior reconstructions, especially during a capsular shift reconstruction.[1104] Richards and associates[1094] presented nine patients sustaining brachial plexus injuries during anterior shoulder repair (three Bristows and six Putti-Platts). Seven involved the musculocutaneous nerve and two the axillary nerve.

Two of the nerves were lacerated, five injured by suture, and two injured by traction. These nerve injuries are relatively more common during reoperation after a previous repair. In this situation, the nerves are tethered by scar tissue and, thus, are more difficult to mobilize out of harm's way. Neurovascular complications can best be avoided by good knowledge of local anatomy (including the possible normal variations), good surgical technique, and a healthy respect for the change in position and mobility of the neurovascular structures after a previous surgical procedure in the area.

Hardware-Related Complications. The next category of complications includes those related to hardware inserted about the glenohumeral joint.[200,499] The screw used to fix the coracoid fragment in Bristow procedures has a particular potential for being problematic.[926,1053] This may be because the coracoid muscles tend to rotate the fragment as the arm is raised and lowered, thereby contributing to screw loosening. Artz and Huffer[54] reported a devastating complication following use of a screw to secure the coracoid process: the screw became loose and caused a false aneurysm of the axillary artery, with a subsequent compression of the brachial plexus and paralysis of the upper extremity.

The axillary artery has been injured by screws placed for Bristow procedures; a false aneurysm of this vessel has been reported as late as 3 years after surgery.[375] In other instances, the screw has damaged the articular surface of the glenoid and humeral head when placed too close to the glenoid lip, irritated the infraspinatus or its nerve when too long, or affected the brachial plexus when it became loose. Staples used to attach the capsule to the glenoid may miss their target, damaging the humeral or glenoid articular cartilage. Staples also may become loose from repeated pull of the muscles and capsule during shoulder use, particularly if they were not well seated in the first place. O'Driscoll and Evans[949] reported an 11% incidence of staple complications after the DuToit procedure. If screws and staples migrate into the intraarticular region, significant damage to the joint surfaces may result. Metal fixation may injure the biceps tendon in a Magnuson-Stack procedure.

Zuckerman and Matsen[1429] reported a series of patients with problems related to the use of screws and staples about the glenohumeral joint; 21 had problems related to the Bristow procedure and 14 to the use of staples (either for capsulorrhaphy or subscapularis advancement). The time between placement and symptom onset ranged from 4 weeks to 10 years. Screws and staples had been incorrectly placed in 10 patients, had migrated or loosened in 24, and had fractured in 3. Almost all patients required reoperation, at which time 41% had a significant injury to one or both of the joint surfaces.

One can only conclude that hardware-free methods of managing glenohumeral instability are safer. The recurrence rates of techniques using screws and staples are no better than with hardware-free repairs. Risks are incurred with hardware that simply do not exist with other repair techniques. The depth and variable orientation of the glenoid at surgery provide substantial opportunity for hardware misplacement (ie, into the joint, under the articular cartilage, subperiosteally, out the back, too high, too low, too medial, too prominent anteriorly, and too insecurely). The large range of motion of the shoulder, with frequent vigorous challenges to its stability, creates an opportunity for hardware loosening and for irreversible surface and neurovascular damage.

Limited Motion. The final category of complications is limited motion. Limited range of motion, especially external rotation, has been reported after the Magnuson-Stack and the Putti-Platt procedures. It has also been noted after the Bristow procedure, which was supposed to be free of this problem.[80,148,533] Hovelius and colleagues[556] reported an average loss of external rotation of 21° with the arm in abduction. This loss of range compromises function. In their series of 46 patients with continuing problems after shoulder reconstruction, Hawkins and Hawkins[491] found that ten had stiffness related to limited external rotation. Excessive

limitation of external rotation has a high association with the subsequent development of osteoarthritis. Angelo and Hawkins[42] reported eight patients with disabling degenerative arthritis presenting an average of 15.1 years after a Putti-Platt procedure. None of the patients had ever developed external rotation beyond zero degrees after their repair.

MATSEN'S PREFERRED METHOD OF SURGICAL TREATMENT FOR RECURRENT TRAUMATIC ANTERIOR SHOULDER INSTABILITY

My approach to traumatic anterior instability (TUBS syndrome) is discussed here.[1290] My nonoperative program for recurrent anterior instability includes vigorous rotator strengthening and coordination exercises (eg, swimming). I present this to the patient as the "four star program" (Table 13-4, Figs. 13-102 through 13-104). Although this program will not cure most cases of traumatic instability, it will frequently enhance function. At a minimum, it introduces the patient to the rehabilitation program used after a surgical repair.

The patient desiring surgical stabilization is presented with a frank discussion of the risks and alternatives. The relative importance to the patient of (1) a full range of motion, and (2) stability is

Table 13-4. Four Star Exercise Program for Optimizing Shoulder Stability

★1. Develop shoulder rotator strength.
  Perform internal and external rotator–strengthening exercises.
    Rubber tubing (Fig. 13-102)
    Decubitus curls (Fig. 13-103)
    Wall weights (Fig. 13-104)
  Perform exercises two to five times per day, selecting a resistance that will allow 20 repetitions.
  Advance until the patient can perform 20 repetitions against 20% of body weight.
★2. Develop shoulder coordination and endurance.
  Swim three to five times per week.
    Avoid breast stroke if it causes symptoms of posterior instability.
    Avoid back stroke and butterfly if they cause symptoms of anterior instability.
  Work up to an average of ½ hour every other day.
★3. Avoid competitive basketball, volleyball, football, kayaking, and other violent overhead sports until goals of Steps 1 and 2 are attained.
★4. Maintain general conditioning with aerobic workouts such as brisk walking, jogging, swimming, biking, and rowing. Sustain these exercises for ½ hour at least four times per week.

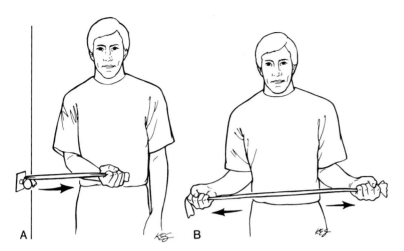

Fig. 13-102. (**A**) Internal and external rotator-strengthening exercises using rubber band. Internal rotator-strengthening exercise with rubber tube secured to the door. The elbow must be maintained close to the patient's side and flexed at 90°. (**B**) External rotator-strengthening exercise. Elbows are held close to the patient's side and in 90° flexion. (*Matsen, F. A., III; Thomas, S. C.; and Rockwood, C. A., Jr.: Anterior Glenohumeral Instability. In Rockwood, C. A., and Matsen, F. A., III (eds.): The Shoulder, Fig. 14-72. Philadelphia, W. B. Saunders, 1990.*)

determined, so the procedure and postoperative care can be biased in the desired direction. Baseball pitchers require more shoulder capsular laxity. Skiers or football linemen require more stability. A preoperative arthrogram is obtained in patients older than 30 years if there is pain between episodes of dislocation or weakness of external rotation.

Electromyograms are obtained if nerve injury is suspected.

Anesthesia and Examination.   After a thorough preoperative evaluation, the patient is taken to the operating room, where either a brachial plexus block or a general anesthetic is administered. The

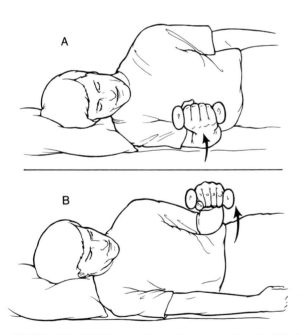

Fig. 13-103. Internal and external rotator-strengthening exercises using free weights. (**A**) Internal rotator strengthening. (**B**) External rotator strengthening. (*Matsen, F. A., III; Thomas, S. C.; and Rockwood, C. A., Jr.: Anterior Glenohumeral Instability. In Rockwood, C. A., and Matsen, F. A., III (eds.): The Shoulder, Fig. 14-73. Philadelphia, W. B. Saunders, 1990.*)

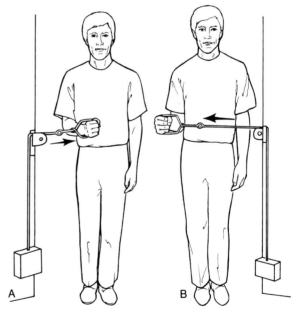

Fig. 13-104. Internal and external rotator-strengthening exercises using wall weights. (**A**) Internal rotator strengthening. The elbow is held close to the side in 90° flexion. (**B**) External rotator strengthening. The elbow is held close to the patient's side and flexed 90°. (*Matsen, F. A., III; Thomas, S. C.; and Rockwood, C. A., Jr.: Anterior Glenohumeral Instability. In Rockwood, C. A., and Matsen, F. A., III (eds.): The Shoulder, Fig. 14-74. Philadelphia, W. B. Saunders, 1990.*)

glenohumeral joint is examined under anesthesia. Although this examination rarely changes the procedure performed, it provides helpful confirmation of the diagnosis. The direction of translation may be documented by axillary and/or anteroposterior roentgenograms taken while the surgeon stresses the glenohumeral joint. Most normal shoulders translate posteriorly for a distance of about 50% of the humeral head diameter.

Positioning. The patient is positioned in a slight head-up position (approximately 20°) with the scapula off the edge of the operating table. This position provides a full range of humeral and scapular mobility, and, if necessary, access to the posterior aspect of the shoulder. The major axillary skin crease is marked with ink or dye. The neck, chest, axilla, and entire arm are prepared with iodine solution. Draping includes application of adherent, transparent plastic to the exposed area to minimize contact with the axillary skin.

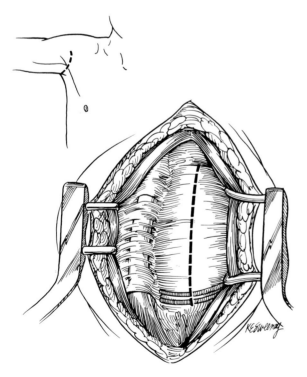

Fig. 13-105. Skin incision and deltopectoral split. Dotted line indicates incision through subscapularis and capsule. *(Matsen, F. A., and Thomas, S. C.: Glenohumeral Instability. In Evarts, C. M. (ed.): Surgery of the Musculoskeletal System, Vol. 2, 2nd ed. p. 1454. New York, Churchill Livingstone, 1989.)*

Skin Incision. The 8-cm skin incision is centered on the inferior border of the pectoralis major tendon and located in the previously marked axillary skin crease.[68] This incision heals with a very good cosmetic result if closed with subcuticular suture and sterile paper tape (Fig. 13-105). The skin and subcutaneous tissue are undermined up to the level of the coracoid process, which is then used as a guide to the cephalic vein and the deltopectoral groove (Fig. 13-106). The groove is opened by spreading with the two index fingers medial to the cephalic vein. A consistent neurovascular bundle (a branch of the thoracoacromial artery and the lateral pectoral nerve) is identified in the upper third of the groove;[457] this bundle is cauterized and transected. The clavipectoral fascia is seen lateral to the coracoid muscles (the coracobrachialis and the short head of the biceps). This fascia is divided up to but not through the coracoacromial ligament, exposing the subjacent subscapularis tendon and lesser tuberosity.

Identification and Protection of the Axillary Nerve. The surgeon's index finger is then passed medially along the subscapularis to palpate the axillary nerve coursing inferolaterally. At this point, it is useful to insert a self-retaining retractor, with one blade on the deltoid muscle and the other on

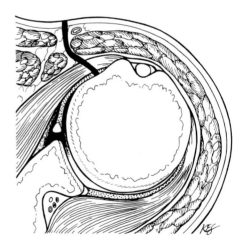

Fig. 13-106. Transverse plane section from a superior view showing the incision and the plane for exposure. Note that the deltopectoral interval is utilized. The subscapularis tendon and the underlying joint capsule are incised as a unit 1 cm medial to the insertion. *(Matsen, F. A., and Thomas, S. C.: Glenohumeral Instability. In Evarts, C. M. (ed.): Surgery of the Musculoskeletal System, Vol. 2, 2nd ed., p. 1456. New York, Churchill Livingstone, 1989.)*

the coracoid muscles (Fig. 13-107). Rotating the arm from internal to external rotation reveals, in succession, the greater tuberosity, the bicipital groove, the lesser tuberosity, and the subscapularis. The anterior circumflex humeral vessels marking the inferior border of the subscapularis may be cauterized, but we prefer to retract them inferiorly.

Division of the Subscapularis With Capsule. The interval between the supraspinatus and subscapularis tendons is identified by palpation, and a blunt elevator is inserted through this interval into the joint. This elevator brings the upper subscapularis into the incision. The subscapularis tendon is tagged with a suture 2 cm medial to the lesser tuberosity. The subscapularis tendon and subjacent capsule are then incised together, approximately 1 cm medial to the lesser tuberosity, beginning at the superior rounded edge of the tendon and extending inferiorly to the anterior circumflex humeral vessels. (See Fig. 13-105.) If necessary for greater exposure, the joint capsule may be further divided along the coracohumeral ligament, just medial to the intra-articular biceps tendon. Without separating them, the subscapularis tendon and anterior shoulder capsule are reflected medially, providing an excellent view of the joint. Visualization of the capsule and glenoid is facilitated by the careful insertion of a humeral head retractor, which leans on the posterior glenoid lip and pushes the humeral head posterolaterally. The capsule is pulled tight by applying traction to its cut edge while the junction of the capsular lig-

aments to the glenoid is palpated. This area is also exposed for inspection using a narrow right-angle retractor (Fig. 13-108). A small (<1 cm) defect is normally found in the capsule just below the coracoid process, the articular opening of the subcoracoid recess. This should not be confused with a Bankart lesion. In the TUBS syndrome, the vast majority of shoulders demonstrate detachment of the glenohumeral ligaments from the anterioinferior bony rim of the glenoid. The labrum usually remains attached to the capsular ligaments, but may remain on the glenoid side of the rupture, may be a separate ("bucket-handle") fragment, or may be absent.

Inspection of the Joint. The glenohumeral joint is inspected thoroughly for loose bodies, defects of the bony glenoid, tears of the glenoid labrum, and tears of the rotator cuff. In traumatic anterior instability, a posterolateral humeral head defect is usually palpable by passing an index finger over the top of the head while putting longitudinal traction on the arm. Approximately 50% of my TUBS patients have moderate to large humeral head defects; this finding does not change my treatment. Massive humeral head defects in this location may require tightening of the anterior structures to keep them from entering the joint on external rotation, but this is highly unusual. The supraspinatus and infraspinatus tendons are palpated to check their integrity, especially in patients past 30 years of age. Finally, the biceps tendon is inspected and note

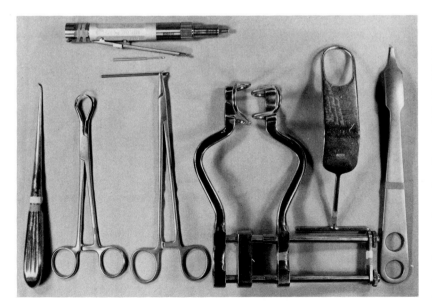

Fig. 13-107. Instruments for surgical repairs of recurrent glenohumeral instability. (**Top**) High-speed drill used for drilling holes in the glenoid rim. (**Bottom, left to right**) Small angled curette and reaming tenaculum used to connect the holes drilled in the glenoid rim; curved-nosed needle holder for passing a No. 5 Mayo needle through the holes; self-retaining retractor; humeral head retractor; and sharp-tipped levering retractor. *(Matsen, F. A., III; Thomas, S. C.; and Rockwood, C. A., Jr.: Anterior Glenohumeral Instability. In Rockwood, C. A., and Matsen, F. A., III (eds.): The Shoulder, Fig. 14-77. Philadelphia, W. B. Saunders, 1990.)*

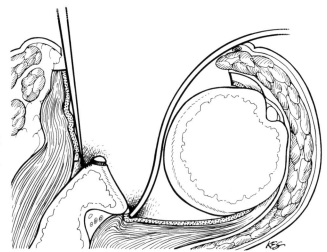

Fig. 13-108. Transverse plane section showing placement of retractors and location of drill holes. Note the area roughened by curette along the anterior glenoid neck; also note the position of the drill hole relative to the anterior glenoid rim. *(Matsen, F. A., and Thomas, S. C.: Glenohumeral Instability. In Evarts, C. M. (ed.): Surgery of the Musculoskeletal System, Vol. 2, 2nd ed. p. 1456. New York, Churchill Livingstone, 1989.)*

taken of the integrity of the transverse humeral ligament. At this point, the surgeon has a complete idea of the anatomical factors contributing to the glenohumeral instability.

In my experience, 97% of patients with the TUBS syndrome have a rupture of the glenoid attachment of the middle and/or inferior glenohumeral ligaments. In my view, the repair of these ligamentous detachments is necessary and sufficient for the repair of the traumatic instability. This repair is carried out from inside the joint, with no need to separate the capsule from the subscapularis muscle and tendon.

Glenoid Exposure and Drill Holes. The glenoid is well exposed by a humeral head retractor laterally

and a sharp-tipped levering retractor is inserted through the capsular defect onto the neck of the glenoid. Bucket-handle or flap tears of the glenoid labrum are excised.[5,84] The anterior, nonarticular surface of the glenoid is prepared by curettage down to bleeding bone. A 1.8-mm drill is used to make holes for the passage of suture. Holes are spaced 6 mm apart; the number of holes is determined by the size of the capsular defect (Fig. 13-109). On the articular side, the holes are placed 4 mm from the anterior edge of the glenoid. On the anterior aspect, corresponding holes are also made 4 mm from the anterior edge of the glenoid edge. These pairs of holes are then connected using a 000 angled curette (Fig. 13-110). No. 2 nonabsorbable suture is then passed through these holes using a No. 5 Mayo

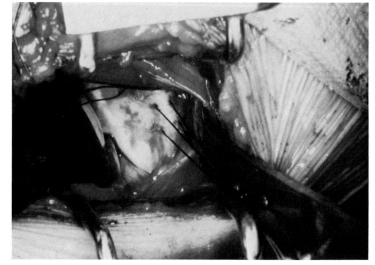

Fig. 13-109. Intraoperative photograph of the Bankart procedure showing the placement of sutures through holes in the glenoid rim. *(Matsen, F. A., III; Thomas, S. C.; and Rockwood, C. A., Jr.: Anterior Glenohumeral Instability. In Rockwood, C. A., and Matsen, F. A., III (eds.): The Shoulder, Fig. 14-79. Philadelphia, W. B. Saunders, 1990.)*

needle and a curved needle holder (Figs. 13-107 and 13-111). Traction is applied to each suture to ensure that it has a firm purchase on the bony glenoid.

Repair of Defect. When sufficient sutures have been placed to repair the capsular defect, the sharp-tipped levering retractor is removed and replaced by a right-angled retractor positioned to show the detached medial edge of the capsule, which is most easily identified by tracing the capsular edge from where it remains attached to the glenoid. The limb of each suture exiting the holes in the anterior glenoid is then passed through the detached medial edge of the capsule, taking just enough tissue to ensure a secure bite. The capsular repair is completed by tying these sutures so the knots lie against the articular surface of the capsule (Fig. 13-112). The capsular repair is checked by palpation and under direct vision to ensure that it is complete and strong.

Approximately 10% of TUBS patients have fractures or deficiencies of the anterior bony lip of the glenoid. Anterior glenoid deficiencies of up to 33% of the articular surface are managed in a similar way with direct repair of capsular ligaments to the edge of the articular surface. I am reluctant to use bone blocks because of the adverse effects of nonphysiologic contact with the articular surface of the humeral head.

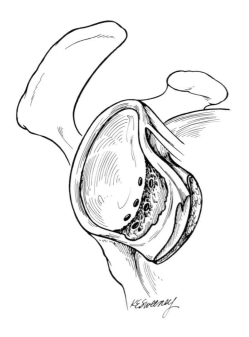

Fig. 13-110. Anteroinferior glenoid rim with holes drilled. The nonarticular edge has been curetted, and the holes have been carefully placed 4 mm from the glenoid rim to afford strong fixation. Note the reflection of the capsule in the typical location of the Bankart lesion, 3 to 6 o'clock. *(Matsen, F. A., and Thomas, S. C.: Glenohumeral Instability. In Evarts, C. M. (ed.): Surgery of the Musculoskeletal System, Vol. 2, 2nd ed. p. 1456. New York, Churchill Livingstone, 1989.)*

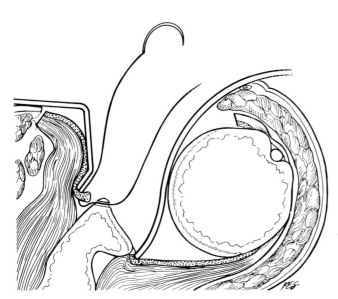

Fig. 13-111. Transverse plane section showing passage of a No. 2 nonabsorbable suture through the drill hole and into the capsule. Note the use of a deep right-angle retractor on the subscapularis and superficial capsule to afford the necessary exposure for proper placement of the suture. *(Matsen, F. A., and Thomas, S. C.: Glenohumeral Instability. In Evarts, C. M. (ed.): Surgery of the Musculoskeletal System, Vol. 2, 2nd ed. p. 1457. New York, Churchill Livingstone, 1989.)*

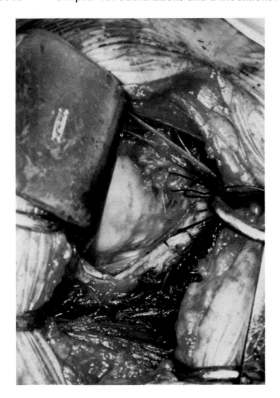

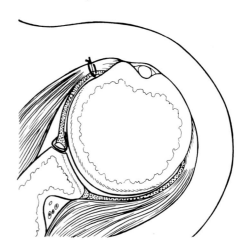

Fig. 13-113. Transverse plane section showing the completed repair of a Bankart lesion and the anatomic repair of an incision through the subscapularis and the capsule. *(Matsen, F. A., and Thomas, S. C.: Glenohumeral Instability. In Evarts, C. M. (ed.): Surgery of the Musculoskeletal System, Vol. 2, 2nd ed. p. 1457. New York, Churchill Livingstone, 1989.)*

Fig. 13-112. Intraoperative photograph during reexploration of a Bankart repair. This patient ruptured his subscapularis tendon repair several months after a Bankart procedure. At the time of reoperation for repair of the subscapularis tendon, the anterior glenoid rim was explored and the Bankart repair was intact. The repair sutures were covered by synovium. *(Matsen, F. A., III; Thomas, S. C.; and Rockwood, C. A., Jr.: Anterior Glenohumeral Instability. In Rockwood, C. A., and Matsen, F. A., III (eds.): The Shoulder, Fig. 14-82. Philadelphia, W. B. Saunders, 1990.)*

Repair of the Subscapularis With Capsule. Once the capsular avulsion is repaired, the lateral capsule and subscapularis tendons are repaired back to the lesser tuberosity in their anatomic positions (Fig. 13-113). This repair minimizes any restriction of external rotation. Once this repair has been completed, shoulder stability is checked. If anterior laxity remains (which is rarely the case), the lateral capsular and subscapularis reattachment may be advanced laterally or superolaterally (Fig. 13-114).

In the rather unusual situation (3% of cases or less) in which a shoulder with the TUBS syndrome is found not to have capsular detachment, the anterior laxity is treated by reefing the anterior capsule and the subscapularis tendon. Shortening these structures by 1 cm limits external rotation of the

humerus by approximately 20°. Generally, restricting external rotation to 30° at the operating table will permit a very functional shoulder once rehabilitation is complete. If the patient has marked anterior ligamentous laxity, proportionately greater anterior tightening may be necessary, although the

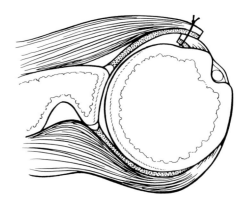

Fig. 13-114. Transverse plane section showing reefing of the subscapularis tendon and capsule in a situation where no Bankart lesion is found with isolated anterior instability. Note the intact anterior glenoid rim and the strong repair of the subscapularis tendon. *(Matsen, F. A., and Thomas, S. C.: Glenohumeral Instability. In Evarts, C. M. (ed.): Surgery of the Musculoskeletal System, Vol. 2, 2nd ed. p. 1458. New York, Churchill Livingstone, 1989.)*

surgeon must be certain the patient does not have multidirectional laxity before a unidirectional tightening is carried out.

Postoperative Management.   After the operation, the shoulder is held for 2 weeks in a conventional sling. The elbow is straightened twice daily to avoid sling soreness. This period of immobilization may be lengthened in young patients, particularly those with generalized ligamentous laxity, or if patients are unreliable. The period is shortened in patients older than 30 years when chronic shoulder stiffness is more likely. During immobilization, the tone of the shoulder musculature is maintained by isometric abduction and external rotation exercises. These are started on the first day after surgery. The repaired subscapularis tendon is protected for 6 weeks by avoiding active internal rotation against resistance. The four star rehabilitation program is initiated 6 weeks after surgery. My goal is near-normal motion within 12 weeks of surgery.

It is important to be observant for excessive anterior tightness. If anterior stiffness appears to be a potential problem (eg, external rotation limited to 0° in a 35-year-old 4 weeks postoperatively), forward flexion and external rotation stretching exercises are started. An axillary roentgenogram should be taken to exclude the possibility of posterior displacement of the humeral head. Patients are allowed to return to sports and vigorous labor after 3 months and after they have regained full forward elevation and excellent rotator strength of the operated shoulder. Patients are advised that maintaining rotator strength will increase the dynamic stability of the glenohumeral joint and decrease the likelihood of further injury. Swimming is routinely recommended to develop and maintain coordination and endurance of the shoulder. This exercise is usually started 6 to 8 weeks after operation.

Results.   In a 5.5-year follow-up of my first group of repairs of this type, I found 97% good to excellent results based on Rowe's[1143] grading system. One of 39 shoulders had a single redislocation, while the patient was practicing karate 4 years after repair. He has been rendered asymptomatic by a strengthening program and is back to full activities, including karate. The average range of motion at follow-up was 171° of elevation, 68° of external rotation with the arm at the side, and 85° of external rotation at 90° of abduction. Ninety-five percent of patients reported that their shoulders felt stable with all activities; 80% had no shoulder pain, while 20%

had occasional pain with activity. None had complications of posterior subluxation due to excessive anterior tightness. None had complications related to hardware.

ROCKWOOD'S PREFERRED METHOD
OF SURGICAL TREATMENT FOR RECURRENT
TRAUMATIC ANTERIOR SHOULDER INSTABILITY

Prior to surgery, all my patients are instructed in a series of exercises designed to strengthen the rotator cuff, deltoid, and the scapular stabilizers. (See Fig. 13-129.) For the past 15 years, my preferred method of surgical repair has been an anatomical reconstruction—that is, repair of the Perthes/Bankart lesion and/or a double-breasting of the capsule. I rarely have to overlap, and thus shorten, the subscapularis tendon.

Surgical Incision.   The standard anterior axillary incision begins in the anterior axillary crease, extending up toward and usually stopping at the coracoid process (Fig. 13-115**A**). In large muscular men, the incision may extend proximally as far as the clavicle. In women, I use the modified axillary incision described by Leslie and Ryan.[715] The skin is undermined subcutaneously in the proximal medial corner and the distal lateral corner to expose the deltopectoral interval (Fig. 13-115**B**). Usually, this interval is identified by the presence of the cephalic vein (Fig. 13-115**C**), which may either be absent or lying deep in the interval out of sight. When the vein is not present I can define the deltopectoral interval proximally, because in this area, it is easier to see the difference in angles of the muscle fibers between the pectoralis major and the deltoid. The interval should be very carefully opened, taking the vein *laterally* with the deltoid muscle. To routinely ligate the vein produces venous congestion in the area and in the upper extremity, and increases the postoperative discomfort. Preservation of the vein contributes to an easier postoperative course (ie, less pain and swelling). I use 8-0 nylon suture to repair an inadvertent nick in the vein. The deltopectoral interval is developed all the way up to the clavicle, and there is no need to detach any of the deltoid from the clavicle. I usually detach the upper 2 cm of the pectoralis major tendon. This allows for better visualization of the inferior capsule and makes it easier to locate and protect the axillary nerve, which passes *just inferior* to the capsule. I do not find it necessary to detach the coracoid process or the conjoined tendons (Fig. 13-115**D**). With the deltopectoral muscles retracted out of the way, the clavipectoral fascia is

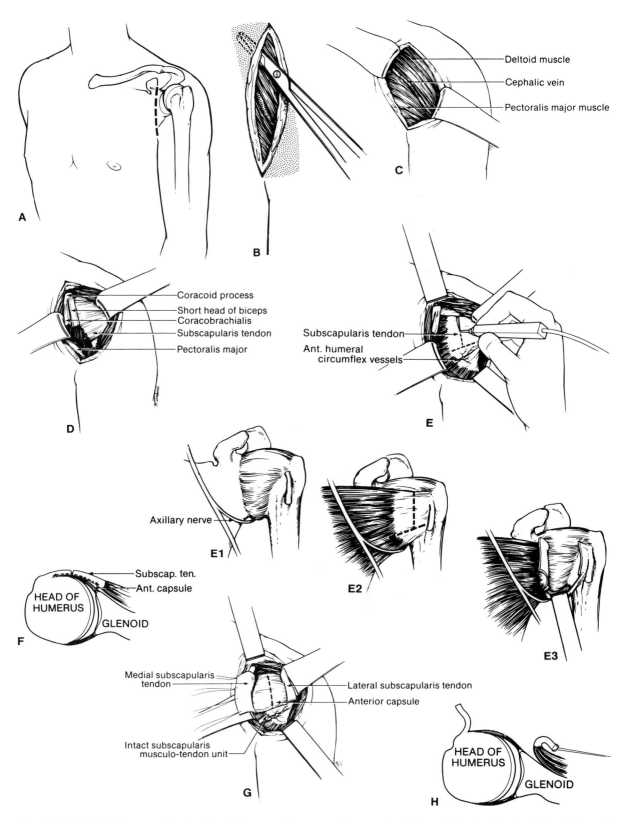

Fig. 13-115. (**A–S**) The precise details of the operative procedure can be followed in the detailed description of the author's preferred method of operative treatment in the text.

Procedure if anterior capsule is stripped off the scapula.

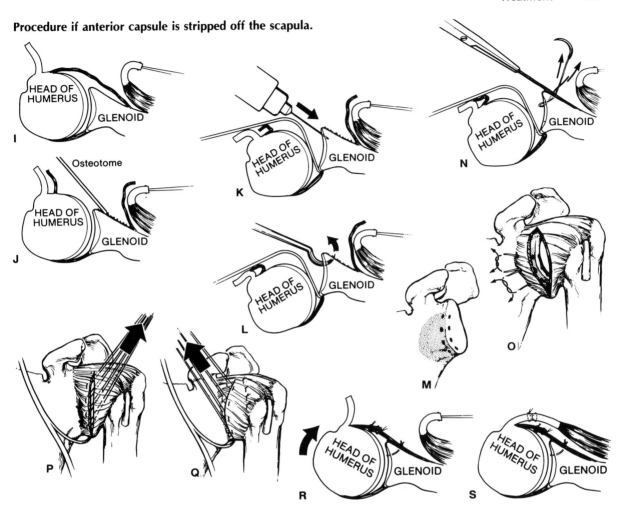

Figure 13-115 *(continued)*

seen covering the conjoined tendons. This fascia is divided vertically along the lateral border of the conjoined tendons. Proximally, the clavipectoral fascia blends into the coracoacromial ligament; I always divide this ligament at the time of a surgical procedure about the shoulder, because it may prevent future symptoms of the impingement syndrome.

Identification of Musculocutaneous Nerve. Before a Richardson retractor is placed in the medial side of the incision to retract the conjoined muscles and pectoralis major muscle, I palpate for the musculocutaneous nerve as it enters the conjoined tendon. Ordinarily, the nerve enters the coracobrachialis and biceps muscles from the medial aspect approximately 5 cm distal to the tip of the coracoid process.

However, it must be remembered that it might penetrate immediately below the tip of the coracoid. I have even seen the nerve visible on the lateral aspect of the conjoined tendon. Usually, by palpating just medial to the conjoined tendon and muscles, one can feel the entrance of the musculocutaneous nerve.

Identification and Protection of the Axillary Nerve. Next, I locate the axillary nerve—an especially important step when performing the capsular shift procedure. This is done by passing the finger down and along the lower and intact subscapularis muscle tendon unit (Fig. 13-115E). The right index finger should be used to locate the nerve in the left shoulder, and the left index finger should be used to locate the nerve in the right shoulder.

When the finger is as deep as it will go, the volar surface of the finger should be on the anterior surface of the muscle. Then, the distal phalanx is flexed and rotated anteriorly, which will hook under the axillary nerve before it dives back posteriorly under the inferior capsule. With the arm in external rotation, the nerve is displaced medially, making it difficult to locate. This large nerve can be easily located with the arm in adduction and in neutral rotation. With the upper 2 cm of the pectoralis major tendon taken down, not only can the nerve be palpated, it also can be visualized. The nerve is at least ⁵⁄₃₂ inch in size.

Division of the Subscapular Tendon and Preservation of the Anterior Humeral Circumflex Vessels.
With the arm in external rotation, the upper and lower borders of the subscapularis tendon can be visualized and palpated. The "soft spot" at the superior border of the subscapularis tendon is the interval between the subscapularis and supraspinatus tendons. The lower border of the tendon is identified by the presence of the anterior humeral circumflex artery and veins (Fig. 13-115E). The upper three fourths of the subscapularis tendon will be vertically transected usually ¾ to 1 inch medial to its insertion into the lesser tuberosity. I cut only the upper three fourths of the subscapularis tendon and prefer to do this with the electric cautery (Fig. 13-115E, F). I am very careful to divide only the tendon. I usually try to leave a little of the subscapularis tendon on the capsule to add to its strength. I avoid transecting the lower fourth of the subscapularis tendon, leaving it in place to prevent injury to the anterior humeral circumflex artery and veins, and to protect the axillary nerve (Fig. 13-115E2 and E3). The anterior humeral circumflex artery is the primary blood supply to the head of the humerus, and I believe it should be preserved. Once the vertical cut in the tendon has been completed, I very carefully reflect the medial part of the tendon off the capsule using curved Mayo scissors, until there are no further connections between the tendon and the capsule. When applying lateral traction on the tendon, it should have a rubbery bounce to it. Three or four stay sutures of No. 2 cottony Dacron are placed in the medial edge of the tendon; these are used initially for retraction and later at the time of tendon repair. The lateral stump of the subscapularis tendon is reflected off the capsule with a small sharp knife. This is rather easy with the capsule intact when the arm is in external rotation, and difficult when the capsule has been divided.

Failure to perform this step will make the two-layer closure of the capsule and the subscapularis tendon more difficult.

With the divided portions of the subscapularis tendon reflected medially *and* laterally, and with the arm in mild external rotation, I use an elevator to gently strip the intact lower fourth of the subscapularis muscle tendon unit off the anteroinferior capsule (Fig. 13-115E3). A narrow deep retractor (ie, Scofield) should be used to retract the lower part of the subscapularis muscle anteriorly and distally, which allows for easy visualization of the inferior capsule. The retractor holds not only the lower part of the subscapularis muscle, but also the axillary nerve anteriorly and distally out of the way, preventing injury when the inferior capsule is opened and divided and repaired (Fig. 13-115E3).

Division of the Capsule. Next, the capsule is divided vertically *midway* between its usual attachment on the glenoid rim and the humeral head (Fig. 13-115G, H). I have found that it is easier to divide the capsule midway between the humeral head and glenoid attachments. This allows for repair of the capsule if there is a Perthes-Bankart lesion. Furthermore, after the medial capsule is reattached to the glenoid rim, I have plenty of room to add strength to the anteroinferior capsule by double-breasting it with the planned capsular reconstruction. This vertical incision begins at the superior glenohumeral ligament and extends all the way down to the most inferior aspect of the capsule. I prefer to insert the horizontal mattress sutures in the medial capsule just as I complete the division of the most interior portion of the capsule. I explore the joint carefully, removing loose bodies and glenoid labrum tears. Close attention should be paid to stripping of the labrum, capsule, and periosteum from their normal attachments on the glenoid rim and neck of the scapula (ie, the Perthes-Bankart lesion (Fig. 13-115I).

Capsular Shift and Reconstruction. If the capsule has a secure fixation on the glenoid rim, the capsular reconstruction can then be performed (Fig. 13-115P, Q). However, if stripping of the capsule and periosteum from the glenoid rim and neck of the scapula has occurred, then the capsule must first be reattached before proceeding to the capsular reconstruction (Fig. 13-115I–O). Formerly, I believed that if there was a stripping of the capsule from the neck of the scapula, all that was needed was to roughen this up with a curette or osteotome to create bleeding and then the capsule would spontaneously reattach or heal itself back to the glenoid rim. However, because of failures on which I had to reoperate, I found this area had not healed and the capsule was still stripped off the glenoid neck. I am sure synovial fluid inhibits the usual healing process and prevents a consistent firm reattachment of the capsule and periosteum to the bony glenoid rim.

In some situations, it may be necessary to horizontally split the medial part of the capsule in its midportion to better visualize and decorticate the anterior rim and neck of the scapula with an osteotome or an air bur. There is a special retractor, developed by Dr. Carter Rowe, that I call the "dinner fork" because of its shape and its three sharp teeth. It is used to retract the capsule and muscles out of the way while the anterior glenoid rim and neck of the scapula are decorticated, and while the drill holes are being placed in the glenoid rim. I have tried a number of devices, including angled dental drills and Hall drills, curved cutting gouges, clamps, and the Ellison glenoid rim punch; no matter what instrument is used, it always seems to be difficult to place these holes in the dense glenoid rim. With the Bowen, Rowe, or Fukuda retractor holding the humeral head out of the way and the "dinner fork" holding the medial capsule and muscles out of the way, I prefer to first use an osteotome to decorticate the anterior surface of the neck of the scapula down to raw cancellous bone. Usually, three holes are then made between 3 and 6 o'clock on the anterior *articular* surface of the glenoid. These holes are made with a small drill bit approximately ⅛ inch in from the rim of the glenoid on the articular surface (Fig. 13-115**K**). Next, a curved Carter Rowe awl and tenaculum are used to connect the drill holes with the decorticated neck of the anterior glenoid (Fig. 13-115**L, M**). I pass the No. 2 nonabsorbable cottony Dacron sutures through these holes so there are two loops of intra-articular sutures through the three holes (the center hole has two sutures through it) (Fig. 13-115**N, O**).

The medial capsule is then pulled laterally and the needles on the intra-articular loops of sutures are passed up and through the medial capsule, so that when they are tied, the capsule is reapproximated to the raw bone of the glenoid rim (Fig. 13-115**N, O**). I believe this step is absolutely critical to eliminate the abnormal pouch in the capsule.

With the medial capsule secured back to the glenoid rim, I proceed with the capsular reconstruction. Prior to closure of the capsule, the joint is thoroughly irrigated with saline. The medial capsule will be double-breasted laterally and superiorly

under the lateral capsule (Fig. 13-115**P**). All sutures should be placed and tied, being sure that the arm is held in neutral to 15° to 20° of external rotation. To carry out this step, the lateral stump of the subscapularis tendon must have been separated from the lateral portion of the capsule. It is critical that the capsular reconstruction sutures be placed under the proper tension so that the arm may easily rotate to the desired position. Next, the lateral capsule is double-breasted by taking it medially and superiorly and suturing it down to the anterior surface of the medial capsule (Fig. 13-115**Q, R**). These sutures are also placed with the arm in the desired rotation. This type of capsular reconstruction not only eliminates all laxity in the anterior and inferior capsular ligaments, but, because of the double-breasting, the capsule is much stronger. The wound is again carefully irrigated with several liters of saline.

With the arm held in 15° to 20° of external rotation or in neutral rotation, the medial subscapularis tendon is brought into view by pulling on the previously placed sutures. The two borders of the tendon are easily approximated with gentle traction, and the tendon is repaired without any overlapping (Fig. 13-115**S**). If the tendon is loose with the arm in neutral rotation, then a double-breasting or overlapping of the tendon can be performed by using a two-layer closure with No. 2 Dacron horizontal mattress sutures.

Wound Closure.   Prior to closure of the wound, I carefully irrigate with antibiotic solution and then infiltrate the joint, muscles, and subcutaneous tissue with about 25 to 30 ml of 0.5% bupivacaine (Marcaine). This aids in decreasing the immediate postoperative pain. I am impressed that the use of bupivacaine prior to wound closure gives the patient an easier postoperative recovery period. The effect of the bupivacaine will last 6 to 8 hours, which allows the patient, as he or she is waking up, to have relatively little pain; later in the day, as the anesthesia begins to wear off, he or she can request pain medications. Care should be taken not to overuse the bupivacaine or to inject it directly into vessels. It is usually unnecessary to put any sutures in the deltopectoral interval. The deep subcutaneous layer is closed with 2-0 nonabsorbable sutures, which help to prevent widening of the scar. The subcutaneous fat is closed with absorbable sutures, and a running subcuticular nylon suture is used in the skin.

Postoperative Management.   Postoperatively, the patient's arm is stabilized in a shoulder immobilizer.

As soon as the patient is awake, I assess and chart the neurovascular status of the extremity. Depending on the anesthesia, this can often be done on the operating room table before the patient is taken to the recovery room. The status of the pulses and the axillary, musculocutaneous, median, ulnar, and radial nerves can be determined and recorded within a few seconds.

I prefer to use a commercial shoulder immobilizer because it is comfortable, quick, and simple to apply, and prevents abduction, flexion, and external rotation. Regardless of the type of immobilization, it is very important to temporarily remove the device when the patient is seen on the afternoon or evening of the day of surgery. For some reason, a patient who awakens from surgery with the arm in the "device" does not want to wiggle any part of the arm—almost as if it were frozen in the sling-and-swathe position. The commercial immobilizer can be easily removed; this allows the patient to move the hand and wrist and then gradually extend the elbow down to the side and lay it on the bed. This almost always relieves the aching pain in the arm and the muscle tension pain. I then tell the patient to flex and extend the elbow several times, which also relieves the generalized arm and shoulder discomfort. In many instances, a patient has related that the vague ache in the shoulder and elbow is more of a problem than pain at the operative site, and this simple release of the immobilizer, allowing movement of the elbow and wrist, eliminates the discomfort. I allow the patient to remove the immobilizer three to four times a day to exercise the elbow, but otherwise I instruct him or her to always keep the immobilizer in place. Specific instructions are given to the patient to avoid abduction, flexion, and external rotation when the device is removed.

Patients are usually dismissed on the second or third postoperative day, and I allow them to remove the immobilizer two or three times a day while at home when sitting, reading, or watching television. The patient can return to school or work any time after discharge from the hospital. At 5 days following surgery, the patient can remove the small dressing, take a shower, and reapply the new bandage. I usually delay removing the running subcuticular nylon stitch for 2 weeks; this seems to help prevent a wide scar.

As a general rule, the older the patient, the shorter the postoperative immobilization; the younger the patient, the longer the immobilization. In patients younger than 20 years, or in competitive, aggressive athletes, I immobilize the shoulder for 3 to 4 weeks; in young, semiathletic people younger than 30 years, shoulders are immobilized for 3 weeks; shoulders of patients younger than 50 years are immobilized for 2 weeks; shoulders of patients older than 50 are immobilized for 1 to 2 weeks. Following removal of the shoulder immobilizer, I allow the patient to gently use the arm for everyday living activities, but do not allow any rough use (eg, lifting, moving furniture, pushing, pulling). At the end of the immobilization period, I start the patient on a stretching exercise program using an overhead pulley and rope set. Following the return of motion, I institute a resisted weight exercise and shoulder-strengthening program to strengthen the deltoid, internal rotators, external rotators and the scapular stabilizers. (See Fig. 13-129.) Athletes are not permitted to return to competitive sports until they have reached a full and functional range of motion and have regained normal muscle strength; this usually requires 4 to 6 months.

Recurrent Posterior Instability

NONOPERATIVE MANAGEMENT

As with anterior glenohumeral instability, strong subscapularis and infraspinatus muscles can significantly augment glenohumeral stability even in the presence of capsular laxity.[900] Voluntary instability is relatively common among patients with recurrent posterior glenohumeral instability;[900] in this population, nonoperative treatment is indicated. These patients may be helped by informing them of the nature of the problem, counseling them to avoid dislocation, and giving them exercises for strengthening the rotator muscles.

OPERATIVE MANAGEMENT

Surgical stabilization of posterior glenohumeral instability may be considered when recurrent involuntary posterior subluxations or dislocations occur in spite of a reasonable effort at rehabilitation. Prior to surgery it is essential to identify all directions of instability and any anatomical factors that may predispose the joint to recurrent instability, such as humeral head or glenoid defects, abnormal glenoid version, rotator cuff tears, neurologic injuries, or generalized ligamentous laxity. It is important to consider the high recurrence and complication rates associated with attempted surgical correction of posterior instability. Hawkins and associates[491,659] reported a 50% failure rate following surgical procedures on recurrent posterior dislocation of the shoulder. Because functional limitations and pain can be minimal, they suggested that some of these patients may do better without reconstructive procedures. Tibone and co-workers[1298] stated that recurrent posterior dislocation of the shoulder is not a definite indication for surgery and stressed the need for careful patient selection prior to surgical reconstruction. They reported a failure rate of 30% following posterior staple capsulorrhaphy. Bayley and Kessel[92] stated that the failure to distinguish between traumatic and habitual (atraumatic) types of instability led to inappropriate surgery and was a major cause of recurrence following the operative repairs.

Several surgical approaches have been described for treatment of recurrent posterior glenohumeral instability. These approaches include scapular osteotomy,[367,435,444,470,662–664,899,1200] posterior bone block,[899] and posterior soft tissue procedures.[444,559,722,897,1133,1334]

Reverse Putti-Platt Procedure.   The infraspinatus muscle and tendon is used in this muscle-shortening or muscle-plication procedure. In some cases the infraspinatus and teres minor tendon may be used together in the plication. Care must be taken not to injure the axillary nerve when the teres minor muscle tendon unit is used.

Boyd-Sisk Procedure.[144]   The long head biceps tendon is transplanted posteriorly around the humerus to the posterior glenoid rim.

Glenoid Osteotomy and Bone Blocks.   Kretzler and co-workers,[662–664] Scott,[1200] English and Macnab,[351] Bestard,[111] Vegter,[1342] and Ahlgren and associates[12] have all reported using an opening, posterior wedge, glenoid osteotomy in recurrent posterior dislocations of the shoulder. In 1966, Kretzler and Blue[662] reported on the use of a posterior opening glenoid osteotomy in six patients with cerebral palsy. They used the acromion as the source of the graft to hold the wedge open. Kretzler[664] reported on 31 cases of the posterior glenoid osteotomy in voluntary (15 cases) and involuntary (16 cases) posterior dislocations with recurrences in 4 patients, 2 from each category. Extreme care must be taken during this procedure to prevent the osteotome from entering into or causing a fracture of the posterior half of the glenoid (Fig. 13-116). The suprascapular nerve above and the axillary nerve below are also at risk. English and Macnab[351] pointed out that there is a tendency for the humeral head to subluxate anteriorly after the osteotomy of the

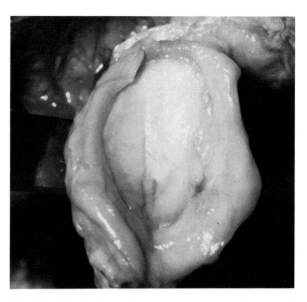

Fig. 13-116. Cadaver dissection showing a fracture of the glenoid created during a posterior opening wedge osteotomy of the glenoid. *(Matsen, F. A., III; Thomas, S. C.; and Rockwood, C. A., Jr.: Anterior Glenohumeral Instability. In Rockwood, C. A., and Matsen, F. A., III (eds.): The Shoulder, Fig. 14-86. Philadelphia, W. B. Saunders, 1990.)*

glenoid. Gerber and associates[429] demonstrated that posterior glenoid osteotomy thrusts the humeral head forward, and potentially causes impingement of the humeral head on the coracoid, producing pain and dysfunction. Their cadaver studies demonstrated that glenoplasty "consistently produced impingement of the subscapularis between the coracoid tip and the humeral head."

The posterior bone block or the glenoid osteotomy has been combined with the various soft tissue reconstructions.[311] Mowery and associates[879] reported five patients having bone blocks for recurrent posterior dislocation; one patient had a subsequent anterior dislocation.

Hawkins and co-workers[497] presented 50 shoulders in 35 patients treated for recurrent posterior instability. Only 11 of the 50 followed a traumatic event; 41 demonstrated voluntary and involuntary instability. Of those operated upon, 17 patients had glenoid osteotomies, 6 had reverse Putti-Platt procedures, and 3 had biceps tendon transfers. The dislocation rate after surgery was 50%; complications occurred in 20% of the operated cases. Two patients developed substantial degenerative osteoarthritis after glenoid osteotomy.

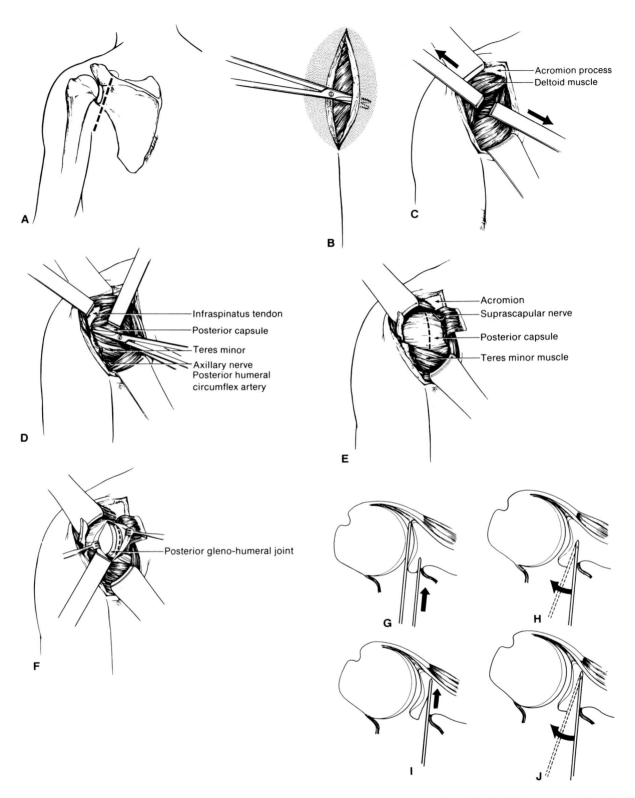

Fig. 13-117. Rockwood's preferred posterior shoulder reconstruction. (See text for a detailed description of each step of the procedure.) *(Matsen, F. A., III; Thomas, S. C.; and Rockwood, C. A., Jr.: Anterior Glenohumeral Instability. In Rockwood, C. A., and Matsen, F. A., III (eds.): The Shoulder, Fig. 14-88. Philadelphia, W. B. Saunders, 1990.)*

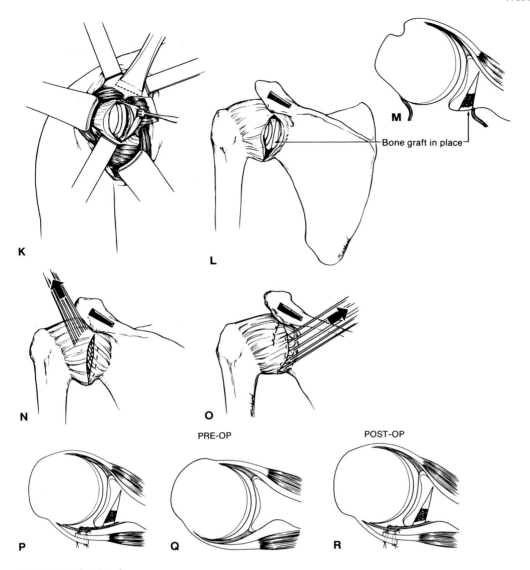

Bone graft in place

Figure 13-117 *(continued)*

ROCKWOOD'S TECHNIQUE OF POSTERIOR RECONSTRUCTION

Positioning the Patient. The patient is placed in the lateral decubitus position with the operative shoulder upward. The best way to support the patient in this position is to use kidney supports and the "bean bag."

Skin Incision. The incision begins 1 inch medial to the posterolateral corner of the acromion and extends downward 3 inches toward the posterior axillary creases[177] (Fig. 13-117**A**). If a bone graft is to be taken from the acromion, the incision extends a little farther superiorly, so the acromion can be exposed (Fig. 13-117**K, L**). Next, the subcutaneous tissues are dissected medially and laterally, so the skin can be retracted to visualize the fibers of the deltoid (Fig. 13-117**B**).

Splitting—Not Detaching—the Deltoid Fibers. A point 1 inch medial to the posterior corner of the acromion is selected, and the deltoid is then split distally 4 inches in the line of its fibers (Fig. 13-117**C**). The deltoid can be easily retracted medially and laterally to expose the underlying infraspinatus and teres minor muscles. This deltoid split can be made down to the midportion of the teres minor muscle. Remember that the axillary nerve exits the quadrangular space at the lower border of the teres minor muscle.

In performing a posterior reconstruction, the teres minor tendon should be reflected inferiorly down to the level of the inferior joint capsule. If the infraspinatus tendon is divided and reflected medially and laterally, care should be taken not to injure the suprascapular nerve. When the infraspinatus tendon is very lax, it can be reflected off the capsule and retracted superiorly without having to divide the tendon (Fig. 13-117**D**).

Capsular Incision and Shift. With the infraspinatus and teres minor muscles retracted out of the way, a vertical incision can be made in the posterior capsule to expose and explore the joint. I prefer to make the incision midway between the humeral and glenoid attachments, so at closure I can double-breast it and make it stronger (Fig. 13-117**E, F**). In doing the posterior capsular shift procedure, it is essential to have the teres minor muscle reflected sufficiently inferior that the vertical cut in the capsule will go all the way down to the most inferior recess of the capsule. If the capsule is thin and friable, and it appears that a capsular shift alone will be insufficient, then the infraspinatus tendon can be divided so it can be double-breasted to shorten it.

With the capsule divided all the way down inferiorly, horizontal mattress sutures of No. 2 cottony Dacron are inserted in the edge of the medial capsule. The arm should be held in neutral rotation, and the medial capsule sutured laterally and superiorly under the lateral capsule (Fig. 13-117**N**). Next, the lateral capsule is reflected and sutured medially and superiorly over the medial capsule, and again held in place with horizontal mattress sutures (Fig. 13-117**O**). This capsular shift procedure effectively eliminates any posterior and inferior capsular redundancy.

Infraspinatus Repair. If the infraspinatus tendon has been denuded, it is repaired with the arm in neutral rotation. If laxity exists, the tendon can be double-breasted (Fig. 13-117**P**). The wound is thoroughly irrigated, and the muscle and subcutaneous tissues are infiltrated with 25 to 30 ml of 0.5% bupivacaine (Marcaine). Care must be taken not to overuse the bupivacaine or inject it directly into vascular channels.

Wound Closure. When the retractors are withdrawn, the deltoid falls nicely together and a subcutaneous closure is performed. Care must be taken throughout the closure of the capsule, infraspinatus tendon, and skin to maintain the arm in neutral rotation. The patient is then gently rolled into the supine position, making sure the arm is in neutral rotation. When the anesthetic is completed, the patient is transferred to a bed, where the arm is maintained in the neutral position and supported by skin traction. Usually within 24 hours of surgery, the patient can stand and a modified shoulder immobilizer cast is applied.

Posterior Glenoid Osteotomy. I do not routinely perform a posterior glenoid osteotomy as part of my posterior reconstruction. Only when there is a posterior glenoid deficiency, or in cases where there is congenital retrotilt of the glenoid (ie, greater than 30°), should a posterior osteotomy be considered. Care must be taken not to overcorrect the retroversion, because it may force the head out anteriorly. However, if a posterior osteotomy is to be performed, it is absolutely essential to know the anatomy and angle of the slope of the glenoid. This can best be determined by placing a straight, blunt instrument into the joint so it lies on the antero-posterior glenoid rim (Fig. 13-117**G**). Next, the osteotome is placed intracapsularly, and directed parallel to the blunt instrument. If one is unsure of the angle and does not have a guide instrument in place, the osteotomy may enter the joint. (See Fig. 13-116.) The osteotomy site is not more than ¼ inch medial to the articular surface of the glenoid. If it is more medial than this, the possibility exists of injuring the suprascapular nerve as it passes around the base of the spine of the scapula to supply the infraspinatus muscle. Each time the osteotome is advanced, the osteotomy site is pried open (Fig. 13-117**H, I**); this helps to create a lateral plastic deformation of the posterior glenoid. The osteotomy should *not* exit anteriorly, but should stop just at the anterior cortex of the scapula (Fig. 13-117**J**). The intact anterior cortex periosteum and soft tissue will act as a hinge, which allows the graft to be secure in the osteotomy without internal fixation. I usually use an osteotome that is 1 inch wide to make the original cut, then use ½-inch osteotomes superiorly and inferiorly to complete the posterior division of bone. Osteotomes are used to open up the osteotomy site, and the bone graft is placed into position (Fig. 13-117**K, L, M**). If the anterior cortex is partially intact, there is no need for any internal fixation of the graft, because it is held securely in place by the osteotomy. The technique of the osteotomy has been described by Kretzler and associates,[662–664] Scott,[1200] and English and Macnab.[351] I prefer to take the bone graft from the acromion (Fig. 13-117**K, L**). Either a small piece (8 × 30 mm) for the osteotomy, or a large piece (15 × 30 mm) for a posteroinferior bone block can be taken from the top or the posterior edge of the acromion. If a larger graft is required, it should be taken from the ilium. Following completion of the osteotomy, the capsular shift, as described above, is performed.

As mentioned, following surgery the patient is supine with the forearm supported by the overhead bed frame, holding the arm in neutral rotation. I usually let the patient sit up on the bed the evening of surgery while maintaining the arm in neutral rotation. I let him or her sit up in a chair the next day, again holding the arm in neutral rotation. Either 24 or 48 hours after surgery, when the patient can stand comfortably, I apply a lightweight, long-arm cast. Next, a well-padded iliac crest band that sits around the abdomen and iliac crest is applied. The arm is then connected to the iliac crest band with a broom-handle support to maintain the arm in 10° to 15° of abduction and in neutral rotation. (See Fig. 13-90.) The cast is left in place for 6 to 8 weeks. Following removal of the plaster, the patient is allowed to use the arm for 4 to 6 weeks for everyday living activities. A rehabilitation program is begun that includes pendulum exercises, isometric exercises, and stretching of the shoulder with the use of an overhead pulley, after which resistive exercises are gradually increased.

Complications.   The principal cause of failure after a posterior repair is recurrent instability.[497,897] As the patient begins to use the shoulder and to regain the normal flexion range, the posterior capsule must stretch out. Unless good dynamic stability is regained, dependence on the repaired capsule will continue and stretch it out. This loosening is hastened if the posterior soft tissues are of poor quality, if the patient voluntarily or habitually tries to translate the shoulder posteriorly, or if large bony defects excessively load the soft tissues.

Occasionally, the opposite outcome can occur—posterior repair may produce a shoulder that is too tight, which may push the joint out anteriorly. Insufficient posterior laxity can limit flexion, cross-body adduction, and internal rotation.

Technical problems may occur in the surgical treatment of posterior glenohumeral instability. Posterior opening-wedge osteotomy of the glenoid is difficult to perform without cracking through the subchondral bone. Posterior glenoid osteotomy may result in avascular necrosis, or may push the humeral head too far anteriorly and give rise to post-surgical degenerative joint disease. Posterior bone blocks placed in an excessively prominent position may cause severe degenerative joint disease. The axillary nerve may be injured as it exits the quadrangular space, or the nerve to the infraspinatus may be injured in the spinoglenoid notch.[578,897]

MATSEN'S PREFERRED METHOD
OF TREATMENT FOR RECURRENT
POSTERIOR GLENOHUMERAL INSTABILITY

Care is taken to identify the circumstances and directions of instability, the presence of generalized ligmentous laxity, and any anatomical factors that might compromise the surgical result. I evaluate the possibilities of atraumatic and voluntary instability in each patient with posterior instability. All patients with posterior instability are placed on the four star rehabilitation program. A substantial number of patients with recurrent posterior instability respond to this program. Only patients who continue to have major symptomatic posterior instability after a reasonable rehabilitation effort are considered for surgery. These patients are told that the risks of surgery include excessive laxity (recurrent instability) and excessive tightness with limited flexion and internal rotation.

Positioning and Skin Incision.   A stress examination under anesthesia is routinely performed to confirm the diagnosis; stress x-ray films frequently are used for documentation.

The patient is placed almost prone with the shoulder off the operating table to allow a full range of humeral and scapular motion. After routine preparation of the arm, shoulder, neck, and back, a 10-cm incision is made in the extended line of the posterior axillary crease (Fig. 13-118**A**). The deltoid muscle is split for a distance of 4 cm between its middle and posterior thirds. If necessary, additional exposure may be obtained by carefully dissecting the muscle for a short distance from the scapular spine and posterior acromion. Retraction of the deltoid muscle inferiorly and laterally reveals the infraspinatus muscle, the teres minor muscle, and the axillary nerve emerging from the quadrangular space. The spinoglenoid notch is palpated to determine the location of the important nerve to the infraspinatus.

Division of Infraspinatus With Capsule.   The infraspinatus, the teres minor, and the attached cap-

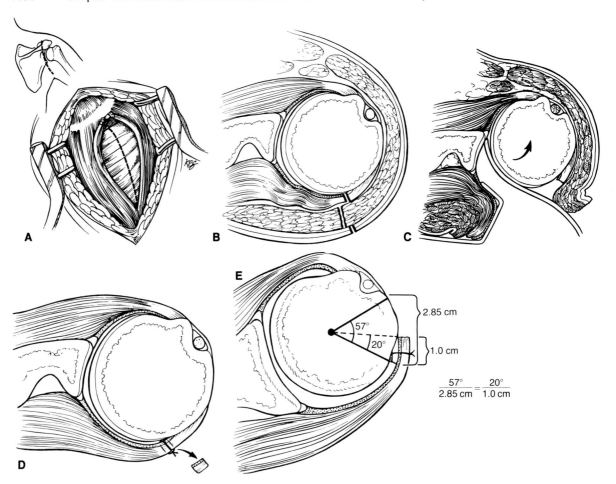

Fig. 13-118. Operative repair for recurrent posterior glenohumeral instability. (**A**) A 10-cm skin incision is made in the extended line of the posterior axillary crease (**inset**). The deltoid muscle is split between its middle and posterior thirds. (**B**) A transverse plane section shows the interval through the deltoid muscle and the infraspinatus tendon. (**C**) A transverse plane section shows placement of the retractors exposing the glenoid. (**D**) A transverse plane section shows repair of the infraspinatus tendon after resecting the desired amount for capsular and tendon advancement. Shortening the posterior capsule and tendon by 1 cm will limit internal rotation by approximately 20°. (**E**) The effect of shortening capsular structures on rotation. The average radius of the humerus is 2.85 cm; this is the length of an arc equal to one radian, or approximately 57°. Shortening the capsule by 2.85 cm would restrict rotation by 57°. Proportionally, a 1-cm shortening of the capsule would restrict rotation by 20°. Shown here is a posterior reefing of approximately 1 cm, decreasing internal rotation by approximately 20°. *(Matsen, F. A., III; Thomas, S. C.; and Rockwood, C. A., Jr.: Anterior Glenohumeral Instability. In Rockwood, C. A., and Matsen, F. A., III (eds.): The Shoulder, Fig. 14-87. Philadelphia, W. B. Saunders, 1990.)*

sule are incised 1 cm from the greater tuberosity to expose the posterior glenohumeral joint (Fig. 13-118A–C). Excessive traction on the axillary nerve and the nerve to the infraspinatus is carefully avoided. The joint is inspected for humeral head defects, wear of the anterior or posterior glenoid, tears in the glenoid labrum, loose bodies, and tears of the rotator cuff. Posterior capsular avulsions are uncommon, but when present, are repaired by a technique similar to that described for anterior repair. In the usual case, the shoulder is stabilized by reefing the capsule, along with the attached infraspinatus and teres minor tendons. This may be accomplished by overlapping the medial and lateral flaps by the desired amount, or by advancing the capsule and tendon into a bony groove at the desired length (Fig. 13-118**D**). We usually try to limit internal rotation of the adducted humerus to 45°. Internal rotation is limited by approximately 20° for each centimeter of shortening of the posterior capsule and tendon (Fig. 13-118**E**). Greater tightening may be used in patients with generalized ligamentous instability.

Capsular Shift and Repair.   If the patient demonstrates posteroinferior capsular laxity, the capsule is released from the inferior neck of the humerus under direct visualization as the humerus is progressively internally rotated. The capsule and muscle tendons are then advanced superiorly, as well as laterally, tightening the axillary recess. If significant multidirectional instability is present, a formal inferior capsular shift may be performed.[900]

Anteromedial humeral head defects of moderate size are managed by tightening the posterior capsule so internal rotation is limited to 30°. A shoulder with an anterior humeral head defect constituting more than a third of the articular surface often cannot be stabilized by soft tissue surgery. In these instances, insertion of a prosthetic head through the anterior approach is required to restore stability and function to the glenohumeral joint. Because it changes the surgical approach, a lesion of this size needs to be identified preoperatively.

Wound Closure and Postoperative Management. When the repair is complete, the deltoid is carefully repaired to the scapular spine and acromion. After surgery, the patient is immobilized in a "handshake" cummerbund cast with the shoulder in adduction, neutral rotation, and slight extension for 3 weeks, during which time internal rotation isometric exercises are instituted. After the cast is removed, the patient is allowed to perform more vigorous rotator-strengthening exercises and to use the shoulder below the horizontal. The patient is encouraged to regain forward flexion strength and range, in concert with increases in external rotation strength, so the repair has the backup of strong posterior cuff muscles. Patients are placed on the four star rehabilitation program (See Table 13-3) 6 to 8 weeks after surgery. Vigorous shoulder activity is prohibited until normal rotator strength is achieved. The patient is advised to continue rotator strengthening-exercises daily to optimize dynamic shoulder stability.

Recurrent Multidirectional Inferior and Voluntary Instability

MATSEN'S APPROACH TO RECURRENT INFERIOR AND MULTIDIRECTIONAL GLENOHUMERAL INSTABILITY

Inferior displacement of the head of the adducted humerus may indicate a torn or lax superior rotator cuff, suprascapular nerve palsy,[298] deltoid atony, or deltoid palsy. These specific lesions must be sought for, because their presence may substantially affect treatment.

Inferior glenohumeral instability is a common component of multidirectional instability (AMBRI syndrome). Inferior instability produces symptoms primarily when loads are carried at the side. This condition may be documented on an anteroposterior x-ray film of each shoulder taken with the shoulders relaxed and a weight of 10 pounds held in each hand (Fig. 13-119). The effects of generalized capsular instability can often be ameliorated by vigorous rotator strengthening. I again use the four star rehabilitation program. (See Table 13-3.) The results are often most satisfying in this group of patients, particularly if they are well informed about the need for dynamic stability in the presence of lax soft tissues about the joint.

When the history and physical examination indicate the shoulder is loose in all directions, and when the patient has failed to respond to vigorous internal and external rotator–strengthening, endurance, and coordination exercises, an inferior capsular shift procedure may be considered.[900] The principle of the procedure is to symmetrically tighten the anterior, inferior, and posterior aspects of the capsule by advancing its humeral attachment. We prefer to carry out this procedure from the anterior approach, advancing the capsular anteriorly on the humerus. In this way, shoulder flexion produces additional posterior capsular tightening (Fig. 13-120). In contrast, when the procedure is performed from a posterior approach, the capsule is advanced posteriorly on the humerus. In this situation, the tightened capsule loosens as the shoulder is flexed (Fig. 13-121).

Skin Incision and Identification of Axillary Nerve. The approach is identical to that used for an anterior repair. The skin incision is made in the anterior axillary crease (Fig. 13-122). The deltopectoral interval is developed, exposing the clavipectoral fascia. This is divided, and the muscles attached to the coracoid process are retracted medially. The axillary

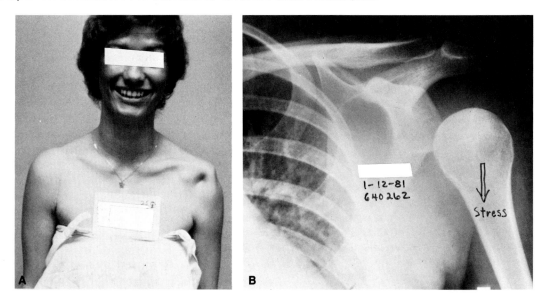

Fig. 13-119. (**A**) Patient with voluntary anteroinferior subluxation of the left shoulder. She can perform this maneuver without any discomfort. The left shoulder has become so unstable that she is unable to carry out her daily activities. The scar on the right shoulder is a result of a successful capsular shift reconstruction. (**B**) Anteroposterior x-ray film taken at the time of her voluntary anteroinferior subluxation.

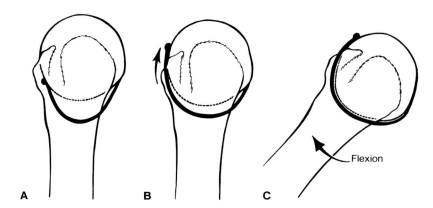

Fig. 13-120. Inferior capsular shift, when performed from the anterior approach, advances the capsule anteriorly on the humerus. This produces additional posterior capsular tightening with shoulder flexion. (**A**) Lax inferior capsule. (**B**) Inferior capsule brought anteriorly on the humerus on an anterior approach. (**C**) With humeral flexion, the posterior and inferior capsule are further tightened. *(Matsen, F. A., III; Thomas, S. C.; and Rockwood, C. A., Jr.: Anterior Glenohumeral Instability. In Rockwood, C. A., and Matsen, F. A., III (eds.): The Shoulder, Fig. 14-90. Philadelphia, W. B. Saunders, 1990.)*

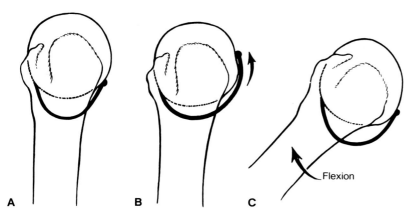

Fig. 13-121. When the inferior capsular shift is performed from the posterior approach and the capsule is advanced posteriorly on the humerus, the tightened capsule loosens with shoulder flexion. (**A**) Lax inferior capsule. (**B**) From the posterior approach the lax inferior capsule is advanced posteriorly on the humerus. (**C**) Humeral flexion loosens the posterior and inferior capsule. *(Matsen, F. A., III; Thomas, S. C.; and Rockwood, C. A., Jr.: Anterior Glenohumeral Instability. In Rockwood, C. A., and Matsen, F. A., III (eds.): The Shoulder, Fig. 14-91. Philadelphia, W. B. Saunders, 1990.)*

nerve is identified and protected during this procedure. The arm is held in external rotation, and the subscapularis tendon is divided near its insertion to the lesser tuberosity, leaving 1 cm of tendon laterally for reattachment. The subscapularis is split from the capsule in the coronal plane, leaving some tendon on the anterior capsule to reinforce it.

Capsular Incision and Shift.   While the arm is progressively externally rotated, the anterior, inferior, and posterior aspects of the capsule are incised from the neck of the humerus up to the midposterior part of the humeral head. The joint is inspected. Capsular detachments from the glenoid and labral tears are uncommon in the AMBRI syndrome. The

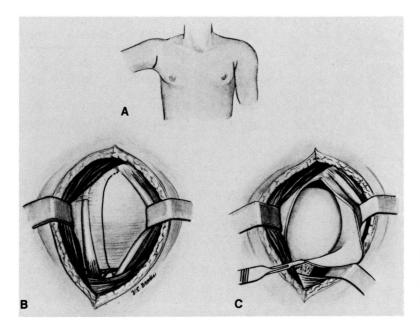

Fig. 13-122. (**A**) Axillary incision. (**B**) Incision through the subscapularis. (**C**) Release of the anterior and inferior capsule from the neck of the humerus. *(Matsen, F. A., III; Thomas, S. C.; and Rockwood, C. A., Jr.: Anterior Glenohumeral Instability. In Rockwood, C. A., and Matsen, F. A., III (eds.): The Shoulder, Fig. 14-92. Philadelphia, W. B. Saunders, 1990.)*

detached lateral margin of the capsule is then rotated from posterior to anterior, reducing the volume of the joint symmetrically (Fig. 13-123). Tension of the capsular flap must reduce the inferior axillary pouch and posterior capsule redundancy until *symmetric* shoulder stability is restored. The advanced capsule is sutured into a bony groove created at the humeral neck. Redundant superior capsule is used to reinforce the anterior repair. The anterior repair must not be excessively tight; a 30° range of external rotation is desired to prevent excessive anterior tightness. The subscapularis tendon is then brought over the capsular repair and reattached at its normal location.

Postoperative Management.   Postoperatively, the arm is held at the side in a sling. If posterior instability was a major problem preoperatively, the

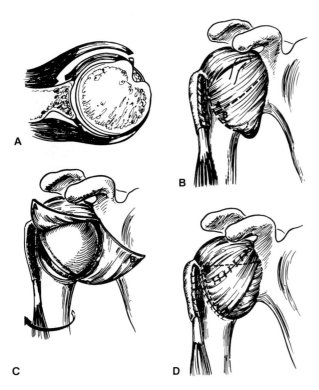

Fig. 13-123. (**A**) The subscapularis split, leaving part of the tendon to reinforce the anterior capsule. (**B**) The split in the rotator internal is closed. (**C**) Capsular flaps A and B are created. (**D**) Flap B is brought superiorly and flap A inferiorly, eliminating capsular redundancy. (*Matsen, F. A., and Thomas, S. C.: Glenohumeral Instability. In Evarts, C. M. (ed.): Surgery of the Musculoskeletal System, Vol. 2, 2nd ed. p. 1439–1470. New York, Churchill Livingstone, 1989.*)

shoulder is held in neutral flexion–extension and neutral rotation, using a "handshake" cast. Immobilization is usually continued for 3 weeks, during which isometric exercises are carried out to prevent atrophy. After immobilization is discontinued, the four star rehabilitation program is instituted. Motion is allowed to progress under active control of strong, coordinated muscles.

ROCKWOOD'S APPROACH TO ATRAUMATIC AND MULTIDIRECTIONAL GLENOHUMERAL INSTABILITY

In 1956 Rowe[1144] carefully analyzed 500 dislocations of the glenohumeral joint, and determined that 96% were caused by trauma and only 4% were atraumatic. However, recent evidence indicates that atraumatic lesions are more common than was previously reported. The patient with atraumatic instability may have instability anteriorly, posteriorly, inferiorly, or in all directions. Atraumatic instability can be voluntary, involuntary, or combined voluntary and involuntary.

In voluntary instability, the patient places the shoulder into the "right" position so that, with selective muscle contraction and relaxation, he or she can subluxate or dislocate the shoulder anteriorly, posteriorly, or inferiorly (see Fig. 13-119). This can become habit-forming. Voluntary subluxation and dislocation can be associated with emotional and psychiatric disorders. Patients with a voluntary problem usually do not have a history of a significant injury, and usually can remember that they have been able to slip one or both shoulders out of position since early childhood. The patient can subluxate or dislocate the shoulder without significant pain.

The involuntary type of subluxation is not quite so obvious and only occurs when the patient puts stress on the shoulder, such as while carrying a suitcase. This type of instability may be associated with congenital abnormalities or developmental problems such as Ehlers-Danlos syndrome, aplasia of the shoulder joint, following a nerve injury to the shoulder, or following a stroke with flail shoulder. The patient notes that when stress is applied, the shoulder will slip out of place; when the stress is removed, the shoulder relocates. There is no history of significant injury, and the patient describes the shoulder slipping in and out of place without significant discomfort.

On physical examination, in both voluntary and involuntary types, the involved shoulder will be quite lax. The patient may demonstrate gross instability (ie, the shoulder may be unstable anteri-

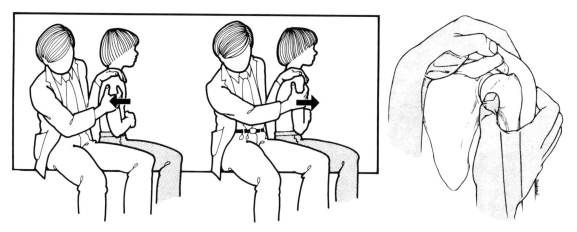

Fig. 13-124. Technique of evaluation of shoulder stability. (**Left**) In examining the right shoulder the physician sits slightly behind the patient's right shoulder on the examining table. The physician's left hand is placed on top of the shoulder so that the fingers grasp the clavicle and the palm of the hand is securely resting on top of the spine of the scapula. (**Right**) By acutely flexing the wrist and placing the forearm on the posterior border of the scapula, the physician can then lean into the scapula and secure the scapula to the thorax. The right hand is then free to push or pull the humeral head in and out of the glenoid fossa.

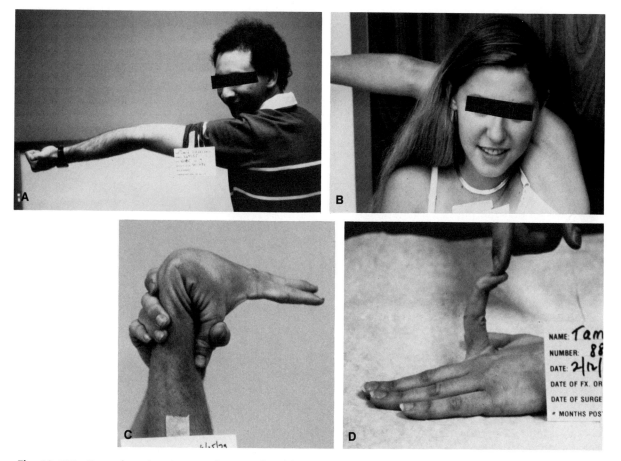

Fig. 13-125. Examples of patients with generalized ligamentous laxity: (**A**) laxity of the elbow, (**B**) the shoulder, (**C**) the wrist, (**D**) the metacarpal phalangeal joints.

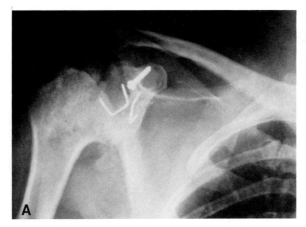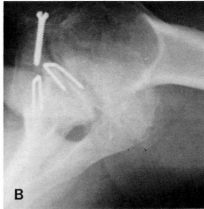

Fig. 13-126. Pitfalls associated with voluntary dislocations. (**A**) Severe traumatic arthritis following six reconstructions of the right shoulder in a patient who had voluntary dislocations of the shoulder. Note the irregularity of the joint, the loose bodies, and the floating metal. (**B**) In the axillary lateral roentgenogram, note the degenerative changes and the irregular contour of the humeral head.

orly, posteriorly, or inferiorly, or may have multi-directional instability) (Fig. 13-124). Not only is the involved shoulder lax to examination, but laxity is also noted in the normal shoulder and in other major joints. The elbows and knees may be hyperextended, and the patient may have extreme laxity of the metacarpophalangeal joints. (Fig. 13-125). Radiographic evaluation of the involved shoulder will be essentially normal; even special x-ray views fail to reveal anterior glenoid rim fractures or compression fractures of the posterolateral humeral head. A stress view with the shoulder voluntarily subluxated, or with weight attached to the wrist, will show displacement of the glenohumeral joint.

The treatment of patients with atraumatic instability requires that the physician differentiate between the voluntary and the involuntary types. Certainly, the patient with voluntary instability who has psychiatric problems should never be treated with surgery (Figs. 13-126 to 13-128). Rowe and Yee[1132] reported on disasters in patients with psychiatric problems who had been treated with surgical reconstructions. Patients with emotional disturbances and psychiatric problems should be referred for psychiatric help. Rowe and Yee[1132] also pointed out that there are patients with voluntary instability who do not have psychiatric problems, and who can be significantly helped with a rehabilitation program. If the emotionally stable patient fails to respond to 6 to 12 months of rehabilitation, a capsular shift reconstruction should be performed. Neer and Foster[896] reported on their capsular shift procedure.

I place all patients with atraumatic instability problems on a very specific rehabilitation program to strengthen the three parts of the deltoid, the rotator cuff, and the scapular stabilizers. If the patient has an obvious psychiatric or emotional problem, I do my best to explain the problem to the patient and family and help them seek psychiatric help.

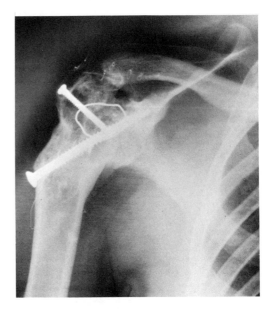

Fig. 13-127. Arthrodesis of the right shoulder was the final operation for a patient who had voluntary anterior dislocations and eight unsuccessful attempts at reconstruction.

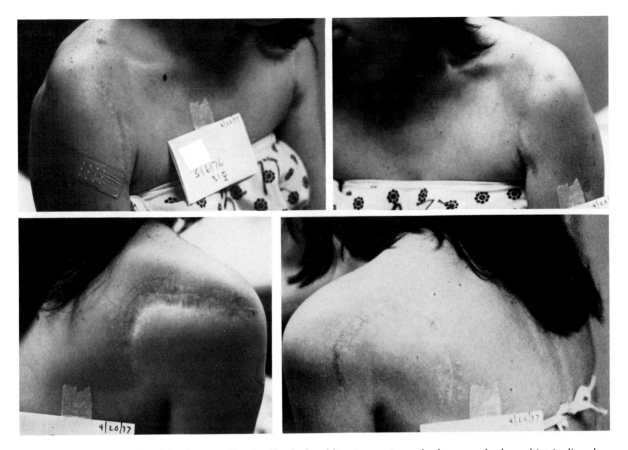

Fig. 13-128. Photographs of the front and back of both shoulders in a patient who has a marked psychiatric disorder. Despite multiple operative procedures, the patient can still displace both shoulders anteriorly and posteriorly. X-ray films reveal severe degenerative changes in both joints.

Under no circumstances do I ever tell the patient or family that surgery is a possibility for the emotionally disturbed patient. When I have ruled out congenital or developmental causes for the instability problem, I personally teach the patient how to perform the shoulder-strengthening exercises and give him or her a copy of the exercise diagrams. (See Fig. 13-129.) I give the patient a set of Therabands, which includes yellow, red, green, blue, and black bands, and the diagrams of the exercises to be performed. Each Theraband is a strip 3 inches wide and 5 feet long that is tied into a loop. The loop can be fastened over a doorknob (or any fixed object) to offer resistance to the pull. The patient does five basic exercises to strengthen the deltoid and the rotator cuff. The yellow Theraband is the weakest and offers 1 pound of resistance; the red, 2 pounds; the green, 3 pounds; the blue, 4 pounds; and, finally, the black offers 5 pounds of resistance to the pull. The patient is instructed to do the five

exercises two to three times a day. Each exercise should be done five to ten times, and each held for a count of five to ten. The patient is instructed to gradually increase the resistance (ie, yellow to red and green, and so on) every 2 to 4 weeks. After the black Theraband becomes easy to use, the patient is given a pulley kit and is instructed to do the same five basic exercises, but now lifting weights, as shown in Figure 13-129. The pulley kit consists of a pulley, an open eye screw hook, a handle, and a piece of rope, all in a plastic bag. The patient begins by attaching 7 to 10 pounds of weight to the end of the rope, and proceeds to the five basic exercises. Over several months, the patient increases the weights of resistance—up to 15 pounds for women and 20 to 25 pounds for men. When we start the basic strengthening of the rotator cuff and the deltoid, I also instruct the patient on how to do the exercises to strengthen the scapular stabilizer muscles. The push-ups (ie, wall push-ups, knee push-

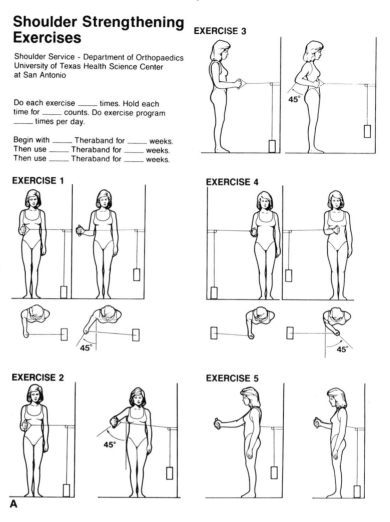

Shoulder Strengthening Exercises

Shoulder Service - Department of Orthopaedics
University of Texas Health Science Center
at San Antonio

Do each exercise _____ times. Hold each
time for _____ counts. Do exercise program
_____ times per day.

Begin with _____ Theraband for _____ weeks.
Then use _____ Theraband for _____ weeks.
Then use _____ Theraband for _____ weeks.

EXERCISE 3

EXERCISE 1

EXERCISE 4

EXERCISE 2

EXERCISE 5

Fig. 13-129. (**A**) Shoulder strengthening exercises. Initially the patient is given rubber Therabands to strengthen the rotator cuff muscles and the three parts of the deltoid. When the patient is proficient with the rubber resistance with exercises 1 to 5, then the patient is given an exercise kit that consists of a pulley, hook, rope, and handle. The pulley is attached to the hook, which is fixed to the wall, and the five exercises are performed. Initially the patient is instructed to use 5 or 10 pounds of weight; this is gradually increased over a period of several months to as much as 25 pounds. The purpose of the five exercises is to strengthen the three parts of the deltoid muscles, the internal rotators, and the external rotators.

(continued) **A**

ups, and regular push-ups) are used to strengthen the serratus anterior, rhomboids, and so forth, and the shoulder-shrugging exercises are done to strengthen the trapezius muscles. We have learned that the rehabilitation program is 80% successful in managing anterior instability problems, and 90% successful in managing atraumatic posterior instability problems.[1103] Regardless of any prior "rehabilitation program" that the patient has participated in, I always start the patient on our strengthening routine.

If the patient still has the signs and symptoms of instability after 6 months of doing the exercises, a very specific capsular shift procedure is performed. One must always remember that it is possible for a patient with laxity of the major joints to have a superimposed traumatic episode, which ordinarily does not respond to a rehabilitation program. A patient with atraumatic instability, who has a history of significant trauma, pain, swelling, and so forth, probably will require a surgical reconstruction, but only after a trial with the rehabilitation program.

The details of the incision, surgical approach, protection of the axillary nerve, and preservation of the anterior humeral circumflex vessels are essentially the same for the management of a recurrent traumatic anterior instability problem. (See Fig. 13-115.) The main difference is that there is no Perthes-Bankart lesion (Fig. 13-130**A**). The deficiency is simply a very redundant capsule anteriorly, inferiorly, or posteroinferiorly. The principle of the capsular shift is to divide the capsule all the way down inferiorly, midway between its attachment on the humerus and on the glenoid rim. The joint is carefully inspected, and then the shift is

Shoulder Strengthening and Stretching Exercises

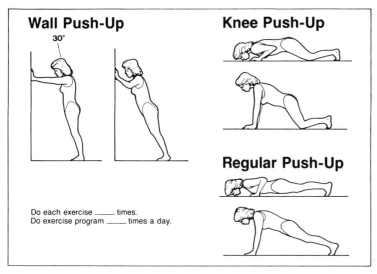

Wall Push-Up

30°

Knee Push-Up

Regular Push-Up

Do each exercise _____ times.
Do exercise program _____ times a day.

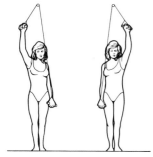

Do each exercise _____ times.
Hold each time for _____ counts.
Do exercise program _____ times a day.

B

Shoulder Shrug

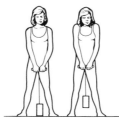

Do each exercise _____ times.
Hold each time for _____ counts.
Use _____ pounds of weight.
Do exercise program _____ times a day.

Fig. 13-129 *(continued)*
(**B**) In addition, the patient is instructed in exercises to strengthen the scapular stabilizer muscles. To strengthen the serratus anterior and rhomboids, the patient is instructed first to do wall push-ups and then is instructed to gradually do knee push-ups and then regular push-ups. The shoulder shrug exercise is used to strengthen the trapezius and the levator scapulae muscles. *(Matsen, F. A., III; Thomas, S. C.; and Rockwood, C. A., Jr.: Anterior Glenohumeral Instability. In Rockwood, C. A., and Matsen, F. A., III (eds.): The Shoulder, Fig. 14-94. Philadelphia, W. B. Saunders, 1990.)*

performed. As is demonstrated in Figure 13-115**P, Q,** I prefer to take the medial capsule superiorly and laterally under the lateral capsule, then take the lateral capsule superiorly and medially over the medial capsule. I am careful that the placement and tying of the sutures are done with the arm in approximately 15° to 20° of external rotation for an anterior reconstruction and in neutral rotation for a posterior reconstruction. Ordinarily, the subscapularis is simply repaired to itself, but should there be laxity of the subscapularis with the arm in 15° to 20° of external rotation, then the subscapularis can be double-breasted (Fig. 13-130**C**). Ordinarily, in doing the posterior capsular shift, the infraspinatus tendon can be reflected superiorly and the teres minor reflected inferiorly off the posterior capsule. As with the anterior shift, the posterior capsule is divided midway between its attachments

(Fig. 13-130**B**), thus allowing a double-breasting or strengthening of the midportion of the capsule (Fig. 13-130**C**). Remember, however, that posterior shifts are rarely required, because most patients do so well with the rehabilitation program.

The surgical management of patients with atraumatic instability demands that the shoulder not be put up too tight, as can be done with the Magnuson-Stack, Putti-Platt, or Bristow procedures. If the surgeon fails to recognize that the patient has an atraumatic instability problem, and if a routine muscle-tightening procedure is performed, the result may be that the humeral head will be pushed out in the opposite direction, leading to early degenerative arthritis. The surgeon must also be careful, even in patients with atraumatic instability, not to perform a capsular shift that is so tight as to force the head out in the opposite direction. As men-

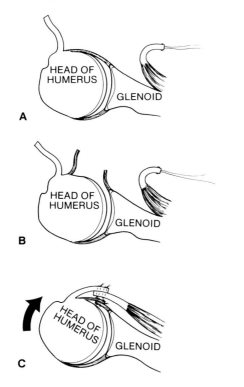

Procedure if anterior capsule is not stripped off scapula.

Capsular Repair

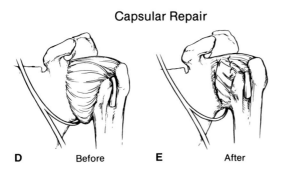

D   Before   **E**   After

Fig. 13-130. Capsular shift reconstruction for atraumatic anterior subluxation or dislocation. The Bankort/Perthes lesion is not present, and the capsule is shifted to eliminate the anteroinferior laxity. *(Matsen, F. A., III; Thomas, S. C.; and Rockwood, C. A., Jr.: Anterior Glenohumeral Instability. In Rockwood, C. A., and Matsen, F. A., III (eds.): The Shoulder, Fig. 14-95. Philadelphia, W. B. Saunders, 1990.)*

tioned, I prefer to place and tie the sutures in the anterior capsular shift procedure with the arm in 15° to 20° of external rotation and held in neutral rotation during the posterior capsular shift reconstruction. The reader must also be warned that it

is essential to isolate and protect the axillary nerve when doing the anterior or posterior capsular shift (Fig. 13-130**D, E**).

INFERIOR AND SUPERIOR DISLOCATIONS

Inferior Dislocations (Luxatio Erecta)

In our experience, inferior dislocation of the shoulder is more common than superior dislocation. We have seen 16 patients with luxatio erecta and have not treated any patient with a superior dislocation. Severe soft tissue injury, or fractures about the proximal humerus, always occur with inferior dislocations. At the time of repair or autopsy, various authors have found avulsion of the supraspinatus and infraspinatus tendons from the humerus; avulsion of the capsule; rupture of the subscapularis, pectoralis major, and teres minor muscles; and fractures of the greater tuberosity.[668,692,754,842,888,1102] Injury to the axillary artery and brachial plexus usually occurs.[418,716,754,828] The clinical picture of a patient with luxatio erecta is so clear that it can hardly be mistaken for any other condition. The humerus is locked in a position somewhere between 110° and 160° of abduction. The elbow is usually flexed, and the forearm is flexed and is lying on or behind the head (Fig. 13-131). The head of the humerus may be palpated on the lateral chest wall. Pain is quite severe. The condition is more common among the elderly. Neurovascular compression is almost always noted with luxatio erecta, and is discussed under Complications.

TREATMENT

Reduction is accomplished by traction and countertraction maneuvers. Traction should be applied in line with the arm (upward and outward), while countertraction is applied through a sheet, folded up over and across the top of the shoulder by an assistant (Fig. 13-132). The line of countertraction is from across the top of the dislocated shoulder, across the chest to the opposite side of the patient, and, in general, is kept in line with the traction being applied to the arm of the dislocated shoulder. Occasionally, because the head and neck of the humerus have ruptured through the inferior capsule, closed reduction cannot be accomplished. The buttonhole rent in the capsule must be enlarged at surgery before reduction can occur.

COMPLICATIONS

Neurovascular compression is usually associated with inferior dislocations, but practically always recovers following reduction.[418,716,754,828] Lev-el and

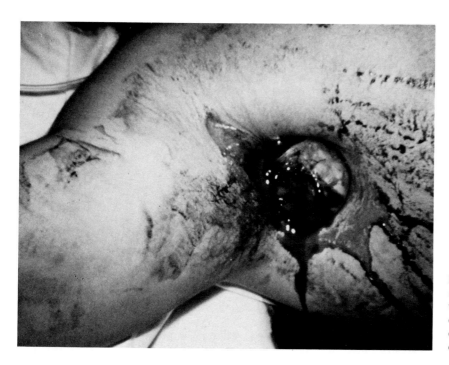

Fig. 13-131. Photograph of the right shoulder and axilla of a patient who had an open inferior dislocation of the humeral head out through the axilla. *(Courtesy of George Armstrong).*

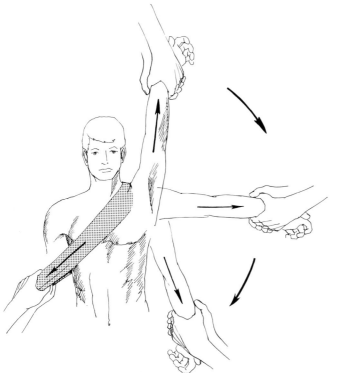

Fig. 13-132. Technique of reduction of an inferior dislocation (luxatio erecta) of the glenohumeral joint. Countertraction is applied by an assistant using a folded sheet across the superior aspect of the shoulder and neck. Traction on the arm is first applied upward and then gradually the arm is brought into less abduction and finally placed at the patient's side as demonstrated.

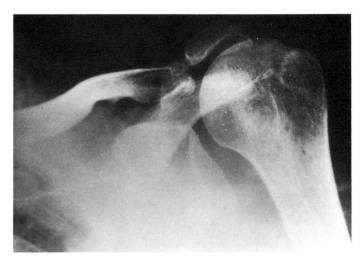

Fig. 13-133. Superior dislocation of the left shoulder. Note that the head of the humerus is displaced superiorly from the glenoid fossa and that the fracture of the acromion process has also been displaced upward.

associates[716] reported a patient who had an injury to the axillary artery and subsequently developed a thrombus that required resection and vein graft. Gardham and Scott[418] reported a case in 1980 in which the axillary artery was damaged in its third part, and was managed by a bypass graft using the saphenous vein. In my series, all 16 patients had brachial plexus injury and some vascular compromise prior to reduction. Fractures may occur to the acromion process or to the inferior glenoid fossa. The greater tuberosity can become detached during displacement of the head, but may be restored at reduction.

Superior Dislocations

Speed[1248] reported that Langier, in 1834, was the first to record a case of superior dislocation of the glenohumeral joint. Stimson[1011] reviewed 14 cases that had been reported in the literature prior to 1912. In current literature, little is mentioned of this type of dislocation, but, undoubtedly, cases occasionally occur. The typical cause is an extreme forward and upward force on the adducted arm. With displacement of the humerus upward, fractures may occur in the acromion, the acromioclavicular joint, the clavicle, the coracoid process, or the humeral tuberosities (Fig. 13-133). Extreme soft tissue damage occurs to the capsule rotator cuff, the biceps tendon, and surrounding muscles. Clinically, the head rides clearly above the level of the acromion and the arm is shortened. The arm is adducted to the side, and shoulder movement is restricted and quite painful. Neurovascular complications are usually present. Treatment consists of closed reduction and restoration of the damaged tissues.

REFERENCES

1. Aamoth, G.M., and O'Phelan, E.H.: Recurrent Anterior Dislocation of the Shoulder: A Review of 40 Athletes Treated by Subscapularis Transfer (Modified Magnuson-Stack Procedure). Am. J. Sports Med., 5:188–190, 1977.
2. Abbott, L.C.; Saunders, J.B.; Hagey, H.; and Jones, E.W.: Surgical Approaches to the Shoulder Joint. J. Bone Joint Surg., 31A:235–255, 1949.
3. Abell, J.M., Jr.: Badgley Combined Repair to Prevent Recurrent Anterior Dislocation of the Shoulder. Personal communication, 1988.
4. Ackermann, C.; Kull, C.; Gachter, A.; and Landmann, J.: [Trillat Procedure in Habitual Shoulder Dislocation.] Helv. Chir. Acta, 54:71–74, 1987.
5. Adams, F.L.: The Genuine Works of Hippocrates, Vols. 1 and 2. New York, William Wood, 1891.
6. Adams, J.C.: Recurrent Dislocations of the Shoulder. J. Bone Joint Surg., 30B:26–38, 1948.
7. Adams, J.C.: The Humeral Head Defect in Recurrent Anterior Dislocations of the Shoulder. Br. J. Radiol., 23:151–156, 1950.
8. Adler, H., and Lohmann, B.: The Stability of the Shoulder in Stress Radiography. Arch. Orthop. Trauma Surg., 103:83–84, 1984.
9. Adler, H.; Schlenkhoff, D.; Kulot, K.H.; Seiler, W.; and Reinert, R.: [Stress X-rays of the Shoulder Joint.] Unfallheilkunde, 84:393–395, 1981.
10. Agerholm-Christensen, J.: A Simple Instrument for a Modified Bankart's Operation for Recurrent Dislocation of the Shoulder. Acta Orthop. Scand., 19:164–165, 1949.
11. Agerholm-Christensen, J.: Recurrent Dislocation of the Shoulder. Acta Orthop. Scand., 16:142–147, 1946.
12. Ahlgren, O.; Hedlund, T.; and Nistor, L.: Idiopathic Posterior Instability of the Shoulder Joint: Results of Operation With Posterior Bone Graft. Acta Orthop. Scand., 49:600–603, 1978.
13. Ahlgren, O.; Lorentzon, R.; Larsson, S.E.: Posterior Dislocation of the Shoulder Associated With General Seizures (abstract). Acta Orthop. Scand., 52:694–695, 1981.

14. Ahmadain, A.M.: The Magnuson-Stack Operation for Recurrent Anterior Dislocation of the Shoulder: A Review of 38 Cases. J. Bone Joint Surg., 69B:111–114, 1987.

15. Albers, W.; Blumlein, H.; and Suhler, H.: [Surgical Treatment of Relapsing Ventral Shoulder Dislocation Using the Rotation Osteotomy Method According to Weber.] Aktuel Traumatol., 16:238–240, 1986.

16. Albert, E.: Arthodese bei einer habituellen Luxation der Schultergelen kes. Int. Klin. Rundschau., 2:281–283, 1888.

17. Aleinikov, A.V.: [A Method of Treatment of Inveterate Posterior Shoulder Dislocations.] Ortop. Travmatol. Protez., 1:51–52, 1988.

18. Alexander, O.M.: Radiography of the Acromioclavicular Articulation. Med. Radiogr. Photogr., 30:34–39, 1954.

19. Alldred, A.: Subscapularis Transplant for Recurrent Dislocation of the Shoulder (abstract). J. Bone Joint Surg., 40B:354, 1958.

20. Allman, F.L., Jr.: Illustration of Bristow Procedure as Modified by Dr. Fred Allman. Contemp. Surg., 7:83, 1975.

21. Allman, F.L., Jr.: Personal communication, 1989.

22. Allman, F.L., Jr.: Upper Extremity in Sports. Presented at AAOS Committee on Continuing Education. Eugene, OR, July 22–24, 1974.

23. Allman, F.L., Jr.: Report of More Than 300 Bristow Procedures in Athletes for Recurrent Dislocation/Subluxation of the Shoulder (abstract). Clin. Orthop., 133:261, 1978.

24. Alnot, J.Y.; Jolly, A.; and Frot, B.: Direct Treatment of Nerve Lesions in Brachial Plexus Injuries by Adults: A Series of 100 Operated Cases. Int. Orthop., 5:151–168, 1981.

25. Altchek, D.W.; Skykar, M.J.; and Warren, R.F.: Shoulder Arthroscopy for Shoulder Instability. Instr. Course Lect., XXXVIII:187–198, 1989.

26. Altchek, D.W.; Warren, R.F.; Wickiewicz, T.L.; Skyhar, M.J.; and Ortiz, G.: Arthroscopic Acromioplasty. Unpublished paper.

27. Altchek, D.W.; Warren, R.F.; and Skykar, M.J.: Shoulder Arthroscopy. *In* Rockwood, C.A., Jr., and Matsen, F.A., III (eds.): The Shoulder. Philadelphia, W.B. Saunders, 1990.

28. Amorth, G., and Lazzari, E.: [Spontaneous Shoulder-Luxation: Therapeutical and Medico-Legal Considerations.] Rivista degli Infortuni e delle Malatti Professionali, 49:494–500, 1962.

29. Anderson, D.; Zvirbulis, R.; and Ciullo, J.: Scapular Manipulation for Reduction of Anterior Shoulder Dislocations. Clin. Orthop., 164:181–183, 1982.

30. Andrews, J.R.; Broussard, T.S.; and Carson, W.G., Jr.: Arthroscopy of the Shoulder in the Management of Partial Tears of the Rotator Cuff: A Preliminary Report. Arthroscopy, 1:117–122, 1985.

31. Andrews, J.R.; Carson, W.G., Jr.; and McLeod, W.D.: Glenoid Labrum Tears Related to the Long Head of the Biceps. Am. J. Sports Med., 13:337–341, 1985.

32. Andrews, J.R.; Carson, W.G., Jr.; and Ortega, K.: Arthroscopy of the Shoulder: Technique and Normal Anatomy. Am. J. Sports Med., 12:1–7, 1984.

33. Andrews, J.R., and Carson, W.G., Jr.: Arthroscopy of the Shoulder. Mediguide to Orthopedics, 5(7):1–5, 1985.

34. Andrews, J.R., and Carson, W.G., Jr.: Shoulder Joint Arthroscopy. Orthopedics, 6:1157–1162, 1983.

35. Andrews, J.R.; Carson, W.G., Jr.; and Hughston, J.C.: Operative Shoulder Arthroscopy. Presented at the Annual Meeting of American Orthopaedic Association, Hot Springs, Va., June 1983.

36. Andrews, J.R., and Gidumal, R.H.: Shoulder Arthroscopy in the Throwing Athlete: Perspectives and Prognosis. Clin. Sports Med., 6:565–571, 1987.

37. Andrews, J.R.; Hughston, J.C.; Carson, W.G., Jr.; et al: Shoulder Arthroscopy: General Principles and Technique. Presented at 47th Annual Meeting of the American Academy of Orthopaedic Surgeons, Hot Springs, Va., June 28, 1983.

38. Andrews, J.R., and Schemmel, S.P.: Arthroscopic Acromioplasty. Surg. Rounds for Orthop., Nov. 1989, pp. 45–50.

39. Andrews, J.R.: Arthroscopy Reveals Overlooked Injuries. Orthopedics Today, 6:1,20, 1986.

40. Andrews, J.R.: Arthroscopic Shoulder Surgery Needs Long-Term Evaluation. Orthopedics Today, 6:12, 1986.

41. Andrzejak, J.R.; Lipski, W.; and Maliszewski, A.: [An Unusual Case of Dislocation of the Shoulder.] Chir. Narzadow. Ruchu. Ortop. Pol., 38:545–548, 1973.

42. Angelo, R.L., and Hawkins, R.J.: Osteoarthritis Following an Excessively Tight Putti-Platt Repair. Presented at the 4th Open Meeting of the American Shoulder and Elbow Surgeons, Atlanta, Ga., Feb. 7, 1988.

43. Anraku, I.; Tsutsui, H.; Mori, Y.; and Yamamoto, R.: Subacromial Bursoscopic Findings in Patients With Painful Shoulders (abstract). J. Bone Joint Surg., 67B:495–496, 1985.

44. Antal, C.S.; Conforty, B.; Engelberg, M.; and Reiss, R.: Injuries to the Axillary Due to Anterior Dislocation of the Shoulder. J. Trauma, 13:564–566, 1973.

45. Antoine, H.A.: De l'Allongement des Membres Luxes Aprés la Reduction de la Luxation. Gaz. Med. Paris, 3:621–622, 1836.

46. Archambault, R.; Archambault, H.A.; and Mizeres, N.J.: Rupture of the Thoracoacromial Artery in Anterior Dislocation of the Shoulder. Am. J. Surg., 97:782–783, 1959.

47. Arden, G.P.: Posterior Dislocation of Both Shoulders: Report of a Case. J. Bone Joint Surg., 38B:558–563, 1956.

48. Arendt, E.A.: Multidirectional Shoulder Instability. Orthopedics, 11:113–120, 1988.

49. Arens, H., and Linden, T.: Arthroscopy of the Shoulder (abstract). Acta Orthop. Scand. 55:481–482, 1984.

50. Arndt, J.H., and Sears, A.D.: Posterior Dislocation of the Shoulder. A.J.R., 94:639–645, 1965.

51. Aronen, J.G., and Regan, K.: Decreasing the Incidence of Recurrence of First Time Anterior Shoulder Dislocations With Rehabilitation. Am. J. Sports Med., 12:283–291, 1984.

52. Aronen, J.G.: Anterior Shoulder Dislocations in Sports. Sports Med., 3:224–234, 1986.

53. Aronen, J.G.: Shoulder Rehabilitation. Clin. Sports Med., 4:477–493, 1985.

54. Artz, T., and Huffer, J.M.: A Major Complication of the Modified Bristow Procedure for Recurrent Dislocation of the Shoulder: A Case Report. J. Bone Joint Surg., 54A:1293–1296, 1972.

55. Asplund, G.: [Bilateral Voluntary Posterior Dislocation of the Shoulder.] Acta Chir. Scand., 87:103–112, 1942.

56. Assmus, H., and Meinel, A.: Schulterverletzung und Axillarparese. Hefte Unfallheilkd, 79:183–187, 1976.

57. Aston, J.W., Jr., and Gregory, C.F.: Dislocation of the Shoulder With Significant Fracture of the Glenoid. J. Bone Joint Surg., 55A:1531–1533, 1973.

58. Aufderheide, T.P.; Frascone, R.J.; and Cicero, J.J.: Simultaneous Bilateral Anterior and Posterior Shoulder Dislocations. Am. J. Emerg. Med., 3:331–333, 1985.

59. Aufranc, O.E.; Jones, W.N.; and Turner, R.H.: Humeral Neck Fracture With Inferior Subluxation of the Shoulder Joint. J.A.M.A., 195:136–138, 1966.

60. Augereau, B.; Leyder, P.; and Apoil, A.: Traitement des Luxations Posterieures Inveterées de l'Epaule par Double Abord et Butee Osseouse Retroglenoidienne. Rev. Chir. Orthop., 69:89–90, 1983.

61. Augustine, R.W.: Repair of the Dislocated Shoulder Using the Modified Magnuson Technic. Am. J. Surg., 91:736–741, 1956.

62. Aupecle, P.; Briet, S.; and Butin, J.: Luxation Antero-Interne de l'Epaule droit: Desinsertion de l'Artere Scapulaire Inferieure Avec Rupture Partielle de l'Artere Axillaire et Hematome Calcifié de l'Aisselle: Reconstitution de l'Axillaire par Greffe Veineuse. Resultat de Deux Ans et Demi. Lyon Chir., 60:101–103, 1964.

63. Babbitt, D., and Cassidy, R.: Obstetrical Paralysis and Dislocation of the Shoulder in Infancy. J. Bone Joint Surg., 50A:1447–1452, 1968.

64. Babcock, J.L., and Wray, J.B.: Analysis of Abduction in a Shoulder With Deltoid Paralysis Due to Axillary Nerve Injury. Clin. Orthop., 68:116–120, 1970.

65. Bacciocchi, C.; Bonacina, P.; Gaetani, G.; Villa, I.; and Zanasi, L.: [Postero-Inferior Shoulder Instability: Surgical Treatment: A Clinical Case.] Minerva Ortop. Traumatol., 39:681–683, 1988.

66. Bach, B.R., Jr.; O'Brien, S.J.; Warren, R.F.; and Leighton, M.: An Unusual Neurological Complication of the Bristow Procedure: A Case Report. J. Bone Joint Surg., 70:458–460, 1988.

67. Bach, B.R., Jr.; Warren, R.F.; and Fronek, J.: Disruption of the Lateral Capsule of the Shoulder: A Cause of Recurrent Dislocation. J. Bone Joint Surg., 70B:274–276, 1988.

68. Badgley, C.E., and O'Connor, G.A.: Combined Procedure for the Repair of Recurrent Anterior Dislocation of the Shoulder (abstract). J. Bone Joint Surg., 47A:1283, 1965.

69. Badgley, C.E.: Sports Injuries of the Shoulder Girdle. J.A.M.A., 172:444–448, 1960.

70. Reference deleted.

71. Bailey, R.W.: Acute and Recurrent Dislocation of the Shoulder. Inst. Course Lect., XVIII:70–74, 1962–1969.

72. Bailey, R.W.: Acute and Recurrent Dislocation of the Shoulder. J. Bone Joint Surg., 49A:767–773, 1967.

73. Baker, L.L., and Parker, K.: Neuromuscular Electrical Stimulation of the Muscles Surrounding the Shoulder. Phys. Ther., 66:1930–1937, 1986.

74. Bankart, A.S.B.: Dislocation of the Shoulder Joints. In Robert Jones' Birthday Volume: A Collection of Surgical Essays, pp. 307–314. London, Oxford University Press, 1928.

75. Bankart, A.S.B.: Recurrent or Habitual Dislocation of the Shoulder Joint. Br. Med. J., 2:1132–1133, 1923.

76. Bankart, A.S.B.: The Pathology and Treatment of Recurrent Dislocation of the Shoulder Joint. Br. J. Surg., 26:23–29, 1938.

77. Banninger, J., and Matter, P.: [Late Results of the Combined Putti-Platt and Bankart Operations for Habitual Shoulder Dislocations.] Ther. Umsch., 31:222–226, 1974.

78. Bárány, I.: [Undiagnosed Posterior Dislocation of the Shoulder.] Magy. Traumatol. Orthop. Helyreallito Sebesz, 31:76–78, 1988.

79. Baratta, J.B.; Lim, V.; Mastromonaco, E.; and Edillon, E.L.: Axillary Artery Disruption Secondary to Anterior Dislocation of the Shoulder. J. Trauma, 23:1009–1011, 1983.

80. Bardenheuer, B.A.: Die Verletzungen der oberen Extremitaten. Dtsch. Chir., 63:268–418, 1886.

81. Barja, R.H., and Reid, R.E.: Brachial Plexus Palsy: A Clinical Evaluation. Milit. Med., 43:464–466, 1978.

82. Barquet, A.; Schimchak, M.; Carreras, O.; Leon, H.; and Masliah, R.: Dislocation of the Shoulder With Fracture of the Ipsilateral Shaft of the Humerus. Injury, 16:300–302, 1985.

83. Barrett, G.R.; Dial, W.W.; and Evins, W.B.: Review of a Modified Bristow Procedure for Recurrent Anterior Dislocation of the Shoulder. J. Miss. State Med. Assoc., 23:254–256, 1982.

84. Barrett, J.: The Clavicular Joints. Physiotherapy, 57:268–269, 1971.

85. Barry, T.P.; Lombardo, S.J.; Kerlan, R.K.; Jobe, F.W.; Carter, V.S.; Shields, C.L., Jr.; Yocum, L.A.; and Tibone, J.E.: The Coracoid Transfer for Recurrent Anterior Instability of the Shoulder in Adolescents. J. Bone Joint Surg., 67A:383–387, 1985.

86. Basmajian, J.V., and Bazant, F.J.: Factors Preventing Downward Dislocation of the Adducted Shoulder Joint. J. Bone Joint Surg., 41A:1182–1186, 1959.

87. Bassey, L.: [Old and Neglected Cases of Shoulder Dislocations as Indication for the Bankart's Operation: Experience in the Tropics and Contribution to Trauma Surgery in the Third World.] Unfallchirurg. 91:85–90, 1988.

88. Bateman, J.E.: Gallie Technique for Repair of Recurrent Dislocation of the Shoulder. Surg. Clin. North Am., 43:1655–1662, 1963.

89. Bateman, J.E.: The Shoulder and Environs. St. Louis, C.V. Mosby, 1955.

90. Bateman, J.E.: The Shoulder and Neck. Philadelphia, W.B. Saunders, 1972.

91. Bateman, J.E.: The Shoulder and Neck, 2nd ed. Philadelphia, W.B. Saunders, 1978.

92. Bayley, I.J.L., and Kessel, L.: Posterior Dislocation of the Shoulder: The Clinical Spectrum (abstract). J. Bone Joint Surg., 60B:440, 1978.

93. Bayley, I.J.L., and Kessel, L.: Shoulder Surgery. New York, Springer-Verlag, 1982.

94. Bazy, M.L.: Les lesions de la Tête Humerale Dans les Luxations Recidivantes de l'Épaule. Soc. Chir., pp. 1961–1964, Dec. 11, 1919.

94A. Beall, M.S., Jr.; Diefenbach, G.; and Allen, A.: Electromyographic feedback in the treatment of voluntary posterior instability of the shoulder. Am. J. Sports Med. 15(2):175–178, 1987.

95. Beattie, T.F.; Steedman, D.J.; McGowan, A.; and Robertson, C.E.: A Comparison of the Milch and Kochner Techniques for Acute Anterior Dislocation of the Shoulder. Injury, 17:349–352, 1986.

96. Bechtol, C.O.: Biomechanics of the Shoulder. Clin. Orthop., 146:37–41, 1980.

97. Beck, E.: [Arthrography in the Prognostic Assessment of the First Shoulder Dislocation.] Unfallchirurgie, 14:22–25, 1988.

98. Beckers, L.: Sub-deltoid Approach to the Shoulder. Acta Orthop. Belg., 51:847–851, 1985.

99. Bell, H.M.: Posterior Fracture–Dislocation of the Shoulder—A Method of Closed Reduction: A Case Report. J. Bone Joint Surg., 47A:1521–1524, 1965.

100. Bellando, R.P.: Treatment of Recurrent Dislocation of the Shoulder in Athletes: Variant of the Bankart-Delitalia Technic. Arch. Putti Chir. Organi. Mov., 66:757–763, 1980.

101. Beller, R.D.; Grana, W.A.; and O'Donoghue, D.H.: Recurrent Posterior Dislocation of the Shoulder: A Method of Reconstruction. Orthopedics, 1:384–388, 1978.

102. Benammar, M.N.; Saragaglia, D.; Legrand, J.J.; Faure, C.; and Butel, J.: [Latarjet Procedure for Recurrent Anterior Dislocation of the Shoulder: 117 Cases With a Mean Follow-up of 8 Years.] Rev. Chir. Orthop., 72:447–454, 1972.

103. Benchetrit, E., and Friedman, B.: Fracture of the Coracoid Process Associated With Subglenoid Dislocation of the Shoulder: A Case Report. J. Bone Joint Surg., 61A:295–296, 1979.

104. Benjamin, A.; Hirschowitz, D.; and Arden, G.P.: The Treatment of Arthritis of the Shoulder Joint by Double Osteotomy. Int. Orthop., 3:211–216, 1979.

105. Bennett, G.E.: Old Dislocations of the Shoulder. J. Bone Joint Surg., 18A:594–606, 1936.

106. Bennett, G.E.: Shoulder and Elbow Lesions of the Professional Baseball Pitcher. J.A.M.A., 117:510–514, 1941.

107. Bermann, M.M., and LeMay, M.: Dislocation of Shoulder: X-ray Signs (letter to the editor). N. Engl. J. Med., 283:600, 1970.

108. Berry, H., and Bril, V.: Axillary Nerve Palsy Following Blunt Trauma to the Shoulder Region: A Clinical and Electrophysiological Review. J. Neurol. Neurosurg. Psychiatry, 45:1027–1032, 1982.

109. Bertolino, D.; Gattullo, G.L.; and Moselli, M.: [Long-Term Result of Bankart's Operation in Habitual or Recurrent Luxation of the Shoulder.] Minerva Ortop. Traumatol., 39:667–669, 1988.

110. Bertrand, J.C.; Maestro, M.; Pequignot, J.P.; and Mouiel, J.: [Vascular Complications in Simple Anterior Dislocations of the Shoulder: Three Cases.] Ann. Chir., 36:329–333, 1981.

111. Bestard, E.A.: Glenoplasty: A Simple, Reliable Method of Correcting Recurrent Posterior Dislocation of the Shoulder. Orthop. Rev., 5:29–34, 1976.

112. Biedermann, H.; Weiman, S.; and Flora, G.: Vascular Lesions of the Upper Extremity in Combination With Fractures and Luxations (abstract). Presented at the International Vascular Workshop II, Obergurge, 1981.

113. Biesold, L., and Irlenbusch, U.: Zur haufigkeit rezidivierender Schulterluxationen nach traumatischen Schulterverrenkungen. Beitr. Orthop. Traumatol., 31:350–355, 1984.

114. Bigliani, L.U.; Endrizzi, D.P.; McIlveen, S.J.; Flatow, E.L.; and Dalsey, R.M.: Operative Management of Posterior Shoulder Instability. Orthop. Trans., 13(2):232, Summer, 1989.

115. Bilbey, D.L.J.: Posterior Dislocation of the Shoulder Joint. Br. Med. J., 1(2):1345–1346, 1957.

116. Billington, R.W.: A New (Plaster Yoke) Dressing for Fracture of the Clavicle. South. Med. J., 24:667, 1931.

117. Biro, A.: [Bilateral Scapulohumeral Luxation: A Complication of Aldrin Intoxication.] Chirurgia, 27:449–451, 1978.

118. Bjelland, J.C., and Freundlich, I.M.: Radiology Case of the Month: Case Number Five. Arizona Med., 32:961–962, 1975.

119. Blackburn, T.A., Jr.: Rehabilitation of the Shoulder and Elbow After Arthroscopy. Clin. Sports Med., 6:587–606, 1987.

120. Blackett, C.W., and Healy, T.R.: Roentgen Studies of the Shoulder. A.J.R., 37:760–766, 1937.

121. Blasier, R.B.; Bruckner, J.D.; Janda, D.H.; and Alexander, A.H.: The Bankart Repair Illustrated in Cross-Section: Some Anatomical Considerations. Am. J. Sports Med., 17:630–637, 1989.

122. Blasier, R.B., and Burkus, J.K.: Management of Posterior Fracture–Dislocations of the Shoulder. Clin. Orthop., 232:197–204, 1988.

123. Blauth, M.; Kujat, R.; and Tscherne, H.: [Modified Capsule-Graft Reconstruction for Recurrent Dislocation of the Shoulder.] Unfallchirurg, 89:429–435, 1986.

124. Blazina, M.E., and Satzman, J.S.: Recurrent Anterior Subluxation of the Shoulder in Athletics—A Distinct Entity (abstract). J. Bone Joint Surg., 51A:1037–1038, 1969.

125. Blom, S., and Dahlback, L.O.: Nerve Injuries in Dislocations of the Shoulder Joint and Fractures of the Neck of the Humerus. Acta Chir. Scand., 136:461–466, 1970.

126. Bloom, M.H., and Obata, W.G.: Diagnosis of Posterior Dislocation of the Shoulder With Use of Velpeau Axillary and Angle-up Roentgenographic Views. J. Bone Joint Surg., 49A:943–949, 1967.

127. Blumensaat, C.: Die Lageabweichungen und Verrenkungen der Kniescheibe. Ergeb. Chir. Orthop., 31:149–223, 1938.

128. Blush, K.: Post-op Therapy for Recurrent Dislocation of the Shoulder. Am. Corr. Ther. J., 30:21–22, 1976.

129. Bocchi, L.; Orso, C.A.; and Bianchini, C.: [Habitual and Recurrent Anterior Dislocation of the Shoulder: A Comparative Analysis of Two Techniques.] Minerva Ortop., 35:555–560, 1984.

130. Boccia, G.; Galante, V.N.; and Cucci, G.: Recurrent Dislocation of the Shoulder: Twenty-five Years Experience With the Delitala Method. Ital. J. Orthop. Traumatol., 14:323–329, 1988.

131. Bodey, W.N., and Denham, R.A.: A Free Bone Block Operation for Recurrent Anterior Dislocation of the Shoulder Joint. Injury, 15:184–188, 1983.

132. Boger, D.; Sipsey, J.; and Anderson, G.: New Traction Devices to Aid Reduction of Shoulder Dislocations. Ann. Emerg. Med., 13:423–425, 1984.

133. Böhler, L.: Die Behandlung von verrenkungsbruchen der Schulter. Dtsch. Z. Chir., 219:238–245, 1929.

134. Böhler, L.: Treatment of Fractures, 4th ed. Bristol, John Wright & Sons, 1935.

135. Boicev, B.: Sulla Lussazione Abituale della Spalla. Chir. Organi. Mov., 23:354–370, 1930.

136. Bonney, G.: Injuries of the Brachial Plexus. Br. J. Hosp. Med., 12:567–578, 1974.

137. Bonnin, J.G.: Transplantation of the Tip of the Coracoid Process for Recurrent Anterior Dislocation of the Shoulder (abstract). J. Bone Joint Surg., 51B:579, 1969.

138. Bonnin, J.G.: Transplantation of the Coracoid Tip: A Definitive Operation for Recurrent Anterior Dislocation of the Shoulder. Proc. R. Soc. Med., 66:755–758, 1973.

139. Boome, R.S.: Brachial Plexus Palsies Following Traumatic False Aneurysms. J. Bone Joint Surg., 64B:143, 1982.

140. Bosso, A.; Marini, S.; and Pollono, F.: [Contribution to the Study of Trillat's Operation in Recurrent Anterior Shoulder Luxation.] Minerva Ortop. Traumatol., 39:695–698, 1988.

141. Bost, F.C., and Inman, V.T.: The Pathologic Changes in Recurrent Dislocation of the Shoulder: A Report on Bankart's Operative Procedure. J. Bone Joint Surg., 24:595–613, 1942.

142. Bowyer, B.L., and Zuelzer, W.A.: Usefulness of Therapeutic Exercise Program in the Management of Shoulder Impingement in Gymnastics (abstract). Arch. Phys. Med. Rehabil., 68:613, 1987.

143. Boyd, H.B., and Hunt, H.L.: Recurrent Dislocation of the Shoulder: The Staple Capsulorrhaphy. J. Bone Joint Surg., 47A:1514–1520, 1965.

144. Boyd, H.B., and Sisk, T.D.: Recurrent Posterior Dislocation of the Shoulder. J. Bone Joint Surg., 54A:779–786, 1972.

145. Boyd, H.B.: Recurrent Posterior Dislocation of the Shoulder (abstract). J. Bone Joint Surg., 54B:379, 1972.

146. Boytchev, B.; Conforty, B.; and Tchokanov, K.: Operatiunaya Ortopediya y Travamatologiya, 2nd ed. Sofia, Meditsina y Fizkultura, 1962.

147. Boytchev, B.: Treatment of Recurrent Shoulder Instability. Minerva Ortop. 2:377–379, 1951.

148. Braly, W.G., and Tullos, H.S.: A Modification of the Bristow Procedure for Recurrent Anterior Shoulder Dislocation and Subluxation. Am. J. Sports Med., 13:81–86, 1985.

149. Braun, R.M.; West, F.; Mooney, V.; Nickel, V.L.; Roper, B.; and Caldwell, C.: Surgical Treatment of the Painful Shoulder Contracture in the Stroke Patient. J. Bone Joint Surg., 53A:1307–1312, 1971.

150. Braunstein, E.M., and Martel, W.: Voluntary Glenohumeral Dislocation. A.J.R., 129:911–912, 1977.

151. Braunstein, E.M., and O'Connor, G.A.: Double-Contrast Arthrotomography of the Shoulder. J. Bone Joint Surg., 64A:192–195, 1982.

152. Brav, E.A., and Jeffress, V.H.: Simplified Putti-Platt Reconstruction for Recurrent Shoulder Dislocation: A Preliminary Report. West. J. Surg. Obstet. Gynecol., 60:93–97, 1952.

153. Brav, E.A.: Evaluation of the Putti-Platt Reconstruction Procedure for Recurrent Dislocation of the Shoulder. J. Bone Joint Surg., 37A:731–741, 1955.

154. Brav, E.A.: Recurrent Dislocation of the Shoulder: Ten Years' Experience With the Putti-Platt Reconstruction Procedure. Am. J. Surg., 100:423–430, 1960.

155. Breederveld, R.S.; Patka, P.; Dwars, B.J.; and Van Mourik, J.C.: Shoulder Injury Caused by Electric Shock. Neth. J. Surg., 39:147–148, 1987.

156. Brennike, P.; Bro-Rasmussen, F.; and Bro-Rasmussen, P.: Dislocation and/or Congenital Malformation of the Shoulder Joint: Observations on a Medieval Skeleton From Denmark. Anthropol. Anz., 45:117–129, 1987.

157. Brewer, B.J.; Wubben, R.C.; and Carrera, G.F.: Excessive Retroversion of the Glenoid Cavity: A Cause of Non-Traumatic Posterior Instability of the Shoulder. J. Bone Joint Surg., 68A:724–731, 1986.

158. Bril, V., and Berry, H.: Axillary (Circumflex) Nerve Palsy Following Blunt Trauma to the Shoulder Region. Can. J. Neurol. Sci., 6:388, 1979.

159. Britt, B.A., and Gordon, R.A.: Peripheral Nerve Injuries Associated With Anesthesia. Can. Anaesth. Soc. J., 11:511, 1964.

160. Broca, A., and Hartmann, H.: Contribution á l'Étude des Luxations de l'Épaule. Bull. Soc. Anat. Paris, 4:312–336, 416–423, 1890.

161. Brockbank, W., and Griffiths, D.L.: Orthopaedic Surgery in the Sixteenth and Seventeenth Centuries: 1. Luxations of the Shoulder. J. Bone Joint Surg., 30B:365–375, 1948.

162. Brodsky, J.W.; Tullos, H.S.; and Gartsman, G.M.: Simplified Posterior Approach to the Shoulder Joint: A Technical Note. J. Bone Joint Surg., 69A:773–774, 1987.

163. Brophy, B.P.: Supraclavicular Traction Injuries of the Brachial Plexus. Aust. N.Z. J. Surg., 48:529–532, 1978.

164. Brostrom, L.A.; Kronberg, M.; and Németh, G.: Muscular Activity in Patients With an Unstable Humeroscapular Joint (abstract). Acta Orthop. Scand., 58:191, 1987.

165. Brostrom, L.A.; Olsson, E.; and Wallensten, R.: Shoulder Function in Patients With Recurrent Anterior Dislocation

of the Shoulder (abstract). Acta Orthop. Scand., 55:95, 1984.

166. Brown, F.W., and Navigato, W.J.: Rupture of the Axillary Artery and Brachial Plexus Palsy Associated With Anterior Dislocation of the Shoulder: Report of a Case With Successful Vascular Repair. Clin. Orthop., 60:195–199, 1968.

167. Brown, J.T.: Nerve Injuries Complicating Dislocation of the Shoulder (abstract). J. Bone Joint Surg., 34B:526, 1952.

168. Brown, R.J.: Bilateral Dislocation of the Shoulders. Injury, 15:267–273, 1984.

169. Brown, W.H.; Dennis, J.M.; Davidson, C.N.; Rubin, P.S.; and Fulton, H.: Posterior Dislocation of Shoulder. Radiology, 69:815–822, 1957.

170. Bryan, R.S.; DiMichele, J.D.; and Ford, G.L., Jr.: Anterior Recurrent Dislocation of the Shoulder: Report of a Series of the Augustine Variation of Magnuson-Stack Repair. Clin. Orthop., 63:177–180, 1969.

171. Budd, F.W.: Voluntary Bilateral Posterior Dislocation of the Shoulder Joint: Report of a Case. Clin. Orthop., 63: 181, 1969.

172. Buhren, V., and Braun, C.: [Displaced Proximal Humeral Fracture With Intrathoracic Dislocation.] Unfallchirurg, 58:789–792, 1987.

173. Burckhardt, A., and Razavi, R.: [The Trillat Procedure in Recurrent Anterior Luxation of the Shoulder.] Helv. Chir. Acta, 48:229–230, 1981.

174. Burkhead, W.Z., Jr., and Box, G.: Musculocutaneous and Axillary Nerve Position After Coracoid Transfer. Orthop. Trans., 13(2):232, Summer, 1989.

175. Burman, M.S.: Arthroscopy or the Direct Visualization of Joints: An Experimental Cadaver Study. J. Bone Joint Surg., 13:669–695, 1931.

176. Burri, C., and Neugebauer, R.: Carbon Fiber Replacement of the Ligaments of the Shoulder Girdle and the Treatment of Lateral Instability of the Ankle Joint. Clin. Orthop., 196:112–117, 1985.

177. Butters, K.P.; Rockwood, C.A., Jr.; and Curtis, R.J., Jr.: Posterior Deltoid Splitting Shoulder Approach. Orthop. Trans., 11:233, 1987.

178. Cain, P.R.; Mutschler, T.A.; Fu, F.H.; and Lee, S.K.: Anterior Stability of the Glenohumeral Joint: A Dynamic Model. Am. J. Sports Med., 15:144–148, 1987.

179. Caird, F.M.: The Shoulder Joint in Relation to Certain Dislocations and Fractures. Edinburgh Med. J., 32:708–714, 1887.

180. Calandriello, B.: Revisione Critica Della Cura Chirugica Della Lussazione Abituale di Spalla. Arch. Putti Chir. Organi. Mov., 1:359–387, 1951.

181. Calandriello, B.: The Pathology of Recurrent Dislocation of the Shoulder. Clin. Orthop., 20:33–39, 1961.

182. Caldwell, C.B.; Wilson, D.J.; and Braun, R.M.: Evaluation and Treatment of the Upper Extremity in the Hemiplegic Stroke Patient. Clin. Orthop., 63:69–93, 1969.

183. Calvet, J.; LeRoy, M.; and Lacroix, L.: Luxations de l'Épaule et Lesions Vasculaires. J. Chir., 58:337–346, 1942.

184. Camargo, J.N., Jr.: [Posterior Fracture–Dislocation of the Shoulder: Case Report.] Rev. Brasil Ortop., 13:137–138, 1978.

185. Cameron, B.M.: Recurrent Posterior Dislocation of the Shoulder: Report of a Case. Texas Med. J., 51:33–35, 1955.

186. Cameron, J.C.; Hall, H.; and Courtenay, B.G.: The Bristow Procedure for Recurrent Anterior Dislocation of the Shoulder (abstract). J. Bone Joint Surg., 67B:327, 1985.

187. Canciani, J.P.: [Traumatic Dislocation of the Shoulder.] Rev. Praticien, 34:2997–3003, 1984.

188. Carew-McColl, M.: Bilateral Shoulder Dislocations Caused by Electric Shock. Br. J. Clin. Prac., 34:251–254, 1980.

189. Carol, E.J.; Falke, L.M.; Kortmann, J.H.; and Roeffen, J.F.W.: Treatment of Recurrent Dislocation of the Shoulder by the Bristow Procedure (abstract). Acta Orthop. Scand., 55:485, 1984.

190. Carol, E.J.; Falke, L.M.; Kortmann, J.H.; Roeffen, J.F.W.; and Van Acker, P.A.M.: Bristow-Latarjet Repair for Recurrent Anterior Shoulder Instability: An Eight-Year Study. Neth. J. Surg., 37:109–113, 1985.

191. Carpenter, G.I., and Millard, P.H.: Shoulder Subluxation in Elderly Inpatients. J. Am. Geriatr. Soc., 30:441–446, 1982.

192. Carter, C., and Sweetnam, R.: Recurrent Dislocation of the Patella and of the Shoulder: Their Association With Familial Joint Laxity. J. Bone Joint Surg., 42B:721–727, 1960.

193. Caspari, R.B.: Arthroscopic Reconstruction for Anterior Shoulder Instability. Techniques Orthop., 3:59–66, 1988.

194. Caspari, R.B.: Shoulder Arthroscopy: A Review of the Present State of the Art. Contemp. Orthop., 4:523–531, 1982.

195. Caspri, I.; Ezra, E.; Oliver, S.; Lin, E.; Lota, G.; and Horoszowski, H.: Treatment of Avulsed Clavicle and Recurrent Subluxations of the Ipsilateral Shoulder by Dynamic Fixation. J. Trauma, 27:94–95, 1987.

196. Cautilli, R.A.; Joyce, M.F.; and Mackell, J.V., Jr.: Posterior Dislocation of the Glenohumeral Joint. Jefferson Orthop. J., 7:15–20, 1978.

197. Cautilli, R.A.; Joyce, M.F.; and Mackell, J.V., Jr.: Posterior Dislocations of the Shoulder: A Method of Postreduction Management. Am. J. Sports Med., 6:397–399, 1978.

198. Cave, E.F. (ed.): Fractures and Other Injuries. Chicago, Year Book Medical Publishers, 1961.

199. Cave, E.F.; Burke, J.F.; and Boyd, R.J.: Posterior Dislocations. *In* Trauma Management, p. 437. Chicago, Year Book Medical Publishers, 1974.

200. Cayford, E.H., and Tees, F.J.: Traumatic Aneurysm of the Subclavicular Artery as a Late Complication of Fractured Clavicle. Can. Med. Assoc. J., 25:450–452, 1931.

201. Cechner, P.E., and Knight, C.D.: Approach to the Canine Shoulder Without Myostomy, Osteotomy, or Tenotomy. J. Am. Animal Hosp. Assoc., 15:753–754, 1979.

202. Chaco, J., and Wolf, E.: Subluxation of the Glenohumeral

Joint in Hemiplegia. Am. J. Phys. Med., 50:139–143, 1971.

203. Chan, K.M.: Arthroscopy of the Shoulder: A Review of 110 Cases (Proceedings). J. Bone Joint Surg., 70B:162, 1988.

204. Chattopadhyaya, P.K.: Posterior Fracture–Dislocation of the Shoulder: Report of a Case. J. Bone Joint Surg., 52B:521–527, 1970.

205. Chaudhuri, G.K.; Sengupta, A.; and Saha, A.K.: Rotation Osteotomy of the Shaft of the Humerus for Recurrent Dislocation of the Shoulder: Anterior and Posterior. Acta Orthop. Scand., 45:193–198, 1974.

206. Chen, S.-K.; Perry, J.; Jobe, F.W.; Healy, B.S.; and Maynes, D.R.: Elbow Flexion Analysis in Bristow Patients: A Preliminary Report. Am. J. Sports Med., 12:347–350, 1984.

207. Cherkes-Zade, D.I.: [A Case of an Open Dislocation of the Shoulder.] Ortop. Travmatol. Protez., 6:45–46, 1984.

208. Chino, N.: Electrophysiological Investigation of Shoulder Subluxation in Hemiplegics. Scand. J. Rehab. Med., 13:17–21, 1981.

209. Christiansen, T.G., and Nielsen, R.: Reduction of Shoulder Dislocations Under Interscalene Brachial Blockade. Arch. Orthop. Trauma Surg., 107:176–177, 1988.

210. Cisternino, S.J.; Rogers, L.F.; Stufflebam, B.C.; and Kruglik, G.D.: The Trough Line: A Radiographic Sign of Posterior Shoulder Dislocation. A.J.R., 130:951–954, 1978.

211. Clairmont, P., and Ehrlich, H.: Ein neues Operations: Verfahren zur Behandlung der habituellen Schulterluxation mittels Muskelplastik. Verh. Dtsch. Ges. Chir., 38:79–103, 1909.

212. Clancy, M.J.: False Aneurysm of the Axillary Artery as a Complication of the Modified Bristow Procedure. Injury, 18:427–428, 1987.

213. Clancy, W.G.; Brand, R.L.; and Bergfield, J.A.: Upper Trunk Brachial Plexus Injuries in Contact Injuries. Am. J. Sports Med., 5:209–216, 1977.

214. Clark, K.C.: Positioning in Radiography, 2nd ed. London, William Heinemann, 1941.

215. Clausen, E.G.: Postoperative Anesthetic Paralysis of the Brachial Plexus. Surgery, 12:933–942, 1942.

216. Cleaves, E.N.: A New Film Holder for Roentgen Examination of the Shoulder. A.J.R., 45:288–290, 1941.

217. Reference deleted.

218. Cleland, J.: On the Actions of Muscles Passing Over More Than One Joint. J. Anat. Physiol., 1:85–93, 1866.

219. Clotteau, J.E.; Premont, M.; and Mercier, V.: [A Simple Procedure for Reducing Dislocations of the Shoulder Without Anesthesia.] Nouv. Presse Med., 11:127–128, 1982.

220. Codman, E.A.: Rupture of the Supraspinatus Tendon and Other Lesions in or About the Subacromial Bursa. In The Shoulder. Boston, Thomas Todd, 1934.

221. Codman, E.A.: The Shoulder. Brooklyn, G. Miller, 1934.

222. Cofield, R.H., and Irving, J.F.: Evaluation and Classification of Shoulder Instability—With Special Reference to Examination Under Anesthesia. Clin. Orthop., 223:32–43, 1987.

223. Cofield, R.H.; Kavanaugh, B.F.; and Frassica, F.J.: Anterior Shoulder Instability. Instr. Course Lect., XXXIV:210–227, 1985.

224. Cofield, R.H., and Simonet, W.T.: The Shoulder in Sports. Mayo Clin. Proc., 59:157–164, 1984.

225. Cofield, R.H.: Arthroscopy of the Shoulder. Presented at American Academy of Orthopaedic Surgeons Sixth Summer Institute, Chicago, IL, July 8–11, 1980.

226. Cofield, R.H.: Arthroscopy of the Shoulder. Mayo Clin. Proc., 58:501–508, 1983.

227. Cofield, R.H.; Kavanaugh, B.F.; and Fressica, F.J.: Anterior Shoulder Instability. Instr. Course Lect. XXXIV:210–231, 1985.

228. Cofield, R.H.: When to Look into a Shoulder. Emerg. Med., 16:71–73, 1984.

229. Cohen, H.H.: Acute Posterior Bilateral Dislocation of the Shoulder. Bull. Hosp. Joint Dis. Orthop. Inst., 26:175–180, 1965.

230. Cohn, B.T., and Froimson, A.I.: Salter 3 Fracture Dislocation of Glenohumeral Joint in a 10-Year-Old. Orthop. Rev., 15:97–98, 1986.

231. Colachis, S.C., and Strohm, B.R.: Effects of Suprascapular and Axillary Nerve Blocks on Muscle Force in Upper Extremity. Arch. Phys. Med. Rehabil. 52:22–29, 1971.

232. Colachis, S.C.; Strohm, B.R.; and Brechner, V.L.: Effects of Axillary Nerve Block on Muscle Force in the Upper Extremity. Arch. Phys. Med. Rehabil., 50:647–654, 1969.

233. Collins, H.R., and Wilde, A.H.: Shoulder Instability in Athletics. Orthop. Clin. North Am., 4:759–774, 1973.

234. Collins, K.A.; Capito, C.; and Cross, M.: The Use of the Putti-Platt Procedure in the Treatment of Recurrent Anterior Dislocation, With Special Reference to the Young Athlete. Am. J. Sports Med., 14:380–382, 1986.

235. Conforty, B.: Boytchev's Procedure for Recurrent Dislocation of the Shoulder (abstract). J. Bone Joint Surg., 56:386, 1974.

236. Conforty, B.: The Results of the Boytchev Procedure for Treatment of Recurrent Dislocation of the Shoulder. Int. Orthop., 4:127–132, 1980.

237. Connolly, J.F.: X-ray Defects in Recurrent Shoulder Dislocations (abstract). J. Bone Joint Surg., 51A:1235–1236, 1969.

238. Connolly, J.F.: Humeral Head Defects Associated With Shoulder Dislocations—Their Diagnostic and Surgical Significance. Instr. Course Lect., XXI:42–54, 1972.

239. Connolly, J.F.: Inferior Shoulder Subluxation Associated With a Surgical Neck Fracture of the Humerus. Nebr. Med. J., 67:11–12, 1982.

240. Connolly, J.F.: Personal communication, 1972.

241. Conwell, H.E., and Reynolds, F.C.: Key and Conwell's Management of Fractures, Dislocations, and Sprains, 7th ed. St. Louis, C.V. Mosby, 1961.

242. Conwell, H.E.: Fractures of the Clavicle. J.A.M.A., 90:838–839, 1928.

243. Cooper, A.: A Treatise on Dislocations and Fractures of the Joints, 2nd American ed. from the 6th London ed. Boston, Lilly & Wait and Carter & Hendee, 1832.

244. Cooper, A.: A Treatise on Dislocations and Fractures of the Joints, p. 391. London, John Churchill, 1842.

245. Cooper, A.: A Treatise on Dislocations and Fractures of the Joints, p. 341. Philadelphia, Lea and Blanchard, 1844.

246. Cooper, A.: On the Dislocation of the Os Humeri Upon the Dorsum Scapulae, and Upon Fractures Near the Shoulder Joint. Guy's Hosp. Report, 4:265–297, 1839.

247. Coover, C.: Double Posterior Luxation of the Shoulder. Penn. Med. J., 35:566–567, 1932.

248. Costello, P.B.; Kennedy, A.C.; and Green, F.A.: Shoulder Joint Rupture in Juvenile Rheumatoid Arthritis Producing Bicipital Masses and a Hemorrhagic Sign. J. Rheumatol., 7:563–566, 1980.

249. Cotton, F.J., and Brickley, W.J.: Treatment of Fracture of Neck of Scapula. Boston Med. Surg. J., 185A:326–329, 1921.

250. Cotton, F.J.: Subluxation of the Shoulder Downward. Boston Med. Surg. J., 185:405–407, 1921.

251. Cozen, L.N.: Congenital Dislocation of the Shoulder and Other Anomalies: Report of a Case and Review of the Literature. Arch. Surg., 35:956–966, 1935.

252. Cozen, L.N.: Pentazocine Injections as a Causative Factor in Dislocation of the Shoulder: A Case Report. J. Bone Joint Surg., 59A:979, 1977.

253. Craig, E.: Importance of Proper Radiography in Acute Shoulder Trauma. Minn. Med., 68:109–112, 1985.

254. Craig, E.V.; Hunter, R.E.; and Kramer, R.S.: Reinforced Cruciate-Capsular Reconstruction for Recurrent Anterior Shoulder Instability. Orthop. Trans., 13(2):231, Summer, 1989.

255. Craig, E.V.: The Posterior Mechanism of Acute Anterior Shoulder Dislocations. Clin. Orthop., 190:212–216, 1984.

256. Cramer, B.M.; Kramps, H.A.; Laumann, U.; and Fischedick, A.R.: [CT Diagnosis of Recurrent Subluxation of the Shoulder.] Fortschr. Rontgenstr., 136:440–443, 1982.

258. Cramer, F.: Resection des Oberarmkopfes wegen habitueller Luxation (nach einem im ärztlichen Verein zu Wiesbaden gehaltenen Vortrage). Berl. Klin. Wochenschr., 19:21–25, 1882.

259. Cranley, J.J., and Krause, R.J.: Injury to the Axillary Artery Following Anterior Dislocation of the Shoulder. Am. J. Surg., 95:524–526, 1958.

260. Crenshaw, A.H. (ed.): Campbell's Operative Orthopaedics, 5th ed., Vols. 1–2. St. Louis, C.V. Mosby, 1971.

261. Cubbins, W.; Callahan, J.J.; and Scuderi, C.S.: The Reduction of Old or Irreducible Dislocations of the Shoulder Joint. Surg. Gynecol. Obstet., 58:129–135, 1934.

262. Curr, J.F.: Rupture of the Axillary Artery Complicating Dislocation of the Shoulder: Report of a Case. J. Bone Joint Surg., 52B:313–317, 1970.

263. Curti, F.; Araldi, R.; Croce, A.; and Bernabe, G.: [Recurring Anterior Dislocation of the Shoulder.] Chir. Ital., 33:787–811, 1981.

264. Curtis, R.J., Jr., and Rockwood, C.A., Jr.: Surgical Treatment of Late Unreduced Posterior Dislocations and Fracture Dislocations of the Shoulder (abstract). Orthop. Trans., 11:246, 1987.

265. Cyprien, J.M.; Vasey, H.M.; Burdet, A.; Bonvin, J.C.; Kritsikis, N.; and Vuagnat, P.: Humeral Retrotorsion and Glenohumeral Relationship in the Normal Shoulder and in Recurrent Anterior Dislocation. Clin. Orthop., 175:8–17, 1983.

266. D'Ambrosia, R.D.: Musculoskeletal Disorders. Philadelphia, J.B. Lippincott, 1977.

267. D'Angelo, D.: [Voluntary Shoulder Dislocation: Report of Four Cases.] Arch. Putti Chir. Organi. Mov., 17:142–147, 1962.

268. D'Aubigne, R.M.: Nerve Injuries in Fractures and Dislocations of the Shoulder. Surg. Clin. North Am., 43:1685–1689, 1963.

269. Dabrowski, W.; Fonseka, N.; Ansell, B.M.; Liyanage, I.S.; and Arden, G.P.: Shoulder Problems in Juvenile Chronic Polyarthritis. Scand. J. Rheumatol., 8:49–53, 1979.

270. Dahmen, G., and Gartner, J.: [Results of Rotational Osteotomy by Weber in the Treatment of Recurrent Shoulder Dislocation.] Z. Orthop., 121:541–546, 1983.

271. Dannaeus, C., and Liedberg, G.: Traumatic Disruption of the Axillary Artery. Acta Chir. Scand., 148:549–550, 1982.

272. Danzig, L.A.; Greenway, G.; and Resnick, D.: The Hill-Sachs Lesion: An Experimental Study. Am. J. Sports Med., 8:328–332, 1980.

273. Danzig, L.A.; Resnick, D.; and Greenway, G.: Evaluation of Unstable Shoulders by Computed Tomography: A Preliminary Study. Am. J. Sports Med., 10:138–141, 1982.

274. Danzl, D.F.; Vicario, S.J.; Gleis, G.L.; Yates, J.R.; and Parks, D.L.: Closed Reduction by Anterior Subcoracoid Shoulder Dislocation: Evaluation of an External Rotation Method. Orthop. Rev., 15:311–315, 1986.

275. Das, S.P.; Ray, G.S.; and Saha, A.K.: Observations on the Tilt of the Glenoid Cavity of Scapula. J. Anat. Soc. India, 15:114–118, 1966.

276. Davidson, W.D.: Traumatic Deltoid Paralysis Treated by Muscle Transplantation. J.A.M.A., 106:2237, 1936.

277. Davis, A.G.: A Conservative Treatment for Habitual Dislocations of the Shoulder. J.A.M.A., 107:1012–1015, 1936.

278. Day, A.J.; MacDonell, J.A.; and Pedersen, H.E.: Recurrent Dislocation of the Shoulder: A Comparison of the Bankart and Magnuson Procedures After 16 Years. Clin. Orthop., 45:123–126, 1966.

279. De Waal Malefijt, J.; Ooms, A.J.A.M.; and Van Rens, T.J.G.: A Comparison of the Results of the Bristow-Latarjet Procedure and the Bankart/Putti-Platt Operation for Recurrent Anterior Dislocation of the Shoulder. Acta Orthop. Belg., 51:831–842, 1985.

280. De Waal Malefijt, J.; Ooms, A.J.A.M.; and Van Rens, T.J.G.: Comparison of the Bristow and Putti-Platt Techniques for Treatment of Recurrent Dislocation of the Shoulder (abstract). Acta Orthop. Scand., 55:485–486, 1984.

281. DeAnquin, C.E., and DeAnquin, C.A.: Comparative Study of Bone Lesions in Traumatic Recurrent Dislocation of

the Shoulder—Their Importance and Treatment. *In* Bateman, J.E., and Welsh, R.P. (eds.): Surgery of the Shoulder, pp. 303–305. Philadelphia, B.C. Decker, 1984.

282. DeAnquin, C.E.: A Reliable Operative Procedure for Recurrent Dislocation of the Shoulder. J. Bone Joint Surg., 43A:26, 1961.

283. DeAnquin, C.E.: Recurrent Dislocation of the Shoulder—Roentgenographic Study (abstract). J. Bone Joint Surg., 47A:1085, 1965.

284. deBaere, G.A.J., and Penterma, H.: Subluxation of the Shoulder (Proceedings). Acta. Orthop. Scand. 55:484, 1984.

285. DePalma, A.F.; Cooke, A.J.; and Prabhakar, M.: The Role of the Subscapularis in Recurrent Anterior Dislocations of the Shoulder. Clin. Orthop., 54:35–49, 1967.

286. DePalma, A.F., and Silberstein, C.E.: Results Following a Modified Magnuson Procedure in Recurrent Dislocation of the Shoulder. Surg. Clin. North Am., 43:1651–1653, 1963.

287. DePalma, A.F.: Factors Influencing the Choice of a Modified Magnuson Procedure for Recurrent Anterior Dislocation of the Shoulder: With a Note on Technique. Surg. Clin. North Am., 43:1647–1649, 1963.

288. DePalma, A.F.: Recurrent Dislocation of the Shoulder Joint. Ann. Surg., 132:1052–1065, 1950.

289. DePalma, A.F.: Recurring Dislocation of the Shoulder: A Symposium. J. Bone Joint Surg., 39B:9–58, 1948.

290. DePalma, A.F.: Surgery of the Shoulder. Philadelphia, J.B. Lippincott, 1950.

291. DePalma, A.F.: Surgery of the Shoulder, 2nd ed. Philadelphia, J.B. Lippincott, 1973.

292. DePalma, A.F.: Surgery of the Shoulder, 3rd ed. Philadelphia, J.B. Lippincott, 1983.

293. DePalma, A.F.: The Management of Fractures and Dislocations, 2nd ed. Philadelphia, J.B. Lippincott, 1973.

294. DePalma, A.F.: The Management of Fractures and Dislocations: An Atlas, 2nd ed., Vol. 1. Philadelphia, W.B. Saunders, 1970.

295. Deane, A.M.: A Neurovascular Traction Injury Involving the Subclavian Artery and Brachial Plexus in a Motorcyclist. Br. J. Clin. Pract., 35:364–366, 1981.

296. Debevoise, N.T.; Hyatt, G.W.; and Townsend, G.B.: Humeral Torsion in Recurrent Shoulder Dislocations: A Technic of Determination by X-ray. Clin. Orthop., 76:87–93, 1971.

297. Dehne, E., and Hall, R.M.: Active Shoulder Motion in Complete Deltoid Paralysis. J. Bone Joint Surg., 41A:745–748, 1959.

298. Dehne, E.: Fractures of the Upper End of the Humerus: A Classification Based on the Etiology of Trauma. Surg. Clin. North Am., 25:28–47, 1945.

299. Delaunay, C.; Lord, G.; Blanchard, J.P.; Marotte, J.H.; and Guillamon, J.L.: [The Present Place of Latarjet's Procedure in the Management of Recurrent Dislocation and Anterior Instability of the Shoulder.] Ann. Chir., 39:293–304, 1985.

300. Delitala, F.: Contributo al Trattamento della Lussazione Abituale della Spalla. *In* Moseley, H.F. (ed.): Recurrent

Dislocation of the Shoulder, p. 92. Montreal, McGill University Press, 1961.

301. Delorme, D.: Die Hemmungsbander des schultergelenks und ihre Bedeutung fur die Schulterluxationen. Arch. Klin. Chir., 92:79–101, 1910.

302. Demos, T.C.: Radiologic Case Study: Bilateral Posterior Shoulder Dislocations. Orthopedics, 3:887–897, 1980.

303. Dempster, W.T.: Mechanisms of Shoulder Movement. Arch. Phys. Med. Rehabil., 46:49–70, 1965.

304. Denti, M., and Marinoni, E.C.: [Notes on the Treatment of Recurrent Dislocation of the Shoulder With Boicev's Procedure.] Ital. J. Sport Traumatol. 10:33–40, 1988.

305. Dericks, G.: Operate First-Time Dislocators to Avoid Shoulder Redislocations. Orthopedics Today, 7:21, 1987.

306. Detenbeck, L.C.: Posterior Dislocations of the Shoulder. J. Trauma, 12:183–192, 1972.

307. Detrisac, D.A.: Indications, Arthroscopic Technique Given for Staple Capsulorrhaphy of the Shoulder. Orthopedics Today, 7:8, 1987.

308. Deutsch, A.L.; Resnick, D.; and Mink, J.H.: Computed Tomography of the Glenohumeral and Sternoclavicular Joints. Orthop. Clin. North Am., 16:497–511, 1985.

309. DiGiovine, N.M., and Ferlic, D.C.: A Long-Term Retrospective Study of the Modified Bristow Procedure. Unpublished Paper.

310. Dias, J.J.: Surgeons's Workshop: A "New" Shoulder Retractor. J. R. Coll. Surg. Edinburgh, 33:216, 1988.

311. Dick, W., and Baumgartner, R.: [Hypermotility and Voluntary Posterior Dislocation of the Shoulder.] Orthop. Praxis, 16:328–330, 1980.

312. Dickson, J.A.; Humphries, A.W.; and O'Dell, H.W.: Recurrent Dislocation of the Shoulder. Baltimore, Williams & Wilkins, 1953.

313. Dickson, J.A., and O'Dell, H.W.: A Phylogenetic Study of Recurrent Anterior Dislocation of the Shoulder Joint. Surg. Gynecol. Obstet., 95:357–365, 1952.

314. Dickson, J.W., and Devas, M.B.: Bankart's Operation for Recurrent Dislocation of the Shoulder. J. Bone Joint Surg., 39B:114–119, 1957.

315. Didiee, J.: Le Radiodiagnostic Dans la Luxation Recidivante de l'Épaule. J. Radiol. Electrol., 14:209–218, 1930.

316. DiGiovanni, C., and Turbacci, F.: [Habitual Posterior Dislocation of the Shoulder: Report of a Case.] Arch. Putti Chir. Organi. Mov., 34:275–279, 1984.

317. Dimon, J.H., III: Posterior Dislocations and Posterior Fracture Dislocation of the Shoulder: A Report of 25 Cases. South Med. J., 60:661–666, 1967.

318. Din, K.M., and Meggitt, B.F.: Bilateral Four-Part Fractures With Posterior Dislocation of the Shoulder: A Case Report. J. Bone Joint Surg., 65B:176–178, 1983.

319. Doege, K.W.: Irreducible Shoulder Joint Dislocations. Lancet, 49:191–195, 1929.

320. Dolk, T., and Gremark, O.: Arthroscopy and Stability Testing of the Shoulder Joint. Arthroscopy, 2:35–40, 1986.

321. Dorgan, J.A.: Posterior Dislocation of the Shoulder. Am. J. Surg., 89:890–900, 1955.

322. Downey, E.F., Jr.; Curtis, D.J.; and Brower, A.C.: Unusual

Dislocations of the Shoulder. A.J.R., 140:1207–1210, 1983.

323. Downing, F.H.: The Operative Treatment for Anterior Dislocation of the Shoulder. J. Bone Joint Surg., 51A: 811–812, 1969.

324. Driessen, A.P.P.M., and Werkman, D.M.: Treatment of Habitual Shoulder Dislocation by Weber's Derotational Osteotomy (abstract). Acta Orthop. Scand., 55:485, 1984.

325. Drury, J.K., and Scullion, J.E.: Vascular Complications of Anterior Dislocation of the Shoulder. Br. J. Surg., 67: 579–581, 1980.

326. Du Toit, G.T., and Roux, D.: Recurrent Dislocation of the Shoulder: A Twenty-Four Year Study of the Johannesburg Stapling Operation. J. Bone Joint Surg., 38A: 1–12, 1956.

327. Du Toit, J.G.: Recurrent Dislocation of the Shoulder. Orthopaedic Correspondence Club Letter, August 1969.

328. Dubs, L., and Gschwend, N.: General Joint Laxity: Quantification and Clinical Relevance. Arch. Orthop. Trauma Surg., 107:65–72, 1988.

329. Dvir, Z., and Berme, N.: The Shoulder Complex in Elevation of the Arm: A Mechanism Approach. J. Biomech., 11:219–225, 1978.

330. Ebel, R.: [The Cause of Axillary Nerve Paresis in Shoulder Luxations.] Monatsschr. Unfallheilkd., 76:445–449, 1973.

331. Ebong, W.W.: The Pattern of Fractures and Dislocations in Western Nigeria. Injury, 9:221–224, 1977.

332. Eckert, R.R.; Richardson, A.B.; and Dericks, G.H.: Arthroscopic Shoulder Stapling for Instability: A Review of 57 Cases Followed for Two Years. Personal communication, 1989.

333. Edeland, H.G., and Stefansson, T.: Block of the Suprascapular Nerve in Reduction of Acute Anterior Shoulder Dislocation: Case Reports. Acta Anesth. Scand., 17:46–49, 1973.

334. Eden, R.: Zur Operation der habituellen Schulterluxation unter mitteilung eines neuen Verfahrens bei Abriss am inneren Pfannenrande. Dtsch. Z. Chir., 144:269–280, 1918.

335. Eden-Hybbinette, R.: Technique of Palmer and Widen. In Crenshaw, A.H. (ed.): Campbell's Operative Orthopaedics, 5th ed., Vol. 1, p. 366. St Louis, C.V. Mosby, 1971.

336. Editorial: Voluntary Dislocation of the Shoulder. Br. Med. J., 4:505, 1973.

337. Ehgartner, K.: [Has the Duration of Cast Fixation After Shoulder Dislocations an Influence on the Frequency of Recurrent Dislocation?] Arch. Orthop. Unfall. Chir., 89: 187–190, 1977.

338. Ehmer, B.; Meeder, P.J.; and Jungeblod, T.: Indikation, Technik und Ergebnisse der operativen Behandlung von Schultergelenksluxationen. Therapiewoche, 32:2350–2358, 1982.

339. El Arjoun, L.; Trafeh, M.; Derfouri, M.; Zryouil, B.; and Benabdenbi, A.: [The Neglected Shoulder Luxation.] Maroc. Med., 7:489–493, 1985.

340. El-Khoury, G.Y.; Kathol, M.H.; Chandler, J.B.; and Albright, J.P.: Shoulder Instability: Impact of Glenohumeral Arthrotomography on Treatment. Radiology, 160: 669–673, 1986.

341. Ellerbroek, N.: Beobachtungen uber Schulterluxationen nach hinten nebst einer Ubersicht uber alle vom 1. januar 1890 bis 1. januar 1907 in der Gottinger chirurgischen Poliklinik beobachteten Luxationen. Dtsch. Ztschr. Chir., 92:453–463, 1908.

342. Ellman, H., and Kay, S.P.: Arthroscopic Treatment of Calcific Tendinitis (abstract). Orthop. Trans., 13(2):240, Summer, 1989.

343. Ellman, H.: Arthroscopic Subacromial Decompression: Analysis of One- to Three-Year Results. Arthroscopy, 3: 173–181, 1987.

344. Ellman, H.: Arthroscopic Subacromial Decompression: New Techniques and Results. Presented at the Arthroscopy Association of North America Instructional Course, 8th Annual Meeting, Seattle, WA, April 14, 1989.

345. Ellman, H.: Arthroscopic Treatment of Impingement of the Shoulder. Instr. Course Lect., 38:177–185, 1989.

346. Ellman, H.: Shoulder Arthroscopy: Current Indications and Techniques. Orthopedics, 11:45–51, 1988.

347. Endo, H.: Loose Shoulder. Personal communication, 1984.

348. Engelhardt, M.B.: Posterior Dislocation of the Shoulder: Report of Six Cases. South. Med. J., 71:425–427, 1978.

349. Engin, A.E.: On the Biomechanics of the Shoulder Complex. Biomech., 13:575–590, 1980.

350. Engle, R.P., and Canner, G.C.: Posterior Shoulder Instability: An Approach to Rehabilitation. J. Orthop. Sports Phys. Ther., 10:488–494, 1989.

351. English, E., and Macnab, I.: Recurrent Posterior Dislocation of the Shoulder. Can. J. Surg., 17:147–151, 1974.

352. Ennker, J., and Gotzen, L.: [Diagnosis of Posterior Dislocations of the Shoulder.] Unfallchirurg, 88:198–203, 1985.

353. Epps, C.H.: Complications in Orthopaedic Surgery. Philadelphia, J.B. Lippincott, 1978.

354. Eriksson, E., and Denti, M.: Diagnostic and Operative Arthroscopy of the Shoulder and Elbow Joint. Ital. J. Sports Traumatol., 7:165–188, 1985.

355. Esch, J.C.; Ozerkis, L.R.; Helgager, J.A.; Kane, N.; and Lilliott, N.: Arthroscopic Subacromial Decompression: Results According to the Degree of Rotator Cuff Tear. Arthroscopy, 4:241–249, 1988.

356. Esch, J.C.; Ozerkis, L.R.; Helgager, J.A.; Kane, N.; and Lilliott, N.: Shoulder Arthroscopy: Basics. (Brochure Prepared in Conjunction With a Scientific Exhibit on Shoulder Arthroscopy.) Annual Meeting of the American Academy of Orthopaedic Surgeons, Las Vegas, Nev., Feb. 1989.

357. Esch, J.C.: Arthroscopic Subacromial Decompression Gets 85% Patient Satisfaction Scores After One Year. Orthopedics Today, 8:15, 1988.

358. Esch, J.C.: Shoulder Arthroscopy: Basic Setup. Techniques Orthop., 3:9–14, 1988.

359. Esch, J.C.: Shoulder Arthroscopy: Treatment of Rotator Cuff Pathology. Presented at the Arthroscopy Association

of North America Instructional Course, 8th Annual Meeting, Seattle, Wa., April 14, 1989.

360. Eve, F.S.: A Case of Subcoracoid Dislocation of the Humerus, With the Formation of an Indentation on the Posterior Surface of the Head, the Joint Being Unopened; With Remarks on the Mode of Production of Fracture of the Anatomical Neck, With Dislocation. MedicoChir. Soc. London Trans., 45:317–321, 1880.

361. Eyre-Brook, A.L.: Posterior Dislocation of the Shoulder (abstract). J. Bone Joint Surg., 54B:760, 1972.

362. Eyre-Brook, A.L.: Posterior Dislocation of the Shoulder (abstract). S. Afr. Orthop. Assoc., 47:2139, 1973.

363. Eyre-Brook, A.L.: Recurrent Dislocation of the Shoulder. Physiotherapy, 57:7–13, 1971.

364. Eyre-Brook, A.L.: Recurrent Dislocation of the Shoulder: Lesions Discovered in Seventeen Cases, Surgery Employed, and Intermediate Report on Results. J. Bone Joint Surg., 30B:39–48, 1948.

365. Eyre-Brook, A.L.: The Morbid Anatomy of a Case of Recurrent Dislocation of the Shoulder. Br. J. Surg., 29:32–37, 1943.

366. Fahey, J.: Anatomy of the Shoulder. Instr. Course. Lect., IV:186–190, 1947.

367. Fairbank, H.A.T.: Birth Palsy: Subluxation of the Shoulder Joint in Infants and Young Children. Lancet, 1:1217–1223, 1913.

368. Fairbank, T.J.: Fracture–Subluxations of the Shoulder. J. Bone Joint Surg., 30B:454–460, 1948.

369. Faletti, C.; Clerico, P.; Indemini, E.; and Crova, M.: [Standard Radiography in Recurrent Dislocation of the Shoulder.] Ital. J. Sports Med., 7:33–40, 1985.

370. Falkner, E.A.: Luxatio Erecta of Shoulder Joint. Med. J. Aust., 1:227–228, 1916.

371. Fanjul-Cabeza, J.M.; Moreno-Guerrero, T.J.; Lopez-Fernandez, P.; and Fernandez-Moral, V.: [Results of Surgery for Recurrent Shoulder Dislocation.] Rev. Ortop. Traumatol., 32:3–9, 1988.

372. Farrugia, P.D.: Superior Glenohumeral Dislocation—A Case Report. Injury, 16:489–490, 1985.

373. Federici, A.; Benvenuti, M.; Siri, R.; and Carbone, M.: [Mobilization of the "T" Nail in Bankart-Delitala Capsulopexy.] Minerva Ortop. Traumatol., 39:671–675, 1988.

374. Federici, A.; Santolini, F.; and Carbone, M.: [Three Cases of Atraumatic Habitual Posterior Subluxations of the Shoulder.] Minerva Ortop. Traumatol., 39:685–688, 1988.

375. Fee, H.J.; McAvoy, J.M.; and Dainko, E.A.: Pseudoaneurysm of the Axillary Artery Following a Modified Bristow Operation: Report of a Case and Review of the Literature. J. Cardiovasc. Surg., 19:65–68, 1978.

376. Ferkel, R.D.; Hedley, A.K.; and Eckardt, J.J.: Anterior Fracture–Dislocations of the Shoulder: Pitfalls in Treatment. J. Trauma, 24:363–367, 1984.

377. Ferlic, D.C., and DiGiovine, N.M.: A Long-Term Retrospective Study of the Modified Bristow Procedure. Am. J. Sports Med., 16:469–474, 1988.

378. Feron, J.M.; Signoret, F.; Bonfait, H.; and Patel, A.: [Treatment of Recurrent Anterior Shoulder Dislocations

379. Féry, A., and Sommelet, J.: [Erect Dislocation of the Shoulder (Luxation Erecta Humeri): General Review Apropos of 10 Cases.] Int. Orthop., 11:95–103, 1987.

380. Fick, R.: Handbuch der Anatomie und Mechanik der Gelenke unter Berucks ichtigung der Bewegenden Muskeln. Jena, Fischer, 1904.

381. Figiel, S.J.; Figiel, L.S.; Bardenstein, M.B.; and Blodgett, W.H.: Posterior Dislocation of the Shoulder. Radiology, 87:737–740, 1966.

382. Finsterbush, A., and Pogrund, H.: The Hypermobility Syndrome: Musculoskeletal Complaints in 100 Consecutive Cases of Generalized Joint Hypermobility. Clin. Orthop., 168:124–127, 1982.

383. Finsterer, H.: Die operative Behandlung der habituellen Schulterluxation. Dtsch. Z. Chir., 141:354–497, 1917.

384. Fipp, G.J.: Simultaneous Posterior Dislocation of Both Shoulders: Report of a Case. Clin. Orthop., 44:191–195, 1966.

385. Fitzgerald, J.F., and Keates, J.: False Aneurysm as a Late Complication of Anterior Dislocation of the Shoulder. Ann. Surg., 181:785–786, 1975.

386. Fitzgerald-Finch, O.P., and Gibson, I.I.J.M.: Subluxation of the Shoulder in Hemiplegia. Age Ageing, 4:16–18, 1975.

387. Fleming, J.: A Working Approach to Brachial Plexus Palsy. J. Bone Joint Surg., 61B:260, 1979.

388. Reference deleted.

389. Flood, V.: Discovery of a New Ligament of the Shoulder Joint. Lancet, 672–673, 1829.

390. Flower, W.H.: On the Pathological Changes Produced in the Shoulder Joint by Traumatic Dislocation, as Derived From an Examination of All the Specimens Illustrating This Injury in the Museums of London. Trans. Path. Soc. London, 12:179–200, 1861.

391. Foster, W.S.; Ford, T.B.; and Drez, D., Jr.: Isolated Posterior Shoulder Dislocation in a Child: A Case Report. Am. J. Sports Med., 13:198–200, 1985.

392. Francis, D.A., and Heron, J.R.: Progressive Muscular Atrophy and Posterior Dislocation of the Humerus Following Electric Shock. Postgrad. Med., 60:143–144, 1984.

393. Franke, G.H.: Dislocations of Shoulder. Dtsch. Z. Chir., 48:399, 1898.

394. Frankel, V.H., and Nordin, M.: Basic Biomechanics of the Skeletal System. Philadelphia, Lea & Febiger, 1980.

395. Freeland, A.E., and Higgins, R.W.: Anterior Shoulder Dislocation With Posterior Displacement of the Long Head of the Biceps Tendon—Arthrographic Findings: A Case Report. Orthopedics, 8:468–469, 1985.

396. Freundlich, B.D.: Luxatio Erecta. J. Trauma, 23:434–436, 1983.

397. Fried, A.: Habitual Posterior Dislocation of the Shoulder Joint: A Report on 5 Operated Cases. Acta Orthop. Scand., 18:329–345, 1949.

398. Frizziero, L.; Zizzi, F.; Facchini, A.; Sgobbi, S.; and Zini, G.L.: Arthroscopy of the Shoulder Joint: A Review of 23 Cases. Rheumatologie, 11:267–276, 1981.

399. Froimson, A., and Alfred, K.S.: Sesamoid Bone of the Subscapularis Tendon: Report of a Case. J. Bone Joint Surg., 43A:881–884, 1961.

400. Fronek, J.; Bowen, M.; Pavlov, H.; and Warren, R.: Posterior Subluxation of the Glenohumeral Joint: Nonsurgical and Surgical Treatment. Orthop. Trans., 10(1):221, Spring, 1986.

401. Fronek, J.; Warren, R.F.; and Bowen, M.: Posterior Subluxation of the Glenohumeral Joint. J. Bone Joint Surg., 71A:205–216, 1989.

402. Fu, F.H., and Klein, A.H.: Shoulder Arthroscopy: Complications and Pitfalls. Techniques Orthop., 3:27–32, 1988.

403. Fullarton, G.M., and MacEwan, C.J.: Bilateral Posterior Dislocations of the Shoulder (letter to the editor). Injury, 16:428–429, 1985.

404. Fusco, E.B.: Procedure to Reduce Dislocation of the Shoulder. J. Bone Joint Surg., 38A:782–786, 1956.

405. Gainor, B.J.; Piotrowski, G.; Puhl, J.; Allen, W.C.; and Hagen, R.: The Throw: Biomechanics and Acute Injury. Am. J. Sports Med., 8:114–118, 1980.

406. Galenus: On the Usefulness of the Parts of the Body, Vol. 2 (Translated by May, M.T.) Ithaca, Cornell University Press, 1968.

407. Galinat, B.J., and Howell, S.M.: Excessive Retroversion of the Glenoid Cavity. A Cause of Non-Traumatic Posterior Instability of the Shoulder (letter to the editor). J. Bone Joint Surg., 69A:632–633, 1986.

408. Galinat, B.J.; Howell, S.M.; and Kraft, T.A.: The Glenoid–Posterior Acromion Angle: An Accurate Method of Evaluating Glenoid Version. Orthop. Trans., 12(3):727, Fall, 1988.

409. Galinat, B.J.; Murphy, J.M.; and MacEwen, G.D.: Shoulder Arthrodesis: A Long-Term Functional Evaluation. Presented at the American Shoulder and Elbow Surgeons 4th Open Meeting, Atlanta, Ga., 1988.

410. Gallen, J.; Wiss, D.A.; Cantelmo, N.; and Menzoin, J.O.: Traumatic Pseudoaneurysm of the Axillary Artery: Report of Three Cases and Literature Review. J. Trauma, 24:350–354, 1984.

411. Gallie, W.E., and LeMesurier, A.B.: An Operation for the Relief of Recurring Dislocations of the Shoulder. Trans. Am. Surg. Assoc., 45:392–398, 1927.

412. Gallie, W.E., and LeMesurier, A.B.: Recurring Dislocation of the Shoulder. J. Bone Joint Surg., 30B:9–18, 1948.

413. Gallie, W.E.: Dislocations. N. Engl. J. Med., 213:91–98, 1935.

414. Gambrioli, P.L.; Magg, F.; and Radelli, M.: Computerized Tomography in the Investigation of Scapulohumeral Instability. Ital. J. Orthop. Traumatol., 11:223–232, 1985.

415. Gandin, J., and Gandin, R.: [Oudard's Operation and its Variants in Recurrent Dislocation of the Shoulder: Statistical Study of 139 Late Results.] Chirurgie, 99:779–786, 1973.

416. Ganel, A.; Horoszowski, H.; Heim, M.; Engel, J.; and Farine, I.: Persistent Dislocation of the Shoulder in Elderly Patients. J. Am. Geriatr. Soc., 28:282–284, 1980.

417. Garcia-Elias, M., and Salo, J.M.: Non-Union of a Fractured Coracoid Process After Dislocation of the Shoulder—A Case Report. J. Bone Joint Surg., 67B:722–723, 1985.

418. Gardham, J.R.C., and Scott, J.E.: Axillary Artery Occlusion With Erect Dislocation of the Shoulder. Injury, 11:155–158, 1980.

419. Gardner, E., and Gray, D.J.: Prenatal Development of the Human Shoulder and Acromioclavicular Joints. Am. J. Anat., 92:219–276, 1953.

420. Gardner, E.: The Prenatal Development of the Human Shoulder Joint. Surg. Clin. North Am., 43:1465–1470, 1963.

421. Gariepy, R.; Derome, A.; and Laurin, C.A.: Brachial Plexus Paralysis Following Shoulder Dislocation. Can. J. Surg., 5:418–421, 1962.

422. Garth, W.P., Jr.; Allman, F.L.; and Armstrong, W.S.: Occult Anterior Subluxations of the Shoulder in Noncontact Sports. Am. J. Sports Med., 15:579–585, 1987.

423. Garth, W.P., Jr.; Slappey, C.E.; and Ochs, C.W.: Roentgenographic Demonstration of Instability of the Shoulder: The Apical Oblique Projection: A Technical Note. J. Bone Joint Surg., 66A:1450–1453, 1984.

424. Gartland, J.J., and Dowling, J.J.: Recurrent Anterior Dislocation of the Shoulder Joint. Clin. Orthop., 3:86–91, 1954.

425. Gartsman, G.M.; Blair, M.; Bennett, J.B.; Tullos, H.S.; and Noble, P.C.: Arthroscopic Subacromial Decompression: An Anatomical Study. Am. J. Sports Med., 16:48–50, 1988.

426. Gartsman, G.M.: Arthroscopic Subacromial Decompression for Advanced Rotator Cuff Disease (abstract). Orthop. Trans., 13(2):240, Summer, 1989.

427. Gartsman, G.M.: Arthroscopic Acromioplasty for Rotator Cuff Lesions. Unpublished paper, 1989.

428. Genovesi, A.: [A Case of Voluntary Shoulder Dislocation in a 14-Year-Old Girl.] Arch. Putti Chir. Organi. Mov., 17:268–275, 1962.

429. Gerber, C.; Ganz, R.; and Vinh, T.S.: Glenoplasty for Recurrent Posterior Shoulder Instability: An Anatomic Reappraisal. Clin. Orthop., 216:70–79, 1987.

430. Gerber, C., and Ganz, R.: Clinical Assessment of Instability of the Shoulder. J. Bone Joint Surg., 66B:551–556, 1984.

431. Gerber, C., and Ganz, R.: [Diagnosis and Casual Therapy in Shoulder Instability.] Unfallchirurg, 89:418–428, 1986.

432. Gerber, C.; Terrier, F.; and Ganz, R.: The Trillat Procedure for Recurrent Anterior Instability of the Shoulder. J. Bone Joint Surg., 70B:130–134, 1988.

433. Gerber, C.: Personal communication, August 24, 1989 re Latarjet, M.: Technique de la Butée Coracoidienne Pre-Glenoidienne Dans le Traitement des Luxations Recidivantes de l'Épaule. Lyon Chir., 54:604–609, 1958.

434. Gerber, C.: Personal communication, November 4, 1985.

435. Ghormley, R.K.; Black, J.R.; and Cherry, J.H.: Ununited Fractures of the Clavicle. Am. J. Surg., 51:343–349, 1941.

436. Giannestras, N.J.: Discussion of Traumatic Posterior (Retroglenoid) Dislocation of the Humerus. J. Bone Joint Surg., 31A:172, 1949.

437. Giannestras, N.J.: The Magnuson-Stack Procedure for Recurrent Dislocations of the Shoulder. Surgery, 23:794–800, 1948.

438. Gibson, A.: Recurrent Dislocation of the Shoulder Joint. Can. Med. Assoc. J., 11:194–199, 1921.

439. Gibson, J.M.C.: Rupture of the Axillary Artery. J. Bone Joint Surg., 44B:114–115, 1962.

440. Gilula, L.A., and Staple, T.W.: Roentgen Rounds #1. Orthop. Rev., 2:53–55, 1973.

441. Gjores, J.E., and Nilsonne, U.: Prognosis in Primary Dislocation of the Shoulder. Acta Chir. Scand., 129:468–470, 1965.

442. Glessner, J.R.: Intrathoracic Dislocation of the Humeral Head. J. Bone Joint Surg., 43A:428–430, 1961.

443. Glousman, R.; Jobe, F.; Tibone, J.; Moynes, D.; Antonelli, D.; and Perry, J.: Dynamic Electromyographic Analysis of the Throwing Shoulder With Glenohumeral Instability. J. Bone Joint Surg., 70A:220–226, 1988.

444. Gold, A.M.: Fractured Neck of the Humerus With Separation and Dislocation of the Humeral Head (Fracture–Dislocation of the Shoulder, Severe Type). Bull. Hosp. Joint Dis. Orthop. Inst., 32:87–99, 1971.

445. Golding, C.: Radiology and Orthopaedic Surgery. J. Bone Joint Surg., 48B:320–332, 1966.

446. Goldman, A.; Sherman, O.; Price, A.; and Minkoff, J.: Posterior Fracture Dislocation of the Shoulder With Biceps Tendon Interposition. J. Trauma, 27:1083–1086, 1987.

447. Goldstone, R.A.: Dislocation of the Shoulder: X-ray Signs (letter to the editor). N. Engl. J. Med., 283:1113, 1970.

448. Goodfellow, J.W., and Boldero, J.L.: Bilateral Synchronous Posterior Dislocation of the Shoulder. Br. J. Surg., 46:413–415, 1959.

449. Goss, T.P., and Costello, G.: Recurrent Symptomatic Posterior Glenohumeral Subluxation. Orthop. Rev., 17:1024–1032, 1988.

450. Goss, T.P.: Anterior Glenohumeral Instability. Orthopedics, 11:87–95, 1988.

451. Goss, T.P.: Factors to Consider in Chronic Symptomatic Shoulder Instability. Orthop. Rev., 14:27–32, 1985.

452. Gosset, J.: Une Technique de Greffe Coraco-Glenordienne Dans le Traitement des Luxations Recidivantes de l'Epoule. Mem. Acad. Chir., 86:445–447, 1960.

453. Gotzen, L., and Ennker, J.: [Bone Block Grafting in Chronic Shoulder Instability.] Unfallheilkd, 170:193–205, 1984.

454. Gould, R.; Rosenfield, A.T.; and Friedlaender, G.E.: Case Report: Loose Body Within the Glenohumeral Joint in Recurrent Anterior Dislocation—CT Demonstration. J. Comput. Assist. Tomogr., 9:404–406, 1985.

455. Gradinger, R.; Flock, K.; Rechl, H.; Scheyerer, M.; and Opitz, G.: [Diagnosis and Treatment of Recurrent Anterior Dislocation of the Shoulder.] Fortschr. Med., 106:44–48, 1988.

456. Graham, B., and Loomer, R.L.: The Anatomical Basis for Axillary Nerve Injury During Inferior Capsular Shift Surgery of the Shoulder (abstract). J. Bone Joint Surg., 69B:502, 1987.

457. Grant, J.C.B.: Grant's Atlas of Anatomy, 6th ed. Baltimore, Williams & Wilkins, 1972.

458. Grant, J.C.B.: Method of Anatomy, 7th ed. Baltimore, Williams & Wilkins, 1965.

459. Grashey, R.: Atlas Typischer Röntgenbilder von Normalen Menschen. München, J.F. Lebmans Verlag, 1923.

460. Green, N.E., and Wheelhouse, W.W.: Anterior Subglenoid Dislocation of the Shoulder in an Infant Following Pneumococcal Meningitis. Clin. Orthop., 135:125–127, 1978.

461. Greenhill, B.J.: Persistent Posterior Shoulder Dislocation: Its Diagnosis and Treatment by Putti-Platt Repair (abstract). J. Bone Joint Surg., 54B:763, 1972.

462. Gregorie, R.: Luxation Recidivante de l'Épaule: Anatomie Pathologique et Pathogenie. Rev. Orthop., 24:15–36, 1913.

463. Greig, D.: On True Congenital Dislocation of the Shoulder. Edinburgh Med. J., 30:157–175, 1923.

464. Griffiths, L.L.: Reducing Dislocated Shoulder (Classic Photographs and Illustrations). J. Bone Joint Surg., 32B:678–679, 1950.

465. Gross, R.M.: Arthroscopic Shoulder Capsulorraphy: Does It Work? Am. J. Sports Med., 17:495–500, 1989.

466. Gryska, P.F.: Major Vascular Injuries: Principles of Management in Selected Cases of Arterial and Venous Injury. N. Engl. J. Med., 266:381–385, 1962.

467. Gugenheim, S., and Sanders, R.J.: Axillary Artery Rupture Caused by Shoulder Dislocation. Surgery, 95:55–58, 1984.

468. Guibe, M.: Des Lesions des Vaisseaux de l'Aisselle qui Compliquent les Luxations de l'Épaule. Rev. Chir., 44:580–614, 1911.

469. Guicciardi, E.; Burroni, L.; and Veronese, M.: [Latarjet Operation in the Treatment of Recurrent Shoulder Luxation.] Minerva Ortop. Traumatol., 39:699–703, 1988.

470. Guilfoil, P.H., and Christiansen, T.: An Unusual Vascular Complication of Fractured Clavicle. J.A.M.A., 200:72–73, 1967.

471. Guney, F.: [Methods in Surgery of Habitual Shoulder Dislocation and Its Results, With Special Reference to the Eden-Brun Method.] Helv. Chir. Acta, 40:329–338, 1973.

472. Guy, D.K.: Shoulder Arthroscopy Does Not Improve Understanding of Disease (letter to the editor). A.O.R.N.J., 49:964, 1989.

473. Ha'Eri, G.B., and Maitland, A.: Arthroscopy Findings in the Frozen Shoulder. J. Rheumatol., 8:149–152, 1981.

474. Ha'Eri, G.B.: Boytchev Procedure for the Treatment of Anterior Shoulder Instability. Clin. Orthop., 206:196–201, 1986.

475. Haas, S.L.: The Treatment of Permanent Paralysis of the Deltoid Muscle. J.A.M.A., 104:99–103, 1935.

476. Hadlow, A.T., and Hardy, A.E.: Recurrent Anterior Dislocation of the Shoulder Treated by Putti-Platt Repair (abstract). J. Bone Joint Surg., 70B:510, 1988.

477. Haley, P.H., and House, J.H.: Recurrent Anterior Dislocation of the Shoulder: Surgical Repair With a Modified Bristow Procedure. Minn. Med., 57:882–885, 1974.

478. Hall, R.H.; Isaac, F.; and Booth, C.R.: Dislocations of the Shoulder With Special Reference to Accompanying Small Fractures. J. Bone Joint Surg., 41A:489–494, 1959.

479. Halley, D.K., and Olix, M.L.: A Review of the Bristow Operation for Recurrent Anterior Shoulder Dislocation in Athletes. Clin. Orthop., 106:175–199, 1975.

480. Hansen, E.B.; Frost, B.; and Jensen, E.M.: [The Arthrographic Picture Following Anterior Dislocation of the Shoulder: A Consecutive Investigation of 71 Outpatients.] Ugeskr. Laeger., 147:4193–4195, 1985.

481. Hardcastle, P.H., and Fisher, T.R.: Intrathoracic Displacement of the Humeral Head With Fracture of the Surgical Neck. Injury, 12:313–315, 1980.

482. Hark, F.W.: Habitual Dislocation of the Shoulder Joint. Arch. Surg., 56:522–527, 1948.

483. Harmon, P.H.: The Posterior Approach for Arthrodesis and Other Operations on the Shoulder. Surg. Gynecol. Obstet., 81:266–268, 1945.

484. Harryman, D.T., II; Sidles, J.A.; Clark, J.M.; McQuade, K.J.; Gibb, T.D.; and Matsen, F.A., III: Humeral Head Translation on the Glenoid Occurs With Passive Glenohumeral Motions. Personal communication, 1989.

485. Hartney-Velazco, K.; Velazco, A.; and Fleming, L.L.: Bilateral Anterior Dislocation of the Shoulder. South. Med. J., 77:1340–1341, 1984.

486. Hastings, D.E., and Coughlin, L.P.: Recurrent Subluxation of the Glenohumeral Joint. Am. J. Sports Med., 9:352–355, 1981.

487. Hauser, E.D.W.: Avulsion of the Tendon of the Subscapularis Muscle. J. Bone Joint Surg., 36A:139–141, 1954.

488. Hawkins, R.B.: Arthroscopic Stapling Capsulorrhaphy for Recurrent Anterior Dislocation of the Shoulder (abstract). Orthop. Trans., 9(1):48, Spring, 1985.

489. Hawkins, R.B.: Arthroscopic Stapling Repair for Shoulder Instability: A Retrospective Study of 50 Cases. Arthroscopy, 5:122–128, 1989.

490. Hawkins, R.H., and Hawkins, R.J.: Failed Anterior Reconstruction for Shoulder Instability (abstract). J. Bone Joint Surg., 69B:502, 1987.

491. Hawkins, R.H., and Hawkins, R.J.: Failed Anterior Reconstruction for Shoulder Instability. J. Bone Joint Surg., 67B:709–714, 1985.

492. Hawkins, R.J.; Belle, R.H.; Hawkins, R.H.; and Koppert, G.J.: Anterior Dislocation of the Shoulder in the Older Patient. Clin. Orthop., 206:192–195, 1986.

493. Hawkins, R.J., and Belle, R.H.: Shoulder Instability—Diagnosis and Management. Can. J. Sports Sci., 12:67–70, 1987.

494. Hawkins, R.J., and Belle, R.H.: Posterior Instability of the Shoulder. Instr. Course Lect., XXXVIII:211–215, 1989.

495. Hawkins, R.J., and Koppert, G.J.: The Natural History Following Anterior Dislocation of the Shoulder in the Older Patient (abstract). J. Bone Joint Surg., 64B:255, 1982.

496. Hawkins, R.J., and Koppert, G.J.: Recurrent Posterior Dislocation of the Shoulder. Orthop. Trans., 4:298, 1980.

497. Hawkins, R.J.; Koppert, G.J.; and Johnston, G.: Recurrent Posterior Instability (Subluxation) of the Shoulder. J. Bone Joint Surg., 66A:169–174, 1984.

498. Hawkins, R.J., and McCormack, R.G.: Posterior Shoulder Instability. Orthopedics, 11:101–107, 1988.

499. Hawkins, R.J.; Neer, C.S., II; Pianta, R.M.; and Mendoza, F.X.: Missed Posterior Dislocations of the Shoulder. Orthop. Trans., 6(1):363, Spring, 1982.

500. Hawkins, R.J.; Neer, C.S., II; Pianta, R.M.; and Mendoza, F.X.: Locked Posterior Dislocation of the Shoulder. J. Bone Joint Surg., 69A:9–18, 1987.

501. Hawkins, R.J.: Failed Shoulder Procedures—Anterior and Posterior Reconstruction. American Academy of Orthopaedic Surgeons Instructional Course Lecture #414, Las Vegas, Nev., Feb. 14, 1989.

502. Hawkins, R.J.: Unrecognized Dislocations of the Shoulder. Instr. Course Lect. XXXIV:258, 1985.

503. Hawkins, R.J.: Posterior Dislocations of the Shoulder. American Academy of Orthopaedic Surgeons Summer Institute, Chicago, July 10–11, 1980.

504. Hawkins, R.J.: Unrecognized Dislocations of the Shoulder. Instr. Course Lect., XXXIV:258–263, 1986.

505. Hawkins, R.J.: Unreduced Dislocations of the Shoulder (handout). American Academy of Orthopaedic Surgeons Instructional Course Lecture #516, Las Vegas, Nev., Jan. 29, 1985.

506. Hays, M.B.: Glenoid Osteotomy for Treatment of Recurrent Dislocation of the Shoulder (abstract). J. Bone Joint Surg., 51A:811, 1969.

507. Heck, C.C.: Anterior Dislocation of the Glenohumeral Joint in a Child. J. Trauma, 21:174–175, 1981.

508. Hehne, H.J.; Meyer, S.; and Hubner, H.: [Treatment of Recurrent Shoulder Dislocation by the Method of Putti-Platt and Bankart and Eden-Hybinette and Lange.] Orthop. Praxis, 16:331–335, 1980.

509. Heisel, J.: Results of Treatment of Fresh Traumatic Dislocation of the Shoulder. Aktuel Traumatol., 12:195–197, 1982.

510. Hejna, W.F., Fossier, C.H.; Goldstein, T.B.; and Ray, R.D.: Ancient Anterior Dislocation of the Shoulder (abstract). J. Bone Joint Surg., 51A:1030–1031, 1969.

511. Helfet, A.J.: Coracoid Transplantation for Recurring Dislocation of the Shoulder. J. Bone Joint Surg., 40B:198–202, 1958.

512. Henderson, M.S.: Habitual or Recurrent Dislocation of the Shoulder. Surg. Gynecol. Obstet., 33:1–7, 1921.

513. Henderson, M.S.: Tenosuspension Operation for Recurrent or Habitual Dislocation of the Shoulder. Surg. Clin. North Am., 5:997–1007, 1949.

514. Henderson, W.D.: Arthroscopic Stabilization of the Anterior Shoulder. Clin. Sports Med., 6:581–586, 1987.

515. Hendry, A.M.: The Treatment of Residual Paralysis After Brachial Plexus Injuries. J. Bone Joint Surg., 31B:42–49, 1949.

516. Henry, A.K.: Exposure of Long Bones and Other Surgical Methods. New York, William Wood, 1927.

517. Henry, J.H., and Genung, J.A.: Natural History of Glenohumeral Dislocation: Revisited. Am. J. Sports Med., 10:135–137, 1982.

518. Henry, J.H.: How I Manage Dislocated Shoulders. Phys. Sports Med., 12:65–69, 1984.

519. Henson, G.F.: Vascular Complications of Shoulder Injuries: A Report of Two Cases. J. Bone Joint Surg., 38B:528–531, 1956.

520. Heppenstall, R.B.: Fracture Treatment and Healing. Philadelphia, W.B. Saunders, 1980.

521. Hermodsson, I.: Rontgenologische Studien uber die traumatischen und habituellen Schultergelenk-Verrenkungen nach vorn und nach unten. Acta Radiol. (Suppl.), 20:1–173, 1934.

522. Hermodsson, I.: Rontgenologische Studien uber die traumatischen und habituellen Schultergelenkverrenkungen nach unten. Moseley, H., and Overgaard, B. (trans.). Montreal, McGill University Press, 1963.

523. Hernandez, A., and Drez, D.: Operative Treatment of Posterior Shoulder Dislocations by Posterior Glenoidplasty, Capsulorrhaphy, and Infraspinatus Advancement. Am. J. Sports Med., 14:187–191, 1986.

524. Hertz, H.; Grundschober, F.; Plenk, H., Jr.; and Weinstabl, R.: Uber die Struktur und Gefassversorgung des Limbus Glenoidalis des Schultergelenkes (abstract). Acta Anat., 120:32, 1984.

525. Hertz, H.; Scharf, W.; Berr, T.; and Wunderlich, M.: [Frequency of Recurrence of Traumatic Anterior Shoulder Dislocation.] Unfallchirurg, 88:437–441, 1985.

526. Hertz, H.; Weinstabl, R.; Grundschober, F.; and Orthner, E.: [Macroscopical and Histological Examinations of the Anatomy of the Limbus Glenoidalis.] Acta Anat., 125:96–100, 1986.

527. Hertz, H.: [The Importance of the Limbus Glenoidalis for the Stability of the Shoulder Joint.] Wien Klin. Wochenschr. (Austria), 96(Suppl. 14):152–175, 1984.

528. Heymanowitsch, Z.: Ein Beitrag zur operativen Behandlung der habituellen Schulterluxationen. Zentralbl. Chir., 54:648–651, 1927.

529. Hildebrand, O.: Zur operativen Behandlung der habituellen Schuterluxation. Arch. Klin. Chir., 66:360–364, 1902.

530. Hill, H.A., and Sachs, M.D.: The Grooved Defect of the Humeral Head: A Frequently Unrecognized Complication of Dislocations of the Shoulder Joint. Radiology, 35:690–700, 1940.

531. Hill, J.A.; Lombardo, S.J.; Kerlan, R.K.; Jobe, F.W.; Carter, V.S.; Shields, C.L.; Collins, H.R.; and Yocum, L.A.: The Modified Bristow-Helfet Procedure For Recurrent Anterior Shoulder Subluxations and Dislocations. Am. J. Sports Med., 9:283–287, 1981.

532. Hill, J.A., and Tkach, L.: A Study of Glenohumeral Orientation in Patients With Anterior Recurrent Shoulder Dislocations Using Computerized Axial Tomography (abstract). Orthop. Trans., 9(1):47, Spring, 1985.

533. Hill, N.A., and McLaughlin, H.L.: Locked Posterior Dislocation Simulating A "Frozen Shoulder." J. Trauma, 3:225–234, 1963.

534. Hindenach, J.C.R.: Recurrent Posterior Dislocation of the Shoulder. J. Bone Joint Surg., 29:582–586, 1947.

535. Hindmarsh, J., and Lindberg, A.: Eden-Hybbinette's Operation for Recurrent Dislocation of the Humero-Scapular Joint. Acta Orthop. Scand., 38:459–478, 1967.

536. Hinton, A.E., and King, D.: Anterior Shoulder Dislocation as a Complication of Surgery for Burns. Burns, 15:248–249, 1989.

537. Hippocrates: The Classic—Injuries of the Shoulder: Dislocations. Clin. Orthop., 246:4–7, 1989.

538. Hippocrates: Works of Hippocrates With an English Translation by W.H.S. Jones and E.T. Withington. London, William Heinemann, 1927.

539. Hodgkinson, J.P., and Case, D.B.: The Modified Staple Capsulorrhaphy for the Correction of Recurrent Anterior Dislocation of the Shoulder. Injury, 18:51–54, 1987.

540. Holmes, T.: A Case of Dislocation of the Humerus Upwards and Inwards, With Fracture of the Coracoid Process of the Scapula. Med. Chir. Trans., 41:447–453, 1858.

541. Honner, R.: Bilateral Posterior Dislocation of the Shoulders. Aust. N.Z. J. Surg., 38:269–272, 1969.

542. Hoofwijk, A.G.M., and Hoogmartens, M.: The Putti-Platt Operation for Recurrent Anterior Dislocation of the Shoulder. Acta Orthop. Belg., 50:481–488, 1984.

543. Hoofwijk, A.G.M., and Vanderwerken, C.: Simultaneous Bilateral Erect Dislocation of the Shoulder (letter to the editor). Neth. J. Surg., 36:175, 1984.

544. Hoover, R.D.: Dislocation of the Shoulder: A Method of Reduction (abstract). Clin. Orthop., 58:296, 1968.

545. Hopkins, G.E., and Pinzur, M.S.: Biceps Tenodesis for Painful Inferior Subluxation of the Shoulder in Adult Acquired Hemiplegia (abstract). Orthop. Trans., 9(1):52, Spring, 1985.

546. Hopkinson, W.J.; Ryan, J.B.; and Wheeler, J.H.: Glenoid Rim Fracture and Recurrent Shoulder Instability. Complications Orthop., March/April:36–45, 1989.

547. Horaguchi, T.: Case Studies: Painless Reduction of Dislocation and Fracture of the Shoulder Joint Utilizing Normal Respiration. J. Orthop. Sports Phys. Ther., 6:296–298, 1985.

548. Horsfield, D., and Stutley, J.: The Unstable Shoulder—A Problem Solved. Radiography, 54:74–76, 1988.

549. Houben, L.M.J., and Hoogmartens, M.: The Putti-Platt Operation for Recurrent Anterior Dislocation of the Shoulder. Acta Orthop. Belg., 50:481–488, 1984.

550. Houben, L.M.J.: Treatment of Old Posterior Dislocation of the Shoulder According to the McLaughlin Technique. Acta Orthop. Belg., 49:247–253, 1983.

551. Hovelius, L.; Akermark, C.; Albrektsson, B.; Berg, E.; Korner, L.; Lundberg, B.; and Wredmark, T.: Bristow-Latarjet Procedure for Recurrent Anterior Dislocation of the Shoulder: A 2–5 Year Follow-Up Study on the Results of 112 Cases. Acta Orthop. Scand., 54:284–290, 1983.

552. Hovelius, L.; Eriksson, K.; Fredin, H.; Hagberg, G.; Hussenius, A.; Lind, B.; Thorling, J.; and Weckstrom, J.: Recurrences After Initial Dislocation of the Shoulder: Results of a Prospective Study of Treatment. J. Bone Joint Surg., 65A:343–349, 1983.

553. Hovelius, L.; Eriksson, K.; Fredin, H.; Hagberg, G.; Lind, B.; Thorling, J.; and Weckstrom, J.: Two-Year Prognosis of Primary Shoulder Joint Dislocation in the Young (abstract). Acta Orthop. Scand., 55:95, 1984.

554. Hovelius, L.; Korner, L.; Lundberg, B.; Akermark, C.; Herberts, P.; Wredmark, T.; and Berg, E.: The Coracoid Transfer for Recurrent Dislocation of the Shoulder: Technical Aspects of the Bristow-Latarjet Procedure. J. Bone Joint Surg., 65A:926–934, 1983.

555. Hovelius, L.; Lind, B.; and Thorling, J.: Primary Dislocation of the Shoulder: Factors Affecting the Two-Year Prognosis. Clin. Orthop., 176:181–185, 1983.

556. Hovelius, L.; Thorling, J.; and Fredin, H.: Recurrent Anterior Dislocation of the Shoulder: Results After the Bankart and Putti-Platt Operations. J. Bone Joint Surg., 61A:566–569, 1979.

557. Hovelius, L.: Anterior Dislocation of the Shoulder in Teen-Agers and Young Adults: Five-Year Prognosis. J. Bone Joint Surg., 69A:393–399, 1987.

558. Hovelius, L.: Incidence of Shoulder Dislocation in Sweden. Clin. Orthop., 166:127–131, 1982.

559. Howard, F.M., and Shafer, S.J.: Injuries to the Clavicle With Neurovascular Complications. J. Bone Joint Surg., 47A:1335–1346, 1965.

560. Howell, A.B.: Speed in Animals. Chicago, Chicago University Press, 1944.

561. Howell, S.M.; Galinat, B.J.; Marone, P.J.; and Renzi, A.M.: Assessment of Glenohumeral Instability in the Actively Positioned Shoulder. Handout: Methodist Hospital, Philadelphia, Pa.

562. Howell, S.M.; Galinat, B.J.; Renzi, A.J.; and Marone, P.J.: Normal and Abnormal Mechanics of the Glenohumeral Joint in the Horizontal Plane. J. Bone Joint Surg., 70A:227–232, 1988.

563. Hoyt, W.A., Jr.: Etiology of Shoulder Injuries in Athletes. J. Bone Joint Surg., 49A:755–766, 1967.

564. Huggler, A.H., and Weidmann, E.: [Treatment of Voluntary Posterior Dislocations of the Shoulder.] Orthopade, 7:189, 1978.

565. Hummel, A.; Bethke, R.O.; and Kempf, L.: [Treatment of Recurrent Dislocation of the Shoulder: Bristow Method.] Unfallheilkunde, 85:482–484, 1982.

566. Humphrey, G.M.: A Treatise on the Human Skeleton (Including the Joints). Cambridge, Macmillan and Co., 1858.

567. Hunter, H.C.: Injuries to the Brachial Plexus: Experience of a Private Sports Medicine Clinic. J. Am. Osteopath. Assoc., 18:757–760, 1982.

568. Hurd, M.M.; Farrell, K.H.; and Waylonis, G.W.: Shoulder Sling for Hemiplegia: Friend or Foe? Arch. Phys. Med. Rehabil., 55:519–522, 1974.

569. Hussein, M.K.: Kocher's Method Is 3,000 Years Old. J. Bone Joint Surg., 50B:669–671, 1968.

570. Huybrechts, A., and Orloff, S.: L'Arthroscopie de l'Épaule. Medica Physica, 9:59–60, 1986.

571. Hybbinette, S.: De la Transplantation d'un Fragment Osseux Pour Remedier aux Luxations Recidivantes de l'Épaule: Constatations et Resultats Operatoires. Acta Chir. Scand., 71:411–445, 1932.

572. Hybbinette, S.: Traite des Fractures et des Luxations, Vol. 2, pp. 433–434. Paris, J.B. Bailliere, 1855.

573. Idrissi, M., and Olivier, C.: [Simple Procedure for Reduction of Anterior Dislocation Without Anesthesia] (letter to the editor). Presse Med., 13:25, 1984.

574. Iftikhar, T.B.; Kaminski, R.S.; and Sliva, I.: Neurovascular Complications of the Modified Bristow Procedure: A Case Report. J. Bone Joint Surg., 66A:951–952, 1984.

575. Ilfeld, F.W., and Holder, H.G.: Recurrent Dislocation of the Shoulder Joint: A Combination Procedure. A Preliminary Report. J. Bone Joint Surg., 25:651–658, 1943.

576. Indemini, E.; Cartesegna, M.; Perotti, G.F.; and Faletti, C.: [Habitual Shoulder Luxation and the Bankart-Delitala Technique.] Minerva Ortop. Traumatol., 39:631–636, 1988.

577. Indemini, E., and Perotti, G.F.: [Anatomical Reconstruction or Bone Barrier in Recurrent Anterior Luxation of the Shoulder.] Minerva Ortop. Traumatol., 39:705–708, 1988.

578. Inman, V.T.; Saunders, J.B.; and Abbott, L.C.: Observations on the Function of the Shoulder Joint. J. Bone Joint Surg., 26:1–30, 1944.

579. Ippolito, E.; Tamburella, G.L.; and Mariani, P.P.: [Recurrent Anterior Dislocation of the Shoulder: Follow-Up of Eighty Operated Cases. Ital. J. Sports Traumatol., 3:3–14, 1981.

580. Irlenbusch, U., and Jager, B.: Arthrographische befunde bei Erkrankungen und Verletzungen des Schultergelenkes. Beitr. Orthop. Traumatol., 33:297–302, 1986.

581. Irlenbusch, U.: Die Subkapitale Humerusdrehosteotomie nach Weber und die Limbusverschraubung nach Muller—2 Verfahren zur Behandlung der rezidivierenden Schulterluxation. Beitr. Orthop. Traumatol., 31: 472–481, 1984.

582. Irlenbusch, U.: Ein Beitrag zur Pathogenese und Therapie der Rezidivierenden Schulterluxation. Beitr. Orthop. Traumatol., 30:12–21, 1983.

583. Ishikawa, M.; Fujimaki, E.; Kobayashi, N.; Hirose, H.; Katagiri, T.; and Nagata, A.: Anterior Dislocation of the Shoulder: Experience With a Modified Clavicular Harness. Int. Orthop., 10:127–130, 1986.

584. Izadpanah, M.: [Habitual Recurrent Dorsal Dislocation or Subluxation of the Shoulder.] Chir. Praxis, 27:245–250, 1980.

585. Jacobs, B.W.; Patterson, R.L., Jr.; and Schultz, T.J.: Shoulder Dislocations Associated With Seizure Disorders (abstract). J. Bone Joint Surg., 52A:824, 1970.

586. Jager, R.: [Problems of Operative Therapy in Posterior Shoulder Dislocations.] Orthopade, 7:203–207, 1978.

587. Jakobsson, A.: On Recurrent Dislocation of the Shoulder Joint: A Contribution to Its Pathomechanics and the Results of Eden-Hybbinette's Bone-Block Operation. Acta Orthop. Scand., 18:284–318, 1949.

588. Jakobsson, A.: Radiography of the Anterior Glenoid Rim in Recurrent Dislocation of the Shoulder Joint. Acta Orthop. Scand., 20:1–7, 1951.

589. Jalovaara, P.; Kortelainen, P.; Paivansalo, M.; and Lindholm, R.V.: Unstable Four-Part Fracture of the Proximal Humerus With Posterior Dislocation of the Shoulder (abstract). Acta Orthop. Scand., 59:603–604, 1988.

590. Jalovaara, P.; Niinimaki, T.; Ramo, J.; and Lindholm,

R.V.: Coracoid Tendon Transposition a.m. Bristow-La-tarjet. Ann. Chir. Gynaecol., 77:103–107, 1988.

591. Jamison, A.M., and Bonney, G.: An Analysis of the Op-erative Findings in Brachial Plexus Traction Lesions Treated Between 1956 and 1978. J. Bone Joint Surg., 61B:516, 1979.

592. Jamison, A.M., and Hughes, S.: The Role of Surgery in the Management of Closed Injuries to the Brachial Plexus. Clin. Orthop., 147:210–215, 1980.

593. Janecki, C.J., and Shahcheragh, G.H.: The Forward Ele-vation Maneuver for Reduction of Anterior Dislocations of the Shoulder. Clin. Orthop., 164:177–180, 1982.

594. Jarde, O.; Staelen, L.; Obry, C.; and Vines, P.: [Traumatic Posterior Dislocations of the Shoulder Treated by Mc-Laughlin's Operation: Report of Twelve Cases.] Ann. Chir., 42:488–491, 1988.

595. Jardon, O.M.; Hood, L.T.; and Lynch, R.D.: Complete Avulsion of the Axillary Artery as a Complication of Shoulder Dislocation. J. Bone Joint Surg., 55A:189–192, 1973.

596. Jeffery, C.C.: Recurrent Dislocation of the Shoulder (ab-stract). J. Bone Joint Surg., 41B:623, 1959.

597. Jekic, M.: The Rare Case of Bilateral Shoulder Dislocation (abstract). Langenbecks Arch. Chir., 334:931, 1973.

598. Jens, J.: The Role of the Subscapularis Muscle in Re-curring Dislocation of the Shoulder (abstract). J. Bone Joint Surg., 46B:780–781, 1964.

599. Jerosch, J.; Castro, W.H.M.; and Colemont, J.: A Lesion of the Musculocutaneous Nerve: A Rare Complication of Anterior Shoulder Dislocation. Acta Orthop. Belg., 55:230–232, 1989.

600. Jerre, T.: A Modification of Nicola's Operation in Re-current Dislocation of the Shoulder. Acta Orthop. Scand., 25:89–96, 1956.

601. Jobe, F.W.; Giangarra, C.E.; Glousman, R.E.; and Kvitne, R.S.: Anterior Capsulolabral Reconstruction in Throwing Athletes (abstract). Orthop. Trans., 13(2):230, Summer, 1989.

602. Jobe, F.W.; Moynes, D.R.; and Brewster, C.E.: Rehabil-itation of Shoulder Joint in Stabilities. Orthop. Clin. North Am., 18:473–482, 1987.

603. Jobe, F.W.; Tibone, J.E.; Perry, J.; and Moynes, D.: An EMG Analysis of the Shoulder in Throwing and Pitching. Am. J. Sports Med., 11:3–5, 1983.

604. Jobe, F.W., and Zeman, B.: How to Detect—and Man-age—an Unstable Shoulder. J. Musculoskeletal Med., 2:60–68, 1985.

605. Jobe, F.W.: Unstable Shoulders in the Athlete. Instr. Course Lect., XXXIV:228–231, 1985.

606. Joessel, D.: Ueber die Recidive der Humerusluxationen. Dtsch. Z. Chir., 13:167–184, 1880.

607. Johner, R., and Roulet, D.: [The Unstable Shoulder: Clinical and Radiological Aspects.] Rev. Med. Swisse Ro-mande, 107:909–917, 1987.

608. Johnson, H.F.: Unreduced Dislocation of the Shoulder. Nebr. State Med. J., 16:220–224, 1931.

609. Johnson, J.R., and Bayley, J.I.L.: Loss of Shoulder Func-tion Following Acute Anterior Dislocation. J. Bone Joint Surg., 63B:633, 1981.

610. Johnson, J.R., and Bayley, J.I.L.: Early Complications of Acute Anterior Dislocation of the Shoulder in the Middle-Aged and Elderly Patient. Injury, 13:431–434, 1982.

611. Johnson, L.L.: Personal communication, 1990.

612. Johnson, L.L.: Arthroscopy of the Shoulder. Orthop. Clin. North Am., 11:197–204, 1980.

613. Johnson, L.L.: Symposium: The Controversy of Arthro-scopic Versus Open Approaches to Shoulder Instability and Rotator Cuff Disease. A New Perspective, a New Opportunity, a New Challenge. American Shoulder and Elbow Surgeons 4th Open Meeting, Atlanta, Ga., Feb. 2, 1988.

614. Johnson, L.L.: The Shoulder Joint: An Arthroscopist's Perspective of Anatomy and Pathology. Clin. Orthop., 223:113–125, 1987.

615. Johnson, P.H.: Recurrent Subluxation of the Shoulder. J. Arkansas Med. Soc., 84:335–337, 1988.

616. Johnston, G.H.; Hawkins, R.J.; Haddad, R.; and Fowler, P.J.: A Complication of Posterior Glenoid Osteotomy for Recurrent Posterior Shoulder Instability. Clin. Orthop., 187:147–149, 1984.

617. Johnston, G.W., and Lowry, J.H.: Rupture of the Axillary Artery Complicating Anterior Dislocation of the Shoul-der. J. Bone Joint Surg., 44B:116–118, 1962.

618. Jones, D.: The Role of Shoulder Muscles in the Control of Humeral Position (an Electromyographic Study). Master's Thesis, Case Western Reserve University, 1970.

619. Jones, F.W.: Attainment of the Upright Posture of Man. Nature, 146:26–27, 1940.

620. Jones, L.: The Shoulder Joint—Observations on the Anatomy and Physiology With an Analysis of a Recon-structive Operation Following Extensive Injury. Surg. Gynecol. Obstet., 75:433–444, 1972.

621. Jones, M.: Bilateral Anterior Shoulder Dislocations Due to the Bench Press (letter to the editor). Br. J. Sports Med., 21:139, 1987.

622. Jones, R.: Injuries to Joints. London, Oxford University Press, 1926.

623. Jones, V.: Recurrent Posterior Dislocation of the Shoul-der: Report of a Case Treated by Posterior Bone Block. J. Bone Joint Surg., 40B:203–207, 1958.

624. Jordan, H.: New Technique for the Roentgen Exami-nation of the Shoulder Joint. Radiology, 25:480–484, 1935.

625. Joseph, K.N.: A Spontaneous Reduction of Persistent Anterior Shoulder Dislocation. Orthop. Rev., 10:85–87, 1981.

626. Kahn, M.L.; Bade, H.A., III; and Stein, I.: Body Surfing as a Cause of Luxatio Erecta: Report of Four Cases. Or-thop. Rev., 16:37–41, 1987.

627. Kaltsas, D.S.: Comparative Study of the Properties of the Shoulder Joint Capsule With Those of Other Joint Cap-sules. Clin. Orthop., 173:20–26, 1983.

628. Kane, W.J.: Bristow Repair in Recurrent Anterior Dis-location of the Shoulder (abstract). J. Bone Joint Surg., 55B:880, 1973.

629. Karadimas, J.; Rentis, G.; and Varouchas, G.: Repair of Recurrent Anterior Dislocation of the Shoulder Using

Transfer of the Subscapularis Tendon. J. Bone Joint Surg., 62A:1147–1149, 1980.

630. Karchinov, K.D., and Karchinov, D.K.: [Etiopathogenetic Factor for Congenital Habitual Shoulder Joint Dislocation.] Zentralbl. Chir., 114:253–254, 1989.

631. Karchinov, K.D.: An Operative Method for Treatment of Recidivans and Habitual Humeral Joint Luxations. Personal communication, 1989.

632. Karpinski, M.R.K., and Porter, K.M.: Bilateral Posterior Dislocation of the Shoulder. Injury, 15:274–276, 1984.

633. Kavanaugh, J.H.: Posterior Shoulder Dislocation With Ipsilateral Humeral Shaft Fracture. Clin. Orthop., 131: 168–172, 1978.

634. Kazar, B., and Relovszky, E.: Prognosis of Primary Dislocation of the Shoulder. Acta Orthop. Scand., 40:216–224, 1969.

635. Keiser, R.P., and Wilson, C.L.: Bilateral Recurrent Dislocation of the Shoulder (Atraumatic) in a Thirteen-Year-Old Girl: Report of an Unusual Case. J. Bone Joint Surg., 43A:553–554, 1961.

636. Kelley, J.P.: Fractures Complicating Electroconvulsive Therapy and Chronic Epilepsy. J. Bone Joint Surg., 36B: 70–79, 1954.

637. Kelly, P.J.; Coventry, M.B.; and Martin, W.J.: Bacterial Arthritis of the Shoulder. Mayo Clin. Proc., 40:695–699, 1965.

638. Kennedy, R.: Complete Atrophy of the Deltoid With Vicarious Restoration of Function. Br. Med. J., 1:1513–1515, 1898.

639. Kerboul, B.; LeSaout, J.; Lefevre, C.; Malingue, E.; Fabre, L.; Roblin, L.; and Courtois, B.: [Latarjet's Operation for Recurrent Antero-Internal Dislocation of Shoulder.] J. Chir. (Paris), 122:371–374, 1985.

640. Kessel, L.: Clinical Disorders of the Shoulder. London, Churchill Livingstone, 1982.

641. Key, J.A., and Conwell, H.E.: The Management of Fractures, Dislocations and Sprains, 5th ed. St. Louis, C.V. Mosby, 1951.

642. Kia-Noury, M.: Axillary Artery Rupture With Dislocated Shoulder. Pa. Med., 83:28, 1980.

643. King, J.M., Jr., and Holmes, G.W.: A Review of Four Hundred and Fifty Roentgen-ray Examinations of the Shoulder. A.J.R., 17:214–218, 1927.

644. King, T.: Recurrent Dislocation of the Shoulder. Med. J. Aust., 1:697–700, 1947.

645. Kingsley, J.S.: Comparative Anatomy of the Vertebrates. Philadelphia, Blakiston, 1917.

646. Kinnard, P.; Gordon, D.; Levesque, R.Y.; and Bergeron, D.: Computerized Arthrotomography in Recurring Shoulder Dislocations and Subluxations. Can. J. Surg., 27:487–488, 1984.

647. Kinnard, P.; Tricoire, J.L.; Levesque, R.Y.; and Bergeron, D.: Assessment of the Unstable Shoulder by Computed Arthrography: A Preliminary Report. Am. J. Sports Med., 11:157–159, 1983.

648. Kinnett, J.G.; Warren, R.F.; and Jacobs, B.: Recurrent Dislocation of the Shoulder After Age Fifty. Clin. Orthop., 149:164–168, 1980.

649. Kirker, J.R.: Dislocation of the Shoulder Complicated by

Rupture of the Axillary Vessels: Report of a Case. J. Bone Joint Surg., 34B:72–73, 1952.

650. Kitano, K.; Tada, K.; and Oka, S.: Congenital Contracture of the Infraspinous Muscle: A Case Report. Arch. Orthop. Trauma Surg., 107:54–57, 1987.

651. Kiviluoto, O.; Pasila, M.; Jaroma, H.; and Sundholm, A.: Immobilization After Primary Dislocation of the Shoulder. Acta Orthop. Scand., 51:915–919, 1980.

652. Klein, A.H.; France, J.C.; Mutschler, T.A.; and Fu, F.H.: Measurement of Brachial Plexus Strain in Arthroscopy of the Shoulder. Arthroscopy, 3:45–52, 1987.

653. Kleinman, P.K.; Goss, T.P.; Kanzaria, P.K.; Pappas, A.M.; and Philbin, A.J.: Injuries of the Glenoid Labrum in Athletic Teenagers (abstract). Pediatr. Radiol., 15:71, 1985.

654. Kleinman, P.K.; Kanzaria, P.K.; Goss, T.P.; and Pappas, A.M.: Axillary Arthrotomography of the Glenoid Labrum. A.J.R., 141:993–999, 1984.

655. Kline, D.G.; Kott, J.; Barnes, G.; and Bryant, L.: Exploration of Selected Brachial Plexus Lesions by the Posterior Subcapsular Approach. J. Neurosurg., 49:872–880, 1978.

656. Kocher, T.: Eine neue Reductionsmethode fur Schulterverrenkung. Berl. Klin. Wochenschr., 7:101–105, 1870.

657. Kohfahl, J.; Stegmann, T.; Muhr, G.; and Tscherne, H.: [Traumatic Dislocation of the Shoulder: Functional Late Results Taking Dislocation Incidence Into Account.] Aktuel Traumatol., 14:164–168, 1984.

658. Kohn, D.: The Clinical Relevance of Glenoid Labrum Lesions. Arthroscopy, 3:223–230, 1987.

659. Koppert, G., and Hawkins, R.J.: Recurrent Posterior Dislocating Shoulder (abstract). J. Bone Joint Surg., 62B: 127–128, 1980.

660. Kreitner, K.F.; Schild, H.; Becker, H.R.; Muller, H.A.; and Ahlers, J.: [Dislocation of the Shoulder—A Clinical and Radiological Follow-Up.] Fortschr. Rontgenstr., 147: 407–413, 1987.

661. Krempen, J.F.; Silver, R.A.; Hadley, J.; and Rivera, V.: The Use of the Varney Brace for Subluxating Shoulders in Stroke and Upper Motor Neuron Injuries. Clin. Orthop., 122:204–206, 1977.

662. Kretzler, H.H., Jr., and Blue, A.R.: Recurrent Posterior Dislocation of the Shoulder in Cerebral Palsy (abstract). J. Bone Joint Surg., 48A:1221, 1966.

663. Kretzler, H.H., Jr., and Scott, D.J., Jr.: Posterior Glenoid Osteotomy for Posterior Dislocation of the Shoulder. In Bayley, I., and Kessel, L. (eds.): Shoulder Surgery. pp. 95–97. New York, Springer-Verlag, 1982.

664. Kretzler, H.H., Jr.: Posterior Glenoid Osteotomy. Presented at the Annual Meeting of the American Academy of Orthopaedic Surgeons, Dallas, Tex., Jan. 17–22, 1974.

665. Kristiansen, B.: [Neglected Shoulder Dislocation.] Ugeskr. Laeger., 147:3901–3902, 1985.

666. Krödel, A., and Melzer, C.: [Usefulness of Heterologous Bone Transplants in Surgical Treatment of Recurrent Shoulder Dislocation.] Z. Orthop., 126:79–84, 1988.

667. Krøner, K.: The Epidemiology of Shoulder Dislocation (abstract). Acta Orthop. Scand., 58:706, 1987.

668. Kubin, Z.: Luxatio Humeri Erecta: Kasuisticke Sdeleni. Acta Chir. Orthop. Traumatol. Czech., 31:565, 1964.

669. Kuhn, K., and Rosman, M.: Traumatic, Nonparalytic Dislocation of the Shoulder in a Newborn Infant: Case Report. J. Pediatr. Orthop., 4:121–122, 1984.

670. Kuhnen, W., and Groves, R.J.: Irreducible Acute Anterior Dislocation of the Shoulder: Case Report. Clin. Orthop., 139:167–168, 1979.

671. Kuhns, L.R.; Sherman, M.P.; Poznanski, A.K.; and Holt, J.F.: Humeral-Head and Coracoid Ossification in the Newborn. Radiology, 107:145–149, 1973.

672. Kujat, R.: The Microangiographic Pattern of the Glenoid Labrum of the Dog. Arch. Orthop. Trauma Surg., 105:310–312, 1986.

673. Kumar, V.P., and Balasubramaniam, P.: The Role of Atmospheric Pressure in Stabilising the Shoulder: An Experimental Study. J. Bone Joint Surg., 67B:719–721, 1985.

674. Kummel, B.M.: Arthrography in Anterior Capsular Derangements of the Shoulder. Clin. Orthop., 83:170–176, 1972.

675. Kummel, B.M.: Fractures of the Glenoid Causing Chronic Dislocation of the Shoulder. Clin. Orthop., 69:189–191, 1970.

676. Kummel, B.M.: Spectrum of Lesions of the Anterior Capsular Mechanism of the Shoulder. Am. J. Sports Med., 7:111–120, 1979.

677. Kummel, B.M.: The Syndrome of Anterior-Capsular Derangement of the Shoulder. Orthop. Rev., 1:7–12, 1972.

678. Kuriyama, S.; Fujimaki, E.; Katagiri, T.; and Uemura, S.: Anterior Dislocation of the Shoulder Joint Sustained Through Skiing: Arthrographic Findings and Prognosis. Am. J. Sports Med., 12:339–346, 1984.

679. Kuster, E.: Ueber habituelle Schulter Luxation. Verh. Dtsch. Ges. Chir., 11:112–114, 1882.

680. L'Episcopo, J.B.: Restoration of Muscle Balance in the Treatment of Obstetrical Paralysis. N.Y. State J. Med., 39:357–363, 1939.

681. Lacey, T., II, and Crawford, H.B.: Reduction of Anterior Dislocations of the Shoulder by Means of the Milch Abduction Technique. J. Bone Joint Surg., 34A:108–109, 1952.

682. Laing, P.G.: The Arterial Blood Supply of the Adult Humerus. J. Bone Joint Surg., 38A:1105–1116, 1956.

683. Lam, S.J.S.: Irreducible Anterior Dislocation of the Shoulder. J. Bone Joint Surg., 48B:132–133, 1966.

684. Lambdin, C.S.; Young, S.B.; and Unsicker, C.L.: A Modified Bankart-Putti-Platt Shoulder Capsulorrhaphy (abstract). J. Bone Joint Surg., 53A:1237, 1971.

685. Lamm, C.R.; Zachrisson, B.E.; and Korner, L.: Radiography of the Shoulder After Bristow Repair. Acta Radiol. Diagn., 23:523–528, 1982.

686. Lance, S., and Putkonen, M.: Positioning of the Painful Patient for the Axial View of the Glenohumeral Joint. Rontgenblatter, 38:380–382, 1985.

687. Landmann, J.; Steenblock, U.; and Allgower, M.: [Results Following Trillat's Surgery in Habitual Shoulder Dislocation.] Helv. Chir. Acta, 47:89–92, 1980.

688. Landsmeer, J.M.F., and Meyers, K.A.W.: The Shoulder Region Exposed by Anatomical Dissection. Arch. Chir. Neerl., 11:274–296, 1959.

689. Lange, M.: Die operative Behandlung der Gewohnheitsmabigen verrenkung an Schulter, Knie und Fub. Z. Orthop., 75:162, 1944.

690. Langford, O., and Rockwood, C.A., Jr.: Posterior Dislocations of the Shoulder. Exhibit at the American Academy of Orthopaedic Surgeons, Annual Meeting, New York, 1965.

691. Langfritz, H.V.: Die doppelseitige traumatische Luxatio humeri erecta eine seltene Verletzungsform. Monatsschr. Unfallheilkd., 59:367, 1956.

692. Laskin, R.S., and Sedlin, E.D.: Luxatio Erecta in Infancy. Clin. Orthop., 80:126–129, 1971.

693. Latarjet, M., and Vittori, P.: Resultat du Traitement des Luxations Recidivantes de l'Épaule par le Procede de Latarjet, à Propos de 42 Cas. Lyon Chir., 64:964–968, 1968.

694. Latarjet, M.: À Propos du Traitement des Luxations Recidivantes de l'Épaule. Lyon Chir., 49:994–997, 1954.

695. Latarjet, M.: Technique de la Butée Coracoidienne Preglenoidienne Dans le Traitement des Luxations Recidivantes de l'Épaule. Lyon Chir., 54:604–607, 1958.

696. Latarjet, M.: Techniques Chirurgicales Dans le Traitement de la Luxation Anteriointerne Recidivante de l'Épaule. Lyon Chir., 61:313–318, 1965.

697. Lavik, K.: Habitual Shoulder Luxation. Acta Orthop. Scand., 30:251–264, 1961.

698. Lawhon, S.M.: Physical Therapy Effective for Dislocations of the Shoulder. News Bulletin, American Academy of Orthopaedic Surgeons, Annual Meeting, 1985.

699. Lawhon, S.M.: Voluntary Dislocations of the Shoulder. Contemporary Orthopedics, 12:13–24, 1986.

700. Lawrence, W.S.: New Position in Radiographing the Shoulder Joint. A.J.R., 2:728–730, 1915.

701. LeClerc, J.: Chronic Subluxation of the Shoulder (abstract). J. Bone Joint Surg., 51B:778, 1969.

702. Leach, R.E.; Corbett, M.; Schepsis, A.; and Stockel, J.: Results of a Modified Putti-Platt Operation for Recurrent Shoulder Dislocations and Subluxations. Clin. Orthop., 164:20–25, 1982.

703. Leach, R.E.; Hunter, S.C.; and Allman, F.L., Jr.: Shoulder Surgery Nixed in Habitual Subluxers. Orthopedics Today, 4:41, 1984.

704. Leborgne, J.; LeNeel, J.C.; Mitard, D.; Monfort, J.; Roy, J.; and Visset, J.: [Lesions of the Axillary Artery and Its Branches Following Closed Trauma of the Shoulder With 10 Case Reports.] Ann. Chir., 27:587–594, 1973.

705. Leffert, R.D., and Seddon, H.: Infraclavicular Brachial Plexus Injuries. J. Bone Joint Surg., 47B:9–22, 1965.

706. Leffert, R.D.: Brachial-Plexus Injuries. N. Engl. J. Med., 291:1059–1067, 1974.

707. Leffert, R.D.: Brachial Plexus Injury Management. Arch. Phys. Med. Rehabil., 63:452, 1982.

708. Leffert, R.D.: Reconstruction of the Shoulder and Elbow Following Brachial Plexus Injury. Rehabilitation, 805–816.

709. Leguit, P.: Recurrent Dislocation of the Shoulder. J. Int. Coll. Surg., 20:741–749, 1953.

710. Leidelmeyer, R.: External Rotation Method of Shoulder Dislocation Reduction (letter to the editor). Ann. Emerg. Med., 10:228, 1981.

711. Leidelmeyer, R.: Reduced! A Shoulder, Subtly and Painlessly. Emerg. Med., 9:233–234, 1977.

712. Leighton, R.L., and Kagan, K.G.: Surgical Repair of Lateral Shoulder Luxation. Mod. Vet. Pract., 57:702–703, 1976.

713. Lemmens, J.A.M., and De Waal Malefijt, J.: Radiographic Evaluation of the Modified Bristow Procedure for Recurrent Anterior Dislocation of the Shoulder. Diagn. Imag. Clin. Med., 53:221–225, 1984.

714. Lescher, T.J., and Andersen, O.S.: Occlusion of the Axillary Artery Complicating Shoulder Dislocation: Case Report. Milit. Med., 144:621–622, 1979.

715. Leslie, J.T., and Ryan, T.J.: The Anterior Axillary Incision to Approach the Shoulder Joint. J. Bone Joint Surg., 44A:1193–1196, 1962.

716. Lev-El, A., and Rubinstein, Z.: Axillary Artery Injury in Erect Dislocation of the Shoulder. J. Trauma, 21:323–325, 1981.

717. Levenets, U.N.: [Treatment of Habitual Shoulder Dislocation.] Ortop. Travmatol. Protez., 4:56–58, 1985.

718. Levick, J.R.: Joint Pressure–Volume Studies: Their Importance, Design and Interpretation. J. Rheumatol., 10: 353–357, 1983.

719. Levy, J.M.; Crowe, J.R.; and Stegman, C.J.: Case of the Month No. 57: Anterior, Subcoracoid Dislocation of the Humerus: "Y" View of the Shoulder. Ariz. Med., 39: 455–456, 1982.

720. Levy, L.J.: Anterior Axillary Incision in the Repair of Recurrent Dislocation of the Shoulder (abstract). J. Bone Joint Surg., 49A:204, 1967.

721. Lewis, W.H.: The Development of the Arm in Man. Am. J. Anat., 1:145–184, 1902.

722. Leyder, P.; Augereau, B.; and Apoil, A.: [Treatment of Old Unreduced Posterior Dislocation of the Shoulder by Double Approach and Posterior Scapular Osteoplasty: Report of Four Cases.] Ann. Chir., 34:806–809, 1980.

723. Liberson, F.: Os Acromiale—A Contested Anomaly. J. Bone Joint Surg., 19A:683–689, 1937.

724. Lichtblau, P.O.: Shoulder Dislocation in the Infant—Case Report and Discussion. J. Fla. Med. Assoc., 64:313–320, 1977.

725. Liebolt, F.L., and Furey, J.G.: Obstetrical Paralysis With Dislocation of the Shoulder Joint: A Case Report. J. Bone Joint Surg., 35A:227–230, 1953.

726. Lilleby, H.: Arthroscopy of the Shoulder Joint. Acta Orthop. Scand., 53:708–709, 1982.

727. Lilleby, H.: Arthroscopic Resection of the Acromion (abstract). Acta Orthop. Scand., 58:452–453, 1987.

728. Lilleby, H.: Intra-Articular Changes in Recurrent Shoulder Dislocation: An Arthroscopic Study (abstract). Acta Orthop. Scand., 57:278, 1986.

729. Lilleby, H.: Shoulder Arthroscopy. Acta Orthop. Scand., 55:561–566, 1984.

730. Lim, T.E.; Ochsner, P.E.; Marti, R.K.; and Holscher, A.A.: The Results of Treatment of Comminuted Fractures and Fracture Dislocations of the Proximal Humerus. Neth. J. Surg., 35:139–143, 1983.

731. Lim, T.E.: Arthroscopic Surgery of the Shoulder (abstract). Acta Orthop. Scand., 57:480, 1986.

732. Linclau, L.A., and Tonino, A.J.: Recurrent Dislocation of the Shoulder. Arch. Chir. Neerland., 26:331–342, 1974.

733. Lindahl, O.: Late Results of Recurrent Dislocation of the Shoulder Joint After Operative Treatment by Orell's Method. Acta Orthop. Scand., 25:281–286, 1956.

734. Lindholm, T.S., and Elmstedt, E.: Bilateral Posterior Dislocation of the Shoulder Combined With Fracture of the Proximal Humerus: A Case Report. Acta Orthop. Scand., 51:485–488, 1980.

735. Lindholm, T.S.: Recurrent Posterior Dislocation of the Shoulder. Acta Chir. Scand., 140:101–106, 1974.

736. Lindholm, T.S.: Results of Treatment for Anterior Recurrent Dislocation of the Shoulder Joint With the Eden-Hybbinette Operation. Acta Orthop. Scand., 45:508–517, 1974.

737. Lippert, F.G., III: Modification of the Gravity Method of Reducing Anterior Shoulder Dislocations. Clin. Orthop., 165:259–260, 1982.

738. Lipscomb, A.B.: Treatment of Recurrent Anterior Dislocation and Subluxation of the Glenohumeral Joint in Athletes. Clin. Orthop., 109:122–125, 1975.

739. List, M.: [Examination and Treatment of Shoulder Joint Disorders.] Krankengymnastik, 36:424–434, 1984.

740. Litchfield, J.C.; Subhedar, V.Y.; Beevers, D.G.; and Patel, H.T.: Bilateral Dislocation of the Shoulders Due to Nocturnal Hypoglycaemia. Postgrad. Med. J., 64:450–452, 1988.

741. Little, M.G.A.: Dislocation of the Shoulder (abstract). J. Bone Joint Surg., 47B:809, 1965.

742. Liveson, J.A.: Nerve Lesions Associated With Shoulder Dislocation: An Electrodiagnostic Study of 11 Cases. J. Neurol. Neurosurg. Psychiatry, 47:742–744, 1984.

743. Löbker, K.: Einige Praparate von habitueller Schulterluxation. Arch. Klin. Chir., 34:658–667, 1887.

744. Lodding, P., and Angeras, U.: Fatal Axillary Artery Injury Following Anterior Dislocation of the Shoulder. Ann. Chir. Gynaecol., 77:125–127, 1988.

745. Lohmann, M., and Jeppesen, D.: [Anterior Dislocation of the Shoulder Caused by Electric Shock.] Ugeskr. Laeger., 151:99–100, 1989.

746. Lombardo, S.J.; Kerlan, R.K.; Jobe, F.W.; Carter, V.S.; Blazina, M.E.; and Shields, C.L., Jr.: The Modified Bristow Procedure for Recurrent Dislocation of the Shoulder. J. Bone Joint Surg., 58A:256–261, 1976.

747. Loomer, R., and Fraser, J.: A Modified Bankart Procedure for Recurrent Anterior/Inferior Shoulder Instability: A Preliminary Report. Am. J. Sports Med., 17:374–379, 1989.

748. Loomer, R., and Graham, B.: Anatomy of the Axillary Nerve and Its Relation to Inferior Capsular Shift. Clin. Orthop., 243:100–105, 1989.

749. Lower, R.F.; McNeish, L.M.; and Callaghan, J.J.: Computed Tomography Documentation of Intra-Articular Penetration of a Screw After Operations on the Shoulder:

A Report of Two Cases. J. Bone Joint Surg., 67A:1120–1122, 1985.

750. Lucas, D.B.: Biomechanics of the Shoulder Joint. Arch. Surg., 107:425–432, 1973.

751. Lucas, G.L., and Peterson, M.D.: Open Anterior Dislocation of the Shoulder: Case Report. J. Trauma, 17:883–884, 1977.

752. Luckey, C.A.: Recurrent Dislocation of the Shoulder: Modification of Bankhart Capsulorrhaphy. Am. J. Surg., 77:220–222, 1949.

753. Lurke, A.S., and Slavutskii, D.A.: Surgical Treatment for Closed Injuries of the Axillary Nerve. Vopr. Neirokhir., 35:43–45, 1971.

754. Lynn, F.S.: Erect Dislocation of the Shoulder. Surg. Gynecol. Obstet., 39:51–55, 1921.

755. Lysholm, J.; Adolfsson, L.; and Hamberg, P.: Arthroscopy of the Shoulder in Evaluation of Patients With Shoulder Instability (abstract). Acta Orthop. Scand., 59:88–89, 1988.

756. Lysholm, J.: Arthroscopy in Evaluation of Shoulder Pain (abstract). Acta Orthop. Scand., 59:89, 1988.

757. Mabrook, A.F.: Primary Dislocation of the Shoulder in a Snooker Player (letter). Arch. Emerg. Med., 6:234–235, 1989.

758. MacArthur, B.J.: Arthroscopy of the Shoulder. Orthop. Nurs., 5:26–28, 1986.

759. MacAusland, W.R.: Recurrent Anterior Dislocation of the Shoulder. Am. J. Surg., 91:323–331, 1956.

760. MacDonald, F.R.: Intra-Articular Fractures in Recurrent Dislocation of the Shoulder. Surg. Clin. North Am., 43:1635–1645, 1963.

761. MacMillan, C.L.: The Many Faces of Posterior Dislocation of the Shoulder. Nova Scotia Med. Bull., 65:90–91, 1986.

762. Macioce, D., and Caruso, S.: [Personal Experience in Habitual Shoulder Luxation Treated Surgically With Latarjet's Technique.] Minerva Ortop. Traumatol., 39:709–712, 1988.

763. Macioce, D., and Caruso, S.: [Use of Cibex II to Assess Scapulo-Humeral Joint Function After Latarjet.] Minerva Ortop. Traumatol., 40:245–248, 1989.

764. Mack, L.A.; Matsen, F.A.; Kilcoyne, R.F.; Davies, P.K.; and Sickler, M.E.: Ultrasound: US Evaluation of the Rotator Cuff. Radiology, 157:205–209, 1985.

765. Mackenzie, A.B.: Recurrent Dislocation of the Shoulder (abstract). J. Bone Joint Surg., 38B:601, 1956.

766. Mackenzie, D.B.: The Bristow-Helfet Operation for Recurrent Anterior Dislocation of the Shoulder (abstract). J. Bone Joint Surg., 62B:273–274, 1980.

767. Mackenzie, D.B.: The Treatment of Recurrent Anterior Shoulder Dislocation by the Modified Bristow-Helfet Procedure. S. Afr. Med. J., 65:325–330, 1984.

768. Mackenzie, D.B.: Treatment of Recurrent Anterior Shoulder Dislocation by the Modified Bristow-Helfet Procedure (reply to letter to the editor). S. Afr. Med. J., 66:436, 1984.

769. Macpherson, I.S.; Crossan, J.F.; and Allister, C.A.: Unstable Fractures of the Greater Tuberosity of the Humerus (abstract). J. Bone Joint Surg., 65B:225, 1983.

770. Madler, M.; Mayr, B.; Baierl, P.; Klein, C.; Habermeyer, P.; and Huber, R.: [The Value of Conventional X-Ray Diagnosis and Computerized Tomography in the Detection of Hill-Sachs Defects and Bony Bankart Lesions in Recurrent Shoulder Dislocations.] Fortschr. Rontgenstr., 148:384–389, 1988.

771. Maggi, G.; Fusaro, I.; and Prioli, L.: [An Uncommon Case of Rupture of the Short Head of Biceps Brachii and Musculocutaneous Nerve Paralysis in Traumatic Shoulder Dislocation.] Arch. Putti Chir. Organi. Mov., 70:389–392, 1985.

772. Magnani, M., and Pardini, P.: [Chronic Dislocation of the Shoulder: Bankart Operation by Means of Arthroscopy.] Minerva Ortop. Traumatol., 39:541–545, 1988.

773. Magnuson, P.B., and Stack, J.K.: Bilateral Habitual Dislocation of the Shoulders in Twins: A Familial Tendency. J.A.M.A., 144:2103, 1940.

774. Magnuson, P.B., and Stack, J.K.: Recurrent Dislocation of the Shoulder. J.A.M.A., 123:889–892, 1943.

775. Magnuson, P.B.: Treatment of Recurrent Dislocation of the Shoulder. Surg. Clin. North Am., 25:14–20, 1945.

776. Majeed, L.: Pulsatile Haemarthrosis of the Shoulder Joint Associated With False Aneurysm of the Axillary Artery as a Late Complication of Anterior Dislocation of the Shoulder. Injury, 16:566–567, 1985.

777. Maki, S., and Gruen, T.: Anthropomorphic Studies of the Glenohumeral Joint. Trans. Orthop. Res. Soc., 1:173, 1976.

778. Makin, M.: Translocation of the Biceps Humeri for Flail Shoulder. J. Bone Joint Surg., 59A:490–491, 1977.

779. Malgaigne, J.F.: Traite des Fractures et des Luxations. Philadelphia, J.B. Lippincott, 1859.

780. Malinovskii, I.L.: [Bilateral Complication of Shoulder Dislocation.] Ortop. Travmatol. Protez., 9:45–46, 1984.

781. Malone, J.M.; Leal, J.M.; Underwood, J.; and Childers, S.J.: Brachial Plexus Injury Management Through Upper Extremity Amputation With Immediate Postoperative Prostheses. Arch. Phys. Med. Rehabil., 63:89–91, 1982.

782. Manes, E.; Trippetta, N.; and Mezzanotte, L.: [The Delitala Technique in the Surgical Treatment of Recurrent Luxation of the Shoulder.] Arch. Putti Chir. Organi. Mov., 71:343–346, 1986.

783. Manes, H.R.: A New Method of Shoulder Reduction in the Elderly. Clin. Orthop., 147:200–202, 1980.

784. Mann, K., and Wellner, F.: [Arc Bone Graft-Plasty in Recurrent Anterior Shoulder Dislocation (1968–1985).] Beitr. Orthop. Traumatol., 34:471–475, 1987.

785. Mansat, M.: Acromial Obstruction and the Rupture of the Rotator Cuff. Ann. Chir., 35:835–841, 1981.

786. Marinoni, E.C.; Denti, M.; Memeo, A.; Simonatti, R.; and Peretti, G.: [The Boicev Procedure.] Minerva Ortop. Traumatol., 39:655–657, 1988.

787. Mariotti, U.; Errichiello, C.; Bellomo, F.; and Indemini, E.: [Habitual Posterior Shoulder Luxation: Remarks on a Bilateral, Dysplasic-Based Case.] Minerva Ortop. Traumatol., 39:689–693, 1988.

788. Mariotti, U.; Graziano, D.; Grillo, P.P.; Peveraro, A.; Sibelli, P.; and Cavallera, S.: [Camera, Bankart, Latarjet: Techniques and Results Compared.] Minerva Ortop. Traumatol., 39:713–716, 1988.

789. Master, R.; Weisman, M.H.; Armbuster, T.G.; Slivka, J.; Resnick, D.; and Goergen, T.G.: Septic Arthritis of the Glenohumeral Joint. Arthritis Rheum., 20:1500–1506, 1977.

790. Matsen, F.A., III, and Zuckerman, J.D.: Anterior Glenohumeral Instability. Clin. Sports Med., 2:319–338, 1983.

791. Matsen, F.A., III: Symposium: Present Management of Shoulder Instability. Contemp. Orthop., 10:77–110, 1985.

792. Matter, P., and Senn, E.: [Recurrence Frequency After Traumatic Shoulder Dislocation: Relation to Treatment?] Schweiz Z. Sportmed., 30:40–41, 1982.

793. Matter, P.; Stromsoe, K.; and Senn, E.: [Traumatic Dislocation of the Shoulder.] Unfallheilkunde, 82:407–412, 1979.

794. Matthews, L.S.; Terry, G.; and Vetter, W.L.: Shoulder Anatomy for the Arthroscopist. Arthroscopy, 1:83–91, 1985.

795. Matthews, L.S.; Vetter, W.L.; and Helfet, D.L.: Arthroscopic Surgery of the Shoulder. Adv. Orthop. Surg., 203–209, 1984.

796. Matthews, L.S.; Vetter, W.L.; Oweida, S.J.; Spearman, J.; and Helfet, D.L.: Arthroscopic Staple Capsulorrhaphy for Recurrent Anterior Shoulder Instability. Arthroscopy, 4:106–111, 1988.

797. Matthews, L.S.; Zarins, B.; Michael, R.H.; and Helfet, D.L.: Anterior Portal Selection for Shoulder Arthroscopy. Arthroscopy, 1:33–39, 1985.

798. Mauck, R.H., and Clements, E.L.: Bilateral Posterior Shoulder Dislocation: An Orthopedic Case Report. Va. Med. Monthly, 93:452–454, 1966.

799. Maxwell, J.S.: Recurrent Shoulder Dislocation (letter to the editor). Lancet, 1:467, 1947.

800. Maxwell, J.S.: Staple Introducer for Recurrent Dislocation (letter to the editor). Br. Med. J., 1:588, 1946.

801. May, H.: Nicola Operation for Posterior Subacromial Dislocation of the Humerus. J. Bone Joint Surg., 25:78–84, 1943.

802. May, H.: The Regeneration of Joint Transplants and Intracapsular Fragments. Ann. Surg., 116:297–310, 1942.

803. May, V.R., Jr.: A Modified Bristow Operation for Anterior Recurrent Dislocation of the Shoulder. J. Bone Joint Surg., 52A:1010–1016, 1970.

804. May, V.R., Jr.: Posterior Dislocation of the Shoulder: Habitual, Traumatic, and Obstetrical. Orthop. Clin. North Am., 11:271–285, 1980.

805. Mayer, L.: Transplantation of the Trapezius for Paralysis of the Abductors of the Arm. J. Bone Joint Surg., 9:412–420, 1927.

806. McAuliffe, T.B., and Dowd, G.S.: Avulsion of the Subscapularis Tendon: A Case Report. J. Bone Joint Surg., 69A:1454–1455, 1987.

807. McAuliffe, T.B.; Pangayatselvan, T.; and Bayley, I.: Failed Surgery for Recurrent Anterior Dislocation of the Shoulder: Causes and Management. J. Bone Joint Surg., 70B:798–801, 1988.

808. McFarland, E.; Perry, J.; Jobe, F.W.; Pink, M.; and Glousman, R.: Electromyography (EMG) Analysis of Pa-

tients With Posterior Shoulder Instability. Orthop. Trans., 13(2):230, Summer, 1989.

809. McFie, J.: Bilateral Anterior Dislocation of the Shoulders: A Case Report. Injury, 8:67–69, 1976.

810. McGlone, R., and Gosnold, J.K.: Posterior Dislocation of Shoulder and Bilateral Hip Fractures Caused by Epileptic Seizure. Arch. Emerg. Med., 4:115–116, 1987.

811. McGlynn, F.J., and Caspari, R.B.: Arthroscopic Findings in the Subluxating Shoulder. Clin. Orthop., 183:173–178, 1984.

812. McGlynn, F.J.; El-Khoury, G.; and Albright, J.P.: Arthrotomography of the Glenoid Labrum in Shoulder Instability. J. Bone Joint Surg., 64A:506–518, 1982.

813. McKenzie, A.D., and Sinclair, A.M.: Axillary Artery Occlusion Complicating Shoulder Dislocation. Ann. Surg., 148:139–141, 1958.

814. McLaughlin, H.L., and Cavallaro, W.U.: Primary Anterior Dislocation of the Shoulder. Am. J. Surg., 80:615–621, 1950.

815. McLaughlin, H.L., and MacLellan, D.I.: Recurrent Anterior Dislocation of the Shoulder: II. A Comparative Study. J. Trauma, 7:191–201, 1967.

816. McLaughlin, H.L.: Discussion of Acute Anterior Dislocation of the Shoulder by Dr. Toufick Nicola. J. Bone Joint Surg., 31A:172, 1949.

817. McLaughlin, H.L.: Dislocation of the Shoulder With Tuberosity Fractures. Surg. Clin. North Am., 43:1615–1620, 1963.

818. McLaughlin, H.L.: Locked Posterior Subluxation of the Shoulder: Diagnosis and Treatment. Surg. Clin. North Am., 43:1621–1622, 1963.

819. McLaughlin, H.L.: On the "Frozen" Shoulder. Bull. Hosp. Joint Dis. Orthop. Inst., 12:383–393, 1951.

820. McLaughlin, H.L.: Posterior Dislocation of the Shoulder. J. Bone Joint Surg., 34A:584–590, 1952.

821. McLaughlin, H.L.: Posterior Dislocation of the Shoulder (Follow-Up Notes on Articles Previously Published in the Journal). J. Bone Joint Surg., 44A:1477, 1962.

822. McLaughlin, H.L.: Recurrent Anterior Dislocation of the Shoulder: I. Morbid Anatomy. Am. J. Surg., 99:628–632, 1960.

823. McLaughlin, H.L.: Trauma. Philadelphia, W.B. Saunders, 1959.

824. McManus, F.: Brachial Plexus Lesions Complicating Anterior Dislocation of the Shoulder Joint. Injury, 8:63–66, 1976–1978.

825. McMaster, W.C.: Anterior Glenoid Labrum Damage: A Painful Lesion in Swimmers. Am. J. Sports Med., 14:383–392, 1986.

826. McMurray, T.B.: Recurrent Dislocation of the Shoulder (abstract). J. Bone Joint Surg., 43B:402, 1961.

827. Mead, N.C., and Sweeney, H.J.: Bristow Procedure (letter). Spectator: July 9, 1964.

828. Meadowcroft, J.A., and Kain, T.M.: Luxatio Erecta—Shoulder Dislocation: Report of Two Cases. Jefferson Orthop. J., 6:20–24, 1977.

829. Meadows, T., and Wallace, W.A.: Missed Posterior Dislocation of the Shoulder (abstract). J. Bone Joint Surg., 69B:152, 1987.

830. Mears, D.C.: Treatment of Shoulder Subluxation in the Hemiplegic (letter to the editor). Br. Med. J., 3:648–649, 1975.

831. Mehta, M.P., and Kottamasu, S.R.: Anterior Dislocation of the Shoulders With Bilateral Brachial Plexus Injury: Case Report. Ann. Emerg. Med., 18:589–591, 1989.

832. Melzer, C.; Krodel, A.; and Refior, H.J.: [Long-Term Clinical and Radiological Results After Surgical Treatment of Recurrent Shoulder Dislocation Using M. Lange's Procedure.] Z. Orthop., 124:703–706, 1986.

833. Melzer, C.; Manz, P.; Krodel, A.; and Sturz, H.: Operative Therapy for Recurrent Shoulder Dislocation With Special Regard to Long-Term Clinical and Radiological Results Using M. Lange Technique. Arch. Orthop. Trauma Surg., 108:107–111, 1989.

834. Menden, J.F.: Reduction of a Dislocated Joint. J. Hist. Med. Allied Sci., 26:204, 1971.

835. Mendoza, F.X.; Nicholas, J.A.; and Reilly, J.P.: Neer Inferior Capsular Shift Repair for Anterior Glenohumeral Instability. Personal communication, 1986.

836. Merrill, V. (ed.): Atlas of Roentgenographic Positions and Standard Radiologic Procedures, 4th ed, Vol. 1. St. Louis, C.V. Mosby, 1975.

837. Messner, D.G.: Posterior Dislocation of the Shoulder: With or Without Associated Fractures. J. Bone Joint Surg., 48A:1220–1221, 1966.

838. Metcalfe, J.W.: The Bankart Operation for Recurrent Dislocation of the Shoulder. U.S. Navy Med. Bull., 47:672–675, 1947.

839. Metges, B.J.; Kleitz, C.; Tellier, P.; Delahaye, R.P.; and Casanova, G.: [Arthropneumotomography in Recurrent Dislocations and Subluxations of the Shoulder: Methods, Results, and Indications in 45 Cases.] J. Radiol., 60:789–796, 1979.

840. Metheny, J.A.: Skiing Orthosis for Recurrent Shoulder Dislocation. Am. J. Sports Med., 12:82–83, 1984.

841. Michaelis, L.S.: Internal Rotation of the Shoulder: Report of a Case. J. Bone Joint Surg., 32B:223–224, 1950.

842. Middeldorpf, M., and Scharm, B.: De Nova Humeri Luxationis Specie. Clinique Europienne, Vol. II. Dissert. Inag. Breslau, 1859.

843. Milch, H.: Treatment of Dislocation of the Shoulder. Surgery, 3:732–740, 1938.

844. Milgram, J.E.: The Shoulder Anatomy. Instr. Course Lect., III:55–68, 1946.

845. Miller, E.R., and Lusted, L.B.: Progress in Indirect Cineroentgenography. A.J.R., 75:56–62, 1956.

846. Miller, L.S.; Donahue, J.R.; Good, R.P.; and Staerk, A.J.: The Magnuson-Stack Procedure for Treatment of Recurrent Glenohumeral Dislocations. Am. J. Sports Med., 12:133–137, 1984.

847. Mills, K.L.G.: Simultaneous Bilateral Posterior Fracture–Dislocation of the Shoulder. Injury, 6:39–41, 1974–1975.

848. Milton, G.W.: The Circumflex Nerve and Dislocation of the Shoulder. Br. J. Phys. Med., 17:136–138, 1954.

849. Milton, G.W.: The Mechanism of Circumflex and Other Nerve Injuries in Dislocation of the Shoulder and the Possible Mechanism of Nerve Injuries During Reduction of Dislocation. Aust. N.Z. J. Surg., 23(1):25–30, 1953.

850. Mirick, M.J.; Clinton, J.E.; and Ruiz, E.: External Rotation Method of Shoulder Dislocation Reduction. Journal of the American College of Emergency Physicians, 8(12):528–531, 1979.

851. Mirkin, L.: Simple Bankhart's Stapling for Recurrent Dislocation of the Shoulder (abstract). J. Bone Joint Surg., 59B:516, 1977.

852. Mital, M.A., and Karlin, L.I.: Diagnostic Arthroscopy in Sports Injuries. Orthop. Clin. North Am., 11:771–785, 1980.

853. Mitton, A.H.: Posterior Staple Capsulorrhaphy Repair of the Shoulder (abstract). J. Bone Joint Surg., 59B:508–509, 1977.

854. Mizak, S.T., and Sennik, V.T.: [Treatment of Habitual Dislocation of the Shoulder.] Voen. Med. Zh., 8:52–53, 1987.

855. Mizuno, K., and Hirohata, K.: Diagnosis of Recurrent Traumatic Anterior Subluxation of the Shoulder. Clin. Orthop., 179:160–167, 1983.

856. Moberg, E.: Traumatic Injuries to the Brachial Plexus. Surg. Clin. North Am., 61:341–351, 1981.

857. Moeller, J.C.: Compound Posterior Dislocation of the Shoulder: Case Report. J. Bone Joint Surg., 57A:1006–1007, 1975.

858. Mohovich, F., and Zanlungo, U.: [Anterior Stabilization in Habitual Shoulder Luxation, According to Trillat.] Minerva Ortop. Traumatol., 39:717–719, 1988.

859. Mollerud, A.: A Case of Bilateral Habitual Luxation in the Posterior Part of the Shoulder Joint. Acta Chir. Scand., 94:181–186, 1946.

860. Montagu, A.: An Introduction to Physical Anthropology. Springfield, Ill., Charles C. Thomas, 1947.

861. Moore, B.H.: A New Operative Procedure for Brachial Birth Palsy—Erb's Paralysis. Surg. Gynecol. Obstet., 61:832–835, 1935.

862. Moran, M.C., and Warren, R.F.: Development of a Synovial Cyst After Arthroscopy of the Shoulder: A Brief Note. J. Bone Joint Surg., 71A:127–129, 1989.

863. Morgan, C.D., and Bodenstab, A.B.: Arthroscopic Bankart Suture Repair: Technique and Early Results. Arthroscopy, 3:111–122, 1987.

864. Morgan, C.D.: Arthroscopic Bankart Suture Repair—2 to 5 Year Results. Orthop. Trans., 13(2):231–232, 1989.

865. Morrey, B.F., and Janes, J.M.: Recurrent Anterior Dislocation of the Shoulder: Long-Term Follow-Up of the Putti-Platt and Bankart Procedures. J. Bone Joint Surg., 58A:252–256, 1976.

866. Morrison, P.D., and Egan, T.J.: Axillary Artery Injury in Erect Dislocation of the Shoulder (Luxatio Erecta): A Case Report. From the Department of Surgery, Limerick Regional Hospital, Limerick, Ireland.

867. Morton, K.S.: The Unstable Shoulder: Recurring Subluxation. Injury, 10:304–306, 1978–79.

868. Morwessel, R.M., and DeHaven, K.: The Allman Modification of the Bristow Procedure in Treatment of Recurrent Anterior Dislocation and Subluxation of the Shoulder. Personal communication, 1989.

869. Moseley, H.F., and Overgaard, B.: The Anterior Capsular Mechanism in Recurrent Anterior Dislocation of the Shoulder: Morphological and Clinical Studies With Special Reference to the Glenoid Labrum and the Gleno-Humeral Ligaments. J. Bone Joint Surg., 44B:913–927, 1962.

870. Moseley, H.F.: Athletic Injuries to the Shoulder Region. Am. J. Surg., 98:401–422, 1959.

871. Moseley, H.F.: Experiences With Recurrent Dislocations of the Shoulder. J. Bone Joint Surg., 38B:780, 1956.

872. Moseley, H.F.: Recurrent Dislocation of the Shoulder. Montreal, McGill University Press, 1961.

873. Moseley, H.F.: Recurrent Dislocation of the Shoulder. Proc. R. Soc. Med., 29:252–256, 1935.

874. Moseley, H.F.: Shoulder Lesions. Springfield, Ill., Charles C. Thomas, 1945.

874a. Moseley, H.F.: Shoulder Lesions. Edinburgh, Churchill Livingstone, 1972.

875. Moseley, H.F.: The Basic Lesions of Recurrent Anterior Dislocation. Surg. Clin. North Am., 43:1631–1634, 1963.

876. Moseley, H.F.: The Use of a Metallic Glenoid Rim in Recurrent Dislocation of the Shoulder. Can. Med. Assoc. J., 56:320–321, 1947.

877. Moskwa, C.A., Jr., and Mendoza, F.X.: Shoulder Arthroscopy. Unpublished paper, Department of Orthopaedics, Lenox Hill Hospital, New York, N.Y., 1988.

878. Moullin, C.W.M., and Keith, A.: Notes on a Case: Backward Dislocation of the Head of the Humerus Caused by Muscular Action. Lancet, 1:496, 1904.

879. Mowery, C.A.; Garfin, S.R.; Booth, R.E.; and Rothman, R.H.: Recurrent Posterior Dislocation of the Shoulder: Treatment Using a Bone Block. J. Bone Joint Surg., 67A:777–781, 1985.

880. Müller, I., and Sklepek, J.: [Bristow-Latarjet's Operation as Another Possibility of Adjustment of Anterior Habitual Dislocation of the Shoulder Joint.] Acta Chir. Orthop. Traumatol. Cech., 52(6):485–488, 1985.

881. Müller, K.H., and Dingels, W.R.: [Development of Habitual Shoulder Dislocation.] Aktuel Traumatol., 14:121–128, 1984.

882. Müller, W.: Uber den negativen Luftdruck im Gelenkraum. Dtsch. Z. Chir., 217:395–401, 1929.

883. Müller-Färber, J., and Müller, K.H.: [Presurgical X-Ray Diagnosis of Recidivating Luxation of the Shoulder Joint.] Unfallheilkunde, 85:369–376, 1982.

884. Müller-Färber, J.; Müller, K.H.; and Scheuer, I.: [Specific Treatment of Recurrent Dislocation of the Shoulder.] Unfallheilkunde, 86:87–95, 1983.

885. Mumenthaler, M., and Schliack, H.: Lasionen Peripherer Nerven. Stuttgart, Georg Thiem Verlag, 1965.

886. Munzinger, U., and Scherrer, H.: [Early and Late Complications in the Operative Treatment of Recurrent Shoulder Dislocations.] Orthopade, 7:190–191, 1978.

887. Murphy, I.D.: Sliding Bone Graft for the Correction of Recurrent Anterior Dislocation of the Shoulder (abstract). J. Bone Joint Surg., 50A:1270, 1968.

888. Murrard, J.: Un Cas de Luxatio Erecta de l'Épaule Double et Symetrique. Rev. Orthop., 7:423, 1920.

889. Mynter, H.: Subacromial Dislocation From Muscular Spasm. Ann. Surg., 36:117–119, 1902.

890. Nagy, E.; Schváb, V.; Balla, I.; and Nemes, J.: [Roentgen Signs of Lateral Dislocation of the Shoulder.] Magy Traumatol. Orthop. Helyreallito. Sebesz., 15:81–86, 1972.

891. Najenson, T., and Pilielny, S.S.: Malalignment of the Glenohumeral Joint Following Hemiplegia: A Review of 500 Cases. Ann. Phys. Med., 8:96–99, 1965.

892. Narakas, A.: Brachial Plexus Surgery. Orthop. Clin. North Am., 12:303–323, 1981.

893. Narakas, A.N.: Surgical Treatment of Traction Injuries of the Brachial Plexus. Clin. Orthop., 133:71–90, 1978.

894. Nash, E.; Soudry, M.; Abrahamson, J.; and Mendes, D.G.: Neuropraxis Secondary to Hemorrhage in a Traumatic Dislocation of the Shoulder. J. Trauma, 24:546–547, 1984.

895. Neal, M.R., and Williamson, J.: Collar Sling for Bilateral Shoulder Subluxation. Am. J. Occup. Ther., 34:400–401, 1980.

896. Neer, C.S., II, and Foster, C.R.: Inferior Capsular Shift for Involuntary Inferior and Multidirectional Instability of the Shoulder: A Preliminary Report. J. Bone Joint Surg., 62A:897–908, 1980.

897. Neer, C.S., II, and Horwitz, B.S.: Fractures of the Proximal Humeral Epiphyseal Plate. Clin. Orthop., 41:24–31, 1965.

898. Neer, C.S., II, and Welsh, R.P.: The Shoulder in Sports: Symposium on Injuries in Sports: Recent Developments. Orthop. Clin. North Am., 8B:583, 1977.

899. Neer, C.S., II: Degenerative Lesions of the Proximal Humeral Articular Surface. Clin. Orthop., 20:116–124, 1961.

900. Neer, C.S., II: Displaced Proximal Humeral Fractures: I. Classification and Evaluation. J. Bone Joint Surg., 52A:1077–1089, 1970.

901. Neer, C.S., II: Fractures of the Distal Third of the Clavicle. Clin. Orthop., 58:43–50, 1968.

902. Neer, C.S., II: Involuntary Inferior and Multidirectional Instability of the Shoulder: Etiology, Recognition, and Treatment. Instr. Course Lect, XXXIV:232–238, 1985.

903. Neer, C.S., II: Multidirectional Instability. Personal communication, 1988.

904. Nelson, C.L., and Razzano, C.D.: Arthrography of the Shoulder: A Review. J. Trauma, 13:136–141, 1973.

905. Nelson, C.L.: The Use of Arthrography in Athletic Injuries to the Shoulder. Orthop. Clin. North Am., 4:775–785, 1973.

906. Nelson, W.E., and Skagerberg, D.: Recurrent Shoulder Dislocations—Modified Magnuson Repair (abstract). J. Bone Joint Surg., 49A:202–203, 1967.

907. Neumark, J., and Niessner, G.: [Regional Block for Reduction of a Dislocated Shoulder.] Anaesthesist, 25:384–386, 1976.

908. Neviaser, J.S., and Tobin, W.J.: Humeral Torsion in Relation to Recurrent Dislocations of the Shoulder. Presented at meeting of the Interurban Club, Washington, D.C., 1959.

909. Neviaser, J.S.: An Operation for Old Dislocation of the Shoulder. J. Bone Joint Surg., 30A:997–1000, 1948.

910. Neviaser, J.S.: Complicated Fractures and Dislocations About the Shoulder Joint. J. Bone Joint Surg., 44A:984–998, 1962.

911. Neviaser, J.S.: Complicated Fractures and Dislocations About the Shoulder Joint. Instr. Course Lect., XL:984–998, 1962.

912. Neviaser, J.S.: Posterior Dislocations of the Shoulder: Diagnosis and Treatment. Surg. Clin. North Am., 43:1623–1630, 1963.

913. Neviaser, J.S.: The Treatment of Old Unreduced Dislocations of the Shoulder. Surg. Clin. North Am., 43:1671–1678, 1963.

914. Neviaser, R.J.; Neviaser, T.J.; and Neviaser, J.S.: Concurrent Rupture of the Rotator Cuff and Anterior Dislocation of the Shoulder in the Older Patient. J. Bone Joint Surg., 70A:1308–1311, 1988.

915. Neviaser, T.J.: Arthroscopy of the Shoulder. Orthop. Clin. North Am., 18:361–372, 1987.

916. Nicholson, J.T.: Recurrent Dislocation of the Shoulder. J. Bone Joint Surg., 32B:510–511, 1950.

917. Nickel, V.L.: Orthopedic Rehabilitation. London, Churchill Livingstone, 1982.

918. Nicola, F.G.; Ellman, H.; Eckardt, J.; and Finerman, G.: Bilateral Posterior Fracture–Dislocation of the Shoulder Treated With a Modification of the McLaughlin Procedure. J. Bone Joint Surg., 63A:1175–1177, 1981.

919. Nicola, T.: Acute Anterior Dislocation of the Shoulder. J. Bone Joint Surg., 31A:153–159, 1949.

920. Nicola, T.: Anterior Dislocation of the Shoulder: The Role of the Articular Capsule. J. Bone Joint Surg., 24:614–616, 1942.

921. Nicola, T.: Recurrent Anterior Dislocation of the Shoulder: A New Operation. J. Bone Joint Surg., 11:128–132, 1929.

922. Nicola, T.: Recurrent Dislocation of the Shoulder: Its Treatment by Transplantation of the Long Head of the Biceps. Am. J. Surg., 6:815, 1929.

923. Nicola, T.: Recurrent Dislocation of the Shoulder. Am. J. Surg., 86:85–91, 1953.

924. Nidecker, A., and Cooke, G.M.: Hill-Sachs Deformity With an Unusually Large Defect. J. Can. Assoc. Radiol., 30:116–117, 1979.

925. Niedzielski, W.: [Simultaneous Chronic Traumatic Dislocation of Both Shoulder Joints.] Chir. Narzadow. Ruchu. Ortop. Pol., 52:490–492, 1987.

926. Nielsen, A.B., and Nielsen, K.: The Modified Bristow Procedure for Recurrent Anterior Dislocation of the Shoulder: Results and Complications. Acta Orthop. Scand., 53:229–232, 1982.

927. Nixon, J.R., and Young, W.S.: Arthrography of the Shoulder in Anterior Dislocation: A Study of African and Asian Patients. Injury, 9:287–293, 1977.

928. Noack, W., and Strohmeier, M.: [On Treatment of Chronic Unreduced Anterior Dislocations of the Shoulder.] Orthop. Praxis, 24:411–415, 1988.

929. Noack, W., and Strohmeier, M.: [Treatment of Unreduced Chronic Anterior Dislocations of the Shoulder.] Unfallchirurgie, 14:184–190, 1988.

930. Nobel, W.: Posterior Traumatic Dislocation of the Shoulder. J. Bone Joint Surg., 44A:523–538, 1962.

931. Nocera, S., and Leo, A.: Lussazione Volontaria Posteriore de Spalla: Contribato Casistico. Minerva Orthop., 33:1–5, 1982.

932. Noesberger, B., and Mader, G.: Die modifizierte Operation nach Trillat bei habitueller Schulterluxation. Z. Unfallchir. Versicherungsmed. Berufskr., 69:34–36, 1976.

933. Noordenbos, W.: Beenplastiek bij habitueele Schouderluxatie. Ned. Tijdschr. Geneeskd., 82:1784, 1938.

934. Norris, T.R., and Bigliani, L.U.: Analysis of Failed Repair for Shoulder Instability: A Preliminary Report. In Bateman, J.E., and Welsh, R.P. (eds.): Surgery of the Shoulder, pp. 111–116, Philadelphia, B.C. Decker, 1984.

935. Norris, T.R.; Bigliani, L.U.; and Harris, E.: Complications Following the Modified Bristow Repair for Shoulder Instability. Presented at the 3rd Open Meeting of the American Shoulder and Elbow Surgeons, San Francisco, Calif., 1987.

936. Norris, T.R.: C-Arm Fluoroscopic Evaluation Under Anesthesia for Glenohumeral Subluxations. In Bateman, J.E., and Welsh, R.P. (eds.): Surgery of the Shoulder, pp. 22–25. Philadelphia, B.C. Decker, 1984.

937. Norris, T.R.: Diagnostic Techniques for Shoulder Instability. Instr. Course Lect., XXXIV:239–257, 1985.

938. Norwood, L.A., Jr.; Del Pizzo, W.; Jobe, F.W.; and Kerlan, R.K.: Anterior Shoulder Pain in Baseball Pitchers. Personal Communication, 1977.

939. Norwood, L.A., and Fowler, H.L.: Rotator Cuff Tears: A Shoulder Arthroscopy Complication. Am. J. Sports Med., 17:837–841, 1989.

940. Norwood, L.A.; Matiko, J.A.; and Terry, G.C.: Posterior Shoulder Approach. Clin. Orthop., 201:167–172, 1985.

941. Norwood, L.A., and Terry, G.C.: Shoulder Posterior Subluxation. Am. J. Sports Med., 12:25–30, 1984.

942. Norwood, L.A.: Treatment of Acute Shoulder Dislocations. Ala. Med., 54:30–36, 1984.

943. Nottage, W.M.; Duge, W.D.; and Fields, W.A.: Computed Arthrotomography of the Glenohumeral Joint to Evaluate Anterior Instability: Correlation With Arthroscopic Findings. Arthroscopy, 3:273–276, 1987.

944. Nottage, W.M.: Shoulder Arthroscopy: Portals and Surgical Techniques. Techniques Orthop., 3:23–26, 1988.

945. O'Brien, S.J.; Warren, R.F.; and Schwartz, E.: Anterior Shoulder Instability. Orthop. Clin. North Am., 18:395–408, 1987.

946. O'Connor, S.J., and Kacknow, A.J.: Posterior Dislocation of the Shoulder. Arch. Surg., 72:479–491, 1956.

947. O'Connor, S.J., and Kacknow, A.J.: Posterior Dislocation of the Shoulder (abstract). J. Bone Joint Surg., 37A:1122, 1955.

948. O'Donoghue, D.H.: Treatment of Injuries to Athletes, 2nd ed. Philadelphia, W.B. Saunders, 1970.

949. O'Driscoll, S.W., and Evans, D.C.: The DuToit Staple Capsulorrhaphy for Recurrent Anterior Dislocation of the Shoulder: Twenty Years of Experience in Six Toronto Hospitals. Orthop. Trans., 12(3):731, Fall, 1988.

950. O'Driscoll, S.W.: Use of Capsulorrhaphy Challenged in Stabilizing Anterior Shoulder. American Academy of Orthopaedic Surgeons Annual Meeting News Bulletin, pp. 7–8, 1988.

951. O'Neill, D.B., and Micheli, L.J.: A Technique for Tendon and Capsule Separation in Shoulder Surgery. Orthop. Rev., 18:504–507, 1989.

952. Ober, F.R.: An Operation to Relieve Paralysis of the Deltoid Muscle. J.A.M.A., 99:2182, 1932.

953. Odgers, S.L., and Hark, F.W.: Habitual Dislocation of the Shoulder Joint. Surg. Gynecol. Obstet., 75:229–234, 1942.

954. Ogilvie, H.: Recurrent Dislocation of the Shoulder: The Johannesburg Staple Driver. Br. Med. J., 1:362, 1946.

955. Ogilvie-Harris, D.J., and Wiley, A.M.: Arthroscopic Surgery of the Shoulder: A General Appraisal. J. Bone Joint Surg., 68B:201–207, 1986.

956. Ogilvie-Harris, D.J.: Arthroscopy and Arthroscopic Surgery of the Shoulder. Semin. Orthop., 2:246–258, 1987.

957. Older, M.W.J.: Arthroscopy of the Shoulder Joint (abstract). J. Bone Joint Surg., 58B:253, 1976.

958. Oliver, J.H.; Hastings, D.E.; and Petrie, D.P.: Glenoid Osteotomy in the Treatment of Recurrent Dislocation of the Shoulder (abstract). J. Bone Joint Surg., 62B:128, 1980.

959. Olsson, O.: Degenerative Changes of the Shoulder Joint and Their Connection With Shoulder Pain: A Morphological and Clinical Investigation With Special Attention to the Cuff and Biceps Tendon. Acta Chir. Scand. [Suppl.], 181:1–130, 1953.

960. Onabowale, B.O., and Jaja, M.O.A.: Unreduced Bilateral Synchronous Shoulder Dislocations: A Case Report. Niger Med. J., 9:267–271, 1979.

961. Oni, O.O.A.: Irreducible Acute Anterior Dislocation of the Shoulder Due to a Loose Fragment From an Associated Fracture of the Greater Tuberosity. Injury, 15:138, 1983.

962. Oppenheim, W.L.; Dawson, E.G.; Quinlan, C.; and Graham, S.A.: The Cephaloscapular Projection: A Special Diagnostic Aid. Clin. Orthop., 195:191–193, 1985.

963. Oretorp, N., and Bassi, P.B.: Arthroscopy of the Shoulder Joint (Technique). Ital. J. Orthop. Traumatol., 9:251–258, 1983.

964. Osmond-Clarke, H.: Habitual Dislocation of the Shoulder: The Putti-Platt Operation. J. Bone Joint Surg., 30B:19–25, 1948.

965. Osmond-Clarke, H.: Recurrent Dislocation of the Shoulder (abstract). J. Bone Joint Surg., 47B:194, 1965.

966. Oster, A.: Recurrent Anterior Dislocation of the Shoulder Treated by the Eden-Hybbinette Operation: Follow-Up on 78 Cases. Acta Orthop. Scand., 40:43–52, 1969.

967. Osterwalder, A., and Huben, R.: [The Use of Dissolvable Fixation Material (PDS-Cord) in the Shoulder Joint.] Helv. Chir. Acta, 54:431–434, 1987.

968. Oswald, T., and Wertsch, J.J.: An Unusual Nerve Injury in Shoulder Dislocation (abstract). Arch. Phys. Med. Rehabil., 69:785, 1988.

969. Oudard, P.: La Luxation Recidivante de l'Épaule (Varieté Antero-Interne): Procede Operatoire. J. Chir. (Paris), 23:13–25, 1924.

970. Oudard, P.: Le Traitement de la Luxation Recidivante de l'Épaule (Varieté Antero-Interne par la Butee Osseuse). Rev. Med., 1:305, 1946.

971. Ovesen, J., and Nielsen, S.: Experimental Distal Subluxation in the Glenohumeral Joint. Arch. Orthop. Trauma Surg., 104:78–81, 1985.

972. Ovesen, J., and Nielsen, S.: Stability of the Shoulder Joint: Cadaver Study of Stabilizing Structures. Acta Orthop. Scand., 56:149–151, 1985.

973. Ovesen, J., and Nielsen, S.: Posterior Instability of the Shoulder. A Cadaver Study. Acta Orthop. Scand., 57:436–439, 1986.

974. Ovesen, J., and Nielsen, S.: Anterior and Posterior Shoulder Instability: A Cadaver Study. Acta Orthop. Scand., 57:324–327, 1986.

975. Ovesen, J., and Söjbjerg, J.O.: Lesions in Different Types of Anterior Glenohumeral Joint Dislocation: An Experimental Study. Arch. Orthop. Trauma Surg., 105:216–218, 1986.

976. Ovesen, J., and Söjbjerg, J.O.: Transposition of Coracoacromial Ligament to Humerus in Treatment of Vertical Shoulder Joint Instability: Clinical Applicability of Experimental Technique. Arch. Orthop. Trauma Surg., 106:323–326, 1987.

977. Ovesen, J., and Söjbjerg, J.O.: Transposition of Coracoacromial Ligament to Humerus in Treatment of Distal Shoulder Joint Instability (discussion). Rev. Chir. Orthop., 74:264, 1988.

978. Ovesen, J., and Söjbjerg, J.O.: Posterior Shoulder Dislocation: Muscle and Capsular Lesions in Cadaver Experiments. Acta Orthop. Scand., 57:535–536, 1986.

979. Ozaki, J.: Glenohumeral Movements of the Involuntary Inferior and Multidirectional Instability. Clin. Orthop., 238:107–111, 1989.

980. Ozaki, J.: Pathogenesis of the Loose Shoulder. Rinsho Shinkeigaku, 16:1161, 1981.

981. Paavolainen, P.; Bjorkenheim, J.M.; Ahovuo, J.; and Slatis, P.: Recurrent Anterior Dislocation of the Shoulder: Results of Eden-Hybbinette and Putti-Platt Operations. Acta Orthop. Scand., 55:556–560, 1984.

982. Pagden, D.; Halaburt, A.S.; Wirpszo, R.; and Karyn, A.: Posterior Dislocation of the Shoulder Complicating Regional Anesthesia. Anesth. Analg., 65:1063–1065, 1986.

983. Paley, D.; Lovet, R.; and Malcolm, B.W.: Bilateral Anterior Fracture Dislocation of the Shoulder With Brachial Plexus and Axillary Artery Injury. Orthop. Rev., 15:45–48, 1986.

984. Palmar, I., and Widen, A.: The Bone Block Method for Recurrent Dislocation of the Shoulder Joint. J. Bone Joint Surg., 30B:53–58, 1948.

985. Palmer, R.S., and Miller, T.A.: Anterior Shoulder Reconstruction With Pectoralis Minor Muscle Flap. Plast. Reconstr. Surg., 81:437–439, 1988.

986. Palumbo, L.T., and Quirin, L.D.: Recurrent Dislocation of the Shoulder Repaired by the Magnuson-Stack Operation. Arch. Surg., 60:1140–1150, 1950.

987. Palumbo, L.T.; Sharpe, W.S.; and Nejdl, R.J.: Recurrent

Dislocation of the Shoulder Repaired by the Magnuson-Stack Operation. Arch. Surg., 81:834–837, 1960.

988. Panaro, V.A.; Tabone, J.; and Barodawala, Y.K.: Diagnostic Approach to Posterior Dislocations (abstract). Invest. Radiol., 18:S34, 1983.

989. Pande, P.; Hawkins, R.; and Peat, M.: Electromyography in Voluntary Posterior Instability of the Shoulder. Am. J. Sports Med., 17:644–648, 1989.

990. Pappas, A.M.; Goss, T.P.; and Kleinman, P.K.: Symptomatic Shoulder Instability Due to Lesions of the Glenoid Labrum. Am. J. Sports Med., 11:279–288, 1983.

991. Paquet, R.; Des Marchais, J.E.; and Benazet, J.P.: Evaluation of Neer Prostheses for Humeral Fractures (abstract). J. Bone Joint Surg., 62B:128, 1980.

992. Parisien, J.S.: Shoulder Arthroscopy Technique and Indications. Bull. Hosp. Joint Dis. Orthop. Inst., 43:56–69, 1983.

993. Parisien, V.M.: Shoulder Dislocation: An Easier Method of Reduction. J. Maine Med. Assoc., 70:102, 1979.

994. Parks, B.J.: Postoperative Peripheral Neuropathies. Surgery, 74:348–357, 1973.

995. Parrish, G., and Skiendzielewski, J.J.: Bilateral Posterior Fracture–Dislocations of the Shoulder After Convulsive Status Epilepticus. Ann. Emerg. Med., 14:264–266, 1985.

996. Parry, C.B.: Pain in Avulsion Lesions of the Brachial Plexus. Pain, 9:41–53, 1980.

997. Parry, C.B.: The Management of Injuries to the Brachial Plexus. Proc. R. Soc. Med., 67:4–6, 1974.

998. Parsons, S.W., and Rowley, D.I.: Brachial Plexus Lesions in Dislocations and Fracture Dislocation of the Shoulder. J. R. Coll. Surg. Edinburgh, 31:85–87, 1986.

999. Parsons, T.: Diagnostic Shoulder Arthroscopy: An Analysis of 55 Cases. (Proceedings) J. Bone Joint Surg., 69B:166, 1987.

1000. Pascoet, G.; Jung, F.; Foucher, G.; and Kehr, P.: [Treatment of Recurrent Dislocation of the Shoulder by Preglenoid Artificial Ridge Using the Latarjet-Vittori Technique.] J. Med. Strasbourg, 6:501–504, 1975.

1001. Pasila, M.; Jaroma, H.; Kiviluoto, O.; and Sundholm, A.: Early Complications of Primary Shoulder Dislocations. Acta Orthop. Scand., 49:260–263, 1978.

1002. Pasila, M.; Kiviluoto, O.; Jaroma, H.; and Sundholm, A.: Recovery From Primary Shoulder Dislocation and Its Complications. Acta Orthop. Scand., 51:257–262, 1980.

1003. Patel, M.R.; Pardee, M.L.; and Singerman, R.C.: Intrathoracic Dislocation of the Head of the Humerus. J. Bone Joint Surg., 45A:1712–1714, 1963.

1004. Paton, D.F.: Posterior Dislocation of the Shoulder: A Diagnostic Pitfall for Physicians. Practitioner, 223:111–112, 1979.

1005. Patra, P.; Hauer, P.; Charbonneau, P.; Duveau, D.; Despins, P.; Letenneur, J.; and Dupon, H.: [Injury to the Axillary Artery in Anterior Dislocation of the Shoulder: Report of a Case.] Rev. Chir. Orthop., 71:333–336, 1985.

1006. Patte, D.; Bernageau, J.; Rodineau, J.; and Gardes, J.C.: [Unstable Painful Shoulders.] Rev. Chir. Orthop., 66:157–165, 1980.

1007. Patterson, J.R.; Zabransky, R.; Grabois, M.; and Ferro, P.: Evaluation of the Effectiveness of Sling Orthoses for the Correction of Glenohumeral Subluxation in the Hemiplegic (abstract). Arch. Phys. Med. Rehabil., 65:635, 1984.

1008. Paulos, L.E.; Harner, C.D.; and Parker, R.D.: Arthroscopic Subacromial Decompression for Impingement Syndrome of the Shoulder. Techniques Orthop., 3:33–39, 1988.

1009. Pavlov, H.; Warren, R.F.; Weiss, C.B., Jr.; and Dines, D.M.: The Roentgenographic Evaluation of Anterior Shoulder Instability. Clin. Orthop., 194:153–158, 1985.

1010. Payne, R.E.: Involuntary Anterior Recurrent Subluxation of the Shoulders (abstract). Clin. Orthop., 126:311, 1977.

1011. Pear, B.L.: Dislocation of the Shoulder: X-Ray Signs (letter to the editor). N. Engl. J. Med., 283:12, 1970.

1012. Peiro, A.; Ferrandis, R.; and Correa, F.: Bilateral Erect Dislocation of the Shoulders. Injury, 6:294–295, 1974–75.

1013. Pelipenko, V.P., and Olexyuk, D.I.: [Outcomes of Operative Treatment of Habitual Shoulder Dislocation.] Ortop. Travmatol. Protez., 4:24–26, 1985.

1014. Percy-Lancaster, R.: Recurrent Posterior Dislocation of the Shoulder (abstract). J. Bone Joint Surg., 42B:863, 1960.

1015. Perkins, G.: Rest and Movement. J. Bone Joint Surg., 35B:521–539, 1953.

1016. Perniceni, B., and Augereau, A.: [Treatment of Old Unreduced Anterior Dislocations of the Shoulder by Open Reduction and a Reinforced Rib Graft: Discussion of Three Cases.] Ann. Chir., 36:235–239, 1983.

1017. Perotti, G.F.; Leonardi, F.; Massetti, P.; and Scagnelli, R.: [Trillat's Technique in the Surgical Treatment of Habitual Anterior Luxation of the Shoulder.] Minerva Ortop. Traumatol., 39:659–662, 1988.

1018. Perthes, G.: Über Operationen bei habitueller Schulterluxation. Dtsch. Z. Chir., 85:199–227, 1906.

1019. Petrucci, F.S.; Morelli, A.; and Raimondi, P.L.: Axillary Nerve Injuries—21 Cases Treated by Nerve Graft Neurolysis. J. Hand Surg., 7:271–278, 1982.

1020. Pettersson, G.: Rupture of the Tendon Aponeurosis of the Shoulder Joint in Antero-Inferior Dislocation: A Study on the Origin and Occurrence of the Ruptures. Acta Chir. Scand. [Suppl.] 77:1–187, 1942.

1021. Pfister, U.; Rohner, H.; and Weller, S.: [Diagnosis and Therapy of Traumatic Posterior Dislocations of the Shoulder.] Unfallchirurgie, 11:12–16, 1985.

1022. Pick, R.Y.: Treatment of the Dislocated Shoulder. Clin. Orthop., 123:76–77, 1977.

1023. Pieper, H.G.: Shoulder Dislocation in Skiing: Choice of Surgical Method Depending on the Degree of Humeral Retrotorsion. Int. J. Sports Med., 6:155–160, 1985.

1024. Pilz, W.: Zur Rontgenuntersuchung der habituellen Schulterverrenkung. Arch. Klin. Chir., 135:1–22, 1925.

1025. Pinzur, M.S., and Hookins, G.E.: Biceps Tenodesis for Painful Inferior Subluxation of the Shoulder in Adult Acquired Hemiplegia. Clin. Orthop., 206:100–103, 1986.

1026. Plummer, D., and Clinton, J.: The External Rotation Method for Reduction of Acute Anterior Shoulder Dislocation. Emerg. Med. Clin. North Am., 7:165–175, 1989.

1027. Plummer, W.W., and Potts, F.N.: Two Cases of Recurrent Anterior Dislocation of the Shoulder. J. Bone Joint Surg., 7:190–198, 1925.

1028. Po, B.T., and Hansen, H.R.: Iatrogenic Brachial Plexus Injury. Anesth. Analg., 48:915–922, 1969.

1029. Poigenfurst, J.; Buch, J.; and Eber, K.: [The Posterior Shoulder Luxation.] Unfallchirurgie, 12:171–175, 1986.

1030. Pollen, A.G.: Successful Surgical Treatment of Bilateral Recurrent Dislocation of the Shoulder. J. R. Soc. Med., 7:331, 1984.

1031. Pollock, L.J.: Accessory Muscle Movements in Deltoid Paralysis. J.A.M.A., 79:526–528, 1922.

1032. Pon, A.; Koob, E.; and Puhlvers, E.: [Operative Treatment of the Habitual Dislocation of the Shoulder.] Orthop. Praxis, 20:704–705, 1984.

1033. Ponseti, I.V., and Shepard, R.S.: Lesions of the Skeleton and of Other Mesodermal Tissues in Rats Fed Sweet-Pea (Lathyrus Odoratus) Seeds. J. Bone Joint Surg., 36A:1031–1058, 1954.

1034. Popke, L.O.A.: Zur Kasuistik und Therapie der inverterirten und habituellen Schulterluxation: Inaugural Dissertation. Halle, 1882. *In* Moseley, H.F. (ed.): Recurrent Dislocation of the Shoulder. Montreal, McGill University Press, 1961.

1035. Poppen, N.K., and Walker, P.S.: Normal and Abnormal Motion of the Shoulder. J. Bone Joint Surg., 58A:195–201, 1976.

1036. Poppen, N.K., and Walker, P.S.: Forces at the Glenohumeral Joint in Abduction. Clin. Orthop., 135:165–170, 1978.

1037. Porter, S.F., and Hersey, S.L.: Supporting the Subluxated Shoulder Joint With a Pajama-Bottom Sling. Nursing, 79:56, 1979.

1038. Post, M.: The Shoulder. Philadelphia, Lea & Febiger, 1978.

1039. Postacchini, F., and Facchini, M.: The Treatment of Unreduced Dislocation of the Shoulder: A Review of 12 Cases. Ital. J. Orthop. Traumatol., 13:15–26, 1987.

1040. Postacchini, F., and Mancini, A.: Anterior Instability of the Shoulder Due to Capsular Laxity. Ital. J. Orthop. Traumatol., 14:175–185, 1988.

1041. Potter, F.A.; Fiorini, A.J.; Knox, J.; and Rajesh, P.B.: The Migration of a Kirschner Wire From Shoulder to Spleen: Brief Report. J. Bone Joint Surg., 70B:326–327, 1988.

1042. Pouget, G.: Recurrent Posterior Dislocation of the Shoulder Treated by Glenoid Osteotomy (abstract). J. Bone Joint Surg., 66B:140, 1984.

1043. Poulsen, S.R.: Reduction of Acute Shoulder Dislocations Using the Eskimo Technique: A Study of 23 Consecutive Cases. J. Trauma, 28:1382–1383, 1988.

1044. Preston, M.F.: Fractures and Dislocations: Diagnosis and Treatment. St. Louis, C.V. Mosby, 1915.

1045. Pridie, K.H.: Bankart's Operation for Recurrent Dislocation of Shoulder (abstract). J. Bone Joint Surg., 38B:589–590, 1956.

1046. Prillaman, H.A., and Thompson, R.C.: Bilateral Posterior Fracture Dislocation of the Shoulder: A Case Report. J. Bone Joint Surg., 51A:1627–1630, 1969.

1047. Pritchett, J.W., and Clark, J.M.: Prosthetic Replacement for Chronic Unreduced Dislocations of the Shoulder. Clin. Orthop., 216:89–93, 1987.

1048. Probst, J.: [Assessment of Rotator Defects and Shoulder Luxation: The Importance of Degeneration and a Predisposition Towards Instability.] Unfallchirurg, 89:436–439, 1986.

1049. Prokin, B.M., and Breigin, E.I.: [Remote Results of the Treatment of Habitual Shoulder Dislocation by a Modified Method.] Ortop. Travmatol. Protez, 1:53–54, 1989.

1050. Protzman, R.R.: Anterior Instability of the Shoulder. J. Bone Joint Surg., 62A:909–918, 1980.

1051. Pushkarsky, V.M.: [Rupture of the Axillary Artery in Dislocation of the Shoulder.] Vest. Khir., 136:99–100, 1986.

1052. Quattrini, M.; Cepparulo, W.; Dezza, O.; and Mottana, S.A.: [Treatment of Habitual Shoulder Luxation According to Putti-Platt.] Minerva Ortop. Traumatol., 39:637–641, 1988.

1053. Quigley, T.B., and Freedman, P.A.: Recurrent Dislocation of the Shoulder: A Preliminary Report of Personal Experience With Seven Bankart and Ninety-Two Putti-Platt Operations in Ninety-Nine Cases Over Twenty-Five Years. Am. J. Surg., 128:595–599, 1974.

1054. Rae, P.J., and Sylvester, B.S.: Luxatio Erecta—Two Cases Without Direct Injury. Injury, 19:361–362, 1988.

1055. Rafii, M.; Firoonzia, H.; Golimbu, C.; Minkoff, J.; and Bonamo, J.J.: CT Arthrography of Capsular Structures of the Shoulder. A.J.R., 146:361–367, 1986.

1056. Rafii, M.; Firoonzia, H.; Bonamo, J.J.; Minkoff, T.; and Golimbu, C.: Athlete Shoulder Injuries: CT Arthrographic Findings. Radiology, 162:559–564, 1987.

1057. Rafii, M., and FiroozNia, H.: Variations of Normal Glenoid Labrum (letter to the editor). A.J.R., 152:201, 1989.

1058. Raju, S., and Carner, D.V.: Brachial Plexus Compression. Arch. Surg., 116:175–178, 1981.

1059. Randelli, M., and Gambrioli, P.L.: Glenohumeral Osteometry by Computed Tomography in Normal and Unstable Shoulders. Clin. Orthop., 208:151–156, 1986.

1060. Randelli, M., and Gambrioli, P.L.: Recurrent Instability of the Glenohumeral Joint. Ital. J. Orthop. Traumatol., 11:107–117, 1985.

1061. Randelli, M., and Odella, F.: [Latarjet Surgical Technique in Recurrent Anterior Luxation of the Shoulder.] Minerva Ortop. Traumatol., 39:643–649, 1988.

1062. Randelli, M.; Odella, F.; and Gambrioli, P.L.: Clinical Experience With Double Contrast Medium Computerized Tomography (Arthro-CT) in Instability of the Shoulder. Ital. J. Orthop. Traumatol., 12:181–158, 1986.

1063. Randelli, M.: Recurrent Instability of the Gleno-Humeral Joint. Ital. J. Orthop. Traumatol., 11:107–117, 1985.

1064. Raney, R.B., and Miller, O.L.: The Nicola Operation for Recurrent Dislocation of the Shoulder: A Review of Twenty-Six Cases. South. Med. J., 35:529–532, 1942.

1065. Raney, R.B.: Andry and the Orthopaedia. J. Bone Joint Surg., 31A:675–682, 1949.

1066. Ransford, A.O., and Hughes, S.P.F.: Complete Brachial Plexus Lesions. J. Bone Joint Surg., 59B:417–420, 1977.

1067. Rao, J.P.; Francis, A.M.; Hurley, J.; and Daczkewycz, R.: Treatment of Recurrent Anterior Dislocation of the Shoulder by duToit Staple Capsulorrhaphy: Results of Long-Term Follow-Up Study. Clin. Orthop., 204:169–176, 1986.

1068. Rao, J.P.; Hurley, J.; and Neviaser, R.J.: Staple Capsulorrhaphy for Recurrent Anterior Dislocation of the Shoulder. Orthop. Consult., 5:1–8, 1984.

1069. Reckling, F.W.: Posterior Fracture–Dislocation of the Shoulder Treated by a Neer Hemiarthroplasty With a Posterior Surgical Approach. Clin. Orthop., 207:133–137, 1986.

1070. Redden, K., and Frankel, C.: Award for Failure to Detect Dislocated Shoulder. Orthop. Digest, August 1976:45–46.

1071. Reeck, C.C.: Grappler's Glenoid (abstract). Clin. Orthop., 165:309, 1982.

1072. Reeves, B.: Acute Anterior Dislocation of the Shoulder: Clinical and Experimental Studies. Ann. R. Coll. Surg. Engl., 43:255–273, 1968.

1073. Reeves, B.: Arthrography of the Shoulder. J. Bone Joint Surg., 48B:424–435, 1966.

1074. Reeves, B.: Arthrography in Acute Dislocation of the Shoulder (abstract). J. Bone Joint Surg., 48B:182, 1968.

1075. Reeves, B.: Experiments on the Tensile Strength of the Anterior Capsular Structures of the Shoulder in Man. J. Bone Joint Surg., 50B:858–865, 1968.

1076. Reeves, B.: Recurrent Posterior Dislocation of the Shoulder (Two Cases). Proc. R. Soc. Med., 56:897–898, 1963.

1077. Refior, H.J.; Plitz, W.; Jager, M.; and Hackenbroch, M.H.: Biomechanik der gesunden und kranken Schulter. Munchner Symposion fur Experimentelle Orthopadie, 1985.

1078. Regan, W.D., Jr.; Webster-Bogaert, S.; Hawkins, R.J.; and Fowler, P.J.: Comparative Functional Analysis of the Bristow, Magnuson-Stack, and Putti-Platt Procedures for Recurrent Dislocation of the Shoulder. Am. J. Sports Med., 17:42–489, 1989.

1079. Reider, B., and Inglis, A.E.: The Bankhart Procedure Modified by the Use of Prolene Pull-Out Sutures: Brief Note. J. Bone Joint Surg., 64:628–629, 1982.

1080. Rierkås, O., and Husby, T.: Arthroscopic Resection of the Acromion (abstract). Acta Orthop. Scand., 59:109–110, 1988.

1081. Rierkås, O.: Posterior Shoulder Dislocation Diagnosed by CT (abstract). Acta Orthop. Scand., 59:109, 1988.

1082. Remmel, E., and Kockerling, F.: Anatomical Study of the Capsular Mechanism in Dislocation of the Shoulder (abstract). J. Biomech., 20:807, 1987.

1083. Rendich, R.A., and Poppel, M.H.: Roentgen Diagnosis of Posterior Dislocation of the Shoulder. Radiology, 36:42–45, 1941.

1084. Renstrom, P.: Swedish Research in Sports Traumatology. Clin. Orthop., 191:144–148, 1984.

1085. Resch, H.; Benedetto, K.P.; Kadletz, R.; and Daniaux, H.: [X-Ray Examination in Recurrent Dislocation of the Shoulder—Value of Different Techniques.] Unfallchirurgie, 11:65–69, 1985.

1086. Resch, H.; Helweg, G.; Nedden, D.; and Beck, E.: [Double-Contrast Computed Tomographic Examination Techniques in Habitual and Recurrent Shoulder Dislocation.] Europ. J. Radiol., 8:6–12, 1988.

1087. Resch, H.; Kadletz, R.; Beck, E.; and Helweg, G.: [Simple and Double-Contrast CT Scanning in the Examination of Recurrent Shoulder Dislocations.] Unfallchirurg., 89:441–445, 1986.

1088. Respet, P.B.: A Practical Technique for Reducing Shoulder Dislocations. J. Musculoskeletal. Med., 6:29–35, 1988.

1089. Restelli, B.; Iapoce, C.; and Graziano, M.: [Habitual Shoulder Luxation: Personal Experience.] Minerva Ortop. Traumatol., 39:677–679, 1988.

1090. Ribbans, W.J.: Bilateral Anterior Dislocation of the Shoulder Following a Grand-Mal Convulsion. Br. J. Clin. Pract., 43:181–182, 1989.

1091. Rice, E.: Experience With the Putti-Platt Shoulder Reconstruction. Presented at Clinical Conference, University of Oklahoma School of Medicine, Oklahoma City, Ok., Nov. 1967.

1092. Richards, R.H., and Clark, N.M.P.: Locked Posterior Fracture–Dislocation of the Shoulder. Injury, 20:297–300, 1989.

1093. Richards, R.R.; Hudson, A.R.; Bertoia, J.T.; Urbaniak, J.R.; and Waddell, J.P.: Injury to the Brachial Plexus During Putti-Platt and Bristow Procedures: A Report of Eight Cases. Am. J. Sports Med., 15:374–380, 1987.

1094. Richards, R.R.; Waddell, J.P.; and Hudson, M.B.: Shoulder Arthrodesis for the Treatment of Brachial Plexus Palsy: A Review of Twenty-Two Patients. Presented at the 3rd Open Meeting of the American Shoulder and Elbow Surgeons, San Francisco, Calif., 1987.

1095. Richardson, A.B.: Arthroscopic Anatomy of the Shoulder. Techniques Orthop., 3:1–7, 1988.

1096. Riel, K.A.; Paar, O.; and Bernett, P.: [Experiences With Derotation of the Humeral Head According to Weber in Recurrent Dislocation of the Shoulder.] Aktuel Traumatol., 14:169–171, 1984.

1097. Rob, C.G., and Standeven, A.: Closed Traumatic Lesions of the Axillary and Brachial Arteries. Lancet, 1:597–599, 1956.

1098. Roberts, A., and Wickstrom, J.: Prognosis of Posterior Dislocation of the Shoulder. Acta Orthop. Scand., 42:328–337, 1971.

1099. Robertson, R., and Stark, W.J.: Diagnosis and Treatment of Recurrent Dislocation of the Shoulder. J. Bone Joint Surg., 29:797–800, 1947.

1100. Robertson, T.S.: Results of the Magnuson-Stack Operation for Recurrent Anterior Dislocation of the Shoulder. Am. J. Surg., 87:761, 1954.

1101. Robertson, W.C.; Eichman, P.L.; and Clancy, W.G.: Upper Trunk Brachial Plexopathy in Football Players. J.A.M.A., 241:1480–1482, 1979.

1102. Roca, L.A., and Ramos-Vertiz, J.R.: Luxacion Erecta de Hombro. Rev. Sanid. Mil. Arg., 61:135, 1962.

1103. Rockwood, C.A., Jr.; Burkhead, W.Z., Jr.; and Brna, J.: Subluxation of the Glenohumeral Joint: Response to Rehabilitative Exercise: Traumatic Versus Atraumatic Instability. Orthop. Trans., 10:220–221, 1986.

1104. Rockwood, C.A., Jr.: Dislocations About the Shoulder. In Rockwood, C.A., Jr., and Green, D.P. (eds.): Fractures, 2nd ed., Vol. 1, pp. 722–985. Philadelphia, J.B. Lippincott, 1984.

1105. Rockwood, C.A., Jr., and Gerber, C.: Analysis of Failed Surgical Procedures for Anterior Shoulder Instability. Orthop. Trans., 9:48, 1985.

1106. Rockwood, C.A., Jr., and Matsen, F.A., III (eds.): The Shoulder. Philadelphia, W.B. Saunders, 1990.

1107. Rockwood, C.A., Jr., and Young, D.C.: Complications and Management of the Failed Bristow Shoulder Reconstructions. Orthop. Trans., 13(2):232, 1989.

1108. Rockwood, C.A., Jr.: Capsular Reconstruction for Shoulder Instability. Orthopedics Today, 6:20, 1986.

1109. Rockwood, C.A., Jr.: Differential Diagnosis of Shoulder Dislocation. Instructional Course Presented at the Annual Meeting of the American Academy of Orthopedic Surgeons, Atlanta, GA, Feb. 9–14, 1984.

1110. Rockwood, C.A., Jr.: Management of Posterior Shoulder Instability. Instructional Course Presented at the Annual Meeting of the American Academy of Orthopaedic Surgeons, San Francisco, CA, Jan. 22–27, 1987.

1111. Rockwood, C.A., Jr.: Posterior Dislocations of the Shoulder (abstract). J. Bone Joint Surg., 62B:271, 1980.

1111a. Rockwood, C.A., Jr.: Shoulder Arthroscopy (editorial). J. Bone Joint Surg., 70A:639–640, 1988.

1112. Rockwood, C.A., Jr.: Shoulder Arthroscopy—A Critical Review. J. Bone Joint Surg., 70A:639–640, 1988.

1113. Rockwood, C.A., Jr.: Subluxation of the Shoulder—The Classification, Diagnosis and Treatment. Orthop. Trans., 4:306, 1979.

1114. Rockwood, C.A., Jr.: The Subluxating Shoulder: The Diagnosis, Classification and Treatment (abstract). J. Bone Joint Surg., 62B:281–282, 1980.

1115. Rockwood, C.A., Jr.: The Diagnosis of Acute Posterior Dislocations of the Shoulder (abstract). J. Bone Joint Surg., 48A:1220–1221, 1966.

1116. Rojvanit, V.: Arthroscopy of the Shoulder Joint—A Cadaver and Clinical Study—Part 1: Cadaver Study. J. Jpn. Orthop. Assoc., 58:1035–1046, 1984.

1117. Rojvanit, V.: Arthroscopy of the Shoulder Joint—A Cadaver and Clinical Study—Part II: Clinical Study. J. Jpn. Orthop. Assoc., 58:1047–1057, 1984.

1118. Rokous, J.R.; Feagin, J.A.; and Abbott, H.G.: Modified Axillary Roentgenogram: A Useful Adjunct in the Diagnosis of Recurrent Instability of the Shoulder. Clin. Orthop., 82:84–86, 1972.

1119. Rollins, C.A., and Robinson, J.L.: Evaluation of Undergraduate Physical Therapy Students' Comprehension of Maitland's Grades (I–IV) for Posterior Mobilization of the Glenohumeral Joint. J. Orthop. Sports Phys. Ther., 1:214–221, 1980.

1120. Rollinson, P.D.: Reduction of Shoulder Dislocations by the Hanging Method. S. Afr. Med. J., 73:106–107, 1988.

1121. Romanes, G.J. (ed.): Cunningham's Textbook of Anatomy, 11th ed. London, Oxford University Press, 1972.

1122. Romanes, G.J.: Upper and Lower Limbs. In Cunningham's Manual of Practical Anatomy, 13th ed., pp. 75–76. London, Oxford University Press, 1966.

1123. Rorabeck, C.H.: Factors Affecting the Prognosis of Brachial Plexus Injuries. J. Bone Joint Surg., 63B:404–407, 1981.

1124. Rosaaen, B.J., and Delisa, J.A.: Voluntary Anterior Dislocation of the Shoulder: Case Study. Arch. Phys. Med. Rehabil., 64:326–328, 1983.

1125. Roston, J.B., and Haines, R.W.: Cracking in the Metacarpophalangeal Joint. J. Anat., 81:165–173, 1947.

1126. Rothman, R.H.; Marvel, P.J.; and Heppenstall, R.B.: Recurrent Anterior Dislocation of the Shoulder. Orthop. Clin. North Am., 6:415, 1975.

1127. Rowe, C.R.; Patel, D.; and Southmayd, W.W.: The Bankart Procedure—A Study of the Late Results (abstract). J. Bone Joint Surg., 59B:122, 1977.

1128. Rowe, C.R.; Patel, D.; and Southmayd, W.W.: The Bankart Procedure: A Long-Term End-Result Study. J. Bone Joint Surg., 60A:1–16, 1978.

1129. Rowe, C.R.; Pierce, D.S.; and Clark, J.G.: Voluntary Dislocation of the Shoulder: A Preliminary Report on a Clinical, Electromyographic, and Psychiatric Study of Twenty-Six Patients. J. Bone Joint Surg., 55:445–460, 1973.

1130. Rowe, C.R., and Pierce, D.S.: The Enigma of Voluntary Recurrent Dislocation of the Shoulder (abstract). J. Bone Joint Surg., 47A:1670, 1965.

1131. Rowe, C.R., and Sakellarides, H.T.: Factors Related to Recurrences of Anterior Dislocations of the Shoulder. Clin. Orthop., 20:40–47, 1961.

1132. Rowe, C.R., and Yee, L.K.: A Posterior Approach to the Shoulder Joint. J. Bone Joint Surg., 26:580–584, 1944.

1133. Rowe, C.R.; Zarins, B.; and Ciullo, J.V.: Recurrent Anterior Dislocation of the Shoulder After Surgical Repair: Apparent Causes of Failure and Treatment. J. Bone Joint Surg., 66A:159–168, 1984.

1134. Rowe, C.R., and Zarins, B.: Chronic Unreduced Dislocations of the Shoulder. J. Bone Joint Surg., 64A:494–505, 1982.

1135. Rowe, C.R., and Zarins, B.: Recurrent Transient Subluxation of the Shoulder. J. Bone Joint Surg., 63A:863–872, 1981.

1136. Rowe, C.R.: A Posterior Approach to the Shoulder Joint. J. Bone Joint Surg., 26:580–584, 1944.

1137. Rowe, C.R.: Acute and Recurrent Dislocations of the Shoulder. J. Bone Joint Surg., 44A:998–1008, 1962.

1138. Rowe, C.R.: Acute and Recurrent Anterior Dislocations of the Shoulder. Orthop. Clin. North Am., 11:253–269, 1980.

1139. Rowe, C.R.: Anterior and Posterior Dislocations of the Shoulder: Pitfalls and Complications. Personal communication, 1987.

1140. Rowe, C.R.: Anterior Dislocations of the Shoulder: Prognosis and Treatment. Surg. Clin. North Am., 43:1609–1614, 1963.

1141. Rowe, C.R.: Complicated Dislocations of the Shoulder: Guidelines in Treatment. Am. J. Surg., 117:549–553, 1969.

1142. Rowe, C.R.: Failed Surgical Repair for Recurrent Dislocations of the Shoulder. Instr. Course Lect., XXXIV:264–267, 1985.

1143. Rowe, C.R.: Instabilities of the Glenohumeral Joint. Bull. Hosp. Joint Dis. Orthop. Inst., 39:180–186, 1978.

1144. Rowe, C.R.: Prognosis in Dislocations of the Shoulder. J. Bone Joint Surg., 38A:957–977, 1956.

1145. Rowe, C.R.: Recurrent Transient Subluxation of the Shoulder: The ''Dead Arm'' Syndrome. Clin. Orthop., 223:11–19, 1987.

1146. Rowe, C.R.: Symposium on Surgical Lesions of the Shoulder. J. Bone Joint Surg., 38A:977–1012, 1956.

1147. Rowe, C.R.: The Results of Operative Treatment of Recurrent Dislocation of the Shoulder. Surg. Clin. North Am., 43:1667–1670, 1963.

1148. Rowe, C.R.: The Surgical Management of Recurrent Anterior Dislocations of the Shoulder Using a Modified Bankart Procedure. Surg. Clin. North Am., 43:1663–1666, 1963.

1149. Royle, G.: Treatment of Acute Anterior Dislocation of the Shoulder. Br. J. Clin. Pract., 27:403–404, 1973.

1150. Rozing, P.M.; DeBakker, H.M.; and Obermann, W.R.: Radiographic Views in Recurrent Anterior Shoulder Dislocation: Comparison of Six Methods for Identification of Typical Lesions. Acta Orthop. Scand., 57:328–330, 1986.

1151. Rubenstein, J.: The Bent Screw: A Sign of Postoperative Recurrent Dislocation. J. Can. Assoc. Radiol., 38:20–22, 1987.

1152. Rubin, S.A.; Gray, R.L.; and Green, W.R.: The Scapular ''Y'': A Diagnostic Aid in Shoulder Trauma. Radiology, 110:725–726, 1974.

1153. Reference deleted.

1154. Rugtveit, A.: Recurrent Posterior Shoulder Dislocation Treated by the Transposition of Pectoralis Minor to the Anterior Bicipital Ridge (abstract). Acta Orthop. Scand., 48:232, 1977.

1155. Rupp, F.: Uber ein vereinfachtes Operationsverfahren bei habitueller Schulterluxation. Dtsch. Z. Chir., 198:70–75, 1926.

1156. Russell, J.A.; Holmes, E.M., III; Keller, D.J.; and Vargas, J.H., III: Reduction of Acute Anterior Shoulder Dislocations Using the Milch Technique: A Study of Ski Injuries. J. Trauma, 21:802–804, 1981.

1157. Ryan, A.J.: Recurrent Dislocation of Shoulder. J.A.M.A., 195:173, 1966.

1158. Saether, J.: The Results of the Bristow and Bristow-Latarjet Procedure for Recurrent Dislocation of the Shoulder (abstract). Acta Orthop. Scand., 56:544, 1985.

1159. Saha, A.K.; Bhadra, N.; and Dutta, S.K.: Latissimus Dorsi Transfer for Recurrent Dislocation of the Shoulder. Acta Orthop. Scand., 57:539–541, 1986.

1160. Saha, A.K.; Das, N.N.; and Chakravarty, B.G.: Treatment of Recurrent Dislocation of Shoulder: Past, Present, and Future—Studies on Electromyographic Changes of Muscles Acting on the Shoulder Joint Complex. Calcutta Med. J., 53:409–413, 1956.

1161. Saha, A.K.: Anterior Recurrent Dislocation of the Shoulder: Treatment by Latissimus Dorsi Transfer With Follow-Up of 22 Cases. J. Int. Coll. Surg., 39:361–373, 1963.

1162. Saha, A.K.: Anterior Recurrent Dislocation of the Shoulder. Acta Orthop. Scand., 38:479–493, 1967.

1163. Saha, A.K.: Dynamic Stability of the Glenohumeral Joint. Acta Orthop. Scand., 42:491–505, 1971.

1164. Saha, A.K.: Mechanics of Elevation of Glenohumeral Joint: Its Application in Rehabilitation of Flail Shoulder in Upper Brachial Plexus Injuries and Poliomyelitis and in Replacement of the Upper Humerus by Prosthesis. Acta Orthop. Scand., 44:668–678, 1973.

1165. Saha, A.K.: Mechanism of Shoulder Movements and a Plea for the Recognition of ''Zero Position'' of Glenohumeral Joint. Indian J. Surg., 12:153–165, 1950.

1166. Saha, A.K.: Recurrent Anterior Dislocation of the Shoulder: A New Concept. Calcutta, Academic Publishers, 1969.

1167. Saha, A.K.: Recurrent Dislocation of the Shoulder, 2nd ed. New York, Thieme-Stratton, 1981.

1168. Saha, A.K.: Surgery of the Paralyzed and Flail Shoulder. Acta Orthop. Scand. [Suppl.] 97:5–90, 1967.

1169. Saha, A.K.: Theory of Shoulder Mechanism. Springfield, Ill., Charles C. Thomas, 1961.

1170. Said, G.Z., and Medbø, I.: Glenoidplasty as a Treatment for Recurrent Anterior Dislocation of the Shoulder. Acta Orthop. Scand., 40:777–787, 1970.

1171. Saillant, G.; Henry, P.; Doursounian, L.; Lazennec, J.Y.; and Roy-Camille, R.: [Extra-Coracoid Axillary Approach to the Humeral Joint.] Presse Med., 16:1649–1652, 1987.

1172. Salem, M.I.: Bilateral Anterior Fracture–Dislocation of the Shoulder Joints Due to Severe Electric Shock. Injury, 14:361–363, 1983.

1173. Salo-Orfila, J.M.: [Glenoid Osteotomy for Bilateral Spontaneous Posterior Dislocation of the Shoulder: A Report of Two Cases.] Rev. Chir. Orthop., 71:51–54, 1985.

1174. Samilson, R.L., and Miller, E.: Posterior Dislocations of the Shoulder. Clin. Orthop., 32:69–86, 1964.

1175. Samilson, R.L., and Prieto, V.: Dislocation Arthropathy of the Shoulder. J. Bone Joint Surg., 65A:456–460, 1983.

1176. Samilson, R.L.: Dislocation Arthropathy of the Shoulder. J. Bone Joint Surg., 65A:456–460, 1983.

1177. Samilson, R.L.: Severe Degenerative Arthritis of the Shoulder Following Repair of Recurrent Anterior Shoulder Dislocations (abstract). J. Bone Joint Surg., 64A:634, 1982.

1178. Sanders, R.J.: Treatment of Recurrent Anterior Dislocation of the Shoulders by the Bankart and Putti-Platt Techniques (abstract). Acta Orthop. Scand., 55:485, 1984.

1179. Sankaran-Kutty, M., and Sadat-Ali, M.: Dislocation of the Shoulder With Ipsilateral Humeral Shaft Fracture. Arch. Orthop. Trauma Surg., 108:60–62, 1989.

1180. Sarkar, M.R.; Nastragelopulos, N.; and Pfister, U.: Luxatio

Erecta: A Rare Variant of Subglenoid Shoulder Dislocation. Unfallchirurg., 92(1):17–20, 1989.

1181. Sarma, A.; Saranchak, H.H.; Levinson, E.D.; and Sigman, R.: Thrombosis of the Axillary Artery and Brachial Plexus Injury Secondary to Shoulder Dislocation. Conn. Med., 45:513–514, 1981.

1182. Savornin, C.; Casanova, G.; Bisserie, P.; Chauvet, J.; and Willems, P.: [The Treatment of Recurrent Antero-Medial Dislocation of the Shoulder: A Report of Eighty-Five Cases Treated by a Variant of Bankart's Operation.] Ann. Chir., 41:216–221, 1987.

1183. Saxena, K., and Stavas, J.: Inferior Glenohumeral Dislocation. Ann. Emerg. Med., 12:718–720, 1983.

1184. Scaglietti, O.: The Obstetrical Shoulder Trauma. Surg. Gynecol. Obstet., 66:868–877, 1938.

1185. Scapinelli, R.: Sul Trattamento Chirurgico Della Lussazione Abituale Posteriore Della Spalla. Clin. Orthop., 24:234–240, 1973.

1186. Schellnack, K.; Buttner, K.; Garz, G.; and Paul, U.: [Operative Treatment of Recurrent Habitual and Permanent Dislocation of the Shoulder.] Beitr. Orthop. Traumatol., 30:512–519, 1983.

1187. Schlemm, F.: Ueber die Verstarkungsbander am Schultergelenk. Arch. Anat. Physiol. Wissenschaft. Med., pp. 45–48, 1853.

1188. Schmidt, G.R.; Dueland, R.; and Vaughan, J.T.: Osteochondrosis Dissecans of the Equine Shoulder Joint. Vet. Med. Sm. Animal Clin., 70:542–547, 1975.

1189. Schmitt, E.; Heisel, J.; and Mittelmeier, H.: [Results of the Operative Treatment of the Recurrent Shoulder Dislocation With a Modified Technique According to Eden-Lange.] Orthop. Praxis, 21:512–520, 1985.

1190. Schobert, W.E.: Shoulder Arthroscopy: Orientation and Landmarks. Techniques Orthop., 3:15–21, 1988.

1191. Schöllner, D.: Habituelle Subluxationen an Schulter und Handgelenken—therapeutische Konsequenzen. Orthop. Praxis, 2:143–145, 1981.

1192. Schrøder, H.A., and Fristed, P.B.: Recurrent Dislocation of the Shoulder: The Alvik Modification of the Eden-Hybinette Operation. Acta Orthop. Scand., 56:396–399, 1985.

1193. Schüller, M.: Berlin Klin. Wochenschr., 33:760, 1896.

1194. Schulz, T.J.; Jacobs, B.; and Patterson, R.L.: Unrecognized Dislocations of the Shoulder. J. Trauma, 9:1009–1023, 1969.

1195. Schwartz, D.I.: Bankart Shoulder Repair Made Easier (abstract). J. Bone Joint Surg., 45A:1334, 1963.

1196. Schwartz, D.I.: Bankart Shoulder Repair Made Easier: A Letter to Dr. Johnson. Clin. Orthop., 56:69–72, 1968.

1197. Schwartz, E.; Warren, R.F.; O'Brien, J.S.; and Fronek, J.: Posterior Shoulder Instability. Orthop. Clin. North Am., 18:409–419, 1987.

1198. Schwartz, R.E.; O'Brien, S.J.; Warren, R.F.; and Torzilli, P.A.: Capsular Restraints to Anterior-Posterior Motion in the Shoulder. Orthop. Trans., 12(3):727, Fall, 1988.

1199. Reference deleted.

1200. Scott, D.J., Jr.: Treatment of Recurrent Posterior Dislocation of the Shoulder by Glenoplasty: Report of Three Cases. J. Bone Joint Surg., 49A:471–476, 1967.

1201. Scott, J.M., and Mackenney, R.D.: Neurological Complications of Dislocation of the Shoulder (abstract). J. Bone Joint Surg., 67:496, 1985.

1202. Scougall, S.: Posterior Dislocation of the Shoulder. J. Bone Joint Surg., 39B:726–732, 1957.

1203. Scovazzo, M.L.; Lombardo, S.J.; and Esposito, R.M.: The Modified Bristow Procedure: A 10–12 Year Follow-Up. Personal communication, May 1989.

1204. Seddon, H.J.: Nerve Lesions Complicating Certain Closed Bone Injuries. J.A.M.A., 135:691–694, 1947.

1205. Seeger, L.L.; Gold, R.H.; and Bassett, L.W.: Shoulder Instability: Evaluation With MR Imaging. Radiology, 168:695–697, 1988.

1206. Segal, D.; Yablon, I.G.; Lynch, J.J.; and Jones, R.P.: Acute Bilateral Anterior Dislocation of the Shoulders. Clin. Orthop., 140:21–22, 1979.

1207. Seiler, H.; Neumann, K.; and Muhr, G.: [Arthroscopy of the Shoulder Joint.] Unfallheilkunde, 87:73–77, 1984.

1208. Self, E.B., Jr.: Ligamentous Laxity. Personal communication, January 18, 1979.

1209. Seltzer, S.E., and Weissman, B.N.: CT Findings in Normal and Dislocating Shoulders. J. Can. Assoc. Radiol., 36:41–46, 1985.

1210. Seradge, H., and Orme, G.: Acute Irreducible Anterior Dislocation of the Shoulder. J. Trauma, 22:330–332, 1982.

1211. Sergio, G.: Recurrent Anterior Dislocation of the Shoulder Joint: A Modification of Bankart's Capsulopexy: Notes on the Surgical Technique. Ital. J. Orthop. Traumatol., 9:469, 1983.

1212. Sever, J.W.: Fracture of the Head of the Humerus: Treatment and Results. N. Engl. J. Med., 216:1100–1107, 1937.

1213. Sever, J.W.: Obstetrical Paralysis. Surg. Gynecol. Obstet., 44:547–549, 1927.

1214. Sever, J.W.: Recurrent Dislocation of the Shoulder Joint: A Mechanical Consideration of Its Treatment. J.A.M.A., 76:925–927, 1921.

1215. Severin, E.: Anterior and Posterior Recurrent Dislocation of the Shoulder: The Putti-Platt Operation. Acta Orthop. Scand., 23:14–22, 1954.

1216. Seyfarth, H., and Irlenbusch, U.: Indikation und Technik unterschiedlicher operationsverfahren bei habituellen und rezidivierenden Schulterluxationen. In Chapchal, G. (ed.): Internationales Symposium uber spezielle Fragen der orthopadischen Chirurgie, pp. 153–155. Stuttgart, Georg Thieme Verlag, 1984.

1217. Shackelford, H.L.: Hydraulic Stretcher Reduction Technique for Anterior Dislocation of the Shoulder. W. Va. Med. J., 78:9, 1982.

1218. Shands, A.R., Jr.: An Analysis of the More Important Orthopedic Information. Surg., 16:569–616, 1944.

1219. Shaw, J.T.: Bilateral Posterior Fracture–Dislocation of the Shoulder and Other Trauma Caused by Convulsive Seizures. J. Bone Joint Surg., 53A:1437–1440, 1971.

1220. Shepherd, E.: Simultaneous Posterior Dislocation of Both Shoulders. J. Bone Joint Surg., 42B:728–729, 1960.

1221. Shively, J., and Johnson, J.: Results of Modified Bristow Procedure. Clin. Orthop., 187:150–153, 1984.

1222. Shuman, W.P.; Kilcoyne, R.F.; Matsen, F.A.; Rogers, J.V.; and Mack, L.A.: Double-Contrast Computed Tomography of the Glenoid Labrum. A.J.R., 141:581–584, 1983.

1223. Shvartzman, P., and Guy, N.: Voluntary Dislocation of Shoulder. Postgrad. Med., 84:265–271, 1988.

1224. Sidles, J.A.; Harryman, D.T.; Simkin, P.A.; et al: Passive and Active Stabilization of the Glenohumeral Joint. J. Bone Joint Surg., (submitted for publication, 1989).

1225. Silfverskiold, N.: On Operative Treatment of Habitual Dislocation of the Shoulder. Acta Orthop. Scand., 4:83–84, 1933.

1226. Sillar, P.: [Surgical Treatment of Habitual Posterior Dislocation of the Shoulder Joint.] Magy Traumatol. Orthop. Helyreallito. Sebesz., 15:146–150, 1972.

1227. Simkin, P.A.: Structure and Function of Joints. In Schumacher, H.R. (ed.): Primer on the Rheumatic Diseases, 9th ed. Atlanta, Ga., Arthritis Foundation, 1988.

1228. Simonet, W.T., and Cofield, R.H.: Prognosis in Anterior Shoulder Dislocation. Am. J. Sports Med., 12:19–23, 1984.

1229. Simonet, W.T.; Melton, L.J., III; Cofield, R.H.; and Ilstrup, D.M.: Incidence of Anterior Shoulder Dislocation in Olmsted County, Minnesota. Clin. Orthop., 186–191, 1984.

1230. Sing, R.F.: Shoulder Injuries in the Javelin Thrower. J.A.O.A., 83:107–111, 1984.

1231. Singson, R.D., and Bigliani, L.U.: CT Arthrographic Patterns in Recurrent Glenohumeral Instability. A.J.R., 149:749–753, 1987.

1232. Singson, R.D.; Feldman, F.; Bigliani, L.U.; and Rosenberg, Z.S.: Recurrent Shoulder Dislocation After Surgical Repair: Double-Contrast CT Arthrography. Radiology, 164:425–428, 1987.

1233. Sisk, T.D., and Boyd, H.B.: Management of Recurrent Anterior Dislocation of the Shoulder: du Toit Type or Staple Capsulorrhaphy. Clin. Orthop., 103:150–156, 1974.

1234. Sisk, T.D.: Campbell's Operative Orthopaedics, 6th ed., pp. 662–670. St. Louis, C.V. Mosby, 1980.

1235. Sjovall, H.: [A Case of Spontaneous Backward Subluxation of the Shoulder Treated by the Clairmont-Ehrlich Operation.] Nord. Med., 21:474–476, 1944.

1236. Skoglund, L.B., and Sundt, P.: Recurrent Anterior Dislocation of the Shoulder: The Eden-Hybbinette Operation. Acta Orthop. Scand., 44:739–747, 1973.

1237. Slawski, D.P.; Rich, M.M.; and Gilula, L.A.: Luxatio Erecta in a 15-Year-Old Boy. Orthop. Rev., 18:481–486, 1989.

1238. Slivka, J., and Resnick, D.: An Improved Radiographic View of the Glenohumeral Joint. J. Can. Assoc. Radiol., 30:83–85, 1979.

1239. Smith, J.F., and Christensen, H.H.: Deltoid-Paralysis Following Shoulder Injuries. Surg. Gynecol. Obstet., 41:451–453, 1925.

1240. Smith, R.G.; Cruikshank, J.G.; Dunbar, S.; and Akhtar, A.J.: Malalignment of the Shoulder After Stroke. Br. Med. J., 284:1224–1226, 1982.

1241. Smith, W.S., and Klug, T.J.: Anterior Dislocation of the Shoulder—A Simple and Effective Method of Reduction. J.A.M.A., 163:182–183, 1957.

1242. Snell, R.W.; Erickson, T.L.; Mess, D.J.; Watt, D.H.; Thomas, L.; Schmitz, N.C.; and Malinick, R.L.: Reduction of Anterior Shoulder Dislocations With Use of a Modified Kocher Maneuver. Orthopedics, 6:1439–1442, 1983.

1243. Snyder, S.J., and Pattee, G.A.: Shoulder Arthroscopy in the Evaluation and Treatment of Rotator Cuff Lesions. Techniques Orthop., 3:47–58, 1988.

1244. Snyder, S.J.: Arthroscopic Acromioclavicular Joint Debridement and Distal Clavicle Resection. Techniques Orthop., 3:41–45, 1988.

1245. Snyder, S.J.: Arthroscopic Diagnosis of Chronic Shoulder Pain. Orthopedics Today, 7:5, 1987.

1246. Spangler, H., and Zwerina, H.: [Treatment of Old Posterior Shoulder Dislocation.] Klin. Med. Osterr. Z. Wiss. Prakt. Med., 22:557–559, 1967.

1247. Speed, K.: A Textbook of Fractures and Dislocations, 2nd ed. Philadelphia, Lea & Febiger, 1928.

1248. Speed, K.: Fractures and Dislocations, 4th ed. Philadelphia, Lea & Febiger, 1942.

1249. Speed, K.: Recurrent Anterior Dislocation at the Shoulder: Operative Cure by Bone Graft. Surg. Gynecol. Obstet., 44:468–477, 1927.

1250. Spence, A.J.: European Travelling Scholarship, 1959 (report). J. Bone Joint Surg., 43B:176–179, 1961.

1251. St. John, F.B.; Scudder, J.; and Stevens, D.L.: Spontaneous Rupture of Axillary Artery. Ann. Surg., 121:882–890, 1945.

1252. Staffel, F.: Verh. Dtsch. Ges. Chir., 24:651–656, 1895.

1253. Staples, O.S., and Watkins, A.L.: Full Active Abduction in Traumatic Paralysis of the Deltoid. J. Bone Joint Surg., 25:89, 1943.

1253A. Steel, J.: Personal communication, 1984.

1254. Steenburg, R.W., and Ravitch, M.M.: Cervicothoracic Approach for Subclavian Vessel Injury From Compound Fracture of the Clavicle: Considerations of Subclavian Axillary Exposures. Ann. Surg., 157:839–846, 1963.

1255. Stein, E.: Case Report 374—Diagnosis: Post-Traumatic Pseudoaneurysm of Axillary Artery. Skeletal Radiol., 15:391–393, 1986.

1256. Stener, B.: Dislocation of the Shoulder Complicated by Complete Rupture of the Axillary Artery: Successful Suture of the Artery in an Eighty-Seven-Year-Old Man. J. Bone Joint Surg., 39B:714–717, 1957.

1257. Steno, M.; Majesky, B.; Kordos, J.; and Blasko, I.: [Our Experience With the Surgical Treatment of Habitual Dislocation of the Shoulder.] Acta Chir. Ortop. Traumatol. Cech., 51:400–403, 1984.

1258. Stevens, J.H.: Brachial Plexus Paralysis. In Codman, E.A.: The Shoulder. Brooklyn, G. Miller, 1934.

1259. Stilli, S.: Spontaneous Anterior and Posterior Subluxation of the Shoulder (Case Presentation). Ital. J. Orthop. Traumatol., 6:293–294, 1980.

1260. Stimson, L.A.: An Easy Method of Reducing Dislocations of the Shoulder and Hip. Med. Record, 57:356–357, 1900.

1261. Stimson, L.A.: Dislocations of the Shoulder. In A Practical

Treatise on Fractures and Dislocations, 7th ed. Philadelphia, Lea Brothers, pp. 607–678, 1912.

1264. Stimson, L.A.: Five Cases of Dislocation of the Hip. N.Y. Med. J., 50:118–121, 1889.

1265. Stimson, L.A.: Fractures and Dislocations, 3rd ed. Philadelphia, Lea Brothers, 1900.

1266. Strauss, M.B.; Wrobel, L.J.; Cady, G.W.; and Neff, R.S.: Radiological Confirmation of Anterior Shoulder Instability (unpublished paper). Dept. of Orthopaedics, Naval Regional Med. Center, San Diego, CA, 1974.

1267. Strauss, M.B.; Wrobel, L.J.; Neff, R.S.; and Cady, G.W.: The Shrugged-Off Shoulder: A Comparison of Patients With Recurrent Shoulder Subluxations and Dislocations. Physician Sports Med., 12:85–97, 1983.

1268. Strauss, M.B.: The Shoulder—Roentgenological Evaluation of Recurrent Anterior Instability (unpublished paper).

1269. Stright, P.A.: How to Help the Patient With a Dislocated Shoulder. Am. J. Nurs., 79:666–669, 1979.

1270. Stromqvist, B.; Wingstrand, H.; and Egund, N.: Recurrent Shoulder Dislocation and Screw Failure After the Bristow-Latarjet Procedure: A Case Report. Arch. Orthop. Trauma Surg., 106:260–262, 1987.

1271. Stromsoe, K.; Senn, E.; Simmen, B.; and Matter, P.: [Recurrent Frequency After the First Traumatic Shoulder Dislocation.] Helv. Chir. Acta, 47:85–88, 1980.

1272. Struhl, S., and Sadler, A.: Shoulder Arthrodesis for End-Stage Multidirectional Instability. Orthop. Grand Rounds, 5(2):2–5, June, 1988.

1273. Stufflesser, H., and Dexel, M.: The Treatment of Recurrent Dislocation of the Shoulder by Rotation Osteotomy With Internal Fixation. Ital. J. Orthop. Traumatol., 39: 191, 1977.

1274. Sturzenegger, M., and Gumppenberg, S.: Bilateral Shoulder Dislocation Fractures, Femoral Neck and Vertebral Fractures: A Remarkable Combination of Injuries During an Epileptic Seizure (abstract). Aktuel Traumatol., 15:180–183, 1985.

1275. Sudarov, Z.: The Results of the Modified Nosske-Oudard-Bazy-Savic Operation for Recurrent Dislocation of the Shoulder (abstract). J. Bone Joint Surg., 48B:855, 1966.

1276. Sutro, C.J., and Sutro, W.: Delayed Complications of Treated Reduced Recurrent Anterior Dislocations of the Humeral Head in Young Adults: With a Pictoral Review of the Components of the Normal Shoulder Joint as a Basis for Comparison. Bull. Hosp. Joint Dis. Orthop. Inst., 42:187–216, 1982.

1277. Sverdlov, I.M.; Arenberg, A.A.; and Ahitnitsky, R.E.: Voluntary Subluxation of the Shoulder. Central Institute of Traumatology and Orthopaedics, 1962.

1278. Sweeney, J.H.; Mead, N.C.; and Dawson, W.J.: Fourteen Years' Experience With the Modified Bristow Procedure. Presented at the Annual Meeting of the American Academy of Orthopaedic Surgeons, San Francisco, Calif., March 1–6, 1975.

1279. Swickard, J.S.: Treatment of Initial Traumatic Anterior Dislocation of the Shoulder in the High School Athlete or Young Athlete (letter to the editor). Am. J. Sports Med., 11:49, 1983.

1280. Symeonides, P.P.: Reconsideration of the Putti-Platt Procedure and Its Mode of Action in Recurrent Traumatic Anterior Dislocation of the Shoulder. Clin. Orthop., 246: 8–15, 1989.

1281. Symeonides, P.P.: The Significance of the Subscapularis Muscle in the Pathogenesis of Recurrent Anterior Dislocation of the Shoulder. J. Bone Joint Surg., 54B:476–483, 1972.

1282. Tagliabue, D., and Esposito, A.: [Latarjet's Operation in Recurrent Dislocation of the Shoulder in Athletes.] Ital. J. Sports Traumatol., 2:91–100, 1980.

1283. Tagliabue, D., and Valsecchi, A.: [Results of the Latarjet Technique in the Treatment of Recurrent Shoulder Luxation.] Minerva Ortop. Traumatol., 39:651–654, 1988.

1284. Taketomi, Y.: Observations on Subluxation of the Shoulder Joint in Hemiplegia. Phys. Ther., 55:39–40, 1975.

1285. Tanzman, M.; Segev, Z.; and Kaufman, B.: [Missed Bilateral Anterior Dislocation of the Shoulder Following Convulsions.] Harefuah, 105:266–295, 1983.

1286. Tavernier, L.: The Recurrent Luxation of the Shoulder (news notes). J. Bone Joint Surg., 12:458–461, 1930.

1287. Taylor, R.G., and Wright, P.R.: Posterior Dislocation of the Shoulder: Report of Six Cases. J. Bone Joint Surg., 34B:624–629, 1952.

1288. Teitge, R.A., and Ciullo, J.V.: CAM Axillary X-Ray Exhibit. Orthop. Trans., 6:451, 1982.

1289. Thomas, M.A.: Posterior Subacromial Dislocation of the Head of the Humerus. A.J.R., 37:767–773, 1937.

1290. Thomas, S.C., and Matsen, F.A., III: An Approach to the Repair of Avulsion of the Glenohumeral Ligaments in the Management of Traumatic Anterior Glenohumeral Instability. J. Bone Joint Surg., 71A:506–513, 1989.

1291. Thomas, T.T.: Habitual or Recurrent Anterior Dislocation of the Shoulder. I. Etiology and Pathology. Am. J. Med. Sci., 137:229–246, 1909.

1292. Thomas, T.T.: Habitual or Recurrent Dislocation of the Shoulder: Forty-Four Shoulders Operated on in Forty-Two Patients. Surg. Gynecol. Obstet., 32:291–299, 1921.

1293. Thomasen, E.: Habitual Dislocation of the Shoulder: A Study on the Nature and Treatment of the Disease Including Remarks on Traumatic Dislocation. Acta Orthop. Scand., 15:206–248, 1944.

1294. Thompson, F.R., and Moga, J.J.: The Combined Operative Repair of Anterior and Posterior Shoulder Subluxation. Audiovisual program, Annual Meeting of the American Academy of Orthopaedic Surgeons, New York, NY, Jan. 10, 1965.

1295. Thompson, F.R., and Winant, W.M.: Unusual Fracture–Subluxations of the Shoulder Joint. J. Bone Joint Surg., 32A:575–582, 1950.

1296. Thompson, F.R., and Winant, W.M.: Comminuted Fractures of the Humeral Head With Subluxation. Clin. Orthop., 20:94–96, 1961.

1297. Thompson, J.E.: Anatomical Methods of Approach in Operations on the Long Bones of the Extremities. Ann. Surg., 68:309–329, 1918.

1298. Tibone, J.E.; Prietto, C.; Jobe, F.W.; Kerlan, R.W.; Carter, V.S.; Shields, C.L., Jr.; Lombardo, S.J.; Collins, H.R.; and

Yocum, L.A.: Staple Capsulorrhaphy for Recurrent Posterior Shoulder Dislocation. Am. J. Sports Med., 9:135–139, 1981.

1299. Tibone, J.E.: Posterior Capsulorrhaphy for Posterior Shoulder Subluxation in Athletes. Techniques Orthop., 3:46–50, 1989.

1300. Tietjen, R.: Occult Glenohumeral Interposition of a Torn Rotator Cuff: A Case Report. J. Bone Joint Surg., 64A:458–459, 1982.

1301. Tijmes, J.; Loyd, H.M.; and Tullos, H.S.: Arthrography in Acute Shoulder Dislocations. South. Med. J., 72:564–567, 1979.

1302. Tkachenko, C.C.: [Modified Nicola Anterior Reconstruction.] Ortop. Travmatol. Protez., 7:57–59, 1979.

1303. Tobis, J.S.: Posthemiplegia Shoulder Pain. N.Y. State J. Med., 57:1377–1380, 1957.

1304. Torg, J.S.; Balduini, F.C.; Bonci, C.; Lehman, R.C.; Gregg, J.R.; Esterhai, J.L.; and Hensal, F.J.: A Modified Bristow-Helfet-May Procedure for Recurrent Dislocation and Subluxation of the Shoulder: Report of Two Hundred and Twelve Cases. J. Bone Joint Surg., 69A:904–913, 1987.

1305. Tos, L.; Bardelli, D.; and Danovaro, M.G.: [Habitual Shoulder Luxation Treated With Weber's Method.] Minerva Ortop. Traumatol., 39:663–666, 1988.

1306. Toumey, J.W.: Posterior Recurrent Dislocation of the Shoulder Treated by Capsulorrhaphy and Iliac Bone Block. Lahey Clin. Bull., 5:197–201, 1946–1948.

1307. Townley, C.O.: Intrinsic Glenohumeral Anatomy and Its Relation to Recurrent Shoulder Dislocation (abstract). J. Bone Joint Surg., 47A:1276, 1965.

1308. Townley, C.O.: Recurrent Shoulder Dislocations: Pathogenesis and Pathology (abstract). Clin. Orthop., 44:280, 1966.

1309. Townley, C.O.: The Capsular Mechanism in Recurrent Dislocation of the Shoulder. J. Bone Joint Surg., 32A:370–380, 1950.

1310. Townley, C.O.: The Dislocating Shoulder: Anatomy, Pathology, Pathogenesis (abstract). J. Bone Joint Surg., 45A:1335–1336, 1963.

1311. Travlos, J., and Boome, R.S.: Axillary Nerve Rupture After Closed Anterior Shoulder Dislocation. Injury, 20:300, 1989.

1312. Trillat, A.; Dejoir, H.; and Roullet, J.: Luxation Recidivante de l'Épaule et Lesions du Bourrelet Glenoidien. Rev. Chir. Orthop., 51:525–544, 1965.

1313. Trillat, A., and Leclerc-Chalvet, F.: Luxation Recidivante de l'Épaule. Paris, Masson, 1973.

1314. Trillat, A.: Traitement de la Luxation Recidivante de l'Épaule: Considerations Techniques. Lyon Chir., 49:986, 1954.

1315. Trimmings, N.P.: Haemarthrosis Aspiration in Treatment of Anterior Dislocation of the Shoulder. J. R. Soc. Med., 78:1023–1027, 1985.

1316. Tronzo, R.G.: Reduction of Dislocated Shoulders Using Methocarbamol. J.A.M.A., 184:1044–1046, 1963.

1317. Truchly, G., and Thompson, W.A.L.: Simplified Putti-Platt Procedure. J.A.M.A., 179:859–862, 1962.

1318. Truchly, G.: Modified Putti Procedure for the Recurrent Dislocation of the Shoulder. American Academy of Orthopaedic Surgeons Scientific Exhibit, 35th Annual Meeting, Chicago, Ill., Jan. 20–25, 1968.

1319. Tullos, H.S.; Bennett, J.B.; and Braly, W.G.: Acute Shoulder Dislocations: Factors Influencing Diagnosis and Treatment. Instr. Course Lect., XXXIII:364–385, 1984.

1320. Tullos, H.S., and King, J.W.: Throwing Mechanism in Sports. Orthop. Clin. North Am., 4:709–720, 1973.

1321. Turek, S.L.: Orthopaedics—Principles and Their Application, 2nd ed. Philadelphia, J.B. Lippincott, 1967.

1322. Turkel, S.J.; Panio, M.W.; Marshall, J.L.; and Girgis, F.G.: Stabilizing Mechanisms Preventing Anterior Dislocation of the Glenohumeral Joint. J. Bone Joint Surg., 63A:1208–1217, 1981.

1323. Tuszynski, W., and Dworczynski, W.: [Anterior Dislocation of the Shoulder Complicated by Temporary Brachial Paresis.] Chir. Narzadow. Ruchu Ortop. Pol., 46:129–131, 1981.

1324. Tzikunov, M.B.: [Functional Rehabilitation Treatment in Traumatic Shoulder Dislocations.] Ortop. Travmatol. Protez, 12:13–17, 1986.

1325. Uhtoff, H.K., and Piscopo, M.: Anterior Capsular Redundancy of the Shoulder: Congenital or Traumatic? An Embryological Study. J. Bone Joint Surg., 67B:363–366, 1985.

1326. Uhtoff, H.K.; Soucy, D.; and Colliou, L.: L'emploi des Fils Metalliques Amovibles Dans la Reparation de la Luxation Recidivante de l'Épaule. Union Med. Can., 104:751–754, 1975.

1327. Uitvlugt, G.; Detrisac, D.A.; and Johnson, L.L.: Arthroscope's Value in Frozen Shoulder Primarily Is in Diagnosis, Not Treatment. Orthopedics Today, 8:16–17, 1988.

1328. Ulrich, C.; Helbing, G.; Worsdorfer, O.; and Lampl, L.H.: [Intrathoracic Luxation of the Humeral Head.] Langenbecks Arch. Chir., 367:197–202, 1986.

1329. Unsworth, A.; Dowson, D.; and Wright, V.: "Cracking Joints": A Bioengineering Study of Cavitation in the Metacarpophalangeal Joint. Ann. Rheum. Dis., 30:348, 1971.

1330. Urban, J.: du Toit Shoulder Arthroplasty (abstract). Clin. Orthop., 144:342–343, 1979.

1331. Uribe, J.W.; Levy, H.J.; and Delaney, L.G.: Arthroscopic Assisted Rotator Cuff Repair: Preliminary Results. Personal communication, 1989.

1332. Urrea, C.L.: Via Axilar Anterior en Luxacion Recidivante de Hombro. VIII Congreso Latinoamericano de Cirugia Ortopedica, Quito, Ecuador, July 3–9, 1971.

1333. Vainionpaa, S.; Kirves, P.; and Laike, E.: The Results of Surgical Treatment for Recurrent Dislocation of the Shoulder (abstract). Acta Orthop. Scand., 54:532, 1983.

1334. Valls, J.: Acrylic Prosthesis in a Case With Fracture of the Head of the Humerus. Bal. Soc. Orthop. Trauma., 17:61, 1952.

1334A. Vander Flier, R.E., and Marti, R.K.: Treatment of Anterior Habitual Shoulder Dislocation by Reefing of the Subscapular Muscle and Weber's Derotational Osteotomy (abstract). Acta Orthop. Scand., 55(4):484, 1984.

1335. Van Der Spek, A.: Rupture of the Axillary Artery as a

Complication of Dislocation of the Shoulder. Arch. Chir. Neerl., 16:113–118, 1964.

1336. Vander Ghirst, M., and Houssa, R.: Acrylic Prosthesis in Fractures of the Head of the Humerus. Acta Chir. Belg., 50:31, 1951.

1337. Vare, V.B., Jr.: The Treatment of Recurrent Dislocation of the Shoulder. Surg. Clin. North Am., 33:1703–1710, 1953.

1338. Varghese, G.: Evaluation and Management: Shoulder Complications in Hemiplegia. J. Kansas Med. Soc., 82:451–453, 1981.

1339. Varmarken, J.E., and Jensen, C.H.: Recurrent Anterior Dislocation of the Shoulder: A Comparison of the Results After the Bankart and the Putti-Platt Procedures. Orthopedics, 12:453–455, 1989.

1340. Vastamaki, M., and Solonen, K.A.: Posterior Dislocation and Fracture–Dislocation of the Shoulder. Acta Orthop. Scand., 51:479–484, 1980.

1341. Vecchini, L.: La Tettoplastica Nella Lussazione Abituale Posteriore Della Spalla (Controllo a 4 Anni Dall' Intervento). Ort. e Traum., 5:199–204, 1985.

1342. Vegter, J., and Marti, R.K.: Treatment of Posterior Dislocation of the Shoulder by Osteotomy of the Neck of the Scapula. J. Bone Joint Surg., 63B:288, 1981.

1343. Velghe, A.; Humblet, P.; Lesire, M.R.; and Liselele, D.: [Recent Posterior Dislocation of the Shoulder: Irreducibility Due to Interposition of the Long Biceps: Observations on Two Cases.] Rev. Chir. Orthop., 74:782–785, 1988.

1344. Verrina, F.: [Para-Articular Ossification Following Simple Dislocation of the Shoulder.] Minerva Ortop., 210:480–486, 1975.

1345. Vestad, E.: Rotational Osteotomy for Recurrent Dislocation of the Shoulder (abstract). Acta Orthop. Scand., 50:803, 1979.

1346. Vezina, J.A., and Beauregard, C.G.: An Update of the Technique of Double-Contrast Arthrotomography of the Shoulder. J. Can. Assoc. Radiol., 36:176–182, 1985.

1347. Vicenzi, G., and Montagnani, A.: [Recurrent Posterior and Atraumatic Dislocation of the Shoulder: A Case Report.] Arch. Putti Chir. Organi Mov., 49:87–90, 1984.

1348. Vichard, P., and Arnould, D.: [Posterior Fracture–Dislocation of the Shoulder: A Study of 11 Cases.] Rev. Chir. Orthop., 67:71–77, 1981.

1349. Vidal, J.; Orst, G.; Denis, P.; Reboul, C.; Marnay, T.; and Deguillaume, P.: The Bankart Procedure: Its Reliability Among Sportsmen (abstract). J. Bone Joint Surg., 66B:140, 1984.

1350. Viek, P., and Bell, B.T.: The Bankart Shoulder Reconstruction: The Use of Pull-Out Wires and Other Practical Details. J. Bone Joint Surg., 41A:236–242, 1959.

1351. Vigliani, F.: [Kocher's Technique for Shoulder Reduction: 120 Years of Signs of Changeability.] Arch. Putti Chir. Organi Mov., 36:11–22, 1986.

1352. Villar, R.N., and Palmer, I.P.: Association of Recurrent Anterior Dislocation of the Shoulder With Free-Fall Parachuting. Injury, 16:15–16, 1984.

1353. Vogel, A.: [Reexaminations of Treatment and Age of Patients at the Time of the First Shoulder Dislocation After Development of Recurrent Dislocations.] Orthopade, 7:145–146, 1978.

1354. Voto, S.J.; Clark, R.N.; and Zuelzer, W.A.: Arthroscopic Training Using Pig Knee Joints. Clin. Orthop., 226:134–137, 1988.

1355. Vukov, V.: Posterior Dislocation of the Shoulder With a Large Anteromedial Defect of the Head of the Humerus: A Case Report. Int. Orthop., 9:37–40, 1985.

1356. Wagner, K.T., and Lyne, E.D.: Adolescent Traumatic Dislocations of the Shoulder With Open Epiphyses. J. Pediatr. Orthop., 3:61–62, 1983.

1357. Wainwright, D.: Glenoidectomy in the Treatment of the Painful Arthritic Shoulder (abstract). J. Bone Joint Surg., 58B:377, 1976.

1358. Walch, G.; Charret, P.; Pietro-Paoli, H.; and Dejour, H.: [Recurrences After Surgical Procedures for Recurrent Dislocation of the Shoulder.] Rev. Chir. Orthop., 72:541–545, 1986.

1359. Walch, G.; Dejour, H.; and Trillat, A.G.: [Recurrent Anterior Dislocation of the Shoulder With Onset After the Age of Forty Years.] Rev. Chir. Orthop., 73:609–616, 1987.

1360. Waldron, V.D.: Dislocated Shoulder Reduction: A Simple Method That Is Done Without Assistants. Orthop. Rev., 11:105–106, 1982.

1361. Ward, W.G.; Bassett, F.H., III; and Garrett, W.E., Jr.: Anterior Staple Capsulorrhaphy for Recurrent Shoulder Dislocation (abstract). South. Med. J., 81:S57, 1988.

1362. Warren, R.F.; Kornblatt, I.B.; and Marchand, R.: Static Factors Affecting Posterior Shoulder Instability. Orthop. Trans., 8:1–89, 1984.

1363. Warren, R.F.: Instability of Shoulder in Throwing Sports. Instr. Course Lect., XXXIV:337–348, 1985.

1364. Warren, R.F.: Beach-Chair for Arthroscope Exam of Shoulder, Personal communication, Aug. 5, 1989.

1365. Warren, R.F.: The Role of Shoulder Arthroscopy. AAOS Instructional Course, Minneapolis, Minn., Feb. 13, 1989.

1366. Warren, R.F.: Watch for Inflammation, Instability in Shoulder Injuries. Orthopedics Today, p. 4, July, 1984.

1367. Warrick, C.K.: Posterior Dislocation of the Shoulder Joint. J. Bone Joint Surg., 30B:651–655, 1948.

1368. Warrick, C.K.: Posterior Dislocation of the Shoulder Joint. Br. J. Radiol., 38:758–761, 1965.

1369. Warwick, R., and Williams, P.L. (eds.): Gray's Anatomy, 35th ed. Philadelphia, W.B. Saunders, 1973.

1370. Watanabe, M.; Takeda, S.; and Ikeuchi, H.: Atlas of Arthroscopy, 3rd ed. New York, Igaku-Shoin, 1978.

1371. Watanabe, M.: Arthroscopy: The Present State. Orthop. Clin. North Am., 10:505–522, 1979.

1372. Watanabe, M.: The Development and Present Status of the Arthroscopy. J. Jpn. Med. Inst., 25:11, 1954.

1373. Watson, D.M.S.: The Evolution of the Tetrapod Shoulder Girdle and Forelimb. J. Anat., 52:1–63, 1918.

1374. Watson-Jones, R.: Dislocation of the Shoulder Joint. Proc. R. Soc. Med., 29:1060–1062, 1936.

1375. Watson-Jones, R.: Fractures and Joint Injuries, 4th ed. Baltimore, Williams & Wilkins, 1957.

1376. Watson-Jones, R.: Fractures and Joint Injuries. London, Churchill Livingstone, 1982.

1377. Watson-Jones, R.: Fractures and Other Joint Injuries, 4th ed, Vol. 2. Baltimore, Williams & Wilkins, 1956.

1378. Watson-Jones, R.: Note on Recurrent Dislocation of the Shoulder Joint: Superior Approach Causing the Only Failure in Fifty-Two Operations for Repair of the Labrum and Capsule. J. Bone Joint Surg., 30B:49–52, 1948.

1379. Watson-Jones, R.: Recurrent Dislocation of the Shoulder (editorial). J. Bone Joint Surg., 30B:6–8, 1948.

1380. Weber, B.G.; Simpson, L.A.; and Hardegger, F.: Rotational Humeral Osteotomy for Recurrent Anterior Dislocation of the Shoulder Associated with a Large Hill-Sachs Lesion. J. Bone Joint Surg., 66A:1443–1450, 1984.

1381. Weber, B.G.: Operative Treatment for Recurrent Dislocation of the Shoulder: Preliminary Report. Injury, 1:107–109, 1969.

1382. Weber, S.C., and Caspari, R.B.: A Biomechanical Evaluation of the Restraints to Posterior Shoulder Dislocation. Arthroscopy, 5:115–121, 1989.

1383. Weber-Laumann, A.: Recurrent Dislocation of the Shoulder Treated by Transposition of the Tendon to Pectoralis Minor: A Follow-Up of Fifteen Patients. Acta Orthop. Scand., 41:161–164, 1970.

1384. Weinstabl, R.; Hertz, H.; and Firbas, W.: [Connections of the Coracoglenoidal Ligament With the Pectoralis Minor Muscle.] Acta Anat., 125:126–131, 1986.

1385. Weinstabl, R.; Hertz, H.; and Firbas, W.: Uber den zusammenhang einzelner Bander des Schultergelenkes mit dem Limbus glenoidalis (abstract). Acta Anat., 120:80, 1984.

1386. Weissman, S.L., and Torok, G.: Bilateral Recurrent Posterior Dislocation of the Shoulder: Report of a Case. J. Bone Joint Surg., 40A:479–482, 1958.

1387. Weitbrecht, J.: Syndesmology; or, a Description of the Ligaments of the Human Body. Kaplan, E.B. (trans.). Philadelphia, W.B. Saunders, 1969.

1388. Welsh, R.P.: Recurrent Dislocation of the Shoulder: Problems Encountered in the Surgically Treated (abstract). J. Bone Joint Surg., 67B:327, 1985.

1389. Wenner, S.M.: Anterior Dislocation of the Shoulder in Patients Over 50 Years of Age. Orthopedics, 8:1155–1157, 1985.

1390. West, E.F.: Intrathoracic Dislocation of the Humerus. J. Bone Joint Surg., 31B:61–62, 1949.

1391. Wheeler, J.H.; Ryan, J.B.; Arciero, R.A.; and Molinari, R.N.: Arthroscopic Versus Nonoperative Treatment of Acute Shoulder Dislocations in Young Athletes. Arthroscopy, 5:213–217, 1989.

1392. White, A.D.N.: Dislocated Shoulder—A Simple Method of Reduction. Med. J. Aust., 2:726–727, 1976.

1393. White, M.: Some Late Results of Dislocation of the Shoulder. Trans. R. Med. Chir. Soc. Glasgow, 22:243–248, 1929.

1394. Wickstrom, J.: Birth Injuries of the Brachial Plexus: Treatment of Defects in the Shoulder. Clin. Orthop., 23:187–196, 1962.

1395. Wiley, A.M., and Austwick, D.H.: Shoulder Surgery Through the Arthroscope. Department of Surgery, University of Toronto and Toronto Wester Hospital, Toronto, Ont., 1982.

1396. Wiley, A.M., and Older, M.W.J.: Shoulder Arthroscopy: Investigations With a Fibro-optic Instrument. Am. J. Sports Med., 8:31–38, 1980.

1397. Wiley, A.M.: Arthroscopy for Shoulder Instability and a Technique for Arthroscopic Repair. Arthroscopy, 4:25–30, 1988.

1398. Wiley, A.M.: Arthroscopy Urged for Surgical Repair of Shoulder Lesions. Orthopedics Today, 3:30–31, 1983.

1399. Wilkinson, J.A., and Thomas, W.G.: Glenoid Osteotomy for Recurrent Posterior Dislocation of the Shoulder (abstract). J. Bone Joint Surg., 67B:496, 1985.

1400. Willard, D.P.: The Nicola Operation for Recurrent Dislocation of the Shoulder. Ann. Surg., 103:438–443, 1936.

1401. Williamson, R.W.: Complication Following Bristow Operation. Personal communication, March, 1981.

1402. Wilson, A.J.: Posterior Dislocation of the Shoulder: A Case for the Lateral Scapula View. Mo. Med., 80:299–303, 1983.

1403. Wilson, J.C., and McKeever, F.M.: Traumatic Posterior (Retroglenoid) Dislocation of the Humerus. J. Bone Joint Surg., 31A:160–172, 1949.

1404. Witvoet, J.; Aubart, F.; and Broutart, J.C.: [Reduction of Old Unreduced Anterior Dislocations of the Shoulder.] Rev. Chir. Orthop., 67:805–809, 1981.

1405. Wolf, E.M.: Arthroscopic Anterior Shoulder Capsulorrhaphy. Techniques Orthop., 3:67–73, 1988.

1406. Wolf, T., and Schauwecker, F.: [Therapy After a Luxation of the Shoulder.] Unfallchirurgie, 13:142–145, 1987.

1407. Wolff, E.F.: Transposition of the Biceps Brachii Tendon to Repair Luxation of the Canine Shoulder Joint: Review of a Procedure. Vet. Med. Sm. Animal Clin., 69:51–53, 1974.

1408. Wong-Chung, J., and Quinlan, W.: Fractured Coracoid Process Preventing Closed Reduction of Anterior Dislocation of the Shoulder. Injury, 20:296–297, 1989.

1409. Wong-Pack, W.K.; Bobechko, P.E.; and Becker, E.J.: Fractured Coracoid With Anterior Shoulder Dislocation. J. Can. Assoc. Radiol., 31:278–279, 1980.

1410. Wood, J.P.: Posterior Dislocation of the Head of the Humerus and the Diagnostic Value of Lateral and Vertical Views. U.S. Navy Med. Bull., 39:532–535, 1941.

1411. Wymenga, A.B., and Morshuis, W.J.: Recurrent Shoulder Dislocation: Comparison of Early Results Obtained by Three Operative Techniques (abstract). Acta Orthop. Scand., 58:202–206, 1987.

1412. Yadav, S.S.: Bilateral Simultaneous Fracture–Dislocation of the Shoulder Due to Muscular Violence. J. Postgrad. Med., 23:137–139, 1977.

1413. Yang, S.O.; Cho, K.J.; Kim, M.J.; and Ro, I.W.: Assessment of Anterior Shoulder Instability by CT Arthrography. J. Korean Med. Sci., 2:167–171, 1987.

1414. Yoneda, B.; Welsh, R.P.; and MacIntosh, D.L.: Conservative Treatment of Shoulder Dislocation in Young Males (abstract). J. Bone Joint Surg., 64B:254–255, 1982.

1415. Zaborowski, R., and Biedrzycki, J.: [Uncommon Traumatic Dislocations.] Chir. Narzadow. Ruchu Ortop. Pol., 42:495–498, 1977.

1416. Zachary, R.B.: Transplantation of Teres Major and Latissimus Dorsi for Loss of External Rotation at the Shoulder. Lancet, 2:757–761, 1947.

1417. Zadik, F.R.: Recurrent Posterior Dislocation of the Shoulder Joint. J. Bone Joint Surg., 30B:531–532, 1948.

1418. Zanoli, R.: Appraisal of the Geriatric Patient. Clin. Orthop., 11:11–13, 1958.

1419. Zarins, B.; Rowe, C.R.; and Stone, J.W.: Shoulder Instability: Management of Failed Reconstructions. Instr. Course Lect., XVIII:217–230, 1989.

1420. Zarins, B., and Rowe, C.R.: An Evaluation of Modifications of the Bankart Procedure. Presented at American Shoulder and Elbow Surgeons 4th International Conference on Surgery of the Shoulder. New York, N.Y., October, 1989.

1421. Zarins, B., and Rowe, C.R.: Current Concepts in the Diagnosis and Treatment of Shoulder Instability in Athletes. Med. Sci. Sports Exerc., 16:444–448, 1984.

1422. Zarins, B.: "Complications in Shoulder Arthroscopy." Personal communication, May, 1989.

1423. Zenni, E.J., Jr.: An Axillary Approach for a Putti-Platt Repair. Clin. Orthop., 136:157–159, 1978.

1424. Ziegler, R.: [X-Ray Examination of the Shoulder in Suspected Luxation.] Z. Orthop., 119:31–35, 1981.

1425. Zimmerman, L.M., and Veith, I.: Great Ideas in the History of Surgery: Clavicle, Shoulder, Shoulder Amputations. Baltimore, Williams & Wilkins, 1961.

1426. Zimmers, T.: Luxatio Erecta: An Uncommon Shoulder Dislocation. Ann. Emerg. Med., 12:716–717, 1983.

1427. Zizzi, F.; Frizziero, L.; Facchini, A.; and Zini, G.L.: Artroscopia Della Spalla: Indicazioni e Limiti. Reumatismo, 33:429–432, 1981.

1428. Zlatkin, M.B.; Bjorkengren, A.G.; Gylys-Morin, V.; Resnick, D.; and Sartoris, D.J.: Cross-sectional Imaging of the Capsular Mechanism of the Glenohumeral Joint. A.J.R., 150:151–158, 1988.

1429. Zuckerman, J.D., and Matsen, F.A., III: Complications About the Glenohumeral Joint Related to the Use of Screws and Staples. J. Bone Joint Surg., 66A:175–180, 1984.

1430. Zych, G.A., and Montane, I.: Acute Fracture of the Proximal Humerus Superimposed on a Chronic Posterior Dislocation of the Humerual Head. South. Med. J., 80:1307–1308, 1987.

14

Injuries to the Acromioclavicular Joint

Charles A. Rockwood, Jr.
Gerald R. Williams
D. Christopher Young

HISTORICAL REVIEW

Dislocation of the acromioclavicular joint, particularly its treatment, has been a subject of controversy from the earliest medical writings. Hippocrates[4] (460–377 B.C.) wrote,

> "Physicians are particularly liable to be deceived in this accident (for as the separated bone protrudes, the top of the shoulder appears low and hollow), so that they may prepare as if for dislocation of the shoulder; for I have known many physicians otherwise not expert at the art who have done much mischief by attempting to reduce shoulders, thus supposing it as a case of dislocation."

Galen[4] (129–199 A.D.) obviously had paid close attention to Hippocrates, because he diagnosed his own acromioclavicular dislocation received from wrestling in the palestra. This famous physician of the Greco-Roman period treated himself in the manner of Hippocrates (ie, tight bandages to hold the projecting clavicle down while keeping the arm elevated). He abandoned the treatment after only a few days because it was so uncomfortable. It is appropriate that one of the earliest reported cases in the literature was related to sports, because today sports participation certainly is one of the most common causes of acromioclavicular dislocations.

From the earliest publications through the time of Paul of Aegina (7th century), dislocations of the acromioclavicular joint have become better recognized. Their treatment, however, has remained essentially unchanged. Hippocrates[4] stated that no impediment, small or great, will result from such an injury. He further stated that there would be a "tumefaction" or deformity, "for the bone cannot be properly restored to its natural situation." This statement apparently was, has been, and will be received by the orthopaedic community as a challenge. There is probably not another joint in the body that has been treated in so many different ways as the acromioclavicular joint in attempts to "properly restore" it to "its natural situation."

SURGICAL ANATOMY

The acromioclavicular joint is a diarthrodial joint located between the lateral end of the clavicle and the medial margin of the acromion process of the scapula (Fig. 14-1). According to Tyurina,[462] the articular surfaces initially are hyaline cartilage. At about 17 years of age, on the acromial side of the joint, and 24 years of age, on the clavicular side, the hyaline cartilage becomes fibrocartilage. Bosworth[76] stated the average size of the adult acromioclavicular joint is 9 × 19 mm. DePalma[128] showed marked variability in the plane of the joint. Viewed from the front, the inclination of the joint may be almost vertical, or it may be inclined from downward medially, with the clavicle overriding the acromion by an angle as large as 50° (Fig. 14-2). Mosely[305] stated that there may be an underriding type of inclination, with the clavicle facet under the acromion process. In his experience, the vertical and underriding joint configurations appear to be most prone to prolonged disability after injury.

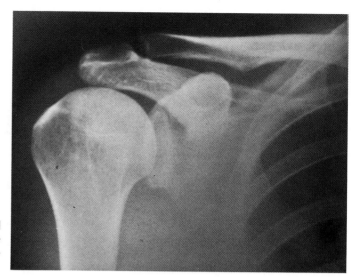

Fig. 14-1. Anteroposterior view of the normal shoulder. Note the acromioclavicular joint, the coracoid process, and the coracoclavicular interspace.

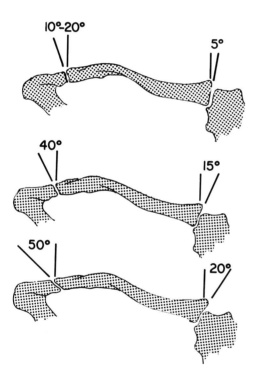

Fig. 14-2. Variations of the inclination of the acromioclavicular and the sternoclavicular joints. *(Redrawn from DePalma, A. F.: Surgery of the Shoulder. Philadelphia, J. B. Lippincott, 1973.)*

Urist[464] studied 100 random x-rays of the shoulder, and found the articular surface of the clavicle overrode the articular surface of the acromion approximately 50% of the time. Additionally, Urist[464] reported that in 21% of acromioclavicular joints, the articular surfaces were incongruent—with the lateral end of the clavicle lying inferior or superior to the acromion. Keats and Pope[236] recently reemphasized the fact that the clavicle may normally lie superior to the acromion. They cautioned against mistaking this normal variant for a traumatic acromioclavicular dislocation.

There are two types of fibrocartilaginous intra-articular disks—complete and partial (meniscoid). The disk has great variation in size and shape. DePalma[130] demonstrated that with age, the meniscus undergoes rapid degeneration until essentially it is no longer functional beyond the fourth decade. Recent work by Petersson[350] and Salter and colleagues[398] substantiated these findings. The nerve supply to the acromioclavicular joint is from branches of the axillary, suprascapular, and lateral pectoral nerves.

ACROMIOCLAVICULAR LIGAMENTS

The acromioclavicular joint is surrounded by a thin capsule reinforced above, below, anteriorly, and posteriorly by the superior, inferior, anterior, and posterior acromioclavicular ligaments (Fig. 14-3). The fibers of the superior acromioclavicular ligament, which is the strongest of the capsular ligaments, blend with the fibers of the deltoid and tra-

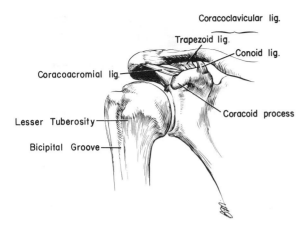

Coracoclavicular lig.
Trapezoid lig.
Conoid lig.
Coracoacromial lig.
Coracoid process
Lesser Tuberosity
Bicipital Groove

Fig. 14-3. Normal anatomy of the acromioclavicular joint.

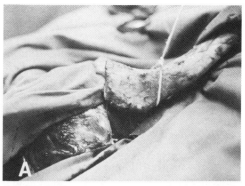

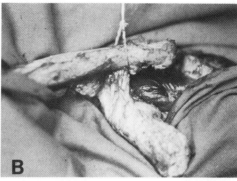

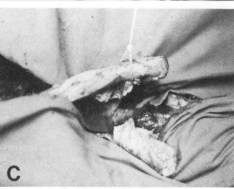

pezius muscles, which are attached to the superior aspect of the clavicle and the acromion process. These muscle attachments are important in that they strengthen the weak and thin ligaments, thereby adding stability to the acromioclavicular joint.

CORACOCLAVICULAR LIGAMENT

The coracoclavicular ligament is a very strong, heavy ligament whose fibers run from the outer, inferior surface of the clavicle to the base of the coracoid process of the scapula (Fig. 14-4). The coracoclavicular ligament has two components: the conoid and the trapezoid ligaments. A bursa may separate these two portions of the ligament. According to Bosworth,[76] the average space between the clavicle and the coracoid process is 1.3 cm. Bearden and co-workers[49] reported a range of values for the coracoclavicular interspace of 1.1 to 1.3 cm. Salter and colleages[398] measured the components of the coracoclavicular ligament in 20 cadavers. They found the trapezoid ligament to vary from 0.8 to 2.5 cm in length and from 0.8 to 2.5 cm in width. The conoid ligament varied from 0.7 to 2.5 cm in length and from 0.4 to 0.95 cm in width.

The conoid ligament[229] is cone shaped, with the apex of the cone attaching on the posteromedial side of the base of the coracoid process. The base of the cone attaches onto the conoid tubercle on the posterior undersurface of the clavicle. The conoid tubercle is located at the apex of the posterior clavicular curve, which is at the junction of the lateral third of the flattened clavicle with the medial two thirds of the triangular-shaped shaft.

Fig. 14-4. The importance of the acromioclavicular and coracoclavicular ligaments for stability of the acromioclavicular joint, using a fresh cadaver. (**A**) With the muscles and acromioclavicular capsule and ligaments resected and with the coracoclavicular ligaments intact, the clavicle can be displaced anteriorly as shown or posteriorly from the articular surface of the acromion. (**B**) However, because the coracoclavicular ligaments are intact, the clavicle cannot be displaced significantly upward. (**C**) Following the transection of the coracoclavicular ligaments the clavicle can be displaced completely above the acromion process. This suggests that the horizontal stability of the acromioclavicular joint is accomplished by the acromioclavicular ligaments, and vertical stability is obtained through the coracoclavicular ligaments.

The trapezoid[229] ligament arises from the coracoid process, anterior and lateral to the attachment of the conoid ligament. This is just posterior to the attachment of the pectoralis minor tendon. The trapezoid ligament extends superiorly to a rough line on the undersurface of the clavicle. This line extends anteriorly and laterally from the conoid tubercle.

Function

The coracoclavicular ligament helps to couple glenohumeral abduction and flexion to scapular rotation on the thorax. Full overhead elevation cannot be accomplished without combined and synchronous glenohumeral and scapulothoracic motion.[104,221,237] Inman and colleagues[221] noted that the clavicle rotates about its longitudinal axis through an arc of 40° to 50° during full abduction. As the clavicle rotates upward, it dictates scapulothoracic rotation by virtue of its attachment to the scapula—the conoid and trapezoid ligaments.

Although the coracoclavicular ligament does mediate "synchronous scapulohumeral" motion, its primary function is to strengthen the acromioclavicular articulation.[3,15,46,49,53,73,94,214,217,228,238,305,] [335,390,395,455] Owing to their medial and downward direction, the fibers of the ligament prevent the acromion process from being driven downward and medially.

The only connection between the upper extremity and the axial skeleton is through the clavicular articulations at the acromioclavicular and sternoclavicular joints. Bearn[50] stressed the importance of the sternoclavicular ligaments in supporting the distal end of the clavicle. Through anatomical dissections and selective divisions of the sternoclavicular ligaments, he demonstrated how these ligaments prevent downward displacement of the distal end of the clavicle. Hence, in the erect position, the strong sternoclavicular ligaments support the clavicles out, away from the body, like the wings off the body of an airplane. Furthermore, just as the jet engines are suspended from the underside of the wings, the upper extremities are suspended from the distal clavicles through the coracoclavicular ligament. Thus, the coracoclavicular ligament is the prime suspensory ligament of the upper extremity.

In addition to the sternoclavicular and coracoclavicular ligaments, the trapezius muscle helps to support the shoulder in the upright position. There must be an important interplay between the trapezius muscle and the sternoclavicular ligaments, because there are patients who have a downward drooping of the entire shoulder complex, including the clavicle, following an injury to the spinal accessory nerve which supplies the trapezius. This presumably would have to occur secondary to progressive elongation of the sternoclavicular ligaments.

Cadenat,[94] in 1917, very carefully studied the importance of the coracoclavicular ligament in stabilizing the acromioclavicular joint. He concluded that a moderate blow to the acromion process would rupture the acromioclavicular ligament and produce an incomplete acromioclavicular dislocation. A heavier blow would then rupture the acromioclavicular and coracoclavicular ligaments, producing a complete dislocation. Cadenat agreed with the studies of Poirier and Rieffel,[359] Delbet,[94] and Mocquot,[94] which confirm that both the trapezoid and conoid portions of the coracoclavicular ligament must be divided to produce a complete dislocation of the acromioclavicular joint. Cadenat further pointed out that before the functional and clinical end results of a given injury can be evaluated, the physician must determine whether the dislocation is incomplete (ie, a mild sprain to the joint) or complete.

Experimental Studies by Urist

Urist[464] concluded from a series of experiments that *complete dislocation* of the acromioclavicular joint can occur without rupture of the coracoclavicular ligament. In a cadaver shoulder with the coracoclavicular ligament intact, he divided the superior acromioclavicular ligament and the entire acromioclavicular joint capsule. He further detached the deltoid and trapezius muscles from the region of the acromioclavicular joint. He then demonstrated that, under these conditions, the distal clavicle could be completely dislocated *anteriorly* and *posteriorly* away from the acromion process (ie, in a horizontal plane). Because the coracoclavicular ligament was intact, upward displacement or subluxation of the acromioclavicular joint was minimal. Only after the coracoclavicular ligament was transsected did a complete upward, or vertical, dislocation of the acromioclavicular joint occur.

The senior author has repeated some of the cadaver studies of Urist[464] and agrees with his anatomical findings, but disagrees with his terminology. Indeed, with the muscles and acromioclavicular ligaments detached, the clavicle can be displaced in a horizontal direction—either anterior or posterior to the acromion process. (See Fig. 14-4A.) However, only a very slight upward displacement is noted in the vertical plane. (See Fig. 14-4**B.**) Only when the conoid and trapezoid ligaments have been divided can the lateral clavicle be vertically and totally dislocated above the acromion process. (See Fig. 14-4**C.**)

Fukuda and colleagues[156] recently studied the individual ligament contributions to acromioclavicular stability. They performed load-displacement tests with a fixed displacement after sequential ligament sectioning. The contribution of the acromioclavicular, trapezoid, and conoid ligaments was determined at small and large displacements. At small displacements, the acromioclavicular ligaments were the primary restraint to both posterior (89%) and superior (68%) translation of the clavicle—the most common failure patterns seen clinically. At large displacements, the conoid ligament provided the primary restraint (62%) to superior translation, while the acromioclavicular ligaments remained the primary restraint (90%) to posterior translation. The trapezoid ligament served as the primary restraint to acromioclavicular joint compression at both large and small displacements. These experiments have led to the following conclusions:

The horizontal stability is controlled by the acromioclavicular ligament.
The vertical stability is controlled by the coracoclavicular ligaments.

The term "dislocation of the acromioclavicular joint" should be (and is) used to describe the upward or vertical displacement of the distal clavicle from the acromion, not the anterior or posterior horizontal displacement.[7,12,20,24,49,73,76,94,98,128,129,214,220,238,263,282,288,305,306,309,311,372,396,443,446]

CORACOCLAVICULAR ARTICULATION

The existence of a joint between the clavicle and the coracoid process is rare. Gradoyevitch[179] reported in 1939 that only 15 cases were known to medical science. Ten had been proven anatomically, and five were demonstrated by radiography. He reported one patient with bilateral coracoclavicular joints. The patient's shoulders exhibited a normal range of motion and were asymptomatic and symmetric. There were no abnormal findings of either the acromioclavicular or sternoclavicular joints.

Radiographic Appearance

X-rays reveal a bony outgrowth from the undersurface of the clavicle. The outgrowth is triangular, with its base oriented toward the inferior surface of the clavicle. The lateral border of the triangle forms the articular surface with a tubercle on the dorsomedial surface of the coracoid process (Fig. 14-5). The radiographic findings are typical for a joint, and Gradoyevitch[179] found a diarthrodial joint (ie, articular surfaces, a true capsule, and an intra-articular synovial membrane) in dissected specimens.

Incidence

Nutter[331] reviewed 1000 random x-rays of adult shoulders and found 12 with coracoclavicular joints—an incidence of 1.2%. Six of the 12 cases were bilateral, and 11 were in men. Liberson[263] reported an incidence of nine patients in 1800 shoulders studied; five had bilateral coracoclavicular joints. According to Wertheimer,[490] Poirier found one case in 2300 shoulders. Frassetto[490] believed a

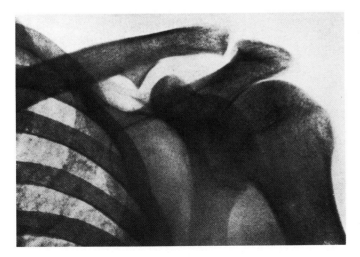

Fig. 14-5. Coracoclavicular articulation. This x-ray demonstrates the triangular bony outgrowth from the inferior clavicle and the general appearance of an articular surface with the dorsomedial aspect of the coracoid process. (Gradoyevitch, B.: Coracoclavicular Joint. J. Bone Joint Surg., 21:918–920, 1939.)

coracoclavicular articulation predisposes to fracture of the neck of the humerus. He suggested a fall on the outstretched hand is normally buffered somewhat by rotation of the scapula about the thorax. Frassetto[490] reasoned that this buffering mechanism is not be possible when there is an extra articulation between the coracoid process and the clavicle. Wertheimer[490] excised the coracoclavicular joint of a manual laborer because of pain. The senior author has seen this anatomical variation on many x-rays of the shoulder, and believes it to be an incidental finding that has little clinical significance.

MOTION OF THE ACROMIOCLAVICULAR JOINT

Inman and colleagues,[221] in their classic 1944 article, suggested the total range of motion of the acromioclavicular joint is 20°. They reported that the motion occurs in the first 30° of abduction and after 135° of elevation of the arm. They also demonstrated that with full elevation of the arm, the clavicle rotates upward 40° to 50°. This was measured by drilling a pin into the clavicle and observing the rotation upward during overhead elevation of the arm. When they manually held the pin, which prevented clavicular rotation, overhead elevation of the arm was restricted to 110°. Inman and colleagues concluded that clavicular rotation was a fundamental feature of shoulder motion. Furthermore, they concluded that a coracoclavicular lag screw or an arthrodesis of the acromioclavicular joint would limit clavicular rotation and, hence, severely limit abduction of the arm. Since 1944, many authors have condemned the use of the coracoclavicular screw because it would produce an extra-articular acromioclavicular arthrodesis. They believed this would prevent normal clavicular rotation and result in significant limitation of elevation or abduction of the arm.

Significant differences of opinion have been reported by Codman,[104] Caldwell,[96] Kennedy and Cameron,[237,238] and Rockwood.[381–384] Codman[104] theorized that approximately 5° of motion occurred at the acromioclavicular joint. He stated that "its [the acromioclavicular joint's] surfaces slide a little, rotate a little, tip apart a little, and act like hinges to some degree." Caldwell[96] reported two cases of acromioclavicular dislocation treated by arthrodesis of the acromioclavicular joint. One patient gained a full, free range of motion of the shoulder and the other had abduction to 165°. Kennedy and Cameron[237,238] demonstrated that patients who

have a coracoclavicular screw in place (essentially an arthrodesis between the clavicle and the coracoid) are capable of almost full overhead motion. They drilled pins into the clavicle and into the spine of the scapula in patients who had a coracoclavicular lag screw in place and noted normal clavicular rotation during overhead elevation of the arm. In further studies of motion of the clavicle and the scapula, Kennedy and Cameron[237] demonstrated that, with the coracoclavicular screw in place, the degree of elevation of the clavicular pins corresponded to the degree of depression of the pins drilled into the scapular spine. In their operative procedure, the clavicle is depressed down to and in contact with the coracoid process by the coracoclavicular screw. The screw is left permanently in place with the hope that a coracoclavicular arthrodesis will be obtained. We have seen patients who developed a solid bar of bone between the clavicle and the coracoid process following acromioclavicular operations. Despite this arthrodesis of the clavicle to the scapula, the patients have had essentially full range of motion (Fig. 14-6). There is no anatomic difference between an arthrodesis of the coracoclavicular area and an arthrodesis of the acromioclavicular area.

The senior author has drilled Kirschner wires into both clavicles of patients who have a coracoclavicular lag screw in place in one shoulder (Fig. 14-7). The degree of upward rotation of each pin during 180° of shoulder abduction and forward flexion was essentially the same—45°. This is in complete agreement with the work of Kennedy and Cameron,[237] who concluded that the clavicle rotates normally in spite of the presence of a coracoclavicular screw. As the clavicle rotates upward, the scapula rotates downward. This is the so called "synchronous scapuloclavicular rotation" (Fig. 14-8).

The senior author has also performed acromioclavicular joint motion studies in young adults with normal shoulders. Kirschner wires were drilled into the superolateral edge of the acromion and into the distal superior aspect of the clavicle. These two pins were placed parallel to each other and were within ½ inch of the acromioclavicular joint (Fig. 14-9). These pins were then observed during range of motion of the upper extremity (ie, flexion, abduction, rotation, and so forth). No matter where or how much the arm was actively moved or rotated by the patient, only 5° to 8° of motion could be detected between the two pins (ie, in the acromioclavicular joint). This finding explains why a coracoclavicular lag screw or a coracoclavicular ar-

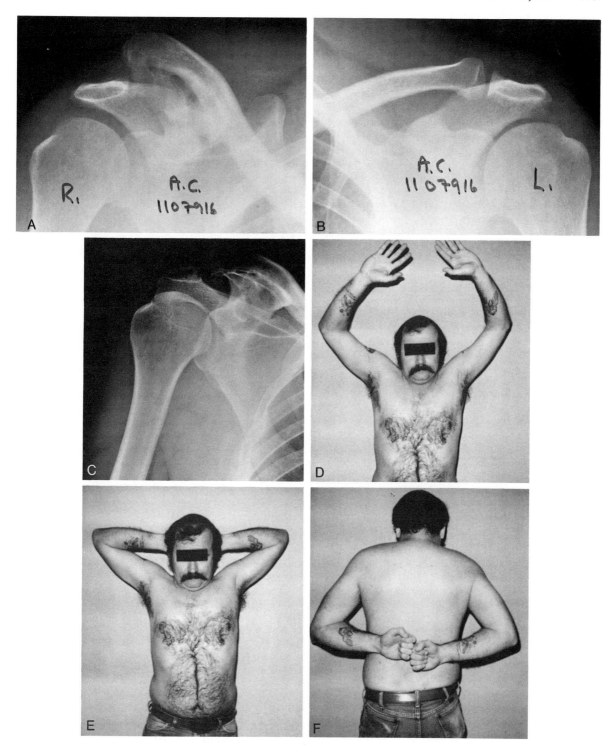

Fig. 14-6. (**A**) Chronic type III dislocation with massive new bone formation between the coracoid and the clavicle of the right shoulder. (**B**) The patient's normal left shoulder. Despite the mass of bone, the patient had essentially a normal range of motion. (**C**) Solid bar of bone between the upper scapula and coracoid and the distal clavicle. (**D–F**) Despite the fusion of the clavicle to the scapula, the patient had essentially a full range of motion with little or no discomfort in the right shoulder.

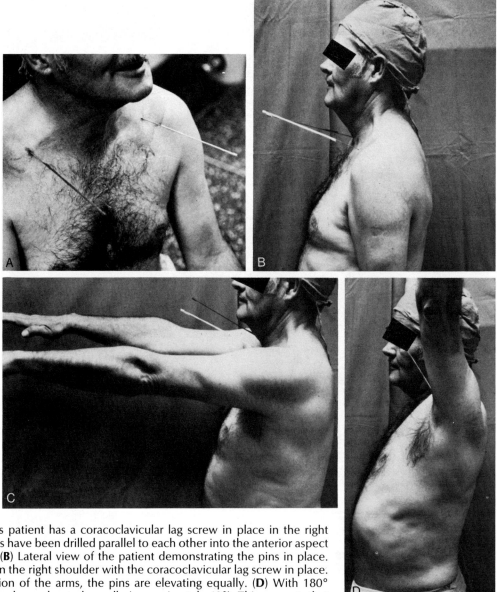

Fig. 14-7. (**A**) This patient has a coracoclavicular lag screw in place in the right shoulder. Two pins have been drilled parallel to each other into the anterior aspect of both clavicles. (**B**) Lateral view of the patient demonstrating the pins in place. The darker pin is in the right shoulder with the coracoclavicular lag screw in place. (**C**) With 90° flexion of the arms, the pins are elevating equally. (**D**) With 180° elevation, both pins have elevated equally (approximately 40°). This suggests that a coracoclavicular lag screw does not limit clavicular rotation.

throdesis does not significantly limit shoulder motion. It also explains why Caldwell's[96] patients, who had arthrodesis of the acromioclavicular joint, had such a surprisingly good range of motion. We completely concur that the clavicle rotates 40 to 50° during full overhead elevation. However, this rotation is combined with simultaneous scapular rotation rather than with pure acromioclavicular joint motion. This "synchronous scapuloclavicular" motion was originally described by Codman[104] and

more recently referred to by Kennedy and Cameron.[237,238]

MECHANISMS OF INJURY
DIRECT FORCE

Injury by direct force is produced by the patient falling onto the point of the shoulder with the arm at the side in an adducted position (Fig. 14-10). This is the most common cause of acromioclavicular in-

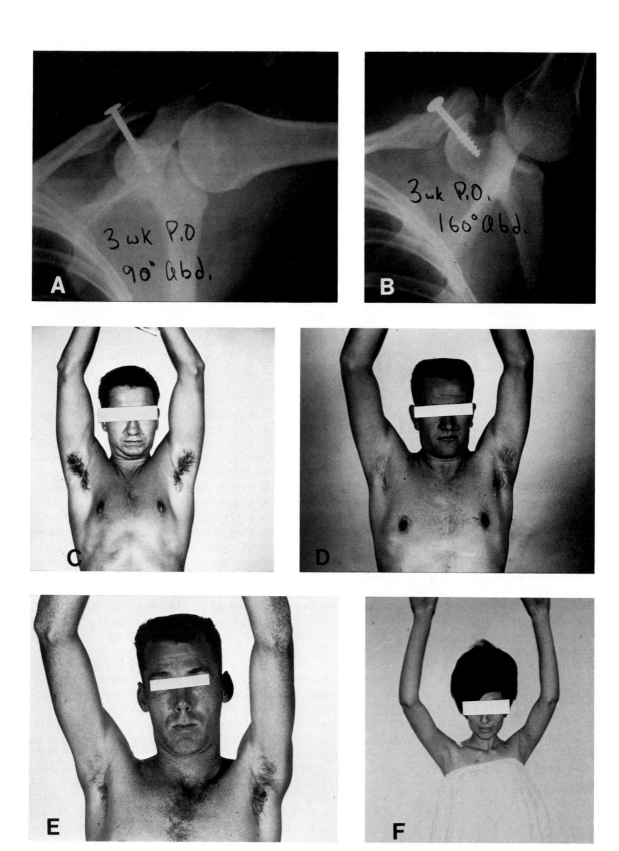

Fig. 14-8. A functional range of motion can be attained with the coracoclavicular screw in place. (**A, B**) Note that the x-ray demonstrates 160° elevation 3 weeks after surgery. (**C–F**) A very functional range of motion is seen in patients with the screw in place.

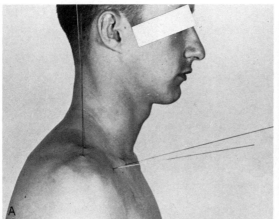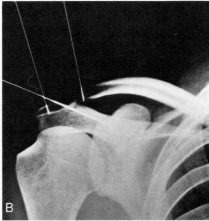

Fig. 14-9. (**A**) Lateral view of a "volunteer" with normal shoulders. Pins have been drilled into the coracoid and clavicle and into the acromion process. (**B**) X-ray with pins in place. When the patient put the shoulder through a full range of motion, the maximum amount of motion in the acromioclavicular joint, as determined by deviation of the pins in the clavicle and in the acromion, was 8°.

jury. The force drives the acromion downward. Bearn[50] showed that downward displacement of the clavicle is primarily resisted through an interlocking of the sternoclavicular ligaments. The end result, then, of a downward force being applied to the superior aspect of the acromion, is acromioclavicular and coracoclavicular ligament injury or clavicle fracture. On rare occasions, there is a disruption of the sternoclavicular ligaments.

If no fracture occurs, the force first sprains the acromioclavicular ligaments (a mild sprain), then tears the acromioclavicular ligaments (a moderate sprain) and stresses the coracoclavicular ligament, and finally—if the downward force continues— tears the deltoid and trapezius muscle attachments from the clavicle and ruptures the coracoclavicular ligament (a severe acromioclavicular sprain, which completes the dislocation). At this point, the upper extremity has lost its suspensory support from the clavicle and droops downward.

The mechanism for the inferior dislocation of the clavicle under the coracoid is thought to be a *very severe* direct force onto the superior surface of the distal clavicle, along with abduction of the arm and retraction of the scapula.[285,346]

Complete Acromioclavicular Dislocation (Type III, IV, or V): Is the Clavicle Up or Is the Shoulder Down?

Classically, the literature indicates that upward displacement of the clavicle is diagnostic of a complete acromioclavicular dislocation. Although there may be a slight upward displacement of the clavicle by the pull of the trapezius muscle, the characteristic anatomical feature is a downward sag of the shoulder and arm.

The clavicle is maintained in its normal anatomic relationship to the body through a linkage system formed by two mechanisms. The first, and probably most important, mechanism is the interlocking of the strong sternoclavicular ligaments, which resist any significant downward displacement of the distal end of the clavicle.[498] The second mechanism is upward support by the trapezius muscle, which attaches onto the distal clavicle.

The scapula and attached upper extremity are suspended from the clavicle primarily by the coracoclavicular ligament, and secondarily through the acromioclavicular ligament and the surrounding musculature. Therefore, when a severe downward force is applied to the point of the shoulder (assuming the sternoclavicular ligaments do not rupture and the clavicle does not fracture), the coracoclavicular ligaments rupture. The suspension system of the scapula and attached upper extremity from the clavicle is lost. Consequently, the arm droops *downward* (Fig. 14-11). Because the weight of the arm is no longer suspended from the clavicle, there may be a slight upward pull by the trapezius muscle on the clavicle. However, the major deformity seen in complete acromioclavicular dislocation is a *downward displacement* of the shoulder.

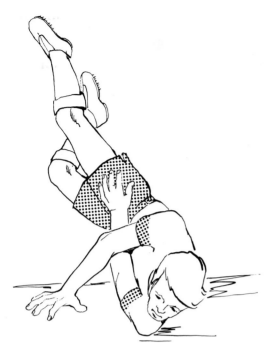

Fig. 14-10. The most common mechanism of injury is a direct force that occurs from a fall on the point of the shoulder.

INDIRECT FORCE

Upward Indirect Force on the Upper Extremity

A force from a fall on the outstretched hand is transmitted up the arm, through the humeral head, and into the acromion process. The strain is referred only to the acromioclavicular ligaments and not to the coracoclavicular ligament, because the coracoclavicular space is actually decreased (Fig. 14-12). This indirect force can then produce mild, moderate, or severe acromioclavicular joint injury. If the force is severe enough, it can fracture the acromion, rupture the acromioclavicular ligaments, and cause a superior dislocation of the glenohumeral joint. This is indeed a very rare mechanism of injury.

Downward Indirect Force Through the Upper Extremity

Forces can be indirectly applied to the acromioclavicular joint by a pull through the upper extremity. Liberson[263] reported a case in which the scapula was forcibly drawn downward and anteriorly by a sudden change in the position of a heavy burden being carried. Again, this is a rare mechanism of injury to the acromioclavicular joint.

CLASSIFICATION OF INJURY

Acromioclavicular joint injuries are best classified according to the extent of damage inflicted by a given force. However, unlike other joints, the differential diagnosis of sprains of the acromioclavicular joint is based on the severity of injury sustained by the capsular ligaments (acromioclavicular ligaments), extracapsular ligaments (coracoclavicular ligament), as well as the supporting musculature (deltoid and trapezius muscles). Therefore, injuries to the acromioclavicular joint are graded according to the amount of injury to the acromioclavicular and coracoclavicular ligaments. Technically, injuries of the acromioclavicular joint should be referred

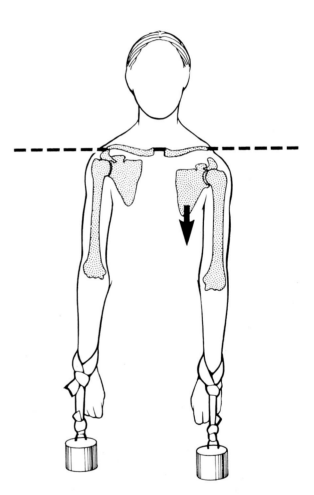

Fig. 14-11. Schematic drawing of a patient with a complete grade III acromioclavicular dislocation. The major deformity seen in this injury is a downward displacement of the scapula and upper extremity—*not* an upward elevation of the clavicle.

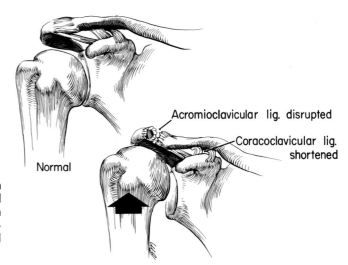

Fig. 14-12. An indirect force applied up through the upper extremity (eg, a fall on the outstretched hand) may superiorly displace the acromion from the clavicle, producing injury to the acromioclavicular ligaments. However, stress is not placed on the coracoclavicular ligaments.

to as "scapuloclavicular injuries." Zaricznyj[502] discussed this in his report. However, because of tradition, subject indexing, and commonly used nomenclature, the injuries in this anatomical area will be referred to as "acromioclavicular joint injuries."

Injuries of the acromioclavicular joint have been referred to as type I, II, or III, depending on the integrity of the acromioclavicular and the coracoclavicular ligaments (Fig. 14-13**A, B, C**).[15,455] *Type I injuries* are characterized by sprained but intact acromioclavicular ligaments and an intact coracoclavicular ligament. In the more severe *type II injuries,* the acromioclavicular ligaments are completely torn and the coracoclavicular ligament is sprained but intact. In *type III injuries,* complete acromioclavicular dislocation occurs when both the acromioclavicular and coracoclavicular ligaments are completely disrupted.

Over the past 15 years, the senior author has encountered three additional types of acromioclavicular dislocation which have been added to the original classification scheme (Fig. 14-13**D, E, F**).[494] In

type IV injuries, the clavicle is grossly displaced posteriorly into or through the trapezius muscle. *Type V injuries* represent an exaggeration of type III injuries, with severe vertical separation of the clavicle from the scapula. In *type VI injuries,* the clavicle is dislocated inferiorly into either a subacromial or a subcoracoid position. Inferior, subcoracoid acromioclavicular dislocation has been described by Patterson,[346] McPhee,[285] Sage,[396] and Schwarz and Kuderna.[409] In 1987, Gerber and Rockwood[165] reported three cases of inferior, subcoracoid dislocation of the distal clavicle—one in a child and two in adults.

The treatment of "complete" acromioclavicular dislocations is controversial. Proponents of both operative and nonoperative management are numerous. However, because the treatment for most type IV, V, and VI injuries is operative, it seems reasonable and practical to remove them from the all-inclusive type III category and to create an expanded, more accurate classification system. The modified classification is described as follows:

→

Fig. 14-13. Schematic drawings of the classification of ligamentous injuries to the acromioclavicular joint. (**Top left**) In the type I injury a mild force applied to the point of the shoulder does not disrupt either the acromioclavicular or the coracoclavicular ligaments. (**Top right**) A moderate to heavy force applied to the point of the shoulder will disrupt the acromioclavicular ligaments, but the coracoclavicular ligaments remain intact. (**Center left**) When a severe force is applied to the point of the shoulder both the acromioclavicular and the coracoclavicular ligaments are disrupted. (**Center right**) In a type IV injury not only are the ligaments disrupted but the distal end of the clavicle is also displaced posteriorly into or through the trapezius muscle. (**Bottom left**) A violent force applied to the point of the shoulder not only ruptures the acromioclavicular and coracoclavicular ligaments, but also disrupts the muscle attachments and creates a major separation between the clavicle and the acromion. (**Bottom right**) This is an inferior dislocation of the distal clavicle in which the clavicle is inferior to the coracoid process and posterior to the biceps and coracobrachialis tendons. The acromioclavicular and coracoclavicular ligaments are also disrupted.

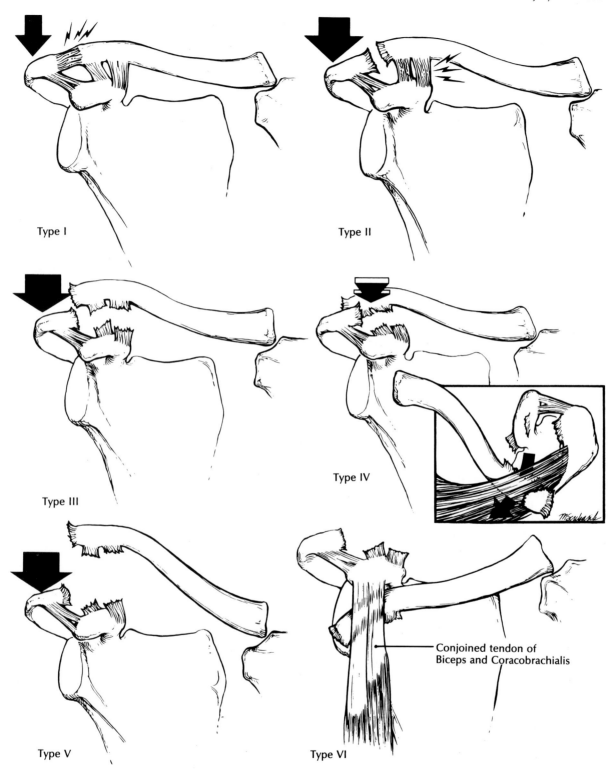

Type I

Type II

Type III

Type IV

Type V

Type VI

Conjoined tendon of
Biceps and Coracobrachialis

Modified Classification of Acromioclavicular Joint Injuries

Type I

Sprain of acromioclavicular ligament
Acromioclavicular joint intact
Coracoclavicular ligaments intact
Deltoid and trapezius muscles intact

Type II

Acromioclavicular joint disrupted
Acromioclavicular joint wider: may be a slight vertical separation when compared with the normal shoulder
Sprain of the coracoclavicular ligaments
Coracoclavicular interspace might be slightly increased
Deltoid and trapezius muscles intact

Type III

Acromioclavicular ligaments disrupted
Acromioclavicular joint dislocated and the shoulder complex displaced inferiorly
Coracoclavicular ligaments disrupted
Coracoclavicular interspace 25% to 100% greater than the normal shoulder
Deltoid and trapezius muscles usually detached from the distal end of the clavicle

TYPE III VARIANTS

"Pseudodislocation" through intact periosteal sleeve
Physeal injury
Coracoid process fracture

Type IV

Acromioclavicular ligaments disrupted
Acromioclavicular joint dislocated and clavicle anatomically displaced posteriorly into or through the trapezius muscle
Coracoclavicular ligaments completely disrupted
Coracoclavicular space may be displaced, but may *appear* same as the normal shoulder
Deltoid and trapezius muscles detached from the distal clavicle

Type V

Acromioclavicular ligaments disrupted
Coracoclavicular ligaments disrupted
Acromioclavicular joint dislocated and gross disparity between the clavicle and the scapula (ie, 100% to 300% greater than the normal shoulder)
Deltoid and trapezius muscles detached from the distal half of the clavicle

Type VI

Acromioclavicular ligaments disrupted
Coracoclavicular ligaments disrupted in subcoracoid type and intact in subacromial type
Acromioclavicular joint dislocated and clavicle displaced inferior to the acromion or coracoid process
Coracoclavicular interspace reversed in the subcoracoid type (ie, clavicle inferior to the coracoid), or decreased

in the subacromial type (ie, clavicle inferior to the acromion)
Deltoid and trapezius muscles detached from the distal clavicle

TYPE I

A mild force to the point of the shoulder produces a minor strain to the fibers of the acromioclavicular ligaments. The ligaments remain intact, and the acromioclavicular joint remains stable. (See Fig. 14-13.)

TYPE II

A moderate force to the point of the shoulder is severe enough to rupture the ligaments of the acromioclavicular joint. (See Fig. 14-13**B**.) The distal end of the clavicle is unstable in the horizontal plane (ie, anteroposterior), but vertical (ie, superoinferior) stability is preserved by virtue of the intact coracoclavicular ligament. The scapula may rotate medially, producing a widening of the acromioclavicular joint. There may be a slight, relative upward displacement of the distal end of the clavicle secondary to a minor stretching of the coracoclavicular ligament. Janecki[227] reported a case of voluntary anterior and posterior subluxation of the acromioclavicular joint in a 19-year-old female with no history of trauma.

TYPE III

When a severe force is applied to the point of the shoulder, "complete" acromioclavicular dislocation occurs. In a "classic" type III injury, the acromioclavicular and coracoclavicular ligaments are disrupted. (See Fig. 14-13**C**.) The distal clavicle appears to be displaced superiorly as the scapula and shoulder complex droop inferomedially. The deltoid and trapezius muscles are detached from the distal clavicle.

Complete acromioclavicular dislocation without disruption of the acromioclavicular and coracoclavicular ligaments has been reported.[57,100,149,297] Children and adolescents occasionally sustain a variant of complete acromioclavicular dislocation in which the clavicle is relatively displaced superiorly through a longitudinal rent in the periosteal sleeve.[149,199,234] Although the clavicle appears displaced superiorly, the acromioclavicular ligaments, the coracoclavicular ligament, and the confluent deltotrapezius fascia are not torn and remain attached to the intact periosteal sleeve. Falstie-Jensen and Mikkelson,[149] as well as Katznelson and colleagues,[234] reported this injury in young adults and children. Havranek[199] reported ten children with relative superior displacement of the clavicle associated with a Salter-Harris II fracture of the distal clavicular physis, rather than with an acromioclavicular dislocation.

Another variation of the type III injury is complete acromioclavicular dislocation associated with coracoid process fracture.[57,100,297,495] Most often, the coracoid process is avulsed at its base by the intact coracoclavicular ligament.[57,100,297] Wilson and Colwill[495] recently reported a case of complete acromioclavicular dislocation associated with a fracture of the tip of the coracoid process in a football player. At the time of operative repair, the acromioclavicular and coracoclavicular ligaments were disrupted and the tip of the coracoid process was attached to the conjoined tendon of the short head of the biceps and coracobrachialis muscles. The presumed mechanism of injury was forcible elbow flexion against resistance combined with a superior blow to the top of the acromion process.

TYPE IV

Posterior dislocation of the distal end of the clavicle, or type IV acromioclavicular dislocation, is relatively rare. The clavicle is posteriorly displaced into or through the trapezius muscle as the force applied to the acromion drives the scapula anteriorly and inferiorly. (See Fig. 14-13**D**.) Posterior clavicular displacement may be so severe that the skin on the posterior aspect of the shoulder becomes tented (See Fig. 14-37). The literature concerning posterior acromioclavicular dislocations consists mostly of small series and case reports.[37,198,274,326,432] While Barber,[37] Malcapi and colleagues,[274] and Sondergard-Petersen and Mikkelsen[432] refer to this injury as a "posterior dislocation of the clavicle," Hastings and Horne[198] and Nieminen and Aho[326] prefer the term "anterior dislocation of the scapula."

TYPE V

Type V acromioclavicular dislocation is a markedly more severe version of the type III injury. The distal clavicle has been stripped of all its soft tissue attachments (ie, acromioclavicular ligaments, coracoclavicular ligament, and the deltotrapezius muscle attachments) and lies subcutaneously near the base of the neck. (See Figs. 14-13 and 14-27.) When combined with superior displacement of the clavicle

owing to unopposed pull of the sternocleidomastoid muscle, the severe downward droop of the extremity produces a grotesque disfiguration of the shoulder.

TYPE VI

Inferior dislocation of the distal clavicle, or type VI acromioclavicular dislocation, is an exceedingly rare injury.[165,285,313,346,396,409] Gerber and Rockwood's series[165] of three patients is the largest one reported in the literature. The injury often is the result of severe trauma and frequently is accompanied by multiple injuries. The mechanism of dislocation is thought to be severe hyperabduction and external rotation of the arm, combined with retraction of the scapula. The distal clavicle occupies either a subacromial[313] or a subcoracoid[165,285,346,396,409] location. (See Figs. 14-13**F** and 14-38.)

In all reported cases of subcoracoid dislocation, the clavicle has become lodged behind an intact conjoined tendon. The acromioclavicular ligaments are disrupted in either a subacromial or subcoracoid dislocation. The coracoclavicular ligament, however, is intact in a subacromial dislocation and completely disrupted in a subcoracoid dislocation. Likewise, the integrity of the deltoid and trapezius muscle attachments depends on the degree of clavicular displacement. Sage[396] reported a case of recurring inferior dislocation; Nauman[313] reported a case of spontaneous, habitual subacromial dislocation.

INCIDENCE

Rowe and Marble[103] retrospectively reviewed the medical records of the Massachusetts General Hospital and found 52 acromioclavicular joint injuries among 1603 shoulder-girdle injuries. Most occurred in the second decade of life. Thorndike and Quigley[453] reported acromioclavicular joint involvement in 223 of 578 athletes with shoulder injuries. Acromioclavicular dislocation is more common in males (5:1 to 10:1) and is more often incomplete than complete (approximately 2:1). In one 5-year period, our institution recorded 520 acromioclavicular injuries.[322] More than 300 of these occurred in the first three decades of life (Table 14-1). The distribution of these injuries according to type is shown in Table 14-2.

Table 14-1. Frequency of Acromioclavicular Injuries by Patient Age*

	Decade of Life								
	1st	*2nd*	*3rd*	*4th*	*5th*	*6th*	*7th*	*8th*	*9th*
Number of Injuries	4	112	226	117	29	5	8	16	3

* Based on a review of 520 acromioclavicular injuries treated at Medical Center Hospital, San Antonio, Texas. Age range 9 to 87 years.

SIGNS AND SYMPTOMS

When acromioclavicular joint injury is suspected, the patient should be examined, whenever possible, in the standing or sitting position. The weight of the arm stresses the acromioclavicular joint and makes a deformity more apparent.

TYPE I INJURY

In a type I injury, there is minimal to moderate tenderness and swelling over the acromioclavicular joint without palpable displacement of the joint. Usually there is only minimal pain with arm movements. Tenderness is not present in the coracoclavicular interspace.

TYPE II INJURY

With subluxation of the acromioclavicular joint, moderate to severe pain is noted at the joint. If the patient is examined shortly after injury, the outer end of the clavicle may be noted to be slightly superior to the acromion. Motion of the shoulder produces pain in the acromioclavicular joint. With gentle palpation, the outer end of the clavicle may appear to be unstable and free-floating. If the mid-clavicle is grasped and the acromion stabilized, a to-and-fro motion of the clavicle in the horizontal plane can be detected. Tenderness is also noted when the physician palpates anteriorly in the coracoclavicular interspace.

Table 14-2. Frequency of Acromioclavicular Injuries by Type*

	Type of Injury					
	I	*II*	*III*	*IV*	*V*	*VI*
Number of Injuries	185	119	204	4	7	1

* Based on a review of 520 acromioclavicular injuries treated at Medical Center Hospital, San Antonio, Texas.

TYPE III INJURY

The patient with type III injury, complete dislocation of the acromioclavicular joint, characteristically presents with the upper extremity held adducted close to the body and supported in an elevated position to relieve the pain in the acromioclavicular joint. The shoulder complex is depressed when compared with the normal shoulder. The clavicle may be prominent enough to tent the skin (Fig. 14-14). Moderate pain is the rule, and any motion of the arm, particularly abduction, increases the pain.

Tenderness is noted at the acromioclavicular joint, the coracoclavicular interspace, and along the superior aspect of the lateral fourth of the clavicle. The lateral clavicle is unstable in both the horizontal and vertical planes. Delbet[94] noted that the clavicle can be so prominent and unstable in this situation that it can be depressed like a piano key.

Cooper,[108] in 1832, described a technique that could be used even by a blind man to detect a complete acromioclavicular dislocation:

> The easiest mode of detecting this accident is to place the finger upon the spine of the scapula and to trace this portion of the bone forward to the acromion in which it ends; the finger is stopped by the projection of the clavicle, and so, as

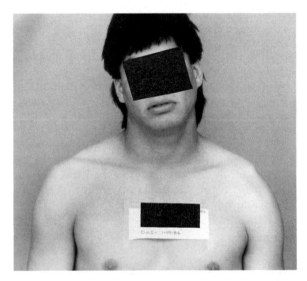

Fig. 14-14. This patient has a complete type III dislocation of the left acromioclavicular joint. The left shoulder is drooping and there is prominence of the left distal clavicle. (*Rockwood, C. A., and Young, D. C.: Disorders of the Acromioclavicular Joint. In Rockwood, C. A., and Matsen, F., III (eds.): The Shoulder, Fig. 12-14. Philadelphia, W. B. Saunders, 1990.*)

the shoulders are drawn back, the point of the clavicle sinks into place, but it reappears when the shoulders let go.

TYPE IV INJURY

The patient with a type IV injury has essentially all the clinical findings of a type III injury. In addition, examination of the seated patient from above reveals that the outline of the posteriorly displaced clavicle is inclined posteriorly compared to the uninjured shoulder (Fig. 14-15; also see Fig. 14-37). Occasionally the clavicle is displaced so severely posteriorly that it becomes "buttonholed" through the trapezius muscle and tents the posterior skin. Consequently, motion of the shoulder is more painful than in a type III injury.

TYPE V INJURY

The type V injury is an exaggeration of the type III injury in which the distal end of the clavicle appears to be grossly superiorly displaced toward the base of the neck (Fig. 14-16). This apparent upward displacement is the result of downward displacement of the upper extremity. The patient has more pain than with a type III injury, particularly over the distal half of the clavicle. This is secondary to the extensive muscle and soft tissue disruption from the clavicle that occurs with this injury. Occasionally, there is so much inferior displacement of the upper extremity that the patient will develop symptoms of traction on the brachial plexus.

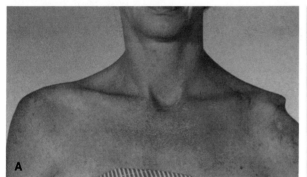

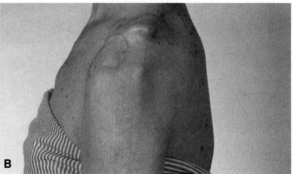

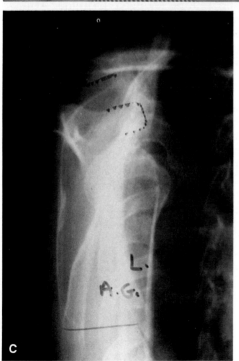

Fig. 14-15. (A, B) A 33-year-old woman with a combined type IV and type V chronic dislocation of the acromioclavicular joint. Note the drooping of the left upper extremity and the prominent distal end of the clavicle. **(C)** The scapulolateral x-ray demonstrates the severe displacement of the acromioclavicular joint.

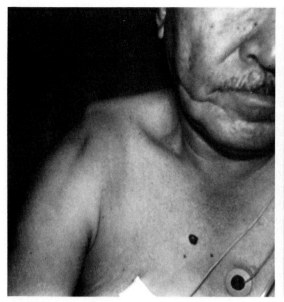 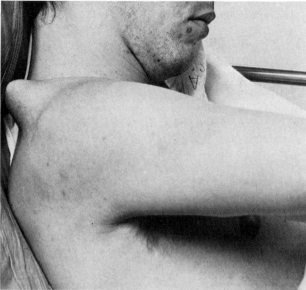

Fig. 14-16. Clinical photographs of patient with grade V acromioclavicular dislocation. (**Left**) A severe upward displacement of the right clavicle into the base of the neck. (**Right**) Note the severe upward displacement of the clavicle in the right shoulder. There was so much tension on the skin that it was becoming necrotic.

TYPE VI INJURY

The superior aspect of the shoulder has a flat appearance, as opposed to the rounded contour of the normal shoulder. With palpation, the acromion is prominent, and there is a definite inferior step-down to the superior surface of the coracoid process. Because of the amount of trauma required to produce a subcoracoid dislocation of the clavicle, there may be associated fractures of the clavicle and upper ribs, or injury to the upper roots of the brachial plexus. These associated injuries may produce so much swelling of the shoulder that the disruption of the acromioclavicular joint may not initially be recognized. Vascular injuries secondary to the dislocation were not present in the patients presented by Patterson,[346] McPhee,[285] Schwarz and Kuderna,[409] and Gerber and Rockwood.[165] However, all the adult cases reported by Patterson,[346] McPhee,[285] and Gerber and Rockwood[165] had transient paresthesias prior to reduction of the dislocation. Following reduction, the neurologic deficits cleared.

RADIOGRAPHIC EVALUATION

The acromioclavicular joint requires one third to one half the x-ray penetration required for the denser glenohumeral joint for good quality radiographs. Radiographs of the acromioclavicular joint taken using routine shoulder technique will be overpenetrated (ie, dark), and small fractures may be overlooked (Fig. 14-17**A**). Therefore, the x-ray technician must be specifically requested to take radiographs of the "acromioclavicular joint," rather than the "shoulder" (Fig. 14-17**B**).

ANTEROPOSTERIOR VIEWS

Routine anteroposterior views should be taken with the patient standing or sitting, with his back against the x-ray cassette and his arms hanging unsupported at his side. Because of significant individual variation in acromioclavicular joint anatomy and because the coracoclavicular interspace will vary with the angle of the x-ray beam and with the distance between the beam and the patient, both acromioclavicular joints should be imaged simultaneously on one large (14 × 17–inch) cassette. Large patients with shoulders too broad to be visualized on a single cassette should have radiographs made with two smaller (10 × 12–inch) cassettes using identical technique.

Zanca[500] reviewed 1000 radiographs of patients with shoulder pain and noted that on a true anteroposterior view of the acromioclavicular joint, the distal clavicle and acromion are superimposed on the spine of the scapula. Therefore, he recommended a 10° to 15° cephalic tilt view to project an unobscured image of the joint (Fig. 14-17**C**, 14-18). This view is useful, particularly when there is suspicion of a small fracture or loose body on routine views (Fig. 14-19).

LATERAL VIEWS

As with any musculoskeletal injury, a radiograph in one plane is not sufficient to classify an acromioclavicular injury. An axillary lateral view should be taken of the injured and normal shoulders when acromioclavicular dislocation is suspected. The cassette should be placed on the superior aspect of the shoulder and medial enough to expose as much of the lateral third of the clavicle as possible. This will reveal any posterior displacement of the clavicle as

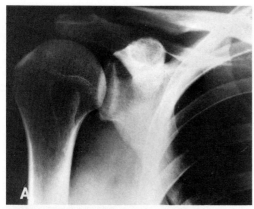
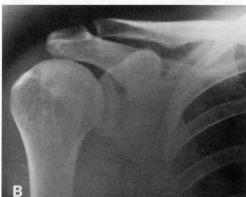
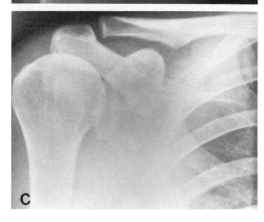

Fig. 14-17. Explanation of why the acromioclavicular joint is poorly visualized on routine shoulder x-rays. (**A**) This routine anteroposterior view of the shoulder shows the glenohumeral joint well. However, the acromioclavicular joint is too dark to interpret, because that area of the anatomy has been overpenetrated by the x-ray technique. (**B**) When the exposure usually used to take the shoulder films is decreased by two thirds, the acromioclavicular joint is well visualized. However, the inferior corner of the acromioclavicular joint is superimposed on the acromion process. (**C**) Tilting the tube 15° upward provides a clear view of the acromioclavicular joint.

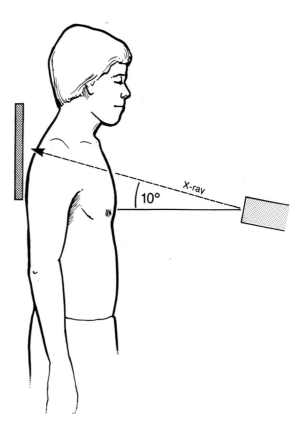

Fig. 14-18. Position of the patient for the Zanca view—a 10° to 15° cephalic tilt of the standard view for the acromioclavicular joint. (*Rockwood, C. A., and Young, D. C.: Disorders of the Acromioclavicular Joint. In Rockwood, C. A., and Matsen, F., III (eds.): The Shoulder, Fig. 12-19. Philadelphia, W. B. Saunders, 1990.*)

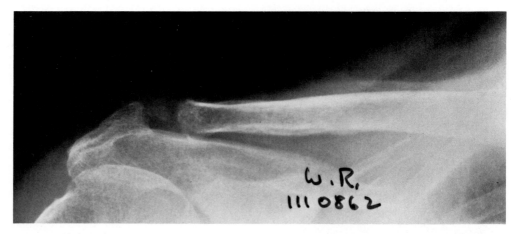

Fig. 14-19. The Zanca x-ray view demonstrates a loose body in the acromioclavicular joint. *(Rockwood, C. A., and Young, D. C.: Disorders of the Acromioclavicular Joint. In Rockwood, C. A., and Matsen, F., III (eds.): The Shoulder, Fig. 12-20. Philadelphia, W. B. Saunders, 1990.)*

well as any small fractures that may have been missed on the anteroposterior view.

STRESS X-RAY STUDIES

Bossart and colleagues[72] reviewed the stress x-rays of 82 patients who did not have obvious type III injury of the acromioclavicular joint. Their study unmasked five cases with type III injuries. Because of this low percentage yield, they did not believe stress x-ray views of the acromioclavicular joint were justified.

Patients who present with a clinically obvious acromioclavicular injury and typical deformity suggestive of complete dislocation (ie, type III, IV, or V), often demonstrate maximal coracoclavicular interspace widening on routine anteroposterior views alone. Occasionally, however, the dislocation will not be apparent on routine radiographs because the patient has supported the injured shoulder with the opposite arm and reduced the acromioclavicular joint (Fig. 14-20). In addition, some type II injuries (ie, subluxations) can be difficult to differentiate from type III, or complete, dislocation on routine views. Therefore, stress films of both shoulders to test the integrity of the coracoclavicular ligament, should be routinely performed when acromioclavicular dislocation is suspected.

Fig. 14-20. Importance of obtaining stress x-ray views of the acromioclavicular joint. (**A**) The patient presents with only a mild deformity in the vicinity of the acromioclavicular joint. (**B**) With weight added to the wrist of the upper extremity, the deformity is exaggerated. (**C**) If the x-ray is taken of the acromioclavicular joint without weights attached to the upper extremity, the patient may, in an effort to relieve the pain, lift the shoulder upward, presenting a view that shows minimal separation of the acromioclavicular joint.

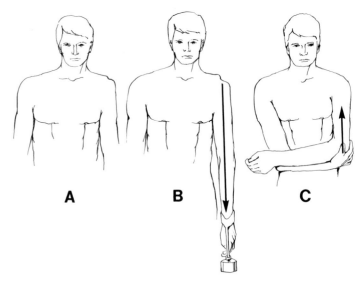

A   **B**   **C**

Anteroposterior Stress Views

The technique for an anteroposterior stress view is similar to that described above for routine anteroposterior radiographs, except that weights (10–15 pounds) are suspended from each arm with wrist straps (Fig. 14-21**A**). The weights should be hanging from the wrists rather than held by the patient, to encourage complete muscle relaxation (Fig. 14-21**B**).

Bannister and colleagues[36] recently described "weight-lifting" in addition to "weight-bearing" stress views. An anteroposterior radiograph is taken with a weight suspended from the arm. After infiltration of the acromioclavicular joint with local anesthetic, the patient is asked to lift the weight by shrugging his shoulders. If, during this "weight-lifting" view, the coracoclavicular distance becomes wider, the patient is thought to have disrupted not only the acromioclavicular and coracoclavicular ligaments, but also the entire deltoid and trapezius

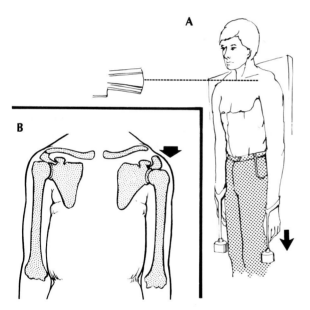

Fig. 14-21. Technique of obtaining stress x-ray views of the acromioclavicular joint. (**A**) Anteroposterior x-rays are made of both acromioclavicular joints with 10 to 15 pounds of weight hanging from the wrists. (**B**) The distance between the superior aspect of the coracoid and the undersurface of the clavicle is measured to determine whether or not the coracoclavicular ligaments have been disrupted. One large horizontal 14 × 17–inch x-ray cassette can be used in small patients to visualize both shoulders on the same film. In large patients it is better to use two horizontal smaller cassettes and take two separate x-rays for the measurements.

attachments. Bannister recommended early surgical repair in such cases. However, this recommendation was based on only six patients, three of whom were treated nonoperatively. Therefore, the significance of this "weight-lifting" radiograph is, as yet, unclear.

Lateral Stress Views

Alexander[9] described a lateral stress view of the acromioclavicular joint to help identify acromioclavicular dislocation. He called it the "shoulder-forward view." The patient is positioned as if a true scapulolateral x-ray is to be taken, as described in the section on posterior glenohumeral dislocations. The patient is then asked to thrust both shoulders forward. Radiographs are taken of both the injured and the normal side for comparison. The acromioclavicular joint on the normal side will maintain its reduced position. However, on the injured side, the acromion will be displaced anteriorly and inferiorly with respect to the distal clavicle (Fig. 14-22). Waldrop and co-workers[477] recommended this view for routine evaluation of all acromioclavicular injuries. However, some type II injuries with significant posterior instability may be difficult to differentiate from complete dislocation using this view.

OTHER MODALITIES

Schmid and Schmid[404] reported the use of ultrasonography in the diagnosis of 22 cases of type III acromioclavicular dislocation. Ultrasound demonstrated visible instability of the distal clavicle, incongruity of the joint, hematoma formation, or visible ligament remnants in all cases. However, in spite of the advent of such sophisticated imaging modalities as ultrasound, CT scan, and magnetic resonance imaging, plain radiography continues to be the most readily available, cost-effective method for routine investigation of injuries to the acromioclavicular joint.

RADIOGRAPHIC FINDINGS

Normal Joints

The width and configuration of the acromioclavicular joint in the coronal plane may vary significantly from individual to individual. In a study of 100 radiographs of normal shoulders, Urist[464] found that nearly half (49%) of the acromioclavicular joints were inclined superolateral to inferomedial, with the articular surface of the clavicle overriding

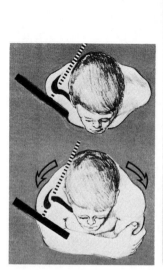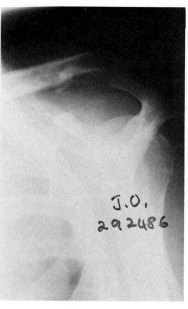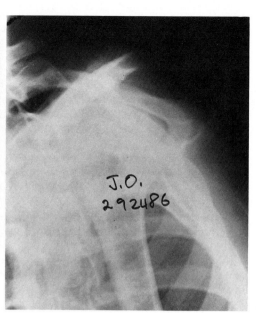

Fig. 14-22. Technique of obtaining the Alexander view or scapular lateral view to evaluate injuries of the acromio-clavicular joint. (**Left**) Schematic drawing illustrating how the shoulders are thrust forward at the time the x-ray is made. (**Center**) Alexander view taken with the shoulder in the relaxed position. Note that the acromioclavicular joint is only minimally displaced. (**Right**) With the shoulders thrust forward there is gross displacement of the acromioclavicular joint with the acromion being displaced anteriorly and inferiorly under the distal end of the clavicle.

the acromion; 27% were vertical and 3% were inclined superomedial to inferolateral, with the articular surface of the clavicle underriding the acromion. Another 21% of the joints were incongruent, with the clavicle lying either superior or inferior to the acromial articular surface. Nguyen[322] reviewed 300 normal acromioclavicular joints at our institution and found that 51% of the joints exhibited an overriding clavicle, 2% had an under-riding clavicle, 18% were vertical in orientation, and 29% were incongruent.

According to Oppenheimer[339] and Zanca,[500] the normal width of the acromioclavicular joint in the coronal plane is 1 to 3 mm. Petersson and Redlund-Johnell[349] radiographically measured acromioclavicular joint width in 151 normal individuals and drew several conclusions: the acromioclavicular joint space normally diminishes with increasing age; a joint space of 0.5 mm in a patient older than 60 years is conceivably normal; and a joint space of greater than 7 mm in men and 6 mm in women is pathologic. In a review of 300 normal subjects at our institution, Nguyen[322] found similar results. The joint widths in these 300 subjects ranged from 0.5 to 7 mm; the latter measurement was recorded in only six patients.

The coracoclavicular interspace also exhibits significant individual variation. Bosworth[76] stated that the average distance between the clavicle and the coracoid process is 1.3 cm. Bearden and colleagues[49] found a range of normal values for the coracoclavicular interspace of 1.1 to 1.3 cm. Bearden and colleagues[49] also stated that an increase in the cor-acoclavicular distance of 50% over the normal side signified complete acromioclavicular dislocation. The senior author has documented complete dislocation with as little as a 25% increase in the cor-acoclavicular distance.

Type I Injury

In a type I injury, the x-rays of the acromioclavicular joint are normal, except for mild soft tissue swelling, as compared to the uninjured shoulder. There is no widening, no separation, and no deformity.

Type II Injury

In a type II injury, the lateral end of the clavicle may be slightly elevated. The acromioclavicular joint, when compared with the normal side, may appear to be widened. The widening probably is the result of a slight medial rotation of the scapula and slight posterior displacement of the clavicle by the pull of the trapezius muscle. Stress films of both shoulders, to test the integrity of the coracoclavicular ligaments, reveal that the coracoclavicular space of the injured shoulder is the same as that of the normal shoulder (Fig. 14-23).

Type III Injury

In obvious cases of complete acromioclavicular dislocations, the joint is totally displaced. The lateral end of the clavicle is displaced completely above the superior border of the acromion and the coracoclavicular interspace is significantly greater than in the normal shoulder (Fig. 14-24). When the case is questionable, which it often is, stress films comparing the injured and normal shoulders will reveal a major discrepancy in the coracoclavicular distances. Fractures may be noted on the distal clavicle, or on the acromion process.

Rarely, complete acromioclavicular dislocation will be accompanied by a fracture of the coracoid process rather than by disruption of the coracoclavicular ligaments. Although the fracture of the coracoid process is difficult to visualize on routine radiographs, its presence should be suspected because of the presence of complete acromioclavicular separation and a normal coracoclavicular distance,

as compared to the uninjured shoulder. (See Fig. 14-51.) The best special view for visualizing the coracoid fracture is the Stryker notch view (Fig. 14-25). The technique for obtaining this view is described in detail in the section on Anterior Glenohumeral Dislocation.

Type IV Injury

Although the radiographic findings associated with a type IV injury include a relative upward displacement of the clavicle from the acromion and an increase in the coracoclavicular interspace, the most striking feature is the posterior displacement of the distal clavicle, as seen on the axillary lateral x-ray (Fig. 14-26). In patients with heavy, thick shoulders, or in patients with multiple injuries in whom an axillary lateral view of the shoulder or a scapulolateral x-ray view cannot be taken, a CT scan may be of great value in helping to confirm clinical suspicions of a posteriorly dislocated acromioclavicular joint.

Type V Injury

The characteristic x-ray feature of type V injuries is a marked increase (ie, two to three times normal) in the coracoclavicular interspace (Fig. 14-27**A,B**). The clavicle appears to be grossly displaced supe-

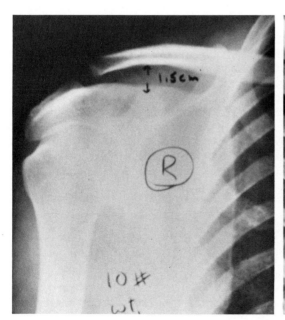
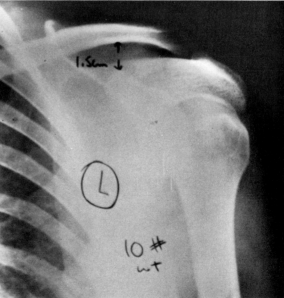

Fig. 14-23. X-ray appearance of a type II acromioclavicular joint injury to the right shoulder. With stress the coracoclavicular distance in both shoulders measures 1.5 cm. However, the injured right shoulder has a widened acromioclavicular joint compared with the normal left shoulder.

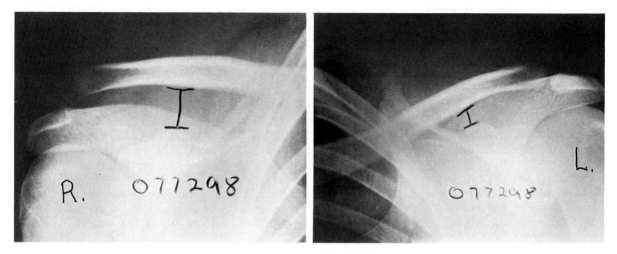

Fig. 14-24. X-ray appearance of a grade III injury to the right shoulder. Stress x-ray films were made to compare the right shoulder with the left. Not only is the right acromioclavicular joint displaced compared with the left, but more significantly notice the great increase in coracoclavicular interspace on the injured right shoulder compared with the normal left shoulder.

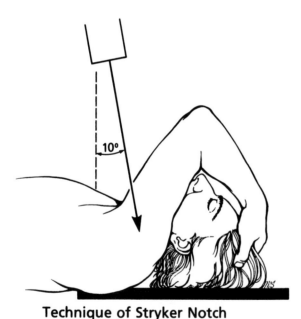

Technique of Stryker Notch

Fig. 14-25. Technique for taking the Stryker notch view to demonstrate fractures of the base of the coracoid. The patient is supine with a cassette placed posterior to the shoulder. The humerus is flexed approximately 120° so the patient's hand can be placed on top of the head. The x-ray beam is directed 10° superior. (Rockwood, C. A., and Young, D. C.: Disorders of the Acromioclavicular Joint. In Rockwood, C. A., and Matsen, F., III (eds.): The Shoulder, Fig. 12-27. Philadelphia, W. B. Saunders, 1990.)

riorly away from the acromion. However, radiographs reveal that the clavicle on the injured side is actually at approximately the same level as the clavicle on the normal side, and the scapula is displaced inferiorly (Fig. 14-27**C,D**).

Type VI Injury

There are two types of inferior acromioclavicular dislocation: subacromial and subcoracoid. In the subacromial type, radiographs reveal a decreased coracoclavicular distance (ie, less than the normal side) and the distal clavicle is in a subacromial location. The subcoracoid dislocation is characterized by a reversed coracoclavicular distance, with the clavicle displaced inferior to the coracoid process (See Fig. 14-38.). Because this injury usually is the result of severe trauma, it often is accompanied by multiple other fractures of the clavicle and ribs.

TREATMENT

In 1917, Cadenat[94] emphasized that the treatment of acromioclavicular injuries depends on whether a complete or an incomplete dislocation has occurred. Although some authors report surgical repair for selected incomplete dislocations, the vast majority of type I and type II injuries do not require surgical intervention. The treatment of complete dislocations, however, is much more controversial.

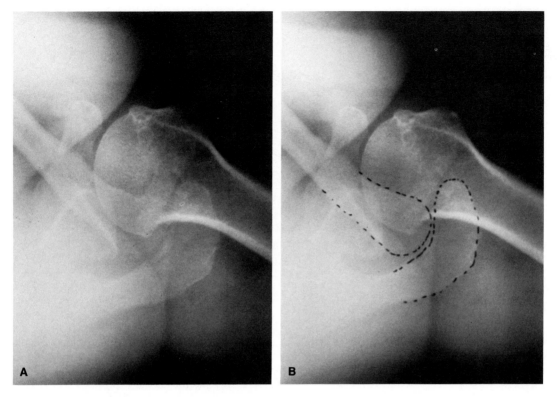

Fig. 14-26. Type IV posterior dislocation of the acromioclavicular joint. (**A**) Axillary lateral x-ray of the right shoulder. (**B**) Axillary view with the distal clavicle and acromion outlined.

Many surgeons adamently recommend operative reduction and repair of all acute, complete acromioclavicular dislocations. Other authors advocate, with equal vigor, routine nonoperative treatment in all cases of complete dislocation. Still other surgeons recommend operative repair in selected circumstances.

The confusion surrounding the treatment of acromioclavicular injuries is not clarified by a review of the literature. Many articles have been written about acromioclavicular injuries. However, there are few, if any, prospective studies comparing the results of operative and nonoperative treatment in two well-matched groups large enough to make statistically significant conclusions. In fact, a review of more than 300 articles pertaining to acromioclavicular injuries reveals that about half have contributed only a new surgical technique or a new twist to an old technique. In addition, some authors include incomplete and complete dislocations together when reporting the results of a given form of treatment. Furthermore, all complete acromioclavicular dislocations are not the same. Complete

dislocations include types III, IV, V, and VI injuries, which have significantly different pathologic findings and prognoses. The treatment of complete acromioclavicular injuries will continue to be controversial until results of different forms of treatment are compared prospectively in truly similar patient groups with comparable types of complete dislocations.

TYPE I INJURY

The type I injury is characterized by sprained, but intact, acromioclavicular ligaments and normal coracoclavicular ligaments. Usually, the symptoms subside after 7 to 10 days of rest. The application of ice bags will help to ease the discomfort. However, the shoulder should be protected from further injury until there is a painless, full range of motion.

TYPE II INJURY

In a type II injury, the acromioclavicular ligaments are torn and the coracoclavicular ligaments are

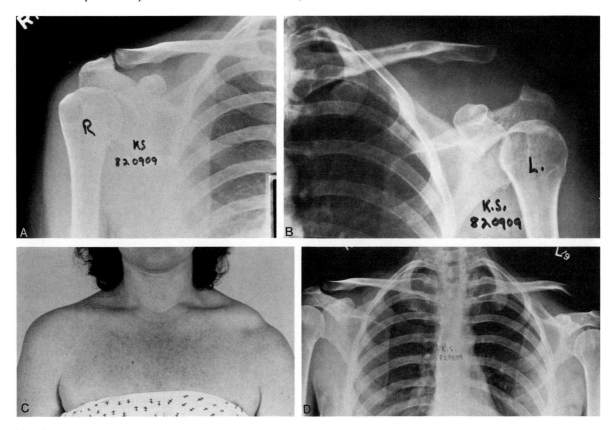

Fig. 14-27. X-rays and clinical photograph of a patient with a type V injury. (**A**) The normal right shoulder. (**B**) The injured left shoulder. Note the gross disparity in the coracoclavicular space interval. (**C and D**) Comparison of the patient's clinical deformity with the x-ray deformity. Note that a line drawn through both clavicles would indicate they are essentially at the same level. The deformity is secondary to the inferior displacement of the upper extremity, which is secondary to the loss of the coracoclavicular suspensory ligaments. (*Rockwood, C. A., and Young, D. C.: Disorders of the Acromioclavicular Joint. In Rockwood, C. A., and Matsen, F., III (eds.): The Shoulder, Fig. 12-29. Philadelphia, W. B. Saunders, 1990.*)

stretched, but intact. There may be some associated partial detachment of the deltoid and trapezius muscles from the clavicle, which increases the pain and discomfort.

Nonoperative Treatment

Most authors agree that nonsurgical measures are indicated to treat type II injuries. However, a report by Bergfeld and colleagues[56] and a study by Cox[115] suggest that untreated type I and II injuries may lead to more chronic disability than previously recognized.

Many types of nonoperative treatment have been reported for type II acromioclavicular dislocation. Some authors attempt to reduce the subluxation through the use of compressive bandages and slings, adhesive tape strapping, braces, harnesses, trac-

tion techniques, and many types of plaster casts. Urist[464–466] reviewed the literature extensively and summarized more than 35 forms of nonoperative management for acromioclavicular dislocation. He advocated the use of a plaster cast device which incorporates an elastic strap to support the arm and depress the clavicle. Allman[15] recommended the use of the Kenny Howard sling or harness (Fig. 14-28) for 3 weeks. Regardless of the method of reduction and immobilization, 3 to 6 weeks of continuous, uninterrupted pressure on the superior aspect of the clavicle is required to allow ligament healing.

Alternatively, many authors recommend a sling for 10 to 14 days, or until the symptoms subside. This is followed by an early and gradual rehabilitation program. With this method of treatment, the subluxation is ignored. Heavy lifting or contact

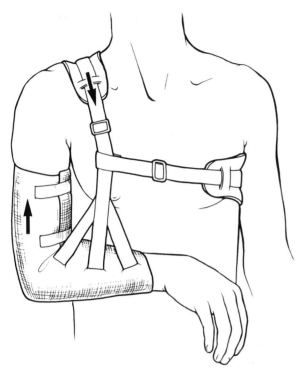

Fig. 14-28. Schematic drawing of shoulder harness (Kenny Howard type) used in the nonoperative treatment of injuries to the acromioclavicular joint. The strap that runs over the top of the shoulder and under the elbow is tightened sufficiently to reduce the clavicle to the acromion. A halter strap around the trunk keeps the harness from slipping off the top of the shoulder.

sports should be avoided for 8 to 12 weeks to allow complete ligament healing. However, a second injury prior to complete ligament healing could convert the subluxation into a complete dislocation.

Operative Treatment

Persistent pain following a type II acromioclavicular injury has been reported.[46] Symptoms can be secondary to post-traumatic osteolysis of the clavicle, torn capsular ligaments trapped within the joint, loose pieces of articular cartilage, or a detached intra-articular meniscus which displaces in and out of the joint like a torn meniscus in the knee. This "internal derangement" has been described by Bateman.[46] Brosgol[84] reported on the use of an arthrogram of the acromioclavicular joint to delineate the pathology associated with persistent acromioclavicular symptoms.

Acromioclavicular joint arthroplasty may be required to relieve persistent pain following type II acromioclavicular injury. If the articular surface of the clavicle is degenerative, then excision of the distal 2 cm of the clavicle, in addition to joint débridement and meniscectomy, is required. Because the coracoclavicular ligament is intact, the scapula does not displace inferiorly and the coracoclavicular interspace is preserved. This procedure has been described by Mumford[309] and Gurd.[186]

TYPE III INJURY

Historical Review

Throughout recorded medical history, both nonoperative and operative methods of treatment of complete acromioclavicular dislocation have enjoyed cyclical popularity. The earliest writings on the subject by Hippocrates, Galen, and Paul of Aegina recommended closed reduction and the use of compressive bandages to maintain the clavicle in the reduced position.[4] Hippocrates[4] stated that the projecting part of the shoulder (ie, the clavicle) should be depressed with compresses while the arm is kept elevated with a sling and bandages (Fig. 14-29). He went on to say that the end result would be good in spite of the inevitable, persistent deformity of the joint. Many of these concepts are still being used today.

Following the discovery of anesthesia by Long and co-workers[505] in 1844, and the development of antiseptic principles of surgery by Lister[505] in 1867, surgical repair of acute acromioclavicular dislocation became popular. Both intra-articular (ie, acromioclavicular) and extra-articular (ie, coracoclavicular) repairs were described. Cadenat,[94] in his classic article in 1917, credited Samuel Cooper of San Francisco with the first acromioclavicular repair. Cooper performed the repair in 1861 with a loop of silver wire. Subsequent to Cooper, many authors reported various techniques of acromioclavicular stabilization for acute, complete acromioclavicular dislocation. Poirier and Rieffel,[359] Tuffier,[94] and Baum[94] used sutures to repair the acromioclavicular ligaments and joint capsule. Baum,[94] in 1886, sutured the acromioclavicular ligaments percutaneously (ie, without an incision). He learned this technique from Volkmann. Bunnell,[90] in 1928, used fascia lata to reconstruct the acromioclavicular joint. Budinger[94] used a screw, and Delbet and Lambotte[94] used a nail for acromioclavicular fixation. Paci,[94] in 1889, and Bauchet and Caldwell[94] performed arthrodesis or ankylosis of the acromioclavicular joint. Morestin[94] resected the outer 2.5 cm of the clavicle.

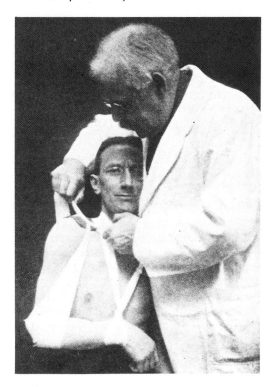

Fig. 14-29. Closed treatment of dislocation of the acromioclavicular joint. Sir Robert Jones is seen applying a sling and bandage that holds the arm elevated while depressing the lateral end of the clavicle. *(Jones, R.: Injuries of Joints, p. 57. London, Oxford University Press, 1917.)*

Although Baum is credited with the first repair of the coracoclavicular ligaments in 1886, he performed the repair as a secondary procedure. He believed repair of the acromioclavicular ligaments was of primary importance. According to Cadenat,[94] Delbet[82] was the first to reconstruct the coracoclavicular ligaments. During his first case, Delbet passed a single strand of silver wire under the coracoid process and through an anteroposterior drill hole in the clavicle. The deformity reappeared 45 days postoperatively. Upon reoperation, Delbet found the wire had broken. Therefore, in two subsequent cases, he used two silk sutures tied over the clavicle. Cadenat[94] used a strip of the short head of the biceps tendon to reconstruct the coracoclavicular ligament in cadavers. He noted the anterior location of the short head of the biceps on the coracoid process resulted in anterior displacement of the clavicle when this tendon was used as a coracoclavicular ligament substitute. Consequently, Cadenat[92] did not perform this operation in any

live patients. Cadenat[92] did, however, report the use of the coracoacromial ligament for coracoclavicular ligament reconstruction in 1917. He noted that the coracoacromial ligament is attached more posteriorly on the coracoid process than the biceps tendon, closer to the attachment of the coracoclavicular ligaments. In addition, he observed detachment of the anteriormost portion of the coracoacromial ligament yielded enough length to suture the ligament to the clavicle, thus establishing a new coracoclavicular ligament. Henry,[203] in 1924, reported on coracoclavicular ligament reconstruction using an autogenous fascia lata graft combined with acromioclavicular fixation using two Kirschner wires.

In the 1930s and 1940s, the trend began to swing away from surgical repairs back toward conservative forms of treatment, both old and new. Plaster casts of all shapes and sizes became particularly popular. Urist,[466] in his 1959 article, stated that "they [the plaster casts] range from the neatest and smallest to the largest and most grotesque seen in the whole field of traumatic and orthopaedic surgery." Additional splints and harnesses were developed in the 1940s by Gibbens,[168] Morrison,[302] Batchelor,[45] Brandt,[81] and Varney and associates.[472]

In spite of this resurgence of nonoperative treatment, many authors in the 1940s still favored surgical repair. Acromioclavicular (intra-articular) procedures continued to be popular. Murray[311] recommended smooth Kirschner wires. Bloom[68] recommended two $\frac{1}{32}$-inch Steinmann pins. Phemister[353] reported the use of heavy, threaded pins through the acromioclavicular joint. Acromioclavicular joint fixation with a screw was described by Stewart.[443] Acromioclavicular arthrodesis was described by Caldwell[96] and distal clavicle excision was described by Mumford[309] and Gurd.[186] Coracoclavicular (extra-articular) fixation was recommended by Bosworth,[73] who described a new technique using a screw inserted blindly from the clavicle into the coracoid process.

During the 1950s, 1960s, and 1970s, surgical repair continued to gain widespread popularity. In 1974, Powers and Bach[364] polled all chairmen of approved residency training programs in the United States and reported the following findings:

The majority of program chairmen treated type III injury by open reduction.
Surgical treatment varied, but 60% used temporary acromioclavicular fixation, and 35% used coracoclavicular fixation.
Nonoperative treatment was rarely advocated, and was often inadequate.

As a result of these findings, Power and Bach[364] concluded surgical repair was the most popular method of treatment for complete acromioclavicular dislocations.

Several recent articles seem to indicate that non-operative treatment is again enjoying a resurgence. Anzel and Streitz[22] reported good results in 31 patients with type II and III acromioclavicular injuries treated with a dynamic splint. Walsh and associates,[478] Glick and co-workers,[172] Sellers and colleagues,[413] and Mac Donald and associates[271] could document little significant strength deficit in patients treated nonoperatively for complete acromioclavicular dislocation. Jakobsen[226] recommended nonoperative treatment over operative treatment for complete acromioclavicular dislocation because of similar functional results in both groups, shorter convalescent time in the nonoperatively treated group, and the association of more easily managed complications with the nonoperatively treated group. However, in none of the strength studies is the question of fatigue, in addition to absolute strength, adequately answered. In addition, in none of these studies has the strength of the trapezius muscle been independently tested.

Nonoperative Treatment

Numerous methods of nonoperative treatment of complete acromioclavicular dislocation have been reported (Table 14-3). The two most commonly used methods are: (1) closed reduction and application of a sling and harness device to maintain reduction of the clavicle; and (2) short-term sling support followed by early range of motion. Multiple studies have reported good functional results, in spite of residual deformity, in patients treated by this manner of "skillful neglect."[200,218,226,271] Although plaster casts are occasionally still used, they are no longer popular. This is undoubtedly owing, in part, to the reported good results with other, more convenient forms of nonoperative management.

SLING AND HARNESS IMMOBILIZATION DEVICE

The sling supports the forearm and arm. A strap or harness is tightened around the top of the shoulder and the elbow to depress the distal clavicle. (See Figs. 14-28 and 14-29.) A separate halter strap around the trunk keeps the harness from slipping off the top of the shoulder. For the reduction to be maintained, the sling and harness must keep continuous pressure under the elbow and on top of the clavicle for 6 weeks. Allman[17] reported that one in five patients will fail this form of treatment because of inability to achieve and maintain a reduction or

Table 14-3. Nonoperative Treatment for Acromioclavicular Disolocation Reported in the Literature

Form of Treatment	Authors
Adhesive strapping	Rawlings,[374] Thorndike and Quigley,[453] Benson,[54] Bakalim and Wilppula[31]
Sling or bandage	Jones,[230] Watson-Jones,[484] Hawkins[200]
Brace and harness	Giannestras,[167] Warner,[479] Currie,[118] Anderson and Burgess,[21] Anzel and Streitz[22]
Crotch loops, stocking, garter, and strap	Darrow and associates,[124] Spigelman,[437] Varney and associates[472]
Figure-of-eight bandage	Usadel[467]
Sling and pressure dressing	Goldberg[174]
Abduction traction and suspension in bed	Caldwell[96]
Casts	Urist,[464,465] Howard,[216] Shaar,[416] Hart,[196] Trynin,[457] Stubbins and McGaw,[446] Dillehunt,[134] Key and Cornwell,[241] Gibbens[168]

because of noncompliance. Additional methods of reduction and immobilization include crotch loops, stockings, garter straps, and special pads.[124,437,472]

"SKILLFUL NEGLECT"

Convenience, shorter rehabilitation times, dissatisfaction with the results of surgical repairs, and reports of good functional outcomes have led some authors to favor "skillful neglect" over other forms of treatment. Nicoll[324] states that operative procedures for acromioclavicular dislocation are unwarranted and that maintenance of reduction by closed means is unattainable. He recommends a sling for 1 to 2 weeks, followed by exercises. Hawkins,[200] Imatani and colleagues,[218] Bjerneld and co-workers,[64] Dias and associates,[133] Sleeswijk and co-workers,[427] and Schwarz and Leixnering[410] all reported 90% to 100% satisfactory results with 5- to 7-year follow-up in patients with type III acromioclavicular dislocations treated by skillful neglect.

This form of treatment is especially popular among physicians who manage athletic injuries. Athletes who sustain an injury to the acromioclavicular joint are very likely to be back in competition within a few days or weeks, subjecting themselves to the same type of violent contact. Glick[171] favors skillful neglect, especially in athletes, because it allows rapid and safe return to competition. Glick and associates[172] reported on 35 athletes with chronic, unreduced type III acromioclavicular dislocations. The results were good and no athlete was disabled. They recommended skillful neglect and emphasized the role of aggressive postinjury strengthening.

Operative Treatment

During the 1800s and early 1900s, practically every conceivable operation for acromioclavicular dislocation was performed. These procedures included acromioclavicular, coracoclavicular, and combined acromioclavicular and coracoclavicular repairs. Currently, four basic types of procedures are performed: (1) acromioclavicular repairs, (2) coracoclavicular repairs, (3) distal clavicle excision, and (4) dynamic muscle transfers (Table 14-4). Many of the specific procedures used today are combinations, modifications, or modifications of modifications of previously described procedures (Fig. 14-30).

INTRA-ARTICULAR
ACROMIOCLAVICULAR REPAIRS

Acromioclavicular repairs and stabilization procedures have enjoyed moderate popularity. Most authors do not use Kirschner wires, because there are only four sizes—0.028-, 0.035-, 0.045-, and 0.062-inch—all of which are small and liable to break and migrate. Most authors use small, smooth or threaded Steinmann pins. These pins can be inserted antegrade from the lateral edge of the acromion through the joint and into the clavicle, or retrograde from the joint out through the acromion and then back across the joint into the clavicle. The portion of the pin that protrudes through the lateral acromion process should always be bent to lessen the possibility of medial migration (Fig. 14-31). Fama and Bonaga[150] reported the use of a smooth wire inserted laterally in the acromion, through the acromioclavicular joint, out the posterior cortex of the clavicle, and through the skin posterior to the clavicle. The wire was then bent back on itself to meet the other end of the wire. The two ends were then fastened together like a safety pin to prevent migration. It must be emphasized that despite the fact that the pin is bent, it can break, migrate, and create serious consequences (Fig. 14-32). (See under Complications to read about pin migration to the

Table 14-4. Operative Techniques for Type III Injuries

Repair	Authors
Primary Acromioclavicular Joint Fixation	
With pins, screws, suture wires, plates, and so forth; or reconstruction, with or without coracoclavicular ligament and/or acromioclavicular ligament repair or reconstruction	Bateman,[46] Bundens and Cook, [89] Southmayd and associates,[435] Dannohl,[123] Ahstrom,[7] DePalma,[128] Dittel and associates,[135] Aderhold,[6] McLaughlin,[282] O'Donoghue,[335] Stephens,[441] Sage and Salvatore,[395] Inman and associates,[220] Zaricznyj,[502] Rowe,[390] Nevaiser,[318] Kaiser and associates,[231] Bartonicek and associates,[43] Bakalim and Wilppula,[31] Schindler and associates,[403] Moshein and Elconin,[307] Fama and Bonaga,[150] Hellmich and Sievers,[202] Augereau and associates,[22] O'Carroll and Sheehan,[296] Barnhart,[31] Smith and Stewart,[383] Bargren and associates,[29] Simmons and Martin,[378] Simeone,[377] Krawzak and associates,[218] Mlasowsky,[294] Holz and Weller,[187] Allman,[13] Schneppendahl and Ludolph,[363] Mikusev and associates,[260] Muller and Schilling,[241] Bednarek and associates,[42] Paavolainen and associates[303]
Primary Coracoclavicular Ligament Fixation	
With screw, wire, fascia, conjoined tendon, or synthetic sutures With or without acromioclavicular ligament repair or reconstruction	Bosworth,[75] Weitzman,[487] Larsen and Peterson,[256] Kennedy and Cameron,[237] Orofinio and Stein,[341] Laing,[249] Batement,[46] Baker and Stryker,[33] Jay and Monnet,[228] Alldredge,[13] Bearden and associates,[49] Mumford,[309] Vargas,[471] Browne and associates,[85] Rockwood,[381–384] Grønmark,[185] Goldberg and associates,[175] Lowe and Fogarty,[268] Heitemeyer and associates,[201] Linke and Moschinski,[265] Graves and Foster,[181] Bargren and associates,[38] Vandekerckhove and associates,[469] Burri and Neugebauer,[92] Burton,[80] Dahl,[121] Augereau and associates,[26] Vargas,[471] Rauschning and associates,[373] Sonnabend and Faithfull,[433] Ganz and associates,[161] Shoji and associates,[419] Kawabe and associates,[235] Moravec and associates,[298] Karlsson and associates[233]
Excision of the Distal Clavicle	
With or without coracoclavicular ligament repair with fascia, suture, or coracoacromial ligament transfer	Gurd,[186] Mumford,[309] Bateman,[46] Weaver and Dunn,[486] Rockwood,[381] Moseley,[305] Urist[465–466]
Dynamic Muscle Transfers	
With or without excision of the distal clavicle	Dewar and Barrington,[131] Bailey and associates,[29,30] Berson and associates,[48] Glorian and Delplace,[173] Brunelli and Brunelli[86]

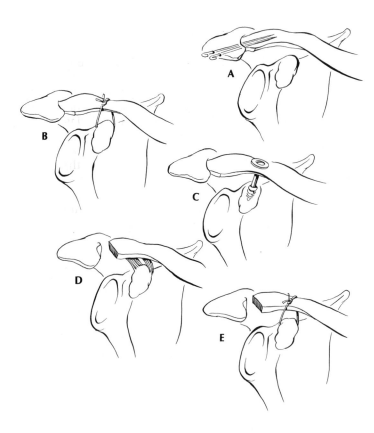

Fig. 14-30. Various operative procedures for injuries to the acromioclavicular joint. (**A**) Steinmann pins across the acromioclavicular joint. (**B**) Suture between the clavicle and the coracoid process. (**C**) A lag screw between the clavicle and the coracoid process. (**D**) Resection of the distal clavicle when the coracoclavicular ligaments are intact. (**E**) Resection of the distal clavicle with suture, fascia, or ligament between the clavicle and the coracoid process when the coracoclavicular ligaments are missing.

spinal cord, lung, subclavian artery, pulmonary artery, mediastinum, heart, and other areas.)

Percutaneous, or blind, pinning of the acromioclavicular joint has been reported (Fig. 14-33).[150,202,291] However, acromioclavicular joint fixation is difficult, even when performed as an open procedure. In addition, the percutaneous technique does not allow either ligament or deltotrapezius fascial repair.

Many methods of internal fixation of the acromioclavicular joint have been reported. Smooth pins of one type or another have been recommended by numerous authors, including Augereau and colleagues,[26] Bartonicek and associates,[43] Bateman,[46] Bundens and Cook,[89] Dannöhl,[123] Fama and Bonaga,[150] Hellmich and Sievers,[202] Inman and co-workers,[220] Mikusev and colleagues,[291] Moshein and Elconin,[307] Neviaser,[316–318] O'Donoghue,[335] Sage and Salvatore,[395] and Zaricznyj.[502] A Stuck nail was advocated by Stephens.[441] Ahstrom[7] advocated the use of a %₄-inch, fully threaded pin. Linke and Moschinski[265] supplemented two smooth pins with a superior acromioclavicular wire, which acted as a tension band. A partially threaded nail was introduced by Simmons and Martin.[424] The shank of the nail was smooth, except near its head. The nail was

inserted percutaneously through a stab wound at the posterolateral edge of the acromion. The smooth portion of the nail was advanced across the acromioclavicular joint and into the clavicle. The threads on the proximal shank then engaged the acromion to prevent medial migration. Vainionpää and colleagues[468] and Paavolainen and associates[342] recommended AO cortical and malleolar screws. Acromioclavicular fixation using the Balser hook plate has been reported by Albrecht,[8] Dittel and colleagues,[135] Dittmer and co-workers,[136] Kaiser and associates,[231] Mlasowsky and co-workers,[294] and Schindler and colleagues.[403]

A comparison of acromioclavicular methods of fixation was reported by Eskola and co-workers.[147] They performed a prospective, randomized trial in 100 patients using three types of acromioclavicular fixation: (1) smooth pins, (2) threaded pins, and (3) cortical screws. Thirteen of the 86 patients available for review developed symptomatic osteolysis of the distal clavicle. Eight of the 13 cases of osteolysis occurred in 25 patients who underwent cortical screw fixation. Smith and Stewart[430] advocated distal clavicle excision in conjunction with acromioclavicular fixation as a means of decreasing degenerative changes in the acromioclavicular joint.

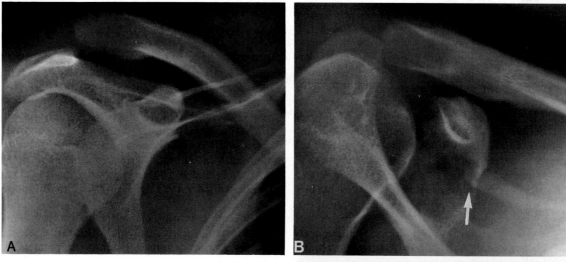

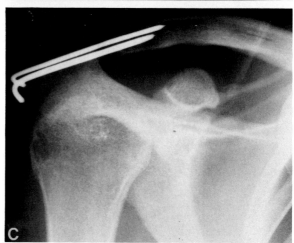

Fig. 14-31. Dislocation of the right acromioclavicular joint associated with an avulsion fracture of the base of the coracoid process. (**A**) The distal end of the clavicle is completely dislocated away from the acromion, but the coracoclavicular distance is about the same as in the normal shoulder. (**B**) A cephalic tilt view of the shoulder reveals a fracture at the base of the coracoid. A Stryker notch view probably would have better defined the fracture of the base of the coracoid. (**C**) Open reduction of the acromioclavicular joint and stabilization of the joint with two pins effectively reduced the fractured coracoid. Note that the distal ends of the pins have been bent to prevent medial migration.

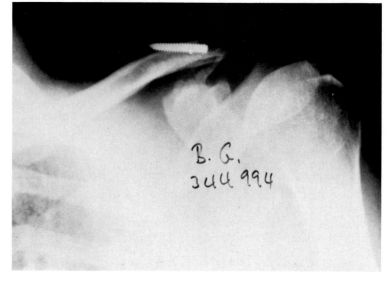

Fig. 14-32. Type III dislocation was previously fixed with a threaded Steinmann pin. The reduction held satisfactorily but the pin broke, leaving the tip embedded in the distal end of the clavicle. (*Rockwood, C. A., and Young, D. C.: Disorders of the Acromioclavicular Joint. In Rockwood, C. A., and Matsen, F., III (eds.): The Shoulder, Fig. 12-35. Philadelphia, W. B. Saunders, 1990.*)

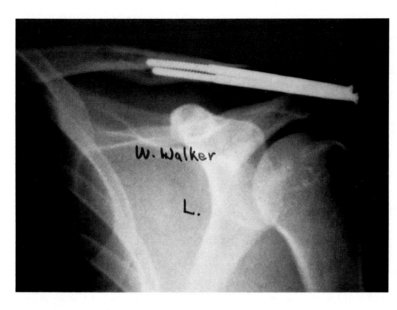

Fig. 14-33. Type III dislocation has been managed by blind pinning of the acromioclavicular joint using two Deyerle hip screws. (Rockwood, C. A., and Young, D. C.: Disorders of the Acromioclavicular Joint. In Rockwood, C. A., and Matsen, F., III (eds.): The Shoulder, Fig. 12-36. Philadelphia, W. B. Saunders, 1990.)

Regardless of the method of fixation, the majority of authors report the use of other procedures as an adjunct to acromioclavicular fixation. Sage and Salvatore[395] advocated acromioclavicular ligament repair and reinforcement of the superior acromioclavicular ligament with the intra-articular, fibrocartilaginous meniscus. Neviaser[316–318] introduced superior acromioclavicular ligament reconstruction through transfer of the coracoid attachment of the coracoacromial ligament to the superior aspect of the clavicle. He did not recommend repair of the coracoclavicular ligament. Ho and colleagues[209] advocated superior acromioclavicular ligament reconstruction using the coracoacromial ligament, and coracoclavicular ligament reconstruction using Marlex tubing between the coracoid and over the clavicle. These procedures were done alone or in combination. Smith and Stewart[430] repaired both the acromioclavicular and coracoclavicular ligaments. Zaricznyj[502] reconstructed the acromioclavicular and coracoclavicular ligaments using the extensor tendon of the fifth toe. O'Donoghue[335] and Inman and associates[220] advocated coracoclavicular ligament repair. Moshein and Elconin[307] reinforced their repair of the coracoclavicular ligament with the coracoacromial ligament. Ahstrom[7] reflected a portion of the conjoined tendon superiorly to reinforce the coracoclavicular ligament. Augereau and colleagues[26] reconstructed the coracoclavicular ligament by transferring the acromial attachment of the coracoacromial ligament through a tunnel in the clavicle, as originally described by Cadenat in 1917.[94] Linke and Moschinski[265] used a Vicryl band

to reconstruct the coracoclavicular ligament. Bateman[46] reconstructed a new suspensory ligament using fascia lata passed under the coracoid, around the clavicle, and attached to the spine of the scapula. Bundens and Cook,[89] as well as Bartonicek and colleagues,[43] emphasized the importance of imbricating the deltotrapezius fascia to reinforce the acromioclavicular fixation.

Postoperative Care. Patients are encouraged to move the hand and elbow, but are discouraged from abducting the shoulder. Motion must be limited to prevent breakage or migration of the pins across the acromioclavicular joint. Rowe[390] recommends abduction motion be limited to 40°, and DePalma[128] recommends no abduction until the pins are removed. Most authors recommend the pins be removed after 6 to 8 weeks. After pin removal, range-of-motion and strengthening exercises are begun.

EXTRA-ARTICULAR CORACOCLAVICULAR REPAIRS

The technique of placing a screw between the clavicle and the coracoid was described by Bosworth[73] in 1941. The screw was placed percutaneously, using local anesthesia and fluoroscopic guidance. With the patient in a seated position, a stab wound was made on the superior aspect of the shoulder, 3.8 cm medial to the distal end of the clavicle. After a drill hole was made in the clavicle, an assistant reduced the acromioclavicular joint by depressing the clavicle and elevating the arm using a special clavicle-depressing instrument. An awl was used to develop a hole in the superior cortex of the base of the coracoid process, which was visualized using fluoroscopy. A regular bone screw was then inserted. The screw was left indefinitely, unless specific indications for removal developed. Bosworth[73-76] did not recommend either repair of the coracoclavicular ligaments or exploration of the acromioclavicular joint. In his original article, Bosworth[73] also described a newly developed lag screw with a broad head, which he preferred to the original regular bone screw. He referred to the procedure as a screw suspension operation, not a fixation, because the screw suspended the scapula from, rather than fixed it to, the clavicle.

Percutaneous insertion of a cannulated coracoclavicular screw was reported by Tsou[458] in 1989. Tsou[458] fluoroscopically placed a guide pin from the clavicle to the coracoid process. After adequate positioning of the pin within the coracoid had been confirmed radiographically, a cannulated drill bit and screw were sequentially passed over the guide pin. Tsou[458] reported a 32% technical failure rate in 53 patients with complete acromioclavicular dislocation using this technique. Accurate insertion of the screw is difficult to perform percutaneously. Furthermore, the percutaneous technique does not allow coracoclavicular ligament repair, deltoid and trapezius reattachment, or acromioclavicular joint débridement.

Several authors have reported good results using coracoclavicular fixation and various modifications of Bosworth's original technique. In 1968, Kennedy and Cameron[237] and Kennedy[238] reported on repair of acromioclavicular dislocation using a coracoclavicular technique. Under general anesthesia, the acromioclavicular joint was thoroughly débrided and the clavicle was brought into contact with the top of the coracoid process (ie, overreduced) using

the Bosworth lag screw. The deltoid and trapezius muscles were then repaired back to the clavicle. The coracoclavicular ligament was preserved, but not repaired. In acute cases, bone dust created by drilling the hole in the clavicle was placed into the coracoclavicular interspace in an effort to gain permanent bone fixation between the clavicle and the coracoid. Kennedy and Cameron[237] stated that screw fixation of the clavicle to the coracoid process combined with ossification in the coracoclavicular interspace created an extra-articular arthrodesis of the acromioclavicular joint. Furthermore, they stated that the procedure produced an essentially normal range of shoulder motion because it did not interfere with the normal "synchronous scapuloclavicular rotation" that occurs during overhead elevation. Weitzman[488] reported good results using open placement of a Bosworth screw under general anesthesia. Although he did not expose or repair the coracoclavicular ligament, he did expose and débride the acromioclavicular joint and imbricated the deltoid and trapezius muscle attachments.

Jay and Monnet[228] reported a modification of Bosworth's technique which they learned from Amspatcher, at the University of Oklahoma Medical Center. They reported a series of 31 cases of acromioclavicular joint dislocation in which the acromioclavicular joint was debrided, the coracoclavicular ligaments were repaired, a Bosworth screw was used to temporarily hold the acromioclavicular joint reduced, and the trapezius and deltoid muscles were repaired back to the clavicle (Fig. 14-34). Jay and Monnet[228] recommended an x-ray be taken on the operating table to ensure the screw was in the vertical position and was engaging both cortices of the coracoid process. Lowe and Fogarty[268] used a similar technique in 21 patients; they noted full

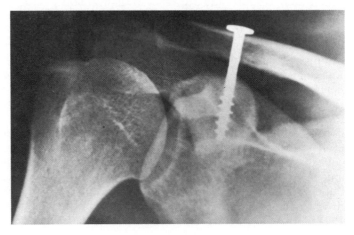

Fig. 14-34. Postoperative anteroposterior x-ray of the shoulder with Bosworth screw in place. Note that the acromioclavicular joint has been reduced and the coarse lag threads of the screw are well seated into the coracoid process.

recovery in all but one patient. In addition, Lowe and Fogarty[268] noted ossification between the clavicle and the coracoid process quite commonly. However, this finding was not correlated with a poor result. In fact, patients had a full range of motion in spite of a bony bridge between the clavicle and the coracoid process. These findings are in agreement with those of Kennedy and Cameron.[237,238]

Coracoclavicular fixation by methods other than a screw has been reported. Bearden and co-workers,[49] as well as Alldredge,[12] recommend the use of two loops of stainless steel wire around the coracoid process and clavicle (Fig. 14-35). Tagliabue and Riva,[449] Park and colleagues,[343] Nelson,[315] Kappakas and McMaster,[232] Fleming and associates,[155] and Goldberg and colleagues[175] all reported on the use of synthetic Dacron arterial graft or velour Dacron graft to repair dislocations of the acromioclavicular joint. Bunnell[90] in 1928, and Lom[267] in 1988, reported the use of fascia lata for reconstruction of the coracoclavicular ligaments. Most of these authors also reported acromioclavicular joint debridement, acromioclavicular joint ligament repair or reconstruction, coracoclavicular ligament repair, and imbrication of the deltotrapezius fascia—either alone or in combination—in addition to the coracoclavicular fixation.

Coracoclavicular fixation using grafts or synthetic material has been associated with various complications. Goldberg and colleagues[175] recognized erosion of the Dacron graft through the distal clavicle in some cases. Dahl[120,121] reported on the use of a synthetic velour or Dacron coracoclavicular loop for fixation, and described marked clavicular erosion by the loop. In one case the prosthesis had eroded through the entire clavicle. In all seven of Dahl's cases, there was significant evidence of clavicular erosion (Fig. 14-36). Moneim and Balduini[296] noted a coracoid fracture following reconstruction of the coracoclavicular ligaments through two drill holes in the clavicle. Park and associates[343] found superior results and no resorption in patients treated with double velour Dacron grafts, compared with the older knitted Dacron vascular grafts.

Other authors have reported extra-articular repairs of the acromioclavicular joint which are combinations of previously reported techniques. Copeland and Kessel[111] transferred the acromial attachment of the coracoacromial ligament, along with a piece of the acromion, to the superior surface of the clavicle. A Bosworth screw was used to hold the graft in place and to hold the acromioclavicular joint reduced. Burton[93] also reported transfer of the coracoacromial ligament to the clavicle. In addition, he recommended meticulous repair of the trapezius and deltoid muscles back to the clavicle, as well as distal clavicle excision. Vargas[471] reported using a part of the conjoined tendon as a substitute for the coracoclavicular ligaments. Laing[249] reported 30 cases of acromioclavicular dislocation in which he reconstructed a new coracoclavicular ligament by transferring the long head of the biceps through a drill hole in the coracoid process and into a drill hole in the clavicle. He stated that this new ligament, with its own nerve and blood supplies, is sensitive to stress and is able to protect itself against stretching.

Postoperative Care. Bosworth[73] recommended a sling until the soft tissues had healed. However, he

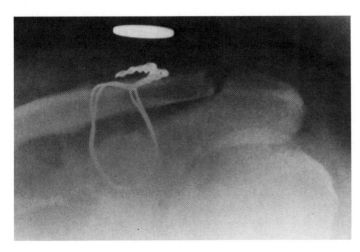

Fig. 14-35. A postoperative anteroposterior x-ray of the acromioclavicular joint shows two loops of wire used to reduce the joint. The loops of wire passed beneath the coracoid process and over the clavicle. Note the coin that has been taped to the skin on the superior aspect of the shoulder to aid in the location of the loop of wire (or screw) when it is to be removed.

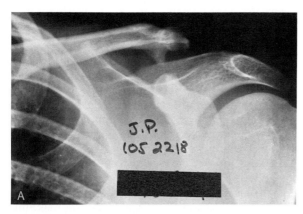 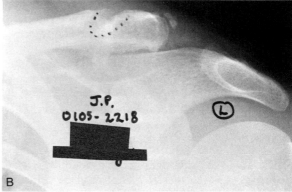

Fig. 14-36. X-rays of patient with a type III injury who was previously treated with a Dacron graft around the coracoid and over the top of the clavicle. At the time of secondary reconstruction, the Dacron graft was noted to be partially eroded down through the clavicle. (*Rockwood, C. A., and Young, D. C.: Disorders of the Acromioclavicular Joint. In Rockwood, C. A., and Matsen, F., III (eds.): The Shoulder, p. 442. Philadelphia, W. B. Saunders, 1990.*)

allowed the patient to perform activities of daily living such as bathing, dressing, and feeding on the first postoperative day. In addition, he encouraged daily removal of the sling to perform pendulum exercises and active assisted range of motion against a wall. Patients were restricted from heavy work for 8 weeks. Kennedy[238] used no form of external splintage and encouraged a gradual range of motion. He anticipated full abduction 7 to 10 days after the operation. The patient was allowed to return to vigorous athletic activities 6 to 8 weeks postoperatively.

Other authors have advocated a slower progression to regular activity to protect the coracoclavicular fixation. Alldredge[12] recommended no postoperative immobilization beyond the second postoperative day. However, he limited the patient's activities for 5 to 6 weeks. Bearden and colleagues[49] supported the arm in a sling for 10 to 14 days following surgery, then instructed the patient to avoid strenuous activity, such as lifting weights. Jay and Monnet[228] recommended a sling for 4 weeks postoperatively, at which time active exercises were started. Weitzman[487] recommended a sling and swathe immediately after surgery. However, on the first postoperative day, a plaster shoulder Velpeau cast was applied. This cast was worn for 4 weeks, then was removed to allow active exercises.

The recommendations concerning removal of fixation devices vary considerably. Neither Bosworth nor Kennedy recommended removal of the coracoclavicular lag screw. Weitzman,[487] on the other hand, recommended coracoclavicular screw removal under local anesthesia after 3 months. Jay

and Monnet[228] removed the screw under local anesthesia at 8 weeks. Bearden and colleagues[49] removed the coracoclavicular wire loops 6 to 8 weeks postoperatively; this was performed under local anesthesia if possible, or general anesthesia if necessary. Bearden and colleagues[49] recommended removing all the fragments of wire, even if they were broken. Alldredge,[12] however, did not remove the coracoclavicular wires if they were broken and the shoulder had a full range of motion. Otherwise, he recommended wire loop removal at 6 to 8 weeks postoperatively.

COMPARISON OF ACROMIOCLAVICULAR
AND CORACOCLAVICULAR REPAIRS

Lancaster and colleagues[251] compared their results with acromioclavicular versus coracoclavicular fixation and found a higher minor complication rate with acromioclavicular fixation, but a higher failure rate with coracoclavicular fixation. However, Bargren and associates[38] had superior results with coracoclavicular versus acromioclavicular fixation. Bargren and associates[38] compared the use of pins across the acromioclavicular joint with the use of the Dacron coracoclavicular loop and favored the latter.

Kiefer and colleagues[242] studied the biomechanics of various surgical procedures used to stabilize the acromioclavicular joint, including: (1) acromioclavicular joint tension band techniques; (2) the Stehli plate; (3) Bosworth screws; (4) Wolter plates; (5) Rahmanzadeh plates; and (6) the Balser plate and carbon fiber ligament. They found the Bosworth screw to provide the most rigid fixation, but noted that it has failed in fatigue clinically. They suggested acromioclavicular fixation either with Kirschner wires and a cerclage wire, or a Wolter plate.

EXCISION OF THE DISTAL CLAVICLE

Exactly who performed the first excision of the outer end of the clavicle is not known. McLaughlin[282] stated that it was first recommended by Facassini in 1902, but gave no reference, and Cadenat[94] stated that it was first performed by Morestin, but gave no reference or date. In 1941, Gurd[186] of Montreal and Mumford[309] of Indiana independently described their results of excision of the distal end of the clavicle. Mumford[309] recommended his operation for the symptomatic, incompletely dislocated (type II) acromioclavicular dislocation. Gurd[186] recommended his procedure for a symptomatic, completely dislocated (type III) acromioclavicular joint.

Excision of the distal end of the clavicle is referred to as the Mumford or the Gurd[186] operation, or by both eponyms combined. Strictly speaking, the simple excision of the distal clavicle is usually used for an old, symptomatic type II injury, and the name associated with this procedure is Mumford. Furthermore, as pointed out by Mumford,[309] if the problem is a symptomatic type III injury in which the supporting coracoclavicular ligaments have been disrupted, then in addition to the excision of the distal clavicle, there must be a reconstruction of the coracoclavicular ligaments. (This is further discussed in the section on operative procedures for chronic symptomatic complete acromioclavicular dislocation.) Weaver and Dunn[486] reported twelve acute and three chronic grade III acromioclavicular joint dislocations. Their procedure was to excise the distal 2 cm of the clavicle and then, rather than use internal fixation, transfer the coracoacromial ligament from its acromial attachment to the intramedullary canal of the clavicle, as recommended by Cadenat[94] in 1917. Rauschning and co-workers[373] performed the Weaver-Dunn procedure in 18 cases and reported stable and painless shoulders.

Although excision of the distal clavicle usually is indicated in a symptomatic, chronic, complete acromioclavicular dislocation—and possibly in an acute injury with severe joint damage—we do not recommend excision of normal clavicle for an acute acromioclavicular dislocation. Browne and co-workers[85] reviewed a series of 25 patients in which 12 had coracoclavicular fixation alone and 13 had coracoclavicular fixation along with resection of the distal 1 inch of the clavicle. They concluded the distal clavicle resection did not offer any significant improvement over coracoclavicular fixation alone.

Postoperative Care. Weaver and Dunn[486] recommended a Velpeau dressing or a sling and the beginning of circumduction exercises on the first day after operation. At the end of 4 weeks, the patient is allowed full active use of the shoulder.

DYNAMIC MUSCLE TRANSFER

Brunelli[86] first reported a technique of transfer of the short head of the biceps with the tip of the coracoid to the clavicle for correction of acromioclavicular dislocations. In 1965, Dewar and Barrington[131] published their results of a procedure for old, complete acromioclavicular dislocations, in which the tip of the coracoid process, along with the muscle attachments of the biceps, coracobrachialis, and a segment of the pectoralis minor tendon, is detached and transferred up and fixed with a screw to the undersurface of the clavicle in the vicinity of the old coracoclavicular ligament attachments. This serves as a dynamic muscle transfer to hold the clavicle down. In two of five chronic acromioclavicular dislocations, they augmented the coracoid transfer with lateral clavicular excision; in the other three, they did not mention whether or not clavicular excision was performed. They recommend a Velpeau dressing after operation, and mobilization of the shoulder starting at 4 weeks.

In 1964, at the annual meeting of the American Academy of Orthopaedic Surgeons, Bailey[30] presented his results on the transfer of the coracoid process with the coracobrachialis and the short head of the biceps to the clavicle in nine patients with acute, complete acromioclavicular dislocation. He reported the operation acted as a dynamic depressor of the clavicle. He did not state whether he excised the lateral end of the clavicle. He noted that in lower vertebrate forms, the coracobrachialis and short head of the biceps muscles arise from the clavicle, and, in a sense, the operation is a step backward in comparative vertebrate anatomy. In 1972, Bailey and associates[30] reported on 38 cases. Berson and co-workers[58] reported satisfactory results in 23 acute and 6 chronic acromioclavicular dislocations. Glorian and Delplace[173] reported satisfactory results in 36 cases, and modified the procedure by temporarily using two pins across the acromioclavicular joint. Recently, Brunelli and Brunelli[87] reported no failures in 51 patients who underwent transfer of the short head of the biceps from 1962 to 1987. Ferris and associates,[152] however, could not recommend coracoid process transfer in acute injuries after their experience with patients, and recommended its use only with caution in patients with chronic acromioclavicular dislocations. They also used a staple to temporarily stabilize the acromioclavicular joint. Skjeldal and colleagues[426] also could not recommend coracoid process transfer after their experience in 17 patients.

CARE OF ACROMIOCLAVICULAR DISLOCATION WITH A FRACTURE OF THE CORACOID PROCESS

Acromioclavicular dislocation with fracture of the coracoid process is not a common injury in adults. The mechanism of injury is essentially the same as for a type III acromioclavicular dislocation, except the coracoclavicular ligaments do not disrupt and a fracture occurs through the base of the coracoid, allowing relative upward displacement of the distal clavicle. It is very difficult to internally stabilize the fracture of the base of the coracoid, and, if surgery is indicated, pins across the acromioclavicular joint are required. (See Fig. 14-31.) Bernard and associates[57] reported four cases and reviewed thirteen cases from the literature. They concluded that although surgery can produce good results, equally satisfactory function and minimal residual deformity could be achieved by immobilization of the shoulder in a sling for 6 weeks. Wilson and Colwill[495] treated a semiprofessional football player with a combined acromioclavicular dislocation and coracoid process fracture and coracoclavicular ligament disruption with screw fixation of both the coracoid process and the acromioclavicular joint. The patient had an excellent result.

Operative Versus Nonoperative Treatment of Type III Injuries to the Acromioclavicular Joint

Clearly, not all patients with complete acromioclavicular dislocation do well with nonoperative management. Larsen and colleagues[254] prospectively studied 84 patients randomized into operative and short-term immobilization treatment. They found a much higher complication rate with surgical management, and recommended surgery be considered in patients with a prominent distal clavicle and in those who do heavy work or frequent overhead work. Larsen and Hede[255] prospectively compared three methods of treatment for acromioclavicular dislocation: (1) reduction of the joint, repair of the coracoclavicular ligaments, imbrication of the deltotrapezius fascia, and acromioclavicular fixation; (2) short-term immobilization followed by early range of motion; and (3) closed reduction and bandaging. Although their patient groups were not well matched, the results are informative. Two of

25 patients in group I required reoperation because of a persistently painful acromioclavicular joint; both underwent distal clavicle excision with excellent results. Three of 29 patients in group II required late operation—two because of pain and one because the distal clavicle was tenting the skin. All three patients underwent distal clavicle excision combined with coracoclavicular ligament reconstruction. There were only two excellent results and one good result. Larson and Hede[255] recommended early surgical repair in patients with extreme prominence of the clavicle and in patients whose occupation demanded prolonged heavy lifting or repeated use of the arm with the shoulder abducted or flexed to 90°. Taft and colleagues[447] retrospectively compared 127 patients managed operatively and nonoperatively. They reported only slightly less good results with nonoperative management at an average followup of 9.5 years. The complication rate was higher with operative management. Hawkins[200] and Imatani and co-workers[218] have done comparative studies of operative and nonoperative treatment, and concluded nonoperative treatment gives an equal, if not better, end result.

Other authors have found operative treatment superior to nonoperative treatment. Indrekvam and colleagues[219] found an equal incidence of good results in a comparative study, but felt operatively treated patients had less pain and could work longer. Park and colleagues[343] found a higher rating in shoulders treated operatively than nonoperatively. Bakalim and Wilppula[31] concluded surgical reconstruction of type III injuries was superior to nonoperative management.

TYPE IV AND V INJURIES

Because of the severe posterior displacement of the distal clavicle in a type IV injury (Fig. 14-37), and the gross superior displacement in the type V injury (see Figs. 14-15 and 14-16), most authors recommend surgical repair.[198,274,326,432] Methods of treatment for pure posterior dislocations of the clavicle vary. Hastings and Horne[198] treated three patients with posterior clavicle dislocations: a 16-year-old hockey player was treated with a figure-of-eight splint with a good result; a 16-year-old girl with an acute injury was treated with a Simmons screw across the acromioclavicular joint; and a 30-year-old man with a 10-year-old injury associated with weakness and pain received nonoperative treatment. Nieminen and Aho[326] treated a 9-week-old posterior dislocation of the clavicle with reconstruction of the coracoclavicular ligaments and the

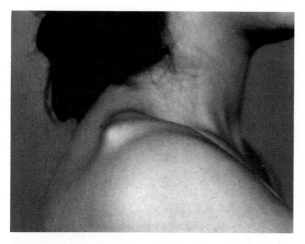

Fig. 14-37. Patient with type IV acromioclavicular joint injury. Note that the distal end of the clavicle is displaced posteriorly back into and through the trapezius muscle. *(Rockwood, C. A., and Young, D. C.: Disorders of the Acromioclavicular Joint. In Rockwood, C. A., and Matsen, F., III (eds.): The Shoulder, Fig. 12-43. Philadelphia, W. B. Saunders, 1990.)*

dorsal acromioclavicular ligament, using the palmaris longus augmented with temporary acromioclavicular Kirschner-wire fixation; this patient was doing well 1 year postoperatively. Malcapi and associates[274] and Sondergard-Petersen and Mikkelsen[432] each reported a case of irreducible dislocation of the distal clavicle; both required excision of the distal clavicle, but no further surgery because the coracoclavicular ligaments were stretched, but still intact. In a type IV injury, the patient is quite symptomatic when the distal end of the clavicle penetrates the trapezius muscle. In an inactive patient where the clavicle can be manipulated out of the trapezius muscle, a nonoperative approach is possible. However, if the clavicle can not be manipulated out of the trapezius muscle, one of the previously described surgical procedures can be performed. In a type V injury, the deformity is so gross that surgical repair usually is indicated.

TYPE VI INJURY

All type VI injuries described in the literature[165,285,346,396] have been treated with surgery. Initial attempts at closed reduction failed. In one instance, following open reduction by lateral retraction of the scapula, the clavicle was stabilized by suturing the deltoid and trapezius muscle avulsion and by repairing the acromioclavicular joint

capsule. In one patient, whose shoulder was operated on 2½ months after injury, a Steinmann pin was used to stabilize the acromioclavicular joint. Following immobilization for 3 to 5 weeks, both these patients had almost full range of motion and good power (Fig. 14-38). One patient with a recurrent subcoracoid dislocation was treated by excision of the distal 1 cm of the clavicle, and at a 5-year follow-up the patient had no complaints or weakness. Gerber and Rockwood[165] reported on using the extra-articular technique with the Rockwood coracoclavicular lag screw, with repair of the ligaments and imbrication of the deltotrapezius fascia over the top of the clavicle.

CHRONIC, SYMPTOMATIC ACROMIOCLAVICULAR INJURIES

Chronic, symptomatic acromioclavicular dislocation has not been extensively discussed in the orthopaedic literature, and only in passing in some articles and textbooks. The usual recommended treatment for a chronic unreduced acromioclavicular dislocation is to excise the distal end of the clavicle, which, in many instances, will give the patient more trouble and more symptoms than prior to the surgery. The excision of the distal clavicle, as reported by Mumford,[309] is indicated for a symptomatic type I or II problem.

Excision of the Distal Clavicle

As previously mentioned, the excision of the distal clavicle has been described by Mumford[309] and Gurd.[186] The simple excision of the distal 1.5 to 2 cm of the clavicle is quite successful for chronic symptomatic type I and II injuries, but as the sole operative treatment, it is not recommended for type III through VI injuries.

Dynamic Muscle Transfer

In 1965, Dewar and Barrington[131] published results of a procedure for chronic complete acromioclavicular dislocations, in which the tip of the coracoid process, along with the muscle attachments of the biceps, coracobrachialis, and a segment of the pectoralis minor tendon, is detached and transferred up and fixed with a screw to the undersurface of the clavicle in the vicinity of the old coracoclavicular ligament attachments. This serves as a dynamic muscle transfer to hold the clavicle down. In two of five chronic acromioclavicular dislocations, they accompanied the coracoid transfer with lateral clavicle excision; in the other three patients, they did not mention whether or not a lateral clav-

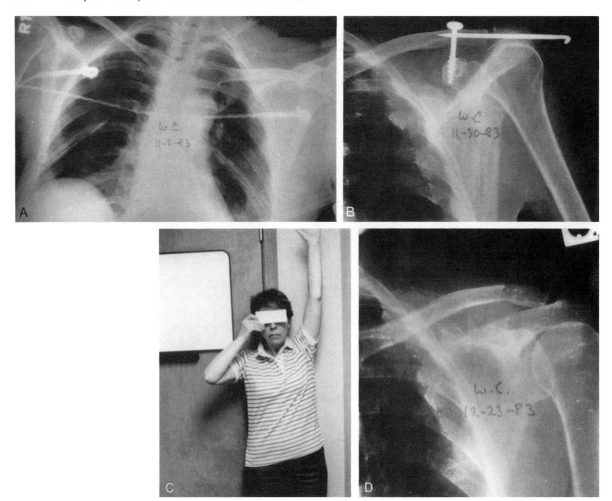

Fig. 14-38. Type VI acromioclavicular dislocation. (**A**) The distal end of the left clavicle is in the subcoracoid position. (**B**) The injury was managed by open reduction and internal fixation with a coracoclavicular lag screw and pins across the acromioclavicular joint. (**C**) Following the surgery, the patient had essentially a full range of motion of the left shoulder. (**D**) X-ray obtained 20 months after injury demonstrates an almost complete bar of bone between the coracoid and the clavicle. *(Rockwood, C. A., and Young, D. C.: Disorders of the Acromioclavicular Joint. In Rockwood, C. A., and Matsen, F., III (eds.): The Shoulder, Fig. 12-44. Philadelphia, W. B. Saunders, 1990. Courtesy of Mrs. R. C. Erickson and D. Massillon of Massillon, OH.)*

icle excision was performed. They recommended a Velpeau dressing after the operation, and mobilization of the shoulder starting at 4 weeks postoperatively. Berson and associates[58] reported satisfactory results of this type of procedure in acute and chronic injuries to the acromioclavicular joint. Ferris and colleagues[152] also performed a similar procedure for acute and chronic injuries, but felt it was only indicated in chronic, symptomatic acromioclavicular dislocations.

Excision of the Distal Clavicle and Transfer of the Coracoacromial Ligament

Weaver and Dunn[486] managed both acute and chronic injuries with distal clavicle excision and transfer of the coracoacromial ligament to the medullary canal of the clavicle. Boussaton and associates[77] performed this procedure for 15 patients with chronic type II and III injuries with 80% good or excellent and 20% poor results. Burton[93]

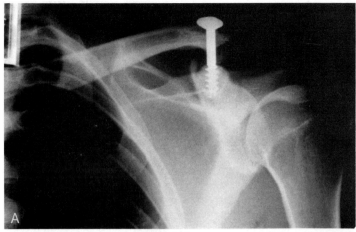

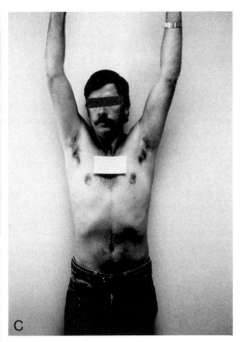

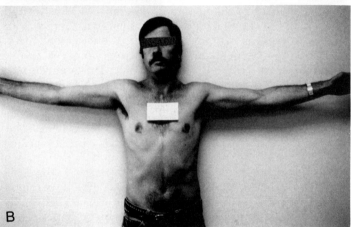

Fig. 14-39. Reconstruction of chronic type III injury of the left acromioclavicular joint. (**A**) The coracoacromial ligament has been transferred into the medullary canal of the distal clavicle. A special coracoclavicular lag screw was inserted to temporarily suspend the upper extremity from the clavicle while the transferred ligament was healing. (**B, C**) The patient had essentially a full range of motion with the screw in place. The screw was removed at 12 weeks. (*Rockwood, C. A., and Young, D. C.: Disorders of the Acromioclavicular Joint. In Rockwood, C. A., and Matsen, F., III (eds.): The Shoulder, Fig. 12-45. Philadelphia, W. B. Saunders, 1990.*)

and Copeland and Kessel[111] described a similar technique. Shoji and co-workers[419] modified the technique by harvesting the coracoacromial ligament with a bone block from the acromion transferred into the medullary canal of the clavicle, and were pleased with their results in three patients. However, Larsen and Petersen[256] were unhappy with transfers of the coracoclavicular ligaments with a bone block to the superior surface of the clavicle, because 50% of their patients had complaints where the flake of bone was attached onto the clavicle. Rockwood and colleagues[381] reported on 25 patients with chronic, symptomatic acro-

mioclavicular type III dislocations. They transferred the coracoacromial ligament according to Cadenat,[94] and stabilized the clavicle to the coracoid with a lag screw for 12 weeks while the transferred ligament healed (Fig. 14-39).

Reconstruction of the Acromioclavicular and/or Coracoclavicular Ligaments

Some authors have recommended reconstructions of the acromioclavicular joint which do not involve excision of the distal clavicle. Zaricznyj[501–503] reconstructed the coracoclavicular and superior acromioclavicular ligament with tendon grafts. He used either the extensor tendon of the fifth toe or the palmaris longus. He supplemented the repair with temporary Kirschner-wire acromioclavicular fixation, and found that 15 of his 16 patients were pain-free an average of 5.1 years postoperatively. Bednarek and associates[52] treated 35 patients with injuries older than 2 weeks with reconstruction of both the coracoclavicular and acromioclavicular ligaments, using an intricate loop of thick fishing line in a Bunnell[90] fashion; all patients were satisfied with the result. Fleming and colleagues[155] used a woven Dacron arterial loop in five patients with 80% good results, although one patient with a good result required distal clavicle excision.

Miscellaneous Reconstructions

Dannöhl[123] advised midclavicular osteotomy with plate fixation for the osteotomy and acromioclavicular fixation with Kirschner wires and a tension band wire.

AUTHORS' PREFERRED METHODS

Type I Injury

We recommend use of an ice pack for the first 12 hours whenever it is convenient, and we give the patient a sling to support the arm and to remind him and others that something is wrong with the shoulder. We encourage the patient to rest the shoulder, but to maintain a gentle, normal range of motion. The symptoms usually subside within 7 days. Heavy stresses, lifting, and contact sports should be delayed until there is a full range of motion and no pain to joint palpation. This usually takes 2 weeks.

Type II Injury

As in a type I injury, rest is an important factor. Ice packs are used during the first 12 hours, followed by moist heat for 12 hours. The patient is given a sling to rest and support the arm. The sling is worn for 1 to 2 weeks, depending on the age of the patient, the symptoms, and the circumstances. We encourage the patient to begin gentle range-of-motion exercises of the shoulder and allow him to use the arm for dressing, eating, and necessary everyday living activities when symptoms permit, which is usually about the seventh day. The average patient is instructed not to use the shoulder for any heavy lifting, pushing, pulling, or contact sports for at least 6 weeks. We do not want the patient to have another injury or stress the acromioclavicular joint to convert a type II problem to a type III prob-

lem. For the average patient who only occasionally puts stress on the acromioclavicular joint, the development of chronic problems is rare and usually can be resolved with anti-inflammatory drugs, moist heat, and maybe one or two injections of steroids into the joint. However, if the patient stresses the shoulder all day with heavy labor (ie, pushes a wheelbarrow, swings a sledge hammer, does a lot of digging), then chronic pain can develop in the acromioclavicular joint secondary to traumatic arthritis. If conservative measures fail, then an arthroplasty may be required. Excision of the distal clavicle should not be skimpy, for we have seen patients who, after excision of 1 cm of the distal clavicle, have continued to have pain in the joint. Films taken with the arm at the side revealed widening of the acromioclavicular joint, but with an x-ray film taken at 90° of abduction, there was impingement of the clavicle into the acromion process. As a general rule, we recommend excision of at least 2 cm of the distal clavicle. This removes most of the trapezoid part of the coracoclavicular ligament, but as long as the conoid ligament remains, the distal clavicle will have a secure anchor to the coracoid process.

After the operation, the arm is carried in a sling until the sutures are removed, and then the patient is instructed in pendulum exercises, followed by range-of-motion exercises, and, finally, strengthening exercises. Laborers and athletes in contact sports usually can return to their activities after 8 to 10 weeks.

Type III Acute Injury

BASIC TREATMENT PHILOSOPHY

Our philosophy is to either restore the anatomy through an operative procedure, or to put the arm into a sling for a few days and gradually allow the patient to begin functional use of the shoulder. We do not use casts, braces, or harnesses, nor do we use adhesive taping or strapping, which has the general tendency to irritate or ulcerate the tender skin on top of the shoulder (Fig. 14-40). Some authors refer to these methods of care as conservative treatment, while others, including ourselves, would call them radical. It seems unreasonable and impractical to immobilize the shoulder and upper extremity in a young, active person for 6 to 8 weeks. However, we do admire the physicians and patients who have the tenacity to achieve a good result with the various shoulder harness devices.

We use an operative repair or a skillful neglect approach. We basically believe that in a person who

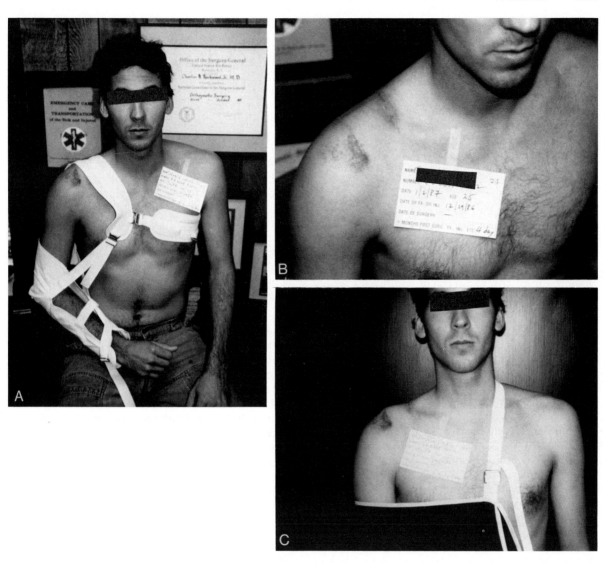

Fig. 14-40. The continuous pressure of the strap over the top of the shoulder, which is used to depress the clavicle, in many instances will cause skin breakdown. (**A**) This patient had been in a shoulder strap harness for a type III acromioclavicular dislocation for 4 days, and said that the burning pain in the top of his shoulder was excessive. (**B**) With the device removed, the skin breakdown on the top of his shoulder was obvious. (**C**) The patient was not involved in any type of heavy-duty labor activities; he was simply placed into a sling and told he could remove the sling and begin to use the arm for everyday living activities whenever the shoulder felt comfortable. (*Rockwood, C. A., and Young, D. C.: Disorders of the Acromioclavicular Joint. In Rockwood, C. A., and Matsen, F., III (eds.): The Shoulder, Fig. 12-47. Philadelphia, W. B. Saunders, 1990.*)

does heavy labor, and in certain young people younger than 25 years of age who have not made up their minds for their future plans for work or sports, a surgical repair should be performed. We also apply this philosophy to active older patients. The senior author recalls a cowboy from one of the large south Texas ranches who was 65 years old, but looked about 45. He worked 12 to 14 hours a day, rode horses, dug post holes, repaired fences, worked cattle, roped and threw calves, and truly demanded a strong, dominant functional shoulder all day long. He had a successful operative repair and returned to his job on the ranch. An exception to the rule for surgical repair in a young athlete would be in the case of a person who regularly subjects his shoulder to violent, unprotected trauma (eg, soccer, rugby, and hockey players). There is no sense in repairing an injury only to have it recur a week later when the patient falls on the point of the shoulder. Thus, we prefer to repair the acutely injured type III injury in many athletes, because we believe this yields a shoulder with more endurance that will stand up to repetitive stresses and heavy loads.

NONOPERATIVE TREATMENT

We recommend a skillful neglect form of treatment for type I and II injuries, and for type III injuries in inactive, nonlaboring patients who have only a mild interest in recreational activities, do not like to work in the yard, or have a desk job—especially when the injury occurs in the nondominant shoulder (Fig. 14-41). In type IV and VI injuries seen early, we recommend attempted closed reduction to dislodge the clavicle from the trapezius muscle or from under the coracoid process. If this is successful, we then apply the same indication as above for a type III problem. If the reduction fails, then an operative reduction and repair are performed. Type V and VI problems are treated with operative repair.

If nonoperative treatment is to be used, we first explain the injury in detail to the patient by describing the ruptured ligaments and why he has the "bump" on the shoulder. We explain that although surgery can correct the problem, he can, without the risks of surgery and anesthesia, end up with a very good functional shoulder. The shoulder is placed in a sling. During the first 12 hours or so, an ice pack is applied to decrease the discomfort. We may give the patient some mild analgesics and tell him that for the first 3 to 4 days he can use the arm in assistive everyday living activities. Usually within 1 week, a functional range of motion is achieved, and by 2 to 3 weeks, the patient has a full range of motion and little, if any, discomfort. (See Fig. 14-41.) It really is amazing to see how fast the symptoms disappear and how fast the range of motion returns following an untreated type III acromioclavicular joint dislocation. The patients are quite pleased with their end results and usually do not complain about the subsequent bump on the shoulder. However, if the patient changes jobs and has to put heavy stress on the acromioclavicular joint, he often will complain of a fatiguing, dull ache in the shoulder after 4 to 6 hours of heavy work. This may require a reconstructive procedure.

OPERATIVE TREATMENT

As noted above, operative procedures are used primarily in people who perform heavy labor and who daily place stress on their shoulders, and in certain patients younger than 25 years who have not made up their minds as to their future careers. The operative technique the senior author has used for the past 22 years was learned from Dr. James Anspacher at the University of Oklahoma Medical Center. The operation encompasses the best ideas and qualities of several operative procedures. The acromioclavicular joint is explored and débrided, the acromioclavicular and coracoclavicular ligaments are reapproximated, and the vertical and horizontal stability of the acromioclavicular joint is restored through the use of temporary, extra-articular screw fixation between the clavicle and the coracoid. The deltoid and trapezius muscles are repaired and imbricated back to the clavicle.

Preoperative Preparation.   A 10 × 12–inch x-ray cassette is placed under the patient's shoulder and the patient is put in the beach-chair position on the operating room table. A special headrest is used so the top of the patient's shoulder is completely free at the top of the corner of the table. The head should be slightly deviated toward the normal shoulder and stabilized to the head rest so there is complete access to the superior aspect of the shoulder. The anesthesiologist and his equipment should be moved over toward the opposite shoulder, so the physician or assistant can stand at the top of the table. Care must be taken during draping to allow access from the top of the shoulder over to the base of the neck.

Skin Incision.   The straplike incision is made in Langer's lines and is approximately 3 inches in length. It begins 1 inch posterior to the clavicle, then crosses the clavicle 1 inch medial to the acromioclavicular joint. It then extends downward to a point medial to the tip of the coracoid process (Fig. 14-42**A**). The incision is then undermined so the acromioclavicular joint, the distal 2 inches of the clavicle, and the anterior deltoid can be visualized. This usually requires a horizontal split, or at least the completion of the horizontal split of the deltotrapezius fascia and periosteum on the superior distal 2 inches of the clavicle.

The Anterior Deltoid.   In some instances, the deltoid and trapezius muscle fascia have been detached from the distal 2 or 3 inches of the clavicle. If not,

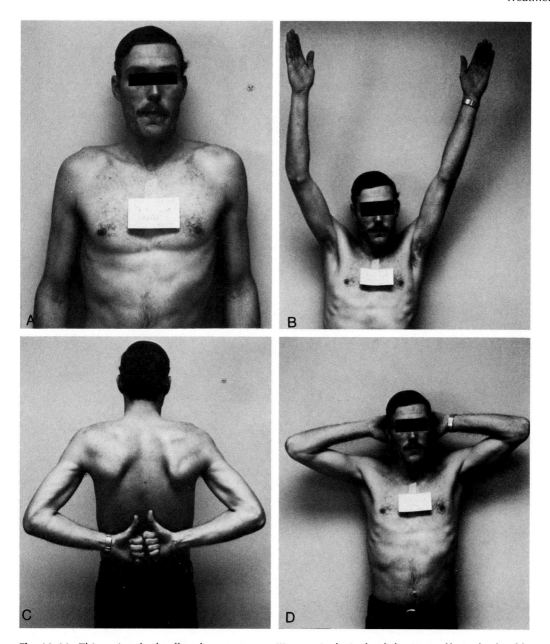

Fig. 14-41. This patient had suffered an acute type III acromioclavicular dislocation of his right shoulder on the previous day. He was initially treated for 4 days in a sling and then allowed to use the arm for everyday living activities. He still has a bump over the top of the right shoulder; however, he has a full range of motion and essentially no pain. He is not involved in heavy physical labor.

this interval must be divided so the clavicle can be grasped with a clamp and lifted upward, while the deltoid muscle is retracted distally to visualize the torn ends of the coracoclavicular ligament and the base of the coracoid process. If the deltoid has been stripped off the clavicle with an intact periosteal tube, then it will be necessary to split the deltoid down 2 inches, in line with its fibers, and detach the distal 2 inches from its insertion into the clavicle. This then will allow exposure of the coraco-

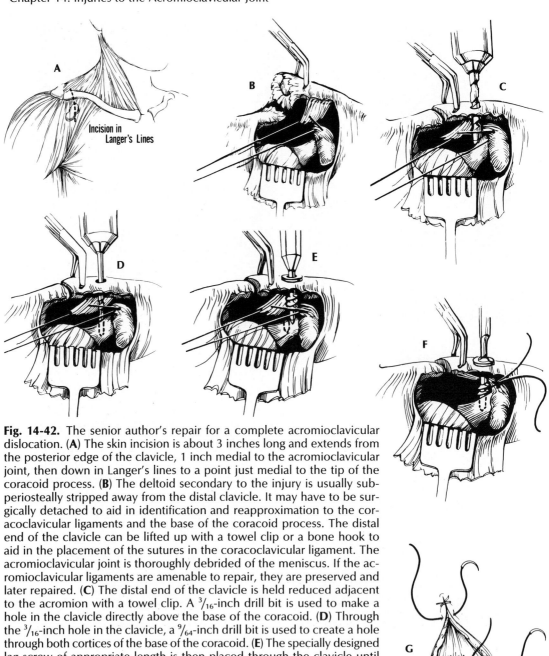

Fig. 14-42. The senior author's repair for a complete acromioclavicular dislocation. (**A**) The skin incision is about 3 inches long and extends from the posterior edge of the clavicle, 1 inch medial to the acromioclavicular joint, then down in Langer's lines to a point just medial to the tip of the coracoid process. (**B**) The deltoid secondary to the injury is usually subperiosteally stripped away from the distal clavicle. It may have to be surgically detached to aid in identification and reapproximation to the coracoclavicular ligaments and the base of the coracoid process. The distal end of the clavicle can be lifted up with a towel clip or a bone hook to aid in the placement of the sutures in the coracoclavicular ligament. The acromioclavicular joint is thoroughly debrided of the meniscus. If the acromioclavicular ligaments are amenable to repair, they are preserved and later repaired. (**C**) The distal end of the clavicle is held reduced adjacent to the acromion with a towel clip. A $^3/_{16}$-inch drill bit is used to make a hole in the clavicle directly above the base of the coracoid. (**D**) Through the $^3/_{16}$-inch hole in the clavicle, a $^9/_{64}$-inch drill bit is used to create a hole through both cortices of the base of the coracoid. (**E**) The specially designed lag screw of appropriate length is then placed through the clavicle until the smooth shank of the screw is in the clavicle. The nonthreaded nipple end of the screw is then passed into the hole of the coracoid, and the screw is tightened home to depress the clavicle down to the level of the acromion. The stay sutures in the coracoclavicular ligaments are then tied and the screw tightened another half turn to take any tension off the reapproximated ligaments. (**G**) The muscle attachments of the deltoid and trapezius are carefully repaired and, if possible, are imbricated over the top of the clavicle and the acromioclavicular joint.

clavicular ligaments and the base of the coracoid process (Fig. 14-42**B**).

The Acromioclavicular Joint. The distal end of the clavicle is grasped with a towel clip, Lewin clamp, or a bone hook and lifted upward so the joint is thoroughly débrided of the intra-articular disk and any loose frays and tags of the acromioclavicular ligament. (See Fig. 14-42**B**.)

Reapproximation of the Coracoclavicular Ligaments. The torn ends of the ligament are freed up and tagged with two or three #1 cottony Dacron sutures. The sutures are not tied at this time. (See Fig. 14-42**B**). This step is important to allow a reapproximation of the ligament ends after the screw is in its position of reducing the acromioclavicular joint. This reapproximation is not like a nice modified Kessler degree stitch that you use to repair a lacerated tendon in the hand: the stitches are secure enough so that when they are tied they do *reapproximate* the torn ends of the ligament. Some authors do not believe this step is important, because with the internal fixation, the whole area fills in with a "dense scar" that secures the distal clavicle down to the coracoid. However, we do not believe this scar will give a consistently good result. Although most coracoclavicular ligaments disrupt in the waist or in the middle of the ligament, we have noted at surgery that on many occasions the coracoclavicular ligament has been stripped off the coracoid and is found lying parallel to and plastered underneath the clavicle, or pulled loose from the clavicle and then curled up in a ball down on the base of the coracoid. The coracoclavicular ligament is a dense, heavy, strong ligament almost the size of your small finger. It has a very definite purpose in the shoulder, and that is to support the scapula and the upper extremity from the clavicle. If you are going to take the time and effort to operate on this joint, you might as well spend a few more minutes to expose the ends of the ligaments and reapproximate them with a few sutures, as opposed to relying on unreliable scar tissue to do the work.

Temporary Internal Fixation. With the superior surface of the clavicle exposed and the base of the coracoid visualized and palpated, the screw should ideally be placed vertically through the clavicle and should then penetrate both cortices of the *base* of the coracoid. With the distal end of the clavicle grasped securely with the clamp and held reduced to the acromion, a vertically placed screw from the

clavicle should enter into the base of the coracoid—*not* the waist of the coracoid. The location of the drill hole in the clavicle is usually more medial to the acromioclavicular joint than you think, because the base of the coracoid is more medial than you think. Usually, the drill hole in the clavicle should be placed 1 to 1½ inches medial to the distal end of the clavicle (Fig. 14-42**C**). While the clavicle is held reduced to the acromion, a $\frac{3}{16}$-inch hole is made through the distal clavicle directly above the base of the coracoid. Next, a $\frac{9}{64}$-inch drill bit is placed through the drill hole in the clavicle, and, either under direct vision by retracting the deltoid out of the way or by palpation, the hole is placed into and through the base of the coracoid (Fig. 14-42**D**). With the acromioclavicular joint still held reduced, a specially adapted screw is inserted through the clavicle down into the coracoid. The screw the senior author currently uses is a modified Bosworth screw.* The Bosworth screw is a lag screw that comes in various lengths and has a rather large head that keeps it from pulling through the clavicle, but also prevents it from being used with a self-retaining screwdriver (Fig. 14-43). It has a smooth shank and large, built-up, grooved threads. The tip end of the screw is quite rounded, and unless the screw-hold in the clavicle and coracoid are exactly perfect, the tip of the screw tends to skid medially or laterally off the coracoid. Without the screw attached to a self-retaining screwdriver, you really do not have much control on the tip of the screw. For that reason, the senior author has modified the Bosworth screw by using a regular screw head that can be attached to a self-retaining screwdriver. We use a self-locking screwdriver that locks the screw rigidly to the screwdriver. We use a washer in place of the large head of the Bosworth screw. To get away from the problem of the rounded tip end of the screw sliding off the coracoid, the senior author has added a ¼-inch smooth nipple, which extends beyond the threads and can be used like a probe to find the hole in the coracoid. (See Fig. 14-42**E**.) Even with these modifications, there still can be some aggravations if the screw holes in the clavicle and coracoid are not lined up in proper position. A depth gauge determines the length of the screw to be used. The screw is then introduced through the clavicle, and once the smooth part of the shank of the screw is in the clavicle, you have some leeway to guide the smooth distal tip of the screw into the hole in the coracoid and twist it. (See Fig. 14-42**F**.)

---

* The screw is produced by the Special Products Division of Howmedica Manufacturing Company.

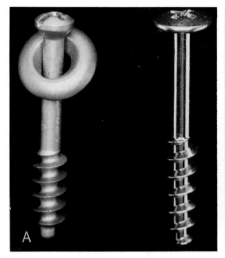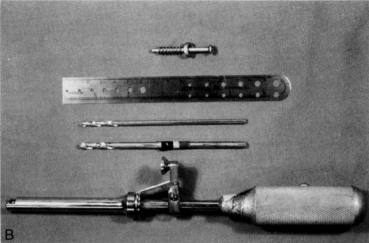

Fig. 14-43. (**A**) Comparison of the modified coracoclavicular lag screw with the original Bosworth screw. The large head of the original screw made it impossible to use the self-retaining screwdriver. Furthermore, the threads extended all the way down to the tip of the screw, making it difficult for the surgeon to place the screw into the hole in the base of the coracoid. The modified screw, which has a washer in place of the large head, can be used with a self-retaining screwdriver. The distal $^1/_4$ inch of the screw, which has no threads and is smooth-tipped, is used to seek out the hole in the base of the coracoid. (**B**) Photograph of the type of self-retaining screwdriver that the senior author uses along with $^3/_{16}$- and $^9/_{16}$-inch drill bits.

Before the final steps of repair are taken, an x-ray using the preoperative positioned cassette under the shoulder is taken to be sure the screw is properly seated in the coracoid (Fig. 14-44). When the screw is placed into the hole in the coracoid under direct vision, it is unlikely that the x-ray will reveal a misdirected screw. However, when the screw is inserted by the palpation or blind technique, it is possible for the screw to skid off medially or laterally and be surprisingly stable because of the purchase of the heavy threads along the side of the coracoid.

As the screw is tightened, the clavicle is gradually reduced down to the level of the upper border of the acromion. At this point, the stay sutures are tied and then another half turn is applied to the screw, which takes any tension off the sutures. The

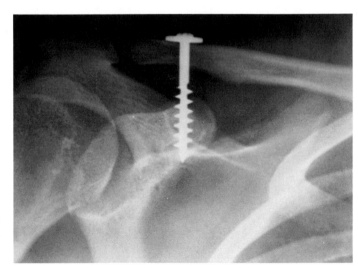

Fig. 14-44. Postoperative x-ray showing the acromioclavicular joint reduced and held temporarily in place with a special modified coracoclavicular lag screw.

primary purpose of the screw is to temporarily hold the clavicle reduced vertically and horizontally to the scapula and to take tension off the coracoclavicular ligament reapproximation until the coracoclavicular ligaments have healed.

Repair and Imbrication of the Deltotrapezius Muscle Fascia.   The deltotrapezius muscle fascia interval must be repaired back to the clavicle. Not only should this be repaired, but also, if possible, the deltotrapezius fascia should be double-breasted or imbricated over the top of the clavicle to help support the shoulder and the repair. (See Fig. 14-42**G**.)

Postoperative Care.   Postoperatively, the arm is supported in a sling for 1 to 2 weeks, but the patient is allowed to use the arm for some daily living activities, such as brushing the teeth, eating, and bathroom care. After 1 to 2 weeks, use of the sling is discontinued and the patient can use the arm for most everyday living activities, but is cautioned to avoid any lifting, pushing, and pulling for 4 to 6 weeks. Ordinarily, by 3 weeks, and certainly by 6 weeks, the patient has a very functional range of motion (ie, up to 150° to 160° of flexion and abduction without significant discomfort. (See Fig. 14-8.) The screw is routinely removed 6 to 8 weeks after surgery under local anesthesia. To aid in the screw removal, a small scratch is made with a 26-gauge hypodermic needle on the skin over the top of the shoulder where you think the screw head is

located. This is usually 1 inch medial to the skin incision. Next, a small coin is taped directly over the scratch mark and an anteroposterior x-ray is made of the shoulder (Fig. 14-45). The location of the coin on the x-ray as compared with the scratch mark on the skin will reveal whether the stab wound was planned in the correct location or whether it needs to be moved medially or laterally to the scratch mark. Following screw removal, the patient is instructed not to perform any heavy lifting, pushing, pulling, or contact sports for 10 to 12 weeks from the initial operative repair. Athletes are not permitted to return to contact sports or undue stress until 12 weeks postoperatively, and only after they have recovered full strength of the shoulder and a full range of motion.

Type IV, V, and VI Injuries

In type IV, V, and VI injuries, because the distal clavicle is so far displaced either posteriorly into the trapezius muscle up toward the base of the neck or under the coracoid process, surgery is usually advised. In a type IV or VI injury in an inactive, nonlaboring person, if we can disengage the distal clavicle from the trapezius muscle or reduce it from under the coracoid process under general anesthesia, we then treat the problem with skillful neglect. If the patient is very young or is a laborer, we surgically repair the problem as described for a type III injury. Most patients with type V injuries whom we have treated have had so much pain and

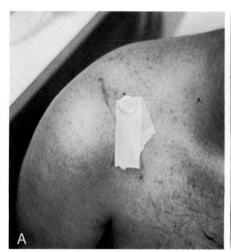
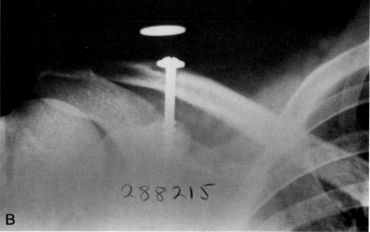

Fig. 14-45. The screw is usually removed 6 weeks after surgery using local anesthesia. A small scratch mark is made on the skin over the top of the shoulder at the approximate location of the head of the screw. A coin is taped over the top of the scratch. An x-ray is then taken to determine the relationship of the scratch mark to the head of the screw.

cosmetic deformity that surgery was almost mandatory. However, if the patient has significant medical problems and is totally uncooperative, we again treat the problem by skillful neglect.

Authors' Comments on Other Operative Procedures

INTRA-ARTICULAR FIXATION

We do not use intra-articular fixation unless there is a complete, symptomatic acromioclavicular dislocation associated with a fracture of the base of the coracoid. We prefer not to place two or more pins or a single large pin across this small joint, because the pins can produce traumatic degenerative changes in the joint. The pins also tend to migrate, and, unless a special pin like the one designed by Simmons and Martin[424] is used, there is a tendency for pins that protrude from the lateral edge of the acromion to irritate the deltoid muscle during movements of the shoulder.

EXTRA-ARTICULAR FIXATION

The use of fascia, suture, tape, vascular synthetic grafts, and other materials that pass under the coracoid and over or through the clavicle are easier to apply than coracoclavicular screws. However, they do tend to displace the clavicle anteriorly away from the acromion. In other words, they reduce the vertical separation of the clavicle away from the acromion, but they do not restore the horizontal alignment of the acromioclavicular joint. Furthermore, if the loop of material is passed over the top of the clavicle, it may erode through the clavicle and produce a fracture. The coracoclavicular lag screw reduces the acromioclavicular joint in the vertical and horizontal planes, only minimally interferes with normal clavicular rotation, and does allow the early restoration of shoulder motion.

DYNAMIC MUSCLE TRANSFERS

The use of dynamic muscle transfers (ie, the coracoid process with the attached conjoined tendon to the clavicle) for an acute injury is bypassing the site of primary pathology (ie, a rupture of the coracoclavicular ligaments). It is a major procedure and appears to us to have more risks involved than are necessary, such as injury to the musculocutaneous nerve, failure of the coracoid to heal to the clavicle, loss of screw fixation or screw breakage.

PRIMARY EXCISION OF THE DISTAL CLAVICLE

Of all the various operative procedures described for an acute injury to the acromioclavicular joint, primary excision of the distal clavicle seems to us to be the most unreasonable. If the distal clavicle is found to be fractured, or if the acromioclavicular joint is arthritic, then a primary excision seems indicated. However, the clavicle, through its articulation at the acromioclavicular joint, is important and should not be indescriminately discarded.

Authors' Treatment of Chronic Problems of the Acromioclavicular Joint

We agree with other authors that excision of the distal clavicle in a patient for a degenerative joint with an old type II injury is appropriate. We recommend excision of a minimum of 2 cm of the distal clavicle. Others have recommended excision of one eighth, one fourth, or one half the distal clavicle, but we do not think that is sufficient. Following excision of only ½ inch of the distal clavicle, the distal clavicle eventually may develop a spur; with abduction, the spur again butts against the acromion, producing symptoms and pain just as before the operation (Fig. 14-46). In many instances, we have had to re-excise the distal clavicle because of recurrence of symptoms. The removal of the distal 1 to 1½ inch of the clavicle essentially removes that part of the clavicle which used to be attached to the coracoid by the trapezoid ligament. The remaining conoid ligament is sufficient to anchor the distal clavicle down to the coracoid process.

It is totally inappropriate to excise only the distal clavicle, even by 1 inch, in a chronic, symptomatic, type III problem; this will not relieve the patient's symptoms. All this does is take a high-riding, *long* clavicle and convert it to a high-riding, *short* clavicle—which will actually increase the patient's symptoms. The remaining stump of the clavicle, without any attachment to the coracoid, is hypermobile, and thus tends to irritate the soft tissues about the shoulder and the base of the neck. We can tell you from personal experience that when our colleagues did not recognize that a patient previously had a type III injury, the symptoms were worse following simple distal clavicle excision (Fig. 14-47). Therefore, we strongly urge you to determine whether or not there is some coracoclavicular ligament fixation *prior* to excising the distal clavicle.

If the clavicle has lost its attachment to the coracoid (ie, a chronic type III, IV, V, or VI injury), you must *reconstruct* a new coracoclavicular ligament. Although fascia, suture, vascular grafts, and other materials can be used, we prefer to use the coracoacromial ligament to replace the coracoclavicular ligament and to temporarily support the reconstruction with a special coracoclavicular lag

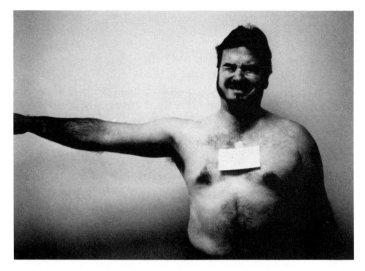

Fig. 14-46. This patient with degenerative arthritis in the right shoulder had the distal 1 cm of the clavicle resected. Four months postoperatively he noted increasing pain with abduction. X-rays confirmed that during the abduction, the distal end of the clavicle again jammed into the acromion process, causing significant pain. *(Rockwood, C. A., and Young, D. C.: Disorders of the Acromioclavicular Joint. In Rockwood, C. A., and Matsen, F., III (eds.): The Shoulder, Fig. 12-46. Philadelphia, W. B. Saunders, 1990.)*

screw. The coracoacromial ligament is ideal for the reconstruction because it already is attached on the coracoid, and because, if left alone, it could later produce an impingement syndrome in the shoulder. In a patient with a chronic dislocation, the use of the coracoacromial ligament alone is insufficient to maintain the reduction. For reconstruction of the joint in a large, strong patient, we have seen so much tension that it caused the screw to bend (Fig. 14-48). Thus, a screw is used to temporarily take the tension off the deforming forces while the new ligament is healing between the clavicle and the coracoid.

If, at the time of reconstruction, the coracoacromial ligament is absent or unsuitable, we use the screw and either 1- or 3-mm cottony Dacron suture, or a strip of conjoined tendons between the coracoid and the clavicle.

Authors' Method to Reconstruct a Chronic, Complete Acromioclavicular Dislocation

The skin incision and much of the surgical approach are the same as described for an acute repair of a type III injury (Fig. 14-49**A**). The distal 2 cm of the clavicle is excised. If a previous surgical procedure has removed part of the distal clavicle, then enough clavicle is removed so the stump of the clavicle is located just at the lateral edge of the base of the coracoid (Fig. 14-49**B**). The medullary canal of the distal clavicle is then drilled and curetted to be able to receive the transferred coracoacromial ligament (Fig. 14-49**C**).

A knife blade is used to remove the acromial attachment of the coracoacromial ligament from the acromion (Fig. 14-49**G**). With the clavicle held re-

duced to just above the base of the coracoid, one should determine if the coracoacromial ligament is long enough to reach into the intramedullary canal of the clavicle. As pointed out by Cadenat,[94] this ligament can be further lengthened by detaching the anterior fasciculus of the coracoacromial ligament from the waist of the coracoid process. A heavy 1-0, nonabsorbable suture is then woven back and forth through the ligament, so both ends of the suture exit through the acromial end of the coracoacromial ligament (Fig. 14-49**E**). Two small drill holes are then placed in the superior cortex of the distal stump of the clavicle, which connects into the medullary canal (Fig. 14-49**D**). A $^3/_{16}$-inch hole is drilled through the distal clavicle, which should be directly above the base of the coracoid. With the clavicle held to its correct position above the *base* of the coracoid, a $^9/_{64}$-inch drill bit is inserted through the hole in the clavicle and drilled through both cortices of the coracoid process. Before the lag screw is inserted into the coracoid, the two ends of the suture through the coracoacromial ligament are passed into the medullary canal and out the two small drill holes in the superior cortex of the clavicle. The special lag screw is then inserted through the clavicle and into the coracoid and tightened to vertically reduce the clavicle down to just above the coracoid process (Fig. 14-49**H**). The two ends of the suture through the coracoacromial ligament are tightened and the coracoacromial ligament is fed into the curetted medullary canal. The suture is tied, thus securing the ligament into the distal clavicle (Fig. 14-49**F**).

Postoperatively, the patient is allowed to use the arm for everyday living activities, but is instructed

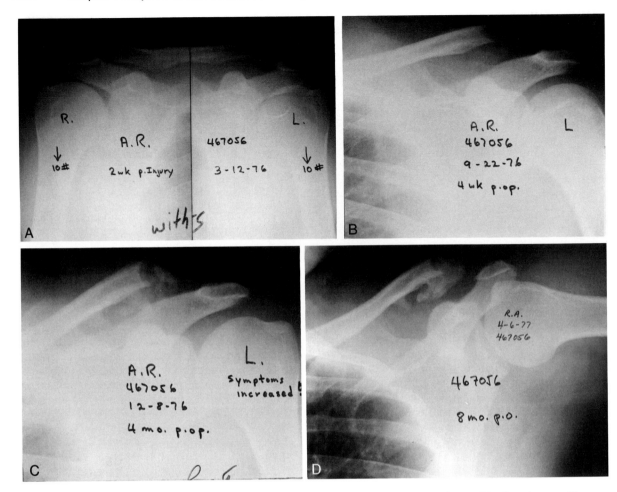

Fig. 14-47. Complications of excising the distal end of the clavicle in a patient with an old, chronic type III acromioclavicular dislocation. (**A**) X-rays comparing the right shoulder with the injured left shoulder. (**B**) Six months later, because of continued discomfort, the distal 2.5 cm of the clavicle was resected. The surgeon did not recognize that this was a type III injury with loss of the coracoclavicular ligaments. Four weeks following surgery, the patient was noting increasing pain. Calcification was beginning to develop around the distal clavicle. (**C**) Four months following the resection of the distal clavicle, the patient was more symptomatic and had more soft tissue calcification; there was greater disparity between the clavicle and the coracoid process. (**D**) Eight months following surgery, the patient continued to have pain.

to avoid any heavy lifting, pushing, or pulling. After 12 weeks, the screw can be removed under local anesthesia.

PROGNOSIS

TYPE I INJURY

In general, the prognosis for a type I injury is excellent. Most patients recover full range of motion and have no pain within 2 weeks. However, Bergfeld and associates[56] and Cox[115] reported that significant symptoms may persist for 6 months to 5 years after a type I injury. Bergfeld and associates[56] reported nuisance symptoms in 30% and significant symptoms in 9% of midshipmen with type I injuries. Cox[115] found nuisance symptoms in 28% and significant symptoms in 8%. Babe and colleagues[27] found that 100% of their patients with type I injuries were asymptomatic.

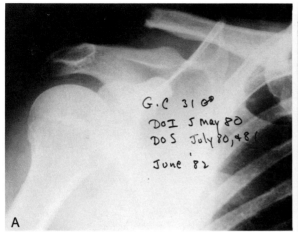

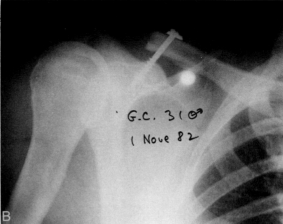

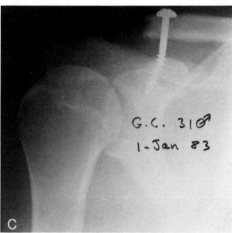

Fig. 14-48. Complications of resecting the distal clavicle without reconstruction of the coracoclavicular ligament. (**A**) Two years following injury and after two resections of the distal clavicle, the patient had continued pain and discomfort in the right shoulder. (**B**) The superiorly and posteriorly displaced clavicle was reduced back to its normal position above the base of the coracoid with great effort. The clavicle was held reduced with a coracoclavicular lag screw, and the coracoacromial ligament was transferred into the medullary canal as described by Cadenat. (**C**) At 2 months after surgery, the screw was removed under local anesthesia. The screw was bent because of the tremendous strain across the coracoclavicular interspace. (*Rockwood, C. A., and Young, D. C.: Disorders of the Acromioclavicular Joint. In Rockwood, C. A., and Matsen, F., III (eds.): The Shoulder, Fig. 12-57. Philadelphia, W. B. Saunders, 1990.*)

TYPE II INJURY

Again, most patients with type II injury recover fully, leaving only a small percentage who require débridement or excision of the outer end of the clavicle because of arthritis in the joint. Bergfeld and associates[56] and Cox[115] reported from the U.S. Naval Academy that 23% to 35% of patients with type II injuries had nuisance symptoms, and 13% to 42% had significant symptoms 6 months to 5 years following injury. Walsh and colleagues[478] also found residual pain and stiffness in some patients with type II injuries, as did Babe and associates.[27] CYBEX-II evaluation of nine patients with type II injuries demonstrated a 24% increase in horizontal abduction strength at fast speeds. All other motions and speeds were not significantly different from the noninjured arm. Bjerneld and associates[64] found 100% good or excellent results in 37 patients with

an average follow-up of 6 years. Park and coworkers[343] found good results in 25 patients with type II injuries treated nonoperatively.

TYPE III, IV, V, AND VI INJURIES

A review of the literature suggests that excellent results can be obtained in patients with type III, IV, V, and VI injuries with both operative and nonoperative treatments. However, we believe that as physicians, we should have more discrimination as to which patients we operate on and which ones we manage by nonoperative techniques. We are quite confident that nonoperative treatment in a white-collar office worker will be successful (ie, will result in minimal pain and allow the patient to carry on with usual activities). However, the senior author is quite certain that a patient whose job involves heavy labor and who is treated by a non-

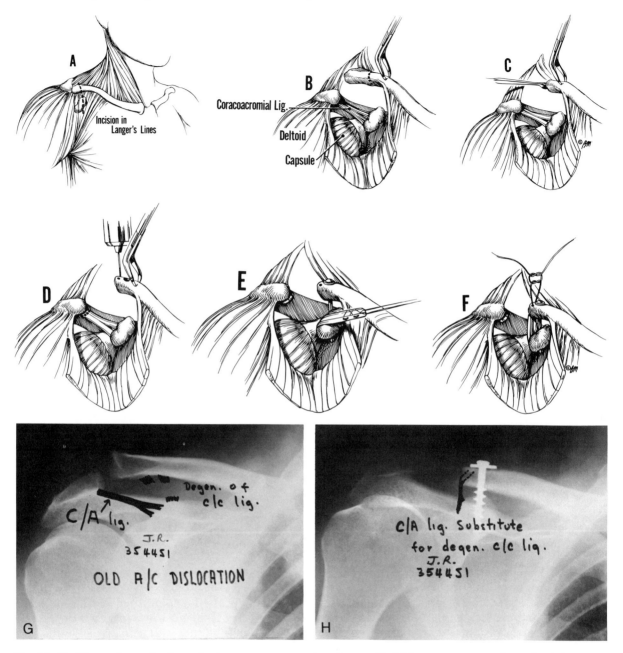

Fig. 14-49. The senior author's method to reconstruct a chronic type III, IV, V, or VI acromioclavicular dislocation. (**A**) The incision is made in Langer's lines. (**B**) The distal end of the clavicle is excised. (**C**) The medullary canal is drilled out and curetted to receive the transferred coracoacromial ligament. (**D**) Two small drill holes are made through the superior cortex of the distal clavicle. The coracoacromial ligament is carefully detached from the acromion process. (**E–H**) With the coracoacromial ligament detached from the acromion, a heavy nonabsorbable suture is woven through the ligament. The ends of the suture are passed out through the two small drill holes in the distal end of the clavicle. The coracoclavicular lag screw is inserted, and when the clavicle is reduced down to its normal position, the sutures used to pull the ligament snugly up into the canal are tied.

operative technique will develop a dull, aching, dragging pain in the shoulder, and will state that this causes difficulty in performing his usual job. In general, given the proper treatment for a specific patient, the end results tend to be completely acceptable in more than 90% of patients.

In patients with type III injuries, Walsh and co-workers[478] found decreased vertical abduction strength in operatively treated patients when compared with nonoperatively treated patients. No other strength parameters were significantly different. However, endurance tests were not performed. Patients with type IV, V, and VI injuries usually require open reduction and internal fixation. In our experience, the end results have been about the same as those in patients with type III injuries.

COMPLICATIONS

COMPLICATIONS OF ACUTE INJURIES

Associated Fractures and Thoracic Injury

Fractures associated with dislocation may include fractures of the midclavicle, the distal clavicle into the acromioclavicular joint, the acromion process, and the coracoid process. Barber[37] reported a patient with a type IV injury associated with contralateral pheumothorax and an ipsilateral pulmonary contusion.

Coracoclavicular Ossification

Coracoclavicular ossification has been referred to as ossification and calcification. Urist[464-466] demonstrated that bone does indeed form in the coracoclavicular interval. Although some authors felt ossification was the result of operative treatment, most have shown that ossification occurs whether the lesion is treated by conservative or operative means. Arner and associates[24] reported that ossification of the acromioclavicular or coracoclavicular ligament is the rule rather than the exception. They reported incidence of mineralization in 14 of 17 patients in their series, and 62 of 109 patients and 15 of 22 patients in other series. Millbourn[292] stated that calcium appears in the mild or severe sprain, whether the treatment is conservative or operative, and that it can be observed as early as the third or fourth week. It may be a bone structure, and it may form a bridge from the coracoid to the clavicle. In our experience, ossification does not seem to affect the late functional results. (See Fig. 14-6.) In Weitzman's[487] series, 16 of 19 patients had min-

eralization, but he could not correlate this with the end results. Alldredge[13] reported calcium in half his operative cases, again with no correlation with the end results.

Osteolysis of the Distal Clavicle

Osteolysis of the distal clavicle may follow an acute injury or may occur in persons who have repeated stress on the shoulder. Madsen[273] reported seven patients with the rare complication known as post-traumatic osteolysis of the distal clavicle. He identified eight cases in the literature at that time (1963), the first of which was reported by Werder in 1950. Ehricht[141] reported a case in a pneumatic tool-worker. Cahill[95] reported 46 patients who were athletes, none of whom had an acute injury, but 45 of whom lifted weights as part of their training. He used technetium bone scans and a 35° cephalic tilt x-ray view to help make the diagnosis. Murphy and associates,[310] Orava and colleagues,[340] and Cooper and Curtis[109] reported this condition in women.

The x-ray findings are osteoporosis, osteolysis, and tapering of the distal clavicle. Usually, bony changes do not occur in the acromion. Changes usually occur only in one shoulder (Fig. 14-50). If changes are noted in both shoulders, then other conditions should be considered, such as rheumatoid arthritis, hyperparathyroidism, and scleroderma. The differential diagnosis of a lesion in one shoulder should include Gorham's massive osteolysis,[177] gout, and a neoplasm such as multiple myeloma.

Most authors believe the symptoms of dull ache, weakness, and pain with flexion and abduction are self-limited within a year or so. They recommend stopping the activities that strain the shoulder, and resting. If the symptoms are not relieved, then excision of the distal clavicle is recommended. Levine and colleagues[262] reported that with rest, the distal clavicle may even reconstitute itself. Microscopic studies of the distal clavicle have been reported by Lamont,[250] Murphy and co-workers,[310] Madsen,[273] and Zsernaviczky and Horst.[507] They described demineralization, subchondral cysts, and erosion of the distal clavicle. Griffiths and Glucksman[183] performed a biopsy 8 months after injury, which showed patches of necrotic and reactive woven bone.

Nonunion of the Coracoid Process

Nonunion of the coracoid process is a rare problem and can be quite disabling. The patient has discomfort when lifting or stressing the arm, and the

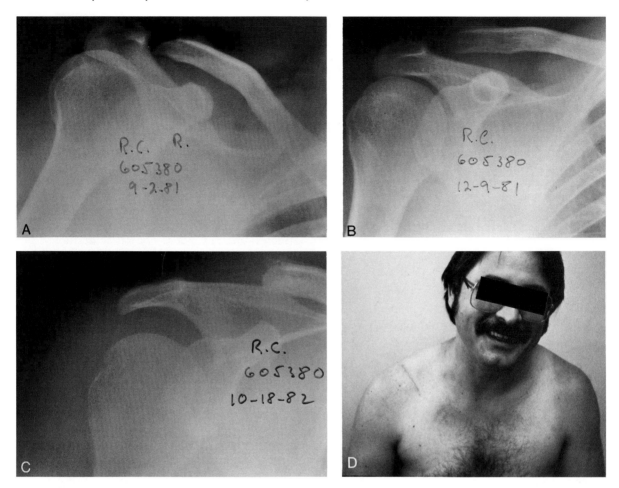

Fig. 14-50. Traumatic osteolysis of the distal clavicle. (**A**) An x-ray taken 3 months after a fall onto the right shoulder reveals resorption of the right distal clavicle and new bone formation on the dorsal aspect of the clavicle. (**B**) An x-ray at 6 months reveals an increase in the resorption and new bone formation; the patient was experiencing pain. (**C**) This x-ray was taken 14 months following the injury and 2 months after resection of the distal 2.5 cm of the clavicle. The remaining clavicle was held securely to the coracoid process through the conoid ligament. (**D**) This skin incision was used for the arthroplasty.

shoulder is weak. Bone graft and stabilization of the nonunion are required (Fig. 14-51).

COMPLICATIONS OF OPERATIVE TREATMENT

The following complications may result from operative treatment:

Wound infection
Osteomyelitis
Acromioclavicular arthritis
Soft tissue ossification
Erosion of bone by metal

Late fracture through the implant holes in the bone
Necessity of a second operative procedure to remove the fixation device
Migration of pins or wires
Metal failure
Unsightly scar
Inadequate purchase of the fixation
Recurrent deformity.

Besides the obvious wound infection and osteomyelitis that might develop from the operative procedure, several other complications can occur (ie, a fracture through a drill hole, loss of purchase of the internal fixation, metal failure, and migration

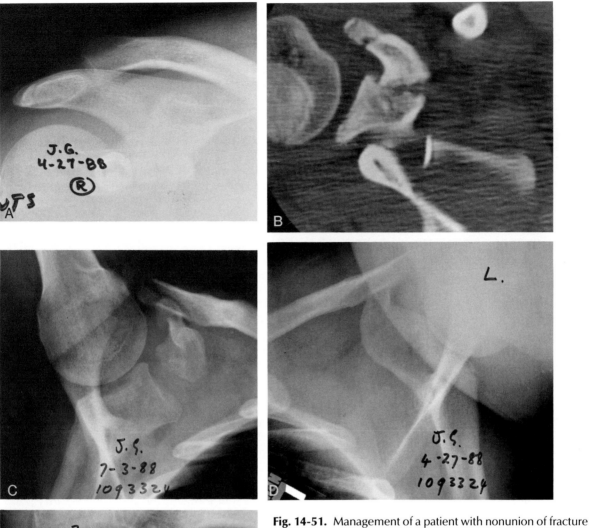

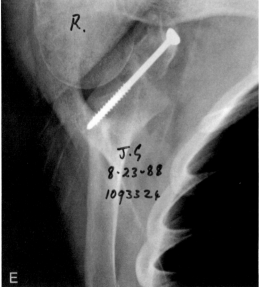

Fig. 14-51. Management of a patient with nonunion of fracture of the base of the coracoid. (**A**) Acromioclavicular subluxation of the right shoulder. (**B**) A CT scan confirms the presence of a fracture of the base of the coracoid. (**C**) Six months following injury, the Stryker notch view clearly demonstrates a nonunion of the fractured coracoid. (**D**) A Stryker notch view compares the appearance of the coracoid of the normal left shoulder. (**E**) Seven months following injury, the coracoid process was exposed, bone was grafted, and the process was held reduced with a lag screw. The patient had an uneventful recovery. (*Rockwood, C. A., and Young, D. C.: Disorders of the Acromio-clavicular Joint. In Rockwood, C. A., and Matsen, F., III (eds.): The Shoulder, Fig. 12-60. Philadelphia, W. B. Saunders, 1990.*)

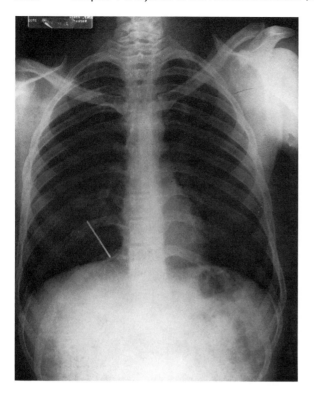

Fig. 14-52. A broken Steinmann pin has migrated into the right lung field from its previous location in the right acromioclavicular joint.

of the fixation device to other parts of the body (Fig. 14-52).

Migration of Pins

Mazet[277] reported migration of a 6-cm Kirschner wire into the lung 76 days after its insertion into the right acromioclavicular joint. Norrell and Llewellyn[330] reported migration of a Steinmann pin from the right acromioclavicular joint into the spinal cord. The pin was found in the subarachnoid space anterior to the spinal cord. It extended transversely across the spinal canal at the level of the first thoracic vertebra. It was easily removed in the direction from which it came.

Lindsey and Gutowski[264] reported migration of a Kirschner wire into the neck posterior to the carotid sheath. The pin was removed uneventfully. They concluded, as did Eaton and Serletti,[140] that CT scan was useful in planning removal of migrated pins. Eaton and Serletti[140] removed a migrated pin that had crossed the midline and was indenting into the pleura posteriorly at the T2 level. Urban and Jaskiewicz[463] reported a case of pin migration into

the ipsilateral pleural cavity 3 months after surgery. Sethi and Scott[414] reported on the migration of a Hagie pin from the acromioclavicular joint, causing a laceration of the subclavian artery. Grauthoff and Klammer[180] reported five cases of migration of pins into the aorta, subclavian artery, or lung. Retief and Meintjes[375] reported a case in which a 12-cm Kirschner wire that had been placed into the acromioclavicular joint had migrated *through* the thoracic cavity and was lodged behind the liver. In the 6-week period between the Kirschner wire insertion and its removal, the patient had suffered a pneumothorax secondary to the wire penetration of the lung.

In most instances, pin migration can be prevented by bending a hook on the portion of the pin that protrudes from the acromion process. However, the pins can break, and then part of the pin is free to migrate. Patients must be prepared and forewarned of the possible necessity of pin removal and the complications of pins that are not removed.

There are no reports of migration of loops of broken wire, and Bosworth[74] states that he knows of no case of migration of a screw into another part of the body. Jay and Monnet[228] reported a Bosworth screw that broke during removal; the tip of the screw was left in the coracoid process.

COMPLICATIONS OF NONOPERATIVE TREATMENT

The following concerns and complications are associated with nonoperative treatment:

Tissues interposed in the acromioclavicular joint
Joint stiffness secondary to immobilization
Required close supervision and adjustments
Immobilization device restrictive and uncomfortable
Skin irritation, maceration, or ulcers on the shoulder secondary to the immobilization device
Patient can independently remove the external device and lose the reduction
Inability of patient to bathe completely or properly
Everyday activities restricted
Pressure sores on other parts of the body in contact with the immobilization device
Deformity
Soft tissue ossification
Acromioclavicular arthritis.

As described, patients with type I or II injuries may develop degenerative changes in the joint severe enough to require excision of the distal clavicle. Following a type III, IV, or V injury, the patient, if he is involved with heavy labor, may well develop a chronic strain and ache in the shoulder and posterior neck muscles. This requires, in addition to an excision of the distal clavicle, reconstruction of the coracoclavicular ligaments. Following a type IV injury, chronic pain is the most likely complication.

REFERENCES

1. Aalders, G.J.; Vroonhoven, T.J.M.V.; Werken, C.; Wijffels, C.C.S.M.: An Expectional Case of Pneumothorax—"A New Adventure of the K Wire." Injury, 16:564–565, 1985.
2. Abbott, L.C., and Lucas, D.B.: The Function of the Clavicle—Its Surgical Significance. Ann. Surg., 140:583–599, 1954.
3. Abbott, L.C.; Saunders, J.B.; Hagey, H.; and Jones, E.W.: Surgical Approaches to the Shoulder Joint. J. Bone Joint Surg., 31A:235–255, 1949.
4. Adams, F.L.: The Genuine Works of Hippocrates, Vols. 1 and 2. New York, William Wood, 1886.
5. Adams, R., and McDonald, M.: Cryptoccal Arthritis of the Acromioclavicular Joint. N.C. Med. J., 45:23–24, 1984.
6. Aderhold, K.: [A New Method of Therapy in Complete Separation of the Acromioclavicular Joint.] Unfallheilkunde, 86:416–422, 1983.
7. Ahstrom, J.P., Jr.: Surgical Repair of Complete Acromioclavicular Separation. J.A.M.A., 217:785–789, 1971.
8. Albrecht, F.: The Balser Plate for Acromioclavicular Fixation. Chirurg., 53:732–734, 1982.
9. Alexander, O.M.: Dislocation of the Acromio-Clavicular Joint. Radiography, 15:260, 1949.
10. Alexander, O.M.: Radiography of the Acromio-Clavicular Joint. Radiography, 14:139, 1948.
11. Alexander, O.M.: Radiography of the Acromio-Clavicular Articulation. Med. Radiogr. Photogr., 30:34–39, 1954.
12. Alldredge, R.H.: Surgical Treatment of Acromioclavicular Dislocations (abstract). J. Bone Joint Surg., 47A:1278, 1965.
13. Alldredge, R.H.: Surgical Treatment of Acromioclavicular Dislocations (abstract). Clin. Orthop., 63:262–263, 1969.
14. Allen, W.C.: Post-Traumatic Osteolysis of the Distal Clavicle. Postgrad. Med., 41:A73, 1967.
15. Allman, F.L., Jr.: Fractures and Ligamentous Injuries of the Clavicle and Its Articulation. J. Bone Joint Surg., 49A:774–784, 1967.
16. Allman, F.L., Jr.: Old Complicated or Symptomatic Untreated Acromioclavicular Sprains. J. Bone Joint Surg., 47A:780–784, 1967.
17. Allman, F.L., Jr.: Personal communication, 1984.
18. Alnor, P.: Die posttraumatische Osteolyse des lateralen Claviculaendes. Fortschr. Rontgenstr., 75:364, 1951.
19. Alpert, M., and Myers, M.M.: Osteolysis of the Acromial End of the Clavicles in Rheumatoid Arthritis. A.J.R., 86:251, 1961.
20. Anderson, M.E.: Treatment of Dislocations of the Acromioclavicular and Sternoclavicular Joints (abstract). J. Bone Joint Surg., 45A:657–658, 1963.

21. Anderson, R., and Burgess, E.: Acromioclavicular Dislocation: A Conservative Method of Treatment. Northwest Med., 38:40, 1939.
22. Anzel, S.H., and Streitz, W.L.: Acute Acromioclavicular Injuries: A Report of Nineteen Cases Treated Non-Operatively Employing Dynamic Splint Immobilization. Clin. Orthop., 103:143–149, 1974.
23. Appell, H.A.: Acromioclavicular Dislocation. Can. Med. Assoc. J., 43:23–25, 1940.
24. Arner, O.; Sandahl, U.; and Ohrling, H.: Dislocation of the Acromioclavicular Joint: Review of the Literature and a Report of 56 Cases. Acta Chir. Scand., 113:140–152, 1957.
25. Aufranc, O.E.; Jones, S.N.; and Harris, W.H.: Complete Acromioclavicular Dislocation. J.A.M.A., 180:681–682, 1962.
26. Augereau, B.; Robert, H.; and Apoil, A.: [Treatment of Severe Acromioclavicular Dislocation: A Coracoclavicular Ligamentoplasty Technique Derived from Cadenat's Procedure.] Ann. Chir., 35:720–722, 1981.
27. Babe, J.G.; Valle, M.; and Couceiro, J.: Treatment of Acromioclavicular Disruptions: Trial of a Simple Surgical Approach. Injury, 19:159–161, 1988.
28. Badgley, C.E.: Sports Injuries of the Shoulder Girdle. J.A.M.A., 172:444–448, 1960.
29. Bailey, R.W.; O'Connor, G.A.; Tilus, P.D.; and Baril, J.D.: A Dynamic Repair for Acute and Chronic Injuries of the Acromioclavicular Area (abstract). J. Bone Joint Surg., 54A:1802, 1972.
30. Bailey, R.W.: A Dynamic Repair for Complete Acromioclavicular Joint Dislocation (abstract). J. Bone Joint Surg., 47A:858, 1965.
31. Bakalim, G., and Wilppula, E.: Surgical or Conservative Treatment of Total Dislocation of the Acromioclavicular Joint. Acta Chir. Scand., 141:43–47, 1975.
32. Baker, C.L.; Wittels, M.; and Curl, W.W.: Avoiding Complications Following Acromioclavicular Injury. Complications Orthop., 4:115–123, 1989.
33. Baker, D.M., and Stryker, W.F.: Acute Complete Acromioclavicular Separations. J.A.M.A., 192:689–692, 1965.
34. Baldrati, L.; Brunetti, L.; Docci, D.; Turci, F.; Bonacini, G.; and Gilli, P.: [Acromioclavicular Subluxation: An Unusual Clinico-Radiological Manifestation of Amyloidosis Due to Dialysis.] Radiologia (Torino), 77:557–559, 1989.
35. Balvanyossy, P., and Devay, K.: [A Case of Acromioclavicular Dislocation, Complicated With Clavicular Fracture.] Magy Traumatol. Orthop. Helyreallito. Sebesz., 31:229–232, 1988.
36. Bannister, G.; Stableforth, P.; and Hutson, M.: The Management of Acute Acromioclavicular Dislocation. Presented at the 4th International Conference on Surgery of the Shoulder, New York, October 4–7, 1989.
37. Barber, F.A.: Complete Posterior Acromioclavicular Dislocation: A Case Report. Orthopedics, 10:493–496, 1987.
38. Bargren, J.H.; Erlanger, S.; and Dick, H.M.: Biomechanics and Comparison of Two Operative Methods of Treatment of Complete Acromioclavicular Separation. Clin. Orthop., 130:267–272, 1978.
39. Barnhart, J.M.; Fain, R.H.; Dewar, F.P.; and Stein, A.H.:

Acromioclavicular Joint Injuries. Clin. Orthop., 81:199, 1970.

40. Barnhart, J.M.: Repair of Acute Acromioclavicular Joint Separation. Am. J. Orthop. Surg., 10:122–123, 1968.

41. Barr, J.S.: Dislocations of the Clavicle. In Wilson, P.D. (ed.): Experience in the Management of Fractures and Dislocations, pp. 387–392. Philadelphia, J.B. Lippincott, 1938.

42. Barrett, J.: The Clavicular Joints. Physiotherapy, 57:268–269, 1971.

43. Bartonicek, J.; Jehlicka, D.; and Bezvoda, Z.: [Surgical Treatment of Acromioclavicular Luxation.] Acta Chir. Orthop. Traumatol. Cech., 55:289–309, 1988.

44. Basmajian, J.V.: Acromioclavicular Joint. In Grant's Method of Anatomy, 8th ed., pp. 160–161. Baltimore, Williams & Wilkins, 1971.

45. Batchelor, J.S.: Splint for Fractured Clavicle and Acromioclavicular Dislocation. Lancet, 2:690, 1947.

46. Bateman, J.E.: Athletic Injuries About the Shoulder in Throwing and Body-Contact Sports. Clin. Orthop., 23:75–83, 1962.

47. Bateman, J.E.: The Shoulder and Neck. Philadelphia, W.B. Saunders, 1972.

48. Bayley, I., and Kessel, L.: Shoulder Surgery. New York, Springer-Verlag, 1982.

49. Bearden, J.M.; Hughston, J.C.; and Whatley, G.S.: Acromioclavicular Dislocation: Method of Treatment. J. Sports Med., 1(4):5–17, 1973.

50. Bearn, J.G.: Direct Observations on the Function of the Capsule of the Sternoclavicular Joint in Clavicle Support. J. Anat., 101:159–170, 1967.

51. Beckman, T.: A Case of Simultaneous Luxation of Both Ends of the Clavicle. Acta Chir. Scand., 56:156–163, 1923.

52. Bednarek, J.; Kaczan, Z.; and Krochmalski, M.: [Results of Treatment in Acromio-Clavicular Dislocations.] Chir. Narzadow. Ruchu. Ortop. Pol., 46:13–16, 1981.

53. Behling, F.: Treatment of Acromioclavicular Separations. Orthop. Clin. North Am., 4:747–757, 1973.

54. Benson, R.A.: Acromioclavicular Dislocation. U.S. Nav. Med. Bull., 34:341–342, 1936.

55. Benton, J., and Nelson, C.: Avulsion of the Coracoid Process in an Athlete. J. Bone Joint Surg., 53A:356–358, 1971.

56. Bergfeld, J.A.; Andrish, J.T.; and Clancy, W.G.: Evaluation of the Acromioclavicular Joint Following First- and Second-Degree Sprains. Am. J. Sports Med., 6:153–159, 1978.

57. Bernard, T.N., Jr.; Brunet, M.E.; and Haddad, R.J.: Fractured Coracoid Process in Acromioclavicular Dislocations: Report of 4 Cases and Review of the Literature. Clin. Orthop., 175:227–232, 1983.

58. Berson, B.L.; Gilbert, M.S.; and Green, S.: Acromioclavicular Dislocations: Treatment by Transfer of the Conjoined Tendon and Distal End of the Coracoid Process to the Clavicle. Clin. Orthop., 135:157–164, 1978.

59. Bertwistle, A.P.: Acromio-Clavicular Dislocation and Sprain. Clinical Journal, 66:76–77, 1937.

60. Besselaar, P.P., and Raaymakers, E.L.F.B.: Operative Treatment of Acromioclavicular Dislocation (abstract). Acta Orthop. Scand., 55:483–484, 1984.

61. Bianchine, J.W.: Acromial Dimples: A Benign Familial Trait (letter to the editor). Am. J. Human Genetics, 26:412–413, 1974.

62. Binet, E.F., and Markarian, B.: Asymptomatic Clavicular Lesion. N.Y. State J. Med., 75:1710–1712, 1975.

63. Birkett, A.N.: The Result of Operative Repair of Severe Acromio-Clavicular Dislocation. Br. J. Surg., 32:103–105, 1944–1945.

64. Bjerneld, H.; Hovelius, L.; and Thorling, J.: Acromio-Clavicular Separations Treated Conservatively: A 5-Year Follow-Up Study. Acta Orthop. Scand., 54:743–745, 1983.

65. Björkenheim, J.M.; Paavolainen, P.; and Slatis, P.: Surgical Treatment of Acromioclavicular Dislocation (abstract). Acta Orthop. Scand., 54:533, 1983.

66. Blankstein, A.; Amsallem, J.L.; Rubinstein, E.; Horoszowski, H.; and Farin, I.: Septic Arthritis of the Acromioclavicular Joint: Current Problem Case. Arch. Orthop. Trauma Surg., 103:417–418, 1985.

67. Blazina, M.E.: Letter to the Editor re: Bearden's Article. Acromioclavicular Dislocation: Method of Treatment. J. Sports Med., 1:5–17, 1973. J. Sports Med., 2:58–59, 1974.

68. Bloom, F.A.: Wire Fixation in Acromioclavicular Dislocation. J. Bone Joint Surg., 27:273–276, 1945.

69. Böhler, L.: Treatment of Fractures, 4th ed. Baltimore, William Wood, 1935.

70. Bonnell, F., and Mirfakhrai, A.M.: [Treatment of Complete Acromioclavicular Luxation by Coracoclavicular Screw.] Acta Chir. Acad. Sci. Hungaricae, 22:69–74, 1981.

71. Bonnin, J.G.: Complete Outline of Fractures. London, William Heinemann, 1941.

72. Bossart, P.J.; Joyce, S.M.; Manaster, B.J.; and Packer, S.M.: Lack of Efficacy of "Weighted" Radiographs in Diagnosing Acute Acromioclavicular Separation. Ann. Emerg. Med., 17:47–51, 1988.

73. Bosworth, B.M.: Acromioclavicular Separation: New Method of Repair. Surg. Gynecol. Obstet., 73:866–871, 1941.

74. Bosworth, B.M.: Acromioclavicular Dislocation: End-Results of Screw Suspension Treatment. Ann. Surg., 127:98–111, 1948.

75. Bosworth, B.M.: Calcium Deposits in the Shoulder and Subacromial Bursitis: A Survey of 12,122 Shoulders. J.A.M.A., 116:2477–2482, 1941.

76. Bosworth, B.M.: Complete Acromioclavicular Dislocation. N. Engl. J. Med., 241:221–225, 1949.

77. Boussaton, M.; Julia, F.; Horvath, E.; Boudet, J.; and Ficat, P.: [Transposition of the Coracoacromial Ligament According to the Technique of Weaver and Dunn in the Treatment of Old Acromioclavicular Luxations: A Report of 15 Cases.] Acta Orthop. Belg., 51:80–90, 1985.

78. Bowers, K.D.: Treatment of Acromioclavicular Sprains in Athletes. Physician Sports Med., 11:79–89, 1983.

79. Bowers, R.F.: Complete Acromioclavicular Separation: Diagnosis and Operative Treatment. J. Bone Joint Surg., 17:1005–1010, 1935.

80. Boyer, D.W.: Trapshooter's Shoulder: Stress Fracture of the Coracoid Process. J. Bone Joint Surg., 57A:862, 1975.

81. Brandt, G.: Die Behandlung der Verrenkung im acro-

miolen Schlusselbeingelenk. Klin. Med., 51:526–528, 1956.

82. Breitner, S., and Wirth, C.J.: [Resection of the Acromial and Sternal Ends of the Clavicula.] Z. Orthop., 125:363–368, 1987.

83. Briggs, J.R.; Laurence, W.; Simurla, M.; Buck, J.E.; Jenkins, S.A.; Bingald, A.C.; Addison, J.: Acromio-Clavicular Dislocation (Proceedings). J. Bone Joint Surg., 44B:227, 1962.

84. Brosgol, M.: Traumatic Acromioclavicular Sprains and Subluxations. Clin. Orthop., 20:98–107, 1961.

85. Browne, J.E.; Stanley, R.F., Jr.; and Tullos, H.S.: Acromioclavicular Joint Dislocations: Comparative Results Following Operative Treatment With and Without Primary Distal Clavisectomy. Am. J. Sports Med., 5:258–263, 1977.

86. Brunelli, G., and Brunelli, F.: The Treatment of Acromioclavicular Dislocation by Transfer of the Short Head of Biceps. Int. Orthop., 12:105–108, 1988.

87. Brunelli, G.: Proposta di un Nuovo Methodo di Correzione Chirurgia Della Lussazione Acromion Clavicolare. Bull. Soc. Med. Chir. Bresciana, 10:95–98, 1956.

88. Brunet, M.E.; Reynolds, M.C.; Cook, S.D.; and Brown, T.W.: Atraumatic Osteolysis of the Distal Clavicle: Histologic Evidence of Synovial Pathogenesis: A Case Report. Orthopedics, 9:557–559, 1986.

89. Bundens, W.D., Jr., and Cook, J.I.: Repair of Acromioclavicular Separations by Deltoid-Trapezius Imbrication. Clin. Orthop., 20:109–114, 1961.

90. Bunnell, S.: Fascial Graft for Dislocation of the Acromioclavicular Joint. Surg. Gynecol. Obstet., 46:563–564, 1928.

91. Burns, S.J., and Zvirbulis, R.A.: A Ganglion Arising Over the Acromioclavicular Joint: A Case Report. Orthopedics, 7:1002–1004, 1984.

92. Burri, C., and Neugebauer, R.: Carbon Fiber Replacement of the Ligaments of the Shoulder Girdle and the Treatment of Lateral Instability of the Ankle Joint. Clin. Orthop., 196:112–117, 1985.

93. Burton, M.E.: Operative Treatment of Acromioclavicular Dislocations. Bull. Hosp. Jt. Dis. Orthop. Inst., 36:109–120, 1975.

94. Cadenat, F.M.: The Treatment of Dislocations and Fractures of the Outer End of the Clavicle. Int. Clin., 1:145–169, 1917.

95. Cahill, B.R.: Osteolysis of the Distal Part of the Clavicle in Male Athletes. J. Bone Joint Surg., 64A:1053–1058, 1982.

96. Caldwell, G.D.: Treatment of Complete Permanent Acromioclavicular Dislocation by Surgical Arthrodesis. J. Bone Joint Surg., 25:368–374, 1943.

97. Caldwell, G.D.: Treatment of Fractures. New York, Paul Hoeber, 1943.

98. Campbell, W.C.: Operative Orthopaedics. St. Louis, C.V. Mosby, 1971.

99. Campos, O.P.: Acromioclavicular Dislocation. Am. J. Surg., 43:287–291, 1939.

100. Carr, A.J., and Broughton, N.S.: Acromioclavicular Dislocation Associated With Fracture of the Coracoid Process. J. Trauma, 29:125–126, 1989.

101. Carrell, W.B.: Dislocation at the Outer End of Clavicle. J. Bone Joint Surg., 10:314–315, 1928.

102. Caspi, I.; Ezra, E.; Nerubay, J.; and Horoszovski, H.: Musculocutaneous Nerve Injury After Coracoid Process Transfer for Clavicle Instability: Report of Three Cases. Acta Orthop. Scand., 58:294–295, 1987.

103. Cave, E.F. (ed.): Fractures and Other Injuries. Chicago, Year Book Medical, 1961.

104. Codman, E.A.: Rupture of the Supraspinatus Tendon. *In* The Shoulder, pp. 123–177. Brooklyn, NY, G. Miller & Co., 1934.

105. Colson, J.H.C., and Armour, W.J.: Sports Injuries and Their Treatment. Philadelphia, J.B. Lippincott, 1961.

106. Conway, A.M.: Movements at the Sternoclavicular and Acromioclavicular Joints. Phys. Ther. Rev., 41:421–432, 1961.

107. Cook, F.F., and Tibone, J.E.: The Mumford Procedure in Athletes: An Objective Analysis of Function. Am. J. Sports Med., 16:97–100, 1988.

108. Cooper, A.: A Treatise on Dislocations and Fractures of the Joints, 2nd Am. ed. from 6th London ed. Boston, Lilly & Wait and Carter & Hendee, 1832.

109. Cooper, D., and Curtis, R.: Traumatic Osteolysis in Women: One Case Report. Personal communication, 1989.

110. Cooper, E.S.: New Method of Treating Long-Standing Dislocations of the Scapulo-Clavicular Articulation. Am. J. Med. Sci., 41:389–392, 1861.

111. Copeland, S., and Kessel, L.: Disruption of the Acromioclavicular Joint: Surgical Anatomy and Biological Reconstruction. Injury, 11:208–214, 1980.

112. Copher, G.H.: A Method of Treatment of Upward Dislocation of the Acromial End of the Clavicle. Am. J. Surg., 22:507–508, 1933.

113. Coues, W.P.: Fracture of the Coracoid Process of the Scapula. N. Engl. J. Med., 212:727, 1935.

114. Cox, J.S.; Hewes, T.F.; Hinckley, J.A.; and Bergfeld, J.A.: Shoulder Separation—The Fate of the Acromioclavicular Joint in Athletic Injuries (pamphlet). Dept. Orthop. Surg., U.S. Naval Hospital, Annapolis, MD.

115. Cox, J.S.: The Fate of the Acromioclavicular Joint in Athletic Injuries. Am. J. Sports Med., 9:50–53, 1981.

116. Craig, E.V.: The Acromioclavicular Joint Cyst: An Unusual Presentation of a Rotator Cuff Tear. Clin. Orthop., 202:189–192, 1986.

117. Crossan, J.F., and Macpherson, I.S.: The Role of the Acromioclavicular Joint in Chronic Shoulder Impingement Syndromes (abstract). J. Bone Joint Surg., 67B:161, 1985.

118. Currie, D.I.: An Apparatus for Dislocation of the Acromial End of the Clavicle. Br. Med. J., 1:570, 1924.

119. D'Ambrosia, R.D.: Musculoskeletal Disorders. Philadelphia, J.B. Lippincott, 1977.

120. Dahl, E.: Follow-Up After Coracoclavicular Ligament Prosthesis for Acromioclavicular Joint Dislocation (abstract). Acta Chir. Scand. [Suppl.] 506:96, 1981.

121. Dahl, E.: [Velour Prosthesis in Fractures and Dislocations in the Clavicular Region.] Chirurg., 53:120–122, 1982.

122. Daniels, S.; Ellis, E., III; and Carlson, D.S.: Histologic Analysis of Costochondral and Sternoclavicular Grafts in the TMJ of the Juvenile Monkey. J. Oral Maxillofac. Surg., 45:675–682, 1987.

123. Dannöhl, C.H.: [Angulation Osteotomy at the Clavicle in Old Dislocations of the Acromioclavicular Joint.] Aktuel Traumatol., 14:282–284, 1984.

124. Darrow, J.C.; Smith, J.A.; and Lockwood, R.C.: A New Conservative Method for Treatment of Type III Acromioclavicular Separations. Orthop. Clin. North Am., 11:727–733, 1980.

125. Dawe, C.J.: Acromioclavicular Joint Injuries. J. Bone Joint Surg., 62B:269, 1980.

126. De Sousa, A., and Veiga, A.: Calcification of the Coraco-Clavicular Ligaments after Acromio-Clavicular Dislocation (abstract). J. Bone Joint Surg., 33B:646, 1951.

127. DePalma, A.F.; Callery, G.; and Bennett, G.A.: Variational Anatomy and Degenerative Lesions of the Shoulder Joint. Instr. Course Lect., VI:255–281, 1949.

128. DePalma, A.F.: Surgery of the Shoulder, 2nd ed. Philadelphia, J.B. Lippincott, 1973.

129. DePalma, A.F.: Surgical Anatomy of the Acromioclavicular and Sternoclavicular Joints. Surg. Clin. North Am., 43:1540–1550, 1963.

130. DePalma, A.F.: The Role of the Disks of the Sternoclavicular and Acromioclavicular Joints. Clin. Orthop., 13:7–12, 1959.

131. Dewar, F.P., and Barrington, T.W.: The Treatment of Chronic Acromio-Clavicular Dislocation. J. Bone Joint Surg., 47B:32–35, 1965.

132. Deyerle, W.M.: Closed Double Rod Fixation of Complete Acromio-Clavicular Separation Using Image Intensifier (abstract). Clin. Orthop., 133:266, 1978.

133. Dias, J.J.; Steingold, R.A.; Richardson, R.A.; Tesfayohannes, B.; and Gregg, P.J.: The Conservative Treatment of Acromioclavicular Dislocation: Review After Five Years. J. Bone Joint Surg., 69B:719–722, 1987.

134. Dillehunt, R.B.: Luxation of the Acromioclavicular Joint. Surg. Clin. North Am., 7:1307–1313, 1927.

135. Dittel, K.K.; Pfaff, G.; and Metzger, H.: [Results After Operative Treatment of Complete Acromioclavicular Separation (Tossy III Injury).] Aktuel Traumatol., 17:16–22, 1987.

136. Dittmer, H.; Jauch, K.W.; and Wening, V.: [Treatment of Acromio-Clavicular Separations With Balser's Hookplate.] Unfallheilkunde, 87:216–222, 1984.

137. Dohn, K.: Luxatio Acromio-Clavicularis Supraspinata. Acta Orthop. Scand., 25:183–189, 1956.

138. Dunlop, J.: Dislocations of the Outer End of the Clavicle. Calif. West. Med., 26:38–40, 1927.

139. Dupus, J.; Badelon, P.; and Dayde, G.: Aspects Radiologiques d'une Osteolyse Essentielle Progressive de la Main Gauche. J. Radiol., 20:383–387, 1936.

140. Eaton, R., and Serletti, J.: Computerized Axial Tomography—A Method of Localizing Steinmann Pin Migration: A Case Report. Orthopedics, 4:1357–1360, 1981.

141. Ehricht, H.G.: Die Osteolyse im lateralen Claviculaende nach Pressluftschaden. Arch. Orthop. Unfallchirurg., 50:576–589, 1959.

142. Eidman, D.K.; Siff, S.J.; and Tullos, H.S.: Acromioclavicular Lesions in Children. Am. J. Sports Med., 9:150–154, 1981.

143. Eikenbary, C.F., and LeCocq, J.F.: The Operative Treatment of Acromioclavicular Dislocations. Surg. Clin. North Am., 13:1305–1314, 1933.

144. Ejeskär, A.: Coracoclavicular Wiring for Acromioclavicular Joint Dislocation: A Ten Year Follow-Up Study. Acta Orthop. Scand., 45:652–661, 1974.

145. Elkin, D.C., and Cooper, F.W., Jr.: Resection of the Clavicle in Vascular Surgery. J. Bone Joint Surg., 28:117–119, 1946.

146. Epps, C.H.: Complications in Orthopaedic Surgery. Philadelphia, J.B. Lippincott, 1978.

147. Eskola, A.; Vainionpää, S.; Korkala, O.; and Rokkanen, P.: Acute Complete Acromioclavicular Dislocation: A Prospective Randomized Trial of Fixation With Smooth or Threaded Kirschner Wires or Cortical Screw. Ann. Chir. Gynaecol., 76:323–326, 1987.

148. Evans, E.T.: Avascular Necrosis—Report of Cases Involving the Distal End of the Clavicle and the Odontoid Process. Minn. Med., 34:970, 1951.

149. Falstie-Jensen, S., and Mikkelsen, P.: Pseudodislocation of the Acromioclavicular Joint. J. Bone Joint Surg., 64B:368–369, 1982.

150. Fama, G., and Bonaga, S.: [Safety Pin Synthesis in the Cure of Acromioclavicular Luxation.] Chir. Organi Mov., 73:227–235, 1988.

151. Ferguson, A.B., Jr., and Bender, J.: The ABC's of Athletic Injuries and Conditioning. Baltimore, Williams & Wilkins, 1964.

152. Ferris, B.D.; Bhamra, M.; and Paton, D.F.: Coracoid Process Transfer for Acromioclavicular Dislocations: A Report of 20 Cases. Clin. Orthop., 242:184–187, 1989.

153. Findlay, R.T.: Fractures of the Scapula and Ribs. Am. J. Surg., 38:489, 1937.

154. Fishkin, V.I., and Vorobyev, A.V.: [Dislocations of the Acromial End of the Clavicle.] Sov. Med., 5:86–89, 1988.

155. Fleming, R.E.; Tomberg, D.N.; and Kiernan, H.A.: An Operative Repair of Acromioclavicular Separation. J. Trauma, 18:709–712, 1978.

156. Fukuda, K.; Craig, E.V.; An, K.N.; Cofield, R.H.; and Chao, E.Y.S.: Biomechanical Study of the Ligamentous System of the Acromioclavicular Joint. J. Bone Joint Surg., 68A:434–439, 1986.

157. Fulton, W.A.: A Treatment for Greenstick Fractures and for Dislocations of the Clavicle. Lancet, 43:383–385, 1923.

158. Gaber, O.; Klima, G.; Lugger, L.J.; and Kostler, G.: Die anatomische Struktur des Ligamentum coracoacromiale als Voraussetzung fur die gestielte bandplastik bei Luxationen de Articulatio acromioclavicularis (abstract). Acta Anat., 120:26, 1984.

159. Gallie, W.E.: Dislocations. N. Engl. J. Med., 213:91–98, 1935.

160. Galpin, R.D.; Hawkins, R.J.; and Grainger, R.W.: A Comparative Analysis of Operative vs. Nonoperative Treatment of Grade III Acromioclavicular Separations. Clin. Orthop., 193:150–155, 1985.

161. Ganz, M.; Gattlen, W.; Laffer, U.; and Regazzoni, P.: [Re-

pair of Acromioclavicular Separation Following Bos-worth's Technique: A Follow-Up Study.] Z. Unfallchir. Versicherungsmed. Berufskr., 79:195–197, 1986.

162. Gardner, E., and Gray, D.J.: Prenatal Development of the Human Shoulder and Acromioclavicular Joints. Am. J. Anat., 92:219–276, 1953.

163. Gartner, W., and Schuier, V.: Die posttraumatische Os-teolyse des Schlusselbeines. Zentralbl. Chir., 80:953, 1955.

164. Gatewood, L.C.: Dislocation of the Outer End of the Clav-icle. Surg. Clin. North Am., 3:1193–1197, 1919.

165. Gerber, C., and Rockwood, C.A., Jr.: Subcoracoid Dislo-cation of the Lateral End of the Clavicle: A Report of Three Cases. J. Bone Joint Surg., 69A:924–927, 1987.

166. Giancola, R.; Torretta, F.; and Burla, S.: [Reviewing of 41 Cases of Third Type Acromioclavicular Luxation, Surgi-cally Treated.] Chir. Ital., 37:345–352, 1985.

167. Giannestras, N.J.: A Method of Immobilization of Acute Acromioclavicular Separation. J. Bone Joint Surg., 26:597–599, 1944.

168. Gibbens, M.E.: An Appliance for the Conservative Treat-ment of Acromioclavicular Dislocation. J. Bone Joint Surg., 28:164–165, 1946.

169. Gillespie, H.S.: Excision of the Outer End of the Clavicle for Dislocation of the Acromioclavicular Joint. Can. J. Surg., 7:18, 1964.

170. Girard, P.M.: Acute Acromioclavicular Dislocation. Bull. U.S. Army Med. Dept., 82:5, 1944.

171. Glick, J.: Acromioclavicular Dislocation in Athletes: Auto-Arthroplasty of the Joint. Orthop. Rev., 1:31–34, 1972.

172. Glick, J.M.; Milburn, L.J.; Haggerty, J.F.; and Nishimoto, D.: Dislocated Acromioclavicular Joint: Follow-Up Study of 35 Unreduced Acromioclavicular Dislocations. Am. J. Sports Med., 5:264–270, 1977.

173. Glorian, B., and Delplace, J.: [Dislocations of the Acro-mioclavicular Joint Treated by Transplant of the Coracoid Process.] Rev. Chir. Orthop., 59:667–679, 1973.

174. Goldberg, D.: Acromioclavicular Joint Injuries: A Modified Conservative Form of Treatment. Am. J. Surg., 71:529–531, 1946.

175. Goldberg, J.A.; Viglione, W.; Cumming, W.J.; Waddell, F.S.; and Ruz, P.A.: Review of Coracoclavicular Ligament Reconstruction Using Dacron Graft Material. Aust. N.Z. J. Surg., 57:441–445, 1987.

176. Goodley, P.H.: The Acromioclavicular Joint and Shoulder Disability: Arthrographic and Anatomic Studies (abstract). Arch. Phys. Med. Rehab., 56:539, 1975.

177. Gorham, L.W., and Stout, A.D.: Massive Osteolysis (Acute Spontaneous Absorption of Bone): Its Relation to Hem-angiomatosis. J. Bone Joint Surg., 37A:985, 1955.

178. Gorham, L.W.; Wright, A.W.; Schultz, H.H.; and Mascon, F.C.: Disappearing Bones: A Rare Form of Massive Os-teolysis. Am. J. Med., 17:674, 1954.

179. Gradoyevitch, B.: Coracoclavicular Joint. J. Bone Joint Surg., 21:918–920, 1939.

180. Grauthoff, V.H., and Klammer, H.L.: [Complications Due to Migration of a Kirschner Wire From the Clavicle.] Fortschr. Rontgenstr., 128:591–594, 1978.

181. Graves, S.E., and Foster, B.K.: Absorbable Suture Lasso in the Treatment of Complete Disruption of the Acro-mioclavicular Joint (abstract). J. Bone Joint Surg., 66B:789–790, 1984.

182. Griffith, P.H., III, and Boyadjis, T.A.: Acute Pyarthrosis of the Acromioclavicular Joint: A Case Report. Ortho-pedics, 7:1727–1728, 1984.

183. Griffiths, C.J., and Glucksman, E.: Posttraumatic Osteolysis of the Clavicle: A Case Report. Arch. Emer. Med., 3:129–132, 1986.

184. Grimes, D.W., and Garner, R.W.: The Degeneration of the Acromioclavicular Joint. Orthop. Rev., 9:41–44, 1980.

185. Grønmark, T.: Surgical Treatment of Acromioclavicular Dislocation. Acta Orthop. Scand., 47:308–310, 1976.

186. Gurd, F.B.: The Treatment of Complete Dislocation of the Outer End of the Clavicle: A Hitherto Undescribed Op-eration. Ann. Surg., 113:1094–1098, 1941.

187. Gyr, U.F.; Leutenegger, A.; and Rüedi, T.: [Results of Bos-worth Procedures for Tossy III Acromioclavicular Luxa-tions.] Z. Unfallchir. Versicherungsmed. Berufskr., 79:171–174, 1986.

188. Haase, H.P.; Sander, E.; and Otto, W.: [Results of Bunnell's Operation for Injuries of Acromioclavicular Joint in Comparison With Those of Conservative Treatment.] Beitr. Orthop. Traumatol., 34:558–564, 1987.

189. Hack, U., and Bibow, K.: [Acromioclavicular Dislocation—Conservative or Surgical Therapy?] Zentralbl. Chir., 113:899–910, 1988.

190. Haggart, G.E.: The Treatment of Acromioclavicular Joint Dislocation. Surg. Clin. North Am., 13:683–688, 1933.

191. Halaby, F.A., and DiSalvo, E.L.: Osteolysis: A Complication of Trauma: Report of 2 Cases. A.J.R., 94:591–594, 1965.

192. Hall, R.H.; Isaac, F.; and Booth, C.R.: Dislocation of the Shoulder With Special Reference to Accompanying Small Fractures. J. Bone Joint Surg., 41A:489–494, 1959.

193. Hamill, R.C.: Acromio-Clavicular Dislocation. Int. Clin., 3:130–132, 1920.

194. Hammond, G.: Complete Acromionectomy in the Treat-ment of Chronic Tendinitis of the Shoulder. J. Bone Joint Surg., 44:494–503, 1962.

195. Harrison, R.B.; Riddervold, H.O.; Willett, E.D.; and Stamp, W.G.: Acromio-Clavicular Separation Masked by Muscle Spasm. Va. Med., 107:377–379, 1980.

196. Hart, V.L.: Treatment of Acute Acromioclavicular Dislo-cation. J. Bone Joint Surg., 23:175–176, 1941.

197. Hasselmann, W.: Die Sogen: Posttraumatische Osteolyse des lat Claviculaendes. Monatsschr. Kinderheilkd., 58:242, 1955.

198. Hastings, D.E., and Horne, J.G.: Anterior Dislocation of the Acromioclavicular Joint. Injury, 10:285–288, 1979.

199. Havranek, P.: Injuries of Distal Clavicular Physis in Chil-dren. J. Pediatr. Orthop., 9:213–215, 1989.

200. Hawkins, R.J.: The Acromioclavicular Joint. Presented at AAOS Summer Institute, Chicago, July 10–11, 1980.

201. Heitmeyer, U.; Hierholzer, G.; Schneppendahl, G.; and Haines, J.: The Operative Treatment of Fresh Ruptures of the Acromioclavicular Joint (Tossy III). Arch. Orthop. Trauma Surg., 104:371–373, 1986.

202. Hellmich, A., and Sievers, U.: [Operative Repair of Ac-romioclavicular Separation Via Transcutaneous Kirschner

Wire Fixation: Results of Follow-Up Examinations in 45 Patients.] Aktuel Traumatol., 18:9–13, 1988.

203. Henry, M.D.: Acromioclavicular Dislocations. Minn. Med., 12:431–433, 1929.
204. Heppenstall, R.B.: Fractures and Dislocation of the Distal Clavicle. Orthop. Clin. North Am., 6:477, 1975.
205. Heppenstall, R.B.: Fracture Treatment and Healing. Philadelphia, W.B. Saunders, 1980.
206. Hierholzer, G., and Caspers, H.D.: [Chronic Dislocation of the Acromioclavicular Joint: Technique and Results of Treatment.] Unfallheilkunde., 170:66–73, 1984.
207. Hill, J.A.: Acromioclavicular Separations Need Conservative Treatment: Same Results Achieved With Surgical Care. Orthopedics Today, 6:25, 1986.
208. Hill, J.A.: Acromioclavicular Dislocations: Conservative Treatment Vindicated (editorial). Lancet, 2:1079, 1986.
209. Ho, W.P.; Chen, J.Y.; and Shih, C.H.: The Surgical Treatment of Complete Acromioclavicular Joint Dislocation. Orthop. Rev., 17:1116–1120, 1988.
210. Hohmann, H.G., and Parhofer, R.: Zur Differentialdiagnose der Erkrankungen des Schlussebeins. Munch. Med. Worchenschr., 102:471, 1960.
211. Holstein, A.; Lewis, G.B.; and Sturtz, H.: Experience in the Treatment of Acromioclavicular Dislocation. J. Bone Joint Surg., 48A:1224, 1966.
212. Holz, U., and Weller, S.: Luxationen im Acromioclavicularen Gelenk. Hefte Unfallheilkd., 160:222–229, 1982.
213. Holz, U.: Acromioclavicular Dislocations. Personal communication, 1984.
214. Horn, J.S.: The Traumatic Anatomy and Treatment of Acute Acromio-Clavicular Dislocation. J. Bone Joint Surg., 36B:194–201, 1954.
215. Horvath, F., and Kerry, L.: Degenerative Deformations of the Acromioclavicular Joint in the Elderly. Arch. Gerontol. Geriatr., 3:259–265, 1984.
216. Howard, N.J.: Acromioclavicular and Sternoclavicular Joint Injuries. Am. J. Surg., 46:284–291, 1939.
217. Hoyt, W.A., Jr.: Etiology of Shoulder Injuries in Athletes. J. Bone Joint Surg., 49A:755–766, 1967.
218. Imatani, R.J.; Hanlon, J.J.; and Cady, G.W.: Acute Complete Acromioclavicular Separation. J. Bone Joint Surg., 57A:328–332, 1975.
219. Indrekvam, K.; Storkson, R.; Langeland, N.; and Hordvick, M.: [Acromioclavicular Joint Dislocation: Surgical or Conservative Treatment?] Tidsskr. Nor. Laegeforen., 106:1303–1305, 1986.
220. Inman, V.T.; McLaughlin, H.D.; Neviaser, J.; and Rowe, C.: Treatment of Complete Acromioclavicular Dislocation. J. Bone Joint Surg., 44A:1008–1011, 1962.
221. Inman, V.T.; Saunders, J.B.; and Abbott, L.C.: Observations on the Function of the Shoulder Joint. J. Bone Joint Surg., 26:1–30, 1944.
222. Inman, V.T., and Saunders, J.B.: Observations on the Function of the Clavicle. Calif. Med., 65:158–166, 1946.
223. Ishizuki, M.; Yamaura, I.; Isobe, Y.; Furuya, K.; Tanabe, I.; and Nagatsuka, Y.: Avulsion Fracture of the Superior Border of the Scapula. J. Bone Joint Surg., 63A:820–822, 1981.

224. Jacobs, B., and Wade, P.A.: Acromioclavicular Joint Injury: An End-Result Study. J. Bone Joint Surg., 48A:475–486, 1966.
225. Jacobs, P.: Post-Traumatic Osteolysis of the Outer End of the Clavicle. J. Bone Joint Surg., 46B:705–707, 1964.
226. Jakobsen, B.W.: [Acromioclavicular Dislocation. Conservative or Surgical Treatment?] Ugeskr. Laeger., 151:235–238, 1989.
227. Janecki, C.J.: Voluntary Subluxation of the Acromioclavicular Joint. Clin. Orthop., 125:29–31, 1977.
228. Jay, G.R., and Monnet, J.C.: The Bosworth Screw in Acute Dislocations of the Acromioclavicular Joint. Presented at Clinical Conference, University of Oklahoma Medical Center, April, 1969.
229. Johnston, T.B.; Davies, D.V.; and Davies, F. (eds.): Gray's Anatomy, 32nd ed. London, Longmans, Green, and Co., 1958.
230. Jones, R.: Injuries of Joints. London, Henry Frowde, Hodder & Stoughton, pp. 56–58, 1917.
231. Kaiser, W.; Ziemer, G.; and Heymann, H.: [Treatment of Acromioclavicular Luxations With the Balser Hookplate and Ligament Suture.] Chururg., 55:721–724, 1984.
232. Kappakas, G.S., and McMaster, J.H.: Repair of Acromioclavicular Separation Using a Dacron Prosthesis Graft. Clin. Orthop., 131:247–251, 1978.
233. Karlsson, J.; Arnarson, H.; and Sigurjonsson, K.: Acromioclavicular Dislocations Treated by Coracoacromial Ligament Transfer. Arch. Orthop. Trauma Surg., 106:8–11, 1986.
234. Katznelson, A.; Nerubay, J.; and Oliver, S.: Dynamic Fixation of the Avulsed Clavicle. J. Trauma, 16:841–844, 1976.
235. Kawabe, N.; Watanabe, R.; and Sato, M.: Treatment of Complete Acromioclavicular Separation by Coracoacromial Ligament Transfer. Clin. Orthop., 185:222–227, 1984.
236. Keats, T.E., and Pope, T.L., Jr.: The Acromioclavicular Joint: Normal Variation and the Diagnosis of Dislocation. Skeletal Radiol., 17:159–162, 1988.
237. Kennedy, J.C., and Cameron, H.: Complete Dislocation of the Acromioclavicular Joint. J. Bone Joint Surg., 36B:202–208, 1954.
238. Kennedy, J.C.: Complete Dislocation of the Acromioclavicular Joint: 14 Years Later. J. Trauma, 8:311–318, 1968.
239. Kery, L., and Wouters, H.W.: Massive Osteolysis. J. Bone Joint Surg., 52B:452, 1970.
240. Kessel, L.: Clinical Disorders of the Shoulder. London, Churchill Livingstone, 1982.
241. Key, J.A., and Conwell, H.E.: The Management of Fractures, Dislocations, and Sprains, 3rd ed. St. Louis, C.V. Mosby, 1942.
242. Kiefer, H.; Claes, L.; Burri, C.; and Holzworth, J.: The Stabilizing Effect of Various Implants on the Torn Acromioclavicular Joint: A Biomechanical Study. Arch. Orthop. Trauma Surg., 106:42–46, 1986.
243. Kleinfeld, F., and Pemsel, W.: [Primary Ligament Replacement With Autologous Corium in the Surgical Treatment of Acromioclavicular Joint Injuries.] Aktuel Traumatol., 10:15–21, 1980.

244. Kolesnikon, I.P., and Dubrovich, G.M.: [Treatment of Dislocation of the Acromial End of the Clavicle.] Orthop. Travmatol. Protez., 12:41–42, 1986.

245. Krawczyk, E.: [Repositoon-Reconstruction in Dislocations of Acromioclavicular Joints.] Chir. Narzadow. Ruchu. Ortop. Pol., 49:335–338, 1984.

246. Krawzak, H.W.; Lindecken, K.D.; Gutgemann, U.; and Schlenkhoff, D.: [Surgical Treatment of Acromioclavicular Separation, Using Balser's Hookplate.] Zentralbl. Chir., 111:1509–1514, 1986.

247. Kurock, W., and Sennerich, T.: Injuries of the Acromioclavicular Joint in Sports (abstract). Int. J. Sports Med., 8:127, 1987.

248. Lagier, R.: [Anatomico-Radiological Study of an Ununited Intracapsular Fracture of the Femoral Neck Dating Back 47 Years: Data Relevant to Osteoarthritis, Bone Infarct, and Paget's Disease of the Bone.] Arch. Orthop. Trauma Surg., 104:155–160, 1985.

249. Laing, P.G.: Transplantation of the Long Head of the Biceps in Complete Acromioclavicular Separations (abstract). J. Bone Joint Surg., 51A:1677–1678, 1969.

250. Lamont, M.K.: Osteolysis of the Outer End of the Clavicle (letter to the editor). N.Z. Med. J., 95:241–242, 1982.

251. Lancaster, S.; Horowitz, M.; and Alonso, J.: Complete Acromioclavicular Separations: A Comparison of Operative Methods. Clin. Orthop., 216:80–88, 1987.

252. Lancourt, J.E.: Acromioclavicular Dislocation With Adjacent Clavicular Fracture (Report of a Case With a Method of Repair). Personal communication, 1985.

253. Landoff, G.A.: Eine Bisher Nicht beschriebene Schadigung am Processus coracoideus. Acta Chir. Scand., 89:401–406, 1943.

254. Larsen, E.; Bjerg-Nielsen, A.; and Christensen, P.: Conservative or Surgical Treatment of Acromioclavicular Dislocation: A Prospective, Controlled, Randomized Study. J. Bone Joint Surg., 68A:552–555, 1986.

255. Larsen, E., and Hede, A.: Treatment of Acute Acromioclavicular Dislocation: Three Different Methods of Treatment Prospectively Studied. Acta Orthop. Belg., 53:480–484, 1987.

256. Larsen, E., and Petersen, V.: Operative Treatment of Chronic Acromioclavicular Dislocation. Injury, 18:55–56, 1987.

257. Lasda, N.A., and Murray, D.G.: Fracture Separation of the Coracoid Process Associated With Acromioclavicular Dislocation: Conservative Treatment—A Case Report and Review of the Literature. Clin. Orthop., 134:222–224, 1978.

258. Lasher, W.W.: Cartilage Injuries: A Clinical Study. Am. J. Surg., 6:493–500, 1929.

259. Lazcano, M.A.; Anzel, S.H.; and Kelly, P.J.: Complete Dislocation and Subluxation of the Acromioclavicular Joint: End Result in Seventy-Three Cases. J. Bone Joint Surg., 43A:379–391, 1961.

260. LeNoir, J.L.: Treatment of Acromioclavicular Separation. Iowa Orthop. J., 4:69–71, 1984.

261. Lei, M.X.; Liu, H.; and Yang, K.H.: [Coracoclavicular Ligamentplasty in the Treatment of Acromioclavicular Dislocation.] Chung Hua Wai Ko Tsa Chih, 25:70–71, 124, 1987.

262. Levine, A.H.; Pais, M.J.; and Schwartz, E.E.: Posttraumatic Osteolysis of the Distal Clavicle With Emphasis on Early Radiologic Changes. A.J.R., 127:781–784, 1976.

263. Liberson, F.: The Role of the Coracoclavicular Ligaments in Affections of the Shoulder Girdle. Am. J. Surg., 44:145–157, 1939.

264. Lindsey, R.W., and Gutowski, W.T.: The Migration of a Broken Pin Following Fixation of the Acromioclavicular Joint: A Case Report and Review of the Literature. Orthopedics, 9:413–416, 1986.

265. Linke, R., and Moschinski, D.: [Combined Method of Operative Treatment of Ruptures of the Acromioclavicular Joint.] Unfallheilkunde, 87:223–225, 1984.

266. Litton, L.O., and Peltier, L.R.: Athletic Injuries. Boston, Little, Brown, 1963.

267. Lom, P.: [Acromioclavicular Disjunction: I. Diagnosis and Classification; II. Surgical Treatment—The Author's Modification.] Rozhl. Chir., 67:253–270, 1988.

268. Lowe, G.P., and Fogarty, M.J.P.: Acute Acromioclavicular Joint Dislocation: Results of Operative Treatment With the Bosworth Screw. Aust. N.Z. J. Surg., 47:664–667, 1977.

269. Lucas, D.B.: Biomechanics of the Shoulder Joint. Arch. Surg., 107:425–432, 1973.

270. Lugger, L.J.; Gaber, O.; and Klima, G.: Structure and Suitability of the Coracoacromial Ligament for the Band Transfer Treating Delayed Acromioclavicular Luxation (abstract). Langenbecks Arch. Chir., 366:718, 1985.

271. MacDonald, P.B.; Alexander, M.J.; Frejuk, J.; and Johnson, G.: Comprehensive Functional Analysis of Shoulders Following Complete Acromioclavicular Separation. Am. J. Sports Med., 16:475–480, 1988.

272. Macey, H.B.: Separation of Acromioclavicular Joint: Report of a Case. Proc. Staff Meet. Mayo Clin., 11:683–684, 1936.

273. Madsen, B.: Osteolysis of the Acromial End of the Clavicle Following Trauma. Br. J. Radiol., 36:822, 1963.

274. Malcapi, C.; Grassi, G.; and Oretti, D.: Posterior Dislocation of the Acromioclavicular Joint: A Rare or an Easily Overlooked Lesion? Ital. J. Orthop. Traumatol., 4:79–83, 1978.

275. Marcove, R.C.; Wolfe, S.W.; Healey, J.H.; Huvos, A.G.; Boskey, A.; and Fleisher, M.: Massive Solitary Tophus Containing Calcium Pyrophosphate Dihydrate Crystals at the Acromioclavicular Joint. Clin. Orthop., 227:305–309, 1988.

276. Mauro, E.: [Fracture of the Clavicle and Acromioclavicular Dislocation: An Unusual Combination of Injuries.] Ital. J. Sports Traumatol., 10:199–203, 1988.

277. Mazet, R.J.: Migration of a Kirschner Wire From the Shoulder Region Into the Lung: Report of Two Cases. J. Bone Joint Surg., 25A:477–483, 1943.

278. McCurrich, H.J.: Calcification of the Bursa of the Coracoclavicular Ligament. Br. J. Surg., 26:329–332, 1938.

279. McLaughlin, H.L., and Cavallaro, W.U.: Primary Anterior Dislocation of the Shoulder. Am. J. Surg., 80:615–621, 1950.

280. McLaughlin, H.L.: On the Frozen Shoulder. Bull. Hosp. Joint Dis. Orthop. Inst., 12:383–393, 1951.
281. McLaughlin, H.L.: Rupture of the Rotator Cuff. J. Bone Joint Surg., 44A:979–983, 1962.
282. McLaughlin, H.L.: Trauma. Philadelphia, W.B. Saunders, 1959.
283. McMurray, T.P.: A Practice of Orthopaedic Surgery. Baltimore, William Wood, 1937.
284. McNealy, R.W.: Dislocations and Fracture–Dislocations Occurring at the Acromioclavicular Articulation. Illinois Med. J., 41:202–205, 1922.
285. McPhee, I.B.: Inferior Dislocation of the Outer End of the Clavicle. J. Trauma, 20:709–710, 1980.
286. McPherson, J.; Black, J.; and Reed, M.H.: Traumatic 'Pseudodislocation' of the Acromioclavicular Joint in Children (abstract). J. Bone Joint Surg., 69B:507, 1987.
287. Meixner, J.: [Dislocations and Juxta-articular Fractures of the Acromioclavicular Joint in Childhood.] Zentralbl. Chir., 108:793–797, 1983.
288. Meyerding, H.W.: The Treatment of Acromioclavicular Dislocations. Surg. Clin. North Am., 17:1199–1205, 1937.
289. Michele, A.A.: New Treatment of Acromioclavicular Dislocation (abstract). Clin. Orthop., 63:245, 1969.
290. Mikhelson, E.R., and Chaika, I.A.: [Surgical Treatment of Dislocations of the Acromial End of the Clavicle.] Ortop. Travmatol. Protez., 6:42–43, 1987.
291. Mikusev, I.E.; Zainulli, R.V.; and Skvortso, A.P.: [Treatment of Dislocations of the Acromial End of the Clavicle.] Vestn. Khir., 139:69–71, 1987.
292. Millbourn, E.: On Injuries to the Acromioclavicular Joint: Treatment and Results. Acta Orthop. Scand., 19:349–382, 1950.
293. Mitchell, A.B.: Dislocation of Outer End of Clavicle. Br. Med. J., 2:1097, 1926.
294. Mlasowski, B.; Brenner, P.; Duben, W.; and Heymann, H.: Repair of Complete Acromioclavicular Dislocation (Tossy Stage III) Using Balser's Hookplate Combined With Ligament Sutures. Injury, 19:227–232, 1988.
295. Moffat, B.M.: Separation of the Acromioclavicular Joint. Surg. Gynecol. Obstet., 41:73–74, 1925.
296. Moneim, M.S., and Balduini, F.C.: Coracoid Fractures as a Complication of Surgical Treatment by Coracoclavicular Tape Fixation. Clin. Orthop., 168:133–135, 1982.
297. Montgomery, S.P., and Loyd, R.D.: Avulsion Fracture of the Coracoid Epiphysis With Acromioclavicular Separation. J. Bone Joint Surg., 59A:963–965, 1977.
298. Moravec, O.; Lexa, C.; Sykora, F.; and Sedivy, J.: [Dynamic Stabilization of Acromioclavicular Luxation.] Acta Chir. Orthop. Traumatol. Cech., 53:225–227, 1986.
299. Mordeja, J.: Die posttraumatische Osteolyse des lateralen Schlusselbeinendes. Arch. Orthop. Unfallchirurg., 49:289, 1957.
300. Morimoto, K.; Mori, E.; and Nakagawa, Y.: Calcification of the Coracoacromial Ligament: A Case Report of the Shoulder Impingement Syndrome. Am. J. Sports Med., 16:80–81, 1988.
301. Morisi, M., and Ferrabosch, P.: Treatment of Acromioclavicular Dislocation With Percutaneous Synthesis of the Axis. Arch. Orthop., 68:1148–1156, 1955.
302. Morrison, G.M.: Cast Treatment of Acromioclavicular Dislocations. J. Bone Joint Surg., 30A:238–239, 1948.
303. Moschinski, D.; Linke, R.; and Druke, V.: [Surgery of Acute Dislocation of the Acromioclavicular Joint Using a Resorbable Implant.] Aktuel Chir., 22:183–186, 1987.
304. Moseley, H.F., and Templeton, J.: Dislocation of Acromio-Clavicular Joint (abstract). J. Bone Joint Surg., 51B:196, 1969.
305. Moseley, H.F.: Athletic Injuries to the Shoulder Region. Am. J. Surg., 98:401–422, 1959.
306. Moseley, H.F.: Shoulder Lesions, 2nd ed. New York, Paul Hoeber, 1953.
307. Moshein, J., and Elconin, K.B.: Repair of Acute Acromioclavicular Dislocation Utilizing the Coracoacromial Ligament (abstract). J. Bone Joint Surg., 51A:812, 1969.
308. Müller, H.W., and Schilling, H.: [Importance of Traction-Wiring Osteosynthesis as Dynamic Stabilization After Acromioclavicular Joint Dislocation: A Critical View.] Aktuel Traumatol., 16:94–96, 1986.
309. Mumford, E.B.: Acromioclavicular Dislocation. J. Bone Joint Surg., 23:799–802, 1941.
310. Murphy, O.B.; Bellamy, R.; Wheeler, W.; and Brower, T.D.: Post-Traumatic Osteolysis of the Distal Clavicle. Clin. Orthop., 109:108–114, 1975.
311. Murray, G.: Fixation of Dislocations of the Acromioclavicular Joint and Rupture of the Coracoclavicular Ligament. Can. Med. Assoc. J., 43:270–273, 1940.
312. Murray, G.: The Use of Longitudinal Wires in the Treatment of Fractures and Dislocations. Am. J. Surg., 67:156–167, 1945.
313. Naumann, T.H.: [The Rare Case of Habitual Lateral Dislocation of the Clavicle in Dorsal Subacromial Direction: A Case Report.] Z. Orthop., 124:34–35, 1986.
314. Nell, W.: Die posttraumatische Osteolyse des Schlusselbeins und ihr Verlauf. Monatsschr. Kinderheilkd., 44:151, 1953.
315. Nelson, C.L.: Repair of Acromio-Clavicular Separations With Knitted Dacron Graft. Clin. Orthop., 143:289, 1979.
316. Neviaser, J.S.: Acromioclavicular Dislocation Treated by Transference of the Coracoacromial Ligament. Bull. Hosp. Joint Dis. Orthop. Int., 12:46–54, 1951.
317. Neviaser, J.S.: Acromioclavicular Dislocation Treated by Transference of the Coracoacromial Ligament. Arch. Surg., 64:292–297, 1952.
318. Neviaser, J.S.: Acromioclavicular Dislocation Treated by Transference of the Coraco-Acromial Ligament: A Long-Term Follow-Up in a Series of 112 Cases. Clin. Orthop., 58:57–68, 1968.
319. Neviaser, J.S.: Complicated Fractures and Dislocations About the Shoulder Joint. J. Bone Joint Surg., 44A:984–998, 1962.
320. Neviaser, J.S.: Injuries of the Clavicle and Its Articulations. Orthop. Clin. North Am., 11:233–237, 1980.
321. Neviaser, R.J.: Injuries to the Clavicle and Acromioclavicular Joint. Orthop. Clin. North Am., 18:433–438, 1987.
322. Nguyen, V.: Personal communication, 1989.
323. Nickel, V.L.: Orthopedic Rehabilitation. London, Churchill Livingstone, 1982.

324. Nicoll, E.E.: Annotation: Miners and Mannequins (editorial). J. Bone Joint Surg., 36B:171–172, 1954.

325. Nielsen, W.B.: Injury to the Acromioclavicular Joint (abstract). J. Bone Joint Surg., 45B:207, 1963.

326. Nieminen, S., and Aho, A.J.: Anterior Dislocation of the Acromioclavicular Joint. Ann. Chir. Gynaecol., 73:21–24, 1984.

327. Nixon, J.R., and Corry, I.S.: Inferomedial Fracture Dislocation of the Acromioclavicular Joint. Injury, 19:211–213, 1988.

328. Norfray, J.F.; Tremaine, M.J.; Groves, H.C.; and Bachman, D.C.: The Clavicle in Hockey. Am. J. Sports Med., 5:275–280, 1977.

329. Norfray, J.F.: Bone Resorption of the Distal Clavicle. J.A.M.A., 241:1922–1934, 1979.

330. Norrell, H., and Llewellyn, R.C.: Migration of a Threaded Steinmann Pin From an Acromioclavicular Joint into the Spinal Canal: A Case Report. J. Bone Joint Surg., 47A:1024–1026, 1965.

331. Nutter, P.D.: Coracoclavicular Articulations. J. Bone Joint Surg., 23:177–179, 1941.

332. Nygaard, Ø.P., and Reikerås, O.: [Acromionectomy in Chronic Shoulder Pain.] Tidsskr. Nor. Laegeforen., 107:560–561, 1987.

333. Nyhuus, P., and Knudsen, L.: [Late Results of Resection of the Lateral End of the Clavicle.] Ugeskr. Laeger., 150:1351–1352, 1988.

334. O'Carroll, P.F., and Sheehan, J.M.: Open Reduction and Percutaneous Kirschner Wire Fixation in Complete Disruption of the Acromioclavicular Joint. Injury, 13:299–301, 1982.

335. O'Donoghue, D.H.: Treatment of Injuries to Athletes. Philadelphia, W.B. Saunders, 1970.

336. Odelberg, A.: Operative Method for Dislocation of the Acromioclavicular Joint. Acta Chir. Scand., 98:507–510, 1949.

337. Oh, W.H., and Garvin, W.: Subluxation of the Distal Clavicle. Orthop. Clin. North Am., 11:813–818, 1980.

338. Olsson, D.: Degenerative Changes of the Shoulder Joint and Their Connection With Shoulder Pain. Acta Chir. Scand. [Suppl.] 181:1–130, 1953.

339. Oppenheimer, A.: Arthritis of the Acromioclavicular Joint. J. Bone Joint Surg., 25:867–870, 1943.

340. Orava, S.; Virtanen, K.; and Holopainen, Y.V.O.: Post-traumatic Osteolysis of the Distal Ends of the Clavicle: Report of 3 Cases. Ann. Chir. Gynaecol., 73:83–86, 1984.

341. Orofinio, C.S., and Stein, A.H., Jr.: Operative Treatment for Recent and Complete Tears of the Acromioclavicular Ligaments. Am. J. Surg., 85:760–763, 1953.

342. Paavolainen, P.; Björkenheim, J.M.; Paukku, P.; and Slätis, P.: Surgical Treatment of Acromioclavicular Dislocation: A Review of 39 Patients. Injury, 14:415–420, 1983.

343. Park, J.P.; Arnold, J.A.; Coker, T.P.; Harris, W.D.; and Becker, D.A.: Treatment of Acromioclavicular Separations: A Retrospective Study. Am. J. Sports Med., 8:251–256, 1980.

344. Paton, D.F.: Complete Acromioclavicular Dislocation Treated by Transfer of the Origin of Coracobrachialis and Short Head of Biceps to the Clavicle (abstract). J. Bone Joint Surg., 62B:117, 1980.

345. Pattee, G.A., and Snyder, S.J.: Synovial Chondromatosis of the Acromioclavicular Joint: A Case Report. Clin. Orthop., 233:205–207, 1988.

346. Patterson, W.R.: Inferior Dislocation of the Distal End of the Clavicle. J. Bone Joint Surg., 49A:1184–1186, 1967.

347. Pearson, G.R.: Radiographic Technic for Acromioclavicular Dislocation. Radiology, 27:239, 1936.

348. Petersson, C.J., and Gentz, C.F.: The Significance of Distally Pointing Acromioclavicular Osteophytes in Ruptures of the Supraspinatus Tendon (abstract). Acta Orthop. Scand., 54:490–491, 1983.

349. Petersson, C.J., and Redlund-Johnell, I.: Radiographic Joint Space in Normal Acromioclavicular Joints. Acta Orthop. Scand., 54:431–433, 1983.

350. Petersson, C.J.: Degeneration of the Acromioclavicular Joint: A Morphological Study. Acta Orthop. Scand., 54:434–438, 1983.

351. Petersson, C.J.: Resection of the Lateral End of the Clavicle: A 3 to 30-Year Follow-Up. Acta Orthop. Scand., 54:904–907, 1983.

352. Petersson, C.J.: The Acromioclavicular Joint in Rheumatoid Arthritis. Clin. Orthop., 223:86–93, 1987.

353. Phemister, D.B.: The Treatment of Dislocation of the Acromioclavicular Joint by Open Reduction and Threaded-Wire Fixation. J. Bone Joint Surg., 24:166–168, 1942.

354. Pilcher, M.: Dislocation of the Acromial End of the Clavicle (abstract). N.Y. State J. Med., 43:419–420, 1886.

355. Pillay, V.K.: Significance of the Coracoclavicular Joint (abstract). J. Bone Joint Surg., 49B:390, 1967.

356. Piterman, L.: Sports Medicine Quiz: "The Dropped Shoulder." Aust. Fam. Physician, 11:469, 1982.

357. Podgorski, M.R.; Ibels, L.S.; and Webb, J.: Case Report 445: Diagnosis—Bilateral Acromioclavicular Gouty Arthritis With Pseudo-Tumor of the Outer End of the Right Clavicle: Saturnine Gout. Skeletal Radiol., 16:589–591, 1987.

358. Poigenfürst, J.: The Infraclavicular Soft Tissue Ossification Following the Tearing of the Shoulder Joint. Personal communication re article in Acta Med. Austriaca, 11:A16, 1984.

359. Poirier, P., and Rieffel, H.: Mechanisme des Luxations sur Acromiales de la Clavicule. Arch. Gen. Med., 1:396–422, 1891.

360. Poletanski, V.Z.: [A Device for Reducing the Dislocation and Fixation of the Acromial End of the Clavicle.] Ortop. Travmatol. Protez., 152:60–61, 1988.

361. Post, M.: Current Concepts in the Diagnosis and Management of Acromioclavicular Dislocations. Clin. Orthop., 200:234–247, 1985.

362. Post, M.: The Shoulder. Philadelphia, Lea & Febiger, 1978.

363. Potter, F.A.; Fiorini, A.J.; Knox, J.; and Rajesh, P.B.: The Migration of a Kirschner Wire From Shoulder to Spleen: Brief Report. J. Bone Joint Surg., 70B:326–327, 1988.

364. Powers, J.A., and Bach, P.J.: Acromioclavicular Separations—Closed or Open Treatment. Clin. Orthop., 104:213–223, 1974.

365. Pridie, K.: Dislocation of Acromio-Clavicular and Sterno-

Clavicular Joints (abstract). J. Bone Joint Surg., 41B:429, 1959.

366. Pritchett, J.W.: Ossification of the Coracoclavicular Ligaments in Ankylosing Spondylitis: A Case Report. J. Bone Joint Surg., 65A:1017–1018, 1983.

367. Protass, J.J.; Stampfli, F.V.; and Osmer, J.C.: Coracoid Process Fracture Diagnosis in Acromioclavicular Separation. Radiology, 116:61, 1975.

368. Pulles, H.J.W.: Operative Treatment of Acromio-Clavicular Dislocation (abstract). Acta Orthop. Scand., 55:483, 1984.

369. Quesada, F.: Technique for the Roentgen Diagnosis of Fractures of the Clavicle. Surg. Gynecol. Obstet., 42:424–428, 1926.

370. Quigley, T.B., and Banks, H.: Progress in the Treatment of Fractures and Dislocations. Philadelphia, W.B. Saunders, 1960.

371. Quigley, T.B.: Correspondence. N. Engl. J. Med., 241:431, 1949.

372. Quigley, T.B.: Injuries to the Acromioclavicular and Sternoclavicular Joints Sustained in Athletics. Surg. Clin. North Am., 43:1551–1554, 1963.

373. Rauschning, W.; Nordesjö, L.O.; Nordgren, B.; Sahlstedt, B.; and Wigren, A.: Resection Arthroplasty for Repair of Complete Acromioclavicular Separations. Arch. Orthop. Traumatol. Surg., 97:161–164, 1980.

374. Rawlings, G.: Acromioclavicular Dislocations and Fractures of the Clavicle: A Simple Method of Support. Lancet, 2:789, 1939.

375. Retief, P.J., and Meintjes, F.A.: Migration of a Kirschner Wire in the Body—A Case Report. S. Afr. Med. J., 53:557–558, 1978.

376. Richards, R.R.; Herzenberg, J.E.; and Goldner, J.L.: Bilateral Nontraumatic Anterior Acromioclavicular Joint Dislocation: A Case Report. Clin. Orthop., 209:255–258, 1986.

377. Richardson, W.F.: "Acromion" in Ancient Greek Medical Writers. Med. History, 20:52–58, 1976.

378. Richter, R.; Hahn, H.; Nubling, W.; and Kohler, G.: [Tuberculosis of the Shoulder Girdle.] Z. Rheumatol., 44:87–92, 1985.

379. Riddel, J.: Dislocation of the Acromioclavicular Joint. Br. Med. J., 1:697, 1926.

380. Roberts, S.M.: Acromioclavicular Dislocation: Anatomical Exposure of the Outer End of the Clavicle and the Coracoid Process. Am. J. Surg., 23:322–324, 1934.

381. Rockwood, C.A., Jr.; Guy, D.K.; and Griffin, J.L.: Treatment of Chronic, Complete Acromioclavicular Dislocation (abstract). Orthop. Trans., 12:735, 1988.

382. Rockwood, C.A., Jr.: Acromioclavicular Dislocation. In Rockwood, C.A. and Green, D.P. (eds.): Fractures in Adults, Vol. 1., pp. 721–756. Philadelphia, J.B. Lippincott, 1975.

383. Rockwood, C.A., Jr.: Acromioclavicular Separations. In Kane, W.J. (ed.): Current Orthopedic Management, pp. 290–311. New York, Churchill Livingstone, 1981.

384. Rockwood, C.A., Jr.: Injuries to the Acromioclavicular Joint. In Rockwood, C.A. and Green, D.P. (eds.): Fractures in Adults, Vol. 1., 2nd ed., pp. 860–910. Philadelphia, J.B. Lippincott, 1984.

385. Rodnan, G.P. (ed.): Primer on the Rheumatic Diseases. J.A.M.A., 224:662–749, 1973.

386. Roper, B.A., and Levack, B.: The Surgical Treatment of Acromioclavicular Dislocations. J. Bone Joint Surg., 64B:597–599, 1982.

387. Rosenørn, M., and Pedersen, E.B.: A Comparison Between Conservative and Operative Treatment of Acute Acromioclavicular Dislocation. Acta Orthop. Scand., 45:50–59, 1974.

388. Rosenørn, M., and Pedersen, E.B.: The Significance of the Coracoclavicular Ligament in Experimental Dislocation of the Acromioclavicular Joint. Acta Orthop. Scand., 45:346–358, 1974.

389. Rounds, R.C.: Isolated Fracture of the Coracoid Process. J. Bone Joint Surg., 31A:662, 1949.

390. Rowe, C.R.: Symposium on Surgical Lesions of the Shoulder: Acute and Recurrent Dislocation of the Shoulder. J. Bone Joint Surg., 44A:977–1012, 1962.

391. Rowe, M.J.: Nylon Bone Suture. Surgery, 18:764–768, 1945.

392. Roy, S.P.: The Nature and Frequency of Rugby Injuries: A Pilot Study of 300 Injuries at Stellenbosch. S. Afr. Med. J., 48:2341, 1974.

393. Ruegger, R.; Bleuler, P.; Schwarz, H.; and Fehr, J.L.: [Primary Surgical Treatment of Fresh Acromioclavicular Dislocation (Tossy III): Results of Treatment in 50 Patients.] Helv. Chir. Acta, 54:425–429, 1987.

394. Ryan, A.J.: Medical Care of the Athlete. New York, McGraw-Hill, 1962.

395. Sage, F.P., and Salvatore, J.E.: Injuries of Acromioclavicular Joint: Study of Results in 96 Patients. South. Med. J., 56:486–495, 1963.

396. Sage, J.: Recurrent Inferior Dislocation of the Clavicle at the Acromioclavicular Joint. Am. J. Sports Med., 10:145–146, 1982.

397. Sage, M.R., and Allen, P.W.: Massive Osteolysis. J. Bone Joint Surg., 56B:130, 1974.

398. Salter, E.G.; Nasca, R.J.; and Shelley, B.S.: Anatomical Observations on the Acromioclavicular Joint and Supporting Ligaments. Am. J. Sports Med., 15:199–206, 1987.

399. Salter, E.G.; Shelley, B.S.; and Nasca, R.: A Morphological Study of the Acromioclavicular Joint in Humans (abstract). Anat. Rec., 211:353, 1985.

400. Sandrock, A.R.: Another Sports Fatigue Fracture: Stress Fracture of the Coracoid Process of the Scapula. Radiology, 117:274, 1975.

401. Saranglia, D.; Julliard, R.; Marcone, L.; and Butel, J.: [The Results of the Modified Cadenat Procedure in Old Acromioclavicular Dislocations: 26 Cases.] Rev. Chir. Orthop., 73:187–190, 1987.

402. Schildhaus, A.I.E., and Meyers, W.J.: Stabilization of the Clavicle in Acromioclavicular Separation. Orthop. Rev., 16:85–87, 1987.

403. Schindler, A.; Schmid, J.P.; and Heyse, C.: [Hookplate Fixation for Repair of Acute Complete Acromioclavicular Separation: Review of 41 Patients.] Unfallchirurg., 88:533–540, 1985.

404. Schmid, A., and Schmid, F.: [Use of Arthrosonography in

Diagnosis of Tossy III Lesions of Acromioclavicular Joints.] Aktuel Traumatol., 18:134–138, 1988.

405. Schneider, C.C.: Acromioclavicular Dislocation: Autoplastic Reconstruction. J. Bone Joint Surg., 15:957–962, 1933.

406. Schneppendahl, G., and Ludolph, E.: [Posttraumatic Chronic Instability of the Shoulder Joint.] Unfallchirurgie, 13:19–21, 1987.

407. Schwarz, B., and Heisel, J.: [Causes, Treatment and Results of Surgery of Fresh and Old Breaks of the Acromioclavicular Joint.] Aktuel Traumatol., 16:97–109, 1986.

408. Schwarz, B., and Heisel, J.: [Late Results of Inverterate Cleavages of the Acromioclavicular Joint.] Orthopödische Praxis., pp. 159–168, March, 1986.

409. Schwarz, N., and Kuderna, H.: Inferior Acromioclavicular Separation: Report of an Unusual Case. Clin. Orthop., 234:28–30, 1988.

410. Schwarz, N., and Leixnering, M.: [Results of Nonreduced Acromioclavicular Tossy III Separations.] Unfallchirurg., 89:248–252, 1986.

411. Scott, J.C., and Orr, M.M.: Injuries to the Acromioclavicular Joint. Injury, 5:13–18, 1973.

412. Seddon, H.J.: Nerve Lesions Complicating Certain Closed Bone Injuries. J.A.M.A., 135:691–694, 1947.

413. Sellers, R.; Tibone, J.; Tonino, P.M.; and Moynes, D.: Strength Testing of Third Degree Acromioclavicular Dislocations. Personal communication, 1988.

414. Sethi, G.K., and Scott, S.M.: Subclavian Artery Laceration Due to Migration of a Hagie Pin. Surgery, 80:644–646, 1976.

415. Seymour, E.Q.: Osteolysis of the Clavicular Top Associated With Repeated Minor Trauma to the Shoulder. Radiology, 123:56, 1977.

416. Shaar, C.M.: Upward Dislocation of Acromial End of Clavicle: Treatment by Elastic Traction Splint. J.A.M.A., 92:2083–2085, 1929.

417. Shands, A.R., Jr.: An Analysis of the More Important Orthopaedic Information. Surgery, 16:569–616, 1944.

418. Shands, A.R., Jr.: Handbook of Orthopaedic Surgery, 2nd ed. St. Louis, C.V. Mosby, 1940.

419. Shoji, H.; Roth, C.; and Chuinard, R.: Bone Block Transfer of Coracoacromial Ligament in Acromioclavicular Injury. Clin. Orthop., 208:272–277, 1986.

420. Sholkoff, S.D., and Cook, J.: Arthrography for Acromioclavicular Joint Cysts (letter to the editor). A.J.R., 151:838, 1988.

421. Siegling, C.W., and Jahn, K.: [Dislocation of the Acromio-Clavicular Joint: Results of Surgical Treatment.] Zentralbl. Chir., 107:858–862, 1982.

422. Silloway, K.A.; McLaughlin, R.E.; Edlich, R.C.; and Edlich, R.F.: Clavicular Fractures and Acromioclavicular Joint Dislocations in Lacrosse: Preventable Injuries. J. Emerg. Med., 3:117–121, 1985.

423. Simeone, L.: Le Lussazioni Acromio-Claveari: Il Cerchiaggio Dinamico. Minerva Ortopedica, 36:805–812, 1985.

424. Simmons, E.H., and Martin, R.F.: Acute Dislocation of the Acromioclavicular Joint. Can. J. Surg., 11:473–479, 1968.

425. Simmons, E.H., and Roscoe, M.W.A.: The Treatment of Complete Acromio-Clavicular Dislocation (abstract). J. Trauma, 23:664, 1983.

426. Skjeldal, S.; Lundblad, R.; and Dullerud, R.: Coracoid Process Transfer for Acromioclavicular Dislocation. Acta Orthop. Scand., 59:180–182, 1988.

427. Sleeswijk-Visser, S.V.; Haarsma, S.M.; and Speeckaert, M.T.C.: Conservative Treatment of Acromioclavicular Dislocation: Jones Strap vs. Mitella (abstract). Acta Orthop. Scand., 55:483, 1984.

428. Smart, M.J.: Traumatic Osteolysis of the Distal Ends of the Clavicles. J. Can. Assoc. Radiol., 23:264–266, 1972.

429. Smith, D.W.: Coracoid Fracture Associated With Acromioclavicular Dislocation. Clin. Orthop., 108:165, 1975.

430. Smith, M.J., and Stewart, M.J.: Acute Acromioclavicular Separations. Am. J. Sports Med., 7:62–71, 1979.

431. Snyder, S.J.: Arthroscopic Acromioclavicular Joint Debridement and Distal Clavicle Resection. Techniques Orthop., 3:41–45, 1988.

432. Søndergard-Petersen, P., and Mikkelsen, P.: Posterior Acromioclavicular Dislocation. J. Bone Joint Surg., 64B:52–53, 1982.

433. Sonnabend, D.H., and Faithfull, D.K.: Operative Repair of Acromioclavicular Dislocation (abstract). J. Bone Joint Surg., 66B:789, 1984.

434. Soule, A.B., Jr.: Ossification of the Coracoclavicular Ligament Following Dislocation of the Acromioclavicular Articulation. A.J.R., 56:607–615, 1946.

435. Southmayd, W.W.; Scheller, A.D.; Tesner, R.J.; and Messinger, B.: Surgical Treatment of Grade III Acromioclavicular Separations. Sportsmed. Clinics, 2(3):1–8, 1985.

436. Speed, K.: A Textbook of Fractures and Dislocations, 4th ed. Philadelphia, Lea & Febiger, 1942.

437. Spigelman, L.: A Harness for Acromioclavicular Separation. J. Bone Joint Surg., 51A:585–586, 1969.

438. Stahl, F.: Considerations on Post-Traumatic Absorption of the Outer End of the Clavicle. Acta Orthop. Scand., 23:9, 1954.

439. Stappaerts, K.H.; Broos, P.L.O.; and Debeer, P.: Surgical Treatment of Complete Acromioclavicular Separations: A Review of 40 Patients. Unfallchirurg., 91:161–164, 1988.

440. Stenlund, B.; Marions, O.; Engstrom, K.F.; and Goldie, I.: Correlation of Macroscopic Osteoarthrotic Changes and Radiographic Findings in the Acromioclavicular Joint. Acta Radiol., 29:571–576, 1988.

441. Stephens, H.E.G.: Stuck Nail Fixation for Acute Dislocation of the Acromio-Clavicular Joint (abstract). J. Bone Joint Surg., 51B:197, 1969.

442. Stewart, C.A.; Siegel, M.E.; King, D.; and Moser, L.: Radionuclide and Radiographic Demonstration of Condensing Osteitis of the Clavicle. Clin. Nucl. Med., 13:177–178, 1988.

443. Stewart, R.: Acute Acromioclavicular Joint Dislocation: Internal Fixation of the Clavicle and Coracoid Process of the Scapula With a Vitallium Screw. Minn. Med., 29:357–360, 1946.

444. Stimson, L.A.: Fractures and Dislocations. Philadelphia, Lea & Febiger, 1941.

445. Strauch, W.: Posttraumatische Osteolysen des lateralen Klavikulaendes. Radiol. Diagn., 11:221–229, 1970.

446. Stubbins, S.G., and McGaw, W.H.: Suspension Cast for Acromioclavicular Separations and Clavicle Fractures. J.A.M.A., 169:672–675, 1959.

447. Taft, T.N.; Wilson, F.C.; and Oglesby, J.W.: Dislocation of the Acromioclavicular Joint: An End-Result Study. J. Bone Joint Surg., 69A:1045–1051, 1987.

448. Taga, I.; Yoneda, M.; and Ono, K.: Epiphyseal Separation of the Coracoid Process Associated With Acromioclavicular Sprain: A Case Report and Review of the Literature. Clin. Orthop., 207:138–141, 1986.

449. Tagliabue, D., and Riva, A.: [Current Approaches to the Treatment of Acromioclavicular Joint Separation in Athletes.] Ital. J. Sports Traumatol., 3:15–24, 1981.

450. Tagliabue, D., and Riva, A.: La Cleidopessi Coraco-Claveare Nella Lussazione Acromion-Claveare. Minerva Ortop., 36: 817–823, 1985.

451. Taylor, G.M., and Tooke, M.: Degeneration of the Acromioclavicular Joint as a Cause of Shoulder Pain. J. Bone Joint Surg., 59B:507, 1977.

452. Thiemeyer, J.S., Jr.: Method of Repair of Symptomatic Chronic Acromioclavicular Dislocation. Ann. Surg., 140: 75–85, 1954.

453. Thorndike, A., Jr., and Quigley, T.B.: Injuries to the Acromioclavicular Joint: A Plea for Conservative Treatment. Am. J. Surg., 55:250–261, 1942.

454. Thorndike, A., Jr.: Athletic Injuries. Philadelphia, Lea & Febiger, 1956.

455. Tossy, J.D.; Mead, N.C.; and Sigmond, H.M.: Acromioclavicular Separations: Useful and Practical Classification for Treatment. Clin. Orthop., 28:111–119, 1963.

456. Toumey, J.W.: Surgery of the Acromioclavicular Joint. Surg. Clin. North Am., 29:905–912, 1949.

457. Trynin, A.H.: Conservative Treatment for Complete Dislocation of the Acromioclavicular Joint. J. Bone Joint Surg., 16:713–715, 1934.

458. Tsou, P.M.: Percutaneous Cannulated Screw Coracoclavicular Fixation for Acute Acromioclavicular Dislocations. Clin. Orthop., 243:112–121, 1989.

459. Tucker, W.E., and Armstrong, J.R.: Injury in Sport. Springfield, Ill., Charles C. Thomas, 1964.

460. Twigg, H.L., and Rosenbaum, R.C.: Duplication of the Clavicle. Skeletal Radiol., 6:281, 1981.

461. Tyler, G.T.: Acromioclavicular Dislocation Fixed by a Vitallium Screw Through the Joint. Am. J. Surg., 58:245–247, 1942.

462. Tyurina, T.V.: [Age-Related Characteristics of the Human Acromioclavicular Joint.] Arkh. Anat. Gistol. Embriol., 89:75–81, 1985.

463. Urban, J., and Jaskiewicz, A.: [Idiopathic Displacement of Kirschner Wire to the Thoracic Cavity After the Osteosynthesis of Acromioclavicular Joint.] Chir. Narzadow. Ruchu. Ortop. Pol., 49:399–402, 1984.

464. Urist, M.R.: Complete Dislocation of the Acromioclavicular Joint: The Nature of the Traumatic Lesion and Effective

465. Methods of Treatment With an Analysis of 41 Cases. J. Bone Joint Surg., 28:813–837, 1946.

465. Urist, M.R.: Complete Dislocation of the Acromioclavicular Joint (Follow-Up Notes). J. Bone Joint Surg., 45A:1750–1753, 1963.

466. Urist, M.R.: The Treatment of Dislocation of the Acromioclavicular Joint: A Survey of the Past Decade. Am. J. Surg., 98:423–431, 1959.

467. Usadel, G.: Zur Behandlung der Luxatio claviculae supraacromialis. Arch. Klin. Chir., 200:621–626, 1940.

468. Vainionpää, S.; Kirves, P.; and Laike, E.: Acromioclavicular Joint Dislocation—Surgical Results in 36 Patients. Ann. Chir. Gynaecol., 70:120–123, 1981.

469. Vandekerckhove, B.; Van Meirhaeghe, J.; Van Steenkiste, M.; De Groote, W.; Verbeke, R.; and Vertongen, P.: Surgical Treatment of Acromioclavicular Dislocations: Long-Term Follow-Up Study. Acta Orthop. Belg., 51:66–79, 1985.

470. van der Werf, G.G.I.M., and Tonino, A.J.: Dacron as Ligament Graft in the Treatment of Acromioclavicular Dislocation (abstract). Acta Orthop. Scand., 55:484, 1984.

471. Vargas, L.: Repair of Complete Acromioclavicular Dislocation, Utilizing the Short Head of the Biceps. J. Bone Joint Surg., 24:772–773, 1942.

472. Varney, J.H.; Coker, J.K.; and Cawley, J.J.: Treatment of Acromioclavicular Dislocation by Means of a Harness. J. Bone Joint Surg., 34A:232–233, 1952.

473. Viehweger, G.: Die posttraumatische Claviculaosteolyse. Chirurg., 30:313, 1959.

474. Vogel, H.; Thomä, J.; and Jungbluth, K.H.: [Plain Film Diagnostic of the Acromioclavicular Dislocation.] Rontgenblatter., 33:564–570, 1980.

475. Wagner, C.: Partial Claviculectomy. Am. J. Surg., 85:259–265, 1953.

476. Wakeley, C.P.G.: Stabilization of the Acromioclavicular Joint. Lancet, 2:708–710, 1935.

477. Waldrop, J.I.; Norwood, L.A.; and Alvarez, R.G.: Lateral Roentgenographic Projections of the Acromioclavicular Joint. Am. J. Sports Med., 9:337–341, 1981.

478. Walsh, W.M.; Peterson, D.A.; Shelton, G.; and Newmann, R.D.: Shoulder Strength Following Acromioclavicular Injury. Am. J. Sports Med., 13:153–158, 1985.

479. Warner, A.H.: A Harness for Use in the Treatment of Acromioclavicular Separation. J. Bone Joint Surg., 19:1132–1133, 1937.

480. Warren-Smith, C.D., and Ward, M.W.: Operation for Acromioclavicular Dislocation: A Review of 29 Cases Treated by One Method. J. Bone Joint Surg., 69B:715–718, 1987.

481. Wasylenko, M.J., and Busse, E.F.: Posterior Dislocation of the Clavicle Causing Fatal Tracheoesophagial Fistula. Can. Med. J., 24:626–627, 1981.

482. Watkins, J.T.: An Operation for the Relief of Acromio-Clavicular Luxations. J. Bone Joint Surg., 7:790–792, 1925.

483. Watson-Jones, R.: Fractures and Joint Injuries, 4th ed, Vol II. Baltimore, Williams & Wilkins, 1956.

484. Watson-Jones, R.: Fractures and Joint Injuries. London, Churchill Livingstone, 1982.

485. Waxman, J.: Acromioclavicular Disease in Rheumatologic Practice—The Forgotten Joint. J. La. State Med. Soc., 129:1–3, 1977.

486. Weaver, J.K., and Dunn, H.K.: Treatment of Acromioclavicular Injuries, Especially Complete Acromioclavicular Separation. J. Bone Joint Surg., 54A:1187–1197, 1972.

487. Weitzman, G.: Treatment of Acute Acromioclavicular Joint Dislocation by a Modified Bosworth Method: Report on Twenty-Four Cases. J. Bone Joint Surg., 49A:1167–1178, 1967.

488. Wenner, S.M.: Dislocation of the Acromioclavicular Joint: A Review of the Literature and a Pathologic Series of Thirteen Joint Dissections. Orthop. Rev., 3:35–42, 1974.

489. Werder, H.: Posttraumatische Osteolyse des Schlusselbeinendes. Schweiz. Med. Wochenschr., 80:912, 1950.

490. Wertheimer, L.G.: Coracoclavicular Joint: Surgical Treatment of a Painful Syndrome Caused by an Anomalous Joint. J. Bone Joint Surg., 30A:570–578, 1948.

491. Weston. W.J.: Arthrography of the Acromio-Clavicular Joint. Aust. Radiol., 18:213–214, 1974.

492. Weston, W.J.: Erosions of the Acromion Process of the Scapula in Rheumatoid Arthritis. Aust. Radiol., 17:219–220, 1973.

493. Wilber, M.C., and Evans, E.B.: Fractures of the Scapula. J. Bone Joint Surg., 59A:358, 1977.

494. Williams, G.R.; Nguyen, V.D.; and Rockwood, C.A., Jr.: Classification and Radiographic Analysis of Acromioclavicular Dislocations. Appl. Radiol., pp. 29–34, Feb. 1989.

495. Wilson, K.M., and Colwill, J.C.: Combined Acromioclavicular Dislocation With Coracoclavicular Ligament Disruption and Coracoid Process Fracture. Am. J. Sports Med., 17:697–327, 1989.

496. Wilson, P.D., and Cochrane, W.A. (eds.): Fractures and Dislocations: Immediate Management, After Care, and Convalescent Treatment, With Special Reference to the Conservation and Restoration of Function. Philadelphia, J.B. Lippincott, 1925.

497. Wolff, E.F.: Transposition of the Biceps Brachii Tendon to Repair Luxation of the Canine Shoulder Joint: Review of a Procedure. Vet. Med. Small Animal Clin., 69:51–53, 1974.

498. Wolin, I.: Acute Acromioclavicular Dislocation: A Simple Effective Method of Conservative Treatment. J. Bone Joint Surg., 26:589–592, 1944.

499. Worchester, J.N., and Green, D.P.: Osteoarthritis of the Acromioclavicular Joint. Clin. Orthop., 58:69–73, 1968.

500. Zanca, P.: Shoulder Pain: Involvement of the Acromioclavicular Joint: Analysis of 1,000 Cases. A.J.R., 112:493–506, 1971.

501. Zaricznyj, B.: Injuries and Treatment of the Acromioclavicular Joint. Orthop. Rev., 10:41–51, 1981.

502. Zaricznyj, B.: Late Reconstruction of the Ligaments Following Acromioclavicular Separation. J. Bone Joint Surg., 58A:792–795, 1976.

503. Zaricznyj, B.: Reconstruction for Chronic Scapuloclavicular Instability. Am. J. Sports Med., 11:17–25, 1983.

504. Zettas, J.P., and Muchnic, P.D.: Fractures of the Coracoid Process Base in Acute Acromioclavicular Separation. Orthop. Rev., 5:77, 1976.

505. Zimmerman, L.M., and Veith, I.: Great Ideas in the History of Surgery. Baltimore, Williams & Wilkins, 1961.

506. Zlotsky, N.A.: Treatment of Acromioclavicular Separations in Athletes. Conn. Med., 40:15–17, 1976.

507. Zsernaviczky, J., and Horst, M.: [Contribution to the Osteolysis in Distal End of the Clavicle.] Arch. Orthop. Unfallchirurg., 89:163–167, 1977.

15

Injuries to the Sternoclavicular Joint
Charles A. Rockwood, Jr.

HISTORICAL REVIEW

A review of the early literature on injuries to the sternoclavicular joint indicates that in the 19th century dislocations of the sternoclavicular joint were managed essentially the same way as fractures of the medial clavicle.[56,132] Sir Astley Cooper,[56] in his 1824 text, recommended that these injuries be treated not only with a clavicle bandage but also with a sling "which through the medium of the os humeri and scapula supports it and prevents the clavicle from being drawn down by the weight of the arm."

Cooper reported that he had never seen an isolated traumatic posterior dislocation of the sternoclavicular joint, but suggested this might occur with excessive force.[56] However, he did describe a posterior dislocation of the sternoclavicular joint in a patient who had such severe scoliosis that as the scapula advanced laterally around the chest wall, it pushed the medial end of the clavicle behind the sternum. The patient finally developed so much pressure on the esophagus and had such difficulty swallowing that Davie, a surgeon in Suffolk, resected the medial end of the clavicle. He must have been an excellent surgeon, for in 1824 he resected one inch of the medial clavicle using a saw! He protected the vital structures in the area from the saw by introducing "a piece of well beaten sole leather under the bone whilst he divided it." The patient recovered and had no more problems with swallowing. This case probably represents the first resection of the medial end of the clavicle, either for trauma or for arthritis.

Rodrigues,[227] in 1843, may have published the first case of traumatic posterior dislocation of the sternoclavicular joint in the literature, "a case of dislocation inward of the internal extremity of the clavicle." The patient's left shoulder was against a wall when the right side of the chest and thorax were compressed and rolled forward almost to the midline by a cart. Immediately, the patient experienced shortness of breath, which persisted for 3 weeks. When first seen by the physician, he appeared to be suffocating and his face was blue. The left shoulder was swollen and painful, and there was "a depression on the left side of the superior extremity of the sternum." Pressure on the depression greatly increased the sensation of suffocation. Rodrigues observed that when the outer end of the shoulder was displaced backward, the inner end of the clavicle was displaced forward, which relieved the asphyxia. Therefore, treatment consisted of binding the left shoulder backward with a cushion between the two scapulas, but only after the patient had been bled twice within the first 24 hours. Rodrigues may have seen other cases of posterior dislocation, since he stated that the patient "retained a slight depression of the internal extremity of the clavicle; such, however, is the ordinary fate of the patients who present this form of dislocation."

In the late 19th century, a number of articles appeared from England, Germany, and France; it was not until the 1930s that articles by Duggan,[70]

Howard and Shafer,[125] and Lowman[163] appeared in the American literature.

SURGICAL ANATOMY

The sternoclavicular joint is a diarthrodial joint and is the only true articulation between the clavicle of the upper extremity and the axial skeleton (Fig. 15–1). The articular surface of the clavicle is much larger than that of the sternum, and both are covered with fibrocartilage. The enlarged bulbous medial end of the clavicle is concave front to back and convex vertically, and therefore creates a saddle-type joint with the clavicular notch of the sternum.[102,103] The clavicular notch of the sternum is curved, and the joint surfaces are not congruent. Cave[46] has demonstrated that in 2.5% of patients there is a small facet on the inferior aspect of the medial clavicle which articulates with the superior aspect of the first rib at its synchondral junction with the sternum.

Because less than half of the medial clavicle articulates with the upper angle of the sternum, the sternoclavicular joint has the distinction of having the least amount of bony stability of the major joints of the body. Grant[102] noted, "The two (make) an ill fit." If a finger is placed in the superior sternal notch, with motion of the upper extremity one can feel that a large part of the medial clavicle is completely above the articulation with the sternum.

LIGAMENTS OF THE STERNOCLAVICULAR JOINT

There is so much joint incongruity that the integrity has to come from its surrounding ligaments—the intra-articular disk ligament, the extra-articular costoclavicular ligament (rhomboid ligament), the capsular ligament, and the interclavicular ligament.

Intra-Articular Disk Ligament

The intra-articular disk ligament is a very dense, fibrous structure that arises from the synchondral junction of the first rib to the sternum and passes through the sternoclavicular joint, which divides the joint into two separate joint spaces (Fig. 15–2).[102,103] The upper attachment is on the superior and posterior aspects of the medial clavicle. De-Palma[63] has shown that the disk is perforated only

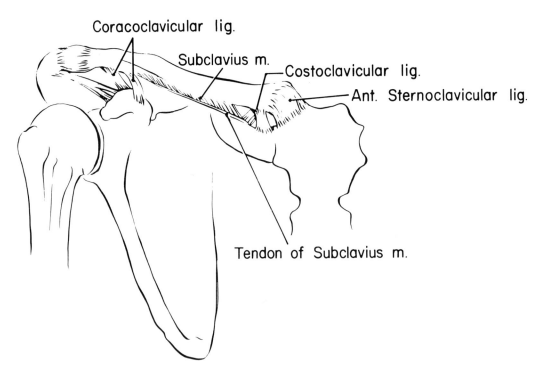

Fig. 15-1. Normal anatomy around the sternoclavicular and acromioclavicular joints. Note that the tendon of the subclavius muscle arises in the vicinity of the costoclavicular ligament from the first rib and has a long tendon structure.

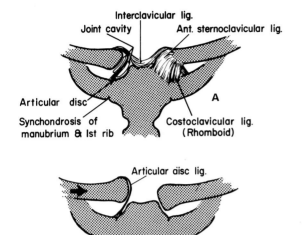

Interclavicular lig.
Joint cavity   Ant. sternoclavicular lig.

Articular disc   A
Synchondrosis of   Costoclavicular lig.
manubrium & 1st rib   (Rhomboid)

Articular disc lig.

B

Fig. 15-2. (**A**) Normal anatomy around the sternoclavicular joint. Note that the articular disk ligament divides the sternoclavicular joint cavity into two separate spaces and inserts onto the superior and posterior aspects of the medial clavicle. (**B**) The articular disk ligament acts as a checkrein for a medial displacement of the proximal clavicle. (*Reprinted with permission from Rockwood, C. A., and Matsen, F., III (eds.): The Shoulder, Fig. 13-2. Philadelphia: W.B. Saunders, 1990.*)

rarely; the perforation allows a free communication between the two joint compartments. Anteriorly and posteriorly, the disk blends into the fibers of the capsular ligament. The disk acts as a checkrein against medial displacement of the inner clavicle. (See Fig. 15–2.)

Costoclavicular Ligament

The costoclavicular ligament, also called the rhomboid ligament, is short and strong and consists of an anterior and a posterior fasciculus (see Fig. 15–1).[21,46,103] Cave[46] reports that the average length is 1.3 cm, the maximum width is 1.9 cm, and the average thickness is 1.3 cm. Bearn[21] has shown that there is always a bursa between the two components of the ligament. Because of the two different parts of the ligament, it has a twisted appearance.[103] The costoclavicular ligament attaches below to the upper surface of the first rib and at the adjacent part of the synchondral junction with the sternum, and above to the margins of the impression on the inferior surface of the medial end of the clavicle, sometimes known as the rhomboid fossa.[102,103] Cave[46] has shown, from a study of 153 clavicles,

that the attachment of the costoclavicular ligament to the clavicle can be any of three types: (1) a depression, the rhomboid fossa (30%); (2) flat (60%); or (3) an elevation (10%).

The fibers of the anterior fasciculus arise from the anteromedial surface of the first rib and are directed upward and laterally. The fibers of the posterior fasciculus are shorter and arise lateral to the anterior fibers on the rib and are directed upward and medially. The fibers of the anterior and posterior components cross and allow for stability of the joint during rotation and elevation of the clavicle. The two-part costoclavicular ligament is in many ways similar to the two-part configuration of the coracoclavicular ligament on the outer end of the clavicle.

Bearn[21] has shown experimentally that the anterior fibers resist excessive upward rotation of the clavicle and that the posterior fibers resist excessive downward rotation. Specifically, the anterior fibers also resist lateral displacement, and the posterior fibers resist medial displacement.

Interclavicular Ligament

The interclavicular ligament connects the superomedial aspects of each clavicle with the capsular ligaments and the upper sternum. (See Fig. 15–2.) According to Grant,[102] this band may be comparable to the wishbone of birds. This ligament helps the capsular ligaments to produce "shoulder poise"—that is, to hold up the shoulder. This can be tested by putting a finger in the superior sternal notch; with elevation of the arm, the ligament is quite lax, but as soon as both arms hang at the sides, the ligament becomes tight.

Capsular Ligament

The capsular ligament covers the anterosuperior and posterior aspects of the joint and represents thickenings of the joint capsule. (See Figs. 15–1 and 15–2.) The anterior portion of the capsular ligament is heavier and stronger than the posterior portion.

According to the original work of Bearn,[21] this may be the strongest ligament of the sternoclavicular joint, and it is the first line of defense against the upward displacement of the inner clavicle caused by a downward force on the distal end of the shoulder. The clavicle attachment of the ligament is primarily onto the epiphysis of the medial clavicle, with some secondary blending of the fibers into the metaphysis. I have demonstrated this, as have Poland,[210] Denham and Dingley,[67] and Brooks and Henning.[35] Although some authors report that

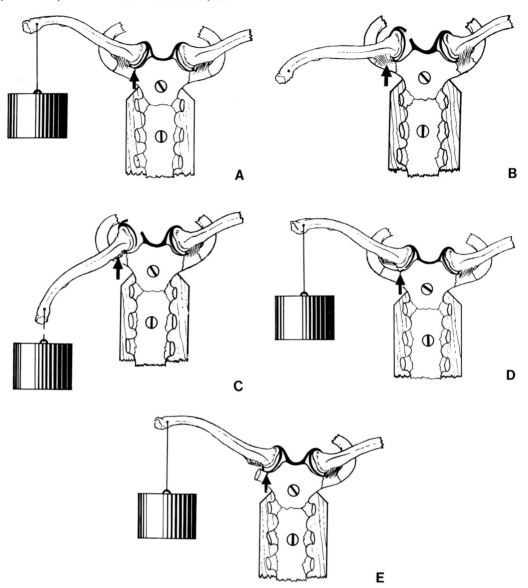

Fig. 15-3. The importance of the various ligaments around the sternoclavicular joint in maintaining normal shoulder poise. (**A**) The lateral end of the clavicle is maintained in an elevated position through the sternoclavicular ligaments. The arrow indicates the fulcrum. (**B**) When the capsule is divided completely, the lateral end of the clavicle descends under its own weight without any loading. The clavicle will seem to be supported by the intra-articular disk ligament. (**C**) After division of the capsular ligament, it was determined that a weight of less than 5 pounds was enough to tear the intra-articular disk ligament from its attachment on the costal cartilage junction of the first rib. The fulcrum was transferred laterally so that the medial end of the clavicle hinged over the first rib in the vicinity of the costoclavicular ligament. (**D**) After division of the costoclavicular ligament and the intra-articular disk ligament, the lateral end of the clavicle could not be depressed, as long as the capsular ligament was intact. (**E**) After resection of the medial first costal cartilage along with the costoclavicular ligament, there was no effect on the poise of the lateral end of the clavicle, as long as the capsular ligament was intact. *(Reproduced with permission from Bearn, J. G.: Direct Observation on the Function of the Capsule of the Sternoclavicular Joint in Clavicular Support. J. Anat., 101:159–170, 1967).*

the intra-articular disk ligament greatly assists the costoclavicular ligament in preventing upward displacement of the medial clavicle, Bearn[21] has shown that the capsular ligament is the most important structure in preventing upward displacement of the medial clavicle. In experimental postmortem studies, he evaluated the strength and the role of each of the ligaments at the sternoclavicular joint to see which one would prevent a downward displacement of the outer clavicle. He attributed the lateral "poise of the shoulder" (ie, the force that holds the shoulder up) to a locking mechanism of the ligaments of the sternoclavicular joint (Fig. 15–3). To accomplish his experiments, Bearn[21] dissected all the muscles attaching onto the clavicle, the sternum, and the first rib and left all the ligaments attached. He secured the sternum to a block in a vise. He then loaded the outer end of the clavicle with 10 to 20 pounds of weight and cut the ligaments of the sternoclavicular joint, one at a time and in various combinations, to determine each ligament's effect on maintaining the clavicle poise, or, thinking of it in another way, which ligament would rupture first when a force was applied to the outer end of the clavicle.

He determined, after cutting the costoclavicular,

intra-articular disk, and interclavicular ligaments, that they had no effect on clavicle poise. However, the division of the capsular ligament alone resulted in a downward depression on the distal end of the clavicle. He also noted that the intra-articular disk ligament tore under 5 pounds of weight once the capsular ligament had been cut. Bearn's article has many clinical implications for the mechanisms of injury of the sternoclavicular joint.

RANGE OF MOTION OF THE STERNOCLAVICULAR JOINT

The sternoclavicular joint is freely movable and functions almost like a ball-and-socket joint in that the joint has motion in almost all planes, including rotation.[30,164] The clavicle, and therefore the sternoclavicular joint, in normal shoulder motion is capable of 30° to 35° of upward elevation, 35° of combined forward and backward movement, and 45° to 50° of rotation around its long axis (Fig. 15–4). It is most likely the most frequently moved joint of the long bones in the body, because almost any motion of the upper extremity is transferred proximally to the sternoclavicular joint.

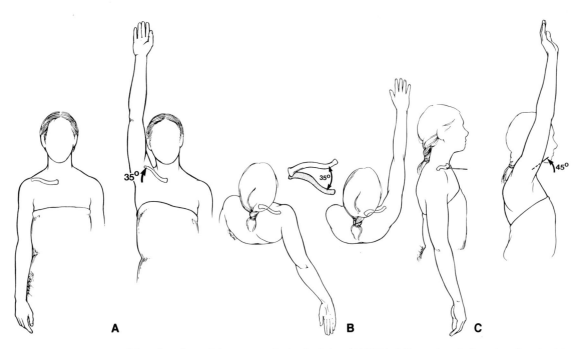

Fig. 15-4. Motions of the clavicle and the sternoclavicular joint. (**A**) With full overhead elevation the clavicle elevates 35°. (**B**) With adduction and extension, the clavicle displaces anteriorly and posteriorly 35°. (**C**) The clavicle rotates on its long axis 45°, as the arm is elevated to the full overhead position.

EPIPHYSIS OF THE MEDIAL CLAVICLE

Although the clavicle is the first long bone of the body to ossify (fifth intrauterine week), the epiphysis at the medial end of the clavicle is the last of the long bones in the body to appear and the last epiphysis to close (Fig. 15–5). The medial clavicular epiphysis does not ossify until the 18th to 20th year, and it fuses with the shaft of the clavicle around the 23rd to 25th year.[102,103,210] Webb and Suchey,[266] in an extensive study of the physis of the medial clavicle in 605 males and 254 females at autopsy, reported that complete unions may not be present until 31 years of age. This knowledge of the epiphysis is important, because I believe that many of the so-called sternoclavicular dislocations are fractures through the physeal plate.

APPLIED SURGICAL ANATOMY

The surgeon who is planning an operative procedure on or near the sternoclavicular joint should be completely knowledgeable about the vast array of anatomic structures immediately posterior to the sternoclavicular joint. There is a "curtain" of muscles—the sternohyoid, sternothyroid, and scaleni—posterior to the sternoclavicular joint and the inner third of the clavicle, and this curtain blocks the view of the vital structures. Some of these vital structures include the innominate artery, innominate vein, vagus nerve, phrenic nerve, internal jugular vein, trachea, and esophagus (Fig. 15–6). If one is considering stabilizing the sternoclavicular joint by running a pin down from the clavicle and into the sternum, it is important to remember that the arch of the aorta, the superior vena cava, and the right pulmonary artery are also very close at hand.

Another structure to be aware of is the anterior jugular vein, which is between the clavicle and the curtain of muscles. The anatomy books state that it can be quite variable in size; I have seen it as large as 1.5 cm in diameter. This vein has no valves, and when it is nicked, it looks like someone has opened up the flood gates.

MECHANISM OF INJURY

Because the sternoclavicular joint is subject to practically every motion of the upper extremity, and because the joint is so small and incongruous, one would think that it would be the most commonly dislocated joint in the body. However, the ligamentous supporting structure is so strong and so designed that it is, in fact, one of the least commonly dislocated joints in the body. A traumatic dislocation of the sternoclavicular joint usually occurs only after tremendous forces, either direct or indirect, have been applied to the shoulder.

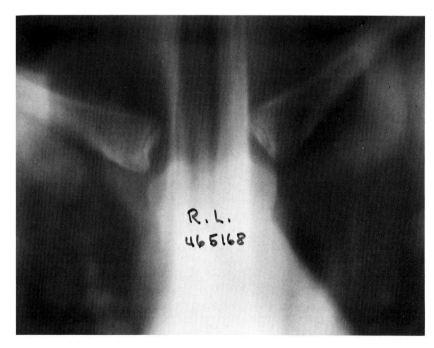

Fig. 15-5. Tomogram demonstrating the thin, waferlike disk of the epiphysis of the medial clavicle.

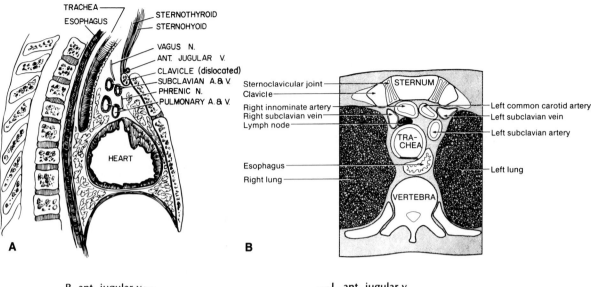

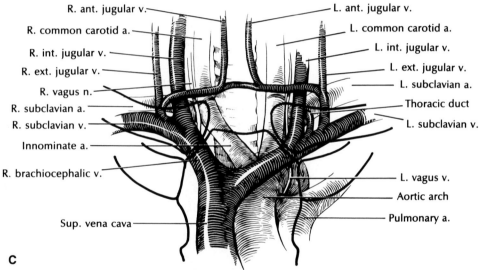

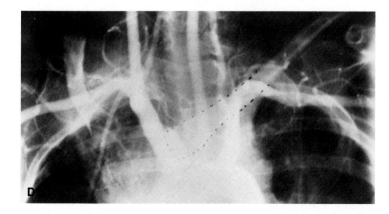

Fig. 15-6. Applied anatomy of the vital structures posterior to the sternoclavicular joint. (**A, B**) Sagittal views in cross section demonstrating the structures posterior to the sternoclavicular joint. (**C**) A diagram demonstrating the close proximity of the major vessels posterior to the sternoclavicular joint. (**D**) An aortogram showing the relationship of the medial end of the clavicle to the major vessels in the mediastinum.

DIRECT FORCE

When a force is applied directly to the anteromedial aspect of the clavicle, the clavicle is pushed posteriorly behind the sternum and into the mediastinum (Fig. 15–7). This may occur in a variety of ways: an athlete lying on his back on the ground is jumped on and the knee of the jumper lands directly on the medial end of the clavicle; a kick is delivered to the front of the medial clavicle; a person is run over by a vehicle; or a person is pinned between a vehicle and a wall. Because of our anatomy, it would be most unusual for a direct force to produce an anterior sternoclavicular dislocation.

INDIRECT FORCE

A force can be applied indirectly to the sternoclavicular joint from the anterolateral or posterolateral aspects of the shoulder. This is the most common mechanism of injury to the sternoclavicular joint. Mehta and coworkers[176] reported that three of four

posterior sternoclavicular dislocations were produced by indirect force, and Heinig[116] reported that indirect force was responsible for eight of nine cases of posterior sternoclavicular dislocations. It was the most common mechanism of injury in our series of 168 patients. If the shoulder is compressed and rolled forward, an ipsilateral posterior dislocation results; if the shoulder is compressed and rolled backward, an ipsilateral anterior dislocation results (Fig. 15–8). One of the most common causes I have seen is a pile-on in a football game. In this instance, a player falls on the ground, landing on the lateral shoulder; before he can get out of the way, several players pile on top of his opposite shoulder, which applies significant compressive force on the clavicle down toward the sternum. If, during the compression, the shoulder is rolled forward, the force directed down the clavicle produces a posterior dislocation of the sternoclavicular joint. If the shoulder is compressed and rolled backward, the force directed down the clavicle produces an anterior dislocation of the sternoclavicular joint. Other types

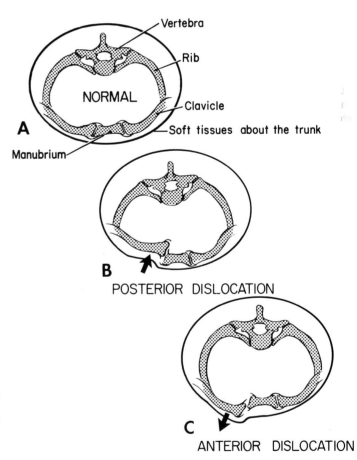

Fig. 15-7. Cross sections through the thorax at the level of the sternoclavicular joint. (**A**) Normal anatomical relations. (**B**) Posterior dislocation of the sternoclavicular joint. (**C**) Anterior dislocation of the sternoclavicular joint.

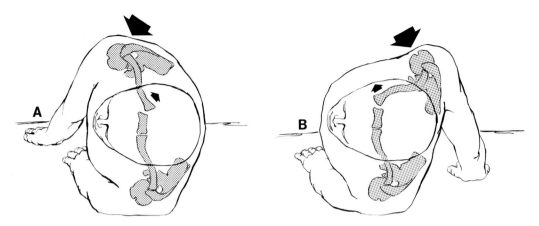

Fig. 15-8. Mechanisms that produce anterior or posterior dislocations of the sternoclavicular joint. (**A**) If the patient is lying on the ground and a compression force is applied to the posterior lateral aspect of the shoulder, the medial end of the clavicle will be displaced posteriorly. (**B**) When the lateral compression force is directed from the anterior position, the medial end of the clavicle is dislocated anteriorly.

of indirect forces that can produce sternoclavicular dislocation are a cave-in on a ditch digger, with lateral compression of the shoulders by the falling dirt; lateral compressive forces on the shoulder when a person is pinned between a vehicle and a wall; and a person's falling on the outstretched abducted arm, which drives the shoulder medially in the same manner as a lateral compression on the shoulder.

MOST COMMON CAUSES OF INJURY

The most common cause of dislocation of the sternoclavicular joint is vehicular accidents; the second is an injury sustained during participation in sports.[185,197,262] Omer,[197] in his review of patients from 14 military hospitals, found 82 cases of sternoclavicular joint dislocations. He reported that almost 80% of these occurred as the result of vehicular accidents (47%) and athletics (31%).

Probably the youngest patient to have a traumatic sternoclavicular dislocation was reported by Wheeler and associates.[269] They described an anterior dislocation in a 7-month-old infant. The injury occurred when she was lying on her left side and her older brother accidentally fell on her, compressing her shoulders together. The closed reduction was unstable, and the child was immobilized in a figure-of-eight bandage for 5 weeks. At 10 weeks she had a full range of motion, and there was no evidence of instability. I have seen an an-

terior injury in a 3-year-old that occurred as a result of an automobile accident (Fig. 15–9).

CLASSIFICATIONS OF STERNOCLAVICULAR DISLOCATIONS

There are two ways to classify sternoclavicular joint dislocations: (1) according to the anatomic position the dislocation assumes; (2) according to etiology.

ANATOMIC CLASSIFICATION

Detailed classifications are confusing and difficult to remember; the following, simple classification is suggested.

Anterior Dislocation

Anterior dislocations are the most common. The medial end of the clavicle is displaced anteriorly or anterosuperiorly to the anterior margin of the sternum. (See Fig. 15–19.)

Posterior Dislocation

Posterior sternoclavicular dislocation is uncommon. The medial end of the clavicle is displaced posteriorly or posterosuperiorly with respect to the posterior margin of the sternum. (See Figs. 15–20 and 15–25.)

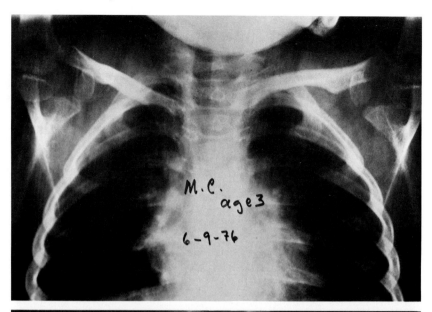

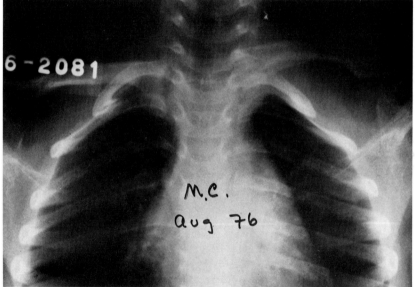

Fig. 15-9. X-ray of a 3-year-old child with traumatic anterior dislocation of the left sternoclavicular joint. The chest film demonstrates that the left clavicle is superior to the right, suggesting an anterior displacement of the left medial clavicle.

ETIOLOGIC CLASSIFICATION

Traumatic Injuries

SPRAIN OR SUBLUXATION

Acute sprains to the sternoclavicular joint can be classified as mild, moderate, or severe. In a *mild* sprain, all the ligaments are intact and the joint is stable. In a *moderate* sprain, there is subluxation of the sternoclavicular joint. The capsular, intra-articular disk, and costoclavicular ligaments may be partially disrupted. The subluxation may be anterior or posterior. In a *severe* sprain, there is complete disruption of the sternoclavicular ligaments, and the dislocation may be anterior or posterior.

ACUTE DISLOCATION

In a dislocated sternoclavicular joint, the capsular and intra-articular ligaments are ruptured. Occasionally, the costoclavicular ligament is intact but stretched out enough to allow the dislocation.

RECURRENT DISLOCATION

If the initial acute traumatic dislocation does not heal, mild to moderate forces may produce recurrent dislocations; this is rare.

UNREDUCED DISLOCATION

The original dislocation may go unrecognized, it may be irreducible, or the physician may decide not to reduce certain dislocations.

Atraumatic Problems

For a variety of nontraumatic reasons, the sternoclavicular joint may subluxate or enlarge.

SPONTANEOUS SUBLUXATION OR DISLOCATION

One or both of the sternoclavicular joints may spontaneously subluxate or dislocate anteriorly during overhead motion. The problem usually is not painful (Fig. 15–10).

CONGENITAL OR DEVELOPMENTAL SUBLUXATION OR DISLOCATION

Newlin[187] reported a 25-year-old man who had bilateral congenital posterior dislocation of the medial ends of the clavicle that simulated an intrathoracic mass. Guerin[105] first reported congenital luxations of the sternoclavicular joint in 1841. Congenital defects with loss of bone substance on either side of the joint can predispose to subluxation or dislocation. Cooper[56] described a patient with scoliosis so severe that the shoulder was displaced forward enough to posteriorly dislocate the clavicle behind the sternum.

ARTHRITIS

Arthritis, with enlargement of the sternoclavicular joint, can occur secondary to osteoarthritis, arthropathies, condensing osteitis of the medial clavicle, sternocostoclavicular hyperostosis, or postmenopausal arthritis.

Osteoarthritis. Osteoarthritis[113,142,144] is characterized by narrowing of the joint space, osteophytes, subchondral sclerosis, and cysts on both sides of the joint (Fig. 15–11). Because most of the wear occurs in the inferior part of the head of the medial clavicle, most of the degenerative changes occur in that region. The sometimes discrete degenerative changes are best seen on tomograms and CT scans.[12,142] Kier and associates[142] correlated the x-ray films and the pathologic specimens of patients with osteoarthritis of the sternoclavicular joint. Sternoclavicular joint arthritis and hypertrophy can develop following radical neck surgery, particularly when the spinal accessory nerve is sacrificed;[45,100] the incidence is reported to be as high as 54%.[45] The reason for the arthritis is the downward and forward droop of the shoulder, which puts an extra stress on the sternoclavicular joint. I followed one patient who had such stress on the sternoclavicular joint following a radical neck and spinal accessory nerve sacrifice that he developed a posterior dislocation of the sternoclavicular joint. The posterior displacement was so severe that the medial end of the clavicle compressed his trachea and esophagus. To swallow he had to hold the right shoulder back

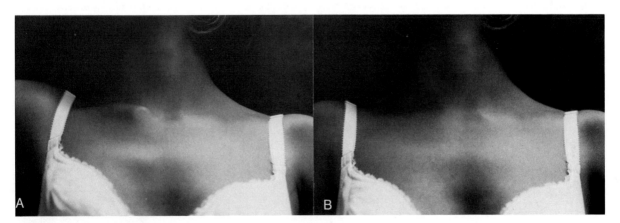

Fig. 15-10. Spontaneous anterior subluxation of the sternoclavicular joint. (**A**) With the arms in the overhead position, the medial end of the right clavicle spontaneously subluxates anteriorly without any trauma. (**B**) When the arm is brought back down to the side, the medial end of the clavicle spontaneously reduces. Usually this is not associated with significant discomfort. *(Reprinted with permission from Rockwood, C. A., and Matsen, F., III (eds.): The Shoulder, Fig. 13-10. Philadelphia: W.B. Saunders, 1990.)*

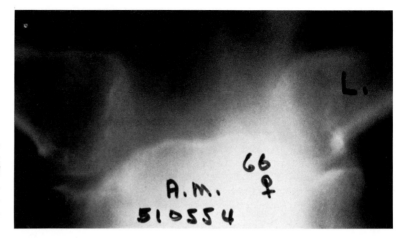

Fig. 15-11. Tomogram of the sterno-clavicular joints in a 66-year-old patient with degenerative arthritis. *(Reprinted with permission from Rockwood, C. A., and Matsen, F., III (eds.): The Shoulder, Fig. 13-11. Philadelphia: W.B. Saunders, 1990.)*

and up, which relieved the pressure on his esophagus. Baker and colleagues[12] reported that the CT scan was very useful in evaluating the pathologic changes in degenerative disease of the sternoclavicular joint.

Arthropathies. Some of the disease processes that produce degenerative changes in the sternoclavicular joint are rheumatoid arthritis (Fig. 15–12),[39,75,277] rheumatoid spondylitis,[217] scleroderma,[75] Reiter's syndrome,[142] psoriasis,[249] polymyalgia rheumatica,[199] secondary hyperparathyroidism,[217,259] gout,[59,170] leprosy,[190] syringomyelia,[61] metastatic carcinoma,[228] condensing osteitis,[36] Friedreich's disease[157] (aseptic necrosis of the medial end of the clavicle), and sternoclavicular hyperostosis.

Condensing Osteitis of the Medial Clavicle. Brower and associates[36] first described in detail the rare condition known as condensing osteitis of the medial clavicle. It usually occurs in women over the age of 40 and may occur secondary to chronic stress on the joint. The joint is swollen and tender, and radionuclide studies reveal an increased uptake of the isotope. X-ray films show sclerosis and slight expansion of the medial third of the clavicle. The inferior portion of the sternal end of the clavicle shows sclerotic changes. Some osteophytes may be present, but the joint space is preserved. The changes of the medial clavicle are best detected with a CT scan. The differential diagnosis includes Paget's disease, sternoclavicular hyperostosis, Friedreich's avascular necrosis of the medial clavicle epiphysis, infection, Tietze's syndrome, and osteoarthritis. The condition has been described by many au-

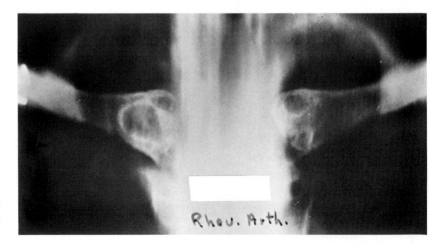

Fig. 15-12. Tomogram of a patient with rheumatoid arthritis with bilateral degenerative changes in the medial clavicles.

thors.[54,87,135,147] Most patients do well with conservative treatment (ie, anti-inflammatory medications). Kruger and associates[147] recommend incisional or excisional biopsy in refractory cases.

Sternocostoclavicular Hyperostosis. According to most authors,[4,52,96,99,134,149,231] sternocostoclavicular hyperostosis was first described by Sonozaki in 1974.[245-247] The majority of cases reported are from Japan.

This condition, usually bilateral, affects adults of both sexes between 30 and 50 years of age. The process begins at the junction of the medial clavicle, the first rib, and the sternum as an ossification in the ligaments and later involves the bones. Lagier and colleagues[149] published an excellent review of the x-ray findings and pathology from an autopsy specimen. In some cases, the hyperostosis is extensive and forms a solid block of bone of the sternum, ribs, and clavicle. Patients may have peripheral arthritis. Subperiosteal bone changes have been noted in x-ray films of other bones (ie, humerus, pelvis, tibia, ribs, and vertebral bodies).[96] The condition has been graded into three stages by Sonozaki.[245-247] Stage I is mild ossification in the costoclavicular ligaments; stage II is characterized by an ossific mass between the clavicle and the first rib; in stage III, a bone mass exists between the clavicle, sternum, and first rib. As might be expected with the fusion of the sternoclavicular joint, shoulder motion is severely restricted. Dohler[69] reported that as a result of the fusion of the sternoclavicular joint, his patient developed compensatory dislocation of the acromioclavicular joint.

Pustular cutaneous lesions of the palmar and plantar surfaces of skin may be seen. There is no specific laboratory test, except for an occasional elevation of the serum alkaline phosphatase.[96]

Postmenopausal Arthritis. Bremner[34] and Bonnin[29] have both reported on "postmenopausal arthritis," so named because it is most often seen in postmenopausal women. Sadr and Swann[230] reported 22 patients with this problem who were seen in a 5-year study; 20 of the cases were in women, and the majority involved the sternoclavicular joint of the dominant arm. Nonoperative treatment was recommended. The condition is the result of normal degeneration of a frequently moved joint. It is almost without symptoms; a lump develops at the sternoclavicular joint and, occasionally, a vague ache (Fig. 15–13). There is no previous history of injury or disease. X-ray studies reveal sclerosis and enlargement of the medial end of the clavicle, re-

active sclerosis of the sternum, and subluxation of the joint. The pathologic changes are those of degenerative arthritis.

INFECTION

Spontaneous swelling with the appearance of joint subluxation may be associated with acute, subacute, or chronic bacterial arthritis. Wohlgethan and Newberg[272] reviewed 39 cases of infection of the sternoclavicular joint; fifteen were in drug addicts. Common causes of the infection in nonaddicts are bacteremia, invasion from surrounding bone, rheumatoid arthritis, alcoholism, and chronic debilitating diseases. Lindsey and Leach[159] reported on sternoclavicular osteomyelitis as a complication of subclavian vein catheterization and in patients undergoing dialysis. There are many case reports of isolated infections of the sternoclavicular joint that have been caused by a variety of microorganisms, including *Staphylococcus aureus,*[60,119,160,172] *Escherichia coli,*[65,160] *Citrobacter diversus,*[89] coliform bacilli,[65] *Pasteurella multocida,*[189] *Streptococcus sanguis,*[189] *Streptococcus anginosus-constellatus,*[128] *Streptococcus pyogenes,*[183] *Pseudomonas aeruginosa,*[88,255] *Brucella,*[14,277] and *Neisseria gonorrhoeae* (Fig. 15–14). Blankstein and associates[26] reported a septic sternoclavicular joint that cultured *Staphylococcus aureus* secondary to bacteremia infection from a paronychia of the finger. Farrer[78] reported a 66-year-old man who had a septic sternoclavicular joint that cultured *Staphylococcus aureus.* Tabatabai and colleagues[257] reported infection of the sternoclavicular joint caused by Group B *Streptococcus.* The CT scan is very helpful in making an early diagnosis of a septic sternoclavicular joint.[159,183,272]

Richter and associates[219] reported nine patients with infection of the sternoclavicular joint secondary to tuberculosis. The average time from onset of the disease until diagnosis was 1.4 years.

For some reason, drug addicts who use the intravenous route seem to have a high incidence of acute gram-negative infection of the sternoclavicular joint.[88,98] Friedman and colleagues[88] reported four cases of sternoclavicular infection in intravenous drug abusers; in three of these *Staphylococcus aureus* was recovered, and in the fourth case *Streptococcus pneumoniae* was isolated.

Higoumenakis[120] reported that unilateral enlargement of the sternoclavicular joint is a diagnostic sign of congenital syphilis. The enlargement of the sternoclavicular joint can be mistaken for an anterior dislocation. He reported the sign to be positive in 170 of 197 cases of congenital syphilis.

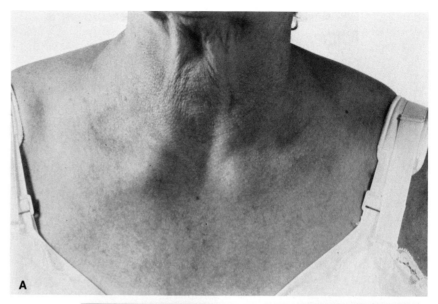

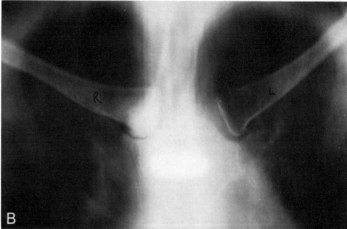

Fig. 15-13. (**A**) Bilateral anterior swelling of the sternoclavicular joints in a 67-year-old female. The right medial clavicle was more prominent because she was right handed. (**B**) The tomogram demonstrates sclerosis and degenerative changes in the right sternoclavicular joint consistent with ordinary degenerative arthritis. *(B reprinted with permission from Rockwood, C. A., and Matsen, F., III (eds.): The Shoulder, Fig. 13-13B. Philadelphia: W.B. Saunders, 1990.)*

Glickman and Minsky[97] reported on the same condition. The enlargement is a hyperostosis of the medial clavicle occurring in the sternoclavicular joint of the dominant extremity, which reaches its permanent stage and size at puberty. The theory of why it affects the sternoclavicular joint relates it to spirochete invasion of the sternal end of the clavicle at the time of early ossification.

INCIDENCE OF INJURY

Sternoclavicular injuries are rare, and many of the authors apologize for reporting only three or four cases. Attesting to this rarity is the fact that some orthopaedists have never treated or seen a dislocation of the sternoclavicular joint.[123,232]

The incidence of sternoclavicular dislocation, based on the series of 1603 injuries of the shoulder girdle reported by Cave and associates,[48] is 3%. (Specific incidences in the study were: glenohumeral dislocations, 85%; acromioclavicular, 12%; and sternoclavicular, 3%). In the series by Cave, and in my own experience, dislocation of the sternoclavicular joint is not as rare as posterior dislocation of the glenohumeral joint.

RATIO OF ANTERIOR TO POSTERIOR DISLOCATIONS

Undoubtedly, anterior dislocations of the sternoclavicular joint are much more common than the posterior type. However, the ratio of anterior to posterior dislocations is only rarely reported. Theo-

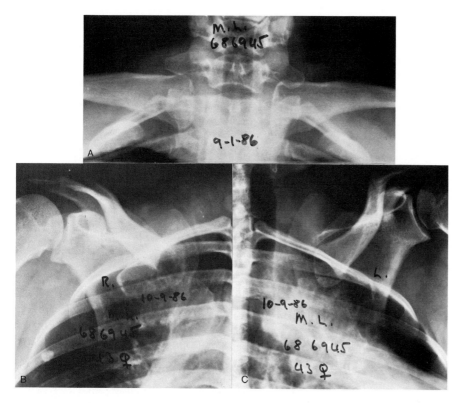

Fig. 15-14. Infection in the right sternoclavicular joint. (**A**) On the initial x-ray there is little difference between the right and left medial clavicles, as seen on the 30° cephalic tilt view. (**B, C**) Thirty-eight days later, the medial end of the right clavicle is seen to be dissolving, compared with the medial end of the left clavicle. The patient had a *Staphylococcus aureus* infection in the right sternoclavicular joint, which was managed by open debridement. *(Reprinted with permission from Rockwood, C. A., and Matsen, F., III (eds.): The Shoulder, Fig. 13-14. Philadelphia: W.B. Saunders, 1990.)*

retically, one could survey the literature and develop the ratio of anterior to posterior dislocations, but most of the published material on sternoclavicular dislocations is on the rare posterior dislocation. Of the references listed at the end of this chapter that deal with injuries of the sternoclavicular joint, more than 60% discuss only posterior dislocations and their various complications. The largest series from a single institution is reported by Nettles and Linscheid,[185] who studied 60 patients with sternoclavicular dislocations (57 anterior and 3 posterior). This gives a ratio of anterior dislocations to posterior dislocations of the sternoclavicular joint of approximately 20 to 1. Waskowitz[262] reviewed 18 cases of sternoclavicular dislocations, none of which was posterior. However, in my series of 273 traumatic sternoclavicular injuries, there have been 121 patients with anterior dislocation and 41 patients with posterior dislocation.

BILATERAL DISLOCATIONS

In 1896, Hotchkiss[124] reported a bilateral traumatic dislocation of the sternoclavicular joint. A 28-year-old man was run over by a cart and suffered an anterior dislocation of the right shoulder and a posterior dislocation of the left one. I have treated four cases of bilateral sternoclavicular dislocation.

SIGNS AND SYMPTOMS

MILD SPRAIN

In a mild sprain, the ligaments of the joint are intact. The patient complains of a mild to moderate amount of pain, particularly with movement of the upper extremity. The joint may be slightly swollen and tender to palpation, but instability is not noted.

MODERATE SPRAIN (SUBLUXATION)

A moderate sprain results in a subluxation of the sternoclavicular joint. The ligaments are either partially disrupted or severely stretched. Swelling is noted and pain is marked, particularly with any movement of the arm. Anterior or posterior subluxation may be obvious to the examiner when the injured joint is compared with the normal sternoclavicular joint.

SEVERE SPRAIN (DISLOCATION)

A severe sprain is analogous to a joint dislocation. The dislocation may be anterior or posterior. The capsular ligament and the intra-articular disk ligament are ruptured. Regardless of whether the dislocation is anterior or posterior, there are characteristic clinical findings of sternoclavicular joint dislocation.

Signs Common to Anterior and Posterior Dislocations

The patient with a sternoclavicular dislocation has severe pain that is increased with any movement of the arm, particularly when the shoulders are pressed together by a lateral force. The patient usually supports the injured arm across the trunk with the normal arm. The affected shoulder appears to be shortened and thrust forward when compared with the normal shoulder. The head may be tilted toward the side of the dislocated joint. The discomfort increases when the patient is placed in the supine position, at which time it will be noted that the involved shoulder will not lie back flat on the table.

Signs and Symptoms of Anterior Dislocations

With an anterior dislocation, the medial end of the clavicle is visibly prominent anterior to the sternum (See Fig. 15–19) and can be palpated anterior to the sternum. It may be fixed anteriorly or be quite mobile.

Signs and Symptoms of Posterior Dislocations

The patient with a posterior dislocation has more pain than a patient with an anterior dislocation. Stankler[251] reported two patients with unrecognized posterior dislocations which developed venous engorgement of the ipsilateral arm. The anterosuperior fullness of the chest produced by the clavicle is less prominent and visible when compared with the normal side. The usually palpable medial end of the clavicle is displaced posteriorly. The corner of the sternum is easily palpated as compared with the normal sternoclavicular joint. Venous congestion may be present in the neck or in the upper extremity. Breathing difficulties, shortness of breath, or a choking sensation may be noted. Circulation to the ipsilateral arm may be decreased. The patient may complain of difficulty in swallowing or a tight feeling in the throat or may be in a state of complete shock or possibly have a pneumothorax.

I have seen six patients who clinically appeared to have an anterior dislocation of the sternoclavicular joint but on x-ray studies were shown to have complete posterior dislocation. The point is that one cannot always rely on the clinical findings of observing and palpating the joint to make a distinction between anterior and posterior dislocations.

X-RAY FINDINGS

ANTEROPOSTERIOR VIEWS

The older literature reflects that routine x-rays of the sternoclavicular joint, regardless of the special views, are difficult to interpret. Special oblique views of the chest have been recommended, but because of the distortion of one clavicle over the other, interpretation is difficult (Fig. 15–15). The older literature also suggests that the diagnosis of dislocation of the sternoclavicular joint is best made from a clinical examination, not from the x-rays. However, it does indicate that tomography offers more detailed information, often showing small fractures in the vicinity of the sternoclavicular joint. Occasionally, the routine anteroposterior or posteroanterior x-rays of the chest or sternoclavicular joint suggest something is wrong with one of the clavicles, because it appears to be displaced as compared with the normal side (Fig. 15–16). It would be ideal to take a view at right angles to the anteroposterior plane, but because of our anatomy, it is impossible to take a true 90° cephalic-to-caudal lateral view. Lateral x-rays of the chest are at right angles to the anteroposterior plane, but they cannot be interpreted because of the density of the chest and the overlap of the medial clavicles with the first rib and the sternum.

Regardless of a clinical impression that suggests an anterior dislocation, x-rays *must* be obtained to confirm one's suspicions.

SPECIAL PROJECTED VIEWS

Kattan[138] has recommended a special projection, as have Ritvo and Ritvo,[220] Schmitt,[237] Fedoseev,[79] and

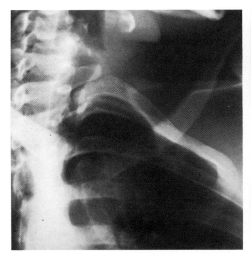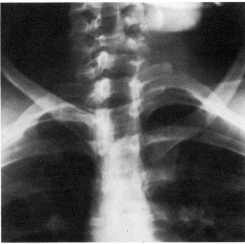

Fig. 15-15. Routine x-rays of the sternoclavicular joint are difficult to interpret, even with a classic posterior dislocation of the joint. (See Fig. 15-34 for further information on this patient.)

Fery and Leonard.[82] Kurzbauer[148] has recommended special lateral projections. Hobbs,[121] in 1968, recommended a view that comes close to being a 90° cephalocaudal lateral view of the sternoclavicular joints.

Hobbs View

In the Hobbs view, the patient is seated at the x-ray table, high enough to lean forward over the table. The cassette is on the table, and the lower anterior rib cage is against the cassette (Fig. 15-17). The patient leans forward so that the nape of his flexed neck is almost parallel to the table. The flexed elbows straddle the cassette and support the head and neck. The x-ray source is above the nape of the neck, and the beam passes through the cervical spine to project the sternoclavicular joints onto the cassette.

Serendipity View

The "serendipity view" is rightfully named because that is the way it was developed. I found, accidentally, that the next best thing to having a true cephalocaudal lateral view of the sternoclavicular joint is a 40° cephalic tilt view. The patient is positioned on his back squarely and in the center of the x-ray table. The tube is tilted at a 40° angle off the vertical and is centered directly on the sternum (Fig. 15-18). A nongrid 11 × 14-inch cassette is placed squarely on the table and under the patient's upper shoulders and neck so that the beam aimed at the sternum will project both clavicles onto the film.

The tube is adjusted so that the medial half of both clavicles is projected onto the film. It is important to note that the cassette should be placed squarely on the x-ray table (ie, not angulated or rotated) and that the patient should be positioned squarely on top of the cassette.

For children, the distance from the tube to the cassette is 45 inches; for adults, whose anteroposterior chest diameter is greater, the distance should be 60 inches. The technical setting of the machine is essentially the same as for a posteroanterior view of the chest.

To understand this view, imagine that your eyes are at the level of the patient's knees and you are looking up toward his clavicles at a 40° angle. If the right sternoclavicular joint is dislocated anteriorly, the right clavicle will appear to be displaced more anteriorly or riding higher on an imaginary horizontal line when compared with the normal left clavicle (Fig. 15-19). The reverse is true if the left sternoclavicular joint is dislocated posteriorly (ie, the left clavicle displaced inferiorly or riding lower on an imaginary horizontal plane than the normal right clavicle) (Fig. 15-20). The idea, then, is to take a 40° cephalic tilt x-ray showing both medial clavicles and compare the injured clavicle to the normal clavicle (Fig. 15-21).

SPECIAL TECHNIQUES

Tomograms

Tomograms can be very helpful in distinguishing between a sternoclavicular dislocation and a frac-

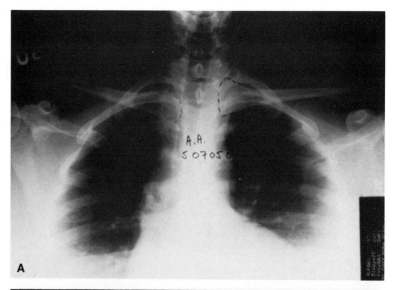

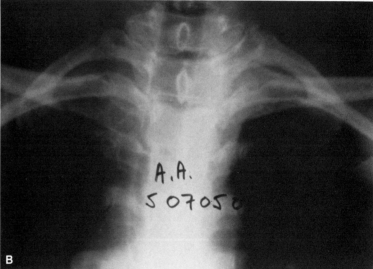

Fig. 15-16. Anteroposterior x-ray of the sternoclavicular joints with anterosuperior displacement of the left medial clavicle. (**A**) The displacement is quite noticeable when the clavicles are outlined. (**B**) However, the displacement is not so noticeable when the clavicles are not outlined.

ture of the medial clavicle. They are also helpful in questionable anterior and posterior injuries of the sternoclavicular joint—to distinguish fractures from dislocations and to evaluate arthritic changes (Fig. 15–22).

In 1959, Baker[12] recommended the use of tomography, which was developed in the late 1920s, and said it was far more valuable than routine films and the fingertips of the examining physician. In 1975, Morag and Shahin[180] reported on the value of tomography, which they used in a series of 20 patients, and recommended that it be used routinely to evaluate problems of the sternoclavicular joint.

From a study of normal sternoclavicular joints, they pointed out the variation in the x-ray appearance in different age groups.

CT Scans

Without question, the CT scan is the best technique to study problems of the sternoclavicular joint (Fig. 15–23). It clearly distinguishes injuries of the joint from fractures of the medial clavicle and defines minor subluxations of the joint. The orthopaedist must remember to ask for CT scans of both sternoclavicular joints and the medial half of both clavicles so the injured side can be compared with the

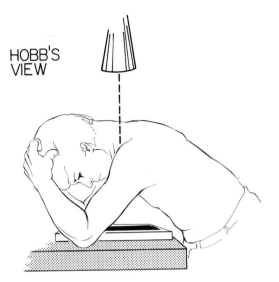

Fig. 15-17. Positioning of the patient for x-ray evaluation of the sternoclavicular joint, as recommended by Hobbs. *(Redrawn from Hobbs, D. W.: The Sternoclavicular Joint: A New Axial Radiographic View. Radiology, 90:801, 1968).*

normal side. The patient should lie flat in the supine position. If one requests a study of the right sternoclavicular joint, the x-ray technician may rotate the patient to the affected side and provide views of only the one joint.

Hartman and Dunnagan[114] reported on the use of CT arthrography to demonstrate capsular dis-

ruption in a patient following a traumatic injury to the joint.

TREATMENT

TRAUMATIC INJURIES

Mild Sprain

The mildly sprained sternoclavicular joint is stable but painful. Application of ice for the first 12 to 24 hours followed by heat is helpful. The upper extremity should be immobilized in a sling for 3 to 4 days, then gradually the patient can regain use of the arm in everyday activities. I recently had a fascinating case of a young woman who after childbirth developed aching pain in both sternoclavicular joints. Her bra size, over a period of 4 weeks, had jumped from a 36B to a 38EE. The increase in weight depressed both shoulders and produced pain while upright in both sternoclavicular joints. I could completely relieve the discomfort by pushing both elbows up, thus elevating the distal clavicles, which in turn took the strain off her sternoclavicular joints. I suggested she consult her gynecologist and surgeon to determine the quickest way to reduce the size of her breasts.

Moderate Sprain (Subluxation)

For subluxation of the sternoclavicular joint, application of ice is recommended for the first 12

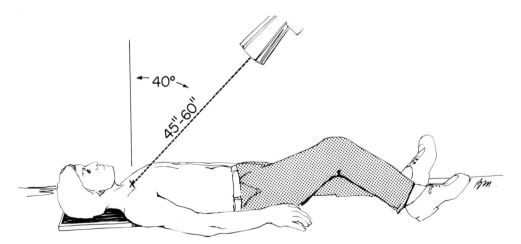

Fig. 15-18. Positioning of the patient to take the "serendipity" view of the sternoclavicular joints. The x-ray tube is tilted 40° from the verticle position and aimed directly at the manubrium. The nongrid cassette should be large enough to receive the projected images of the medial halves of both clavicles. In children the tube distance from the patient should be 45 inches; in thicker-chested adults the distance should be 60 inches.

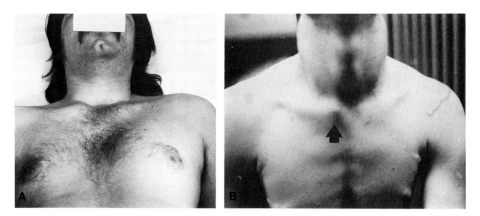

Fig. 15-19. (**A**) Clinically an anterior dislocation of the right sternoclavicular joint is evident (*arrow*). (**B**) When the clavicles are viewed from around the level of the patient's knees, it is apparent that the right clavicle is dislocated anteriorly.

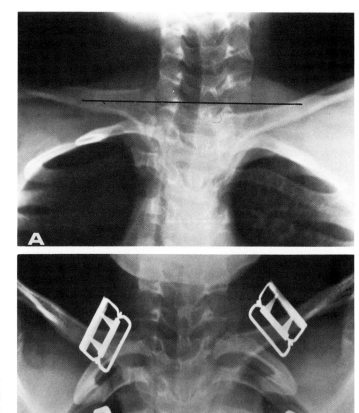

Fig. 15-20. (**A**) Posterior dislocation of the left sternoclavicular joint as seen on a 40° cephalic tilt x-ray in a 12-year-old boy. The left clavicle is displaced inferiorly to a line drawn through the normal right clavicle. (**B**) Following closed reduction, the medial ends of both clavicles are in the same horizontal position. The buckles are part of the figure-of-eight clavicular harness used to hold the shoulders back after reduction.

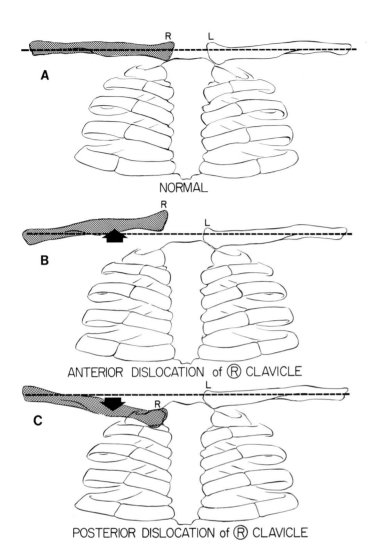

NORMAL

ANTERIOR DISLOCATION of Ⓡ CLAVICLE

POSTERIOR DISLOCATION of Ⓡ CLAVICLE

Fig. 15-21. Interpretation of the cephalic tilt x-rays of the sternoclavicular joints. (**A**) In the normal person, both clavicles appear on the same imaginary line drawn horizontally across the film. (**B**) In a patient with anterior dislocation of the right sternoclavicular joint, the medial half of the right clavicle is projected above the imaginary line drawn through the level of the normal left clavicle. (**C**) If the patient has a posterior dislocation of the right sternoclavicular joint, the medial half of the right clavicle is displaced below the imaginary line drawn through the normal left clavicle.

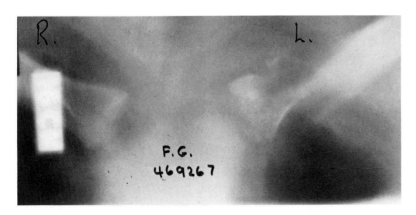

Fig. 15-22. Tomogram demonstrating a fracture of the left medial clavicle. The clinical pre–x-ray diagnosis was an anterior dislocation of the left sternoclavicular joint.

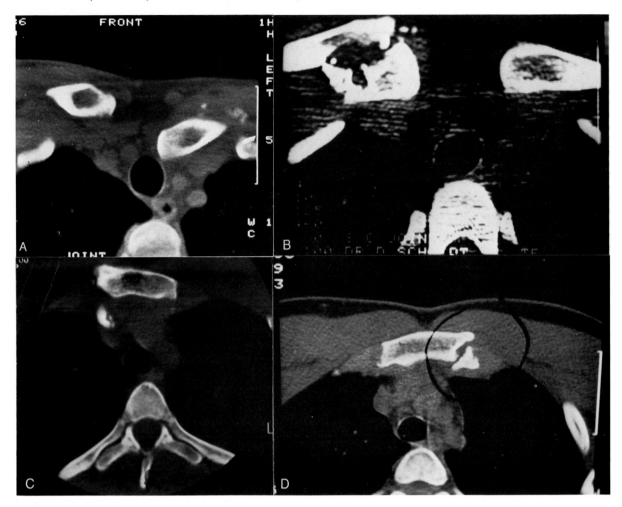

Fig. 15-23. CT scans of the sternoclavicular joint demonstrating various types of injuries. (**A**) A posterior dislocation of the left clavicle compressing the great vessels and producing swelling of the left arm. (**B**) A fracture of the medial clavicle that does not involve the articular surface. (**C**) A fragment of bone displaced posteriorly into the great vessel. (**D**) A fracture of the medial clavicle into the sternoclavicular joint. *(Reprinted with permission from Rockwood, C. A., and Matsen, F., III (eds.): The Shoulder, Fig. 13-22. Philadelphia: W.B. Saunders, 1990.)*

hours, followed by heat for the next 24 to 48 hours. The joint may be subluxated anteriorly or posteriorly, which may be reduced by drawing the shoulders backward as if reducing and holding a fracture of the clavicle. A clavicle strap can be used to hold the reduction. A sling and swath should also be used to hold up the shoulder and to prevent motion of the arm. The patient should be protected from further injury for 4 to 6 weeks. DePalma[64] suggests a plaster figure-of-eight dressing, and McLaughlin[179] recommended the same type of treatment that would be used for fracture of the clavicle, with the addition of a sling to support the arm.

Allman[7] prefers the use of a soft figure-of-eight bandage with a sling and occasionally uses adhesive strapping over the medial end of the clavicle. When in certain circumstances the subluxation cannot be reduced, some authors[19,64] have recommended repair of the ligaments and temporary internal fixation of the sternoclavicular joint with pins drilled from the clavicle into the sternum. Postoperatively, DePalma[64] applies a plaster figure-of-eight cast and, in addition, supports it with a sling and swath; the pins and the cast are removed after 6 weeks.

As will be pointed out in the section on author's preferred method of treatment, I believe the placement of pins across the sternoclavicular joint has too many serious complications to ever be used.

Occasionally, following conservative treatment of a type II sternoclavicular injury, the pain lingers on and the symptoms of popping and grating persist. This may require joint exploration. Bateman[19] has commented on the possibility of finding a tear of the intra-articular disk, which should be excised.

Duggan[70] reported a case in which, several weeks after an injury to the sternoclavicular joint, the patient still had popping in the joint. Through a small incision, Duggan exposed the capsule and out through the capsule popped the intra-articular disk, which looked like "an avulsed fingernail." Following repair of the capsule, the patient had no more symptoms. If degenerative changes become severe in the sternoclavicular joint, excision of the medial end of the clavicle may be required.

Severe Sprain (Dislocation)

NONOPERATIVE TREATMENT

Anterior Dislocation. There still is some controversy regarding the treatment of acute or chronic anterior dislocation of the sternoclavicular joint. Most acute anterior dislocations are unstable following reduction, and many operative procedures have been described to repair or reconstruct the joint.

Method of Closed Reduction. Closed reduction of the sternoclavicular joint may be accomplished with local or general anesthesia or, in stoic patients, without anesthesia. Most authors recommend the use of narcotics or muscle relaxants. The patient is placed supine on the table, lying on a 3- to 4-inch-thick pad between the shoulders. In this position, the clavicle may reduce with direct gentle pressure over the anteriorly displaced clavicle. However, when the pressure is released, the clavicle usually dislocates again.

Occasionally, the clavicle will remain reduced. Sometimes, the physician will need to push both shoulders back to the table while an assistant applies pressure to the anteriorly displaced clavicle. Laidlaw[150] treated an interesting case of a patient who had a dislocated clavicle. The sternoclavicular joint was dislocated anteriorly and was mildly symptomatic. The acromioclavicular joint was most symptomatic and was treated by excision of the distal clavicle. Surprisingly, the anteriorly dislocated sternoclavicular joint reduced and became pain-free.

Postreduction Care. If, with the shoulders held back, the sternoclavicular joint remains reduced,

the shoulders can be stabilized with a soft figure-of-eight dressing, a commercial clavicle strap harness, or a plaster figure-of-eight cast. Some authors recommend a bulky pressure pad over the antero-medial clavicle that is held in place with elastic tape. A sling might be used because it holds up the shoulder and prevents motion of the arm. Immobilization should be maintained at least 6 weeks, and then the arm should be protected for another 2 weeks before strenuous activities are undertaken. If the sternoclavicular joint again dislocates when the reduction pressure is released, as it usually does, a figure-of-eight dressing or a sling can be used until the patient's symptoms subside. Most anterior closed reductions of the sternoclavicular joint are unstable, and even with the shoulders held back, the joint is unstable. Although some authors have recommended operative repair of anterior dislocations of the sternoclavicular joint, I believe that the operative complications are too great and the end results are too unsatisfactory to consider an open reduction. Certainly in children, in whom many if not most of the injuries are physeal fractures, a nonoperative approach should be strongly considered.

Posterior Dislocation. *A careful examination of the patient is extremely important.* Complications are common with posterior dislocation of the sternoclavicular joint, and the patient should receive prompt attention.

A very careful history and physical examination should be done to rule out damage to the pulmonary and vascular systems. The sternoclavicular joint must be carefully evaluated by all available x-ray techniques including, when indicated, combined aortogram–CT scan for potential vascular injuries. If specific complications are noted, appropriate consultants should be called in before reduction is performed. Worman and Leagus[274] reported a posterior dislocation of the sternoclavicular joint in which it was noted at surgery that the displaced clavicle had put a hole into the right pulmonary artery. The clavicle had prevented exsanguination, because the vessel was still impaled by the clavicle. Had a closed reduction been performed in the emergency department, the result could have been disastrous.

General anesthesia is usually required for reduction of a posterior dislocation of the sternoclavicular joint because the patient has so much pain and muscle spasm. However, for the stoic patient, some authors have performed the reduction under intravenous narcotics and muscle relaxants. Heinig[116] has successfully used local anesthesia in a posterior dislocation reduction.

From a review of the earlier literature, it would appear that the treatment of choice for posterior sternoclavicular dislocation was by operative procedures. However, since the 1950s, the treatment of choice has been closed reduction.[43,53,58,81,107,116,174,175,178,203,232,253] Some authors[203,253] who had previously done open reductions reported that they were amazed at how easily the dislocation reduced under direct vision, and thereafter they used closed reductions with complete success.

Methods of Closed Reduction.   Many different techniques have been described for closed reduction of a posterior dislocation of the sternoclavicular joint.

ABDUCTION TRACTION TECHNIQUE.   For the abduction traction technique,[63,81,174,178,222,232] the patient is placed on his back with the dislocated shoulder near the edge of the table. A 3- to 4-inch-thick sandbag is placed between the shoulders (Fig. 15–24). Lateral traction is applied to the abducted arm, which is then gradually brought back into extension. This may be all that is necessary to accomplish the reduction. The clavicle usually reduces with an audible snap or pop, and it is almost always stable. Too much extension can bind the anterior surface of the dislocated medial clavicle on the back of the manubrium. Occasionally, it may be necessary to grasp the medial clavicle with one's fingers to dislodge it from behind the sternum. If this fails, the skin is prepared, and a sterile towel clip is used to grasp the medial clavicle to apply lateral and anterior traction (Fig. 15–25).

ADDUCTION TRACTION TECHNIQUE.   In this technique,[40] the patient is supine on the table with a 3- to 4-inch bolster between the shoulders. Traction is then applied to the arm in adduction, while a downward pressure is exerted on the shoulders. The clavicle is levered over the first rib into its normal position. Buckerfield and Castle[40] reported that this technique has succeeded when the abduction traction technique has failed. Butterworth and Kirk[43] used a similar adducted position, except they applied lateral traction on the upper humerus.

OTHER TECHNIQUES.   Heinig[116] and Elting[73] have reported that they accomplished reduction by placing the patient supine on the table with three or four folded towels between the two shoulders. Forward pressure is then applied on both shoulders, which accomplished the reduction. Other authors have put a knee between the shoulders of the seated patient and, by pulling back on both shoulders, have accomplished a reduction. Stein[253] used skin trac-

tion on the abducted and extended arm to accomplish the reduction gently and gradually. Many authors have reported that closed reduction usually cannot be accomplished after 48 hours. However, others[40,153] have reported closed reduction as late as 4 and 5 days after the injury.

Postreduction Care.   After reduction, to allow ligament healing, the shoulders should be held back for 4 to 6 weeks with a figure-of-eight dressing or one of the commercially available figure-of-eight straps used to treat fractures of the clavicle.

OPERATIVE TREATMENT

The operative procedure should be performed in a manner that disturbs as few of the anterior ligament structures as possible. If the procedure can be performed with the anterior ligaments intact, then, with the shoulders held back in a figure-of-eight dressing, the reduction may be stable. If all the ligaments are disrupted, a significant decision has to be made to try to stabilize the sternoclavicular joint or to resect the medial 1 to 1.5 inches of the medial clavicle and stabilize the remaining clavicle to the first rib.

Some of the literature from the 1960s and 1970s recommended stabilization of the sternoclavicular joint with pins. Elting[73] used Kirschner wires to stabilize the joint and supplemented ligament repairs with a short-toe extensor tendon. Denham and Dingley[67] and Brooks and Henning[35] used Kirschner wires. DePalma[64] and Brown[37] recommended repair of the ligaments and stabilized the sternoclavicular joint with one or two Steinmann pins.

Habernek and Hertz,[110] Nutz,[193] Pfister and Weller,[208] Kennedy,[139] Tagliabue and Riva,[258] Hartman and Dunnagan,[114] Bankart,[13] Ecke,[72] and Stein[253] avoided the use of pins across the sternoclavicular joint and used loops of various types of suture wires across the joint. Burri and Neugebauer[41] recommended the use of a figure-of-eight loop of carbon fiber. Maguire,[167] Booth and Roper,[30] Barth and Hagen,[16] and Lunseth and associates[166] reconstructed the sternoclavicular joint using local tendons of the sternocleidomastoid, subclavius, or pectoralis major tendons for repair. Haug[115] reported on the use of a special plate to stabilize the joint. The complications of fixation of the sternoclavicular joint with Kirschner wires or Steinmann pins are horrendous and are discussed in the section on complications.

In recent years (ie, since 1982), various authors have recommended open reduction and internal fixation for acute injuries, as well as for chronic problems.[76,77,80,83,207,208,278]

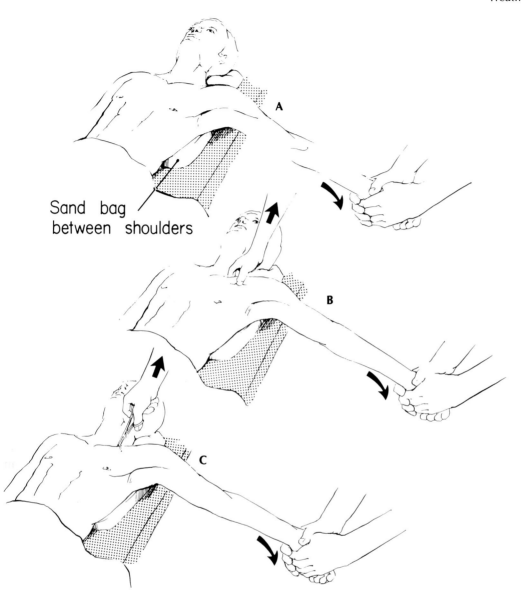

Fig. 15-24. Technique for closed reduction of the sternoclavicular joint. (**A**) The patient is positioned supine with a sandbag placed between the two shoulders. Traction is then applied to the arm against countertraction in an abducted and slightly extended position. In anterior dislocations, direct pressure over the medial end of the clavicle may reduce the joint. (**B**) In posterior dislocations, in addition to the traction it may be necessary to manipulate the medial end of the clavicle with the fingers to dislodge the clavicle from behind the manubrium. (**C**) In stubborn posterior dislocations, it may be necessary to sterilely prepare the medial end of the clavicle and use a towel clip to grasp *around* the medial clavicle to lift it back into position.

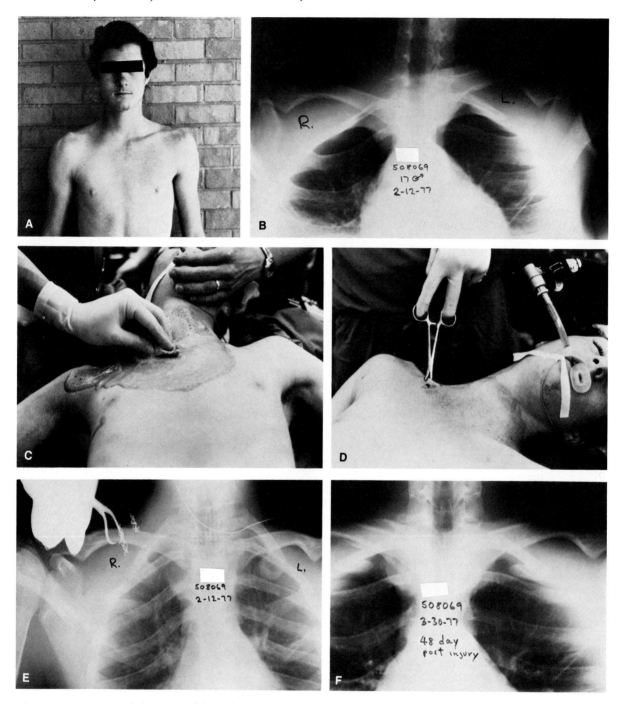

Fig. 15-25. Posterior dislocation of the right sternoclavicular joint. (**A**) A 16-year-old boy has a 48-hour-old posterior displacement of the right medial clavicle that occurred from direct trauma to the anterior right clavicle. He noted immediate onset of difficulty in swallowing and some hoarseness in his voice. (**B**) A 40° cephalic tilt x-ray confirmed the posterior displacement of the right medial clavicle as compared with the left clavicle. Because of the patient's age, this was considered most likely to be a physeal injury of the right medial clavicle. (**C**) Because the injury was 48 hours old, we were unable to reduce the dislocation with simple traction on the arm. The right shoulder was surgically cleansed so that a sterile towel clip could be used. (**D**) With the towel clip securely around the clavicle

In 1982, Pfister and associates[207,208] recommended open reduction and repair of the ligaments over nonoperative treatment. In symptomatic chronic dislocation or nontraumatic cases, they recommended the use of autogenous grafts between the sternum and the first rib without placing Kirschner wires across the sternoclavicular joint. In 1988 Fery and Sommelet[83] reported 49 cases of dislocations of the sternoclavicular joint. In these patients, if closed reduction was not successful, they performed open reduction. In symptomatic chronic unreduced dislocations, they either performed a myoplasty or excised the medial end of the clavicle if the articular surfaces were damaged. They were able to follow 55% of their patients, with an average follow-up of more than 6 years. They had 42% excellent results in the operative cases. Of those patients who were treated with closed reduction, 58% were satisfied. Krenzien[146] reported that a closed reduction of a posterior dislocation was difficult if not impossible and recommended an open reduction over conservative treatment. He reported that the use of Kirschner wires is not without risk and recommended that they be used only by experienced surgeons. He said use of the fascial plasties of Bunnel, Steindler, and Bankart are more suitable for fixation. Ferrandez and colleagues[80] reported 17 subluxations and dislocations of the sternoclavicular joint. Seven had moderate sprains and 11 had dislocations. Of the three patients with posterior dislocation, all had symptoms of dysphagia. All of the subluxations were treated nonoperatively with excellent results. The remaining ten patients with dislocations were treated with surgery (ie, open reduction with suture of the ligaments and Kirschner wires between the clavicle and the sternum). The wires were removed 3 to 4 weeks following surgery. At follow-up at 1 to 4 years, most of the operative cases had a slight deformity. In two patients, migration of the Kirschner wires was noted but was without clinical significance. Eskola and associates[76,77] strongly urged operative repair of dislocations of the sternoclavicular joint. In 1989, they reported on 12 patients treated for painful sternoclavicular joints. The average time from in-

jury was 1.5 years, and the average follow-up after surgery was 4.7 years. In five patients, the sternoclavicular joint was stabilized with a tendon graft from either the palmaris tendon or the plantaris tendon between the first rib and the manubrium; in four patients, the medial 2.5 cm of the clavicle was resected without any type of stabilization; and in three patients, the clavicle was fixed to the first rib with a fascia lata graft. They reported good results in four patients, three treated with tendon grafts and one with a fascia lata graft. They had four fair results and four poor results in those patients who had only resection of the medial clavicle. There was little discussion of the preoperative symptoms, work habits, range of motion, or the degree of joint reduction following the surgery.

Recurrent or Unreduced Dislocation. *Nonoperative Approach.* Should closed maneuvers fail in the adult, an operative procedure should be performed, because most adult patients cannot tolerate posterior displacement of the clavicle into the mediastinum. Holmdahl,[123] Louw and Louw,[162] and Borrero[32] have reported complications following unreduced posterior dislocations. Gangahar and Flogaites[91] reported a case of late thoracic outlet syndrome following an unreduced posterior dislocation, and Borrero[32] reported late and significant vascular problems. I recently was asked to evaluate a patient who, following a significant injury, complained of swelling and bluish coloration of his left arm after any type of physical activity. He really did not have many local sternoclavicular joint symptoms, but by physical examination, the left clavicle was displaced posteriorly. The CT scan demonstrated a major posterior displacement of the left clavicle (Fig. 15–26). Because of the marked displacement and the vascular compromise, arteriography combined with the CT scan was performed, which did not reveal any vascular leak. With the help of the chest surgeon, the clavicle was removed from the mediastinum, the medial 1.5 inches were removed, and the shaft was stabilized to the first rib. The greatest displacement I have seen was in a patient with a posteroinferior dislo-

and with continued lateral traction, a visible and audible reduction occurred. (**E**) Postreduction x-rays showed that the medial clavicle had been restored to its normal position. The reduction was quite stable, and the patient's shoulders were held back with a figure-of-eight strap. (**F**) The right clavicle has remained reduced. Note the periosteal new bone formation along the superior and inferior borders of the right clavicle. This is the result of a physeal injury, whereby the epiphysis remains adjacent to the manubrium while the clavicle is displaced out of a split in the periosteal tube.

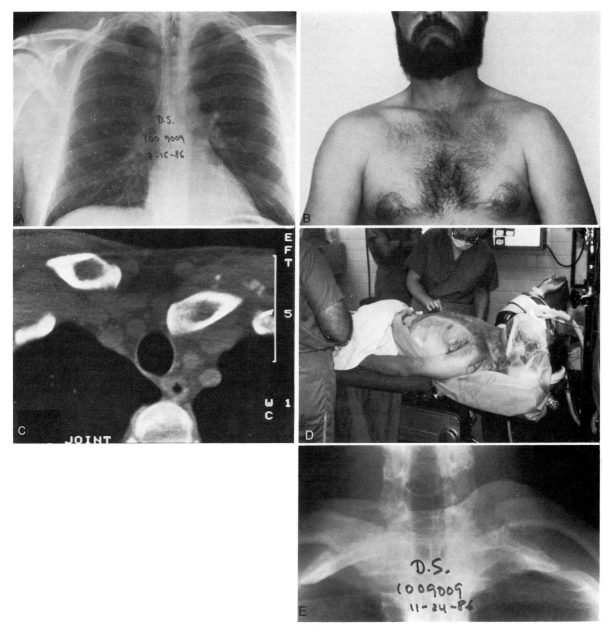

Fig. 15-26. Open reduction of a posterior dislocation of the left sternoclavicular joint causing compression of the great vessels in the mediastinum and resultant swelling in the patient's left arm. (**A**) Chest film does not suggest any serious problem with the left medial clavicle. (**B**) Clinically the patient had a depressed medial end of the left clavicle compared with the right. (**C**) The CT scan reveals posterior displacement of the medial clavicle back into the mediastinum, compressing the great vessels and slightly displacing the trachea. (**D**) The patient was carefully prepared for a surgical repair in cooperation with a cardiovascular surgeon. The patient was prepared from the base of his neck down to the umbilicus so that we could manage any type of vascular problem or complication. Open reduction was accomplished without any vascular incident. The medial end of the clavicle was totally unstable, so the medial 2 cm was resected and the remaining clavicle stabilized to the first rib. (**E**) Four months following surgery, the slight anterior displacement of the clavicle was essentially asymptomatic and the remaining clavicle was stable. (*Reprinted with permission from Rockwood, C. A., and Matsen, F., III (eds.): The Shoulder, Fig. 13-25. Philadelphia: W.B. Saunders, 1990.*)

cation of the medial clavicle down into an intrathoracic position (Fig. 15–27).

However, Louw and Louw[162] reported a 30-year-old patient with a T3–T4 paraplegia and posterior dislocation of the left sternoclavicular joint who had essentially no problems. He underwent an extensive rehabilitation program and could lower himself from his wheelchair to the floor and back again without assistance, and he could transfer from his wheelchair to the bed, bath, and car without difficulty.

If children and adults younger than 25 years of age have symptoms from the pressure of the posteriorly displaced clavicle into the mediastinum, and closed reduction was unsuccessful, an operative procedure should be performed. However, children may have no symptoms, and the physician can wait to see if the physeal plate remodeling process removes the posteriorly displaced bone.

Surgical Reconstructions. There are several basic procedures to maintain the medial end of the clavicle in its normal articulation with the sternum. Fascia lata, suture, internal fixation across the joint, subclavius tendons, osteotomy of the medial clavicle, and resection of the medial end of the clavicle have been advocated.

FASCIA LATA. Bankart[13] and Milch[177] used fascia lata between the clavicle and the sternum. Low-man[163] used a loop of fascia in and through the sternoclavicular joint so that it acts like the ligamentum teres in the hip. Speed[250] and Key and Conwell[141] reported on the use of a fascial loop between the clavicle and the first rib. Allen[6] used fascia lata to reconstruct a new sternoclavicular ligament.

SUBCLAVIUS TENDON. Burrows[42] recommended that the subclavius tendon be used to reconstruct a new costoclavicular ligament. The origin of the subclavius muscle is from the first rib just 6 mm lateral and 1.3 mm anterior to the attachment of the costoclavicular ligament.[102,103] The insertion of the tendon is to the inferior surface of the junction of the middle third with the outer third of the clavicle, and the muscle fibers arising from the tendon insert into the inferior surface of the middle third of the clavicle (Fig. 15–28). The muscle fibers coming off the tendon look like feathers on a bird's wing. Burrows detaches the muscle fiber from the tendon, does not disturb the origin of the tendon, and then passes the tendon through drill holes in the anterior proximal clavicle.

In comparing his operation with the use of free strips of fascia, Burrows said that it is "safer and easier to pick up a mooring than to drop anchor; the obvious mooring is the tendon of the subclavius separated from its muscle fiber and suitably re-

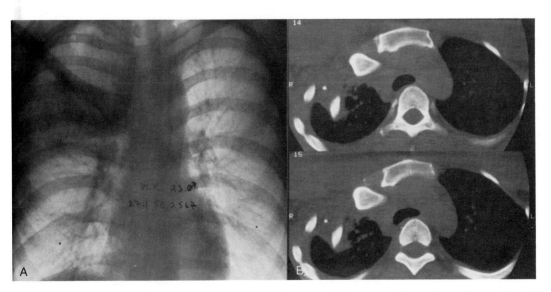

Fig. 15-27. A most unusual posterior, inferior, intrathoracic dislocation of the right medial clavicle. (**A**) On the chest film the clavicle is displaced behind the manubrium down into the parenchyma of the lung. (**B**) The CT scan shows the clavicle down into the lung field with partial collapse of the lung. (Courtesy of Roberto Barja, M.D.) *(Reprinted with permission from Rockwood, C. A., and Matsen, F., III (eds.): The Shoulder, Fig. 13-26. Philadelphia: W.B. Saunders, 1990.)*

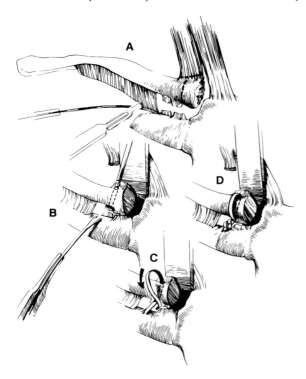

Fig. 15-28. The technique of Jackson Burrows using the subclavius tendon to reconstruct the coracoclavicular ligament. *(Redrawn from Burrows, H. J.: Tenodesis of the Subclavius in the Treatment of Recurrent Dislocation of the Sternoclavicular Joint. J. Bone Joint Surg., 33B:240–243, 1951.) (Reprinted with permission from Rockwood, C. A., and Matsen, F., III (eds.): The Shoulder, Fig. 13-27. Philadelphia: W.B. Saunders, 1990.)*

aligned.'' Lunseth and associates[166] have reported a modified Burrows procedure with the additional use of a threaded Steinmann pin across the joint.

OSTEOTOMY OF THE MEDIAL CLAVICLE. As previously described, Omer,[197] following repair or reconstruction of the ligaments, creates a step-cut osteotomy lateral to the joint and detaches the clavicular head of the sternocleidomastoid muscle from the proximal fragment.

RESECTION OF THE MEDIAL END OF THE CLAVICLE. McLaughlin,[175] Breitner and Wirth,[33] Pridie,[212] Bateman,[18,19] and Milch[177] all have recommended excision of the medial clavicle when degenerative changes are noted in the joint. If the medial end of the clavicle is to be removed because of degenerative changes, the surgeon should be careful not to damage the costoclavicular ligament.

ARTHRODESIS. Arthrodesis was once reported[218] in the treatment of a habitual dislocation of the sternoclavicular joint. However, this procedure should *not* be done because it prevents the previously described normal elevation, depression, and rotation of the clavicle. The end result would be a severe restriction of shoulder movement (Fig. 15–29).

PHYSEAL INJURIES

As has been described earlier in the chapter, the epiphysis on the medial end of the clavicle is the last epiphysis in the body to appear on x-ray and the last one to close. The epiphysis on the medial end of the clavicle does not appear on x-rays until about the 18th year and does not unite with the clavicle until the 23rd to 25th year (Fig. 15–30; see also Fig. 15–5).[102,103,266]

This is important to remember because many so-called dislocations of the sternoclavicular joint are not dislocations but physeal injuries. Most of these injuries will heal with time, without surgical intervention. In time, the remodeling process eliminates any bone deformity or displacement. Anterior physeal injuries can certainly be left alone without problem. Posterior physeal injuries should be reduced. If the posterior dislocation cannot be reduced closed and the patient is having no significant symptoms, the displacement can be observed while remodeling occurs. If the posterior displacement is symptomatic and cannot be reduced closed, the displacement must be reduced during surgery.

In 1967, Denham and Dingley[62] reported three cases of medial clavicle physeal injury in patients aged 14 to 16 years. They demonstrated at surgery that the pathology was indeed a physeal fracture of the medial clavicle. In 1972, Brooks and Henning[35] presented a paper in which they concluded from a review of nine cases that many ''sternoclavicular dislocations'' and ''fractures of the medial clavicle'' were indeed medial clavicle physeal injuries. In 1984, Lemire and Rosman[154] reported a ''double fracture'' of the medial clavicle in a 15-year-old patient. One fracture was through the physis and the other through the medial third of the clavicle. They surgically restored the clavicle into the periosteal tube, and the patient returned to normal activity without any further problems. Winter and associates[271] reported two cases of posterior physeal injuries in children, one 9 years and the other 12 years old. One had displacement against the trachea. The other as seen on the CT scan, had compression of the subclavian vein, which was associated with a carotid artery bruit. Krenzein[146] reported on luxations of the sternocla-

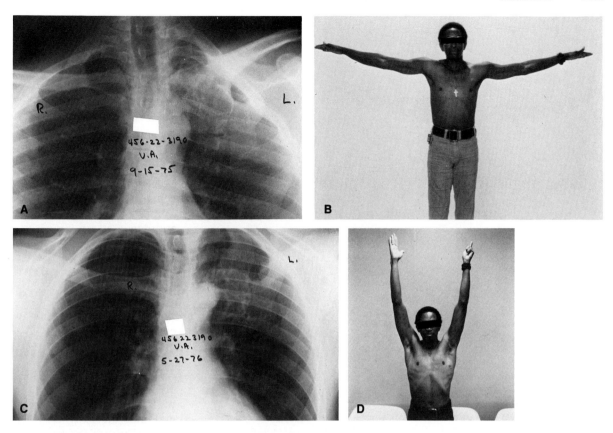

Fig. 15-29. The effect of an arthrodesis of the sternoclavicular joint on shoulder function. (**A**) As a result of a military gunshot wound to the left sternoclavicular joint, this patient had a massive bony union of the left medial clavicle to the sternum and the upper three ribs. (**B**) Shoulder motion was limited to 90° flexion and abduction. (**C**) An x-ray following resection of the bony mass, freeing up the medial clavicle. (**D**) Function of the left shoulder was essentially normal following the elimination of the sternoclavicular arthrodesis.

vicular joint but did not comment on whether they were physeal injuries.

Anterior Displacement of the Medial Clavicle

For an anterior displacement of the medial clavicle, if the physeal injury is recognized or if the patient is younger than 25 years, closed reduction, as described for anterior dislocation of the sternoclavicular joint, should be performed. The shoulders should be held back in a clavicular strap or figure-of-eight dressing for 3 to 4 weeks, even if the reduction is stable. Healing is prompt, and remodeling will occur at the site of the deformity.

Posterior Displacement of the Medial Clavicle

Closed reduction of a posterior displacement of the medial clavicle should be performed in the manner described for posterior dislocation of the sternocla-

vicular joint. The reduction is usually stable with shoulders held back in a figure-of-eight dressing or strap. Immobilization should continue for 3 to 4 weeks. If the posterior physeal injury cannot be reduced, the patient is not having symptoms, and the patient is younger than 23 years, the physician can wait to see if remodeling eliminates the posterior displacement of the clavicle (Fig. 15–30C).

ATRAUMATIC PROBLEMS

Spontaneous Subluxation or Dislocation

Spontaneous subluxations and dislocations of the sternoclavicular joint are seen most often in patients younger than 20 years and more often in females. Without significant trauma, one or both of the medial clavicles spontaneously displace anteriorly

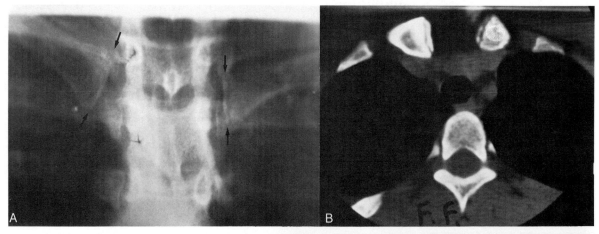

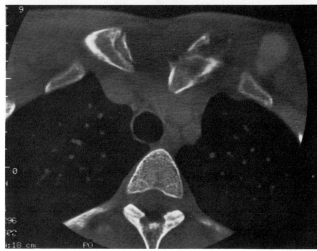

Fig. 15-30. An anteroposterior view of the medial ends of both clavicles demonstrates the thin, waferlike appearance of the epiphysis of the medial clavicle. (**B**) A CT scan of the sternoclavicular joints demonstrates the epiphyses of both medial clavicles. (**C**) Posterior sternoclavicular physeal injury of right medial clavicle. The patient is 18 years old and has no symptoms of the dislocation. Note that the physeal plate has remained in its normal position. Remodeling will eliminate the posteriorly displaced metaphysis. (*A, B reprinted with permission from Rockwood, C. A., and Matsen, F., III (eds.): The Shoulder, Fig. 13-29A, B. Philadelphia: W.B. Saunders, 1990.*)

during abduction or flexion to the overhead position. (See Fig. 15–10.) The clavicle reduces when the arm is returned to the side. This usually is associated with laxity in other joints of the extremities. Odor and I reviewed 37 cases and found it to be a self-limiting condition.[226] The conditions should not be treated with *attempted* surgical reconstruction, because the joint will continue to subluxate or dislocate and surgery may indeed cause more pain, discomfort, and an unsightly scar (Fig. 15–31). The condition should be carefully explained to the patient and the family, and they should be told that ultimately it will not be a problem and the symptoms may disappear.

Congenital or Developmental Problems

Congenital or developmental problems (eg, absence or partial absence of bone or muscles) can produce subluxation or dislocation of the sternoclavicular joint. Specific rehabilitation or surgical procedures are usually unnecessary.[105,187]

Arthritis

The management of patients with osteoarthritis or postmenopausal osteoarthritis can usually be done with conservative nonoperative treatment (ie, heat, anti-inflammatory agents, and rest).[29,34] However, the patient must be thoroughly evaluated to rule out other conditions that mimic the changes in the sternoclavicular joint (eg, tumor, metabolic, infectious, collagen disorders). Patients with post-traumatic arthritic changes in the sternoclavicular joint, which follow fractures of the sternoclavicular joint and previous attempts at reconstruction, may require formal arthroplasty of the joint and careful stabilization of the remaining clavicle to the first rib.

Patients with collagen disorders, such as rheu-

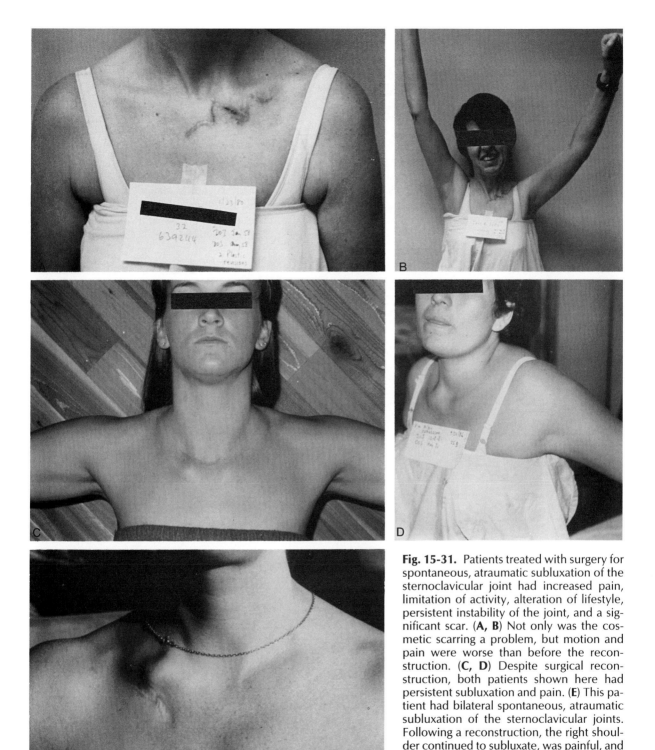

Fig. 15-31. Patients treated with surgery for spontaneous, atraumatic subluxation of the sternoclavicular joint had increased pain, limitation of activity, alteration of lifestyle, persistent instability of the joint, and a significant scar. (**A, B**) Not only was the cosmetic scarring a problem, but motion and pain were worse than before the reconstruction. (**C, D**) Despite surgical reconstruction, both patients shown here had persistent subluxation and pain. (**E**) This patient had bilateral spontaneous, atraumatic subluxation of the sternoclavicular joints. Following a reconstruction, the right shoulder continued to subluxate, was painful, and significantly altered the patient's lifestyle. The left shoulder had minimal subluxations and was essentially asymptomatic. (*Reprinted with permission from Rockwood, C. A., and Matsen, F., III (eds.): The Shoulder, Fig. 13-30. Philadelphia: W.B. Saunders, 1990.*)

matoid arthritis, and some patients with condensing osteitis of the medial clavicle may require arthroplasty. In operating on the sternoclavicular joint, care must be taken to evaluate the residual stability of the medial clavicle. It is the same analogy as used when resecting the distal clavicle for an old acromioclavicular joint problem. If the coracoclavicular ligaments are intact, an excision of the distal clavicle is indicated. If the coracoclavicular ligaments are gone, then in addition to excision of the distal clavicle, you must reconstruct the coracoclavicular ligaments. If the costoclavicular liga-

ments are intact, the clavicle medial to the ligaments should be resected and beveled smooth (Fig. 15–32). If the ligaments are gone, the clavicle must be stabilized to the first rib. If too much clavicle is resected, or if the clavicle is not stabilized to the first rib, an increase in symptoms can occur (Fig. 15–33).

Sternocostalclavicular hyperostosis is a very difficult problem to manage.[4,52,96,99,134,149,231,245–247] The condition cannot be arrested with medication. Treatment is largely dependent on pain and anti-inflammatory medications and physical therapy.

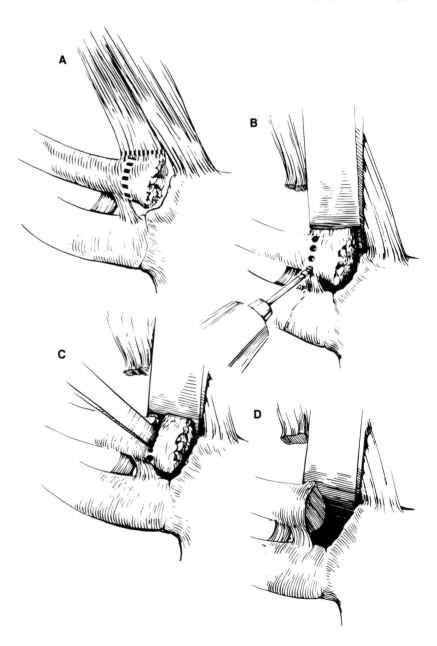

Fig. 15-32. Technique for resecting the medial clavicle for degenerative arthritis. (**A**) Care must be taken to remove only that part of the clavicle medial to the costoclavicular (rhomboid) ligaments. There must be adequate protection for the vital structures that lie posterior to the medial end of the clavicle. (**B, C**) An air drill with a side-cutting burr can be used to perform the osteotomy. (**D**) When the fragment of bone has been removed, the dorsal and anterior borders of the clavicle should be smoothed down to give a better cosmetic appearance.

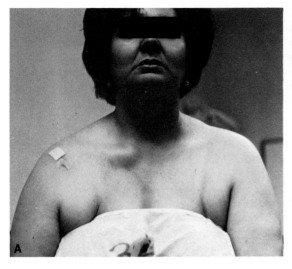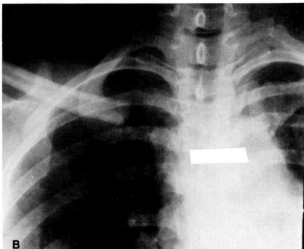

Fig. 15-33. (**A**) This postmenopausal, right-handed woman had a resection of the right medial clavicle because of preoperative diagnosis of "possible tumor." The postoperative microscopic diagnosis was degenerative arthritis of the right medial clavicle. Following surgery, the patient complained of pain and discomfort, marked prominence, and gross instability of the right medial clavicle. (**B**) An x-ray confirms that the excision of the medial clavicle extended lateral to the costoclavicular ligaments, hence, the patient had an unstable medial clavicle.

Occasionally, surgical excision of the bony mass to allow an increase in function of the upper extremity is indicated.

Infection

Infections of the sternoclavicular joint should be managed as they are in other joints, except that during aspiration and surgical drainage, great care and respect must be directed to the vital structures that lie posterior to the joint. If aspiration or a high index of suspicion demonstrates purulent material in the joint, a formal arthrotomy should be carried out. The anterior sternoclavicular ligament will need to be removed, but the posterior and interclavicular ligaments should be spared. Occasionally, the infection will arise in the medial end of the clavicle or the manubrium, which will necessitate the resection of some of the dead bone. Depending on the status of the wound following debridement, one can either close the wound loosely over a drain or pack the wound open and close it later.

AUTHOR'S PREFERRED METHODS OF TREATMENT

TRAUMATIC INJURIES

Mild Sprain

For mild sprains (type I injuries), I recommend the use of cold packs for the first 12 to 24 hours and a

sling to rest the joint. Ordinarily, after 5 to 7 days, the patient can use the arm for everyday activities.

Moderate Sprain (Subluxation)

In addition to the cold pack, for subluxations (type II injuries), I may use a soft, padded figure-of-eight clavicle strap to gently hold the shoulders back to allow the sternoclavicular joint to rest. The harness can be removed after a week or so; then the arm is placed in a sling for about another week, or the patient is allowed to return gradually to everyday activities.

Severe Sprain (Dislocation)

In general, I manage almost all dislocations (type III injuries) of the sternoclavicular joint in children and in adults by either a closed reduction or by "skillful neglect." The acute traumatic posterior dislocations are reduced closed and become stable when the shoulders are held back in a figure-of-eight dressing. Most of the anterior dislocations are unstable, but I accept the deformity since I believe it is less of a problem than the potential problems of operative repair and internal fixation.

ANTERIOR DISLOCATION

Method of Reduction. In most instances, knowing that the anterior dislocation will be unstable, I still try to reduce the anterior displacement. Muscle relaxants and narcotics are administered intravenously, and the patient is placed supine on the table with a stack of three or four towels between the shoulder blades. While an assistant gently applies downward pressure on the anterior aspect of both shoulders, I push the medial end of the clavicle backward where it belongs. On some occasions, rare as they may be, the anterior displacement may stay adjacent to the sternum. However, in most cases, either with the shoulders still held back or when they are relaxed, an anterior displacement promptly recurs. I explain to the patient that the joint is unstable and that the hazards of internal fixation are too great, and I prescribe a sling for a couple of weeks and allow the patient to begin using the arm as soon as the discomfort is gone.

Most of the anterior injuries that I have treated in patients up to 25 years of age are not dislocations of the sternoclavicular joint but type I or II physeal injuries, which heal and remodel without operative treatment. Patients older than 23 to 25 years with anterior dislocations of the sternoclavicular joint do have persistent prominence of the anterior clavicle. However, this does not seem to interfere with usual activities and, in some cases, has not even interfered with heavy manual labor.

I wish to reemphasize that *I do not recommend open reduction* of the joint, and I would *never* recommend transfixing pins across the sternoclavicular joint.

Postreduction Care. If the reduction is stable, I place the patient in either a figure-of-eight dressing or in whatever device or position the clavicle is most stable. If the reduction is unstable, the arm is placed into a sling for a week or so, and then the patient can begin to use the arm for gentle everyday activities.

POSTERIOR DISLOCATION

It is important to take a very careful history and to perform a very careful physical examination in the patient with a posterior sternoclavicular dislocation. The physician should obtain x-rays, tomograms or CT scans, or angio–CT scans to document whether there is any compression of the great vessels in the neck or arm or any difficulty in swallowing or breathing. It is also important to determine if the patient has a feeling of choking or hoarseness. If any of these symptoms are present, indicating pressure on the mediastinum, the appropriate specialist should be consulted.

I do not believe that operative techniques are usually required to reduce acute posterior sternoclavicular joint dislocations. Furthermore, once the joint has been reduced closed, it is usually stable (Fig. 15–34).

Although I used to think that I could always make the diagnosis of anterior or posterior injury of the sternoclavicular joint on physical examination, I know now that one cannot rely on the anterior swelling and firmness as being diagnostic of an anterior injury. I have been fooled on six occasions when, from physical examination, the patient appeared to have an anterior dislocation, but x-rays documented a posterior problem. Therefore, I recommend that the clinical impression *always* be documented with appropriate x-ray studies before a decision to treat or not to treat is made.

Method of Closed Reduction. The patient is placed in the supine position with a 3- to 4-inch-thick sandbag or three to four folded towels between the scapulas to extend the shoulders. The dislocated shoulder should be over toward the edge of the table so that the arm and shoulder can be abducted and extended. If the patient is having extreme pain and muscle spasm and is quite anxious, I use general anesthesia; otherwise, narcotics, muscle relaxants, or tranquilizers are given through an established intravenous route in the normal arm. First, gentle traction is applied on the abducted arm in line with the clavicle while countertraction is applied by an assistant who steadies the patient on the table. The traction on the abducted arm is gradually increased while the arm is brought into extension.

Reduction of an acute injury usually occurs with an audible pop or snap and the relocation can be noted visibly. If the traction in abduction and extension is not successful, an assistant grasps or pushes down on the clavicle in an effort to dislodge it from behind the sternum. Occasionally, in a stubborn case, especially in a thick-chested person or a patient with extensive swelling, it is impossible to obtain a secure grasp on the clavicle with the assistant's fingers. The skin should then be surgically prepared and a sterile towel clip used to gain purchase on the medial clavicle percutaneously. (See Fig. 15–25.) The towel clip is used to grasp completely around the shaft of the clavicle. The dense cortical bone prevents the purchase of the towel clip into the clavicle. Then the combined traction through the arm plus the anterior lifting force on the towel clip will reduce the dislocation. Following the reduction, the sternoclavicular joint is stable, even with the patient's arms at the side. However, I always hold the shoulders back in a well-padded figure-of-eight clavicle strap for 3 to 4 weeks to allow for soft tissue and ligamentous healing.

I have not used the technique described by Butterworth and Kirk[43] of traction on the arm in adduction, but I believe this technique is valid and

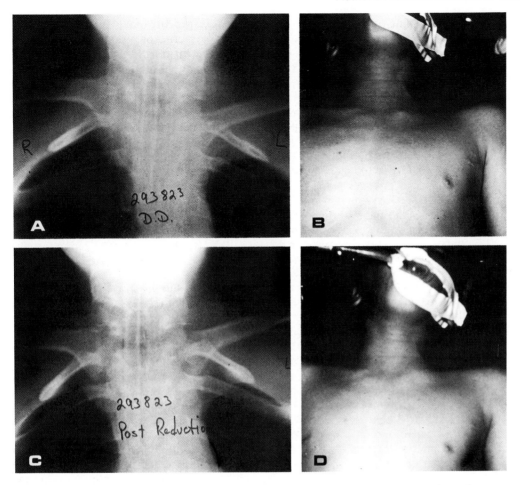

Fig. 15-34. Posterior dislocation or type I epiphyseal separation of the left sternoclavicular joint in a 12-year-old boy. (**A**) The 40° cephalic tilt "serendipity" x-ray reveals that the left clavicle is significantly lower on the horizontal plane than the normal right clavicle. Prior to reduction, the medial end of the left clavicle was displaced posteriorly compared with the normal right clavicle. The only remaining prominence of the left sternoclavicular joint was the prominence of the superomedial corner of the manubrium. (**C**) Under general anesthesia, a closed reduction was performed by traction on the arm out into abduction and extension. The clavicle reduced with an audible "pop" back into position. It was restored to the same horizontal level as the normal right clavicle. (**D**) Clinically, both clavicles were palpable at the same level following reduction.

will use it should the traction abduction technique fail.

Method of Open Reduction.   The complications of an unreduced posterior dislocation are numerous—thoracic outlet syndrome,[91] vascular compromise,[32] and erosion of the medial clavicle into any of the vital structures that lie posterior to the sternoclavicular joint. Therefore, in adults, if closed reduction fails, an open reduction should be performed.

The patient is supine on the table, and the three

to four towels or sandbag should be left between the scapulae. The upper extremity should be draped out free so that lateral traction can be applied during the open reduction. In addition, a folded sheet around the patient's thorax should be left in place so that it can be used for countertraction during the traction on the involved extremity. An anterior incision is used that parallels the superior border of the medial 3 to 4 inches of the clavicle and then extends downward over the sternum just medial to the involved sternoclavicular joint. As previously described, this should usually be done with a thoracic surgeon. The trick is to remove sufficient soft tissues to expose the joint but to leave the anterior capsular ligament intact. The reduction can usually be accomplished with traction and countertraction while lifting up anteriorly with a clamp around the medial clavicle. Along with the traction and countertraction, it may be necessary to use an elevator to pry the clavicle back to its articulation with the sternum. When the reduction has been obtained, and with the shoulders held back, the reduction will be stable because the anterior capsule has been left intact. If the anterior capsule is damaged or is insufficient to prevent anterior displacement of the medial end of the clavicle, I recommend excision of the medial 1 to 1.5 inches of the clavicle and securing the residual clavicle to the first rib with 1-mm Dacron tape. Postoperatively, the patient should be held with the shoulders back in a figure-of-eight dressing for 4 to 6 weeks to allow for healing of the soft tissues.

I *do not* recommend the use of Kirschner wires, Steinmann pins, or any other type of metallic pins to stabilize the sternoclavicular joint. The complications are horrendous, as will be discussed in the section on complications.

PHYSEAL INJURIES OF THE MEDIAL CLAVICLE

I believe many anterior and posterior injuries of the sternoclavicular joint in patients younger than 25 years which are thought to be "dislocations" are, in fact, injuries to the medial physis of the clavicle. Many authors have observed at the time of surgery that the intra-articular disk ligament stays with the sternum, and I agree with them. In addition, I submit that the unossified or ossified epiphyseal disk, depending on the age of the patient, also stays with the sternum. Anatomically, the epiphysis is lateral to the articular disk ligament, and it is held in place by the capsular ligament and can be mistaken for the intra-articular disk ligament.

As previously described, the medial epiphysis does not ossify and thus does not appear on the x-ray until the age of 18. Therefore, the diagnosis cannot be "documented" until after ossification occurs. However, I still perform the closed reduction maneuvers as described above for a suspected anterior or posterior injury. Open reduction of the physeal injury is seldom indicated, except for an irreducible posterior displacement in a patient with significant symptoms of compression of the vital structures in the mediastinum. After reduction, the shoulders are held back with a figure-of-eight strap or dressing for 3 to 4 weeks.

In 1966, I first treated a 16-year-old boy with a fracture of the medial third of the clavicle and a "dislocation" of the sternoclavicular joint which turned out to be a type I epiphyseal injury (Fig. 15-35). I thought then that it might be an original observation. Since I could not find any references on the problem, I was ready to publish my observation when my good friend Lee Rogers, M.D. (now Professor and Chairman of the Department of Radiology at Northwestern Medical School) recommended I review a text written by John Poland in 1898. As happens with most "new" ideas in orthopaedics, my observation was not new. Poland,[210] in his text entitled *Traumatic Separation of Epiphyses of the Upper Extremity*, described the same entity in detail. He reviewed several French articles that evaluated more than 60 cases of fracture of the medial epiphysis of the clavicle that clinically appeared as

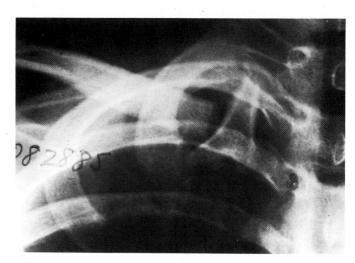

Fig. 15-35. Type I epiphyseal separation of the right medial clavicle associated with fracture of the shaft of the clavicle, with 90° rotation of the segment.

sternoclavicular dislocations. He discussed the anatomy of the joint and the classifications of the injury and described methods of treatment. He described in detail an article by Verchere, written in 1886, which probably represents the first published report of a death caused by posterior dislocation of the sternoclavicular joint:

> A 20-year-old man, following a severe crushing injury, died on the seventh day, of subcutaneous emphysema. Autopsy revealed that the inner third of the right clavicle was detached of its periosteum, and its smooth rounded end was displaced posteriorly and had produced a perforation of the pleural sac about the size of a 2-franc piece. The hole was in the left lung, whereas the ipsilateral lung escaped injury.

The report very clearly described that the sternoclavicular joint was not injured and that the 5-mm-wide epiphyseal plate was held firmly in place by the ligaments about the joint. The specimen of the separated epiphysis was placed in the Dupuytren Museum.

Poland went on to describe that the capsular ligament is primarily attached to the epiphysis of the medial clavicle and stated that with injury the epiphysis is held by the capsular ligament and stays with its articulation with the sternum.

In treating the 16-year-old boy with the fracture of the medial clavicle and the "dislocation" of the sternoclavicular joint, I figured that I needed to, at least, line up the clavicle and put the sternoclavicular joint in better approximation. (See Fig. 15–38.) The fragment was 3.7 cm long and had rotated 90° from the long axis of the clavicle. In my eagerness to explore the anatomy, the fragment of clavicle, which had been completely stripped of its periosteum, fell onto the floor. However, the sternal end of the fragment did not have a smooth cartilaginous articular surface. It was rough and had the appearance of the end of a chicken leg, when the last bite had taken off the epiphysis. The costoclavicular ligaments were intact to the periosteum inferiorly, and in the most medial corner of the periosteal tube was a dense structure that could be taken for the intra-articular disk ligament—or it could have been the unossified epiphysis.

Treatment consisted of closing the periosteal tube

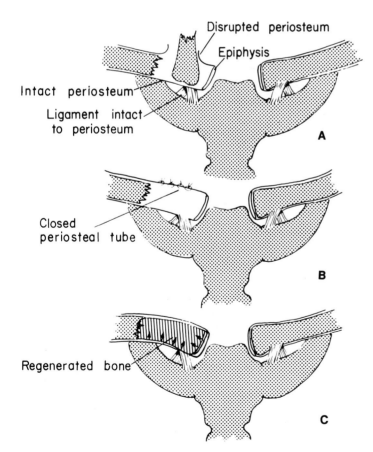

Fig. 15-36. Schematic of the injury and healing of the patient in Fig. 15-35. (**A**) The fragment, with its metaphysis, has been separated from the epiphyseal plate and partially displaced out of the periosteal tube. (**B**) The fragment was removed, and the defect in the periosteal tube was closed. The coracoclavicular ligaments were intact and were attached inferiorly to the periosteal tube. The epiphysis remained in its normal anatomic position by the sternoclavicular capsular ligaments. (**C**) At 18 months, the medial end of the clavicle was replaced by new bone formation from the epiphysis and the periosteum.

and hoping that the epiphysis was still present adjacent to the sternum (Fig. 15–36). Later, microscopic studies of the most medial end of the fragment revealed the provisional zone of calcification of the metaphysis, indicating that indeed there had been a separation through the physeal plate and that it had occurred through the zone of hypertrophy (Fig. 15–37). Serial x-rays revealed a gradual replacement of the medial clavicle, and after 18 months the entire defect had been replaced with bone (Fig. 15–38**A**). The patient returned to his former job as a manual laborer (Fig. 15–38**B,C**).

Since 1966, in other cases of "dislocation of the sternoclavicular joint," I have been able to document with the 40° cephalic tilt x-ray view and CT scans that the injury really was a physeal fracture, because the thin, wafer-like disk has remained in

its normal articulation with the sternum, while the metaphysis and shaft were displaced. Some of the physeal fractures have been type II injuries, with a small fragment of the metaphysis remaining with the epiphysis. Obviously, before the epiphysis ossifies at the age of 18, one cannot be sure whether a displacement about the sternoclavicular joint is a dislocation of the sternoclavicular joint or a fracture through the physeal plate.

Despite the fact that there is significant displacement of the shaft with either a type I or type II physeal fracture, the periosteal tube remains in its anatomic position and the attaching ligaments are intact to the periosteum (ie, the costoclavicular ligaments inferiorly and the capsular and interarticular disk ligaments medially) (Fig. 15–39).

RECURRENT TRAUMATIC DISLOCATION

Recurrent anterior or posterior dislocation of the sternoclavicular joint following an acute injury is extremely rare; I have not seen or read of such a case. Usually the joint is stable following reduction, or it remains permanently anteriorly or posteriorly displaced. This entity should not be confused with the problem of spontaneous subluxation or dislocation.

UNREDUCED TRAUMATIC DISLOCATION
OF THE STERNOCLAVICULAR JOINT

Anterior Dislocation. As previously described, most patients with an unreduced and permanent anterior dislocation of the sternoclavicular joint are not very symptomatic, have almost a complete range of motion, and can work and even perform manual labor without many problems (Fig. 15–40). Because the joint is so small and incongruous and because the results I have seen in patients who have had attempted reconstructions are so miserable, I usually recommend skillful neglect. In patients who have had a previous failed sternoclavicular operative procedure, I perform a repeat arthroplasty with a resection of the medial clavicle in an attempt to reduce and stabilize the joint with suture, fascia, tendons, and so on.

If the patient has persistent symptoms of traumatic arthritis for 6 to 12 months following a dislocation, and if the symptoms can be completely relieved by injection of local anesthesia into the sternoclavicular joint region, I perform an arthroplasty of the sternoclavicular joint. This includes a resection of the medial 1 inch of the clavicle with a beveling of the superoanterior corner for cosmetic purposes, a debridement of the intra-articular disk ligament, and stabilization of the remaining clavicle

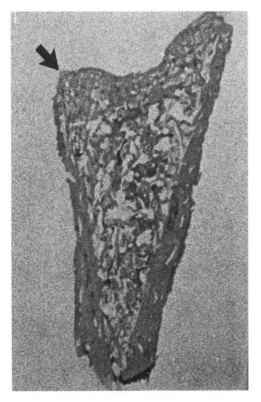

Fig. 15-37. Microscopic examination of the fragment of clavicle that was removed from the patient in Fig. 15-35. The medial end of the fragment revealed the provisional zone of calcification of the metaphysis. This indicates that the epiphysis of the medial clavicle was still in its normal position adjacent to the manubrium. The physeal injury occurred through the zone of hypertrophy.

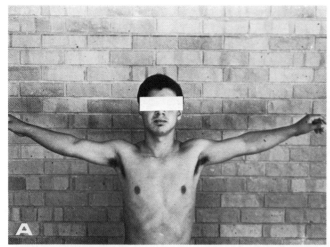

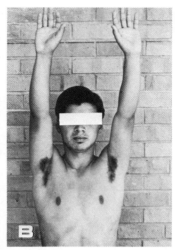

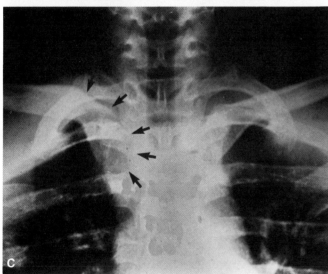

Fig. 15-38. (**A, B**) Eighteen months after the injury shown in Fig. 15-35, the patient had a full range of motion, was asymptomatic, and was performing manual labor. (**C**) X-ray of the sternoclavicular joint taken 18 months after the removal of the medial clavicle. There has been total regeneration of the medical clavicle by the periosteal tube and the retained epiphysis.

to the first rib with either 1-mm or 3-mm cotton Dacron tape. If the costoclavicular ligaments do not stabilize the medial clavicle, it is essential to construct a ligament-like structure between the clavicle and the first rib. I also detach the clavicular head of the sternocleidomastoid to temporarily resist the upward pull of the clavicle by this muscle.

Posterior Dislocation.   In the adult, because of the potential problems that can be associated with the clavicle remaining displaced posteriorly into the mediastinum, an open reduction is usually indicated. This requires excision of the medial 1 inch of the clavicle and stabilization to the first rib as described above.

ATRAUMATIC PROBLEMS

Spontaneous Subluxation or Dislocation

I have seen 37 patients with spontaneous subluxation or dislocation of the sternoclavicular joint. About the only symptom they have is that the medial end of the clavicle subluxates or dislocates anteriorly when they raise their arms over their heads.[226] This occurs spontaneously and without any significant trauma (Fig. 15–41). Many of these patients have the characteristic finding of generalized ligamentous laxity (ie, hyperextension of the elbows, knees, and fingers as well as hypermobility of the glenohumeral joints). This problem might be

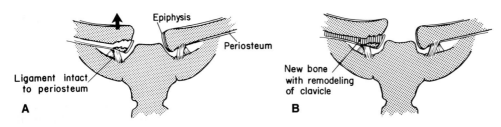

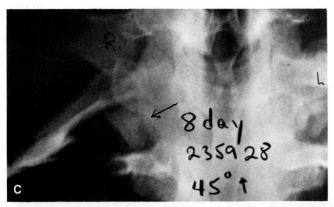

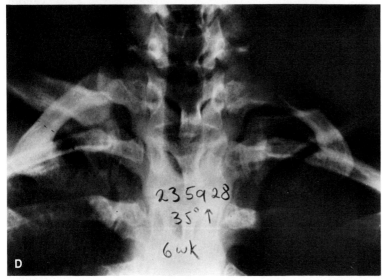

Fig. 15-39. A type II physeal injury of the right medial clavicle. (**A**) A schematic of the healing process with a type II physeal injury to the medial clavicle. The medial clavicle splits out of the periosteal tube, leaving a small fragment (Thurston-Holland sign) behind. The costoclavicular ligaments are intact to the inferior periosteal tube. (**B**) Through remodeling from the retained epiphysis and the periosteal tube, the fracture heals itself. (**C**) The x-ray at 8 days reveals that the right medial clavicle is displaced superiorly from the left clavicle. The inferior medial corner of the clavicle is still located in its normal position adjacent to the epiphysis. (**D**) The x-ray at 6 weeks reveals new bone formation along the inferior periosteal tube. Note the thin epiphyseal plate of the normal left medial clavicle. (**E, F**) Clinically, at 8 weeks the physeal injury was healed and the patient had a full range of motion. (*Reprinted with permission from Rockwood, C. A., and Matsen, F., III (eds.): The Shoulder, Fig. 13-38. Philadelphia: W.B. Saunders, 1990.*)

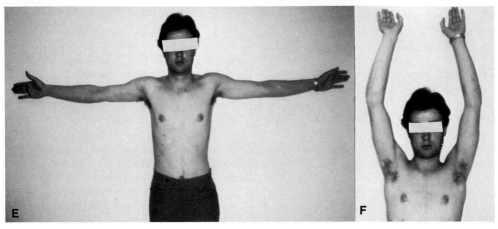

considered voluntary or involuntary, because it occurs whenever the patient raises the arms to the overhead position. Some patients seen for another shoulder problem are completely unaware that with the overhead motion the medial end of the clavicle subluxates or dislocates. I have never seen a spontaneous posterior subluxation of the sternoclavicular joint. Only occasionally does the patient with atraumatic anterior displacement complain of pain during the displacement. Because I do not believe that I can stabilize the joint and prevent the subluxation or dislocation and end up with a pain-free range of motion, I manage the problem with skillful neglect. I very carefully explain the anatomy of the problem to the patient and the family. I explain further that surgery is of little benefit, that they should discontinue the voluntary aspect of the dislocation, and that in time either the symptoms will disappear or they will completely forget that the dislocation is a problem.

In the review by Odor and me of 37 patients with spontaneous atraumatic subluxation, 29 were managed without surgery and 8 were treated (elsewhere) with surgical reconstruction.[226] With an average follow-up of more than 8 years, all 29 nonoperated patients were doing just fine without limitations of activity or lifestyle. The eight patients treated with surgery had increased pain, limitation of activity, alteration of lifestyle, persistent instability, and significant scars. In many instances, before reconstruction or resection, these patients had minimal discomfort, excellent range of motion, and only complained of a "bump" that slipped in and out of place with certain motions. Postoperatively, these patients still had the bump, along with scars and painful range of motion. (See Fig. 15–31.)

Arthritis

Most patients with simple degenerative arthritis or postmenopausal osteoarthritis can be managed with rest, moist heat, and anti-inflammatory medications (See Figs. 15–12 and 15–13.) As previously described, it is very important to do a good work-up of the patient with arthritis of the sternoclavicular joint to rule out tumor, arthropathies, condensing osteitis of the medial clavicle, and sternocostoclavicular hyperostosis. Patients with posttraumatic osteoarthritis or sternocostoclavicular hyperostosis may require resection of the medial clavicle. Care must be taken to remove enough, but not too much, of the medial clavicle (Fig. 15–42).

Infection

I believe that pus in the sternoclavicular joint should be managed by arthrotomy and exploration. If the procedure is done soon after the onset of the infection, the arthrotomy and joint clean-out usually are sufficient. If the infection is long-standing and there is destruction of the cartilage and bone, a resection of the medial clavicle or the involved manubrium should be performed. Care should be taken to preserve the posterior, interclavicular, and costoclavicular ligaments. (See Fig. 15–14.)

COMPLICATIONS OF INJURIES TO THE STERNOCLAVICULAR JOINT

The serious complications that occur at the time of dislocation of the sternoclavicular joint are primarily limited to the posterior injuries. About the only complications that occur with the anterior dislocation of the sternoclavicular joint are a "cosmetic bump" or late degenerative changes.

Many complications have been reported secondary to the retrosternal dislocation: pneumothorax and laceration of the superior vena cava;[201] venous congestion in the neck; rupture of the esophagus with abscess and osteomyelitis of the clavicle;[31] pressure on the subclavian artery in an untreated patient;[125,251] occlusion of the subclavian artery late in a patient who was not treated;[251] compression of the right common carotid artery by a fracture–dislocation of the sternoclavicular joint;[125] brachial plexus compression;[174] and hoarseness of the voice, onset of snoring, and voice changes from normal to falsetto with movement of the arm (Fig. 15–43; see also Fig. 15–26).[31,139,178,232,261] Wasylenko and Busse[263] reported a posterior dislocation of the medial clavicle that caused a fatal tracheoesophageal fistula. Gangahar and Flogaites[91] reported a posterior dislocation of the clavicle that produced a severe thoracic outlet syndrome with swelling and cyanosis of the upper extremity. Gardner and Bidstrup[92] reported three patients who had severe great-vessel injuries following blunt chest trauma and posterior dislocation of the sternoclavicular joint; two cases involved the innominate artery, and one the carotid and subclavian arteries.

Several of my patients have had unusual complications from traumatic injuries to the sternoclavicular joint. One patient, as the result of a posterior dislocation and rupture of the trachea, developed massive subcutaneous emphysema (Fig. 15–44). Another patient had an anterior dislocation on the right and a posterior dislocation on the left. When first seen, his blood pressure was very low. Following reduction of the posterior dislocation, his blood pressure, as recorded on his monitor, instantly returned to normal (Fig. 15–45). It was theorized that the posteriorly displaced clavicle was irritating some

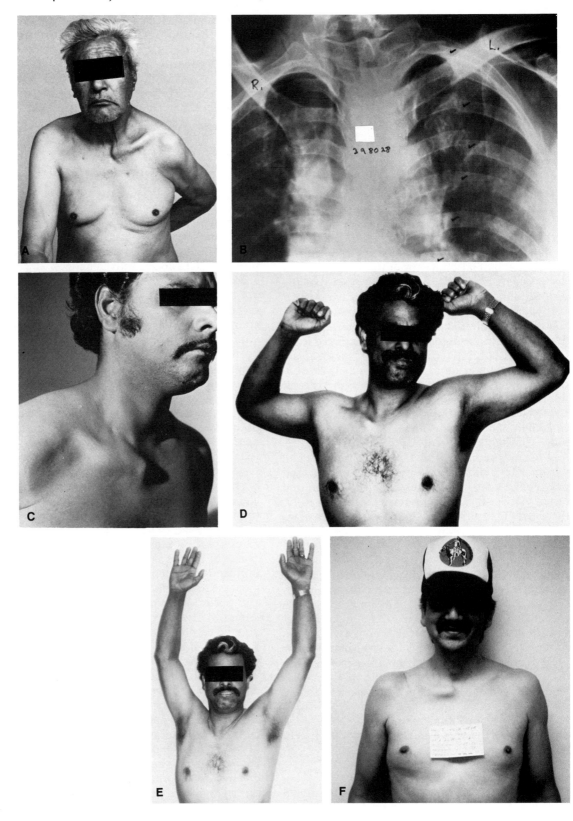

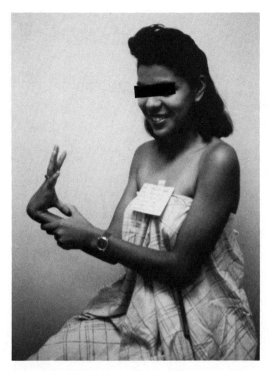

Fig. 15-41. This patient has developed spontaneous subluxation of her sternoclavicular joints. She also has generalized ligamentous laxity of the wrists, fingers, and elbows.

of the vital structures of the mediastinum. Another patient, who had vascular compromise, was already discussed. (See Fig. 15–26.) Another patient had a traumatic injury to both sternoclavicular joints— the left was posterior and the right was anterior. Following reduction of the left posterior dislocation, the right side remained unstable. However, he developed a painless full range of motion (Fig. 15–46).

Worman and Leagus,[274] in an excellent review of the complications associated with posterior dislocations of the sternoclavicular joint, reported that 16 of 60 patients reviewed from the literature had suffered complications of the trachea, esophagus, or great vessels. I should point out that even though the incidence of complications was 25%, only four deaths have been reported as a result of this injury.[104,139,210]

COMPLICATIONS OF OPERATIVE PROCEDURES

Through 1984, six deaths[50,95,155,185,232] and three near deaths[37,200,274] from complications of transfixing the sternoclavicular joint with Kirschner wires or Steinmann pins were reported. The pins, either intact or broken, migrated into the heart, pulmonary artery, innominate artery, or aorta. Tremendous leverage force is applied to pins that cross the sternoclavicular joint, and fatigue breakage of the pins is common. Most of the deaths or near deaths were reported in the 1960s;[37,155,185,200,232,274] one was reported in 1974.[50] To my knowledge, there were no deaths reported that occurred as a result of migrating pins from the sternoclavicular joint, until the report in 1984 by Gerlach and associates[95] from West Germany. They reported two deaths from migrating nails that caused cardiac tamponade. The physicians were charged with manslaughter by negligence. *I do not recommend use of any transfixing pins—large or small, smooth or threaded, bent or straight—across the sternoclavicular joint.*

Brown[37] has reported three complications in ten operative cases: two from broken pins which had to be removed from a window in the sternum; and one a near death, in which the pin penetrated the back of the sternum and entered the right pulmonary artery. Nordback and Markkula[192] removed a

←————————————————————————————————

Fig. 15-40. Unreduced anterior traumatic dislocations of the sternoclavicular joint. (**A**) This patient has an anterior unreduced dislocation of the left sternoclavicular joint. He works as a laborer and has few, if any, complaints. (**B**) The injury occurred 5 years prior to the photograph, when he had a dislocation and multiple fractures of his ribs. (**C**) The patient suffered an unreduced traumatic anterior dislocation in his right shoulder following an automobile accident. At the time of the injury the medial clavicle could be manually reduced, but it would not stay in position. (**D, E**) Fifteen years later the patient continues to have prominence of his right medial clavicle, but he works as a day laborer unloading and loading 50-pound sacks of cement. (**F**) Following a traumatic total dislocation of this patient's right clavicle, he persisted in having symptoms secondary to a posterior dislocation of the acromioclavicular joint, which required a reconstruction. However, despite his anterior dislocation of the sternoclavicular joint, he had a full range of motion and no pain in the sternoclavicular joint. (*D–F reprinted with permission from Rockwood, C. A., and Matsen, F., III (eds.): The Shoulder, Fig. 13-39. Philadelphia: W.B. Saunders, 1990.*)

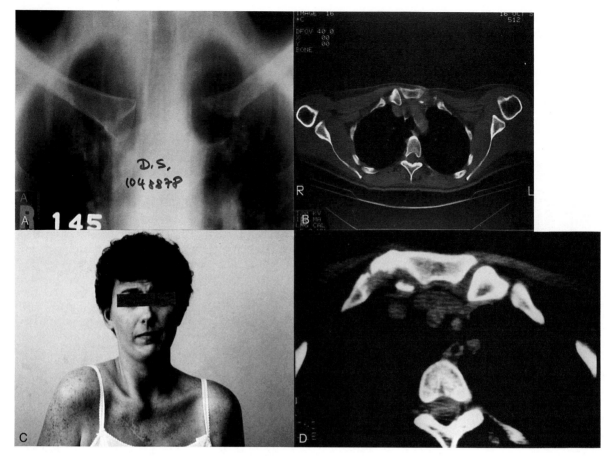

Fig. 15-42. In performing sternoclavicular joint arthroplasty, care must be taken to remove sufficient bone. **(A, B)** Following resection of the left medial clavicle, this patient continued to have pain with shoulder motion. The CT scan confirms fragments of bone in the site of the arthroplasty. **(C)** Following arthroplasty of the right sternoclavicular joint, the medial clavicle was still quite prominent and painful. **(D)** A CT scan confirms the medial right clavicle butting into the manubrium and a loose fragment of bone in the joint. *(Reprinted with permission from Rockwood, C. A., and Matsen, F., III (eds.): The Shoulder, Fig. 13-40. Philadelphia: W.B. Saunders, 1990.)*

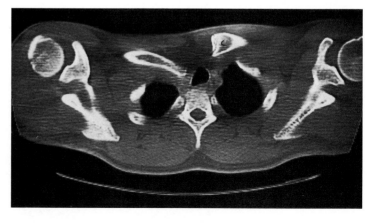

Fig. 15-43. A CT scan demonstrates posterior dislocation of the clavicle back into the mediastinum, displacing the trachea. *(Reprinted with permission from Rockwood, C. A., and Matsen, F., III (eds.): The Shoulder, Fig. 13-41. Philadelphia: W.B. Saunders, 1990.)*

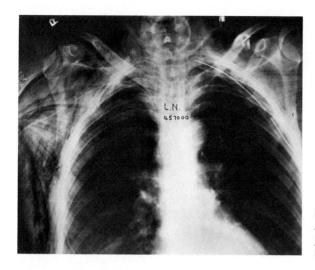

Fig. 15-44. Complications of sternoclavicular dislocation. As a result of posterior dislocation of the sternoclavicular joint, the patient had a lacerated trachea and developed massive subcutaneous emphysema.

pin that migrated completely inside the aorta. Jelesijevic and associates,[131] Pate and Wilhite,[200] Rubenstein and colleagues,[229] and Schechter and Gilbert[236] reported cases where the pin migrated into the heart. Leonard and Gifford[155] reported migration to the pulmonary artery. Sethi and Scott[239] reported migration of the pin to lacerate the subclavian artery. Clark and associates,[50] Gaston (in the report by Nettles and Linscheid,[115] and Salvatore[232] reported migration of pins into the aorta and resultant death. Grabski[101] reported migration of the pin to the opposite breast in a 37-year-old female. In addition, I personally have

treated patients in whom the pin has migrated into the chest and up into the base of the neck.

Omer,[197] in a review of 14 military hospitals, reported 15 patients who had elective surgery for reduction and reconstruction of the sternoclavicular joint. Eight patients were followed by the same house staff for more than 6 months with the following complications: of the five patients who had internal fixation with metal, two developed osteomyelitis, two had fracture of the pin with recurrent dislocation, and one had migration of the pin into the mediastinum with recurrent dislocation. Of the three patients who had soft tissue reconstructions,

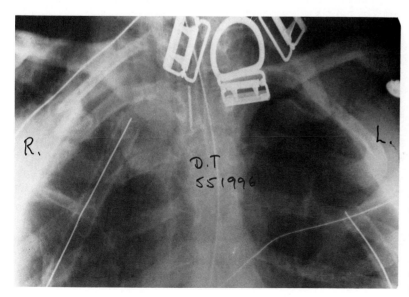

Fig. 15-45. Complications of sternoclavicular joint dislocation. This patient had an anterior dislocation on the right and a posterior dislocation on the left. As a result of the posterior dislocation, he had sufficient pressure on the mediastinal structures to cause significant hypotension. When the posterior dislocation was reduced, the blood pressure on the continuous monitor promptly returned to normal.

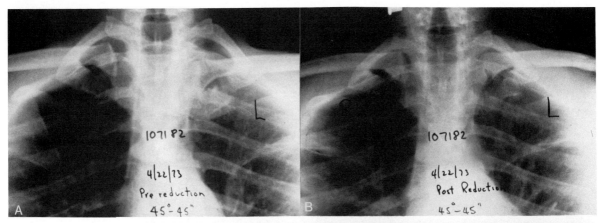

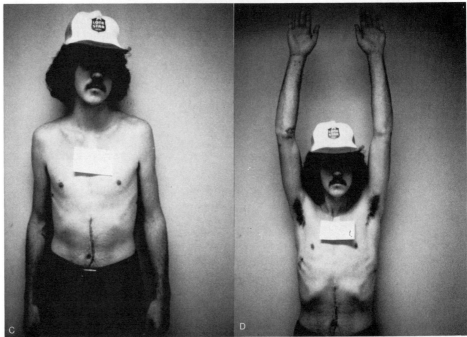

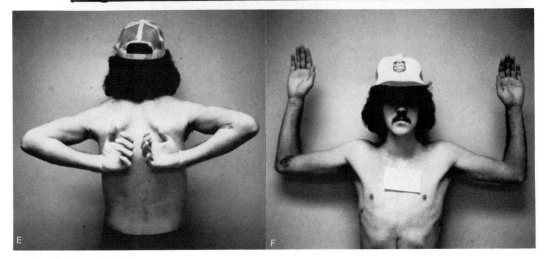

1300

Fig. 15-46. **(A)** Anterior dislocation of the right sternoclavicular joint and posterior dislocation of the left sternoclavicular joint. **(B)** Following reduction, the posterior dislocation was stable and the right remained slightly anteriorly displaced. **(C–F)** Despite this serious injury, the patient had a full recovery and a normal range of motion of both shoulders. *(Reprinted with permission from Rockwood, C. A., and Matsen, F., III (eds.): The Shoulder, Fig. 13-44. Philadelphia: W.B. Saunders, 1990.)*

←

two developed recurrent dislocation (one with drainage), and the third developed arthritis and extremity weakness and was discharged from military service. Omer commented on this series of complications: "It would seem that complications are common in this rare surgical problem." To Omer's comment I can only add, "Amen."

REFERENCES

1. Abbott, L.C.; and Lucas, D.B.: The Function of the Clavicle: Its Surgical Significance. Ann. Surg., 140:583–599, 1954.
2. Abbott, L.C.; Saunders, J.B.; Hagey, H.; and Jones, E.W.: Surgical approaches to the Shoulder Joint. J. Bone Joint Surg., 31A:235–255, 1949.
3. Abel, M.S.: Symmetrical Anteroposterior Projections of the Sternoclavicular Joints With Motion Studies. Radiology, 132:757–759, 1979.
4. Aberle, D.R.; Milos, M.J.; Aberle, A.M.; and Bassett, L.W.: Case Report 407: Diagnosis: Sternocostoclavicular Hyperostosis Affecting the Sternum, Medial Ends of the Clavicles and Upper Segments of the Anterior Ribs. Skeletal Radiol., 16:70–73, 1987.
5. Adunsky, A.; Yaretzky, A.; and Klajman, A.: Malignant Lymphoma Presenting as Sternoclavicular Joint Arthritis (letter to the editor). Arthritis Rheum., 2:1330–1331, 1980.
6. Allen, A.W.: Living Suture Grafts in the Repair of Fractures and Dislocations. Arch. Surg., 16:1007–1020, 1928.
7. Allman, F.L.: Fractures and Ligamentous Injuries of Clavicle and Its Articulations. J. Bone Joint Surg., 49A:774–784, 1967.
8. Anderson, M.E.: Treatment of Dislocations of the Acromioclavicular and Sternoclavicular Joints (abstract). J. Bone Joint Surg., 45A:657–658, 1963.
9. Bachmann, M.: Swelling of the Sternoclavicular Joint. Isr. J. Med. Sci., 17:65–72, 1958.
10. Badgley, C.E.: Sports Injuries of the Shoulder Girdle. J.A.M.A., 172:444–448, 1960.
11. Baker, E.C.: Tomography of the Sternoclavicular Joint. Ohio State Med. J., 55:60, 1959.
12. Baker, M.E.; Martinez, S.; Kier, R.; and Wain, S.: Computed Tomography of the Cadaveric Sternoclavicular Joint: Technique, Findings, and Significance in Degenerative Disease. Presented at the 33rd Annual Meeting, of the Association of University Radiologists, Nashville, TN, 1985.
13. Bankart, A.S.B.: An Operation for Recurrent Dislocation (Subluxation) of the Sternoclavicular Joint. Br. J. Surg., 26:320–323, 1938.
14. Baranda, M.M.; Pascual, J.B.; Gomez-Escolar, I.A.; Abaitua, L.G.; and Errasti, C.A.: Sternoclavicular Septic Arthritis as First Manifestation of Brucellosis (letter to the editor). Br. J. Rheumatol., 25:322, 1986.
15. Barrett, J.: The Clavicular Joints. Physiotherapy, 57:268–269, 1971.
16. Barth, E., and Hagen, R.: Surgical Treatment of Dislocations of the Sternoclavicular Joint. Acta Orthop. Scand., 54:746–747, 1983.
17. Basmajian, J.V.: Joints of the Upper Limb. *In* Grant, JCB (ed.): Grant's Method of Anatomy, 8th ed., pp. 158–159. Baltimore, Williams & Wilkins, 1971.
18. Bateman, J.E.: The Shoulder and Neck. Philadelphia, W.B. Saunders, 1972.
19. Bateman, J.E.: The Shoulder and Neck, 2nd ed. Philadelphia, W.B. Saunders, 1978.
20. Bayley, I.; and Kessel, L.: Shoulder Surgery. New York, Springer-Verlag, 1982.
21. Bearn, J.G.: Direct Observations on the Function of the Capsule of the Sternoclavicular Joint in Clavicular Support. J. Anat., 101:159–170, 1967.
22. Beckman, T.: A Case of Simultaneous Luxation of Both Ends of the Clavicle. Acta Chir. Scand., 56:156–163, 1923.
23. Beller, R.D.; Grana, W.A.; and O'Donoghue, D.H.: Recurrent Posterior Dislocation of the Shoulder: A Method of Reconstruction. Orthopedics, 1:384–388, 1978.
24. Berkhina, F.O.: [Traumatic Dislocations of Clavicle.] Orthop. Traumatol., 9:11–26, 1935.
25. Bernard, T.N. Jr., and Haddad, R.J. Jr.: Enchondroma of the Proximal Clavicle: An Unusual Cause of Pathologic Fracture–dislocation of the Sternoclavicular Joint. Clin. Orthop., 167:239–247, 1982.
26. Blankstein, A.; Nerubay, J.; Lin, E.; Keren, G.; Friedman, B.; and Horoszowski, H.: Septic Arthritis of the Sternoclavicular Joint. Orthop. Rev., 15:41–43, 1986.
27. Bloom, F.A.: Wire Fixation in Acromioclavicular Dislocation. J. Bone Joint Surg., 27:273–276, 1945.
28. Bohler, L.: The Treatment of Fractures, Vol. 1, pp. 540–545. New York: Grune & Stratton, 1956.
29. Bonnin, J.G.: Spontaneous Subluxation of the Sternoclavicular Joint. Br. Med. J., 2:274–275, 1960.
30. Booth, C.M., and Roper, B.A.: Chronic Dislocation of the Sternoclavicular Joint: An Operative Repair. Clin. Orthop., 140:17–20, 1979.
31. Borowiecki, B.; Charow, A.; Cook, W.; Rozycki, D.; and Thaler, S.: An Unusual Football Injury (Posterior Dislocation of the Sternoclavicular Joint). Arch. Otolaryngol., 95:185–187, 1972.
32. Borrero, E.: Traumatic Posterior Displacement of the Left Clavicular Head Causing Chronic Extrinsic Compression

of the Subclavian Artery. Physician Sports Med., 15:87–89, 1987.

33. Breitner, S., and Wirth, C.J.: [Resection of the Acromial and Sternal Ends of the Clavicula.] Z. Orthop., 125:363–368, 1987.

34. Bremner, R.A.: Nonarticular, Non-infective Subacute Arthritis of the Sterno-clavicular Joint. J. Bone Joint Surg., 41B:749–753, 1959.

35. Brooks, A.L., and Henning, G.D.: Injury to the Proximal Clavicular Epiphysis (abstract). J. Bone Joint Surg., 54A:1347–1348, 1972.

36. Brower, A.C.; Sweet, D.E.; and Keats, T.E.: Condensing Osteitis of the Clavicle: A New Entity. A.J.R., 121:17–21, 1974.

37. Brown, J.E.: Anterior Sternoclavicular Dislocation: A Method of Repair. Am. J. Orthop., 31:184–189, 1961.

38. Brown, R.: Backward and Inward Dislocation of Sternal End of Clavicle: Open Reduction. Surg. Clin. North Am., 7:1263, 1927.

39. Buchmann, M.: Swelling of the Sternoclavicular Joint. Acta Med.Orient, 17:65–72, 1958.

40. Buckerfield, C.T., and Castle, M.E.: Acute Traumatic Retrosternal Dislocation of the Clavicle. J. Bone Joint Surg., 66A:379–385, 1984.

41. Burri, C., and Nuegebauer, R.: Carbon Fiber Replacement of the Ligaments of the Shoulder Girdle and the Treatments of Lateral Instability of the Ankle Joint. Clin. Orthop., 196:112–117, 1985.

42. Burrows, H.J.: Tenodesis of Subclavius in the Treatment of Recurrent Dislocation of the Sterno-clavicular Joint. J. Bone Joint Surg., 33B:240–243, 1951.

43. Butterworth, R.D., and Kirk, A.A.: Fracture Dislocation Sterno-clavicular Joint: Case Report. Va. Med., 79:98–100, 1952.

44. Camus, J.P.; Prier, A.; and Cassou, B.: [Sternocostoclavicular hyperostosis.] Rev. Rhum. Mal. Osteoartic., 47:361–363, 1980.

45. Cantlon, G.E., and Gluckman, J.L.: Sternoclavicular Joint Hypertrophy Following Radical Neck Dissection. Head Neck Surg., 5:218–221, 1983.

46. Cave, A.J.E.: The Nature and Morphology of the Costoclavicular Ligament. J. Anat., 95:170–179, 1961.

47. Cave, E.F.: Fractures and Other Injuries. Chicago, Year Book Medical Publishers, 1958.

48. Cave, E.R.; Burke, J.F.; and Boyd, R.J.: Trauma Management, pp. 409–411. Chicago, Year Book Medical Publishers, 1974.

49. Christensen, E.E., and Dietz, G.W.: The Supraclavicular Fossa. Radiology, 118:37–39, 1976.

50. Clark, R.L.; Milgram, J.W.; and Yawn, D.H.: Fatal Aortic Perforation and Cardiac Tamponade Due to a Kirschner Wire Migrating From the Right Sternoclavicular Joint. South. Med. J., 67:316–318, 1974.

51. Codman, E.A.: The Shoulder. Boston, Thomas Todd, 1934.

52. Colhoun, E.N.; Hayward, C.; and Evans, K.T.: Inter-Sterno-Costo-Clavicular Ossification. Clin. Radiol., 38:33–38, 1987.

53. Collins, J.J.: Retrosternal Dislocation of the Clavicle (abstract). J. Bone Joint Surg., 54B:203, 1972.

54. Cone, R.O.; Resnick, D.; Goergen, T.G.; Robinson, C.; Vint, V.; and Haghighi, P.: Condensing Osteitis of the Clavicle. A.J.R., 141:387–388, 1983.

55. Conway, A.M.: Movements at the Sternoclavicular and Acromioclavicular Joints. Phys. Ther. Rev., 41:421–432, 1961.

56. Cooper, A.: A Treatise on Dislocations and Fractures of the Joints, 2nd Am. ed. (from the 6th London ed.). Boston, Lilly & Wait & Carter & Hendee, 1832.

57. Cooper, AP: The Lectures of Sir Astley Cooper on the Principles and Practices of Surgery, p 559. Philadelphia, E.L. Carey & A. Hart, 1935.

58. Cope, R., and Riddervold, H.O.: Posterior Dislocation of the Sternoclavicular Joint: Report on Two Cases, With Emphasis on Radiologic Management and Early Diagnosis. Skeletal Radiol., 17:247–250, 1988.

59. Currey, H.: Primary Gout Affecting the Sternoclavicular Joint (letter to the editor). Br. Med. J., 1:583–584, 1976.

60. D'Ambrosia, R.D.: Musculoskeletal Disorders. Philadelphia, J.B. Lippincott, 1977.

61. Daffner, R.H., and Gehweileer, J.A. Jr.: Case Report 236: Diagnosis: Neuropathic Arthropathy of the Sternoclavicular Joint, Secondary to Syringomyelia. Skeletal Radiol., 10:113–116, 1983.

62. DePalma, A.F.: The Role of the Disks of the Sternoclavicular and the Acromioclavicular Joints. Clin. Orthop., 13:222–233, 1959.

63. DePalma, A.F.: Surgical Anatomy of Acromioclavicular and Sternoclavicular Joints. Surg. Clin. North Am., 43:1541–1550, 1963.

64. DePalma, A.F.: Surgery of the Shoulder, 2nd ed., pp. 328–240, Philadelphia, J.B. Lippincott, 1973.

65. Delevette, A.F., and Monahan, D.T.: Acute Arthritis of the Sternoclavicular Joint Due to Coliform Bacillus. Conn. Med., 34:629–630, 1970.

66. Deluca, S.A.: Sternoclavicular Dislocation. Am. Fam. Physician, 37:137–138, 1988.

67. Denham, R.H., Jr., and Dingley, A.F., Jr.: Epiphyseal Separation of the Medial End of the Clavicle. J. Bone Joint Surg., 49A:1179–1183, 1967.

68. Destouet, J.M.; Gilula, L.A.; Murphy, W.A.; and Sagel, S.S.: Computed Tomography of the Sternoclavicular Joint and Sternum. Radiology, 138:123–128, 1981.

69. Dohler, J.R.: [Ankylosing hyperostosis of the sternoclavicular joint.] Dtsch. Med. Wochenschr., 112:304–305, 1987.

70. Duggan, N.: Recurrent Dislocation of Sternoclavicular Cartilage. J. Bone Joint Surg., 13:365, 1931.

71. Duthie, R.B., and Ferguson, A.B., Jr. (eds.): Mercer's Orthopaedic Surgery, 7th ed., pp. 958–959. Baltimore, Williams & Wilkins, 1973.

72. Ecke, H.: Sternoclavicular Dislocations. Personal communication, 1984.

73. Elting, J.J.: Retrosternal Dislocation of the Clavicle. Arch. Surg., 104:35–37, 1972.

74. Epps, C.H.: Complications in Orthopaedic Surgery. Philadelphia, J.B. Lippincott, 1978.

75. Epstein, B.S.: Sternoclavicular Arthritis in Patients With

Scleroderma and Rheumatoid Arthritis. A.J.R., 89:1236–1240, 1963.

76. Eskola, A.: Sternoclavicular Dislocation: A Plea for Open Treatment. Acta Orthop. Scand., 57:227–228, 1986.

77. Eskola, A.; Vainionpaa, S.; Vastamaki, M.; Slatis, P.; and Rokkanen, P.: Operation for Old Sternoclavicular Dislocation: Results in 12 Cases. J. Bone Joint Surg., 71B:63–65, 1989.

78. Farrer, W.E.: Case Report: Sternoclavicular Pyarthrosis. J. Med. Soc. N.J., 82:735–737, 1985.

79. Fedoseev, V.A.: [Method of Radiographic Study of the Sternoclavicular Joint.] Vestn. Rentgenol. Radiol., 3:88–91, 1977.

80. Ferrandez, L.; Yubero, J.; Usabiaga, J.; No, L.; and Martin, F.: Sternoclavicular Dislocation, Treatment and Complications. Ital. J. Orthop. Traumatol., 14:349–355, 1988.

81. Ferry, A.M.; Rook, F.W.; and Masterson, J.H.: Retrosternal Dislocation of the Clavicle. J. Bone Joint Surg., 39A:905–910, 1957.

82. Fery, A., and Leonard, A.: [Transsternal sternoclavicular projection: Diagnostic Value in Sternoclavicular Dislocations.] J. Radiol., 62:167–170, 1981.

83. Fery, A., and Sommelet, J.: [Dislocation of the Sternoclavicular Joint: A Review of 49 Cases.] Int. Orthop., 12:187–195, 1988.

84. Fisk, G.H.: Some Observations of Motion at the Shoulder Joint. Can. Med. Assoc. J., 50:213–216, 1944.

85. Fitchet, S.M.: Cleidocranial Dysostosis: Hereditary and Familial. J. Bone Joint Surg., 11:838–866, 1929.

86. Foucher, J.T.E.: The Classic: Separations of the Epiphyses (1867). Clin. Orthop., 188:3–9, 1984.

87. Franquet, T.; Lecumberri, F.; Rivas, A.; Inaraja, L.; and Idoate, M.A.: Condensing Osteitis of the Clavicle: Report of Two New Cases. Skeletal Radiol., 14:184–187, 1985.

88. Friedman, R.S.; Perez, H.D.; and Goldstein, I.M.: Septic Arthritis of the Sternoclavicular Joint Due to Gram-Positive Microorganisms. Am. J. Med. Sci., 282:91–93, 1981.

89. Fuxench-Chiesa, Z.; Mejias, E.; and Ramirez-Ronda, C.H.: Septic Arthritis of the Sternoclavicular Joint Due to Citrobacter Diversus (letter to the editor). J. Rheumatol., 10:162–164, 1983.

90. Gallie, W.E.: Dislocations. N. Engl. J. Med., 213:91–98, 1935.

91. Gangahar, D.M., and Flogaites, T.: Retrosternal Dislocation of the Clavicle Producing Thoracic Outlet Syndrome. J. Trauma, 18:369–372, 1978.

92. Gardner, N.A., and Bidstrup, B.P.: Intrathoracic Great Vessel Injury Resulting From Blunt Chest Trauma Associated With Posterior Dislocation of the Sternoclavicular Joint. Aust. N.Z. J. Surg., 53:427–430, 1983.

93. Gartland, J.J.: Fundamentals of Orthopaedics, 3rd ed., pp. 249–250. Philadelphia, WB Saunders, 1979.

94. Gazak, S., and Davidson, S.J.: Posterior Sternoclavicular Dislocations: Two Case Reports. J. Trauma, 24:80–82, 1984.

95. Gerlach, D.; Wemhoner, S.R.; and Ogbuihi, S.: [On Two Cases of Fatal Heart Tamponade Due to Migration of Fracture Nails From the Sternoclavicular Joint.] Z. Rechtsmed., 93:53–60, 1984.

96. Gerster, J.C.; Lagier, R.; and Nicod, L.: Case Report 311: Open-Quiz Solution. Skeletal Radiol., 14:53–60, 1985.

97. Glickman, L.G., and Minsky, A.A.: Case Reports—Enlargement of One Sternoclavicular Articulation: A Sign of Congenital Syphilis. Radiology, 28:85–86, 1937.

98. Goldin, R.H.; Chow, A.H.; Edwards, J.E. Jr.; Louie, J.E.; and Guze, L.B.: Sternoarticular Septic Arthritis in Heroin Users. N. Engl. J. Med., 289:616–618, 1973.

99. Goossens, M.; Vanderstraeten, C.V.; and Claessens, H.: Sternoclavicular Hyperostosis: A Case Report and Review of the Literature. Clin. Orthop., 194:164–168, 1985.

100. Gorman, J.B.; Stone, R.T.; and Keats, T.E.: Changes in the Sternoclavicular Joint Following Radical Neck Dissection. A.J.R., 111:584–587, 1971.

101. Grabski, R.S.: [Unusual Dislocation of a Fragment of Kirschner Wire After Fixation of the Sternoclavicular Joint.] Wiad. Lek., 40:630–632, 1987.

102. Grant, J.C.B.: Method of Anatomy, 7th ed. Baltimore, Williams & Wilkins, 1965.

103. Gray, H.; Goss, C.M. (ed.): Anatomy of the Human Body, 28th ed., pp. 324–326. Philadelphia, Lea & Febiger, 1966.

104. Greenlee, D.P.: Posterior Dislocation of the Sternal End of the Clavicle. J.A.M.A., 125:426–428, 1944.

105. Guerin, J.: Recherchés sur les Luxations Congenitales. Gaz. Med. Paris, 9:97, 1841.

106. Gunson, E.F.: Radiography of Sternoclavicular Articulation. Radiog. Clin. Photog., 19:20–24, 1943.

107. Gunther, W.A.: Posterior Dislocation of the Sternoclavicular Joint: Report of a Case. J. Bone Joint Surg., 31A:878–879, 1949.

108. Gurd, F.B.: Surplus Parts of the Skeleton: A Recommendation for the Excision of Certain Portions as a Means of Shortening the Period of Disability Following Trauma. Am. J. Surg., 74:705–720, 1947.

109. Haas, S.L.: The Experimental Transplantation of the Epiphysis: With Observations on the Longitudinal Growth of Bone. J.A.M.A., 65:1965–1971, 1915.

110. Habernek, H., and Hertz, H.: [Origin, Diagnosis and Treatment of Traumatic Dislocation of Sternoclavicular Joint.] Aktuel. Traumatol., 17:25–28, 1987.

111. Haenel, L.C.; Bradway, W.R.; and Costantini, P.J.: Thrombophlebitis Complicating Sternoclavicular Hyperostosis: Case Report. Postgrad. Med. J., 68:113–118, 1980.

112. Hallas, J., and Olesen, K.P.: Sterno-costo-clavicular Hyperostosis: A Case Report With a Review of the Literature. Acta Radiol., 29:577–579, 1988.

113. Hamilton-Wood, C.; Hollingworth, P.; Dieppe, P.; Ackroyd, C.; and Watt, I.: The Painful Swollen Sterno-clavicular Joint. Br. J. Radiol., 58:941–945, 1985.

114. Hartman, T.J., and Dunnagan, W.A.: Cinearthrography of the Sternoclavicular Joint. Personal communication, November 1979.

115. Haug, W.: Retention Einer Seltenen Sterno-clavicular-luxationsfraktur Mittels Modifizierter Y-Platte der AO. Aktuel. Traumatol., 16:39–40, 1986.

116. Heinig, C.F.: Retrosternal Dislocation of the Clavicle: Early Recognition, X-ray Diagnosis, and Management (abstract). J. Bone Joint Surg., 50A:830, 1968.

117. Heppenstall, R.B. (ed.): Fracture Treatment and Healing, pp. 417–419. Philadelphia: W.B. Saunders, 1980.

118. Hermann, G.; Rothenberg, R.R.; and Spiera, H.: The Value of Tomography in Diagnosing Infection of the Sternoclavicular Joint. Mt. Sinai J. Med., 50:52–55, 1983.

119. Hernandez, L.A.; Watson, J.D.; and Sturrock, R.D.: Septic Arthritis of the Sternoclavicular Joint: Complicated by Fistula Formation. Rheumatol. Rehabil., 15:292–294, 1976.

120. Higoumenakis, G.K.: Neues Stigma der kongenitalen Lues: Die Vergrosserung des sternalen Endes des rechten Schlusselbeins, seine Beschreibung, Deuting und Atiologie. Dtsche. Ztschr. Nervenh., 114:228, 1930.

121. Hobbs, D.W.: Sternoclavicular Joint: A New Axial Radiographic View. Radiology, 90:801–802, 1968.

122. Hollinshead, W.H.: Anatomy for Surgeons, Vol. 3, pp. 265–268. Philadelphia, Harper & Row, 1958.

123. Holmdahl, H.C.: A Case of Posterior Sternoclavicular Dislocation. Acta Orthop. Scand., 23:218–222, 1953–1954.

124. Hotchkiss, L.W.: Double Dislocation of the Sternal End of the Clavicle. Ann. Surg., 23:600, 1896.

125. Howard, F.M., and Shafer, S.J.: Injuries to the Clavicle With Neurovascular Complications: A Study of Fourteen Cases. J. Bone Joint Surg., 47A:1335–1346, 1965.

126. Howard, N.J.: Acromioclavicular and Sternoclavicular Joint Injuries. Am. J. Surg., 46:284–291, 1939.

127. Hoyt, W.A.: Etiology of Shoulder Injuries in Athletes. J. Bone Joint Surg., 49A:755–766, 1967.

128. Hynd, R.F.; Klofkorn, R.W.; and Wong, J.K.: Case Report: *Streptococcus Anginosus-Constellatus* Infection of the Sternoclavicular Joint. J. Rheumatol., 11:713–715, 1984.

129. Inman, V.T., and Saunders, J.B.: Observations on the Function of the Clavicle. California Med., 65:158–166, 1946.

130. Inman, V.T.; Saunders, J.B.; and Abbott, L.C.: Observations on the Function of the Shoulder Joint. J. Bone Joint Surg., 26:1–30, 1944.

131. Jelesijevic, V.; Knoll, D.; Klinke, F.; Sine, K.; and Dittrich, H.: [Penetrating injuries of the heart and intrapericardial blood vessels caused by migration of a Kirschner pin after osteosynthesis.] Acta Chir. Iugosl., 29:274–276, 1982.

132. Jones, R.: Injuries of Joints, 2nd ed., pp. 53–55. London, Oxford University Press, 1917.

133. Jonsson, G.: A Method of Obtaining Structural Pictures of the Sternum. Acta Radiol., 18:336–340, 1937.

134. Jurik, A.G., and De Carvalho, A.: Sterno-clavicular Hyperostosis in a Case With Psoriasis and HLA-B27 Associated Arthropathy. Fortschr. Rontgenstr., 142:345–347, 1985.

135. Jurik, A.G.; De Carvalho, A.; and Graudal, H.: Sclerotic Changes of the Sternal End of the Clavicle. Clin. Radiol., 36:23–25, 1985.

136. Kalliomaki, J.L.; Viitanen, S.M.; and Virtama, P.: Radiological Findings of Sternoclavicular Joints in Rheumatoid Arthritis. Acta Rheum. Scand., 14:233–240, 1969.

137. Kanoksikarin, S., and Wearne, W.M.: Fracture and Retrosternal Dislocation of the Clavicle. Aust. N.Z. J. Surg., 48:95–96, 1978.

138. Kattan, K.R.: Modified View for Use in Roentgen Examination of the Sternoclavicular Joints. Radiology, 108:8, 1973.

139. Kennedy, J.C.: Retrosternal Dislocation of the Clavicle. J. Bone Joint Surg., 31B:74–75, 1949.

140. Kessel, L.: Clinical Disorders of the Shoulder. London, Churchill Livingstone, 1982.

141. Key, J.A., and Conwell, H.E. (eds.): The Management of Fractures, Dislocations, and Sprains, 5th ed., pp. 458–461. St. Louis, C.V. Mosby, 1951.

142. Kier, R.; Wain, S.; Apple, J.; and Martinez, S.: Osteoarthritis of the Sternoclavicular Joint: Radiographic Features and Pathologic Correlation. Invest. Radiol., 21:227–33, 1986.

143. King, J.M. Jr., and Holmes, G.W.: A Review of Four Hundred and Fifty Roentgen Ray Examinations of the Shoulder. A.J.R., 17:214–218, 1927.

144. Kofoed, H.; Thomsen, P., and Lindenbergs, S.: Serous Synovitis of the Sternoclavicular Joint: Differential Diagnostic Aspects. Scand. J. Rheumatol., 14:61–64, 1985.

145. Kohler, H.; Uehlinger, E.; Kutzner, J.; and West, T.B.: Sternoclavicular Hyperostosis: Painful Swelling of the Sternum, Clavicles, and Upper Ribs: Report of Two New Cases. Ann. Intern. Med., 87:192–194, 1977.

146. Krenzien, J.: Acromioclavicular and Sternoclavicular Luxations. Personal Communication, July 1987.

147. Kruger, G.D.; Rock, M.G.; Munro, T.G.: Condensing Osteitis of the Clavicle: A Review of the Literature and Report of Three Cases. J. Bone Joint Surg., 69A:550–557, 1987.

148. Kurzbauer, R.: The Lateral Projection in Roentgenography of the Sternoclavicular Articulation. A.J.R., 56:104–105, 1946.

149. Lagier, R.; Arroyo, J.; and Fallet, G.H.: Sternocostoclavicular Hyperostosis: Radiological and Pathological Study of a Specimen With Ununited Clavicular Fracture. Pathol. Res. Pract., 181:596–603, 1986.

150. Laidlaw, J.T.: Treatment of Dislocated Clavicle. Personal Communication, 1985.

151. Lasher, W.W.: Cartilage Injuries: A Clinical Study. Am. J. Surg., 6:493–500, 1929.

152. Lee, H.M.: Sternoclavicular Dislocations: Report of a Case. Minn. Med., 20:480–482, 1937.

153. Leighton, R.K.; Buhr, A.J.; and Sinclairs, A.M.: Posterior Sternoclavicular Dislocations. Can. J. Surg., 29:104–106, 1986.

154. Lemire, L., and Rosman, M.: Sternoclavicular Epiphyseal Separation With Adjacent Clavicular Fracture: A Case Report. J. Pediatr. Orthop., 4:118–120, 1984.

155. Leonard, J.W., and Gifford, R.W.: Migration of a Kirschner Wire From the Clavicle Into Pulmonary Artery. Am. J. Cardiol., 16:598–600, 1965.

156. Levinsohn, E.M.; Bunnell, W.P.; and Yuan, H.A.: Computed Tomography in the Diagnosis of Dislocations of the Sternoclavicular Joint. Clin. Orthop., 140:12–16, 1979.

157. Levy, M.; Goldberg, I.; Fischel, R.E.; Frisch, E.; and Maor, P.: Friedrich's Disease: Aseptic Necrosis of the Sternal End of the Clavicle. J. Bone Joint Surg., 63B:539–541, 1981.

158. Lewin, K.W.: Rhomboid Fossa or Inflammation? (letter to the editor). Arch. Intern. Med., 138:658–659, 1978.

159. Lindsey, R.W., and Leach, J.A.: Sternoclavicular Osteo-

myelitis and Pyoarthrosis As a Complication of Subclavian Vein Catheterization: A Case Report and Review of the Literature. Orthopedics, 7:1017–1021, 1984.

160. Linscheid, R.L.; Kelly, P.J.; Martin, W.J.; and Fontana, R.S.: Monarticular Bacterial Arthritis of the Sternoclavicular Joint. J.A.M.A., 178:421–422, 1961.

161. Lourie, J.A.: Tomography in the Diagnosis of Posterior Dislocations of the Sterno-Clavicular Joint. Acta Orthop. Scand., 51:579–580, 1980.

162. Louw, J.A., and Louw, J.A.: Posterior Dislocation of the Sternoclavicular Joint Associated With Major Spinal Injury: A Case Report. S. Afr. Med. J., 71:791–792, 1987.

163. Lowman, C.L.: Operative Correction of Old Sternoclavicular Dislocation. J. Bone Joint Surg., 10:740–741, 1928.

164. Lucas, D.B.: Biomechanics of the Shoulder Joint. Arch. Surg., 107:425–432, 1973.

165. Lucas, G.L.: Retrosternal Dislocation of the Clavicle. J.A.M.A., 193:850–853, 1965.

166. Lunseth, P.A.; Chapman, K.W.; and Frankel, V.H.: Surgical Treatment of Chronic Dislocation of the Sterno-clavicular Joint. J. Bone Joint Surg., 57B:193–196, 1975.

167. Maguire, W.B.: Safe and Simple Method of Repair of Recurrent Dislocation of the Sternoclavicular Joint (abstract). J. Bone Joint Surg., 68B:332, 1986.

168. Marsh, H.O.; Shellito, J.G.; and Callahan, W.P. Jr.: Synovial Sarcoma of the Sternoclavicular Region. J. Bone Joint Surg., 45A:151–155, 1963.

169. Martinez, S.; Khoury, M.B.; and Harrelson, J.: Imaging of Condensing Osteitis of the Clavicle: New Observations. Presented at the 33rd Annual Meeting of the Association of University Radiologists, Nashville TN, 1985.

170. Mathews, J.G.: Primary Gout Affecting the Sternoclavicular Joint. Br. Med. J., 1:262, 1976.

171. Mazet, R. Jr.: Migration of a Kirschner Wire From the Shoulder Region Into the Lung: Report of Two Cases. J. Bone Joint Surg., 25A:477–483, 1943.

172. McCarroll, J.R.: Isolated Staphylococcal Infection of the Sternoclavicular Joint. Clin. Orthop., 156:149–150, 1981.

173. McCaughan, J.S., and Miller, P.R.: Migration of Steinmann Pin From Shoulder to Lung (letter to the editor). J.A.M.A., 207:1917, 1969.

174. McKenzie, J.M.M.: Retrosternal Dislocation of the Clavicle: A Report of Two Cases. J. Bone Joint Surg., 45B: 138–141, 1963.

175. McLaughlin, H.: Trauma, pp. 291–292. Philadelphia, W.B. Saunders, 1959.

176. Mehta, J.C.; Sachdev, A.; and Collins, J.J.: Retrosternal Dislocation of the Clavicle. Injury, 5:79–83, 1973.

177. Milch, H.: The Rhomboid Ligament in Surgery of the Sternoclavicular Joint. J. Int. Coll. Surg., 17:41–51, 1952.

178. Mitchell, W.J., and Cobey, M.C.: Retrosternal Dislocation of the Clavicle. Med. Ann. D.C., 29:546–549, 1960.

179. Moncada, R.; Matuga, T.; Unger, E.; Freeark, R.; and Pizarro, A.: Migratory Traumatic Cardiovascular Foreign Bodies: Case Reports. Circulation, 57:186–189, 1978.

180. Morag, B., and Shahin, N.: The Value of Tomography of the Sterno-clavicular Region. Clin. Radiol., 26:57–62, 1975.

181. Moseley, H.F.: Athletic Injuries to the Shoulder Region. Am. J. Surg., 98:401–422, 1959.

182. Mouchet, A.: Luxation Sterno-claviculaire en Avant: Reduction Sanglante. Rev. Orthop., 28:99–100, 1942.

183. Muir, S.K.; Kinsella, P.L.; Trevilcock, R.G.; and Blackstone, I.W.: Infectious Arthritis of the Sternoclavicular Joint. Can. Med. Assoc. J., 132:1289–1290, 1985.

184. Nair, V.: Case Report—Sternoclavicular Arthritis: An Unusual Complication of Drug Abuse. J. Med. Soc. N.J., 72: 519–520, 1975.

185. Nettles, J.L., and Linscheid, R.: Sternoclavicular Dislocations. J. Trauma, 8:158–164, 1968.

186. Neviaser, J.S.: Injuries of the Clavicle and Its Articulations. Orthop. Clin. North Am., 11:233–237, 1980.

187. Newlin, N.S.: Congenital Retrosternal Subluxation of the Clavicle Simulating an Intrathoracic Mass. A.J.R., 130: 1184–1185, 1978.

188. Nickel, V.L.: Orthopedic Rehabilitation. London, Churchill Livingstone, 1982.

189. Nitsche, J.F.; Vaughan, J.H.; Williams, G.; and Curd, J.G.: Septic Sternoclavicular Arthritis With *Pasteurella multocida*, and *Streptococcus sanguis.* Arthritis Rheum., 25:467–469, 1982.

190. Nittis, S.: Prominence of the Right Sterno-clavicular Junction in Lepers. Urol. Cutan. Rev., 41:625–630, 1937.

191. Noonan, T.R.: Sternoclavicular Dislocation. Personal Communication, July 30, 1984.

192. Nordback, I., and Markkula, H.: Migration of Kirschner Pin From Clavicle Int. Ascending Aorta. Acta Chir. Scand., 151:177–179, 1985.

193. Nutz, V.: [Fracture dislocation of the sternoclavicular joint.] Unfallchirurg., 89:145–148, 1986.

194. O'Donoghue, D.H.: Treatment of Injuries to Athletes, 2nd ed. Philadelphia, W.B. Saunders, 1970.

195. O'Donoghue, D.H.: Treatment of Injuries to Athletes, 3rd ed., pp. 144–151. Philadelphia, W.B. Saunders, 1976.

196. Ogden, J.A.; Conlogue, G.J.; and Bronson, M.L.: Radiology of Postnatal Skeletal Development: III. The Clavicle. Skeletal Radiol., 4:196–203, 1979.

197. Omer, G.E.: Osteotomy of the Clavicle in Surgical Reduction of Anterior Sternoclavicular Dislocation. J. Trauma, 7:584–590, 1967.

198. Orsini, G.; Guercio, N.; and Paschero, B.: Retrosternal Dislocation of the Clavicle: Observations on Three Cases. Ital. J. Orthop. Traumatol., 10:533–539, 1984.

199. Paice, E.W.; Wright, F.W.; and Hill, A.G.S.: Sternoclavicular Erosions in Polymyalgia Rheumatica. Ann. Rheum. Dis., 42:379–383, 1983.

200. Pate, J.W., and Wilhite, J.: Migration of a Foreign Body From the Sternoclavicular Joint to the Heart: A Case Report. Am. Surg., 35:448–449, 1969.

201. Paterson, D.C.: Retrosternal Dislocation of the Clavicle. J. Bone Joint Surg., 43B:90–92, 1961.

202. Pauleau, J.L., and Baux, S.: [Sternoclavicular dislocations: a case report of a posterior dislocation and review of the published literature.] J. Chir., 117:453–456, 1980.

203. Peacock, H.K.; Brandon, J.R.; and Jones, O.L.: Retrosternal Dislocation of the Clavicle. South. Med. J., 63:1324–1328, 1970.

204. Pendergrass, E.P., and Hodes, P.J.: The Rhomboid Fossa of the Clavicle. A.J.R., 38:152–155, 1937.

205. Percy, E.C.: Sternoclavicular Dislocation (Case P55). Can. Med. Assoc. J., 104:1016–1017, 1971.

206. Persoons, D.; Copin, G.; and Dosch, J.: [Retrosternal Dislocation of the Clavicle: Contribution of Computertomography in Diagnosis and Treatment—Case Report.] Acta Orthop. Belg., 51:103–109, 1985.

207. Pfister, U., and Ode, E.: Die Luxation im sterno-clavicular-gelenk. Unfallmed Arbeit, October 1983.

208. Pfister, U., and Weller, S.: [Luxation of the Sternoclavicular Joint.] Unfallchirurgie, 8:81–87, 1982.

209. Pierce, R.O. Jr.: Internal Derangement of the Sternoclavicular Joint. Clin. Orthop., 141:247–250, 1979.

210. Poland, J.: Traumatic Separation of Epiphyses of the Upper Extremity, pp. 135–143. London, Smith, Elder, & Co., 1898.

211. Post, M.: The Shoulder. Philadelphia, Lea & Febiger, 1978.

212. Pridie, K.: Dislocation of Acromio-clavicular and Sternoclavicular Joints (abstract). J. Bone Joint Surg., 41B:429, 1959.

213. Quigley, T.B.: Injuries to the Acromioclavicular and Sternoclavicular Joints Sustained in Athletics. Surg. Clin. North Am., 43:1551–1554, 1963.

214. Raney, R.B.; Brashear, H.R.; and Shands, A.R. Jr.: Shands' Handbook of Orthopaedic Surgery, p. 421. St. Louis, C.V. Mosby, 1971.

215. Reeves, B.D.: Postpartum Sternoclavicular Joint Pain. J.A.M.A., 248:3030–3031, 1982.

216. Resnick, D.: Sternocostoclavicular Hyperostosis. A.J.R., 135:1278–1280, 1980.

217. Reuler, J.B.; Girard, D.E.; and Nardone, D.A.: Sternoclavicular Joint Involvement in Ankylosing Spondylitis. South. Med. J., 71:1480–1481, 1978.

218. Rice, E.E.: Habitual Dislocation of the Sternoclavicular Articulation: A Case Report. J. Okla. State Med. Assoc., 25:34–35, 1932.

219. Richter, R.; Hahn, H.; Nubling, W.; and Kohler, G.: [Tuberculosis of the Shoulder Girdle.] Z. Rheumatol., 44:87–92, 1985.

220. Ritvo, M., and Ritvo, M.: Roentgen Study of the Sternoclavicular Region. A.J.R., 53:644–650, 1947.

221. Rockwood, C.A. Jr.: Dislocations of the Sternoclavicular Joint. Instr. Course Lect., 24:144–159, 1975.

222. Rockwood, C.A. Jr.: Dislocation of the Sternoclavicular Joint. In Rockwood, C.A. Jr., and Green, D.P. (eds.): Fractures, 1st ed. Vol. 1, pp. 756–787. Philadelphia, J.B. Lippincott, 1975.

223. Rockwood, C.A. Jr.: Injuries of the Sternoclavicular Joint (abstract). Orthop. Trans., 1:96, 1977.

224. Rockwood, C.A. Jr.: Management of Fractures of the Clavicle and Injuries of the Sternoclavicular Joint (abstract). Orthop. Trans., 6:422, 1982.

225. Rockwood, C.A. Jr.: Injuries to the Sternoclavicular Joint. In Rockwood, C.A. Jr., and Green, D.P. (eds.): Fractures, 2nd ed. Vol. 1, pp. 910–948. Philadelphia, J.B. Lippincott, 1984.

226. Rockwood, C.A. Jr., and Odor, J.M.: Spontaneous Atraumatic Anterior Subluxations of the Sternoclavicular Joint in Young Adults: Report of 37 Cases (abstract). Orthop. Trans., 12:557, 1988.

227. Rodrigues, H.: Case of Dislocation, Inwards, of the Internal Extremity of the Clavicle. Lancet, 1:309–310, 1843.

228. Rozboril, M.B.; Good, A.E.; Zarbo, R.J.; and Schultz, D.A.: Sternoclavicular Joint Arthritis: An Unusual Presentation of Metastatic Carcinoma. J. Rheumatol., 10:499–502, 1983.

229. Rubenstein, Z.R.; Moray, B.; and Itzchak, Y.: Percutaneous Removal of Intravascular Foreign Bodies. Cardiovasc. Intervent. Radiol., 5:64–68, 1982.

230. Sadr, B., and Swann, M.: Spontaneous Dislocation of the Sternoclavicular Joint. Acta Orthop. Scand., 50:269–274, 1979.

231. Sala, R.S., and Gomez, J.M.: [Sterno-costo-clavicular Hyperostosis: Presentation of One Case and Review of the Literature.] Medicina Clinica, 84:483–486, 1985.

232. Salvatore, J.E.: Sternoclavicular Joint Dislocation. Clin. Orthop., 58:51–54, 1968.

233. Sante, L.R.: Manual of Roentgenological Technique, 9th ed., pp. 160–161. Ann Arbor, Edwards Brothers, 1942.

234. Sartoris, D.J.; Schreiman, J.S.; Kerr, R.; Resnick, C.S.; and Resnick, D.: Sternocostoclavicular Hyperostosis: A Review and Report of 11 Cases. Radiology, 158:125–128, 1986.

235. Savastano, A.A., and Stutz, S.J.: Traumatic Sternoclavicular Dislocation. Int. Surg., 63:10–13, 1978.

236. Schechter, D.C., and Gilbert, L.: Injuries of the Heart and Great Vessels Due to Pins and Needles. Thorax, 24:246–253, 1969.

237. Schmitt, W.G.H.: Articulatis Sternoclavicularis: Darstellung in Einer Zweiter Ebene. Rontgenpraxis, 34:262–267, 1981.

238. Selesnick, F.H.; Jablon, M.; Frank, C.; and Post, M.: Retrosternal Dislocation of the Clavicle: Report of Four Cases. J. Bone Joint Surg., 66A:287–291, 1984.

239. Sethi, G.K., and Scott, S.M.: Subclavian Artery Laceration Due to Migration of a Hagie Pin. Surgery, 80:644–646, 1976.

240. Silberberg, M.; Frank, E.L.; Jarrett, S.R.; and Silberberg, R.: Aging and Osteoarthritis of the Human Sternoclavicular Joint. Am. J. Pathol., 35:851–865, 1959.

241. Silverman, M.: Sternocostoclavicular Hyperostosis (letter to the editor). Ann. Intern. Med., 87:797, 1977.

242. Simurda, M.A.: Retrosternal Dislocation of the Clavicle: A Report of Four Cases and a Method of Repair. Can. J. Surg., 11:487–490, 1968.

243. Snyder, C.C.; Levine, G.A.; and Dingman, D.L.: Trial of a Sternoclavicular Whole Joint Graft as a Substitute for the Temporomandibular Joint. Plast. Reconstr. Surg., 48:447–452, 1971.

244. Sokoloff, L., and Gleason, I.O.: The Sternoclavicular Articulation in Rheumatic Diseases. Am. J. Clin. Pathol., 24:406–414, 1954.

245. Sonozaki, H.; Azuma, A.; Okai, K.; Kaminuma, S.; Nakamura, K.; Kukuoka, S.; Fukuoka, S.; and Mannoji, T.: Inter-sterno-costo-clavicular Ossification With a Special Reference to Cases of Unilateral Type. Kanto J. Orthop. Traumatol., 9:196–200, 1978.

246. Sonozaki, H.; Azuma, A.; Okai, K.; Nakamura, K.; Fu-

kuoka, S.; Tateishi, A.; Kurosawa, H.; Mannoji, T.; Kabata, K.; Mitsui, H.; Seki, H.; Abe, I.; Furusawa, S.; Matsura, M.; Kudo, A.; and Hoshino, T.: Clinical Features of 22 Cases With Inter-sterno-costo-clavicular Ossification. Arch. Orthop. Trauma Surg., 95:13–22, 1979.

247. Sonozaki, H.; Furusawa, S.; Seki, H.; Kurokawa, T.; Tateishi, A.; and Kabata, K.: Four Cases With Symmetrical Ossifications Between the Clavicles and the First Ribs of Both Sides. Kanto J. Orthop. Traumatol., 5:244–247, 1974.

248. Southworth, S.R., and Merritt, T.R.: Asymptomatic Innominate Vein Tamponade With Retromanubrial Clavicular Dislocation: A Case Report. Orthop. Rev., 17:789–791, 1988.

249. Spar, I.: Psoriatic Arthritis of the Sternoclavicular Joint. Conn. Med., 42:225–226, 1978.

250. Speed, K.: A Textbook of Fractures and Dislocations, 4th ed., pp. 282–290. Philadelphia, Lea & Febiger, 1942.

251. Stankler, L.: Posterior Dislocation of Clavicle: A Report of 2 Cases. Br. J. Surg., 50:164–168, 1962.

252. Stapelmohr, S.V.: Ueber die habituelle Luxation sternoclavicularis und eine neue operative Behandlungsmethode Dersleben. Acta Orthop. Scand., 3:1–42, 1932.

253. Stein, A.H.: Retrosternal Dislocation of the Clavicle. J. Bone Joint Surg., 39A:656–660, 1957.

254. Stimson, L.A.: Fractures and Dislocations, pp. 588–589. Philadelphia, Lea & Febiger, 1912.

255. Streifler, J.; Gartz, M.; Rosenfeld, J.B.; Pitlik, S.; and Grosskopf, I.: Sternoclavicular Arthritis and Osteomyelitis Due to *Pseudomonas Aruginosa*, Not Related to Drug Abuse. Isr. J. Med. Sci., 21:458–259, 1985.

256. Szilvasy, J.: Age Determination of the Sternal Articular Faces of the Clavicula. J. Human Evol., 9:609–610, 1980.

257. Tabatabai, M.F.; Sapico, F.L.; Canawati, H.N.; and Harley, H.A.J.: Sternoclavicular Joint Infection With Group B Streptococcus (letter to the editor). J. Rheumatol., 13:466, 1986.

258. Tagliabue, D., and Riva, A.: Le lussazioni sterno-claveari. Minerva Orthop., 36:876–871, 1985.

259. Teplick, J.G.; Eftekhari, F.; Haskin, M.E.: Erosion of the Sternal Ends of the Clavicles: A New Sign of Primary and Secondary Hyperparathyroidism. Radiology, 113:323–326, 1974.

260. Turek, S.L.: Orthopaedics: Principles and Their Application, 2nd ed., pp. 568–570. Philadelphia, J.B. Lippincott, 1967.

261. Tyler, H.D.D.; Sturrock, W.D.S.; and Callow, F.M.: Retrosternal Dislocation of the Clavicle. J. Bone Joint Surg., 45B:132–137, 1963.

262. Waskowitz, W.J.: Disruption of the Sternoclavicular Joint: An Analysis and Review. Am. J. Orthop., 3:176–179, 1961.

263. Wasylenko, M.J., and Busse, E.F.: Posterior Dislocation of the Clavicle Causing Fatal Tracheoesophageal Fistula. Can. J. Surg., 24:626–627, 1981.

264. Watson-Jones, R.: Fractures and Joint Injuries, 4th ed., Vol. 2, pp. 462–463. London, E & S Livingstone, 1956.

265. Watson-Jones, R.: Fractures and Joint Injuries, 6th ed. New York, Churchill Livingstone, 1982.

266. Webb, P.A., and Suchey, J.M.M.: Epiphyseal Union of the Anterior Iliac Crest and Medial Clavicle in a Modern Multiracial Sample of American Males and Females. Am. J. Phys. Anthropol., 68:457–466, 1985.

267. Weiner, S.N.; Levy, M.; Bernstein, R.; and Morehouse, H.: Condensing Osteitis of the Clavicle: A Case Report. J. Bone Joint Surg., 66A:1484–1486, 1984.

268. Weingarten, M.; Tash, R.; Klein, R.M.; and Kearns, R.J.: Posterior Dislocation of the Sternoclavicular Joint. N.Y. State J. Med., 85(5):225–226, 1985.

269. Wheeler, M.E.; Laaveg, S.J.; and Sprague, B.L.: S-C Joint Disruptions in an Infant. Clin. Orthop., 139:68–69, 1979.

270. Williams, H.H.: Oblique Views of the Clavicle. Radiog. Clin. Photog., 5:191–194, 1929.

271. Winter, J., Sterner, S.; Maurer, D.; Varecka, T.; and Zarzycki, M.: Retrosternal Epiphyseal Disruption of Medial Clavicle: Case and Review in Children. J. Emerg. Med., 7:9–13, 1989.

272. Wohlgethan, J.R., and Newberg, A.H.: Clinical Analysis of Infection of the Sternoclavicular Joint (abstract). Clin. Res., 32:666A, 1984.

273. Wolford, L.M., and Smith, B.R.: Sternoclavicular Grafts for Temporomandibular Joint Reconstruction (abstract). J. Oral Maxillofac. Surg., 45:M3, 1987.

274. Worman, L.W., and Leagus, C.: Intrathoracic Injury Following Retrosternal Dislocation of the Clavicle. J. Trauma, 7:416–423, 1967.

275. Worrell, J., and Fernandez, G.N.: Retrosternal Dislocation of the Clavicle: An Important Injury Easily Missed. Arch. Emerg. Med., 3:133–135, 1986.

276. Yang, S.O.; Cho, K.J.; Kim, M.J.; and Ro, I.W.: Assessment of Anterior Shoulder Instability by CT Arthrography. J. Korean Med. Sci., 2:167–171, 1987.

277. Yood, R.A., and Goldenberg, D.L.: Sternoclavicular Joint Arthritis. Arthritis Rheum., 23:232–239, 1980.

278. Zucman, J.; Robinet, L.; and Aubart, J.: [Treatment of Sternal Dislocations of the Clavicle.] Rev. Chir. Orthop., 64:35–44, 1978.

Index
Volumes 1 and 2

The letter f *after a page number indicates a figure;*
t *following a page number indicates tabular material.*

Muscle(s). *See also specific muscle and region*
   composition of, 210–211
   débridement of, 235–236, 284
   exercise of, 161
   fatigue of, stress fractures in, 7–8
   gunshot wound of, 226
   healing of, 210–213
   injury of
     classification of, 212
     mechanisms of, 212–213
   ischemia of. *See* Compartment syndrome
   regeneration of, after ischemia, 391
   structure of, 210–211
   transfer of
     in acromioclavicular joint dislocations, 1217–1220, 1230
     functional, 272, 273t
Muscle fibers, 211
Muscle flaps. *See under* Flaps
Muscle-pedicle bone graft, in femoral neck fractures, 1505, 1506f, 1507–1508
   diagnosed late, 1519
   in young adult, 1521–1522
Muscle relaxants, in tetanus, 374
Musculocutaneous nerve, of shoulder
   anatomy of, 874f, 875, 1029–1030
   injury of, 875
     in dislocations, 1084
     in surgery, 1111
   protection of, in surgery, 1121
Myelography, in spinal injury, 1321, 1377
Myeloma, laboratory evaluation in, 420–421, 421t
Myelomere, anatomy of, 1359, 1359f
Myofibrils, 211
Myonecrosis, clostridial. *See* Gas gangrene
Myositis ossificans
   in acetabular fractures, 1623
   in elbow dislocations, 789–791, 792f
   in hip dislocations, 1612, 1623
   in humeral fractures, 867, 913
   in muscle trauma, 212
Myotubes, in muscle healing, 211

Nafcillin, in osteomyelitis, 382t
Nail(s) (digital)
   injury of, in finger fractures, 446, 447f, 483
   traction on, in phalangeal fractures, 461f, 462–463
Nail-plates, in femoral fractures
   intertrochanteric, 1547–1548, 1550–1551, 1556, 1556f
   subtrochanteric, 1565–1566
Nail(s)/rod(s)
   in acromioclavicular joint repairs, 1211
   AO/ASIF universal, 122, 123f, 126f

Brooker-Wills, 122, 126f, 1948
centromedullary, 1942–1943, 1944f
cloverleaf, 1671–1672. *See also subhead*: Küntscher
Ender. *See* Ender nail/rod
in femoral fractures
   intertrochanteric, complications with, 1559
   neck, 1482, 1503–1505, 1507–1509
in femoral head, placement location of, 1554–1555
fixed-angle, in femoral neck fractures, 1503
gamma locking, 1553, 1553f
Grosse-Kempf, 121, 123f, 1673f
   in femoral fractures, 1567, 1568f
   locking system for, 1704
   in tibial fractures, 1944–1945
Hackethal, 855
Halder (gamma locking), 1553, 1553f
Hansen-Street, 1670
Harris, 1553
Huckstep, 123, 1671
interlocking, 121–123, 122f–127f
   in femoral shaft-intercondylar fractures, 1688, 1690f–1693f
   in humeral shaft fractures, 857, 857f, 859
   second-generation, 1686–1688
intramedullary, 119–139
   advancement in canal, 133–134
   in ankle fractures, 2015
   bending of, 138
   biomechanics of, 126–131
   bone weakening from, 129–130
   breakage of, 138
   with cerclage, 94–95, 94f
   in clavicular fractures, 976, 978
   in clavicular nonunion, 968–969, 969f
   closed technique for, 131–137, 135f–137f
   complications of, 131–139, 135f–137f, 140f–141f, 1552–1553, 1570–1571
   delayed insertion of, 1695
   distal locking of, 1704, 1705f–1706f
   distal screw locking and, 134–135, 137f
   in dynamic fixation, 130–131
   entry portal for, 132, 136f
   equipment for, 1701–1702, 1702f, 1704
   failure of, 1712f–1716f, 1715–1716
   fat embolism syndrome and, 342, 349
   in femoral fractures, 256, 430–431, 432f
     intertrochanteric, 1552–1553, 1552f–1553f, 1556, 1556f
     neck, 11486

shaft. *See under* Femoral fractures, shaft
   subtrochanteric, 1567–1572, 1567f–1569f, 1677, 1679f–1680f
   supracondylar, 1789, 1791f
gripping strength of, 128
guide pin for, 1556, 1556f, 1701, 1702f
guide wire for, 132
in gunshot fractures, 1689, 1697f
historical review of, 1653–1654, 1669–1670
history of, 119, 121
in humeral shaft fractures, 855, 857, 857f, 859, 865–866, 866f
in humeral shaft nonunion, 864, 865f
infection from, 138, 1708, 1710, 1709f
interlocking, in tibial fractures, 1944–1945, 1944f, 1948, 1948f
locking, 1567–1568, 1568f, 1672, 1673f
malunion and, 1711
in massive trauma, 252–253
in metacarpal neck fractures, 487
migration of, 1716
multiple flexible, 1941–1942, 1941f
nail insertion in, 1702–1703
nerve injury from, 1707
nonunion and, 1710
in olecranon fractures, 799, 800f
in open fractures, 245
open technique for, 137, 139, 140f–141f
in pathologic fractures, 1689, 1695f–1696f
patient positioning for, 131–132, 135f
in phalangeal fractures, 468–469, 471f
planning for, 1695, 1698
vs. plating, 151
proximal locking of, 1703–1704, 1703f
proximal screw insertion and, 134
in radius-ulna fractures, 688–695, 689f–694f
reaming procedure, 133, 1700–1703, 1700f–1702f
reduction loss with, 138
reduction with, 132
refracture and, 1715
removal of, 1570–1571, 1710
revascularization and, 1656
rigidity of, 128–129
size of, 133
in static fixation, 131
in tibial fractures, 288, 288f, 1940–1945, 1941f, 1943f–1944f

Packed red cells, in transfusion therapy, 339

Paget's disease
femoral fractures in, 1689
intertrochanteric, 1556
neck, 1526, 1529
prosthesis in, 1510, 1515–1516
laboratory evaluation in, 420, 421t
pathologic fractures in, 436

Pain. *See also specific injury,* signs and symptoms of
in bone metastasis, 423–424
in calcaneal fractures, 2130–2131, 2130f–2131f
in causalgia, 389–390
in compartment syndrome, 391–392
in dislocations, 22
in fractures, 21
negligence involving, 166
in reflex sympathetic dystrophy, 384–385, 656–657
in shoulder-hand syndrome, 388–389, 389t

Pain dysfunction syndrome, in carpal injuries, 656–657
prevention of, 663–664

Pallor, in compartment syndrome, 392

Palmar arches, anatomy of, 572–573, 574f

Palmer method, for calcaneal fracture reduction, 2124, 2125f

Panclavicular dislocation, 938, 945

Papineau graft
in osteomyelitis, 311, 314
in tibial fractures, 292, 292f

Papineau technique, in tibial defects, 1955

Paralysis, in compartment syndrome, 392

Paramysium, 211

Paré, Ambroise, on cervical spine injuries, 1309

Paresthesia, in compartment syndrome, 392

Parham's bands, 94, 96

Parham support, in clavicular fractures, 963f

Parkinson's disease, femoral fractures in
intertrochanteric, 1556
neck, 1529–1530
prosthesis in, 1510, 1514–1515

Partridge bands, in internal fixation, 96–97

Parvin gravity technique, of elbow dislocation reduction, 782, 784, 784f

Passive motion machine, 160–161

Patella
anatomy of, 1762–1763, 1763f, 1801–1802, 1802f
bipartite, 1762, 1763f, 1825, 1827f
blood supply of, 1763, 1901–1802, 1801f, 1807

dislocations of. *See under* Patellofemoral joint
fractures of, 1762–1777
anatomic considerations in, 1762–1763
arthritis after, 1775
avascular necrosis in, 1775
bilateral, 1764
classification of, 1765, 1765f–1766f
comminuted, 1764–1765, 1765f, 1768, 1770–1772, 1772f–1774f
displaced, 1769–1770, 1771f
distal, 1770
historical review of, 1763–1764
incomplete, 1764
indirect reduction of, 1770–1772, 1772f–1773f
infection in, 1775
inferior pole, 1765, 1765f, 1768, 1768f
internal fixation of, 97f, 1767–1772, 1767f–1768f, 1771f–1773f
mechanism of injury in, 1764, 1764f
nonunion of, 1775
open, 1769
open reduction in, 1764, 1767–1772, 1767f–1768f, 1771f–1773f
osteochondral, 1765, 1765f
patellectomy in, 1762, 1768–1769, 1768f, 1772, 1774f, 1775
radiography of, 1765–1766, 1765f
refracture of, 1775
retained hardware problems in, 1775
signs and symptoms of, 1765
stellate, 1764, 1765
traction, 14f
transverse, 1765, 1765f, 1768, 1770
treatment of, 1766–1776
comminuted, 1768, 1770–1772, 1772f–1774f
complications of, 1775–1776
controversy over, 1762
displaced, 1769–1770, 1771f
distal, 1770
historical review of, 1763–1764
nonoperative, 1766, 1769
in open fractures, 1769
operative, 1766–1772, 1767f–1768f, 1771f–1774f
postoperative care in, 1772
prognosis for, 1772, 1775
transverse, 1770
undisplaced, 1769
undisplaced, 1765, 1765f, 1769
vertical, 1765, 1765f
function of, 1762

osteochondritis dissecans of, 1829–1830, 1830f, 1842
refracture of, 1775
tripartite, 1825, 1826f

Patella alta, 1820, 1820f, 1825–1826

Patella baja, 1822

Patellar tendon
in cruciate ligament reconstruction, 1882–1884, 1883f, 1886, 1890, 1890f–1891f
inflammation of, 1825
iatrogenic injuries of, 1892
reconstruction of, 1821–1822, 1822f
rupture of, 1820–1822, 1820f–1822f, 1892

Patellar tendon-bearing brace, in talar neck fractures, 2084

Patellar tendon-bearing cast
application of, 35–36, 36f
biomechanics of, 40
in tibial fractures, 1928, 1928f, 1963

Patellectomy
complications of, 1772, 1775
historical review of, 1762
partial, 1768, 1768f
technique for, 1772, 1774f
total, 1768–1769

Patellofemoral joint
anatomy of, 1762, 1802–1803
arthritis of, in patellar fractures, 1775
biomechanics of, 1823, 1823f–1824f
chondromalacia of, 1826–1830, 1827f–1830f
dislocations of, 1825
immobilization of, 1835, 1838
injury of, 1823–1839
classification of, 1824–1830, 1825f–1830f
mechanism of, 1824
with no cartilage damage, 1824–1825, 1825f–1827f
radiography of, 1826f, 1830–1833, 1830f–1834f
with significant cartilage damage, 1826–1830, 1827f–1829f
treatment of, 1834–1839, 1836f–1839f
with variable cartilage damage, 1825–1826
subluxation of, 1825

Patellofemoral ligament, function of, 1823, 1824f

Patellotibial ligament, function of, 1823, 1824f

Pathologic fractures, 1, 417–439
of acetabulum, 431, 433f
biopsy of, 422–423, 422t–423t
of clavicle, 940–941, 941f
clinical course of, 1531
definition of, 417
diagnosis of, 422–423, 422t–423t

shaft, 849–850, 850f
supracondylar, 747–748, 748f–749f
Neufeld, 1662, 1662f
ninety-ninety, 1662, 1663f
in open fractures, 244–246, 245f–246f
in pelvic fractures, 1434, 1436t, 1438f, 1459, 1459f, 1461
in phalangeal fractures, 463–464
Thomas splint with Pearson attachment, 1661
in tibial fractures
plafond, 1970, 2031, 2033
plateau, 1743–1744, 1750–1751
skin, 42–43, 42f–43f
in femoral fractures, 1561, 1659–1660, 1660f
in hip dislocations, 1594
anterior, 1591
posterior, 1604, 1604f, 1606
in humeral fractures
intercondylar, 754
supracondylar, 747–748, 749f
in phalangeal fractures, 462
soft tissue interlocking in, 29, 29f
"split Russell's," 46
in sternoclavicular joint reduction, 1276, 1277f–1278f
temporary (skin), 41–43, 42f–43f
in tibial fractures, 1931
in toe fractures, 2166f, 2167
well-leg, in femoral fractures, 1495, 1545
Traction fractures, 9f, 12–13, 14f
"Traction unit," in femoral fracture, 44
Transcondylar (dicondylar) fractures, of elbow, 751–752
Transforming growth factor beta, in healing, 183
Transfusion
in hemophilia, 355
in shock, 336–339, 337f–338f
Transiliac bar technique, in pelvic fractures, 1433, 1433f, 1437f, 1438
Translation motion, of spine, 1363–1364, 1364f
Transplantation
of bilaterally amputated parts, 302
of cartilage, in knee injury, 1844
Transtrochanteric approach, in acetabular fractures
posterior, 1466, 1471f
triradiate, 1464t, 1466, 1472f
Transverse fractures
of glenoid, 1002
of metacarpal shaft, 490–491, 490f–491f
of olecranon, 797, 803–804
of phalanx, 465, 466f
distal, 445, 445f
proximal, 474–475
in stress, 8

of thumb metacarpal, 499, 499f
Transverse ligament, in cervical spine, rupture of, 1326, 1328f, 1329, 1346
Transverse tarsal joint. See Midfoot/midtarsal joints
Trapeziotrapezoidal joint, anatomy of, 570f
Trapezium
anatomy of, 568–569, 569f–570f
fractures of, 631f, 632, 634f
Trapezius muscle, scapular attachment of, 991, 992f
Trapezoid
anatomy of, 568–569f, 570f
fractures of, 636–637
Trapezoid ligament, anatomy of, 1183f, 1184
TraumaFix apparatus, 69f, 72
Trauma series
in humeral fracture radiography, 880f, 881–882, 882f–883f
in scapular fracture radiography, 994, 995f
Triangular fibrocartilage, of wrist, 569–570, 570f, 586
anatomy of, 657–658
injury of, 592, 659–661, 662f
Triangulate triple (Chalet) frame, in external fixation, 72, 75f
Trigger finger, vs. metacarpophalangeal joint locking, 524
Trillat procedure, in shoulder dislocations, 1103
Triple arthrodesis
in calcaneal fractures, 2127
in midtarsal joint injuries, 2135
in talar head fractures, 2089
Triple frame, in external fixation, 71, 75f
Triquetrum
anatomy of, 568–569, 568f
fractures of, 631–632, 631f, 633f
Triradiate transtrochanteric approach, to acetabular fractures, 1464t, 1466, 1472f
Triscaphe (scaphotrapeziotrapezoidal) fusion, in scapholunate dissociation, 617, 618f–619f, 619
Trispiral tomography
in lunate fractures, 652, 653f
in scaphoid fractures, 639
of wrist, 582
Trochanter
fractures between. See Femoral fractures, intertrochanteric
greater, fractures of, 1560–1562, 1561f
Trochlea
anatomy of, 740–741, 741f, 761, 762f
fractures of, 766, 768, 774–775
vs. medial condyle, 761, 762f

"Trough line," in shoulder radiograph, 1061, 1062f
Tscherne-Gotzen classification, of tibial fractures, 1924
Tuber angle (Böhler's), of calcaneus, 2104, 2104f
in intra-articular fractures, 2119, 2129
in sustenaculum tali fractures, 2113–2114, 2114f
TUBS acronym, in shoulder dislocation, 1042, 1097–1098, 1098t
Matsen procedure and, 1112–1119, 1112t, 1113f–1118f
Tumors. See also Malignancy; Metastasis
benign, 435
biopsy of, 422–423, 422t–423t
laboratory evaluation in, 420–422, 421t
pathologic fractures in. See under Pathologic fractures
primary malignant, 435–436
radiography of, 418–420, 418t–419t, 420f, 425, 425f
staging of, 422, 422t–423t
"Turf toe" (great toe sprain), 2160
Two-point gait, 162

Ulna
anatomy of, 679–681, 742–743
fractures of
bracing of, 163
displaced, 720, 720f
Monteggia, 679, 701f–702f, 720–728, 721f, 725f–727f
nightstick (without radial injury), 679, 719–720, 720f
open, 248, 257
with radial fractures. See under Radial fractures, shaft
with radial radial head dislocations, 679, 701f–702f, 720–728, 721f, 725f–727f
undisplaced, 719–720
head of. See also Radioulnar joint
anatomy of, 657–658, 658f
dislocations of, 787–788
excision of, in distal radioulnar joint injury, 661, 662f
motion of, 679–680
plastic deformation of, 685
shortening of, in radial translation, 824f, 825
styloid of, anatomy of, 567, 567f
synostosis of, after fracture, 717–718, 718f
Ulnar collateral ligament injury, of thumb, 531–537, 531f–537f
Ulnar deviation, of wrist, 577–578, 578f

ISBN 0-397-51230-9

90000

9 780397 512300